Care of childbearing women and neonates demands a nurse's best skills.
Give your students the clear visual instruction they need to succeed!

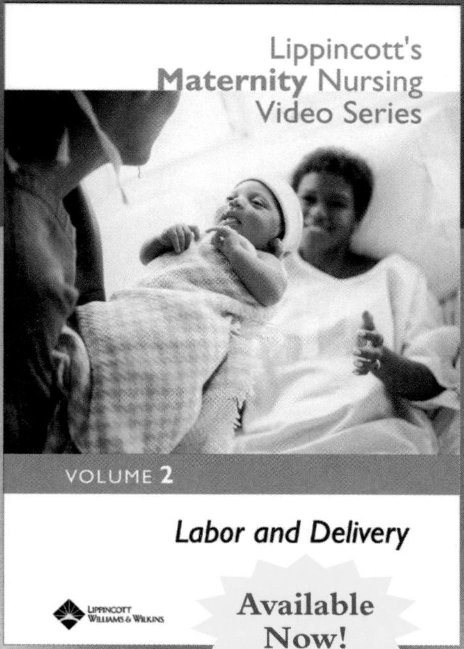

Available Now!

Lippincott's Maternity Nursing

Video Series

Created with today's visual learners in mind, each of these documentary-style videos guides users through a specific phase of maternity nursing—from prenatal care, through labor and delivery, to postpartum care—while broadening their clinical expertise and enhancing your decision-making ability.

Begin your students' journey to understanding...

- **Several scenarios** address a range of pregnancy experiences, types of labors and deliveries, and postpartum experiences to prepare students for any challenge.
- **Nurse, patient, and family interviews** help users maximize their communication skills and establish therapeutic relationships.
- **A range of formats**—VHS, DVD, or Streaming Video—lets you choose the one that's best for you.

They'll build' skill and confidence each step of the way...

- **Volume 1: Prenatal Care** addresses family adaptations to pregnancy, ways to promote a healthy pregnancy, and nursing management of at-risk pregnancies.
  VHS: ISBN: 0-7817-8250-3 • DVD: ISBN: 0-7817-9778-0
- **Volume 2: Labor and Delivery** begins from the moment of admission and addresses the nurse's role in assessment, monitoring, pain management, emotional support, stabilization of the newborn, and maternal-neonatal bonding.
  VHS: ISBN: 0-7817-7590-6 • DVD: ISBN: 0-7817-9547-8
- **Volume 3: Cesarean Delivery** covers several labor scenarios, including nursing care during an emergency C-section, and planned C-section.
  VHS: ISBN: 0-7817-9532-X • DVD: ISBN: 0-7817-6599-4
- **Volume 4: Postpartum Care** presents three normal range cases, from 12 hours to 6 weeks postpartum, with emphasis on maternal and newborn assessment, pain management, and family teaching.
  VHS: ISBN: 0-7817-7511-6 • DVD: ISBN: 0-7817-6545-5

2006 • Set of 4 VHS tapes: ISBN: 0-7817-6071-2 • Set of 4 DVDs: ISBN: 0-7817-8626-6

Add these skill-building videos to ...

ORDER TODAY

Call TOLL FREE 1-800-638

Visit us on the Web at **LWW.com/nursing** o

Or visit your local health science bookstore

D1218206

D5G311ZZ

Brief Contents

MATERNITY, NEWBORN, AND WOMEN'S HEALTH NURSING

Comprehensive Care Across the Lifespan

Susan A. Orshan, PhD, RN, BC
University of Phoenix On-Line Education
Phoenix, Arizona

Healthy Matters, LLC
Rocky Hill, New Jersey

Wolters Kluwer | Lippincott Williams & Wilkins
Health
Philadelphia • Baltimore • New York • London
Buenos Aires • Hong Kong • Sydney • Tokyo

Acquisitions Editor: Elizabeth Nieginski
Development Editor: Renee Gagliardi
Senior Production Editor: Marian A. Bellus
Director of Nursing Production: Helen Ewan
Senior Managing Editor / Production: Erika Kors
Art Director, Design: Joan Wendt
Art Director, Illustration: Brett MacNaughton
Senior Manufacturing Manager: William Alberti
Manufacturing Coordinator: Karin Duffield
Indexer: Alexandra Nickerson
Compositor: Circle Graphics
Printer: R. R. Donnelley-Willard

9 8 7 6 5 4 3 2 1

Library of Congress Cataloging-in-Publication Data

Orshan, Susan A.
Maternity, newborn, and women's health nursing : comprehensive care across the lifespan / Susan A. Orshan.
p. ; cm.
Includes bibliographical references and index.
ISBN-13: 978-0-7817-4254-2
ISBN-10: 0-7817-4254-4
1. Maternity nursing. 2. Gynecologic nursing. I. Title.
[DNLM: 1. Maternal–Child Nursing. 2. Women's Health.
WY 157.3 O76m 2007]
RG951.O774 2007
618.2'0231—dc22

2006025353

Care has been taken to confirm the accuracy of the information presented and to describe generally accepted practices. However, the authors, editors, and publisher are not responsible for errors or omissions or for any consequences from application of the information in this book and make no warranty, express or implied, with respect to the content of the publication.

The authors, editors, and publisher have exerted every effort to ensure that drug selection and dosage set forth in this text are in accordance with the current recommendations and practice at the time of publication. However, in view of ongoing research, changes in government regulations, and the constant flow of information relating to drug therapy and drug reactions, the reader is urged to check the package insert for each drug for any change in indications and dosage and for added warnings and precautions. This is particularly important when the recommended agent is a new or infrequently employed drug.

Some drugs and medical devices presented in this publication have Food and Drug Administration (FDA) clearance for limited use in restricted research settings. It is the responsibility of the health care provider to ascertain the FDA status of each drug or device planned for use in his or her clinical practice.

LWW.com

Dedication

This edition is dedicated to all the children (and grandchildren) born to the many people involved in this project during its development. Several of their pictures can be found throughout this textbook.

I especially wish to acknowledge and dedicate this edition to my children, Aaron, Samuel, and Aviva Orshan and my nephews, Ryan, Justin, Matthew, and Mitchell Kramer, for their love and support during this experience. I appreciate their reminders that sometimes the best way to complete a project is to spend some time away from it with those you love.

Memorial

In memory of my parents, Miriam and Martin Orshan, and my grandmother, Minnie Orshan.

Acknowledgments

When I began working on this project, friends who had given birth to both textbooks and babies (although not always simultaneously) warned me that the textbook is the more challenging experience! Having welcomed two children into my family since the start of this textbook endeavor, I have to agree that childbirth and book publishing are very similar: both challenging—and wonderful—in their own ways.

I would like to acknowledge:

- My students and colleagues who helped to shape the vision for this textbook.
- The contributors who shared their expertise and persevered through the many temporal and physical challenges inherent in a first edition.
- The editorial staff at Lippincott Williams and Wilkins, who thought the time was right for a book with a new vision and supported its development. In particular, Elizabeth Nieginski, Senior Acquisitions Editor, believed in this project since its inception and provided the support, guidance, and humor necessary for it to reach this point (and also adopted Gordon during the process). Renee Gagliardi, Senior Developmental Editor, entered into this project with extraordinary enthusiasm that helped to transform my "fantasy textbook" into a reality, and chose to "own" the content throughout the process, which included the birth of her son William.
- Katie Carangelo and her family, without whose help this book would never have come into reality.

From the Author

The joy I felt when Lippincott Williams & Wilkins asked me to provide an outline of my fantasy textbook still reverberates whenever I think of it. Having both clinical and academic experience in maternity, newborn, and women's health nursing, I had many ideas about where we needed to be heading and what was important. I was thrilled to learn that many other educators and practitioners shared my thoughts—and thus, this text was born!

I began my formal nursing education at the University of Pennsylvania in Philadelphia, where I earned my BSN. After working in various areas of maternity-newborn nursing, I found myself at New York University, where I earned my master's and doctoral degrees in the Division of Nursing. I also became certified as a perinatal nurse, Lamaze instructor, and Feldenkrais practitioner. I recently earned certification in Distance Education and almost completed certification as the handler of a pet therapy dog. (My last pregnancy actually put a stop to that, but we may take it up again!)

While initially these educational milestones may seem very diverse, in reality they have helped me to achieve a level of professional expertise that has allowed me to continue as a nurse-educator of both professional and nonprofessional students. They have accommodated my needs as the single mother of two very active boys, as well as providing the personal flexibility I needed to coordinate and provide care for my grandmother, who died at 104 years, two months after my oldest son was born.

I am fortunate that I was able to create an environment in which my personal and professional needs could be met. As a health care professional, I realized that many women, regardless of whether they were in the process of childbearing, were not having most of their health care needs met within the health care system of the last century. This textbook, through its innovative approach to nursing care of women and their families, will help to educate students to provide care that reflects the changing needs of women and their significant others, resulting in a healthier population ready to face the challenges of the 21st century—and beyond!

Susan A. Orshan, PhD, RN, BC

Contributors

Louise A. Aurilio, PhD, RNC, CAN
Assistant Professor, Nursing Department
Youngstown State University
Youngstown, Ohio

Lisa Marie Bernardo, PhD, MPH, RN
Associate Professor and Director of Continuing Education
University of Pittsburgh School of Nursing
Pittsburgh, Pennsylvania

Jennifer Black, MS, RNC
Clinical Instructor, Maternal Child Nursing
Virginia Commonwealth School of Nursing
Richmond, Virginia

Christine Bradway, PhD, RN
Assistant Professor of Gerontological Nursing and John A. Hartford Foundation Building Academic Geriatric Nursing Capacity Scholar
University of Pennsylvania School of Nursing
Philadelphia, Pennsylvania

Wendy C. Budin, PhD, RN, BC
Associate Dean, Graduate Nursing Programs and Research
Seton Hall University, College of Nursing
South Orange, New Jersey

Rebecca Cahill, RN, MSN
Assistant Professor of Nursing
University of Saint Mary
Leavenworth, Kansas

Della Campbell, PhD(c), APRN-C, CNA, BC
Seton Hall University, College of Nursing
South Orange, New Jersey

Sylvia Escott-Stump, MA, RD, LDN
Dietetic Programs Director
East Carolina University
Greenville, North Carolina

Robin Evans, RN, PNC(C), BScN, MSA, PhD
Assistant Professor, College of Nursing
University of Saskatchewan, Regina Site
Saskatchewan, Canada

Evelyn S. Farrior, PhD, RD, LDN, FADA
Professor Emeritus, Department of Nutrition and Hospitality Management
East Carolina University
Greenville, North Carolina

Faye A. Gary, EdD, RN, FAAN
Medical Mutual of Ohio Professor of Nursing for Vulnerable and At-Risk Populations
Frances Payne Bolton School of Nursing
Case Western Reserve University
Cleveland, Ohio

Barbara Hotelling, BSN, CD (DONA), LCCE, FACCE
President, Lamaze International
Rochester Hills, Michigan

Michelle Johnson, RD, LD
Neonatal and Pediatric Nutritionist
Bel Air, Maryland

Shirley L. Jones, PhD, RNC
Chief Executive Officer
Planned Parenthood of Louisville, Inc.
Louisville, Kentucky

Mary F. King, RN, MS
Level Coordinator, Instructor
Phillips Community College of the University of Arkansas, Helena Campus
Helena, Arkansas

Judith A. Lewis, PhD, RNC, FAAN
Professor, Maternal Child Nursing Department
School of Nursing
Virginia Commonwealth University
Richmond, Virginia

Deborah A. Raines, PhD, RN
Professor and Director; Christine E. Lynn College of Nursing
Florida Atlantic University
Boca Raton, Florida

Gayle Roux, PhD, RN, CNS, NP-C
Associate Professor
Associate Dean for Faculty
Loyola University Chicago Marcella Niehoff School of Nursing
Chicago, Illinois

Susan Scanland, MSN, APRN, BC-GNP
President
GeriScan Geriatric Consulting
Clarks Summit, Pennsylvania

Eileen Scaringi
Women's Health Nurse Practitioner
Dundee, Scotland, UK

Judy Kaye Smith, MSN, MN, RN, BC
Assistant Professor
Lamar University
Beaumont, Texas

Thelma Sword, RN, MSN
Assistant Professor of Nursing
Graceland University
Online Nursing Facilitator
University of Phoenix

Nancy Watts, RN, MN, PNC [C]
Clinical Nurse Specialist, Perinatal Program
London Health Sciences Centre
London, Ontario

Vi Wilkes, MS, EdD Candidate
Faculty
University of Phoenix On-Line

Jeanette Zaichkin, RNC, MN
Neonatal Consultant
Olympia, Washington

Reviewers

Violeta Aguilar-Figuly
Miami Dade College
Miami, Florida

Tracy Anderson
University of Michigan, Ann Arbor
Ann Arbor, Michigan

Bridget Bailey
Iowa Lakes Community College
Emmetsburg, Iowa

Linda Bennington
Old Dominion University
Norfolk, Virginia

Rosemarie Berman
The Catholic University of America
Washington, District of Columbia

Johnett Benson-Soros
Kent State University Ashtabula Campus
Ashtabula, Ohio

Gary Berringer
Gannon University
Erie, Pennsylvania

Donna Bohmfalk
University of Texas
Friendswood, Texas

Therese Bower
Firelands Regional Medical Center
Sandusky, Ohio

Michele Brimeyer
University of Florida
Gainesville, Florida

Beverly Bye
Towson University
Towson, Maryland

Lizabeth Carlson
Delta State University
Cleveland, Mississippi

Marsha Conroy
Cuyahoga Community College
Cleveland, Ohio;
Kent State University
Kent, Ohio

E. (Tina) Cuellar
University of Texas Medical Branch
Galveston, Texas

Carrie Davis
Norfolk State University
Suffolk, Virginia

Schenita Davis
North Carolina Agricultural and Technical University
Greensboro, North Carolina

Adele Dean
Northern Kentucky University
Highland Heights, Kentucky

Susan Dickey
Temple University
Philadelphia, Pennsylvania

Holly Diesel
Barnes-Jewish College of Nursing and Allied Health
St. Louis, Missouri

Laurie Downes
Springfield Technical Community College
Springfield, Massachusetts

Emily Drake
University of Virginia
Charlottesville, Virginia

Susan Dudek
Erie Community College
Erie, Pennsylvania

Carmen Escoto-Lloyd
California State University, Los Angeles
Los Angeles, California

Carolyn Fong
California State University, Hayward
Concord, California

Sherry Foran
University of Western Ontario
London, Ontario

Bunny Forgione
Texas A&M University—Corpus Christi
Corpus Christi, Texas

Sandra Founds
University of Pennsylvania
Philadelphia, Pennsylvania

Karolyn Givens
Radford University
Radford, Virginia

Enid Gorman
University of New England
Portland, Maine

Gay Goss
California State University, Dominguez Hills
San Francisco, California

Ronald Graf
DePaul University
North Riverside, Illinois

Laura Greenfield
University of Phoenix
Phoenix, Arizona

Susan Groth
University of Rochester
Rochester, New York

Pam Hamre
College of St. Catherine
St. Paul, Minnesota

Mary Hickey
Adelphi University
Garden City, New York

Daisy Hines
Long Beach Community College
Long Beach, California

Melissa Holcomb
Truman State University
Kirksville, Missouri

Jean Ivey
University of Alabama at Birmingham
Birmingham, Alabama

M. Regina Jennette
West Virginia Northern Community College
Lansing, Ohio

Wendy Keezer
Central Community College, Grand Island
Grand Island, Nebraska

Joan Keller-Maresh
Viterbro University
La Crosse, Wisconsin

JoAnne Kirk
University of Texas, Tyler
Whitehouse, Texas

Kathleen Krov
Raritan Valley Community College
Milford, New Jersey

Mary Lynd
Wright State University
Dayton, Ohio

Marilyn Marquardt
Marion College, Fond du Lac
Fond du Lac, Wisconsin

Rhonda Martin
University of Tulsa
Tulsa, Oklahoma

Lucy Martinez-Schallmoser
Loyola University Chicago
Chicago, Illinois

Janet Massoglia
Delta College
University Center, Michigan

Shelly Moore
Clarion University
Oil City, Pennsylvania

Cindy Morgan
University of South Alabama
Mobile, Alabama

Patricia Morgan
University of New England
Portland, Maine

Catherine Muskus
University of Vermont
Burlington, Vermont

Donna Paulsen
North Carolina Agricultural and Technical State University
Greensboro, North Carolina

Michelle Patterson
Nichols State University
Houma, Louisiana

Deborah Pollard
University of North Carolina, Wilmington
Wilmington, North Carolina

Julie Pope
Georgian College
Barrie, Ontario

Susan Salazar
University of Florida
Jacksonville, Florida

Jane Savage
Louisiana State University
New Orleans, Louisiana

Gayle Sewell
North Central Kansas Technical College
Beloit, Kansas

Marilyn Simons
Indiana Wesleyan University
Marion, Indiana

Ualetta Singhu
Northwestern State University
Keithville, Louisiana

Ida Slusher
Richmond, Kentucky

Jennifer Spann
Middle Tennessee State University
Smyrna, Tennessee

Sharon Thompson
Gannon University
Erie, Pennsylvania

Gerry Walker
Park University
St. Joseph, Missouri

Mary Walker
Lamar University
Beaumont, Texas

Maureen Waller
College of DuPage
Tinley Park, Illinois

Judy Wika
University of Kansas
Osage City, Kansas

Anne Woods
Johns Hopkins University
Baltimore, Maryland

Preface

For most of recorded time, a woman's life was defined by her ability to bear and raise children. By 20 years old, many women were mothers and continued to bear children for a significant portion of what remained of their lives. That began to change in the latter half of the 20th century. Scientific advances resulting in better nutrition, improved health, and a longer lifespan have ensured that the duration of a woman's life spent childbearing is significantly shorter than the other phases of her life. Additionally, societal shifts and evolving attitudes toward gender roles have expanded roles and opportunities for women, adding new dimensions to their lives while still maintaining certain expectations for them relative to their childbearing capacity.

At the beginning of this new millennium, the nursing profession continues to ensure that women are knowledgeable about their health choices and actively participate with their health care providers in setting goals and choosing strategies to achieve optimal health. Continued progress in this endeavor requires nurses to have a knowledge base from which they can identify expected findings, normal variations, and abnormalities in women's health throughout the life cycle. Additionally, nurses need technical skills to implement appropriate nursing interventions and collaborative and delegation skills to work with other members of the health care team (including the client and her family) as needed to effectively manage care.

To date, many nursing textbooks have focused primarily on the health of women during or between pregnancies. This new textbook for the new millennium presents comprehensive knowledge that nurses need to provide evidence-based practice in the area of reproductive health. It provides detailed coverage of the aspects nurses need to understand to give effective care during pregnancy, labor and birth, and the postpartum period. Unlike many other textbooks, however, this book presents those processes within a larger context of women's health and related concerns beyond reproductive issues. It approaches the comprehensive care of women from adolescence through older adulthood, viewing the reproductive process as part of that life cycle continuum.

PURPOSE

This textbook provides a comprehensive resource for nursing students and registered professional nurses that can be used to help plan nursing care for women throughout the life cycle. The text and its supporting products:

1. Disseminate up-to-date knowledge within a practical context for use in today's multifaceted health care environment
2. Elucidate the influence of sociocultural beliefs and practices in understanding and identifying health care needs (when interacting with a client of the same or different sociocultural group than the nurse)
3. Clarify the importance of understanding gender-specific issues including physical and emotional development

This product has a major emphasis on sociocultural aspects of client care when working with women and their families at various points throughout the lifespan. In recognizing the importance and uniqueness of the female experience from menarche to post-menopause, the text includes information about every phase from adolescence through older adulthood. While other texts touch on different stages in a woman's life, this text provides more detail on areas outside of the average maternity text. For example, the entire last unit focuses on the experience of women at and after menopause.

ORGANIZATION

The organization of this text reflects a progressive, life-cycle orientation toward the care of women. The book is divided into six units, each of which emphasizes unique aspects of the client's experience.

Unit 1—Foundations of Maternal, Newborn, and Women's Health Care

Unit 1 covers foundational content with applications throughout every stage of a woman's life. Chapter 1, "Philosophy and Framework for Women's Reproductive and Sexual Health," introduces women's reproductive and sexual health throughout the life cycle within a broad cultural perspective. It emphasizes the current state of women's health care in the United States and Canada and explores current issues of significant concern to nurses. Chapter 2, "Health Promotion," encompasses major areas for preserving and optimizing wellness in women. Chapter 3, "Nutrition for Adolescent and Adult Women," presents nutritional guidelines for different female life stages within a multicultural framework. A particular focus is women's reproductive years, with emphasis given to nutritional screening, the nurse's role in providing nutritional guidance, and practical applications. Chapter 4, "Medical Alterations in Women During Adolescence and Adulthood," gives comprehensive coverage of physiological issues commonly (or increasingly) occurring in women that affect quality of life. While it includes significant information about breast disorders, reproductive problems, and sexually transmitted infections, this chapter differs from many other books by addressing diseases with serious implications for or different manifestations in women. Examples include autoimmune diseases and cardiovascular disease. Chapter 5, "Mental Health Concerns for Women in Adolescence and Adulthood," provides an overview of potential changes in women's psychological health. The unit concludes with chapters focusing on two topics relevant to every stage of a woman's life: Chapter 6, "Sexuality and Reproduction" and Chapter 7, "Family Formation."

Unit 2—Special Reproductive Health and Concerns

This unit covers those issues of special importance to women during their childbearing years separate from the actual experience of pregnancy, labor, birth, and postpartal care. Chapter 8, "Fertility Control and Contraception," focuses on mechanisms for preventing or timing pregnancy and related nursing care. Chapter 9, "Voluntary Pregnancy Termination," examines abortion from a political, social, cultural, and medical perspective. It emphasizes historical and current controversies surrounding the issue as well as providing information for nurses when working with clients contemplating or making this choice, regardless of personal viewpoints. Chapter 10, "Fertility Challenges" covers care for families struggling with infertility, a problem of increasing significance. Finally, Chapter 11 "Genetics, Embryology, and Preconceptual/Prenatal Assessment and Screening" describes the developmental processes at various stages in utero, threats to embryonic and fetal health, and screening measures prospective parents can take before conception or birth to prevent or manage problems in their children.

Unit 3—Pregnancy

Unit 3 covers the unique experience of pregnancy in both normal and high-risk circumstances. Chapter 12, "Process of Pregnancy," lays a foundation for nursing practice that reflects the influence of pregnancy on a woman and her significant others from cultural, psychological, and physiologic perspectives. The focus is pregnancy without complications and associated care. Chapter 13, "High-Risk Pregnancy," assists students to differentiate and apply knowledge regarding expected changes of pregnancy. It also presents detailed information about preexisting or gestational-onset conditions and associated collaborative management. Chapter 14, "Educational Preparation for Pregnancy, Childbirth, and Parenthood," provides knowledge regarding the meaning and position of today's methods of childbirth education. It compares various types of preparation and their applications.

Unit 4—Labor and Childbirth

In Unit 4, the reader becomes familiar with normal and high-risk labor and childbirth, as well as pharmacological methods of managing pain during this time. Chapter 15, "Labor and Childbirth," covers the physiologic and psychological aspects of labor, the mechanisms and stages of normal vaginal childbirth, and collaborative care for each crucial point of this phenomenal experience. Chapter 16, "High-Risk Labor and Childbirth," covers those conditions or problems that can interfere with normal labor outcomes and their collaborative management. It also presents detailed information about common obstetrical interventions used to assist labor and childbirth, including labor augmentation and induction, operative obstetrics, and cesarean birth. Chapter 17, "Pharmacologic Pain Management of Labor," covers the etiology of pain during childbirth and the various pharmacologic methods commonly implemented during normal and high-risk labor and birth.

Unit 5—Postpartum Period and Newborn Care

This unit presents postpartal care for the mother, her family/support people, and the newborn. Chapter 18, "Fourth Stage of Labor and Postpartum Period," emphasizes expected maternal physiologic and psychological changes, as well as collaborative care provisions for the new family throughout the first 6 weeks after childbirth. Chapter 19, "The High-Risk Postpartum Woman," explores care for women and families experiencing maternal postpartal complications or deviations. The content covers both physiological problems and psychological maladjustments with serious ramifications. Chapter 20, "The Healthy Newborn," enhances students' understanding of the newborn's adjustment to extrauterine life, including assessment findings. It presents comprehensive collaborative care during the immediate postpartal period and extensive areas for family teaching throughout the newborn's first few months of life. Chapter 21, "Newborn Nutrition," promotes nursing knowledge to facilitate parental decision-making concerning newborn nutrition. It emphasizes interventions to assist both breastfeeding and bottle-feeding families, describes measures for newborns needing special adjustments, and explores the management of common newborn feeding-related difficulties. Finally, Chapter 22, "The High-Risk Newborn," covers collaborative strategies for newborns experiencing challenges transitioning to extrauterine life. It covers problems related to birth weight, gestational age, acquired conditions, and congenital factors, as well as measures to address them.

Unit 6—Menopause and Beyond

Unit 6 explores the experience of the largest-growing segment of today's population—women who are at the end of or are past their reproductive years. Chapter 23, "The Menopausal Experience," enhances the reader's understanding of the physiologic, psychological, and cultural factors inherent in the gradual cessation of the menstrual cycle and its effects on women and their significant others. Chapter 24, "The Older Postmenopausal Woman," focuses on health promotion, screening, assessment, common concerns, and common abnormalities for middle-aged and older women. The discussion emphasizes normal female physiology related to aging, along with psychological and sociocultural variations and dimensions for nurses to consider when working with this increasingly influential demographic group.

SPECIAL FEATURES

This book's unique framework reflects emerging views of and attitudes toward women's health. Several key features emphasize the modern approach and student-oriented focus woven throughout this text and its associated products:

Progressive Case Studies

Each chapter begins with two or more illustrated scenarios related to the content found within the chapter. Accompanying questions there begin the student's thought process about the scenarios and the topics he or she will be exploring. Throughout the chapter, the student will find ongoing questions at relevant points related to the opening case studies. Photographic reminders assist visual learners to recall the scenario and its circumstances when shaping responses. Answers to the questions are provided in the back of the book. Additionally, associated care for the clients in these scenarios are explored in detailed Nursing Care Plans found within the chapters as well.

Learning Objectives

Objectives at the start of each chapter outline the fundamental goals. They are linked to the summary points at the end of each chapter and provide a framework for instructors to organize their teaching.

Key Terms

Essential vocabulary is presented at the beginning of each chapter. Terms are bolded with their explanations in the chapters themselves and reinforced in the book's Glossary.

Quotable Quotes

At key points in each chapter, quotes from real women, historical figures, and nurses are found. These sayings and statements underscore the relevance of the accompanying discussions and provide a real-life context to which students can relate.

Collaborative Care

Collaborative Care sections throughout the book are presented in a different text color and review the steps of assessment, diagnosis, planning, implementation, and evaluation relative to the content under consideration. The collaborative care focus emphasizes the nurse's need to work in partnership with the client and her family. It also underscores those areas in which nurses coordinate care with other care team members, emphasizing both independent and cooperative interventions.

Nursing Care Plans

As mentioned earlier, more than 40 care plans relate to the progressive case studies found throughout each chapter. These scenarios and their care plans were designed to cover common women's health issues and concerns, with their appropriate diagnoses, interventions, rationales, and expected outcomes.

NIC/NOC Boxes

Throughout the book, NIC/NOC boxes summarize those interventions and outcomes commonly related to conditions, problems, or considerations found within each chapter. The labels are from the latest version of the approved Nursing Interventions and Nursing Outcomes Classifications.

Nursing Procedures

Significant skills and techniques are outlined in illustrated procedures throughout the text. Each procedure has a clearly articulated purpose and explains needed equipment. The steps are organized around the nursing process, providing areas for assessment and planning, relevant interventions and their rationales, and desired outcomes for evaluation. Additionally, these procedures emphasize variations needed for different life stages or age groups, as well as considerations needed for implementing the skill in community-based settings.

Complementary and Alternative Medicine

Boxes reviewing special issues related to CAM modalities are found throughout the text. Additionally, text coverage of issues related to CAM are indicated in the following accompanying icon: 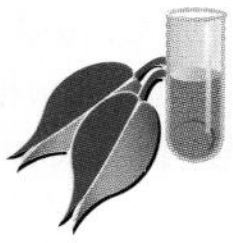.

Teaching Tips

Client and family education is essential for health promotion, disease prevention, and illness management. Appropriate areas for instruction are reviewed in boxes of bulleted points throughout the book.

Pharmacology Boxes

Medications of importance are presented in boxes throughout the book. Such boxes review mechanisms of action, usual dosages, common side effects, and implications for nurses.

Assessment Tools

Throughout the book, tools to assist nurses with health history and physical examination are found. These Assessment Tools include well-known instruments like the "Cage Questionnaire" as well as original approaches related to the different topics found across the text.

Research Highlights

Up-to-date, evidence-based research studies are summarized within most chapters to reinforce students' familiarity with the literature and to link results with interventions and best practices as much as possible.

Review Questions

At the end of each chapter, 8 to 10 NCLEX-style Review Questions help students to integrate previous learning and test their understanding. Answers with comprehensive rationales are found at the end of the book.

Summary

Bulleted end-of-chapter summaries review pertinent content and help distill coverage into the most important considerations. The points link to the objectives found at the beginning of the book.

Questions to Ponder (Critical Thinking)

These scenarios ask students to apply their knowledge to possible scenarios or developments related to the topics at hand. Guidelines for discussion related to these scenarios are found as part of the accompanying Instructor's Resource package.

References and Resources

Each chapter has been written based on the most current articles, textbooks, Web sites, and other sources available. Detailed lists of the appropriate citations are found at the end of each chapter. Additionally, several chapters contain information on Resources helpful for students, nurses, and clients.

Art

One goal of this text was to present a highly visual learning experience for the reader. Beautiful drawings and photos throughout the book underscore important content, highlight complicated issues or care components, and crystallize pertinent information in a way that words alone cannot convey.

TEACHING-LEARNING PACKAGE

Instructor's Resource CD-ROM

This free resource for teachers is compatible with WebCT and Blackboard and includes the following valuable materials to assist with instruction in Women's Health Nursing, Maternal/Newborn Nursing, and similar courses:

- Test Generator, containing hundreds of questions within a dynamic tool that permits sorting and additional personalization for examinations and quizzes of all levels
- PowerPoint presentations for each chapter in the book, with capabilities for use as overheads, handouts, on-line posting, and supplementation
- Searchable Image Bank containing the library of illustrations and photographs found in the text
- Guidelines to Answers to end-of-chapter Critical Thinking Exercises, to facilitate class discussion and other projects

Student CD-ROM

The free CD-ROM for students packaged with this textbook includes the following materials:

- 25 minutes of video footage reviewing the following core concepts:
  - Pregnancy Development in Each Trimester
  - Vaginal Labor and Birth
  - Scheduled Cesarean Birth
  - Breastfeeding
- Tutorial for NCLEX Alternate Items, to help prepare students to approach innovative questions on their upcoming licensing examination
- Spanish-English Audio Glossary, to facilitate the student's communication with Spanish-speaking clients

thePoint Web Site*

Visit *http://thePoint.lww.com* for on-line versions of many of the aforementioned educational supplements, as well as additional material, including, but not limited to, the following:

- Course Syllabi
- Strategies for Effective Teaching
- Learning Objectives
- Pre-Lecture Quizzes
- Journal Articles
- Additional Lecture Notes, Questions, Discussion Topics, and Assignments

Electronic Study Guide

This for-sale resource helps students master their understanding of core textbook content in a dynamic, interactive, electronic environment. Content for each chapter is divided into the following sections:

- **Learning Objectives.** These objectives summarize the chapter's essential goals and provide a quick mechanism for review.
- **Assessing Your Understanding.** These sections focus on broadening the student's knowledge base in multiple exercise formats, such as matching, fill-in-the-blank, and short answers.
- **Applying Your Knowledge.** These sections contain additional case studies and corresponding questions in a style consistent with the main textbook. Additionally, students will find video clips with following review questions to ensure their mastery of topics in practice.
- **Practicing for NCLEX.** Each chapter ends with more NCLEX-style review questions exclusive to this study guide, for a total across the product of 300 more examination preparation questions.

MARKET INVOLVEMENT/FOCUS

This book reflects a strong desire to include experts in various components of women's health and to use feedback from prospective instructors to improve and to refine not only the text itself, but also the design, art program, and ancillary products. More than 20 contributors from institutions throughout the United States and Canada supplied content for chapters, reflecting their expertise and knowledge. A team of subject matter experts who teach women's health, maternity, and obstetrics courses provided feedback and original content for supplemental materials and support components. More than 150 instructors gave feedback on elements of this product suite from its earliest stages up to initial publication. All these measures were implemented to ensure that this book involved its intended market as much as possible to create a teaching–learning package that would successfully enable students to excel in the relevant content areas and provide the best caregiving possible for women and their families.

---

*thePoint is a trademark of WKHealth.

Contents

MATERNITY, NEWBORN, AND WOMEN'S HEALTH NURSING

Comprehensive Care Across the Lifespan

FOUNDATIONS OF MATERNAL, NEWBORN, AND WOMEN'S HEALTH CARE

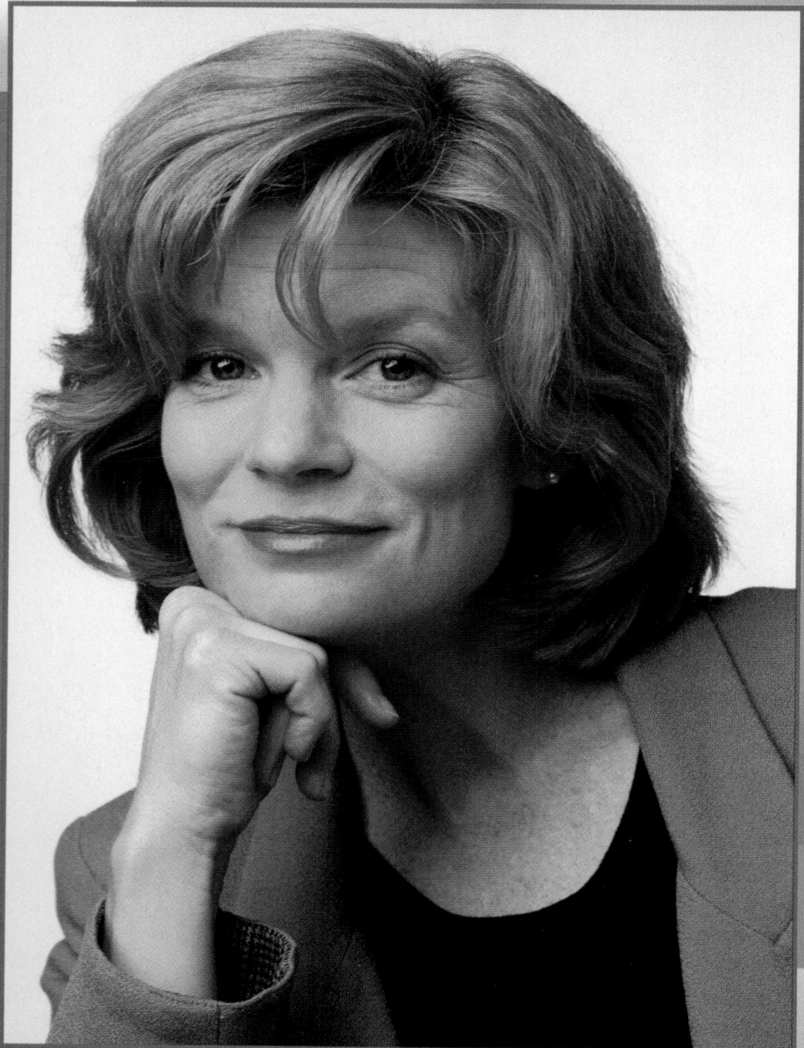

UNIT 1

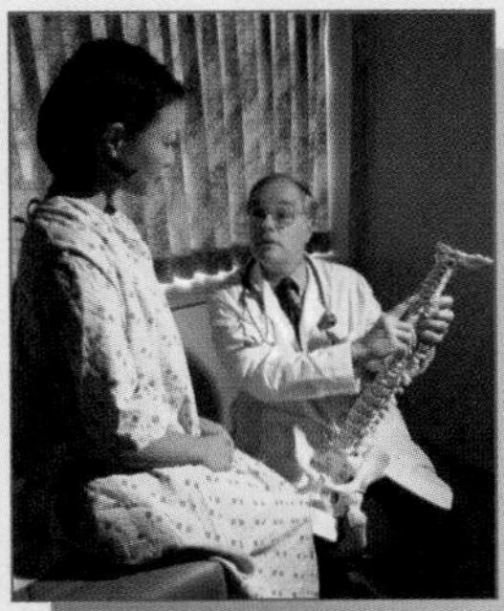
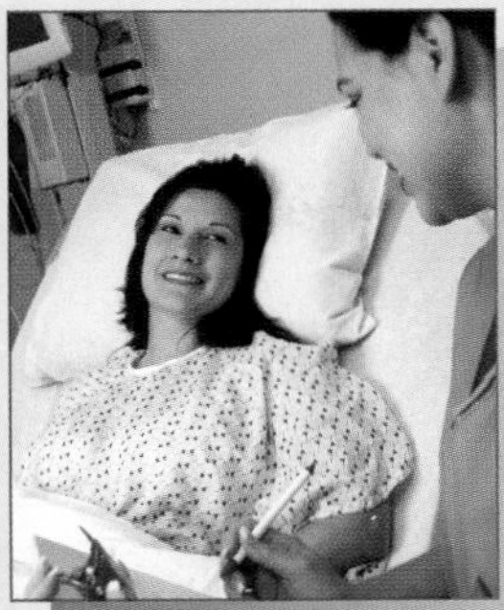
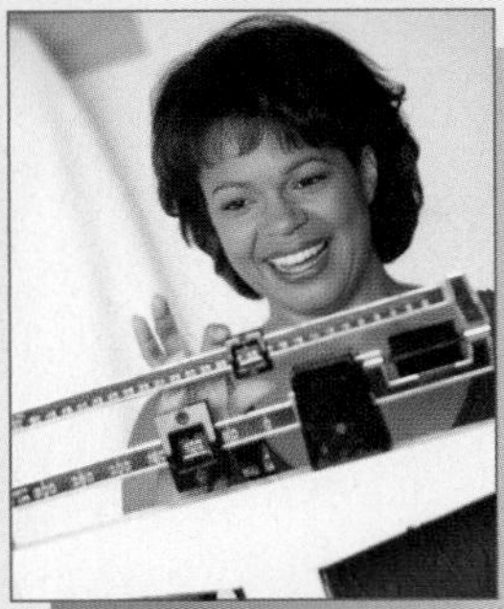
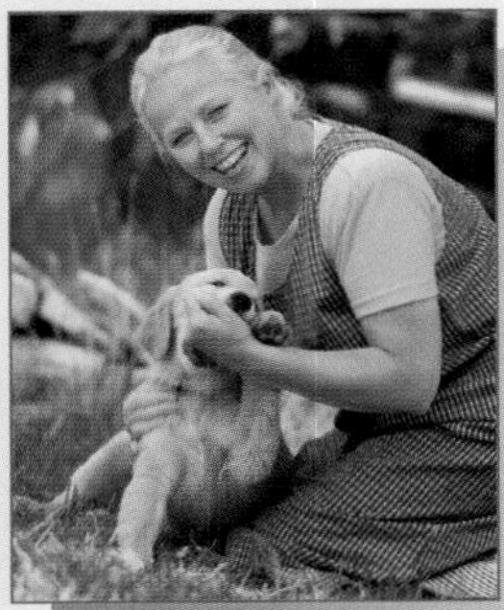

This unit focuses on fundamental components of women's health across the lifespan. The topics covered are relevant for women of all ages and stages of life. In the 21st century, health care providers need to educate women about how their choices can influence their own and their families' well-being. Nurses need to form partnerships with clients to outline goals and to plan strategies that will maximize wellness, prevent illness, and manage any problems that do develop as effectively as possible.

While past paradigms for women's health focused mainly on care during or between pregnancies, this unit fully reflects today's philosophy of promoting and optimizing a woman's health from adolescence through the end of life. The section begins with a framework for current maternal, newborn, and women's health care that provides a context informing the rest of the textbook. Then, the focus moves to health promotion and nutrition, including modifications that may be necessary according to life stage, sociocultural variables, and other factors. Next are covered common medical and mental health alterations, along with relevant collaborative care strategies. Unit 1 ends with chapters on two topics relevant to every stage of a woman's life: (1) sexuality and reproduction and (2) the family.

CHAPTER 1

Philosophy and Framework for Women's Reproductive and Sexual Health

Susan A. Orshan

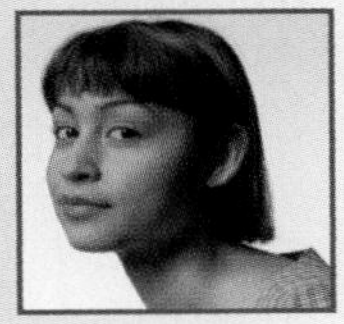

Georgia, 22 years old, is a Hispanic woman who has been brought to the clinic by an older aunt named Esperanza. Georgia has been experiencing lower abdominal pain and menstrual irregularities for the past few months. Esperanza says, "I've been urging her to see a doctor, but she says she's embarrassed." Georgia refuses to say anything unless her aunt leaves the room.

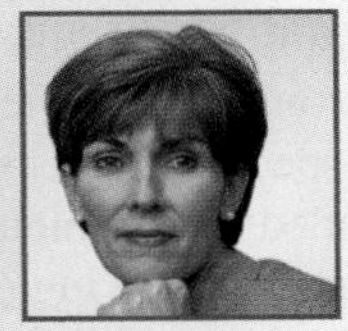

Elaine, 45 years old, has three children and works part-time as an office assistant. She has developed hypertension, and her blood glucose level is elevated. The nurse practitioner discusses the need for lifestyle changes and prescribes medications to help bring her problems under control. Elaine rolls her eyes and says, "I'll try to keep up with the diet and exercise, but I don't know how we're going to afford these prescriptions. My job doesn't provide any insurance, and my husband's plan isn't very good."

These women are a few examples of the wide-ranging experiences found in the realm of women's health nursing. Both clients and nurses have stories to draw on and circumstances that shape their attitudes and feelings about wellness, reproduction, motherhood, and aging. You will learn more about these stories as the chapter progresses. For now, consider the following points:

- How might age, ethnicity, parenthood, socioeconomic status, fertility, illness, and family relationships shape women's health experiences?
- What aspects of Elaine's situation might be less concerning if she had adequate health insurance coverage?
- What are the implications for her family if Georgia turns out to have a serious health problem?
- What current issues are reflected in these stories?
- How can nurses provide ethically based responses to their clients, while also demonstrating caring and concern?

LEARNING OBJECTIVES

On completion of this chapter, the reader should be able to:

- Discuss demographic and sociopolitical changes during the past decades that have influenced women's health care.
- Examine the ramifications of lack of access to health care for uninsured women and children in the United States.
- Explore the significance of critical thinking in nursing, particularly as related to addressing women's reproductive and sexual concerns.
- Discuss the role of ethics and ethical decision making in women's health nursing.
- Evaluate the significance of informed consent in practice and research. Identify procedures and problems for which informed consent is needed when working with women.
- Explore the role of nursing in women's health research.
- Evaluate the significance of evidence-based practice in nursing and women's health care.

KEY TERMS

critical thinking
ethically based practice
evidence-based decision making
evidence-based health care
evidence-based practice
fertility rate
informed consent
maternal morbidity
maternal mortality

At the dawn of the new millennium, there are new realities to experience and multiple potentials to be realized. The only constant at this new dawn is that change is inevitable and continuous. To understand better where women's health, maternal, and newborn nursing are going, it is necessary to recognize where these areas have been and where they are now.

This chapter discusses current issues affecting women's health and nursing care. It examines the foundational context within which today's women's health care is provided and on important issues currently influencing practice and interactions. The topics discussed in this chapter have implications for and are connected to the content found throughout this book and its supplements. Many of the issues touched on here are described in detail in other sections of this text.

SHIFTING PARADIGMS AND CURRENT CONTEXT

QUOTE 1-1

"I can remember as a child my mother saying that she was 'unwell.' It was only after I myself began to menstruate that I realized she used that terminology in reference to having her period."

A 44-year old woman of Russian-Polish descent

When the 20th century began, most North American families were "nuclear." Men and women in families and communities generally adhered to specific gender roles, and heavy involvement with extended family members was normal, with two or more generations living either together in the same house or in close proximity to one another. The dominant perspective in the United States was that of the white Christian male. Women did not have the right to vote, contraceptives were not readily available, abortion was illegal, and laws prohibited some types of nonheterosexual sexual intercourse. (Some of these laws remain active in some states today.)

The world is changing. The next paragraphs demonstrate the enormous changes that have occurred during the past 100 years. Individuals may agree or disagree regarding whether changes are for the better or for the worse. What all people can generally accept is that understanding the realities of today's women and their families will enable nurses and other health professionals to better help clients to achieve their health care goals.

Changes in Family Structures and Relationships

At the beginning of the 21st century, many families in the United States and Canada are headed by married heterosexual couples; however, the percentage of "traditional" families is decreasing, from 40% in 1970 to 23% in 2003 (U.S. Census Bureau, 2004) (Fig. 1.1). During the same period, families headed by single mothers increased from 12% to 26%; those headed by single fathers grew from 1% to 6% (U.S. Census Bureau, 2004). The increase in single-parent families is not related to adolescent pregnancy, which in fact has decreased during this time, but may be related to divorce, delayed marriages, or both (U.S. Census Bureau, 2004). Although multiple publications regarding childbearing and fertility are available from the U.S. Census Bureau, no information specific to lesbian childbearing and family development is currently available; this information would affect the statistical findings.

In terms of gender roles, options for both men and women are much more diverse than they were 100 years ago, although such potentials are not always actualized. "Mommy and Me" classes have evolved into "Mommy, Daddy, Grandma, Grandpa, and/or Nanny and Me" classes. Between 1967 and 2001, the percentage of wives in heterosexual marriages who were the sole wage earner of the family almost tripled (1.7% vs. 4.8%), and the number of families in which both husband and wife were employed outside the home increased from 43.6% in 1967 to 59.3% in 2001, with 24.1% of wives earning more than their husbands (Bureau of Labor Statistics, 2004). More fathers are assuming caretaking responsibilities for their young offspring, with 26% of fathers providing caretaking responsibilities for their children younger than 15 years while the children's mother worked outside the home and 20% of fathers reporting having the role of primary caretaker of a preschooler, although both percentages are lower than they were in the 1990s (Overturf Johnson, 2005). Regardless of wage earner status, however, women continue to perform most household and family-focused responsibilities (Casper & Bianchi, 2002).

In addition to the changes in the "traditional" family structure, the number of couples with children has been decreasing in both the United States and Canada. In 1981, 55% of all families in Canada were deemed "traditional"—that is, two adults (married or common-law) with children (Statistics Canada, 2002). In 2001, this type of family group represented only 44% of Canadian families (Statistics Canada, 2002). See Chapter 7.

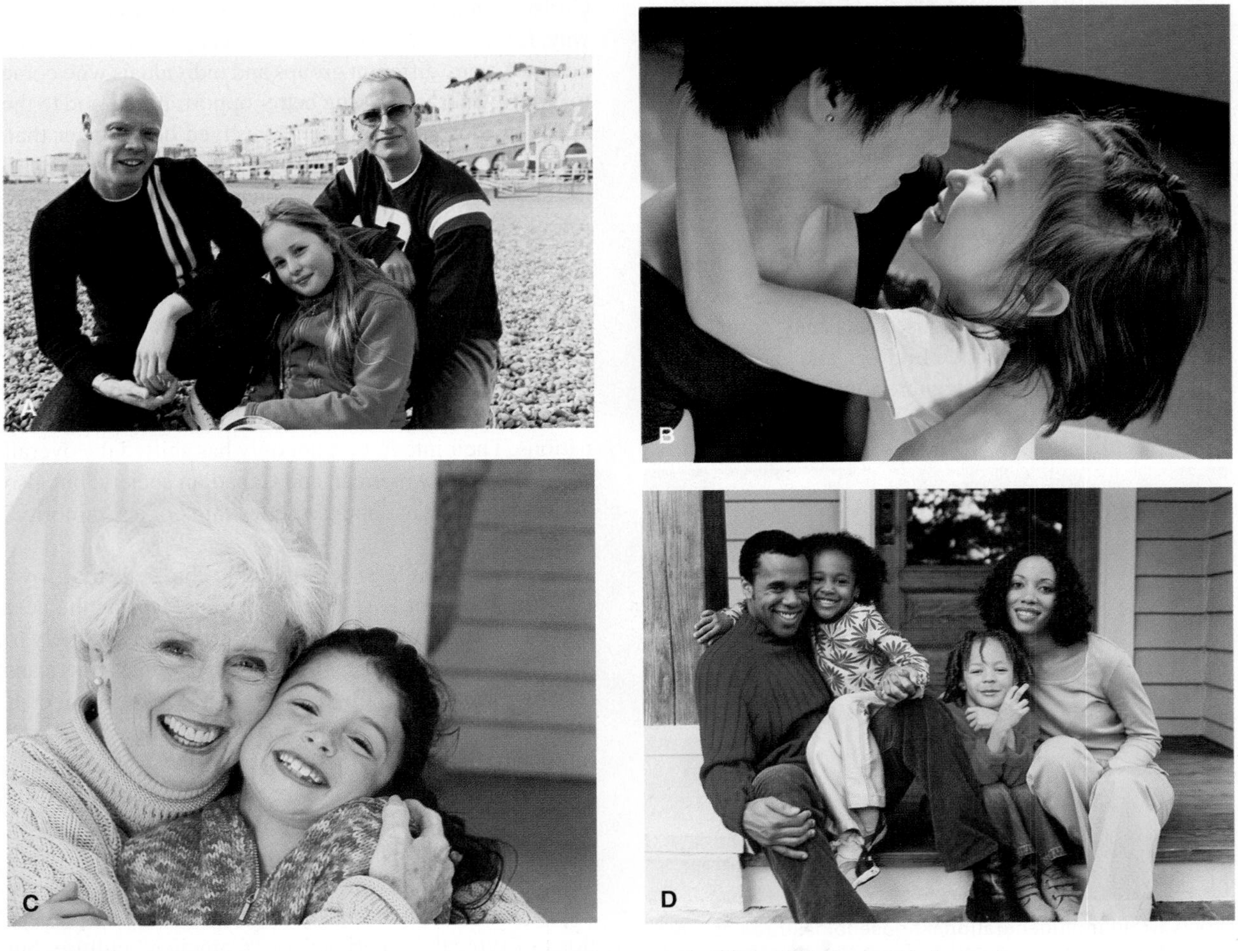

FIGURE 1.1 Notions of what constitutes a family continue to change. Families might be headed by same-sex parents (**A**), single parents (**B**), grandparents (**C**), or heterosexual couples living together who are not married (**D**).

Previous generations of children tended to remain with their parents (and possibly their grandparents) at home until marrying at a relatively young age, and starting a family of their own. An increasingly larger number of people in their 20s, however, have either never left home or have returned home after living independently at college or in other circumstances (Statistics Canada, 2002). Forty-one percent of adults in their 20s were living with their family of origin in Canada, with 33% of men and 28% of women returning home after being independent (Statistics Canada, 2002).

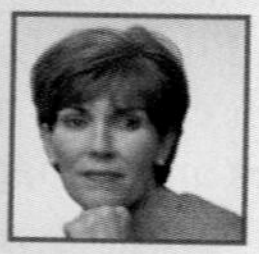

The nurse practitioner tries to explore Elaine's situation in more detail. "I've just started this job, now that my youngest is in middle school. Being back to work has increased my stress level, although we need the extra money. We're ordering out more because I don't have the time to plan meals and cook. I know I have to take better care of myself and ask for help, but my husband has never done much around the house." What suggestions might the nurse offer to help Elaine manage her lifestyle dynamics better to improve her health?

The shape of extended families has changed as well. In the United States, 3.7% of all families have more than two generations living in the same household (Fields, 2004). The most common manifestation (65%) of the multiple-generation family is that of parents, children, and grandchildren living under the same roof, whereas 2% of multigenerational households may contain parents, the parents' parents, children, and the children's children (Fig. 1.2). Multigenerational households may vary in accordance with geographic location, availability of affordable housing, and prevalence among new immigrants (Fields, 2004). Of course, for those families who do not reside in a single home, a multitude of recently developed communication devices—from cell phones to video phones—can help them to "stay in touch."

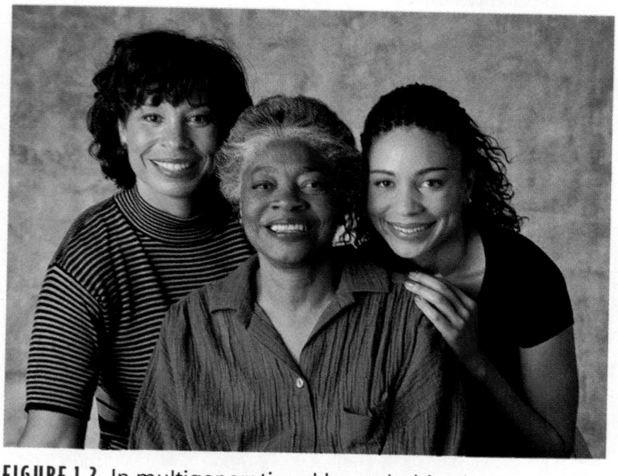

FIGURE 1.2 In multigenerational households, three or more generations are represented as living together under one roof.

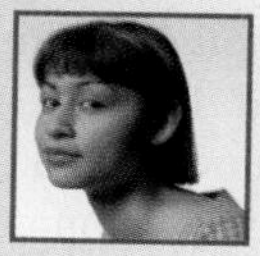

Think back to Georgia, the 22-year-old woman who comes to the clinic with her aunt. The nurse learns that Georgia recently moved in with her grandmother and Esperanza after a short time living in her own apartment. Georgia's mother is dead, and she has not seen her father in 15 years. What influences might these circumstances have on Georgia's state of health and ability to care for herself adequately?

Changes in Sociocultural Influences

North America no longer is dominated primarily by white Christian male views. Diversity is increasing in every way. Health care has become increasingly sensitive to the needs of many different groups and individuals who come to North America seeking better opportunities, and to the needs of those people who have lived here longer than people from the dominant culture. Many changes are still needed, however, to obtain equal access to health care for all.

Recent demographic shifts reflect the growing diversity of populations. During the 1990s, new arrivals to the United States numbered 12 million, a number that exceeded the previous largest wave of immigration in the early 1900s. Current immigration has largely been by people from Asia, Latin America, and Middle Eastern nations. Their integration not only has shifted the overall components of American and Canadian society, but also has influenced what both societies think of as "minority" orientations.

A significant U.S. demographic change is the growing importance of Hispanic Americans. During the next 50 years, the number of Hispanic Americans is likely to more than double, whereas the number of white Americans should decrease by approximately 25% and the number of African Americans should remain about the same. Based on such trends, Hispanic Americans will surpass African Americans as the second largest cultural group in the United States by 2050. Additionally, the number of white Americans will approximately equal that of all "minority" populations combined. These changes are important, not only because of their influence on perceptions of typical "American" or "Canadian" culture, but also because of their effects on health indicators and overall national wellness. For example, currently, rates of infant mortality are higher for African American, Hispanic American, and Native American infants than for white infants (Fig. 1.3). Maternal mortality rates are four times higher for minority women than for white women (Keefe, 2003). If current minority groups continue to grow at their expected rates and such health disparities persist, overall national health will be further compromised, and higher rates of various diseases will lead to more economic and social problems.

Changes in Political Viewpoints

Politically, sexual and reproductive issues have seen various shifts. Unlike in the year 1900, contraceptives are available now to people who desire them, although not all types of contraception are accessible to those who want them (see Chap. 8). Voluntary abortions are currently considered legal in the United States and Canada, but access to an abortion service provider varies geographically in both countries. Trained providers are becoming less common, and those who are available often are physically threatened by people who do not support abortion (Health Canada, 2004d). See Chapter 9 for a fuller discussion. Although homosexuality is not universally accepted, marriage among same-sex couples is being debated in many locations. In some places, such unions have been legally sanctioned.

QUOTE 1-2

"As part of our undergraduate maternity clinical, I always had the students do a day at Planned Parenthood in either the abortion or contraceptive clinics. One year, we literally had to step over people lying on the sidewalk in front of the door. It really brought the controversy surrounding these issues home to the students!"

A nursing instructor recounting her experiences related to politically charged issues

NORTH AMERICAN HEALTH CARE SYSTEMS

Perspectives on the provision of health care vary greatly around the world. In most industrialized countries, these perspectives fall mainly into two categories: (1) government-sponsored care that is accessible to all citizens independent of their ability to pay for it, and (2) health care provided based on each health care consumer's ability to pay for services individually.

This dichotomous approach is represented through the two diverse systems found in North America. The Canadian health care system is government funded and predicated on the belief that all Canadians should have access to needed health care services on a prepaid basis (Health Canada, 2005b). Recently, however, Canada seems to be moving toward adding privatization of health care

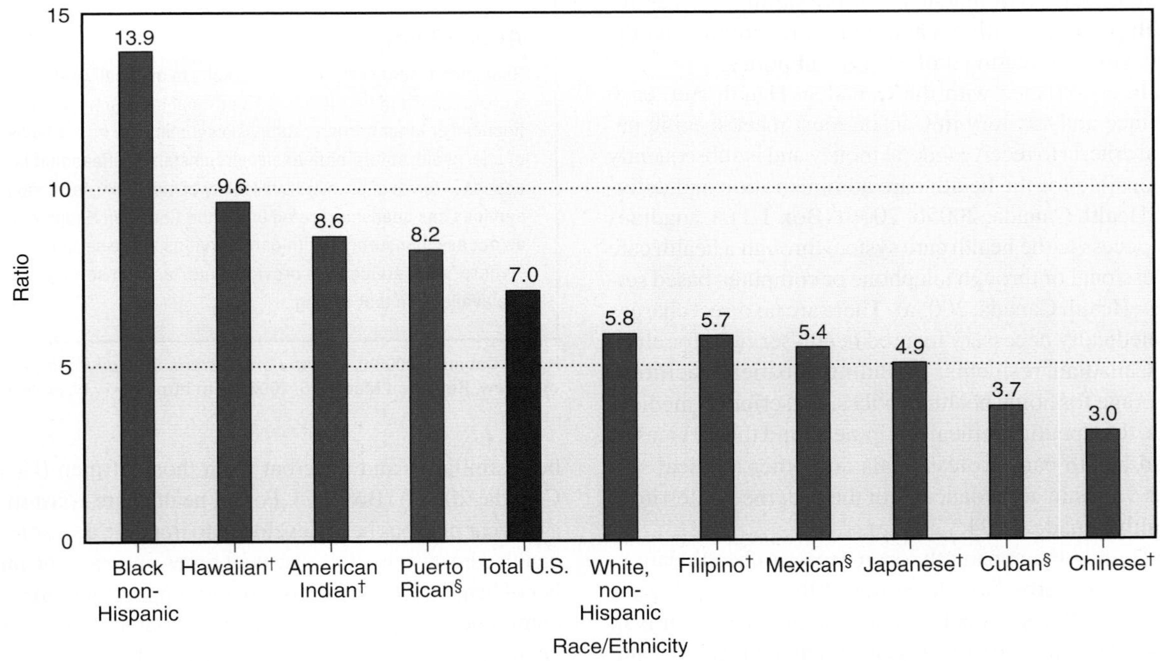

* Per 1,000 live births.
† Can include persons of Hispanic and non-Hispanic origin.
§ Persons of Hispanic origin may be of any race.

FIGURE 1.3 Infant mortality rates by selected racial and ethnic groups, United States, 2002. (From http://www.cdc.gov.)

to its present system. In the United States, the health care system is primarily for-profit, with access to high quality care related to the ability to pay for services.

The issue of access to and affordability of care is significant for women, who often must negotiate care not only for themselves, but also for children, spouses, parents, and other family members. In the United States, a significant number of women do not have insurance coverage, and with today's emphasis on controlling health care costs, current insurance programs often provide only limited coverage, placing the burden of paying for prescriptions, office visits, and follow-up care on the consumer. These circumstances can be especially challenging for women of low to middle socioeconomic status. The implications are especially concerning when one considers the number of uninsured or underinsured women likely to become pregnant, raise children, and require services that their families simply cannot afford.

Canadian Health Care System

Canada's health care system is based on the premise that all eligible residents of the various provinces and territories should have reasonable access to specific health care services on a prepaid basis (2005b). The primary health care model is used as the delivery method of health care within the system (Health Canada, 2005a). As defined by Health Canada (2004b), providing primary health care includes recognizing the centrality of income, housing, education, and environment when providing services for health promotion, illness and injury prevention, and the diagnosis and treatment of illness and injury.

In accordance with the Canadian Health Act, each province and territory in Canada must meet specific national criteria to receive federal money and is subsequently responsible for the health care administration and delivery (Health Canada, 2005b, 2006) (Box 1.1). Canadians gain access to the health care system through a health care professional or through telephone or computer-based services (Health Canada, 2005a). There are no direct charges for medically necessary insured health services for eligible Canadian residents, including inpatient facilities. Coverage for home health services, prescription medications, therapeutic medical equipment, and the services of allied health care professionals and other medical services varies in accordance with the province or territory (Health Canada, 2004c, 2005a).

Despite the apparently open access to health care in Canada, concerns have been raised that access to good quality health care is not as available in reality as it is in theory. To change that reality, a formal Women's Health Strategy was developed to enhance the ability of the Canadian health care system to meet the unique needs of women (Health Canada, 2004a). Integral to this plan is the recognition that women's health care needs include more than just reproductive health and that women's health needs are both similar to and different from those of men (Health Canada, 2004a) (Box 1.2). For all health care consumers, a 10-year plan has been developed to improve access to the health care system, decrease wait times, increase the number of health care providers, provide support for home- and community-based services, increase programs focusing on health promotion, and improve accessibility of needed medications (Office of the Prime Minister, 2004).

BOX 1.1 Principles of the Canadian Health Act

Public Administration

The administration and operation of the health care insurance plan of a province or territory must be carried out on a non-profit basis by a public authority, responsible to the provincial or territorial government and subject to audits of their accounts and financial transactions.

Comprehensiveness

The health insurance plans of the provinces and territories must insure all medically necessary health services (insured services—hospital, physician, surgical-dental) and, where permitted, services rendered by other health care practitioners.

Universality

All insured persons in the province or territory must be entitled to public health insurance coverage on uniform terms and conditions. Provinces and territories usually require that residents register with the plans to establish entitlement.

Portability

Residents moving from one province or territory to another must continue to be covered for insured health services by the "home" province during a minimum waiting period, not to exceed 3 months, imposed by the new province or territory of residence. Residents temporarily absent from their home provinces or territories, or from the country, must also continue to be covered for insured health care services.

Accessibility

Reasonable access by insured persons to medically necessary hospital and physician services must be unimpeded by financial or other barriers, such as discrimination on the basis of age, health status, or financial circumstances. Reasonable access in terms of physical availability of medically necessary services has been interpreted under the Canadian Health Act as access to insured health care services at the setting "where" the services are provided and "as" the services are available in that setting.

Health Canada. (2005b). *Health Care System. Canada Health Act: overview.* Retrieved March 26, 2006, from http://www.hc-sc.gc.ca.

The U.S. Health Care System

Unlike the public health systems of Canada and many other industrialized countries, the U.S. health care system

BOX 1.2 Objectives of Health Canada's Women's Health Strategy

Health Canada's Women's Health Strategy, an integrated framework for addressing major women's health issues, has seven main attributes:

- Balanced
- Respectful of diversity
- Egalitarian
- Evidence-based
- Coherent
- Multisectorial
- Incremental

The strategy has four objectives with key activities undertaken to fulfill them:

1. **Ensure that policies and programs are responsive to sex and gender differences and to women's health needs.** The government is committed to ensuring that all legislation and policies include, where appropriate, an analysis of the potential for different impacts on women and men. It represents Health Canada's commitment to doing business in a way that is sensitive to women's health needs and concerns.
2. **Increase knowledge and understanding of women's health and women's health needs.** Health Canada plays a significant role in the collection and analysis of data and the support of several research programs and activities. The Strategy will make this research more relevant to women's health concerns. Findings will be widely shared, evidence based, and in simple and straightforward language.
3. **Support the provision of effective health services to women.** Health Canada supports groups and jurisdictions with direct responsibility for the delivery of health services. The Department is responsible for interpreting and enforcing the **Canada Health Act** whose principles constitute the framework for Canada's publicly financed health care system. In addition to strengthening knowledge, the federal government provides leadership and support for public awareness, health practices, and educational aids.
4. **Promote good health through preventive measures and the reduction of risk factors that most imperil the health of women.** Health Canada has a responsibility to reach women before they adopt health-threatening lifestyles and to assist them in avoiding high-risk situations, behaviors, and products that lead to health conditions or disease.

is primarily private, with access to good quality care related largely to one's ability to pay for services. People who are uninsured and cannot pay for health care out-of-pocket are not guaranteed health care (American Public Health Association, 2003). Government-sponsored programs are available to facilitate access to health care for qualified people, such as those with low incomes, the elderly, or those on active military status (Organisation for Economic Cooperation and Development, 2002). Nevertheless, these programs do not cover all the needs of the people who participate.

More than 15% of the U.S. population does not have health insurance (Mills & Bhandoff, 2003). Among all women, women of Hispanic/Latina (38%), Native American (30%), African American (23%), and Asian (20%) origin are less likely than whites (13%) to be insured (March of Dimes, 2003). Pregnant women are more likely to be insured than all women, either through private insurers (71.2% vs. 65.9%) or through Medicaid (18.4% vs. 7.6%) (Thorpe, 2001). Among pregnant women, women of Hispanic/Latina background (65.4%) are less likely than African Americans (80.1%) or whites (87.1%) to have any type of health insurance coverage (Thorpe, 2001).

People without health insurance may be fortunate enough to participate in a prenatal health care program that provides care regardless of ability to pay, but these programs do not meet the needs of all the women who require them. Additionally, many women who need the programs may not be able to participate because of child care issues, inability to take off from work, difficulty in obtaining or paying for transportation, or prolonged wait times to obtain an appointment.

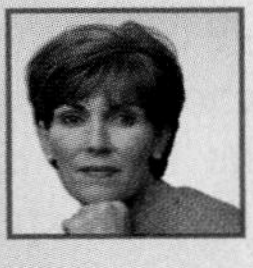

The nurse practitioner suggests to Elaine that she come back to visit in 3 weeks to follow up with some teaching suggestions, recheck her blood pressure, and evaluate the effectiveness of some interventions to manage stress. Elaine looks discouraged. "This is going to cost more money. I have to make sure we can do this appointment on a day I'm not working—I can't afford to miss!" How might the nurse help Elaine with these problems?

Regardless of health insurance status, most women in the United States give birth to their children as inpatients in a hospital facility. In 1980, the average woman could anticipate a hospital stay after childbirth of 3.8 days. By 1995, the length of stay following childbirth had decreased to 2.1 days (Dennison & Pokras, 2000). The Newborns' and Mothers' Health Protection Act of 1996 (NMHPA) was passed to ensure that new mothers had the benefit of a minimum of 48 hours hospitalization after a vaginal birth and 96 hours after a cesarean birth (Center for Medicare and Medicaid, 2002). The effects of the NMHPA vary, however, depending on the state in which the plan exists, the type of health care insurance a person holds, and the primary health care provider's beliefs about the new mother's eligibility for early discharge. Although not a component of the act, community-based programs have been implemented to facilitate the transition to home for parents and their newborns (American Nurses Association, 1997). This type of innovative program is an excellent example of the creativity of health care providers in meeting the changing needs of health care consumers.

HEALTH PROMOTION AND HEALTH STATISTICS

The United States is facing many problems in the arena of women's health. According to the 2004 edition of *Making the Grade on Women's Health: A National and State-by-State Report Card,* the nation as a whole, as well as each state, is failing to meet the health needs of U.S. women, as outlined by *Healthy People 2010* (Box 1.3). Some of the desired goals of *Healthy People 2010* and current progress toward those goals are listed in Table 1.1.

In today's complex, fast-paced society, it sometimes seems that health takes a back seat to other aspects of life. One role of nursing is to help health care consumers to recognize the positive effects that being healthy can have on all aspects of their lives; another is to help them to develop strategies to improve their health. Although nursing care needs to be individualized for each client and family, it is important to be aware of the trends and patterns of health care and to be cognizant of where the client potential fits in the pattern. This knowledge can help the nurse to help clients in health promotion choices, anticipate potential challenges in ensuring that health care needs of clients are met, and improve the overall experience of the client and family in the health care system.

One way that nursing can promote health is by helping health care consumers to understand the importance of participating in a variety of health-promoting behaviors. An example is teaching women how to perform monthly breast self-examinations (Fig. 1.4). Some health promotion activities have diverse and wide-ranging effects on quality of life and health. An excellent example is facilitating the achievement and maintenance of good periodontal (oral) health. For women of childbearing age, good oral health is particularly important because research suggests a potential relationship between poor periodontal health and preeclampsia (Bogess et al., 2003), premature birth, and low birth weight in newborns (Carta et al., 2004; Offenbacher et al., 2001). For people of all ages, periodontal health is related to the potential for achieving a healthy nutritional intake and a healthy body weight.

Another important aspect of providing quality nursing care is an understanding of key statistics for specific groups. For women, such statistics include awareness of risks for specific diseases, common fertility rates, and maternal morbidity and mortality data. Knowledge of these factors can help nurses look for certain indicators or problems when working with women of certain ages or ethnic groups.

Nutritional Status and Body Weight

Most U.S. women do not have a healthy nutritional intake from food sources, in accordance with the U.S. Department of Agriculture's Food Guide Pyramid (see Chaps. 2 and 3). Approximately 27% of adult U.S. women have been identified as overweight, whereas 31.6% were classified as obese, with the highest rate of both overweight and obesity occurring in women 65 to 74 years (U.S. Department of Health and Human Services [USDHHS], 2005, p. 46). When viewed in accordance with ethnic and cultural groups, Hispanic women were found to have the highest rates of being overweight (32.7%), whereas black women had the highest rate of obesity (45.3%). When viewed together, black women had the greatest likelihood of being either overweight or obese (72.6%). It is important to note that obesity has been linked with infertility and increases risks during pregnancy (see Chaps. 10 and 13).

Exercise

Obesity is linked not only to nutritional intake but also to lack of adequate physical activity—an important component in promoting a healthy lifestyle. Thirty percent of women of all ages participate in less than the recommended minimum of 30 minutes of physical activity on most days, although the percentage of women who exercise has increased slightly since 2001 (USDHHS, 2003, 2005). The percentage varies by age, with the highest percentage (36.8%) being between 18 to 24 years, gradually decreasing to 14.3% of women 75 years or older. Exercise is not only important in achieving or maintaining a healthy weight, but is also related to reducing the risk for disease (USDHHS, 2003, 2005) and can be an important component of a healthy pregnancy (American College of Obstetricians and Gynecologists, 2002c).

A wide variety of exercise programs can meet the needs of various population groups, from chair- and water-based exercise programs, to weight lifting and aerobics, to specific prenatal and postnatal exercises classes. What is important is to ensure that the client who is healthy enough to participate in an exercise program chooses the program that reflects any physical limitations she may have and enhances her health status. See Chapter 2 for further details.

Prenatal Care

Of women who become pregnant, 83.4% begin prenatal care within the first trimester of pregnancy (National Women's Law, 2004) (Fig. 1.5). This statistic is far more meaningful and practical when considered in relation to subgroups of women. When viewed by ethnic and cultural subgroups, the percentage of women who began prenatal care during the first trimester varies considerably. Among

BOX 1.3 Leading Health Indicators

Physical Activity

Regular physical activity throughout life is important for maintaining a healthy body, enhancing psychological well-being, and preventing premature death. The objectives selected to measure progress in this area are:

- Increase the proportion of adolescents who engage in vigorous physical activity that promotes cardiorespiratory fitness 3 or more days per week for 20 or more minutes per occasion.
- Increase the proportion of adults who engage regularly, preferably daily, in moderate physical activity for at least 30 minutes per day.

Overweight and Obesity

Overweight and obesity are major contributors to many preventable causes of death. The objectives selected to measure progress in this area are:

- Reduce the proportion of children and adolescents who are overweight or obese.
- Reduce the proportion of adults who are obese.

Tobacco Use

Cigarette smoking is the single most preventable cause of disease and death in the United States. Smoking results in more deaths each year in the United States than AIDS, alcohol, cocaine, heroin, homicide, suicide, motor vehicle crashes, and fires—combined. The objectives selected to measure progress in this area are:

- Reduce cigarette smoking by adolescents.
- Reduce cigarette smoking by adults.

Substance Abuse

Alcohol and illicit drug use are associated with many of this country's most serious problems, including violence, injury, and HIV infection. The objectives selected to measure progress in this area are:

- Increase the proportion of adolescents not using alcohol or any illicit drugs during the past 30 days.
- Reduce the proportion of adults using any illicit drug during the past 30 days.
- Reduce the proportion of adults engaging in binge drinking of alcoholic beverages during the past month.

Responsible Sexual Behavior

Unintended pregnancies and sexually transmitted diseases (STDs), including infection with the human immunodeficiency virus that causes AIDS, can result from unprotected sexual behavior. The objectives selected to measure progress in this area are:

- Increase the proportion of adolescents who abstain from sexual intercourse or use condoms if currently sexually active.
- Increase the proportion of sexually active persons who use condoms.

Mental Health

Approximately 20% of the U.S. population is affected by mental illness during a given year; no one is immune. Of all mental illnesses, depression is the most common disorder. More than 19 million adults in the United States suffer from depression. Major depression is the leading cause of disability and is the cause of more than two thirds of suicides each year. The objective selected to measure progress in this area is:

- Increase the proportion of adults with recognized depression who receive treatment.

Injury and Violence

More than 400 Americans die each day from injuries, due primarily to motor vehicle crashes, firearms, poisonings, suffocation, falls, fires, and drowning. The risk for injury is so great that most persons sustain a significant injury at some time during their lives. The objectives selected to measure progress in this area are:

- Reduce deaths caused by motor vehicle crashes.
- Reduce homicides.

Environmental Quality

An estimated 25% of preventable illnesses worldwide can be attributed to poor environmental quality. In the United States, air pollution alone is estimated to be associated with 50,000 premature deaths and an estimated $40 billion to $50 billion in health-related costs annually. The objectives selected to measure progress in this area are:

- Reduce the proportion of persons exposed to air that does not meet the U.S. Environmental Protection Agency's health-based standards for ozone.
- Reduce the proportion of nonsmokers exposed to environmental tobacco smoke.

Immunization

Vaccines are among the greatest public health achievements of the 20th century. Immunizations can prevent disability and death from infectious diseases for individuals and can help control the spread of infections within communities. The objectives selected to measure progress in this area are:

- Increase the proportion of young children who receive all vaccines that have been recommended for universal administration for at least 5 years.
- Increase the proportion of noninstitutionalized adults who are vaccinated annually against influenza and ever vaccinated against pneumococcal disease.

Continued

BOX 1.3 Leading Health Indicators *(Continued)*

Access to Health Care

Strong predictors of access to quality health care include having health insurance, a higher income level, and a regular primary care provider or other source of ongoing health care. Use of clinical preventive services, such as early prenatal care, can serve as indicators of access to quality health care services. The objectives selected to measure progress in this area are:

- Increase the proportion of persons with health insurance.
- Increase the proportion of persons who have a specific source of ongoing care.
- Increase the proportion of pregnant women who begin prenatal care in the first trimester of pregnancy.

From Department of Health and Human Services. (2000). Leading health indicators. *Healthy People 2010.* Washington, DC: DHHS.

American Indian/Alaska Native women, only 69.3% receive first-trimester prenatal care—a number that represents an increase of 20% to 26% since 1990 (USDHHS, 2003). This is in contrast with non-Hispanic white and black women, of whom 88.5% and 74.5%, respectively, receive first-trimester prenatal care (USDHHS, 2003).

Since 1990, the percentage of women who received prenatal care during the first trimester (84.1% vs. 75.5%) has increased steadily, along with a corresponding decrease in the percentage of women who received late or no prenatal care (61.5% vs. 3.5%), although the actual amounts varied in accordance with ethnic and racial groups (USDHHS, 2005, p. 50). In decreasing order, non-Hispanic white (89%), Asian/Pacific Islander (85.4%), Hispanic (77.4%), non-Hispanic black (76%), and American Indian women (70.9%) received care in the first trimester of pregnancy. American Indian/Alaska Native women were also most likely to receive late or no prenatal care (7.6%), followed by non-Hispanic black women (6.0%) and Hispanic women (5.3%).

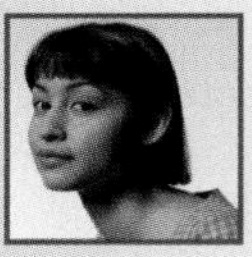

The nurse convinces Esperanza to let her speak with Georgia alone. Once they have privacy, Georgia says, "I'm pretty sure that I am pregnant. My boyfriend and I had unprotected sex a few times, and I've missed two periods. I don't want my family to know what's going on. I'm not sure what I want to do about this yet, and I don't need their opinions." How can the nurse respond with sensitivity, but help Georgia to receive the prenatal care she needs if she decides to continue with the pregnancy?

TABLE 1.1 Healthy People 2010 Indicators and U.S. Progress

INDICATOR	BENCHMARK	NATIONAL AVERAGES
Health insurance	100% coverage for all women	84%
Receive first-trimester prenatal care	At least 90% of all pregnant women	83.4%
Pap test within the past 3 years	At least 90% of all women 18 years or older	86.6%
Mammograms within the past 2 years	100% of all women 40 years or older	76.1%
Sigmoidoscopy	At least 50% of all women 50 years or older at least once in their lives	48.1%
Leisure-time physical activity	At least 80%	73.1%
Obesity	No more than 15%	21.3%
Smoking	No more than 12% of women 18 years or older	20.8%
Binge drinking	No more than 6%	8.2%
Death rates (per 100,000) from:		
Coronary heart disease	84.5	154.8
Stroke	38.8	58.5
Lung cancer	16.6	41
Breast cancer	22.3	26.5
Incidence of:		
Hypertension	No more than 16%	26.1%
Diabetes	No more than 2.5%	6.4%
Chlamydia	No more than 3%	5.6%

From National Women's Law Center and Oregon Health & Science University. (2004). *Making the grade on women's health: A national and state-by-state report card.* Washington, DC: National Women's Law Center.

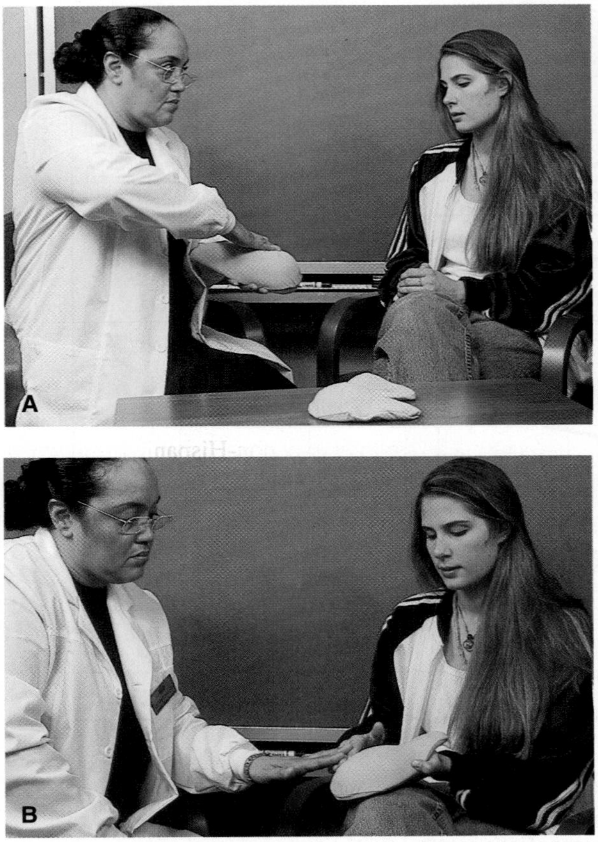

FIGURE 1.4 An important health-promotion behavior is teaching clients the correct way to perform breast self-examinations. (**A**) The nurse may use a prosthetic model to show the right procedure. (**B**) She can then ask the client to perform a return demonstration to check under-

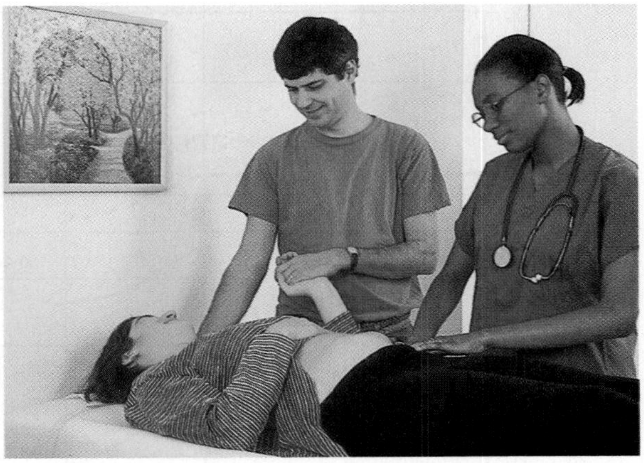

FIGURE 1.5 Prenatal care within the first trimester of pregnancy optimizes the chances for successful maternal and neonatal outcomes.

Birth and Fertility Rates

Figure 1.6 reflects birth rates by age of mother from 1960 to 2004. Thirty years ago, approximately 90% of women had had at least one child by the age of 44. By 2002, the number of women without children had almost doubled to 17.9% (U.S. Census Bureau, 2003). Those women who have children bear fewer children than their counterparts 30 years ago. In 2002, less than 30% of women had three or more children, as compared with 1976, when approximately 60% of women had three or more children (U.S. Census Bureau, 2003). Most women having children were married at the time of the child's birth; however, 22.8% of women who had never been married had given birth to at least one child (U.S. Census Bureau, 2003).

Between 2002 and 2003, the overall birth rate increased among non-Hispanic white and American Indian/Alaska Native women (1%), Hispanic (4%), and Asian/Pacific Islander women (5%), but not among non-Hispanic black women, who experienced a slightly decreased birth rate of less than 1% (USDHHS, 2005, p. 51). **Fertility rate** compares births to the number of women in their childbearing years within a specific group. Hispanic women in 2002 had the highest rate of fertility, with 86.9% of Hispanic women reporting to have borne at least one child by the age of 44, as compared with Asian and Pacific Islander women, who had the lowest rate of fertility at 83.2% (U.S. Census Bureau, 2003). When viewed in terms of "replacement, the rate at which a given generation can exactly replace itself," only Hispanic women exceeded the minimal level for replacement, and no other group of women achieved the minimum level needed (Hamilton et al., 2003, p. 5).

Within the Hispanic megaculture, fertility rates vary widely. In 2001, the average birth rate among all Hispanics was 96 per 1000 population (Hamilton et al., 2003). Women of Mexican background had the highest rate of fertility, with 105.7 births per 1000 population, followed by Puerto Rican women (72.2 of 1000 population) and women of Cuban origin (56.7 per 1000 population). Although the previous paragraph indicated that Hispanic women had a higher rate of fertility than that of non-Hispanic white women, when viewed from the specific cultures, it is revealed that women of Cuban origin have lower birth rates than non-Hispanic women (60.1 per 1000 population).

Maternal Morbidity

Maternal morbidity is defined as a condition outside of normal pregnancy, labor, and childbirth that negatively affects a woman's health during those times and is reported in terms of 1000 live births. Each year, 1.7 million U.S. women experience some level of maternal morbidity (Martin et al., 2002).

Pregnancy-associated hypertension (37.7%), diabetes (31.1%), and anemia (25%) are reported most frequently as risk factors during pregnancy (Martin et al., 2002).

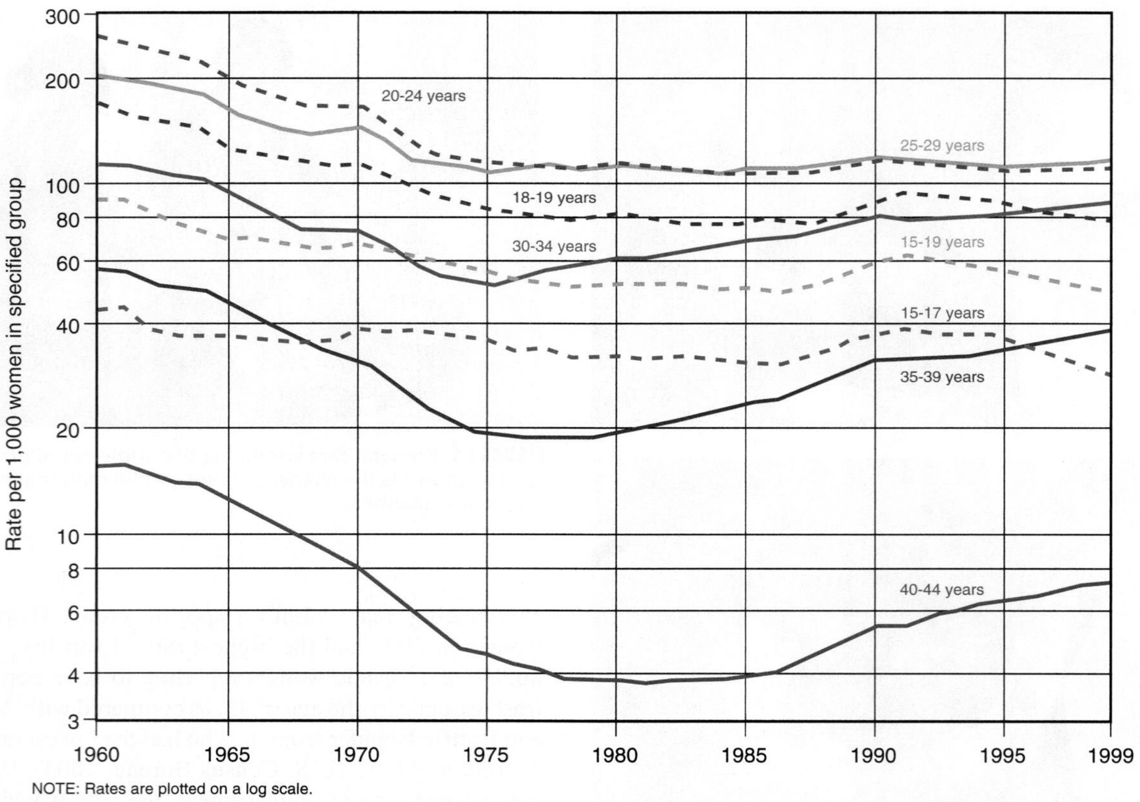

FIGURE 1.6 Birth rates by age of mother: United States, 1960–2004. (From National Center for Health Statistics. [2004]. Births, marriages, divorces, and deaths. *National Vital Statistics Report, 49*[1], 6.)

Between 1993 and 1997, 9.5% of women who had a caesarean birth and 21.2% of women who had a vaginal birth experienced at least one type of maternal morbidity during labor and childbirth. These included obstetrical traumas (10.6%), including third- or fourth-degree lacerations (5%), hypertensive disorders of pregnancy (3%), and gestational diabetes (2.8%), along with preexisting medical conditions such as hypertension (1.5%), cardiac disease (0.9%), and diabetes (0.6%). Native American women had the highest rate of reported medical risk factors.

Maternal Mortality

Maternal mortality is defined as pregnancy-related deaths that occurred during or within 1 year after pregnancy and resulted from (1) complications of pregnancy itself; (2) a chain of events initiated by pregnancy; or (3) aggravation of an unrelated condition by the physiologic effects of pregnancy-related deaths (Centers for Disease Control and Prevention [CDC], 2001, p. 361). The risk for maternal mortality varies according to ethnic and racial groups and age (Fig. 1.7), with younger women of all groups having the lowest mortality overall. Pregnancy-related mortality ratios (PRMRs) are defined as the number of pregnancy-related deaths per 1000 live births (CDC, 2001, p. 361). Black women have the highest PRMR, followed distantly by American Indian/Alaska Native women, Asian/Pacific Islander women, Hispanic women, and white women, who had the lowest mortality rate—approximately three times lower than that of black women.

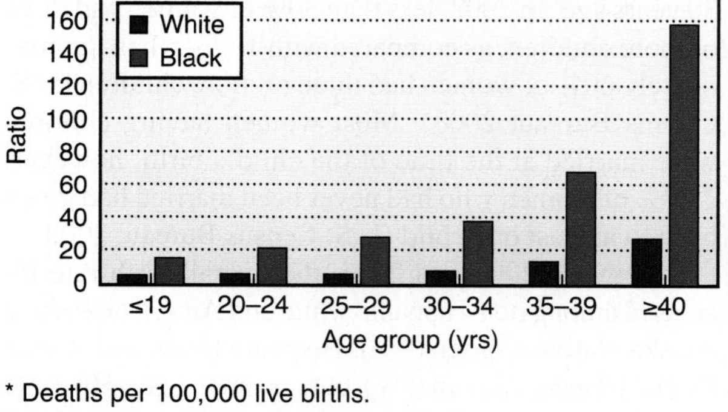

FIGURE 1.7 Pregnancy-related maternal mortality ratios according to age and race, United States, 1991–1999. (From http://www.cdc.gov.)

Using a definition of *maternal death* that limited the time interval to a maximum of 42 days following pregnancy termination, Hoyert and colleagues (2000) found that both the United States and Canada experienced an overall long-term decrease in maternal mortality, followed by a plateau, with Canada experiencing a lower maternal mortality rate than the United States. Women experiencing direct obstetrical complications, such as amniotic and thrombotic embolisms, pregnancy-induced hypertension, and hemorrhage, were at highest risk for maternal mortality.

CRITICAL THINKING, ETHICALLY BASED PRACTICE, AND EVIDENCE-BASED CARE

Certain aspects of care are crucial to the provision of quality client care. These aspects include such dimensions as critical thinking, **ethically based practice,** and evidence-based practice. Although these aspects of caregiving are important for all clients, certain components emerge when working in the areas of maternal, newborn, and women's health nursing and are discussed subsequently.

Critical thinking is inherent in nursing practice; in fact, without critical thinking, there would be no professional nursing. **Critical thinking** is a higher-level, complex thought process through which competent, comprehensive decision making and problem solving can result in informed, intelligent, decisions. Critical thinking is holistic: it requires more than just rote knowledge to make a decision, or solve a problem. Inherent in critical thinking is an understanding of people, situations, and phenomena, along with recognizing the potential for each situation, both perceived and actualized. It is creative.

Participating in critical thinking involves awareness and acknowledgement of personal values and attitudes, the ability to evaluate each aspect, and the potential actualization of the different possibilities of the situation. It also requires knowing when personal knowledge limitations have been met and additional information is required (Green, 2000; Wilkinson, 2001). For example, knowing that, according to statistics, a woman from a specific ethnic background may be likely to choose early prenatal care is an important piece of information to have in promoting client health. Although it may not translate into an observed action by a specific client, it can provide some additional insights that will help in understanding the client's overall culture and belief system. The important factor is applying the information in a meaningful way for the specific client, and that is accomplished through using critical thinking.

Nursing practice is grounded in both informal and formal ethical beliefs (Wilkinson, 2001). An informal ethical code is "based on conventional moral principles—unwritten values rooted in nurses' more general moral views, experiences, and the history of the profession" (Wilkinson, 2001, p. 41). For example, the belief that nurses have theoretical knowledge that they can apply correctly in various settings would be an unwritten value.

In addition to the informal code of ethics, both the Canadian and the American Nurses' Associations have formally codified ethical values for use in practice and decision making (American Nurses Association, 2001; Canadian Nurses Association, 2002a) (Boxes 1.4 and 1.5). The codes also may clarify expectations within the profession for both professional and client (Beauchamp & Childress, 2001), and between professions. Ethical principles provide guidance for practice and most likely formed the bases for the codes of ethics. The guiding principles include autonomy, beneficence, nonmaleficence, and justice (Beauchamp & Childress, 2001).

BOX 1.4 American Nurses Association Code of Ethics for Nurses With Interpretive Statement

1. The nurse, in all professional relationships, practices with compassion and respect for the inherent dignity, worth, and uniqueness of every individual, unrestricted by considerations of social or economic status, personal attributes, or the nature of health problems.
2. The nurse's primary commitment is to the patient, whether an individual, family, group, or community.
3. The nurse promotes, advocates for, and strives to protect the health, safety, and rights of the patient.
4. The nurse is responsible and accountable for individual nursing practice and determines the appropriate delegation of tasks consistent with the nurse's obligation to provide optimum patient care.
5. The nurse owes the same duties to self as to others, including the responsibility to preserve integrity and safety, to maintain competence, and to continue personal and professional growth.
6. The nurse participates in establishing, maintaining, and improving health care environments and conditions of employment conducive to the provision of quality health care and consistent with the values of the profession through individual and collective action.
7. The nurse participates in the advancement of the profession through contributions to practice, education, administration, and knowledge development.
8. The nurse collaborates with other health professionals and the public in promoting community, national, and international efforts to meet health needs.
9. The profession of nursing, as represented by associations and their members, is responsible for articulating nursing values, for maintaining the integrity of the profession and its practice, and for shaping social policy.

Adapted from American Nurses Association. (2001). *Code of ethics for nurses with interpretive statements.* Washington, DC: American Nurses Association Publications.

BOX 1.5 Canadian Code of Ethics for Registered Nurses

Nursing values defined: A value is something that is prized or held dear; something that is deeply cared about. This code is organized around eight primary values that are central to ethical nursing practice:

1. *Safe, competent, and ethical care.* Nurses value the ability to provide safe, competent, and ethical care that allows them to fulfill their ethical and professional obligations to the people they serve.
2. *Health and well-being.* Nurses value health promotion and well-being and assisting persons to achieve their optimum level of health in situations of normal health, illness, injury, disability, or at the end of life.
3. *Choice.* Nurses respect and promote the autonomy of persons and help them to express their health needs and values, and also to obtain desired information and services so that they can make informed decisions.
4. *Dignity.* Nurses recognize and respect the inherent worth of each person and advocate for respectful treatment of all persons.
5. *Confidentiality.* Nurses safeguard information learned in the context of a professional relationship, and ensure it is shared outside the health care team only with the person's informed consent, or as may be legally required, or where the failure to disclose would cause significant harm.
6. *Justice.* Nurses uphold principles of equity and fairness to assist persons in receiving a share of health services and resources proportionate to their needs and in promoting social justice.
7. *Accountability.* Nurses are answerable for their practice, and they act in a manner consistent with their professional responsibilities and standards of practice.
8. *Quality practice environments.* Nurses value and advocate for practice environments that have the organizational structures and resources necessary to ensure safety, support, and respect for all persons in the work setting.

From Canadian Nurses Association. (2002a). *Nursing ethics: Code of ethics for Registered Nurses.* Retrieved March 29, 2006, from http://www.cna-aiic.ca.

Autonomy is the right of the individual to make personal choices and decisions independent of the beliefs of others. Beneficence is doing good; nonmaleficence is doing no harm. Justice is providing the person with what he or she deserves. Justice is widely regarded as the most complex ethical principle; from it derived the imperatives of equal treatment for all as well as the allocation of limited health care resources (American College of Obstetricians and Gynecologists [ACOG], 2002a).

Although both the codes and principles seem to provide a very clear directive for nursing practice, the reality is that there are situations in which it is difficult to support them equally (ACOG, 2002a). For example, a postpartum client asks the nurse for assistance in breastfeeding her 1-hour-old newborn. The nurse, a breastfeeding advocate, is aware that the client is HIV positive and has refused treatment with AZT. Breastfeeding will increase the likelihood of the newborn being permanently HIV positive. In this situation, simultaneously upholding the principles of autonomy, beneficence, and nonmaleficence *seems* impossible.

Ethical Decision Making

Through the introduction of new technologies and practices, particularly in the areas of women's health and maternity nursing, the potential need for ethical decision making has increased dramatically (ACOG, 2002b). Situations requiring ethical decision making may be as diverse as client care decisions, application of institutional philosophical beliefs, or, as in a previous example, resource allocation. Nurses, as well as other members of the health care team, can use professionally based codes of ethics along with ethical principles to promote decision making. A growing number of health care institutions have formed ethics committees to assist health care clients, families, and professionals in ethically based decision making (Fig. 1.8). Membership in ethics committees should reflect the demographics of the community and health care facility (ACOG, 2002b) and may include physicians, registered professional nurses, social workers, and other health care professionals, along with representatives from the community and religious groups.

Advances in health care technology have brought with them numerous ethical decision-making challenges

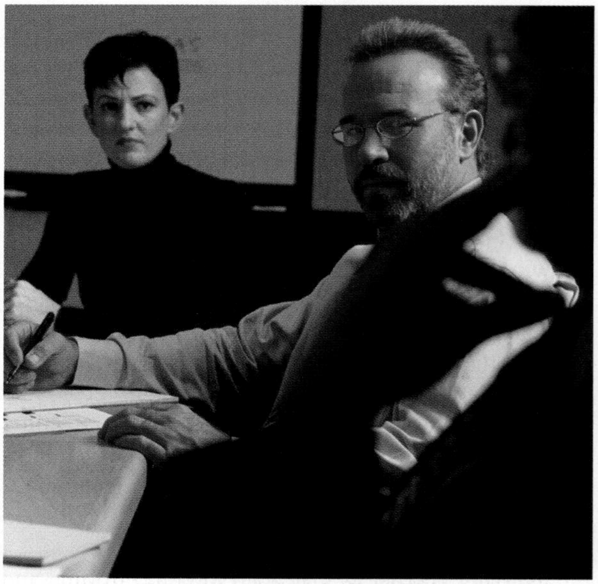

FIGURE 1.8 Ethics committees in health care facilities and institutions can provide assistance with difficult choices and decisions in all areas, including maternal, newborn, and women's health care.

that require examination of personal beliefs, along with religious beliefs and legal boundaries. One area in which this becomes very apparent is that of infertility. Nurses specializing in infertility care are frequently working with women who may have infertility based on maternal age. Is there a specific age at which infertility treatments should be denied? What about marital status? Socioeconomic status? Who should decide or be involved in the decision? (Some insurance companies actually do use age and marital status as parameters for funding infertility treatments.) Suppose a multifetal pregnancy has been achieved, but the woman wants to have only one baby (either for personal or practical reasons). What are the issues surrounding multifetal pregnancy reduction? Continuing on with this scenario, what if the pregnancy was achieved through in vitro fertilization (IVF) and multiple embryos remain that have been frozen but are not desired by the woman or her partner and they do not wish to donate them to another infertile couple? What should happen to the embryos? Should they remain frozen in case the woman changes her mind? Should they be donated for practice? What if the woman and her partner wish to donate them for stem cell research?

For some people, and in some, but not all, religions, stem cell research is viewed as destroying a human life and is not supported (National Bioethics Advisory Commission, 1999). The issue is in this situation a question of the genesis of personhood. It is the same issue that emerges for some individuals when faced with participating in a multifetal pregnancy reduction (Box 1.6).

On the other side of fertility—undesired pregnancy—the issue of personhood is also a dilemma, and one that is becoming more complex than ever with the advances in technology that have resulted in a blurring of the boundary between second-trimester abortion and fetal viability. Box 1.7 contains a partial list of areas of potential ethical concern and controversy identified by the Canadian Nurses Association. See also Chapter 9.

Resolving ethical dilemmas requires the implementation of critical thinking. One of the most important aspects of applying a decision-making guideline to an ethical dilemma is that personal thoughts, beliefs, biases, and values need to be identified and acknowledged if the ethical dilemma is to be resolved in an appropriate and professional manner. A dilemma is ethical when knowledgeable, thoughtful individuals, faced with the same ethical dilemma, can come to different conclusions and both are correct (Murphy & Murphy, 1976, p. 13). There are numerous structured decision-making strategies that have been developed specifically for, or that can be applied to, ethical decision-making, including the nursing process. One strategy that has been useful was developed by Murphy and Murphy (1976) for health-related ethical decision making. The strategy does not include a focus on resolving the health issue. Rather, the

BOX 1.6 Embryonic Stem Cell Research

Many scientists and lay people believe that embryonic stem cell research may hold the cure for multiple disorders, including Parkinson's disease, type 1 diabetes mellitus, cardiac disease, and cellular impairment, such as in injuries to the spinal cord (National Bioethics Advisory Commission, 1999). Stem cells are harvested at the blastocyst stage of embryonic development (see Chap. 11) (Fischbach & Fischbach, 2004). Sources for the embryos include elective abortion or in vitro fertilization (IVF) procedures. IVF-generated embryos may have been generated for reproductive purposes, but are no longer needed for the fertility treatment, or the embryos may have been purposely developed for stem cell research (National Bioethics Advisory Commission, 1999). Although adult tissue does contain stem cells, the stem cells thus harvested do not have the same potential as those originating from an embryo (Fischbach & Fischbach, 2004).

Embryonic stem cells are unique among cells because they are pluripotent—that is, they have the ability to develop into multiple types of cell types. For people who believe that human life begins at conception, the ethical dilemma involves destroying a potential human life to improve an existing life (Fischbach & Fischbach, 2004). For those people who do not hold that belief, the ethical dilemma may be related to the perceived waste of the opportunity to find treatments to help improve the health of those with chronic illnesses or injuries. In either case, there are also legal issues regarding the use of stem cells.

In 2001, President George W. Bush (2001) mandated that U.S. federal funds could be used to support research only on existing stem cell lines that met specific criteria, such as being generated from excess embryos that were created but not used for reproductive purposes. Because no additional stem cell lines can be created using federal funds, stem cell research has been curtailed in the United States, although that is not the case internationally (Fischbach & Fischbach, 2004).

In Canada, controversies regarding stem cell research were acknowledged along with the important potential benefit of research in this area. Legislation and guidelines were established that would support stem cell research using human embryonic tissue as well as other stem cell sources, including the development of stem cell lines using government research funds. The guidelines were derived from the following principles:

- Research undertaken should have potential health benefits for Canadians.
- Materials were harvested in situations involving free and informed consent, provided voluntarily and with full disclosure of all information relevant to the consent.
- Respect for privacy and confidentiality is maintained.
- No direct or indirect payment for tissues is collected for stem cell research, with no financial incentives.
- Embryos are not created specifically for research purposes.
- Respect is shown for individual and community notions of human dignity and physical, spiritual, and cultural integrity (Canadian Institutes of Health Research, 2005).

BOX 1.7 Key Areas of Ethical Concern and Controversy

- The moral status of the embryo, fetus, and organisms created by cloning, as a function of selective reduction of pregnancy, use of spare embryos not needed in IVF for purpose of research, and creating embryos for research purposes
- The protection of the child as a function of reproduction through donor insemination, surrogacy, duplicate identity through cloning, right to know genetic heritage and to have genetic heritage protected by privacy legislation
- Access to sound reproductive technologies by all citizens
- The integrity of family relationships when reproductive and genetic technologies such as surrogacy, cloning, and genetic alteration are employed
- The safety of products developed for therapeutic cloning and the lack of evidence to know longer-term effects
- The potential for abuse of genetic testing, such as denying individuals life insurance and abuse of testing in the workplace leading to job loss, stigmatization
- The morality of presymptomatic genetic testing in cases in which no therapeutic treatment can yet be provided (ie, Huntington's chorea)
- The morality of sex selection and genetic enhancement (eg, creating the perfect child)
- The commercialization of reproductive technologies (eg, infertility as a business) and genetic technologies, including cloning techniques (eg, treating body parts and processes as items that can be bought and sold)
- The potential benefits of stem cell research versus the protection of the human embryo
- The claims for patents on living organisms in order to realize future profits versus the protection of human embryos
- The claims for patents on living organisms in order to realize future profits versus the human genome as a public treasure
- The need for valid information available to the public on all these issues for informed public and personal choices

From Canadian Nurses Association. (2002b). *Position statement: The role of the nurse in reproductive and genetic technologies.* Retrieved January 23, 2005, from http://www.cna-nurses.ca.

focus is simply deciding how to resolve the dilemma. Table 1.2 contains the steps of the Murphy and Murphy decision-making guide, along with the analogous nursing process steps.

Another method the nurse can use to gain knowledge about a situation in which ethical concerns may be raised is to view the situation from a trilevel perspective: societal, institutional, and individual (Canadian Nurses Association, 2000, p. 1). By implementing this method of critical thinking, the multiple influences that affect decision making and outcomes in the specific situation will be illuminated, along with a possible direction regarding the most appropriate action for resolving the situation (Box 1.8).

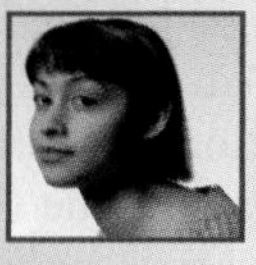

Examination has shown that Georgia, the 22-year-old from the beginning of the chapter, is pregnant. Georgia does not seem upset or surprised by this news. She says, "My aunt doesn't like my boyfriend, but I know he'll help me out. I wish she'd mind her own business, but I need her help financially right now. I'm just going to tell her nothing's wrong and let her know what's happening once Freddy and I have made our decision." What dilemmas might this pose for the nurse providing care?

TABLE 1.2 Comparison of Murphy and Murphy's Method of Ethical Decision Making with the Nursing Process

MURPHY & MURPHY'S STEP	COMPONENT OF THE NURSING PROCESS
1. Identify the health problem.	Assessment
2. Identify the ethical problem.	Assessment
3. State who is involved in making the decisions.	Assessment
4. Identify your role, if any, in the decision-making process.	Assessment
5. Consider as many possible alternative decisions as you can.	Diagnosis
6. Consider the long- and short-range consequences of each alternative decision.	Planning
7. Reach your decision.	Implementation
8. Consider how this decision fits in with your general philosophy of client care.	Evaluation
9. Follow the situation until you can see the actual results of your decision and use this information to help in making future decisions.	Evaluation

Adapted from Murphy & Murphy (1976), p. 13.

BOX 1.8 Trilevel Decision Making

The Tristate Health Care Center is the primary facility for women who have chosen to give birth in a hospital. Eighty-five percent of women who give birth in the facility are without health insurance and return home with their newborns with minimum to no support (*individual level*). During an interdisciplinary staff meeting, data are presented that indicate a need for a home visit from an RN following discharge from the inpatient facility. Subjective data supporting the need for a visit include a number of the women stating they had a need for someone to come to their home and help them to adapt to caring for a baby. The objective data included the nurses' observations that a number of the women required two to three attempts to correctly return-demonstrate infant care before discharge, along with multiple postdischarge phone calls requesting clarification of infant care.

To meet these needs, the staff generate a potential home care program that includes inpatient RN staff rotating to the community to perform home visits to women discharged to home with their newborns (*institutional level*). The staff provide both education and material support, such as extra diapers, wipes, and so forth.

Because most of the women who would be recipients of this program do not have health insurance coverage, external funding sources would need to be used to support the program (*societal level*).

Sample questions that need to be considered for each level:

- *Individual level:* Are the individual women and their newborns who would benefit from this program able to access the proposed services or similar ones in a more cost-effective or more easily accessible manner?
- *Institutional level:* Does the Tristate Health Care Center have the resources (personnel as well as physical) to effectively administer and implement the program?
- *Societal level:* Is the cost per individual served by this program make it fiscally viable? Does the program represent the most optimal use of the limited funds available?

Informed Consent

In the 21st century, the belief that health care consumers have a right to make informed decisions about their health care, and health care providers have an obligation to ensure that their clients are informed at a level in which active, informed decision making is possible, seems routine. Yet, although **informed consent** appears to have evolved from ethical principles, in fact, its origin is legal (Nelson-Marten & Rich, 1999). From the middle 1700s in England through the 1950s in the United States and elsewhere, there were several legal cases in which physicians were sued for not providing reasonable care—either through physical action (battery) or by not providing adequate verbal information about a medical procedure (as cited in Nelson-Marten & Rich, 1999). In the 1970s, informed consent began to emerge in the United States as a means for client autonomy in health care decisions. During the next decade through the present, the importance of collaborative decision making with the client and health care providers has been emphasized (Association of Women's Health, Obstetric and Neonatal Nurses, 2003; Brazell, 1997).

In clinical settings, there are several types of consent, some of which require a signature on a specific informed consent form, and others that are more informal and do not require written documentation (Beauchamp & Childress, 2001). For example, a health care professional may assume that a client who gives permission for a specific routine procedure automatically gives permission for additional procedures. That assumption, however, may be incorrect and result in violation of the client's rights. Encouraging the client to make an informed decision about a procedure will ensure that the client's rights are upheld. For example, educating a client about postpartum assessment, including the nurse's actions, and the benefits and risks of having the assessment completed at specific intervals, followed by an assessment of client understanding and verbal permission or denial to perform the assessment, will help to ensure that the client has made an informed decision. If the client refuses, the nurse has no right or authority to proceed. The nurse should document the intervention with the client very clearly in the chart, and follow protocol in ensuring that the appropriate personnel, including the primary health care provider, are aware of the refusal to ensure the client's safety and rights (Fig. 1.9).

Informed Consent for Interventions

One of the difficulties in achieving true informed consent—either verbal or written—is that many health care consumers are unaware of their basic rights in health care. Nurses are responsible for ensuring that clients understand their rights, and then confirming

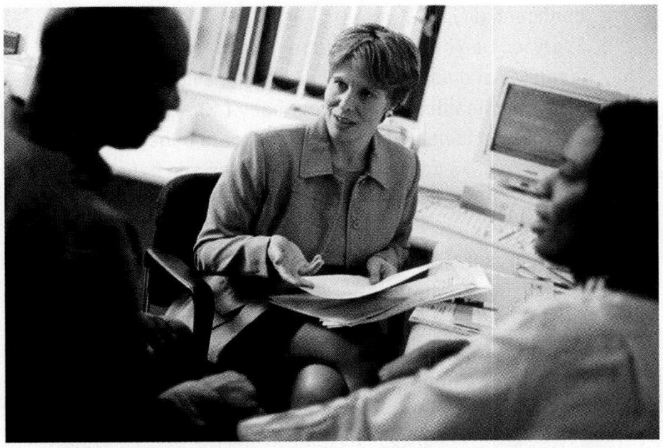

FIGURE 1.9 Nurses must carefully explain and obtain informed consent, as well as document that they have done so, to protect themselves, clients, colleagues, and employers.

that their rights have been upheld. Empowering clients to ask the questions that will get the answers they need is one way in which clients can initiate being active participants in their care decisions. Box 1.9 contains a series of questions adapted from the Childbirth Connection (2004) Web site that guides health care consumers in gathering the needed information to make informed decisions about their health care. Although the questions were originally generated to assist women with maternity choices, they are broad and applicable to all nonemergency health

BOX 1.9 Every Woman's Rights

Consideration and respect for every woman under all circumstances is the foundation of this statement of rights.

1. Every woman has the right to health care before, during, and after pregnancy and childbirth.
2. Every woman and infant has the right to receive care that is consistent with current scientific evidence about benefits and risks.* Practices that have been found to be safe and beneficial should be used when indicated. Harmful, ineffective, or unnecessary practices should be avoided. Unproven interventions should be used only in the context of research to evaluate their effects.
3. Every woman has the right to choose a midwife or a physician as her maternity care provider. Both caregivers skilled in normal childbearing and caregivers skilled in complications are needed to ensure quality care for all.
4. Every woman has the right to choose her birth setting from the full range of safe options available in her community, on the basis of complete, objective information about benefits, risks, and costs of these options.*
5. Every woman has the right to receive all or most of her maternity care from a single caregiver or a small group of caregivers, with whom she can establish a relationship. Every woman has the right to leave her maternity caregiver and select another if she becomes dissatisfied with her care.* (Only second sentence is a legal right.)
6. Every woman has the right to information about the professional identity and qualifications of those involved with her care, and to know when those involved are trainees.*
7. Every woman has the right to communicate with caregivers and receive all care in privacy, which may involve excluding nonessential personnel. She also has the right to have all personal information treated according to standards of confidentiality.*
8. Every woman has the right to receive maternity care that identifies and addresses social and behavioral factors that affect her health and that of her baby.† She should receive information to help her take the best care of herself and her baby and have access to social services and behavioral change programs that could contribute to their health.
9. Every woman has the right to full and clear information about benefits, risks, and costs of the procedures, drugs, tests, and treatments offered to her, and of all other reasonable options, including no intervention.* She should receive this information about all interventions that are likely to be offered during labor and birth well before the onset of labor.
10. Every woman has the right to accept or refuse procedures, drugs, tests, and treatments, and to have her choices honored. She has the right to change her mind.* (Please note that this established legal right has been challenged in a number of recent cases.)
11. Every woman has the right to be informed if her caregivers wish to enroll her or her infant in a research study. She should receive full information about all known and possible benefits and risks of participation, and she has the right to decide whether to participate, free from coercion and without negative consequences.*
12. Every woman has the right to unrestricted access to all available records about her pregnancy, her labor, and her infant; to obtain a full copy of these records; and to receive help in understanding them, if necessary.*
13. Every woman has the right to receive maternity care that is appropriate to her cultural and religious background, and to receive information in a language in which she can communicate.*
14. Every woman has the right to have family members and friends of her choice present during all aspects of her maternity care.†
15. Every woman has the right to receive continuous social, emotional, and physical support during labor and birth from a caregiver who has been trained in labor support.†
16. Every woman has the right to receive full advance information about risks and benefits of all reasonably available methods for relieving pain during labor and birth, including methods that do not require the use of drugs. She has the right to choose which methods will be used and to change her mind at any time.*
17. Every woman has the right to freedom of movement during labor, unencumbered by tubes, wires, or other apparatus. She also has the right to give birth in the position of her choice.*
18. Every woman has the right to virtually uninterrupted contact with her newborn from the moment of birth, as long as she and her baby are healthy and do not need care that requires separation.†
19. Every woman has the right to receive complete information about the benefits of breastfeeding well in advance of labor, to refuse supplemental bottles and other actions that interfere with breastfeeding, and to have access to skilled lactation support for as long as she chooses to breastfeed.†
20. Every woman has the right to decide collaboratively with caregivers when she and her baby will leave the birth site for home, based on their condition and circumstances.†

*At this time in the United States, childbearing women are legally entitled to these rights.

†The legal system would probably uphold these rights.

From Childbirth Connection. (2004). *The rights of childbearing women.* New York: Maternity Center Association. Retrieved March 29, 2006, from http://www.childbirthconnection.org/article.asp?ck=10084&ClickedLink=0&area=27.

care situations. The questions can be handed to the client when she enters the health care system, or at any time during her interactions. The client should be assured that she has the right to be involved in a knowledgeable way in her health care. Although the questions are directed at health care consumers, they can also serve as a guide to ensure that nurses have provided clients with the tools they need to be informed consumers of health care. Barriers to informed consent are listed in Box 1.10.

For written informed consent, the health care provider who will be performing a medical or surgical procedure is responsible to ensure that informed consent is obtained. This includes education regarding the procedure, including the risk and benefits of the procedure, alternatives, and potential side effects (see Chap. 17). Yet, despite the legal obligation of the primary health care provider, frequently it is the staff nurse who accepts responsibility for providing the necessary education as well as witnessing the client's signature on the consent form (Curtin, 1993).

Providing informed consent is a form of personal empowerment. The nurse can facilitate this empowerment through providing the information needed by the client to make an informed decision, and helping the client recognize her personal knowledge level about the procedure. Box 1.11 contains five questions that can help the client to assess her ability to provide an informed consent.

Informed consent evolved to protect the client; however, the written form evolved to protect the health care provider by providing concrete evidence that informed consent was obtained (Curtin, 1993). When the staff nurse who is not the primary provider in the situation provides informed consent, the reality of the informed consent is in question because it is a contract between the health care provider responsible for the specific procedure and the client (Curtin, 1993).

A client who has given informed consent has the right to change her mind and refuse a treatment or procedure at any time during the process, including before it is initiated. Her decision must be shared with the health care provider who is implementing the treatment or procedure. Concurrently, if the client states confusion or misinformation about the treatment or procedure, the nurse is responsible for informing the health care provider who is to implement the action that further information is needed by the client before proceeding (Curtin, 1993).

BOX 1.10 Barriers to Informed Consent

Client-Focused Barriers

- Age, either very young or old
- Education level, which may relate to the client's ability to process the information in the informed consent document
- Illness, both presence and degree, which may affect ability to process the information needed for informed consent
- Relationship between the client and the primary health care provider, which may be construed as having coercive elements

Process-Centered Barriers to Informed Consent

- Timing of the discussion related to the informed consent. For example, opening a discussion about a research protocol during the same meeting as receiving a devastating diagnosis will hinder informed consent.
- Time allocated for the prospective participant/subject to discuss the informed consent with the person responsible for the study
- Reading level and the actual wording of the information in the informed consent document

Adapted from Taylor, H. A. (1999). Barriers to informed consent. *Seminars in Oncology Nursing, 15*(2), 89–95.

BOX 1.11 Making Informed Decisions

1. What are the possible choices that I have?
2. What does the best available research tell me about the safety and effectiveness of each of these choices?
3. What are my needs and preferences and those of other family members who may be affected by my choice?
4. What choices are available and supported in my care setting and through my care providers?
5. If I want an option that will not or may not be available to me, would I consider switching to a care setting or care provider that does offer me preferred care?

Adapted from Childbirth Connection. (2005). Vision, mission, and beliefs: Informed decision making, informed consent or refusal. Retrieved March 29, 2006, from http://www.Childbirthconnection.org/article.asp?ck=10081.

Informed Consent for Research

Unlike informed consent for health care interventions, informed consent for research grew out of the ashes of the Holocaust. Among the atrocities of the Nazi regime, physicians performed horrible "experiments" involving pain, mutilation, and death on innocent men, women, and children imprisoned in the concentration camps. Following World War II, these physicians were brought to trial by the world in Nuremberg, and the need for ethically based research was brought to the awareness of the world (E. Weisel, as cited in Nelson-Marten & Rich, 1999).

The U.S. government officially recognized the need for formal guidelines and peer review of research on human subjects in 1953 (Nelson-Marten & Rich, 1999), although this recognition did not concurrently result in ethical research in the United States (Faden & Beauchamp, 1986). Today, multiple operating mechanisms are in place to help ensure that ethical principles are upheld. Institutional Review Boards (IRBs) composed of health care professionals, including registered professional nurses, physicians, social workers, and possibly community members, were developed as a peer review mechanism for research studies and now have an active mandate to ensure that research studies achieve ever greater ethical standards before being implemented.

Frequently, a client who is a recipient of nursing care is also approached to participate in a research study. It is imperative that the nurse as a client advocate—regardless of whether he or she is involved in the research itself or is focused on providing nursing care to the client—ensures that the client receiving health care does not feel coerced to participate in the study. The client needs to be assured that regardless of whether she becomes or remains a study participant, the level of care that she experiences will be completely independent of her decision regarding research participation. It is of equal importance to determine that the client does indeed understand the study enough to provide true informed consent.

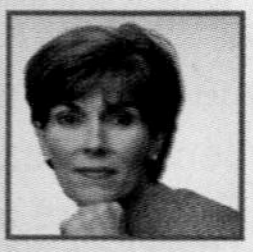

As Elaine is leaving the nurse practitioner's office, she sees a flyer on the bulletin board recruiting participants for a research study on the effects of a new exercise program. Elaine points to the flyer and asks, "Does this study pay money? If I agree to participate, can we postpone starting one of these drugs you've prescribed?" How should the nurse respond?

Nursing and Women's Health Research

Historically, women of reproductive age were excluded from participating in most clinical research studies (Legato & Dean, 1999). As women's voices became stronger, through grassroots organizations such as the Boston Women's Health Collective and the Black Women's Health Network, the need to include women in research along with their male counterparts became increasingly obvious, resulting in a mandate from the National Institutes of Health for the inclusion of women in all research studies (Pinn, 1999). (Of course, women would be omitted from studies focusing on specific male issues, such as cancer of the male prostate gland.)

Not only are women being included in research, it is now recognized that research needs to include women throughout the life cycle (Pinn, 1999). And women are more than just biological organisms. Both physiologic research, such as women's unique responses to medications or illness, and research on women's psychological experiences are significant areas of study (Pinn, 1999). Because the health of women throughout the life cycle reflects racial, ethnic, and socioeconomic diversity (Canadian Institute for Health Information, 2003; Williams, 2002), research should reflect the importance of understanding these differences, as well as the similarities.

The focus of nursing is to promote client health. Understanding the responses and experiences of women throughout the life cycle is imperative for safe and effective nursing care. The very nature of nursing practice places nurses in the optimal position to be participants in research. In fact, abstracts of nursing research articles are integrated throughout this textbook. By using critical thinking skills along with clinical expertise and theoretical knowledge, nurses can make a real difference in the health of their clients through research. The level at which participation should occur depends on the practice site as well the educational background of the individual nurse, although this may vary with professional experience (Table 1.3).

TABLE 1.3 Research Roles for Nursing

LEVEL	RESEARCH ROLES
Associate degree nurse	• Helping to identify clinical problems in nursing practice • Assisting with data collection • Using research findings in practice in conjunction with nurses who hold more advanced nursing degrees
Baccalaureate degree nurse	• Identifying clinical problems requiring investigation • Assisting experienced investigators to gain access to clinical sites • Influencing the selection of appropriate methods of data collection • Collecting data and implementing research findings for nursing research (as well as interdisciplinary research and research originating in other health care professions)
Master's degree nurse	• Collaborating with experienced investigators in all aspects of the research process • Appraising the clinical relevance of research findings • Creating a practice environment supporting scholarly inquiry • Providing leadership for integrating research findings in clinical practice
Doctoral degree nurse	• Designing research for theory generation or theory testing • Conducting research • Disseminating research

Adapted from the American Nurses Association (1994). *Position statements: Education for participation in nursing research.* Retrieved on March 30, 2006, from http://nursingworld.org/readroom/position/research/resdat.htm.

Evidence-Based Practice

Evidence-based practice represents a paradigm shift in nursing and other health care professions (Jennings & Loan, 2001; Pape, 2003). Nursing has historically been viewed as both an art and a science. This has translated into practice based on a combination of clinical research, expert opinion, and "nursing intuition," but not necessarily reflective of the most up-to-date information available.

Several reasons for this discrepancy with the most current information exist. Comfort with evaluating research varies greatly among nurses. Plus, research may not be easily available in a practice setting, or research may be used inappropriately to guide practice changes—for example, implementing a practice change based on a single study that additional research has not validated.

Many health care providers, within and outside of nursing, view the information that they received in their academic programs as the pinnacle of knowledge—regardless of the interval of time between their graduation and their present clinical practice. Although expert opinions are an important source of valuable information, different experts frequently hold different opinions in specific areas. For example, a nurse who asks several colleagues their opinions on a health-related issue is likely to receive different expert opinions from each of them. Nursing intuition, although valuable, is not always accurate or scientifically based.

Evidence-based decision making "is a continuous interactive process involving the explicit, conscientious and judicious consideration of the best available evidence" (Canadian Nurses Association, 2002b, p. 1) along with "individual clinical experience" (Sackett et al., 1996, p. 71) to provide optimal health care choices through evidence-based practice. **Evidence-based health care** occurs "when decisions that affect the care of patients are taken with due weight accorded to all valid, relevant information" (Hicks, 1997). Within the paradigm, nurses use critical thinking to evaluate sources of evidence, transform them to meet the needs and desires of their individual clients, and evaluate the outcomes of the intervention (Simon, 1999; Tanner, 1999).

But isn't nursing already scientifically based? Surprisingly, the answer is no (Pape, 2003). Evidence-based practice offers nurses the opportunity to eliminate the wide variations in practice that exist (Tanner, 1999), while accessing the most universally effective interventions, individualizing them through clinical expertise and client input, with the result of better client outcomes and improved use of health care resources (Jennings & Loan, 2001). Although it can be anticipated that evidence-based practice will eventually result in economic benefits, in the short term, there is a possibility it will be more costly because of the multiple steps required to initiate evidence-based practice.

Many health care facilities, along with some of the nurses and other health care providers, may object to the implementation of evidence-based practice (Grol & Grimshaw, 2003). Reasons for the objections may include the lack of the computer hardware and software needed to search and analyze the evidence, lack of knowledge regarding literature reviews and research evaluation, resource allocation that does not incorporate the time needed to perform the needed steps, difficulty in transforming the results from the aggregate of evidence to the individual client, and the desire to continue to practice in a familiar manner (Grol & Grimshaw, 2003; O'Rourke, 1998; Rosenberg & Donald, 1995).

Several of these objections can be eliminated through the use of completed systematic reviews of research, known as evidence reports, that include the meta-analysis of research studies, or actual evidence-based practice guidelines that different organizations have developed focusing on specific client needs (Fig. 1.10). The Cochrane Collaboration (2005) is an international organization with the primary focus of ensuring the availability of the outcomes of health care intervention research, while producing and disseminating "systematic reviews of healthcare interventions" and "promoting the search for evidence in the form of clinical trials and other studies of the effects of interventions." Although this endeavor provides the most accurate and up-to-date studies of practice evidence available, it is unlikely that it could be accessed by many of the people in need of the information.

Professional organizations, such as the Association of Women's Health, Obstetric and Neonatal Nurses (AWHONN, 2003), have developed evidence-based

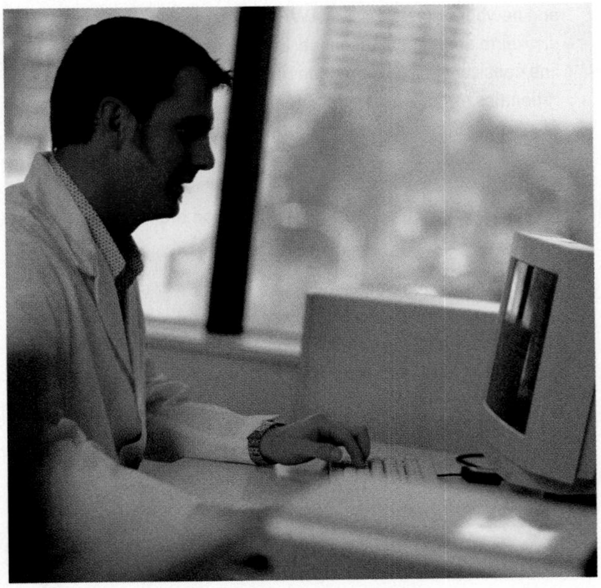

FIGURE 1.10 This nurse is studying evidence-based research findings to provide the best advice and care for clients.

practice guidelines that can be adapted for a specific practice site (Box 1.12). These guidelines, however, are not updated regularly—in fact, at this writing, the AWHONN guidelines are several years old. According to Health Canada (2004c), some of the challenges of implementing evidence-based practice are the lack of easily understood or accessible information. One way that AWHONN updates information on evidence-based practice is through a monthly column in the organization's journal, *The Journal of Obstetric, Gynecologic, and Neonatal Nursing (JOGNN),* which identifies resources for evidence-based practice.

Learning how to access the existing guidelines for evidence-based practice along with related updates can help to alleviate some of the objectives individuals and institutions may have to evidence-based practice. Implementation of these guidelines can help nursing and health care in general to develop more effective interventions because they will be evaluated in multiple sites by multiple individuals caring for different clients. And, the more effective the intervention, the more cost-effective it is for the institution—and the more likely it is that the organization will support evidence-based practice.

BOX 1.12 AWHONN Evidence-Based Clinical Practice Guidelines

To help ensure that clinical nursing practice is implemented according to the strongest and most reliable scientific evidence, AWHONN has designed a process for developing clinical practice guidelines within accepted evidence-based frameworks. As research studies in women's health, maternal, and newborn nursing grow, AWHONN plans to create and distribute additional guidelines. Each evidence-based guideline consists of clinical practice recommendations, referenced rationales, ratings for each statement, a detailed background describing the scope and importance of the clinical issue addressed, and a quick reference to the guideline for the clinician.

Currently, guidelines are available on the following topics:

- Continence for women
- Nursing management of the second stage of labor
- Breastfeeding support: prenatal care through the first year
- Nursing care of the woman receiving regional analgesia/anesthesia in labor
- Neonatal skin care
- Promotion of emotional well-being in midlife
- Cardiovascular health for women

From AWHONN. (n.d.). *Evidence-based clinical practice guidelines.* Retrieved April 2, 2006, from http://www.awhonn.org/awhonn/pg=0-873-5580.

Questions to Ponder

1. A nursing student is at the grocery when she runs into a former classmate from high school who is visibly pregnant. The two women catch up on old times for a while, and then the student asks how far along in her pregnancy the other woman is. The classmate replies "About 5 months. I'm not really sure because I haven't seen a doctor yet. I'll probably go this month, but my mom and aunts give me lots of advice."
   - What is the nursing student's role in this scenario? What questions might she want to ask?
   - How can the nursing student help her acquaintance and begin acting as an advocate and teacher?
   - How can nurses better emphasize in the community the importance of early prenatal care?
2. Two nurses are presenting an initiative to begin incorporating more evidence-based protocols and approaches for women's health in their public health clinic. A few of the nurses seem skeptical. One nurse questions the quality of studies and findings in this area. Another nurse says that she thinks the idea is good, but that the clinic is too busy to implement this in the best way possible.
   - How might the nurses be able to confront the skepticism and reluctance shown by their colleagues?
   - How might the nurses incorporate such an initiative in an efficient and organized way that may be better received by their associates?

SUMMARY

- Demographic and sociopolitical changes in North America over the past several decades have resulted in more diverse roles for women and their significant others, along with changes in family structure and dynamics and in fertility.
- Two diverse health care systems are found in North America. The Canadian system is supported by its federal government; at least in theory, it guarantees health care access to all Canadian citizens. The U.S. health care system is primarily for-profit, and access is not guaranteed for anyone, including pregnant women. The importance of increasing health promotion activities is becoming apparent within both systems.
- Critical thinking is integral to nursing practice. It requires the ability to see beyond the obvious and view a situation from multiple perspectives. The nursing process is one method by which critical thinking can be implemented in an organized manner.
- Ethical principles guide nursing practice in both formal and informal ways. Formalized nursing codes have been developed to promote ethical values within

nursing. Informally, nurses practice within an informal ethical code based on unwritten values held by nurses that have been generated through moral views, experiences, and the history of the profession.

- Ethical decision making is becoming more prevalent in nursing practice and can be facilitated through the use of formal strategies.
- Informed consent in clinical practice evolved from legal auspices, despite its apparent connection to ethical principles. In research, informed consent emerged from a history of unethical practices on subjects who were forced to participate in research.
- Informed consent ensures that the client or research subject is aware of the risks and benefits of the health intervention or research study. Written consent provides legal support for the primary health care provider responsible for the intervention or the principal investigator of the research study. Informed consent is not a mandate for the client or research subject to complete, or even begin, the intervention or study. The client may change her mind at any time and revoke the informed consent.
- Although historically women were not included in research, it is now recognized that women need to be included in all aspects of research and that the inclusion needs to encompass women throughout the life cycle. The role that nurses have in the research process will reflect their professional experience as well as their educational backgrounds.
- Evidenced-based practice, through the use of evidence-based decision making, promotes the integration and implementation of scientifically based practice into nursing and health care in general. Evidence-based practice is based on transforming scientifically sound evidence into individualized clinical interventions with measurable outcomes. It requires critical thinking skills as well as an understanding of research and the ability to access pertinent information. The result of evidence-based practice is evidence-based health care.

REFERENCES

American College of Obstetricians and Gynecologists. (2002a). Ethical decision making in obstetrics and gynecology. In *Ethics in obstetrics and gynecology* (pp. 1–6). Washington, DC: Author.

American College of Obstetricians and Gynecologists. (2002b). Ethical dimensions of informed consent. In *Ethics in obstetrics and gynecology* (pp. 19–27). Washington, DC: Author.

American College of Obstetricians and Gynecologists. (2002c). *Committee opinion: Exercising during pregnancy and the postpartum period.* Retrieved April 2, 2006, from http://www.acog.com.

American Nurses Association. (1994). *Position statements: Education for participation in nursing research.* Retrieved March 30, 2006, from http://nursingworld.org/readroom/position/research/resdat/htm.

American Nurses Association. (1997). *Position statements: Home care for mother, infant and family following birth.* Retrieved December 11, 2003, from http://nursingworld.org/readroom/position/social/scnnat.htm.

American Nurses Association. (2001). *Code of ethics for nurses with interpretive statements.* Washington, DC: Author.

American Public Health Association. (2003). *Fact sheet: Access to care.* Retrieved January 4, 2004, from http://www.apha.org/legislative/factsheets.

Association of Women's Health, Obstetric and Neonatal Nurses. (n.d.). Evidence-based clinical practice guidelines. Retrieved April 2, 2006, from http://www.awhonn.org/?pg=0-873-5580.

Association of Women's Health, Obstetric and Neonatal Nurses. (2003). *Standards for professional practice in the care of women and newborns* (6th ed.). Washington, DC: Author.

Beauchamp, T. L., & Childress, J. F. (2001). *Principles of biomedical ethics* (5th ed.). New York: Oxford University Press.

Bogess, K. A., Lieff, S., Murtha, A. P., Moss, K., Beck, J., & Offenbacher, S. (2003). *Maternal periodontal disease is associated with an increased risk for preeclampsia, 101*(2), 227–231.

Brazell, N. E. (1997). The significance and application of informed consent. *Association of Perioperative Registered Nurses Journal, 65*(2), 377–386.

Bureau of Labor Statistics. (2004). *Women in the labor force: A databook.* Washington, DC: U.S. Department of Labor.

Bush, G. W. (2001). Radio address by the President to the Nation. Retrieved January 21, 2005, from http://www.whitehouse.gov/news/releases/2001/08/20010811-1.html.

Canadian Institute for Health Information. (2003). *Women's health surveillance report.* Ottawa, Ontario: Author.

Canadian Institutes of Health Research. (2005). Updated guidelines for human pluripotent stem cell research, June 7, 2005. Retrieved March 29, 2006, from http://www.cihr-irsc.gc.ca/cgi-bin/print-imprimer.pl.

Canadian Nurses Association. (2000). Working with limited resources: Nurses' moral constraints. *Canadian Registered Nurses: Ethics in Practice.* Retrieved December 14, 2003, from http: www.cna-nurses.ca.

Canadian Nurses Association. (2002a). *Nursing ethics: Code of ethics for Registered Nurses.* Retrieved March 29, 2006, from http://www.cna-aiic.ca/CAN/documents/pdf/publications/CodeofEthics2002_e.pdf.

Canadian Nurses Association. (2002b). *Position statement: Evidence-based decision-making and nursing practice.* Retrieved April 2, 2006, from http://www.cna-aiic.ca.

Canadian Nurses Association. (2002c). *Position statement: The role of the nurse in reproductive and genetic technologies.* Retrieved January 25, 2005, from http://www.cna-nurses.ca.

Casper, L. M., & Bianchi, S. M. (2002). *Continuity and change in the American family.* Thousand Oaks, CA: Sage Publications.

Carta, G., Persia, G. Falciglia, K., & Iovenitti, P. (2004). Periodontal disease and poor obstetrical outcome. *Clinical and Experimental Obstetrics and Gynecology, 31*(1), 47–49.

Centers for Disease Control and Prevention. (2001). Pregnancy-related deaths among Hispanic, Asian/Pacific Islander, and American Indian/Alaskan Native women-United States, 1991–1997. *Morbidity and Mortality Weekly Report, 50*(18), 361–364.

Center for Medicare and Medicaid Services (2002). *HIPAA insurance reform: The newborns and mothers health protection act.* Retrieved December 11, 2003, from http://www.cms.hhs.gov.hipaa/hipaa1/content/nmhpa.asp.

Childbirth Connection. (2004). *The rights of childbearing women.* New York: Author. Retrieved March 29, 2006, from http://www.childbirthconnection.org/article.asp?ck=10084&ClickedLink=0&area =27.

Childbirth Connection. (2005). Vision, mission, and beliefs: Informed decision making, informal consent or refusal. Retrieved March 29, 2006, from http://www.childbirthconnection.org/article.asp?ck=10081.

Cochrane Collaboration. (2005). *Newcomer's guide.* Retrieved April 2, 2006, from http://www.cochrane.org/docs/newcomersguide.htm.

Curtin, L. (1993). Informed consent: Cautious, calculated candor. *Nursing Management, 24*(3), 18–19.

Dennison, C., & Pokras, R. (2000). Design and operation of the national hospital discharge survey: 1988 Redesign. *Vital Health Statistics, 1*(39).

Faden, R. R., & Beauchamp, T. L. (1986). *A history and theory of informed consent.* New York: Oxford University Press.

Fields, J. (2004). *America's families and living arrangement—2003: Current population reports.* Washington, DC: Author.

Fischbach, G. D., & Fischbach, R. L. (2004). Stem cells: Science, policy, and ethics. *Journal of Clinical Investigation, 114*(10), 1364–1370.

Green, C. (2000). *Critical thinking in nursing: Case studies across the curriculum.* Upper Saddle River, NJ: Prentice Hall Health.

Grol, R., & Grimshaw, J. (2003). From best evidence to best practice: Effective implementation of change in patients' care. *Lancet, 362,* 1225–1230.

Hamilton, B. E., Sutton, P. D., & Ventura, S. J. (2003). Revised birth and fertility rates for the 1990s and new rates for Hispanic populations, 2001 and 2001: United States. *National Vital Statistics Reports, 51*(12). Hyattsville, MD: National Center for Health Statistics.

Health Canada. (2004a). *About health Canada: Women's health strategy.* Retrieved March 27, 2006 from http://www.hc-sc.gc.ca/ahc-asc/pubs/strateg-women-femmes/strateg_e.html.

Health Canada. (2004b). *Health care system: About primary health care.* Retrieved March 26, 2006, from http://www.hc-sc.gc.ca/hcs-sss.

Health Canada. (2004c). *Health care system: Home and community care.* Retrieved March 26, 2006, from http://www.hc-sc.gc.ca/hcs-sss.

Health Canada. (2004d). *Health care system: Canada Health Action—building on the legacy. Vol. II: Synthesis reports and issues papers.* Retrieved April 2, 2006, from http://www.hc-sc.gc.ca/hcs-sss/pubs/care-soins/1997-nfoh-fnss-v2/legacy_heritage8_e.html.

Health Canada. (2005a). *Health care system: Health care system delivery.* Retrieved March 26, 2006, from http://www.hc-sc.gc.ca/hcs-sss.

Health Canada. (2005b). *Health care system: Canada Health Ac—overview.* Retrieved March 26, 2006, from http://www.hc-sc.gc.ca/hcs-sss.

Health Canada (2006). *Health care system: Canada's health care system (Medicare).* Retrieved March 26, 2006, from http://www.hc-sc.gc.ca/hcs-sss.

Hicks, N. (1977). Evidence-based health care. *Bandolier,* 39, 9. Retrieved April 4, 2006, from http://www.jr2.ox.ac.uk/bandolier/band39/b39-9.html.

Hoyert, D. L., Danel, I., & Tully, P. (2000). Maternal mortality, United States and Canada, 1982–1997. *Birth, 27*(1), 4–11.

Jennings, B. M., & Loan, L. A. (2001). Misconceptions among nurses about evidence-based practice. *Journal of Nursing Scholarship, 33*(2), 121–127.

Keefe, C. (2003). *Overview of maternity care in the U.S.* [Online]. Retrieved April 3, 2006, from www.efmidwifery.org/pdf/OverviewofMatCareApr2003.pdf.

Legato, M., & Dean, D. (1999). Overview and perspectives of the task force cochairs. In *U.S. Department of Health and Human Services, Pubic Health Service, National Institutes of Health. Agenda for Research on Women's Health for the 21st Century* (Vol. 2, pp. 9–14). Bethesda, MD: National Institutes of Health.

March of Dimes. (2003). *March of Dimes Data Book for policy makers: Maternal, infant, and child health in the United States.* Wilkes-Barre, PA: Author.

Martin, J. A., Hamilton, B. E., Ventura, S. J., Menacker, F., Park, M. M., & Sutton, P. D. (2002). Births: Final data for 2001. *National Vital Statistics Report, 51*(2). Hyattsville, MD: National Center for Health Statistics.

Maternity Center Association. (2001) *Making informed decisions.* Retrieved December 14, 2003, from http://www.maternitywise.org/mw/mid.html.

Mills, R. J., & Bhandoff, S. (2003). Health insurance coverage in the United States: 2002. *Current Population Reports.* Washington, DC: U.S. Census Bureau.

Murphy, M., & Murphy, J. (1976). Making ethical decisions—systematically. *Nursing76, 6*(5), 13–14.

National Bioethics Advisory Commission. (1999). *Ethical issues in human stem cell research.* Rockville, MD: National Bioethics Advisory Commission.

National Women's Law Center and Oregon Health & Science University. (2004). *Making the grade on women's health: A national and state-by-state report card.* Washington, DC: National Women's Law Center.

Nelson-Marten, P., & Rich, B. A. (1999). A historical perspective of informed consent in clinical practice and research. *Seminars in Oncology Nursing, 15*(2), 81–88.

Offenbacher, S., Lieff, S., Boggess, K. A., Murtha, A. P., Madianos, P. N., et al. (2001). Maternal periodontitis and prematurity. Part I: Obstetric outcomes . . . prematurity and growth restriction. *Annals of Periodontology, 6*(1), 167–174.

Office of the Prime Minister. (2004). A ten year plan to strengthen health care. Retrieved February 17, 2005, from http://www.pm.gc.ca/english/news.

Organisation for Economic Cooperation and Development (2002). *OECD economic surveys: United States.* Paris: Author.

O'Rourke, A. (1998). *Seminar 3: An introduction to evidence-based practice.* Sheffield, UK: Wisdom Centre, The University of Sheffield. Retrieved December 21, 2003, from http://www.shef.ac.uk/uni/projects/wrp/sem3.html.

Overturf Johnson, J. (2005). Who's minding the kids? Child care arrangements: Winter 2002. *Current Population Reports* (pp. 70–101). Washington, DC: U.S. Census Bureau.

Pape, T. M. (2003). Evidence-based nursing practice: To infinity and beyond. *Journal of Continuing Education in Nursing, 34*(4), 154–161.

Pinn, V. (1999). Introduction. In U.S. Department of Health and Human Services, Public Health Service, National Institutes of Health, *Agenda for Research on Women's Health for the 21st Century* (Vol. 2, pp. 3–7). Bethesda, MD: National Institutes of Health.

Rosenberg, W., & Donald, A. (1995). Evidence based medicine: An approach to clinical problem-solving. *British Medical Journal, 310*(6987), 1122.

Rosse, P. A., & Krebs, L. U. (1999). The nurse's role in the informed consent process. *Seminars in Oncology Nursing, 15*(2), 116–123.

Sackett, D., Rosenberg, W., Gray, J., Haynes, R., & Richardson, W. (1996). Evidence based medicine: What it is and what it isn't. *British Medical Journal, 312*(7023), 71–72.

Simon, J. M. (1999). Evidence-based practice in nursing. *International Journal of Nursing Terminologies and Classifications, 10,* 3.

Statistics Canada. (2002). Profile of Canadian families and households. Retrieved August 10, 2006, from http://www.statcan.ca.

Tanner, C. A. (1999). Evidence-based practice: Research and critical thinking. *Journal of Nursing Education, 38*(3), 99.

Taylor, H. A. (1999). Barriers to informed consent. *Seminars in Oncology Nursing, 15*(2), 89–95.

Thorpe, K. (2001). *The distribution of health insurance coverage among pregnant women, 1999.* White Plains, NY: March of Dimes. Retrieved December 12, 2003, from www.marchofdimes.com/files/2001FinalThorpeReport.pdf.

U.S. Census Bureau. (2003). *Fertility of American women: June 2002.* Washington, DC: Author.

U.S. Department of Health and Human Services. (2003). *Women's health USA 2003.* Rockville, MD: Author.

U.S. Department of Health and Human Services. (2005). *Women's health USA 2005.* Rockville, MD: Author.

Wilkinson, J. M. (2001). *Nursing process and critical thinking.* Upper Saddle River, NJ: Prentice Hall.

Williams, D. R. (2002). Racial/ethnic variations in women's health: The social embeddedness of health. *American Journal of Public Health, 92*(4), 588–597.

CHAPTER 2

Health Promotion

Gayle M. Roux

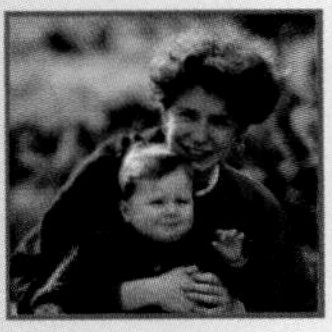

Renee is a 33-year-old married woman with a 20-month-old son. During an annual checkup, the nurse discusses with Renee nutrition, exercise, and lifestyle. Renee says, "I've lost almost all the weight I gained during my pregnancy, but I was 15 pounds heavier than I wanted to be before I became pregnant! Now I'm so busy, I'm worried I'll never get into shape. I don't have a specific number of pounds I want to be; I just want to be a healthy weight."

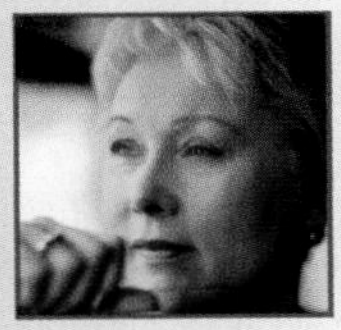

Linda, a 53-year-old single accountant, comes to the clinic complaining of hot flashes. She has not menstruated for the past 9 months. She works approximately 50 hours a week, spending at least 7 hours each day at the computer. She does not like milk but tries to eat fruits and vegetables.

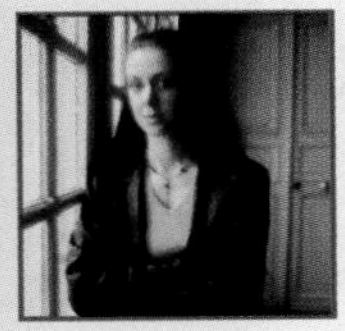

Jill, 25 years old, comes to the health care facility for her first vaginal examination and Pap smear. She looks very apprehensive when the nurse begins to take her health history. The nurse asks if anything is wrong. Jill responds, "I'm really scared about what will happen during the exam."

Nurses working with such clients need to understand this chapter to promote health effectively and to address each issue appropriately. You will learn more about these clients' circumstances as the chapter continues. Before beginning, consider the following points:

- What health issues are similar for each woman? What concerns are different?
- How do age, lifestyle, and other circumstances influence health and illness?
- How can nurses help active and busy women prevent health-related issues from becoming sources of stress?
- How can nurses help women become motivated to manage their self-care effectively?

LEARNING OBJECTIVES

On completion of this chapter, the reader should be able to:

- Define health promotion from a multidimensional perspective.
- Discuss history-taking parameters for nutritional, psychological, physical, sexual, reproductive, and breast health.
- Summarize health promotion issues of special concern for Latina and African American women.
- Describe physical examination for women across the lifespan, discriminating expected findings from alterations.
- Identify collaborative health promotion strategies in women during the reproductive years.
- Explain methods of early detection of common health issues in women during the reproductive years.
- Identify health-screening guidelines for women during the reproductive years.
- Identify immunization recommendations for women during the reproductive years.

KEY TERMS

alternative therapies
body mass index (BMI)
bone-density scan
breast cancer 1 and breast cancer 2 genes (*BRCA1* and *BRCA2*)
breast self-examination (BSE)
clinical breast examination (CBE)
complementary therapies
health
health promotion
inner strength
mammogram
menarche
menopause
metabolic rate
osteoporosis
perimenopause
postmenopause
risk factor
self-management
ultrasound
women's health

Health promotion encompasses all areas of a woman's life. Choices related to health reflect her place in the world, including cultural, social, and spiritual perspectives. These perspectives help form the basis for the woman's actualization of her choices.

Nurses are in a strong position to understand the complexity of beliefs and behaviors related to health promotion, and to assume leadership positions in the primary care of women and their families. Health promotion is as important, if not more so, as secondary and tertiary health care measures. Nurses have the distinct opportunity to interact with consumers in key settings, including family practice sites, communities, schools, and places of employment. They are accountable for working to reduce preventable health problems such as obesity, diabetes, domestic violence, and heart disease by communicating and teaching women and their families about these issues. Health promotion and disease prevention can decrease these public health epidemics and provide cost-effective approaches to community health.

Economic resources for health care will grow scarcer with an increasing aging population (see Chap. 24). Strategies to prevent chronic health conditions and maintain optimum functioning for women across the lifespan and their families are critical challenges for nurses. Nurses are obligated to be aware of current research and evolving evidence-based protocols. Translating research findings into practice helps to ensure that nurses remain at the forefront of changing health promotion strategies.

This chapter addresses common health promotion issues in women, including information on healthy lifestyles, risk factors for health problems, assessment and physical examination, and interventions for preventing and early screening for common health problems. Important areas of focus include nutrition, exercise, psychological health, physical health, and sexual, reproductive, and breast health.

HEALTH PROMOTION

Health is one of the key concepts of nursing. Definitions of health, health promotion, and women's health have evolved based on the current philosophy that clients should control their bodies and act as partners with health care providers in decision making. For this reason, nurses no longer characterize health as the absence of illness or disability. Rather, they consider **health** to be total physical, psychological, and social well-being (World Health Organization [WHO], 2006a). Health is a resource for living.

Health promotion is the process that allows people to increase control over and thus improve health and its determinants (WHO, 2006b). Choices and actions related to health promotion reflect the person's cultural, educational, social, and spiritual perspectives. In this transformative process, the nurse functions as a partner with the client and family in education, consciousness raising, and advocacy. She or he should show respect for the client's autonomy and acknowledge the dynamic relationship between client and environment. The goals of health promotion are to maintain and to improve health. Health promotion requires highly complex professional practice and has evolved in recent years as scholars, researchers, and practitioners have addressed its complexities (Young, 2002).

The Association of Women's Health, Obstetric, and Neonatal Nursing (AWHONN) defines **women's health** as "the health care of nonpregnant women across the lifespan from adolescence to senescence with a focus on health issues distinctive to women" (1998). This view reflects the expansion of women's health beyond its original focus primarily on reproduction.

Many of today's health problems are amenable to community and public health approaches. Nurses can make a difference. Sharing their concerns about issues that affect women's health is a prerequisite to changing nursing practice. Nurses also should use information as resource material for teaching plans. For example, one study showed that more than 90% of women with localized (stage I) cervical cancer at diagnosis were alive 5 years later, whereas only 14% of those with metastatic disease (stage IV) at diagnosis were alive within that same period (Stekler & Elmore, 2002). Screening for cervical cancer is less frequent among minorities, older women, and those without insurance (Bazargan, Bazargan, Farooq, & Baker, 2004; National Institutes of Health [NIH], 1996). This is just one example that demonstrates the need for increased health education and comprehensive preventive programs to improve access to and quality of health care for women of all ages (Fig. 2.1).

Nursing Approaches to Health Promotion

Nursing views women holistically. From this perspective, the individual woman, her family, and her community are a single, complex entity. Nursing within this philosophy of care provides a means for growth and change. Whether women are confronting psychological and physiologic stresses associated with substance abuse or domestic violence, developmental events such as menopause, or everyday decisions regarding exercise and nutrition, nurses should offer holistic approaches, support, and advocacy to improve and maintain health. Health promotion concepts include developments of nursing theory in relation to empowerment, collaboration, participation, and equity (MacDonald, 2002).

Health promotion includes the complex dimensions of providing health education, marketing health messages, encouraging necessary lifestyle modifications, engaging in social and environmental changes, and incorporating the client's values. During health history interviews, nurses should elicit each woman's beliefs about her health and her values as related to health behaviors and choices.

Health promotion includes both self-management strategies and interventions implemented by health care

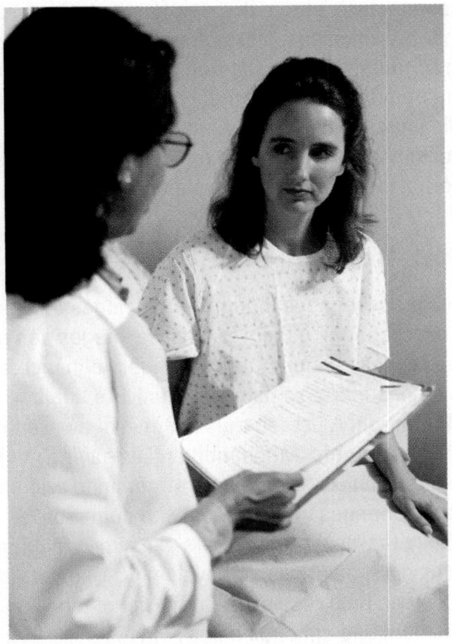

FIGURE 2.1 Screening measures and appropriate teaching are essential components of health promotion and disease prevention. Not only do women need to be encouraged to undergo routine screening, but also they must understand the importance of such examinations.

professionals. Therapies to promote and to maintain health include both traditional and complementary or alternative therapies. **Complementary therapies** are nontraditional or integrative therapies that underscore or interface with traditional therapies, whereas **alternative therapies** are those used in place of traditional choices (National Center for Complementary and Alternative Medicine, 2006). Complementary/Alternative Medicine (CAM) 2.1 provides a classification system with examples of common modalities.

● COMPLEMENTARY/ALTERNATIVE MEDICINE 2.1

Classification System of Techniques With Examples

ALTERNATIVE SYSTEMS OF MEDICAL PRACTICE

- **Acupuncture:** Practitioners treat illnesses by applying needles to specific points on the body. The needles draw energy away from organs with excesses and redirect it to organs with deficits. Rebalanced energy flow relieves pain and restores health.
- **Ayurvedic medicine:** This comprehensive approach focuses on daily living in harmony with the laws of nature to achieve a clear mind, sturdy body, and peaceful spirit. Practitioners prescribe meditation, herbal therapy, yoga, and massage to maintain health or reverse disease.
- **Homeopathy:** Homeopathy means to "treat like with like." Practitioners believe that a substance that causes symptoms of illness in a healthy person may, in minute doses, also cure similar symptoms resulting from an illness.
- **Naturopathy:** This all-encompassing term refers to "natural health" modalities alone or in combination: acupuncture, herbal therapy, homeopathy, hydrotherapy, massage, nutrition, and osteopathy.
- **Traditional Chinese medicine:** This system is based on the principle of internal balance and harmony (Qi). Measures such as acupuncture, acupressure, moxibustion, exercise, advice on diet and lifestyle, and herbal medicines restore, maintain, or improve Qi.

MIND–BODY INTERVENTIONS

- **Imagery:** Negative thoughts and images can lead to illness; changing them to positive images can reverse the process. Regular use of imagery can increase relaxation, decrease pain, and facilitate healing.
- **Meditation:** A person tries to achieve awareness without thought. Meditation entails paying nonjudgmental, moment-to-moment attention to bringing about changes in perception and cognition.
- **Music therapy:** Practitioners use music to change behaviors, emotions, or physiology. Musical vibrations can help regulate a body "out of tune" and help maintain and enhance a body "in tune."

BIOLOGICALLY BASED THERAPIES

- **Aromatherapy:** Practitioners use essential oils to treat symptoms and for physiologic and psychological benefits.
- **Herbal therapies:** Practitioners use plant parts (including barks, roots, stems, flowers, leaves, fruits, seeds, or sap) as medicines.

MANIPULATIVE AND BODY-BASED METHODS

- **Massage:** Benefits of this systematic and scientific manipulation of soft tissues may include decreased stress and anxiety; enhanced mental clarity, energy, and performance; promotion of vitality, energy, and personal growth; and emotional release.
- **T'ai Chi and Qigong:** T'ai chi blends exercise and energy with choreographed movements performed with mental concentration and coordinated breathing. Qigong, a therapeutic Chinese practice, includes gentle exercises for the breath, body, mind, and voice. These modalities often are combined.
- **Yoga:** Yoga teaches basic principles of spiritual, mental, and physical energy to promote health and wellness. It uses proper breathing, movement, meditation, and postures to promote relaxation and enhance energy flow.

ENERGY THERAPIES

- **Bioelectromagnetic-based therapies:** Practitioners use magnetic fields to prevent and treat disease and as first aid for injuries.
- **Biofield therapies**
  - **Reflexology:** Reflexology involves massaging specific points on the hands or feet to relieve stress or pain in corresponding related body areas.
  - **Reiki:** This ancient Buddhist healing modality focuses on giving the body direct access to transcendental, universal, radiant, and light energies. Practitioners hold their hands in 12 basic positions on the client's head, chest, and back to access universal energy and help the client's body to rebalance and heal.
  - **Therapeutic touch and healing touch:** These two methods of energetic healing derive from the ancient practice of "the laying on of hands." Practitioners focus on the client's energy field to promote health.

From National Center for Complementary and Alternative Medicine. Retrieved February 2, 2006, from http://nccam.nih.gov.

Health Theories and Models

QUOTE 2-1

"Your success and happiness lie in you."

Helen Keller

In many ways, the U.S. and Canadian health care systems remain disease oriented. Researchers, theorists, and major public health movements have promoted a shift to valuing health promotion and fitness. In this framework, nurses form partnerships with women to blend professional therapeutic management with self-management of lifestyle and behavior. This view conceptualizes health as an active process involving motivation, an ability to assume responsibility for health, respect for sociocultural values and economic issues, and integration of the entire person. The process is abstract and fluid. Theories evolve and are updated based on changing perspectives and research findings.

Initially, health promotion theories were criticized for being too individualistic and not designed to address broad contextual factors. For example, people may have difficulty changing behavior not because they are "noncompliant," but because of challenges in finding access, resources, and services to support behaviors, as well as economic and cultural factors. Using a holistic approach, nurses assist clients to promote growth toward health by focusing on strengths and facilitating clients' acceptance or overcoming of physical and sociopolitical challenges.

The educational background of nurses ideally suits them to apply theoretical concepts in clinical settings. The next section focuses on three models: the Health Promotion Model, the Transtheoretical Model, and the Theory of Inner Strength in Women. Nurses can use these and other approaches to identify assessment parameters and clinical interventions to enhance a client's strengths and promote her health. Nurses are encouraged to read further to apply techniques based on these theories to help clients and make meaningful lifestyle choices.

Health Promotion (Pender) Model

Nola Pender developed her Health Promotion Model (HPM) in the early 1980s, with subsequent revisions (Pender, 1996). The HPM integrates nursing and behavioral sciences with a focus on health behaviors and decisions. Based on extensive research, it depicts health-promoting behaviors in relationship to influences of individual characteristics and experiences, behavior-specific cognitions and affect, commitment to a plan of action, and immediate competing demands (Fig. 2.2). Women

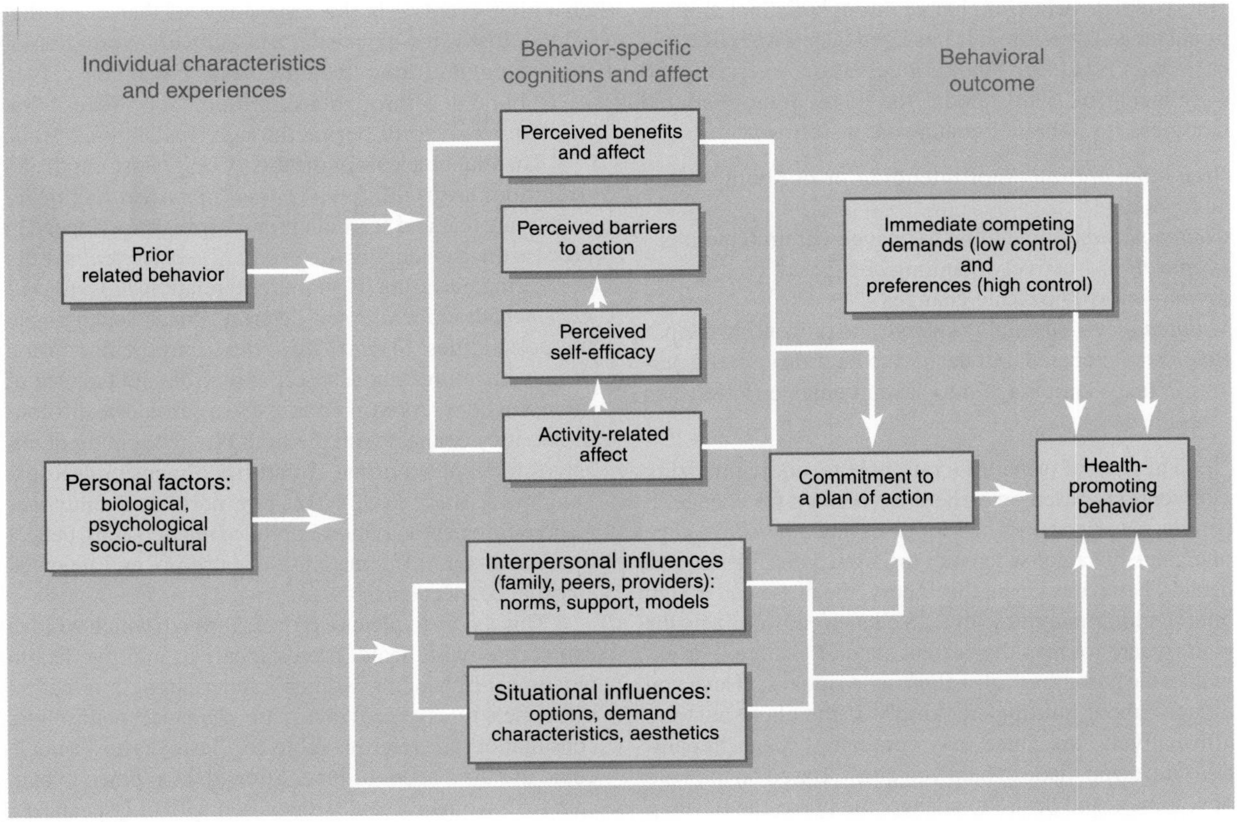

FIGURE 2.2 Pender's Health Promotion Model.

must take responsibility for their own lifestyle choices. Nurses can assist clients to facilitate change, but only when both nurse and client explore the meaning of health promotion to the client and pinpoint the client's expectations. Nurses can use the HPM to shift thinking from blaming clients for weaknesses to empowering clients by building on strengths and promoting positive lifestyle changes.

Pender (1996) reports the "behavior-specific cognitions and affect" category to contain the major motivational factors for health promotion and a focus for nursing intervention. The nurse should explore and discuss these variables with the client and family to modify health behaviors and lifestyle choices through nursing interventions. The HPM takes an approach of partnership with the client that includes building strengths, using community resources, and fostering actualization of health potentials.

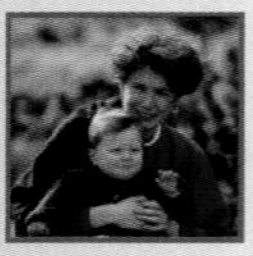

Consider Renee, the 33-year-old with a toddler who wants to be a healthy weight. Applying the HPM, what information would be important to determine with her?

Transtheoretical Model

The Transtheoretical Model (Prochaska & DiClemente, 1983) depicts behavior change through distinct motivational stages over time. It has been tested with lifestyle behaviors including smoking cessation, exercise, and weight control. In this model, the stages of motivational readiness for behavior change are as follows:

Precontemplation—not intending or not being ready to change
Contemplation—intending to change within 6 months
Preparation—actively planning change
Action—overtly making changes
Maintenance—sustaining change and preventing relapse
Relapse—expected, but desired to be transient; the person takes action again to sustain change (Prochaska et al., 1994).

This model provides a rationale for individualizing interventions based on a client's readiness for change. It continues to be researched for assessing a person's stage of change behavior when moving from a detrimental to a healthy behavior. Using this theory, the nurse can design intervention strategies with each client by customizing the plan of care to meet the current state of change. For example, the nurse may ask a client who smokes, "Have you thought about quitting smoking?" If the client answers affirmatively, the nurse may continue, "What preparations have you made to help you quit?" Based on the state of readiness and desire to change, the nurse can develop effective interventions grounded in the client's experience and with a nonjudgmental approach.

Theory of Inner Strength in Women

A large body of literature explores health strengths and the interrelationship of a life-threatening or otherwise demanding situation with the human biobehavioral response. The Theory of Inner Strength in Women (Dingley, Roux, & Bush, 2000; Roux, Dingley, & Bush, 2002) is a gender-specific theory based on health strengths as the woman interacts with her environment during a challenging event or illness. The theory has been researched with women with breast cancer, heart disease, transplantation, and multiple sclerosis.

Inner strength is a positive healing force in healthy as well as ill people. It underscores the desire to make changes to live as fully as possible. The middle-range theory of inner strength in women examines the woman's health needs from a model of strength as opposed to deficits. In a concept analysis of inner strength, Dingley, Roux, and Bush (2000) described attributes as a component of spirituality, facet of quality of life, contributor to overcoming problems, and dimension of empowerment. A life-changing event or challenging experience initiates tapping into inner strength and its display. The essence of inner strength is an intrinsic human resource that promotes well-being and healing.

Although inner strength exists before the life-changing event, it is the *experience* of that event that often initiates the expansion and outward expression of inner strength. **Inner strength** means having the capacity to build self through a developmental process that positively moves the person through challenging events.

The four concepts of the theory of inner strength and definitions are as follows: (1) *anguish and searching* describes the fear and searching for meaning experienced to process the challenging life event; (2) *connectedness* describes the nurturing of supportive relationships; (3) *engagement* describes the self-determinism and engaging in life possibilities; (4) *movement* describes the dimension of movement, rest, honest self-appraisal, and balance of mind and body. As women adjust to a chronic health condition, they connect with the future by reorienting themselves to a "new normal" in all life dimensions (Roux, Dingley, & Bush, 2002). This new normal encompasses responses to new activities, improved relationships, deeper understanding, different sense of purpose, and renewed spiritual connectedness.

This theory explains a process through which women can partner with health professionals to improve health outcomes. Enhancing women's inner strength is within the nurse's roles of providing care, guidance, counseling, consultation, and referral. Table 2.1 illustrates how a nurse could use the Theory of Inner Strength in Women to plan care for a woman recently diagnosed with breast cancer.

TABLE 2.1 Applying the Theory of Inner Strength in Women to a Client With Breast Cancer

THEORETICAL CONCEPT	NURSING INTERVENTIONS
Anguish and searching: transition from shock and fear to acceptance	● Provide information about breast cancer. ● Answer the client's questions. ● Explore the meaning of the diagnosis to the client. ● Encourage the client to voice her fears.
Movement: a realistic appraisal of one's abilities and limitations; awareness of life's possibilities	● Discuss exercise, sleep, and fatigue. Plan strategies for these areas based on the client's particular needs. ● Encourage activity and balance.
Engagement: reframing circumstances to engage with life as a source of strength	● Encourage the client to put herself first, and to make treatment decisions that are right for her. ● Assist the client to ensure that her lifestyle includes time for reflection and relaxation. ● Discuss economic and cultural concerns. ● Suggest appropriate resources or referrals.
Connectedness: nurturing relationships with self, family, friends, and a Greater Source of Strength	● Assess the client's support systems. ● Encourage the client to ask for help and to allow herself to experience support and caring from others. ● Suggest outlets such as keeping a journal or meditating. ● Assess and encourage spiritual outlets.

HEALTH ASSESSMENT AND SCREENING

Successful assessment and screening programs for women involve many criteria and sociocultural considerations.

The first criterion for screening is that the condition has high incidence, morbidity, and mortality. An example is the need to evaluate diet, exercise, and lifestyle patterns for early detection of obesity, an epidemic that increases risks for morbidity and mortality from diabetes, heart disease, and some cancers (Centers for Disease Control and Prevention [CDC], 2006b).

A second criterion is that testing is sensitive, inexpensive, and widely available. For example, practice settings can assess for alcoholism and domestic violence at essentially no cost by screening with easily administered, valid tools that identify high-risk women.

The third criterion is that early detection and treatment affect morbidity and mortality. Screening for cervical cancer is a good example. Some screening endeavors (eg, assessing psychological health, examining cultural beliefs about health behaviors) are invaluable to the treatment and well-being of women, but outcomes may be more difficult to measure in terms of morbidity and mortality.

The fourth criterion for screening includes assessment of unique sociocultural and behavioral patterns.

This section includes information on assessment and screening of common health conditions in women encompassing these four screening criteria.

Diet, Exercise, and Lifestyle

In April 2005, the U.S. Department of Agriculture (USDA) unveiled *MyPyramid,* which updates and replaces the familiar Food Guide Pyramid, introduced by the USDA in 1992. *MyPyramid* can be individualized based on age, gender, and activity level to provide guidance on healthy nutritional choices. The nutritional recommendations of the pyramid are based on the "2005 Dietary Guidelines for Americans," issued jointly by the USDA and the Department of Health and Human Services. Information tailored to both consumers and health professionals is available at www.MyPyramid.gov. See Chapter 3 for more detailed information.

Nutritional education also should emphasize positive methods of cooking. For example, broiling is preferred to frying because broiling decreases fat intake. Steaming vegetables retains more vitamins than does boiling them in water.

Although a balanced diet provides adequate vitamins and minerals, nurses should give special consideration to each woman's health history and developmental circumstances. For example, the menopausal woman needs to balance cholesterol and calcium needs by consuming low-fat dairy products for a daily calcium intake of 1000 to 1500 mg (Moore, 2003). The woman with heavy menstrual periods is at increased risk for iron-deficiency anemia (Grund, 2004). The nurse who performs a thorough health and diet history to identify nutritional risks for various stages can adapt dietary guidelines to meet special needs for specific clients (see Chap. 3).

Overweight, Obesity, and Body Mass Index

Results from the 1999–2002 National Health and Nutrition Examination Survey indicate that approximately 64% of U.S. adults are overweight (CDC, 2002c). In *Healthy People 2010,* the U.S. Department of Health and Human Services (USDHHS, 2000) identified overweight and obesity as a major public health epidemic. It grouped together overweight and obesity as a leading health indicator with specific objectives for the nation to achieve during the first decade of the 21st century. Although the terms overweight and obesity often are used interchangeably, they are distinct conditions of varying magnitude.

Body mass index (BMI) is a calculated measure of weight in relation to height (Kealy, 2003). It is one assessment parameter, along with height, weight, body measurements, hip-to-waist ratio, and percentage of body fat, used to determine overweight and obesity. Overweight is defined as a BMI between 25 and 30, obesity is defined as a BMI of 30 or greater, and extreme obesity is defined as a BMI of 40 or greater (Kealy, 2003). Figure 2.3 depicts methods by which nurses can calculate a client's BMI and an accompanying scale for determining BMI status.

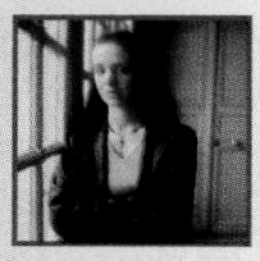

Recall Jill, the 25-year-old undergoing her first vaginal examination. As part of her evaluation, the nurse measures her height and weight. What would be Jill's BMI if she is 5 feet, 5 inches tall and weighs 136 pounds?

Body-Mass Index Calculation and Interpretation

CALCULATION

1. Divide pounds by 2.2 = kilograms (kg).
2. Divide height in inches by 39.4 = meters (m).
3. Square the answer in step 2 by multiplying the number times itself.
4. Divide weight in kg by m^2.

Interpretation	BMI (kg/m^2)
Underweight	<18.5
Normal	18.5 to 24.9
Overweight	25.0 to 29.9
Obese	30.0 to 34.9
Severely Obese	35.0 to 39.9
Extremely Obese	≥40

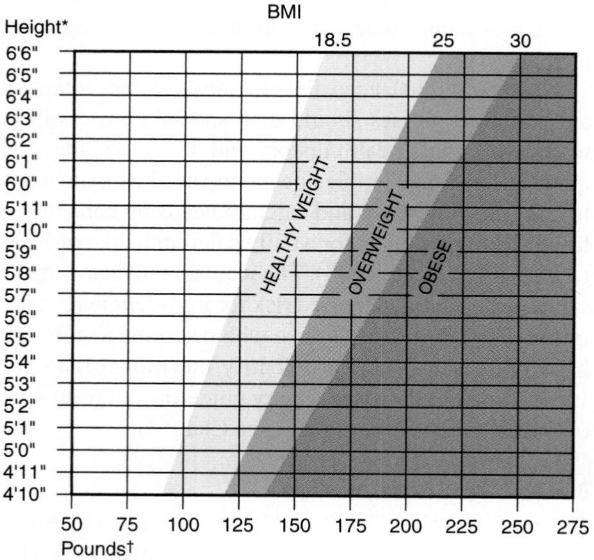

* Without shoes.
† Without clothes. The higher weights apply to people with more muscle and bone, such as many men.
Source: Report of the Dietary Guidelines Advisory Committee on the Dietary Guidelines for Americans, 2000, pages 3-4. http://www.health.gov/dietaryguidelines

FIGURE 2.3 Measures to calculate and to interpret body mass index.

Fat and Cholesterol

All fats are composed of fatty acids; their attributes are determined by the amounts and mixtures of fatty acids they contain. Fatty acids may be saturated, monosaturated, or polyunsaturated, depending on their amount of hydrogen. *Saturated fatty acids* are found mainly in animal foods (eg, meat, poultry, butter, milk). *Monosaturated fatty acids* are found in plant foods (eg, canola, peanut, and olive oils; nuts; avocados). *Polyunsaturated fatty acids* are found in plant foods (eg, corn and sesame oils, fish and seafood). Through hydrogenation, polyunsaturated fatty acids can be made more saturated, resulting in a more stable semisolid form, called *trans fat* (International Food Information Council, 2002). *Trans fats* are in a wide range of foods, including most foods made with partially hydrogenated oils: baked goods, fried foods, and some margarine. High consumption of trans fats can lead to elevated cholesterol levels and subsequent cardiovascular and other problems (see later discussions).

Vitamins and Minerals

Vitamins and minerals are essential for life, and a balanced, nutritious diet can provide them in sufficient amounts (see Chap. 3). Because women do not always have the time, education, or finances to eat a balanced diet, however, nurses must be aware of common deficiencies in women. Two of the most important considerations are calcium and iron.

Calcium. Calcium needs vary with age (Table 2.2). Dairy products probably account for most calcium in the average U.S. diet. Currently, however, the average daily calcium intake for women from dietary sources is only 50%

TABLE 2.2 Recommendations for Calcium Intake in Women

DEMOGRAPHIC GROUP	DAILY CALCIUM NEEDS
11–18 years	1,300 mg
19–50 years	1,000 mg
Pregnant or lactating, 14–18 years	1,300 mg
Pregnant or lactating, 19–50 years	1,000 mg
51 years or older	1,200 mg

From National Institutes of Health. (2006). *Dietary supplements fact sheet: Calcium.* Bethesda, MD: Author. Retrieved February 2, 2006, from http://ods.od.nih.gov/factsheets/calcium.asp#h2.

of the recommended amount (NIH, 1994) (Research Highlight 2.1).

Dietary calcium sources are milk products, calcium-fortified foods (orange and grapefruit juice, cereals, breads), and fish and shellfish (salmon and sardines). To balance calories and cholesterol, clients should opt for nonfat and low-fat dairy foods. It takes only three 10-oz glasses of milk to supply 1,000 mg of calcium. Women who need more dietary calcium may choose to take supplements. Because vitamin D is needed for proper calcium absorption, 400 to 800 IU of vitamin D must be added with calcium supplementation to ensure adequate metabolism and absorption of calcium (Moore, 2003).

Daily calcium intake should not exceed 2,000 mg, including dietary sources and supplements. Most commercial calcium supplements come in pills of 200 to 500 mg. A woman taking three of these pills can take divided doses during the day or a single bedtime dose. Gastrointestinal upset is the most common side effect. Constipation, flatulence, gastric distention, and nausea also may be experienced.

Iron. Losses of iron from menstruation and the increased demands during pregnancy place women at increased risk for iron-deficiency anemia (see Chap. 4). Nurses are alert to the following situations in which even a balanced diet may not supply enough iron:

- Women with very heavy menstruation
- Women on a low-calorie diet (particularly consuming fewer than 1,500 calories/day)
- Pregnant women
- Vegetarians and women who do not eat red meat
- Adolescents

Iron absorption is a complex process that varies with the food combinations consumed. Eating foods high in vitamin C facilitates the body's absorption of iron. Therefore, nurses encourage vitamin C intake from fruits, fruit juices, or vegetables at meals in combination with the selected iron food source. Although moderate amounts of lean meat contribute to iron status, consumption of meat is not essential for adequate iron. Vegetarians need to consume legumes and nuts for iron as well as protein. Breads, cereals, and pasta enriched with iron also supply a fair amount of iron for women.

Exercise

QUOTE 2-1

"I am much more consistent with exercise when I have a friend to walk with. I just get too distracted with everything going on at work and home to do it myself. When I make a commitment to walk with my neighbor, we make each other stick to it."

A 38-year-old woman

Regular exercise has many benefits, including, but not limited to, weight control, reduced stress, improved mood, and increased bone mass. Exercise is an area of special consideration for women who work continually to control their weight. Walking, stair climbing, low-impact aerobic exercising, and hiking contribute to cardiovascular health as well as to bone mass, muscle strength, balance, and flexibility (Moore, 2003) (Fig. 2.4). Nurses should emphasize the relationship between diet and exercise in the teaching plans for clients.

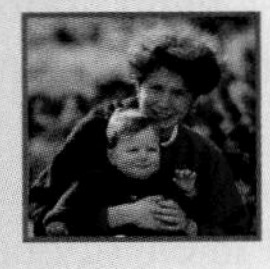

Renee wants to be a healthy weight and is busy with a 20-month-old son. What suggestions might be appropriate for Renee about exercise?

● RESEARCH HIGHLIGHT 2.1 Dietary Calcium Intake and Supplement Use Among Older African American, White, and Native American Women in a Rural Southeastern Community

Bell, R. A., Quandt, S. A., Spanler, J. G., & Case, L. D. (2002). *Journal of the American Dietetic Association, 102*(6).

PURPOSE: Calcium intake below recommended levels, whether through dietary or supplemental intake, has been associated with osteopenia, or low bone mass, which can lead to osteoporosis. The Robeson Osteoporosis Screening Study was performed to assess the calcium intake of an ethnically diverse group of older women living in a low socioeconomic area.

DESIGN: The study was performed in Robeson, North Carolina, which was found to have substantial ethnic diversity, as well as a high poverty rate. The area's population is two-thirds African American and Native Indian, with 22.8% of the population living at or below the poverty line. Calcium intake was assessed using the Oregon Dairy Council Score Sheet, which categorizes 25 foods by seven levels of calcium content. Calcium supplement use also was considered.

RESULTS: The study found that 94% of the women surveyed consume less than 1000 mg/day of calcium. Although it has been shown that white women are at greater risk for osteoporosis, this study found that all three ethnic groups were deficient in calcium intake.

Practitioners need to be aware of this greater risk in women of low socioeconomic status. When encountering these women in practice, it is necessary to discuss the importance of calcium intake and to devise a plan to overcome the barriers each client is facing.

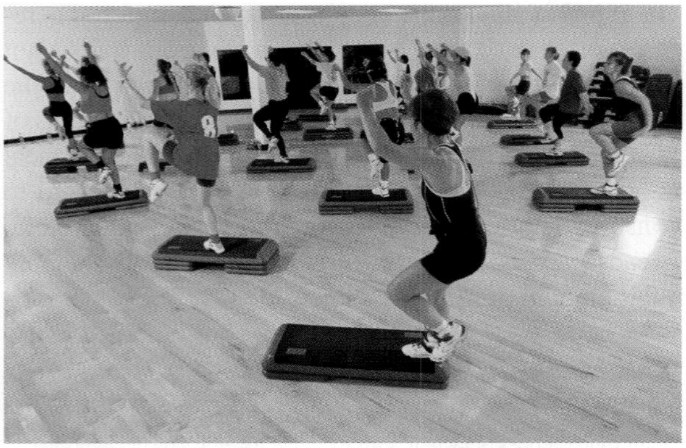

FIGURE 2.4 The benefits of exercise for overall health cannot be overestimated. In addition to assisting with weight control, exercise helps to prevent cardiovascular disease, diabetes, and other leading contributors to morbidity and mortality.

Exercise has definite effects on **metabolic rate** (a measure of energy production, or how fast the body burns calories). Factors that affect metabolic rate include sex, age, heredity, food intake, body composition, activity level, and frequent cycles of weight loss. Frequent weight loss through severe caloric restriction, followed by increased caloric intake and weight gain, seems to slow metabolic rate in many people. Commonly, this is called *starvation metabolism* or *yo-yo dieting.* It is as though the body fears starvation and becomes more efficient at conserving and storing energy. This weight loss cycling can be discouraging and potentially harmful. Clients should avoid excessive over-exercising. Like restrictive dieting, it can give the body the same starvation message.

Numerous genetic, physiologic, environmental, and psychological causes have been proposed in energy balance and weight control. Increasing evidence suggests that overweight and obesity is not a simple problem, but a complex disorder of appetite regulation and energy metabolism. The *set-point theory* states that some areas of the brain might control body composition. According to this theory, severe dietary restriction will cause the body to fight to maintain the set point by decreasing energy expenditure and increasing appetite. Set point is thought to be one factor controlling metabolic rate, probably through hormonal and nervous system connections. The set point is not really "set" but changes in response to diet components and calories.

Aerobic exercise burns calories, lowers set point, and promotes good health. Other theories include fat cell theories, insulin response, and genetic theories. Health professionals are encouraged to do further reading by visiting the Web site of the National Heart, Lung, and Blood Institute (www.nhlbi.nih.gov). It contains clinical guidelines, executive summary, BMI calculations, treatment plans, and other resources for nutrition and weight management.

Osteoporosis

Osteoporosis is a condition resulting from decreased density, or thinning, of the bone. Imbalances in bone resorption (osteoclastic activity) and bone formation (osteoblastic activity) result in a decreased bone density. Most commonly, osteoporosis develops as a consequence of aging. U.S. women typically reach menopause at 51 or 52 years, and the most bone loss occurs during the first 5 to 7 years after menopause (Moore, 2003). Osteoporosis promotes the development of fractures and is the most common of all skeletal disorders. With poor calcium intake in childhood and adolescence, osteoporosis is now considered a pediatric problem. Factors that affect bone development adversely during childhood and adolescence include low calcium intake, poor general nutrition, sedentary lifestyle, carbonated beverage intake, and smoking.

Osteoporotic bone is more porous and weaker than normal bone, allowing fractures to happen more easily. Fractures in postmenopausal women contribute to long-term disability, frailty, and enormous expense. A woman loses 2% to 5% of bone tissue per year immediately before and for approximately 8 years after menopause (Moore, 2003). Common fracture sites are the spine, wrists, forearms, and hips. With the exception of arthritis, osteoporosis is the leading cause of musculoskeletal disturbances in older adults (National Osteoporosis Foundation, 2006a). Women are at higher risk for osteoporosis than are men, primarily as a result of differences in bone mass and density (National Osteoporosis Foundation, 2006a).

Osteoporosis commonly is called the "silent epidemic" because early stages have no symptoms. Without improved preventive care for girls and women during the growth years and throughout the lifespan, osteoporosis will not be recognized until it is too late and fractures are likely. An early prediction of which clients are at risk is helpful.

Risk Factors. In simple terms, a **risk factor** is an action or behavior that increases a person's chances to develop a condition. In complex human terms, clients have combinations of social, psychological, cultural, physical, and addictive behaviors that lead to negative results.

Risk factors contributing to osteoporosis are important to emphasize in educating and motivating women to practice preventive screening and positive lifestyle behaviors. Such risk factors are as follows (National Osteoporosis Foundation, 2006a):

Family history of osteoporosis. This is learned primarily through health history information, especially if any female relatives have had a broken wrist or hip or a hump in the cervical spine caused by compression of the vertebrae from osteoporosis.

Hysterectomy, surgical removal of ovaries, or both before 50 years of age. Secondary osteoporosis is used to define reduced bone mass that develops from reasons other than aging. Young women who have had their ovaries surgically removed have the same risk for osteoporosis as do postmenopausal women.

Smoking. Women who smoke increase their odds of developing osteoporosis.

Alcohol. Women who consume excessive alcohol lose more calcium, which can result in osteoporosis. Women who drink wine, beer, or other alcoholic beverages daily increase their risk for osteoporosis.

Small, thin body frame. Slender women of European and Asian descent have osteoporosis more often than African American women, largely because of differences in peak bone mass and density.

Caffeinated soft drinks and coffee. Women who drink soft drinks and more than a few cups of coffee with caffeine daily increase their chances for osteoporosis as a result of calcium loss. Dietary items that interfere with calcium absorption include fiber, sodium, protein, iron, caffeine, and oxalates (Moore, 2003).

Inactivity. Weight-bearing exercise improves bone density. With the approval of their health care providers, women should engage in weight-bearing exercise (eg, walking, jogging, low-impact aerobics) for at least 1 hour per week.

Eating disorders and strenuous exercise causing amenorrhea. Anorexia nervosa and bulimia nervosa increase the likelihood of osteoporosis through general poor nutrition and low calcium intake (see Chap. 5). Exercise that is so strenuous that a woman's periods become irregular or absent is just as harmful as inactivity (see Chap. 4). Excessive exercise causing amenorrhea is also a form of bulimic activity that leads to bone loss. A balanced exercise and diet program is the key to health promotion habits to prevent osteoporosis.

Low-calcium dietary intake. Many factors in a woman's background can influence her intake of calcium. Nurses should determine during the health history any milk allergies or lactose intolerance, eating disorders, or continued dieting for weight management that often excludes dairy products. Most women do not consume adequate calcium in their young adult years to achieve peak bone mass (Nicklas, 2003).

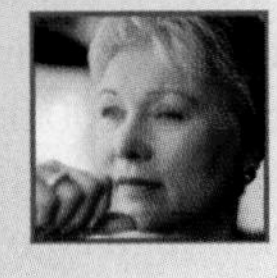

Remember Linda, the 53-year-old accountant described at the start of the chapter. What factors in the scenario might place Linda at risk for osteoporosis?

Prevention. Because women are at increased risk for osteoporosis, nurses should teach preventive health measures. Dietary instruction on calcium intake requires special attention when developing teaching plans for girls and women because preventive measures are the primary defense. Optimum calcium intake and exercise during growth years enhances peak bone mass (National Osteoporosis Foundation, 2006b). Measures that have been identified as helpful in preventing further bone loss include increasing calcium intake; taking vitamin D supplements; avoiding excessive caffeine, soft drinks, and alcohol; not smoking; increasing physical activity; and undergoing bone density screening for appropriate women at risk (National Osteoporosis Foundation, 2006b).

COLLABORATIVE CARE: DIET, EXERCISE, AND HEALTHY LIFESTYLE

The nursing response to the public health epidemic of overweight and obesity involves educating clients and supporting their efforts to change behaviors through diet and exercise. Nurses should advise women to consume most dietary fat as polyunsaturated and monosaturated fat, while reducing saturated and trans fats (Teaching Tips 2.1). The best results in weight management have been with nutritional programs that decrease both fat and calories and focus on exercise and remaining active (Kealy, 2003; Wing & Phelan, 2005).

Assessment

When working with clients in the area of diet, exercise, and healthy lifestyles, the nurse should perform a thorough health history. He or she should ask the client to keep an exercise log and a diet diary that covers typical eating patterns. The client should record her fat, iron, and calcium intake for 2 weeks to increase awareness of her choices. The nurse should ask the client about the type, amount, and frequency of exercise, along with satisfaction with routines.

Select Potential Nursing Diagnoses

Nursing diagnoses that may apply in the area of diet, exercise, and lifestyle management include, but are not limited to, the following (NANDA, 2006):

- Imbalanced Nutrition: More Than Body Requirements
- Health-Seeking Behaviors
- Deficient Knowledge
- Readiness for Enhanced Knowledge
- Readiness for Enhanced Nutrition

Planning/Intervention

Discussing concerns such as weight control, lowering cholesterol, and food preferences is essential. If the woman is allergic to milk products, she needs information about other sources of dietary calcium and calcium supplementation. Ways to balance cholesterol and calcium include consuming low-fat yogurt, skim milk, pudding made with skim milk, and low-fat cheese. Nursing Care

TEACHING TIPS 2.1 Nutrition and Weight Management

Nurses should share with clients the following points about nutrition:

- Ensure that your diet contains a variety of foods.
- Limit fat intake to 30% of daily calories. Most calories should come from grains, fruits, and vegetables.
- Monitor the *types* of fat consumed. Choose foods low in saturated and trans fats and cholesterol and moderate in monosaturated fat:
  - Choose vegetable oils rather than solid fats.
  - Trim fat from meat; remove skin from poultry.
  - Limit intake of bacon, sausages, salami, and bologna.
  - Use egg whites and egg substitutes.
  - Choose fat-free or low-fat milk, yogurt, and cheese.
  - Always check Nutrition Facts labels to determine saturated fat and cholesterol in prepared foods.
  - When eating out, choose lean meats, limit intake of creamy sauces, and select fruit as dessert.
- Use moderate sugar and salt.
- Drink at least 8 glasses of water per day.
- Recommended servings of the food groups include the following:
  - Sparing amounts of fats, oils, and sweets
  - 6 to 11 servings of bread, cereal, rice, and pasta
  - Small servings of whole wheat breads, nonsweetened cereals, oatmeal, brown rice, and pasta to obtain 20 to 35 mg/day of fiber and according to individual weight management
  - 5 to 9 servings of fruits and vegetables
  - 2 to 3 servings of milk, yogurt, and cheese
  - 2 to 3 servings of meat, poultry, fish, dry beans, eggs, and nuts
- Obtain 1000 to 1500 mg/day of calcium and 400 to 800 IU/day of vitamin D. Sources of calcium include the following:
  - Vitamin supplement
  - Low-fat yogurt
  - Low-fat milk
  - Soy-based beverages with added calcium
  - Breakfast cereals with added calcium
  - Fruit juices with added calcium
  - Dark green, leafy vegetables
- Obtain 400 μg/day (0.4 mg/day) of folate. Sources of folate include the following:
  - Vitamin supplement (folic acid)
  - Cooked dry beans and peas, peanuts
  - Oranges, orange juice
  - Dark green, leafy vegetables: spinach, mustard greens, romaine lettuce
  - Green peas
- Obtain 15 mg/day of iron. Sources of iron include the following:
  - Vitamin supplement
  - Shellfish: shrimp, clams, mussels, and oysters
  - Lean meats, especially beef, liver, and other organ meats
  - Cereals with added iron
  - Turkey dark meat with skin removed
  - Sardines
  - Spinach
  - Cooked dry beans, peas, and lentils
  - Enriched and whole grain breads
- Obtain 20 to 35 g/day of fiber. Sources of fiber include the following:
  - Fruits
  - Vegetables
  - Whole grains
  - Cereals
  - Dried beans and peas

References

Dietary Guidelines for Americans. (2000). 5th ed.
Erickson, J. D. (2002). Folic acid and prevention of spinal bifida and anencephaly 10 years after the U.S. Public Health Service recommendation. *Morbidity and Mortality Weekly Report, 51,* s1–s3.
Iron deficiency: Latest guidelines for controlling and preventing a common problem. (1998). *Consultant, 38,* 2127–2131.
McBean, L. D. (1999). Emerging dietary benefits of dairy foods. *Nutrition Today, 31,* 47.

Plan 2.1 provides a sample scenario of a client seeking to improve her health habits. NIC/NOC Box 2.1 provides common interventions and outcomes related to healthy lifestyles.

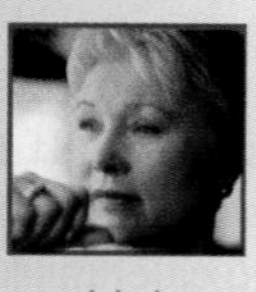

Think back to Linda, who came to the clinic for help with her hot flashes. History taking reveals that Linda does not like milk. What other suggestions could the nurse give to ensure that Linda consumes enough calcium?

Controlling Fat Intake

Experts no longer recommend following a diet low in *total* fat only; instead, they emphasize being aware of the *types* of fat and reducing intake of saturated and trans fats and cholesterol (American Heart Association [AHA], 2006b). The nurse should teach the client that fats are essential for health but must be consumed moderately. Although enjoyment of the appealing qualities and satiety of high-fat items is normal, clients should balance their intake with low-fat choices such as fresh fruits, vegetables, grains, and lean meats. Also, clients need to monitor the type of fats they consume. The AHA (2006b) recommends eating at least two servings of fatty fish with omega-3 oil (eg, tuna,

NURSING CARE PLAN 2.1

A Client Making Nutrition, Exercise, and Lifestyle Choices

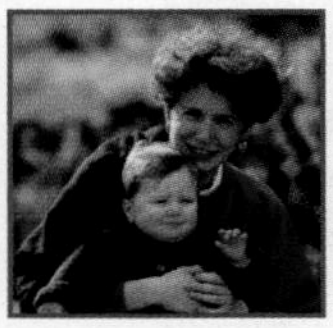

Consider Renee from the beginning of the chapter. During the interview, Renee mentions a history of heart disease and type 2 diabetes in her family. She states that she is motivated to maintain physical activity and a weight-control program. She does not smoke. Renee's BMI is 25.4. She wants to bring that number down from overweight to within normal.

NURSING DIAGNOSIS

Health-Seeking Behaviors related to weight control and exercise

EXPECTED OUTCOMES

1. The client will verbalize areas of daily routine that may contribute to unhealthy behaviors leading to weight gain.
2. The client will identify measures that promote weight control and gradual weight loss.
3. The client will participate in an exercise routine for approximately 20 to 30 minutes three to four times each week.

INTERVENTIONS	RATIONALES
Question the client about her daily routine and activities, including child care and home demands.	This information provides a baseline to identify problem areas and develop suggestions for healthy behaviors.
Review the client's daily eating patterns, including frequency of eating and types of foods and fluids consumed. Ascertain the client's likes and dislikes.	Knowledge of current dietary patterns provides clues to nutritional status and amount and types of calories and nutrients ingested. Information about the client's likes and dislikes aids in individualizing suggestions for proper food selection.
Encourage the client to eat small, frequent meals throughout the day and not to skip meals. Provide suggestions to replace empty calories with nutritious ones.	Small frequent meals throughout the day maintain metabolism and proper insulin secretion and prevent starvation metabolism.
Reinforce the need to limit consumption of fats and to select vegetables, fruits, whole grains, legumes, fish, poultry, and lean meats low in saturated and trans fats and cholesterol. Instruct the client in methods of cooking such as broiling and steaming.	Because of the client's family history, the client should avoid intake of foods high in trans fat and cholesterol to reduce her risk. Consumption of diets high in saturated fats, elevated lipid levels, and obesity are associated with type 2 diabetes. Positive methods of cooking promote the intake of healthier, more nutritious foods.
Offer suggestions about how to incorporate healthy eating into her daily routine.	Incorporating healthy habits into the routine enhances the chances for success and adherence to the plan.
Reinforce the need for portion control; show how to estimate or visualize portions in terms of concrete objects.	This measure aids in compliance with the regimen.

Continued

NURSING CARE PLAN 2.1 ● A Client Making Nutrition, Exercise, and Lifestyle Choices *(Continued)*

INTERVENTIONS	RATIONALES
Encourage the client to keep a food diary or log of her intake for review on the next visit.	Keeping a food diary or log helps the client to visualize the amount and types of food consumed and possible patterns of intake that need adjustment or correction.
Investigate the types of activities that the client enjoys.	Doing exercise that the client enjoys promotes adherence and increases the chances for success.
Encourage the client to exercise with someone else.	Women with exercise partners may feel safer participating in outdoor activities. Research has shown that people with partners are more likely to maintain consistent exercise patterns.
Advise the client to start slowly. Recommend a 5-minute warm-up and cool-down at the beginning and end of each exercise session. Encourage her to exercise approximately three to four times a week for 20 to 30 minutes. If she cannot afford a health club, she may find walking to be an economical and rewarding sport.	Consistency, not speed, is the key to aerobic exercise. For women, it is very important to select an exercise that will fit easily into their schedule and responsibilities.
Emphasize the need to vary exercise routines and gradually increase intensity as tolerated.	Varying exercise decreases boredom and works different muscle groups. Increasing intensity helps strengthen muscles and increase endurance.
Instruct the client to avoid weighing herself daily; suggest that she weigh herself approximately twice a week, at the same time and wearing approximately the same amount of clothing at each measure.	Weight fluctuates throughout the day and daily. Too frequent weighing may lead to discouragement. Improved fitness and a gradual sustained weight loss are key.

EVALUATION

1. The client reports that she is engaging in brisk walks of 1 to 1½ miles three times a week.
2. The client states that her energy level has increased and that she feels "healthier."
3. The client verbalizes the intake of a healthy, nutritious diet low in saturated and trans fat and cholesterol.
4. The client demonstrates a weight loss of approximately 2 pounds by return visit in 3 to 4 weeks.

salmon, mackerel, lake trout, herring, sardines, and albacore) every week. In a guideline issued from a publication in *Circulation: Journal of the American Heart Association* (Kris-Etherton et al., 2002), the AHA reported that omega-3 fatty acids are not just good fats but also affect health by making the blood less likely to clot and protect against irregular heartbeats that cause sudden cardiac death (Box 2.1).

Emphasizing Portion Control

Portion control is a major component in weight management. New trends in portion control that have been

NIC/NOC Box 2.1 Healthy Behaviors

Common NIC Labels

- Behavior Management
- Decision-Making Support
- Exercise Promotion
- Health Education
- Health Screening
- Learning Facilitation
- Learning Readiness Enhancement
- Nutritional Counseling
- Risk Identification
- Self-Awareness Enhancement
- Self-Modification Assistance
- Teaching: Individual
- Teaching: Prescribed Diet
- Weight Management
- Weight Reduction Assistance

Common NOC Labels

- Adherence Behavior
- Health Beliefs
- Health Orientation
- Health Promoting Behavior
- Health Seeking Behavior
- Knowledge: Diet
- Knowledge: Health Behaviors
- Knowledge: Health Promotion
- Knowledge: Health Resources
- Weight Control
- Well-Being

successful include having the woman visualize her portion in terms of a concrete object. For example, the nurse may recommend that the client take a portion of rice or vegetables the size of a tennis ball. Another example is for the nurse to show apples of various sizes so that the client fully understands what is meant by a "medium-sized" apple.

BOX 2.1 Benefits of Omega-3 Fatty Acids

Although the mechanisms are not totally known and are currently being researched, consumption of omega-3 fatty acids has been shown to contribute to:

- Decreased thrombosis
- Decreased risk for sudden death and dysrhythmia
- Decreased growth of atherosclerotic plaque
- Improved arterial health
- Lower blood pressure
- Decreased triglyceride levels

From Kris-Etherton, P. M., Harris, W. S., Appel, L. J., for the American Heart Association, Nutrition Committee. (2002). Fish consumption, fish oil, omega-3 fatty acids, and cardiovascular disease. *Circulation, 106*(21), 2747–2757.

Developing Exercise Routines

The client should slowly increase the intensity of her exercise routine. The nurse should focus exercise guidelines on process—a healthy lifestyle across the lifespan. Focusing on the end result—weight control or weight loss—can become counterproductive. Fitness and fun are more important than are being thin. Nurses need to reinforce exercise measures in teaching plans that promote the idea of exercise being a life habit.

Evaluation

Nurses should conduct follow-up discussions to evaluate progress. One method that they may use is to ask the client to complete a daily food intake and exercise diary and bring it to the nurse for evaluation. If necessary, the nurse should ask the client to suggest alternatives when current plans do not seem to be working. Consultation with a dietitian, physician, or both should be initiated if the client requires additional assistance.

Psychosocial Health

Psychological health includes factors in every woman's life related to balancing work, home, stress, relationships, family, and sense of meaning and healing. In this chapter, psychological health promotion focuses on the woman, her family, and her community; it applies to all women, including those with diagnosed psychiatric conditions. Therefore, this section briefly summarizes health history and assessment parameters for psychological health promotion and common mental health concerns for women, including depression, anxiety, domestic violence, substance abuse, and gun safety. Chapter 5 explores these issues in more detail.

Mental Health Promotion

The Center for Health Promotion (1997) defines *mental health promotion* as the process of enhancing the capacity of individuals and communities to take control of their lives and improve their mental health. Mental health promotion uses strategies that foster support, empowerment, resilience, and inner strength (Roux, Dingley, & Bush, 2002). Some experts debate whether mental health promotion focuses exclusively on the "well" population; others feel that mental health promotion includes the mentally ill and issues specific to their environment and conditions (Willinsky & Pape, 2002).

Women fulfilling multiple roles often need support from health providers to ensure that they attend to their own psychological needs. Teaching Tips 2.2 provides some general strategies for nurses to communicate to their clients.

TEACHING TIPS 2.2 Taking Care of You—Personal Action Steps

Nurses share the following points with clients when teaching about self-care:

- Find time for yourself each day. Focus on what your body/mind is telling you. Try to take at least 15 minutes a day to do something special and relaxing for you.
- Exercise every day. It increases endorphins in the body and improves emotional and physical health. Risk for coronary artery disease (CAD) almost doubles in a sedentary person. Walking 30 minutes a day, three to five times a week is beneficial. Exercise has more cardiovascular benefits if the pace is brisk enough to elevate heart rate.
- Eat a nutritious diet. Studies have shown a connection between early and continued consumption of fruits and vegetables and reduced risk for chronic health conditions such as obesity and heart disease. Overweight women have been shown to have higher rates of morbidity and mortality than lean women.
- Get your annual examination. This is an opportunity for screening for common conditions such as hypertension, breast and cervical cancer, and depression. Most importantly, it is also a time to address your concerns with a nurse practitioner or physician. During the annual examination, you can get answers and discuss how to modify lifestyle as necessary.
- Get enough sleep. Don't eat, exercise, or do stimulating activity right before bedtime. Have a ritual every night to promote a relaxed sleeping pattern. Sleep will allow you to be more equipped to deal with everyday stressors.
- Quit smoking (if you are a smoker). Smoking does not just affect the lungs. It is associated with diseases that affect every organ in the body. Smoking affects and can harm not only the smoker but also those exposed to secondhand smoke.
- Reduce your risk for injury.
- Practice safer sex.
- Avoid violence and contact with violent people.
- Be aware of safety principles at home and when traveling.
- Always wear a seatbelt.
- Never drive under the influence of alcohol or drugs.

Health history questions to assess the woman's environment and mental health needs include the following:

Do you pay attention to your inner feelings?
How many hours of sleep do you get per night? Do you feel rested?
What activities do you do to relax? What are your hobbies?
Do you take at least 15 minutes out for yourself each day?
Do you have anyone close to you to confide in?
Do you have an outlet that satisfies your spiritual needs?
Do you have anything that lifts your spirits?

Mental health promotion facilitates healing by restoring harmony and balance between mind and body. Mind–body and CAM therapies can alleviate stress-related health problems. Nursing interventions to promote psychological health include touching, listening, praying, caring, music, humor, counseling, pharmacotherapeutics, and story telling.

Depression

Physical and psychological symptoms of depression can cause significant distress and impairment to the woman and her family. Clients with depression either have a depressed mood or express a lack of interest in all or most routine activities. They develop a constellation of the following: significant weight loss or gain or alterations in appetite; sleep disturbances manifested by insomnia or hypersomnia; psychomotor agitation or retardation; fatigue or loss of energy; feelings of worthlessness or inappropriate guilt; diminished ability to concentrate; poor concentration or difficulty making decisions; feelings of hopelessness; and recurrent thoughts of death. These symptoms must represent a change in recent functioning and be present and persistent (almost every day) for at least 2 consecutive weeks (American Psychiatric Association [APA], 2000). Depression can be a single episode or periodically recur, but it remains independent of life events. Loss of a loved one or a life-changing event may act as a catalyst to depression, but in the category of mood disorders, depression remains a psychiatric diagnosis distinct from grief.

Depression may occur with or without comorbid conditions. Close monitoring includes assessment for anxiety, panic disorder, posttraumatic stress disorder, substance abuse, or grief reactions.

Risk Factors. Risk factors for depression include family or personal history of depression, family or personal history of postpartum depression, poor self-concept or low self-esteem, female gender, other chronic health conditions, substance abuse, loss or death, and stressful life occurrences (APA, 2000). Risk factors for suicide include previous attempts at suicide, depression, dysfunctional family, abuse, domestic violence, alcoholism and other substance abuse, and chronic illness (Berg, 2002; Youngkin & Davis, 2004).

Screening Tools. Depressive disorders are more common in women than in men (Youngkin & Davis, 2004). Screening for depression as a component of the annual comprehensive examination can enhance early detection and treatment. The U.S. Preventive Services Task Force (USPSTF, 2002b) recommends screening adults for depression in clinical practices that have systems in place to ensure accurate screening, diagnosis, and follow-up (Berg, 2002). The following tools are used widely:

- *Beck Depression Inventory:* contains 21 items with four statements each; all items apply to "the past week, including today." A short version is available. Emphasis is on cognitive symptoms.
- *Zung Self-Rating Scale:* 20 items, rated by duration of each depressive symptom. Zung describes the scale as a "depression thermometer."
- *Geriatric Depression Scale:* 15 yes/no questions; scale takes 5 to 7 minutes to complete. It is one page and easy to understand.
- *Center for Epidemiological Studies Depression Scale (CES-D):* 30 items; screens for depressed mood, psychomotor retardation and somatic complaints, lack of well-being, and interpersonal difficulties.

Health care providers follow all positive results on screening tests with an extensive interview, health history, and physical examination along with a full diagnostic workup. Sample tools and expanded discussions, including treatment, are found in Chapter 5.

Anxiety Disorders

Anxiety differs from fear, in that anxiety is a response to an unknown, internal, vague, or conflictual threat (Running & Berndt, 2003), whereas fear is a response to a known or definite threat. Anxiety may be temporary or a persistent health issue. When anxiety escalates beyond healthy functioning and interferes with quality of life, assessment for anxiety disorders and potential treatment are indicated.

Anxiety disorders are characterized by symptoms of physiologic arousal (eg, palpitations, sweating) and excessive worry that persist over time and interfere with normal functioning (Uphold & Graham, 2003). They are classified further as panic attacks, phobias, generalized anxiety disorder, obsessive-compulsive disorder, posttraumatic stress disorder, and acute stress disorder (APA, 2000). The most common risk factors for anxiety disorders are physical and mental illness, stressful life situations or crises, family history of anxiety disorders, abuse, and domestic violence (APA, 2000).

Women with potential anxiety disorders require a thorough examination and history with diagnostic testing to rule out other medical, neurologic, or endocrine disorders (Running & Berndt, 2003). The nurse can refer clients to psychiatrists or psychologists for follow-up. A woman with an anxiety disorder may need pharmacologic treatment. Nonpharmacologic treatments include therapy, biofeedback, relaxation therapies, meditation, journaling, and yoga. CAM Box 2.2 discusses the use of kava for anxiety. Support groups and family therapy may be beneficial, as well as establishing normal eating, sleeping, and exercise patterns tailored to the woman's lifestyle. See Chapter 5 for more information.

Domestic Violence

"I really wanted the nurse to ask me about what was going on at home. He always seemed too busy. I get the feeling he didn't ask me because he did not want to deal with my problems."

Domestic violence occurs when there is relationship abuse, violence, or both. One person physically, sexually, verbally, or emotionally abuses another, destroys the person's property, or some combination (see Chap. 5). Economic control, stalking, and control of social contacts are other forms of violence against women. Experiencing fear in a relationship is characteristic of abuse, regardless of whether there is physical violence. Fear of physical harm is enough to characterize a relationship as abusive (Hawkins, Roberto-Nichols, & Stanley-Haney, 2000).

Nurses assess clients for risks for or presence of domestic violence at each visit. Assessment Tool 2.1 presents the "SAFE" screening tool, which helps identify victims of abuse. Chapter 5 provides a more detailed discussion of this important topic.

● COMPLEMENTARY/ALTERNATIVE MEDICINE 2.2
Use of Kava for Anxiety

Kava is an herb that has shown great promise in the treatment of anxiety. In seven double-blind, placebo-controlled, randomized trials, researchers found kava consistently better than placebo at treating symptoms of anxiety (Cauffield & Forbes, 1999; Pittler & Ernst, 2000). Findings also indicated that kava had results equivalent to those of benzodiazepines, with the added benefit of fewer side effects.

The client should not take kava if she is using other substances that act on the central nervous system, such as antidepressants, alcohol, and barbiturates. As with all complementary/alternative medicine products, the nurse should urge the client to discuss the use of kava with her primary health care provider before initiating any therapy independently.

ASSESSMENT TOOL 2.1 "SAFE" Questions That Can Help Identify Victims of Abuse

STRESS/SAFETY

- What stresses do you have in your relationship with your partner?
- How do you handle disagreements?
- Do you feel safe in your relationship with (name spouse/partner)?
- Should I be concerned for your safety?

AFRAID

- Are there situations in which you feel afraid?
- Have you ever been threatened or abused?
- Has your partner forced you to have sexual intercourse that you did not want?

FRIENDS/FAMILY

- If positive responses to items above: Ask "Are your friends/family aware that this is happening?"
- If negative responses to items above: Ask "Do you think you could tell them if it did happen?"
- Would they help you?

EMERGENCY PLAN

- Do you have a safe place to go in an emergency situation?
- If you are in danger now, would you like me to help you find a shelter?
- Would you like to talk with a social worker/counselor to help you develop a plan?

Follow any questions answered affirmatively with additional questions to determine the following:

- How and when mistreatment occurs
- Who perpetrates it
- How the woman copes with it
- What she plans to do to protect herself (and children)

From Uphold, C. R., & Graham, M. V. (2003). *Clinical guidelines in family practice* (3rd ed.). Gainesville, FL: Barmarrae Books.

Substance Abuse

Alcohol, drug, and tobacco abuse are prominent public health issues for women and their families. Consequences of addictive use of alcohol, drugs, and tobacco include liver disease, heart disease, breast and lung cancer, violence, sexual victimization, and auto accidents. Factors that may increase women's risk for substance abuse or dependence include genetic influences, early initiation of smoking and substance use, and victimization. Some increased risks for substance abuse in women compared with men may be gender-related differences in metabolism, brain chemistry, genetic risk factors, or entirely different factors still undiscovered. Because of the increased consequences of substance abuse in women, early assessment and treatment are key to increasing awareness and preventing serious consequences.

Nurses assess adolescents and women for alcohol and substance use during the health history. Assessment Tools 2.2, 2.3, and 2.4 have wide screening applicability for high-risk clients. Women and girls whose scores indicate a problem require extensive interviews and medical follow-up. The nurse provides community resources and referrals to these clients and their families.

Adolescent girls are the most rapidly increasing population of new smokers (CDC, 2006a). Frequently, girls report they initiate smoking to lose weight and maintain the weight loss. Other factors that contribute to adolescent smoking are peer pressure and stress relief. Nurses adapt smoking cessation programs for adolescents to points that teens view as meaningful to their development. Adolescents may be more likely to stop smoking if providers relate the effects to body image and attractiveness such as bad breath, smelly clothes, and wrinkles (Teaching Tips 2.3).

Gun Safety

When examining violence as a public health promotion issue, nurses must consider gun safety as a variable. Between 1994 and 1998, 23,776 children 19 years or younger died from a gun-related injury (CDC, 2002b).

ASSESSMENT TOOL 2.2 CAGE Questionnaire for Alcoholism Screening

Have you ever felt you should **C**ut down on your drinking?
Have people **A**nnoyed you by criticizing your drinking?
Have you ever felt **G**uilty about your drinking?
Have you ever had a drink first thing in the morning (**E**ye-opener) to steady your nerves or get rid of a hangover?

Two or more "yes" answers indicate probable alcoholism. Any one "yes" answer deserves further evaluation.

Source: Ewing, J. A. (1984). Detecting alcoholism: The CAGE questionnaire. *Journal of the American Medical Association, 252,* 1905–1907.

● ASSESSMENT TOOL 2.3 Primary Screening Tools for Alcohol Problems

HALT

1. Do you drink to get **H**igh?
2. Do you drink **A**lone?
3. Do you **L**ook forward to drinking (instead of going to an event)?
4. Has your **T**olerance for alcohol increased or decreased?

BUMP

1. Have you had **B**lackouts?
2. Is your drinking **U**nplanned (you drink when you said you would not or drink more than you thought)?
3. Do you drink **M**edicinally (when depressed, sad, anxious)?
4. Do you **P**rotect your supply (so that you will always have enough)?

FATAL DTs

Family history of alcohol problems?
Alcoholics Anonymous attendance?
Thoughts or attempts at suicide?
Alcoholism. Ever thought you might have it?
Legal problems, such as driving under the influence or assault?
Depression, feeling down, low, or sad?
Tranquilizer or disulfiram use?

Source: Martin, A., Schaeffer, S., & Campbell, R. (1999). Managing alcohol-related problems in the primary care setting. *The Nurse Practitioner,* 23(8), 14–39.

Having a firearm in the home makes it 43% more likely that a family member or friend, not an intruder, will be killed (CDC, 2002b). The American Academy of Pediatrics (AAP, 1999) now recommends inclusion of gun safety education in each visit to the pediatrician.

Nurses must increase awareness of safety and specific rules of gun safety in the home. Key points for gun safety education to emphasize with girls, adolescents, parents, and grandparents are given in Teaching Tips 2.4.

Cardiovascular Health

Although some still believe the myth that heart disease is a man's disease, cardiovascular diseases are the leading cause of mortality in women (AHA, 2006a; CDC, 2001). The incidence of cardiovascular disease in women continues to rise markedly in perimenopause and menopause. Natural and surgically induced menopause are associated with changes in serum lipid profiles, with a decline in high-density lipoprotein (HDL) cholesterol and an increase in low-density lipoprotein cholesterol. These cholesterol changes may be factors in the development of a woman's increased risk for postmenopausal heart disease (see Chaps. 4, 23, and 24).

Deposition of cholesterol in plaque-laden arterial walls is the primary pathologic risk for heart disease. *Angina pectoris* occurs when the client experiences a deficit of oxygen being infused through the myocardium itself. The actual pain sensation is thought to result from a state of anaerobic physiology. *Myocardial infarction* occurs with an actual necrosis, or "death," of the myocardial cells from anaerobic insult. A clot, spasm, or atherosclerotic plaque in the coronary arteries can cause these anaerobic conditions (Fig. 2.5). The most common cause is atherosclerosis. Contrary to common belief, many women who die suddenly of coronary heart disease (CHD) have no prior symptoms. This highlights the need for preventive screening with blood pressure monitoring, lipid profiles, weight management, smoking cessation, and prevention and management of diabetes mellitus.

Risk Factors for Heart Disease

Many women and practitioners do not think of CHD, especially myocardial infarction, as a "woman's disease." Nurses can play a key role in educating their professional peers and clients about the facts of CHD in

● ASSESSMENT TOOL 2.4 CRAFFT Substance Abuse Screening Tool

This tool has been tested recently in adolescent clinic patients.

1. Have you ever ridden in a **C**ar driven by someone (including yourself) who was "high" or had been using alcohol or drugs?
2. Do you ever use alcohol or drugs to **R**elax, feel better about yourself, or fit in?
3. Do you ever use alcohol or drugs when you are **A**lone.
4. Do your family or **F**riends ever tell you that you should cut down on your drinking or drug use?
5. Do you ever **F**orget things you did while using alcohol or drugs?
6. Have you gotten in **T**rouble while using alcohol or drugs?

Two or more "yes" answers indicate a significant problem (Knight, Sherritt, Shrier, Harris, & Chang, 2002).

For more information, visit www.SAMHSA.gov. Substance Abuse and Mental Health Services Administration (SAMHSA) is an agency of the United States Department of Health and Human Services.

TEACHING TIPS 2.3 Prevention of Adolescent Smoking

Nurses share the following points with adolescent clients when discussing smoking:

- Adolescent women who smoke:
  - May have more painful menstruation
  - May stop menstruating all together
  - May have menstrual irregularity
  - Have less oxygen available to their lungs, making playing sports difficult
  - Run slower and not as far as nonsmokers
  - Have bad breath, cracked lips, sores, and bleeding in the mouth from tobacco
  - Have an increased risk for ectopic pregnancies and spontaneous abortions
- Babies born to women who smoke are at an increased risk for sudden infant death syndrome (SIDS).
- Women smokers who die of a smoking-related disease lose approximately 14 years of potential life.

Know the truth. Despite all the tobacco use on TV and in movies, music videos, billboards, and magazines, most teens, adults, and athletes DON'T use tobacco!

TEACHING TIPS 2.4 Gun Safety

Nurses share the following points with clients when teaching about gun safety:

GENERAL GUIDELINES

- Learn the characteristics of your firearm.
- Treat the firearm as if it were loaded at all times.
- Point the muzzle in a safe direction.
- Keep your finger off the trigger, unless you intend to fire it.
- Never rely on mechanical safety features to protect you or someone else.
- Keep the gun unloaded and action open until you are ready to shoot.
- Know your target and what is beyond it.
- Use only the correct ammunition for your firearm.
- Know what to do in case of a misfire.
- Wear protective eye and ear equipment.
- Keep the firearm free from obstructions and keep it well maintained.
- Do not modify your firearm.
- Do not mix guns with alcohol, drugs, or fatigue.

SAFETY FOR PARENTS AND GRANDPARENTS

If there is a gun in your home:

- When to teach the child about gun safety: when the child starts to ask questions or acts out gun play. Keep your lessons simple, but credible. Repeat, repeat, and repeat.
- Teach facts, not fear: The first rule for small children is DON'T TOUCH! Once the child is older, taking him or her to a gun range may take away the "forbidden fruit" attraction. Consider having the older child take a gun safety course.
- Distinguish between fantasy and reality. Many parents establish their home as a "no gun zone," meaning no real or pretend guns allowed. If children are allowed to play with pretend guns, teach them the difference between real and pretend. Tell them to always assume a gun is real first! They should be taught to play with their pretend guns as if they were real.
- Options for safe storage: vaults, safes, and locked metal storage boxes. Store ammunition and the firearm in separate safes. Think about gun storage from your child's point of view. Children will climb up onto areas that you think they cannot reach! Consider using trigger, action-blocking locks for additional safety.
- Practice what you preach:
  - Follow the rules you have set for your children! Remember, you are their role model!
  - Don't leave firearms lying around.

If your child encounters a gun not in your home:

- If your child discovers a gun outside the home or in the home of a friend, he or she should know the four steps of the Eddie Eagle gun safety program, including:
  STOP!
  DON'T TOUCH.
  LEAVE THE AREA.
  TELL AN ADULT.
- Discuss gun safety with other parents of family members if your child spends time in their homes. It is not enough to assume that if they do have guns in the house, they have them stored properly.

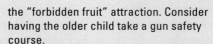

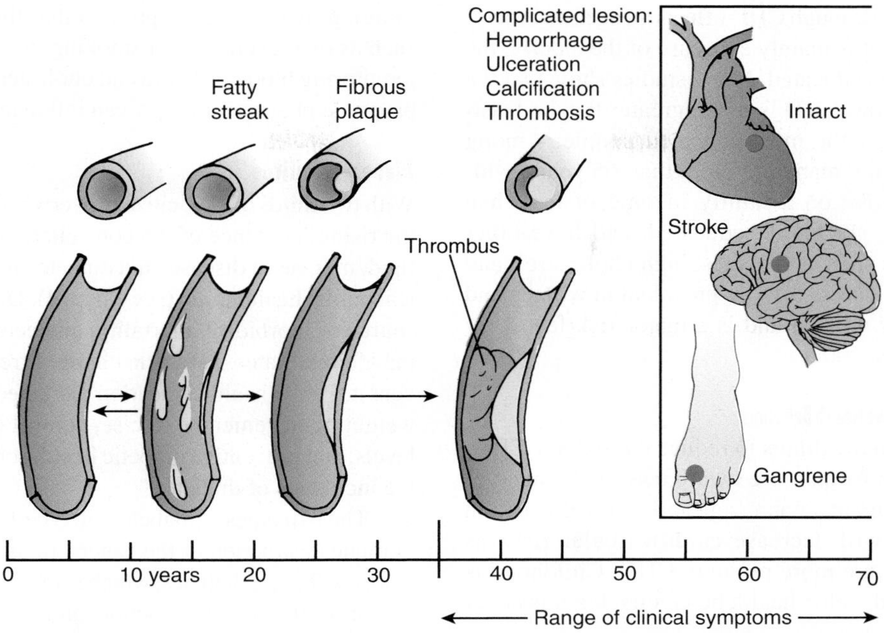

FIGURE 2.5 In atherosclerosis, the process begins with fatty streaks, which can progress to form fibrous plaque. The plaque can progress to cause hemorrhage, ulceration, calcification, or thrombosis. The result can be a myocardial infarction or a cerebrovascular accident.

women. The following are major risk factors for CHD in women (Joint National Committee on Prevention, Detection, Evaluation and Treatment of High Blood Pressure, 2003; Kealy, 2003):

- Cigarette smoking
- Hypertension (blood pressure > 130/80 mm Hg) or poor control of blood pressure with the prescribed antihypertensive medications. (The treatment goal is < 130/80 mm Hg with diabetes mellitus.)
- HDL < 50 mg/dL; LDL < 100; triglycerides > 150
- Family history of CHD
- Age 55 years or older
- BMI greater than 25 (see Fig. 2.3)
- Diabetes mellitus
- Large waist-to-hip ratio; central or abdominal obesity; waist greater than 35 inches is an independent risk factor

The major modifiable risk factors for CHD are cigarette smoking, dyslipidemia, hypertension, diabetes, physical inactivity, excessive alcohol consumption, stress, and excessive weight. The risk for developing heart disease in a person with high blood pressure, high blood cholesterol, and history of smoking is eight times that of a person who has none of those factors (Grundy et al., 1997). In women with diabetes, mortality from CHD is 4 to 6 times that of women without diabetes (Allen & Phillip, 1997).

The following are key points regarding gender differences in CHD that require consideration for nursing practice.

Age. Women tend to show signs of cardiovascular disease later than men. Between 25 to 35 years, men have 3 times the incidence of CHD as women. Even though menopause decreases a woman's protection from heart disease, this biologic advantage persists until 65 to 70 years. With advanced aging, about 90% of women die of CHD and related complications. At older ages, women who have heart attacks are twice as likely as men to die from them within a few weeks. Therefore, although rates of CHD mortality are higher in men than women throughout the lifespan, there are almost as many CHD deaths in women as men because of the dramatic rise in older women who die from the disease (USDHHS, 2002a).

Signs and Symptoms. Previously, women were not included in major CHD research and treatment, greatly compromising the known facts regarding early identification and treatment for women. Often the signs and symptoms of CHD in women differ significantly from those of men. Women also may have unspecified pain and vague symptoms, which can lead physicians and women themselves to look for other causes. Nurses need to begin to suspect heart attack in a woman the same as they would for a man. They should ask women how the symptoms respond or change in response to exercise, extremes in temperature, and heavy meals.

Social Factors. Although CHD affects all ages and socioeconomic strata, it is mainly a disease of the elderly, the poor, and the less educated. Many studies show that the risk for death from CHD is much greater for the least-educated than for the most-educated people. Among women with CHD, many are older than 65 years, widowed, living alone on a family income of less than $25,000 a year, not highly educated, and have other health problems such as diabetes, high cholesterol, and hypertension. Diabetes is more prevalent in women and also in minority women and is a major risk factor for CHD (USDHHS, 2002a).

Cardiovascular Preventive Health Behaviors

Clients can do many things to reduce the risk for CHD. The first step is to increase awareness of the need to take responsibility at a young age and to develop health behaviors that will decrease cardiovascular risks as women age and are more prone to CHD. Childhood is the best time to develop health behaviors, but it is never too late (Fig. 2.6).

Although heart attacks are uncommon in premenopausal women, the factors after menopause that lead to increased incidence are not exactly clear. Because women present with CHD at different ages and with different signs and symptoms, providers may take them less seriously than their male counterparts. Women eventually may be diagnosed with CHD when they are in the older age cohort, are more likely to be taking other medications, and have other conditions such as diabetes, hypertension, and osteoporosis.

Nurses, women, and the general community must recognize that a higher risk for CHD in women accompanies the years surrounding menopause; however, nurses need to emphasize that CHD is not an inevitable consequence of aging. It is a disease process that lifestyle behaviors such as diet, exercise, not smoking, maintaining weight, monitoring blood pressure and cholesterol, and using appropriate pharmacotherapy can influence greatly.

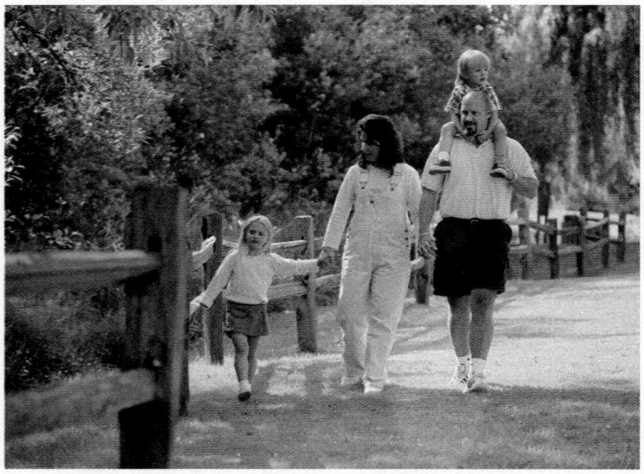

FIGURE 2.6 Families should try to instill good health and exercise habits in their children from the earliest ages. A healthy lifestyle from childhood on helps prevent problems like cardiovascular disease, diabetes, and obesity later in life.

Diabetes Mellitus

With two thirds of U.S. citizens overweight (CDC, 2002c), the rising incidence of the constellation of obesity, dyslipidemia, heart disease, and diabetes in women is a critical public health issue (see Chap. 4). Diabetes is a major source of morbidity, mortality, and economic burden in the United States. Lifestyle changes frequently can prevent it. Public health education marketed toward women, weight management, exercise, control of blood glucose levels, and preventive diabetic health services can reduce the incidence of diabetes.

The two types of diabetes are type 1 and type 2. Autoimmune destruction of the pancreatic islets causes type 1 diabetes. Type 2 diabetes, which is more prevalent, is a defect of insulin secretion, action, and resistance. Although type 2 diabetes was previously commonly seen in those older than 40 years, its prevalence is increasing among children and adolescents as more of them become overweight or obese (Reasner, 2002). Previously, almost 100% of children and adolescents newly diagnosed with diabetes had the type 1 form, but today, approximately 20% of new pediatric cases of diabetes are type 2 (Ward, 2002).

Risk Factors

Risk factors for type 2 diabetes mellitus include the following:

- Hypertension (≥130/80 mm Hg in adults on at least two separate occasions and measured in both arms)
- Family history (parents or siblings) of diabetes
- Overweight (BMI ≥ 25) (see Fig. 2.3)
- Race/ethnicity (African American, Hispanic American, Native American, Asian American, Pacific Islanders)
- Habitual physical inactivity
- HDL cholesterol ≤ 40 mg/dL men, < 50 mg/dL women; triglyceride level >150 mg/dL; or both
- History of gestational diabetes or delivery of a baby weighing more than 9 pounds
- Polycystic ovary syndrome

Screening

People presenting with any of the listed risk factors should be screened for diabetes yearly. Any person presenting with frequent urination, extreme thirst, unexplained weight loss, or repeated infections also should be screened. Screening consists of a comprehensive health history and physical examination along with taking blood glucose levels, both fasting and 2 hours postprandial. A fasting blood glucose level of 100 mg/dL or below is within the normal range. A blood glucose level above 126 mg/dL on more than one occasion supports a medical diagnosis of diabetes mellitus. Diabetes treatment goals for management of plasma glucose include a hemoglobin A1c level of less than 7, a preprandial plasma glucose level of 90 to 130 mg/dL, and a peak prandial glucose level less than 180 mg/dL (American Diabetes Association, 2006). See Chapter 4 for more information on the pathophysiology and management of diabetes.

Education and Prevention

Education and prevention are of great importance in decreasing incidence of diabetes in women and promoting **self-management** practices to reduce complications when it is diagnosed. Clients take self-management decisions and actions in response to their environment and situation to improve their health status. Women need the skills, information, and community and financial resources for effective self-management.

The importance of prevention in high-risk clients is substantiated in the alarming increase in diabetes in women and in minority women. Although genetic susceptibility has a role in the development of type 2 diabetes, the current epidemic is associated primarily with particular lifestyle behaviors. Such behaviors include lack of regular exercise, consumption of diets high in saturated fat, dyslipidemia, obesity, and smoking. Moderate sustained weight loss and regular moderate to vigorous exercise can decrease the risk for developing type 2 diabetes.

The role of the nurse and other health care providers is to prevent the disease, promote early detection, and encourage preventive services to reduce short and long-term complications. These interventions can improve client outcomes and ultimately reduce health care costs. To accomplish these objectives, providers must adopt a multifaceted management approach that consists of education, promotion of self-management, well-established communication between the providers and client, and regular feedback on the client's outcomes.

Evidence is mounting that early preventive interventions can reduce the morbidity, mortality, and economic burden of diabetes (Buse, 1999; Diabetes Control and Complications Trial Research Group, 1993). Many preventive interventions can achieve this balance. Table 2.3 provides a quick reference of specific interventions for the prevention of selected long-term complications of diabetes.

● **TABLE 2.3 Recommendations to Prevent Complications of Diabetes**

POTENTIAL COMPLICATIONS	RECOMMENDATIONS
Cardiovascular disease	Blood pressure every visit
A. Maintain BP ≤ 130/80.	Orthostatic BP every visit
B. LDL cholesterol < 100 mg/dL	Early lifestyle interventions
C. HDL cholesterol > 40 mg/dL (men); > 50 mg/dL (women)	Serum lipids yearly
D. Triglycerides < 150 mg/dL	Smoking cessation counseling
E. Smoking cessation	
F. Plasma glucose:	
HgA1c < 7%	HgA1c every 3 months
Preprandial plasma glucose 90–130 mg/dL Peak prandial glucose < 180 mg/dL	SMBG several times daily before meals, peak prandial, and bedtime. The American Diabetes Association recommends more than 3 times per day for patients with type 1 diabetes or pregnant women taking insulin. Greater frequency of SMBG is needed when adding to or changing therapy.
Renal disease	BP every visit Maintain BP at < 130/80 mmHg Yearly testing for microalbuminuria
Retinopathy	Annual dilated eye exam by ophthalmologist Glasses for sun protection Optimal glycemic control Optimal BP control
Foot ulcers with high potential for amputations	Yearly comprehensive foot exam by a podiatrist Visual foot inspection every visit Daily skin care Appropriate footwear
Influenza, pneumococcal disease	Yearly flu vaccine Limit exposures during high incidence times Pneumococcal vaccine at age 65 years or older. Revaccinate if a dose was given ≥ 5 years before 65 years of age.

BP, blood pressure; HDL, high-density lipoprotein; LDL, low-density lipoprotein; SMBG, self-monitoring of blood glucose.

Menstrual Health

The discipline of women's health views the care of young girls to aging women comprehensively. The menstrual cycle can serve as a developmental parameter for specific health promotion needs focused on specific age cohorts. For example, school-age girls and adolescents need information to prepare them for their bodily changes. This developmental phase highlights decision making regarding initiation of sexual activities, birth control, and peer pressure regarding sex, alcohol, and drugs. Aging women need health education on the transition of perimenopause and education on prevention of specific health risks such as osteoporosis, heart disease, and diabetes. The following section discusses phases of the menstrual cycles and health promotion needs for women in various cohorts.

Menarche

On average, girls begin menstruating at approximately 12 years, with a normal age of onset ranging from 8 to 18 years (Youngkin & Davis, 2004). **Menarche,** initiation of menses, begins when the brain, ovaries, and adrenal glands are mature and when the percentage of body fat is adequate. Initial menstrual cycles usually are irregular and unpredictable because hormonal communications may be erratic. Pregnancy can occur at any time, even before a girl's first menstrual period, if she has ovulatory cycles.

The nurse's health promotion focus for girls is to provide health education on how the body functions, changes to expect (including breast enlargement and secondary sexual characteristics), and what happens with initiation of menses. It is also important that young girls understand the relationship between ovulation and their beginning fertility (see Chap. 6). Health education details on sexual intercourse and how pregnancy occurs are essential to promote positive sexuality and safer sexual practices and to prevent unplanned adolescent pregnancies and sexually transmitted infections (STIs).

Folic acid is essential to normal cell development and the formation of major fetal structures. Many women do not consume adequate folate in their diets before they know they are pregnant. This is the time when the need for folate is most critical. For that reason, the March of Dimes, following recommendations from the U.S. Public Health Service, posits that all adolescents and women who can become pregnant should consume a multivitamin containing 400 μg of folic acid daily, in addition to eating foods that contain folate (March of Dimes, 2006). Good sources of folate include leafy dark-green vegetables, legumes, citrus fruits and juices, peanuts, whole grains, and some fortified breakfast cereals. Since January 1998, grain products have been fortified with 140 μg per gram of folic acid. The Daily Value is 400 μg; pregnant women need more (600 to 800 μg/day).

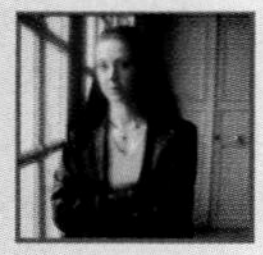

Consider Jill, the young woman who is to have her first pelvic examination. Because this is her first experience, what information would be critical for the nurse to assess?

Perimenopause and Menopause

QUOTE 2-2

"Women may be the one group that grows more radical with age."

Gloria Steinem

Perimenopause refers to the period during which ovarian function regresses, which can last as long as 7 to 10 years. This time begins with the last menstrual cycle leading to menopause and extends to 1 year after the last menses. Thereafter, the woman is considered postmenopausal. Menstrual periods stop because the ovaries no longer produce progesterone and estrogen.

The simplest definition of menopause is the end of menstruation. Although menopause literally means cessation of menses, it is actually a process rather than a discrete, single event. Referring only to the cessation of menses is a narrow definition, and menopause is now being defined as a transition of biologic and cultural events over months to years, and not purely the single event of absence of menses (see Chap. 23).

The major source of estrogen before menopause is the ovarian follicle, which accounts for more than 90% of the body's total production. Estrogen deficiency that accompanies menopause can result in symptoms such as hot flashes, vaginal dryness, emotional changes, and weight gain. Some women experience no symptoms at all. Menopause is a gradual process and does not occur suddenly unless it is surgically or medically induced (eg, chemotherapy, radiation) (Research Highlight 2.2).

To work most effectively, sensitively, and practically with midlife women, nurses should recognize that menopause takes months to years: it is not merely the absence of menses. Although "perimenopause" is correct usage of a term to define the entire change-of-life process, women themselves do not always use this term. Therefore, to avoid further confusion when counseling women, it is often best to explain the change of life as a process. Nurses should teach women about the entire process, in addition to the cessation of menses, and counsel women regarding the maintenance of contraceptives. Women and their partners need advice about contraception because ovulation may be sporadic during perimenopause. Many physicians and nurse practitioners advise women 50 years or older to continue contraception for 1 year after the last period.

In Western culture, with its strong emphasis on female youth and beauty, menopause may be a difficult adjustment for some women. Some women find symptoms

● RESEARCH HIGHLIGHT 2.2 Risks and Benefits of Estrogen Plus Progestin in Healthy Postmenopausal Women: Principal Results from the Women's Health Initiative Randomized Controlled Trial

Writing Group for the Women's Health Initiative Investigators. (2002). *Journal of the American Medical Association, 288*(3).

BACKGROUND: For decades, hormone replacement therapy (HRT) had been used routinely for perimenopausal and menopausal women. In addition to alleviating bothersome symptoms of menopause such as hot flashes and vaginal dryness, HRT also had been advised as a primary prevention measure for more serious conditions affecting postmenopausal women such as cardiovascular disease, osteoporosis, and even Alzheimer's disease. Despite widespread use of HRT, however, the risk-to-benefit ratio had remained uncertain.

PURPOSE: The purpose of the Women's Health Initiative study was to assess the risk-to-benefit ratio of HRT.

DESIGN: The study was designed as a randomized controlled primary prevention trial to last 8.5 years. Eligible women were recruited from 40 participating U.S. clinical centers over a 5-year period. Eligibility was defined as age 50 to 79 years, postmenopausal, intact uterus, probability of remaining in the area for at least 3 years, and written informed consent. An equal number of women were selected randomly to receive HRT versus placebo, respectively. HRT initially was started as equine estrogen, 0.625 mg/d, plus medroxyprogesterone acetate, 5.2 mg/d, given as a single pill, with dose adjustments permitted to allow for the treatment of side effects such as breast tenderness and vaginal bleeding. Data from each client were collected concerning incidences of breast cancer, hip fractures related to osteopenia or osteoporosis, and coronary artery disease, including myocardial infarction, stroke, and thrombosis.

RESULTS: In 2002, 3 years before the scheduled end of the trial, the data and safety monitoring board recommended terminating the trial because of the risks for breast cancer exceeding the original boundary set to stop the study. In addition, the board also determined that overall risks of HRT exceeded its benefits. Although hip fractures decreased among those women on HRT, incidences of breast cancer, stroke, cardiovascular disease, and pulmonary embolus increased significantly.

At this time, the board's recommendation is not to initiate or continue HRT in the primary prevention of cardiovascular disease. In addition, providers must weight the substantial risks for breast cancer and cardiovascular disease against the benefit of decreased hip fractures when choosing pharmacotherapy for clients with osteoporosis. When prescribing HRT to treat menopausal symptoms, providers should use the lowest dose feasible along with annual reassessment. When used for menopause, optimal duration of HRT is less than 5 years.

Based on the results of the Women's Health Initiative and further studies, the current recommendation is not to initiate or continue HRT in the primary prevention of cardiovascular disease. In addition, providers must weigh the substantial risks for breast cancer and cardiovascular disease against the benefit of management of vasomotor symptoms. Currently, the management of hot flashes and other menopausal symptoms is the only recommended first-line therapy for HRT. Choosing other pharmacotherapy options for clients with osteoporosis is suggested. When prescribing HRT to treat menopausal symptoms, providers should use the lowest dose feasible along with annual reassessment. When used for menopause, optimal duration of HRT is less than 5 years.

bothersome or emotions unexpected. Nurses can assist women in dealing with this transition. Generally, however, the perimenopausal years now often are looked upon as "time left to live," and women are finding meaning in their lives in a wide variety of roles (George, 2002). Historically, the negative stereotypes surrounding "change of life" probably began when a woman's life expectancy was short. Generations ago, many women didn't live past menopause. Women who did live long enough to reach menopause were so few that they were considered old if they survived to 50 years! Naturally, menopause came to be associated with all the undesirable attributes of extreme old age. Also, when female life expectancy was low, women were valued primarily for their reproductive capacity.

As nurses, conveying positive attitudes toward sexuality, sexual expression, intercourse, and the maturing adult is important. With an average life expectancy of 78 years, many women will live one third of their lives after menopause. Along with changes in women's rights and roles in society, many women and health care providers want to replace negative stereotypes of menopause with a realistic and positive outlook. This new viewpoint is easier to achieve as women learn more about how to live through the changes of middle age with good health and peace of mind. Her own understanding and expectations of menopause, marital or relationship stability, financial resources, family views, physical health, and sociocultural expectations influence a woman's adjustment to menopause.

Cessation of menses frees women from periods, fear of pregnancy, and contraceptive concerns. Many women see menopause as a time of fewer child care responsibilities and increased opportunities to pursue

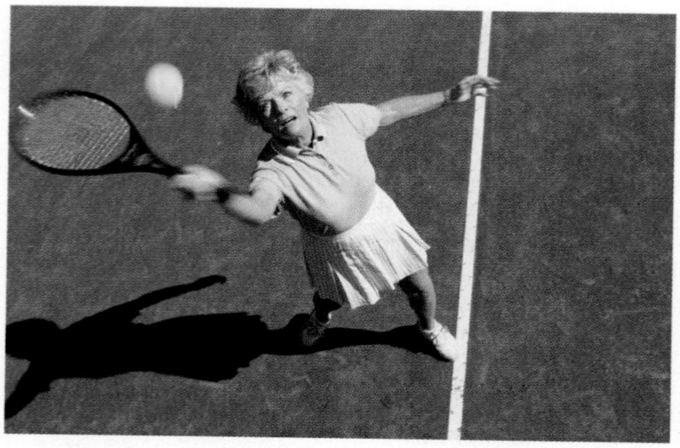

FIGURE 2.7 Many women today are using the time after menopause to pursue hobbies and activities they may not have had time to enjoy in younger years. They also are maintaining health and wellness through exercise and physical activity.

other goals (Fig. 2.7). This combination often is energizing for women seeking added dimensions to their careers or relationships. The transition to menopause often provides more leisure time as well as increased opportunities for self-expression and community involvement. Despite a strong cultural message that youth is better than age, women who maintain a positive image and value themselves adapt well to menopause.

The perimenopausal years can be eased for women if they have information about normal anticipated changes. Menopause can be used as a time to make some important health or lifestyle changes. Preventive health behaviors are suggested for aging women to decrease the incidence of chronic or fatal illnesses such as osteoporosis, heart disease, and diabetes (Research Highlight 2.3). For further details, refer to Nursing Care Plan 2.2 and Chapter 23.

Sexual and Reproductive Health

Increasingly, experts are recognizing environmental factors and lifestyle patterns as crucial variables affecting individual, family, and public health. This is especially true in the areas of sexual and reproductive health. Lifestyle-related diseases are influenced not only by diet, smoking, alcohol consumption, and exercise, but also by emotional relationships and sexuality. Nurses should never underestimate the importance of sexual health and conducting a sexual history in girls and women of all ages. Nursing care involves developing competency in conducting a thorough and sensitive health history and assessment of sexual and reproductive health (see Chap. 6).

Participation by women in screening programs for STIs, in addition to breast and cervical cancer, is far from optimal. Because these conditions sometimes are not detected until they have reached advanced stages, many lives are lost or adversely affected when such consequences could have been prevented. Therefore, nurses should increase health education and improve availability of screening programs for optimum sexual and reproductive health. It is particularly important that nurses put effort into reaching women in the lower socioeconomic or minority groups who have a disproportionate burden of breast and cervical cancer. Nurses must provide support, information, and a caring attitude as women make difficult and emotional health care decisions.

Sexual History and Risk Factors

Through a sexual health history, the nurse and client are better equipped to mutually identify risk factors and discuss sexual behaviors that may be placing the client at risk for STIs or pregnancy. This health history should be conducted at the annual examination with a nurse practitioner, nurse-midwife, or physician, and when the woman presents with a sexual health or contraceptive concern. Health history questions include the following objective data:

Are you sexually active? At what age did you begin intercourse? With men? With women? With both?
How many partners have you had in the last year?
What type of contraceptive do you use? Are you satisfied with this contraceptive?
Do you use condoms? Do you use them with every sexual encounter?
When was your last Pap smear? Have you ever had an abnormal Pap? If so, when and what treatment was performed?
How many times have you been pregnant? Have you had any term births, preterm births, elective abortions, or miscarriages? If you have had a miscarriage, what was the gestational age? Was the cause known? Were births vaginal or cesarean? Were births normal or were there complications?
Do you have living children? If so, what are their ages?
Are you satisfied with your sexual relationship?

Sexual and reproductive health is not always a comfortable topic for discussion. Consequently, women, their families, and health care professionals sometimes minimize or hide the full effects of sexual health. An appreciation and understanding of the magnitude of adjustments for the woman and for the people who care about them is essential.

Concerns about gynecologic problems, sexuality, and childbearing are common. With the diagnosis of any gynecologic condition (eg, STIs) or breast or cervical cancer, guilt, embarrassment, shame, and body image disturbances are common feelings. Women also may feel their personal privacy is being invaded. They may feel defensive and angry with the health care team having to treat such an innermost private part of them. Some women associate problems in the genital area with forms

● RESEARCH HIGHLIGHT 2.3 An Evaluation of Choose to Move 1999: An American Heart Association Physical Activity Program for Women

Koffman, D. M., Bazzarre, T., Mosca, L., Redberg, R., Schmid, T., & Wattigney, W. A. (2001). *Archives of Internal Medicine, 161,* 2193–2199.

BACKGROUND: The leading cause of death in U.S. women is heart disease. Sedentary lifestyle, obesity, and dietary intake of foods containing high amounts of saturated fat are major risk factors. A national study based on self-report found that 31% of U.S. women had no leisure physical activity in the previous month (Centers for Disease Control and Prevention, 1999). Another study revealed that only 25% of U.S. women 20 years or older are meeting the Healthy People 2010 recommendation to limit dietary fat intake to 30% of daily calories or less (U.S. Department of Health and Human Services, 2000).

PURPOSE: To address the epidemic of physical inactivity, obesity, and poor dietary practices among U.S. women, in 1999 the American Heart Association (AHA) launched *Choose to Move,* a free, 12-week, self-help lifestyle intervention program. The purpose was to increase the proportion of women who met AHA's recommendations for physical activity and consumption of low-fat foods. The study was to determine the effects of *Choose to Move* on women's physical activity, diet, and knowledge about heart disease and stroke.

DESIGN: The study was a descriptive, prospective design using a nonrandomized sample without a control group. The program targeted women 25 years or older recruited through local AHA offices, physicians, nurse practitioners, physical therapists, occupation therapists, exercise instructors, and other community sources. Women registered for the program by calling a toll-free number or e-mailing the AHA's Web site (http://www.women.americanheart.org) to request a registration packet. The theoretical approaches of the program were the Transtheoretical Stages of Change Model (Prochaska & DiClemente, 1983; Prochaska et al., 1994) and social marketing theory, which states that health promotion programs should reach a specific audience, satisfy consumer needs, and meet organization objectives (Kotler & Andreasen, 1987; Lefebvre & Flora, 1988).

RESULTS: More than 50% of the initial 23,171 registered participants (called the *registration cohort*) were between 35 and 54 years. Almost 50% had two or three risk factors for heart disease or stroke. Ninety percent were white, whereas 5.7% were African American, 2.1% Hispanic, 1.0% Asian, and 0.3% Native American. Educational level was not reported. The program consisted of 12 weekly behavioral modification topics designed to teach women how to incorporate daily physical activity into their lives and address eating behaviors. These materials were mailed to preregistered participants, along with encouraging newsletters, postcards, and e-mails.

The program was evaluated through biweekly self-reported questionnaires sent by mail to participants. The questionnaires asked about the participant's physical activity, diet, and knowledge of heart disease, stroke, and related symptoms. Continuing follow-up evaluations were returned from 6389 women at 2 weeks, 5338 women at 4 weeks, 4209 women at 8 weeks, 3916 at 10 weeks, and 3775 (called the *evaluation cohort*) at 12 weeks.

The registration cohort differed significantly from the evaluation cohort. Thirty-two percent of participants who completed the baseline evaluations reported moderate exercise at least 5 times per week, whereas 67% of participants who completed the 12-week evaluation reported moderate exercise at least 5 times per week. The evaluation cohort was more knowledgeable about heart disease and its effects on women. Women who completed the program reported using more strategies to improve nutrition than the registration cohort. The evaluation cohort reported more physical activity, and had more confidence about improving their physical activity.

The main finding of the study is that *Choose to Move,* a mail-mediated lifestyle intervention program, significantly improved self-reported physical activity levels, heart healthy food choices, and increased knowledge about heart disease among a cohort of women. Results show that a social marketing approach promoting a targeted, self-help lifestyle intervention program designed to reduce risk for heart disease and stroke can reach a large number of women and help them to change behaviors positively within 12 weeks.

of punishment for real or imagined sexual expression. Health care providers can diminish shame and guilt associated with the diagnosis if they communicate an accepting and nonjudgmental approach.

Assessment of a woman's self-image is necessary. Providers should discuss with the client the potential for some conditions to interfere with sexual function. Feelings of guilt, anger, and shame may prevent women from asking questions or initiating a discussion on the subject of sexual activity. Nursing Care Plan 2.3 addresses these issues in more detail.

Papanicolaou Test (Pap Smear)

Regular pelvic examinations and Pap smears are the best way to assess and to detect various conditions in the reproductive system early (Nursing Procedure 2.1). The Papanicolaou (Pap) test, or smear, is a safe and inexpensive tool for the early detection of cervical cancer. Developed

NURSING CARE PLAN 2.2

A Client Experiencing Perimenopause

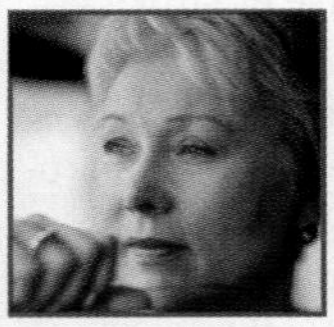

Recall Linda, the 53-year-old perimenopausal accountant. Further questioning reveals that Linda became aware only recently of how much time had passed since her last menstrual cycle. "I didn't realize it. Am I starting menopause? Work has been so crazy over the last several years. Where has the time gone?" Her last visit to her primary care physician was almost 5 years ago; she has gained 20 pounds since then. When questioned about exercise, she states, "I hate it. Who has time for it? I can't even think about it. I realize that exercise might help me manage my stress better, but I'm so drained when I get home."

NURSING DIAGNOSIS

Deficient Knowledge related to normal body changes associated with perimenopause and menopause and healthy lifestyle

EXPECTED OUTCOMES

1. The client will describe perimenopause and menopause and the associated normal body changes.

INTERVENTIONS	RATIONALES
Assess the client's knowledge about her body and typical changes in perimenopause and menopause.	Assessment of knowledge provides a baseline from which to develop appropriate teaching strategies.
Define perimenopause and menopause. Review the typical accompanying body changes and correlate them with what the client is experiencing.	Accurate descriptions are essential to understanding the changes. Correlating the client's signs and symptoms promotes her understanding of these events.
Assess the client's interpretation of the relationship between her womanhood and perimenopause/menopause.	Some women view menopause as a loss of female youth and beauty; others view it as a time of increased opportunities.
Emphasize that the client can use this time to make important health and lifestyle changes.	Such changes can reduce the incidence of heart disease and osteoporosis, which can be chronic or fatal.

EVALUATION

1. The client identifies typical normal body changes associated with perimenopause and menopause.

NURSING DIAGNOSIS

Ineffective Health Maintenance related to demands of work, sedentary lifestyle, and weight gain

EXPECTED OUTCOMES

1. The client will identify appropriate strategies to deal with body changes.
2. The client will verbalize measures that contribute to a healthy lifestyle.
3. The client will identify the required screening and examinations needed to promote health.

Continued

NURSING CARE PLAN 2.2 ● A Client Experiencing Perimenopause

INTERVENTIONS	RATIONALES
Review the client's daily routine, including diet, activity level, and rest.	Knowledge of the routine aids in developing an individualized program to fit the client's lifestyle, thereby enhancing the chances for success.
Encourage exercise. Suggest aerobic, weight-bearing exercise 3 to 4 times a week for at least 20 minutes.	Aerobic weight-bearing exercise helps slow down bone loss, keep weight down, and improve sense of well-being.
Recommend the American Heart Association balanced diet, which consists of 66% complex carbohydrate, 20% fat, and 15% protein. Also encourage adequate vitamin D (400–800 IU/day) and calcium (1200–1500 mg/day) intake. Provide the client with a list of foods that would promote adequate intake.	A diet low in saturated fats and cholesterol reduces the client's risk for heart disease. Adequate vitamin D (400–800 IU/day) and calcium (1200–1500 mg/day) help prevent osteoporosis. Maintaining ideal body weight with BMI less than 25 decreases incidence of type 2 diabetes.
Instruct the client about the need for appropriate screenings: annual Pap smear, mammogram, cholesterol testing, clinical breast examination, fecal occult blood and digital rectal examination, and blood pressure checks; biannual or annual dental care; annual fasting blood glucose screening (if at risk for diabetes).	Routine screenings are necessary for early detection and treatment of health problems.
Assist the client to determine her priorities. Work with her to develop a written plan for exercise, diet, and health screenings. Provide positive reinforcement for changes.	Midlife adjustment can be a time to reflect on future goals and development of new roles. Positive reinforcement promotes adherence to the plan.

EVALUATION

1. The client demonstrates appropriate self-management strategies to promote health during perimenopause and menopause.
2. The client collaborates with the health care provider to devise a healthy lifestyle plan, demonstrating healthy behaviors.
3. The client participates in setting up a schedule for appropriate screenings and examinations.

by the Greek physician Dr. George Papanicolaou in the 1940s, the Pap smear became a regular component of gynecologic examinations during the 1950s. Since then, the incidence of invasive cervical cancer and the death rate from cervical cancer have declined, but the number of women with cervical intraepithelial neoplasia (CIN) has increased alarmingly (Allen & Phillips, 1997). When diagnosed early, the cure rate is almost 100%.

The Pap smear involves scraping the endocervix with a swab, brush, or spatula to obtain a sample of cells. Computerized analysis of the Pap smears, such as "Papnet," is now available at an additional laboratory cost of approximately $20. This technique holds promise of decreasing false-positive or false-negative Pap reports. Most women barely feel the "scraping" of the cervix during the Pap smear. Barriers to gynecologic checkups and Pap smears include fear, denial, lack of information, cultural beliefs, social status, embarrassment, absence of symptoms experienced, lack of access to health care, and cost.

NURSING CARE PLAN 2.3

A Client With Sexual and Reproductive Concerns

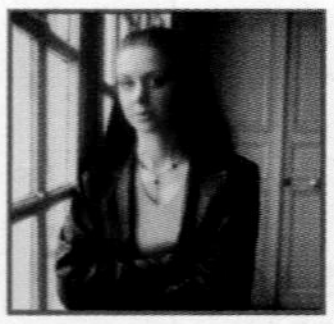

Jill is about to undergo her first vaginal examination and Pap smear. She is nervous and scared. The nurse asks Jill to identify specifically what is frightening her most. Jill sighs and says, "I've just put off doing this for so long. I'm worried that I have a tumor or an infection. What will I do if something is wrong?"

NURSING DIAGNOSES

Anxiety related to fear and lack of information about reproductive and sexual health

Deficient Knowledge related to vaginal examination, Pap smear, and preventive measures for reproductive health

EXPECTED OUTCOMES

1. The client will verbalize fears and concerns openly.
2. The client will identify positive methods to cope with fears.
3. The client will identify what will happen during the examination, including possible findings.

INTERVENTIONS	RATIONALES
Use a nonjudgmental approach and establish rapport with the client. Maintain this approach throughout the visit and care of the client.	Establishing a nonjudgmental and caring relationship with the woman will enhance the therapeutic relationship, foster honesty, and communicate respect.
Provide as much privacy and comfort as possible. Explore the woman's feelings of privacy and how you can meet her needs within the scope of the examination.	Privacy communicates respect of the client's personal boundaries and comfort zone.
Perform a complete nursing assessment of the woman's sexual and reproductive history.	The data provide a baseline from which to develop a plan of care; they also give clues to potential problems.
Encourage the client to discuss the "causes" of any real or perceived problems. Communicate accurate facts; answer questions honestly. Reinforce facts. Provide brochures. Encourage the client not to blame herself if problems are found.	Information about possible causes provides clues to the client's anxiety. Facts help dispel unfounded fears, myths, misconceptions, and guilt.
Review the steps of the vaginal examination and Pap smear. Show the client the various pieces of equipment that may be used (eg, the speculum).	Providing the client with information about the procedure aids in alleviating fear of the unknown.
Instruct the client to take slow deep breaths during the examination.	Slow deep breaths aid in relaxing the client, which facilitates the examination.
Warm the speculum before insertion; drape the client appropriately.	Warming the speculum and proper draping provide comfort and privacy for the client.

Continued

NURSING CARE PLAN 2.3 ● A Client With Sexual and Reproductive Concerns

INTERVENTIONS	RATIONALES
Perform the vaginal examination and Pap smear, explaining each step before doing it (see Nursing Procedure 2.1).	Explaining what is to happen helps prepare the client for what to expect and aids in alleviating anxiety.
After the examination, openly and sensitively discuss any issues of fertility, sexual expression, body image, and safer sexual practices.	Open discussion alleviates anxiety and provides facts to promote health.
Encourage the woman to follow-up with future examinations, Pap smears, and contraceptive planning as necessary. Reinforce the use of safer sexual practices.	Follow-up is important to promote positive health-seeking behaviors, empowering the client to protect her safety and health.
Provide the client with information about support services in the community. Encourage their use as appropriate.	Community services provide additional means of support in dealing with reproductive and sexual health concerns.

EVALUATION

1. The client states that her anxiety about the vaginal examination is decreased.
2. The client uses positive methods to cope with the procedures.
3. The client demonstrates knowledge of the examination and possible findings, verbalizing information and questions related to reproductive health.

Screening Schedule and Guidelines. Recommendations regarding how frequently women should have Pap smears vary. Previously, national health organizations such as the American Cancer Society (ACS), National Cancer Institute (NCI), and American Medical Association had adopted a consensus recommendation. In late 2002, the ACS released new guidelines (Box 2.2). These guidelines all address the *Pap test only.* It is critical for nurses to emphasize to clients that women need health care appointments to discuss sexual questions, risk factors related to sexual behavior, STIs, contraception, blood pressure, weight control, clinical breast examination, and any other issues that concern the woman.

Classification of Pap Tests. In many women, cervical cells go through a series of changes. Cervical intraepithelial neoplasia (CIN) is the term used to encompass all epithelial abnormalities. An older classification system had described two separate entities (dysplasia and carcinoma in situ); this classification also influenced different treatment techniques. The newer classification system, the Bethesda System, is preferred because it indicates more of a single neoplasia continuum, and it is more descriptive of actual cellular changes (see Chap. 4). The newer classification, although still having subgroups, indicates more of a continuum of preinvasive cervical cancer.

What do these changes in classification mean from the client's perspective? Nurses should inform women that the changes were implemented to improve identification and treatment of changes in cervical cells before they become invasive cancer. Also, researchers are beginning to understand the pattern of changes that cervical cells undergo as a continuum over months to years. The woman needs to know that if the Pap test shows any abnormality, the physician or nurse practitioner will do more tests to discover the problem. When a vaginal infection is the suspected cause of an abnormal result, the practitioner will treat the infection and then repeat the test, usually in 3 months. If an infection is not the reason, the practitioner often will perform a colposcopy and biopsy.

Risk Factors for Cervical Cancer. Most risk factors for cervical cancer are ultimately related to sexual behavior and can be identified through a sexual history. Although the exact etiology is unknown, the general cause is thought to be cellular changes in the cervix that result from "insult" caused by viruses and multiple partners. Women with

(text continues on page 62)

NURSING PROCEDURE 2.1

Performing a Pelvic Examination and Pap Smear

PURPOSE

To evaluate the condition of the internal female reproductive structures and to obtain specimens for cytologic screening

ASSESSMENT AND PLANNING

- Assess client's knowledge of and previous exposure to the procedure.
- Determine the date of the client's last menstrual period. (Ideally, the Pap smear should be taken approximately 2 weeks after the first day of the last menstrual period to enhance obtaining the best specimen possible.)
- Ask the client if she has abstained from sexual intercourse and douching for the past 48 hours.
- Question the client about the use of tampons; contraceptive foams, jellies, or creams; or vaginal medications within the last 72 hours.
- Check for evidence of current vaginal bleeding, which would require rescheduling the Pap smear. (Blood cells interfere with examination of the sample).
- Gather the necessary equipment.
  - Examination gloves
  - Speculum
  - Sheet or bath blanket for draping
  - Specimen collection devices such as Cytobrush and plastic spatula
  - Properly labeled specimen container (liquid based preservative) or slide and spray fixative
  - Completed laboratory request form
  - Adequate light source
  - Water-soluble lubricant (only if not performing Pap smear)

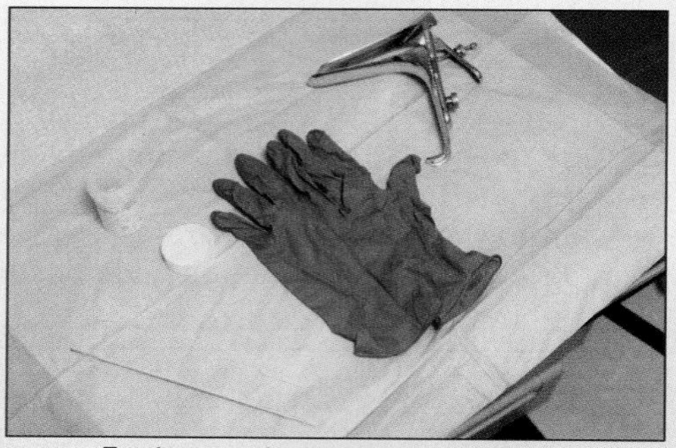

Equipment for pelvic examination and Pap smear.

IMPLEMENTATION

1. Explain the procedure to the client and answer any questions *to help allay her anxiety.*
2. Have the client empty her bladder *to minimize discomfort during the procedure.*
3. Wash hands thoroughly.
4. Have client position herself on the examination table with her feet in stirrups or foot pedals (or flat on the examination table) so that her legs fall outward. Ask the client to move herself down on the table so that her buttocks are just past the bottom edge of the table. *This positioning ensures adequate access to the perineum.*

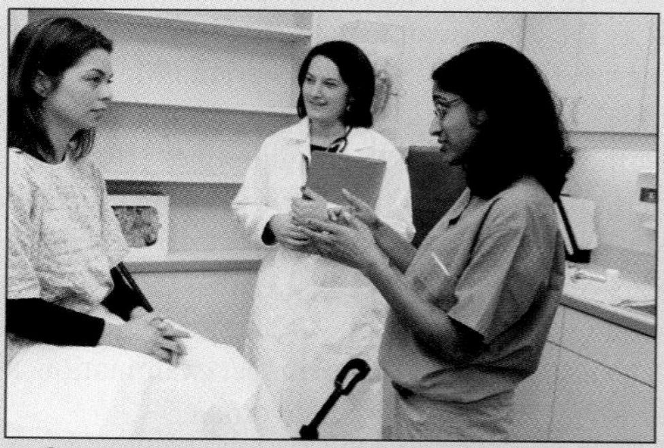

Step 1: Explain the procedure to the client.

5. Place sheet or bath blanket over the client, keeping the area over the perineum exposed *to ensure privacy and allow access to the perineum.* Adjust the light source as necessary.
6. Put on gloves.
7. Warm the speculum with warm water *to avoid chilling the client.*
8. Tell the client that you are about to touch her *to prevent startling her.*
9. Using a gloved hand, spread the labia, inspecting and palpating the area to check for abnormalities; throughout encourage the woman to take deep breaths *to aid in relaxation.*

Continued

NURSING PROCEDURE 2.1

Performing a Pelvic Examination and Pap Smear

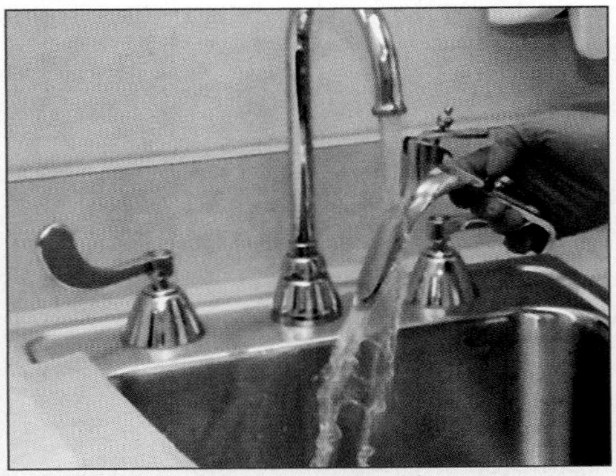

Step 7: Warm the speculum with warm water.

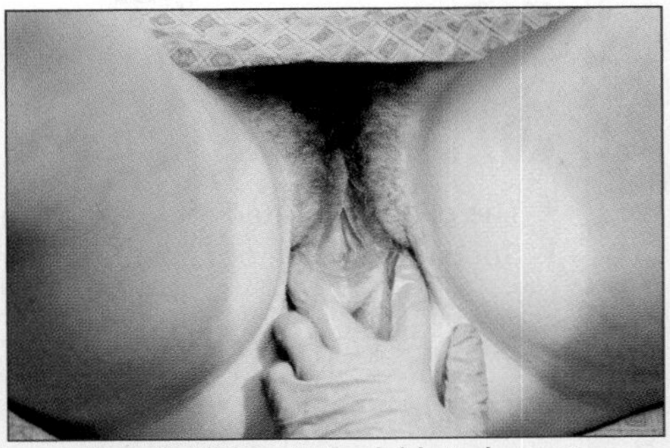

Step 9: Separate the labia to inspect and palpate the vaginal area.

10. Insert the warmed speculum into the vagina and slowly open the blades *to allow clear visualization of the cervix;* once in place, lock the blades.
11. Obtain samples for Pap smear; use the Cytobrush or sterile cotton tipped applicator and swab the endocervix, using one full circular motion.
12. Use the plastic curved spatula to gently and firmly scrape the cervix os.
13. Swab the posterior fornix or vaginal pool using the opposite end of the cervical spatula or a sterile cotton-tipped applicator.
14. Immediately after collecting each specimen, place the specimen in the appropriately labeled container or the slide and spray with a fixative.
15. Unlock the blades of the speculum and remove it gently *to reduce the risk for trauma to the client.*
16. Remove the glove from the nondominant hand and place on lower abdomen; insert a lubricated gloved finger of the dominant hand into the vagina *to perform the bimanual examination.*

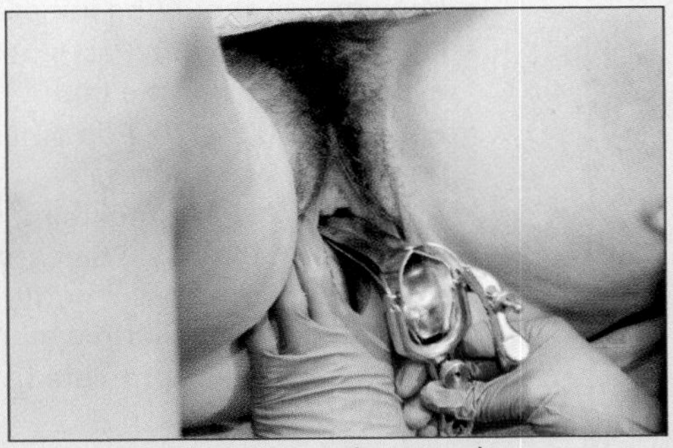

Step 10: Insert the speculum.

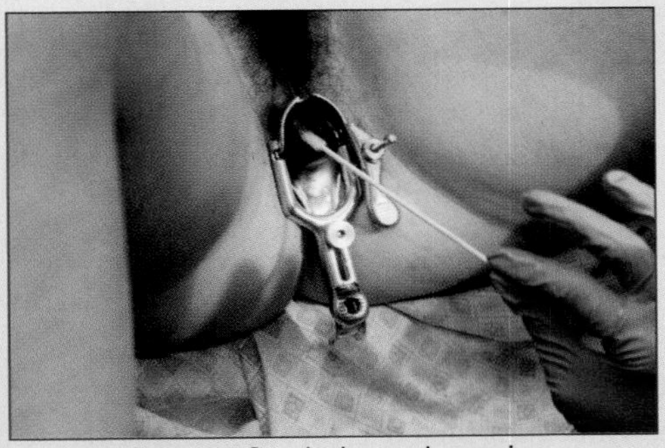

Step 11: Swab the endocervix.

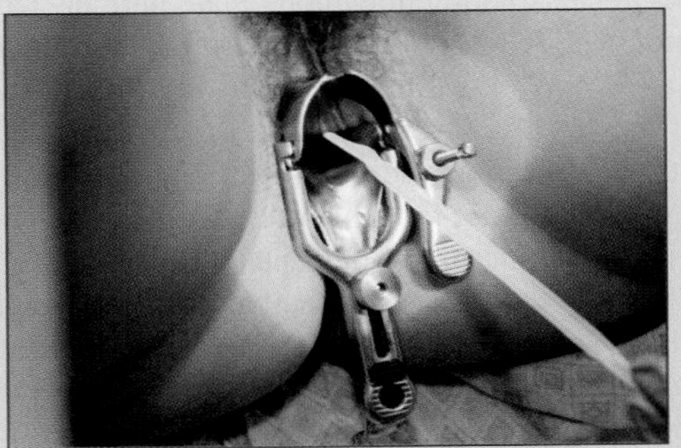

Step 12: Scrape the cervical os.

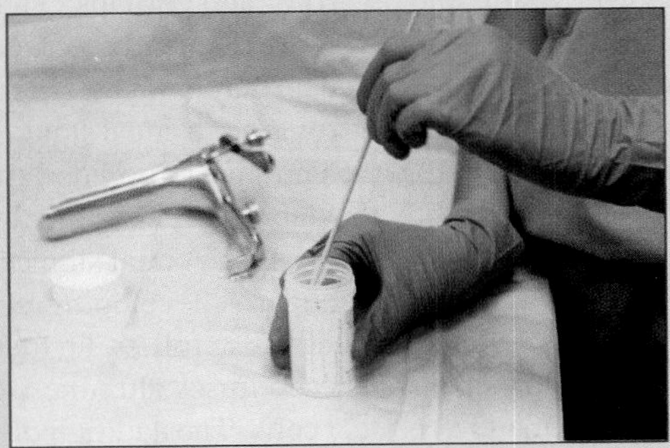

Step 14: Appropriately preserve the specimen.

Continued

NURSING PROCEDURE 2.1 CONTINUED

Performing a Pelvic Examination and Pap Smear

17. On completion, remove the glove from the dominant hand and discard appropriately.
18. Assist the client to sitting position and allow her to get dressed.

EVALUATION

- The client tolerated the procedure without difficulty.
- Specimens were obtained and sent to the laboratory.

AREAS FOR CONSIDERATION AND ADAPTATION

Lifespan Considerations

- If this is the client's first experience with pelvic examination, ensure that an additional person is available to support the client and reinforce any explanations or instructions.
- Keep in mind that Pap smear recommendations vary with age groups:
    - Pap smears should be initiated at age 21 or within 3 years of the first sexual intercourse.
    - Up to the age of 30, Pap smears should be done every year (for the slide method) or every 2 years (for the liquid-based method).
    - From ages 30 to 70, Pap smears are recommended every 2 to 3 years as long as the last three tests were normal.
    - After age 70, Pap smears may be discontinued if the last three tests were normal and tests within the past 10 years were all normal.
- Remember that some older adult women may experience atrophic vaginitis; be sure to lubricate the speculum well with water.
- If the client has had a complete hysterectomy, obtain the specimen for the Pap smear from the vaginal pool.

Community-Based Considerations

- Most pelvic examinations and Pap smears are done on an outpatient basis as part of the routine gynecologic examination. Private offices, clinics, and community-based health centers offer this service.
- Education about the risk factors and techniques to prevent cervical cancer is key to primary prevention programs.

cervical cancer often report a history of cervical infections. Infections linked to cervical carcinoma are caused by herpes simplex virus 2; human papillomavirus (HPV) types 16, 18, 45, and 58; HIV; and perhaps cytomegalovirus. HPV 16 is linked most frequently to squamous cancers and HPV 18 to adenocarcinomas. HPV DNA testing can be performed from the residual liquid of the ThinPrep solution from the Pap smear, provided arrangements are made with the laboratory. Women whose high-risk HPV infection persists in genital skin cells are at greatest risk for subsequently developing cervical cancer. These women require close follow-up treatment and repeat Pap smears. These viruses alter the DNA of nuclei of immature cervical cells. The addition of sperm from many different partners is also thought to promote the process that ends in dysplasia (Grund, 2005).

Risk factors for cervical cancer are multiple sexual partners, early age (before 18 years) of sexual intercourse, history of STIs, HPV, lack of access or use of health care, a nonmonogamous male partner, DES exposure, cigarette smoking, and lower socioeconomic status (Grund, 2005). Most predisposing factors relate to patterns of sexual activity, which could lead to barriers for early detection and treatment. Nurses need to discuss psychosexual factors and the implications for risk for cervical cancer nonjudgmentally. They must be sensitive to women to decrease any embarrassment. Communication should convey that nurses regard sexual health as a basic component of total health, and a normal physiologic function. Societal norms today differ from 40 years ago. Today, women often marry later. Divorce and remarriage are relatively frequent, and many women have more than one

BOX 2.2 Pap Smear Guidelines

American Cancer Society Guidelines

A panel of experts from the ACS issued new guidelines for Pap tests in late 2002.

- Pap tests should begin approximately 3 years after the woman begins having vaginal intercourse or at 21 years. (Previous guidelines recommended 18 years.)
- Regular Pap test should be done annually, but the newer liquid-based tests may be done every 2 years.
- At or after 30 years, women who have had three or more normal Pap results in a row for 3 years need screening only once every 2 or 3 years. More frequent screening may be recommended for women with certain risks (eg, HIV) that raise risk of cervical cancer.
- Women 70 years or older who have had three normal Pap tests and no abnormal findings for the last 10 years may stop Pap tests.
- Most women who have had a total hysterectomy with removal of the cervix do not need Pap tests. They still need these tests, however, if the hysterectomy was done as treatment for cervical cancer or precancerous conditions.
- The ACS emphasizes that cervical pre-cancers grow slowly, and having a test every 2 or 3 years will find pre-cancers that can be treated successfully. Most cases of cervical cancers are caused by HPV, and this condition warrants close follow-up and treatment. Currently, separate vaccines for cervical cancer and genital herpes are under clinical trials. Very promising initial results offer hope for immunizing young women against HPV in the future. In the first large trial, the HPV vaccine worked in 100% of the women, but it is unsure how long the vaccine will provide protection.

U.S. Preventive Services Task Force Guidelines

Circumstance	Schedule
First Pap smear	At age 18 or at age of first intercourse (if before the age of 18)
18 to 64 years	Yearly, or every 3 years after three consecutive yearly normal results
Age 65	Yearly, or every 3 years after two consecutive yearly normal results

Adapted from American Cancer Society. (2003). *ACS cancer detection guidelines.* Retrieved December 27, 2004, from http://www.cancer.org/docroot/PED/content/PED_2_3X_ACS_Cancer_Detection_Guidelines_36.asp and U.S. Preventive Services Task Force Guidelines. (2003). *Screening for cervical cancer.* Retrieved December 27, 2004, from http://www.ahcpr.gov/clinic/uspstf/uspscerv.htm.

sexual partner in their lifetime. Nurses should consider these changes as a social norm, and not a stigma associated with a risk factor for cervical cancer. They should educate themselves and their clients regarding both sexual health and risk factors for cervical cancer. The best approach is to encourage any sexually active woman to participate in regular gynecologic checkups and Pap smears, and to use safer sex practices such as limiting sexual partners and using latex condoms.

Perineal Hygiene and Infection Prevention

Organisms, transmission, and complications of perineal infections and STIs are known and in many cases preventable. Despite efforts, however, these problems continue. The rate of STIs has increased during the past few decades; they are one of the most common reasons for outpatient, community-based treatment of women (CDC, 2004). The spread of STIs dramatically demonstrates the need to address the social determinants of disease. Nurses need to be informed regarding the pathophysiology, transmission, and social dimensions of perineal infections and STIs, and provide education and anticipatory guidance to clients of all ages at each stage of the lifespan. Chapter 4 discusses STIs in more detail.

In addition, some infections during pregnancy may cause additional risk to the fetus or newborn, and require special care. In the near future, widespread administration of the HPV vaccine to both male and female adolescents before initiation of sexual activity offers the best hope for preventing cervical cancer. By immunizing adolescents against HPV, the epidemiologic profile of cervical cancer could dramatically change. At present, the AAP is promoting educational information to foster informed choices by parents and young adolescents. Health professionals also are addressing the ethical concerns of some groups over an immunization linked to sexual activity.

Nurses should provide women with a teaching plan for perineal hygiene. The goal is to prevent organisms such as *Escherichia coli* from spreading from the rectum to the vagina and urethra. Nurses should instruct women to wash their hands before and after genital contact and after using the restroom. It also is important to instruct women to wipe the perineum from front to back each time they void or defecate, as well as after sex and during menstruation. Women should also be instructed to avoid products that may disturb the normal vaginal flora, or cause irritation and allergic reaction of the genital area, such as routine douching or use of other vaginal "cleansers." In truth, the vagina is normally a clean organ and does not need special "cleanliness" attention.

Women prone to vaginitis should use only white, unscented toilet tissue and unscented pads or tampons (Cottrell, 2003). They should not use feminine hygiene or other sprays near the perineum. They should avoid deodorized tampons and pads; if using tampons, they must be sure that the string does not slip to the rectal area. If it does, the tampon should be changed immediately.

Women are often at risk for genital infections or vaginitis because of the warm, moist vaginal environment, which promotes microbial growth. Wearing cotton underpants with a cotton crotch, especially under panty hose, girdles, and Lycra shorts, can decrease this risk. Cotton pants are best during any exercise such as aerobics, jogging, or biking. Women should avoid nonabsorbent clothes as much as possible, especially when exercising. Showers are preferable to tub baths. Women prone to vaginitis and urine infections need to avoid bubble bath and other bath additives. If a lubricant is necessary during sexual intercourse, women can use a water-soluble lubricant such as K-Y jelly, Replens, or Astroglide (over-the-counter products). Vaseline is a less effective vaginal lubricant because it is not water-soluble and may not be compatible with some contraceptives. Allowing time for sexual stimulation (foreplay) before intercourse often is the only lubrication technique necessary. Vaginal dryness may occur, however, with perimenopausal changes.

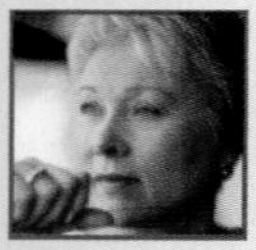

Recall Linda, the 53-year-old with hot flashes. During the interview, she mentions that she has noticed increased vaginal dryness, especially during sexual intercourse. How can she minimize this dryness?

Douches are rarely necessary. Douching washes out the normal balance of bacteria in the vagina, increasing the risk for bacterial vaginosis (Cottrell, 2003; Youngkin & Davis, 2004). Women do not need to douche, unless otherwise instructed by a health care provider (Cottrell, 2003; Youngkin & Davis, 2004). When a nurse practitioner or physician recommends a douche, distilled white vinegar (two tablespoons per quart of water) is more economical and efficacious than commercial products. Women should avoid perfumed or flavored douches. Vaginal deodorants, sprays, gels, or powders are not recommended for routine hygiene (Cottrell, 2003).

Changes in vaginal physiology or a rise in pH makes women more vulnerable to vaginal infections. The nurse should caution women that risk factors include pregnancy, use of high-estrogen oral contraceptives, antibiotic therapy, and uncontrolled diabetes. Women in these situations should follow the suggested techniques in addition to a protocol for care for that specific risk factor. If the woman is taking antibiotics, eating yogurt or sour cream may help to prevent vaginal infections. Some women need prophylactic antifungal therapy in conjunction with antibiotic therapy. If a woman has itching, irritations, burning, sores, or odor, she should be examined to determine the exact cause. There are many different types of vaginal infections, each with different treatments (see Chap. 4).

During any treatment for vaginal infections, the woman should refrain from sexual contact or use a condom. If the woman develops irritations easily, she should check with her partner because his soap or other personal products could be inadvertently promoting infection.

Breast Health

The outlook for breast cancer diagnosis, treatment, and survival remains promising. The most important research breakthrough, however, will be when researchers find the key to preventing breast cancer. This section focuses on risk factors, screening, and diagnostic testing for breast health. Detailed information on the breast cancer diagnosis, treatment, and nursing management is found in Chapter 4.

Risk Factors for Breast Cancer. The cause of breast cancer remains essentially unknown and continues to elude investigators. Although researchers have identified some clear risk factors, the significance of many is still controversial. The greatest risk factor for breast cancer is being a woman. Other strongly accepted risk factors are age and personal and family history of breast cancer. Most women with breast cancer do not have any known risk factors (DiSaia & Creasman, 2002).

In 1994, **breast cancer 1 and breast cancer 2 genes (*BRCA1* and *BRCA2*)** were discovered and found to correlate with increased risk for breast, ovarian, and other cancers. *BRCA1* is located on chromosome 17; *BRCA2* is located on chromosome 13. Mutations of *BRCA1* and *BRCA2* impair production of tumor-suppressor proteins. Although alterations in these genes may increase the risk for cancer, they certainly do not explain fully the history of breast or ovarian cancer in every family. *BRCA1* and *BRCA2* account for approximately 15% to 20% of all inherited cancers, and inherited cancers account for only 3% to 5% of cases of breast cancer (Barton, Harris, & Fletcher, 1999).

An understanding of breast health and breast cancer is important for all women. Breast cancer is the most common cancer in women. It is also one of the most treatable cancers if detected early. The risk to U.S. women of developing breast cancer in their lifetime is reported as one in eight. Risk increases with age, meaning that if a woman lives to be 85 years old, her risk is one in eight. Nodal involvement remains the single most prognostic criterion for long-term survival. The ACS (2003) reported the 5-year survival rate as 99% for no invasion, 90% for local invasion, and 68% for regional spread. Clearly, early detection underscores the importance of rigorous screening for all women.

More than half of all women who menstruate regularly go through, at one time or another, the frightening experience of finding a breast lump; less than 10% of these lumps are malignant or need treatment (ACS, 2003). Nevertheless, few conditions in women create as much concern as breast cancer. Understanding breast health, screening protocols, and options for treatment are important dimensions of women's health. Although breast cancer remains a concern for many women, early detection and treatment remain the best hopes for improving both quality of life and survival. Nurses have a vitally important role as educators and advocates in shaping the woman's and family's experiences during all aspects of breast health and breast cancer. Women with breast cancer that is detected early are living full and productive lives.

Individualized Screening Information. Screening information is based on standards from the ACS and the NCI. Table 2.4 provides a general guideline for a screening schedule. Each woman must make informed choices with her health care provider regarding her individual and family risk factors and personal screening schedule choices. Nurses must communicate to women and their families that these recommendations are just that: recommendations based on the generalized population of women. Individual risk factors and informed choice should still guide each woman.

Breast Self-Examination. **Breast self-examination** (BSE) is a method for women to check their own breasts by methodically palpating the breast tissue for changes and lumps. BSE also includes observation in a mirror for any changes in the appearance of the breast. The ACS (2003) recommends that women older than 20 years begin BSE; other sources suggest starting earlier if women seek care for family planning. Generally speaking, all women 20 years or older should establish a pattern of monthly BSE. Early detection of potential malignancies continues to be the single most important factor in the successful treatment of breast cancer. Because professional breast examination occurs only periodically (yearly), each woman is advised to perform BSE monthly. The best time to examine the breasts is a few days after the menstrual period, when hormonal changes have the least influence on the breasts. After the menstrual period, women find they are more accurate in detecting lumps, because then swelling and fibrocystic changes have the fewest effects. Also, BSE is most comfortable after the menstrual period because the breasts are least tender. If the woman is menopausal, or does not have regular periods, she should do BSE on the same day every month, such as the first day of the month. By performing BSE monthly, the woman becomes familiar with the usual feel and appearance of her breasts, making it easier to notice any changes from 1 month to the next.

The following signs and symptoms require follow-up:

- Lump
- Pain (breast cancer may or may not be painful)
- Discharge
- Skin changes
- Lymphadenopathy, with or without other symptoms
- Any change the woman finds as personally unusual

Women get to know their breasts best and are more likely to find a change. When performed correctly and consistently, BSE enables women to detect palpable masses that a mammogram may not visualize. Although mammography has significantly increased the number of breast cancers identified, it does fail to detect some malignancies. Few diagnostic tests are 100% sensitive. Proportions of breast cancers found by clinical breast examination (CBE) but missed by mammography reported in studies range from 5.2% to 29% (Barton, Harris, & Fletcher, 1999). If the woman finds a change in the breast, she should not try to diagnose it herself. There is no substitute for a practitioner's evaluation and further diagnostic tests.

The number of women performing BSE remains low. Women often lack confidence or simply do not remember or take the time to do it. Shower cards illustrating BSE technique have been helpful (Fig. 2.8). Nurses should encourage and educate women on performing BSE regardless of the field of nursing in which they are employed.

Clinical Breast Exam. The **clinical breast examination** (CBE) is an important part of ACS and NCI breast cancer detection guidelines. Overall, the CBE has a dual purpose. First, experienced professionals may find changes that the woman has missed. The CBE thus reinforces the woman's monthly BSE. Second, the CBE is the golden opportunity to demonstrate and explain a thorough breast examination. Modeling of the correct technique is the best way to reinforce the pattern the woman should follow at home each month. The effectiveness of the CBE

TABLE 2.4 Breast Cancer Screening Recommendations

PROCEDURE	RECOMMENDATIONS
Breast self-examination	Monthly at 20 years
Clinical breast examinations	Every 3 years from 20–40 years Yearly after 35 years if at risk Yearly after 40 years
Mammography	35 years if at risk Every 1 to 2 years from 40 to 50 years Every year after 50 years

Data from the American Cancer Society (ACS) and the National Cancer Institute (NCI).

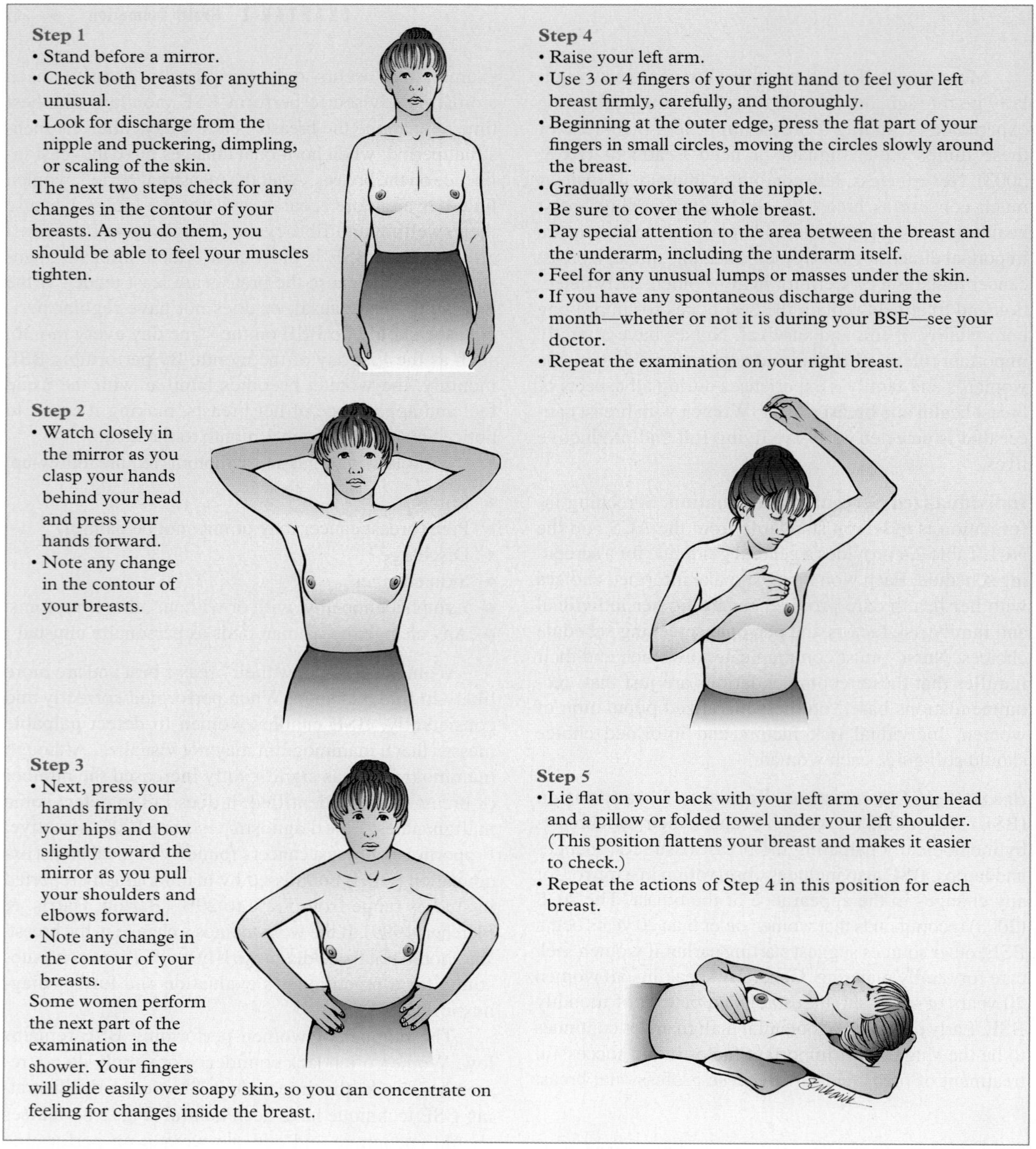

Step 1
• Stand before a mirror.
• Check both breasts for anything unusual.
• Look for discharge from the nipple and puckering, dimpling, or scaling of the skin.
The next two steps check for any changes in the contour of your breasts. As you do them, you should be able to feel your muscles tighten.
Step 2
• Watch closely in the mirror as you clasp your hands behind your head and press your hands forward.
• Note any change in the contour of your breasts.
Step 3
• Next, press your hands firmly on your hips and bow slightly toward the mirror as you pull your shoulders and elbows forward.
• Note any change in the contour of your breasts.
Some women perform the next part of the examination in the shower. Your fingers will glide easily over soapy skin, so you can concentrate on feeling for changes inside the breast.
Step 4
• Raise your left arm.
• Use 3 or 4 fingers of your right hand to feel your left breast firmly, carefully, and thoroughly.
• Beginning at the outer edge, press the flat part of your fingers in small circles, moving the circles slowly around the breast.
• Gradually work toward the nipple.
• Be sure to cover the whole breast.
• Pay special attention to the area between the breast and the underarm, including the underarm itself.
• Feel for any unusual lumps or masses under the skin.
• If you have any spontaneous discharge during the month—whether or not it is during your BSE—see your doctor.
• Repeat the examination on your right breast.
Step 5
• Lie flat on your back with your left arm over your head and a pillow or folded towel under your left shoulder. (This position flattens your breast and makes it easier to check.)
• Repeat the actions of Step 4 in this position for each breast.

FIGURE 2.8 How to perform breast self-examination. (Adapted from U.S. Department of Health and Human Services, Public Health Service. [2004]. *What you need to know about breast cancer.* Bethesda, MD: National Institutes of Health.

depends on its precision and accuracy (Barton, Harris, & Fletcher, 1999). Controversy exists on CBE because of the lack of strong research evidence linking its effectiveness to screening for breast cancer (Barton, Harris, & Fletcher, 1999). Until new techniques and diagnostic tests provide strong research evidence as proven alternatives, CBE and mammograms are still commonly conducted for breast cancer screening (Fig. 2.9).

Mammography. Depending on the source of the guideline, mammogram schedules vary slightly. Some guidelines recommend mammograms every year after 40 years; the USPSTF (2002b) suggests every 2 years from 40 to 49 years. As with CBE, the U.S. Preventive Services Task Force (USPSTF) thought that strong research evidence was lacking to mandate mammograms every year from 40 to 49 years. Most breast lesions are present

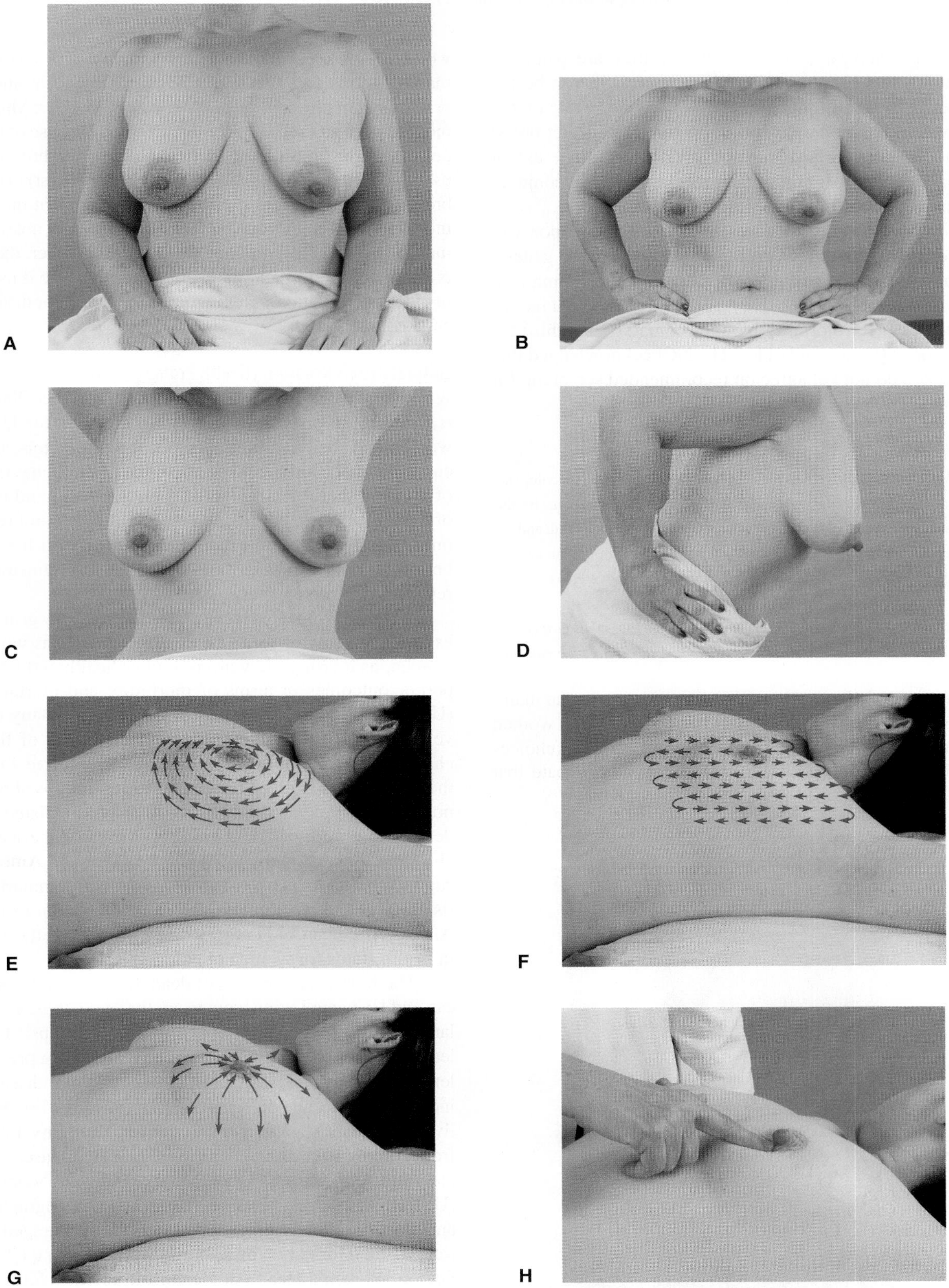

FIGURE 2.9 Steps in the clinical breast examination. (**A**) The nurse inspects the client's breasts for general appearance while the client keeps her arms at her sides. For the nurse to look for masses, retraction, dimpling, or other problems, the client (**B**) places her hands on the hips, (**C**) raises her arms, and (**D**) puts her hands on her hips and leans forward. The client lies on the table while the nurse palpates each breast using one of three patterns: (**E**) spiral, (**F**) vertical strip, or (**G**) pie-shaped. (**H**) The nurse uses the index finger to palpate the nipple for discharge or masses.

for several years, however, before they are palpable. Lumps that cannot yet be felt through BSE can be detected by **mammogram,** the soft tissue x-ray of the breast. Mammography has the potential to detect breast cancer at its earliest stage of development. The use of mammography is still usually recommended in conjunction with BSE and CBE (Fig. 2.10).

The NCI released a statement in 1993 in response to the controversy of mammogram schedules. The general consensus among experts was that routine screening with mammography and CBE every 1 to 2 years could reduce breast cancer mortality by approximately one third for women 50 years and older. The NCI acknowledged that experts do not yet agree on recommended screening for women 40 to 49 years.

QUOTE 2-3

"When I was 50, I went in for a routine checkup to the gynecologist and went through everything. I actually said to the physician, 'By the way, don't you think I should have a mammogram?' So I did, and they discovered it. I cannot sing the praises of a mammogram any higher. The cancer could not be felt, and it was discovered as a result of the mammogram."

From a woman diagnosed with early stage breast cancer following a screening mammogram.

Ultrasound. Experts agree that women need regular mammograms every 1 to 2 years after 50 years. For women younger than 50 years, risk factors and informed choices will determine the schedule. There is little debate that women with special risk factors should begin routine mammograms and breast examinations by their nurse practitioner or physician at approximately 35 years. Mammograms are less reliable in young women because of the density of the breast tissue. **Ultrasound** of the breast is useful to differentiate a solid or fluid structure (cyst) in the breast. Although recent statistics demonstrate that mammograms for women younger than 50 years might not dramatically affect the overall picture of breast cancer, there is a woman behind every number. Ultrasound also is used in older women after mammography to confirm or differentiate findings.

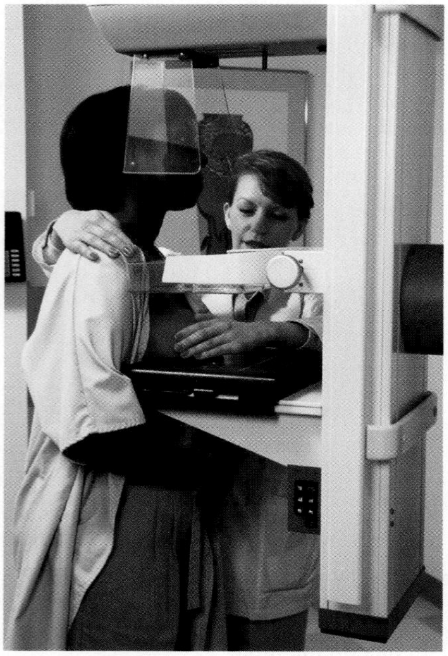

FIGURE 2.10 Mammography can help detect cancerous breast lumps and masses and is an important screening tool for women.

Cultural Beliefs Regarding Health Promotion Issues

A primary goal of *Healthy People 2010* (USDHHS, 2000) is to decrease disparities in health outcomes for U.S. women and their families. Socioeconomic factors and cultural beliefs and practices affect the health behaviors of women, thereby influencing their access to and use of health services, confidence in practitioners and recommended prevention guidelines, and general health beliefs. Nurses assess cultural beliefs and demonstrate respect for diverse belief systems.

Although women in racial and ethnic minority groups experience many of the same health problems as white women, as a group, they are in poorer health and have poorer outcomes in terms of morbidity and mortality (USDHHS, 2000). Women of color represent many diverse populations, and it is beyond the scope of this chapter to provide an extensive cultural perspective. Further information is given on the two largest groups of minorities. In the United States, the four groups listed in descending order of population are African American, Hispanic, Asian American/Pacific Islander, and American Indian/Alaska Native. Tables 2.5 and 2.6 summarize risk factors and recommended screening procedures for African American and Latina women to decrease the gap in health status for women of color.

The four leading causes of death for African American and Hispanic/Latina women are the same; thus, similar screening procedures apply to these groups. The leading causes of death in these women, in order of prevalence, are heart disease, cancer, cerebrovascular disease including stroke, and diabetes (USDHHS, 2005). For Native American/Alaskan Native women, mortality rates from chronic liver disease, cirrhosis, kidney disease, suicide, and homicide are higher than those of white women (USDHHS, 2005). Therefore, depending on geographic and practice settings, individual readers are encouraged to refer to the information on minority women from the Office on Women's Health at Health Information for Minority Women (www.4woman.gov/minority/index.cfm) and the Minority Health Report www.4woman.gov/owh/pub/minority/index.htm).

Many important health promotion issues are of special concern to African American and Hispanic women. Women from these groups are at higher risk than white

TABLE 2.5 Health Promotion Strategies Among African-American Women

HEALTH CONCERN	SCREENING TEST	RISK FACTORS	HEALTH PROMOTION
Diabetes	Blood glucose test with annual examination if abnormal follow-up with PCP/NP	Family history Obesity Race/ethnicity Genetics/environmental factors HTN History of gestational DM Sedentary lifestyle	Preventive measures for type II DM: ● Eat a healthy diet. ● Exercise regularly. ● Maintain ideal weight (BMI < 25).
High Blood Pressure	BP checked with annual examination. If normal, get BP checked every 1–2 years; if abnormal, follow-up with PCP/NP.	Smoking Dyslipidemia DM Older age Family history of cardiovascular disease Diet high in sodium Alcohol consumption	Eat a healthy diet. Exercise regularly. Weight reduction. Decrease sodium and alcohol intake. Yearly physical examinations with BP check.
Obesity	BP check Blood glucose test Weight check	Sedentary lifestyle Diet high in saturated fat and cholesterol Alcohol intake	Eat a healthy diet. Engage in regular exercise for at least 30 minutes most days of the week.
HIV/AIDS	Oral examination, vision examination, Pap smear and pelvic examination, TB test, thyroid test (TSH), sexually transmitted infection (STI) tests	Unprotected sex, sharing needles, coming in contact with blood or body fluids of an infected person	Do not have unprotected sex. Use condoms. Don't share needles or syringes. Limit sexual partners.
Breast Health: Breast Examination	Yearly clinical breast exam (CBE); monthly breast self-examination (BSE)	Older age Early age at menarche Late age of first birth History of prior breast biopsy Family history	There are no preventive measures, but lifestyle modifications (healthy diet, weight control, smoking cessation) can minimize risk factors.
Heart Health: Minimizing Heart Disease and Stroke	Discuss with your primary health care provider if family history of problems. Screen blood pressure and lipid profile. Undergo exercise stress test.	HTN Increased cholesterol Sedentary lifestyle or smoking Excessive alcohol intake	Eat a healthy diet. Exercise regularly. Have regular physical examinations. Stop smoking.
Autoimmune Disease (Lupus, Arthritis)	Thyroid test (TSH) Autoimmune screening test TB test	Stress Smoking Poor diet Excess alcohol intake	Exercise regularly. Eat a healthy diet: calcium, vitamin D. Stop smoking.
General Health	Discuss with your primary health care provider.	Discuss with your primary health care provider.	Discuss with your primary health care provider.

BMI, body mass index; BP, blood pressure; DM, diabetes mellitus; HTN, hypertension; TB, tuberculosis; TSH, thyroid-stimulating hormone.

women for such conditions as diabetes, hypertension, obesity, heart disease, stroke, kidney disease, arthritis, HIV/AIDS, lupus, and advanced cervical and breast cancer. The importance of health education, assessment and early screening, and self-management with health-promoting behaviors can minimize or prevent these conditions.

African American and Latina women have a higher prevalence of diabetes and diabetes-related complications and death. Approximately 25% of African American women older than 55 years have diabetes, nearly twice the rate of white women (USDHHS, 2005). Improving the lipid profile, weight management, and exercise patterns of women with diabetes could decrease their risk for diabetes-related cardiovascular disease and other complications. Maintaining a blood pressure less than 130/80 mm Hg also will help minimize heart disease and stroke, which are more common in African Americans.

Of all U.S. women, African Americans have the highest death rates from heart disease (USDHHS, 2005). African American women may have atypical symptoms when suffering from angina or myocardial infarction. They often present with shortness of breath, rather than angina, as their chief complaint; often, their results on electrocardiogram are normal as well. African American

TABLE 2.6 Health Promotion Strategies for Latina Women

COMMON HEALTH CONDITIONS	HEALTH STRATEGIES
Diabetes DID YOU KNOW? Hispanics are nearly twice as likely to have diabetes and die than non-Hispanics of the same age (Brewington, 2002).	Begin screening at 40 years of age with yearly fasting glucose levels. If a client is diagnosed with diabetes: Encourage diet changes and exercises before initiating medications. Refer client to dietitian or diabetic educator for assistance with meal planning. Discuss importance of routine foot care. Discuss symptoms of hypoglycemia/hyperglycemia and how to treat episodes. Encourage routine follow-up care with health care provider or nurse practitioner. Explain and demonstrate importance of daily home glucose monitoring. Encourage a yearly eye examination with ophthalmologist. Distribute any and all pamphlets and written information to reinforce education. Discuss resources and financial means to follow health plan.
Breast Cancer DID YOU KNOW? Cases of breast cancer for Latina women are rising. The risk is nearly double for women with obesity (www.4woman.gov).	Explain the importance of performing BSE every month; demonstrate multiple techniques. Encourage yearly breast examinations by health care provider or nurse practitioner. Begin yearly mammogram screening at 40 years of age (sooner if there is a positive family history of breast cancer or if health care provider or nurse practitioner believe it necessary). Encourage moderate exercise and weight loss; obesity may contribute to the development of breast cancer.
AIDS and Sexually Transmitted Illnesses DID YOU KNOW? Latinas are at higher risk for rape and domestic abuse and three times more likely to acquire AIDS than other U.S. women (Newcomb et al., 1998).	Initial discussion should begin between 10 and 12 years of age and may be easier if parent is not in room. Recognize and acknowledge that this topic is very sensitive and personal but one that must be discussed. Explore level of knowledge regarding topic. Clarify any misconceptions or myths. Discuss transmission of AIDS/STIs. Discuss safe sex, abstinence, condom use, "buddy system" for parties, and general safety measures. Encourage client to voice concerns or questions at any time during discussion. Periodically reaffirm information with clients.
Glaucoma and Vision Disorders DID YOU KNOW? Open-angle glaucoma is the leading cause of blindness among U.S. Hispanics. Hispanic women are more likely to suffer vision impairment from cataracts, glaucoma, and diabetic retinopathy than men (*Angiogenesis* Weekly, 2002).	Report any visual changes immediately to a health care provider or nurse practitioner. Encourage use of safety gear, including sunglasses and protective eye wear, during activities. Begin yearly ophthalmology examinations at 50 years of age, sooner if any visual changes occur or positive family history of diabetes or glaucoma exist.

women are less likely than others to be referred for cardiac catheterization, which is necessary to diagnose congestive heart failure.

In its beginning years, the HIV/AIDS epidemic was thought to be a disease of homosexual men. Now, however, it is a leading cause of death in young African American and Latina women. Nurses must improve culturally sensitive health education and screening programs to increase awareness of HIV risks and to promote safer sexual practices among women of color.

Although age-adjusted rates of breast cancer are higher in white women, particularly those of Ashkenazic Jewish ancestry, African American women have higher mortality rates because cancer tends to be in a more advanced stage when these women are diagnosed. Access to care and social, cultural, economic, and educational factors play a major role in the health behaviors of African American women regarding BSE, CBE, mammography, and other preventive care practices.

Cultural and religious beliefs of Latina women affect their use of the health care industry. These women are frequently the primary caregivers for their extended families, as well as for community members. Latina women often use traditional folk medicine and home remedies passed down over generations as treatments against common illnesses. Because they are busy caring for their families, Latina women may not take time or use limited financial resources to care for themselves. In addition, when they seek medical care, it may not be until their illness or disease is more advanced. A further complication is that their religious beliefs may include perceptions that disease is viewed as punishment for sins committed or is caused by the will of their god. As health care providers, nurses must recognize the cultural and religious diversity within this ethnic group and the effects their beliefs have on their health decisions. Nurses must educate Latina women on health care practices within a cultural framework that communicates respect for their value system. The nurse and client should explore ways to promote seeking preventive care and early medical treatment consistent with the client's value system.

Environmental Factors Related to Health Issues

Nurses need to recognize that many women frequently and unknowingly are exposed to unseen health threats in the environment. Table 2.7 contains a wide variety of environmental risks of concern to women that can pose serious health concerns. For each risk, the table lists specific steps to avoid exposure and to minimize any harm from exposure to that potentially serious health hazard.

PHYSICAL EXAMINATION

With an overwhelming amount of health information available to women, nurses must focus strongly on identifying risk factors based on the woman's health history, assessment, and physical examination. Table 2.8 discusses body systems and organ changes in relation to normal and alterations in normal across the woman's life cycle.

TABLE 2.7 Environmental Risks and Protective Measures

POTENTIAL RISKS	PREVENTIVE OR CORRECTIVE ACTION
Allergies	Keep environment free of known allergens. Consider allergy-free pets. Use HEPA filters. If exposure is unavoidable, consider antihistamine use.
Asbestos	Have a qualified contractor check old homes and remove any existing asbestos. Avoid handling or working with asbestos-containing materials (eg, patching compounds, ceiling tiles, pipe insulation, vinyl floors, brake shoes, clutch pads). Vigorously wash hands and shower after use of these materials.
Benzene	Avoid breathing cigarette smoke, gasoline fumes, and vehicular emissions.
Carbon monoxide	Ensure appliances are installed and operating correctly. Perform annual automobile and home heating inspections. Do not burn charcoal or operate gasoline engines in confined areas (home, garage, camper). Install detectors with audible alarms in home and garage. Avoid cigarette smoke.
Cigarette smoke	Avoid cigarette and cigar smoking and secondhand smoke.
Dioxins	These are fat-soluble and cross the placenta into breast milk. They are found in meats, fish, eggs, and dairy products. Reduce fat consumption. Broil food instead of frying. Limit use of chlorine-bleached products (eg, toilet paper, tampons).
Food poisoning	Use proper handwashing technique when preparing food. Refrigerate food at adequate temperatures. Thoroughly cook meat, fish, poultry, and eggs. Disinfect countertops and utensils that come in contact with uncooked food. Wash thoroughly all fruits and vegetables to be eaten uncooked.
Hair solutions and products	Read labels carefully. Avoid direct inhalation and prolonged exposure. Use pump instead of aerosolized products.
Histoplasmosis	Avoid areas that may harbor the disease-causing fungus (eg, areas with accumulated bird or bat droppings, such as caves).
Lead	Have old homes tested before renovations. Ensure lead removal when feasible. Cover lead paint in good condition with lead-free paint or wallpaper. Pregnant women should avoid contact with lead-contaminated water, soil, and paint. Keep yard well vegetated to reduce contamination from soil. Clean floors and sills regularly with wet mop or cloth. Run faucet for 15 seconds before drawing drinking water.
Lightning	Seek shelter during storms; avoid open fields and trees. Unplug appliances not on a surge protector. Avoid phone and water use during thunderstorms.
Mercury	Avoid eating large, long-lived fish (eg, shark, swordfish, king mackerel, tilefish). It is safe for pregnant women to eat an average of 12 oz of cooked shellfish, canned fish, or small ocean or farm-raised fish weekly. The US Food and Drug Administration Center for Food Safety and Applied Nutrition food information line is open 24 hr/day at 1-888-SAFE FOOD.
Motor vehicle collisions	Wear seatbelts. Ensure proper airbag functioning. Children 12 years or younger should sit in the back. Use appropriate car seats for infants, toddlers, and young children. Use headlights and turn signals. Avoid speeding (leave early). Conduct annual automobile inspections.

Continued

TABLE 2.7 Environmental Risks and Protective Measures *(Continued)*

POTENTIAL RISKS	PREVENTIVE OR CORRECTIVE ACTION
Radon	Have home inspected or buy test kit from local grocery or hardware store. If radon is detected, arrange for a qualified radon-reduction contractor to visit the home. (The government hotline for info is 1-800-SOS-RADON.)
Teratogenic medications	Read warnings on medication labels carefully. Avoid ingesting or handling any medication shown to cause birth defects. Discuss risks with physician or pharmacist.
Toluene	Use toluene-containing substances (eg, glue, paint, paint thinner, nail polish, adhesives) in well-ventilated areas.
Ultraviolet (UV) radiation	Avoid sun exposure between 10 AM and 4 PM. Wear sunscreen with minimum SPF 15, using approximately 1 oz per application. Wear wide-brimmed hats, pants, and long sleeves (wear white clothing to avoid overheating). Wear sunglasses with UV protection year round.
Viral infections	Vaccinate against infections such as rubella and hepatitis B before pregnancy. Practice strict hand-washing and personal hygiene. Avoid unprotected sexual contact.
Xenoestrogens	Avoid pesticides (eat organic foods; wash fruits and vegetables thoroughly before eating). Avoid microwaving plastics and reusing plastic containers (eg, margarine or butter tubs).

Internet Resources for Environmental Health Issues:

American Lung Association Fact Sheet: Carbon Monoxide
http://www.lungusa.org/air/carbon_factsheet99.html

American Lung Association Fact Sheet: Radon
http://www.lungusa.org/air/radon_factsheet99.html

Consumer Advisory: Center for Food Safety and Applied Nutrition, U.S. Food and Drug Administration, March 2001
http://vm.cfsan.fda.gov/~dms/admehg.html

National Safety Council Fact Sheet: Lead
http://www.nsc.org/library/facts/lead.htm

National Safety Council Fact Sheet: Asbestos
http://www.nsc.org/library/facts.asbestos.htm

National Institute of Environmental Health Sciences
http://www.cdc.gov/ncidod/dbmd/diseaseinfo/histoplasmosis.htm

U.S. Department of Health and Human Services: Agency for Toxic Substance and Disease Registry
http://www.atsdr.cdc.gov

U.S. Environmental Protection Agency: Staying Healthy in the Sun
http://epa.gov/sunwise/stayheal.html

U.S. Environmental Protection Agency National Center for Environmental Research
http://es.epa.gov/ncer

NURSING AND COLLABORATIVE CARE ROLES RELATED TO HEALTH PROMOTION

QUOTE 2-4

"When you cease to make a contribution you begin to die."

Eleanor Roosevelt

Health behaviors involve complex variables and decisions. Examples include issues such as weight control, smoking cessation, obesity, and domestic violence. Decisions related to these areas are best made within a partnership of equity and support from health professionals.

When working with clients to make needed changes in the area of health promotion, nursing interventions address the following health needs:

- Social support
- Strengths of the woman and her family
- Need for culturally sensitive education and expression of questions
- Sexuality and relationship concerns
- Spirituality and psychological needs
- Financial needs

Box 2.3 represents a model for the woman making health-related decisions or lifestyle changes in each of the areas listed previously. The nurse focuses on a multidisciplinary model to ensure that the woman and her family have referrals to dietitians, counselors, specialists, and community health resources, as needed. Box 2.4 provides a list of Internet resources for women.

Health Screening

As providers collaborating with other health care and community professionals, nurses must be knowledgeable regarding proper health screening for women. In educating women and conducting health screenings,

(text continues on page 76)

TABLE 2.8 Physical Examination Guidelines

CONSIDERATIONS, FINDINGS, AND LIFE CYCLE PERSPECTIVES	THERAPEUTIC INTERVENTIONS
Dermatologic System	
Skin should be dry, warm, and smooth. *Wrinkles* are a natural part of aging, determined mostly by genetics and sun exposure. Normal facial expressions ultimately cause crease lines. Smiling, squinting, and frowning all contract the facial muscles, causing accordion-like lines to develop. *Dry skin* increases with age, mostly from sun exposure, which thins the skin and decreases moisture retention. *Acne* may appear for the first time or worsen in midlife from hormonal fluctuations. Some women experience alopecia, but to a much lesser extent than men. *Excessive hair growth,* especially on the upper lip or along the jaw line, can result from hormones as menopause approaches.	Check sun-exposed areas well, especially head, neck, and hands. Use sunscreen with a broad spectrum that protects from ultraviolet A and B (UVA and UVB) rays. Apply enough; apply frequently; reapply immediately after swimming or every 2 hours if out of the water. Apply sunscreen 15 to 30 minutes before going into the sun. Wear clothing made from tight-weave fabrics or those that absorb UV light. Avoid the sun from 10 AM to 4 PM when rays are most intense. A wide-brimmed hat will protect the client's face. Advise client to avoid cigarettes, which cause cancer *and* wrinkles. Certain medications cause a photosensitivity reaction; check adverse reactions for all medications the client uses. Add moisture to the air with humidifiers or a pan of water set on the radiator to help prevent dry skin. Instruct clients to use lukewarm water instead of hot water, which strips away natural oils, when showering. Advise clients to use nondrying soaps without abrasives or irritants. Cleansing bars and super-fatted soaps are less drying. Clients should pat, not rub, the skin dry. Instruct clients to apply moisturizer immediately after a bath or shower to retain the water absorbed.
Eyes, Ears, Nose, Throat	
Sclera may look buff-colored at the extreme periphery. Visual acuity is fairly constant between 20 and 50 years. Near vision begins to blur for almost everyone. As the lens loses its elasticity, it increasingly cannot focus on nearby objects. This presbyopia becomes noticeable after 40 years of age (Bickley, 2007).	
Cardiovascular System	
Heart sounds: assess for regular rate and rhythm, murmurs, JVD, carotid bruits, and pulses. *Heart rate* may be as low as 50 beats/min in a woman who regularly engages in aerobic activity. A *split S2* can be normal in women 20 to 30 years of age. The split may widen on inspiration. *Spider veins* are groups of blood vessels close to the skin surface that have dilated. They may appear on thighs, calves, and ankles as part of aging, heredity, hormonal changes, or external injuries. *Varicose veins* may result from pooled blood as veins lose elasticity and the valves malfunction.	Regular exercise, such as walking, jogging, biking, and swimming, will help prevent varicose veins. The American Heart Association and the American College of Cardiology suggest screening for cardiovascular risk with the tool from the Framingham Heart Study, recommended by the National Cholesterol Education Project, available at: http://hin.nhlbi.hih.gov/.
Pulmonary System	
A healthy person typically breathes effortlessly and automatically 20,000 times a day.	To keep lungs healthy, instruct clients to avoid irritants, such as chemical and gas fumes, smoke, and asbestos, as much as possible. Encourage them to consider installing a particulate air filter, especially if they have asthma or respiratory problems or live with a smoker. Encourage clients to eat a diet rich in antioxidants: fruits and vegetables, carotenes (found in carrots, yellow squash), and dark leafy greens. Antioxidants may help protect against cancer. Regular aerobic exercise strengthens the muscles of breathing. Advise clients to breathe consciously: practice breathing more deeply, slowly, quietly, and regularly, working to extend each exhalation to squeeze out more air. Advise clients to alert the nurse right away for a cough that lasts longer than 1 month, frequent chest colds, shortness of breath with limited exertion, difficulty breathing, wheezing, or coughing up blood.

Continued

● **TABLE 2.8** **Physical Examination Guidelines *(Continued)***

CONSIDERATIONS, FINDINGS, AND LIFE CYCLE PERSPECTIVES	THERAPEUTIC INTERVENTIONS
Gastrointestinal System	
Inspect abdomen, noting posture, contour, masses, bulging, distention, scars, venous patterns, lesions, and striae. Note the abdominal contour after asking the client to take a deep breath and raise her head. Listen for bowel sounds in all four quadrants; they should be high pitched. The skin of the abdomen is subject to the same color variations as the rest of the body. Venous patterns may be more prominent in thin clients. Striae result from stretched tissue: obesity or pregnancy. The abdomen may be symmetrically distended from a heavy meal, obesity, or gas. No bulges should appear. Clicks or gurgles are normal. Bowel sounds may last from 1/2 second to several seconds.	Educate clients regarding diet, which greatly influences risk for colorectal cancer. A diet that is generally ● High in fresh fruits and vegetables ● Modest in calories ● Modest in alcohol consumption and ● Low in red meat and animal fat is cancer protective. Eating foods high in fiber and low in fat, exercising regularly, drinking plenty of water, and avoiding foods that cause problems can help keep the digestive system healthy. Research by the Department of Oncological Studies at the Salt Lake City Medical Center (Slattery et al., 1998) found that a "Western" dietary pattern is associated with: ● Higher body mass index ● Greater intake of total energy and dietary cholesterol The "prudent" pattern is associated with ● Higher levels of vigorous leisure time physical activity ● Smaller body size, and ● Higher intakes of dietary fiber and folate The "Western" dietary pattern is associated with an increased risk for colon cancer in both men and women. The "prudent" diet is protective, and although "substituters" (people who substituted low-fat dairy products for high-fat dairy products, margarine for butter, poultry for red meat, and whole grains for refined grains) are at reduced risk for colon cancer, the reduction in risk is not statistically significant. These data support the hypothesis that overall dietary intake pattern is associated with colon cancer and that the dietary pattern associated with the greatest increase in risk is the one that typifies a Western-style diet (Slattery, Boucher, Caan, Potter, & Ma, 1998). Counsel the client about hepatitis B, a type of hepatitis virus that attacks and damages the liver. Advise immunizations if appropriate.
Urologic	
	Educate clients about factors that contribute to infection of the urinary tract: ● Sexual activity can introduce bacteria into the urethra. ● Poor hygiene habits, such as not bathing or showering routinely, or changing underwear and sanitary pads infrequently, can introduce bacteria from the rectum into the urethra. ● Excessive use of caffeine can cause urinary irritation and diuresis. ● Excessive stress can reduce the immune response. ● Using a diaphragm may press on the bladder and cause stasis of urine. Spermicides inhibit growth of lactobacilli. ● Waiting long periods between urinations results in stasis of urine and decreases flushing of bacteria from bladder (Carcio, 1999).
Breasts	

Inspect breasts and nipples with the client sitting, disrobed to the waist.
Look for skin changes, symmetry, contours, and retraction. Also examine the woman's breasts with the client's hands over head, and hands on hips. Some difference in the size of the breasts, including the areolas, is common. Long-standing inversion of a nipple is usually normal. Normal tissue varies widely. Nodularity may increase premenstrually. A firm transverse ridge of breast tissue is often found along the lower edge of the breast, especially in large breasts. Tenderness is common premenstrually.
	Educate clients about breast cancer screening and breast self-examination (BSE):
	● Ideal time for BSE is just after menses.
	● All women 40 years of age or older should have a clinical examination and baseline mammography.
	● With increased risk factors, the examination should begin sooner.
	  ● Family history of a first-degree relative with breast cancer
	  ● Menstrual history: age at menarche younger than 12 years, age at menopause older than 55 years
	  ● Pregnancy: nulliparous
	  ● Breast conditions such as atypical hyperplasia or lobular carcinoma in situ
	Further counsel clients about the relationship between obesity, diet, and breast cancer:
	● In premenopausal women, obesity is not associated with increased risk for breast cancer, presumably because it decreases the number of ovulatory cycles, reducing exposure to estrogen between menarche and menopause.

Continued

● **TABLE 2.8 Physical Examination Guidelines**

CONSIDERATIONS, FINDINGS, AND LIFE CYCLE PERSPECTIVES	THERAPEUTIC INTERVENTIONS
	• Obesity may increase breast cancer risk because body fat is critical in the early initiation of menarche, expanding the period between menarche and menopause, thereby increasing total exposure to estrogen. • Obese postmenopausal women show a greater risk for breast cancer. • A positive correlation between alcohol consumption and breast cancer risk was observed in premenopausal but not in postmenopausal women. • Isothiocyanates found in broccoli and watercress have been found to have antitumor activity in mammary tissue.
Reproductive System	
Lesbians are women who are mainly emotionally and sexually attracted to other women. They need the same health care as other women, including screening for sexually transmitted infections (STIs).	Counsel clients about various aspects of reproductive health. • Birth control (or contraception) helps a woman plan her pregnancies. Some methods of birth control also help protect against STIs, including AIDS. The more the client knows about birth control and her own needs, the easier it will be for her to choose a method that's right for her. • There are many methods of birth control. The birth control pill, implants, injections, intrauterine device (IUD), diaphragm, and cervical cap require a prescription. • The most used method of hormonal birth control is the birth control pill (oral contraceptive). One injection of hormonal birth control provides birth control for 3 months. • If a woman has sex without any type of birth control, she may be able to use a type of backup birth control called *emergency contraception.* In this method, high doses of certain birth control pills are taken within 72 hours (3 days) of sex without birth control. • Most birth control failures result from not using birth control correctly each time. • Barrier methods are some of the oldest and safest forms of contraception (birth control). These methods work by acting as barriers to keep the man's sperm from reaching the woman's egg. Some methods also may protect against certain STIs. Barrier methods are effective when used correctly and every time the client has sex. Today, barrier methods are safe and effective ways to prevent pregnancy. The diaphragm, cervical cap, sponge, and condom (male and female) act as physical barriers. • Spermicides act as chemical barriers. The best results are achieved when spermicides are used along with a physical barrier method, such as a condom, diaphragm, sponge, or cervical cap. Use of latex condoms, especially those with spermicide, can help protect against the spread of some STIs, including HIV infection, the virus that causes AIDS. If a woman has sex without any type of birth control or if she thinks her barrier method has failed (for instance, a condom broke), she may use emergency birth control. • The nurse counsels her client to begin good care and a healthy lifestyle before pregnancy to increase the odds that the client will have a healthy baby. • If the client is planning to become pregnant, the nurse counsels her to have a prepregnancy checkup. • As a part of this visit, the nurse practitioner asks the client about her medical and family history, medications she takes, any past pregnancies she has had, and her diet and lifestyle. Her answers will help her nurse practitioner decide whether she needs special care during pregnancy. • Some women have medical conditions, such as diabetes, high blood pressure, and seizure disorders, that can cause problems during pregnancy. Instruct the client to let your primary health care provider know if a past pregnancy was complicated by diabetes, high blood pressure, premature labor, preterm birth, or birth defects. • Folic acid, taken before pregnancy and for the first 3 months of pregnancy, can reduce the risk for neural tube defects. • Three types of providers offer medical care for pregnancy and birth: obstetrician-gynecologists (ob-gyns), family practitioners, and certified nurse-midwives (CNMs). Labor and delivery nurses help care for women and their babies during labor, during delivery, and right after birth.

Continued

TABLE 2.8 Physical Examination Guidelines *(Continued)*

CONSIDERATIONS, FINDINGS, AND LIFE CYCLE PERSPECTIVES	THERAPEUTIC INTERVENTIONS
	The nurse counsels the client on safe sex practices, including common STIs. ● Human papillomavirus (HPV) is a virus that causes warts. HPV is one of the most common STIs. ● Infection with gonorrhea and chlamydia causes two of the most common STIs. ● Gonorrhea and chlamydia often have no symptoms. When symptoms do occur, they may show up 2 days to 3 weeks after infection. ● Syphilis, another STI, occurs less often, but can be serious if it is not treated. ● If the client thinks she may be at risk for gonorrhea, chlamydia, or syphilis, the nurse encourages her to see her primary health care provider to get tested. ● Pregnant women also may be offered testing for gonorrhea and chlamydia. ● Women who douche at least once a month have higher rates of bacterial vaginosis (BV) infections than do women who don't douche. The nurse should also counsel her lesbian clients to see their primary health care provider regularly for preventive health care. Such care includes routine tests and exams that all women need, regardless of their sexual orientation. STIs, including HIV, although potentially less common in lesbians than in heterosexual women, still occur in the lesbian population; therefore, the nurse should include them in the health history. The nurse counsels her client about premenstrual syndrome (PMS), including educating the client on how the menstrual cycle works: ● During the menstrual cycle, estrogen and progesterone—two hormones made by the ovaries—cause changes in the lining of the uterus (endometrium). Women with PMS have symptoms in the second half of the cycle (after they ovulate on about day 14). ● As many as 85% of women who menstruate report some symptoms of PMS in the days or weeks before menstruation.
Nervous System	
An estimated 45 million people in the United States suffer from chronic headaches serious enough to interfere with daily life. The most common type is tension headache. Most headaches are minor and can be treated with over-the-counter pain relievers.	Counsel clients that limiting stress, avoiding triggers, and exercising regularly can help control headaches.
Psychological	
Each year, more than 11 million people in the United States (approximately 5%) suffer from depression, which disrupts daily life. A family history of depression may increase a client's risk; such clients should tell nurse practitioners about symptoms.	Counsel clients that depression is a treatable medical problem, similar to diabetes, hypertension, and heart disease.

nurses play a key role in preventing illness and optimizing health. As advocates for clients, nurses are obligated to help them truly understand and integrate the need for routine screening as a preventive strategy. Within these general guidelines, the nurse collaborating with other professionals must consider each woman's history and risk factors. The objectives of *Healthy People 2010* (USDHHS, 2000) are the focus of the overall health guidelines for American women. Table 2.9 summarizes health screening guidelines, laboratory and diagnostic tests, and immunization recommendations for client education, referral, and clinical practice.

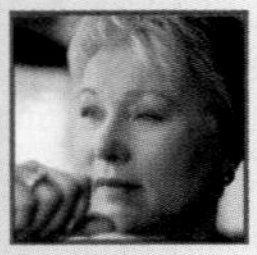

Linda, the 53-year-old perimenopausal woman from the beginning of the chapter, asks how often she should have a mammogram and Pap smear. What response is appropriate?

Immunizations

Each year, vaccine-preventable diseases have costly effects, resulting in doctor visits, hospitalizations, and premature deaths (CDC, 2006). Immunizations are rec-

BOX 2.3 Nursing Interventions to Encourage Health-Promoting Behavior Changes

Social Support

- Give the woman time and space to adjust to the lifestyle change.
- Encourage networking with other women with a similar situation.
- Encourage women to ask for help and to allow themselves to experience others' expressions of support and caring.

Strengths of Woman and Family

- Focus on current strengths in making the decisions and lifestyle changes.
- Explore what skills and strengths work for this client and her family.

Need for Culturally Sensitive Education and Expression of Questions

- Give the information needed or requested. Offer brochures and Internet resources.
- Encourage sharing of thoughts and feelings on barriers to the lifestyle change.
- Explore and clarify misconceptions or unrealistic fears.
- Educate about any medication regimen prescribed for treatment. Include medication, dosage, side effects, and desired benefit. Review any over-the-counter medications or herbal therapies being used.
- Educate the client regarding risk factors, screening guidelines, and recommended diagnostic or laboratory test and follow-up plan.

Sexuality and Relationship Concerns

- Encourage client to seek support from spouse/partner as well as others.
- Spouses or partners may not be able to fulfill all the woman's connections needs. Suggest outlets to connect with oneself, such as journaling, poetry, and meditation.

Spirituality and Psychological Needs

- Discuss the need to fight to keep a positive outlook. Explain that relapse is expected.
- Encourage the client to do what is important to her. Promote self-nurturing activities and positive self-talk.
- Suggest journaling, music, imagery, or yoga for relaxation and to enhance maintaining health-promoting behaviors.
- Encourage release of energy through humor and playful activities.
- Encourage church activities or personal expressions and prayer with their "spiritual power."

Financial Needs

- Discuss behavior changes and treatment options in relation to expense, financial circumstances, and insurance reimbursement.
- Discuss alternative behaviors or treatments when the client has financial burdens.

Community Resources and Collaborative Care

- Offer the resource of a support group, counselor, or specialist, as needed.
- Offer community resources and validation of experiences with others in the community.

BOX 2.4 Internet Resources for Women's Health

http://www.americanheart.org
http://www.niaaa.nih.gov/publications/aa13.htm
http://www.niaaa.nih.gov/publications/aa46.htm
http://www.niaaa.nih.gov/publications/aa10.htm
http://www.cdc.gov/tobacco/christy/women.htm
http://www.osteo.org/newfile.asp?doc=r705i&doctitle=Smoking+and+Bone+Health&doctype=HTML+Fact+Sheet
http://www.acsh.org/publications/reports/tobacco2001.html
http://www.cdc.gov/wisewoman/
http://www.cdc.gov/tobacco/sgr/sgr_forwomen/factsheet_tobaccouse.htm
http://www.cdc.gov/tobacco/sgr/sgr_forwomen/factsheet_use.htm
http://www.cdc.gov/nccdphp/sgr/women.htm
http://www.cdc.gov/ncbddd/folicacid/folicfaqs.htm
http://www.4woman.gov/faq/preg-nutr.htm
http://www.youngwomenshealth.org/healthyeating.html
http://www.nap.edu/catalog/6035.html
http://www.ahrq.gov/research/womenh1.htm
http://www.ncbi.nlm.nih.gov/

TABLE 2.9 Health Screening for Women During the Reproductive Years

SCREENING TESTS	18 TO 39 YEARS	40 TO 49 YEARS	50 TO 64 YEARS
General Health			
Full checkup, including height, weight, and BMI	Dependent on risk factors	Yearly	Yearly
Thyroid test (TSH)	Starting at 35 years, then every 5 years; sooner if symptomatic	Every 5 years	Every 5 years
Heart Health			
Blood pressure measurement	Begin testing at 21 years, then every 1 to 2 years depending on risk factors	Every 1–2 years depending on risk factors	Every 1 to 2 years depending on risk factors
Cholesterol screening	Begin at 20 years, then every 5 years	Every 5 years; more frequently with CAD, DM, obesity, or dyslipidemia	Every 5 years; more frequently with CAD, DM, obesity, or dyslipidemia
Bone Health			
Bone mineral density test	Only if significant risk factors (anorexia, multiple fractures)	Dependent on risk factors	Dependent on risk factors
Diabetes			
Blood glucose test	Only if significant risk factors (family history, obesity, symptomatic)	Begin testing at 45 years, then every 3 years	Every 3 years
Breast Health			
Breast examination	Yearly by a health care provider; monthly BSE recommended	Yearly by a health care provider; monthly BSE recommended	Yearly by a health care provider; monthly BSE recommended
Mammogram	Only if significant risk factors (family history, mass noted in breast)	Every 1–2 years depending on risk factors	Yearly
Reproductive Health			
Pap smear and pelvic examination	Yearly with the option of every 1–3 years after three consecutive normal results and minimal risk factors	Yearly with the option of every 1–3 years after three consecutive normal results and minimal risk factors	Yearly with the option of every 1–3 years after three consecutive normal results and minimal risk factors
Chlamydia test	If sexually active, yearly until 25 years. Continue to perform if high risk (multiple sexual partners, recent change in partner)	If high risk for contracting an STI, continue testing yearly; otherwise, according to risk factors	If at high risk for contracting an STI, continue testing yearly; otherwise, according to risk factors
STI tests	Yearly if client has multiple sexual partners, a partner with multiple sexual partners, a partner with an STI, or a personal history of STI	Yearly if client has multiple sexual partners, a partner with multiple sexual partners, a partner with an STI, or a personal history of STI	Yearly if client has multiple sexual partners, a partner with multiple sexual partners, a partner with an STI, or a personal history of STI
Colorectal Health			
Colonoscopy	Only if significant risk factors or rectal bleeding	Only if significant risk factors or rectal bleeding	Every 5–10 years
Double contrast barium enema	Only if significant risk factors or rectal bleeding	Only if significant risk factors or rectal bleeding	Every 5–10 years only if not having colonoscopy every 10 years
Flexible sigmoidoscopy	Only if significant risk factors or rectal bleeding	Only if significant risk factors or rectal bleeding	Every 5 years
Rectal examination	Only if significant risk factors or rectal bleeding	Only if significant risk factors or rectal bleeding	Yearly
Fecal occult blood test	Only if symptomatic	Only if symptomatic	Yearly

Continued

TABLE 2.9 Health Screening for Women During the Reproductive Years

SCREENING TESTS	18 TO 39 YEARS	40 TO 49 YEARS	50 TO 64 YEARS
Eye and Ear Health			
Vision examination	Examination with an eye care provider once initially between 20 and 39 years and then as recommended by provider	Every 2–4 years	Every 2–4 years
Hearing test	Initial examination at 18 years, then every 10 years unless hearing changes	Every 10 years	Dependent on symptoms and risk factors (employed with loud machinery)
Skin Health			
Mole examination	Monthly self-examination starting by 20 years; every 3 years by a health care provider	Monthly self-examination; every year by a health care provider	Monthly self-examination; every year by a health care provider
Oral Health			
Dental examination	One to two times a year	One to two times a year	One to two times a year
Mental Health Screening	Abuse and depression screen with office visits based on risk factors and symptoms	Abuse and depression screen with office visits based on risk factors and symptoms	Abuse and depression screen with office visits based on risk factors and symptoms
Nutrition Supplements	Teens to age 24, 1,200–1,500 mg calcium; age 25–50 years, 1,000 mg calcium daily; pregnant or lactating, 1200–1500 mg calcium; vitamin D, 400 to 800 IU; 15 mg iron daily; 0.4 mg folic acid daily	1000 mg calcium daily; vitamin D, 400–800 IU; 15 mg iron daily; 0.4 mg folic acid daily	1500 mg calcium daily; vitamin D, 400–800 IU; 10 mg iron daily; 0.4 mg folic acid daily
Safety	Wear a seatbelt and bike helmet. Use smoke and carbon monoxide detectors. Wear sunscreen and UV-protected sunglasses. Practice safe sex.	Wear a seatbelt and bike helmet. Use smoke and carbon monoxide detectors. Wear sunscreen and UV-protected sunglasses. Practice safe sex.	Wear a seatbelt and bike helmet. Use smoke and carbon monoxide detectors. Wear sunscreen and UV-protected sunglasses. Practice safe sex.

BMI, body mass index; BSE, breast self-examination; CAD, coronary artery disease; DM, diabetes mellitus; STI, sexually transmitted infection; TSH, thyroid-stimulating hormone.

Information adapted from The National Women's Health Information Center (NWHIC). Available at http://www.4woman.gov and *Healthy People 2010.*

ommended for adults as well as children. Nurses collaborating with other health care providers must ensure the well-being of clients by following immunization recommendations. Figure 2.11 lists the 2005–2006 CDC recommendations for adult immunizations.

Questions to Ponder

1. How can you understand and respect the relational nature of women's health beliefs and health promotion behaviors?
2. How can you educate women on risk factors and promote improved health-seeking behaviors in women?
3. What culturally sensitive health promotion interventions can you implement in your nursing practice with women?

SUMMARY

- Health promotion for each woman is situated in a complex sociopolitical context. Health promotion strategies are an interdisciplinary activity, of which the nurse is a key professional team member. The focus of health promotion is based on the woman's own perspective.
- Health promotion includes health education, marketing the health message, lifestyle modification, engaging in social and environmental change, and encompassing the client's cultural values. In partnership with the woman, the nurse can support physical and mental health promotion strategies to improve health outcomes for the woman, her family, and the community.

(text continues on page 82)

Recommended Adult Immunization Schedule (by vaccine and age group)

United States, October 2005 - September 2006

Vaccine	Age: 19-49 years	50-64 years	65 years
Tetanus, diphtheria (Td)[1]*	1-dose booster every 10 years		
Measles, mumps, rubella (MMR)[2]*	1-2 doses	1-dose	
Varicella[3]*	2 doses: 0, 4-8 weeks	2 doses: 0, 4-8 weeks	
Vaccines below broken line are for selected populations			
Influenza[4]*	1 dose annually	1 dose annually	
Pneumococcal (polysaccharide)[5,6]	1-2 doses		1 dose
Hepatitis A[7]*	2 doses: 0, 6-12 months, or 0, 6-18 months		
Hepatitis B[8]*	3 doses: 0, 1-2 months, 4-6 months		
Meningococcal[9]	1 or more doses		

Note: These recommendations must be read along with the footnotes.
*Covered by the Vaccine Injury Compensation Program.

For all persons in this category who meet the age requirements and who lack evidence of immunity (e.g., lack documentation of vaccination or have no evidence of prior infection)

Recommended if some other risk factor is present (e.g., based on medical, occupational, lifestyle, or other infections)

This schedule indicates the recommended age groups and medical indications for routine administration of currently licensed vaccines for persons aged 19 years. Licensed combination vaccines may be used whenever any components of the combination are indicated and when the vaccine's other components are not contraindicated. For detailed recommendations, consult the manufacturers' package inserts and the complete statements from the ACIP (www.cdc.gov/nip/publications/acip-list.html).

Report all clinically significant postvaccination reactions to the Vaccine Adverse Event Reporting System (VAERS). Reporting forms and instructions on filing a VAERS report are available by telephone: 800-822-7967, or from the VAERS website at www.vaers.hhs.gov.

Information on how to file a Vaccine Injury Compensation Program claim is available at www.hrsa.gov/osp/vicp or by telephone: 800-338-2382. To file a claim for vaccine injury, contact the U.S. Court of Federal Claims, 717 Madison Place, N.W., Washington, D.C. 20005, telephone: 202-357-6400.

Additional information about the vaccines listed above and contraindications for vaccination is also available at www.cdc.gov/nip or from the CDC-INFO Contact Center at 800-CDC-INFO (232-4636) in English and Spanish, 24 hours a day, 7 days a week.

Recommended Adult Immunization Schedule, UNITED STATES, OCTOBER 2005–SEPTEMBER 2006

1. **Tetanus and Diphtheria (Td) vaccination.** Adults with uncertain histories of a complete primary vaccination series with diphtheria and tetanus toxoid-containing vaccines should receive a primary series using combined Td toxoid. A primary series for adults is 3 doses; administer the first 2 doses at least 4 weeks apart and the third dose 6–12 months after the second. Administer 1 dose if the person received the primary series and if the last vaccination was received ≥10 years previously. Consult ACIP statement for recommendations for administering Td as prophylaxis in wound management (www.cdc.gov/mmwr/preview/mmwrhtml/00041645.htm). The American College of Physicians Task Force on Adult Immunization supports a second option for Td use in adults: a single Td booster at age 50 years for persons who have completed the full pediatric series, including the teenage/young adult booster. A newly licensed tetanus-diphtheria-acellular pertussis vaccine is available for adults. ACIP recommendations for its use will be published.
2. **Measles, Mumps, Rubella (MMR) vaccination.** *Measles component:* adults born before 1957 can be considered immune to measles. Adults born during or after 1957 should receive ≥1 dose of MMR unless they have a medical contraindication, documentation of ≥1 dose, history of measles based on healthcare provider diagnosis, or laboratory evidence of immunity. A second dose of MMR is recommended for adults who 1) were recently exposed to measles or in an outbreak setting, 2) were previously vaccinated with killed measles vaccine, 3) were vaccinated with an unknown type of measles vaccine during 1963–1967, 4) are students in postsecondary educational institutions, 5) work in a healthcare facility, or 6) plan to travel internationally. Withhold MMR or other measles-containing vaccines from HIV-infected persons with severe immunosuppression. *Mumps component:* 1 dose of MMR vaccine should be adequate for protection for those born during or after 1957 who lack a history of mumps based on healthcare provider diagnosis or who lack laboratory evidence of immunity. *Rubella component:* administer 1 dose of MMR vaccine to women whose rubella vaccination history is unreliable or who lack laboratory evidence of immunity. For women of childbearing age, regardless of birth year, routinely determine rubella immunity and counsel women regarding congenital rubella syndrome. Do not vaccinate women who are pregnant or might become pregnant within 4 weeks of receiving the vaccine. Women who do not have evidence of immunity should receive MMR vaccine upon completion or termination of pregnancy and before discharge from the healthcare facility.
3. **Varicella vaccination.** Varicella vaccination is recommended for all adults without evidence of immunity to varicella. Special consideration should be given to those who 1) have close contact with persons at high risk for severe disease (healthcare workers and family contacts of immunocompromised persons) or 2) are at high risk for exposure or transmission (e.g., teachers of young children; child care employees; residents and staff members of institutional settings, including correctional institutions; college students; military personnel; adolescents and adults living in households with children; nonpregnant women of childbearing age; and international travelers). Evidence of immunity to varicella in adults includes any of the following: 1) documented age-appropriate varicella vaccination (i.e., receipt of 1 dose before age 13 years or receipt of 2 doses [administered at least 4 weeks apart] after age 13 years; 2) born in the United States before 1966; 3) history of varicella disease based on healthcare provider diagnosis or self- or parental report of typical varicella disease for non–U.S.-born persons born before 1966 and all persons born during 1996–1997 (for a patient reporting a history of an atypical, mild case, healthcare providers should seek either an epidemiologic link with a typical varicella case or evidence of laboratory confirmation, if it was performed at the time of acute disease); 4) history of herpes zoster based on healthcare provider diagnosis; or 5) laboratory evidence of immunity. Do not vaccinate women who are pregnant or might become pregnant within 4 weeks of receiving the vaccine. Assess pregnant women for evidence of varicella immunity. Women who do not have evidence of immunity should receive dose 1 of varicella vaccine upon completion or termination of pregnancy and before discharge from the healthcare facility. Dose 2 should be given 4–8 weeks after dose 1.
4. **Influenza vaccination.** *Medical indications:* chronic disorders of the cardiovascular or pulmonary systems, including asthma; chronic metabolic diseases, including diabetes mellitus, renal dysfunction, hemoglobinopathies, or immunosuppression (including immunosuppression caused by medications or by HIV); any condition (e.g., cognitive dysfunction, spinal cord injury, seizure disorder or other neuromuscular disorder) that compromises respiratory function or the handling of respiratory secretions or that can increase the risk of aspiration; and pregnancy during the influenza season. No data

FIGURE 2.11 Recommended Adult Immunization Schedule by Vaccine and Age Group, United States, October 2005–September 2006. (Courtesy of the Department of Health and Human Services Centers for Disease Control and Prevention.) Continued on page 81.

Recommended Adult Immunization Schedule (by vaccine and other indications)
United States, October 2005 - September 2006

Vaccine	Age: Pregnancy	Congenital immunodeficiency; leukemia[10]; lymphoma; generalized malignancy; cerebrospinal fluid leaks; therapy with alkylating agents, antimetabolites, radiation, or high-dose, long-term corticosteroids	Diabetes; heart disease; chronic pulmonary disease; chronic liver disease, including chronic alcoholism	Asplenia[10] (including elective splenectomy and terminal complement component deficiencies)	Kidney failure, end-stage renal disease, recipients of hemodialysis or clotting factor concentrates	Human immunodeficiency virus (HIV) infection[2,10]	Healthcare workers
Tetanus, diphtheria (Td)[1]*	1-dose booster every 10 years						
Measles, mumps, rubella (MMR)[2]*			1 or 2 doses				
Varicella[3]*			2 doses: 0, 4-8 weeks				2 doses
Influenza[4]*	1 dose annually			1 dose annually	1 dose annually		
Pneumococcal (polysaccharide)[5,6]	1-2 doses	1-2 doses					1-2 doses
Hepatitis A[7]*	2 doses: 0, 6-12 months, or 0, 6-18 months						
Hepatitis B[8]*	3 doses: 0, 1-2 months, 4-6 months			3 doses: 0, 1-2 months, 4-6 months			
Meningococcal[9]	1 dose			1 dose	1 dose		

Note: These recommendations must be read along with the footnotes.
*Covered by the Vaccine Injury Compensation Program.

- For all persons in this category who meet the age requirements and who lack evidence of immunity (e.g., lack documentation of vaccination or have no evidence of prior infection)
- Recommended if some other risk factor is present (e.g., based on medical, occupational, lifestyle, or other infections)
- Contraindicated

Approved by the Advisory Committee on Immunization Practices (ADIP), the American College of Obstetricians and Gynecologists (ACOG), and the American Academy of Family Physicians (AAFP)

exist on the risk for severe or complicated influenza disease among persons with asplenia; however, influenza is a risk factor for secondary bacterial infections that can cause severe disease among persons with asplenia. *Occupational indications:* healthcare workers and employees of long term-care and assisted living facilities. *Other indications:* residents of nursing homes and other long-term care and assisted living facilities; persons likely to transmit influenza to persons at high risk (i.e., in-home household contacts and caregivers of children birth through 23 months of age, or persons of all ages with high-risk conditions); and anyone who wishes to be vaccinated.

For healthy nonpregnant persons aged 5–49 years without high-risk conditions who are not contacts of severely immunocompromised persons in special care units, intranasally administered influenza vaccine (FluMist®) may be administered in lieu of inactivated vaccine.

5. **Pneumococcal polysaccharide vaccination.** *Medical indications:* chronic disorders of the pulmonary system (excluding asthma); cardiovascular diseases; diabetes mellitus; chronic liver diseases, including liver disease as a result of alcohol abuse (e.g., cirrhosis); chronic renal failure or nephrotic syndrome; functional or anatomic asplenia (e.g., sickle cell disease or splenectomy [if elective splenectomy is planned, vaccinate at least 2 weeks before surgery]); immunosuppressive conditions (e.g., congenital immunodeficiency, HIV infection [vaccinate as close to diagnosis as possible when CD4 cell counts are highest], leukemia, lymphoma, multiple myeloma, Hodgkin disease, generalized malignancy, organ or bone marrow transplantation); chemotherapy with alkylating agents, antimetabolites, or high-dose, long-term corticosteroids; and cochlear implants. *Other indications:* Alaska Natives and certain American Indian populations; residents of nursing homes and other long-term care facilities.
6. **Revaccination with pneumococcal polysaccharide vaccine.** One-time revaccination after 5 years for persons with chronic renal failure or nephrotic syndrome; functional or anatomic asplenia (e.g., sickle cell disease or splenectomy); immunosuppressive conditions (e.g., congenital immunodeficiency, HIV infection, leukemia, lymphoma, multiple myeloma, Hodgkin disease, generalized malignancy, organ or bone marrow transplantation); or chemotherapy with alkylating agents, antimetabolites, or high-dose, long-term corticosteroids. For persons aged ≥65 years, one-time revaccination if they were vaccinated ≥5 years previously and were aged <65 years at the time of primary vaccination.
7. **Hepatitis A vaccination.** *Medical indications:* persons with clotting factor disorders or chronic liver disease. *Behavioral indications:* men who have sex with men or users of illegal drugs. *Occupational indications:* persons working with hepatitis A virus (HAV)-infected primates or with HAV in a research laboratory setting. *Other indications:* persons traveling to or working in countries that have high or intermediate endemicity of hepatitis A (for list of countries, visit www.cdc.gov/travel/diseases.htm#hepa) as well as any person wishing to obtain immunity. Current vaccines should be given in a 2-dose series at either 0 and 6–12 months, or 0 and 6–18 months. If the combined hepatitis A and hepatitis B vaccine is used, administer 3 doses at 0, 1, and 6 months.
8. **Hepatitis B vaccination.** *Medical indications*: hemodialysis patients (use special formulation [40 μg/mL] or two 20-μg/mL doses) or patients who receive clotting factor concentrates. *Occupational indications:* healthcare workers and public-safety workers who have exposure to blood in the workplace; and persons in training in schools of medicine, dentistry, nursing, laboratory technology, and other allied health professions. *Behavioral indications:* injection-drug users; persons with more than one sex partner in the previous 6 months; persons with a recently acquired sexually transmitted disease (STD); and men who have sex with men. *Other indications:* household contacts and sex partners of persons with chronic hepatitis B virus (HBV) infection; clients and staff of institutions for the developmentally disabled; all clients of STD clinics; inmates of correctional facilities; or international travelers who will be in countries with high or intermediate prevalence of chronic HBV infection for >6 months (for list of countries, visit www.cdc.gov.travel/diseases.htm#hepa).
9. **Meningococcal vaccination.** *Medical indications:* adults with anatomic or functional asplenia, or terminal complement component deficiencies. *Other indications:* first-year college students living in dormitories; microbiologists who are routinely exposed to isolates of *Neisseria meningitidis;* military recruits; and persons who travel to or reside in countries in which meningococcal disease is hyperendemic or epidemic (e.g., the "meningitis belt" of sub-Saharan Africa during the dry season [Dec–June]), particularly if contact with the local populations will be prolonged. Vaccination is required by the government of Saudi Arabia for all travelers to Mecca during the annual Hajj. Meningococcal conjugate vaccine is preferred for adults meeting any of the above indications who are aged ≤55 years, although meningococcal polysaccharide vaccine (MPSV4) is an acceptable alternative. Revaccination after 5 years may be indicated for adults previously vaccinated with MPSV4 who remain at high risk for infection (e.g., persons residing in areas in which disease is epidemic).
10. **Selected conditions for which *Haemophilus influenzae* type b (Hib) vaccine may be used.** *Haemophilus influenzae* type b conjugate vaccines are licensed for children aged 6 weeks–71 months. No efficacy data are available on which to base a recommendation concerning use of Hib vaccine for older children and adults with the chronic conditions associated with an increased risk of Hib disease. However, studies suggest good immunogenicity in patients who have sickle cell disease, leukemia, or HIV infection, or have had splenectomies: administering vaccine to these patients is not contraindicated.

- The major U.S. public health epidemics, including heart disease, obesity, diabetes, substance abuse, and domestic violence, are all amenable to change through health promotion strategies. Nurses are in a leadership position to engage with the client in motivating and regulating health-promoting behaviors.
- Nurses should obtain specific health history data and perform assessment parameters to care for the woman based on her unique health needs.
- Health promotion issues and risk factors are embedded in cultural beliefs and barriers for women.
- Nurses should conduct physical examinations of women to identify normal and alterations in normal for women in relation to their stage of the life cycle.
- Nursing interventions for health promotion involve collaboration with multidisciplinary professionals to implement recommended traditional and complementary therapies.
- Evidence-based health screening guidelines and immunization recommendations should be implemented in care of women throughout their reproductive years.

REVIEW QUESTIONS

1. In developing a teaching plan for a woman who is to initiate an exercise program, the nurse emphasizes that people who are successful at integrating exercise into their routine find that
   A. focusing on a long-term goal is helpful.
   B. having an exercise partner helps with motivation.
   C. exercising alone helps them to focus on the process.
   D. doing the same exercise each day helps maintain consistency.
2. When designing an exercise program with a client, it is important to consider the client's
   A. basal metabolic rate.
   B. daily caloric and calcium intake.
   C. priorities in changing her appearance.
   D. preferences regarding the type of movement she enjoys.
3. When providing counseling to a client on avoiding osteoporosis, the nurse should include
   A. limiting alcoholic beverages.
   B. increasing proteins from nonanimal sources into the diet.
   C. exercising for short periods of time a few times a day.
   D. integrating non–weight-bearing exercises into the daily routine.
4. The nurse's teaching plan for a woman experiencing osteoporosis should include that an important source of dietary calcium is
   A. beef.
   B. chicken.
   C. fatty fish.
   D. fresh orange juice.
5. The nurse is reviewing the laboratory results of a number of clients before the beginning of the shift. Which of these women would be *least* likely to have iron-deficiency anemia?
   A. A 27-year-old primigravida woman
   B. A 40-year-old woman with menorrhagia
   C. A 54-year-old woman who is 2 years postmenopausal
   D. A 16-year-old woman who reached menarche 6 months earlier
6. The nurse is reviewing the health history of a woman who has come to the clinic complaining of a yeast infection. A risk factor for a yeast infection that the woman identified during the health history is that she
   A. has been diagnosed with osteopenia.
   B. has been breastfeeding her newborn.
   C. has difficulty controlling her diabetes.
   D. had a normal vaginal delivery 8 weeks earlier.
7. Which of the following statements, if made by an adolescent who has just received education by the nurse regarding health promotion strategies, would indicate that further education is needed?
   A. "I will participate in low-impact aerobic classes a few times a week."
   B. "I will make sure to eat or drink foods containing dietary calcium every day."
   C. "I will get my first Pap smear once I begin to have sex, regardless of my age."
   D. "I will perform breast self-examinations at the same time in my cycle every month."
8. When reviewing the health history of a client diagnosed with cervical carcinoma, the nurse notes that the most likely causative agent is
   A. *Candida albicans.*
   B. *Neisseria gonorrhoeae.*
   C. Herpes simplex virus 2.
   D. Human papillomavirus (HPV) 18.
9. Which of the following statements, if made by a client who has just received education by the nurse regarding risk factors associated with cervical cancer, indicates a need for additional teaching?
   A. "Oral contraceptives increase my risk for cervical cancer."
   B. "Having sex before I was 16 increases my risk for cervical cancer."
   C. "Multiple sexual partners increase my risk for cervical cancer."
   D. "I will quit cigarette smoking because it could cause cervical cancer."
10. When developing a teaching plan on breast self-examination (BSE), the nurse should include that the *best* time to perform BSE is

A. during ovulation.
B. a few days after ovulation.
C. on the first day of menstruation.
D. a few days after the beginning of menstruation.

Acknowledgment

The family nurse practitioner students who contributed to the development of this chapter are greatly appreciated: C. Bickett Cupp, C. Dufner, A. Dunn, L. Gambito, Y. Gazoni, J. Gray, V. Hamilton, T. Hedspeth, A. Hirsch, T. Markwalter, R. Grubbs, A. Schaefer, J. Shelton, J. Shepherd, E. Spiker, and W. Sweeney-Rodriguez.

REFERENCES

Allen, K., & Phillips, J. (1997). *Women's health across the lifespan.* Philadelphia: Lippincott Williams & Wilkins.

American Academy of Pediatrics. (1999). The role of the pediatrician in youth violence prevention in clinical practice and at the community level. *Pediatrics, 103*(1), 173–181.

American Cancer Society (2006). *ACS: Pap Test. The ACS recommends the following guidelines for early detection.* Retrieved May 24, 2006 from http://www.cancer.org/docroot/PED/content/PED_2_3X_Pap_Test.asp

American Diabetes Association (2006). *Checking Your Blood Glucose.* Retrieved May 24, 2006 from http://www.diabetes.org/type-2-diabetes/blood-glucose-checks.jsp.

American Heart Association (AHA). (2006a). *Women and cardiovascular disease.* Retrieved February 6, 2006, from http://www.americanheart.org/presenter.jhtml?identifier=1200011.

American Heart Association (AHA). (2006b). *Trans fat overview.* Retrieved February 6, 2006, from http://www.americanheart.org/presenter.jhtml?identifier=4776.

American Psychiatric Association (APA). (2000). *Diagnostic and statistical manual of mental disorders* (4th ed., text revision). Washington, DC: Author.

Angiogenesis Weekly. (2002, May 10). Glaucoma the leading cause of blindness among a sample of US Hispanics. Available at: http://80-web3.infotrac.galegroup.com.

Association of Women's Health, Obstetric, and Neonatal Nurses. (1998). *Standards and guidelines for professional nursing practice in the care of women and newborns* (5th ed.). Washington, DC: Author.

Barton, M., Harris, R., & Fletcher, S. (1999). Does this patient have breast cancer? The screening clinical breast examination: Should it be done? How? *Journal of the American Medical Association, 282*(13), 1270–1280.

Bazargan, M., Bazargan, S. H., Farooq, M., & Baker, R. S. (2004). Correlates of cervical cancer screening among underserved Hispanic and African-American women. *Preventive Medicine, 39*(3), 465–473.

Bell, R. A., Quandt, S. A., Spanler, J. G., & Case. L. D. (2002). Dietary calcium intake and supplement use among older African American, white, and Native American women in a rural southeastern community. *Journal of the American Dietetic Association, 102*(6).

Berg, A., Corresponding author for USPTF (2002). Screening for depression: Recommendations and rationale. *American Journal for Nurse Practitioners* 6(2), 27–31.

Bickley, L. S. (2007). *Bates' guide to physical examination and history taking* (9th ed.). Philadelphia: Lippincott Williams & Wilkins.

Bradlow, H. L., & Sepkovic, D. W. (2002). Diet and breast cancer. *Annals of the New York Academy of Sciences.* New York: New York Academy of Sciences.

Brewington, K. (2002, Aug. 21). Hispanics organize to fight diabetes. *Knight Ridder/Tribune News Service.* Available at: http://80-web3.infotrac.galegroup.com.

Buse, J. (1999). Overview of current therapeutic options in type 2 diabetes: Rational for combining oral agents with insulin. *Diabetes Care, 22*(Suppl. C), 65–70.

Carcio, H. (1999). *Advanced health assessment of women: Clinical skills and procedures.* Philadelphia: Lippincott Williams & Wilkins.

Cauffield, J. S., & Forbes, H. J. (1999). Dietary supplements used in the treatment of depression, anxiety, and sleep disorders. *Lippincott's Primary Care Practitioner, 3*(3), 290–304.

Center for Health Promotion (1997, June). *Proceedings from the International Workshop on Mental Health Promotion.* University of Toronto, Toronto, Canada.

Centers for Disease Control and Prevention (CDC). (2001). *Chronic diseases and their risk factors: The nation's leading causes of death.* Atlanta, GA: National Center for Chronic Disease Prevention and Health Promotion.

Centers for Disease Control and Prevention (CDC). (2002a). *Diabetes surveillance report.* Atlanta, GA: USDHHS. Retrieved October 14, 2002, from http://www.cdc.gov/diabetes/statistics/index.htm.

Centers for Disease Control and Prevention (CDC). (2002b). *National injury mortality statistics.* Atlanta, GA: USDHHS. Retrieved March 28, 2003, from http://www.cdc.gov/std/guidelines/index.htm.

Centers for Disease Control and Prevention (CDC). (2002c). Prevalence of overweight and obesity among adults: United States, 1999–2000. Atlanta, GA: USDHHS. Available at: http://www.hhs.gov.

Centers for Disease Control and Prevention (CDC). (2002d). *Sexually transmitted disease treatment guidelines.* Atlanta, GA: USDHHS. Retrieved September 1, 2002, from http://www.cdc.gov/std/guidelines/index.htm.

Centers for Disease Control and Prevention (CDC). (2004). *Sexually transmitted disease surveillance 2003.* Atlanta, GA: USDHHS.

Centers for Disease Control and Prevention, National Center for Chronic Disease Prevention and Health Promotion. Behavioral Risk Factor Surveillance Survey. Retrieved May 24, 2006 from http://www.cdc.gov/nccdphp/behavior.htm.

Centers for Disease Control and Prevention (CDC). (2006a). *Tobacco information and prevention source.* Atlanta, GA: Author. Retrieved February 6, 2006, from http://www.cdc.gov/tobacco/sgr/sgr_forwomen/factsheet_tobaccouse.htm.

Centers for Disease Control and Prevention (CDC). (2006b). *Overweight and obesity.* Atlanta, GA: Author. Retrieved February 2, 2006, from http://www.cdc.gov/nccdphp/dnpa/obesity/.

Chan, P., & Johnson, S. (2004). *Current clinical strategies. Gynecology and obstetrics, ACOG 2004 treatment guidelines.* Laguna Hills, CA: Current Clinical Strategies Publishing.

Cottrell, B. (2003). Vaginal douching. *Journal of Obstetric, Gynecologic, and Neonatal Nursing, 32*(1), 12–18.

Diabetes Control and Complications Trial Research Group. (1993). The effect of intensive treatment of diabetes on the development and progression of long-term complications of insulin-dependent diabetes mellitus. *New England Journal of Medicine 329,* 977–986.

Dingley, C., Roux, G., & Bush, H. (2000). Inner strength: A concept analysis. *Journal of Theory Construction and Testing, 4*(2), 30–35.

DiSaia, P. J., & Creasman, W. T. (2002). *Clinical gynecologic oncology* (rev. ed.). St. Louis: Mosby.

Erickson, J. D. (2002). Folic acid and prevention of spina bifida and anencephaly 10 years after the U.S. Public Health Service recommendation. *Morbidity and Mortality Weekly Report, 51,* s1–s3.

George, S. (2002). The menopause experience: A woman's perspective. *Journal of Obstetric, Gynecologic, and Neonatal Nursing, 31*(1), 77–85.

Grund, S. (2004). Iron-deficiency anemia. *Medline Plus.* Available at: http://www.nlm.nih.gov.

Grund, S. (2005). Cervical cancer. *Medline Plus.* Available at: http://www.nlm.nih.gov.

Grundy, S., Balady, G. J., Criqui, M. H., et al. (1997). Guide to primary prevention of cardiovascular diseases: A statement for healthcare professionals from the Task Force on Risk Reduction. American Heart Association Science Advisory and Coordinating Committee. *Circulation, 95,* 2329–2331.

Hawkins, J. W., Roberto-Nichols, D. M., & Stanley-Haney, J. L. (2000). *Protocols for nurse practitioners in gynecologic settings* (7th ed.). New York: The Tiresias Press.

International Food Information Council. (2002). *Healthy eating during pregnancy and folic acid.* Retrieved April 6, 2003, from http://www.ific.org.

JNC 7 (2003). *Seventh Report of the Joint National Committee on Prevention, Detection, Evaluation, and Treatment of High Blood Pressure (JNC 67).* Retrieved May 24, 2006 from http://www.nhlbi.nih.gov/guidelines/hypertension/jnc7full.htm

Kealy, M. (2003). Preventing obesity. *AWHONN Lifelines 7*(1), 24–27.

Knight, J., Sherritt, L., Shrier, L., Harris, S., & Chang, G. (2002). Validity of CRAFFT substance abuse screening test among adolescent clinic patients. *Archives of Pediatric Adolescent Medicine, 156,* 607–614.

Koffman, D. M., Bazzarre, T., Mosca, L., Redberg, R., Schmid, T., & Wattigney, W. A. (2001). An evaluation of *Choose to Move 1999:* An American Heart Association physical activity program for women. *Archives of Internal Medicine, 161,* 2193–2199.

Kotler, P., & Andreasen, A. R. (1987). *Strategic marketing for nonprofit organizations* (3rd ed.). Englewood Cliffs, NJ: Prentice-Hall International.

Kris-Etherton, P. M., Harris, W. S., Appel, L. J., for the American Heart Association. Nutrition Committee. (2002). Fish consumption, fish oil, omega-3 fatty acids, and cardiovascular disease. *Circulation, 106*(21), 2747–2757.

Lefebre, R. C., & Flora, J. A. (1988). Social marketing and public health intervention. *Health Education Quarterly, 15,* 299–315.

Liaschenko, J. (2002). Health promotion, moral harm, and the moral aims of nursing. In L. E. Young & V. Hayes (Eds.), *Transforming health promotion practice* (pp. 136–147). Philadelphia: F. A. Davis.

MacDonald, M. A. (2002). Health promotion: Historical, philosophical and theoretical perspectives. In L. E. Young & V. Hayes (Eds.), *Transforming health promotion practice* (pp. 22–45). Philadelphia: F. A. Davis.

March of Dimes (2006). *Quick Reference and Fact Sheet: Folic Acid.* Retrieved May 24, 2006 from http://search.marchofdimes.com/cgi-bin/MsmGo.exe?grab_id=54%page_id=4457472%query=folic+acid&hiword=ACIDITY+ACIDO+ACIDS+FOLICO+acid+folic+

Martin, A., Schaeffer, S., & Campbell, R. (1999). Managing alcohol-related problems in the primary care setting. *Nurse Practitioner, 23*(8), 14–39.

Moore, A. (2003). Menopausal health strategies: Focus on osteoporosis. *American Journal for Nurse Practitioners 7*(2), 9–21.

NANDA (North American Nursing Diagnosis Association International 2006). Retrieved May 24, 2006 from www.nanda.org.

National Center for Complementary and Alternative Medicine. (2006). *Get the facts: What is complementary and alternative medicine?* Bethesda, MD: Author. Retrieved February 2, 2006, from: http://nccam.nih.gov/health/whatiscam/.

National Institutes of Health. (1994, June 6–8). Optimal calcium intake. *NIH Consensus Statement, 12*(4), 1–31.

National Institutes of Health. (1996). Cervical cancer. *NIH Consensus Statement, 14*(1), 1–38.

National Osteoporosis Foundation. (2006a). *Fast facts on osteoporosis.* Retrieved February 6, 2006, from http://www.nof.org/osteoporosis/diseasefacts.htm.

National Osteoporosis Foundation. (2006b). *Osteoporosis prevention.* Retrieved February 6, 2006, from http://www.nof.org/prevention/index.htm.

National Women's Health Information Center (NWHIC). Health information for minority women and minority health report. Retrieved March 28, 2003, from http://www.4woman.gov/owh/pub/minority/index.htm.

Newcomb, M., Wyatt, G. E., Romero, G. J., Tucker, M.B., et al. (1998). Acculturation, sexual risk taking, and HIV health promotion among Latinas. *Journal of Counseling Psychology, 4*(45), 454.

Nicklas, T. (2003). Calcium intake trends and health consequences from childhood through adulthood. *Journal of the American College of Nutrition, 22*(5), 340–356.

Noble, J. (Ed.) (2001). *Textbook of primary care medicine* (3rd ed.). St. Louis: Mosby.

Pender, N. J. (1996). *Health promotion in nursing practice* (3rd ed.). Stamford, CT: Appleton & Lange.

Pittler, M. H., & Ernst, E. (2000). Efficacy of kava extract for treating anxiety: Systematic review and meta-analysis. *Journal of Clinical Psychopharmacology, 20*(1), 84–89.

Prochaska, J. O., & DiClemente, C. C. (1983). Stages and processes of self-change of smoking: Toward an integrative model of change. *Journal of Consulting Clinical Psychology, 51,* 390–395.

Prochaska, J. O., Velicer, W. F., Rossi, J. S., Goldstein, M. G., Marcus, B., Rakowski, W., Fiore, C., Harlow, L., Redding, C., Rosenbloom, D., & Rossi, S. (1994). Stages of change and decisional balance for 12 problem behaviors. *Health Psychology, 13,* 39–46.

Reasner, C. (2002). Aggressive control of type 2 diabetes using oral agents. *Clinician Reviews Supplement, Oct.,* 2–11.

Roux, G., Dingley, C., & Bush, H. (2002). Inner strength in women: Metasynthesis of qualitative findings in theory development. *Journal of Theory Construction and Testing 6*(1), 86–92.

Running, A., & Berndt, A. (2003). *Management guidelines for nurse practitioners.* Philadelphia: F. A. Davis.

Slattery, M. L., Boucher, K. M., Caan, B. J., Potter, J. D., & Ma, K. N. (1998). Eating patterns and risk of colon cancer. *American Journal of Epidemiology, 148*(1), 4–16.

Stekler, J., & Elmore, J. (2002). Cervical cancer screening. Who, when, why? *Clinical Advisor, 5*(10), 107–115.

Substance Abuse and Mental Health Services Administration of the United States Department of Health and Human Services. Retrieved October 18, 2002, from http://www.samhsa.gov.

Uphold, C. R., & Graham, M. V. (2003). *Clinical guidelines in family practice* (3rd ed.). Gainesville, FL: Barmarrae Books.

U.S. Department of Agriculture (USDA). (2006). Steps to a healthier you. Washington, DC: Author. Retrieved February 6, 2006, from http://www.mypyramid.gov/.

U.S. Department of Health and Human Services (USDHHS). (2000). *Healthy people 2010* (Conference ed., Vols. 1 and 2). Washington, DC: Author.

U.S. Department of Health and Human Services (USDHHS). (2002). Frequently asked questions about coronary artery disease. Available at: http://www.4woman.gov.

U.S. Preventive Services Task Force. (2002a). *Screening for breast cancer: Recommendations and rationale.* Rockville, MD: Agency for Healthcare Research and Quality. Available at: http://www.ahrq.gov.

U.S. Preventive Services Task Force. (2002b). Systematic evidence review for depression. *Screening for depression.* File Inventory, Systematic Evidence Review Number 6. AHRQ Publication No. 02-S002. Rockville, MD: Agency for Healthcare Research and Quality. Available at: http://www.ahrq.gov.

U.S. Department of Health and Human Services (USDHHS). (2005). *Health Disparities Experienced by Black or African Americans.* Retrieved May 24, 2006 from http://www.cdc.gov/mmwr/preview/mmwrhtml/mm5401a1.htm

Ward, J. (2002). Type 2 diabetes in children and adolescents. *Advance for Nurse Practitioners, 10*(2), 62–64.

Willinsky, C., & Pape, B. (2002). Mental health promotion. In L. E. Young & V. Hayes (Eds.), *Transforming health promotion practice* (pp. 162–173). Philadelphia: F. A. Davis.

Wing, P. R., & Phelan, S. (2005). Long-term weight loss maintenance. *American Journal of Clinical Nutrition, 82*(1 Suppl), 222S–225S.

World Health Organization (WHO). (2006a). *Frequently asked questions.* Retrieved February 2, 2006, from http://www.who.int/suggestions/faq/en/.

World Health Organization (WHO). (2006b). *Health promotion and education: About HPE.* Retrieved February 2, 2006, from http://w3.whosea.org/EN/Section1174/Section1458/Section2057.htm.

Writing Group for the Women's Health Initiative Investigators. (2002). Risks and benefits of estrogen plus progestin in healthy postmenopausal women: Principal results from the women's health initiative randomized controlled trial. *Journal of the American Medical Association, 288*(3).

Young, L. (2002). Transforming health promotion practice: Moving toward holistic care. In L. E. Young & V. Hayes (Eds.), *Transforming health promotion practice* (pp. 3–21). Philadelphia: F. A. Davis.

Youngkin, E. Q., & Davis, M. S. (2004). *Women's health: A primary care clinical guide* (3rd ed.). Stamford, CT: Appleton & Lange.

CHAPTER 3

Nutrition for Adolescent and Adult Women*

Sylvia Escott-Stump and Evelyn S. Farrior

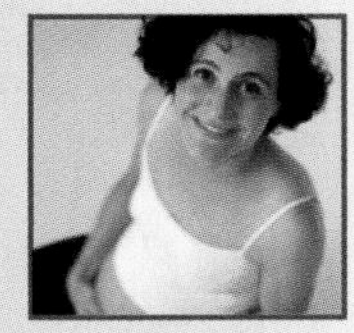

Sheila, 37 years old and in her third trimester of pregnancy, comes to the clinic for a routine visit. She is planning to breastfeed her newborn. During the interview, Sheila tells the nurse, "I've been trying to follow the nutritional suggestions for pregnancy that you gave me as best as I can, but I'm having trouble drinking enough milk."

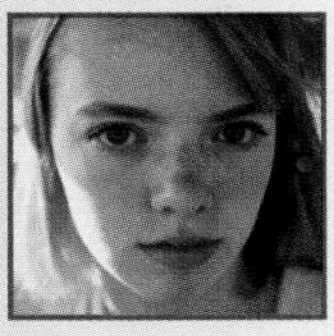

Betsy, 14 years old, is at the nurse practitioner's office for a checkup. Betsy is 5 feet, 6 inches tall and weighs 115 lbs; she started menstruating 3 months ago. Betsy mentions feeling uncomfortable with the changes in her body over the past year. "Every day, something new is happening," she says. "My hips and thighs are thicker than they used to be, and I'm still not used to having a chest!" During assessment of her diet habits, Betsy reports that she skips breakfast and doesn't like fish or vegetables. When the nurse asks why she doesn't eat breakfast, Betsy replies, "I don't want to get fat."

You will learn more about Sheila's and Betsy's care later. Nurses working with such clients need to understand the material in this chapter to promote solid nutrition and to address issues appropriately. Before beginning, consider these points:

- What information from these scenarios may pose concerns for each client's immediate and long-term health?
- How can nurses provide instruction that helps these clients develop and maintain solid dietary habits?
- What nutritional issues related to pregnancy and lactation are priorities in Sheila's case? What nutritional issues related to adolescence are priorities in Betsy's case?
- What external influences might be different for these clients? How might these influences affect their feelings about food?
- How can nurses lead by example relative to nutrition?

*Portions of this chapter have been derived from Escott-Stump, S. (2002). *Nutrition and diagnosis-related care* (5th ed.). Philadelphia: Lippincott Williams & Wilkins.

LEARNING OBJECTIVES

On completion of this chapter, the reader should be able to:

- Explain why nurses need to understand nutrition and modifications necessary for different age groups and life circumstances.
- Describe the roles of various nutrients in the maintenance of overall health.
- Identify components of nutritional assessment for women.
- Discuss individual factors that can influence food selection and how nurses can work with clients to incorporate unique preferences.
- Identify special nutritional needs and adjustments required in pregnancy, lactation, and adolescence.
- Describe collaborative care strategies related to nutrition and the pregnant teen.
- Discuss nutritional concerns of special interest to adult and older adult women.

KEY TERMS

coenzyme
cofactor
complementary proteins
complete proteins
fortified
glycemic index
incomplete proteins
macronutrients
macrosomia
nutrient density
nutritional assessment
nutritional screening
phytochemicals
pica
vegan

Food can supply the nutrients necessary to build and to maintain healthy bodies. In the United States and Canada, a generous food supply, the proliferation of restaurants and packaged and fast foods, and food-related marketing and advertising have contributed to an overabundance of some nutrients and general overconsumption (Guthrie, Lin, & Frazao, 2002; Kant & Graubard, 2004). Consequently, many women suffer from imbalanced nutrient intake (Bartley, Underwood, & Deckelbaum, 2005). Another problem is the growing number of women who are overweight or obese and the subsequent chronic diseases related to these states (Freedman et al., 2006; Li et al., 2006).

This chapter emphasizes nutritional information and strategies to promote women's health and to assist with dietary management at various developmental stages. It reviews the function, recommended intake, sources, and consequences of overconsumption or underconsumption of each major nutrient. It presents how nurses can assess nutritional status and assist clients to make food choices appropriate for their circumstances. Because of the correlation between solid nutrition and positive gestational and postpartal outcomes, this chapter contains detailed sections on dietary adjustments and considerations related to pregnancy and lactation. (A comprehensive exploration of newborn nutrition is found in Chapter 21.) It also explores nutritional considerations for adolescent, adult, and older adult females.

QUOTE 3-1

"Food = joy . . . guilt . . . anger . . . pain . . . nurturing . . . friendship . . . hatred . . . the way you look and feel. Food = everything you can imagine."

Susan Powter

NUTRIENTS

For nutritional counseling and advice to be effective, nurses need to work as partners with their clients. Nurses can facilitate women's involvement by carefully assessing dietary needs and preferences, involving them in meal planning, answering questions, and giving thorough explanations of the reasons for nutritional recommendations (Fig. 3.1).

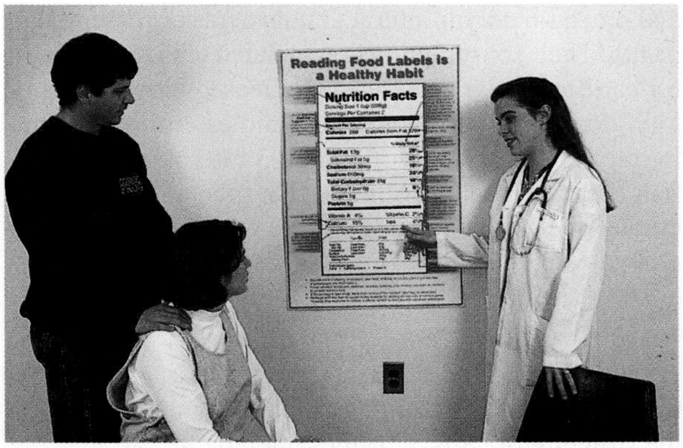

FIGURE 3.1 Involving the client in nutrition and diet planning will enhance the chances for successful outcomes.

To do these things effectively, nurses need general knowledge of each nutrient's contribution to health. Additionally, a baseline familiarity with nutrients and their functions is essential when a client's circumstances dictate a need for dietary changes. Scientists work continually to delineate nutrient requirements for specific groups based on age, sex, and race. The task is daunting because each person is unique and has individualized nutrient requirements. Recommendations for optimal nutrient intakes change as research reveals new information. Health professionals should keep abreast of changes as they happen.

The Institute of Medicine (IOM, 1997, 2000a, 2000b, 2001, 2002) has published recommended Dietary Reference Intakes (DRIs) for nutrients to promote health and prevent chronic disease in most people. The DRIs come in several forms, the definitions of which are summarized in Box 3.1.

● **BOX 3.1 Definitions of Dietary Reference Intakes**

- *Recommended dietary allowance (RDA):* The average daily dietary nutrient intake level that meets the nutrient requirement for nearly all (97%–98%) healthy people of a particular life stage and gender.
- *Adequate intake (AI):* The recommended average daily intake level based on observed or experimentally determined approximations of nutrient intake by a group (or groups) of apparently healthy people; assumed to be adequate and used when an RDA cannot be determined.
- *Tolerable upper intake level (UL):* The highest average daily nutrient intake level likely to pose no risk for adverse effects to almost all people. As intake rises above the UL, the potential for adverse effects may increase.
- *Estimated average requirement (EAR):* The average daily nutrient intake level estimated to meet the requirement of half the healthy people of a particular life stage and gender.
- *Estimated energy requirement (EER):* The average dietary energy intake predicted to maintain energy balance in a healthy adult of a defined age, gender, weight, height, and level of physical activity. In children and pregnant and lactating women, the EER includes the needs associated with the deposition of tissues or the secretion of milk at rates consistent with good health.

From Institute of Medicine. (2002). Dietary reference intakes for energy, carbohydrate, fiber, fat, fatty acids, cholesterol, protein, and amino acids. Retrieved February 7, 2006, from http://www.iom.edu.

Macronutrients

Macronutrients are those nutrients that provide energy: carbohydrates, fats, and proteins (Table 3.1). The recommended distribution for adults is for 45% to 65% of total calories to come from carbohydrates, 20% to 35% to come from fat, and 10% to 35% to come from protein (IOM, 2002).

Overconsumption of macronutrients and lack of exercise frequently are associated with increased risk for such chronic diseases as obesity, coronary heart disease, diabetes, hypertension, and cancer (Freedman et al., 2006; Li et al., 2006; Tsai, Donnelly, & Wendt, 2006). An overall public health goal is to decrease the risk for such diseases (U.S. Department of Health and Human Services [USDHHS], 2000). When assisting clients with weight management, nurses should emphasize the need to balance the total number of calories consumed and expended. The amount of calories and duration or frequency of exercise can be adjusted to promote weight loss or gain. See Chapter 2 for more discussion.

Carbohydrates

Sources of carbohydrates include fruits, vegetables, breads, pasta, cereals, and grains. The minimum intake level for adolescents and adults is 130 g/day (IOM, 2002).

Carbohydrates come in various forms, the most common of which are sugar, starch, and fiber (Harvard School of Public Health, 2005). The digestive system breaks down sugar and starch into single molecules and converts them to glucose (blood sugar), which the body's cells use for energy. Fiber is different because the digestive system cannot break it down, and it passes through the body undigested (Harvard School of Public Health, 2005). Fiber helps prevent constipation and decrease blood glucose and cholesterol levels (Brown et al., 1999; McKeown et al., 2002; Pereira et al., 2004). Recommended intake of total fiber is 25 g/day for women younger than 50 years and 21 g/day for women 50 years or older (IOM, 2002). The recommendation for girls 9 to 18 years is 26 g/day (IOM, 2002).

Recently, low-carbohydrate diets have been a trend for weight loss; their effectiveness over low-fat, reduced-calorie, and other types of diets remains under investigation (Volpe, 2006). Current explorations related to carbohydrates are focusing on **glycemic index,** or the

● **TABLE 3.1 Dietary Reference Intakes: Macronutrients for Adolescent and Adult Females**

NUTRIENT	LIFE STAGE GROUP	RDA OR AI
Carbohydrate: total digestible	9 to >70 y	**130**
	Pregnancy	**175**
	Lactation	**210**
Total fiber	9 to 18 y	26*
	19 to 50 y	25*
	51 to >70 y	21*
	Pregnancy	28*
	Lactation	29*
Total fat	9 to 18 y	25–35
	19 to >70 y	20–35
	Pregnancy and lactation	20–35
n-6 Polyunsaturated fatty acids	9 to 13 y	10*
	14 to 18 y	11*
	19 to 50 y	17*
	51 to >70 y	14*
	Pregnancy and lactation	13*
n-3 Polyunsaturated fatty acids	9 to 13 y	1.0*
	14 to >70 y	1.1*
	Pregnancy	1.4*
	Lactation	1.3*
Protein and amino acids	9 to 13 y	**34**
	14 to >70 y	**46**
	Pregnancy and lactation	**71**

Bold, recommended daily allowance (RDA); *, adequate intake (AI); Adapted from *Dietary Reference Intakes for Energy, Carbohydrate, Fiber, Fat, Fatty Acids, Cholesterol, Protein, and Amino Acids.* (2002). Retrieved December 28, 2004, from http://www.iom.edu/Object.File/Master/7/300/0.pdf.

measure of how quickly and how high blood sugar increases after a certain food is eaten (Jenkins, Kendall, Augustin, et al., 2002). Diets with many high-glycemic-index foods (eg, white bread, potatoes) are linked to increased risks for diabetes and heart disease (Liu & Willett, 2002; Pereira & Liu, 2003; Schulze et al., 2004; Willett, Manson, & Liu, 2002). Other factors that influence glycemic index include fiber, fat, and acid contents; ripeness; and type of starch contained (Harvard School of Public Health, 2005). The use of glycemic index is controversial because there are so many variables.

Fat

Fat is a concentrated source of energy and comes in several forms: saturated, monounsaturated, trans, polyunsaturated, and cholesterol. High intakes of foods with saturated and trans fats and cholesterol are associated with increased health risks (Harvard School of Public Health, 2005).

Polyunsaturated fatty acids can be subdivided further based on the location of their double bonds. Omega-3 and omega-6 polyunsaturated fatty acids are essential to health. Their consumption is associated with reduced risk for cardiovascular disease and increased blood levels of high-density lipoprotein (HDL) cholesterol (good cholesterol). Food sources of omega-3 fatty acids are fatty fish (salmon, tuna, sardines), fish oils, and some vegetable oils (eg, canola, soy, flax). Food sources of omega-6 fatty acids are nuts, seeds, and vegetable oils.

Proteins

Proteins and their components, amino acids, are essential for building and maintaining the body. Amino acids form the structure of cells, enzymes, membrane carriers, and hormones. Recommended daily protein intake is 0.8 g/kg body weight for adults, 1.1 g/kg body weight during pregnancy and lactation, and a level that correlates with growth needs in children and teens (IOM, 2002). The newest recommendations add age-based levels for each of the nine essential amino acids and scoring procedures to account for protein quality (IOM, 2002).

Sources of **complete proteins** (foods that provide all nine essential amino acids) are animal foods: meat, poultry, fish, eggs, milk, cheese, and yogurt. Combinations of **incomplete proteins** (foods lacking one or more of the nine essential amino acids) can be selected to meet complete protein needs. Examples of foods with incomplete proteins are legumes, grains, nuts, seeds, and vegetables.

Micronutrients

Vitamins and minerals are considered micronutrients (Craven & Hirnle, 2007). Vitamins help regulate carbohydrate, fat, and protein metabolism and other reactions that maintain body tissues. Minerals make up body materials and also assist with internal body processes.

Water-Soluble Vitamins

Water-soluble vitamins are eliminated with body fluids, not stored to any extent, and require daily replacement. Consequently, their average intakes over several days should meet the recommended level to avoid depletion. They include biotin, choline, folate, niacin, pantothenic acid, riboflavin, thiamin, B_6, B_{12}, and C. See Table 3.2.

Biotin and Choline. Two vitamins with emerging evidence to support requirements are biotin and choline. *Biotin* is a **coenzyme** (a small organic molecule that increases enzyme activity) in the synthesis of fat, glycogen, and amino acids. *Choline* is a precursor for acetylcholine, phospholipids, and betaine. An intake level was established in 2001. Because adverse effects from high intake are possible, a upper limit (UL) for choline has been established (IOM, 2000a). Meats, especially liver, provide both biotin and choline.

Folate. *Folate,* an important coenzyme in nucleic and amino acid metabolism, is required to prevent

TABLE 3.2 Dietary Reference Intakes: Water-Soluble Vitamins for Adolescent and Adult Females

NUTRIENT	LIFE STAGE GROUP	RDA OR AI
Biotin		(μg/d)
	9 to 13 y	20*
	14 to 18 y	25*
	19 to >70 y	30*
	Pregnancy	30*
	Lactation	35*
Choline		(mg/d)
	9 to 13 y	375*
	14 to 18 y	400*
	19 to >70 y	425*
	Pregnancy	450*
	Lactation	550*
Folate		(μg/d)
	9 to 13 y	**300**
	14 to >70 y	**400**
	Pregnancy	**600**
	Lactation	**500**
Niacin		(mg/d)
	9 to 13 y	**12**
	14 to >70 y	**14**
	Pregnancy	**18**
	Lactation	**17**
Pantothenic acid		(mg/d)
	9 to 13 y	4*
	14 to >70 y	5*
	Pregnancy	6*
	Lactation	7*
Riboflavin (vitamin B_2)		(mg/d)
	9 to 13 y	**0.9**
	14 to 18 y	**1.0**
	19 to >70 y	**1.1**
	Pregnancy	**1.4**
	Lactation	**1.6**
Thiamin (vitamin B_1)		(mg/d)
	9 to 13 y	**0.9**
	14 to 18 y	**1.0**
	19 to >70 y	**1.1**
	Pregnancy and lactation	**1.4**
Vitamin B_6		(mg/d)
	9 to 13 y	**1.0**
	14 to 18 y	**1.2**
	19 to 50 y	**1.3**
	51 to >70 y	**1.5**
	Pregnancy	**1.9**
	Lactation	**2.0**
Vitamin B_{12}		(μg/d)
	9 to 13 y	**1.8**
	14 to >70 y	**2.4**
	Pregnancy	**2.6**
	Lactation	**2.8**
Vitamin C		(mg/d)
	9 to 13 y	**45**
	14 to 18 y	**65**
	19 to >70 y	**75**
	Pregnancy	
	≤ 18 y	**80**
	19 to 50 y	**85**
	Lactation	
	≤ 18 y	**115**
	19 to 50 y	**120**

Bold, recommended daily allowance; *, adequate intake (AI).

From Institute of Medicine (IOM). (2001). Dietary reference intakes for vitamin A, vitamin K, arsenic, boron, chromium, copper, iodine, iron, manganese, molybdenum, nickel, silicon, vanadium, and zinc. Retrieved July 30, 2003, from http://www.iom.edu; IOM. (2000a). Dietary reference intakes for vitamin C, vitamin E, selenium, and carotenoids. Retrieved February 8, 2006, from http://www.iom.edu.; IOM. (2000b). Dietary reference intakes for thiamin, riboflavin, niacin, vitamin B6, folate, vitamin B12, pantothenic acid, biotin, and choline. Retrieved July 30, 2003, from http://www.iom.edu; and IOM. (1997). Dietary reference intakes for calcium, phosphorous, magnesium, vitamin D, and fluoride. Retrieved July 30, 2003, from http://www.iom.edu.

megaloblastic anemia. In addition, neural tube defects in newborns are prevented when women enter pregnancy with adequate folate levels (see Chap. 11). The recommended dietary allowance (RDA) for folate is 400 μg for women of childbearing age (IOM, 2000a). The recommendation increases to 600 μg for pregnant women and 500 μg for lactating women (IOM, 2000a).

Folate typically is present in small amounts in foods; it often is removed during processing. Thus, folate usually is added to foods to prevent deficiencies or improve nutrient balance. Sources of folate are **fortified** (nutrient-added) cereals, grains, dark green leafy vegetables, and orange juice.

Niacin and Pantothenic Acid. *Niacin* (vitamin B_3) is required for the oxidation and reduction reactions of energy metabolism; thus, niacin requirements are related directly to total energy intake, as reflected in the RDAs for each age group and sex (IOM, 2000a). A UL has been established because high intakes cause flushing and gastrointestinal distress (IOM, 2000a). Sources include meats, fish, poultry, and enriched or whole grains.

Pantothenic acid functions as a coenzyme in fatty acid metabolism. A variety of foods provide pantothenic acid: chicken, beef, potatoes, oats, cereals, tomato, liver, egg, broccoli, and whole grains.

Other B Vitamins. *Riboflavin (vitamin B_2)* functions as a coenzyme in many oxidation and reduction reactions.

Food sources are organ meats, milk, breads, and fortified cereals. *Thiamin (vitamin B_1)* functions as a coenzyme in carbohydrate and branched-chain amino acid metabolism. Fortified and whole-grain foods provide this nutrient.

Vitamin B_6 functions in amino acid, glycogen, and sphingoid base metabolism. Foods that contain B_6 are fortified cereals, organ meats, and fortified soy-based meat substitutes. *Cobalamin (vitamin B_{12})*, an important coenzyme in nucleic and amino acid metabolism, helps prevent megaloblastic anemia. Sources include meat, fish, poultry, and fortified cereals. Supplements of B_{12} may be prescribed for those who do not eat meat, as well as those older than 50 years, who may experience decreased absorption of the nutrient.

Vitamin C. *Vitamin C* (ascorbic acid) functions as an antioxidant and in reactions that require reduced copper or iron. A UL has been established because excess intake of vitamin C can cause gastrointestinal distress, kidney stones, and excess iron absorption (IOM, 2000b). The need for vitamin C increases in clients who smoke (IOM, 2000b). Citrus fruits, tomatoes, potatoes, Brussels sprouts, cauliflower, broccoli, strawberries, cabbage, and spinach are sources.

Fat-Soluble Vitamins

Fat-soluble vitamins are stored in the body. Thus, inadequate intakes present later than those of water-soluble vitamins. At the same time, the danger of toxicity increases. The fat-soluble vitamins are A, D, E, and K. See Table 3.3.

Vitamin A. *Vitamin A* is required for vision, gene expression, reproduction, embryonic development, and immune function. Good sources of vitamin A are liver, dairy products, and fish. A UL is based on the danger of teratogenic effects and liver toxicity, mainly from preformed vitamin A (IOM, 2001). Carotene, the precursor form, is considered safe. Dark-colored and leafy vegetables provide carotene.

Vitamin D. *Vitamin D* (calciferol) functions in calcium and phosphorus metabolism. People with adequate sunlight exposure convert a precursor compound in skin to this vitamin. Sunlight exposure can substitute for dietary intake. Food sources of vitamin D are fish liver oil, fatty fish, fortified milk products, and fortified cereals.

Vitamin E. *Vitamin E* (α-tocopherol) functions as an antioxidant. Toxicity is related to overuse of supplements, not overconsumption of food (Henry & Schalch, 2005). Vegetable oils, whole grains, nuts, creamy salad dressings, and meats are food sources of vitamin E.

Vitamin K. *Vitamin K* functions as a coenzyme in protein synthesis related to blood clotting and bone metabolism. For those taking anticoagulant therapy, daily intake of vitamin K from all sources should remain constant. Inconsistent intake alters blood-clotting time, which can have adverse effects (Aschenbrenner & Venable, 2006). Foods that provide vitamin K are green vegetables, plant oils, and margarine.

TABLE 3.3 Dietary Reference Intakes: Fat-Soluble Vitamins for Adolescent and Adult Females

NUTRIENT	LIFE STAGE GROUP	RDA OR AI
Vitamin A		(μg/d)
	9 to 13 y	**600**
	14 to >70 y	**700**
	Pregnancy	
	≤18 y	**750**
	19 to 50 y	**770**
	Lactation	
	≤18 y	**1200**
	19 to 50 y	**1300**
Vitamin D		(μg/d)
	9 to 50 y	5*
	51 to 70 y	10*
	>70 y	15*
	Pregnancy and lactation	5*
Vitamin E	9 to 13 y	**11**
	14 to > 70 y	**15**
	Pregnancy	**15**
	Lactation	**19**
Vitamin K		(μg/d)
	9 to 13 y	60*
	14 to 18 y	75*
	19 to >70 y	90*
	Pregnancy and lactation	
	≤ 18 y	75*
	19 to 50 y	90*

Bold, recommended daily allowance (RDA); *, adequate intake (AI).

From Institute of Medicine (IOM) (2001). Dietary reference intakes for vitamin A, vitamin K, arsenic, boron, chromium, copper, iodine, iron, manganese, molybdenum, nickel, silicon, vanadium, and zinc. Retrieved July 30, 2003, from http://www.iom.edu; IOM. (2000a). Dietary reference intakes for vitamin C, vitamin E, selenium, and carotenoids. Retrieved February 8, 2006, from http://www.iom.edu.; IOM. (2000b). Dietary reference intakes for thiamin, riboflavin, niacin, vitamin B6, folate, vitamin B12, pantothenic acid, biotin, and choline. Retrieved July 30, 2003, from http://www.iom.edu; and IOM. (1997). Dietary reference intakes for calcium, phosphorous, magnesium, vitamin D, and fluoride. Retrieved July 30, 2003, from http://www.iom.edu.

Minerals

Minerals can be subclassified based on the quantity needed in the body (Table 3.4). Macrominerals are required in large amounts and generally make up body structures. Microminerals are needed in small amounts and serve as **cofactors** (small inorganic or organic substances that work with enzymes to promote chemical re-

TABLE 3.4 Dietary Reference Intakes: Minerals for Adolescent and Adult Females

NUTRIENT	LIFE STAGE GROUP	RDA OR AI
Calcium		(mg/d)
	9 to 13 y	1,300
	19 to 50 y	1,000
	51 y or older	1,200
	Pregnancy and lactation	
	≤ 18 y	1,300
	19 to 50 y	1,000
Phosphorous		(mg/d)
	9 to 18 y	1,250
	19 to > 70 y	700
	Pregnancy and lactation	
	≤ 18 y	1,250
	19 to 50 y	700
Magnesium	9 to 13 y	240
	14 to 18 y	360
	19 to 30 y	310
	31 to > 70 y	320
	Pregnancy	
	≤ 18 y	400
	19 to 30 y	350
	30 to 50 y	360
	Lactation	
	≤ 18 y	360
	19 to 30 y	310
	30 to 50 y	320
Iron		(mg/d)
	9 to 13 y	8
	14 to 18 y	15
	19 to 50 y	18
	51 to >70 y	8
	Pregnancy	
	≤18 to 50 y	27
	Lactation	
	≤18 y	10
	19 to 50 y	9
Iodine		(µg/d)
	9 to 13 y	120
	14 to >70 y	150
	Pregnancy	220
	Lactation	290
Zinc		(mg/d)
	9 to 13 y	8
	14 to 18 y	9
	19 to >70 y	8
	Pregnancy	
	≤18 y	12
	19 to 50 y	11
	Lactation	
	≤18 y	13
	19 to 50 y	12

Bold, recommended daily allowance (RDA); *, adequate intake (AI).

From Institute of Medicine (IOM). (2001). Dietary reference intakes for vitamin A, vitamin K, arsenic, boron, chromium, copper, iodine, iron, manganese, molybdenum, nickel, silicon, vanadium, and zinc. Retrieved July 30, 2003, from http://www.iom.edu; IOM. (2000a). Dietary reference intakes for vitamin C, vitamin E, selenium, and carotenoids. Retrieved February 8, 2006, from http://www.iom.edu.; IOM. (2000b). Dietary reference intakes for thiamin, riboflavin, niacin, vitamin B6, folate, vitamin B12, pantothenic acid, biotin, and choline. Retrieved July 30, 2003, from http://www.iom.edu; and IOM. (1997). Dietary reference intakes for calcium, phosphorous, magnesium, vitamin D, and fluoride. Retrieved July 30, 2003, from http://www.iom.edu.

actions). The body of knowledge about some of these elements is evolving.

Macrominerals. *Calcium* functions in blood clotting, muscle contraction, nerve transmission, and bone and tooth formation. Overconsumption potentially can cause kidney stones, hypercalcemia, milk alkali syndrome, and renal insufficiency. Underconsumption is largely responsible for osteoporosis in women (see Chaps. 2 and 24). Food sources of calcium are dairy products (milk, cheese, and yogurt), corn tortillas, calcium-set tofu, Chinese cabbage, kale, and broccoli.

Phosphorus plays a vital role in acid–base balance, energy transfer, and nucleotide synthesis. Foods that provide phosphorous include dairy products, meat, eggs, and some cereals and grains.

Sodium regulates extracellular fluid volume, helps maintain acid–base balance, and functions in nerve transmission and muscle contraction. The RDA for healthy people 19 to 50 years is 1.5 g/day (IOM, 2004). Many processed foods supply sodium. Overconsumption is more common than underconsumption (IOM, 2004).

Potassium regulates intracellular fluid volume, functions in nerve transmission and muscle contraction, and regulates heartbeat. This element is important in prevention of hypertension. The adult RDA is 4.7 g/day (IOM, 2004). Potassium is found in fresh fruits and vegetables.

Chloride is the major anion in extracellular fluids. With sodium and potassium, it functions to maintain electrolyte balance. Chloride is part of the acid in gastric juice. Salt or sodium chloride is the main food source. The RDA is 2.3 g/day (IOM, 2004).

Sulfur functions as part of the amino acids methionine and cysteine and as part of thiamin. A recommended intake has not been established (IOM, 2004).

Microminerals. *Chromium* helps maintain normal blood glucose levels. An adequate intake (AI) is given, but no UL has been set, even though excessive consumption can lead to chronic renal failure (IOM, 2002). Meat, fish, poultry, and some cereals are food sources of chromium.

Copper is a component of enzymes in iron metabolism. Intakes above the UL can lead to gastrointestinal distress and liver damage (IOM, 2001). Organ meats, seafood, nuts, seeds, wheat bran cereals, whole grains, and cocoa are sources.

Fluoride hardens tooth enamel and stimulates new bone formation. Excessive intake can cause fluorosis of the skeleton and tooth enamel. Fluoridated water, beverages made with fluoridated water, and marine fish are sources.

Iodine regulates metabolism through production of thyroid hormone. Excessive intakes can lead to elevated thyroid-stimulating hormone (TSH) concentrations. Food sources are iodized salt, seafood, and processed foods with iodine added.

Iron is an essential component of hemoglobin and numerous enzymes. Anemia can result from an iron deficiency. Vegetarian diets do not provide iron in its most absorbable form; thus, vegetarians need approximately twice the RDA for iron (Craig, 1994). Excessive intakes of iron can lead to gastrointestinal distress, iron overload, or both. Meat and poultry provide the most absorbable (heme) form. Fruits, vegetables, and fortified grain products provide less absorbable (nonheme) sources.

Magnesium is a cofactor in some enzyme systems. The UL applies to supplemental forms only. Green leafy vegetables, whole grains, nuts, meat, starches, and milk are food sources.

Manganese functions in bone formation and as a cofactor with enzymes required for amino acid, cholesterol, and carbohydrate metabolism. The UL is set to decrease the possibility of elevated blood concentrations and neurotoxicity. Nuts, legumes, tea, and whole grains are the food sources.

Molybdenum is a required cofactor for catabolic reactions involving sulfur amino acids, purines, and pyridines. Legumes, grains, and nuts supply this element.

Selenium functions as an antioxidant, to regulate thyroid hormone action, and to maintain the reduction/oxidation status of vitamin C and other molecules. The best food sources are organ meats, seafood, and plants grown in soil that contains selenium.

Zinc is a component of enzyme systems and specific proteins that regulate gene expression. Fortified cereals, red meat, and some seafood are food sources. Vegetarians, are at risk for deficiency.

Several elements are listed in the DRIs as having no known biologic function in humans (IOM, 2002). Those elements are *arsenic, boron, nickel, silicon,* and *vanadium.* Because high intakes pose a danger of adverse effects, ULs have been set for boron, nickel, and vanadium (IOM, 2002).

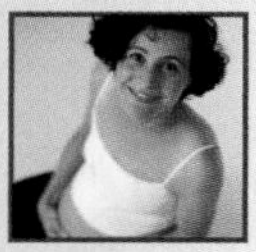

Consider Sheila, the 37-year-old woman in her third trimester of pregnancy. What if Sheila were a vegetarian? What specific nutrients might be inadequate in her diet?

NUTRITIONAL ASSESSMENT

Morbidity and mortality are related closely to behavioral choices: eating habits, exercise, smoking, alcohol consumption, and stress. Choosing a healthy diet can reduce the risk for chronic disease. To successfully address clients' health needs, nurses should complete a **nutritional assessment.** In such an assessment, the health care provider evaluates general state of health, educational background, weight history, and current body mass index (BMI) (see Chap. 2). A nutritionally oriented health history and physical examination are effective tools for identifying real or potential problems (Assessment Tool 3.1). Chronic problems with nausea, vomiting, diarrhea, constipation, edema, or anemia should cause concern and require more investigation. Findings may warrant laboratory testing or referrals to specialists to rule out conditions, such as eating disorders or cancer, that require intervention.

Activity and exercise patterns affect overall nutritional status. Many people in the United States and Canada assume that they lead a moderately active lifestyle; however, their usual patterns are actually sedentary. Numerous software programs are available by which a person can complete a self-assessment of dietary intake and exercise patterns, thereby determining an effective course of action to improve health status. Box 3.2 provides some general guidelines related to what types of activity qualify as very light, light, moderate, or heavy.

QUOTE 3-2

"Walking is the very best exercise. Habituate yourself to walk very far."

Thomas Jefferson

Assessing Dietary Intake

A **nutritional screening** helps to identify risk factors that can be ameliorated through appropriate nutritional counseling. Once problems are identified, the diet can be adjusted to prevent or decrease the likelihood of later complications. See Research Highlight 3.1.

● ASSESSMENT TOOL 3.1 Adult Nutritional Assessment Form

Name: **Medical Record:**

Date of Birth: **Age:** **Gender:**

Physician:

Date of Assessment:

Ethnic or Cultural Background:

Notes About Family Involvement:

Current Medical Diagnoses:

Prior Medical History:

Weight Record:

Height: Current weight: Usual weight:

Recent weight changes:

Possible causes:

Occupation:

Activity level: Sedentary_____ Moderately Active______ Very Active_________

NOTED PROBLEMS (CHECK ALL THAT APPLY)

Chewing: **Swallowing:** **Vision:** **Hearing:** **Ambulation:**

Feeding Self: **Anorexia:** **Chronic Vomiting:** **Chronic Diarrhea (over 5 days):**

Food Allergies: **Foods Not Tolerated:**

Current Diet Prescribed: **How Long?**

Snacks between meals? (If yes, list what and when)

Relevant Laboratory Values:

Glucose: **BUN:** **Albumin:**

Other:

Medications with Potential Nutrient Interactions (laxatives, diuretics, insulin, coumadin, etc.):

Other:

Regular Use of Vitamins/Minerals (list):

Regular Use of any Herbs/Botanical Products (list):

Estimated Needs: (To be done by Dietitian or Dietetic Technician)

Protein ____ g/kg/day =_____ **kcals**/kg/day=______ **Fluid:**____cc/kg/day=______

Provider Name and Credentials: **Date:**

BOX 3.2 Examples of Activities and Their Corresponding Levels

- **Very light:** Cooking, driving, ironing, laboratory work, painting, playing cards, playing a musical instrument, sewing, typing
- **Light:** Carpentry, child care, electrical work, garage work, golf, housecleaning, sailing, table tennis, walking on a level surface at 2.5 to 3 miles per hour
- **Moderate:** Carrying a load, cycling, dancing, skiing, tennis, walking 3.5 to 4 miles per hour, weeding
- **Heavy:** Basketball, carrying a load uphill, climbing, football, heavy manual digging, soccer

Adapted from http://www.fda.gov.

The U.S. Department of Agriculture's *MyPyramid* (USDA, 2005) can be individualized based on sex, age, and level of activity to assist clients to make healthy nutritional decisions (Fig. 3.2). The pyramid's recommendations derive from the "2005 Dietary Guidelines for Americans," issued jointly by the USDA and the USDHHS.

MyPyramid was designed to emphasize several concepts. Personalization is key, and the pyramid can be individualized at the Web site. A client can enter her age, gender, and activity level, and the site provides a food plan based on the appropriate number of calories. For a more in-depth personal assessment and analysis of diet and activity, consumers can go to MyPyramid Tracker (www.mypyramidtracker.gov). The pyramid also emphasizes gradual improvement, symbolized by the "Steps to a Healthier You" slogan at the bottom. Along with healthy nutrition choices, the pyramid is meant to encourage daily physical activity, symbolized by the person walking up the stairs on one side of the pyramid. It stresses the selection of a variety of foods with the differently colored bands representing different food groups. It encourages moderation and limiting fats by the narrowing of each color band as it goes toward the top of the pyramid. Finally, the pyramid shows moderation of portions by the varying widths of the different bands, indicating that more foods from some groups are needed than from others.

To assess usual intake, an interview for 24-hour dietary recall is often useful. Inclusion of all food groups from *MyPyramid* is recommended. Those clients who omit whole food groups may be at risk for nutrient inadequacies. For example, clients who do not include five or more servings of fruits, vegetables, or their juices may consume low amounts of vitamins A and C in particular. Low intake of breads and cereals may place clients at risk for inadequate intake of B-complex vitamins, carbohydrates, and iron. Low intake from the protein-rich group may lead to low serum levels of zinc and iron, with poor wound healing and delayed growth. Dairy foods are rich in calcium and riboflavin, as well as protein and carbohydrate. Low levels of essential fatty acids fats may be problematic. Oils and mayonnaise are good sources of natural vitamin E, which has preventive factors against some cancers and cardiovascular disease (Rao, 2002; Fairfield & Fletcher, 2002).

RESEARCH HIGHLIGHT 3.1 Introducing a Nutrition Screening Tool: An Exploratory Study in a District General Hospital.

Jordan, S., Snow, D., Hayes, C., & Williams, A. (2003). *Journal of Advanced Nursing, 44*(1), 12–24.

BACKGROUND: Concerns have been raised that the nutrition of clients is a neglected aspect of care. Accordingly, "nutrition screening tools" have been devised to ensure that nurses assess all clients and, as appropriate, refer them to dietitians. The tool adopted in this study was the Nursing Nutritional Screening Tool.

PURPOSE: The purpose of the study was to investigate the effects of the Nursing Nutritional Screening Tool on nutrition-related nursing documentation, client care at mealtimes, and dietitian referral.

DESIGN: This study was conducted on two similar general medical wards in a United Kingdom (UK) district general hospital, with the help of staff and clients (n = 175) admitted during May 1999 and January 2000. Researchers collected data over 28 days before and after introducing the screening tool on one of the wards. For both wards, in each study stage, collected data included review of clients' notes and nonparticipant observations of mealtimes. Researchers used cross-tabulations to compare frequencies of dietitian referral and documentation of weight. Nine months later, the researchers discussed the findings with ward sisters in a group interview.

RESULTS: Use of the screening tool affected the process but not the outcomes of screening. The tool increased the frequency of nutrition-related documentation: the proportion of clients with weights recorded increased on the intervention ward ($p < 0.001$) and decreased on the comparator ward. Frequency of dietitian referral decreased on both wards, but differences were statistically insignificant. No change in client care at mealtimes was observed. The nurses in charge of the wards felt that introduction of the screening tool had raised awareness of nutrition-related care.

Meeting the nutritional needs of clients is a complex aspect of nursing that may benefit from use of structured guidelines. Diverse factors that require more exploration seem to limit the potential of screening to improve care.

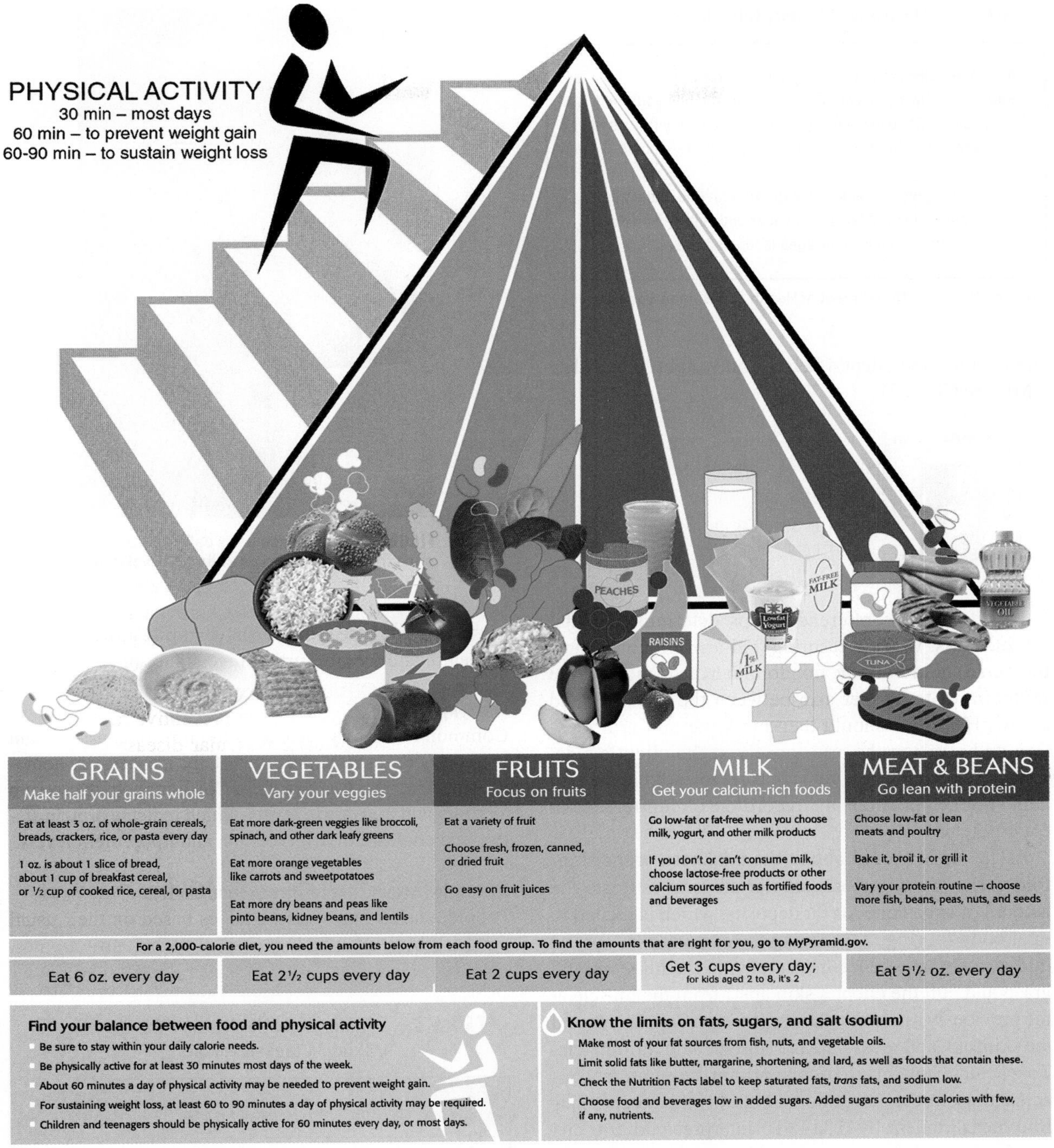

PHYSICAL ACTIVITY
30 min – most days
60 min – to prevent weight gain
60-90 min – to sustain weight loss
PEACHES
RAISINS
FAT-FREE MILK
Lowfat Yogurt
1% MILK
TUNA
VEGETABLE OIL
GRAINS
Make half your grains whole
Eat at least 3 oz. of whole-grain cereals, breads, crackers, rice, or pasta every day
1 oz. is about 1 slice of bread, about 1 cup of breakfast cereal, or ½ cup of cooked rice, cereal, or pasta
VEGETABLES
Vary your veggies
Eat more dark-green veggies like broccoli, spinach, and other dark leafy greens
Eat more orange vegetables like carrots and sweetpotatoes
Eat more dry beans and peas like pinto beans, kidney beans, and lentils
FRUITS
Focus on fruits
Eat a variety of fruit
Choose fresh, frozen, canned, or dried fruit
Go easy on fruit juices
MILK
Get your calcium-rich foods
Go low-fat or fat-free when you choose milk, yogurt, and other milk products
If you don't or can't consume milk, choose lactose-free products or other calcium sources such as fortified foods and beverages
MEAT & BEANS
Go lean with protein
Choose low-fat or lean meats and poultry
Bake it, broil it, or grill it
Vary your protein routine – choose more fish, beans, peas, nuts, and seeds
For a 2,000-calorie diet, you need the amounts below from each food group. To find the amounts that are right for you, go to MyPyramid.gov.
Eat 6 oz. every day
Eat 2½ cups every day
Eat 2 cups every day
Get 3 cups every day; for kids aged 2 to 8, it's 2
Eat 5½ oz. every day
Find your balance between food and physical activity
Be sure to stay within your daily calorie needs.
Be physically active for at least 30 minutes most days of the week.
About 60 minutes a day of physical activity may be needed to prevent weight gain.
For sustaining weight loss, at least 60 to 90 minutes a day of physical activity may be required.
Children and teenagers should be physically active for 60 minutes every day, or most days.
Know the limits on fats, sugars, and salt (sodium)
Make most of your fat sources from fish, nuts, and vegetable oils.
Limit solid fats like butter, margarine, shortening, and lard, as well as foods that contain these.
Check the Nutrition Facts label to keep saturated fats, trans fats, and sodium low.
Choose food and beverages low in added sugars. Added sugars contribute calories with few, if any, nutrients.

FIGURE 3.2 The USDA 2005 Food Guide Pyramid: Steps to a Healthier You.

Another useful guide to planning healthy meals is the Dietary Guidelines for Americans. Box 3.3 briefly summarizes important points from those guidelines.

Assessing Nutritional Status

More information about the client's nutritional status can be ascertained by performing specific physical examinations and certain laboratory tests.

Anthropometric Measurements

Anthropometric data consist of measurements pertaining to body size and composition and include height, weight, BMI, midarm circumference, and triceps skinfold thickness (Bickley, 2007). The nurse should measure the client's height with the client wearing no shoes. For weight, actually weighing the client on a scale, rather than relying on a client's report, is essential. The nurse

BOX 3.3 The ABCs of Dietary Guidelines

Aim for fitness: Include regular physical activity.
Build a healthy base. Let the Food Pyramid guide your food choices. Choose a variety of foods, especially fruits and vegetables. Keep foods safe during preparation and service.
Choose sensibly. A diet low in saturated fat and cholesterol, moderate in total fat, low in sugar and salt, and moderate in use of alcoholic beverages is recommended.

Adapted from U.S. Department of Health and Human Services, 2000.

can then use the client's height and weight to calculate BMI (see Chap. 2).

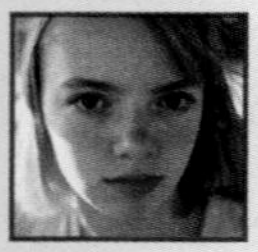

Betsy is 5 feet, 6 inches tall and weighs 115 lbs. Refer to Chapter 2 for the formula for calculating BMI. What is Betsy's BMI?

Mid-arm circumference helps determine skeletal muscle mass. When measuring mid-arm circumference, the nurse should use the nondominant arm and find the midpoint of the upper arm between the shoulder and elbow. He or she should then mark the mid-arm location and position the arm loosely at the client's side. The nurse should use a tape measure to encircle the arm at the marked position and record the circumference in centimeters.

The nurse should obtain the thickness of the skinfold at the triceps or subscapular areas to estimate the amount of subcutaneous fat deposits, which is related to total body fat (Fig. 3.3). Using the same arm as for the mid-arm circumference measurement, the nurse should grasp and pull the client's skin apart from the muscle at the previously marked location, place the calipers around the skinfold, and record the measurement in millimeters. To calculate how much of the mid-arm circumference is actual muscle, the nurse should multiply the triceps skinfold measurement by 0.314. To interpret mid-arm circumference and triceps skinfold thickness measurements, the nurse should compare the findings with averages provided in standardized charts (Table 3.5).

Other Physical Evaluations

Additional information from the physical examination that is central to a nutritional assessment includes the client's general appearance, characteristics of skin and hair, mouth integrity, teeth condition, ability to chew and swallow, gag reflex, joint flexibility, hand strength, and attention and concentration (Bickley, 2007). Abnormalities in any of these areas can have implications for overall health and require further investigation.

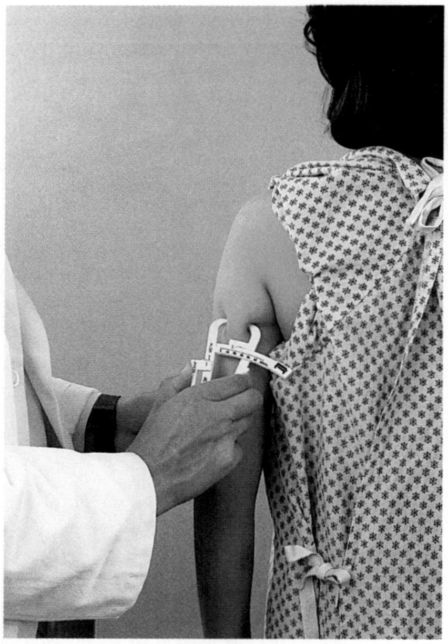

FIGURE 3.3 The nurse uses calipers to measure the client's triceps skinfold thickness.

Laboratory Data

Common laboratory tests used in nutritional assessment include a complete blood count (CBC), especially hemoglobin, hematocrit, and number of lymphocytes; serum albumin and transferrin levels, which indicate protein status; and cholesterol, triglyceride, and lipoprotein levels.

Assessing Factors That Influence Food Choices

People tend to make food choices based on their usual patterns, most of which started in their family homes.

TABLE 3.5 Findings of Mid-Arm and Triceps Skinfold Measurements

MEASUREMENT*	GENDER	NORMAL RANGE*
Mid-arm circumference	Male	29.3–17.6 cm
	Female	28.5–17.1 cm
Mid-arm muscle circumference	Male	25.3–15.2 cm
	Female	23.2–13.9 cm
Triceps skinfold	Male	12.5–7.3 mm
	Female	16.5–9.9 mm

*If measurements are below the lowest range for normal, nutritional support may be indicated.

Adapted from Jelliffe, D. B. (1986). *The assessment of the nutritional status of the community.* World Health Organization Monograph No. 53. Geneva, World Health Organization.

Differences in nutrient intake, knowledge, and attitudes about diet and health can influence women's willingness and ability to choose foods for a more healthful diet (Gates & McDonald, 1997).

The client's *cultural or religious* background may influence the foods she likes or considers acceptable to eat. Table 3.6 provides information about various cultural groups and common issues related to food and nutritional patterns. The nurse should remember, however, not to make assumptions about dietary habits or preferences based solely on a client's identified ethnicity or religion.

Vegetarian diets can be healthy if planned carefully. Omission of any of the key food groups should be concerning to the practitioner. Dairy foods provide B-complex vitamins, especially riboflavin, vitamin D, calcium, potassium, protein, and other key nutrients. The meat group provides excellent sources of iron, niacin, thiamin, protein, zinc, and vitamin B_{12}. When either of these food groups is limited or severely restricted, the potential exists for nutrient deficiencies. A full nutritional assessment by a dietetics professional is suggested whenever a client states that she follows a vegetarian pattern.

The nurse should analyze the client's *resources to procure nutrition.* Economic insecurity usually leads to food insecurity and an inability to guarantee access to a nutrient supply that is predictable over time. Transportation also may be a problem, and local supermarkets may charge more for food than larger stores, compounding the problem. Where possible and necessary, nurses should refer eligible pregnant or breastfeeding women, infants, and children younger than 5 years to the Women, Infants, and Children's (WIC) supplemental feeding program. In cases of economic and medical need, eligible participants may receive either monthly vouchers for food and infant formula or the actual products on site. Nurses can refer other family members who need food to local Food Stamps programs and related commodity programs or farmers' markets.

TABLE 3.6 Cultural Variations on Nutrition

CULTURE	FOOD PATTERNS	ADDITIONAL COMMENTS
African American	• Favorite meats are pork and chicken. • Intake of milk and dairy foods is low. • Intake of dark green, leafy vegetables.	• Diet tends to be high in fat and sodium. • Frying is a common method of preparation. • Obesity is common.
Chinese	• Little milk or cheese is used. • Rice is consumed with most meals. • Fresh foods are used and stir-fried before serving. • Unsweetened green tea is a common drink.	• Diet is high in fiber, low in fat, and may be deficient in protein. • Moderation is valued, and obesity is rare.
Greek	• Cheese is a favorite food. • Yogurt is a popular source of calcium. • Lamb is the favorite meat.	• Relatively large quantities of sweets and snacks are consumed. • Consumption of meat is on the increase. • A meal is a family ritual.
Italian	• Bread and pasta are basic foods. • Olive oil is used to prepare meats. • Cheese is main source of calcium.	• Milk is rarely consumed as a beverage. Red or white wine is consumed with dinner.
Japanese	• Rice may be eaten with every meal. • Seafood, especially raw fish, is the main protein source. • Main seasoning is soy sauce. • Tea is main beverage.	• Diet is low in fat but high in sodium. • Common methods of food preparation include broiling, steaming, boiling, and stir-frying.
Latino	• Many varieties of beans are consumed; little meat is used. • Milk intake is small but large quantities of coffee are consumed. • Corn is the basic grain.	• Selection of hot and cold foods plays a role in body equilibrium. • Lactose intolerance is possible. • Diet is high in fiber and starch. • Lard is a basic cooking fat, and obesity is common.
Puerto Rican	• Steamed white rice is a staple. • Starchy vegetables (eg, breadfruit and viandas) and fruits such as plantains are popular. • Legumes are a good source of protein.	• Milk is rarely consumed as a beverage. • Food is frequently fried and cooked for a long period of time.

Adapted from Dudek, S. G. (2006). *Nutrition handbook for nursing practice* (5th ed.). Philadelphia: Lippincott Williams & Wilkins; Purnell, L., & Paulanka, B. (1998). *Transcultural health care.* Philadelphia: F. A. Davis.

One of the most influential factors related to client nutrition involves *developmental stage* and *life circumstances*. Considerations related to specific life stages are discussed in the next part of this chapter.

NUTRITIONAL VARIATIONS FOR VARIOUS GROUPS

Dietary needs, behaviors, and habits vary depending on whether a client is just beginning to menstruate, pregnant, lactating, or experiencing menopause. Her place in her family, peer group, and significant others can influence her food choices greatly. The following sections focus on specific nutrition considerations for various developmental stages in the woman's life cycle.

Pregnancy

During pregnancy, changes must occur to ensure that gestation progresses and that both mother and fetus remain healthy (Ford, 2004). These changes involve synthesis of new tissues and hormonal variations to regulate essential processes. Nutrition has a critical role in pregnancy outcomes—maternal nutritional status at conception and throughout gestation greatly influences not only the mother's health, but also that of the fetus. Although solid nutrition cannot guarantee a healthy pregnancy, it can certainly minimize problems.

Ideally, the woman's nutrition is optimal before she becomes pregnant. Two conditions demonstrate the importance of optimal health before pregnancy: adequate folate status, which helps prevent neural tube defects, and control of blood glucose level, which improves the abilities to conceive and to give birth to a healthy newborn. Even if a woman's nutritional behaviors before pregnancy were less than adequate, pregnancy can provide an excellent opportunity for nurses to teach women the importance of making sound nutritional choices and to encourage them to develop habits they will continue into the postpartum period and beyond.

QUOTE 3-3

"I always tried to follow a proper diet. Now that I am pregnant, there's so much more to consider. I'm always hungry, but some foods that I crave are not really good for me. I guess it's better to have an appetite than not, like my sister, who had morning sickness throughout her pregnancy."

A woman pregnant for the first time, adapting to related nutrition and appetite changes

Weight Gain

One indicator of a healthy pregnancy is adequate weight gain, which is necessary to ensure optimal fetal outcomes. Suggested weight gain during pregnancy varies depending on the maternal prepregnancy BMI. For women with a normal BMI, the suggested timing for weight gain during pregnancy is 2 to 4 lbs in the first trimester, 10 to 11 lbs in the second trimester, and 12 to 13 lbs in the last trimester (Kaiser, Allen, & American Dietetic Association, 2002). Extra weight gain may be beneficial to women who were underweight before pregnancy. Women who were overweight before pregnancy should gain approximately two thirds of a pound per week and avoid more weight gain (Baeten et al., 2001). See Table 3.7 for recommendations for total weight gain based on prepregnancy BMI.

Weight gained during pregnancy is distributed among various tissues essential to both fetus and mother. See Figure 3.4 for the components of maternal weight gain and its distribution.

Although women who were overweight before pregnancy have a decreased risk for giving birth to a small-for-gestational-age (SGA) infant, obesity is associated with an increased risk for gestational hypertension, giving birth to a baby with **macrosomia** (birth weight of 9 lbs [4000 g] or more), and perinatal mortality (Cnattingius et al., 1998; Dawson et al., 2000; Robinson et al., 2005; Surkan, et al., 2004). These women need to be monitored closely to facilitate positive outcomes.

Nutritional Requirements

Pregnancy requires energy to support growth and activity. The general recommendation is for the woman to add 300 kcal/day to her normal daily requirements in the second and third trimesters (IOM, 2002). A well-balanced diet should supply this energy so there is ample carbohydrate to spare protein and prevent formation of ketones. High levels of ketones in the blood can lead to fetal neurologic damage (Fowles, 2002). If the rate of weight gain follows the normal pattern, then health care providers can assume that energy intake is adequate.

The pregnant woman's diet should follow these recommendations for numbers of servings from each food group represented on *MyPyramid* (Women's Health.gov, 2005):

- Nine servings from the grains group
- Four servings from the vegetable group

TABLE 3.7 Recommendations for Weight Gain in Pregnancy Based on Prepregnancy Body Mass Index

BODY MASS INDEX (KG/M^2)	RECOMMENDED WEIGHT GAIN
Low (<19.8)	12.5–18 kg (28–40 lb)
Normal (19.8–26)	11.5–16 kg (25–35 lb)
High (26–29)	7–11.5 kg (15–25 lb)
Obese (>29)	6+ kg (15+ lb)

From Kaiser, L. L., Allen, L., & American Dietetic Association. (2002). Position of the American Dietetic Association: Nutrition and lifestyle for a healthy pregnancy outcome. *Journal of the American Dietetic Association, 102*(10), 1479–1490.

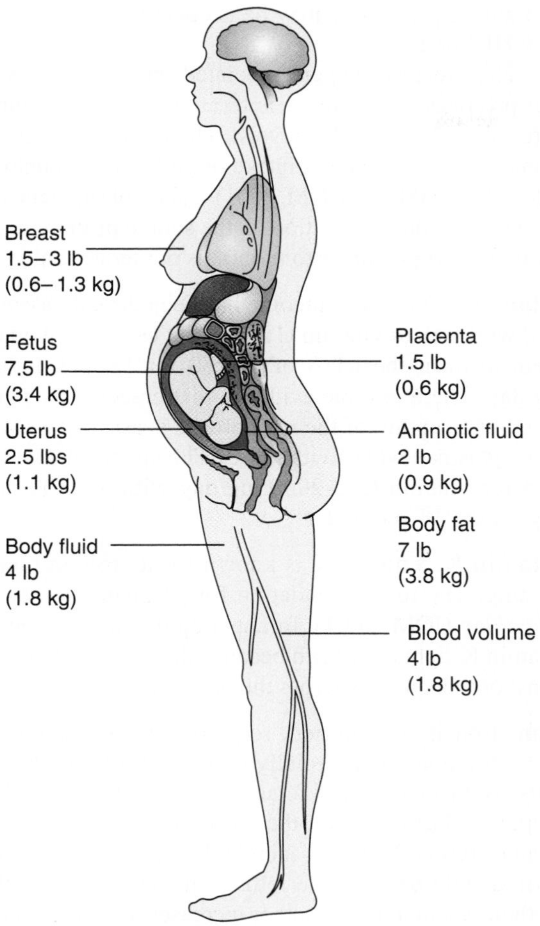

FIGURE 3.4 Distribution and amount of maternal weight gain.

- Three servings from the fruit group
- Three servings from the milk group
- Three servings from the meat and beans group

These servings of milk, vegetables, and meat provide the extra protein, calcium, zinc, folate, and iron needed for successful maternal and fetal outcomes.

Supplements

When a woman is planning pregnancy, her primary health care provider usually prescribes a prenatal vitamin to help ensure adequate levels of nutrients essential to embryonic and fetal development (eg, folic acid). If a pregnancy is unplanned, the provider should prescribe a prenatal vitamin as soon as a woman knows that she is pregnant (Florida Department of Health, 2003). To promote the best use of nutrients, the woman should take the supplement between meals with water or liquids other than milk or caffeinated beverages. If just an iron supplement is prescribed, bedtime is a good time to take it; the woman should not take iron supplements with antacids because the antacids decrease absorption. See Pharmacology Box 3.1 for information on common nutritional supplements prescribed in pregnancy.

Role of Specific Nutrients in Pregnancy

The RDA for each major nutrient in pregnancy can be found in Tables 3.1 to 3.4. The following paragraphs describe those nutrients of special significance during pregnancy.

Protein. Each woman's body processes protein uniquely, but generally most dietary protein is used to form new tissue. Because the woman's body is producing tissues not only for herself but also for the growing fetus, the RDA

● PHARMACOLOGY 3.1 Prenatal Vitamins (Natalins)

ACTION: Supplements nutrition to ensure adequate intake of vitamins and minerals during pregnancy. The folic acid content helps prevent megaloblastic anemia in the mother and neural tube defects in the fetus (Karch, 2004).

INGREDIENTS: Vitamin A (4,000 U), vitamin D (400 U), vitamin E (15 U), vitamin C (80 mg), vitamin B_1 (1.5 mg), vitamin B_2 (2.0 mg), vitamin B_6 (4 mg), vitamin B_{12} (2.5 µg), niacin (17 mg), folic acid (1.0 mg), pantothenic acid (7 mg), calcium (200 mg), iron (54 mg), copper (3 mg), zinc (25 mg), and magnesium (100 mg)

DOSAGE: One tablet daily

POSSIBLE ADVERSE EFFECTS: None known. Folic acid may mask the signs of pernicious anemia.

NURSING IMPLICATIONS

- Encourage women to take the medication exactly as prescribed; caution women not to exceed the recommended dosage.
- Assist with ways to remind women to take the medication, such as a note on the refrigerator.
- Advise women to keep vitamins, like all medications, out of the reach of small children to prevent accidental poisoning.

Source: Karch, A. M. (2006). 2005 *Lippincott's nursing drug guide.* Philadelphia: Lippincott Williams & Wilkins.

for protein in pregnancy is 71 g/day or an additional 15 g (IOM, 2002). The principal sources that provide this level of protein are dairy products and meat. Getting enough energy from other sources is essential so that the body reserves protein for tissue synthesis.

Fat. Fats supply energy and essential fatty acids (linoleic and α-linolenic acids) necessary for adequate fetal brain and nervous system development and function. Although specific recommendations have yet to be established, severe lack of essential fatty acids may be associated with placental abnormalities and subsequent newborn complications (see Chap. 22).

Folate. One poor pregnancy outcome considered preventable through nutrition is neural tube defect (NTD). The two main forms of NTD are *anencephaly* and *spina bifida* (see Chap. 22). The first condition usually results in stillbirth or early neonatal death; the second results in problems with paralysis or bowel and bladder control. Prevention is accomplished by folic acid supplementation from 1 month before through at least the first 3 months of pregnancy (Karch, 2004). The supplementation level is much higher for the woman who has previously given birth to a child with NTD (IOM, 2000a).

Recommended folate intakes are as follows:

- 400 μg/day for all women of childbearing age
- 600 μg/day for all pregnant woman
- 4 mg/day for prevention of recurrence of a child with NTD (IOM, 2000a)

B Vitamins. Riboflavin, thiamin, and niacin are necessary for cellular energy production. Because energy intake increases during pregnancy, the need for these vitamins also is greater. As long as the woman's diet contains whole grains, legumes, dark green vegetables, meats, and dairy products, these nutrients probably are adequate. A diet predominantly consisting of fat and sugar necessitates B vitamin supplementation. Niacin is the one vitamin for which a UL has been set during pregnancy (35 mg/day, or 30 mg/day in women 18 years or younger) (IOM, 2000a).

The other two vitamins necessary for protein synthesis are B_{12} and B_6. The interrelationship between B_{12} and folic acid in the synthesis of new protein is well established. B_{12} deficiency is rare during pregnancy because most women's diets usually supply an adequate level. The possible exception is the woman who is a **vegan** (a type of vegetarian who eats and uses no meat or meat products, such as eggs or milk) or the fetus diagnosed with methylmalonic acidemia, an inborn error of metabolism. B_6 has a vital role in protein metabolism. Evidence of specific poor pregnancy outcomes related to this vitamin is lacking.

Vitamin A. The role of vitamin A in tissue development is well defined. Because the body stores vitamin A, deficiencies are rare. Two situations in which supplementation during pregnancy may be necessary are in women with HIV or anemia.

The greatest danger associated with vitamin A is that preformed vitamin A is teratogenic (causes birth defects) at high intake levels. Therefore, a pregnant woman needs to limit her intake of preformed vitamin A to less then 3000 μg/d (IOM, 2001). Labels of supplements need to provide information on the source of vitamin A. Carotene, the precursor to retinol, is not teratogenic.

Vitamin C. No poor outcome has been directly associated with lack of vitamin C in the diet and most women seem to meet the RDA of 85 (80 for 18 and under) mg/day. There is some evidence that preeclampsia and premature rupture of the membranes is associated with a low plasma level of vitamin C. The upper limit of intake for vitamin C is 2000 mg/day with a 1,800 mg/day for the 18 and under.

Vitamin K. Vitamin K is known for its role in blood clotting. The recommendation for pregnant women is 90 μg/day (IOM, 2001). Infants require an injection of vitamin K right after birth because the vitamin does not transport adequately across the placenta.

Iron. Iron is one nutrient required for production of heme compounds, especially hemoglobin in red blood cells. Both mother and fetus produce red blood cells; during the last trimester, the fetus absorbs more iron to produce blood. Maternal anemia does not result in newborn anemia because the fetus removes iron from the mother. Anemia in the mother increases her risk for cardiac arrest, causes fatigue, and can result in a preterm or low-birth-weight infant (Scholl & Reilly, 2000).

Anemia is common during pregnancy. Although lack of folate, B_6, or B_{12} could be the cause, the most common reason is lack of iron (Scholl, 2005). One protective mechanism during pregnancy is increased absorption of iron from the diet. Because the RDA (27 mg/day) during pregnancy increases greatly over normal, the woman needs ferrous salt supplements. The recommended supplementation level is 30 mg/day in the second and third trimesters (IOM, 2001). The upper limit of 45 mg/day is not to be exceeded (IOM, 2001). Supplements may cause nausea and constipation, so women require counseling on how to reduce these problems.

Diagnosis of anemia is based on hematocrit and hemoglobin levels. Another clue that should trigger a close look at these laboratory data is **pica** (eating or craving nonfood substances such as starch, clay, dirt, or ice). It is not known whether pica causes anemia or anemia causes pica, but the two are related closely. With a diagnosis of anemia, the supplement level recommended is 60 to 120 mg/day. Even though 45 mg/day is considered the UL, anemia regulates the amounts absorbed to prevent overload. Supplements are given in divided doses.

High hemoglobin levels (greater than 13.2 g/dL) are detrimental to mother and fetus. Failure of the blood to expand, poor circulation to the fetus through the placenta, and placental infarcts are thought to contribute to associated poor outcomes. Women with such hemoglobin levels should not use iron supplements.

Calcium. The fetus needs calcium for skeletal formation. The placental hormones of human chorionic somatomammotropin and estrogen increase bone turnover rates and maintain calcium balance by enhancing intestinal calcium absorption and decreasing urinary excretion. Increased retention of calcium throughout pregnancy helps supply the high demand needed for skeleton and tooth formation during the last trimester. The AI for pregnant women is the same as for nonpregnant women (1,000 mg/day; 1,300 mg/day for women 18 years and younger) (IOM, 1997). These levels are higher than those set by other countries, largely because the high phosphorus and protein intake in the United States causes urinary loss of calcium.

Some researchers have theorized that high calcium intake protects against hypertension in adults (Alonso et al., 2005). Encouraging selection of foods to provide calcium is valid. Some health professionals recommend calcium supplements routinely. More testing is needed before standard bodies will issue a general recommendation for calcium supplementation during pregnancy.

Other Minerals. *Magnesium* is stored in bone and functions in nerve and muscle metabolism. Supplementation may reduce leg cramps for pregnant women with low serum levels of magnesium.

Zinc is necessary for growth and development, but conclusive evidence that zinc deficiency results in poor pregnancy outcomes is lacking. Iron supplementation may increase the need for zinc because iron inhibits zinc absorption.

More research is needed on *copper* needs during pregnancy. Copper deficiency is teratogenic in animals. Iron supplementation decreases absorption of copper, and the U.S. diet tends to be low in copper.

Fluoride is necessary for healthy tooth formation as early as the 10th week of pregnancy. Research has not yet shown the importance of fluoride to development during pregnancy.

Phosphorus is important to bone formation, meeting the adequate intake recommendation of 700 mg/d, 1250 mg/d if 18 or under, is not a problem for most women. The U.S. diet is high in phosphorus. Calcium balance and bone formation involves phosphorus, vitamin D, calcium, and hormones. Calcium and vitamin D are the nutrients that are likely to be limiting. An upper limit has been set for phosphorus at 3.5 g/d.

Sodium restriction for edema during pregnancy is not recommended. Some degree of fluid retention is expected during pregnancy and sodium is needed to balance the electrolytes. Therefore, an intake of 2–3 grams per day is suggested. The only evidence we have of restriction causing problems is that women on sodium restrictions tend to deliver infants with hyponatremia.

Nutritional Deficits and Problems

Nutritional deficits in pregnancy are significant and should be avoided as much as possible. Continuous dietary monitoring of pregnant women is critical; nutrients that require special emphasis include calcium, magnesium, zinc, iron, fiber, folate, and vitamins D and E (Bienz, Cori, & Hornig, 2003).

Pregnant females with poor eating habits (eg, skipping meals) or a history of eating disorders place their fetuses and infants at risk for malnutrition and its associated consequences. Women who have had previous pregnancy complications, including miscarriages, or previous poor fetal or obstetrical outcomes may be at risk as well (Swan & Apgar, 1995). Women with insufficient funds to purchase foods during pregnancy; those who smoke, take drugs, or consume alcoholic beverages; those with chronic diseases (eg, diabetes, renal disease); and those with chronic anemia are at risk for poor pregnancy outcomes (Rainville, 1998; Shaw & Lammer, 1999). These clients need increased attention from health care providers and appropriate referrals to specialists, nutritionists, social workers, and other resources for assistance.

Isotretinoin (Accutane) is an acne medication prescribed to some women and currently under enhanced management by the U.S. Food and Drug Administration. This drug is related to preformed vitamin A, which can cause birth defects if levels in the mother exceed the UL. Women should stop using isotretinoin before becoming pregnant. In addition, all pregnant women should consume no more than 5000 IU of vitamin A each day in the diet and supplements (Azais-Braesco & Pascal, 2000).

Similarly, pregnant women should not use herbs and botanical supplements without checking with their health care provider first. Women using such supplements should stop immediately when they discover they are pregnant. Pregnant women should *not* take kava, chasteberry, dong quai, Asian ginseng, licorice root, and Saw Palmetto (American Pregnancy Association, 2004).

Pregnant women who experience hyperemesis gravidarum may require enteral feedings to alleviate nausea and to prevent or correct weight loss. Careful attention to recovery of lost weight is an important aspect in this group of pregnant women. See Chapter 13 for more information.

COLLABORATIVE CARE: NUTRITION IN PREGNANCY

Assessment

During the initial prenatal visit, the nurse should perform a detailed nutritional assessment (see earlier discussion). The nurse and client should analyze habits and pinpoint concerns for ongoing monitoring as the pregnancy progresses. During that visit and subsequent appointments, the assessment of a pregnant woman should include body weight measurement and plotting on a weight gain grid. The nurse then should use this information along with other laboratory data to determine the status of the pregnant woman's nutrition (Fig. 3.5).

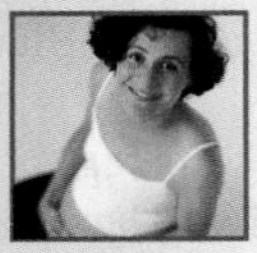

When reviewing the client's medical record, the nurse finds that Sheila's prepregnancy weight was 144 lbs, and that her BMI was 27. What would the nurse expect the client approximately to weigh at this visit?

Select Potential Nursing Diagnoses

The following nursing diagnoses related to nutritional issues and concerns may apply to the pregnant woman:

- **Health-Seeking Behaviors** related to desire to have a healthy baby
- **Deficient Knowledge** related to appropriate weight gain during pregnancy
- **Ineffective Health Maintenance** related to control of weight during pregnancy and appropriate food selection

Planning/Intervention

The nurse should discuss the relationship of weight gain to a healthy pregnancy and show the woman the weight gain grid with her weight plotted on it. The nurse should then suggest ways to manage weight gain and food intake to ensure that the client meets nutrient needs while avoiding either weight loss or excessive gain. If nutritional problems are extensive, the nurse may refer the woman to a registered dietitian for in-depth assistance with food selection. See NIC/NOC Box 3.1 and Nursing Care Plan 3.1.

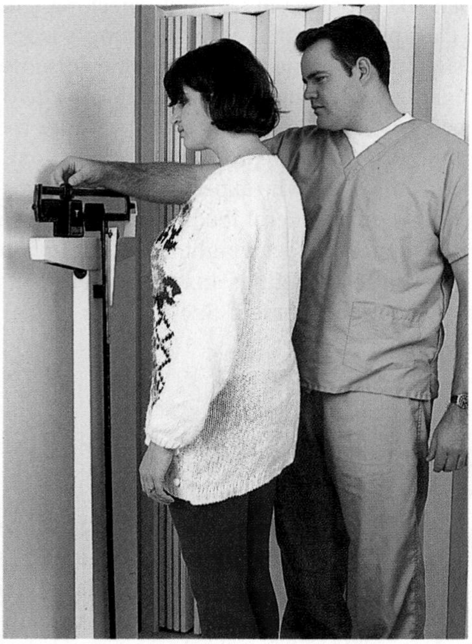

FIGURE 3.5 Monitoring the progress of weight gain in pregnancy is an essential nursing activity.

Evaluation

The nurse should weigh the woman at the next clinic visit, plot the weight on the grid, and evaluate changes to determine the next education steps to take. After being weighed, some women show signs of anxiety or depression because their weight is higher than what they normally experience. Such clients may need reassurance that they can lose the weight gained during pregnancy after the baby is born.

Lactation

Breastfeeding confers important immunologic, physiologic, economic, social, and hygienic effects to mother and infant. Infants digest and absorb human milk more efficiently than they do other forms of milk (cow's milk, goat's milk). The composition of breast milk adapts over time to meet the human infant's changing needs, whereas the composition of cow's milk or formula is stable and not adaptive (see Chap. 21).

Some research has indicated that asthma and associated problems are decreased in children who were

NIC/NOC Box 3.1 Optimal Nutrition

Common NIC Labels

- Behavior Management
- Decision-Making Support
- Health Education
- Learning Facilitation
- Learning Readiness Enhancement
- Nutritional Counseling
- Self-Modification Assistance
- Teaching: Individual
- Teaching: Prescribed Diet
- Weight Management
- Weight Reduction Assistance

Common NOC Labels

- Adherence Behavior
- Health Beliefs
- Health Orientation
- Health Promoting Behavior
- Health Seeking Behavior
- Knowledge: Diet
- Knowledge: Health Behaviors
- Knowledge: Health Promotion
- Knowledge: Health Resources
- Weight Control
- Well-Being

NURSING CARE PLAN 3.1

A Teen With Nutritional Issues

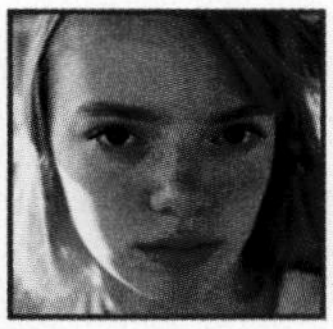

The nurse asks Betsy, the 14-year-old who mentions fear of weight gain, to provide more information about her typical diet and food preferences. Betsy mentions that she enjoys eating at fast-food restaurants, consumes about two cans of carbonated soda per day, and frequently skips breakfast.

NURSING DIAGNOSES

- **Imbalanced Nutrition, Less Than Body Requirements** related to inadequate intake secondary to desire for weight control
- **Deficient Knowledge** related to importance of nutrition

EXPECTED OUTCOMES:

1. The client will verbalize an understanding of nutritional needs during adolescence.
2. The client will state the rationale for why additional calories are essential.
3. The client will identify appropriate nutritional choices.
4. The client will participate in developing a nutritional plan to foster growth and development.

INTERVENTIONS	RATIONALES
Assess the client's level of understanding about nutrition and nutritional requirements of adolescence.	This information provides a baseline to identify specific client needs and to develop an individualized teaching plan.
Review the nutritional needs of adolescence, describing what the needs are and why.	The client needs this basic knowledge.
Complete a 24-hour dietary recall.	Dietary recall provides information about client's typical intake during a day and helps identify eating patterns.
Ask the client about foods that she likes and dislikes; determine any cultural influences on her choices.	Knowledge of food likes and dislikes and cultural influences provides a baseline for dietary suggestions and menu planning.
Encourage client to identify foods in her diet that are nutritionally inadequate. Work with client to identify suggestions for replacing non-nutritious foods with foods that are nutritionally sound.	Client participation in evaluating her own nutrition and identifying appropriate suggestions promotes control over the situation and fosters positive self-esteem.
Arrange for consultation with dietitian about meal planning. Provide the client with menus and teaching pamphlets.	Collaborative care can ensure that diets are sound and will optimize health; printed materials can reinforce learning.
Plan with the client to keep a journal outlining her food choices and selections over the next few weeks. Schedule an appointment to monitor the client's progress within 2 weeks.	The journal can provide objective evidence of the client's behaviors. Follow-up is critical to ensure that selections and behaviors are improving.

Continued

NURSING CARE PLAN 3.1 ● A Teen With Nutritional Issues *(Continued)*

EVALUATION

1. The client expresses accurate understanding of the reasons that enhanced nutrition during adolescence is important.
2. The client commits to keeping a food journal and following the menus designed by the nurse and dietitian.
3. The client schedules and keeps her 2-week follow-up appointment and shows compliance with the recommended dietary plan.
4. The client demonstrates adequate weight gain at follow-up appointments.

NURSING DIAGNOSIS

Disturbed Body Image related to lack of understanding the difference between a healthy body and an overweight body

EXPECTED OUTCOMES

1. The client will verbalize feelings about her maturing body and its effect on her view of herself.
2. The client will identify body changes as reflective of her developmental stage.

INTERVENTIONS	RATIONALES
Assess the client's beliefs about her current body image, developmental stage, and self-esteem. Explore with the client her feelings about her changing body.	Assessment provides a baseline from which to develop appropriate strategies for teaching and care. Exploration of client's feelings provides insight into the client's thinking to ensure planning of appropriate individualized interventions.
Communicate accurate facts and answer questions honestly; clarify any misconceptions or misinformation about weight gain and being overweight.	Clear communication helps to provide accurate information to aid in alleviating fears and clarifying misinformation. Honesty promotes the development of trust in the relationship.
Question client about how her friends view her.	Adolescence focuses on the development of a sense of identity, with a strong emphasis on body image and peer influence.
Assess the client's stress level associated with her current situation and measures used to cope with similar stressful situations in the past; ask client to identify people who have been a source of support.	Identification of the client's stress level, previous coping strategies, and support people helps determine effective strategies for use in this situation.
Reassess client's view of self on next visit.	Reassessment provides information about client's progress in understanding the changes of pregnancy and her adaptation to her changing body image.

EVALUATION

1. The client states positive feelings about herself.
2. The client demonstrates acceptance of her changing body.

exclusively breastfed (Oddy et al., 1999). Other researchers have reported opposite results (Sears et al., 2002). An analysis of data from studies conducted from 1966 to 2001 supports the claim that breastfeeding protects infants from atopic diseases (Odijk et al., 2003). Other documented breastfeeding benefits include protections against diarrhea (Carver, 1999), respiratory illnesses, ear infections, and allergies (Wright et al., 2001).

Breastfeeding is an ethical dilemma in mothers with HIV, which can be transmitted to infants through the breast milk. The position of the American Academy of Pediatrics Committee on Pediatric AIDS (1995) is that mothers with HIV should not breastfeed.

Chapter 21 provides a comprehensive discussion of breastfeeding and newborn nutrition. The following paragraphs provide a brief summary of nutritional issues during this life stage for women.

Nutrient Needs

The nutrient needs of the lactating woman are related to the energy required to produce approximately 25 oz/day of breast milk. Recommendations are for the woman to consume 500 kcal/day above the requirements for her age group (IOM, 2002). Most nursing mothers need a total of 2500 to 3300 kcal/day, which should come from a varied diet to supply the vitamins and minerals recommended.

If the woman's diet is balanced, supplementation of nutrients is unnecessary, with the possible exception of iron to replete maternal stores. Food selections should include five dairy servings to ensure adequate calcium. Other foods that provide calcium are broccoli, sesame seeds, tofu, and kale.

Fluids are important to keep the mother hydrated. A good way to ensure that a woman consumes enough fluid is to drink milk or water with every meal and every time the baby nurses. Lactating women should be encouraged to fill a sports bottle with water or another liquid and have it within reach each time they breastfeed.

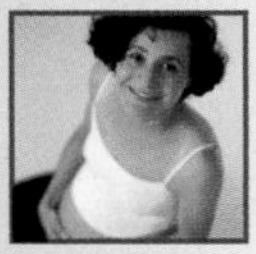

Remember Sheila, the woman in her third trimester who is planning to breastfeed her newborn. She reported that she is having difficulty drinking milk. What other suggestions could the nurse make to ensure that her calcium intake is adequate?

Counseling Issues

The American Academy of Pediatrics (Work Group on Breastfeeding, 1997) recommends that infants nurse for at least 12 months and continue as long thereafter as both mother and infant desire. This period maximizes the infant's benefits from breast milk and allows time for the child to transition successfully to table foods. All health care personnel should support the mother as much as possible to continue breastfeeding for as long as possible.

A woman's milk supply usually remains adequate unless she is poorly nourished. Weight loss during the lactation period is not recommended because too few nutrients and calories to produce milk results in decreased quantity of breast milk (American Dietetic Association [ADA], 2001; McCrory, 2001). Women who have difficulty with a poor milk supply should rest frequently; avoid caffeinated beverages, medications, and smoking; increase fluid intake; and correct any underlying illnesses. Increasing the number of feedings per day (supply responds to demand) and not giving the infant supplemental bottles or solid food are additional ways to increase milk supply.

Nutrient Problems in Breastfeeding

Breast milk alone can meet the infant's nutrient needs in the first 6 months, with the exception of vitamin D (Kreiter et al., 2000). The American Academy of Pediatrics (Work Group on Breastfeeding, 1997) recommends that breastfed infants may need vitamin D, iron, and fluoride supplements beginning at 6 months. Iron and fluoride may be supplied through iron-fortified baby cereal mixed with fluoridated water. Vitamin D can be supplied by exposure to sunlight.

Women can transmit alcohol, nicotine, and many drugs through breast milk to infants. Practitioners should discourage the use of such products. The list of drugs that transfer from the mother's breast milk to the infant and cause adverse effects is long. For many more drugs, the effects are currently unknown (Committee on Drugs, 1989). Breastfeeding women should consult their practitioners for the safety of both over-the-counter medications and prescription drugs before taking them. Most drugs should not be taken during breastfeeding.

Herbs and botanical products have not been proved safe for breastfeeding mothers and their infants. Women should *not* consume kava kava, chasteberry, dong quai, Asian ginseng, or licorice root during lactation. There is a danger of liver damage with kava kava (Mayo Clinic Staff, 2003). Dong quai interacts with antibiotics, St. John's wort, and blood-thinning medications to increase the danger of excessive bleeding. Asian ginseng interacts with other drugs to cause several problems: excessive bleeding with blood thinners; headache and manic behavior with antidepressants; heart problems with digoxin; and low blood glucose levels with antidiabetic medications. Natural licorice can increase problems with control of hypertension.

Adolescence

Sociocultural influences may affect adolescent eating patterns and behaviors, leading to trends such as using laxatives or diuretics to decrease weight, fasting, skipping meals, eating snacks at unusual hours, and self-inducing vomiting. Teens require increased nutrients to allow for accelerated growth; nutritional deficiencies in adolescence may decrease height, lead to osteoporosis, or delay sexual maturation (Herbold & Frates, 2000).

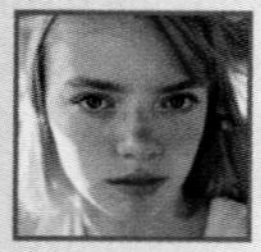

Think back to Betsy, the teen described at the beginning of the chapter. Consider her statement, "I don't want to get fat." How might the nurse interpret this statement based on Betsy's developmental stage?

Food intake in adolescence often varies, especially during growth spurts and different stages of physical maturation. Dietary intake and body size influence age at menarche and growth patterns. Age at menarche also is related inversely to percentage of energy intake from dietary protein at 3 to 5 years and fat intake at 1 to 2 years; the percentage of energy from animal protein at 6 to 8 years influences age at peak growth (Berkey et al., 2000). These factors (body weight and protein intake) may be related to later development of diseases, including breast cancer and heart disease. Controlling weight through exercise and a balanced diet becomes important to health in later life. Risks for breast cancer include younger age at menarche, older age at menopause, and older age at first child's birth. As body fat percentage increases, the age at menarche decreases (Freeman et al., 2003). Prevention of obesity is one measure to reduce risks for heart disease, hypertension, and type 2 diabetes (Whitney, Cataldo, & Rolfes, 2002). Calcium intake and exercise throughout life may help prevent osteoporosis in later life (Whitney et al., 2002).

Dietary modifications in adolescence are needed to meet ongoing or potential growth spurts and to prevent or correct anemia. Nurses should address unusual eating patterns, emphasizing caring and concern. In some cases, family counseling may be useful, especially in cases of obesity or a tendency toward eating disorders.

More information about healthy eating during the adolescent years can be found at the ADA Web site (www.eatright.org).

Nutrient Needs

Vegetarian teens should be encouraged to consume adequate sources of vitamin B_{12}, riboflavin, zinc, iron, calcium, protein, and energy for growth (Messina & Reed Mangels, 2001). Teen diets should include the following servings from *MyPyramid:*

- Four cups of milk or equivalent source of calcium
- Two to three servings of meat or equivalent
- Six to twelve servings from the bread group
- Two to four servings of fruit or juices
- Three to five servings from the vegetable group

Fruit and vegetable juices are acceptable, but nurses should encourage teens to consume the real item for fiber and other **phytochemicals** (plant-based nutrients that may have protective health properties).

In general, teens who consume healthy diets do not need vitamin and mineral supplements. Pregnant teens or those with inadequate nutrition need dietary modifications, supplements, or both. Intake of vitamins A and E, calcium, and zinc tend to be low among all teens, regardless of use of supplements (Stang, 2000). Excesses of nutrients such as vitamins A and D, however, are not recommended, because they may lead to toxicity.

Teen use of nonprescription medications (eg, aspirin, cold remedies), alcohol, and illegal drugs should be monitored carefully. Side effects of the use of such items may include poor oral intakes of several nutrients. Smoking tends to decrease serum levels of vitamin C.

As much as possible, the nurse should support the adolescent to make independent choices. Autonomy is part of the developmental process that teens must experience. Choices in meal planning, snacking, timing, and **nutrient density** (a variable used to assess the quality of a food choice) may be ways in which the teen can actively provide input. Rather than assuming that a teen will not be willing to include fruits and vegetables, the nurse should discuss the client's preferences and provide guidance about the value of specific foods to empower the adolescent while educating her about nutrition.

Because adequate calcium intake during childhood, adolescence, and early adulthood helps prevent later problems with osteoporosis, the nurse should encourage the adolescent's consumption of low-fat dairy products throughout the day (Fig. 3.6). Some examples are low-fat milk at breakfast; low-fat yogurt, low-fat

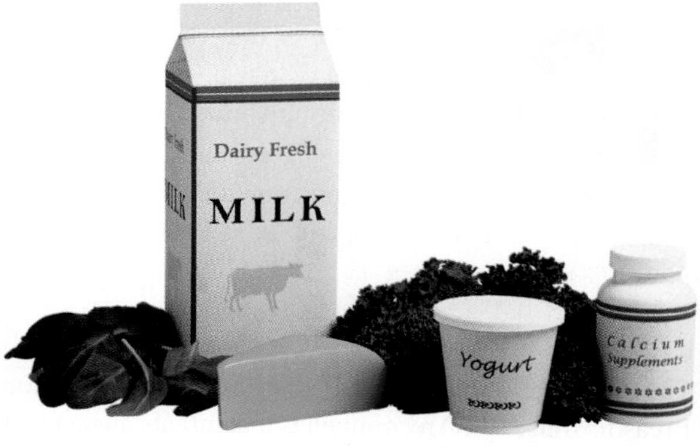

FIGURE 3.6 Calcium is enormously important for girls and adolescent females. Nurses, parents, teachers, and other influential adults should encourage teens to eat strong sources of calcium, including milk, yogurt, cheese, and green leafy vegetables.

flavored milk beverages, or low-fat cheese for snacks; and low-fat cottage cheese with fruit at meals or for snacks. Nondairy sources such as greens are less effective in meeting calcium requirements but can be part of the overall plan.

In addition, teens can consume other nutrient-dense foods:

- Vitamin A from cantaloupe, mango, spinach, and apricots
- Vitamin C from oranges, grapefruit, citrus juices, broccoli, spinach, melon, and strawberries
- Iron from liver, enriched rice, whole milk, raisins, and baked potatoes
- Vitamin B_6 from pork, bananas, potatoes, and egg yolks
- Folate from wheat germ, spinach, asparagus, and strawberries
- Zinc from meats and poultry, peanut butter, and tuna

Vitamin B_{12} is available only from meats and milk (animal foods); a true vegan diet may not suffice and cause some difficulty in learning effectively (Louwman et al., 2000). Foods acceptable to vegetarians that supply B_{12} are fortified soy milk, miso (soybean paste), yeast grown on B_{12} medium, and supplements.

Guidance for being active is also important for this population, especially with the current inactive status of many young people. Obesity should be managed early, and family interventions are often effective.

Overall, working with teens on their nutritional intake can be rewarding and challenging. See Nursing Care Plan 3.2.

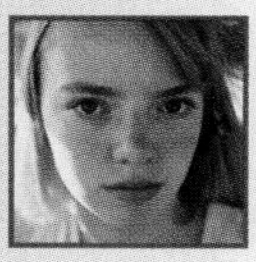

Consider Betsy, the adolescent from the beginning of the chapter. What areas would be important to assess specifically related to Betsy's nutrition?

Nutritional Concerns for Pregnant Adolescents

In general, the nutritional needs of pregnant adolescents are those for pregnancy plus those for the age group. Because growth spurts and maturation rates determine needs, the health care provider also must consider the adolescent's gynecologic age (years since start of menses). If the woman is gynecologic age 4 years or greater, then she probably is finished growing and her nutritional needs will be less than those of a teen who is still growing.

Pregnancy in adolescence can pose significant dietary challenges for those adolescents who are still growing because the fetus must compete with the mother for nutrients. Height measures during pregnancy may not reflect ongoing growth because spine and postural changes during pregnancy may appear to decrease the teen's stature.

To ensure a healthy infant and mother at time of birth, weight gain recommendations for pregnant teens are 0.9 to 1.3 lbs (0.41–0.59 kg) per week in the second and third trimesters, for a total of 28 to 40 lbs (12.7–18.1 kg) during gestation. Individualizing weight gain recommendations to each teen is advisable. Some evidence supports gaining to the middle but not to the top of weight gain ranges for these women; the concern is that high weight gain could result in excess body fat, macrosomia, need for cesarean birth, and birth asphyxia.

Energy needs vary greatly among pregnant teens—actual needs seem related to activity level, with needs increasing with the gestation. Protein intakes generally meet the estimated need for females who consume enough total energy to spare protein for tissue building. Because the recommended iron intake is difficult to achieve through diet alone, a supplement is recommended to prevent depletion and provide for stores. Calcium is needed to accrue bone mass and to form the fetal skeleton. If calcium intake is insufficient to meet these needs, then the calcium is absorbed from the maternal skeletal system. Diets often do not supply the needed calcium; a 600-mg supplement is prescribed.

Often the adolescent has not consumed adequate sources of folate and enters pregnancy with a deficit that increases the danger of neural tube defects. Supplementation as soon as possible to meet needs is recommended, even though pregnancy is too late to prevent most neural tube defects.

COLLABORATIVE CARE: NUTRITION AND THE PREGNANT TEEN

Assessment

A nutritional assessment with a pregnant adolescent should include all of the following areas:

- Dietary intake
  - Source of animal or **complementary proteins** (two or more proteins that in combination supply all essential amino acids, but alone lack at least one essential amino acid)
  - Vitamin C
  - Fresh fruits and vegetables
  - Fiber
  - Calcium sources
  - Iron sources
  - Empty calorie foods
  - Dietary fats
- Physical characteristics
  - Gynecologic age
  - Height and weight before pregnancy
  - Weight changes during pregnancy
  - Signs and symptoms of malnutrition
- Laboratory data
- Activity

NURSING CARE PLAN 3.2

Nutrition for Pregnancy and Breastfeeding

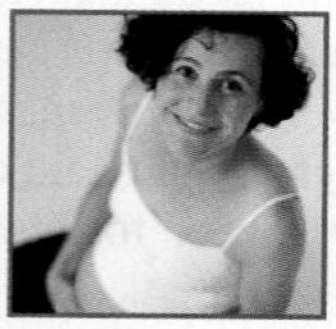

The nurse asks Sheila, the 37-year-old in her third trimester from the beginning of the chapter, about her milk intake. Sheila states, "I just don't like the taste of milk. I never have." Her weight gain has been within acceptable ranges for gestation, height, and weight. Sheila reports that she has been taking her prescribed prenatal vitamins every day.

NURSING DIAGNOSES

- **Imbalanced Nutrition, Less Than Body Requirements** related to inadequate intake of calcium rich foods
- **Deficient Knowledge** related to nutritional needs for breastfeeding and foods high in calcium

EXPECTED OUTCOMES

1. The client will identify the need for increased consumption of calories and fluid to promote breastfeeding.
2. The client will verbalize appropriate sources of foods to meet increased nutritional needs.
3. The client will identify options for calcium rich foods in addition to milk.

INTERVENTIONS	RATIONALES
Assess the client's knowledge of nutrition and breastfeeding.	This information provides a baseline from which to develop appropriate strategies.
Review the nutritional requirements for the current stage of pregnancy and for breastfeeding.	Ongoing education is essential to promote healthy outcomes.
Review the client's daily eating patterns, including frequency and types of foods consumed. Ascertain the client's likes and dislikes.	Knowledge of current dietary patterns provides clues to nutritional status and to the amount and types of calories and nutrients ingested. Information about likes and dislikes aids in individualizing suggestions for proper food selection.
Discuss the need to eat 2,500 to 3,300 kcal/day, emphasizing the importance of a varied diet.	Increased calories ensure an adequate production of breast milk. A varied diet ensures ingestion of necessary nutrients.
Review food sources that are high in calcium, including dairy options such as cheese and yogurt. Also instruct the client about other calcium-rich foods (eg, broccoli, sesame seeds, tofu, kale).	This information helps the client to understand the options available other than milk that can help ensure adequate calcium consumption.
Provide the client with a written list of appropriate foods for intake.	A written list promotes learning and provides a means of reference for the client.
Assess daily intake of fluid, including types consumed, amounts, and frequency.	This information gives clues to daily patterns and establishes a baseline for additional teaching and suggestions.

Continued

NURSING CARE PLAN 3.2 ● Nutrition for Pregnancy and Breastfeeding

INTERVENTIONS	RATIONALES
Encourage the client to ingest adequate fluids each day, including water. Suggest that she drink water with meals and carry water with her throughout the day.	Adequate fluid intake is essential for production of adequate breast milk.
Encourage the client to keep a diary or log of food and fluid intake for review on the next visit.	Keeping a diary or log helps the client visualize the amount and types of food and fluid consumed and possible patterns of intake that need adjustment or correction.

EVALUATION

1. The client demonstrates intake of the required amount of calories and fluid.
2. The client identifies appropriate alternative food sources for calcium with the recommended dietary plan.

- Medications
- Chronic diseases or infections

The results of the previous quick screen can help the provider identify important issues. Some indications of nutritional problems are identifiable by height, weight, and weight changes. The nurse should look for sudden weight gain or loss before or during pregnancy. Dietary habits that indicate eating disorders or unusual eating patterns are another indicator requiring follow-up. The nurse also should consider unhealthy social or economic dynamics: substance abuse, low income, homelessness, physical abuse, and psychological stress.

Select Potential Nursing Diagnoses

The following nursing diagnoses related to nutritional issues and concerns may apply to the pregnant adolescent:

- **Deficient Knowledge** related to nutrition during pregnancy
- **Situational Low Self-Esteem** related to immaturity and social situations created by the pregnancy
- **Disturbed Body Image** related to the physical changes taking place during both adolescence and the pregnancy

Planning/Intervention

Although the nutritional assessment will reveal each client's specific nutritional issues, some of the more common concerns to address with pregnant teens include excessive reliance on fast foods, which results in a diet high in fat and low in folate, and meal skipping or irregular eating. The nurse should address the adolescent's nutritional knowledge, providing education and psychological support as necessary. Teens who show significant nutritional deficits, financial or psychosocial problems, or other high-risk factors should be referred to a registered dietitian for additional information.

Evaluation

Follow-up at each visit should reveal adequate weight gain, improved food intake, and resolution of any social or psychological problems. The ideal outcome is for the adolescent to give birth to a healthy baby.

Adulthood and Older Adulthood

Leading causes of death in women include heart disease, cancer, cerebrovascular diseases, and diabetes mellitus. Osteoporosis and extremes in body weight are approaching epidemic proportions. Nutritional habits are a factor in all these illnesses. Additionally, a woman's diet and nutritional habits can influence her menstrual cycles and contribute to reproductive and breast problems. The ADA has numerous resources for women's health and nutrition available at www.eatright.org. The following paragraphs focus on special ways for adult and older adult women to practice sound nutritional habits to promote health and prevent illness and guidance that nurses can provide in these areas.

Weight Management

When planning meals with adult and older adult women, the nurse should emphasize the nutrient density of meals.

These clients have fewer natural energy requirements than found in pregnant, lactating, or adolescent women. Actual energy requirements depend on the woman's level of activity and exercise and other factors such as illness and stress. The nurse should teach these clients ways to avoid a sedentary lifestyle and subsequent obesity. He or she should encourage clients to seek 30 to 60 minutes or more of reasonable physical activity (eg, brisk walking) most days of the week.

Bone Density Preservation

To promote adequate bone mass density, which peaks at 25 to 30 years, women should include good sources of calcium and vitamin D each day in the diet. In addition, they need sufficient but not excessive iron in the diet to prevent anemia with its resulting fatigue, irritability, and related symptoms. Chapters 2 and 24 provide detailed discussion of osteoporosis prevention and management.

Women's Health Concerns

For common complaints related to women's health, there are several reasonable nutrition-related suggestions but insufficient evidence. The use of herbs and botanicals often increases with age to treat problems related to menstruation. See Complementary/Alternative Medicine 3.1 for more discussion.

Premenstrual Syndrome. For premenstrual syndrome (PMS), use of a low-fat vegetarian diet is associated with reductions in body weight, duration and intensity of dysmenorrhea, and duration of overall symptoms (Barnard et al., 2000). Calcium has been found to be of benefit to clients with PMS; limited evidence suggests that vitamins E and B_6 and carbohydrate supplements may be useful (Bendich, 2000). A daily magnesium supplement reduces symptoms associated with PMS (Walker et al., 1998). Use of herbals for PMS has no supporting evidence; black cohosh in large doses may cause hypotension, vomiting, headache, dizziness, gastrointestinal distress, and limb pain. The health care practitioner may recommend a general multivitamin and mineral capsule.

Fibrocystic Breast Disease. Randomized controlled studies of caffeine restriction have failed to support nutritional interventions recommended for fibrocystic breast disease. Likewise, use of evening primrose oil, vitamin E, or pyridoxine treatments have not proven effective for this condition. Use of a low-fat (15% to 20% of kcal), adequate fiber (30 g/day) diet and soy products shows some promise by reducing some markers related to this condition, but enough evidence is not available to make a recommendation without further evidence (Horner & Lampe, 2000).

Fertility Problems. The average U.S. woman has sufficient levels of body fat for reproduction. For women with fertility problems, nutritional assessment should include caffeine intake and client weight. Dietary changes that may help enhance fertility include reducing high intake of caffeine (Bolumar et al., 1997; Klebanoff et al., 1999). For obese women, losing weight may result in the achievement of successful pregnancy (Clark et al., 1998.)

Menopause and Beyond

Nutritional needs during menopause change because of declining levels of estrogen and other hormones and because of cessation of menstrual periods, which decreases needs for extra iron. Exogenous estrogen may be a concern in the development of adenoma of the endometrium. Postmenopausal osteoporosis may lead to bone fractures. Nurses should encourage regular physical examinations for aging women to help address such concerns.

Researchers are examining exercise, calcium, and hormonal therapy for their roles in preventing fractures. Although some women use alfalfa, licorice, and red clover to relieve symptoms of menopause, these supplements have not been thoroughly studied for efficacy, and health care providers should not promote their use. Black cohosh, which some women use for menopausal symptoms, may cause undesirable side effects if taken in large doses or for a long time.

Vitamins C and E and soy may be useful to lessen hot flashes and vaginal dryness, although not yet proved. In addition, women older than 50 years must carefully select diets that provide sufficient calcium and vitamin D. Weight-bearing activity such as walking is often recommended.

● COMPLEMENTARY/ALTERNATIVE MEDICINE 3.1

Herbal Supplements for Menstrual Problems

The use of herbs and botanicals often increases with age. Dong Quai is a Chinese women's tonic for menstrual cramps and other symptoms; clients should not take it with warfarin, aspirin, or ticlopidine because Dong Quai has blood-thinning attributes. Nurses counsel clients to avoid use of evening primrose oil with antiseizure medications, antiepileptics, chlorpromazine, fluphenazine, and mesoridazine. If a client uses valerian as an antianxiety or sleep aid, she should not mix it with other sedatives, alcohol, and other central nervous system depressants because of the risk of additional sedation (Houghton, 1999).

Questions to Ponder

1. A 28-year-old woman who is 5 feet, 5 inches tall and has a prepregnancy weight of 180 lbs is seeing the nurse for the first time at approximately 12 gestational weeks. This is her first pregnancy. As a result of morning sickness, she has lost 5 lbs and tells the nurse she is thrilled.
   - What recommendations for weight gain are appropriate for this woman based on her baseline weight?
   - What problems are associated with lack of weight gain during pregnancy?
   - List some approaches to take during counseling sessions that would help this woman have a healthy pregnancy outcome.

SUMMARY

- Macronutrients that provide energy are carbohydrate, fat, and protein. Nutrients that function as coenzymes are usually vitamins. Cofactors are usually microminerals; some macrominerals help form the skeleton. All these nutrients coordinate their functions to help keep the body healthy.
- The level of intake of each nutrient needed to keep the body healthy is found in the Dietary Reference Intake publications.
- Culture, religion, and other factors influence food selection. Careful planning and choices designed to take advantage of the plusses of the cultural pattern and counteract the minuses can result in healthy, culturally acceptable meals.
- Nutritional needs of women vary with stage in life.
- Solid nutrition in pregnancy is vital to positive maternal and fetal outcomes.
- Breastfeeding benefits both mother and infant.
- Pregnancy increases needs by 300 kcal/day, whereas lactation increases needs by 500 kcal/day. All other increased needs are provided when women select foods wisely.
- Adult and older adult women need to control weight by regulating intake of energy nutrients while getting adequate folate, iron, and calcium.

REVIEW QUESTIONS

1. The nurse is teaching a pregnant woman of normal prepregnancy weight for height about appropriate weight gain during pregnancy. The nurse determines that instruction has been effective when the client states
   A. "A weight gain of about 16 lbs per trimester is recommended."
   B. "I shouldn't gain any more than 15 to 20 lbs for the total pregnancy."
   C. "I should eat whatever I want and not worry about my total weight."
   D. "An average weight gain between 25 to 35 lbs is considered appropriate."
2. A client reports that she and her husband are considering starting a family within the next year. The nurse should advise the client to increase intake of folic acid
   A. immediately.
   B. if she misses her period.
   C. if pregnancy is confirmed.
   D. one week before her period.
3. The nurse is conducting a quantitative assessment of a client's food intake. Which of the following techniques would *not* be appropriate in such an evaluation?
   A. Interview of the client for recall of food intake
   B. Evaluation of foods using the Food Guide Pyramid
   C. Analysis of foods eaten to determine quantities of nutrients
   D. Comparison of quantities of nutrients to Dietary Reference Intakes
4. A nurse is working with a breastfeeding woman who has low milk production. Which of the following interventions should the nurse recommend?
   A. Increase the frequency of nursing.
   B. Give the infant supplemental feedings.
   C. Replace breastfeeding with formula feeding.
   D. Increase fluid intake with more caffeinated beverages.
5. A nurse is working with a client to choose a suitable contraceptive device. The client selects an intrauterine device. The nurse should advise the client to be sure to increase consumption of
   A. iron and vitamin C.
   B. folate and magnesium.
   C. riboflavin and protein.
   D. vitamin A and calcium.
6. Assessment findings reveal an elevated total cholesterol level in a menopausal client. When assisting the client to take appropriate management measures, the nurse is correct in advising the client to consume which of the following percentages of calories from fat?
   A. 15%
   B. 20%
   C. 30%
   D. 45%
7. Following surgery, the nurse notes that an expected outcome is that the client will increase protein intake. Which of the following dietary choices would the nurse encourage?
   A. Frozen yogurt
   B. Dry cereal

C. Apples
D. Nachos

8. The nurse is conducting a teaching session with a group of women about iron needs. Which of the following clients would the nurse expect to have the lowest iron needs?
A. A 15-year-old gymnast
B. A 24-year-old pregnant woman
C. A 38-year-old smoker
D. A 60-year-old with arthritis

9. A client reports that she has been following a vegan diet over the past few years. When working with the client to review dietary intake and needs, which of the following sets of the nutrients would the nurse expect to be potentially deficient?
A. B_{12}, iron, zinc
B. Vitamins A, B, and C
C. Vitamins D, E, and K
D. Vitamin B_6, folate, and calcium

REFERENCES

Alonso, A., Beunza, J. J., Delgado-Rodriguez, M., Martinez, J. A., & Martinez-Gonzalez, M. A. (2005). Low-fat dairy consumption and reduced risk of hypertension: The Seguimiento Universidad de Navarra (SUN) cohort. *American Journal of Clinical Nutrition, 82*(5), 972–979.

American Academy of Pediatrics. (2000). Breastfeeding and your diet. Medem, Inc. Retrieved October 1, 2003, from http://www.medem.com/medlb/article_detaillb.cfm?article_ID=ZZZNIUQXQ7C&sub_cat=20.

American Academy of Pediatrics. (2003). A woman's guide to breastfeeding. Retrieved October 1, 2003, from http://www.aap.org/family/brstguid.htm.

American Academy of Pediatrics Committee on Pediatric AIDS. (1995). Human milk, breastfeeding, and transmission of human immunodeficiency virus in the United States. *Pediatrics, 96*(5), 977–980.

American Dietetic Association. (1999). Position of the American Dietetic Association and Dietitians of Canada: Women's health and nutrition. *Journal of the American Dietetic Association, 99,* 738.

American Dietetic Association. (2001). Position of the American Dietetic Association: Breaking the barriers to breast feeding. *Journal of the American Dietetic Association, 101,* 1213.

American Dietetic Association. (2002). The role of dietetics professionals in health promotion and disease prevention: Position of ADA. *Journal of the American Dietetic Association, 102,* 1680–1687.

American Pregnancy Association. (2004). Natural herbs and vitamins to avoid during pregnancy. Retrieved February 10, 2006, from http://www.americanpregnancy.org/pregnancyhealth/herbstoavoid.html.

Anderson, R. N. (2001). Deaths: Leading causes for 1999. *National Vital Statistics Reports, 49*(11), 1–87.

Aranceta, J., Serra-Majem, L., Perez-Rodrigo, C., Llopis, J., Mataix, J., Ribas, L., Tojo, R., & Tur, J. A. (2001). Vitamins in Spanish food patterns: The eVe Study. *Public Health Nutrition, 4*(6A), 1317–1323.

Aschenbrenner, D., & Venable, S. (2006). *Drug therapy in nursing* (2nd ed.). Philadelphia: Lippincott Williams & Wilkins.

Azais-Braesco, V., & Pascal, G. (2000). Vitamin A in pregnancy: Requirements and safety limits. *American Journal of Clinical Nutrition, 71,* 1325S.

Baeten, J. M., et al. (2001). Pregnancy complications and outcomes among overweight and obese nulliparous women. *American Journal of Public Health, 91,* 436.

Barnard, N. D., et al. (2000). Diet and sex-hormone binding globulin, dysmenorrhea, and premenstrual symptoms. *Obstetrics and Gynecology, 95,* 245.

Bartley, K. A., Underwood, B. A., & Deckelbaum, R. J. (2005). A life cycle micronutrient perspective for women's health. *American Journal of Clinical Nutrition, 81*(5), 1188S–1193S.

Bendich, A. (2000). The potential for dietary supplements to reduce premenstrual syndrome (PMS) symptoms. *Journal of the American College of Nutrition, 19,* 3.

Berkey, C. S., et al. (2000). Relation of childhood diet and body size to menarche and adolescent growth in girls. *American Journal of Epidemiology, 152,* 446.

Bienz, D., Cori, H., & Hornig, D. (2003). Adequate dosing of micronutrients for different age groups in the life cycle. *Food and Nutrition Bulletin, 24*(3 Suppl), S7–S15.

Bolumar, F., et al. (1997). Caffeine intake and delayed conception: A European multicenter study on infertility and subfecundity. *American Journal of Epidemiology, 145,* 324.

Braunschweig, C., et al. (2000). Impact of declines in nutritional status on outcomes in adult patients hospitalized for more than 7 days. *Journal of the American Dietetic Association, 100,* 1316.

Brown, L., Rosner, B., Willett, W. W., & Sacks, F. M. (1999). Cholesterol-lowering effects of dietary fiber: A meta-analysis. *American Journal of Clinical Nutrition, 69,* 30–42.

Carver, J. D. (1999). Dietary nucleotides: Effects on the immune and gastrointestinal systems. *Acta Paediatr Suppl, 88,* 83.

Clark, A. M., et al. (1998). Weight loss in obese infertile women results in improvement in reproductive outcomes for all forms of fertility treatment. *Human Reproduction, 13,* 1505.

Cnattingius, S., et al. (1998). Prepregnancy weight and the risk of adverse pregnancy outcomes. *New England Journal of Medicine, 338,* 147.

Committee on Drugs. (1989). Transfer of drugs and other chemicals into human milk. *Pediatrics, 84*(5), 924–936.

Committee on Nutritional Status During Pregnancy and Lactation, Institute of Medicine. (1990). *Nutrition during pregnancy: Part I: Weight gain, Part II: Nutrient supplements.* Washington, DC: The National Academies Press.

Committee on Substance Abuse. (1990). Drug-exposed infants. *Pediatrics, 86*(4), 639–642.

Craig, W. J. (1994). Iron status of vegetarians. *American Journal of Clinical Nutrition, 59,* 1233–1237.

Craven, R. C., & Hirnle, C. J. (2007). *Fundamentals of nursing: Human health and function* (5th ed.). Philadelphia: Lippincott Williams & Wilkins.

Dawson, E. B., et al. (2000). Blood cell lead, calcium, and magnesium levels associated with pregnancy-induced hypertension and preeclampsia. *Biological Trace Element Research, 74,* 107.

Dewey, K. G. (2001). Nutrition, growth and complementary feeding of the breastfed infant. *Pediatric Clinics of North America, 48,* 87.

Fairfield, K. M., & Fletcher, R. H. (2002). Vitamins for chronic disease prevention in adults: Scientific review. *Journal of the American Medical Association, 287*(23), 3116–3126.

FANSA. Retrieved May 8, 2003, from http://www.eatright.com/folicacid.html.

Finn, S. Women in the new world order: Where old values command new respect. *Journal of the American Dietetic Association, 97,* 475.

Florida Department of Health. (2003). *Prenatal and postpartum nutrition module.* Bureau of WIC and Nutritional Services. Tallahassee, FL: Author.

Ford, F. (2004). A guide to nutrition in pregnancy. *Practicing Midwife, 7*(11), 24, 26.

Fowles, E. (2002). Comparing pregnant women's nutritional knowledge to their actual diet intake. *The American Journal of Maternal Child Nursing, 27*(3), 171–177.

Freedman, D. M., Ron, E., Ballard-Barbash, R., Doody, M. M., & Linet, M. S. (2006). Body mass index and all-cause mortality in a nationwide US cohort. *International Journal of Obesity, 30.*

Freeman, D. S., Khan, L. K., Serdula, M. K., Dietz, W. H., Srinivasan, S., et al. (2003). The relation of menarcheal age to obesity in childhood and adulthood: the Bogalusa heart study. *BMC Pediatrics, 3*(1), 3.

Gates, G., & McDonald, M. (1997). Comparison of dietary risk factors for cardiovascular disease in African-American and white women. *Journal of the American Dietetic Association, 97*(12), 1394–1400.

Guthrie, J. F., Lin, B-H., & Frazao, E. (2002). Role of food prepared away from home in the American diet, 1977–78 versus 1994–96: Changes and consequences. *Journal of Nutrition Education and Behavior, 34,* 140–150.

Harvard School of Public Health. (2005). *Carbohydrates.* Retrieved February 6, 2006, from http://www.hsph.harvard.edu/nutrition source/carbohydrates.html.

Harvard School of Public Health. (2005). *Fats and cholesterol.* Retrieved February 6, 2006, from http://www.hsph.harvard.edu/nutritionsource/fats.html#references.

Henry, C. L., & Schalch, D. S. (2005). Vitamin E toxicity. E-Medicine. [On-line]. Retrieved February 8, 2006, from http://www.emedicine.com/med/topic2384.htm.

Herbold, N. H., & Frates, S. E. (2000). Update of nutrition guidelines for the teen: Trends and concerns. *Current Opinion in Pediatrics, 12,* 303.

Horner, N. K., & Lampe, J. W. (2000). Potential mechanisms of diet therapy for fibrocystic breast conditions show inadequate evidence of effectiveness. *Journal of the American Dietetic Association, 100,* 1368.

Houghton, P. J. (1999). The scientific basis for the reputed activity of Valerian. *Journal of Pharmacology, 51*(5), 505–512.

Institute of Medicine. (1997). Dietary reference intakes for calcium, phosphorous, magnesium, vitamin D, and fluoride. Retrieved July 30, 2003, from http://www.iom.edu.

Institute of Medicine. (2000a). Dietary reference intakes for vitamin C, vitamin E, selenium, and carotenoids. Retrieved February 8, 2006, from http://www.iom.edu.

Institute of Medicine. (2000b). Dietary reference intakes for thiamin, riboflavin, niacin, vitamin B6, folate, vitamin B12, pantothenic acid, biotin, and choline. Retrieved July 30, 2003, from http://www.iom.edu.

Institute of Medicine. (2001). Dietary reference intakes for vitamin A, vitamin K, arsenic, boron, chromium, copper, iodine, iron, manganese, molybdenum, nickel, silicon, vanadium, and zinc. Retrieved July 30, 2003, from http://www.iom.edu.

Institute of Medicine. (2002). Dietary reference intakes for energy, carbohydrate, fiber, fat, fatty acids, cholesterol, protein, and amino acids. Retrieved July 30, 2003, from http://www.iom.edu.

Institute of Medicine. (2004). Dietary reference intakes: Water, potassium, sodium, chloride, and sulfate. Retrieved February 7, 2006, from http://www.iom.edu.

Jenkins, D. J., Kendall, C. W., Augustin, L. S., et al. (2002). Glycemic index: Overview of implications in health and disease. *American Journal of Clinical Nutrition, 76,* 266S–273S.

Kaiser, L. L., Allen, L., & American Dietetic Association. (2002). Position of the American Dietetic Association: Nutrition and lifestyle for a healthy pregnancy outcome. *Journal of the American Dietetic Association, 102*(10), 1479–1490.

Kant, A. K., & Graubard, B. I. (2004). Eating out in America, 1987–2000: Trends and nutritional correlates. *Preventive Medicine, 38,* 243–249.

Karch, A. M. (2004). *Lippincott's nursing drug guide.* Philadelphia: Lippincott Williams & Wilkins.

Klebanoff, M. A., et al. (1999). Maternal serum paraxanthine, a caffeine metabolite, and the risk of spontaneous abortion. *New England Journal of Medicine, 341,* 1639.

Kreiter, S. R., et al. (2000). Nutritional rickets in African American breast-fed infants. *Journal of Pediatrics, 137,* 153.

Lenders, C. M., McElrath, T. F., & Scholl, T. O. (2000). Nutrition in adolescent pregnancy. *Current Opinion in Pediatrics, 12,* 291–296.

Li, T. Y., Rana, J. S., Manson, J. E., Willett, W. C., Stampfer, M. J., Colditz, G. A., Rexrode, K. M., & Hu, F. B. (2006). Obesity as compared with physical activity in predicting risk of coronary heart disease in women. *Circulation, 113*(4), 499–506.

Liu, S., & Willett, W. C. (2002). Dietary glycemic load and atherothrombotic risk. *Current Atherosclerosis Report, 4,* 454–461.

Louwman, M. W., et al. (2000). Signs of impaired cognitive function in adolescents with marginal cobalamin status. *American Journal of Clinical Nutrition, 72,* 762.

Mattison, D. (2003). Herbal supplements: Their safety, a concern for health care providers. March of Dimes. Retrieved October 1, 2003, from http://www.marchofdimes.com/professionals/681_1815.asp.

Mayo Clinic Staff. (2003, April 1). Herb and drug interactions: "Natural" products not always safe. Retrieved October 1, 2003, from http://www.mayoclinic.com/invoke.cfm?id=SA00039.

McCrory, M. A. (2001). Does dieting during lactation put infant growth at risk? *Nutrition Review, 59,* 18.

McKeown, N. M., Meigs, J. B., Liu, S., Wilson, P. W., & Jacques, P. F. (2002). Whole-grain intake is favorably associated with metabolic risk factors for type 2 diabetes and cardiovascular disease in the Framingham Offspring Study. *American Journal of Clinical Nutrition, 76,* 390–398.

Messina, V., & Reed Mangels, A. (2001). Considerations in planning vegan diets: Children. *Journal of the American Dietetic Association, 101,* 661.

Oddy, W. H., Holt, P. G., Sly, P. D., Read, Q. W., Landau, L. I., Stanley, F. J., et al. (1999). Association between breast feedings and asthma in 6-year-old children: Findings of a prospective birth cohort study. *British Medical Journal, 319,* 815–819.

Odijk, J., Kull, I., Borres, M. P., Brandtzaeg, P., Edberg, U., Hanson, L. A., et al. (2003). Breastfeeding and allergic disease: A multidisciplinary review of the literature (1966–2001) on the mode of early feeding in infancy and its impact on later atopic manifestations. *Allergy, 58,* 833–843.

Okasha, M., McCarron, P., McEwen, J., & Smith, G. D. (2001). Age at menarche: Secular trends and association with adult anthropometric measures. *Annals of Human Biology, 28*(1), 68–78.

Pereira, M. A., O'Reilly, E., Augustsson, K., et al. (2004). Dietary fiber and risk of coronary heart disease: A pooled analysis of cohort studies. *Archives of Internal Medicine, 164,* 370–376.

Pereira, M. A., & Liu, S. (2003). Types of carbohydrates and risk of cardiovascular disease. *Journal of Women's Health, 12,*115–122.

Rainville, A. (1998). Pica practices of pregnant women are associated with lower maternal hemoglobin level at delivery. *Journal of the American Dietetic Association, 98,* 293.

Rao, A. V. (2002). Lycopene, tomatoes, and the prevention of coronary heart disease [review]. *Experimental Biology and Medicine, 227*(10), 908–913.

Robinson, H. E., O'Connell, C. M., Joseph, K. S., & McLeod, N. L. (2005). Maternal outcomes in pregnancies complicated by obesity. *Obstetrics & Gynecology, 106*(6), 1357–1364.

Scholl, T. O. (2005). Iron status during pregnancy: Setting the stage for mother and infant. *American Journal of Clinical Nutrition, 81*(5), 1218S–1222S.

Scholl, T. O., & Reilly, T. (2000). Anemia, iron and pregnancy outcome. *Journal of Nutrition, 130,* 443S–447S.

Schulze, M. B., Liu, S., Rimm, E. B., Manson, J. E., Willett, W. C., & Hu, F. B. (2004). Glycemic index, glycemic load, and dietary fiber intake and incidence of type 2 diabetes in younger and middle-aged women. *American Journal of Clinical Nutrition, 80,* 348–356.

Sears, M. R., Greene, J. M., Willan, A. R., Taylor, D. R., Flannery, E. M., Cowan, J. L., et al. (2002). Long-term relation between breastfeeding and development of atopy and asthma in children and young adults: A longitudinal study. *Lancet, 360,* 901–907.

Shaw, G. M., & Lammer, E. J. (1999). Maternal periconceptional alcohol consumption and risk for orofacial clefts. *Journal of Pediatrics, 134,* 298.

Stang, J., et al. (2000). Relationships between vitamin and mineral supplement use, dietary intake, and dietary adequacy among adolescents. *Journal of the American Dietetic Association, 100,* 905.

Surkan, P. J., Hsieh, C. C., Johansson, A. L., Dickman, P. W., & Cnattingius, S. (2004). Reasons for increasing trends in large for gestational age births. *Obstetrics & Gynecology, 104*(4), 720–726.

Swan, L. L., & Apgar, B. S. (1995). Preconceptual obstetric risk assessment and health promotion. *American Family Physician, 51*(8), 1875–1885.

Tsai, S. P., Donnelly, R. P., & Wendt, J. K. (2006). Obesity and mortality in a prospective study of a middle-aged industrial population. *Journal of Occupational and Environmental Medicine, 48*(1), 22–27.

Turner, R. E., Langkamp-Henken, B., et al. (2003). Comparing nutrient intake from food to the estimated average requirements shows middle- to upper-income pregnant women lack iron and possibly magnesium. *Journal of the American Dietetic Association, 103*(4), 461–466.

U.S. Department of Health and Human Services (USDHHS). (2000). *Healthy people 2010.* Washington, DC: Author.

Volpe, S. L. (2006). Popular weight reduction diets. *Journal of Cardiovascular Nursing, 21*(1), 34–39.

Walker, A. F., et al. (1998). Magnesium supplementation alleviates premenstrual symptoms of fluid retention. *Journal of Women's Health, 7,* 1157.

Weinberg, G. A. (2000). The dilemma of postnatal mother-to-child transmission of HIV: To breastfeed or not? *Birth, 27,* 199.

Whitney, E. N., Cataldo, C. B., & Rolfes, S. R. (2002). *Understanding normal and clinical nutrition* (6th ed.). Belmont, CA: Wadsworth/ Thomson Learning.

Willett, W., Manson, J., & Liu, S. (2002). Glycemic index, glycemic load, and risk of type 2 diabetes. *American Journal of Clinical Nutrition, 76,* 274S–280S.

Women's Health.gov. (2005). *Pregnancy and a healthy diet.* Retrieved February 7, 2006, from http://www.womenshealth.gov/faq/ preg-nutr.htm#2.

Work Group on Breastfeeding. (1997). Breastfeeding and the use of human milk. *Pediatrics, 100*(6), 1035–1039.

Worthington-Roberts, B. S., & Roberts, S. R. (1997) *Nutrition in pregnancy and lactation* (6th ed.). Boston: McGraw-Hill.

Wright, A. L., et al. (2001). Factors influencing the relation of infant feeding to asthma and recurrent wheeze in childhood. *Thorax, 56,* 192.

CHAPTER 4

Medical Alterations in Women During Adolescence and Adulthood

Louise Aurilio

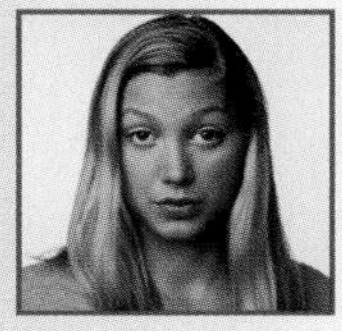

Lela, 33 years old, comes to the clinic for evaluation of vaginal discharge. She states, "It started about 2 days ago, and it seems to be getting worse. My vagina also feels sore and itchy. I've been wearing a thin sanitary pad so that the drainage doesn't get on my clothes."

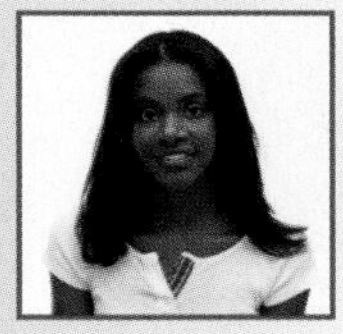

Jade, a 21-year-old woman, arrives at the clinic for a prenatal visit. Health history taking reveals that Jade experienced menarche at 11 years old and a previous full-term pregnancy at 19 years old. Jade denies any use of drugs, alcohol, or cigarettes. Her body mass index is 23. When questioned about her family history, Jade states, "My grandmother on my mother's side just died of breast cancer. Could I be at risk now, too?"

You will learn more about Lela's and Jade's stories later. Nurses working with these clients and others like them need to understand the material in this chapter to manage care and address issues appropriately. Before beginning, consider the following points related to the above scenarios:

- Does anything about either case present any issues of immediate concern or worry? Explain your answer.
- How might each client's circumstances influence the nurse's approach to care?
- How are the clients similar? How are they different?
- What details will the nurse need to investigate with Lela? What about Jade?
- What areas of concern would the nurse need to address with each client?

LEARNING OBJECTIVES

On completion of this chapter, the reader should be able to:

- Identify risk factors for the various alterations addressed in this chapter.
- Discuss strategies that promote and enhance the health and well-being of women experiencing health alterations.
- Review common genetic disorders with special implications for women.
- Identify common autoimmune disorders in women and their implications for childbearing.
- Describe the different types of diabetes mellitus, as well as effective prevention and management strategies.
- Describe cardiovascular and pulmonary problems addressed in this chapter and the implications of these disorders for women.
- Compare and contrast common sexually transmitted infections (STIs), including risk factors and prevention strategies.
- Identify the different types of hepatitis and the problems posed by each one.
- Summarize common benign and malignant breast disorders.
- Outline specific risk factors, treatment strategies, and collaborative care for the client with breast cancer.
- Explain disorders, infections, and cancers of the female reproductive tract.
- Discuss risks for pelvic relaxation alterations and urinary tract disorders as addressed in this chapter.

KEY TERMS

amenorrhea
bacterial vaginosis
BRCA1
BRCA2
candidiasis
carcinoma in situ
cervical dysplasia
condylomata
cystitis
diabetes mellitus
dysfunctional uterine bleeding
dysmenorrhea
endometriosis
fibroadenoma
genital herpes
hepatitis
inflammatory breast cancer
leiomyoma (fibroid tumor)
leukorrhea
lumpectomy
lymphedema
mastalgia
mastectomy
mastitis
menorrhagia
pelvic inflammatory disease
premenstrual syndrome
rheumatoid arthritis
sexually transmitted infections
sickle cell crisis
sickle cell disease
systemic lupus erythematosus
trichomoniasis

During the past several decades, women's health has grown as a distinct specialty in the field of health care. Additionally, women themselves are becoming more active participants in their own well-being, demanding more information about prevention and treatment to assist them with important health-related decisions, as well as issues of well-being and quality of life. This chapter reflects a comprehensive view of women's health beyond a traditional focus on reproduction. It does so by examining sexually transmitted infections (STIs), problems with the reproductive organs, and disorders of the breasts, as well as several alterations in other body systems that affect women in great numbers or that have different implications or manifestations in women than in men. The content incorporates information on illness, factors that affect health status, and trends in research, prevention, diagnosis, and collaborative care. Discussions of those medical conditions that emerge during pregnancy or with dangerous implications in pregnancy are found in Chapter 13.

GENETIC DISORDERS

The field of genetics has burgeoned in recent years, largely as a result of the human genome project (see Chap. 11). Genetic disorders often influence women's reproductive capabilities and caregiver roles. Nurses must work to understand how to prevent, reduce, and overcome the adverse effects caused by genetic disorders in women. Additionally, women themselves need knowledge about inherent genetic risks for illness and to understand how such risks can affect their quality of life.

SICKLE CELL DISEASE

Sickle cell disease (SCD; sickle cell anemia) is an autosomal recessive genetic disorder found primarily in African Americans, but also in people of Mediterranean, Arabic, East Indian, and South and Central American heritage. This serious, chronic hemolytic anemia is incurable and may be fatal by midlife. SCD results from a mutation in hemoglobin (Hb), in which sickled Hb (HbS) replaces normal adult Hb (HbA) and has a reduced oxygen-carrying ability. As a result, the red blood cells (RBCs) have a decreased lifespan (Fig. 4.1). The sickling of RBCs leads to obstruction of small blood vessels and causes infarcts of the lungs, kidneys, spleen, and bones.

Assessment Findings

Symptoms of SCD vary. Pediatric clients with SCD exhibit general delays and impairments in growth and development. Typically, clients are healthy most of the time. The anemia causes fatigue, pallor of mucous membranes, and decreased exercise tolerance. The skin may appear gray; jaundice is common. Clients may have

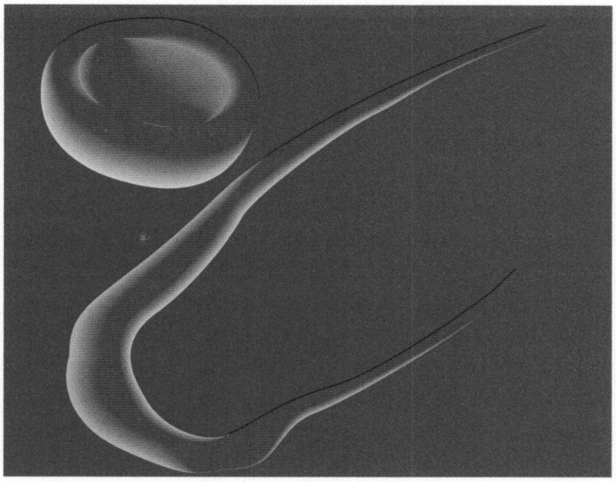

FIGURE 4.1 A normal red blood cell (*upper left*). A sickled red blood cell (*bottom*).

frequent infections. The heart may be enlarged, leading to congestive heart failure. The median survival age for clients with SCD is 40 to 50 years (Smeltzer & Bare, 2008).

People with SCD are *homozygous* for the disease. This means that they carry two genes for the disorder at the given locus on a homologous chromosome. Some people, however, have *sickle cell trait* (SA), a milder and potentially asymptomatic form of SCD. Usually, those with SA are *heterozygous,* meaning that they carry two different genes at the given locus on a pair of homologous chromosomes. In clients with SA, up to 75% of Hb is normal (HbA) (Smeltzer & Bare, 2008). Thus, they display milder symptoms than clients with SCD.

In clients with SCD, conditions that lead to hypoxia, deoxygenated RBCs, and dehydration can result in acute and sudden episodes of **sickle cell crisis** (exacerbations of sickling). The most common type of sickle cell crisis results from vaso-occlusion, in which tissues become hypoxic, leading to tissue death and pain. Sickle cell crisis can be fatal depending on the part of the body affected and the amount of occlusion. Commonly affected parts of the body include the chest, abdomen, and extremities. Precipitating factors include viral or bacterial infections, activities in high altitudes, emotional or physical stress, surgery, vomiting, diarrhea, and diaphoresis (Smeltzer & Bare, 2008).

Pregnant clients with SA or SCD can experience complications such as pyelonephritis, pregnancy-induced hypertension, urinary tract infections, congestive heart failure, and life-threatening cardiopathology (James et al., 2006). Women considering pregnancy, a contributor to sickle cell crisis, should seek counseling to understand health risks and the possibility of fetal loss. See Chapter 13 for discussion of SA and SCD in pregnancy.

Collaborative Management

The most common problem in clients with SA and SCD is inadequate oxygen. Thus, regular monitoring of Hb and hematocrit counts is essential. Oxygen administration should occur as ordered. Clients may need to maintain bedrest to help control their metabolic requirements.

Acute painful episodes are the most common reason for seeking medical care; often, clients with pain related to SCD are undertreated (Labbe et al., 2005). Thus, pain assessment and evaluation of these clients are extremely important. To promote comfort, clients with SCD usually receive large doses of continuous narcotic analgesics; continuous narcotic administration is the mainstay of pain management during an acute phase (Jacob & American Pain Society, 2001). Patient-controlled analgesia also may be used.

Nursing interventions and outcomes can be wide ranging (NIC/NOC Box 4.1). Client teaching focuses on measures to prevent sickle cell crises and to control the condition as much as possible. The nurse should instruct the client to avoid high altitudes and infections and encourage the client to obtain vaccines that prevent influenza and pneumonia. Adequate rest and sleep and stress reduction techniques may be beneficial. The nurse should ensure that the client maintains adequate fluid intake. Use of oral contraceptives is contraindicated, but the client should take measures to avoid unplanned pregnancy, which can precipitate life-threatening sickle cell crisis. Women may need counseling about sterilization options and alternative contraceptive measures to decrease the risk for pregnancy. See Chapter 13 for more discussion of SCD in pregnant women.

NIC/NOC Box 4.1 Sickle Cell Anemia

Common NIC Labels

- Analgesic Administration
- Circulatory Care
- Health Education
- Medication Administration
- Medication Management
- Oxygen Therapy
- Pain Management
- Patient-Controlled Analgesia (PCA) Assistance
- Teaching: Disease Process
- Vital Sign Monitoring

Common NOC Labels

- Comfort Level
- Knowledge: Disease Process
- Knowledge: Health Behaviors
- Pain Control
- Pain: Disruptive Effects
- Pain Level
- Respiratory Status: Gas Exchange
- Tissue Perfusion (specify peripheral, cerebral, abdominal organs)
- Vital Signs Status

THALASSEMIA

Thalassemia (Mediterranean or Cooley's anemia) is the name given to a group of autosomal recessive disorders associated with defective synthesis of hemoglobin (Smeltzer & Bare, 2008). Clients with thalassemia have problems involving the alpha or beta globin proteins in blood. As a result, RBCs neither form properly nor carry sufficient oxygen, which leads to potential hemolysis.

Heterozygous carriers of *thalassemia minor* (thalassemia trait) usually are asymptomatic or have acquired chronic anemia with normal or elevated RBCs. Usually, no systemic problems ensue, even though the anemia does not respond to iron therapy. Prolonged iron therapy can lead to harmful, excessive storage of iron in the body. Clients with thalassemia minor usually have a normal lifespan and normal pregnancies (Yaish, 2005).

Homozygous clients usually experience the more severe *thalassemia major,* a life-threatening disorder with general symptoms of anemia and retarded physical and mental growth. Clients with thalassemia major usually display pronounced splenomegaly, hepatomegaly, jaundice, RBC hemolysis, and chronic bone marrow hyperplasia with expansion of the marrow space (Yaish, 2005). Thalassemia major also causes complications in pregnancy such as pregnancy-induced hypertension, low birth weight, and increased fetal mortality (Yaish, 2005). Women with this disorder usually have larger than normal placentas, increased risk for chronic infection, and progressive hepatic or cardiac failure that may lead to death (Yaish, 2005). Additionally, iron is contraindicated in these women because this type of anemia does not respond to iron therapy, and administration of iron could lead to excessive iron storage and toxicity (see Chap. 13).

Diagnosis is determined through an evaluation of complete blood count (Yaish, 2005). Thalassemia trait can be diagnosed by looking at the size of the blood cell and mean corpuscular volume (MCV). Trait carriers have an MCV reading of less than 75 (Yaish, 2005). Often, this reading is lower and more varied in children.

Hemoglobin electrophoresis is used to identify β-thalassemia trait; α-thalassemia trait (silent carrier) is difficult to diagnose and can be found only using DNA testing (Cooley's Anemia Foundation, 2001). Treatment consists of folic acid, regular transfusions if needed, and splenectomy in cases of spleen enlargement and pain.

CYSTIC FIBROSIS

Cystic fibrosis (CF), a chronic and progressive autosomal recessive genetic disease, affects people of both sexes and of all races and ethnicities, with the highest prevalence found in Northern European whites. Approximately 30,000 people in the United States have CF, with more than 10 million asymptomatic carriers of the gene for CF. To inherit CF, a person must inherit two defective CF genes—one from each parent. Each time two carriers of CF conceive, a 25% chance exists that the child will have CF, and a 50% chance exists that the child will be an asymptomatic carrier. Although CF once was considered fatal in childhood, today nearly 40% of people living with CF are 18 years or older (Cystic Fibrosis Foundation, 2005).

With CF, excessive viscous secretions interfere with digestion and respiration. As a result, endocrine functioning is impaired, with subsequent manifestations affecting the lungs, pancreas, and sweat glands. Most clients with CF have exocrine pancreatic insufficiency, and their sweat glands excrete increased sodium and chloride. Furthermore, many of them develop chronic obstructive diffuse pulmonary disease, decreased lung volume, and shunting that result in arterial hypoxemia, possible respiratory failure, and early death.

The most common test for CF is the pilocarpine sweat test and application of electric current. This test may not work well in newborns, who may undergo an immune reactive test instead. Other tests assess lung and pancreatic function and genetic structure. See Box 4.1.

Major treatment goals include clearance of secretions, control of infection, and provision of adequate nutrition. Clients with CF must receive preconception counseling. Well-nourished women with mild forms of the disease usually tolerate pregnancy well (McMullen et al., 2006). In cases of severe CF, pregnancy complications include chronic hypoxia and frequent pulmonary problems. Severe pulmonary infections lead to increased risk for maternal and fetal mortality. Because of the risks involved, female clients with severe CF need information about contraceptive options and, should pregnancy occur, counseling about potential termination as concurrent with the client's value system. See Chapter 13 for considerations related to CF and pregnancy.

BOX 4.1 Common Diagnostic Tests for Cystic Fibrosis

- Sweat test (adults): a positive finding is greater than 65 mEq/L for both sodium and chloride
- Immunoreactive (infant) blood test for protein (IRT) measures for protein trypsinogen
- Gene markers (fetal) and analysis from chorionic villi tissue sampling
- Lung function
- Chest x-ray
- Sputum cultures
- Pulmonary function studies
- Pancreatic function
- Fecal analysis for fat
- Duodenoscopy for quantitative determination of pancreatic enzymes

TAY-SACHS DISEASE

Tay-Sachs disease is an incurable, autosomal recessive metabolic disease that occurs primarily in newborns of Ashkenazi (Eastern European) Jewish descent. Approximately 1 in 27 Ashkenazi Jews are carriers (heterozygous) of Tay-Sachs disease (National Tay-Sachs and Allied Diseases Association, 2006). Incidence of TSD also is notable in Sephardic Jews and non-Jewish French Canadians living near the St. Lawrence River and in the Cajun community of Louisiana (National Tay-Sachs and Allied Diseases Association, 2006).

Clients with Tay-Sachs disease exhibit a deficiency of the β-hexosaminidase enzyme, normally responsible for decomposing the naturally occurring fatty substance GM2-ganglioside. Toxic buildup of GM2-ganglioside affects the cells of the nervous system. Symptoms include progressive deterioration of both motor and mental function, with diminished vision. They generally manifest at 4 to 6 months of age, with death occurring at 3 to 4 years.

To determine carrier status, clinicians measure hexosaminidase activity in plasma or white blood cells; they also may use gene mutation analysis. Prenatal diagnosis by chorionic villi sampling or amniocentesis can identify couples at risk. Available counseling can help couples identify options for having unaffected children. See Chapter 11 for more information on genetic counseling and screening for Tay-Sachs and other similar conditions.

AUTOIMMUNE DISORDERS

Autoimmune disorders develop when the immune system responds inappropriately to and attacks the body's natural tissues. Although multiple theories abound, the etiology of autoimmune disorders remains unknown. Multiple environmental and genetic factors likely contribute, with the incidence of some types increasing with age. These disorders seem to occur in clusters; a client may present with more than one type. They are more common in women than in men and affect approximately 5% to 8% of the U.S. population (U.S. Department of Health and Human Services [USDHHS], Health Resources and Services Administration, Maternal Child Health Bureau, 2002).

Generally, autoimmune disorders are classified as organ specific or systemic (Box 4.2). With organ-specific autoimmune disorders, tissue damage is localized; with systemic autoimmune disorders, tissue damage is widespread. Regardless of classification, these debilitating and chronic disorders increase health care costs and decrease quality of life. The goals of treatment include (1) restoration of normal immune response, (2) prevention of further tissue and organ damage, and (3) limitation or prevention of complications (USDHHS, Health Resources and Services Administration, Maternal Child Health Bureau, 2002).

RHEUMATOID ARTHRITIS

Rheumatoid arthritis (RA) affects approximately 2 million people in the United States, 70% of whom are women (Arthritis Foundation, 2006). Onset is most common between 30 and 50 years of age (Arthritis Foundation, 2006). RA generally develops as symmetrical inflammation in the joints, which may extend to other tissues and cause erosion of bone and cartilage (Fig. 4.2). Signs and symptoms include fatigue, anorexia, generalized weakness, symmetrical polyarthritis or multiple joint inflammation, joint swelling, pain, and fever (Smeltzer & Bare, 2008). Periods of remission and exacerbation are characteristic. Because RA often affects the wrists, hands, knees, and feet, clients may complain of significant pain with movement.

Risk factors for RA include age, obesity, joint injuries, infections such as Lyme disease, and repetitive joint use. Complications include infection, osteoporosis, and amyloidoses with the possibility of spinal cord compression (Smeltzer & Bare, 2008).

BOX 4.2 Common Autoimmune Disorders

Organ-Specific

Central nervous system
- Guillain-Barré syndrome
- Multiple sclerosis

Endocrine
- Hypothyroidism
- Thyroiditis
- Type 1 diabetes

Gastrointestinal
- Ulcerative colitis

Musculoskeletal
- Fibromyalgia
- Myasthenia gravis

Systemic

Rheumatoid arthritis
Systemic lupus erythematosus

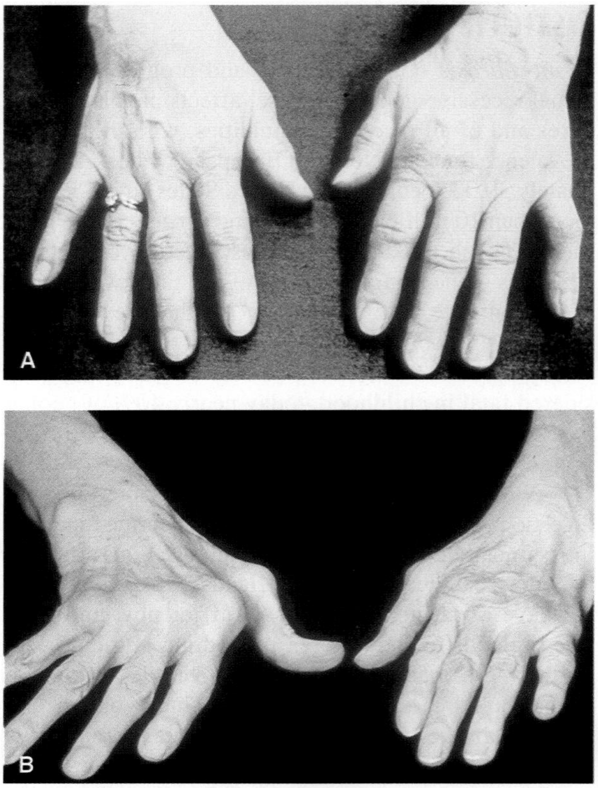

FIGURE 4.2 Joint appearance in rheumatoid arthritis. (**A**) Early. (**B**) Advanced.

Clinicians usually diagnose RA through physical examination of joints, especially muscle strength evaluation; medical and family history study; elevated rheumatoid factor reading; and synovial fluid analysis. Radiography and magnetic resonance imaging (MRI) can identify the extent of joint involvement and the disease's progression.

Collaborative management involves a comprehensive program of drug therapy and education to prevent joint destruction. Several emerging medications for RA include leflunomide, tumor necrosis factor inhibitors, and anakinra (Rindfleisch & Muller, 2005). Nonsteroidal anti-inflammatory drugs (NSAIDs) help reduce pain and inflammation, whereas antimetabolic and immunomodulating drugs can prevent joint destruction and improve comfort and functioning (Rindfleisch & Muller, 2005). Education should focus on compliance with drug therapy, including proper administration, correct dosing, reporting of side effects, and frequent medical and laboratory follow-up. Physical therapy and acupuncture also may assist with maintenance of joint motion and muscle strength. Splinting and assistive devices are recommended to ensure joint protection. Because food allergies have been associated with RA, testing for food allergy, elimination of nonallergy food intolerances, and proper nutrition are recommended to help alleviate symptoms (Condon,

2004). Proper balance between rest and activity and therapies can improve quality of life.

Nursing interventions include client education, pain management, increased range-of-motion exercises, promotion of daily activities, careful monitoring of mental functions and sleep, and assessment of psychological wellness (Martin, 2004). NIC/NOC Box 4.2 highlights some common nursing interventions and outcomes for a client with RA.

MYASTHENIA GRAVIS

Myasthenia gravis (MG) is a chronic disorder characterized by fluctuating weakness of the voluntary musculoskeletal groups. It affects women more than men, usually peaking between 20 and 30 years of age. MG occurs among all races. It may be found in more than one member of a family, but it is neither inherited nor contagious. The cause might rest in an autoimmune process that produces antibodies directed against acetylcholine (ACh) receptor sites and reduces ACh receptors cells at the neuromuscular junction. The result is lost muscle strength and increased muscle weakness.

The muscles most frequently affected are those that control eye and eyelid movements, chewing, swallowing, coughing, and facial expressions. The illness can change speech patterns; the voice may become faint during long conversations. It also affects upper torso muscles more than it affects trunk and limb muscles. Weakness in the muscles that control breathing can cause dyspnea. No other indications of neurologic deficits appear. Reflexes and sensory perception remain normal, and muscle atrophy is rare. Rest usually can restore muscle strength.

The disease affects people differently. Certain conditions, such as emotional stress, pregnancy, menses, secondary illness, trauma, temperature extremes, injection with neuromuscular blocking drugs, surgery, and trauma, may cause exacerbations. Clients may encounter complications such as respiratory infection aspiration and respiratory insufficiency, possibly necessitating hospitalization. They also may experience periods of remission.

An electromyelogram (EMG), fatigability, Tensilon, and blood tests to detect abnormal antibodies can confirm MG. Many people tested, however, have negative or equivocal results. Therefore, clinical findings always take precedence over negative conformity tests. During a Tensilon test, atropine should always be available to counteract any effects detrimental to the client (Table 4.1).

No known cure for MG exists. Treatments such as medications, thymectomy, and plasmaphereses allow clients with MG to lead normal lives. Current treatments differ according to severity of weakness, age, sex, and degree of impairment. Ultimate goals include a return of normal muscle endurance and strength, avoidance of complications, and maintenance of quality of life commensurate to the disease's cause.

When clients with MG are admitted to the hospital, management involves monitoring for respiratory infection, providing adequate ventilation and drug therapy, and observing for side effects caused by medications. An important issue is distinguishing cholinergic crisis from myasthenia crisis. Cholinergic crisis occurs when a client overdoses on anticholinesterase drugs, which will result in an increase in ACh receptor sites. Clients in cholinergic crisis develop symptoms of increased weakness of the skeletal muscles, especially 1 hour after ingesting anticholinesterase; dyspnea; salivation; diarrhea; nausea and vomiting; abdominal cramps; increased bronchial secretions; sweating; and lacrimation. Myasthenia crisis occurs when the dose of medication is too low or the client forgets to take medication as prescribed. Symptoms of myasthenia crisis include muscle weakness in areas that affect swallowing and breathing, aspiration, respiratory insufficiency, and respiratory infection. Intravenous (IV) injection of ACh agent (Tensilon) improves muscle contractility in women who are in myasthenia crisis.

The nurse makes accurate, detailed assessments about the client's fatigue, body area affected, and severity of affliction. Physical examination should include respiratory rate, oxygen saturation levels, arterial blood gas analysis, and pulmonary function studies. The nurse also should evaluate the client's lifestyle and coping skills,

NIC/NOC Box 4.2 Rheumatoid Arthritis

Common NIC Labels

- Analgesic Administration
- Body Mechanics Promotion
- Exercise Promotion: Strength Training
- Exercise Therapy: Joint Mobility
- Health Education
- Medication Administration
- Medication Management
- Pain Management
- Patient-Controlled Analgesia (PCA) Assistance
- Teaching: Disease Process
- Teaching: Prescribed Activity/Exercise

Common NOC Labels

- Comfort Level
- Joint Movement: Active
- Knowledge: Disease Process
- Knowledge: Health Behaviors
- Mobility Level
- Muscle Function
- Pain Control
- Pain: Disruptive Effects
- Pain Level

TABLE 4.1 Diagnostic Tests for Myasthenia Gravis*

TEST	POSITIVE FINDING
Blood test	Look for presence of abnormal antibody.
Fatigability; upward gaze for 2 to 3 minutes	Client with myasthenia gravis cannot hold eyes open. He or she shows increased drooping of the eyelids.
Electromyogram	Decrementing response to repeated stimulation of hand muscles, which indicates muscle fatigue.
Tensilon test (Edrophonium chloride)	Improvement of strength after injected into vein

*Many people have negative or equivocal results. Clinical findings take precedence over negative results on confirmatory tests.

swallowing, speaking volume and clarity, and coughing and gagging reflexes. Client and family education focuses on the importance of following the treatment plan, recognizing potential adverse reactions to medications, planning daily activities to avoid fatigue, investigating community resources and support groups, avoiding infections, and gaining awareness of complications of the disease and therapy. Dietary education includes information about foods that the client can chew and swallow easily. The client should schedule doses of medication so that peak action occurs during meals.

SYSTEMIC LUPUS ERYTHEMATOSUS

Systemic lupus erythematosus (SLE), a chronic inflammatory disorder of the connective tissue, affects the skin, joints, serous membranes, blood, kidneys, and central nervous system. Its effects range from mild to severe, with exacerbations and remissions. SLE ranks as a leading cause of morbidity among women. The Centers for Disease Control and Prevention (CDC, 2002) report that SLE has contributed to a 6% increase in the death rate during the past 20 years. Women have a higher incidence of SLE than do men; 90% of all women with SLE are of childbearing age (Gill et al., 2003). The disorder appears three times more commonly in African American than white women (Office on Women's Health, 2000).

Heredity, environmental factors, infections, drugs, antibiotics (especially sulfa and penicillin groups), ultraviolet light, extreme stress, and hormones may cause or contribute to SLE. Ten percent of clients with SLE have a parent or sibling with the condition; only 5% of children born to people with SLE also develop the disease (Lupus Foundation of America, 2006). Although SLE can occur for no apparent reason, sun exposure, infection, medication, and pregnancy can serve as catalysts.

In this disorder of immunoregulation, antibodies conflict with the client's nuclear antigens, cytoplasmic antigens, and platelets. Autoantibodies then bind with their specific antigens, resulting in an accumulation of immune complexes in blood vessel walls. Lupus vasculitis, ischemia with thickened lining of the vessels, fibrinoid degeneration, and thrombus formation ensue.

In pregnant women with SLE, miscarriage and fetal damage are common (Condon, 2004). Estrogens and hormonal changes may stimulate enhanced immune reactivity, whereas antigens suppress immune reactivity, a factor that contributes to a woman's increased risk for acquiring this disorder. See Chapter 13 for more discussion of SLE and other autoimmune problems in pregnancy.

Assessment Findings

Symptoms usually have no characteristic pattern of organ or system involvement (Box 4.3). They initially may include fatigue, nausea, anorexia, weight loss, generalized pain, anemia, and skin photosensitivity (Lupus Foundation of America, 2006). Joint pain and skin rashes are the most common symptoms. Approximately 75% of people with SLE develop skin rashes, including a butterfly-shaped rash on the face (Lupus Foundation of America, 2006) (Fig. 4.3). Symptoms of pneumonia, pleurisy, and mental dysfunction sometimes occur; many clients with SLE display nephritis (Austin & Balew, 1999).

BOX 4.3 Common Symptoms of Lupus

- Achy joints (arthralgia) (95%)
- Frequent fevers, with temperatures higher than 100°F (37.7°C) (90%)
- Arthritis (swollen joints) (90%)
- Prolonged or extreme fatigue (81%)
- Skin rashes (74%)
- Anemia (71%)
- Kidney involvement (50%)
- Pain in the chest on deep breathing (pleurisy) (45%)
- Butterfly-shaped rash across the cheek and nose (42%)
- Sun or light sensitivity (photosensitivity) (30%)
- Hair loss (27%)
- Abnormal blood clotting problems (20%)
- Raynaud's phenomenon (fingers turning white and/or blue in the cold) (17%)
- Seizures (15%)
- Mouth or nose ulcers (12%)

From Lupus Foundation of America. (2006). *Lupus fact sheet.* Retrieved March 21, 2006, from http://www.lupus.org/education/factsheet.html.

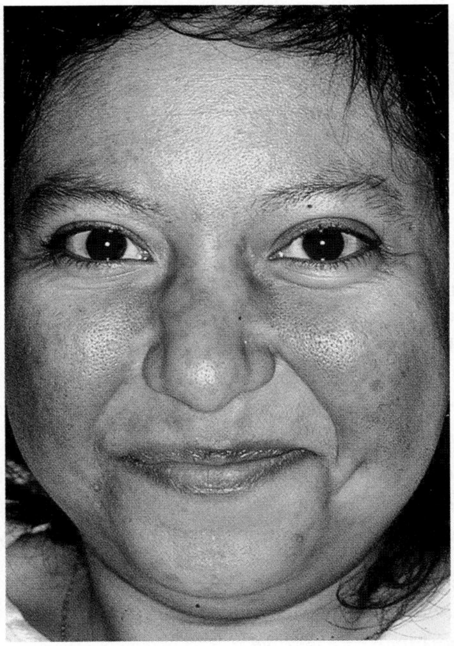

FIGURE 4.3 The characteristic facial butterfly rash of systemic lupus erythematosus.

Diagnosis of SLE includes a review of symptoms and medication history. Clients may exhibit abnormal C-reactive protein (CRP) levels or elevated erythrocyte sedimentation levels (ESR), suggesting inflammation (Gill et al., 2003). Results of laboratory testing, however, may be within normal limits. A complete blood count (CBC) and urinalysis are used to detect kidney and blood vessel involvement. Anti–double-stranded DNA and Smith antibodies specific for SLE appear positive in 30% to 60% of cases (Gill et al., 2003). Although not unique to SLE, an antinuclear antibody test (ANA) can usually diagnose this disease. This test also can return positive findings in people with other inflammatory, as well as general, disorders. Clinicians also may use biopsies of the skin and kidney to diagnose SLE.

Collaborative Management

SLE has no known method of prevention or cure. Current treatment includes medications, nontraditional therapies, and dietary supplements. Antimalarial agents (eg, Plaquenil, ARALEN), NSAIDs, corticosteroids, immunosuppressive drugs, and methotrexate can ease symptoms and improve quality of life (Lupus Foundation of America, 2006). Nontraditional therapies include massage, therapeutic touch, transcendental meditation, and faith-based approaches (Condon, 2004).

Preventive measures are important in reducing exacerbations of SLE. Clients should avoid excessive sun exposure and use sunscreen regularly to prevent rashes. The nurse should encourage stress reduction modalities and exercise to prevent muscle weakness and fatigue. In addition, the nurse should refer the client to support groups, review the benefits of dietary changes, and explore the use of nontraditional therapies. The nurse also should ask about the use of herbal therapies that may affect the immune system and increase inflammatory symptoms (Condon, 2004).

DIABETES MELLITUS

Diabetes mellitus, a metabolic disorder of the pancreas that affects carbohydrate, fat, and protein metabolism, is reaching epidemic proportions in the United States (see Chap. 2). Because the condition is chronic, affected clients can experience many debilitating and life-threatening complications. Risk factors, screening, and prevention measures for diabetes mellitus are discussed in detail in Chapter 2.

Classification

The major classifications of diabetes are as follows:

- Type 1 diabetes (previously referred to as insulin-dependent diabetes)
- Type 2 diabetes
- Gestational diabetes
- Diabetes mellitus associated with other conditions or syndromes

In *type 1 diabetes,* the body fails to produce any insulin. As a result, the immune system attacks and destroys insulin-producing β cells in the pancreas. Type 1 diabetes accounts for 5% to 10% of all cases of diabetes and usually develops in clients younger than 35 years (CDC, 2005a). It is 1.5 to 2 times more common in whites than in nonwhites (Harvard Medical School, 2003).

Approximately 90% of cases of diabetes in the United States are type 2 (American Diabetes Association [ADA], 2005; CDC, 2005a). In this type, the body still produces some insulin, although it displays cellular resistance to its action. The cause of type 2 diabetes remains unknown, but studies show a strong association with obesity (Hu et al., 2003).

Gestational diabetes develops or is discovered during pregnancy. It usually disappears when the pregnancy is over; however, women with this condition are at increased risk for developing type 2 diabetes later in life (National Women's Health Information Center [NWHIC], 2003). Chapter 13 discusses gestational diabetes in detail.

Assessment Findings

Table 4.2 compares the signs and symptoms of types 1 and 2 diabetes. For both types, early signs and symptoms include polyuria, polydipsia, polyphagia, fatigue, weakness, sudden vision changes, tingling and numbness in the hands or feet, dry skin, nonhealing sores, and recurrent infections, especially vulvovaginitis in women (Condon, 2004).

TABLE 4.2 Signs and Symptoms in Types 1 and 2 Diabetes Mellitus

TYPE 1	TYPE 2
Short and sudden development of symptoms Increased thirst and urination Constant hunger Weight loss Blurred vision Extreme tiredness	Less noticeable, often "silent" symptoms Frequent urination Unusual thirst Weight loss Blurred vision Fatigue or feeling "ill" Frequent infections, especially vaginal in women Slow healing of sores Tingling or numbness in feet and hands Dry skin

Diagnostic testing for diabetes is relatively simple. Blood tests include a random blood glucose test, a fasting blood glucose test, a postprandial glucose test, and the oral glucose tolerance test (Table 4.3). Another method of testing is with a glucometer (Fig. 4.4), which measures capillary blood glucose from blood sampled from a finger stick or through the skin on the arm.

Collaborative Management

Treatment of all types of diabetes mellitus requires a daily commitment from the client to healthy lifestyle patterns. Usual treatment includes a balanced combination of diet, exercise, drug therapy, frequent blood glucose monitoring, and stress management (Condon, 2004). Health care providers must educate clients and families about diabetes to enhance their understanding of the following:

- The etiology of the disorder
- Associated dietary needs
- Importance of exercise
- Relevant drug therapies and administration of insulin as needed
- Symptoms of hypoglycemia and hyperglycemia (Box 4.4)
- Signs of infection
- Foot care

TABLE 4.3 Diagnostic Tests for Diabetes Mellitus

TEST	IMPLEMENTATION	DIAGNOSTIC RESULT
Random blood glucose	Blood specimen is drawn without preplanning.	≥200 mg/dL in the presence of symptoms is suggestive of diabetes mellitus.
Fasting blood glucose	Blood specimen is obtained after 8 hours of fasting.	In the nondiabetic client, the glucose level will be between 70 and 110 mg/dL. In the diabetic client, glucose is ≥ 110 mg/dL but <126 mg/dL.
Postprandial glucose	Blood sample is taken 2 hours after a high-carbohydrate meal.	In the nondiabetic client, the glucose level will be between 70 and 110 mg/dL. In the client with diabetes mellitus, the result is ≥140 mg/dL but <200 mg/dL.
Oral glucose tolerance test	Diet high in carbohydrates is eaten for 3 days. Client then fasts for 8 hours. A baseline blood sample is drawn, and a urine specimen is collected. An oral glucose solution is given and time of ingestion recorded. Blood is drawn at 30 minutes and 1, 2, and 3 hours after the ingestion of glucose solution. Urine is collected simultaneously. Drinking water is encouraged to promote urine excretion.	In the nondiabetic client, the glucose returns to normal in 2 to 3 hours, and urine is negative for glucose. In the diabetic client, blood glucose level returns to normal slowly; urine is positive for glucose.
Glycosylated hemoglobin or hemoglobin A1c	Single sample of venous blood is withdrawn.	The amount of glucose stored by the hemoglobin is elevated above 7.0% in the newly diagnosed client with diabetes mellitus, in one who is noncompliant, or in one who is inadequately treated.

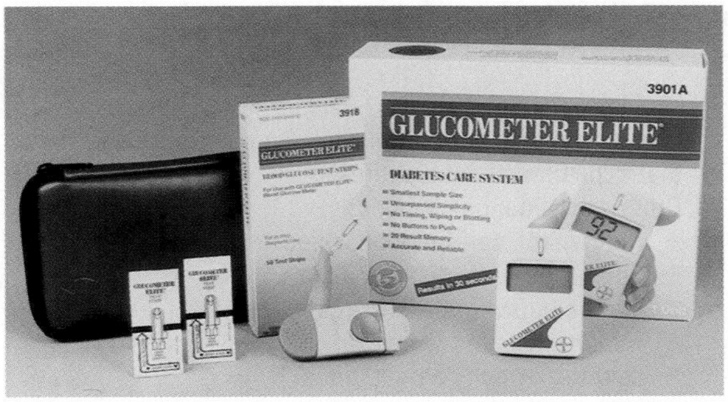

FIGURE 4.4 Clients with diabetes can take regular readings of their blood glucose level with a glucometer.

A thorough discussion of complications arising from unchecked diabetes is essential. Teaching Tips 4.1 provides information nurses can share with clients to help them understand the risks associated with diabetes and the reasons that aggressive prevention and management of the illness are vital.

CARDIOVASCULAR DISEASE

As discussed in Chapter 2, cardiovascular disease (CVD) is the number one cause of death across all races and ethnicities. Traditionally, research about CVD often excluded women, even though 500,000 women die from the condition annually (American Heart Association [AHA], 2006). African American women are more likely to die from CVD than are white women, although the incidences of morbidity are similar (AHA, 2006). Death rates from CVD are higher in white women older than 65 years than in African American women in this same age group (AHA, 2006; Condon, 2004).

Doctors define *arteriosclerosis* as thickening or hardening of the arteries. *Atherosclerosis,* a form of arteriosclerosis and the major cause of CHD, causes the heart vessels to narrow or clog. Plaque or fat deposits accumulate on the inner lining of blood vessels, impeding blood flow to the heart and leading to a myocardial infarction (heart attack) of the heart muscle. Embolus also can cause blockages in the vessel.

Risk factors for CVD are often classified as modifiable and nonmodifiable (Table 4.4). Chapter 2 presents further discussion of measures to control risk, along with associated health screening. The following paragraphs focus on assessment and interventions in clients with cardiovascular illness.

Assessment Findings

Women may experience different signs and symptoms of CVD than do men (AHA, 2005). The most common symptom for all clients is chest pain; however, women may be more likely to have vague symptoms like nausea, sweating, shortness of breath, and dizziness, especially during physical activity (AHA, 2005). Often, clients ignore such symptoms and do not seek medical care for them in a timely manner. Health care providers sometimes misdiagnose coronary chest pain in premenopausal women as stress or anxiety.

Collaborative Management

When a client is diagnosed with CVD, she needs to be informed of the risks and benefits of various medical and surgical interventions so that she can make informed decisions about her health. Treatment is based on the extent and location of occlusions. Medications used include nitrates, aspirin, and β-adrenergic receptor antagonists (β blockers) to control hypertension and ischemic heart disease. Calcium channel blockers decrease vascular resistance and increase blood flow (Youngkin & Davis, 2004). Surgical interventions usually include cardiac catheterization with percutaneous transluminal coronary angioplasty (PTCA) or coronary artery bypass surgery (CABG) (Youngkin & Davis, 2004).

All clients need education and counseling about reducing modifiable risks for CVD (see Chap. 2). Women can lower their chances primarily by educating themselves about risk factors and making the appropriate modifications, knowing the symptoms of a heart attack, and adjusting their lifestyle and behaviors (see Chap. 2). Widespread knowledge and appropriate responses can improve women's awareness of CVD and decrease incidence of the illness. The nurse can explain that a low-fat diet and regular aerobic exercise can significantly reduce

● BOX 4.4 Signs and Symptoms of Hypoglycemia and Hyperglycemia

Hypoglycemia

- Anxiety
- Diaphoresis
- Dizziness
- Headache
- Hunger
- Impaired vision
- Irritability
- Shaking
- Tachycardia
- Weakness and fatigue

Hyperglycemia

- Blurred vision
- Drowsiness or increased sleep
- Dry skin
- Extreme thirst
- Frequent urination
- Nausea

TEACHING TIPS 4.1 Diabetes-Related Complications

The nurse shares with the client and family the following information about diabetes mellitus:

- Heart disease is more common in and more serious in women with diabetes than in men.
- Death rates from heart disease have increased 23% in women with diabetes. In women without the disorder, heart disease has decreased by 27%.
- Women are 50% more likely than are men to be at risk for diabetic ketoacidosis (DKA), which is the most prominent cause of diabetes-related deaths.
- Women with diabetes are 7.6 times more likely to develop peripheral vascular disease (PVD) than women without diabetes.
- Other complications include:
  - Congenital malformations, macrosomia
  - End-stage renal disease
  - Greater susceptibility to infections and illnesses
  - Hypertension
  - Lower-extremity amputations
  - Neuropathy
  - Retinopathy
  - Stroke

From American Diabetic Association. Retrieved June 3, 2003, from http://www.diabetes.org.

risks. He or she also can arrange for the client to consult with a dietitian about a heart-healthy diet, in addition to referring clients to smoking cessation programs.

The nurse should assess signs and symptoms of chest pain and administer prescribed drugs as ordered. He or she should encourage rest and administer oxygen to improve the available supply to the heart. The nurse needs to teach clients about the side effects of any drugs and that severe, unrelieved chest pain indicates a need for immediate examination. The nurse should advise the client to report changes in the usual pattern of angina.

NIC/NOC Box 4.3 highlights some of the more common nursing interventions and outcomes for clients with CVD.

CEREBROVASCULAR ACCIDENT

Cerebrovascular accident (CVA), also called *stroke* or *brain attack,* can result in death and serious long-term disability. More women than men die as a result of stroke yearly (AHA, 2000). While stroke affects people of all ages, older adults account for most stroke-related fatalities. Among middle-aged people, stroke is the third leading cause of death (Condon, 2004). Mortality rates from stroke remain higher among African American women than among white women.

The two major types of stroke are ischemic and hemorrhagic. Mortality rates are lower for ischemic than for hemorrhagic strokes (AHA, 2000). Ischemic stroke accounts for approximately 75% of all cases and occurs if a thrombus or embolus occludes blood supply to the brain (AHA, 2000). With hemorrhagic stroke, a defective artery bursts in the brain, usually resulting in death. Other factors relevant to hemorrhagic stroke include head trauma, cocaine use, and, most commonly, hypertension.

TABLE 4.4 Cardiovascular Risk Factors

MODIFIABLE	NONMODIFIABLE
Hypertension	Increasing age
Smoking	Family history
Hyperlipidemia	Gender
Obesity	Race
Sedentary lifestyle	Type 2 diabetes
Menopause	

NIC/NOC Box 4.3 Cardiovascular Disease

Common NIC Labels

- Cardiac Care: Acute
- Circulatory Care
- Energy Management
- Fluid Monitoring
- Hemodynamic Regulation
- Risk Identification
- Teaching: Individual

Common NOC Labels

- Activity Tolerance
- Cardiac Pump Effectiveness
- Circulation Status
- Health-Seeking Behaviors
- Knowledge: Health Promotion
- Tissue Perfusion: Cardiac
- Tissue Perfusion: Pulmonary
- Vital Signs Status

Assessment Findings

Major symptoms of stroke, related to the area of the brain affected, include motor, sensory, and cognitive deficits. Early warning signs are dizziness; loss or difficulty of speech; vision loss, especially in one eye; and unexplained weakness of the face or extremities (AHA, 2000). A computed tomography (CT) scan or MRI can diagnose a stroke. Quick instillation of therapy often determines survival chances and extent of recovery.

Collaborative Management

If a blood clot causes an ischemic stroke, the clinician uses thrombolytic agents and, in acute stages, antiplatelet and antithrombotic drugs (eg, aspirin, warfarin sodium [Coumadin]) to break up the causative clot. Aspirin given within 48 hours of onset of stroke has proved helpful to clients of both genders (Mosca et al., 1997). The primary goal of treatment for hemorrhagic stroke is to stop the bleeding. Usual treatment consists of drug administration to lower blood pressure and to increase clot formation.

The nurse's primary focus should be to assess a woman for stroke accurately. Following assessment, the nurse focuses client and family education on risk prevention and modification of lifestyle behaviors that may contribute to stroke (see Chap. 2).

SEXUALLY TRANSMITTED INFECTIONS

Sexually transmitted infections (STIs) are infections of the reproductive tract resulting from microorganisms transmitted during vaginal, oral, or anal intercourse. They pose a significant public health problem, with an estimated 19 million new cases in the United States annually (Condon, 2004). Many STIs are asymptomatic; others manifest with minor or nonspecific symptoms in early stages (Table 4.5). Consequently, many STIs are not diagnosed until late stages, when significant damage already has resulted. Complications of STIs include infertility (see Chap. 10), high-risk and tubal pregnancy (see Chap. 13), and pelvic inflammatory disease (PID; discussed later in this chapter). Pregnant women pass STIs to their fetuses in approximately 33% to 66% of pregnancies (CDC, 2003a). Maternal–fetal transmission of STIs can lead to premature birth, low birth weight, or both. See Teaching Tips 4.2 and Chapters 13 and 22 for more information.

CHLAMYDIA

Chlamydia is the most common and fastest spreading STI in the United States (CDC, 2005b). Treating this infection costs approximately $2 billion annually (National Institute of Allergies and Infectious Disease [NIAID], 2002a). Most cases occur in clients 15 to 25 years old; chlamydia also is more prevalent in large urban areas and among lower socioeconomic groups (CDC, 2005b; USDHHS, 2002).

The causative bacterium *Chlamydia trachomatis* is transmitted through oral, vaginal, or anal sexual contact with an infected person. *C. trachomatis* can invade women's reproductive structures and urethra. Tissue irritation may be permanent despite successful eradication of the bacteria and can increase a client's risks for other STIs. Untreated infection can cause serious complications for men, women, and newborns of infected mothers.

Assessment Findings

Clients may not know that they have chlamydia because this infection may be dormant and asymptomatic. Early mild symptoms include abnormal purulent or mucus discharge from the vagina during urination 1 to 3 weeks after exposure. The infection, usually located in the endocervix in women, can spread to the endometrium, uterine tubes, peritoneum, rectum, and urethra, and can lead to inflammation, ulceration, and scarring (Adler et al., 2005). Chlamydia can reside in the cervix for many years, damaging uterine tubes and resulting in PID. Consequently, PID can lead to problems with fertility (Cohen, 2004).

Infection with chlamydia can inflame the lining of the eye. Approximately 10% to 20% of newborns develop pneumonia from infection with chlamydia acquired at birth (NIAID, 2002a). Symptoms of congenitally acquired chlamydia arise within the first 10 days of life. Because of the risk to the newborn, all pregnant women should be tested for chlamydia infection (Adler et al., 2005; NIAID, 2002a).

Most commonly, diagnosis involves examination of a specimen removed from the endocervix, vagina, or penis. A client also can also undergo a urine test, which yields results within 24 hours. All sexually active reproductive women should pursue recommended screening. Although the test is expensive, the cost of treating infertility remains even more expensive.

Collaborative Management

Usual treatment of infection with chlamydia consists of the following:

1. Taking azithromycin 1 g for 1 day
2. Ingesting 100 mg of doxycycline twice a day for 7 days
3. Taking 500 mg of erythromycin or amoxicillin four times a day for 7 days if a client is pregnant or lactating
4. Tracing sexual contacts; examining and treating partners with medication
5. Abstaining from sexual intercourse until a sexual partner receives examination or medication, or using condoms if partner has not received examination or medication

Infected clients do not require follow-up testing unless their sexual partners do not receive treatment.

● **TABLE 4.5 Common Sexually Transmitted Infections**

	CAUSATIVE ORGANISM	SYMPTOMS IN WOMEN	DIAGNOSTIC TESTING	TREATMENT
Chlamydia	Bacteria: *Chlamydia trachomatis*	Frequently asymptomatic Vaginal discharge Burning on urination	Specimen examination Urine test	Azithromycin, doxycycline, and erythromycin or amoxicillin
Gonorrhea	Bacteria: *Neisseria gonorrhoeae*	Frequently asymptomatic Pain or burning on urination Yellow and sometimes bloody vaginal discharge Bleeding between menstrual periods Pain during vaginal sexual intercourse Lower abdominal pain	Endocervical cultures	Cefixime, ceftriaxone, ciprofloxacin, ofloxacin, or levofloxacin
Syphilis	Bacteria: *Treponema pallidum*	May be asymptomatic Painless sores (chancres) and skin rashes Mild fever Fatigue Headache Sore throat Hair loss Swollen lymph glands throughout the body	Recognition of signs and symptoms Microscopic identification of the bacteria Examinations of blood samples	Penicillin by injection Tetracycline or doxycycline for clients with penicillin allergy
Genital herpes	Herpes simplex virus	May be asymptomatic Small red bumps, blisters, or open sores on the vagina or surrounding areas Vaginal discharge Fever, headache, and muscle aches Pain on urination Itching, burning, or swollen glands in genital area Pain in legs, buttocks, or genital area	Clinical examination Study of rectal cultures Exclusion of other STIs	Acyclovir (Zovirax) Famciclovir (Famvir) Valacyclovir (Valtrex)
Genital warts	Human papillomavirus (HPV)	May be asymptomatic Genital warts that sometimes are difficult to see	Visual inspection Application of vinegar-like solution to the suspected area, which causes warts to turn white Pap smear Colposcopy Tissue sampling	Imiquimod cream Podophyllin and podofilox solutions 5-Fluorouracil cream Trichloroacetic acid (TCA) Cryosurgery Electrocautery Laser surgery Surgical removal
Bacterial vaginosis (BV)	*Gardnerella vaginalis* or mixed anaerobes	May be asymptomatic White or gray thin and malodorous vaginal discharge Burning or pain on urination Itching around the vulva	Microscopic examination of vaginal fluid, either in stained or special lighting	Oral metronidazole or clindamycin cream

Continued

TABLE 4.5 Common Sexually Transmitted Infections

	CAUSATIVE ORGANISM	SYMPTOMS IN WOMEN	DIAGNOSTIC TESTING	TREATMENT
Trichomoniasis	Protozoan parasite: *Trichomonas vaginitis*	Yellow, green, or gray discharge with strong odor Discomfort during vaginal sexual intercourse and urination Irritation and itching of the genitals Lower abdominal pain (rare)	Wet smear of vaginal or penile secretions	Single-dose metronidazole
Candidiasis	Fungus: *Candida albicans*	Itching, burning, and irritation of the vagina Pain during urination Cottage cheese–like vaginal discharge	Culture and microscopic examination	Antifungal medications

Health care professionals should screen clients for STI risk, perform comprehensive historical and physical assessment, and provide education about STIs. They should recommend testing if mucopurulent vaginal drainage appears, if an STI or PID is suspected, before termination of pregnancy, before insertion of intrauterine contraceptive devices, and for all sexually active teenagers. Anyone who has more than one sexual partner, especially women younger than 25 years, should be tested routinely for chlamydia, even when no symptoms appear. Infection rates can diminish with the correct use of male latex condoms during all sexual encounters (see Chap. 8).

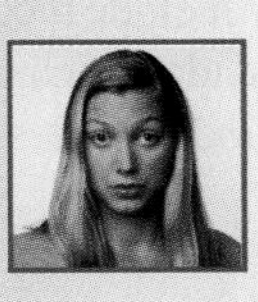

Think back to Lela, the young client described at the beginning of the chapter complaining of a vaginal discharge. Would the nurse suspect a STI? Why or why not?

GONORRHEA

Gonorrhea, the second most frequently reported communicable disease in the United States, is caused by the bacterium *Neisseria gonorrhea* (CDC, 2005b). It commonly affects the cervix, urethra, rectum, and oropharynx (Fig. 4.5). Rectal infections can develop from vaginal secretions, anal sex, or both. The incubation period lasts 3 to 7 days. Many clients are asymptomatic and may be infected for several months without knowing it (NIAID, 2002b). When symptoms occur, the most common include purulent vaginal discharge, dysuria and urinary frequency, urethral discharge, cervicitis, and intermenstrual bleeding. The usual method of diagnosis is procuring vaginal cultures from the cervix, urethra, and rectum. Ninety percent of cases are diagnosed by endocervical cultures (Adler et al., 2005).

Antibiotic therapy consists of single doses of cefixime, ceftriaxone, ciprofloxacin, ofloxacin, or levofloxacin. Ciprofloxacin or ofloxacin should not be prescribed

TEACHING TIPS 4.2 Preventing Sexually Transmitted Infections

- Abstinence is the best protection against STIs. Monogamous sexual relationships increase protection against STIs.
- Refrain from engaging in sex with anyone you suspect may have an STI.
- Know the signs and symptoms of STIs. Observe sexual partners closely for rashes and discharge.
- Use latex condoms when having vaginal, oral, or anal sex. (If you have a latex allergy, use plastic polyurethane condoms.)
- If you have an STI, your partner also must be tested and receive treatment.
- If you have an STI, don't have sex until your treatment is complete.
- Avoid wearing nylon pants, tights, and tight jeans.
- Refrain from using vaginal deodorants, perfumed soap, and bubble bath.
- Do not wear others' underwear.

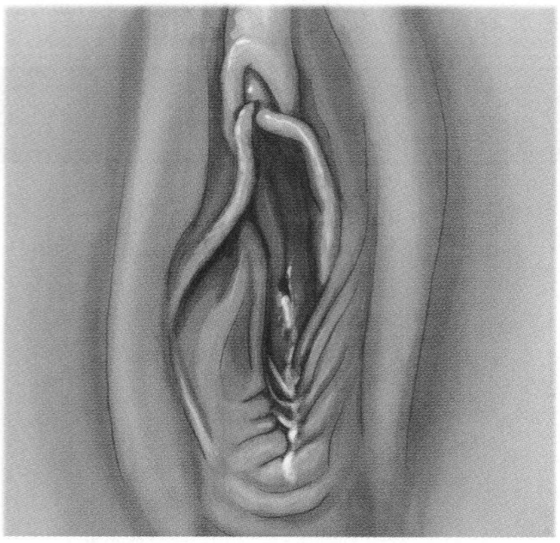

FIGURE 4.5 Gonorrhea.

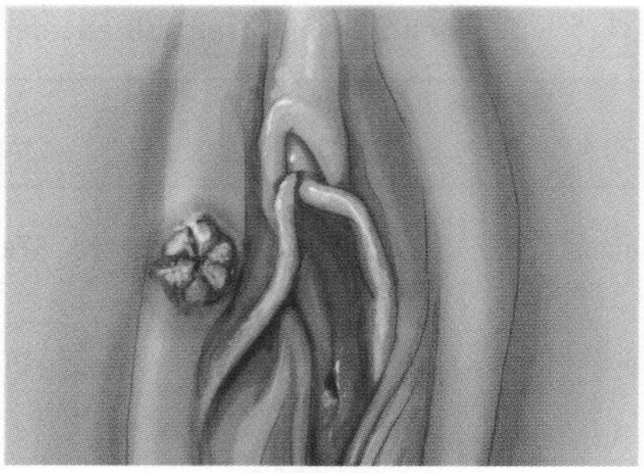

FIGURE 4.6 The painless ulcer (chancre) of primary syphilis.

for or administered to pregnant women. Treatment considerations should include a review of drug resistance patterns, pregnancy, allergies, and other infections. Clients with gonorrhea should refrain from sexual activity until effectiveness of treatment has been confirmed. Sexual partners of infected clients should be contacted, screened, and treated appropriately.

SYPHILIS

Syphilis is caused by the bacterium *Treponema pallidum.* From 1990 to 2004, the number of U.S. cases decreased by 89% (CDC, 2005b). Syphilis always is transmitted through sexual intercourse. Initially, the infection appears as a localized ulcer. Over time, however, the infection can become systemic, damage other organs, and display severe symptoms. Many cases are fatal.

Maternal–fetal transmission of syphilis is high, with 40% to 70% of pregnant women with syphilis passing the infection to their fetuses (NIAID, 2002c). In such cases, the risks for stillbirth or neonatal death shortly after birth are high. How the newborn is affected depends on how long the mother has had the infection. Symptoms of congenital syphilis include skin ulcers, rashes, fever, hoarse crying sounds, swollen liver and spleen, anemia, deformation, and jaundice. An asymptomatic newborn who is not treated immediately can develop serious mental and physical handicaps, which usually manifest 2 to 3 months after birth.

Assessment Findings

Syphilis has four stages: primary, secondary, latent, and tertiary (late):

- **Primary syphilis.** The initial symptom is a painless ulcer or chancre, which usually appears within 2 to 6 weeks of exposure. The ulcer can occur internally, but it more frequently is found on the body part that was exposed to the bacterium (Fig. 4.6). Additional ulcers may develop on the cervix, tongue, lips, and other body parts. The client is contagious.
- **Secondary syphilis.** During this chronic stage, the client has a skin rash and brown sores 3 to 6 weeks after the initial ulcer. The rash may cover small areas or the entire body. The client also may experience mild fever, fatigue, headache, sore throat, hair loss, and swollen lymph glands. These symptoms occur sporadically over 1 to 2 years (NIAID, 2002c). The client is contagious.
- **Latent syphilis.** During this stage, no symptoms appear, and the client is not contagious.
- **Tertiary syphilis.** In the final stage, syphilis spreads to many body systems, such as the heart, eyes, brain, nervous system, bones, and joints. Clients may show signs of mental illness, blindness, neurologic disorders, and heart problems. This stage can last years to decades (NIAID, 2002c), although the client is no longer contagious.

Methods of diagnosing syphilis usually include recognition of signs and symptoms, microscopic identification of the bacterium, and examinations of blood samples.

Collaborative Management

Penicillin by injection remains the customary treatment for primary and secondary syphilis. Clients allergic to penicillin receive other antibiotics, usually tetracycline or doxycycline. Clients normally can no longer transmit this infection 24 hours after receiving treatment. Frequent monitoring through blood tests, however, is recommended (NIAID, 2002c). Those with tertiary syphilis require larger doses of penicillin. The response is poor in those with cardiovascular syphilis. Treatment plans always should include instructional screening, with disease prevention as the ultimate goal.

GENITAL HERPES

Herpes is a highly contagious STI affecting at least 45 million Americans (CDC, 2004a). The disease is controllable, but not curable. Although herpes simplex virus type 2 (HSV-2), also known as **genital herpes,** is primarily responsible for genital and perineal lesions, herpes simplex virus type 1 (HSV-1), associated with cold sores around the nose and lips, also can cause anogenital lesions. Up to 30% of first-episode cases of genital herpes are caused by HSV-1, but recurrences are much less frequent than for HSV-2 genital infection (CDC, 2005b). The distinction between HSV stereotypes is based on laboratory and virologic tests, the results of which influence treatment, prognosis, and counseling (CDC, 2004a).

Assessment Findings

Early symptoms include itching and burning in the genital and anal areas; pain in the legs, buttocks, or genitals; vaginal discharge; and abdominal pressure. The virus incubates for 7 days and can be shed from ulcers for approximately 12 days or until healing occurs. An ulcer's cycle lasts approximately 3 weeks (Fig. 4.7). Clients also may experience fever and malaise. Approximately 50% of those with HSV experience less severe recurrences with milder symptoms of shorter duration. Itching, tingling, or numbness in the genital area usually occurs for 24 to 48 hours before recurrence. Factors associated with recurrence include sexual intercourse, stress, hormonal changes, menstruation, and climatic changes (Adler et al., 2005). Diagnosis is through clinical examination, study of rectal cultures, and exclusion of other STIs.

Collaborative Management

Presently, acyclovir (Zovirax), famciclovir (Famvir), and valacyclovir (Valtrex) are used to treat symptoms and prevent recurrences (CDC, 2004a). Clients should maintain cleanliness and dryness in the infected area and avoid touching sores. If contact with sores does occur, the client should wash her hands. In addition, an infected person should avoid sexual contact until sores heal completely and new skin forms. Health care personnel should screen the sexual partners of the infected client and treat them appropriately. Infected clients may require counseling; ongoing support can prove helpful. Instruction on the need for condom use during sexual intercourse between attacks is imperative (Adler et al., 2005).

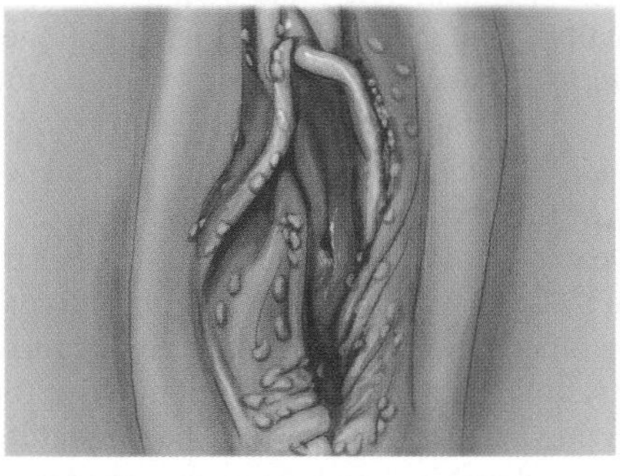

FIGURE 4.7 Ulcers in genital herpes simplex virus.

Genital herpes increases the risk for cervical cancer and HIV infection. Transmission also can occur from mother to infant during a vaginal birth and carries a neonatal mortality rate of 50% (CDC, 2004a).

The client may take oral antiviral medications episodically for 3 to 5 days or continuously to suppress the frequency of outbreaks. Episodic therapy begins within 1 day of the onset of lesions or during the period immediately before an outbreak, when the client is aware of early symptoms. Intravenous acyclovir is used when there is a severe episode of HSV-2 or when the client is immunocompromised. Cesarean birth is indicated for pregnant clients with active lesions. Infected clients receiving drug therapy remain contagious. See Teaching Tips 4.3 for appropriate education measures for clients with genital herpes.

HUMAN PAPILLOMAVIRUS (GENITAL WARTS)

Human papillomavirus (HPV) is a group of more than 100 viruses, most of which are harmless, that cause warts (papilloma). Different types of viruses cause warts to grow on different parts of the body, such as the hands and soles. The types of viruses that cause warts on the hands and feet do not cause genital warts (**condylomata**). Genital warts are spread easily during oral, vaginal, or anal sex with infected people. Almost two thirds of women who have sex with infected people develop warts within 3 months of the encounter (NWHIC, 2002a).

Thirty types of HPV are spread through sexual contact and cause genital warts. High-risk HPV causes abnormal results on Pap testing and can lead to cervical or other types of cancer. Low-risk viruses also have been associated with abnormal Pap test results and genital warts. Approximately 5.5 million new cases are reported annually; 20 million people in the United States are infected (NIAID, 2004). Seventy-five percent of infected women have no symptoms (NWHIC, 2002a).

Assessment Findings

Clients may develop condylomata both inside and around the outside of the vagina, as well as on the vulva, cervix, and anus (Fig. 4.8). Genital warts are less common in men and usually develop on the tip of the penis but also may be present on the shaft of the penis, scrotum, or anus. Rarely, warts grow in the mouth or throat of a person who has had oral sex with an infected person (NWHIC, 2002a). Warts vary in size, appear flat and flesh colored or take on a cauliflower look, occur in clusters, and can spread in large masses throughout the anal and vaginal areas (NWHIC, 2002a).

A health care provider usually diagnoses genital warts during a pelvic examination. Clients also may

● TEACHING TIPS 4.3 Genital Herpes

The nurse instructs clients with genital herpes infections as follows:

- Alert all past and current sexual partners of the HSV infection, even if it is inactive. Urge them to undergo appropriate screening and diagnosis.
- Tell all potential sexual partners of the infection before participating in any sexual activities with them.
- Use condoms during sexual activity, even if the infection is dormant. Refrain from sexual contact if the infection is or may be active. Condoms will not protect skin and mucous membranes that remain exposed.
- Check with a health care provider about bathing with Epsom salts or baking soda to relieve discomfort.
- Use alcohol, witch hazel, peroxide, and warm air from a hair dryer to keep lesions dry.
- Wear loose clothing and underwear that promotes air circulation.
- Thoroughly wash your hands after contact with lesions.
- Separate your personal hygiene articles (eg, towels) to avoid inadvertent use by others.
- Use a different towel to pat lesions dry.
- Have annual Pap tests.
- Reduce stress and follow other general health promotion strategies.

notice warts in their genital area. Sometimes warts are hard to see. Differential diagnosis can be made using a vinegar-like solution applied to the suspected area. This solution causes the warts to turn white, making them easier to identify. Pap smear, colposcopy, and tissue sampling are additional diagnostic measures (NIAID, 2004; NWHIC, 2002a).

Collaborative Management

HPV is incurable. There is no way to predict whether the warts will disappear without treatment, although occasionally this happens. Several treatments are used; options depend on the size and location of the warts. Topical methods include imiquimod cream, podophyllin and podofilox solutions (contraindicated in pregnant women), 5-fluorouracil cream (contraindicated in pregnancy), and trichloroacetic acid (TCA). Cryosurgery, electrocautery, and laser surgery are used to remove small warts. Surgical removal of large warts is an option when warts do not respond to other measures (NIAID, 2004).

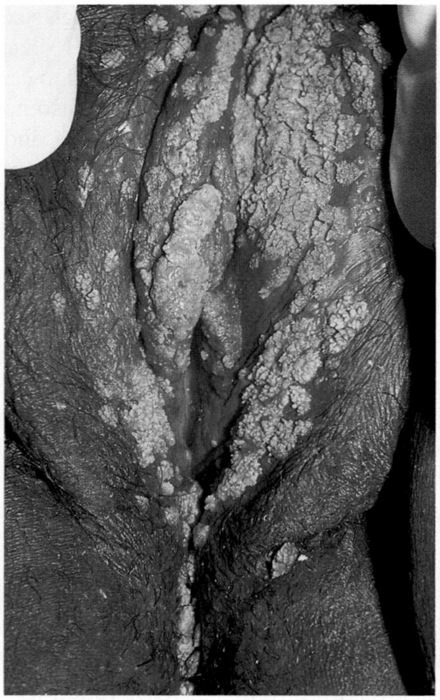

FIGURE 4.8 Genital warts.

Clients need education and counseling regarding prevention and transmission of HPV. Adolescent and young women need encouragement to delay first-time sex because younger people are at increased risk for all STIs. Risk for HPV grows with time, especially as the number of sex partners increases. Safe sex helps reduce a client's risk for HPV. Education regarding the common symptoms of HPV, as well as other STIs, is important for preventing this serious infection. As with all STIs, infected clients should receive prompt treatment, finish all medications, avoid sex until treatments are completed, inform sex partners and encourage them to be tested and treated, and practice safe sex (NWHIC, 2002b).

BACTERIAL VAGINOSIS

Bacterial vaginosis (BV) develops when harmful bacteria in the vagina increase and outnumber those bacteria normally found in the vagina (Fig. 4.9). For example, *G. vaginalis* or mixed anaerobes eventually outnumber normal vaginal lactobacilli such as *Mobiluncus* and *Mycoplasma hominis.* The pH of the vaginal ecosystem changes, with concomitant symptoms.

Researchers have not determined whether BV qualifies as an STI. Any woman can get BV, but it is more common in women who have had sexual intercourse (CDC, 2004b). Activities that increase a client's risk for BV include having a new sexual partner, having multiple sexual partners, douching, and using an intrauterine device (IUD) (CDC, 2004b).

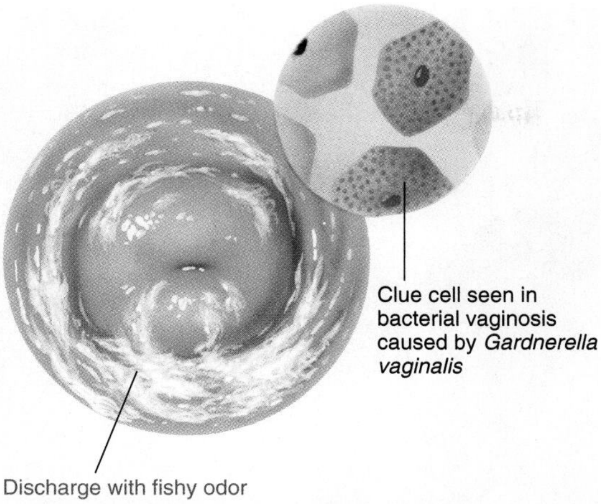

FIGURE 4.9 Bacterial vaginosis. (From Anatomical Chart Company. [2002]. *Atlas of pathophysiology.* Springhouse, PA: Springhouse.)

Assessment Findings

Many clients with BV are asymptomatic. Primary symptoms include abnormal vaginal odor and vaginal discharge. A fish-like odor may be noticeable, especially after intercourse. In addition, some clients experience itching in or around the vagina.

Diagnosis involves microscopic examination of vaginal fluid, either in stained or special lighting. Classic indicators of BV include decreased vaginal acidity (pH > 4.5); cells from the vaginal lining coated with BV organisms; thin, gray-white, or watery vaginal discharge; and fish-like vaginal odor.

Collaborative Management

Oral metronidazole or clindamycin cream usually is prescribed to treat BV (Pharmacology Box 4.1). Clients in the first trimester of pregnancy should be treated with clindamycin because metronidazole is contraindicated. BV has been linked to premature rupture of membranes, premature labor and birth, and postpartum endometriosis. It also is associated with increased risk for gonorrhea and HIV infection (CDC, 2004b).

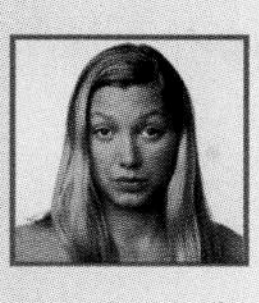

Recall Lela, the young woman described at the beginning of the chapter who is complaining of a vaginal discharge. What information would the nurse need to obtain to determine whether Lela is experiencing BV?

TRICHOMONIASIS

Trichomoniasis is the most common curable STI in young, sexually active women (CDC, 2004c). The cause is the protozoan parasite *Trichomonas vaginitis.* Often, trichomoniasis is silent and asymptomatic. When symptoms occur in men, the penis has a thin, whitish discharge; urination is painful and difficult. Symptomatic women emit a vaginal odor 4 to 20 days after infection and exhibit a thick, yellow-green or gray discharge (Fig. 4.10). Other symptoms may include painful urination, genital irritation and itching, discomfort after intercourse, and occasional abdominal pain. A wet smear of vaginal or penile secretions can confirm diagnosis.

Both sexual partners should receive treatment, even if no symptoms appear. Single-dose metronidazole remains the preferred regimen. Clients should abstain from alcohol consumption during treatment because the combination of metronidazole and alcohol can cause severe nausea and vomiting. To avoid recurrence, partners engaging in sex should use condoms during the first 4 to 6 weeks after treatment.

Pregnant clients commonly experience recurrences of trichomoniasis, which can result in premature rupture of the membranes and preterm birth. Low birth weight and

● PHARMACOLOGY 4.1 Metronidazole (Flagyl)

ACTION: Metronidazole inhibits Dopamine synthesis in obligate anaerobes, leading to cell death.

PREGNANCY CATEGORY: B

DOSAGE: For bacterial vaginosis, 500 mg bid PO for 7 days. For trichomoniasis, 2g PO in 1 day (1-day treatment) or 250 mg tid PO for 7 days.

POSSIBLE ADVERSE EFFECTS:
Headache, dizziness, ataxia, unpleasant metallic taste, anorexia, nausea, vomiting, diarrhea, and dark urine.

NURSING IMPLICATIONS

- Teach the client to take the medicine with food.
- Emphasize the importance of completing the full medication regimen.
- Caution the client to avoid alcohol while using this drug.
- Prepare the client for the possibility of darkened urine.
- Instruct the client to avoid sexual intercourse without a condom during treatment.

Source: Karch, A. (2005). *2005 Lippincott's nursing drug guide.* Philadelphia: Lippincott Williams & Wilkins.

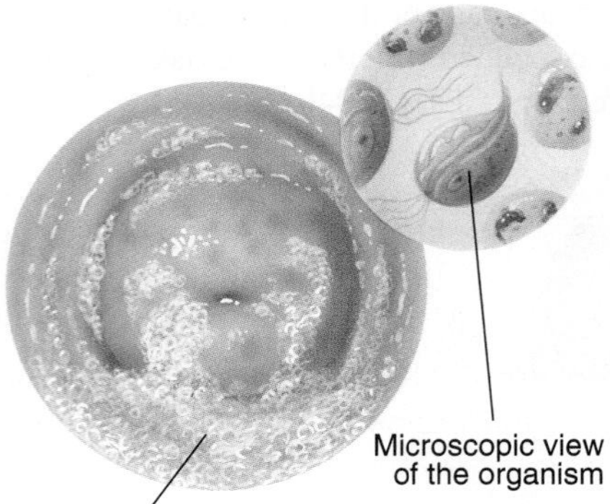

FIGURE 4.10 Trichomoniasis. (From Anatomical Chart Company. [2002]. *Atlas of pathophysiology*. Springhouse, PA: Springhouse.)

genital and lung infection in the newborn also can result. Some researchers link trichomoniasis to increased transmission of HIV and suggest that using male condoms during sex can prevent both problems (CDC, 2004c). More studies are needed to confirm this opinion.

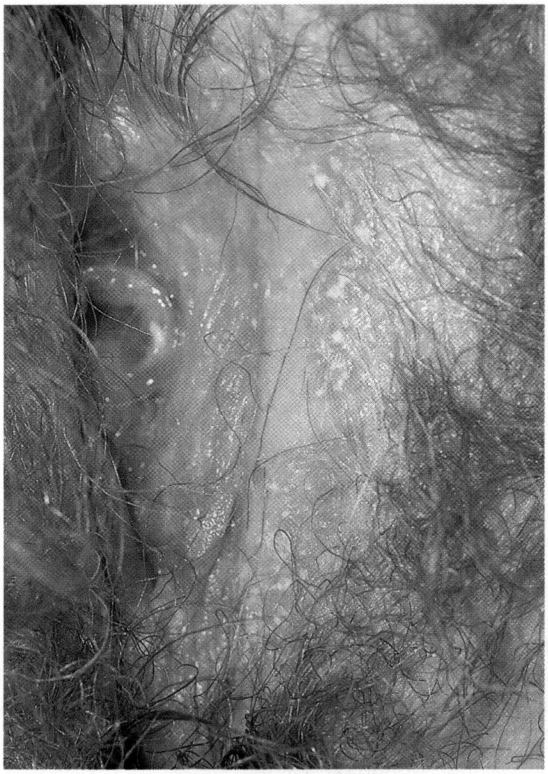

FIGURE 4.11 Overgrowth of *Candida albicans.*

YEAST INFECTION (CANDIDIASIS)

Yeast infections commonly cause vaginal irritation in women. Almost all women have *Candida albicans* in the vagina in small numbers; symptoms develop only when there is overgrowth. Approximately 75% of all women experience at least one symptomatic episode (CDC, 2005c).

This disorder has proved rather difficult to study. Debate continues on whether to define **candidiasis** as an STI because so many women have candida as normal vaginal flora.

Overgrowth of *C. albicans* follows a disruption of the normal vaginal ecosystem. Candida or thrush also can appear in the mouth and gut. Factors contributing to yeast infection include pregnancy; use of antibiotics, corticosteroids, or immunosuppressive treatments; diabetes; STIs; immunodeficiency; use of oral contraceptives, douches, and perfumed feminine hygiene sprays; and wearing tight, poorly ventilated clothes or underwear.

Assessment Findings

The most common symptoms in women include itching, burning, and irritation of the vagina and vulva. Minimal thick or watery vaginal discharge resembling cottage cheese appears (Fig. 4.11). Clients also may display dysuria and dyspareunia. Men with this disorder do not exhibit major symptoms but may experience transient rash and a limited burning sensation.

History and physical examination usually are not sufficient to diagnose this infection. Culture and microscopic examination of a swab sampling from the upper vagina or cervix may diagnose and confirm yeast forms. Home screening kits also can test for yeast infections.

Collaborative Management

Treatment is recommended only for symptomatic clients and their sexual partners. Several over-the-counter (OTC) oral and suppository antifungal vaginal medications can serve as remedies. Nevertheless, it is important for infected people to visit their clinician because some OTC products contain antihistamines that can mask the disorder. Clients with HIV may have serious yeast infections that do not respond to treatment.

Recurrent candidiasis is difficult to manage. Infected clients must avoid other infections and their catalysts. Those with chronic recurring infections may require extended treatment.

To prevent candidiasis, all women should wipe their genitalia from front to back and ensure that the genital area remains clean and dry. They also should avoid wearing nylon pants, tights, pantyhose, and tight jeans, and refrain from using vaginal deodorants, perfumed soap, and bubble bath. Moreover, when douching, using vaginal tampons, and engaging in sexual intercourse, clients should avoid vaginal trauma. Treatment also may include the use of oral contraceptives in low dosages.

Nursing Care Plan 4.1 highlights the care of a client with a yeast infection. NIC/NOC Box 4.4 highlights

NURSING CARE PLAN 4.1

The Client With a Vaginal Infection

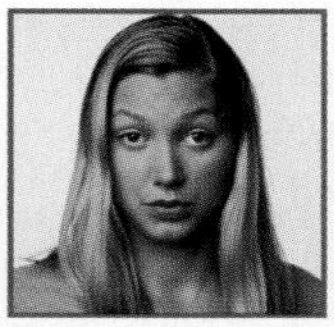

Think back to Lela, the 33-year-old client who comes to the clinic for evaluation of her vaginal discharge. She reports douching daily since the discharge started. Further assessment reveals a white vaginal discharge of cottage cheese consistency. The vulva and vaginal area are red and irritated. Lela complains of burning and some pain on urination. "It's been a terrible week. First I had gone to the dentist for an abscessed tooth and he gave me a prescription for an antibiotic which I've been taking. Now this." Specimen obtained for culture reveals *Candida albicans.*

NURSING DIAGNOSES

- **Impaired Tissue Integrity** related to vaginal infection and resultant irritation and redness
- **Deficient Knowledge** related to measures to prevent infection and reduce the risk for recurrent infection

EXPECTED OUTCOMES

1. The client will experience no further vaginal irritation.
2. The client will report that redness and irritation have decreased, rating it as a 5 out of 10.
3. The client will exhibit signs and symptoms of resolving infection.
4. The client will state situations that increase the risk for yeast infection.
5. The client will identify measures to maintain vaginal integrity and health.

INTERVENTIONS	RATIONALES
Assess the client's perineal area for redness, irritation, and drainage.	Assessment provides a baseline from which to develop an individualized plan of care.
Ask the client to rate her level of discomfort on a scale of 1 to 10.	Quantifying the level of discomfort helps determine measures to relieve it.
Assist the client in cleaning the perineal area with warm soap and water. Instruct her to perform frequent perineal care.	Cleaning the area removes vaginal discharge that irritates the mucosa.
Encourage the client to wipe the area using a front to back motion.	This motion prevents contamination of the vaginal area.
Discuss with the client factors that can contribute to yeast infections such as medications, douching, perfumed feminine hygiene sprays, and tight poorly ventilated clothing.	Knowledge of contributing factors helps the client begin measures to control them.
Instruct the client to wear cotton underwear and avoid nylon pants, tights, and jeans. Encourage her to refrain from using vaginal deodorants, perfumed soaps, and bubble baths.	Cotton underwear allows air to circulate, reducing the risk for a dark, moist environment conducive to organism growth. Nylon pants, pantyhose, tights, and tight jeans interfere with air circulation. Substances such as vaginal deodorants and soaps contain ingredients that can irritate the mucosa.
Instruct the client to avoid douching.	Douching can alter the vaginal pH, which could lead to an overgrowth of organisms.

Continued

NURSING CARE PLAN 4.1 ● The Client With a Vaginal Infection (*Continued*)

INTERVENTIONS	RATIONALES
Encourage the client to have her sexual partner treated.	Recurrent infection can occur if the client engages in sex with an infected partner.
Administer antifungal agent as ordered; teach client about antifungal agent prescribed and how to administer.	Antifungal agents typically are used to treat symptomatic women and their infected partners.
Advise the client to monitor the amount and characteristics of her vaginal discharge. Instruct her to report an increase in drainage amount or odor, an increase in irritation, or continued burning or pain on urination.	Candidiasis can become a recurrent or chronic infection that requires extended treatment.
Arrange for a follow-up visit in 1 to 2 weeks.	A follow-up visit allows for evaluation of the infection and adherence to the treatment regimen.

EVALUATION

1. The client reports that redness and irritation have subsided, rating the discomfort at a level of 3 or less.
2. The client states that vaginal discharge has ceased.
3. The client accurately identifies situations that increase her risk for infection.
4. The client demonstrates appropriate measures to keep vaginal area free of infection.

some common nursing interventions and outcomes associated with vaginal infections.

HUMAN IMMUNODEFICIENCY VIRUS (HIV)

Acquired immunodeficiency syndrome (AIDS) is an infectious disorder that profoundly weakens the immune system. It is acquired from a specific virus called *human immunodeficiency virus* (HIV). It can take 10 years or longer for an initial infection with HIV to develop into AIDS. During that time, infected people can give HIV to others through sexual contact, pregnancy, breastfeeding, organ transplants, sperm donation, IV drug use, and blood transfusions. Often, HIV is associated with other STIs because it is transferred more easily with coexistent infections.

Estimates are that 900,000 people in the United States are currently living with HIV, with 19% of these cases being women (CDC, 2003b). Worldwide, women account for approximately 50% of the more than 40 million adults with HIV/AIDS (NIAID, 2004). Although African American and Hispanic women make up 21% of the U.S. female population, they represent 75% of all new cases of AIDS in women (CDC, 2003b). African American women have higher mortality rates and are 9 times more likely to die from AIDS than are white women (CDC, 2003b). Cases of HIV in women continue to rise, and pregnant clients can spread the virus to their fetus (see Chap. 13).

HIV kills CD4 cells (helper T cells), which help the body fight off infection and disease. The CD4 cells in an infected person decrease as the number of HIV-infected

NIC/NOC Box 4.4 Vaginal Infections

Common NIC Labels

- Infection Control
- Infection Protection
- Medication Administration: Vaginal
- Perineal Care
- Risk Identification

Common NOC Labels

- Knowledge: Health Behaviors
- Knowledge: Infection Control
- Knowledge: Medication
- Risk Control: Sexually Transmitted Diseases
- Tissue Integrity: Skin and Mucous Membranes

cells increases (National Center for HIV, STD and TB Prevention, 2003). AIDS is diagnosed when a client tests positive for antibodies to HIV, has a low T-lymphocyte count, or develops an opportunistic infection (National Center for HIV, STD and TB Prevention, 2003).

Assessment Findings

Symptoms include lack of energy or fatigue, weight loss, frequent low-grade fevers or night sweats, skin rashes, and flaky skin that fails to heal. Many clients with HIV/AIDS experience vaginal yeast infections and other STIs, PID, and menstrual cycle changes (NWHIC, 2002b).

Tests for HIV include the *enzyme-linked immunosorbent assay* (ELISA) test, which gives a positive result when HIV antibodies appear in sufficient numbers. Because the ELISA test can be positive when the client has antibodies from other infectious diseases, the test is repeated if results are positive. If a second ELISA test gives positive results, the *Western blot* diagnostic test is performed. A positive Western blot result confirms diagnosis, although this test also can have false-positive results.

Total T-cell count, T4 and T8 count, and T4/T8 ratio determine the status of T lymphocytes. A T4 cell count below 500/mm^3 indicates immune suppression; a T4 cell count at or below 200/mm^3 indicates AIDS. The *p24 antigen test* and *polymerase chain reaction test* measure viral loads and can chart progression of the illness to guide drug therapy. These tests and T4-cell counts may be performed every 2 to 3 months after HIV status is confirmed.

Collaborative Management

Clients with HIV/AIDS receive antiretroviral medications, adjunct immune-enhancing drugs, and supportive care during opportunistic infections. They should receive pneumococcal, hepatitis B, and yearly influenza vaccines. Additional treatment measures involve managing anorexia, diarrhea, weight loss, and side effects of medications.

Antiretroviral Drug Therapy

The primary care provider selects an antiretroviral drug for treatment based on the client's circumstances. These medications are expensive. For clients who lack insurance coverage and cannot afford them independently, some agencies and pharmaceutical companies have programs that supply these medications.

Opinions about when to initiate drug therapy vary. Resistance over time is common with the use of HIV drugs; thus, some researchers promote delaying the initiation of medication therapy for as long as possible while the client remains relatively healthy. The standard guideline is to treat symptomatic clients, and otherwise to start the medications when the client's viral load is more than 30,000 copies/mL or the T4-cell count is less than 350/mm^3 (Daar, 2002).

Initial drug therapy usually involves a combination of two *reverse transcriptase inhibitors* (which interfere with the viral genetic replication) and one *protease inhibitor* (which inhibits the ability of HIV to leave its host). *Fusion inhibitors* also may be prescribed. These drugs interfere with HIV's ability to fuse with and enter CD4 cells. Fusion inhibitors are not commonly used as monotherapy. The combination approach has several benefits:

- Various mechanisms work to suppress HIV replication.
- The viral load is lowered rapidly, halting disease progression and prolonging survival.
- The rate of viral mutations is delayed.
- Chances for drug resistance or cross-resistance are minimized because different drugs are working together at one time.

Adjunct Drug Therapy

Other drugs are used in tandem with antiretroviral drugs. For example, hydroxyurea (Hydrea) combined with antiretroviral therapy interferes with HIV replication. The use of interleukin-2 boosts the body's immune defenses against HIV.

Care of Opportunistic Infections

Many opportunistic infections that develop as a consequence of the weakened immunity that is secondary to HIV/AIDS are fatal. For example, HIV-positive clients are at increased risk for *Pneumocystis carinii* pneumonia, which can lead to respiratory failure. Mechanical ventilation may be necessary, as well as deep suctioning and aerosol therapy to clear the lungs of thick sputum. Trimethoprim-sulfamethoxazole (Bactrim, Septra), monthly aerosolized pentamidine isethionate (NebuPent), or both may be prescribed for prevention or treatment. Another common problem is candidiasis (see earlier discussion).

Another opportunistic infection in HIV is cytomegalovirus (CMV), which may infect the eyes, leading to blindness, as well as the gastrointestinal system. Foscarnet (Foscavir), cidofovir (Vistide), and ganciclovir (Cytovene) are used aggressively to treat acute CMV infections and as maintenance drug therapy.

Client Teaching

Nurses provide health teaching and counseling to high-risk populations about HIV/AIDS. They should emphasize prevention strategies such as abstinence and safe sex (sexual activities in which body fluids are not exchanged). They should encourage testing among clients with a history of risky behaviors. Nurses also should help clients interpret diagnostic test results and assist with ongoing monitoring in the months after potential exposure.

For clients with HIV, nurses should explain the mechanisms of each drug and help clients to develop a schedule for self-administration. Nurses need to emphasize the importance of rigidly adhering to the particulars of the medication regimen to avoid contributing to drug resistance. Because many of these medications have challenging and debilitating side effects, the nurse should warn clients of what to expect, while stressing the necessity of never discontinuing any prescribed drugs without first consulting the primary care provider. Further educational components for clients living with HIV are found in Teaching Tips 4.4.

HEPATITIS

Hepatitis, an inflammation of liver, results from different viruses that can be transmitted sexually, especially hepatitis B. This section focuses on types A, B, and C.

Hepatitis A

Thirty-three percent of the U.S. population is infected with the hepatitis A virus (HAV) (CDC, 2006a). HAV is found in contaminated food or water and the feces of infected people. Uncooked shellfish from contaminated water, oral or anal sexual contact, infected clothes and linen, and household-item cross-contamination can transmit hepatitis A and expedite its spread. Infected clients develop future immunity against this infection. The incubation period lasts 3 to 4 weeks.

Signs and symptoms include anorexia, low-grade fever, nausea or vomiting, upper abdominal pain, and jaundice. Clients with HAV neither develop chronic liver disease nor become carriers. Blood tests are used for diagnosis.

Treatment consists of rest, safe hygiene practices (eg, handwashing after toilet use), adequate hydration, and the avoidance of alcohol and medications metabolized in the liver. The primary care provider may administer immune globulin prophylactically to uninfected family members and other frequent contacts of the client. A series of vaccine administrations can provide long-term immunity. Vaccination is recommended for people traveling to countries such as Africa or Asia where HAV is common, those engaging in anal or oral sex, IV drug users, daycare and institutional workers, and people with chronic liver diseases (CDC, 2006a).

Hepatitis B

According to the CDC, approximately 1 in 20 people in the United States will be infected with the highly contagious hepatitis B virus (HBV) in their lifetime (CDC, 2006b). HBV is transmitted primarily through sexual contact, which accounts for 30% to 70% of the 73,000 new HBV infections in the United States annually (CDC, 2006b). Other modes of transmission include shared contaminated drug needles and accidental needle pricks. Transfusions of infected blood also can transmit HBV. Women can transmit HBV to their newborns during childbirth.

In some clients, HBV is asymptomatic; others display a low-grade fever, fatigue, headache, generalized aches, appetite loss, nausea, vomiting, abdominal pain, and jaundice. Clients may exhibit mild disease or develop chronic liver disease, liver cancer, liver failure, or death (CDC, 2006b). Blood tests can detect the infection and identify the virus.

HBV has no cure. Usually, treatment is symptomatic. Researchers are developing preventive antiviral agents. The CDC recommends that sexual partners of infected clients receive hepatitis B immune globules (CDC, 2006b). Health care workers, households with infected people, sexually active homosexuals and bisexuals, people with multiple sexual partners, staff and residents of institutions such as prisons, clients receiving hemodialysis or frequent blood products, clients with recent STIs, and all infants born in the United States should receive vaccination (CDC, 2006b).

Hepatitis C

Hepatitis C is rapidly becoming an epidemic in the United States. This RNA virus is often transmitted percuta-

● TEACHING TIPS 4.4 Living With HIV

For clients with HIV who are managing their conditions on an outpatient basis, the nurse should emphasize the following educational points:

- Strictly follow the medication schedule. Never omit, decrease, or increase doses without receiving approval from your primary care provider.
- Take the antiviral medications around meals. Eat small, frequent, and well-balanced meals. Drink plenty of water.
- Check your weight weekly, and report any weight loss or appetite loss promptly.
- Avoid people with infections, including colds.
- Notify the primary care provider if you show any signs of infection.
- Wash food before cooking. Do not eat any raw meat, fish, or vegetables, which may carry dangerous pathogens.
- Separate your laundry from others, especially if the bedding and clothes are soiled with body secretions.
- Avoid smoking.
- Maintain high standards of personal hygiene.
- Avoid extreme temperatures and environmental conditions.
- Rest frequently.
- Do not share needles or donate blood.

neously and is spread through exposure to contaminated blood transfusions, blood products, injection of drugs, hemodialysis, tattooing, and ear and body piercing. The disease also spreads through high-risk sexual behavior, organ transplants, and mishandling of blood and blood products by health care workers. Infrequently, the disease is transmitted through sexual contact and from mother to fetus during gestation. Prognosis remains generally poor because this disorder is incurable.

Hepatitis C is the most common cause of liver disease in the United States. It is generally a silent disease, with 80% of affected people showing no signs or symptoms. When symptoms occur, they include jaundice, fatigue, dark-colored urine, abdominal pain, loss of appetite, and nausea (National Center for Infectious Diseases, 2004).

Diagnosis is based on presenting symptoms and laboratory blood test analysis that confirms three types of virus present (virology studies). Liver function studies also help with determining the extent of the disease and liver functioning.

Although there is no biomedical cure for hepatitis, options are available to control the disease. Clients who are positive for hepatitis C generally are evaluated for liver disease. Pharmacologic treatment consists of interferon and riboflavin and is used for those with chronic hepatitis C (CDC, 2006c). These drugs may be given alone or in combination, with combination therapy being the treatment of choice. Combination therapy has successfully eliminated the virus in up to 5 of 10 people with genotype 1 and in up to 8 of 10 people with genotypes 2 and 3 (CDC, 2006c). Symptoms are treated with rest and supportive care. Clients should be counseled to maintain a healthy diet, get adequate rest, employ stress reduction techniques, and especially to avoid alcohol. Those receiving hormonal therapy (estrogen) or oral contraceptives also may be advised to discontinue use until normal liver function returns. Complementary/Alternative Medicine Box 4.1 discusses some herbal treatments used in clients with hepatitis C.

BENIGN BREAST DISORDERS

Women experience breast changes throughout their lives, beginning with gestation and continuing past menopause. In many cultures, breasts symbolize femininity and help to form each woman's self-image. Throughout history, female breasts have been associated with sexuality, erotica, fashion, beauty, and art. Breasts also have associations related to their important role in nourishing babies. As Sloane indicates (2002), it is no wonder that threats or injury to or loss of a breast creates stress, anxiety, and fear in women.

Breast disorders can affect both physical and psychological health (Meechan et al., 2005; Woodward & Webb, 2001). They can cause problems with body image and self-esteem.

Breast assessments during routine health care visits and routine physical examination are an important part of a woman's health maintenance. Clients who practice proper BSE techniques are in a better position to detect lumps early in their progression, which enhances rates of breast cancer detection, early treatment, and survival (Vahabi, 2003). Dienger (1998) found that many women with breast self-examination (BSE) anxiety performed BSEs less frequently than women with less anxiety. See Chapter 2 for more information on breast health promotion and screening strategies.

Common benign breast conditions in women include pain (**mastalgia**), infections, fibrocystic changes, fibroadenoma, and nipple discharge.

BREAST PAIN (MASTALGIA)

Breast pain is usually nonspecific. It is common, occurring in approximately two thirds of women at some point

● COMPLEMENTARY/ALTERNATIVE MEDICINE 4.1

Selected Treatments for Hepatitis C

- ***Milk thistle*** (*Silybum marianum*) is an aster-like plant that has been used in Europe to treat liver disease and jaundice since the 1500s. To date, research findings have not definitively supported benefits of milk thistle in treating hepatitis C. Animal studies have suggested that silymarin may help the liver by promoting cell growth, protecting existing liver cells, fighting oxidation damage, and minimizing inflammation. These studies, however, did not specifically focus on hepatitis C. A 2002 study of milk thistle as treatment for liver disease found no difference in mortality reduction or other effects. The National Center for Complementary and Alternative Medicine currently is sponsoring a clinical trial on use of milk thistle for hepatitis C.
- ***Licorice root*** has been used since ancient times. Cellular laboratory studies suggest that licorice root may have antiviral properties. Research findings on the effectiveness of licorice root for hepatitis C have been conflicting.
- ***Ginseng*** may have some beneficial effects on the liver and strengthen glandular systems and immunity. One study found ginseng to be beneficial in older adults with liver problems similar to hepatitis.

Data from the National Center for Complementary and Alternative Medicine.

in their reproductive lives (Olawaiye et al., 2005). Clients with mastalgia usually complain of diffuse breast tenderness or heaviness. They may experience pain cyclically or continuously. Cyclic pain suggests hormonal sensitivity and often coincides with the menstrual cycle. Continuous pain usually is unilateral and may be felt specifically in one section of the breast. This type of pain is usually anatomic in nature.

The etiology may be trauma, fat necrosis, or duct ectasia; often, the cause is unknown. Both cyclic and continuous pain can be related to a mass, cyst, or thickening in the breast. All complaints and findings should be evaluated with mammogram or ultrasound (Cady et al., 1998).

Once cancer has been ruled out, treatment may consist of reliving the pain with NSAIDs, hormonal therapy (eg, oral contraceptives), evening primrose oil, tamoxifen, or danazol. Reduced intake of caffeine, chocolate, sodium, and dietary fat, as well as use of a good supporting bra, also has been found to help alleviate symptoms (Olawaiye et al., 2005).

BREAST INFECTIONS

Breast infection (**mastitis**) usually occurs in a localized area (Fig. 4.12). Many lactating women experience mastitis (see Chaps. 19 and 21). The etiology usually is staphylococci, which enter the breast through cracked or fissured nipples. Signs and symptoms include redness, pain, and tenderness on palpation.

Mastitis usually is treated with antibiotics. Lactating women are encouraged to continue to nurse. Nurses should instruct them to use a breast shield or hand pump until the pain subsides. Those with a breast abscess or purulent drainage should discard their milk and discontinue nursing until the infection clears.

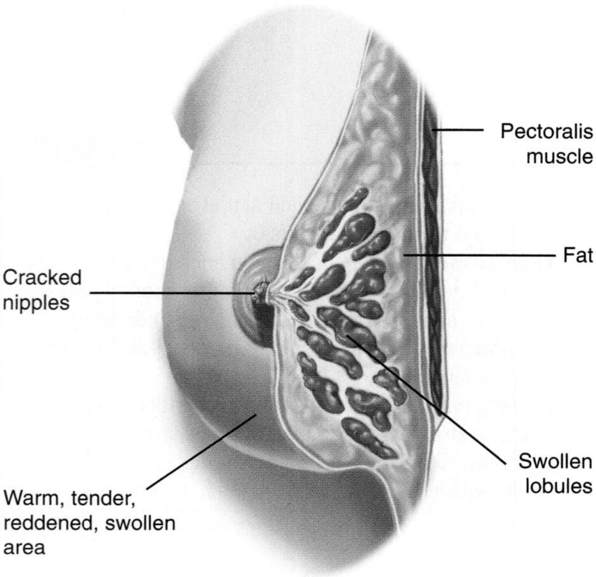

FIGURE 4.12 Mastitis.

Lactating women should receive breastfeeding education before beginning nursing so that they can be prepared for this potential complication. They should be aware that they should seek medical attention at the first sign of any infection. In the event that the woman does not respond to antibiotic therapy and the infection continues, she should be evaluated for inflammatory breast cancer.

FIBROCYSTIC CHANGES

Several changes occur in women's breasts that create anxiety, most of which are noncancerous. Many such changes are age related and include the development of excess fibrous tissue (thickening of breast tissue), cyst formation, hyperplasia of the epithelial lining of the mammary ducts, and proliferation of the primary ducts resulting in lumpy breasts (Smeltzer & Bare, 2008) (Fig. 4.13).

Assessment Findings

Pain or tenderness on a cyclic or episodic basis may result from nerve irritation caused by connective tissue edema and fibrous nerve pinching. Most masses or nodular ties are bilateral and found in the upper outer quadrant (maxilla area). The incidence is higher in perimenopausal women 35 to 50 years old and is related to changes and imbalances in estrogen and progestin. Most of these changes subside after menopause if women do not receive estrogen replacement therapy (Hindle & Gonzales, 2001; Hughes et al., 2000).

Screening methods may include clinical breast examination, mammography, and ultrasound evaluation when the breast tissue is very dense to differentiate cystic masses from solid masses. Often, the fluid in the cysts is aspirated and examined for neoplastic cell changes. Most women with fibrocystic changes are not at increased risk for breast cancer. A small percentage of women with fibrocystic changes that result from hyperplasia, however, appear to be at increased risk for breast cancer (Smeltzer & Bare, 2008).

Collaborative Management

Treatment may include surgical removal of the mass if indicated. Medical management consists of using good support bras and dietary and medicinal therapies. Dietary management may include restriction of sodium and methylxanthines (found in coffee, chocolate, and caffeinated beverages) (Smeltzer & Bare, 2008).

Pharmacologic management may consist of vitamin E, analgesics, danazol, diuretics, and hormone therapy. Other nonpharmacologic treatments include stress reduction measures because stress has been associated with breast changes and discomfort (Smeltzer & Bare, 2008).

Client education is a primary nursing intervention in the care of women with mastalgia and fibrocystic

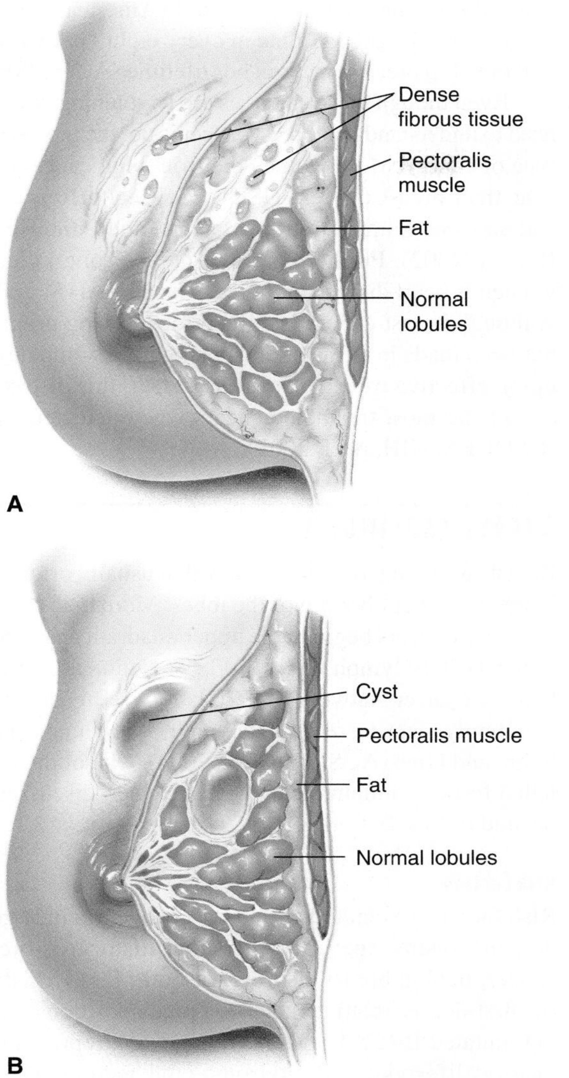

FIGURE 4.13 (**A**) Fibrocystic breast changes. (**B**) Breast cysts. (From Anatomical Chart Company. [2002]. *Atlas of pathophysiology.* Springhouse, PA: Springhouse.)

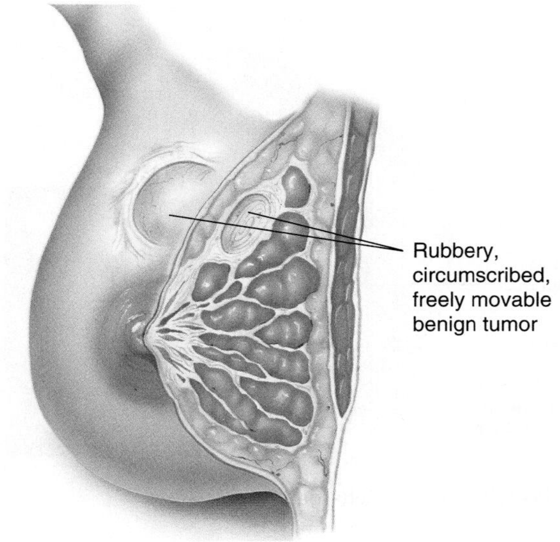

FIGURE 4.14 Fibroadenoma. (From Anatomical Chart Company. [2002]. *Atlas of pathophysiology.* Springhouse, PA: Springhouse.)

breast changes. Women should be encouraged to have regular clinical breast examinations throughout their lives. Education should include reassurance that cysts do not increase risk for breast cancer and that most women experience recurrences of fibrocystic changes until menopause. Nurses should teach BSE techniques and clarify points about medical therapies (Condon, 2004; Smeltzer & Bare, 2008).

FIBROADENOMA

Fibroadenoma occurs frequently in women between 20 and 30 years of age. A **fibroadenoma** is a firm, mobile, solitary, painless breast tumor with well-defined borders (Smeltzer & Bare, 2008) (Fig. 4.14). These masses usually are found during physical examination or are noted during mammography. Biopsy and tissue examination confirm the diagnosis. Screening techniques include mammography, ultrasound, and fine-needle aspiration.

Nursing care should include client education regarding procedures and tests and reassurance about the benign nature of these masses. Once again, women should be encouraged to perform regular BSEs and have their health care practitioner perform regular routine clinical breast examinations as a follow-up measure (Smeltzer & Bare, 2008).

NIPPLE DISCHARGE

Nipple discharge (fluid emission from the mammary nipple) is a common complaint that may be a manifestation of a more serious underlying disorder, such as a pituitary lesion, hypothyroidism, or substance abuse (Fig. 4.15). Usually, the woman reports nipple discharge to her primary health care provider, who must identify the type and rule out pathology, especially cancer (Hussain et al., 2006).

With *lactation* during pregnancy and the postpartum period, milk is discharged from the breasts naturally from hormonal stimulation to provide nutrition for the infant. It is not considered harmful.

Also called *galactorrhea, physiologic discharge* results from drug therapy, endocrine problems, and neural disorders. It is bilateral and may be milky white or multicolored. Usually, galactorrhea is not part of a disease and requires reassurance and counseling. Treatment includes identifying the underlying cause (Smeltzer & Bare, 2008).

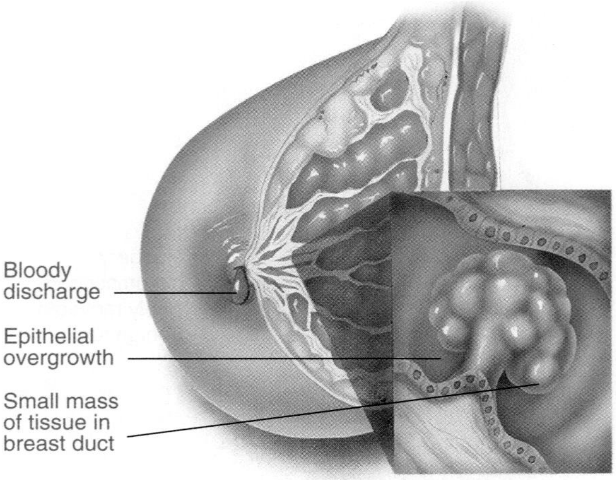

FIGURE 4.15 Nipple discharge.

Benign pathologic discharge may be related to cystic disease, intraductal papilloma, and ductal ectasia, which are related to inflammatory responses caused by stagnation of breast duct secretions and breast infections. *Intraductal papillomas* are growths in the mammary ducts that often emit a bloody discharge. They usually occur in women 40 to 60 years old. Treatment for them consists of surgical excision. *Ductal ectasia* occurs in both premenopausal and postmenopausal women and is not associated with malignancy. The discharge can be bloody, brown, cream colored, gray, green, purulent, or white; it may be sticky, thick, or thin. It usually is painless, but some women complain of burning, itching, and pain around the nipple. Some women also experience swelling in the alveolar area. Symptoms may become more pronounced with advanced disease. Treatment consists of warm compresses, antibiotic therapy, and close follow-up. Surgical excision of the involved ducts also may be indicated.

Pathologic discharge may be related to tumors of the pituitary gland, Addison's disease, and hypothyroidism. Discharge may be bilateral and of thin milky white color but generally is unilateral and is emitted from one duct orifice. The color can be serous, pink, serosanguineous, or bloody. It is spontaneous in nature and not emitted. About 8% to 15% of cases are related to underlying cancer (Sickles, 2000). These lesions are small and are usually not detected on mammography. Diagnosis usually begins with collecting fluid specimens on slides to detect the specific pathologic process. Treatment depends on the underlying cause (Smeltzer & Bare, 2008).

MALIGNANT BREAST DISORDERS

Breast cancer is one of the most frightening conditions for women. Estimates are that in 2006 approximately 40,000 U.S. women will die from breast cancer, with more than 200,000 new cases diagnosed (American Cancer Society [ACS], 2006a). One in every eight U.S. women will develop breast cancer in her lifetime (ACS, 2006a).

Even though these statistics are frightening, women need to understand that breast cancer is not the most lethal type of cancer. More women die from lung cancer each year than breast cancer (USDHHS, Health Resources and Services Administration, Maternal and Child Health Bureau, 2002). Furthermore, the number one killer of women is heart disease, not breast cancer (AHA, 2006). Although breast cancer is still serious, strong progress has been made in terms of diagnosing it early and developing effective treatments for it. In fact, this disease is one of the most treatable cancers when detected early (USDHHS, NIH, NCI, 2003).

BREAST CARCINOMA

Breast carcinoma is a malignancy that usually originates in the duct or epithelium of the lobes. More than 50% of all breast cancers begin in the upper quadrant and spread to the axillary lymph nodes (ACS & National Comprehensive Cancer Network [NCCN], 2004). Breast cancer commonly metastasizes to the lymph nodes, lungs, liver, brain, and bone (ACS & NCCN, 2004). One of the most lethal forms is inflammatory breast cancer, discussed at the end of this section.

Risk Factors

Risk factors associated with breast cancer include gender; increasing age; race; personal history of breast cancer, benign breast disorder, or both; family history (ie, first-degree relatives); genetic predisposition (carrying mutated BRCA1 and BRCA2 genes); reproductive history; lifestyle; and environmental factors (DiSaia & Creasman, 2002; NCI, 2003). Some risk factors are modifiable and can be avoided; others, such as family history, cannot. Most women who have these risk factors, however, do not get cancer (NCI, 2003). Approximately 85% of women who develop breast cancer have no known family history (DiSaia & Creasman, 2002; NCI, 2003).

Although certain factors have been identified as posing risk, many women who develop breast cancer have no known risk factor other than growing older (NIC, 2003). Modifying lifestyle patterns by increasing physical activity, reducing excess weight, avoiding environmental factors, and making dietary changes can help lower a woman's risk (Fitzgibbon et al., 2005). Early identification of risk factors can help women assume an active role in preventing breast cancer. Early detection of breast cancer is lifesaving; prognosis often is related to the stage at which the cancer is identified (ACS, 2006a; Facione et al., 2002; Meechan et al., 2003; NCI, 2003).

Age and Race

Age is probably the most important risk factor because risk is especially high for women older than 60 years. Many cases occur in women older than 50 years (NCI, 2003). Breast cancer incidence is higher in white women than in Latina, Asian, or African American women (USDHHS, Health Resources and Services Administration, Maternal and Child Health Bureau, 2002). Although overall rates of breast cancer have decreased since 1990, mortality rates have remained constant among African American women (Research Highlight 4.1). This finding may be related to the fact that aging African American women tend to develop less aggressive forms of breast cancer than younger women. When discovered early, the lesions are usually smaller (less than 2 cm). Thus, older African American women with more advanced forms of breast cancer may not have the same opportunities for access to health care that white women do. Another factor is that African American women often seek medical attention at a later stage of the disease, which carries a higher mortality rate (Condon, 2004). Even though the incidence of breast cancer is higher in aging women, they usually have no lymph node involvement (Condon, 2004). Previous benign breast disorders, such as atypical hyperplasia, also increase risk. Women who had biopsies that showed proliferative breast changes are also at increased risk for breast cancer (Forshee et al., 2003; Morgan et al., 1998).

Genetics

Two genes identified as associated with breast cancer are the **BRCA1** and **BRCA2** genes (see Chap. 2). Alterations of these genes have been implicated in approximately 5% to 10% of all breast cancers (Martin & Weber, 2000). This risk factor should be investigated when incidence of breast cancer in families is increased. Ovarian cancer also is associated with these genetic marker alterations (see later discussion).

These BRCA1 and BRCA2 genetic alterations have been found in 2.3% of women with Ashkenazi Jewish heritage (NCI, 2003). Women of Ashkenazi Jewish ancestry are five times more likely to present with breast cancer than women in the general population (NCI, 2003). Genetic testing can be used to determine whether women are carriers of these abnormal genes. Although positive test results for BRCA1 and BRCA2 genes identify a person's risk for developing cancer, these results cannot affirm whether a person will actually develop breast cancer (NCI, 2003).

Reproductive History

Reproductive history also contributes to risk for breast cancer. Morgan and colleagues (1998) reported that women who experienced their first full-term pregnancy before 22 years are at decreased risk, whereas women who experienced a full-term pregnancy later in life may be at increased risk. Nulliparous women are at increased risk. Researchers also have established age at menarche and age at menopause as potential risk factors. Women who experience menarche before 12 years, menopause after 55 years, or both appear to be at increased risk (Morgan et al., 1998).

Breastfeeding and breast cancer risk continue to be investigated because study results have been inconsistent.

● RESEARCH HIGHLIGHT 4.1 A Combined Breast Health and Weight Loss Intervention for Black Women

Fitzgibbon, M. L., Stolley, M. R., Schiffer, L., Sanchez Johnson, L. A., Wells, A. M., & Dyer, A. (2005). *Preventive Medicine, 40*(4), 373–383.

OBJECTIVE: Overall incidence of breast cancer is slightly lower in black women than in white women. Nevertheless, mortality rates from breast cancer are higher in black women than in white women. Possible contributors to this disparity may include higher body mass index (BMI), sedentary lifestyle, and decreased compliance with recommended breast health behaviors.

DESIGN: A randomized pilot intervention trial was conducted to assess the feasibility and efficacy of a combined breast health and weight loss intervention for 64 overweight or obese black women, 35 to 65 years old. The primary objectives were to determine whether a 20-week intervention (twice weekly) could decrease weight and dietary fat intake and increase physical activity and proficiency with breast self-examination (BSE).

RESULTS: The project was implemented in two cohorts; retention was high for both (96% and 86%, respectively). Both cohorts showed increased proficiency with BSE in the intervention versus the control group (2.4 vs. –0.4, $p < 05$; 3.3 vs. –0.2, $p < 0.001$, respectively), but only one cohort showed decreased body weight (4.0% decrease vs. 0.9% increase, $p < 0.01$).

CONCLUSION: Few studies have documented weight loss among black women, and no combined breast health and weight loss intervention has been conducted. This study documents the feasibility of recruiting, randomizing, and retaining women in a combined intervention and demonstrates weight loss and associated lifestyle changes.

Some findings suggest that increased duration of breastfeeding may reduce risk in premenopausal women, whereas others show little or no association between breastfeeding and cancer risk (Morgan et al., 1998).

Other reproductive factors associated with the development of breast cancer include estrogen and diethylstilbestrol (DES) exposure. Women exposed to estrogen for a longer period are at increased risk for breast cancer. Therefore, estrogen and hormone replacement therapy have been called into question, with research providing evidence that these hormones place women at greater risk for developing breast cancer (Morgan et al., 1998; NIC, 2003). DES was used in the 1940s until the early 1970s to reduce spontaneous abortions in women with pregnancy complications. It appears that women who were exposed to DES may be at slightly higher risk for developing cancer, but there is still not enough information available to apply to daughters who may have been exposed to DES in utero (NIC, 2003). Morgan's group (1998) has suggested that more research is needed in this population of women and their daughters.

Some have suggested that phytoestrogens may reduce cancer risk. Phytoestrogens are estrogen-like substances (isoflavone constituents of soy) and plant compounds that exhibit some estrogenic proprieties. These dietary compounds appear to act as estrogen antagonists and may protect against breast cancer (Briese, 2000). Research to date has been inconclusive as to the relationship between phytoestrogens and cancer risk (Morgan et al., 1998).

Twenty-four independent studies have investigated the relationship between induced abortion and breast cancer risk. Meta-analysis of these studies reported a weak increase in risk for breast cancer following induced abortion. Lack of reliable population data limits the availability of information on this topic (Morgan et al., 1998). Current data regarding breast augmentation and long-term health risks do not support the idea that breast augmentation increases cancer risk (Morgan et al., 1998).

It has been reported that women with dense breasts (ie, breasts with a lot of lobular or ductal tissue) are at increased risk for breast cancer. This makes sense in light of the fact that breast cancer generally always develops in these tissue types. It is also more difficult to identify abnormal areas on mammograms of dense breasts (NCI, 2003).

Several researchers have studied the use of oral contraceptives versus nonoral contraceptives and breast cancer incidence. Consistent findings from these researchers have shown no strong association between oral contraceptives and breast cancer. Data to date do not support oral contraceptive use as a strong risk factor for the development of breast cancer; however, further research in this area is warranted (Morgan et al., 1998).

Lifestyle

Lifestyle patterns also have been investigated as risk factors. In the past, assumptions were that high dietary fat intake increased breast cancer risk; however, during the past decade, epidemiologic investigations have not supported this premise. Most studies have failed to support dietary fat as an independent risk factor for breast cancer (Morgan et al., 1998). Many researchers continue to debate this issue, however, and some evidence suggests a link between diet and breast cancer. The National Institute of Cancer (2003) reported that women who consume diets rich in fruits and vegetables and low in fat are at decreased risk for breast cancer. Research on physical activity and breast cancer incidence has been more positive. Increased physical activity has been associated with decreased risk for breast cancer (Bernstein et al., 1994; Morgan et al., 1998; Patel et al., 2003). Women who drink alcohol also may be at slightly higher risk (NCI, 2003). Viel and others (1997) reported that risk of breast cancer increases with consumption of alcohol.

Women who have been exposed to chest and breast radiation therapy are also at risk for breast cancer later in life (NIC, 2003).

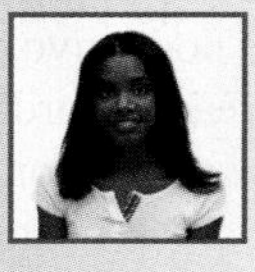

Remember Jade, the woman described at the beginning of the chapter who stated that her grandmother recently died of breast cancer. What other risk factors are present with Jade?

Assessment Findings

Signs and Symptoms

The most common sign of breast cancer is a painless breast mass, often in the upper outer quadrant. A breast mass can develop for as long as 2 years before becoming palpable. Other signs and symptoms include bloody nipple discharge, skin dimpling over the site of the lesion, nipple retraction, an orange appearance to the affected area (peau d'orange), and bilateral difference in breast size. The lesion may be movable or fixed; lymph node enlargement in the adjacent axilla is possible.

Diagnostic Testing

Clinical breast examination can provide information about the size, mobility, and texture of the lump, as well as the status of the surrounding tissue and underarm lymph nodes. If results indicate suspicious lesions, additional diagnostic mammography examinations or biopsy may be necessary to assess for abnormal cell growth (NCI, 2003). Invasive diagnostic breast tests include fine-needle aspiration, stereotactic core biopsy, needle localization biopsy, excisional biopsy, incisional biopsy, and hormone receptor assays (Youngkin & Davis, 2004).

Mammography. Mammograms often detect breast lumps before they are palpable; they also can detect microcalcifications, which may be early signs of cancer (NCI, 2003) (Fig. 4.16). See Chapter 2 also.

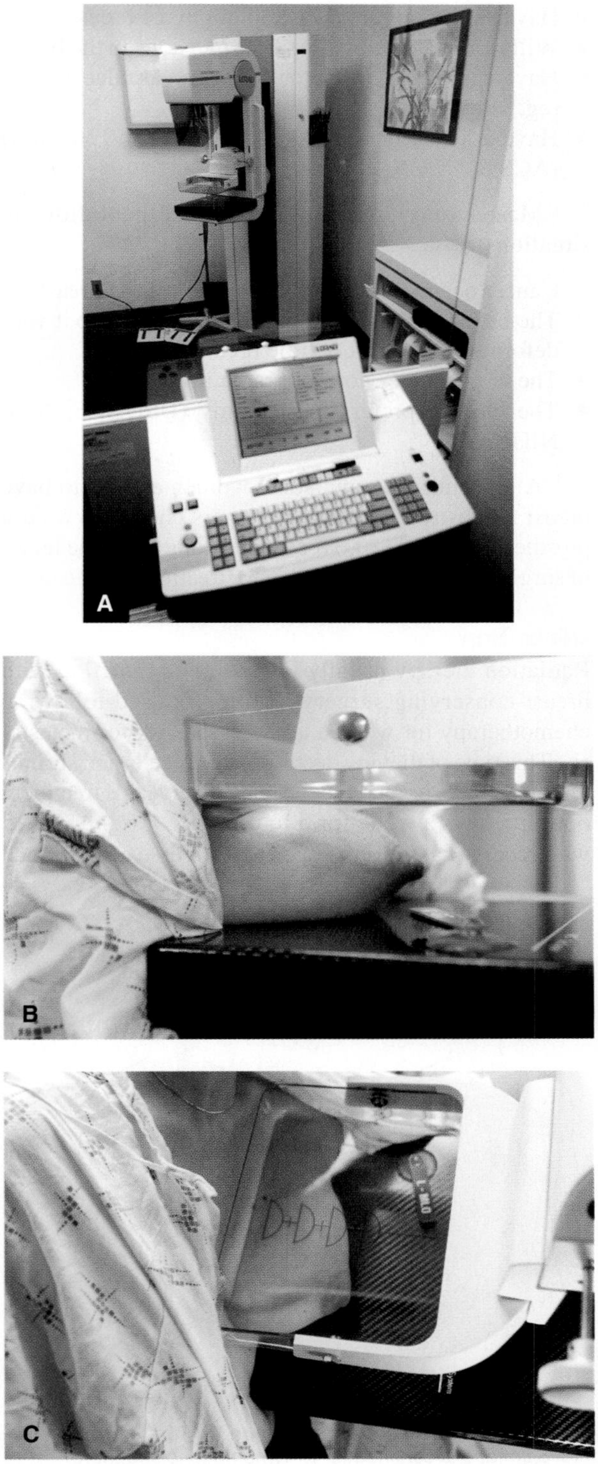

FIGURE 4.16 Mammography. (**A**) Equipment. (**B**) Top-to-bottom view of breast. (**C**) Side view of breast.

Fine-Needle Aspiration. A fine needle is inserted into the lump to remove fluid and cells. Usually, if the fluid is clear, it is sent to the laboratory for further analysis (NCI, 2003).

Stereotactic Core Biopsy. Stereotactic core biopsy is a three-dimensional computerized view of the breast used to identify breast abnormalities. A biopsy is done on the identified area; specimens are sent to the laboratory for histologic diagnosis. This procedure has been reported as highly sensitive (98% in detecting breast cancers when used in women who meet procedure criteria). Clients with difficulty lying prone or who experience frequent coughing spells often cannot tolerate the procedure, which affects results. Another factor is location of the mass or lump. When tumors are close to the nipple or chest wall, obtaining a specimen often is difficult. Usually, this procedure can be done with local anesthesia. Although clients may experience some pain, scarring is minimal, and most women can resume routine activities within 24 hours (Youngkin & Davis, 2004).

Needle Biopsy. When mammography reveals a nonpalpable mass or lesion, a needle biopsy can be performed. This is usually an outpatient procedure done with local anesthesia. The benefits are that the procedure removes less normal tissue and provides more precise identification of lesions (NCI, 2003; Youngkin & Davis, 2004).

Excisional Biopsy. Excisional biopsy usually includes removal of all of the lump or suspicious tissue, as well as an area of healthy tissue surrounding the lesion edges (rim). The tissue is sent for microscopic histologic examination to check for cancer cells. This method is the usual treatment of small, mobile, benign lesions. As with any surgical procedure, it can carry the usual risk for postoperative complications, including hematoma, stitch abscess, anesthetic reaction, and infection (NCI, 2003; Youngkin & Davis, 2004).

Incisional Biopsy. Incisional biopsy is the procedure used for diagnostic purposes because it provides rapid determination of malignancy status. It also is used to confirm a diagnosis of advanced cancer. Usually, this procedure is done before surgical removal of the lump or breast tissue. Only the suspicious area or lump is removed; histologic examination is performed immediately to provide a rapid diagnosis (NCI, 2003; Youngkin & Davis, 2004).

Hormone Receptor Assay. Often, when cancer is diagnosed, a hormone receptor assay test follows. This test is used to determine the tumor's dependency on estrogen and progesterone. It identifies the tumor's response to endocrine therapy and also may be used to determine the client's prognosis. Hayes (2000) suggests that estrogen appears to stimulate normal ductal growth and that progesterone is responsible for lobular-alveolar growth. Classifying and diagnosing tumors with high estrogen or progesterone receptors are easier because clients with these types of breast tissue usually have a better prognosis.

Treatment

A wide range of treatment options is available to clients diagnosed with breast cancer. Providers usually suggest an individualized approach based on specific prognostic indicators. Factors that assist with clinical decisions include lymph node status, tumor size, histologic classification, and subtype identification. Each of these factors is used to stage the breast cancer (Fig. 4.17). Treatment options are then offered based on the clinical stage classification.

Surgery

Surgical options, which collectively constitute the primary treatment method, are varied and wide ranging (NCI, 2002, 2003). Clients are presented with choices for breast surgery immediately following a positive rapid biopsy, which avoids the need for an additional second round of anesthesia, or a two-step procedure that includes surgical biopsy and an additional second surgery to treat the cancer later (NCI, 2003). The next decision is either **lumpectomy** (breast-conserving option) with radiation or **mastectomy** (removal of the entire affected breast). Research has shown that clients who choose lumpectomy with radiation can expect the same survival rate as those who choose mastectomy (ACS & NCCN, 2004).

Lumpectomy with radiation is not always a viable option. It is not recommended for women who:

- Have had previous radiation to the chest wall or breast
- Are pregnant
- Have cancer in several areas of the breast
- Have suspicious areas of calcium in the breast
- Will need to have two separate incisions in the breast
- Have connective tissue or collagen vascular disease (eg, scleroderma, lupus)
- Have a lesion or tumor larger than 5 cm (2 inches) (ACS & NCCN, 2004)

Mastectomy is recommended in the following situations:

- Cancer occurs in more than one part of the breast.
- The breast is small, and removal would leave it very deformed or with very little breast tissue.
- The woman does not want radiation.
- The woman prefers mastectomy (USDHHS, NCI, NIH, 2003).

After a mastectomy, some women choose to have breast reconstruction surgery; others choose to wear a prosthesis. See Table 4.6 for more details about the levels of surgical procedures available for treating breast cancer.

Radiation Therapy

Radiation therapy usually is used in conjunction with breast-conserving surgery. It often is used following chemotherapy for women at increased risk for metastasis. This type of therapy destroys cancer cells and shrinks tumors before surgery. Clients may receive this treatment option 5 days a week for 5 to 6 weeks. Often, women who receive radiation experience adverse effects such

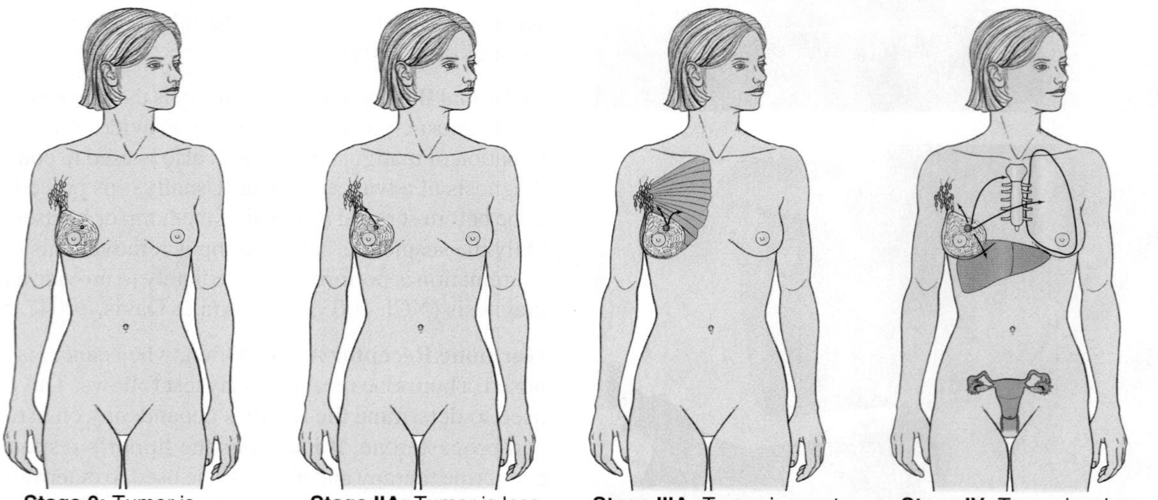

Stage 0: Tumor is confined to the milk duct or lobule.
Stage I: Tumor is less than 2 cm in diameter and confined to the breast.

Stage IIA: Tumor is less than 5 cm, or tumor is smaller with 1, 2, or 3 axillary lymph node involvement.
Stage IIB: Tumor is greater than 5 cm. Up to 3 axillary lymph nodes may be involved.

Stage IIIA: Tumor is greater than 5 cm and is confined to 4 to 10 lymph nodes.
Stage IIIB: Tumor, regardless of size, has spread to the chest wall or skin.
Stage IIIC: Tumor of any size with involvement of 10 or more lymph nodes, but no distant metastases.

Stage IV: Tumor involves lymph nodes and there are distant metastases.

FIGURE 4.17 Staging of breast cancer.

TABLE 4.6 Surgical Procedures for Breast Cancer

PROCEDURE	DESCRIPTION	ILLUSTRATION
Lumpectomy	Only the tumor is removed; some axillary lymph nodes may be excised at the same time for microscopic examination.	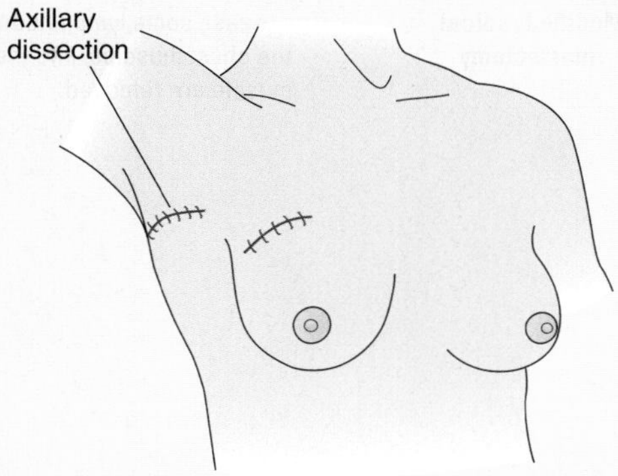
Partial or segmental mastectomy	The tumor and some breast tissue and some lymph nodes are removed.	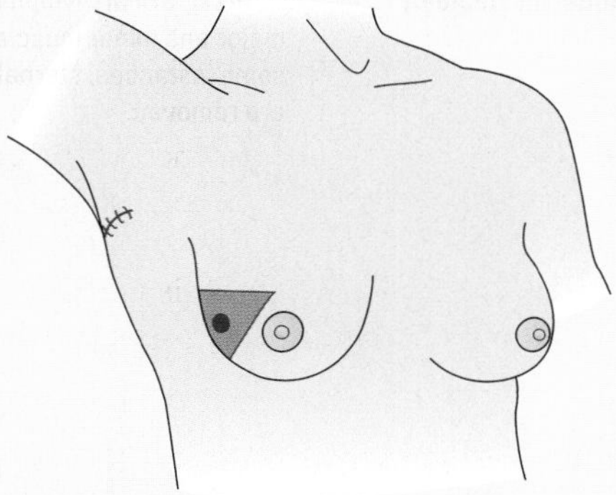
Simple or total mastectomy	All breast tissue is removed. No lymph node dissection is performed.	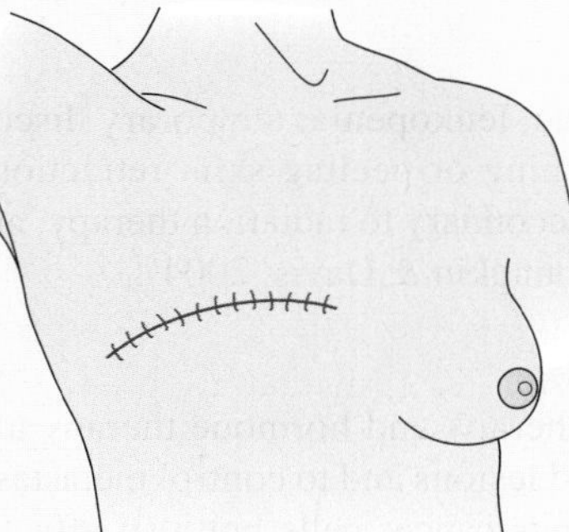
Subcutaneous mastectomy	All breast tissue is removed, but the skin and nipple are left intact.	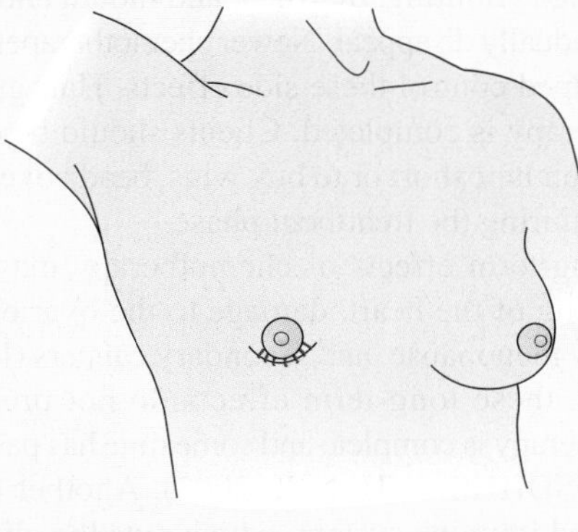

Continued

TABLE 4.6 Surgical Procedures for Breast Cancer *(Continued)*

PROCEDURE	DESCRIPTION	ILLUSTRATION
Modified radical mastectomy	The breast, some lymph nodes, the lining over the chest muscles, and the pectoralis minor muscle are removed.	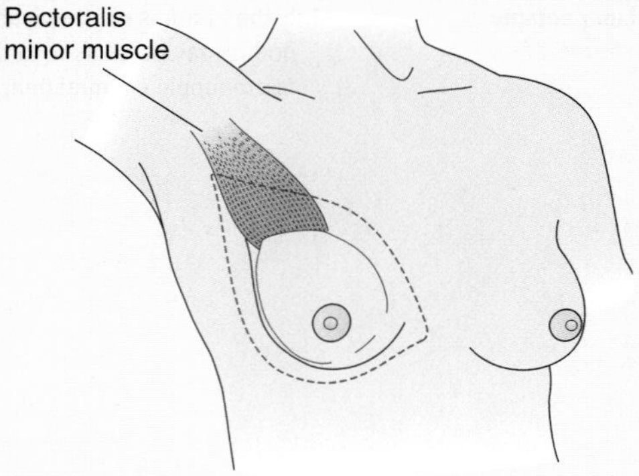
Radical mastectomy	The breast, axillary lymph nodes, and pectoralis major and minor muscles are removed. In some instances, sternal lymph nodes also are removed.	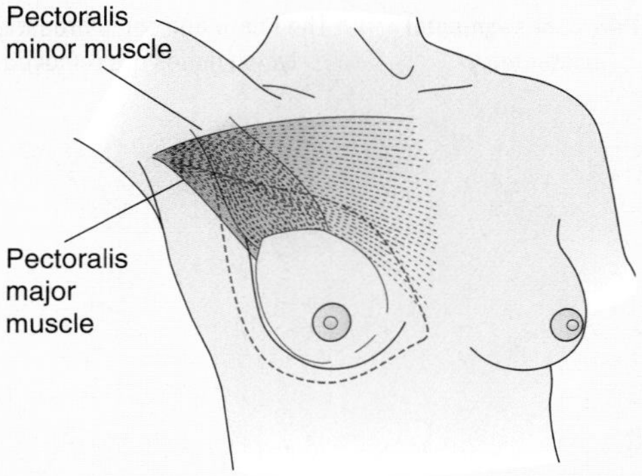

as fatigue, leukopenia, temporary discoloration of the skin, itching or peeling skin, retraction of the breast, cancer secondary to radiation therapy, and pleural effusion (Youngkin & Davis, 2004).

Chemotherapy

Chemotherapy and hormone therapy are used to treat localized lesions and to control metastasis. Chemotherapy targets cancer cells but also affects normal cells. Short-term side effects include hair loss, loss of appetite, nausea and vomiting, diarrhea, and mouth and lip sores. They gradually disappear. Newer chemotherapeutic agents have helped control these side effects. Hair grows back after therapy is completed. Clients should be counseled to cut their hair short or to buy wigs, head coverings, and scarves during the treatment phase.

Long-term effects of chemotherapy may result in weakening of the heart, damage to the ovaries, infertility, early menopause, and secondary cancers (leukemia). Usually, these long-term effects do not present until chemotherapy is complete and some time has passed (NCI, 2003; USDHHS, NIH, NCI, 2003). Another effect is a weakened immune system, which puts the client at risk for infection. Women should receive counseling about avoiding infections and seeking medical attention promptly when they suspect one. Counseling and education also needs to be provided regarding pregnancy risks. Women should avoid pregnancy during treatment because the effects of chemotherapy on the unborn child are unknown. Pregnancy after a course of chemotherapy depends on the client's age and type of drugs received. Women older than 35 years are likely to experience permanent infertility (NCI, 2003).

Hormonal Therapy

Cyrus-David and Strom (2001) have reported that acceptance of breast cancer hormone therapy depends on the woman's knowledge of her breast cancer risk factors and her perceptions of the barriers to and benefits of this type of therapy. Hormone therapy prevents growth of cancer cells and controls metastasis and recurrence (NIH & NCI, 1998). Selective estrogen receptor modulators (SERMs) have been shown to reduce the incidence of breast cancer in high-risk women. This type of therapy is used to block the effects of estrogen when hormone receptor assays show that the breast tissue receptors are estrogen positive (Jordon, 2000a, 2000b, 2000c). Tamoxifen and raloxifene have been used to successfully reduce the risk for cancer in high-risk women and to treat breast cancer (Jordan 2000b, 2000c) (Pharmacology Box 4.2). Nevertheless, hormone therapy carries risks and adverse effects (Box 4.5). It has been associated with increased endometrial cancer, cataracts, and blood clots. Raloxifene has not been shown to increase endometrial cancer (Breslin & Lucas, 2003; Goldstein, 2000).

Aromatase inhibitors, a new drug therapy, are gaining in popularity. They appear to reduce and improve side effects by antagonizing estrogen and blocking its synthesis from androgens. This therapy offers another option for preventing the effects of estrogen on the breast (Weipple-Strasser & Goss, 2003).

Biologic Therapy

Biologic therapy is used to strengthen and improve the immune system to fight infections and cancer (NCI, 2003). These agents produce various side effects that depend on the agent used and on individual differences. Side effects associated with these agents may include rashes, swelling at the injection site, flu-like symptoms, fever, chills, fatigue, digestive tract problems, and allergic reactions (NIH & NCI, 1998).

Herceptin has been used to fight advanced cancers that contain the HER-2 gene. This drug can lead to heart failure and lung damage resulting in breathing problems. Clients receiving this therapy need to be monitored closely (NCI, 2003). Although it appears promising, more study is needed to support its efficacy (Condon, 2004).

COLLABORATIVE CARE: THE CLIENT WITH BREAST CANCER

Assessment

For all clients, health care providers must identify their current knowledge level regarding BSE, previous experience with BSE, and understanding of breast cancer knowledge and risks. When breast cancer is suspected or procedures for treatment have been established as necessary, the nurse needs to discuss the client's medical, drug, allergy, and family history. He or she should take the client's vital signs and weight, determine the location of the breast lesion, and establish what diagnostic tests were performed before admission (if any). The nurse also should review information the client has received about the type and extent of surgery or other treatment.

Select Potential Nursing Diagnosis

The following are examples of commonly applicable NANDA diagnoses:

- **Fear** related to situational crisis (cancer), threat to health/socioeconomic status, role functioning, interaction patterns
- **Risk for Impaired Tissue Integrity** related to surgical removal of tissues, altered circulation, edema, drainage, changes in skin elasticity, sensation, effects of chemotherapy and radiation, immunologic deficit, altered nutritional status, or anemia
- **Pain (Acute)** related to surgical procedure, tissue trauma, disease process, side effects of various cancer therapy
- **Risk for Situational Low Self-Esteem** related to disfiguring surgical procedure and concern about sexual attractiveness
- **Risk for Impaired Physical Mobility** related to pain/discomfort, edema formation, neuromuscular impairment
- **Deficient Knowledge** related to BSE, breast cancer risks, breast disorder, prognosis, treatment, self-care, and discharge needs
- **Risk for Imbalanced Nutrition, Less Than Body Requirements** related to hypermetabolic state associated with cancer, side effects of chemotherapy, radiation, surgery, nausea

PHARMACOLOGY 4.2 Tamoxifen

ACTION: Tamoxifen has potent antiestrogen effects, competing with estrogen for binding sites in the breast and other target tissue organs.

PREGNANCY CATEGORY: D

DOSAGE: For breast cancer, 20 to 40 mg/day orally for 5 years taken in divided doses, morning and evening.

POSSIBLE ADVERSE EFFECTS: Hot flashes, rash, nausea, vomiting, vaginal bleeding and discharge, menstrual irregularities.

NURSING IMPLICATIONS

- Arrange for periodic blood counts.
- Counsel client to use contraception while taking tamoxifen, because of the risk of congenital fetal effects.
- Alert the client to avoid taking this medication with grapefruit juice, which dilutes the drug's effects.
- Instruct the client to have regular reproductive examinations while on this therapy.
- Caution the client to report any marked sleepiness, weakness, confusion, leg pain or swelling, dyspnea, or blurry vision.

Source: Karch, A. (2005). *2005 Lippincott's nursing drug guide.* Philadelphia: Lippincott Williams & Wilkins.

BOX 4.5 Hormonal Therapy Potential Adverse Effects

Common

Hot flashes
Nausea
Vaginal spotting
Increased fertility

Less Common

Depression
Vaginal itching
Vaginal bleeding and discharge
Loss of appetite
Eye problems
Headache
Weight gain

NIC/NOC Box 4.5 Breast Cancer

Common NIC Labels

- Body Image Enhancement
- Chemotherapy Management
- Health Screening
- Radiation Therapy Management
- Risk Identification
- Teaching: Disease Process
- Teaching: Preoperative

Common NOC Labels

- Health-Seeking Behavior
- Knowledge: Treatment Regimen
- Risk Control: Cancer
- Risk Detection

- **Anticipatory Grieving** related to loss of psychosocial well-being, perceived potential death
- **Risk for Deficient Fluid Volume** related to impaired intake of fluids, hypermetabolic state, excessive body fluid loss
- **Fatigue** related to altered body chemistry; side effects of pain, medications, and chemotherapy; overwhelming psychological/emotional demands
- **Risk for Infection** related to inadequate secondary defenses and immunosuppression, malnutrition, invasive procedures, and chronic disease processes
- **Risk for Impaired Oral Mucous Membranes** related to chemotherapy side effects, dehydration, malnutrition
- **Risk for Ineffective Sexuality Patterns** related to lack of understanding of alternative responses to health-related transitions, altered body functioning/structure, illness, medical treatment, fatigue, fear, and anxiety

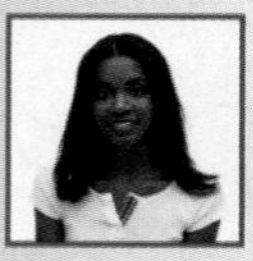

Review Jade's statements at the beginning of the chapter related to her risk for breast cancer. Which nursing diagnoses might be priorities for her?

Planning/Intervention

Nursing goals, interventions, and outcomes depend on the client's diagnoses and treatment plan. Universal goals should include active participation in decision making for treatment options, compliance with treatment plans, and management of the side effects of adjunct therapy. NIC/NOC Box 4.5 highlights some of the major nursing interventions and outcomes associated with breast cancer.

Preventing Breast Cancer

Important strategies to prevent breast cancer include maintaining and adopting a healthy lifestyle. As discussed in detail in Chapter 2, women can reduce their risk by eating a healthy diet rich in vegetables, fruits, and whole grains; exercising daily; avoiding obesity; limiting alcohol consumption; avoiding hormone replacement therapy; performing monthly BSE; and receiving mammograms as recommended by health care providers (Condon, 2004).

Clients at high risk need to work with their health care provider and discuss the use of chemoprevention options (Condon, 2004). The nurse should encourage anyone who detects breast changes to see a health care provider immediately for evaluation. Nursing Care Plan 4.2 presents more information on teaching and follow-up for high-risk clients.

Assisting With Surgery

When a client needs to undergo surgical treatment for breast cancer, the nurse should prepare her and assist with her safe recovery. When a client undergoes breast-conserving surgery, care focuses on wound management and discharge instructions. Clients also need reassurance that their skin will return to normal appearance after 1 or more months. They should be counseled to use protective clothing to prevent further damage to their skin.

Usually, clients are discharged from the health care facility soon after mastectomy. Important nursing measures thus include early discharge instructions and arrangements for home care. Common interventions for the client who has undergone mastectomy include the following:

- Explain care of the wound and drain or arrange for home care nursing.
- Explore availability of assistance from family and friends at home.

NURSING CARE PLAN 4.2

The Client at Risk for Breast Cancer

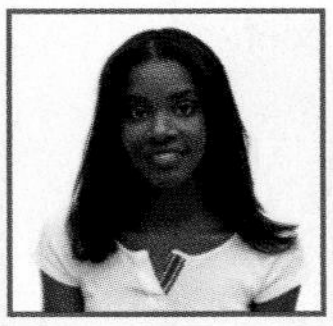

Recall Jade, the 21-year-old client from the beginning of the chapter. Further discussion with Jade reveals that she had planned to breastfeed her first child but had difficulty. "I became so frustrated that I decided it was better for everyone if I used the bottle." Jade reports that although she tries to exercise regularly, she really doesn't have time because her 2-year-old keeps her busy. Review of Jade's health history reveals that she doesn't perform breast self-examination (BSE) and has not had a mammogram. "I really don't know how to check my breasts."

NURSING DIAGNOSIS

Deficient Knowledge related to BSE and health promotion behaviors to reduce the risk for breast cancer.

EXPECTED OUTCOMES

1. The client will identify possible risk factors for development of breast cancer.
2. The client will verbalize the steps of a BSE.
3. The client will state warning signs of breast abnormalities to report to her health care provider.

INTERVENTIONS	RATIONALES
Assess the client's knowledge of breast cancer and associated risks.	This information provides a baseline from which to develop a teaching plan.
Explore the client's exposure to breast examination and breast cancer; correct any misconceptions or myths; allow time for questions.	Information about exposure provides additional foundation for teaching and provides opportunities to clarify or correct misinformation and teach new information.
Review the health history for evidence of risk factors; teach the client measures to reduce her risk, such as increasing activity level and eating a nutritious diet. Discuss the need for regular breast examinations.	Identification of risk factors provides a basis for developing appropriate measures to modify risks.
Assess the client's level of comfort with touching her breasts.	BSE requires touching the breasts. Discomfort or embarrassment may affect the client's ability to perform BSE.
Teach the client about BSE, including when and how to do it, the importance of early detection, and signs to report to a health care provider. Provide the client with brochures, pamphlets, and other materials on BSE and breast cancer as indicated. Reinforce the need for mammograms.	Early detection leads to positive outcomes. Most breast changes or lumps are benign, but only a health care provider can tell for sure. Use of additional teaching materials helps foster learning and provides the client with a reference for later information. Mammograms are the best way to find breast cancer early and to enhance chances for recovery.
Demonstrate each step of BSE, explaining each action before performing it.	Demonstration coupled with explanation facilitates learning.

Continued

NURSING CARE PLAN 4.2 ● The Client at Risk for Breast Cancer *(Continued)*

INTERVENTIONS	RATIONALES
Encourage the client's participation with the demonstration.	Client participation promotes feelings of confidence and helps to reduce anxiety.
Have the client return-demonstrate the procedure, including verbalization of any findings that should be reported.	Return demonstration helps evaluate the client's degree of learning.
Review with the client any possible changes in her breasts because of the pregnancy. Advise her to report these findings during her prenatal examinations.	During pregnancy, breasts increase in size; they may become tender, and sebaceous glands enlarge. Reporting these findings is important to ensure that the changes are normal and not suggestive of cancer.
Instruct the client to choose a time each month to examine her breasts (typically during the week after the menstrual period ends when not pregnant) and to record the findings. Encourage her to bring this information to each health care visit.	Performing BSE at the same time each month ensures consistency with examination findings. The breasts are less tender and swollen the week after the menstrual period ends.
Arrange for follow-up visits as scheduled.	Ongoing visits provide an opportunity to evaluate the client's learning and understanding of the teaching and compliance with the procedure. It also provides opportunities for additional teaching and feedback.

EVALUATION

1. The client lists personal risk factors associated with the development of breast cancer.
2. The client demonstrates BSE technique correctly.
3. The client states that she will perform BSE each month and report any unusual findings.

- Identify and report any signs of infection or impaired healing. Examples include drainage or a pale or dusky appearance to the skin surrounding the incision.
- Emphasize the need to continue performing arm exercises.
- Arrange for follow-up examinations by the surgeon.
- Teach the client the particulars of self-administration of prescribed medications.
- Explain to the client that she likely will feel numbness or tingling on the chest wall and inner side of the arm for up to 1 year after the surgery.
- Remind the client to apply cream or lotion to the skin in the incision location if it tends to be dry.
- Caution against carrying or lifting anything that weighs more than 15 lbs; additionally, the client should not make repetitive or stressful movements with the affected arm.
- Alert the client not to wear tight garments around or sleep on the affected arm; these measures could impair circulation.
- Teach the client that blood pressure measurements, infusions, injections, and so forth are contraindicated in the affected arm.

Managing Chemotherapy

The nurse should assist the client receiving chemotherapy to anticipate and to deal with the common side effects: nausea and vomiting, hair loss, changes in taste, dermatitis, weight gain, and fatigue (Teaching Tips 4.5). Some clients also experience mild memory loss and unclear thinking, a syndrome commonly referred to as "chemo-brain." The nurse should explain the particulars of medication administration to relieve nausea and mouth sores and to boost white blood cell or RBC production. If alopecia is likely, the nurse may offer a list of wig sup-

TEACHING TIPS 4.5 Chemoprevention Adverse Effects

Infection

- Avoid infections.
- Avoid dental work during chemotherapy.
- Maintain a healthy diet.
- Get plenty of rest.
- Avoid large crowds and anyone with colds, infections, and contagious diseases.
- Maintain good hygiene habits (bathe daily, good oral care, wash hands frequently).
- Protect hands against cuts, burns, and irritations (use work gloves).
- Clean all cuts and wounds; keep them covered and seek medical attention immediately when infections are suspected.

Nausea

- Eat small meals often.
- Fast for 3 to 4 hours before treatment.
- Eat whatever you can tolerate.
- Chew food thoroughly.
- Relax during mealtime.
- Practice stress reduction techniques such as deep breathing exercises, meditation, yoga, acupuncture, and visualization strategies.

pliers or catalogs with scarves, turbans, or hats to camouflage hair loss. Such resources are available through the American Cancer Society.

Managing Lymphedema

Both radiation and surgery may change the normal lymph drainage pattern, leaving clients with complications of **lymphedema** of the arm. Treatment options include using elastic sleeves, arm pumps, arm massage, and Ace bandaging (NCI, 2003). Teaching Tips 4.6 provide more information about preventing and reducing the effects of lymphedema (NIH & NCI, 1998).

Providing Client Teaching

Nursing care should include client education and counseling about the course of treatment, expected reactions, and tips for dealing with and relieving untoward effects. It is also helpful to refer the client to support programs such as Reach to Recovery or local cancer survivor and support programs in their community (Youngkin & Davis, 2004).

INFLAMMATORY BREAST CANCER

Inflammatory breast cancer (IBC) is a rare type of breast cancer in which cancer cells block lymph vessels in the skin and breast. This most aggressive form of breast cancer accounts for approximately 1% to 6% of all cases; however, it kills at least 30% of clients who receive this diagnosis (DuVal, 2004). It is most common in postmenopausal women and often is misdiagnosed as mastitis. Because it usually is diagnosed after it has spread to the lymphatic system, 90% of women with IBC die within 1 year unless they receive prompt treatment (DuVal, 2004). Overall survival rates have increased because of improved breast cancer treatments (DuVal, 2004).

Assessment Findings

IBC usually begins with a painless portion of the breast enlarging. Women notice a sensation of heaviness and mild burning. Following this initial change, the skin of the breast becomes mottled with a pink color that progresses to a diffuse erythema. This redness usually occurs on the lower portion of the breast. Usually, no mass is palpable. The breasts then become tender and painful because the lymphatic pathways become affected. The nipple may retract and become swollen and crusted. The woman will begin to see dimpling of the skin (DuVal, 2004).

Collaborative Management

Clients do not usually seek attention when this process begins. Often, cases are first treated as mastitis. If a

TEACHING TIPS 4.6 Preventing Lymphedema

- Do not carry packages or handbags on the affected side.
- Avoid sunburn and burns to the affected arm or hand.
- Do not use the affected arm for blood pressure tests, blood draws, or injections.
- Avoid cuts when shaving underarms by using an electric shaver.
- Avoid infections in the affected arm, wash cuts promptly, apply antibacterial medication, and cover with a bandage. Seek out medical attention promptly at the first sign of infection.
- Wear gloves when gardening or using strong detergents.
- Avoid elastic cuffs on blouses and nightgowns or anything tight on the affected arm.
- Avoid cutting cuticles; be extremely cautious when manicuring fingernails.

suspected case of mastitis does not respond to a 10- to 14-day antibiotic regimen, more thorough immediate investigation is necessary (DuVal, 2004).

Most clients with this disorder are diagnosed at stage IIIB (see Fig. 4.17). Usual treatment is chemotherapy to reduce the tumor and control metastases, followed by modified radical mastectomy. Once healing has occurred, the client also will receive radiation therapy and possibly additional chemotherapy (DuVal, 2004).

MENSTRUAL DISORDERS

Normally, monthly menstruation poses few concerns for women, with cycles beginning and ending each month around the same time, lasting for an expected duration, and remaining a consistent amount and quality. Nevertheless, some women develop menstrual problems. Such problems can involve frequency, amount, or symptoms related to menstruation.

AMENORRHEA

Amenorrhea is the term used for the absence of menses during the woman's reproductive years. *Primary amenorrhea* is the term used when a woman has never experienced a menstrual cycle. It is used in the following cases:

- By 14 years of age, the adolescent has not had menses and shows no growth and development of secondary sexual characteristics.
- By 16 years of age, the adolescent has not had menses, but growth and development of secondary sexual characteristics are normal.

Secondary amenorrhea is the term used when menses are absent for three or more cycles or for 6 months or longer in women with previously established menstruation.

Etiology and Pathophysiology

The most common causes of primary amenorrhea include structural abnormalities (eg, imperforate hymen and gonadal dysgenesis); endocrine problems (eg, prepubertal ovarian failure, hypopituitarism, congenital adrenal hyperplasia, androgen insensitivity syndrome); and congenital disorders (eg, absent uterus or vagina). Eating disorders or extreme weight gain or loss can lead to primary amenorrhea, as can excessive stress or chronic illness.

Secondary amenorrhea can develop for numerous reasons. The most common and normal causes are pregnancy, lactation, and menopause. Menses also may cease as a consequence of stress, thyroid problems, endocrine tumors, excessive exercise, malnutrition, and kidney failure.

Assessment Findings

The nurse first should determine whether the client is experiencing primary or secondary amenorrhea. Health history taking should begin with finding out whether the client has ever had a regular and cyclic menstrual pattern. If the client reports that such a pattern once existed, the nurse should follow up to learn more about the pattern, when amenorrhea began, and what events during that time may have precipitated the problem. The nurse should explore any past illnesses or hospitalizations, pregnancy history, medication history, lifestyle, nutrition, and diet.

During the physical examination, the nurse should take the client's weight and height and compare findings with previous measurements to determine whether changes are substantial. He or she should look for any visible signs of a genetic problem or endocrine disease. The nurse should take vital signs and look for abnormalities (eg, hypothermia, hypotension) that may indicate an eating disorder or thyroid dysfunction. If the nurse suspects primary amenorrhea in a teen, the nurse should look for characteristics of secondary sex development and perform evaluation of the reproductive tract.

Diagnostic evaluations may include karyotyping (see Chap. 11), pregnancy testing, and thyroid function tests. Ultrasound, CT scans, and laparoscopy may be ordered if a tumor is suspected as the cause. Hormonal studies may include evaluations of levels of prolactin, follicle-stimulating hormone, and luteinizing hormone.

Collaborative Management

Treatment measures vary depending on the cause. For primary amenorrhea, interventions focus on correcting the underlying problems. If necessary, estrogen therapy can be administered to induce the development of secondary sex characteristics. In cases of severe or irreversible problems, health care providers will need to focus on helping the woman to accept the condition and what it means for future infertility.

DYSMENORRHEA

Dysmenorrhea (painful menstruation) may affect more than 50% of menstruating women (Alzubialdi & Calais, 2004). It is characterized by pain shortly before or during menstruation. *Primary dysmenorrhea* refers to pain accompanying menstruation for which no accompanying pelvic disorder or other problem exists. *Secondary dysmenorrhea* is the term used when painful menstruation is the result of an underlying pelvic or uterine disorder.

Etiology and Pathophysiology

Increased production of prostaglandins is the main cause of primary dysmenorrhea. Their levels are highest during the first 2 days of menses, when symptoms are most prevalent (Hart, 2005). Prostaglandins contribute to an increase in uterine contractions, which leads to pain.

Secondary dysmenorrhea can result from numerous causes: pelvic infection, endometriosis, uterine fibroids, or congenital reproductive abnormalities.

Assessment Findings

Women report sharp and intermittent suprapubic pain that may radiate to the back and legs. Pain may be accompanied by headache, nausea and vomiting, fatigue, dizziness, or other symptoms. The pain usually begins with the menses and worsens as the menstrual flow increases, improving as the amount of bleeding tapers off (Clark & Steele, 2004).

The history and physical examination should enable the health care team to determine whether the dysmenorrhea is primary or secondary to better facilitate treatment. With primary dysmenorrhea, the physical examination should reveal no underlying pathology contributing to the menstrual pain. With secondary dysmenorrhea, the health history may reveal fertility problems, menstrual irregularities, pelvic abnormalities, or other problems. The client will undergo a bimanual pelvic examination and laboratory testing, including blood count, urinalysis, cervical cultures for STIs, erythrocyte sedimentation rate, and ultrasound of the pelvis.

Collaborative Management

Treatment focuses on managing the pain and, with secondary dysmenorrhea, eliminating or controlling the underlying cause. The client may be prescribed NSAIDs or COX-2 inhibitors. Management with oral contraceptives also is common.

DYSFUNCTIONAL UTERINE BLEEDING

Dysfunctional uterine bleeding (DUB) is considered abnormal or irregular bleeding not related to pregnancy, infection, or tumor (Bradley, 2005). The most common cause is a hormonal disturbance leading to anovulatory menstrual cycles. DUB can be part of or overlap with other menstrual problems (see Fig. 4.18).

The client will need thorough evaluation of her health history, physical examination, and diagnostic testing to identify the cause. Treatment will focus on elimination or control of the cause. If no cause can be found, management efforts emphasize ways to minimize the bleeding problems so that they do not disrupt the client's lifestyle.

PREMENSTRUAL SYNDROME

Premenstrual syndrome (PMS) is defined as regular premenstrual physical or emotional symptoms that inter-

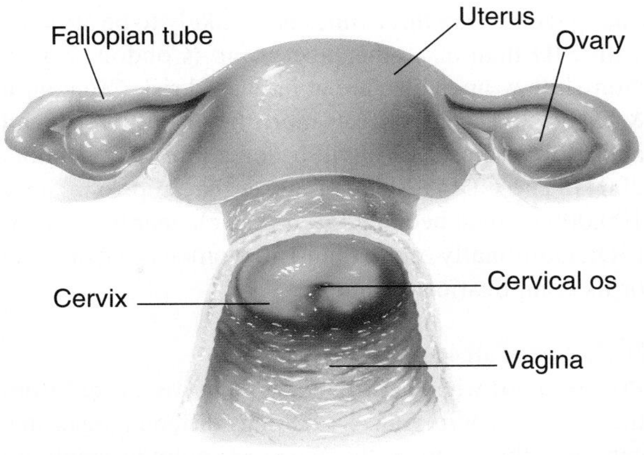

FIGURE 4.18 Dysfunctional uterine bleeding.

fere with daily living and functioning at home and work. PMS occurs during the luteal phase of the menstrual cycle, when estrogen and progesterone initially rise and then fall if no pregnancy occurs. Common symptoms include anxiety, irritability, mood swings, fatigue, palpitations, crying, forgetfulness, fluid retention, weight gain, and breast tenderness.

Despite the prevalence of PMS, much remains unknown about its cause. Several theories involve imbalances of hormones or neurotransmitters. Popular theories also include vitamin deficiency, mineral deficiency, and prostaglandin imbalance. Therefore, treatments often seek to balance levels of hormones or serotonin and to address potential lifestyle conditions. Medical treatment may include trying to balance hormones with oral contraceptives or balancing serotonin with antidepressants. Lifestyle changes that may help include decreased sodium and refined sugar content, decreased alcohol and caffeine intake, increased B vitamins and calcium, exercise, relaxation techniques, and increased rest. Aerobic exercise during the luteal phase is thought to be beneficial to decrease anxiety, depression, and anger.

REPRODUCTIVE TRACT ALTERATIONS

PELVIC INFLAMMATORY DISEASE

Infection is one of the most prevalent reproductive problems, experienced by most women at some point in their lives. Infections can have serious health threats and cause significant sequelae, such as chronic pelvic pain, scarring, infertility, and pelvic inflammatory disease (Condon, 2004).

Pelvic inflammatory disease (PID), a serious complication stemming from previous infections (STIs), can result from infection of the internal upper reproductive tract, uterus (*endometritis*), fallopian tubes (*salpingitis*), ovaries (*oophoritis*), or peritoneum. Adolescents and young women are three times more likely to be affected with PID than any other age group (Condon, 2004). Nonwhite women also are at increased risk (Youngkin & Davis, 2004). PID affects more than 1 million women annually; of those, 12% will become infertile (Condon, 2004). The CDC (2004d) reports that approximately 100,000 women become infertile each year because of PID; additionally, more than 150 women die from PID or its complications annually.

Etiology and Pathophysiology

PID develops when harmful bacteria move upward from the vagina or cervix (Fig. 4.19). Many different organisms can cause this disorder; the two most common agents are chlamydia and gonorrhea (CDC, 2004d). They lead to infection that often results in pelvic scarring and obstruction of the fallopian tubes.

Common risk factors associated with PID are young age, low income, unemployment, low educational status, history of PID or STIs, recent IUD insertion, nulliparity, and cigarette smoking. Risk is increased in single sexually active women and women with more than one male sexual partner in the previous 30 to 60 days. Other factors include intercourse during menstruation and frequent douching. Use of IUDs in women with multiple partners also has been identified as a risk factor.

PID often occurs during the first 5 days of the menstrual cycle. Because of the nature of PID and its consequences, accurate diagnosis and early treatment are crucial (CDC, 2002; Youngkin & Davis, 2004).

Assessment Findings

Symptoms can range from mild to severe; many women are asymptomatic. The most frequent symptom is abdominal pain. The CDC (2002) has established minimum criteria for diagnosis and treatment of PID without a competing diagnosis (eg, pregnancy, acute appendicitis, urinary tract infection [UTI]). These minimum criteria are lower abdominal tenderness, bilateral adnexal tenderness, and cervical motion tenderness.

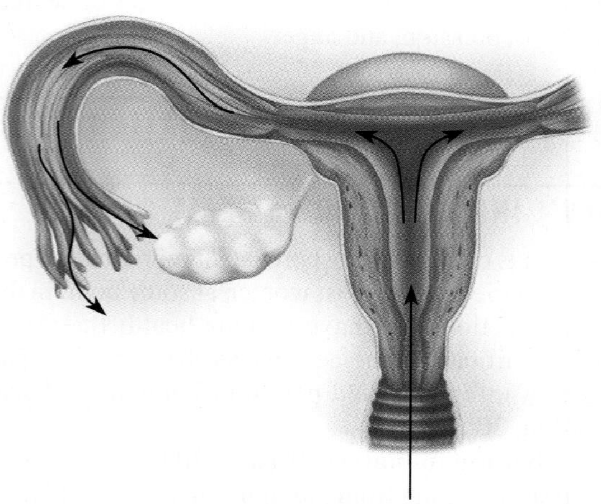

FIGURE 4.19 Progression of pelvic inflammatory disease. A sexually transmitted infection (eg, chlamydia, gonorrhea) moves up into the uterus, progressing to the fallopian tubes and ovaries.

Mild symptoms include vaginal discharge (may or may not be purulent), mild persistent abdominal or back pain, and pain with intercourse (CDC, 2002). Severe symptoms include sudden and severe pelvic pain, high fever, chills, heavy vaginal discharge or bleeding, pain on movement of the cervix, feeling of abdominal fullness, and abdominal mass (when abscess is present) (CDC, 2002).

Chlamydial infections are usually insidious and asymptomatic or mild. Gonorrheal infections are more likely to present with serious symptoms. Peritonitis and abdominal abscess are high when bacteria and purulent drainage escape from the fallopian tubes into the pelvic cavity (CDC, 2002).

Often, diagnosis is difficult because the symptoms are similar to many other diseases. Health care experts have concluded that many cases of PID go undetected, which leads to serious sequelae in young women. Confirmation depends on presenting symptoms and findings from physical and pelvic examinations. Bacterial vaginal smears and cervical cultures are used to identify the causative organism. Blood analysis includes erythrocyte sedimentation rate (ESR), C-reactive protein, and complete blood count with emphasis on white blood cell analysis. Pelvic sonogram is used when pelvic abscess is suspected. When clients are treated and fail to respond to therapy, a laparoscopy may be performed for further diagnostic evaluation to evaluate infertility, occlusions, and masses (Youngkin & Davis, 2004).

Collaborative Management

Treatment options depend on the presenting symptoms. Women with abscess and severe symptoms are hospitalized and treated with IV antibiotics for 24 to 48 hours. Examples of common regimens are cefotetan, 2 g every 12 hours, or cefoxitin, 2 g every 6 hours, and IV or oral doxycycline, 100 mg every 12 hours. Laparoscopy is performed to drain the abscess (Youngkin & Davis, 2004). Women with mild symptoms and suspected infection are treated as outpatients and also receive antibiotic therapy. An example of an outpatient treatment regimen is 500 mg of oral levofloxacin twice a day for 14 days with or without 500 mg of oral metronidazole twice a for 14 days. Women must be counseled to complete all prescriptions and to receive follow-up evaluation 48 to 72 hours after starting the medication and again in 7 to 10 days. Levofloxacin and ofloxacin are contraindicated in women 17 years or younger, as well as in all pregnant women because of the serious side effects. In these situations, alternative medications should be used. Sexual partners also should be treated (Youngkin & Davis, 2004).

Nurses should educate and counsel clients about modifiable risk factors for PID, such as multiple sexual partners and sex without condoms. They should instruct clients to seek medical attention for any unusual vaginal discharge or possible signs of infection. Education also must emphasize the need for sexual partners to be treated and should include methods for decreasing risk for STIs and ways to recognize infection in partners (Smeltzer & Bare, 2008).

Open discussion regarding the client's feelings and concerns about PID is important and can assist her to cope effectively with outcomes. The nurse's role for hospitalized women also includes medication administration and monitoring; comfort measures to reduce pain; assessment of status, vital signs, and characteristics of vaginal discharge (amount, color, odor); and documentation (Smeltzer & Bare, 2008).

ENDOMETRIOSIS

Endometriosis is a benign uterine condition in which endometrial tissue attaches to sites outside the endometrial cavity. This disorder affects approximately 5.5 million women and is one of the top three causes of infertility in women (NIH, 2004) (see Chap. 10).

Endometrial tissue is found most commonly in and near the ovaries, the uterosacral ligaments, and peritoneum; however, it also may appear in the stomach, lungs, spleen, and intestines. This tissue responds to hormones during the menstrual cycle and undergoes changes similar to normally sited uterine endometrial tissue. Each month, estrogen causes all the endometrial tissue, regardless of location, to swell, become inflamed, and cause pain.

Endometriosis occurs in all ethnic groups, although Asians appear to be at increased risk. It is seen most frequently in women 20 to 45 years and in those who report a family history (sisters and mothers), suggesting a genetic predisposition (Corwin, 1997). It usually is not found in women who have borne more than one child. Although endometriosis is not life-threatening, it interferes with a client's ability to work and can cause much pain and discomfort.

Etiology and Pathophysiology

Several theories have been suggested as to the cause of endometriosis, but to date it remains unknown. Corwin (1997) has suggested that during the menstrual cycle, tissue backs up through the fallopian tubes and attaches and implants in the peritoneal cavity (retrograde menstruation theory). Others have suggested that this disorder may be associated with an immune or hormonal problem, or that the tissue travels from the uterus to the lymphatic or blood system to reach other sites in the body (Endometriosis Association, 2002).

Assessment Findings

Symptoms vary and often do not reflect the extent of this disorder. Many clients are asymptomatic. Common symptoms reported include dysmenorrhea, infertility, pelvic pain, dyspareunia, and irregular or heavy bleeding. Symptoms may be associated with menstrual cycles. Other signs are premenstrual back pain, abdominal pain, rectal pain, diarrhea or bleeding, upset stomach or nausea, fatigue, abdominal bloating, and urinary problems (Condon, 2004).

A complete history, physical examination, and pelvic examination usually are warranted when clients present with symptoms. Although the CA-125 assay is a marker for clients with endometriosis, it is not useful in diagnosis because so many other conditions also elevate this marker (Youngkin & Davis, 2004). Diagnostic laparoscopy or laparotomy can be used to visually inspect and identify this disorder for definitive diagnosis. Tissue biopsy and pathologic studies are used for further confirmation (Condon, 2004; Youngkin & Davis, 2004).

Collaborative Management

Treatment often depends on the extent and location of the endometrial growths, the client's age, her desire for pregnancy, and the severity of the symptoms. Although, to date, endometriosis has no cure, several treatment options are available. The goals of management are to relieve or reduce pain, shrink or slow endometrial growths, preserve and restore fertility, and prevent or delay recurrence (Endometriosis Association, 2002). Drug therapy consists of NSAIDs to reduce symptoms and relieve pain. When pain is not relieved with NSAIDs, stronger prescriptions may be necessary. Hormonal therapy also is an option to interrupt or stop ovulation and menstrual cycles. Drugs used for this purpose are oral contraceptives, progesterone drugs, danazol, and gonadotropin-releasing hormone agonists (Endometriosis Association, 2002).

An additional option is surgery. The first-line surgical treatment is conservative and aims to destroy and remove the endometrial growth and preserve reproductive functioning. This option is used in clients who fail to respond to drug therapy and desire to become pregnant. Often, drug therapy and conservative surgical therapy are used together. In cases of extensive and severe endometriosis, more radical surgery may be necessary, such as hysterectomy with removal of all growths and the ovaries (Endometriosis Association, 2002).

The nurse's primary role is to develop a plan of care that incorporates education and counseling about endometriosis. Teaching should include reassurance that the disorder is not life-threatening. The nurse should provide information about the use of nonpharmacologic comfort measures, as well as about OTC pain relievers and hormonal drugs and their side effects.

Nurses need to be aware of the strong association between reported pelvic pain and sexual abuse. Youngkin and Davis (2004) recommend that women with endometriosis be assessed for the possibility of past or present physical or emotional abuse, as well as reactive depression. Nursing plans of care also should include psychological referrals as necessary, especially for women experiencing sexual difficulties and infertility issues.

Preoperative teaching and postoperative nursing care are required for women who undergo conservative or radical surgery. Possible adverse effects are similar to those of other surgical procedures and can include bleeding, infection, and damage to nearby organs. Postoperative discharge education should include information regarding activity, expected vaginal discharge changes (from bleeding to clear drainage), signs of infection, resumption of sexual activity, and diet (Youngkin & Davis, 2004).

The following referral resources may be helpful: the Endometriosis Association, RESOLVE, and the American Association of Reproductive Specialists. Follow-up is important for dealing effectively with this disorder: the woman should be encouraged to see her health provider routinely and to maintain a healthy lifestyle that includes a proper diet, physical activity, adequate sleep, and stress management (Youngkin & Davis, 2004).

LEIOMYOMAS (UTERINE FIBROIDS, MYOMAS)

One of the most common benign gynecologic tumors is a **leiomyoma (fibroid tumor).** Leiomyomas are composed of muscle and connective fibrous tissue in the uterus. Approximately 80% of all women have uterine fibroids, but only 25% have symptoms that warrant treatment (National Uterine Fibroid Foundation, 2004). Many leiomyomas are asymptomatic.

Etiology and Pathophysiology

The etiology of these tumors is unknown. They cause the uterus to enlarge abnormally and are the most common reason hysterectomy is performed. Fibroids usually become symptomatic in women between 35 and 50 years of age. Approximately 30% of African American women have uterine leiomyomas (National Uterine Fibroid Foundation, 2004). These women usually experience this disorder at an earlier age and are 3 to 4 times more likely to present with symptomatic fibroids than the rest of the population of women with fibroids (National Uterine Fibroid Foundation, 2004).

Fibroids are classified according to location: subserosal, intramural, or submucosal (Youngkin & Davis, 2004) (Fig. 4.20). Leiomyomas appear to be dependent on ovarian hormones because they grow slowly during the reproductive years and atrophy during menopause (Smeltzer & Bare, 2008).

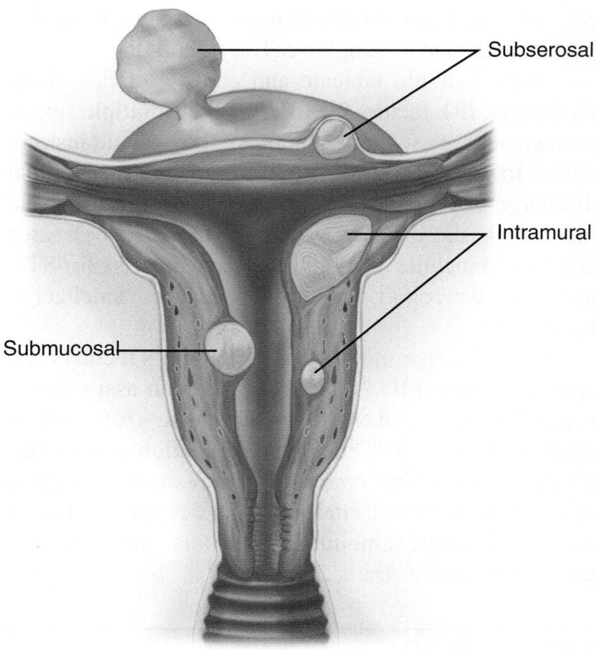

FIGURE 4.20 Leiomyomas (fibroid tumors).

Assessment Findings

The most common symptoms are **menorrhagia** (heavy prolonged vaginal bleeding) and frequent vaginal bleeding. Women may present with complaints of dysmenorrhea or dyspareunia, with large tumors causing expansion of the lower abdomen. When located in the uterine cavity, these tumors also are associated with miscarriage and infertility. They can compromise pregnancy outcomes because during pregnancy they typically grow and become quite large (Condon, 2004). Severe anemia can occur when women experience frequent episodes of copious vaginal bleeding. Often, these symptoms are so incapacitating that women cannot participate in activities outside the home during their menstrual periods and are forced to plan their lives around their cycles. These tumors also can put pressure on surrounding organs and cause frequent urination, pelvic pressure, abdominal discomfort, and constipation.

A complete physical assessment with a pelvic examination may reveal an abnormally shaped uterus. Accurate diagnosis usually is made through the use of transvaginal ultrasound, hysterosalpingogram, MRI, hysteroscopy, and endometrial biopsy (National Uterine Fibroid Foundation, 2004; Youngkin & Davis, 2004).

Collaborative Management

Many treatment options are available for symptomatic fibroids. Some clients choose to treat the increased vaginal bleeding with oral contraceptives, Depo-Provera injections, NSAIDs, vitamins, herbal remedies, or dilation and curettage (D&C). Iron supplements often are recommended to treat anemia related to blood loss. A diet rich in green vegetables, fruit, and fish may afford some protection against fibroids and also may help prevent constipation and hemorrhoids associated with fibroid pressure.

In clients 35 years or younger, surgical treatment focuses on myomectomy (removal of the fibroid without removing the uterus). Types include laparoscopic myomectomy, hysteroscopic myomectomy, laparotomy myomectomy, laparoscopic myomectomy with mini-laparotomy, and laparoscopic-assisted vaginal myomectomy. One of the newest measures is uterine artery embolization (ablation) (UFE), which appears to be quickly becoming the treatment of choice. In this minimally invasive nonsurgical procedure, an interventional radiologist places a catheter into the artery that feeds the fibroid and occludes it. The fibroid is thus deprived of its blood supply. Condon (2004) reports that approximately 85% to 95% of women have reduced symptoms, but long-term effects are still being researched (National Uterine Fibroid Foundation, 2004).

A final treatment option is hysterectomy, which some physicians recommend for symptomatic women who do not desire to have any or additional children. Hysterectomy carries the risks inherent with any surgery and potential long-term physical and psychological effects, such as depression and loss of sexual pleasure. When the ovaries also are removed, the woman is at risk for osteoporosis and possible heart disease (National Uterine Fibroid Foundation, 2004). Postoperative risks also include complications such as blood clots, infection, adhesions, hemorrhage, bowel obstruction, and urinary tract injury or infection.

ENDOMETRIAL HYPERPLASIA

Endometrial hyperplasia is a benign condition in which the cells lining the uterus grow too much. It is most common in women older than 40 years and sometimes develops into cancer. Heavy menstrual periods, DUB, and bleeding after menopause are common symptoms. Clients at highest risk are those who are perimenopausal or menopausal, skip menstrual periods or have no periods at all, are overweight, have diabetes, have polycystic ovary syndrome, or take unopposed estrogen (without progesterone) to relieve the symptoms of menopause (American College of Obstetricians and Gynecologists [ACOG], 2001; NCI, 2001).

Diagnosis is made when the client presents with symptoms. Physical examination including a pelvic examination is routine. Definitive diagnosis is made with ultrasound, endometrial biopsy, D&C, and hysteroscopy (ACOG, 2001).

Treatment focuses on prevention of hyperplasia and includes administration of hormones (progesterone) and regular follow-up examinations. The physician may recommend hysterectomy to prevent endometrial hyperplasia from developing into cancer.

UTERINE CANCER

One of the most common types of uterine cancer is endometrial cancer (cancer in the uterine lining). Usual sites of metastasis are the lungs, bones, liver, and, eventually, the brain (Smeltzer & Bare, 2008). The ACS (2006b) reported that more than 7000 U.S. women will die of uterine cancer in 2006. Although this type of cancer has a 5-year survival rate of 84%, prognosis really depends on the stage of cancer at diagnosis, as well as other risk factors (Box 4.6).

Etiology and Pathophysiology

Women between 55 and 70 years of age are at highest risk (Smeltzer & Bare, 2008). White women are more likely to have uterine cancer than African American women. Risk is increased in clients with obesity, diabetes, hypertension, or all these factors. The number of years that a woman is exposed to estrogen is also a factor. Clients who experience increased bleeding during the perimenopausal years are four times more likely to develop uterine cancer than are women who did not have this problem (ACS, 2006b). Risk factors include the following:

- Early menarche (before 12 years)
- Increasing age (older than 50 years)
- Delayed menopause
- Prolonged total duration of years menstruating
- Endometrial hyperplasia
- Use of hormone replacement therapy, especially long term
- Obesity
- Infertility or nulliparity
- Use of tamoxifen
- White race
- Family history of colorectal cancer

Endometrial cancer usually grows slowly, exhibits late metastasis, and is responsive to treatment (Smeltzer & Bare, 2008).

BOX 4.6 Uterine Cancer Five-Year Survival Rates by Stage

- Stage I: 90%–95%
- Stage II: 75%
- Stage III: 60%
- Stage IV: 15%–26%

Note: More than 75% of clients are diagnosed at either stage I or II.
Data from the American Cancer Society.

Assessment Findings

Abnormal bleeding is the most common symptom. Many women incorrectly assume that abnormal bleeding in menopause is normal, which is a major contributor to late diagnosis. Other symptoms include unusual discharge, difficult or painful urination, pain during sexual intercourse, and pelvic pain. The last symptom usually develops late in the disease (NCI, 2001).

Transvaginal ultrasound is an excellent screening test for endometrial cancer. All clients at increased risk should be screened routinely; those at high risk should undergo an endometrial biopsy at menopause. Pelvic examination and Pap tests are only partially effective in diagnosing endometrial cancer (Smeltzer & Bare, 2008). Definitive diagnosis usually is made after histologic examination of endometrial tissue obtained by endometrial biopsy or during D&C.

Collaborative Management

Treatment depends on several factors, with emphasis on the stage of the disease at diagnosis (Table 4.7). Early-stage disease involves removal of the uterus, fallopian tubes, and ovaries to prevent rapid spread. When cancer is advanced or involves the lymph nodes, radiation is offered as an added therapy.

Usually, prognosis is good because this cancer often is detected early (stages I and II) (Condon, 2004; NCI, 2001). If the cancer recurs, it does so in less than 3 years and usually presents in the vagina (Condon, 2004).

Advanced metastatic endometrial cancer has a poor prognosis but usually is treated with progesterone, which has been shown to improve survival rate but not cure this disease. Additionally, surgical intervention may include not only radical hysterectomy but also removal of the cervix, part of the vagina, and lymph nodes (Smeltzer & Bare, 2008).

Nurses can provide emotional support and reassurance as well as education about this disease. They should counsel women on preventive lifestyle practices such as maintenance of a healthy body weight, increased physical activity, and medication regimens that prevent endometrial cancer. Often, oral contraceptives or progesterone is used for 10 to 14 days a month to help facilitate normal shedding of the uterine lining (Condon, 2004). Women with advanced cancer will need pain control and comfort measures initiated and also should be referred to local cancer support groups (NCI, 2001).

BENIGN OVARIAN CYSTS

Ovarian cysts are fluid-filled benign growths that can vary from small to large (Fig. 4.21). They are common and rarely cause symptoms such as pain or discomfort. Types of cysts include follicular, luteal, epithelial, and dermoid

TABLE 4.7 International Federation of Gynecology and Obstetrics (FIGO) Endometrial Cancer Staging System

STAGE	CHARACTERISTICS
Stage I	Cancer is limited to the body of the uterus. There is no spread to lymph system or distant sites.
Stage IA	Cancer is in an early form and limited to the inner lining of the uterus (endometrium).
Stage IB	Cancer has spread to less than halfway through the uterine myometrium.
Stage IC	Cancer has spread halfway through the myometrium but not beyond the body of the uterus.
Stage II	Cancer has spread from the body of the uterus to another part of the uterus next to the cervix. There is no spread to lymph system or distant sites.
Stage IIA	Cancer is in the body of the uterus and glands forming the inner lining of the cervix (endocervical glands).
Stage IIB	Cancer is in the body of the uterus and supporting connective tissue of the cervix.
Stage III	Cancer has spread beyond or outside the uterus, but remains confined to the pelvis.
Stage IIIA	Cancer has spread to layers of tissue on the outer surface of the uterus or to tissues near the sides of the uterus. Or, cancer cells are found in fluid from the pelvis or abdomen.
Stage IIIB	Cancer has spread to the vagina but not to lymph nodes or distant sites.
Stage IIIC	Cancer is of any size and has spread to the lymph system near the uterus. There is no spread to distant parts.
Stage IV	Cancer has spread to the inner surface of the urinary bladder or the lower part of the large intestine. Or, it has spread to the lymph system in the groin and to other organs such as the bones or lungs.
Stage IVA	Cancer has spread to the inner lining of the rectum or bladder. It may or may not have spread to the lymph system. There is no spread to distant sites.
Stage IVB	Cancer has spread to organs away from the uterus, such as the bone or lungs. It may be of any size and may or may not have spread to the lymph system.

Adapted from American Cancer Society. (2004). Detailed guideline: Endometrial cancer. How is endometrial cancer staged? Retrieved November 26, 2004, from www.cancer.org/docroot/CRI/content/CRI_2_4_3X_How_is_Endometrial-cancer_s.'

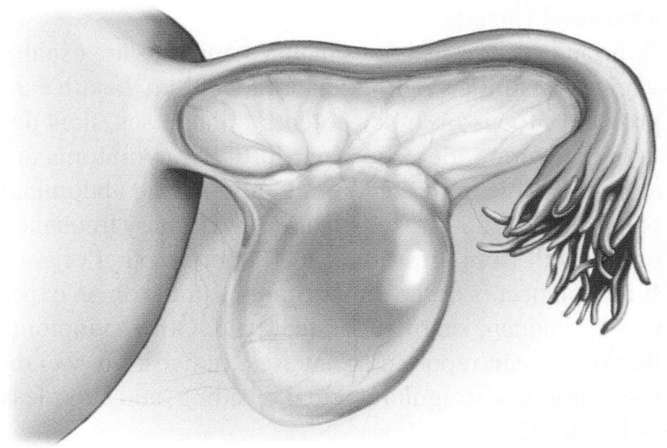

FIGURE 4.21 Ovarian cyst.

and are differentiated by their tissue makeup. *Follicular cysts,* the most common type, form when the follicle that surrounds an ovum does not rupture to release the egg during ovulation. This follicle continues to grow and eventually forms a cyst. *Luteal (hemorrhagic) cysts* form when bleeding from the ovulation site enters the ovarian capsule. *Epithelial cysts* form from the epithelium of the ovary. *Dermoid cysts* form from skin precursor cells and develop when cells of the ovary not associated with reproduction itself begin to multiply (Condon, 2004). Dermoid cysts contain fat, hair, and even teeth.

Ovarian cysts are common during the childbearing years and are generally noncancerous in this age group. Even though most cysts are benign, however, postmenopausal women with ovarian cysts are at increased risk for ovarian cancer. It is imperative for women 50 to 70 years of age to have these cysts evaluated by their health care providers. Most clinicians will recommend surgical removal of ovarian cysts for older women (NWHIC, 2001).

Assessment Findings

Many clients have ovarian cysts that cause no symptoms. When cysts become large, they can cause pelvic discomfort and pain because they tend to put pressure on nerves and other organs. Cysts pressing on the urinary tract are likely to cause problems with urinary flow. Women also may complain of pain during sexual intercourse. A rare but serious complication is that cysts can rupture, causing sudden, severe, and sharp pain. Large cysts also can become twisted and cut off the blood vessels supplying the cyst and ovary (torsion). In such cases, the client may experience nausea, fever, and severe abdominal pain. If women also have endometriosis, ovarian cysts can cause pelvic pain, painful menstruation, abnormal bleeding, and painful sexual intercourse (NWHIC, 2001).

Most ovarian cysts are discovered on routine pelvic examination when the health care provider palpates a swelling or mass. When this finding is seen, an ultrasound is done to identify the characteristics and location of the cyst.

Collaborative Management

Because most ovarian cysts shrink and resolve on their own, the first-line treatment for childbearing women is usually a "wait and see" approach with follow-up examination in 2 to 3 months. Additional treatment strategies are used when the cyst persists, has grown, or causes increasing pain. Treatment consists of additional blood testing and CA-125 assay (ovarian cancer marker). Often, surgical removal is recommended. A laparoscopy will be used to remove small cysts; a laparotomy with biopsy will be used when the cyst is large (NWHIC, 2001). Although surgery may be recommended, usually the ovary can be spared. Often, oral contraceptives are ordered for the woman to prevent the formation of additional cysts. The low-dose formulations are not appropriate because they do not contain enough hormones to affect regression of the existing cysts (Condon, 2004).

Women need education and counseling regarding this disorder as well as reassurance that most of these cysts are benign. Standard preoperative and postoperative nursing care is required for women who undergo surgical treatment.

OVARIAN CANCER

According to the ACS (2006c), more than 20,000 new cases of ovarian cancer are diagnosed in U.S. women annually; this disorder is the fifth most common cancer found in U.S. women (Fig. 4.22). Incidence of ovarian cancer has decreased since 1991, and it accounts for 4% of all cancers found in women. Nevertheless, this cancer is the fourth leading cause of death in U.S. women (ACS, 2006c).

Only 78% of women diagnosed with ovarian cancer survive 1 year after diagnosis; only 50% survive longer than 5 years (ACS, 2006c). Usually, diagnosis is late, with

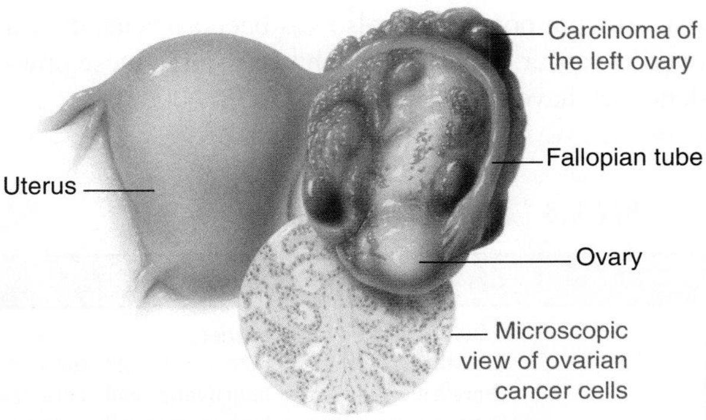

FIGURE 4.22 Ovarian cancer. (From Anatomical Chart Company. [2002]. *Atlas of pathophysiology.* Springhouse, PA: Springhouse.)

only 29% of cases found during the early stage. When ovarian cancer is found early and has not spread outside the ovary, the chances for success of treatment are optimized. Five-year survival rates when treatment begins early are 90% to 95% (ACS, 2006c).

Etiology and Pathophysiology

Women have a 1 in 58 chance of developing ovarian cancer in their lifetime and a 1 in 98 chance of dying from it (ACS, 2006c). Women of North American, North European, or Ashkenazi Jewish heritage are at higher risk for ovarian cancer than African American women. Women between 55 and 65 years of age are more likely to present with this disorder than younger women; 50% of all cases of ovarian cancer are found in those older than 63 years (ACS, 2006c). Many clients diagnosed with ovarian cancer have no risk factors.

One of the strongest risk factors for ovarian cancer is family history. Women are at increased risk if their mother, sister, or daughter has had ovarian cancer. This risk can be inherited from both the mother's and the father's side of the family. Approximately 10% of cases of ovarian cancer result from an inherited factor. Women with a family history of BRCA1 and BRCA2 gene mutation are at very high risk for this disorder but also have a better prognosis than women without this gene mutation (ACS, 2006c) (see Chap. 2).

Age is a risk factor because clients are more likely to be diagnosed with ovarian cancer after menopause. Obesity has been associated with ovarian cancer, with obese women having an increased death rate from ovarian cancer. Reproductive history also plays a part: women who started menses before 12 years, had no children, had their first child after 30 years, or experienced menopause after 50 years are at increased risk for ovarian cancer (ACS, 2006c).

Clients who take infertility drugs for long periods and do not become pregnant are also at increased risk for ovarian cancer. Hormone replacement and estrogen therapy for more than 10 years also can increase a woman's risk. Clients who have had breast cancer are at increased risk. Talcum powder use also has been associated with ovarian cancer; asbestos, which was used in these powders, may have been responsible (ACS, 2006c).

Assessment Findings

Ovarian cancer is insidious in that symptoms are usually vague and similar to other disorders. Often, health care providers focus on other potential diagnoses, thus delaying accurate identification. Initially, symptoms are abdominal swelling or bloating, fatigue, and abdominal pain (Condon, 2004). Constipation and urinary frequency often result from pressure of the tumor on other organs. If torsion occurs or the tumor ruptures, the woman experiences sudden, sharp abdominal pain. Other symptoms that have been reported are nausea, indigestion, weight loss, anorexia, irregular vaginal bleeding, and shortness of breath (Condon, 2004).

Pelvic examination can reveal ovarian cancer when the health care provider palpates an enlargement or mass in the ovarian area. Usually, ultrasound is used to identify the characteristics and location of the enlargement. MRI of the pelvis is used when a mass looks suspicious. A CA-125 may be ordered, although this blood test may not be able to reflect ovarian cancer accurately. If diagnostic evidence remains inconclusive, a laparoscopy with biopsy will be done to confirm the diagnosis (NCI, 2000).

Currently no good screening test is available to identify ovarian cancer in women; therefore, many women must undergo surgery for diagnosis. Both CA-125 and ultrasound are currently used as screening tests for high-risk women as a means of identifying ovarian cancer earlier (Condon, 2004; NCI, 2000). Because insurance plans may not pay for this screening, high-risk women often enroll in clinical studies to obtain free screening. Researchers are attempting to find out more about the etiology, diagnostic methodology, and treatments to provide women with better care and prognosis (Condon, 2004; NCI, 2000).

Collaborative Management

Treatment of ovarian cancer depends on the stage of the disease and the woman's general health (Table 4.8). Usually, a team approach involves many health care providers. In general, treatment includes surgery, chemotherapy, and radiation (ACS, 2006c). The client also may have the option of enrolling in ovarian cancer clinical trials. By doing so, she may have access to new, promising treatments. Clients may experience preopera-

TABLE 4.8 Ovarian Cancer Staging

STAGE	CHARACTERISTICS
I	Growth is limited to the ovaries.
II	Growth involves one or both ovaries with pelvic extension.
III	Growth involves one or both ovaries with metastases outside the pelvis or positive retroperitoneal or inguinal nodes.
IV	Growth involves one or both ovaries with distant metastases.

tive and postoperative side effects and complications, as well as side effects from chemotherapy and radiation (ACS, 2006c; Condon, 2004).

Women with ovarian cancer experience many of the same problems and issues faced by women with breast cancer. They have to adapt and cope with physical, emotional, and medical challenges. Nursing support and client-to-client networks (support groups) can help improve quality of life. Nursing interventions are similar to those used for women with breast cancer and focus on teaching, counseling, giving support, and meeting the woman's physical care needs.

BENIGN CERVICAL ALTERATIONS

Cervical polyps are benign growths that often develop in the mucosa of the endocervical canal. They usually are discovered during a speculum examination and may even protrude through the cervical os. Polyps are usually bright red, small (a few millimeters to several centimeters) and may be single or multiple (Fig. 4.23). They are most common in women in their 30s or 40s (Youngkin & Davis, 2004).

The cause of these growths is unknown, but they are rarely cancerous. Chronic cervical inflammation may be responsible for cervical polyps. These polyps also have been found with endometrial hyperplasia and hyperestrogen states (Youngkin & Davis, 2004).

Assessment Findings

Clients are usually asymptomatic; occasionally, they complain of spotting between periods and after sexual intercourse, profuse thick vaginal drainage (**leukorrhea**), menorrhagia, postmenopausal bleeding, and purulent or blood-tinged vaginal discharge (Condon, 2004; Youngkin & Davis, 2004). Polyps usually are found during examination of the cervix with a speculum. They are purple-red, friable (bleed easily when touched), and prone to infection.

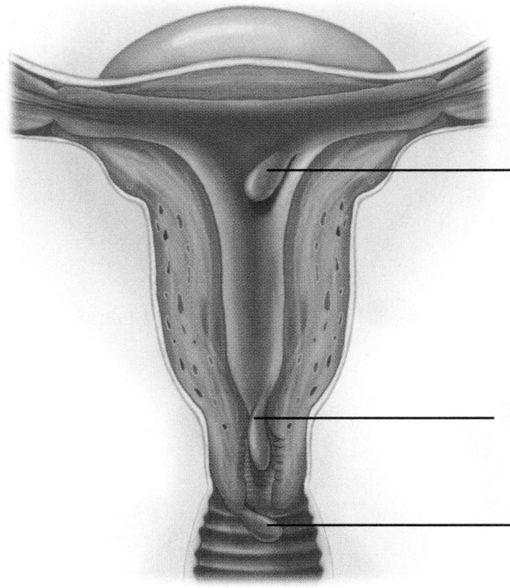

FIGURE 4.23 Endometrial, endocervical, and cervical polyps.

Collaborative Management

Surgical removal and cauterization is the usual treatment. Small polyps are excised and sent to the laboratory for tissue analysis. This is usually done as an outpatient procedure or in the office at the time of the examination and followed with cautery. Laboratory analysis is required because polyps occasionally undergo malignant changes. Clients should receive education and counseling regarding the procedure and reassurance that most polyps are benign.

Postoperative education for women must address the need to rest the pelvic area (ie, avoid sexual intercourse) for at least 24 hours to prevent irritation and bleeding. The client also will need to inform the health care provider of any excessive bleeding or vaginal discharge. Follow-up examination and evaluation are necessary to determine the need for additional endometrial sampling (Youngkin & Davis, 2004).

CERVICAL DYSPLASIA

Cervical dysplasia is a benign condition that involves abnormal changes in the cells of the cervix. Cervical tissue changes are classified as mild, moderate, or severe. Cervical dysplasia usually is asymptomatic and does not present an immediate health risk; however, it is considered a precancerous condition. Untreated cervical dysplasia can progress to cervical carcinoma in situ or invasive cervical cancer. This abnormal progression to cancer is slow and can take 10 years or longer. Early detection and monitoring can prevent this condition from becoming cancerous.

Assessment Findings

Routine gynecologic examinations that include Pap testing can detect dysplasia. Pap testing is the most important method of diagnosing this disorder and preventing cancer. Abnormal cervical cells are classified as squamous intraepithelial lesions (SILs). *Lesion* means an area of abnormal cells and *intraepithelial* means that the abnormal cells are found only in the surface layer of cells (NCI, 1994).

Collaborative Management

Low-grade or mild dysplasia, usually seen in women 25 to 35 years, is the most common type and detected during Pap testing. Approximately 70% of affected women will have their cervical tissue return to normal without treatment (Smeltzer & Bare, 2008). High-grade moderate or severe dysplasias usually require treatment because they are more likely to develop into cancer. Severe dysplasia is also referred to as **carcinoma in situ** because it is likely to become cancerous but can be cured if treated promptly.

Treatment varies with severity and may include conization, cautery, cryosurgery, or laser treatment to remove and destroy the abnormal cells. Health care providers will require women who present with this disorder to have frequent Pap smears and gynecologic examinations to monitor for recurrences (Smeltzer & Bare, 2008).

CERVICAL CANCER

Before cancer appears in the cervix, the cells of the cervix go through changes known as *dysplasia,* in which abnormal cells begin to appear in the cervical tissue. If cervical dysplasia is not treated, the woman will develop cervical cancer. This cancer affects the lower portion of the uterus, commonly referred to as the cervical canal. Even though Pap testing has helped to reduce U.S. mortality rates from cervical cancer (see Chap. 2), the number of cases of cervical cancer has remained constant (Andersen & Runowicz, 2002). Paley (2001) reported that 50% of diagnoses of cervical cancer were found in women who had never had a Pap test. Incidence in women 50 years or younger may be on the rise. A primary reason may be that a growing number of U.S. women have never had a Pap smear, especially Latina immigrants (Gerbera & Chiasson, 2004).

Cervical cancer is the third most common cancer in U.S. women (Fig. 4.24). Incidence is increased in Hispanics, Native Americans, African Americans, and Filipinas. African American women are twice as likely to be affected as white women (ACS, 2006d). Most cases begin in the cells lining the cervix. When abnormal cells spread deeper into the cervix or into other tissue, it is called invasive cervical cancer. Each year, more than 4000 women die from invasive cervical cancer (Youngkin & Davis, 2004). Invasive cervical cancer occurs most often in women older than 40 years.

Cervical cancer is classified using a staging system that ranges from stage 0 (carcinoma in situ) to stage IV (invasive cervical cancer) (Table 4.9). Cervical cancer generally develops slowly over time.

Etiology and Pathophysiology

Human papillomavirus (HPV; especially types 16 and 18) has been associated with cervical cancer and is considered one of the major risk factors for its development. Clients who forego regular Pap testing to detect HPV or other cell abnormalities are at increased risk for cervical cancer. Other risk factors are as follows:

- Long-term persistent HPV infection and history of other STIs
- Smoking
- Weakened immune system and immunocompromised state
- Being a daughter of a woman who took DES
- Multiple sex partners
- First intercourse at an early age

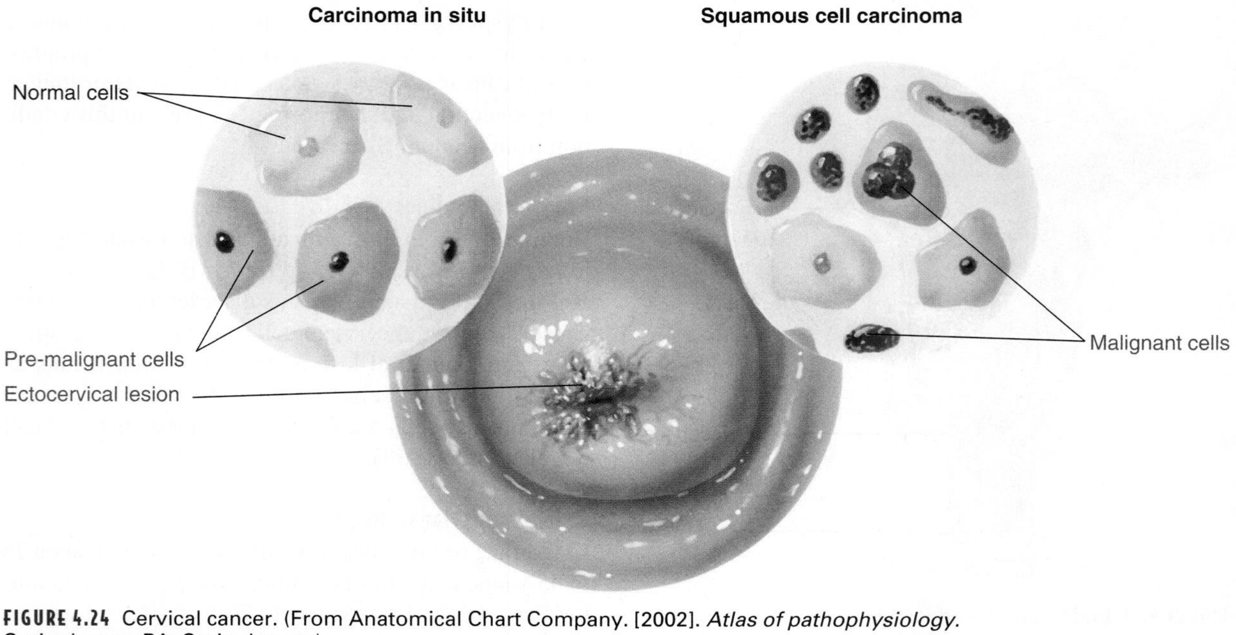

FIGURE 4.24 Cervical cancer. (From Anatomical Chart Company. [2002]. *Atlas of pathophysiology.* Springhouse, PA: Springhouse.)

TABLE 4.9 Cervical Cancer Staging

STAGES	CHARACTERISTICS
Stage 0 carcinoma in situ	Cancer is found in the first layer of cells lining the cervix only.
Stage I	Cancer is found in the cervix only.
Stage IA	A very small amount of cancer in cervical tissue is found only with a microscope and is not deeper than 5 mm and not wider than 7 mm.
Stage IB	Cancer is seen only with a microscope but is more than 5 mm deep and 7 mm wide. *Or* Cancer can be seen without a microscope and is larger than 4 cm.
Stage II	Cancer has spread beyond the cervix but not into the pelvic wall.
Stage IIA	Cancer has spread beyond the cervix to the upper two thirds of the vagina but not to the tissue around the uterus.
Stage IIB	Cancer has spread beyond the cervix to the upper two thirds of the vagina and to the tissue around the uterus.
Stage III	Cancer has spread to the lower third of the vagina and may have spread to the pelvic wall and lymph nodes.
Stage IIIA	Cancer has spread to the lower part of vagina but not the pelvic wall.
Stage IIIB	Cancer has spread to the pelvic wall, and the tumor has become large enough to block the ureters; cells may have spread to the pelvic lymph nodes.
Stage IV	Cancer has spread to the bladder, rectum, or other parts of the body.
Stage IVA	Cancer has spread to the bladder or rectal wall; it may have spread to the pelvic lymph nodes.
Stage IVB	Cancer has spread beyond the pelvis and pelvic lymph nodes to other parts of the body.

Adapted from National Cancer Institute. (2004). *Stages of cervical cancer.* Retrieved November 28, 2004, from http://www.cancer.gov/cancertopics/pdq/treatment/cervical/patient/allpages.

- First childbirth before 20 years
- Low socioeconomic status
- Diet lacking in vitamin A and C
- Oral contraceptive use (NCI, 2004; Youngkin & Davis, 2004).

Assessment Findings

Many women are asymptomatic in the early stages. Symptomatic women may notice and present with vague problems often associated with other conditions, such as vaginal bleeding, unusual vaginal discharge, pelvic pain, and pain during intercourse (NCI, 2004). Clients should be advised to consult their health care provider when they have such symptoms.

Routine regular Pap screening has proved reliable in identifying women with cervical dysplasia (see Chap. 2). Cells are analyzed using the 2001 Bethesda system, which has proved useful in classifying dysplasia. The ACS recommends that all women who are sexually active or have reached 21 years should have a conventional Pap test every year, or a liquid Pap test every 2 years along with a pelvic examination (Saslow et al., 2002). For women older than 30 years, usual screening is a Pap test and HPV test; if both results are normal, follow-up screenings every 3 years is appropriate (Saslow et al., 2002; Wright et al., 2002).

The Pap test is inexpensive and has helped decrease the incidence of cervical cancer. Many new technologies also are being used clinically to diagnosis cervical cancer. Examples include the automated slide thin-layer preparation (thin Prep), computer-assisted automated Pap test prescreening, and HPV-DNA typing (Youngkin & Davis, 2004).

Collaborative Management

When an abnormal Pap result is obtained, a colposcopy, biopsy, or endocervical curettage is used to further analyze the abnormal cells. Treatment varies and depends on the findings and the cervical cancer stage. The most common treatments used are cryosurgery, loop electrosurgical excision procedure (LEEP), cone biopsy, and laser cone biopsy (Youngkin & Davis, 2004). When the woman has invasive cervical cancer, treatment consists of radical hysterectomy (removal of all organs and affected lymph nodes) and possible chemotherapy and radiation, which depends on the degree and amount of invasion (Condon, 2004).

VULVAR CANCER

Cancer of the vulva is rare. It can develop at any age, but the most invasive form affects older women (Smeltzer & Bare, 2008). Associated risk factors include chronic vulvitis, vulvar dermatosis, STIs, cervical cancer, immunosuppression, hypertension, diabetes mellitus, and a few subtypes of HPV.

Clients usually present with symptoms of vulvar itching, burning, and pain. Clinical examination may identify scaly lesions that present as red or white with irregular pigmentation. Lesions can vary in size and shape and can be raised or flat, small or large. A diagnosis of vulvar cancer is based on biopsy and pathologic analysis of the tissue.

Treatment usually involves surgery to remove the tissue or tumor. Surgery type depends on the extent of the cancer. More extensive surgery with skin grafting is required for large tumors. Complications from radical vulvectomy can include scarring and wound breakdown. More conservative surgical techniques, such as radical hemivulvectomy, are being used to prevent complications and loss of function.

PELVIC RELAXATION ALTERATIONS

Muscles of the pelvic floor support the abdominal and pelvic organs, and the ligaments, muscles, and connective tissues support the pelvis itself. Sometimes, these structures become stretched or damaged. Pregnancy, damage from childbirth, chronic coughing or straining, surgery, and aging usually cause pelvic support problems (ACOG, 2004; Youngkin & Davis, 2004). Associated risk factors are obesity, Caucasian race, multiparity, and menopause (with its associated loss of estrogen) (Youngkin & Davis, 2004). These disorders are expected to be more frequent because of the increasing aging population of women. The median age for women seeking care for these disorders is 61 years; more than 50% of women seeking care for pelvic relaxation alterations are between 30 and 60 years (Youngkin & Davis, 2004).

Organs affected include the urethra, bladder, small intestine, rectum, uterus, and vagina (ACOG, 2004). The vaginal wall weakens and descends, and the pelvic organs begin to protrude into the vaginal canal. The most common disorders associated with these changes are cystocele, rectocele, and uterine prolapse (Youngkin & Davis, 2004) (Fig. 4.25). All these disorders are discussed in detail in Chapter 19.

URINARY TRACT DISORDERS

Bacteria in the urinary tract can result in urinary infections. Usually, the body removes these bacteria without symptoms; when the body cannot protect itself, a urinary infection ensues. *Escherichia coli* is a common causative organism in healthy women. Women are more likely to get UTIs than are men. UTIs are especially dangerous for older people and pregnant women. Sexual activity also places women at risk (National Kidney and Urologic Diseases Information Clearinghouse, 2004).

CYSTITIS

Cystitis is an infection of the bladder. Bacterial growth in a woman's urinary tract is related primarily to sexual intercourse and urethral manipulation during oral sex or masturbation (Youngkin & Davis, 2004). The relationship between vaginal intercourse and cystitis has led to the colloquial terminology of "honeymoon cystitis." Women should be advised that voiding after intercourse helps decrease rates of infection. Use of diaphragms and spermicide increases the risk for cystitis (see Chap. 8) (Youngkin & Davis, 2004).

Approximately 20% of women experience lower UTIs; among these women, 25% usually have a recurrence (National Kidney and Urologic Diseases Information Clearinghouse, 2004; Youngkin & Davis, 2004). UTIs can occur throughout the woman's lifetime, but aging is associated with increased prevalence. Factors contributing to higher rates in older women may include

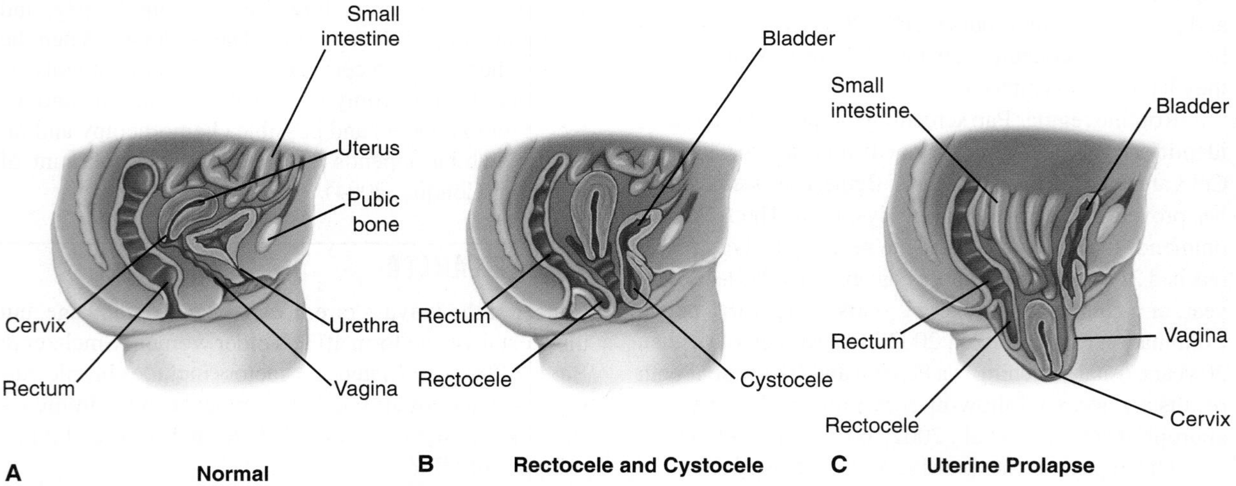

FIGURE 4.25 (**A**) Normal appearance and positioning of the uterus. (**B**) Rectocele and cystocele. (**C**) Uterine prolapse.

decreased estrogen levels, bladder emptying problems, concurrent diseases, bowel incontinence, and poor nutrition (Youngkin & Davis, 2004).

Assessment Findings

Health care providers must decide whether a woman's presenting symptoms are vaginal or urinary. When a UTI is suspected, the health care provider must determine whether it is a lower or upper UTI (National Kidney and Urologic Diseases Information Clearinghouse, 2004). Common presenting symptoms include burning on urination; a frequent and intense urge to urinate, often with little urine to pass; pain in the back or lower abdomen; cloudy, dark, or bloody urine with an unusual smell; fever; and chills (Youngkin & Davis, 2004).

Diagnostic testing includes a complete health history and physical examination, as well as a urine dipstick test, urinalysis, urine culture and sensitivity, vaginal wet smears, and various cultures (Youngkin & Davis, 2004).

Collaborative Management

Treatment goals are to eradicate the invading bacteria; thus, antibiotics are prescribed. Two of the most common types used are cephalosporins and sulfa drugs. They are prescribed for 7 to 10 days; women should be counseled to complete the entire prescription (Condon, 2004; National Kidney and Urologic Diseases Information Clearinghouse, 2004).

Increasing fluid intake is controversial and should be discussed with the health care provider. Drinking cranberry juice has been found to decrease recurrent UTIs, especially in older women; some health care providers also suggest applying estrogen topical cream to the urinary tissue (Condon, 2004). Recurrences must be treated promptly and thoroughly to prevent development of an upper UTI (kidney infection) (Condon, 2004; National Kidney and Urologic Diseases Information Clearinghouse, 2004).

INTERSTITIAL CYSTITIS

Interstitial cystitis (IC) is a chronic and painful inflammatory bladder disorder that primarily affects women 40 to 60 years old. Ninety percent of the 700,000 U.S. cases each year affect women; this disorder is three times more common in the United States than in Europe (Condon, 2004). Often, IC is misdiagnosed as a psychiatric disorder. The condition seriously affects quality of life by interfering with the ability to work, maintain a home, attend to family responsibilities, and engage in sexual relations (Youngkin & Davis, 2004).

The etiology of IC is unknown. Various theories and factors have been suggested, such as a neurogenic inflammatory response, allergies, autoimmune disease, defects in or damage to the urinary bladder, obstruction of the blood vessels and lymph system of the bladder, and most recently, hereditary organic factors (Condon, 2004; National Kidney and Urologic Diseases Information Clearinghouse, 2003; Youngkin & Davis, 2004).

Assessment Findings

Women with IC complain of urinary frequency and urgency, nocturia, and pain. Other reported symptoms are severe pain with intercourse, lower back and thigh pain, sleep deprivation, and depression (Condon, 2004; Youngkin & Davis, 2004).

On physical examination, the health provider may note lower abdominal tenderness. Laboratory testing of the urine reveals no infection; microscopic examination of the urine may show RBCs when the bladder is overdistended. Hemorrhages (Hunner's ulcers) noted during cystoscopy confirm a diagnosis of IC (National Kidney and Urologic Diseases Information Clearinghouse, 2003).

Collaborative Management

The goal of treatment is to alleviate and relieve symptoms. Women must take an active role in the management of the problem and understand that healing may take a long time. Pharmacologic agents are used to treat most symptoms. Inflammation and pain are relieved with NSAIDs. Anticholinergic drugs can relieve bladder spasms. Pentosan polysulfate sodium, which has demonstrated effectiveness in restoring the bladder lining, also is used to treat IC.

Another treatment option is regular weekly drug instillations into the bladder using dimethyl sulfoxide (DMSO). Transcutaneous electrical nerve stimulation (TENS) may be used to relieve pain. Laser therapy has been used to treat Hunner's ulcers.

Nursing interventions include education, counseling, and support. Clients need to undergo lifestyle changes, follow bladder-training programs, use stress reduction strategies, and increase physical activity to manage symptoms. Avoidance of caffeine and artificial sweeteners, alcohol, and tobacco can also help. Dietary changes that have proved helpful in alleviating symptoms include restriction of salt, sugar, yeast, acidic foods, and the amino acids tyrosine and tryptophan (Condon, 2004).

URINARY INCONTINENCE

Urinary incontinence means the inability to control urination (involuntarily loss of urine). More than 13 million people in the United States have this problem, which is twice as common in women as in men (Condon, 2004; National Kidney and Urologic Disease Information Clearinghouse, 2004). This gender-associated difference may be attributable to pregnancy, childbirth, menopause, and the structures of the female urinary tract. Older women are more likely than younger women to be affected with urinary incontinence; estimates are that approximately 45% of women older than 65 years experience this problem (Condon, 2004; National Kidney and Urologic Disease Information Clearinghouse, 2004). For detailed discussion of this problem and its treatment, see Chapter 24.

SUMMARY

- Women's health care is moving from focusing only on those conditions that affect the breasts and reproductive organs to also emphasizing those conditions with greater prevalence in women, different courses and manifestations in women, or both.
- Sickle cell disease, thalassemia, cystic fibrosis, and Tay-Sachs disease are genetic disorders in women that can have difficult outcomes in pregnancy.
- In autoimmune disorders, the body attacks its own tissues. Examples of such conditions with high prevalence in women include rheumatoid arthritis, myasthenia gravis, and systemic lupus erythematosus.
- Incidence of diabetes mellitus is growing at alarming rates.
- Cardiovascular disease is the leading killer of U.S. women. Preventive measures can do much to avert this problem.
- Common STIs include chlamydia, gonorrhea, syphilis, genital herpes, and genital warts. Bacterial vaginosis, trichomoniasis, and yeast infections may be transmitted sexually. Preventive measures can be taken to avoid all these problems; once they occur, rapid screening and management are necessary to preserve fertility and control transfer of the problem to others.
- HIV and hepatitis are viral illnesses often transmitted sexually. Management approaches for both are aggressive. These diseases pose chronic difficulties for affected clients.
- Common benign breast disorders include mastalgia, infections, fibrocystic changes, and fibroadenomas.
- A diagnosis of breast malignancy can be threatening to a client's sense of womanhood and emotionally devastating. Nevertheless, breast cancer is one of the most treatable forms of cancer, and new management modalities are being created every day.
- Diagnostic testing for breast cancer can include mammography, fine-needle aspiration, sterotactic core biopsy, needle biopsy, excisional biopsy, incisional biopsy, and hormone receptor assay.
- Treatment of breast cancer may involve surgery, radiation therapy, chemotherapy, hormonal therapy, biologic therapy, or a combination of these approaches. Nursing measures focus on cancer prevention, assisting with any treatments and their side effects, and providing client teaching about expected side effects and their management, resources for assistance, and long-term outcomes.
- Menstrual problems are common complaints for women and may develop chronically or episodically throughout a woman's childbearing years. Examples include amenorrhea, dysmenorrheal, dysfunctional uterine bleeding, and premenstrual syndrome.
- Pelvic inflammatory disease and endometriosis are two reproductive tract problems that often require aggressive management because they have long-term consequences on a woman's fertility.
- Problems of the female reproductive tract can be benign or malignant disorders. Examples of benign conditions include leiomyomas, endometrial hyperplasia, ovarian cysts, cervical polyps, and cervical dysplasia. Malignancies include cancers of the uterus, ovaries, cervix, and vulva.

REVIEW QUESTIONS

1. A 30-year-old client is suspected of having systemic lupus erythematosus (SLE). Which of the following assessment findings would the nurse be least likely to expect to see for this client?
   A. Butterfly-shaped facial rash
   B. Elevated erythrocyte sedimentation rate
   C. Positive antinuclear antibody titer
   D. Multiple-joint inflammation and swelling
2. After teaching a group of young women about chlamydia, which statement by the group indicates that the nurse's teaching was successful?
   A. "Chlamydia can be detected early on because of a characteristic vaginal discharge."
   B. "A painless ulcer forms on the area of the body that was exposed to the organism."
   C. "Infertility can occur if the infection damages the fallopian tubes."
   D. "An injection of penicillin commonly is used to treat the infection."
3. When assessing a woman with HIV, the nurse should suspect AIDS if the client's T4-cell count is
   A. $725/mm^3$.
   B. $550/mm^3$.
   C. $375/mm^3$.
   D. $195/mm^3$.
4. The pharmacologic agent that the nurse should expect the health care provider to prescribe for a woman diagnosed with genital herpes is
   A. azithromycin.
   B. ofloxacin.
   C. metronidazole.
   D. acyclovir.
5. Which of these topics should the nurse include in preparing a presentation about breast cancer for a local woman's group?

A. Breast cancer is the most lethal type of cancer for women.
B. Most breast cancers begin in the upper quadrant of the breast.
C. Most women who get breast cancer have a family history of it.
D. Women younger than 40 years are at highest risk for breast cancer.

6. The nurse is preparing a client who has undergone a mastectomy of her right breast for discharge from the hospital. Which statement, if made by the client indicates the need for additional teaching?
A. "I'll immediately report any tingling on the inner side of my right arm."
B. "I'll ask my husband for help if a package feels heavy."
C. "I won't allow any blood pressures to be taken in my right arm."
D. "I should avoid sleeping on my right side."

7. A young client comes to the health clinic for an evaluation. During the visit, she asks, "When I get my period, sometimes I get cramps that can really hurt. What causes this?" Which of the following responses, if made by the nurse, would be most appropriate?
A. "You probably have an underlying infection that is causing the pain."
B. "An increase in a hormone makes the uterus contract more, causing pain."
C. "It's absolutely normal to have cramps with your period."
D. "I will get you a prescription to help with the pain."

8. When caring for a A 45-year-old woman diagnosed with uterine leiomyoma, the nurse should expect the client to manifest
A. high fever with complaints of pain on cervical movement
B. dysmenorrhea and irregular vaginal bleeding
C. abnormal bleeding in menopause with pelvic pain
D. menorrhagia and reports of pelvic pressure

9. When teaching a client with cervical dysplasia about this disorder, the nurse would emphasize the importance of which of the following?
A. Regular Pap smears
B. Yearly CA-125 testing
C. Strict condom use
D. Frequent perineal hygiene

10. Which of the following instructions should the nurse not include in a teaching plan for an older woman diagnosed with cystitis?
A. "Be sure to urinate after you engage in sexual intercourse."
B. "If your symptoms reappear, call the office as soon as possible."
C. "You will take medication for 5 days and then stop."
D. "Try drinking cranberry juice during the day."

Resources

American Academy of Family Physicians
913-906-6000
http://familydoctor.org

American Cancer Society
1599 Clifton Road, NE
Atlanta, GA 30329
202-4-CANCER
http://www.cancer.org

American College of Nurse Midwives
818 Connecticut Avenue, NW
Suite 900
Washington, DC 20006
202-728-9860
http://www.midwife.org

American College of Obstetricians and Gynecologists (ACOG)
409 12th Street, SW
Washington, DC 20024
800-762-2264
http://www.acog.org

American Diabetes Association
Diabetes Information Service Center
1660 Duke Street
Alexandria, VA 22314
800-342-2383
http://www.diabetes.org

American Heart Association
Women's Heart Information
888-694-3278
800-242-8721
http://www.americanheart.org

American Nurses Association
600 Maryland Avenue, SW
Suite 100W
Washington, DC 20024
800-274-4262
http://www.ana.org

American Social Health Association
P.O. Box 13827
Research Triangle Park, NC 27709-9940
919-361-8400
http://www.ashastd.org

American Society of Colon and Rectal Surgeons (ASCRS)
85 West Algonquin Road
Suite 550
Arlington Heights, IL 60005
800-791-0001
http://www.ascrs.org

Association of Women's Health, Obstetric and Neonatal Nurses (AWHONN)
2000 L Street, NW
Suite 740
Washington, DC 20036
800-673-8499 (U.S.)
800-245-0231 (Canada)
http://www.awhonn.org

Centers for Disease Control and Prevention (CDC)
1600 Clifton Road
Atlanta, GA 30333
888-232-3228
http://www.cdc.gov

CDC National Prevention Information Network
P.O. Box 6003
Rockville, MD 20849-6003
800-458-5231
301-562-1098 (international)
http://www.cdcnpin.org

CDC National STD and AIDS Hotline
800-227-8922
http://www.ashastd.org/NSTD/index.html

National Breast and Cervical Cancer Early Detection Program
888-842-6355 (option7)
http://www.cdc.gov/cancer/nbccedp/index.htm

National Cancer Institute (NCI)
800-4-CANCER (800-422-6257)
http://www.nci.nih.gov
http://breasthealth.cancer.gov

National Institute of Allergy and Infectious Diseases
National Institutes of Health
31 Center Drive, MSC 2520
Bethesda, MD 20892-2530
301-496-5717
http://www.niaid.nih.gov

National Women's Health Information Center
800-994-9662
http://www.4women.gov

National Women's Health Resource Center (NWHRC)
157 Broad Street
Suite 315
Red Bank, NJ 07701
http://www.healthywomen.org

Planned Parenthood Federation of America
810 Seventh Street
New York, NY 10019
800-230-7526
http://plannedparenthood.org

REFERENCES

Adler, M., Cowan, F., French, P., Mitchell, H., & Richens, J. (2005). *ABC of sexually transmitted infections* (5th ed.). London: BMJ Publishing.

Alzubialdi, N., & Calis, K. A. (2004). Dysmenorrhea. *Emedicine.* [Online]. Retrieved April 1, 2006, from http://www.emedicine.com/med/topic606.htm.

American Cancer Society. (2006a). *Estimated new cancer cases and deaths by sex for all sites, US, 2006.* Retrieved April 1, 2006, from http://www.cancer.org/downloads/stt/CAFF06EsCsMc.pdf.

American Cancer Society. (2006b). *Detailed guide: Uterine sarcoma.* Retrieved April 1, 2006, from http://www.cancer.org/docroot/CRI/CRI_2_3x.asp?dt=63.

American Cancer Society. (2006c). *Detailed guide: Ovarian cancer.* Retrieved April 1, 2006, from http://www.cancer.org/docroot/CRI/CRI_2_3x.asp?rnav=cridg&dt=33.

American Cancer Society. (2006d). *Detailed guide: Cervical cancer.* What are the key statistics about cervical cancer? Retrieved January 13, 2006, from http://www.cancer.org/docroot/CRI/content/CRI_2_4_1X_What_are_the_key_statistics_for_cervical_cancer_8.asp?sitearea.

American Cancer Society & National Comprehensive Cancer Network (NCCN). (2004). *Breast cancer treatment guidelines for patients* (vers. VI). Atlanta, GA: Author.

American College of Obstetricians and Gynecologists. (2001). *Medical library endometrial hyperplasia.* Retrieved November 26, 2004, from http://medem.com/MedLB/article_detaillb_for printer.cfm?article_ID=ZZZ7Z2G.

American College of Obstetricians and Gynecologists. (2004). *Pelvic support problems.* Retrieved November 29, 2004, from http://www.medem.com/MedLB/article_detaillb.cfm?article_ID=ZZZ68BWD27C&sub_.

American Diabetes Association. (2005). *National diabetes fact sheet.* Retrieved July 20, 2006, from www.diabetes.org/uedocuments/NationalDiabetesfactsheetRev.pdf

American Heart Association. (2000). *Heart and stroke: Statistical update.* Dallas, TX: Author.

American Heart Association. (2005). *Heart attack, stroke, and cardiac arrest warning signs.* Retrieved March 21, 2006, from http://www.americanheart.org/presenter.jhtml?identifier=3053.

American Heart Association. (2006). *Women and coronary heart disease.* Retrieved April 1, 2006, from http://americanheart.org/presenter.jhtml?identifier=2859.

Andersen, P. S., & Runowicz, C. D. (2002). Beyond the Pap test: New techniques for cervical cancer screening. *Women's Health, 2,* 37–43.

Arnold, G. C., & Neiheisel, M. B. (1997). A comprehensive approach to evaluating nipple discharge. *Nurse Practitioner, 22*(7), 96, 98–102, 105–111.

Arthritis Foundation. (2006). Rheumatoid arthritis. Retrieved March 21, 2006, from http://www.arthritis.org/conditions/DiseaseCenter/RA/ra_who.asp.

Austin, H. A., & Balow, J. E. (1999). Natural history and treatment of lupus nephritis. *Seminars in Nephrology, 19*(1), 2–11.

Bernstein, L., Henderson, B. E., & Hanish, R., et al. (1994). Physical exercise and reduced risk of breast cancer in young women. *Journal of National Cancer Institute, 1994*(18), 1403–1408.

Bradley, L. D. (2005). Abnormal uterine bleeding. *Nurse Practitioner, 30*(10), 38–51.

Breslin, E. T., & Lucas, V. A. (2004). *Women's health nursing: Toward evidence-based practice.* St. Louis: W. B. Saunders.

Briese, V. (2000). Prevention of breast cancer and menopausal symptoms by phyto-oestrogen. *Der Gynakologe, 33*(1), 28–35.

Cady, B., Steele, G. D., Morrow, M., Gardner, B., Smith, B. L., Lee, N. C., et al. (1998). Evaluation of common breast problems: Guidance for primary care providers. *CA—Cancer Journal for Clinicians, 48*(1), 49–63.

Centers for Disease Control and Prevention. (2002). Trends in death from systemic lupus erythematosus—United States, 1979–1998. *Morbidity and Mortality Weekly Report, 51*(17), 371–374.

Centers for Disease Control and Prevention. (2003a). *Trends in reportable sexually transmitted diseases in the United States, 2003.* Atlanta, GA: U.S. Department of Health and Human Services.

Centers for Disease Control and Prevention. (2003b). *Fact sheet—HIV and AIDS.* Retrieved April 1, 2006, from http://www.cdc.gov/hiv/pubs/facts/transmission.htm.

Centers for Disease Control and Prevention. (2004a). *STD facts—genital herpes.* Retrieved April 1, 2006, from http://www.cdc.gov/std/Herpes/STDFact-Herpes.htm.

Centers for Disease Control and Prevention. (2004b). *STD facts—bacterial vaginosis.* Retrieved April 1, 2006, from http://www.cdc.gov/std/bv/STDFact-Bacterial-Vaginosis.htm.

Centers for Disease Control and Prevention. (2004c). *STD facts—trichomoniasis.* Retrieved April 1, 2006, from http://www.cdc.gov/std/trichomonas/STDFact-Trichomoniasis.htm.

Centers for Disease Control and Prevention, Division of STD Prevention (DSTRP). (2004d). *CDC pelvic inflammatory disease.* Retrieved November 23, 2004, from DSTRP Web site: http://www.cdc.gov/std.

Centers for Disease Control and Prevention. (2005a). *National diabetes fact sheet: General information and national estimates on diabetes in the United States, 2005.* Atlanta, GA: U.S. Department of Human Health and Services.

Centers for Disease Control and Prevention. (2005b). *Sexually transmitted disease surveillance, 2004.* Atlanta, GA: U.S. Department of Health and Human Services.

Centers for Disease Control and Prevention. (2005c). *Genital candidiasis. Frequently asked questions.* Retrieved April 1, 2006, from http://www.cdc.gov/ncidod/dbmd/diseaseinfo/candidiasis_gen_g.htm.

Centers for Disease Control and Prevention, National Center for HIV, STD, and TB Prevention. (2006a). *Viral hepatitis A fact sheet.* Retrieved April 1, 2006, from http://www.cdc.gov/ncidod/diseases/hepatitis/a/fact.htm.

Centers for Disease Control and Prevention, National Center for HIV, STD, and TB Prevention. (2006b). *Hepatitis B: Frequently asked questions.* Retrieved April 1, 2006, from http://www.cdc.gov/ncidod/diseases/hepatitis/b/faqb.htm.

Centers for Disease Control and Prevention, National Center for HIV, STD, and TB Prevention. (2006c). *Hepatitis C: Frequently asked questions.* Retrieved April 1, 2006, from http://www.cdc.gov/ncidod/diseases/hepatitis/c/faq.htm#1a.

Clark, A. D., & Steele, T. (2005). Dysmenorrhea. *EMedicine.* [Online]. Retrieved April 1, 2006, from http://www.emedicine.com/emerg/topic156.htm.

Condon, M. C. (2004). *Women's health: An integrated approach to wellness and illness.* Upper Saddle River, NJ: Prentice Hall.

Cooley's Anemia Foundation, Inc. (2001). *About thalassemia.* Retrieved April 1, 2006, from: http://www.thalassemia.org.

Corwin, E. J. (1997). Endometriosis: Pathophysiology, diagnosis and treatment. *Nurse Practitioner, 22*(10), 35–51, 55.

Cyrus-David, M. S., & Strom, S. S. (2001). Chemoprevention of breast cancer with selective estrogen receptor modulators: Views from broadly diverse focus groups of women with elevated risk for breast cancer. *Psycho-Oncology, 10,* 521–533.

Cystic Fibrosis Foundation. (2005). What is CF? Retrieved March 21, 2006, from http://www.cff.org/about_cf/what_is_cf/.

Daar, E. S. (2002). Treatment of primary HIV infection. *Medscape General Medicine, 4*(4), 15.

Dienger, M. J. (1998). Anxiety and performance of breast self-examination (Doctoral dissertation, Rush University, Department of Nursing, 1998). *Dissertation Abstracts International, #AA19910815,* 92. Abstract retrieved November 17, 2004, from http://olc3.ohiolink.edu:20080/bin/gate.exe?f=doc&state=feo89u.8.6.

DiSaia, P. J., & Creasman, W. T. (2002). *Clinical gynecologic oncology* (6th ed.). St. Louis: Mosby.

DuVal, S. (2004). Inflammatory breast cancer. *RN, 67*(2), 43–44.

Endometriosis Association. (2002). *What causes endometriosis.* Retrieved April 1, 2006, from http://endometrosisassn.org/endo.html.

Facione, N. C., Miaskowski, C., Dodd, M. I., & Paul, S. M. (2002). The self-report likelihood of patient delay in breast cancer: New thoughts for early detection. *Preventive Medicine, 34,* 397–407.

Fitzgibbon, M. L., Stolley, M. R., Schiffer, L., Sanchez-Johnson, L. A., Wells, A. M., & Dyer, A. (2005). A combined breast health/weight loss intervention for black women. *Preventive Medicine, 40*(4), 373–383.

Forshee, R. A., Storey, M. L., & Ritenbaugh, C. (2003). Breast cancer risk and lifestyle differences among perimenopausal and postmenopausal African-American women. *Cancer, 97*(S1), 280–288.

Gerbera, S., & Chiasson, M. A. (2004). *Inadequate functional health literacy in Spanish as a barrier to cervical cancer screening among immigrant Latinas in New York City.* Retrieved April 1, 2006, from http://www.cdc.gov/pcd/issues/2004/oct/03 0038.htm.

Gill, J. M., Quisel, A. M., Rocca, P. V., & Walters, S. R. (2003). Diagnosis of systemic lupus erythematosus. *American Family Physician, 68*(11), 2179–2189.

Goldstein, S. R. (2000). Update on Raloxifene to prevent endometrial-breast cancer. *European Journal of Cancer, 36*(4), 54–56.

Hart, J. A. (2005). Painful menstrual periods. *Medline Plus.* [Online]. Retrieved April 1, 2006, from http://www.nlm.nih/gov/medlineplus/ency/article/003150.htm.

Harvard Medical School. (2003). *Type I diabetes mellitus.* Retrieved April 1, 2006, from http://www.intelihealth.com/IH/ihtIH/EMIHC256/9888/9820.html.

Hayes, D. E. (2000). *Atlas of breast cancer* (2nd ed.). New York: Mosby.

Hindle, W. H., & Gonzales, S. (2001). Breast disease: What to do when it's not cancer. *Women's Health in Primary Care, 4*(1), 21–34.

Hu, F. B., Li, T. Y., Colditz, G. A, Willett, W. C., & Manson, J. E. (2003). Television watching and other sedentary behaviors in relation to risk of obesity and type 2 diabetes mellitus in women. *Journal of American Medical Association, 289*(14), 1785–1791.

Hughes, L. E., Mansel, R. E., & Webster, D. J. T. (2000). *Benign disorders and diseases of the breast* (2nd ed.). London: Balliere Tindall.

Hussain, A. N., Policarpio, C., & Vincent, M. T. (2006). Evaluating nipple discharge. *Obstetric and Gynecologic Survey, 61*(4), 278–2783.

Jacob, E., & American Pain Society. (2001). Pain management in sickle cell disease. *Pain Management in Nursing, 2*(4), 121–131.

James, D., Steer, P., Weiner, C., & Gonik, B. (Eds.) (2006). *High-risk pregnancy* (3rd ed.). Philadelphia: W. B. Saunders.

Jordon, V. C. (2000a). Antiestrogens: Clinical application of pharmacology. *Journal of the Society for Gynecologic Investigation, 7*(1S), s47–s48.

Jordon, V. C. (2000b). Tamoxifen personal retrospective. *Lancet Oncology, 1,* 43–49.

Jordon, V. C. (2000c). Progress in the prevention of breast cancer: Concept to reality. *Journal of Biochemistry & Molecular Biology, 74,* 269–277.

Labbe, E., Herbert, D., & Haynes, J. (2005). Physicians' attitude and practices in sickle cell disease pain management. *Journal of Palliative Care, 21*(4), 246–251.

Lupus Foundation of America. (2006). *Lupus fact sheet.* Retrieved April 1, 2006, from http://www.lupus.org/education/factsheet.html.

Marrow, M. (2000, April 15). Retrieved July 5, 2004, from American Academy Family Physicians Web Site: http://www.aafp.org/afp/20000415/2371.html.

Martin, A. M., & Weber, B. L. (2000). Genetic and hormonal risk factors in breast cancer. *Journal of the National Cancer Institute, 92*(14), 1126–1135.

Martin, L. (2004). Rheumatoid arthritis: Symptoms, diagnosis, and management. *Nursing Times, 100*(24), 40–44.

McMullen, A. H., Pasta, D. J., Frederick, P. D., Konstan, M. W., Morgan, W. J., Schechter, M. S., & Wagener, J. S. (2006). Impact of pregnancy on women with cystic fibrosis. *Chest, 129*(3), 706–711.

Meechan, G. T., Collins, J. P., Moss-Morris, R. E., & Petrie, K. J. (2005). Who is not reassured following benign diagnosis of breast symptoms? *Psychooncology, 14*(3), 239–246.

Meechan, G., Collins, J., & Petrie, K. J. (2003). The relationship of symptoms and psychological factors to delay in seeking medical care for breast cancer. *Preventive Medicine, 36,* 374–378.

Morgan, J. W., Gladson, J. E., & Rau, K. S. (1998). Position paper of the American Council on Science and Health on risk factors for breast cancer: Established, speculated, and unsupported. *Breast Journal, 4*(3), 177–197.

Mosca, L., Manson, J. E., Sutherland, S. E., Langer, R. D., Manolio, T., & Barrett-Connor, E. (1997). Cardiovascular disorders in women: A statement for healthcare professionals from the American Heart Association writing group. *Circulation, 96,* 2468–2482.

Mosure, D. J., Berman, S., Fine, D., Delisele, S., Cates, W., & Boring, J. R. III (1997). Genital chlamydia infections in sexually active female adolescents: So we really need to screen everyone? *Journal of Adolescent Health, 20,* 6–13.

Murray, M., & Pizzorno, J. (1998). *Encyclopedia of natural medicine.* Rockin, CA: Prima Health.

Myasthenia Gravis Foundation of America, Inc. (2001). *Facts about autoimmune myasthenia gravis for patients and families.* Minneapolis, MN: Author.

Nash, J. (1997). Sexual health and sexually acquired infection. In G. Andrews (Ed.), *Women's sexual health.* London: Bailliere Tindall.

National Cancer Institute. (2000). *What you need to know about ovarian cancer.* Bethesda, MD: U.S. Department of Health and Human Services.

National Cancer Institute. (2001). *What you need to know about cancer of the uterus* [Brochure]. Bethesda, MD: Author.

National Cancer Institute. (2004). *Stages of cervical cancer.* Retrieved November 28, 2004, from http://www.cancer.gov/cancertopics/pdq/tretment/cervical/patient/all pages.

National Center for HIV, STD and TB Prevention. (2003). *HIV and AIDS: Are you at risk?* Retrieved December 1, 2004, from http://www.cdc.gov/hiv/pubs/brochure/atrisk.htm.

National Center for Infectious Diseases. (2004). *Viral hepatitis C fact sheet.* Retrieved December 1, 2004, from http://cdc.gov/ncidod/diseases/hepatitis/c/fact.htm.

National Institute of Allergies and Infectious Disease. (1998). *Vaginitis due to vaginal infections.* Retrieved June 12, 2003, from http://www.niaid.nih.gov/factsheets/stdvag.htm.

National Institute of Allergy and Infectious Diseases. (2002a). *Chlamydial infection.* Retrieved June 12, 2003, from http://www.niaid.nih.gov/factsheets/stdclam.htm.

National Institute of Allergy and Infectious Diseases. (2002b). *Gonorrhea.* Retrieved June 12, 2003, from http://www.niaid,niH.gov/factsheets/stDgon.htm.

National Institute of Allergy and Infectious Diseases. (2002c). *Syphilis.* Retrieved June 12, 2004, from http://www.niaid.nih.gov/factsheets/sdtsyph.htm.

National Institute of Allergy and Infectious Diseases. (2004). *Human papillomavirus and genital warts.* Retrieved December 8, 2004, from http://www.niaid.nih.gov/factsheets/stdhpv.htm.

National Institutes of Health. (2004). *Uterine prolapse.* Retrieved November 29, 2004, from http://www.nlm.nih.gov./medlineplus/ency/article/001508.htm.

National Institutes of Health. (n.d.). *Fast facts about endometriosis.* Retrieved November 26, 2004, from http://nichd.nih.gov/publications/pubs/endometriosis/index.htm.

National Institutes of Health, National Heart, Lung, and Blood Institute (2002). Facts about cystic fibroses. [Data File]. Retrieved February 5, 2003, from http://www.cdc.gov.

National Kidney and Urologic Diseases Information Clearinghouse. (2003). *Interstitial cystitis.* Retrieved February 14, 2006, from http://kidney.niddk.nih.gov/kudiseases/pubs/interstitialcystitis/index.htm.

National Kidney and Urologic Diseases Information Clearinghouse. (2004). Urinary tract infections in adults. Retrieved February 14, 2006, from http://kidney.niddk.nih.gov/urinary_tract_infection/index/htm.

National Tay-Sachs and Allied Diseases Association, Inc. (2006). *What every family should know.* Retrieved March 21, 2006, from http://www.ntsad.org/pages/t-sachs.htm#What%20is%20Tay-Sachs%20Disease?.

National Uterine Fibroid Foundation. (2004). *About uterine fibroids.* Retrieved September 1, 2005, from http://nuff.org/health_statistics.htm.

National Women's Health Information Center. (2001). *Ovarian cysts.* Bethesda, MD: Author.

National Women's Health Information Center. (2002a). *Frequently asked questions about human papillomavirus and genital warts.* Bethesda, MD: Author.

National Women's Health Information Center. (2002b). *Frequently asked questions about sexually transmitted diseases: Overview.* [Brochure]. Bethesda, MD: Author.

National Women's Health Information Center. (2003). *Frequently asked questions about diabetes: Overview.* Bethesda MD: Author.

Office on Women's Health. (2000). *Lupus and women.* Retrieved June 6, 2005, from http://www.4women.gov/owh/pub/factsheets/fslupus.htm.

Olawaiye, A., Withiam-Leitch, M., Danakas, G., & Kahn, K. (2005). Mastalgia: A review of management. *Journal of Reproductive Medicine, 50*(12), 933–939.

Paley, P. J. (2001). Screening for the major malignancies affecting women. *American Journal of Obstetrics and Gynecology, 184,* 1021–1030.

Patel, A. V., Calle, E. E., Bernstein, L., Wu, A. H., & Thun, M. J. (2003). Recreational physical activity and risk of postmenopausal cancer in a large cohort of U.S. women. *Cancer Causes and Control, 14*(6), 519–529.

Rindfleisch, J. A., & Muller, D. (2005). Diagnosis and management of rheumatoid arthritis. *American Family Physician, 72*(6), 1037–1047.

Roe, B., Watson, N. M., Palmer, M. H., Mueller, C., Vinsnes, A. G., & Wells, M. S. (2004). Translating research on incontinence into practice. *Nursing Research, 53*(6S), S56–S60.

Saslow, D., et al. (2002). American Cancer Society Guidelines for the early detection of cervical neoplasia and cancer. *CA: A Cancer Journal for Clinicians, 52,* 342–362.

Sickles, E. A. (2000). Galactography and other imaging investigations of nipple discharge. *Lancet, 356,* 1622–1623.

Sloane, E. (2002). *Biology of women* (4th ed.). Albany, NY: Delmar Thomson Learning.

Smeltzer, S. C., Bare, B. G., Hinkle, J. L., & Cheever, K. H. (2008). *Brunner and Suddarth's textbook of medical-surgical nursing* (11th ed.). Philadelphia: Lippincott Williams & Wilkins.

U.S. Department of Health and Human Services, Health Resources and Services Administration, Maternal and Child Health Bureau. (2002). *Women's health USA 2002.* Rockville, MD: Author.

U.S. Department of Health and Human Services, National Institutes of Health, and National Cancer Institute. (1998). *Understanding breast cancer treatment: A guide for patients* (NIH No. 98-4251). Washington, DC: U.S. Government Printing Office.

U.S. Department of Health and Human Services, National Institutes of Health, and National Cancer Institute. (2003). *What you need to know about breast cancer* (NIH Publication No.03-1556). Washington, DC: U.S. Government Printing Office.

U.S. Department of Health and Human Services, Natural Journal of Health. (2002). *Women's health in the U.S.: Research on health issues applying to women.* NIH Publication No. 02-46 97. Washington, DC: U.S. Government Printing Office.

Vahabi, M. (2003). Breast cancer screening methods: A review of the evidence. *Health Care of Women International, 24*(9), 773–793.

Viel, J-F, Perarnau, J-M, Challier, B., & Faivre-Nappez, I. (1997). Alcoholic calories, red wine consumption and breast cancer among perimenopausal women. *European Journal of Epidemiology, 13*(6), 639–643.

Weipple-Strasser, K., & Goss, P. (2003). Prevention of breast cancer using SERMS and aromatase inhibitors. *Journal of Mammary Gland Biology and Neoplasia, 8*(1), 5–18.

Woodward, V., & Webb, C. (2001). Women's anxieties surrounding breast disorders: A systematic review of the literature. *Journal of Advanced Nursing, 33*(1), 28–41.

Wright, T. C., Cox, J. T., Massad, L. S., Twiggs, L. B., & Wilkinson, F. J. (2002). 2001 Consensus guidelines for the management of women with cervical cytological abnormalities. *Journal of the American Medical Association, 287,* 2120–2129.

Yaish, H. M. (2005). Thalassemia. Retrieved March 11, 2006, from http://www.emedicine.com/ped/topic2229.htm.

Youngkin, E. Q., & Davis, M. S. (2004). *Women's health: A primary care clinical guide* (3rd ed.). Upper Saddle River, NJ: Pearson Prentice Hall.

CHAPTER 5

Mental Health Concerns for Women in Adolescence and Adulthood

Faye Gary

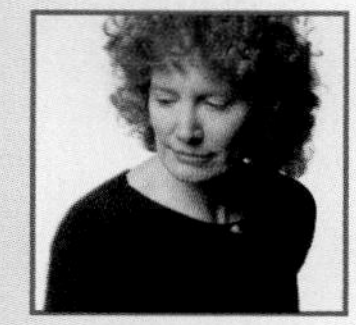

Gladys, a 35-year-old multigravida in her 23rd week of pregnancy, comes to the emergency department (ED) accompanied by a male friend. She reports difficulty sleeping, periodic dizziness, and late-day swelling in her feet. She states, "Sometimes, I hear voices telling me to 'watch out for the baby inside . . . it might just jump out at any minute.' " The nurse notes that Gladys seems easily distracted and frequently looks away, making some statement irrelevant to the conversation at hand and appearing annoyed. She murmurs, "My friend and I are in a hurry to move things along."

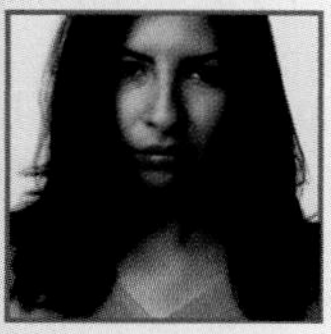

Maria, a 30-year-old multipara, is making her first visit to the neighborhood prenatal clinic at 6 months' gestation. She and her husband moved to the United States approximately 12 years ago. Although she classifies herself and her husband as Hispanic, she states that she frequently tells people that she is white for fear of rejection and prejudice, including from health care professionals. She has two children younger than 5 years. She works approximately 60 hours a week at a local bakery. She reports that her unemployed husband has difficulty keeping a job because of his "red pepper temper."

Nurses working with such clients need to understand this chapter to manage care and address issues appropriately. You will read more about the nurse's interactions with these clients later. Before beginning this chapter, consider the following points related to the above scenarios:

- How will the nurse working with both clients tailor care to best suit the needs of the women and their families?
- What aspects of teaching do these women require? What issues are similar for the women? What issues are different?
- What mental health issues or concerns might be relevant for each of these women?
- How might each client's current situation affect her health literacy? What factors might be important to assess?

LEARNING OBJECTIVES

On completion of this chapter, the reader should be able to:

- Describe conceptual models of mental health and illness pertinent to women's health care.
- Discuss common psychiatric disorders in women, including signs and symptoms, treatment, and pertinent nursing issues.
- Explore the societal problems of suicide and intimate partner violence.
- Discuss the therapeutic benefits and potential side effects of psychotropic medications to manage psychiatric disorders, particularly in the care of pregnant or lactating women.
- Discuss the nurses' responsibilities for overall health care when a pregnant or lactating woman has past or current mental illness.
- Describe a health literacy plan for women with mental illness.

KEY TERMS

anorexia nervosa
attachments
bingeing
bulimia nervosa
dysthymic disorder
learned helplessness
mental health literacy
postpartum blues
postpartum depression

This chapter provides information about mental health and illness in women throughout adolescence and adulthood. The content has a special focus on pregnant or lactating women facing mental health challenges. The discussions in this chapter are pertinent to all health care settings and based on the assumption that all health professionals, especially nurses who provide health services to women and their children, are in a unique position to assist families.

Encounters between nurses and women experiencing mental health challenges abound. Common examples include the following (Schatzberg & Nemeroff, 2004; Usher et al., 2005):

- A woman experiencing her first episode of mental illness
- A woman experiencing an exacerbation of signs and symptoms of an established mental illness
- A woman who uses psychotropic medications needing consultation for family planning
- A woman using psychotropic drugs who conceives and likely needs her medications throughout the gestation
- A woman who plans to breastfeed but is at risk for postpartum mental illness and needs psychotropic drugs to prevent or treat her condition

Early identification and prompt and efficient treatment remain the cornerstones of quality health care. The information in this chapter is designed to assist nurses in providing such care.

The chapter is divided into four sections. The first section summarizes common conceptual models in mental health. The second section covers major psychiatric and social problems affecting women. It discusses risk factors and common conditions for women of all age groups and circumstances. A special emphasis is placed on pregnant or lactating women. The third section explores psychopharmacologic treatment and its related risk-to-benefit ratio during pregnancy or lactation. The fourth section provides recommendations germane to nursing management and nursing interventions for women experiencing psychosocial health concerns.

CONCEPTUAL MODELS IN MENTAL HEALTH CARE

This section briefly reviews psychoanalytic, behavioral, sociocultural, feminist, and biologic conceptual models of mental health. Those desiring more content on these theoretical foundations should consult psychiatric–mental health nursing textbooks.

Psychoanalytic Models

Psychoanalytic models explore unconscious motivations and seek to explain behaviors related to these shielded motivations. Although many of their tenets have been called into question over time, they can be useful for understanding women's mental health because of their focuses on the motivations for behaviors, the way in which attachments are formed in early life, and developmental progression of the personality. Two important theorists of this model are Sigmund Freud and Erik Erikson.

Freud

Freud postulated that the mind was divided into two parts: the small conscious segment, and the much larger *unconscious* part. The powerful and driving unconscious mind contains hurtful memories, forbidden desires, and other repressed experiences, or things that a person has pushed from awareness. Unconscious material seeks expression, which may be reflected in a woman's dreams or fantasies; according to Freud, it also may lead to irrational and maladaptive behavior (Brenner, 1957; Mohr, 2006).

Freud also proposed a topography of the mind consisting of id, ego, and superego:

- The entirely selfish *id* consists of instinctual drives (ie, aggression and sexuality). It demands immediate gratification, regardless of external constraints. The id supplies all the power for the other two subsystems.
- The *ego* emerges during childhood and controls the id by supplying mechanisms for reality testing, judgment formation, and other functions essential to daily living. The ego enables the person to meet the id's demands, but in a way that allows her to function normally in society.
- The *superego,* which develops gradually, regulates and sanctions behavior by providing a conscience for decision making. It provides a way of distinguishing right from wrong.

Freud postulated that attachments in early life lay the foundation for future relationships. **Attachments** are those significant relationships between an infant or child and his or her caregivers. Optimal attachments provide security, trust, warm and affectionate exchanges, satisfaction of physical and emotional needs, and psychological and physical comfort (Fig. 5.1) (Zeanah et al., 2003).

Erikson

Erikson built on the concepts of attachment and its consequences, focusing on physiologic and cognitive influences on child development (Mohr, 2006). His approach is grounded on the *epigenetic principle,* dominant in embryology (see Chap. 11), that human development proceeds in an organized, sequential, and defined manner. His framework emphasizes the particular tasks that a person should master at each specific stage if growth and development are to continue without tension and conflict (Sadock & Sadock, 2003) and those elements that can help or hinder the person on the road to task achievement (Table 5.1).

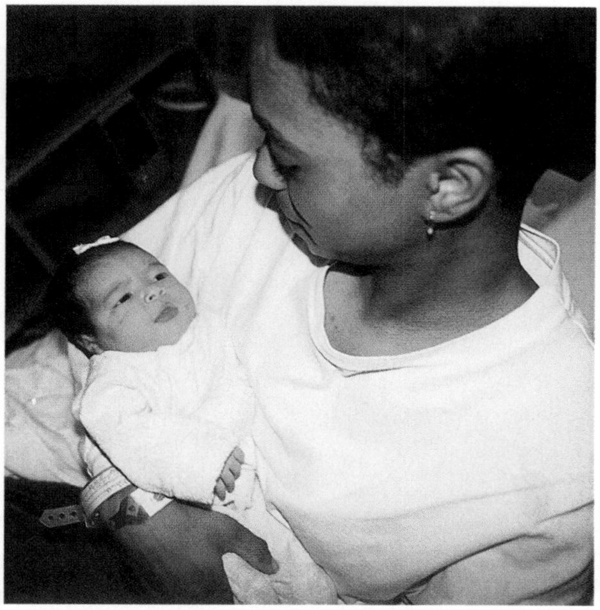

FIGURE 5.1 Attachments in early life provide lifelong foundations for each person's sense of security, trust, affection, and comfort.

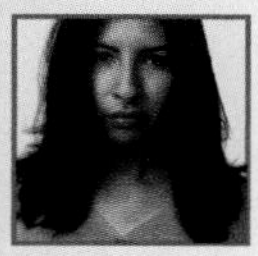

Consider Maria, the 30-year-old Hispanic woman from the beginning of the chapter. Using Table 5.1, at which of Erikson's stages would the nurse expect Maria to be? What tasks would be of chief concern?

Behavioral Models

Behavioral models emphasize that all behavior is learned from the environment through timed reinforcement and gradual conditioning. Many psychological therapies are based on behavioral models; examples include substance abuse treatments, management of hallucinations, and enhancement of school performance.

Learned helplessness, a behavioral theory proposed by Martin Seligman (1975), deserves comment. Seligman posited that negative thought patterns, as often observed in depressed and suicidal clients, are learned. A client's perception of her control over her life affects how she feels about herself and her ability to act. Low self-esteem, negative self-concepts, and self-critical commentary typically

(text continues on page 178)

TABLE 5.1 Erikson's Developmental Stages

STAGE	APPROXIMATE AGE RANGE	DESCRIPTION	
Basic Trust vs. Mistrust	Birth to 18 months	The person experiences a reliable or unreliable world in which needs are met or unmet.	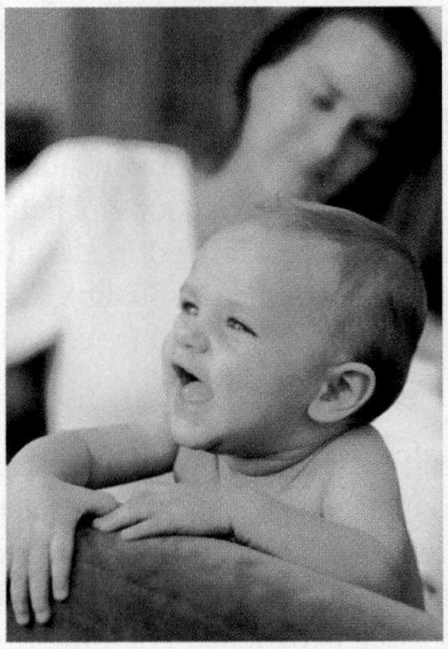
Autonomy vs. Shame and Doubt	18 months to 3 years	The person learns about body and thought control and confronts realities about how she will satisfy others and herself.	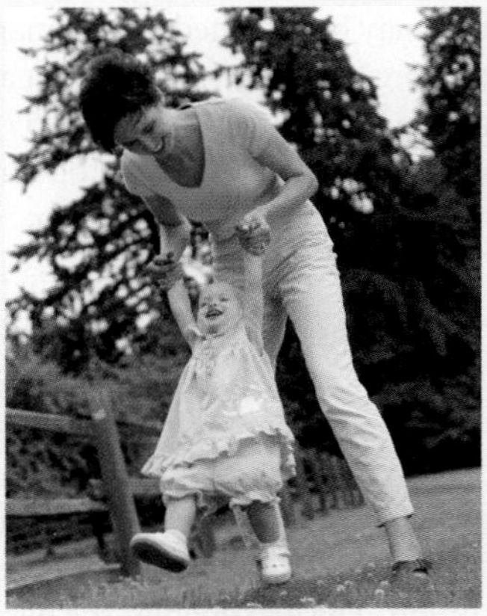
Initiative vs. Guilt	3 to 5 years	The person struggles with wanting to take over relationships with loved ones and exclude others from their affection.	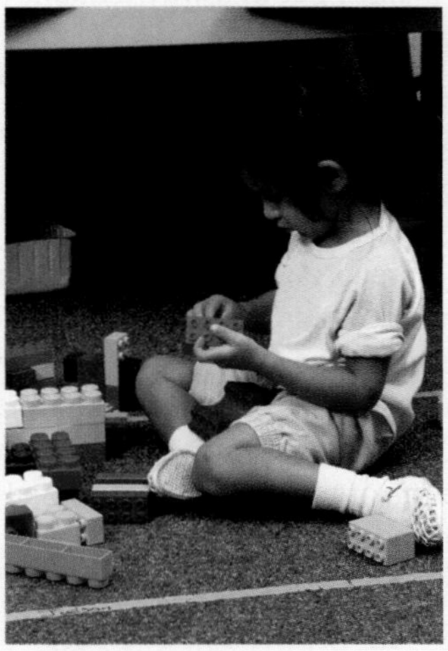

Continued

TABLE 5.1 Erikson's Developmental Stages

STAGE	APPROXIMATE AGE RANGE	DESCRIPTION	
Industry vs. Inferiority	5 to 13 years	Major concerns relate to self-identify, peers, and academic demands. The person begins to understand the nature of work and should learn skills associated with goal attainment.	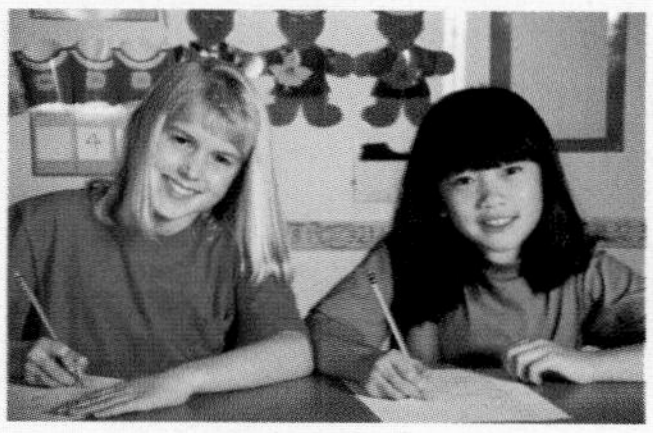
Identity vs. Role Confusion	13 to 21 years	The person deals with many new growth phenomena; additional demands at school and home related to self-management, identity, and career choices; and independence.	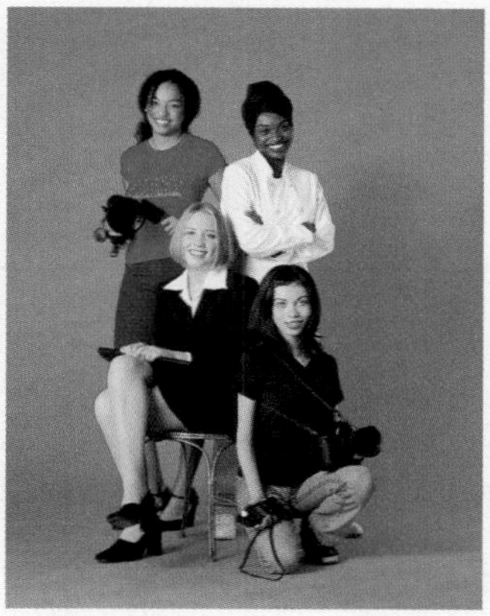
Intimacy vs. Isolation	21 to 40 years	The person is concerned with developing mature attachments and making commitments. Being in love has responsibilities; decision making could have far-reaching consequences into midlife.	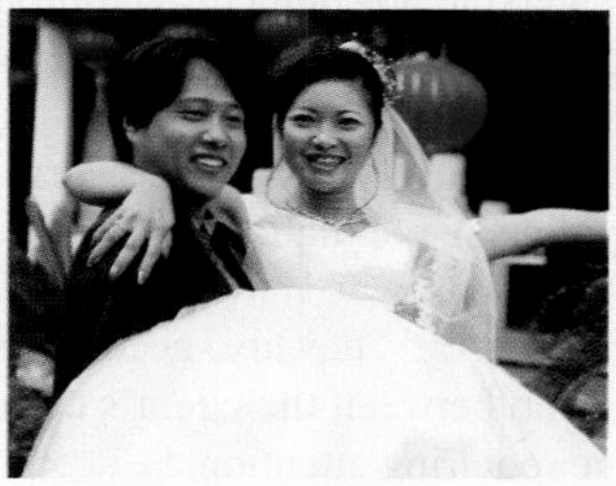
Generativity vs. Stagnation	40 to 60 years	The person focuses on a vocation and career and experiences continued growth and development through intellectual and emotional stimulation. Attachments to others should be evident; needs for intimacy, belonging, and a sense of self ought to be solidified.	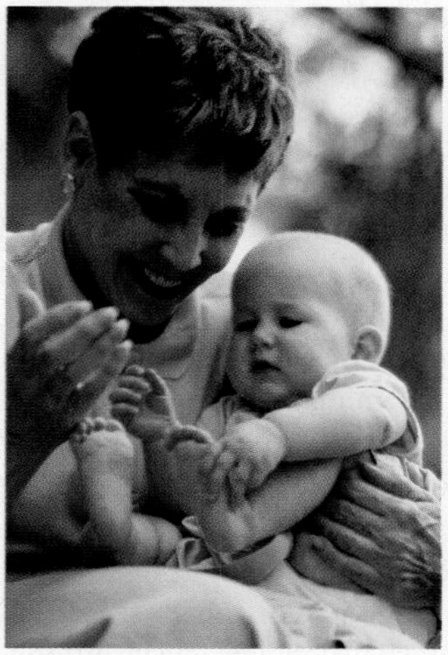

Continued

● **TABLE 5.1 Erikson's Developmental Stages *(Continued)***

STAGE	APPROXIMATE AGE RANGE	DESCRIPTION
Ego Integrity vs. Despair	60 years to death	The person engages in reflective self-appraisal, with the outcome being a sense of accomplishment or despair/anguish about the previous years. The person must accept responsibilities and decisions related to life's outcomes. 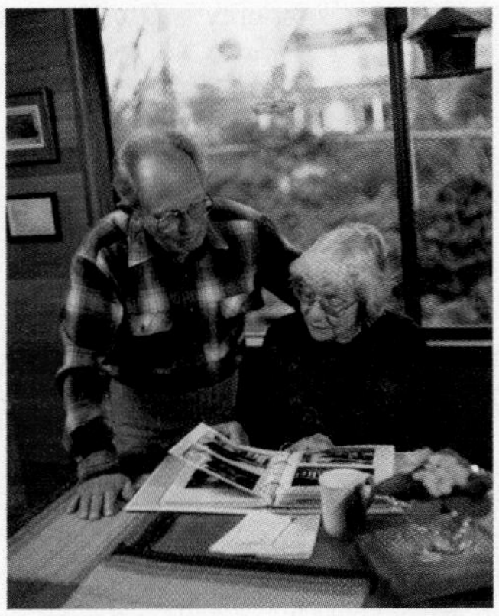

are evident in the thought processes of those with depression as well as victims of domestic violence (Kuehner & Buerger, 2005; Saint Arnault et al., 2005; Seligman, 1975).

Sociocultural Models

Heterogeneous societies (e.g., the United States, Canada) include numerous cultural groups. Acculturation occurs when continuous interactions among the different groups change the original cultural patterns of all the groups involved over time. Nurses working with culturally diverse populations must understand the perspective of the client, who may be struggling with his or her cultural identity. They also need to always consider the relationship between the client's culture and the health care issue requiring attention.

Feminist Models

Feminism and feminist movements have helped raise awareness in some societies that tradition, history, and necessity largely have dictated women's various roles and functions. Demographic realities such as diversity among women, socioeconomic differences, health and education disparities, and environmental factors require in-depth thinking about, and perhaps the repositioning of, feminist theory (Hale, 2002).

Feminist models shed light on the contextual variables in a woman's life. They include the building of knowledge related to such concepts as power and powerlessness, egalitarianism, self-determination, and control over reproduction.

One feminist theorist is Carol Gilligan, who studied moral development and its differences in girls and women. Gilligan stressed that women often emphasize the effects of caring on human relationships, which tends to be different from a male focus on individual rights and rules. She emphasized that neither approach was necessarily right or wrong, and that both viewpoints needed to be considered, not one at the expense of another. Gilligan also diverged from feminist colleagues who posited that no differences exist between men and women. According to Gilligan, moral and psychological tendencies are gender oriented, and Western societies traditionally have limited women by valuing "male" morality over female.

Biologic Models

Biologic models that explain mental illness are based on relatively recent findings indicating a link between mental disorders and neurochemical alterations and imbalances in the brain. Biologically oriented treatments for mental illness did not begin until the 1940s, when researchers discovered that some drugs could reduce the intensity and frequency of hallucinations and other devastating psychiatric symptoms. In recent years, scientists have given additional attention to the promise of neurotransmitters in the treatment of mental disorders. For example, increased levels of dopamine have been implicated in schizophrenia. Consequently, researchers have developed drug therapies to decrease the effects of dopamine on the disease process (Schatzberg & Nemeroff, 2004; Wilcox et al., 1998). Use of drugs to treat psychiatric disorders is the major focus of the third section of this chapter.

COMMON PSYCHIATRIC CHALLENGES IN WOMEN

This section introduces readers to major psychiatric and social problems in women. It contains detailed presentations on common psychiatric illnesses, suicide, and intimate partner violence. Most of this section is relevant to women across the lifespan. The effects of disorders on pregnant or lactating women receive special focus. Although the risk for untreated mental illness during pregnancy has not been documented definitively, certain negative associations have been established. For example, untreated schizophrenia is linked to increased perinatal deaths; untreated depression may contribute to low-birth-weight infants; and maternal stress can cause elevated maternal serum concentrations of cortisol, which may be deleterious to fetal brain development (Hales & Yudofsky, 2003; Nillson et al., 2002; Patel & Prince, 2006; Schatzberg & Nemeroff, 2004).

Depression and Related Disorders

Clients with depression have either a sad, depressed mood or a loss of interest or inability to derive pleasure from previously enjoyed activities. Symptoms include recurrent suicidal thoughts, appetite changes, lack of concentration, faulty decision making, feelings of worthlessness, poor energy, sleep problems, substance abuse, and social withdrawal. These symptoms cause significant distress or impair functioning nearly every day for at least 2 weeks. Typically, episodes last many weeks or months, followed by periods of normal mood and behavior.

Dysthymic disorder differs from major depression in terms of intensity and duration. Its course can be persistent or intermittent. The client with dysthymic disorder has a sad or irritable mood and feelings of inadequacy, guilt, anger, and difficulty experiencing joy and elation on most days for at least 2 years. During this time, no more than 2 months pass without symptoms; however, the client has no manic or depressive episodes (American Psychiatric Association [APA], 2000). The chronic nature of dysthymic disorder often manifests as a lifelong struggle, which can cause significant distress (Mohr, 2006). Negative feelings, lack of energy, and pessimism impair occupational functioning and interrupt activities of daily living.

Both depression and dysthymia are more prevalent in women than in men (Hales & Yudofsky, 2003). Genetics, reactions to stress, interpersonal relationships, and other factors may contribute to this disparity. Other possible risk factors that lead to the preponderance of depression and dysthymia in women include the following:

- Hormonal influences (eg, premenstrual syndrome, pregnancy, postpartal adjustments) (Kornstein et al., 2005)
- Financial disparities or poverty
- Insufficient social supports
- History of sexual or physical abuse
- Traditional caretaking roles of women in caring for elderly or sick family members (Mazure et al., 2002; Pinquart & Sorensen, 2006)
- Chronic medical conditions (Brown & Prigerson, 2000; Brown & Schulberg, 1998; Brown et al., 1995)

As discussed in Chapter 2, nurses should incorporate assessment of a woman's mental health into the overall assessment of her physical and reproductive health. Each health care appointment provides an opportunity to screen for depression and dysthymic disorder. A brief mental health history assessment can help prevent or identify these serious problems (Lolak et al., 2005; Moline et al., 2001; Perfetti et al., 2004).

Evidence has shown that women with depressive disorders respond best to combined treatment with psychotherapy and psychopharmacology (Mazure et al., 2002). The most common antidepressants used are the selective serotonin reuptake inhibitors (SSRIs). Examples of SSRIs include citalopram (Celexa), fluoxetine (Prozac), sertraline (Zoloft), and nefazodone (Serzone) (Schatzberg et al., 2003). Other commonly prescribed classes of drugs for depressive disorders include cyclic antidepressants and monoamine oxidase inhibitors.

Pregnancy

Approximately 10% of pregnant women experience a depressive disorder, a rate similar to that among nonpregnant women (Hales & Yudofsky, 2003). Depression in pregnancy is associated with compromised prenatal care, insufficient nutrition, and poor overall health status. If a woman becomes depressed during pregnancy, her chances of experiencing postpartum depression increase (Hales & Yudofsky, 2003). Extreme stress during pregnancy leads to elevated maternal serum concentrations of cortisol, which are detrimental to fetal brain development. Infants and children born to women with untreated depression could experience complications and long-range problems (Campbell et al., 2004; Rahman et al., 2004).

General guidelines for treatment of depression during pregnancy have been difficult to establish. As much as possible, the health care provider should avoid prescribing antidepressants for women during the first trimester, when organogenesis occurs. If symptoms are severe (eg, mood lability, disorganization, inability to care for self, cognitive deficits) or the woman has a history of chronic relapse without medication, then the primary health care provider should consider medication. Fluoxetine (Prozac) in the smallest dosage that will control florid symptoms is one potential agent (Hales & Yudofsky, 2003). Other options include tricyclic and tetracyclic antidepressants. Although these drugs are considered relatively safe, the literature has not yet substantiated these findings. They are known to cause perinatal toxicity near the end of pregnancy, resulting in maternal urinary retention, jitteriness, irritability, and other symptoms (Schatzberg et al., 2003) (see Chap. 13).

Postpartum

Postpartum depressive disorders can affect mother, infant, and other family members. Depending on the extent of the problem, the client may require attention from a health care provider. Support from partner or spouse, family, and friends is key in helping the woman regain and strengthen her sense of stability (Fig. 5.2).

QUOTE 5-1

"While I was pregnant, I couldn't wait for the baby to arrive. I had no idea how demanding taking care of him would be. I am so exhausted, and I look terrible. I wonder how I'm ever going to be able to care for my son appropriately. Then, I feel guilty and wonder what kind of mother I am for feeling like this. Shouldn't I be joyful?"

A woman who gave birth 10 days ago

Postpartum Blues. Postpartum blues ("maternity blues") is a mild condition of short duration that affects approximately 30% to 75% of all women who give birth (Seyfried & Marcus, 2003). Symptoms include tearfulness, moodiness, irritability, and anxiety. They worsen progressively over the first 3 to 4 days postpartum and improve by approximately the 12th postpartum day. Approximately 20% of cases progress to postpartum depression (Moline et al., 2001). Unlike postpartum depression and postpartum psychosis, postpartum blues typically resolves without professional intervention.

During prenatal teaching and before discharge from the health facility following childbirth, nurses should caution women and their support people about postpartum blues. Health care professionals might not see clients before or while symptoms emerge, since most clients return home 2 to 3 days after birth. Hence, teaching and enhancing the health literacy of the client and her support people are essential roles for nurses in maternal and child health settings (APA, 2000; Hales & Yudofsky, 2003). Nurses should teach clients the early signs and symptoms of postpartum blues and give clear instructions about how to access treatment should the need arise (Hales & Yudofsky, 2003). See Teaching Tips 5.1 for more information.

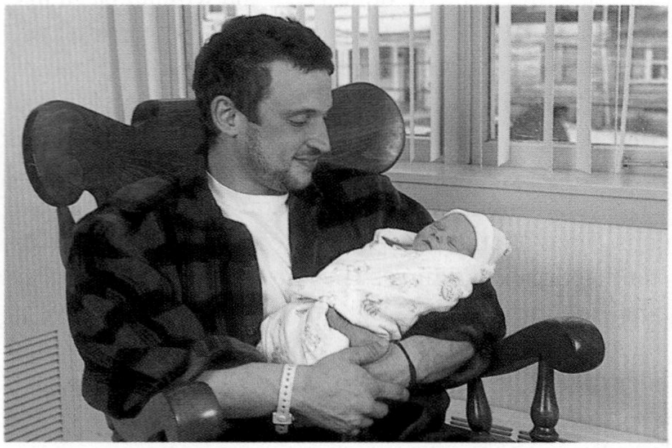

FIGURE 5.2 Support from others can assist the new mother to avoid or to manage symptoms of postpartum "blues" or depression.

Postpartum Depression. Postpartum depression develops within the first 4 weeks after delivery (APA, 2000). Clients typically complain of being tired; they are irritable and find care for themselves and the newborn difficult. The infant is likely to experience a poor quality of mothering and be exposed to behavioral, emotional, and cognitive deficits because of the mother's depression. If a woman has a history of major depression, previous postpartum depression, or depression during pregnancy, her odds of experiencing postpartum depression are increased (Bloch et al., 2006). Women without adequate support from others are also at risk (Hales & Yudofsky, 2003).

The woman with postpartum depression loses pleasure in things that once brought satisfaction. She typically feels tired, down, guilty, hopeless, and worthless; in some cases, she has thoughts of death or suicide. Health care professionals, family, and friends might not recognize immediately that the client is experiencing depression, believing instead that she is tired or exhausted from caring for her new infant (Moline et al., 2001).

A multimodal treatment approach is best. Interpersonal therapies typically are helpful with their focus on transitional roles, new demands, and expectations that the woman must confront. Individual, group, family, and couples therapies are examples of interpersonal interventions. Appropriate medications administered under the supervision of a knowledgeable primary care provider or mental health specialist may be indicated (Mazure et al., 2002). See Chapter 19 for more information.

Postpartum Psychosis. In this most severe disorder, the client develops psychotic symptoms: hallucinations, delusions, and feelings of unreality. Postpartum psychosis affects approximately 1 in 1500 women (Seyfried & Marcus, 2003). These clients usually require hospitalization and are at risk for suicide, infant neglect, self-neglect, failed reality testing, and poor judgment. They need several therapies, including supportive therapy, individual and group therapy, and medication. Pharmacologic treatment usually involves several classes of medications, including antipsychotics and antidepressants (Schatzberg et al., 2003).

Nurses need to understand and educate others regarding this severe disorder. Family, particularly the client's partner or spouse, should be involved in planning care. The partners and spouses of women with postpartum psychosis need support and understanding from immediate and extended family members and friends (MacKey et al., 2000). See Chapter 19 for more information.

Older Women and Depression

Epidemiologic studies suggest that the risk for depression does *not* increase as women enter perimenopause and beyond (Hales & Yudofsky, 2003). The current thinking is that women who experience depression later in life

TEACHING TIPS 5.1 Postpartum Blues

The nurse teaches the client about to give birth or who has recently given birth the following information related to mood changes that frequently develop in the early postpartal period:

- Feeling sad, anxious, tired, and irritable in the days and weeks after giving birth is normal. The combination of fluctuating hormone levels and sleep deprivation is challenging alone, in addition to providing constant care for a helpless and utterly dependent human being. Many women find the adjustment to motherhood (whether with a first or subsequent baby) difficult. Talk about your feelings with a supportive person.
- Plan for and ask for help with child care, chores, cooking, and errands. Use this assistance to rest and find some time for yourself apart from taking care of the baby. Try reading, taking a bath, or getting out of the house for a short walk and some fresh air.
- Keep a journal of your feelings to explore your frustrations and concerns. As time moves on, you can reread your entries to see how you have progressed and what has changed.
- Accept that you will have days in which you cannot get anything done other than caring for your baby. Let go of the "supermom" myth. Set small goals, and don't be shy about asking others to help you.
- If your feelings do not improve with time, talk with your doctor about how you feel.

The nurse teaches the client's partner or spouse as follows:

- Help ensure that the woman gets as much sleep as possible. Encourage her to nap and to sleep when the baby sleeps.
- Assume responsibility for some feedings (of either pumped breast milk once nursing is well established or formula). Sharing feedings not only gives the mother a break but promotes your bonding with the infant.
- See that the new mother has opportunities to spend time outside the house, even for brief breaks. Arrange babysitting so that you and she can spend some time together without the baby.
- Help make arrangements for you, family, friends, paid help, and volunteers to assume duties and household chores. People can assist with tasks from cleaning and cooking, to writing thank-you notes, to caring for older children and pets.
- Each day, ask the new mother what is most important and with what she needs your help specific to baby care. She needs to be in control of the situation as much as possible, even if it means mainly giving orders for some time!
- Remember to praise the woman and encourage her repeatedly if she feels she is not doing a "good job" as a mom. Love and admiration from her significant other will likely mean more to her than all the kind words of other people combined.

may have had previously neglected signs and symptoms of depression, vasomotor symptoms, or other health-related and socioeconomic problems that were troublesome stressors (Mazure et al., 2002).

Nurses caring for women across all settings must be aware that distinguishing depression from other psychiatric conditions, such as dementia and cognitive decline, can be difficult as women age. Physical health problems may precipitate depression. Contributing factors also may include side effects from medications to treat physical problems, pain, and compromised activities of daily living (Mazure et al., 2002; Moline et al., 2001). For more information on psychological health in menopausal and older women, see Chapters 23 and 24.

Suicide

Suicide, a serious public health problem, ranks 11th among the leading U.S. causes of death (Arias et al., 2003). The suicide rate has not changed over the past 2 decades (Hales & Yudofsky, 2003). Approximately 90% of all people who commit suicide have been diagnosed with a mental illness, primarily depression or alcoholism. Hence, if a woman has a mental disorder, especially depression or alcoholism, health care providers must be alert at all times to her risk for suicide.

Clients who are suicidal display common characteristics. One core element is a sense of hopelessness. Another is desperation, or a feeling that life is too difficult and that change is unlikely. Guilt, too, is dominant and associated with self-hatred. Feelings of shame and humiliation also are common. Some clients elect suicide as a reaction against shame or humiliation related to past or current overwhelming events (Hales & Yudofsky, 2003). An example might be sexual abuse, child abandonment, or prostitution.

Suicide and its implications present difficult challenges for health care providers. Completed suicides cause enormous pain and suffering for millions of Americans who endure the loss of a loved one. When the nurse suspects that a woman is experiencing tremendous stress or feeling hopeless, he or she should complete a suicide assessment of the client. Clinical scales useful for promptly and effectively identifying suicidal clients include the modified SAD PERSONS scale, the revised Beck Depression Inventory, the Beck Anxiety Inventory, the Beck Hopelessness Scale, and the Beck Scale for Suicidal Ideation (BSS). Positive results on any of these scales should prompt the nurse to refer the client to a mental health specialist.

QUOTE 5-2

"I felt like I was drowning in a pool of nothingness. Every day was harder to get through than the next. Some nights, I would just lie awake until morning, going over and over in my mind how hopeless everything was. I finally tried to kill myself so I wouldn't have to feel or think about anything anymore. It was a way to get some rest and peace."

A 48-year-old woman recovering from depression and attempted suicide

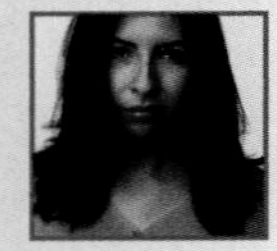

Maria, the young Hispanic woman pregnant with her third child, states, "I feel so alone. I don't speak English well. I'm worried about my baby and my two young children, money, and my husband's temper. Sometimes I wonder if it is worth trying to carry on." How would the nurse interpret Maria's statements?

Anxiety, Stress, and Anxiety Disorders

Anxiety needs to be differentiated from fear. Anxiety alerts a person to impending danger, but the source of that danger is unknown. Thus, anxiety is internal, vague, conflictual, and insidious. With fear, the danger is known, identifiable, and sudden (Sadock & Sadock, 2003).

Anxiety presents with many symptoms expressed in two ways. First, the client becomes aware of associated physiologic sensations, such as sweating and palpitations (Box 5.1). Second, the client experiences nervousness, fright, or upset. Others observe that she is experiencing anxiety even if the client herself is unaware. Anxiety also affects thinking, perception, and learning.

BOX 5.1 Common Manifestations of Anxiety

- Diarrhea
- Dizziness, lightheadedness
- Hyperreflexia
- Hypertension
- Nausea and vomiting
- Palpitations
- Restlessness
- Tachycardia
- Tingling in the extremities
- Tremors
- Upset stomach
- Urinary frequency, hesitancy, urgency

Anxiety disorders are among the most common psychiatric illnesses, affecting one in four people at any given time (Sadock & Sadock, 2003). Their prevalence decreases with increased socioeconomic status (Sadock & Sadock, 2003). Recent studies have implicated anxiety in the etiology and exacerbation of numerous physiologic problems, including heart disease.

Many disorders, reactions to medications and other substances, and exposure to real trauma and stressors can cause signs and symptoms of anxiety disorders. Examples include cardiac disease, thyroid disorders, lupus, blood disorders, and the effects of caffeine or nicotine. Herbal medicines, decongestants, steroids, and appetite suppressants can induce anxiety. Violent events in a woman's past, such as rape or sexual assault, increase her chances of experiencing anxiety problems (Schatzberg et al., 2003; Schatzberg & Nemeroff, 2004). The health care team must rule out such problems before establishing a diagnosis of an anxiety disorder.

COLLABORATIVE CARE: THE CLIENT WITH ANXIETY

When working with anxious clients, nurses may find it useful to conceptualize the level of anxiety (Mohr, 2006; Peplau, 1963):

- *Mild.* The client experiences and manages tension related to activities of daily living. She sees, hears, and is aware of environmental stimuli. This level of anxiety acts as a motivator, helping the woman accomplish tasks.
- *Moderate.* The client's attention focuses on immediate concerns. What she hears, sees, and perceives is compromised.
- *Severe.* The client's perceptual field is restricted significantly, narrowing her awareness. The intent is to relieve or reduce anxiety to a more reasonable or comfortable level, at which functioning can be restored.
- *Panic.* The client experiences awe, dread, and terror. Even when directed by others, she may be unable to follow simple commands. She experiences increased motor activity, loses the capacity to think and reason, and could become a danger to herself and others.

Assessment

The nurse should ask the client if she is anxious or worried or has experienced such feelings lately. If the client answers positively, the nurse should continue to discuss feelings and use observation and interview techniques to gauge whether the client has had or is having the signs and symptoms of anxiety presented in Box 5.1. The nurse should suspect an anxiety disorder when the client shows evidence of anxiety that she cannot dismiss, reports anxiety that interferes with her daily life, or both.

The nurse should ask the client about worrying, obsessive thinking, repetitive activity, specific phobias, and exposure to trauma. If the client's responses to any of these questions are affirmative, the nurse should elicit details about the behavior or response.

If a pregnant client experiences anxiety, an especially important aspect of assessment is to determine associated risks to the fetus. The nurse should take necessary action to prevent the client from harming herself or her fetus. Teaching about the woman's changing body and the growing fetus, alcohol and nicotine use during pregnancy, nutrition, rest, family support, and self-care are some areas for discussion.

Select Potential Nursing Diagnoses

Three major nursing diagnoses are associated with anxiety disorders (Mohr, 2006):

- Anxiety
- Ineffective Coping
- Ineffective Breathing Pattern

Other nursing diagnoses may apply based on the client's specific circumstances.

Planning/Intervention

The nurse should plan interventions based on the client's level of anxiety. Also, he or she should determine whether the level is appropriate to the client's specific situation and consider whether the client's thought patterns seem logical and rational. NIC/NOC Box 5.1 presents common interventions and outcomes for clients with anxiety disorders.

To help the client meet established goals, the nurse should display the hallmarks of the therapeutic relationship: trust, empathy, respect, and calmness. He or she should help the client identify those thoughts and behaviors related to anxiety, as well as effective coping strategies to deal with them. Therapeutic questioning techniques and reflective listening can make the client feel understood and supported.

A quiet environment is important. The nurse should provide facts to negate any misconceptions. By doing so, the client can objectively appraise her situation. If the client is breathing rapidly, the nurse should assist with slow or controlled breathing exercises. See Teaching Tips 5.2.

The nurse should encourage a healthy lifestyle that can help limit or control stress (see Chap. 2). Examples of suggestions include getting sufficient aerobic exercise, eating a well-balanced diet (see Chap. 3), and minimizing use of alcohol, tobacco, drugs, and caffeine.

Coping strategies help determine the client's overall mental health status. Moreover, constructive or useful

NIC/NOC Box 5.1 Anxiety Management

Common NIC Labels

- Anticipatory Guidance
- Anxiety Reduction
- Behavior Modification: Social Skills
- Calming Technique
- Cognitive Restructuring
- Complex Relationship Building
- Coping Enhancement
- Decision-Making Support
- Emotional Support
- Impulse Control Training
- Security Enhancement
- Self-Awareness Enhancement
- Simple Guided Imagery
- Simple Relaxation Therapy

Common NOC Labels

- Aggression Control
- Anxiety Control
- Coping
- Decision Making
- Impulse Control
- Information Processing
- Role Performance
- Sleep
- Social Interaction Skills

TEACHING TIPS 5.2 Controlling Breathing

The nurse instructs the client how to perform a slow-breathing exercise to help deal with symptoms of anxiety. Although such exercises have variations, a common approach to use is to:

1. Hold the breath and count to 5.
2. On 5, breathe out, slowly and calmly saying the word *relax.*
3. Then breathe in for 3 seconds and out for 3 seconds, saying the word *relax* with each exhalation.
4. After 1 minute, hold the breath for 5 seconds again and then continue breathing using the 6-second cycle (3-second inhalation, 3-second exhalation).
5. Continue until hyperventilation is under control and all symptoms have subsided.

Adapted from Mohr, W. K. (2006). *Psychiatric mental health nursing* (6th ed.). Philadelphia: Lippincott Williams & Wilkins.

coping mechanisms help protect the client and give her direction for problem solving. The nurse should assist the client to identify maladaptive coping strategies (eg, alcohol use) and to replace them with positive techniques. Two common examples of positive coping strategies are the use of relaxation and reliance on problem solving (Mohr, 2006).

Relaxation

Regular use of relaxation techniques can reduce autonomic arousal, which in turn decreases oxygen demands, heart rate, blood pressure, and metabolic rate. Common methods of relaxation include visualization, meditation, yoga, progressive muscle relaxation, and hypnosis. The nurse and client should together identify the most acceptable method; the nurse can then teach the selected technique or refer the client to a professional who can do so.

Problem Solving

The nurse also may assist the client to develop or enhance problem-solving skills. In this way, the client learns to replace avoidance and worry with clear and effective thought and reflection. Problem-solving skills may include learning to first identify the specific problem, as well as all possible solutions, followed by identifying the pros and cons of each solution, and ultimately arriving at one solution or a combination of solutions that best addresses her circumstances and helps eliminate the original conundrum. Importantly, the client devises a way to implement the solution. After doing so, she also reviews the effectiveness of her solution. Thus, even when the client's actions don't completely resolve the original problem, she learns how to connect feelings, thoughts, and actions, rather than allowing anxiety to paralyze and overwhelm her.

Evaluation

Successful care is based on the client's report of improved feelings and observable changes in behavior. Examples of positive outcomes include the following:

- The client reports use of one or more relaxation techniques.
- The client reports decreased anxiety or panic.
- The client uses problem-solving techniques in difficult situations (Mohr, 2006).

Schizophrenia

Schizophrenia, a debilitating psychiatric disorder affecting approximately 1% of the population, occurs in all societies and among people of all socioeconomic levels (Sadock & Sadock, 2003). The peak age of onset in women is 25 to 35 years (Sadock & Sadock, 2003), which coincides with the woman's optimal childbearing years. The number of women diagnosed with schizophrenia and becoming pregnant is increasing (Inhorn & Whittle, 2001). Factors associated with this trend include deinstitutionalization (placement of people with psychiatric illnesses in the community rather than in long-term health care facilities), psychopharmacologic agents with fewer side effects, and improved perinatal care strategies for women with chronic illness (see Chap. 13).

No one theory explains the cause of schizophrenia; biologic, environmental, and psychosocial etiologies have been posited. Women with schizophrenia present with various clinical symptoms, experience the illness in numerous ways, and respond to treatment and rehabilitation diversely. Table 5.2 reviews the subtypes of schizophrenia.

Assessment Findings

This chronic, complex, and potentially devastating illness has a plethora of signs and symptoms. Prominent characteristics include numerous changes in mood, cognition, perception, motivation, interpersonal relations, and motor function (APA, 2000; Gary et al., 2003; Sadock & Sadock, 2003; Schatzberg et al., 2003; Wallerstein, 2002). Each group of symptoms can change in intensity, wax and wane, or become stable with treatment.

Mood Changes. The client experiences anxiety, depression, tension, and irritation. She may isolate herself and withdraw from events and people. One example is *blunted affect,* in which the person appears emotionless. Another example is *anhedonia,* in which the client seems

● COMPLEMENTARY AND ALTERNATIVE MEDICINE 5.1
Visualization

Visualization can be an effective technique to manage anxiety. The client starts by practicing techniques such as focused breathing or progressive muscle relaxation. Another person, an audiotape, or the woman herself may then guide the client to imagine a calm and peaceful environment where she can work through a problem or stress. The client may choose to focus on an inspirational person, event, or deity to provide guidance and wisdom.

TABLE 5.2 Subtypes of Schizophrenia

The five subtypes of schizophrenia demonstrate the variety in symptom formation and expression related to the condition (APA, 2000; Sadock & Sadock, 2003):

SUBTYPE	CHARACTERISTICS
Paranoid	Preoccupation with one or more delusions Frequent hallucinations (usually auditory) Organized speech and behavior, with appropriate affect
Disorganized	Disorganized speech Disorganized behavior Flat and inappropriate affect
Catatonic	At least two of the following: ● Motor immobility with *waxy flexibility* (allowing others to move the limbs, but then holding them for hours in the position in which they are placed) or stupor ● Purposeless but excessive motor activity not influenced by external stimuli and demand ● *Negativism* (resistance to all instructions or guidance) ● Maintenance of a rigid posture that continues even with attempts by others to move or reposition the client ● Mutism Peculiar movements such as posturing and excessive grimacing Strange speech patterns
Undifferentiated	Delusions, hallucinations, and disorganized speech, but no symptoms that meet the predetermined criteria for paranoid, disorganized, or catatonic
Residual	No prominent delusions, hallucinations, disorganized speech, or disorganized or catatonic behavior Negative signs, odd thought content and form, and unusual perceptual experiences

to experience continuous apathy and cannot experience joy or happiness.

Cognitive Changes. The cognitive changes of schizophrenia can make life strange and difficult for the woman. Disordered thoughts make up the core component of the condition. The client loses the capacity to concentrate. Sometimes, health care providers confuse this symptom with intellectual impairment or another organic disorder. On the contrary, the client's energy and interest are centered elsewhere.

Objective observations of cognitive changes are evident in speech and written communication. The client's conversation may shift from one topic to another irrelevantly and sometimes incoherently. The client may make up new words and phrases with no meaning to others but highly significant definitions for her. For example, a woman, upset with her nurse, makes this statement: "The nurse is meaquous and has vinlengenge, and she will get a hyptismytous statement from me about her behavior."

Disturbances in thought content manifest themselves primarily through delusions or false beliefs. The woman expresses her ideas and interpretations about stimuli in a manner different from those of others in the same environment. Delusions are the most frequently observed phenomena in this category.

Perceptual Changes. Hallucinations in schizophrenia can affect any of the five senses. In addition, nurses also should be aware of kinesthetic hallucinations (altered bodily states affecting different organ systems). Among clients of childbearing age, the nurse might encounter those who think they are pregnant but are not. Conversely, nurses also could encounter women who are pregnant but who state, emphatically, that they are not and attribute accompanying physical changes to some other process. Some might deny any changes whatsoever.

Clients with schizophrenia also can misinterpret things in the environment. For instance, they may perceive string on the clinic floor to be a snake. Such a phenomenon is referred to as an *illusion.*

Physical Changes. During the early stage of schizophrenia, clients might present with sweaty palms, dilated pupils, and mild tachycardia. Other changes may include psychomotor activity (eg, restlessness), which often occurs in those who have been taking psychotropic medications over an extended period.

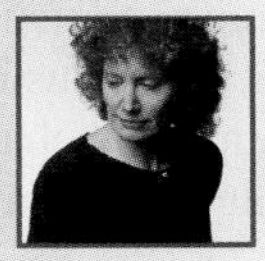

Gladys says she hears voices. What evidence would the nurse identify as suggesting that Gladys is experiencing disturbances in thought perception and content?

Interpersonal Disturbances. Various behaviors in schizophrenia can be bizarre and inappropriate for social norms. For example, a client might interrupt conversations, mutilate body parts with knives, bang her head repeatedly, or attempt suicide. She might pick her nose in public, cough over others, introduce inappropriate topics, or laugh about things that typically provoke sadness and remorse in others.

Disturbances in Motor Function. The client might no longer interact with others. With *catatonia* (see Table 5.2), the client becomes rigid and unresponsive to the environment. This rare condition is an extreme response to crisis, such as when a woman with schizophrenia experiences a miscarriage or stillbirth.

Collaborative Management

Primary assessment for schizophrenia includes interviewing and direct observation. The interview focuses on signs and symptoms, degree of impaired thought processes, risk for injury or violence toward self or others, and available support. If the client's reports are unreliable because of the severity of the illness, a family member or friend may be called on to supply pertinent information about the client's health history.

Treatment for clients with schizophrenia requires collaboration from all members of the health care team, as well as the client, family, and other support people. Nursing Care Plan 5.1 highlights the care of a pregnant woman with schizophrenia. The team individualizes the plan for the particular client's needs, strengths, and limitations.

In the early stages of treatment, health care providers should focus on improving the client's sense of reality. The nurse should involve the woman in conversations and activities about real events, particularly in the event of hallucinations and delusions. The nurse should not engage in arguments about such content. Rather, he or she should gently introduce doubt and attempt to shift the client's focus to other activities (eg, taking a walk, looking at a magazine).

Because the client's language can be confusing and disorganized, the nurse should listen and try to clarify meaning. He or she should be alert for any behavior or speech that indicates mounting aggression or agitation. Such manifestations usually require an emergency response.

One of the most difficult aspects of schizophrenia for clients is the social isolation it tends to impose. The chronic and inconsistent nature of the illness, even when controlled with medication, can make forming and maintaining friendships and social outlets difficult. By using therapeutic communication, the nurse can model behaviors to help the client improve social skills and learn ways to build rapport with others.

The nurse should assess the knowledge of the woman's family regarding schizophrenia. Relatives may require teaching about the illness, its symptom management, the necessity of following the therapeutic regimen, signs of relapse, and lifestyle accommodations. Schizophrenia imposes not only enormous physical and psychological difficulties but also challenges relative to employment, finances, social support, and ability for self-care. The client's support from others is pivotal, particularly in terms of helping her to follow the treatment plan and to assist with monitoring for signs of relapse or exacerbation.

Eating Disorders

QUOTE 5-3

"I was totally immersed in self-starvation . . . I kept running into people who hadn't seen me in awhile. They all looked shocked . . . 'You're so thin. You don't look like yourself any more!' "

Annie Ciseaux, 1980

In the past 30 years, the number of reported cases of bulimia nervosa and anorexia nervosa has increased (Mitchell-Gielegham et al., 2002). Currently, 5% to 10% of women have an eating disorder; 90% of these women are in the childbearing years (Little & Lowkes, 2000). Pregnant women with a history of eating disorders seem to be at high risk for birth and neonatal complications (Kouba et al., 2005).

Several theories exist about the etiology of eating disorders; most researchers believe that they result from complex interactions among biologic, environmental, and sociocultural factors. Additional contributors may include family functioning style and stress.

Assessment Findings

Anorexia nervosa is characterized by disturbed body image, extreme fear about being fat, and emaciation. The primary indicators are a refusal to eat and weight below 85% of normal for age and height (APA, 2000). Despite objective evidence, these women view their extremely thin bodies as fat. Preoccupation with food and dieting may extend to fixating on particular body parts these clients see as "defective"; obsessions with cooking for others; and extreme exercise. Women with anorexia tend to be compliant, obedient perfectionists, achieving in school, sports, employment, and other objectively measured endeavors. Physiologic consequences of self-starvation are severe and often life-threatening. They include hypotension, bradycardia, hypothermia, chronic constipation, and electrolyte imbalances. Many of these clients experience amenorrhea (cessation of menstruation).

Bulimia nervosa is characterized by the consumption of extreme amounts of food (*bingeing*), with subsequent behaviors to eliminate the excess calories (*purging*). Many women with bulimia binge and purge secretly; their weights may be normal. Clients with bulimia consume incredible calories in short periods (2000 to 3000 per episode), called **bingeing.** To prevent associated

NURSING CARE PLAN 5.1

The Pregnant Client With Psychoses

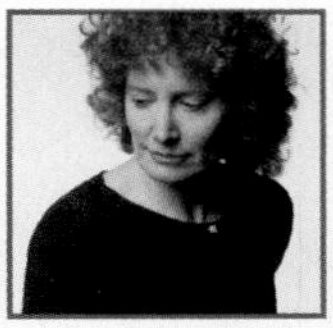

Recall Gladys, the 35-year-old client from the beginning of the chapter. Further assessment reveals slightly elevated blood pressure and pulse; history of cigarette smoking, approximately 1 pack/day for the past 15 years; and client reports that something is aggravating her. Review of the health history reveals remissions and exacerbations of schizophrenia over several years. Assessment of pregnancy status indicates that gestation is progressing normally; however, the client has not yet received any prenatal care. The physician assigned to the case prescribes chlorpromazine (Thorazine) to manage the client's schizophrenic symptoms.

NURSING DIAGNOSES

- **Disturbed Sensory Perception, Auditory** related to hearing voices.
- **Disturbed Thought Processes** related to underlying schizophrenia and hallucinations
- **Risk for Injury** related to auditory hallucinations and medication therapy and possible associated extrapyramidal side effects and dystonic reactions

EXPECTED OUTCOMES

1. The client will verbalize an accurate interpretation of her environment.
2. The client will report fewer episodes of hearing voices.
3. The client will use appropriate measures to deal with voices.
4. The client will experience minimal to no adverse effects of drug therapy.

INTERVENTIONS	RATIONALES
Use active listening, knowledge, and skills; accept the client as she presents herself. Develop a trusting relationship with her.	Listening helps elicit more information to use during overall treatment. Avoiding approaches that the client does not understand or cannot implement facilitates trust. The therapeutic relationship allows the client to attain basic health goals for herself and the fetus.
Determine the intensity and frequency of hallucinations and whether they have ever been commanding.	Close observation of the client's behavior provides information about how she is responding and the degree to which hallucinations control her behavior.
Review changes and sensations associated with pregnancy. Discuss hallucinations with the client and help her gain control over them. Request that the client take notice of the frequency, duration, and intensity of the sensations.	Knowledge about pregnancy's physical progression helps the client understand the changes and sensations that she experiences. Teaching her to identify reality from sensations could help her feel "in charge," enhance her health literacy, and empower her to take control of the situation.
If the client is hearing voices, do not argue about whether the experience is real.	Arguing could increase the client's anxiety, disrupt the therapeutic relationship, and decrease the chances that she will return to the clinic.

Continued

NURSING CARE PLAN 5.1 ● The Pregnant Client With Psychoses *(Continued)*

INTERVENTIONS	RATIONALES
Communicate understanding of the client's feelings and sensations as real. Provide reality testing, assuring the client that the fetus is not talking to her or threatening to jump out.	Honest, clear communication fosters trust, promotes the therapeutic relationship, and enhances the effectiveness of the interventions.
Assess the client for drug and alcohol use and abuse; include over-the-counter medications and herbal preparations.	Substances can alter sensory, perceptual, and cognitive functioning. Substance abuse can have deleterious effects on both mother and fetus.
Assist client with referral to mental health services.	Mental health services aid in providing necessary therapy to treat the underlying disorder.
Administer drug therapy as prescribed; instruct the client in the specifics of the drug regimen, including the need to comply with therapy.	Antipsychotic drug therapy is a primary mode of treatment. Compliance with therapy is essential to control the client's signs and symptoms.

EVALUATION

1. The client verbalizes a realistic view of her environment, stating that the fetus is not communicating with her.
2. The client reports that episodes of hearing voices have decreased to approximately once per week.
3. The client uses appropriate strategies to deal with voices.
4. The client demonstrates no signs and symptoms of extrapyramidal effects or dystonic reactions.

NURSING DIAGNOSIS

Deficient Knowledge related to prenatal care and underlying schizophrenia

EXPECTED OUTCOMES

1. The client will verbalize understanding of teaching and instructions.
2. The client will return for scheduled follow-up appointments.
3. The client will identify danger signs and symptoms that need to be reported immediately.

INTERVENTIONS	RATIONALES
Assess the client's knowledge about pregnancy, labor, and birth.	This information provides a baseline from which to develop an individualized plan of care based on the client's needs.
Instruct the client in prenatal care measures, including strategies to promote optimal fetal growth and development and methods to cope with common discomforts of pregnancy. Review the progression of pregnancy and signs and symptoms of labor, including true and false labor and danger signs and symptoms to report.	Adequate knowledge of care measures enhances the client's sense of control over the situation, thereby promoting a positive self-image.

Continued

NURSING CARE PLAN 5.1 ● The Pregnant Client With Psychoses

INTERVENTIONS	RATIONALES
Instruct the client in her medication regimen; teach her the signs and symptoms of adverse effects to report immediately.	Adherence to the medication regimen is key. Prompt reporting of adverse effects minimizes the risk for injury.
Create a written schedule of follow-up appointments; stress the need to keep them.	A written schedule serves as a reminder for the client and reinforces what is discussed.
Have the client repeat teaching information.	Repeating information aids in determining the effectiveness of teaching.
Assist with referral to social services as appropriate.	Social service referral can help meet the client's needs and ensure follow-up.

EVALUATION

1. The client states that she understands the teaching and instructions.
2. The client adheres to the schedule of follow-up visits.
3. The client states which signs and symptoms are dangerous and need to be reported immediately.

weight gain, they induce vomiting, use laxatives, exercise obsessively, or employ a combination of these methods. Like their counterparts with anorexia, typical clients with bulimia are high achievers. Physiologic complications include changes in heart rate and rhythm, gastric dilation, menstrual irregularities, and electrolyte imbalances. The tooth enamel of these clients frequently becomes eroded from frequent contact with gastric fluids, leading to excessive cavities.

Collaborative Management

Treatment of eating disorders is often difficult (Mohr, 2006). Many of these clients deny their problems. Most require a combination of therapies: individual and group psychotherapy, behavioral therapy, cognitive-behavioral therapy, and family therapy. Medications generally are not a primary treatment measure; however, antidepressants, antianxiety drugs, lithium, and anticonvulsants have been reported useful.

The client requires a thorough physical examination. The nurse should obtain weight, history of previous high and low weights, and chronology of recent weight fluctuations. He or she should question the rate of weight loss or gain and any associated circumstances. The nurse also should ask the client to describe typical food and fluid intake, any problems related to elimination (eg, constipation, diarrhea), and whether she regularly menstruates. He or she should question the client about types of exercise, difficulty sleeping, and energy level. Additionally, laboratory and cardiac testing can be done to look for electrolyte abnormalities and cardiac dysfunction.

Interventions focus largely on measures to restore nutritional balance. Other measures are geared toward encouraging realistic thinking processes, improving the client's self-esteem and body image, and assisting the client to develop effective coping and problem-solving strategies. In extreme cases of self-starvation, the client is hospitalized and receives intravenous or enteral feedings until nutritional balance is restored.

Intimate Partner Violence

Intimate partner violence (IPV) is real or threatened physical, sexual, emotional, or psychological abuse perpetrated against a spouse or life partner; it includes measures to control another person's actions. Women who experience intimate partner violence are at risk for depression, anxiety, eating disorders, alcoholism, posttraumatic stress disorder, and numerous other maladies (Coker et al., 2005).

Approximately 4 million U.S. women experience IPV each year (CDC, 2004; Greenfeld et al., 1998). This total includes pregnant women, who are most likely to be struck in the abdomen. Such abuse places the fetus at risk for low birth weight and other detrimental conditions such as brain damage and broken limbs (Boy & Salihu, 2004; Curry & Harvey, 1998).

IPV occurs in both heterosexual and homosexual relationships. Because the overwhelming majority of cases are perpetrated by men against women, however, the following discussions focus on heterosexual relationships.

Cycle of IPV

The woman in an abusive relationship is conflicted. On the one hand, she is satisfied with and accepts the good aspects of her partner and does not want to lose him. On the other hand, she must endure abuse to remain with him. Nurses who have researched the interpersonal components of IPV have proposed that it is a dynamic process with several phases: binding, enduring, disengaging, and recovering (Landenburger, 1998). The long process from binding to recovery is not linear but involves a series of triggers, maintenance behaviors, disturbances in identity, and eventually, the regaining of identity and recovery.

Binding Phase. During this phase, the woman believes that the support and love of her partner can fill her dreams for romance and commitment. She makes concerted efforts to satisfy the partner and to do what will make him happy. There may be warning signs, however, characterized by disconcerting behaviors. Nevertheless, the woman overlooks them and continues to try to please her partner.

Enduring Phase. Abuse begins to dominate more of the relationship. The woman continues to highly value the relationship while enduring the abuse. Frequently, she blames herself, thinking that her own behavior justifies the partner's reaction. She begins to lose her identity; her self-esteem wanes. The partner treats her as if she is an object or invisible, except when he needs her to satisfy his needs. The conflict intensifies: if she tries to leave, there is the possibility that the partner will kill or harm her. If she stays, the partner might kill her, she could kill herself, or she might kill herself and her partner.

Disengaging Phase. This phase begins when the abused woman identifies with other women who are being or have been abused. Conflict abides, but this time it is related to struggles over loyalty to the relationship and loyalty to self. The woman is likely to be amenable to professional help and might actually seek counseling or report to others that she is unsafe. She begins to communicate with herself about the abusive situation, thinking that if she remains in the relationship, she will not survive. When feelings of empowerment begin to emerge, the woman actually might become frightened and overwhelmed.

Recovering Phase. The women will need to readjust to life away from the abusive partner and regain balance. At this point, she is focused on self-survival and the continued existence of any children. Moreover, the woman is aware that her experiences of abuse have influenced her attitudes toward and behaviors in the world. Here recovery will continue, as she struggles to derive meaning from the experiences and search for meaning in her new existence. This process can take years. It also requires the help of supportive and informed professionals, family members, and friends.

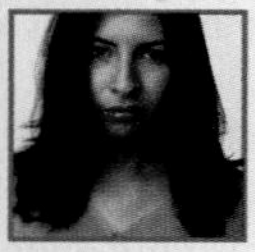

Suppose that Maria reports that her husband has hit her on numerous occasions after drinking. She states, "I've really been pushing him to find a job lately so that we'd have more money, especially when the baby comes. I guess he's been under a lot of stress." Maria is in which phase of the process?

Collaborative Management

When a nurse suspects that a client is experiencing abuse, he or she performs an assessment to detect this problem (Assessment Tool 5.1). Time is a persistent problem in such cases; however, screening can be simple. Two basic questions are, "Has a past or current partner ever caused you to be afraid?" and "Has a past or current partner ever physically hurt you?" (Hinderliter et al., 1998). Nursing Care Plan 5.2 highlights the care of a woman experiencing IPV.

Landenburger (1998) has developed interventions for each phase of IPV:

- **Binding:** The woman, at this time, does not perceive herself as abused and is not willing to use this concept to define her predicament. The nurse should help the client identify what she wants for herself; however, he or she must tell the client that she is being abused. The nurse should assist the woman to identify those behaviors exhibited by the partner that are abusive. The nurse also should help the woman strengthen her self-esteem and self-concept.
- **Enduring:** In cases of IPV, psychological and physical abuse can become the essence of the relationship. The good sense of self that the woman once experienced slips away. The nurse should help the client understand that the abuse will not end and that the partner will continue to blame her for the situation. The nurse also should support the client to deal with shame about the abuse and help her move beyond covering for her partner. In these ways, the woman can realize that she is confronted with danger and needs intervention and support.
- **Disengaging:** At this time, the woman constantly deals with her feelings of fear and shame. The nurse should reinforce that the partner can be dealt with within the legal, health care, and social systems. The

(text continues on page 195)

ASSESSMENT TOOL 5.1 Intimate Partner Violence Documentation Form

INTIMATE PARTNER VIOLENCE DOCUMENTATION FORM

Explain to Client: The majority of what you tell me is confidential and cannot be shared with anyone without your written permission. However, I am required by law to report information pertaining to child or adult abuse and gunshot wounds or life-threatening injuries.

STEP 1–Establish total privacy to ask screening questions. Safety is the first priority. Client must be alone, or if the client has a child with her, the child must not be of verbal age. ONLY complete this form if YOU CAN assure the client's safety, privacy, and confidentiality.

STEP 2–Ask the client screening questions.

"Because abuse is so common, we are now asking all of our female clients:

Are you in a relationship in which you are being hurt or threatened, emotionally or physically?
___Yes ___ No

Do you feel unsafe at home?"
___Yes ___ No

If both screening questions are NO in STEP 2, and you are not concerned that the client may be a victim, sign and date the form in the signature block directly below. Provide information and resources as appropriate.

Signature ______________________ **Title** ______________________ **Date** ____________

If both screening answers are NO and you are concerned that the client may be a victim, go to STEP 5. If the client answers YES to either question, proceed to STEP 3 below. Sign and date the signature block on the back of the form after completing STEP 6.

STEP 3–Assess the abuse and safety of the client and any children

Say to client: "From the answers you have just given me, I am worried for you."

"Has the relationship gotten worse, or is it getting scarier?" ___Yes ___ No

"Does your partner ever watch you closely, follow you, or stalk you?" ___Yes ___ No

Ask the following question in clinic settings only. Do not ask in home settings:

"If your partner is here with you today, are you afraid to leave with him/her?" ___Yes ___ No

"Is there anything else you want to tell me?" ____
____
____
____

Name: ______________________
ID No: ______________________
Date of Birth: ______________________

DH 3202, 2/03
Stock Number: 5744-000-3202-2

Continued

ASSESSMENT TOOL 5.1 Intimate Partner Violence Documentation Form *(Continued)*

"Are there children in the home?" ___Yes ___ No

If the answer to the question above is "yes," say to client: "I'm concerned for your safety and the safety of your children. You and your children deserve to be at home without feeling afraid."

"Have there been threats of abuse or direct abuse of the children?" ___Yes ___ No

STEP 4–Assess client's physical injuries and health conditions, past and present

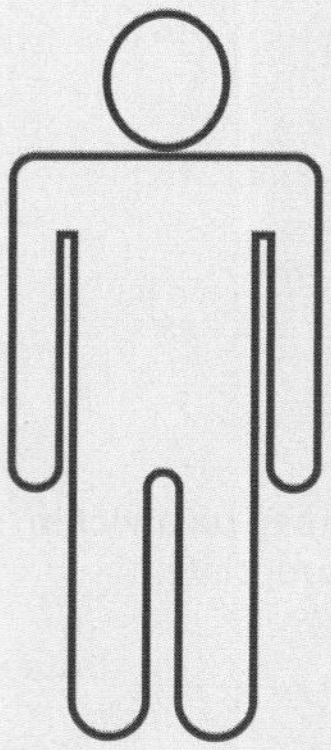

Observations/Comments/Interventions:

____
____
____
____
____
____
____
____
____

STEP 5–If both screening answers are NO, and you ARE CONCERNED that the client may be a victim:

a. Say to the client: "All of us know of someone at some time in our lives who is abused. So, I am providing you with information in the event you or a friend may need it in the future."

b. Document under comments in Step 6.

STEP 6–Information, referrals, or reports made

Yes No

___ ___ 1. Client given domestic violence information including safety planning
___ ___ 2. Reviewed domestic violence information including safety planning
___ ___ 3. State Abuse Hotline (1-800-96-ABUSE) and State Domestic Violence Hotline number (1-800-500-1119) given to the client
___ ___ 4. Client called hotline during visit
___ ___ 5. Client seen by advocate during visit
___ ___ 6. Report made. If yes, to whom: ______________________________

Comments

____
____
____
____
____
____

Signature ______________________ Title ______________ Date ____________

NURSING CARE PLAN 5.2

The Client Who Is Being Abused

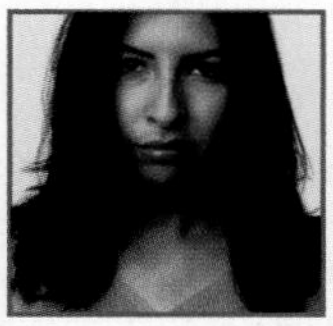

Recall Maria, the 30-year-old multipara in her 6th month of gestation. During the visit, Maria complains about feeling tired. She says that she thinks that she needs vitamins and, maybe, some food vouchers. At one point in the interview, she quietly mentions a concern about her husband hitting her when he is "drinking and drugging." She states, "When he is sober, he doesn't remember it. And he doesn't believe me either, even when I show him the bruises. I've thought about leaving him, but I have no money."

Further assessment reveals frequent awakening during the middle of the night with the inability to return to sleep; intermittent crying during the day; and decreased appetite with a failure to gain weight over the past 2 months. "I don't know if I have the strength to take care of two small children and a new baby. I'm worried about everything. Sometimes I wonder if it is worth trying to carry on."

NURSING DIAGNOSES

- **Ineffective Coping** related to current life stressors, overwhelming demands of situation, and lack of support
- **Situational Low Self-Esteem** related to feelings of inferiority secondary to cultural background and current life stressors
- **Risk for Injury** (self and fetus), related to husband's episodes of violence, failure to gain weight in pregnancy, and difficulty sleeping
- **Fear** related to husband's violent episodes

EXPECTED OUTCOMES

1. The client will identify stressors affecting her life.
2. The client will identify positive methods for dealing with current stressors.
3. The client will verbalize at least one positive aspect of herself by the end of the visit.
4. The client will identify possible sources of support and assistance.
5. The client (and fetus) will remain safe.
6. The client will identify appropriate measures to deal with husband's violent episodes.

INTERVENTIONS	RATIONALES
Assess the client's level of understanding about pregnancy and its associated changes, intimate partner violence, and the effects of stress on herself and her fetus.	This information provides a baseline for identifying specific client needs and developing an individualized plan.
Discuss with the client her concerns, feelings, and perceptions related to pregnancy, her family (including her husband's violent episodes), and how they are affecting the current family situation.	Discussion provides opportunities to emphasize positive aspects of the current situation; verbalization of concerns aids in establishing sources of stress and problem areas to address.
Inquire about methods used to cope with past stressful situations; encourage the client to use positive methods that were successful; provide additional suggestions for ways to cope with the current situation.	Use of past successful methods enhances the chance of current success. Additional suggestions to deal with the current situation aid in relieving stress associated with outside variables and events, provide more options, and thereby promote a greater feeling of control.

Continued

INTERVENTIONS	RATIONALES
Review with the client measures to ensure a healthy pregnancy, including the need for adequate nutrition and sleep and rest.	Pregnancy places added demands on the woman's body; adequate nutrition, sleep, and rest are essential for fetal growth and development.
Arrange for the client to speak with nutritionist to aid in meal planning.	Adequate nutritional intake is necessary for optimal fetal growth and development as well as for prevention of complications that would compound the client's current stress.
Review with the client known behaviors associated with intimate partner violence; help the client correlate the husband's behaviors with them; assist the client to acknowledge that she is being abused.	Identification of known behaviors provides a base for comparison, giving support to the fact that the client is being abused. Acknowledging the reality of the abuse is a first step in stopping it.
Assist the client to identify her desires and goals for her own life.	Identification of client's wishes is important in developing strategies appropriate for her.
Provide the client with accurate facts and communicate openly; answer questions honestly.	Open honest communication promotes trust and helps to correct any misconceptions or misinformation.
Review and reinforce the client's positive attributes about her self and her abilities; reinforce with the client that husband's violent episodes are not "her fault."	Targeting positive attributes provides a foundation for enhancing self-esteem and aids in the realization that the client has an identity, can care for herself and her children, and is worthy of assistance.
Assist the client in measures to promote her safety; help her develop a plan for leaving the partner, including strategies for safe departure. Provide suggestions for storing resources such as money, clothing, and keys in a safe place and for places to go such as shelters or houses of friends.	The client's safety is paramount. Preplanning aids in minimizing risks and enhances the chances of a successful, safe departure.
Discuss with the client available community services. Inquire about any friends or family who could help.	Additional support can alleviate the stress of the client's current situation and provide her with options should problems arise.
Assist with referral to social services for additional support in areas such as finances; arrange for possible referral to Women, Infants, and Children (WIC) program.	Social services can provide additional mechanisms for support and guidance. The WIC program aids in promoting adequate nutrition for the mother and her children.
Provide the client with emergency contact numbers, with instructions to call at any time.	Having emergency contact numbers readily available promotes safety.
Institute a referral for home care services; arrange for a follow-up visit in 1 week.	Follow-up with home care and return visits aids in evaluating the effectiveness of interventions and changes in the client's situation. Such measures provide an opportunity for additional teaching, support, and guidance.

EVALUATION

1. The client accurately identifies the multiple stressors affecting her life.
2. The client demonstrates at least two positive coping strategies for dealing with stressors.
3. The client identifies positive attributes in herself.
4. The client states that she will use available sources of support.
5. The client and fetus exhibit no further evidence of injury, with the client's pregnancy progressing without incident.
6. The client implements strategies to protect herself and children from further violence.

nurse should assist the client to realize that she can successfully leave the partner. Careful assessment of the client's safety is essential; the nurse should outline strategies to ensure a safe departure. Together, the nurse and client should consider safe places, shelters, and housing with family members. The focus is on helping the client to achieve a sense of self-worth and to realize that she has an identity, is competent to care for herself, and is worthy of the help that she has and will receive.

- **Recovering:** During this phase, the woman assumes control of her own life. She needs employment and perhaps therapy to sort out the nature and components of the previous relationship. With time, she must assign the abuse that she experienced to the source (her partner) and let go of feeling like she caused the abuse. Then, the woman needs to perceive the abusive partner as a person once, but no longer, in her life. The nurse can help the woman work through feelings of worthlessness, self-doubt, depression, and vulnerability, lest she become involved in another abusive relationship.

Nurses who provide care for women should always be aware of local resources in the community from which women can receive help. The National Clearing House number is 1-800-799-SAFE. Other strategies for assisting clients are outlined in Box 5.2.

BOX 5.2 Protecting Safety in Intimate Partner Violence

- Identify safe retreats for the client when the potential for violence exists. If she cannot escape, alert her to avoid rooms where no exit is possible and rooms that may hold weapons (eg, kitchen).
- Alert the client to memorize phone numbers of people who can help during violent episodes. Advise her to develop a code with phone contacts to alert them to the need for assistance.
- Give the client contact information for one or more domestic shelters. Such shelters house women and children for 1 to 2 months and provide food and counseling for employment, finances, and new residences.
- Explain how to obtain a *personal protection order* (a document that forbids contact between the abuser and victim for a specified period) or a *temporary restraining order* (a legal document that requires the abuser to avoid all contact with the victim).
- Encourage the client to press charges against the abuser.
- Suggest that police or a friend photograph physical injuries for use in future court cases.
- Offer phone numbers of community mental health therapists available for crisis intervention and family counseling.
- Recommend discussing personal safety with employer security.

Substance Abuse

Substance abuse contributes significantly to rates of morbidity and mortality. Problems with alcohol and drugs contribute to physical illnesses such as cardiovascular disorders, liver disease, and infections; they also are associated with domestic violence, crime, and accidents. Commonly abused drugs include alcohol, marijuana, cocaine, heroin, hallucinogens, and amphetamines.

Causes

Substance abuse often starts with experimentation, progresses to psychological and physical dependence, and finally becomes an addiction. Some people abuse drugs in a dysfunctional effort to cope with psychosocial stressors or other disorders. For example, many women with depression or anxiety turn to alcohol or drugs to mitigate the effects of their primary psychiatric illness. That is to say, these women use substances to "self-treat" their depression. Potentially, however, the reverse is also true. Women who use substances may become depressed because of their use.

Concerns Related to Pregnancy

Use of drugs, alcohol, or both during pregnancy poses serious risks, regardless of the reasons for use. Among such dangers are premature labor, abruptio placentae, stillbirth, and numerous other complications (Mazure et al., 2002). Alcohol-related teratogenic effects put the fetus at risk for various disorders. *Fetal alcohol syndrome* includes the problems of mental retardation, microcephaly, hypoplastic philtrum and maxilla, and attention deficit hyperactivity disorder during childhood (see Chap. 22) (Hales & Yudofsky, 2003). Maternal use of cocaine causes intrauterine growth retardation and organ malformations. Moreover, preterm labor, abruptio placentae, and numerous other conditions are likely because of cocaine's ability to constrict normal blood flow. The neonate could experience withdrawal symptoms lasting for months, a time when growth and development are important to overall survival (Ness et al., 1999).

Much like cocaine, heroin has potentially devastating fetal effects. Withdrawal symptoms for mother, infant, or both include irritability, poor feeding, respiratory complications, tremulousness, and other neuropsychological difficulties. Heroin use also is linked to sudden infant death syndrome (SIDS). Women can be treated with methadone, and those women who receive treatment will have a better chance of having a positive pregnancy outcome than those women who are not treated (Hales & Yudofsky, 2003).

Collaborative Management

Initiating treatment is one of the most difficult hurdles. Clients rationalize or deny their addiction, or blame other people or external circumstances for their habits.

Often, they must "hit bottom" before getting help. Clients in recovery need to learn new methods of coping with stressors, repair relationships, and develop interests and activities to fill the time once devoted to alcohol or drugs.

Many clients benefit from treatment plans that involve abstinence, counseling, and peer support. Twelve-step programs are free and provide specific guidelines for becoming and remaining free from substance abuse. Frequent attendance at meetings where members share their experiences and discuss topics related to recovery is essential.

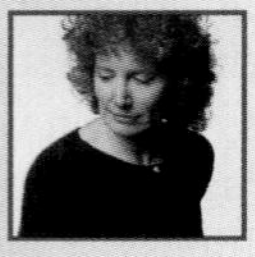

Think back to Gladys, the woman at the beginning of the chapter who reports hearing voices. What if she states, "With all this commotion, I could really use a drink." How should the nurse respond?

PSYCHOPHARMACOLOGIC THERAPY DURING PREGNANCY OR LACTATION

The use of pharmacologic agents to manage psychiatric problems during pregnancy and lactation poses challenges for both health care providers and clients (Allison, 2004; Usher et al., 2005). Such agents can be detrimental to fetal or newborn development and health; some of these medications are totally contraindicated during pregnancy. At the same time, many women who stop taking these medications when they are trying to conceive or after they become pregnant suffer relapses or exacerbations of their conditions. In some cases, maternal health or safety is compromised because of a lack of psychotropic medication, which, in turn, also can compromise fetal and newborn health.

Primary health care providers must always remember that medicating a pregnant woman is a serious undertaking requiring great caution. During pregnancy, a basic assumption is that all psychotropic medications cross the blood–placenta barrier. Placental transport occurs through simple diffusion; the amount of diffusion is linked to the drug's molecular size, amount of protein binding, polarity, lipid solubility, and frequency and duration of exposure. For the most part, a drug's safety during pregnancy is based on outcomes from monitoring therapeutic plasma levels of nonpsychotropic medications (Schatzberg & Nemeroff, 2004). Even though the mother and fetus share the same blood circulation, fetal characteristics could increase the fetus's risk for exposure to the psychotropic medication, resulting in increased drug concentrations in the developing central nervous system. Potential outcomes are increased cardiac output, augmented blood–brain barrier permeability, decreased plasma protein and plasma-binding activity, and reduced hepatic enzyme activity (Schatzberg & Nemeroff, 2004).

The use of psychotropic agents during lactation, too, requires special attention. First, the newborn hepatic system is still evolving after birth and does so with great variability among infants. Delay of hepatic development is likely among premature and low-birth-weight infants. Second, the neonate's glucuronidation and oxidation systems are immature. The potential for high serum concentrations and metabolites of any drug needs careful and deliberate clinical consideration (Schatzberg & Nemeroff, 2004). Third, glomerular filtration and tubular secretions in neonates are 30% to 40% and 20% to 30% lower, respectively, than those in adults. The American Academy of Pediatrics (AAP) Committee on Drugs (2001) has published important information on drugs and other chemicals in breast milk. Knowledge about a drug's specific risk classification is helpful in making determination about the safety of its use in pregnancy or lactation (Box 5.3).

BOX 5.3 Risk–Benefit Assessment for Lactation

The information is divided into three sections: what is known, what is being considered, and what is unknown.

Known Knowledge

- Breastfeeding is beneficial for the infant.
- All professional organizations consider breastfeeding to be the best form of nutrition for the infant.
- Less than 60% of women plan to breastfeed during the puerperium.
- Approximately 5% to 17% of all nursing women take a prescription drug during their breastfeeding activities.
- Approximately 12% to 20% of nursing mothers smoke cigarettes.
- The postnatal period is a high-risk time for onset or relapse of psychiatric illness.
- All psychotropic medications with scientific data available are considered to be excreted in breast milk.

Increasing Data

- Untreated maternal mental illness has an adverse effect on mother–infant attachment and later infant development.
- The adverse effects of psychotropic agents on infants are limited to case reports.
- The nursing infant's daily dose of psychotropic agents is less than the maternal daily dose.
- Psychotropic medications are excreted into breast milk with a specific time course, allowing the minimization of infant exposure with continuation of breastfeeding.

Unknown

- The long-term neurobehavioral effects of infant exposure to psychotropic medications through breastfeeding are unknown.

Adapted from Schatzberg, A. F., & Nemeroff, C. B. (2004). *The American Psychiatric Publishing textbook of clinical pharmacology* (3rd ed.). Washington, DC: American Psychiatric Publishing.

Determining Risks and Benefits

The health care provider and client need to evaluate the risks and benefits of maternal drug therapy during pregnancy or lactation, even though, to date, little empirical research exists to inform clinicians (Schatzberg & Nemeroff, 2004). Limited large-scale epidemiologic studies addressing the adverse effects of untreated mental illness among pregnant or lactating women leaves many questions unexplored, among which are the potential adverse effects of psychopharmacologic treatment and the short-term and long-term outcomes for the infant. The nurse should be alert to mental illness during pregnancy or lactation. It is important to be especially cautious for psychotic disorders, such as schizophrenia and schizoaffective disorders (a subtype of schizophrenia that involves features of a thought disorder and mood disturbances), and depression, all of which are likely to worsen during pregnancy.

The U.S. Food and Drug Administration (FDA) has not approved psychotropic agents for the treatment of mental illness during pregnancy or lactation. The FDA has, however, developed a classification system for clinicians to use as a guide when prescribing medications (Table 5.3). This system and current research have helped with the creation of three categories of somatic risk to the fetus or newborn with the use of psychotropic agents during pregnancy or lactation (Altshuler et al., 1996):

1. Teratogenicity and organ malformation
2. Neonatal toxicity
3. Neurobehavioral and developmental teratogenic effects (Schatzberg & Nemeroff, 2004)

Clearly, all these outcomes would be deleterious to the infant and the family.

Commonly Used Agents for Psychiatric Disorders

National trends suggest that people are receiving more psychopharmacologic treatment and less psychotherapy or interpersonal therapy for psychiatric disorders, although nonpharmacologic treatments remain important. Family therapy, individual therapy, cognitive therapy, and relaxation therapy, and so forth are viable options and should be considered appropriate. Nevertheless, an additional resource is medications. The intent of the following discussion is to acquaint nurses with the options in treatment and at the same time to alert all health providers to the potential dangers associated with the agents.

Antidepressants

The marketing of effective antidepressants with few side effects and enhanced therapeutic benefits is one major reason for the shift away from nonpharmacologic treatment modalities for the various types of depression (Olfson et al., 2002). For pregnant or lactating women, however, management of mood disorders may require exclusive reliance on nonpharmacologic methods, such as psychotherapy, for the safety of both mother and fetus.

Tricyclic Antidepressants (TCAs). TCAs have been on the market for some time. No clear-cut relationship has been established between their maternal use and congenital malformations (Eberhard-Gran et al., 2005). During labor, it is not yet established clearly if these drugs affect woman or infant.

The AAP Committee on Drugs (2001) has suggested that clinicians proceed with caution because support for the use of TCAs for lactating women is not documented clearly. Agents such as amitriptyline (Elavil, Endep), desipramine (Norpramin), and trazodone (Desyrel) are known to reach a peak in breast milk 4 to 6 hours after dosing. Should the infant develop health problems, the pediatrician might consider obtaining a blood sample to determine the level of medication that is in the infant's system. If the mother with depression experiences psychotic symptoms, including hallucinations, delusions, or a sense of unreality, her provider should consider antipsychotic medications (Moline et al., 2001; Schatzberg & Nemeroff, 2004; Stahl, 1996).

Monoamine Oxidase Inhibitors (MAOIs). MAOIs are listed in the FDA's C category, indicating that providers cannot rule out their risks and that human studies are

TABLE 5.3 U.S. Food and Drug Administration (FDA) Use-in-Pregnancy Ratings

CATEGORY	INTERPRETATION
A	Controlled studies show no risk: Adequate, well-controlled studies in pregnant women have failed to demonstrate risk to the fetus.
B	No evidence of risk in humans: Either animal findings show risk, but humans do not; or, if no adequate human studies have been done, animal findings are negative.
C	Risk cannot be ruled out: Human studies are lacking, and animal studies are either positive for fetal risk or lacking as well. However, potential benefits may justify the potential risk.
D	Positive evidence of risk: Investigational or postmarketing data show risk to the fetus. Nevertheless, potential benefits may outweigh risks.
X	Contraindicated in pregnancy: Studies in animals or humans, or investigational or postmarketing reports, have shown fetal risk that clearly outweighs any possible benefit to the patient.

lacking to provide the needed evidence to support or rule out definitively their use during pregnancy or lactation. Therefore, MAOIs should not be used in pregnancy or during lactation (Schatzberg et al., 2003; Stahl, 1996). Use of MAOIs also requires dietary restrictions associated with preventing hypertensive crisis, which could be dangerous during pregnancy and lactation (Schatzberg & Nemeroff, 2004). Such dangerous foods are beer, red wine, aged cheese, smoked fish, brewer's yeast, beef and chicken livers, yogurt, bananas, soy sauce, chocolate, caffeine-based beverages, and raisins (Schatzberg et al., 2003).

Selective Serotonin Reuptake Inhibitors (SSRIs). Breastfeeding mothers can be treated for depression with relative safety with SSRIs. The drug sertraline (Zoloft) is considered a safe choice for these women (Whitby & Smith, 2005). Traces of this drug enter the breast milk, but little evidence is shown in the infant's body. No detrimental side effects have been reported (Whitby & Smith, 2005).

Paroxetine (Paxil) is also a choice for use in lactating women because it is not detectable in breast milk or nursing infants. Fluoxetine (Prozac) and citalopram (Celexa) are known to enter the mother's breast milk but in small amounts. Breast milk will contain different levels of SSRIs, as determined by time between the mother taking the medications and the infant's actual nursing (Schatzberg & Nemeroff, 2004; Stahl, 1996). In a research study conducted by Stowe and associates (1997), the highest concentration of antidepressant agents in the mothers' milk occurred approximately 7 to 10 hours after maternal dosing. When the dose of sertraline was increased, sertraline and desmethylsertraline were found in breast milk. Identified infant serum concentrations were below the levels typically detected in commercial laboratories.

Mood Stabilizers

Mood stabilizers are another group of psychotropic agents used to treat mental illness, particularly bipolar disorder. Lithium carbonate (Eskalith, Lithobid, Lithonate) is the major mood stabilizer; however, lithium is contraindicated during pregnancy and lactation (Schatzberg et al., 2003). The main alternatives to lithium in pregnancy and lactation are anticonvulsant drugs. Commonly used examples are carbamazepine (Tegretol), valproic acid (Depakote), and clonazepam (Klonopin). Evidence suggests that these drugs do pose teratogenic risks (Hunt & Morrow, 2005).

Anxiolytics

Anxiolytics are a commonly used class of drugs. Benzodiazepines are the most frequently prescribed drugs for anxiety disorders; this class of drugs can accumulate in the fetus if given to the mother for a prolonged period. The half-life of benzodiazepines is longer in infants than in adults (Schatzberg & Nemeroff, 2004). These drugs should not be withdrawn abruptly from the mother; they should be tapered significantly before birth, if at all possible, to prevent infant withdrawal. Research data regarding this class of drugs are scarce, but clinicians have posited that benzodiazepines produce infant withdrawal syndromes that can last as long as 3 months (Eberhard-Gran et al., 2005).

Because such limited data are available about the use of anxiolytics during pregnancy and lactation, the clinician always uses caution when prescribing any medications for the expectant mother. During lactation, benzodiazepines administered to the woman in small doses are considered relatively safe; this class of drugs has a low milk-to–maternal serum ratio (Schatzberg & Nemeroff, 2004).

Antipsychotics

Antipsychotic drugs are used to manage schizophrenia and other thought disorders in women. Most antipsychotic medications fall in the FDA's C category of drugs, indicating that they are associated with rare anomalies, such as fetal jaundice and anticholinergic effects at birth (Schatzberg et al., 2003). The risk of administering these drugs is related to teratogenesis, and during the first trimester, the woman and infant are at risk. Again, it is assumed that all psychotropic drugs, to some degree, cross the placenta, predisposing the infant to potential problems (Usher et al., 2005). Three antipsychotics, haloperidol (Haldol), perphenazine (Trilafon), and chlorpromazine (Thorazine), have received attention from researchers, who have determined no direct link between these agents and major congenital malformations (McKenna et al., 2005; Schatzberg & Nemeroff, 2004).

Aside from teratogenic risks, several antipsychotic drugs pose potential problems for the woman, including extrapyramidal side effects and neuroleptic malignant syndromes (Schatzberg et al., 2003; Schatzberg & Nemeroff, 2004; Stahl, 1996). Table 5.4 outlines the extrapyramidal side effects and neuroleptic problems associated with antipsychotics.

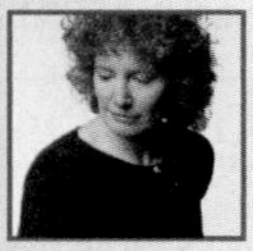

Suppose Gladys is started on chlorpromazine (Thorazine). She comes to the clinic for a visit 2 weeks later. During the visit, the nurse notices akathisia. What behaviors might the nurse observe?

NURSING CARE AND MENTAL HEALTH AND ILLNESS IN WOMEN

Nurses have many opportunities to ensure that women are knowledgeable about their own health as well as health-related concerns linked to pregnancy, lactation, and aging.

TABLE 5.4 Antipsychotic-Induced Side Effects

CONDITION INDUCED BY THE PSYCHOTROPIC MEDICATION	SIDE EFFECTS
Akathisia: a continuous, observable restlessness	● Fidgety movements ● Swinging of the legs and arms ● Foot-to-foot rocking when standing ● Pacing ● Inability to sit or stand still for more than a few minutes
Dystonia: abnormal postures and muscle spasms	● Torticollis: abnormal positioning of the head and neck ● Trismus: spasms of the jaw muscles ● Laryngeal: pharyngeal spasm, which may impair swallowing or breathing ● Macroglossia: slurred or thick speech because of enlarged tongue ● Protrusion of the tongue that is not under voluntary control ● Oculogyric crisis: eyes are positioned upward, downward, or to the side ● Abnormal positions: the limbs or trunk in abnormal positions
Parkinsonism: involuntary movements	● Parkinsonian tremor: rhythmic, intermittent oscillating movements, which may be unilateral or bilateral and affect the head, mouth, tongue, or limbs ● Muscular rigidity: extreme firmness and tensing of muscles, which may affect all skeletal muscles or discrete muscle groups ● Lead pike-like rigidity or cogwheel rigidity: forms of resistance ● Akinesia: decreased spontaneous motor activity, such as expression in facial gestures, speech, and other body movements
Tardive dyskinesia	● Involuntary movements of the tongue, jaw, trunk or extremities, which persist for 4 weeks or more and include activities such as jerky, choreiform movements; athetoid movements; rhythmic movements; typically, the condition is irreversible but treatable with varying degrees of therapeutic response
Neuroleptic malignant syndrome	● Triad of rigidity, hyperthermia, and autonomic instability ● Elevated serum creatinine kinase activity ● Risk factors include being young, preexisting neurologic disability, physical illness, dehydration, rapid advance of dosage
Sedation	● Most common side effect, most evident during the initial phase of treatment ● May cause daytime drowsiness beyond initial treatment
Anticholinergic and antiadrenergic effects	● Dry mouth, blurred vision, constipation, tachycardia, and urinary retention, which range from mild to other complications such as ileus of the bowel and others ● Impaired memory and cognition, confusion, delirium, somnolence, and hallucinations ● Tachycardia related to anticholinergic effects as well as postural hypotension
Weight gain	● Slightly less than 50% of clients experience weight gain.
Ophthalmologic effects	● Pigmentary retinopathies and corneal opacities can occur with administration of antipsychotics over time.

Adapted from Schatzberg, A. F., & Nemeroff, C. B. (2004). *The American Psychiatric Publishing textbook of clinical pharmacology* (3rd ed.). Washington, DC: American Psychiatric Publishing; and American Psychiatric Association. (1997). Practice guideline for the treatment of patients with schizophrenia. *American Journal of Psychiatry, 154*(4), 1–62.

The discussions in this section describe some basic roles and functions of nurses in these practice areas as related to women experiencing alterations in mental health and illness.

Discussing Informed Consent

Many risks are associated with psychotropic medications; these risks usually increase when a woman is pregnant or lactating. One major nursing responsibility is to ensure that the woman and her family (when appropriate) are knowledgeable about the risks of using psychotropic medications during pregnancy and lactation; this is also true for aging clients (Bonari et al., 2005). A thorough discussion of the risks versus the benefits of medications is essential. Exploring and discussing other available treatment alternatives to medications is also essential (Usher et al., 2005). See Chapter 2.

Documenting Risks Versus Benefits

Another important nursing responsibility is to document potential risks if an illness is untreated, including risks to the woman and the fetus and, eventually, to the infant as well (Schatzberg & Nemeroff, 2004). The nurse should discuss these concerns with the woman and her family. Critical decisions must be based on scientific knowledge, the client's clinical history, cultural considerations, and personal preferences. It may be helpful if the woman is pregnant or lactating to include the pediatrician in the discussion because maternal medication decisions may affect the infant.

Promoting Community and Psychosocial Interventions

The current approach to treatment for women with mental illness is to maintain them in the community as much as possible. Many women with chronic and severe mental illness are sexually active, and motherhood is either a present or future reality for them. These women require integrative mental health and physical health services, including information about sexual health, pregnancy prevention, and prenatal health. They also might need added help and support to care for children appropriately. Several community-focused interventions exist, including case management, rehabilitation, self-help groups, and day hospitalization.

QUOTE 5-4

"I really look forward to my group discussions. They help reinforce what I've learned, and I'm always finding out new information and being reminded that I am not alone."

A 57-year-old woman who has attended a self-help group for recovering alcoholics for the past 3 years

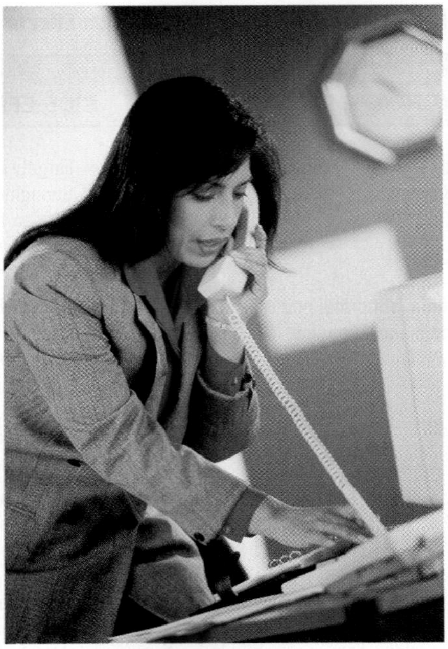

FIGURE 5.3 Everyday frustrations and pressures can accumulate and compromise the mental health of women of all ages. Effective stress management techniques can assist clients to avoid some triggering factors for psychiatric problems.

Teaching Stress Management

Most women face stress daily. Both happy and unhappy events have stress-related consequences. Planning for an extensive vacation or getting married can produce the same stress as caring for an ill relative or having financial difficulties. The plethora of obligations and responsibilities that women confront daily can produce stress in their lives (Fig. 5.3). Each type of stress causes reactions within the psyche and human body. The body typically responds with "fight or flight" techniques. Common physical reactions to stress include increased blood pressure, palpitations, tense muscles, poor or excessive appetite, and disturbed sleep. As stress increases, so do the hormones that the stress produces. Ever-present stress is not congruent with a healthy immune system, and the body reacts with colds, fatigue, sluggishness, and other warning signs. Common symptoms of stress also include being short-tempered, feeling tired frequently, eating too much or too little, sleeping too much or too little, changes in the menstrual cycle, forgetfulness, anxiety, frustration, irritability, difficulty concentrating, angering easily, crying easily, and sleep disturbances. Heart disease, diabetes, irritable bowel syndrome, depression, urinary tract infections, and asthma are some illnesses linked to stress.

Effective ways to manage stress require behavioral changes. Women must make it a priority to stay healthy and to take care of their bodies. Specific strategies such as prioritizing responsibilities, taking time to relax, exercising, becoming involved in a social support system, and having a healthy perspective on life are a few simple but powerful strategies to improve quality of life. A regular sleep routine is extremely helpful; going to bed and getting up at the same time every day is a good habit to develop. Chapter 2 discusses health promotion strategies that are beneficial to all components of the woman's life: physical, spiritual, emotional, and psychological.

Assisting With Access to Health Care

The nurse is responsible for helping clients to obtain access to the mental health care system. Doing so, however, can be challenging. Mental health clinics are typically open from 9 AM to 5 PM and closed on weekends. After hours, people with mental illness and experiencing crisis must go to emergency departments or jails, where they get whatever help these facilities make available (National Council on Disability, 2002).

Rural dwellers have few opportunities for adequate mental health services; many of them also lack health insurance. They live too far from providers, and stigma can function as a distancing mechanism (National Council on Disability, 2002; U.S. Department of Health and Human Services [USDHHS], 1999). The implementation of managed care in rural areas has helped to diminish the availability of quality services to rural women who may need mental health services.

Language and culture also can serve as barriers to mental health care. Mental health systems in the public domain lack the necessary resources required to serve some ethnic minorities, in part because clients may not speak English and the culture of clients may not be Eurocentric. The Surgeon General has described mental health disparities as striking in ethnic minorities, and these disparities impose a greater burden on people of color than their white counterparts experience (National Council on Disability, 2002; USDHHS, 1999). These burdens directly influence the potential for women of color to have a healthy pregnancy and infant. Women of color bear the greatest burden of most health and mental health disorders. They are more likely to live in poverty, not have access to health insurance, have inadequate housing or live in shelters or on the streets, experience poor health status, and have less desirable pregnancy outcomes (O'Malley et al., 2003; Taylor et al., 1991; Zimmer-Gembeck & Helfand, 1996).

There may be times when nurses need to visit jails, women's shelters, and other facilities to provide services to women and their children. In some communities, jails are the "new mental hospitals," serving thousands of people who are incarcerated and mentally ill. The number of mentally ill men and women in U.S. jails ranges from 600,000 to 1,000,000, representing about 8 times more people in jails than in psychiatric hospitals (National Council on Disability, 2002). Women who are incarcerated and mentally ill need special attention from nurses and other health care providers (Fig. 5.4).

Promoting Health Literacy: A Critical Role for Nurses

Mental health literacy means knowledge and beliefs about mental illness that help the person to recognize, manage, and prevent such disorders. This information assists women to provide self-care, facilitates treatment compliance, and provides a sense of control over personal well-being.

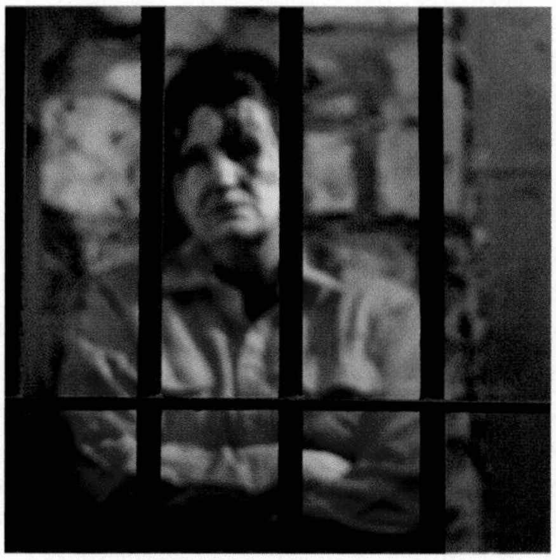

FIGURE 5.4 The number of women with mental illness and incarcerated is increasing steadily in the United States. With the push away from hospitalization and toward community-based psychiatric care, prison is the only housing alternative for some women with chronic and persistent psychiatric disorders.

A client's health literacy can be viewed as the currency she needs to negotiate with the nation's complex health system. According to "Health Literacy: Report of the Council on Scientific Affairs," health literacy is "the ability to read and understand the basic requirements in health care that will allow the person to successfully function as a patient. Such requirements include being able to read prescription bottles, understand appointment slips, and the other essential health-related materials required to better understand the illness, methods of treatment and self care responsibilities" (Health literacy, 1999, 552). Nurses are always mindful that approximately 90 million Americans have limited literacy skills. Most health-related materials are written at the 10th-grade level or above; health care literacy problems incur heavy costs, estimated to be between $50 and $73 billion dollars annually (Health literacy, 1999). Health systems also have a highly specialized language. A woman could accurately understand familiar concepts and written material but struggle to grasp content and information with new vocabulary and concepts, as in health care. Teaching Tips 5.3 provide steps to help nurses improve communications with clients and consumers.

As the demands for self-care are placed continually on women, problems with health literacy are expected to increase. It is not atypical for nurses to be in situations in which a woman receiving care cannot read health literature, accurately comprehend the directions for taking prescribed medications, or understand information about scheduled appointments or the rights and responsibilities sections of the Medicaid application form. Many clients fail to understand the standard informed consent (Williams et al., 1995). Given these findings, it is clear that nurses will need to discuss and explain those components that other providers may previously have taken for granted, erroneously assuming that clients understood and could comprehend without assistance. Nursing Care Plan 5.1 and Box 5.4 present more information related to health literacy in the care of a client experiencing hallucinations.

Questions to Ponder

1. Provide a synthesis of the theories used to explain mental health and illness. Select one theory, and detail its strengths and limitations for providing a framework for your clinical practice. Does it account for variables such as poverty, abuse, access to care, ethnicity, race, and socioeconomic status? If not, how do

TEACHING TIPS 5.3 Improving Clinician–Client Communication

Nurses should consider the following steps to improve communications with women regarding mental health and to promote mental health literacy:

- Provide written information at the appropriate reading level for the client.
- Use easy-to-follow layouts and simple pictures, especially diagrams that clarify written concepts and instructions.
- Focus discussions on desired behaviors and outcomes, not on medical terms, facts, and jargon.
- Ensure that information is culturally and personally meaningful and relevant to the woman.

Adapted from Doak, L. G., & Doak. C. C. (Eds.) (2003). *Pfizer principles for clear health communication* (2nd ed.). Potomac, MD: Pfizer Inc. Retrieved January 11, 2005, from http://www.pfizerhealthliteracy.com/improving.html.

BOX 5.4 Sample Health Literacy Approach

- Make the client comfortable; offer milk, juice, or water.
- Ask the client to update her address and to share two telephone numbers of people who would know how to get in touch with her, in case she moves to another location.
- Schedule the next clinic appointment with her; write the time on the large envelope used to store the health materials given to the client.
- Include the telephone number of the clinic, the nurse's name, and the clinic's name.
- Encourage the client to phone the clinic if she feels ill or experiences an increase in any of the symptoms of which she complained (eg, swollen feet, difficulty sleeping).
- Draw out and illustrate as much health literacy content as possible during this contact (eg, smoking, high blood pressure). Give the client copies of all materials used for teaching.
- Succinctly teach the client about her blood pressure and methods of controlling it; give her a colorful pamphlet with pictures that explains high blood pressure.
- Demonstrate feet elevation; assist the client to elevate the feet during the teaching.
- Offer a referral to the smoking cessation program located at the clinic; explain to the client the potential dangerous effects of cigarette smoking on her infant and herself.
- Discuss nutrition; give simple, matter-of-fact written information about foods that she should be eating.
- Discuss the current stage of pregnancy and present to her the physiologic changes that will occur over the next 2 months.
- Schedule a psychiatric consult for further evaluation; underscore the major concern about the voices and the thoughts about the fetus's threatening behaviors.
- Discuss the necessity of rest. Review with the client basic strategies that would help increase her chances of rest.
- Make a preliminary plan for the client's labor and delivery, and orient her to the facility while she is at the clinic. Provide the names of clinic personnel to increase the sense of belonging and connectedness.

these factors influence your plan of care, and to what extent is the theory helpful to you?

2. Of the psychiatric disorders presented, develop a grid that portrays the signs, symptoms, and predominant behaviors associated with each of the disorders. List the reasons for treating or referring the woman for specialty care. Determine the desired outcomes for treating the woman and the potential deleterious consequences for not treating her. Include the fetus or child in all comments. Can you create a scenario in which the woman with a serious mental disorder should not be treated? Why? Why not?
3. What would the nurse need to know when assessing a woman for suicide? Outline the major components for determining whether the women is actively suicidal, and develop a plan of action that will address her immediate needs, future mental health and maternal health care, and other family needs.

SUMMARY

- When caring for pregnant or lactating women, the nurse has great responsibilities and obligations. When a woman is at risk for or develops a mental illness, the nurse's responsibility expands.
- Nurses and other clinicians must recognize the unique characteristics of the woman, her culture, and her wishes.
- Psychological, physiologic, and psychopharmacologic treatments should address the women's specific needs at the particular time in her life that she seeks or needs care.
- Nurses who provide health care to women and children are uniquely positioned to query the woman about violence in her relationship. Assessment tools should be available to aid in getting important information quickly.
- Engaging the women in her care will enhance the level of care that she receives and is likely to increase her level of health literacy.

REVIEW QUESTIONS

1. The nurse has just completed discussing stress management techniques with a client. Which of the following statements, if made by the client, would indicate the need for further information?
   A. "I will begin to practice some relaxation techniques regularly."
   B. "I need to eat a diet high in protein and yellow or orange vegetables."
   C. "I plan to exercise several times a week for at least 3 minutes each time."
   D. "I will schedule some time during the week to work on my hobbies."
2. Which of these interventions should the nurse perform *first* when caring for a client experiencing intimate partner violence?
   A. Help the client to formulate a realistic escape plan.
   B. Share with the client that she is being abused.
   C. Document with pictures the client's physical injuries.
   D. Provide the client with the location of a local battered women's shelter.
3. A 24-year-old client is being treated as an outpatient for anorexia nervosa. Assessment reveals that the 5′8″ client weighs 100 lb. She describes eating certain foods only on specific days of the week and cutting food into cubes before eating. Which of the following expected outcomes is most appropriate for this client?
   A. The client will learn to identify situations that trigger anxiety.
   B. The client will gain 4 lb per week until she reaches 140 lb.
   C. The client will acknowledge that she looks ill and is emaciated.
   D. The client will eliminate ritualistic behaviors within 1 month.
4. The nurse is teaching an expectant couple about psychoactive medications in pregnancy. Which of the following statements from the couple indicates successful teaching?
   A. "The drugs help the symptoms of mental illness but may lead to other problems."
   B. "The drugs act solely on specific target sites and pose limited risks."
   C. "The effects of drugs on the fetus usually are minimal."
   D. "Drug therapy has limited effectiveness for psychiatric problems."
5. A nurse is assessing a 42-year-old client who was brutally beaten and raped by her ex-husband. The client has fractures, lacerations, and bruises. She states, "This has happened before." The client cooperates with the examination and shows little emotion. The nurse attributes the client's affect to which of the following explanations?
   A. The client may have an underlying psychological problem.
   B. The client is handling the assault well emotionally.
   C. The client may be struggling internally to regain control.
   D. The client is concerned about her physical injuries at this time.
6. A client who has been diagnosed with general anxiety disorder shares with the nurse, "I'm worried about my finances. I'm afraid I will go bankrupt." Which of the following responses would be most therapeutic for the nurse to use in this situation?
   A. "Do you have health insurance?"
   B. "You think that you will lose all your money."
   C. "Has there been a change in your life recently?"
   D. "It sounds as if you have managed your money responsibly."
7. A client with depression who recently lost her job shares with the nurse, "I think that my family would be better off without me. I am only a burden to them." Which of these possible responses by the nurse would be appropriate?
   A. "Does your family share your feelings?"
   B. "Have you considered career counseling?"
   C. "Are you thinking about hurting yourself?"
   D. "When did you first start to feel like a burden?"
8. The community nurse is reviewing the health assessment form of a client who is to receive a follow-up home visit later in the day. Which of this information would suggest that the woman may be experiencing postpartum depression?
   A. The client is a primipara.
   B. The client is 5 weeks postpartum.
   C. The client has shared that she feels tired all the time.
   D. The client has shared that she had no newborn experience before giving birth.
9. Which of the following observations by the nurse would suggest that the plan of care developed for a client who has been diagnosed with a mood disorder was successful?
   A. The client has a strong social support network.
   B. The client follows a healthy, well-balanced diet.
   C. The client is dressed in a clean, coordinating outfit.
   D. The client is exercising on average three times a week.
10. Which of the following outcomes in a client with schizophrenia best supports effectiveness of the care plan?
    A. The client is taking her medications and attending therapy sessions.

B. The client reports that she no longer has hallucinations.
C. The client has resumed work and attends community center social functions.
D. The client no longer believes that she has special powers.

REFERENCES

Allison, S. K. (2004). Psychotropic medication in pregnancy: Ethical aspects and clinical management. *Journal of Perinatal and Neonatal Nursing, 18*(3), 194–205.

Altshuler, L., Cohen, L., & Szuba, M. (1996). Pharmacologic management of psychiatric illness during pregnancy: Dilemmas and guidelines. *American Journal of Psychiatry, 153,* 592–606.

American Academy of Pediatrics Committee on Drugs. (2001). Transfer of drugs and other chemicals into human milk. *Pediatrics, 108*(3), 776–789.

American Psychiatric Association. (2000). *Diagnostic and statistical manual of mental disorders* (4th ed., text rev.). Washington, DC: American Psychiatric Publishing.

Arias, E., Anderson, R. N., Kung, H. C., Murphy, S. L., & Kochanek, K. D. (2003). Deaths: Final data for 2001. *National Vital Statistics Report, 52*(3), 1–115.

Bloch, M., Rotenberg, N., Koren, D., & Klein, E. (2006). Risk factors for early postpartum depressive symptoms. *General Hospital Psychiatry, 28*(1), 3–8.

Bonari, L., Koren, G., Einarson, T. R., Jasper, J. D., Taddio, A., & Einarson, A. (2005). Use of antidepressants by pregnant women: Evaluation of perception of risk, efficacy of evidence-based counseling and determinants of decision making. *Archives of Women's Mental Health, 8*(4), 214–220.

Boy, A., & Salihu, H. M. (2004). Intimate partner violence and birth outcomes: A systematic review. *International Journal of Fertility and Women's Medicine, 49*(4), 159–164.

Brenner, C. (1957). *An elementary textbook of psychoanalysis.* New York: Doubleday Anchor Books.

Brown, C. S. H., & Prigerson, H. G. (2000). Factors associated with symptomatic improvement and recovery from major depression in primary care patients. *General Hospital Psychiatry, 22*(4), 242–250.

Brown, C., & Schulberg, H. (1998). Diagnosis and treatment of depression in primary medical care practice: The application of research findings to clinical practice. *Journal of Clinical Psychology, 54*(3), 303–314.

Brown, D., Ahmed, F., Gary, L., & Milburn, N. (1995). Major depression in a community sample of African Americans. *American Journal of Psychiatry, 152*(3), 373–378.

Campbell, S. B., Brownell, C. A., Hungerford, A., Spieker, S. I., Mohan, R., & Blessing, J. S. (2004). The course of maternal depressive symptoms and maternal sensitivity as predictors of attachment security at 36 months. *Developmental Psychology, 16*(2), 231–252.

Ciseaux, A. (1980). Anorexia nervosa: A view from the mirror. *American Journal of Nursing, 80*(8), 1468–1470.

Coker, A. L., Smith, P. H., & Fadden, M. K. (2005). Intimate partner violence and disabilities among women attending family practice clinics. *Journal of Women's Health, 14*(9), 829–838.

Curry, M., & Harvey, S. (1998). *Stress related to domestic violence during pregnancy and infant birth weight.* Thousand Oaks, CA: Sage Publications.

Eberhard-Gran, M., Eskild, A., & Opjordsmoen, S. (2005). Treating mood disorders during pregnancy. Safety considerations. *Drug Safety, 28*(8), 695–706.

Gary, F., Yarandi, H., & Scruggs, F. (2003). Suicide among African Americans: Reflections and a call to action. *Issues in Mental Health Nursing, 24*(3), 353–375.

Greenfeld, L. A., Rand, M. R., Craven, D., Klaus, P. A., Perkins, C. A., Ringel, C., et al. (1998). *Violence by intimates: Analysis of data on crimes by current or former spouses, boyfriends, and girlfriends. Bureau of Justice Statistics factbook.* Washington, DC: U.S. Department of Justice. NCJ-167237.

Hale, B. (2002). Shifting the frame: Teaching feminist psychologics. *Transformations—A Resource for Curriculum Transformation and Scholarship, 13*(1), 61–72.

Hales, R. E., & Yudofsky, S. C. (2003). *The American Psychiatric Publishing textbook of clinical psychiatry* (4th ed.). Washington, DC: American Psychiatric Publishing.

Health Literacy: Report of the Council on Scientific Affairs. Ad Hoc Committee on Health Literacy for the Council on Scientific Affairs, American Medical Association. (1999). *Journal of the American Medical Association, 281*(6), 552–557.

Hinderliter, D., Pitula, C., & Delaney, K. R. (1998). Partner violence. *American Journal for Nurse Practitioners, 2,* 32–40.

Hunt, S. J., & Morrow, J. L. (2005). Safety of antiepileptic drugs during pregnancy. *Expert Opinions on Drug Safety, 4*(5), 869–877.

Inhorn, M., & Whittle, L. (2001). Feminism meets the "new" epidemiologies: Toward an appraisal of antifeminist biases in epidemiological research on women's health. *Social Science and Medicine, 53,* 553–567.

Keeling, J. (2004). A community-based perspective on living with domestic violence. *Nursing Times, 100*(11), 28–29.

Kornstein, S. G., Harvey, A. T., Rush, A. J., Wisniewski, S. R., Trivedi, M. H., Svikis, D. S., et al. (2005). Self-reported premenstrual exacerbation of depressive symptoms in patients seeking treatment for major depression. *Psychological Medicine, 35*(5), 683–692.

Kouba, S., Hallstrom, T., Lindholm, C., & Hirschberg, A. L. (2005). Pregnancy and neonatal outcomes in women with eating disorders. *Obstetrics & Gynecology, 105*(2), 255–260.

Kuehner, C., & Buerger, C. (2005). Determinants of subjective quality of life in depressed patients: The role of self-esteem, response styles, and social support. *Journal of Affective Disorders, 86*(2–3), 205–213.

Landenburger, K. (1998). *Exploration of woman's identity—clinical approaches with abused women.* Thousand Oaks, CA: Sage Publications.

Lolak, S., Rashid, N., & Wise, T. N. (2005). Interface of women's mental and reproductive health. *Current Psychiatry Report, 7*(3), 220–227.

MacKey, M., Williams, C., & Tiller, C. (2000). Stress, pre-term labour and birth outcomes. *Journal of Advanced Nursing, 32*(3), 666–674.

Mazure, C., Keita, G., & Blehar, M. (2002). *Summit on women and depression: Proceedings and recommendations.* Washington, DC: American Psychological Association.

McKenna, K., Koren, G., Tetelbaum, M., Wilton, L., Shakir, S., Diav-Citrin, O., et al. (2005). Pregnancy outcome of women using atypical antipsychotic drugs: A prospective comparative study. *Journal of Clinical Psychiatry, 66*(4), 444–449.

Mitchell-Gielegham, A., Mittelstaedt, M. E., & Bulik, C. M. (2002). Eating disorders and childbearing: concealment and consequences. *Birth* 29(3), 182–191.

Mohr, W. K. (2006). *Psychiatric mental health nursing* (6th ed.). Philadelphia: Lippincott Williams & Wilkins.

Moline, M. L., Kahn, D. A., Ross, R. W., Altshuler, L. L., & Cohen, L. S. (2001). Postpartum depression: A guide for patients and families. *Postgraduate Medicine, Mar*(Spec No), 112–113.

National Council on Disability. (2002). *An inter-generational vision of effective mental health services and supports.* Washington, DC: Author.

Ness, R., Grisso, J., & Hirshchinger, N. (1999). Cocaine and tobacco use and the risk of spontaneous abortion. *New England Journal of Medicine, 340,* 333–339.

Nilsson, E., Lichtenstein, P., Cnattingius, S., Murray, R. M., & Hultman, C. M. (2002). Women with schizophrenia: Pregnancy outcome and infant death among their offspring. *Schizophrenia Research, 58*(2–3), 221–229.

Olfson, M., Marcus, S., Druss, B., Elinson, L., Tanielian, T., & Pincus, H. (2002). National trends in the outpatient treatment of depression. *Journal of the American Medical Association, 287*(2), 203–209.

O'Malley, A. S., Forrest, C. B., & Miranda, J. (2003). Primary care attributes and care for depression among low-income African American women. *American Journal of Public Health, 93*(8), 1328–1334.

Patel, V., & Prince, M. (2006). Maternal psychological morbidity and low birth weight in India. *British Journal of Psychiatry, 188,* 284–285.

Peplau, H. (1963). A working definition of anxiety. In S. Burd & M. Marshall (Eds.), *Some clinical approaches to psychiatric nursing.* New York: Macmillan.

Perfetti, J., Clark, R., & Fillmore, C. M. (2004). Postpartum depression: Identification, screening, and treatment. *Wisconsin Medical Journal, 103*(6), 56–63.

Pinquart, M., & Sorensen, S. (2006). Gender differences in caregiver stressors, social resources, and health: An updated meta-analysis. *Journals of Gerontology, 61*(1), P33–45.

Rahman, A., Iqbal, Z., Bunn, J., Lovel, H., & Harrington, R. (2004). Impact of maternal depression on infant nutritional status and illness: A cohort study. *Archives of General Psychiatry, 61*(9), 946–952.

Sadock, B., & Sadock, V. (2003). *Kaplan and Sadock's synopsis of psychiatry.* Philadelphia: Lippincott Williams & Wilkins.

Saint Arnault, D., Sakamoto, S., & Moriwaki, A. (2005). The association between negative self-descriptions and depressive symptomatology: Does culture make a difference? *Archives of Psychiatric Nursing, 19*(2), 93–100.

Schatzberg, A. F., & Nemeroff, C. B. (2004). *The American Psychiatric Publishing textbook of clinical pharmacology* (3rd ed.). Washington, DC: American Psychiatric Publishing.

Schatzberg, A., Cole, J., & DeBattista, C. (2003). *Manual of clinical psychopharmacology* (4th ed.). Washington, DC: American Psychiatric Publishing.

Seligman, M. (1975). *Helplessness: On depression, development, and death.* San Francisco: Freeman & Co.

Seyfried, L. S., & Marcus, S. M. (2003). Postpartum mood disorders. *International Review of Psychiatry, 15*(3), 231–242.

Stahl, S. (1996). *Essential psychopharmacology—neuroscientific basis and practical applications.* Cambridge, UK: Cambridge University Press.

Stowe, Z., Owen, C., Landry, J., Kilts, C., Ely, T., Llewellyn, A., et al. (1997). Sertraline and desmethylsertraline in human breast milk and nursing infants. *American Journal of Psychiatry, 154*(9), 1255–1260.

Taylor, J., Henderson, D., & Jackson, B. (1991). A holistic model for understanding and predicting depressive symptoms in African American women. *Journal of Community Psychology, 19,* 306–321.

U.S. Department of Health and Human Services. (1999). *Mental health: A report of the Surgeon General.* Washington, DC: Author.

Usher, K., Foster, K., & McNamara, P. (2005). Antipsychotic drugs and pregnant or breastfeeding women: The issues for mental health nurses. *Journal of Psychiatric and Mental Health Nursing, 12*(6), 713–718.

Wallerstein, R. (2002). The growth and transformation of American ego psychology. *Journal of the American Psychoanalytic Association, 50*(1), 135–169.

Whitby, D. H., & Smith, K. M. (2005). The use of tricyclic antidepressants and selective serotonin reuptake inhibitors in women who are breastfeeding. *Pharmacotherapy, 25*(3), 411–425.

Wilcox, R., Gonzales, R., & Miller, J. (1998). *Introduction to neurotransmitters, receptors, signal transduction, and second messenger.* Washington, DC: American Psychiatric Press.

Williams, M. V., Parker, R. M., Baker, D. W., Parikh, N. S., Pitkin, K., Coates, W. C., & Nurss, J. R. (1995). Inadequate functional health literacy among patients at two public hospitals. *Journal of the American Medical Association, 274*(21), 1677–1682.

Zeanah, C. H., Satfford, B., Boris, N. W., & Scheeringa, M. (2003). Infant development: The first 3 years of life. In A. Tasman, J. Kay, & J. Lieberman (Eds.), *Psychiatry* (2nd ed., Vol. 1, pp. 91–117). New York: Wiley.

Zimmer-Gembeck, M. J., & Helfand, M. (1996). Low birthweight in a public prenatal care program: Behavioral and psychosocial risk factors and psychosocial intervention. *Social Science and Medicine, 43*(2), 187–197.

CHAPTER 6

Sexuality and Reproduction

Vi Wilkes

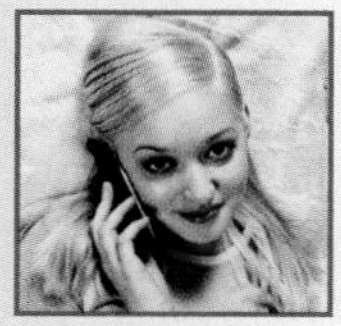

Rochelle, 42 years old, brings her 14-year-old daughter, Kendra, to the facility for a yearly examination. Kendra is wearing makeup, platform shoes, and other items that make her appear several years older. While Kendra is getting changed in the examination room, Rochelle quietly states, "These teenage years are tough. I know girls my daughter's age are already having sex. I just hope Kendra isn't."

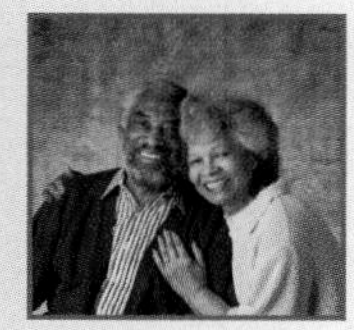

Patti is a 54-year-old married woman who has made an appointment to discuss problems related to fatigue and a "personal sexual issue." During the interview, the nurse asks Patti to describe her concerns. Patti looks down and quietly responds, "My sex life with my husband just isn't what it used to be. We haven't had sex for several months because I no longer enjoy it. Frankly, it's really become painful. Do you have any suggestions about what might help us?"

You will learn more about these stories later in this chapter. Nurses working with these clients and others like them need to understand the material in this chapter to manage care and address issues appropriately. Before beginning, consider the following points:

- What behaviors and approaches from nurses are especially important when dealing with aspects of sexuality for clients?
- What other information from both clients is needed to fully address the concerns?
- How might age and developmental stage be influencing Kendra's scenario? What about Patti?
- How would the nurse need to modify care when working with a parent and child together? What about when working with a husband and wife?

LEARNING OBJECTIVES

On completion of this chapter, the reader should be able to:

- Discuss issues related to sexuality and reproduction across the lifespan.
- Summarize assessment factors related to the anatomic, physiologic, and psychological aspects of sexuality development in both genders across the lifespan.
- Identify the effects of sociocultural and economic issues on sexuality and reproduction.
- Discuss positive and negative outcomes of heterosexuality and minority sexual orientations.
- Discuss ethno-sociocultural rites of passage associated with sexual and reproductive milestones.
- Identify nursing strategies to promote positive sexual and reproductive outcomes.

KEY TERMS

adolescence
androgen
androgyny
andropause
bisexual
conception
corpus luteum
cultural identity
dyspareunia
estrogen
gender constancy
gender identity
gender role development
hermaphroditism
masturbation
menarche
menopause
menstrual cycle
menstrual phase
minority sexual orientation
nocturnal emission
ovulation
proliferative phase
pseudohermaphroditism
puberty
rites of passage
secretory phase
sex compatibility
stigma
testosterone

Development of sexuality is an important part of each person's psychosocial identity, integrated sense of self, reproductive capacity, and ability to fulfill role functions in society. Although sexuality is separate and different from reproduction, the two concepts are linked inherently. Nevertheless, sexual behavior and function are separate from reproductive function in that reproduction is not the aim of all sexual activity. Engagement in sexual activity is often for pleasure (Berman, 2005; Levin, 2002).

The purpose of this chapter is to differentiate and discuss manifestations of sexuality and reproduction within a sociocultural and economic perspective. The content presents male and female sexual anatomy, development, and responses. It explores sexual orientation and sexual and reproductive rites of passage. Nurses should understand the issues in this chapter so that they can identify variations from normal, design nursing care plans that address accompanying manifestations, and promote sexual and reproductive health for all women and families.

SEXUAL AND REPRODUCTIVE DEVELOPMENT ACROSS THE LIFESPAN

Sexual development and reproductive development are aligned closely, demonstrating their interdependence in forming the mature sexual being. The sections that follow emphasize the anatomic, physiologic, and psychological aspects of sexual and reproductive development.

A discussion of the concept of **gender identity** (a person's sense of maleness or femaleness, acceptance of the roles associated with that gender, and internalization of the gender and gender roles [Woelfle et al., 2002]) is an essential precursor to subsequent content. Physiologic and genetic forces determine whether a person is biologically male or female; however, many other factors contribute to gender identity. Children proceed through predictable stages in which they achieve **sex compatibility** or comfort with a certain sex (gender role development), affirm their gender identity (labeling themselves male or female), adopt the stereotypical roles or behaviors associated with that gender (gender role behavior), and express an attitude of gender superiority (Egan & Perry, 2001; Yunger et al., 2004). By the time most children are 6 or 7 years old, parents, peers, and others have socialized them to assume and accept the gender identity and roles that match their biologic gender. Nevertheless, some children, regardless of biologic sex determination, identify with the opposite sex and adopt its associated sexual behaviors.

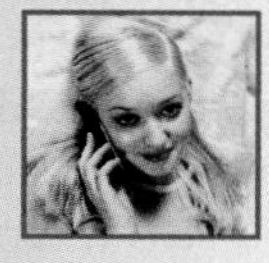

Recall Rochelle and Kendra described at the beginning of the chapter. What findings would provide some evidence that Kendra has adopted a female gender identity?

It is important to note that a conflict over gender identity is *not* the same as homosexuality. Although gay men and lesbians are attracted sexually to people of the same sex, they recognize and accept themselves as men or women. They have no desire to change their gender or assume behaviors and roles commonly associated with the opposite sex. Those with conflicted gender identity may be attracted sexually to people of the same sex, the opposite sex, or both. There are males who identify with and may wish to become females, and females who identify with and may wish to become males.

Conception Through Infancy

Genes determine the gender of the new organism. Briefly, an ovum always has an X chromosome; a sperm can have an X or a Y chromosome. When a sperm with an X chromosome fertilizes an ovum, a female (XX) is produced. Likewise, when a sperm with a Y chromosome unites with an ovum, a male is produced (XY).

While in utero, the human goes through three distinct stages, each of which is marked by increasing and rapid cell division and differentiation (Fig. 6.1). The pre-embryonic (also called germinal) stage of a fertilized ovum (zygote) lasts from gestational days 1 to 14, the embryonic stage lasts from gestational day 15 to the end of gestational week 8, and the fetal stage lasts from the beginning of gestational week 9 until birth. Chapter 11 discusses associated genetic processes and fully outlines pre-embryonic, embryonic, and fetal development in detail.

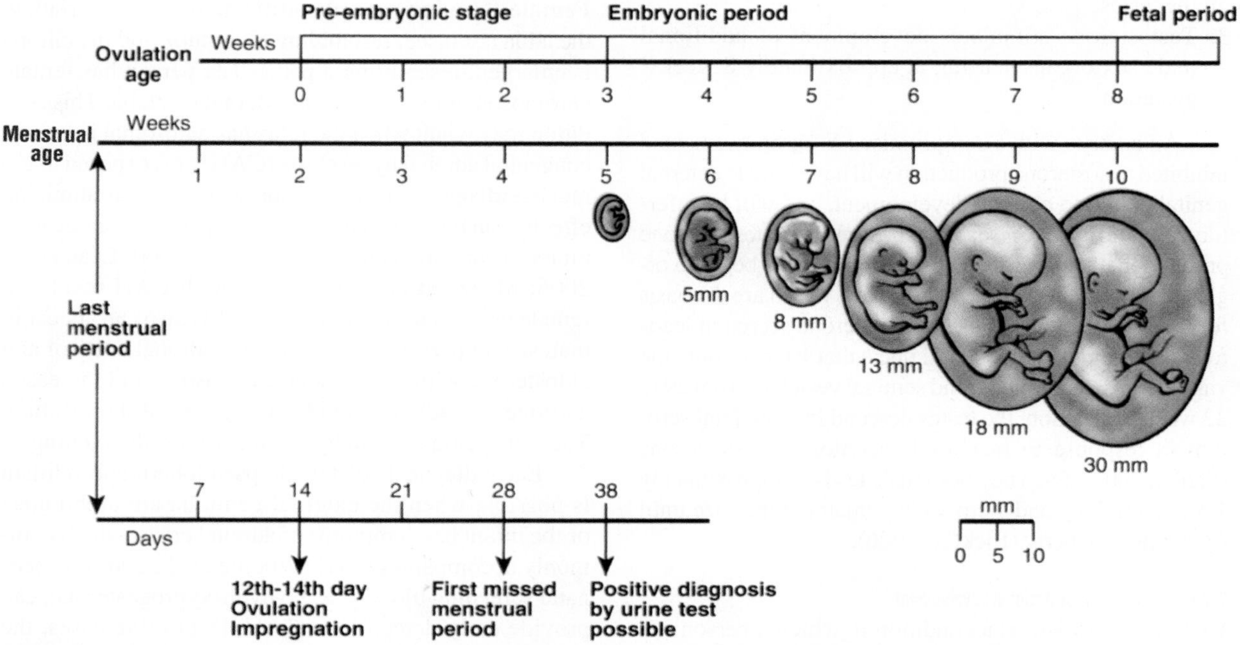

FIGURE 6.1 Stages of in utero development: pre-embryonic, embryonic, and fetal. The fetal period continues until the birth of the baby, normally at approximately gestational week 40.

In Utero Sex Organ Differentiation

Initially, the human organism shows no physical characteristics specific to either gender. The anatomic rudiments of the genetically determined sex organs begin to differentiate in the embryo at approximately gestational day 14 (coinciding with the start of the embryonic stage). Clinicians can distinguish gender with high-resolution ultrasound as early as the first trimester (Krone et al., 2000; Michailidis et al., 2003). Figure 6.2 depicts the differentiation of both external and internal genitalia from the embryonic stage to birth.

Female. In an embryo with normal XX sex chromosomes, the ovaries begin to develop between gestational weeks 11 and 12. The ovaries give rise to oocytes by gestational week 16; hormone-producing cells and associated ovarian tissues also begin to emerge by this time. It is important to note that in biologically female organisms, the sex organs differentiate independently of hormonal influences. External genital structures emerge, and their development progresses even in cases of ovarian impairment or absence. Thus, an embryo with only one sex chromosome of X is considered and has the sexual characteristics of a female. She will be infertile in adulthood, however, because she lacks ovarian function and, subsequently, produces no ova for fertilization.

Male. Because the male embryo has X and Y chromosomes, an extra step is necessary for development of the sex organs. The sequence of events is as follows:

1. The maternal placenta secretes human chorionic gonadotropin (hCG) hormone during pregnancy.
2. The hCG stimulates the secretion of testosterone from the testes.
3. Testosterone stimulates development of additional male sex organs starting at approximately 8 weeks' gestation.

An embryo with a compromised Y chromosome and inhibited testosterone production will have female external genitalia, but no ovarian development, and will be infertile. With normal XY sex chromosomes and testosterone production, the testes begin to grow, and cells begin to organize to form the seminiferous cords, which are the basis for the seminiferous tubules. Testosterone secretion leads to the development of several ducts that later become the vas deferens, epididymis, and seminal vesicles. From 29 to 32 weeks' gestation, the testes descend into the fetal scrotum in response to increased secretion of testosterone (Sadler, 2004). Each newborn male testis is approximately 1.5 to 2 cm long and 1 cm wide, remaining this size until right before puberty (Bickley, 2006).

Variations in Normal Gestational Development

Hermaphroditism is a condition in which a person has both ovarian and testicular tissue. Sometimes the external genitalia are ambiguous; in many cases, they present as female. In **pseudohermaphroditism,** the appearance of the outer genitalia fails to match the internal sex organs. The person may have ambiguous genitalia, male-appearing genitalia with internal ovarian tissue, or female-appearing genitalia with internal testicular tissue (Sadler, 2004).

When external genitalia are ambiguous at birth, identifying the baby as male or female is difficult or impossible. This development prompts investigation and testing, which help establish an early diagnosis. In such cases, sex assignment is usually consistent with the internal rather than the external organs. Prompt treatment can be relatively uneventful and facilitate a consistent gender identity for the child: optimally, he or she has no recollection of the experience.

Sometimes, the condition is not recognized until the person is well into childhood or adolescence. In such cases, the person's gender identity and sexual role development already have been established. Attempts to change these elements are fraught with difficulty and can have challenging psychological and emotional ramifications, not only for the person but also for family, friends, and peers. Research indicates that sex reassignment should be completed before the child is 18 months old to avoid problems with gender identity and **gender role development** (the process by which children come to know and accept the social implications of their sex) (Perrin, 2002; Woelfle et al., 2002). In cases of diagnosis delayed beyond 18 months, sex assignment usually is based on the external organs (which have dictated the gender role that the person has been following to that point).

Female Pseudohermaphroditism. With this variation, the labia are fused, resembling a scrotum, and the clitoris is enlarged, resembling a penis. The person has female chromosomes (XX) but male external genitalia. This condition may result when the fetus has autosomal recessive congenital adrenal hyperplasia (CAH) or is exposed to too much **androgen** (any steroid hormone with masculinizing effects), such as when the mother experiences an ovarian tumor during pregnancy (Krone et al., 2000; Lean et al., 2005; Mazza et al., 2002). Although CAH results in female pseudohermaphroditism, CAH also can appear in males. The person has insufficient adrenal cortisol and aldosterone with consequent salt wasting and increased androgens, leading to rapid bone aging and short stature. The salt wasting and dehydration are life-threatening.

Early diagnosis of female pseudohermaphroditism is possible when the external genitalia are ambiguous or the infant has symptoms of adrenal crisis, which commonly accompanies CAH (Woelfle et al., 2002). A neonatal screening blood test, 17-hydroxyprogesterone, can provide early detection of CAH. In positive cases, the level of 17-hydroxyprogesterone is elevated.

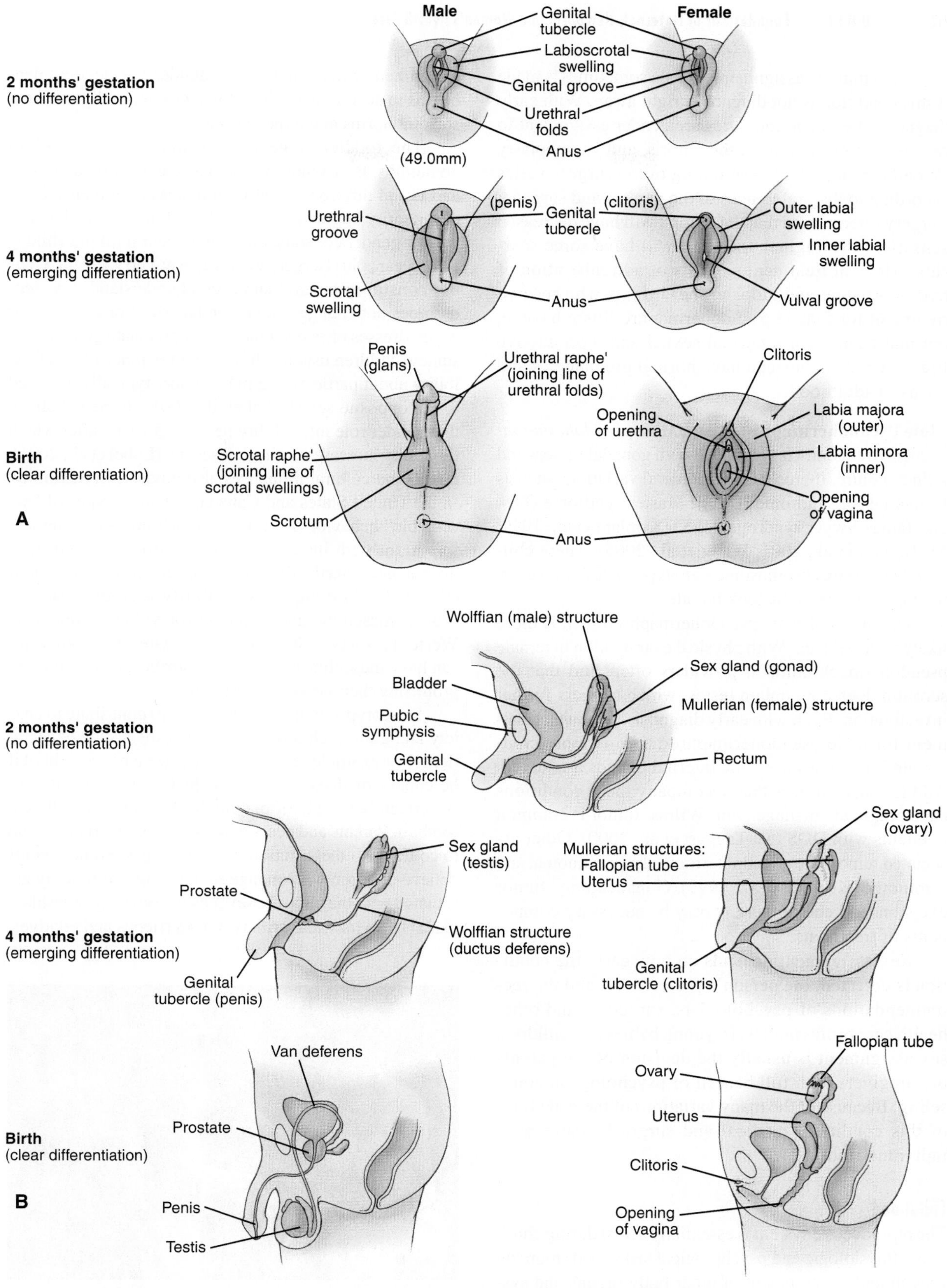

FIGURE 6.2 Differentiation of male and female genitalia. (**A**) The external genitalia are identical until gestational week 7, when differentiation begins. By birth, the genitalia clearly indicate whether the infant is a boy or girl (except in rare cases of gender ambiguity). (**B**) The same process of differentiation occurs in the internal genitalia.

An initial sex assignment of male sometimes is made if this condition is not diagnosed right away. With early diagnosis, treatment measures are gender assignment to female, surgery to reduce the clitoris, and vaginoplasty (Woelfle et al., 2002). The timing of the surgery varies according to the preferences of the parents and surgeon. Surgery often means that the clitoris will have decreased sensation; the vaginal wall also will have some scarring. Medical treatment consists of administration of hydrocortisone and aldosterone. Infants who receive treatment for female pseudohermaphroditism have an optimal chance for a normal sexual and reproductive life as females; they can have normal pregnancies and births in adulthood.

Male Pseudohermaphroditism. *Male pseudohermaphroditism* frequently is associated with gonadal tumors and kidney failure. It presents with several variations such as Denys-Drash syndrome (DDS), Frasier syndrome (FS), and James-Swyer syndrome (JSS) (Kriplani et al., 1999; McTaggart et al., 2001; Wang et al., 2005). These children have a sex chromosome genotype of XY; however, their external genitalia look female.

Diagnosis of male pseudohermaphroditism is more likely to be delayed. With physical examination in female pseudohermaphroditism, providers often find that the scrotum does not contain testes, which triggers further investigation. Even with early diagnosis, however, treatment for male pseudohermaphroditism is more complicated. In some cases, the internal gonads are mixed. Additionally, tumors that accompany these conditions can complicate management. Wilms' tumor is common in clients with DDS (McTaggart et al., 2000). Other associated tumors are gonadoblastoma, dysgerminoma, and seminoma (Kriplani et al., 1999). Gonadectomy, tumor excision, and chemotherapy may be necessary components of treatment.

Sex assignment depends on how early the condition is detected, the person's preferences, and the recommendations of psychologists, surgeons, and other health care professionals. In young babies and children, sex assignment is usually the decision of the parents or caregivers with full benefit of psychological counseling. Because of the many variations of the male form of this condition, medical and surgical treatment is individualized.

Childhood

The reproductive system is essentially at rest during childhood. Physiologic and psychological tasks focus more on growth and development of other body organs and systems, cognition, and language (see Chap. 5). Nevertheless, an important task of childhood related to sexual development is socialization to the gender role. Once gender assignment is made in infancy, gender role development begins in accordance with ethnic, cultural, religious, and societal norms and expectations.

The toddler stage is from approximately 12 to 36 months. By 24 months, toddlers can identify anatomic and visual differences between males and females. Gender identity begins to be established; however, the concept of gender constancy does not occur until the child is 5 or 6 years old (Berger, 2004; Egan & Perry, 2001). **Gender constancy** means that the child understands that gender does not change if a person has short or long hair or wears dresses or pants. Once they appreciate gender constancy, children usually show more tolerance of and flexibility about participating in behaviors typically assigned to the opposite sex (Lobel et al., 2001). Experts believe that gender role inflexibility peaks at 5 years, after which flexibility increases until adolescence (Lobel et al., 2001). Social and cultural influences also guide such flexibility. In the United States and Canada, old stereotypes of "acceptable" behaviors for boys and girls are becoming less important with increased understanding that activities do not necessarily dictate or belong to either gender (Fig. 6.3). **Androgyny** (flexibility regarding stereotypical masculine and feminine roles) has increased in Western society as it has become clearer that both sexes can have masculine and feminine attributes without compromising their gender (Perrin, 2002).

Stereotyped beliefs about sex roles contribute to anxiety and guilt in children who do not meet such expectations. For example, peers may ostracize a boy in school if he cannot or does not want to fit into the typical "all-American boy" role of playing basketball, baseball, and football. Parents and peers may exert pressure on the child to conform to these masculine stereotypes. Some parents believe children who engage in behaviors commonly associated with the opposite sex may become gay or lesbian; parents also may fear criticism from friends and relatives.

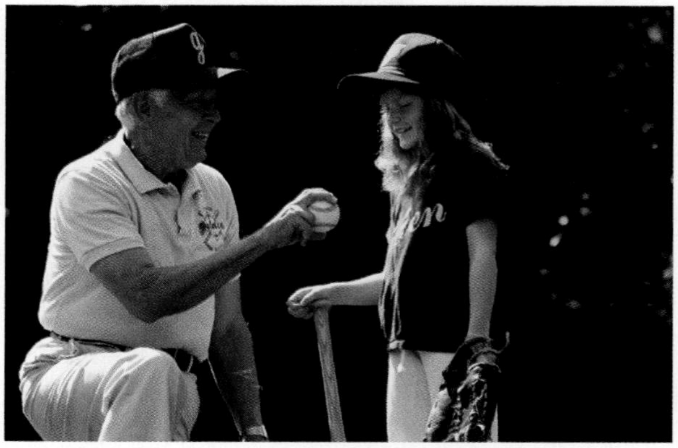

FIGURE 6.3 Expectations related to gender roles for children have changed and are continuing to evolve. Girls are increasingly participating in sports, with involvement from parents and extended family.

Origins in sex-role behaviors can be traced to historical, cultural, social, and religious influences. The more traditionally stereotypical the masculine and feminine roles are in a culture, the more that parents, schools, churches, and peers will enforce those stereotypical behaviors (Lobel et al., 2001). See Research Highlight 6.1.

Pubescence and Adolescence

"While the onset of puberty can vary by as much as six years, every adolescent wants to be right on the 50-yard line, right in the middle of the field. One is always too tall, too short, too thin, too fat, too hairy, too clear-skinned, too early, too late. Understandably, problems of self-image are rampant."

Joan Lipsitz, U.S. educator,
"Easing the Transition From Child to Adult,"
Education Week *(May 16, 1984).*

Puberty is when reproduction becomes physically possible. Experts differ on the average age of when puberty begins. Generally, puberty starts between 8 and 14 years, depending on ethnicity, sex, health, nutrition, genetics, and activity level (Pinyerd & Zipf, 2005). **Adolescence** is the developmental stage that begins with puberty and lasts 8 to 10 years (Berger, 2004). Tasks associated with adolescence include developing relationships, preparing for careers, and participating in family life (see Chap. 5).

Those going through puberty and adolescence often are preoccupied with sexual issues and concerns as a result of increased hormones and changes in body appearance and functioning. **Masturbation** (self-manipulation of the genitals for sexual pleasure) is common and normal for both boys and girls during this time. In addition, some adolescents periodically engage in sexual activity with same-sex partners, even if they do not consider themselves homosexual or engage in homosexual behavior later in life. Dating activity prepares teens for mature relationships and helps them learn social skills they will need upon entering young adulthood.

Adolescents often feel conflicted about sex. On the one hand, peers and internal feelings are pushing them toward physical relationships. On the other hand, parents and society are pulling them back, asking them to delay sexual gratification until they have reached maturity and are accountable for the consequences. Satisfactory relationships are built on self-confidence, self-esteem, trust in and concern for the partner, open communication skills, and dexterity. Preteens and adolescents are still developing these skills required for satisfactory, positive, and mature sexual relationships.

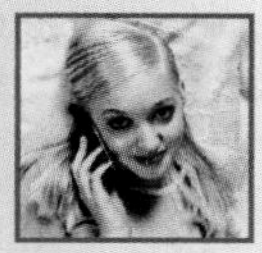

Recall Rochelle and Kendra from the beginning of the chapter. Rochelle states, "Kendra has all these magazines in her room that talk about boys, dating, and sex. And she's been talking a lot about this boy at school who is 16 years old. I remember what I was like at her age. But I was a late bloomer and things are so different now." How should the nurse respond to Rochelle?

In 2002, a representative research sample showed that 45.6% of U.S. students in grades 9 through 12 had engaged in sex, 14.2% with four or more partners, and 6% before 13 years old (Grunbaum et al., 2002). Hispanic American students were significantly more likely to have had intercourse than white American students; African American students were significantly more likely to have

● RESEARCH HIGHLIGHT 6.1 Children's Gender-Related Inferences and Judgments: A Cross-Cultural Study

OBJECTIVES: The authors studied the effects of culture on gender specificity and gender flexibility. The authors assumed that there is no justifiable reason for children to hold role and sex behavior stereotypes; they posited that the strength and rigidity of the culture maintain these stereotypes. There were several hypotheses, one of which was that children would associate feminine activities with females and male activities with males, and that differences would be based on known characteristics of the culture.

DESIGN: The study sample included 542 third-grade and fifth-grade Israeli, Taiwanese, and Chinese students. The authors developed and administered a questionnaire to the children about activities, occupations, and emotional traits stereotypical for male and female.

RESULTS: The more traditional the culture, the more strongly the children associated with male and female stereotypical activities, occupations, and emotional traits. The Taiwanese children held stronger, more rigid, and more traditional stereotypes of characteristics of masculine and feminine roles, activities, and emotional traits.

CONCLUSION: The strength of the study favors the possibility that culture defines many activities as being typically feminine or masculine.

Lobel, T. E., Gruber, R., Govrin, N., & Mashraki-Pedhatzur, S. (2001). *Developmental Psychology, 37*(6), 839–846.

had intercourse than Hispanic or white American students (Grunbaum et al., 2002). Male teens had significantly higher rates than females of both sexual intercourse and number of partners. Nationwide, 4.7% stated that they had experienced unwanted pregnancies, 34.4 % had used condoms, and 18.2 % had used oral contraceptives (Grunbaum et al., 2002).

These statistics make it clear that many people begin sexual activity at an early age. Many youth are at risk for unwanted pregnancy, sexually transmitted infections (STIs), interrupted schooling, delayed careers, changes in career or educational goals, and lowered social and economic status. These risks pose tremendous potential and actual costs to society in terms of lost wages, increased health care costs, and increased use of public assistance programs. Parents and children need sex education before children enter puberty. Such education requires discussion of the changes inherent in puberty, along with the consequences of unprotected sex, as well as methods of contraception (see Chap. 8).

Nurses can play important roles in teaching related to sexual activity for teens and their families by identifying the existing knowledge base of each involved individual, supplementing the knowledge as appropriate, and identifying and promoting strategies uniquely individualized to each specific situation. For example, the nurse might assist the adolescent to explore the consequences of sexual activity and the effects on the teen's personal life in the home, school, and community. The nurse should also consider, when appropriate, encouraging adolescents and their parents or other adult caretakers to communicate about sexual issues. This may require that the nurse assist the parents or caretakers in learning not only information, but also ensuring that important strategies are culturally and religiously specific and will promote positive interactions with their adolescents. Nursing Care Plan 6.1 addresses some of these issues of adolescence and sexuality.

Teaching Tips 6.1 provides recommendations for encouraging healthy and honest communication between children and their adult caregivers about sex. The American Academy of Pediatrics (AAP, 2001) has published guidelines of topic areas to address with families relative to sex education; a summary is found in Box 6.1.

Male Pubescent Changes

Anatomy and Physiology. The major organs of the male sexual and reproductive system are the penis, scrotum, testes, prostate gland, and seminal vesicles (Fig. 6.4). The penis is composed of the shaft and glans. The shaft

NURSING CARE PLAN 6.1

A Family With Concerns Related to Adolescent Sexual Activity

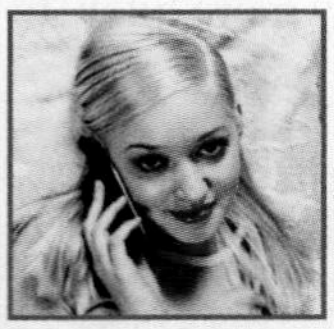

Recall Kendra, a 14-year-old whose mother voices concerns about her potential sexual behavior. Kendra's history reveals that she experienced menarche at 12 years old. She reports that her menstrual cycle is somewhat irregular, ranging in frequency from every 28 to 35 days and lasting anywhere from 3 to 6 days. She states that her flow is heaviest on the first day but then gradually subsides.

During the physical examination, Kendra states, "I've been dating this boy who is about 2 years older than me for a few months now. Some of my friends have had sex with their boyfriends. I really like him a lot. I'm afraid that he'll break up with me if I don't sleep with him."

NURSING DIAGNOSES

- **Decisional Conflict** related to participation in sexual activity and fear of loss
- **Deficient Knowledge** related to consequences of engaging in unprotected sex

EXPECTED OUTCOMES

1. The client will identify information necessary to make an informed decision about sexual activity.
2. The client will identify the positive and negative aspects of engaging in sexual activity.

Continued

NURSING CARE PLAN 6.1 ● A Family With Concerns Related to Adolescent Sexual Activity

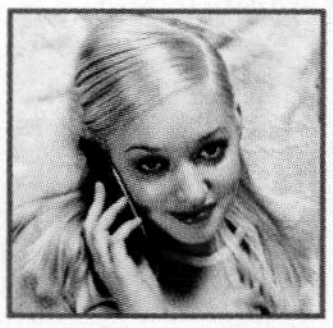

INTERVENTIONS	RATIONALES
Assess the client's beliefs about her current body image, developmental stage, and self-esteem. Explore her feelings about herself and her peers.	These data provide a baseline from which to develop appropriate strategies for teaching and care. Exploration of feelings provides insight into the client's thinking to ensure appropriate planning of individualized interventions.
Question the client about her understanding of the menstrual cycle, sexual activity, pregnancy, and STIs. Communicate accurate facts and answer questions honestly; clarify any misconceptions or misinformation.	Clear communication helps provide accurate information to aid in alleviating fears and clarifying misinformation. Honesty promotes the development of trust in the relationship.
Review the developmental changes common during adolescence, including the search for identity and independence from parents and strong influence of peers.	Adolescence focuses on the development of a sense of identity, emphasizing body image and peer influence. An understanding of developmental changes helps to promote understanding of the client's feelings as normal.
Teach the client about safer sex practices and contraceptive methods as appropriate. Provide the client with written material.	Knowledge of safer sex practices and contraception help reduce risks for pregnancy and STIs should she decide to engage in sexual activity. Written material promotes learning and allows for later review and reference.
Explore with the client the consequences of sexual activity and how it might affect her life at home, at school, and in the community.	Exploration of the consequences helps to promote awareness in teens who are self focused and present oriented and believe that "it won't happen to me."
Ask the client to identify person(s) with whom she can openly discuss her concerns, fears, and beliefs, such as her mother, a teacher, an older sibling, or friend.	Open discussion of fears and concerns aids in reducing anxiety and promotes clear decision making.
Offer nonjudgmental support throughout the client's care.	Nonjudgmental support fosters trust and promotes effective decision making.

EVALUATION

1. The client makes an informed decision about engaging in sexual activity based on sound rationales.
2. The client demonstrates understanding of the consequences of unprotected sexual activity.
3. The client employs safer sex behaviors.

contains the urethra, which allows urine to flow from the bladder. The glans is cone shaped and covered with loose skin called the *foreskin* or *prepuce.* In men who are circumcised, removal of the foreskin exposes the glans.

The scrotum is a loose sac that contains the testes. It is within the testes that sperm and testosterone are produced (Fig. 6.5). The prostate gland and seminal vesicles produce and store most of the seminal fluid. Together, seminal fluid and spermatozoa form semen, which is discharged during male orgasm.

Sperm develop in the seminiferous tubules in the testes. The process of sperm maturation is complex. The testes form approximately 120 million sperm per day; along with the epididymis and vas deferens, they are capable of storing sperm for 1 month (Guyton & Hall, 2001). During fertilization, approximately 120 million

TEACHING TIPS 6.1 Promoting Family Communication About Sex

The nurse provides the following recommendations to assist parents and other adult caregivers to communicate with their children about sex and related issues:

- Be aware of and clear about your own sexual attitudes and values. Reflect on your own beliefs about how to set realistic sexual limits. Consider when you became sexually active and how you feel about your past choices. Decide what advice you want to give to your child about abstinence, contraception, or both.
- Talk about sex with your child early and frequently. Avoid relying on one conversation (eg,, "the talk," "the birds and the bees"). Parents and children need to discuss love, sex, and relationships often throughout the preteen and teen years. Regular conversations help correct mistakes and misperceptions. Initiate honest and respectful conversations in which you confidently outline and explain your beliefs. Ask also what your children think and why.
- Monitor your child's activities. Establish and enforce age-appropriate curfews, rules, and standards. Know where your child is when not with you and what he or she is doing. Get to know your child's friends and, ideally, their families.
- Avoid hurtful teasing or ridicule related to relationships and crushes. Embarrassing or upsetting your child in this sensitive area may compromise his or her desire to talk with or confide in you.
- Make sure that an older adolescent dates people close to his or her own age (within 2 to 3 years of difference at most).
- Discuss future plans with your child: college, employment, and other goals. Reinforcing a positive focus on the future can increase the chances that your child will postpone sex, particularly if he or she appreciates that pregnancy and parenthood can derail these plans.
- Focus on and promote education. Set high expectations for academic performance; intervene early when a child shows signs of not performing to his or her potential. Be aware of homework assignments, tests, and projects. Be involved in your child's school.
- Acquaint yourself with the music, films, books, Web sites, and other information your child enjoys. The media sends children mixed messages and can espouse poor values. If elements offend you, tell your child and explain why. Encourage your child to think critically about his or her media exposures.
- Express your love and affection clearly and often. Tell your children how much you value them. Praise accomplishments, discipline them as needed, but always reinforce your unconditional love for them.

Adapted from The National Campaign to Prevent Teen Pregnancy. (2002). *Ten tips for parents to help their children avoid teen pregnancy* [Online]. Available at: http://www.teenpregnancy.org/whycare/sowhat.asp. Washington, DC: Author.

sperm cells mix with fluid from the seminal vesicles, prostate gland, and vas deferens. The man ejaculates this mixture through the penis to deposit sperm into the woman's vaginal canal, where they travel through the cervix and uterus up to the fallopian tubes and the released ovum. Only one sperm fertilizes the female ovum to create a new organism.

Box 6.2 describes pubescent physical changes in boys. The testes enlarge first, followed by growth of facial, axillary, and pubic hair, followed by enlargement of

BOX 6.1 Guidelines for Sexuality Education for Children and Adolescents

- Actively encourage families to provide sex education and contraceptive information in accordance with their values and beliefs. Guide or refer families to clinicians who can assist.
- Encourage families to discuss sexuality issues at appropriate times (eg, birth of a sibling or pet). Provide resource information.
- Obtain a comprehensive sexual history and encourage open communication in an atmosphere that ensures privacy and confidentiality. The history would include asking about sexual partners, sexual relationships, sexual identity, contraceptive practices, and specific worries about sex or sexually transmitted infections.
- Discuss high-risk behaviors leading to sexually transmitted infections, unwanted pregnancies, and contraceptive methods (eg, condom use).
- Provide acceptance and guidance to youths with special sexual issues (eg, gay and lesbian identities). Encourage parents to accept their gay and lesbian children.
- Identify youths at risk for sexual abuse. Examples include children who have previously been victimized sexually or have witnessed sexual abuse in the family or community. Others at risk are children with a history of alcohol or drug use, antisocial behavior, and learning disabilities.
- Investigate the curriculum of sex education that is given in the schools and reinforce instruction.
- Provide written material such as brochures and other handouts.

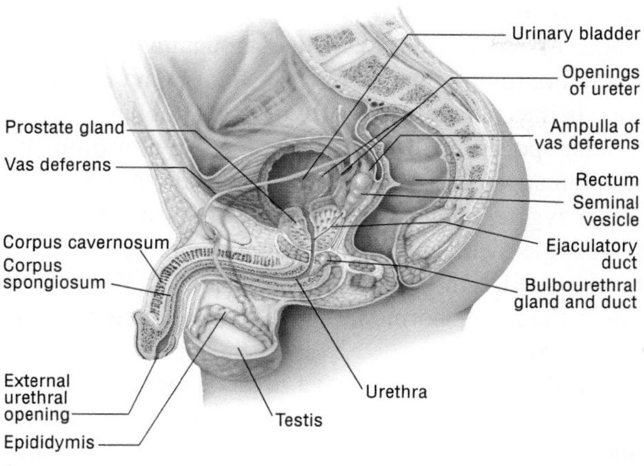

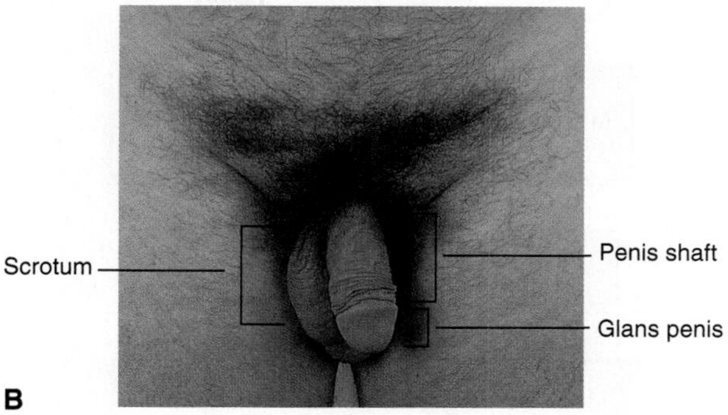

FIGURE 6.4 (**A**) Lateral view of the internal male reproductive system. (**B**) The external male genitalia. (**A** from The Anatomical Chart Company. [2001]. Atlas of human anatomy. Springhouse, PA: Springhouse.)

the penis. Approximately 1 year after the penis begins to grow, the adolescent male experiences a **nocturnal emission** (ejaculation of semen during sleep). The first nocturnal emission (commonly referred to as a "wet dream") is considered the hallmark of male puberty.

Male Hormones. Hormones are responsible for the maturation of the sexual organs (Fig. 6.6). **Testosterone** is the major androgen responsible for development and maintenance of male sex characteristics, muscle mass, and bone density. Testosterone also is found in females, but only in small amounts. Essentially, the hypothalamus controls the onset of puberty by secreting gonadotropin-releasing hormone (GnRH), which in turn stimulates the anterior pituitary gland to secrete luteinizing hormone (LH). LH then stimulates the testes to produce testosterone and follicle-stimulating hormone (FSH), which stimulates the production of sperm. Secretion of GnRH coincides and is coordinated with the growth spurt of adolescence, specifically growth of the long bones (Guyton & Hall, 2001). The timing of the increase in GnRH and testosterone production are executed carefully in the male body so that he attains a maximum height before closure of the epiphysis of the long bones (which in turn stops growth).

Any significant secretion of testosterone during preadolescence causes premature closure of the epiphyses. In such cases, these males are sexually precocious and short in stature.

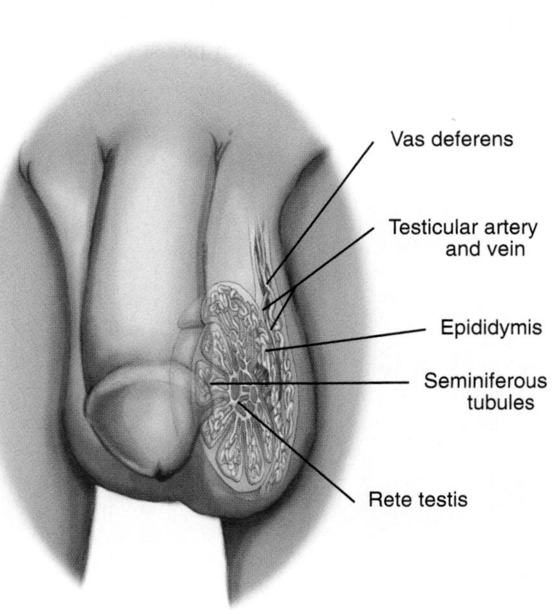

FIGURE 6.5 Internal testicular structures.

Female Pubescent Changes

Anatomy and Physiology. External female genitalia include the mons pubis, labia majora, labia minora, clitoris, urethral meatus, Skene's and Bartholin's glands, and the vaginal orifice (Fig. 6.7). Collectively, these parts are called the *vulva.*

The mons pubis consists of fatty tissue that covers the bony prominence called the symphysis pubis. The

BOX 6.2 Physical Changes in Male Puberty

- Enlargement of the testes and scrotum (first major event)
- Appearance of facial, axillary, and pubic hair (second major event)
- Enlargement of the penis (third major event)
- Thickening of larynx and deepening of voice
- Thickening of skin over body
- Roughening of scrotal skin
- Deeper pigmentation of scrotum
- Excessive secretion of the sebaceous glands
- Increase in long bone width and length

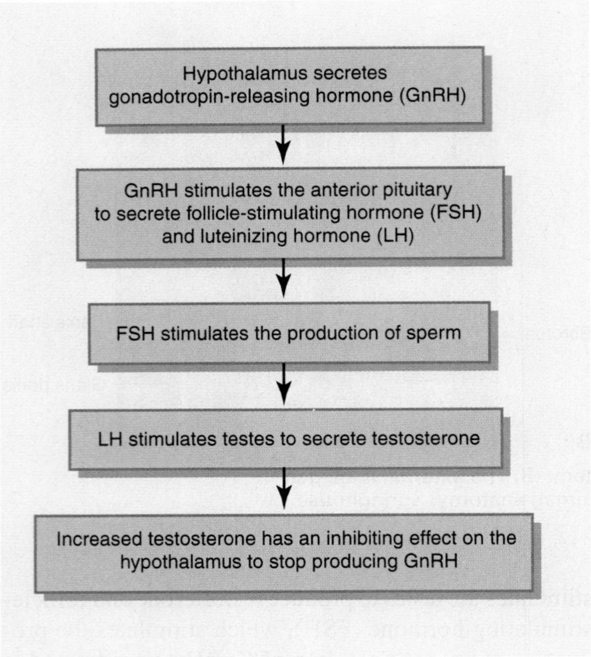

FIGURE 6.6 Summary of male reproductive hormones.

labia majora surround the external genitalia; the labia majora lie on either side of the vaginal opening. Stimulation of the *clitoris* is generally responsible for female orgasm. The Skene's and Bartholin's glands provide some lubrication.

The internal genitalia include the ovaries, fallopian tubes, uterus, and vagina (Fig. 6.8). The ovaries are two almond-shaped bodies, one on each side of the woman's pelvic cavity. The ovaries hold ova (female sex cells), **estrogen,** and progesterone. The narrow fallopian tubes are approximately 4.5 inches (11.4 cm) long and extend laterally along the sides of the uterus. They end with finger-like projections near but not touching the ovaries. Each month, the ovaries release a single ovum, which travels into the uterus by way of the fallopian tubes. If a male sperm fertilizes the ovum, the ovum implants (implantation) into the uterus and develops progressively into a zygote, embryo, and fetus. If the ovum is not fertilized, the ovum and preparatory lining (endometrium) are expelled as the female menstrual period. Box 6.3 reviews the major hormonally dependent changes of puberty in females.

Unlike male sperm, ova are not replenished. At birth, the two ovaries of the female newborn contain approximately 2,000,000 ova. By puberty, this number has declined to 300,000 to 400,000 ova, and by menopause, the number of ova is very small (Guyton & Hall, 2001). Women in developed countries can expect to release 400 ova and have approximately 400 menstrual cycles over their reproductive lives (Critchley et al., 2001). In contrast, women in developing countries experience fewer menstrual cycles because of many factors, some of which include poorer nutrition, many pregnancies, and prolonged lactation periods (Critchley et al., 2001).

The pear-shaped uterus lies between the sacrum and symphysis pubis. This muscular and expandable organ can be divided into three parts: the fundus (upper portion), the cavity, and the cervix (lower portion). The cervix connects the uterus to the vagina (Fig. 6.9).

The vagina, which lies between the urinary bladder and rectum, serves as a passageway from the uterus to the vulva. The walls of the vagina stretch during sexual intercourse and the birth of a baby.

The breasts (mammary glands) are directly influenced by estrogen and progesterone. They are the primary organs of lactation. Each breast consists of fatty

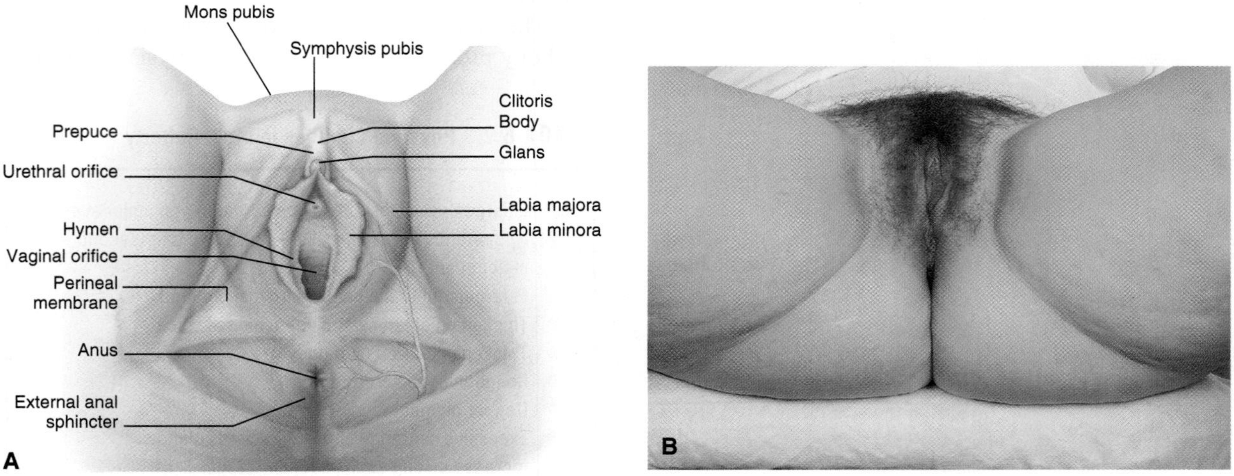

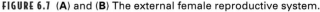

FIGURE 6.7 (**A**) and (**B**) The external female reproductive system.

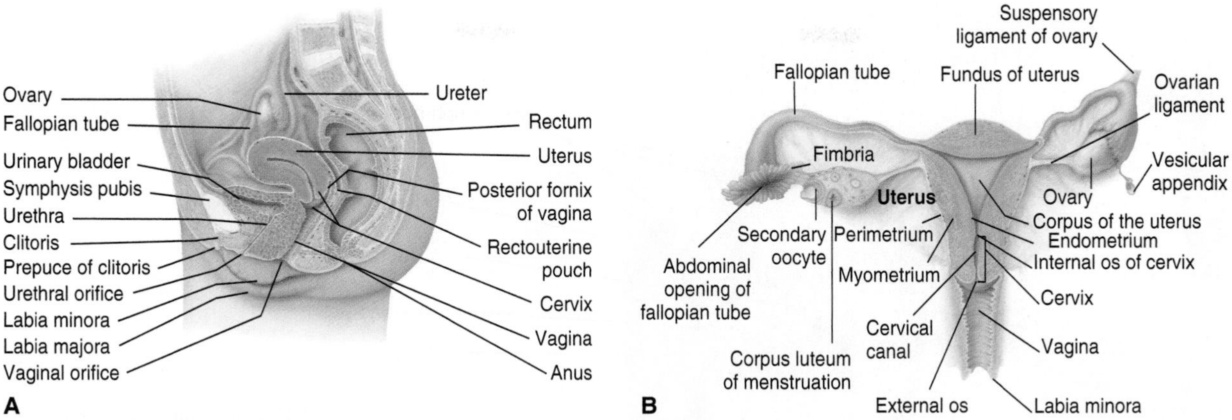

FIGURE 6.8 Internal female reproductive organs. (**A**) Lateral view. (**B**) Anterior view. (From The Anatomical Chart Company. [2001]. Atlas of human anatomy. Springhouse, PA: Springhouse.)

and glandular tissue (Fig. 6.10). The lobes of the breasts drain through ducts that open on the nipple. The round areola surrounds the nipple; its color depends on the rest of the woman's pigmentation. Breast size varies, not only among different clients, but also in the same client at different parts of her life.

Menstrual Cycle. Hormones control both the release of the unfertilized ovum at ovulation and the preparation of the uterus for the fertilized ovum in cases of pregnancy. These hormones are secreted at various times throughout the **menstrual cycle** (also called the *endometrial, ovarian,* and *sexual cycle*). The menstrual cycle lasts an average of 28 days, but it can vary normally in women from 21 to 40 days. It starts with the first day of menstruation (day 1) and ends the day before the beginning of the next period (approximately day 28) (Fig. 6.11). From **menarche** (the first ovulation and menstrual period) to **menopause,** the menstrual cycle continues monthly.

Figure 6.12 summarizes the role of hormones in the menstrual cycle. The **proliferative phase** (estrogen phase) of the menstrual cycle lasts from approximately day 5 to day 13. The hypothalamus secretes GnRH, which stimulates the anterior pituitary to secrete both FSH and LH. FSH causes several follicles to grow on both ovaries. At a given size, the follicles secrete **estrogen** (the primary female hormone), which stimulates further follicular growth and sensitivity to LH. Secreted estrogen also is responsible for the increased proliferation of epithelial cells in the endometrium (uterine lining), which thickens in preparation to house a fertilized ovum (Guyton &

BOX 6.3 Physical Changes in Female Puberty

Estrogen

- Increase in size of external genitals at puberty
- Development of mature ovaries, uterus, and fallopian tubes
- Development of the breasts
- Growth of long bones and closure of the epiphysis
- Development and maintenance of bone matrix
- Development and maintenance of secondary sex characteristics
- Development and maintenance of fat deposition patterns
- Development and maintenance of skin thickness and texture

Progesterone

- Preparation of the uterus for implantation
- Development of secretory function of the fallopian tubes
- Development of secretory function in the breasts

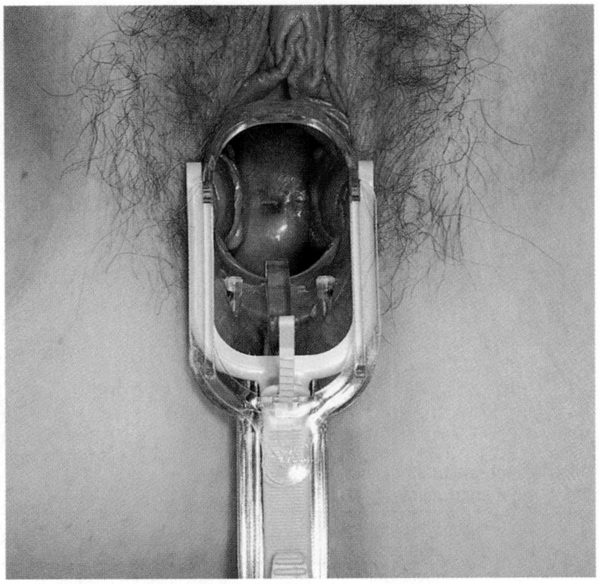

FIGURE 6.9 Appearance of the normal cervix in a multipara.

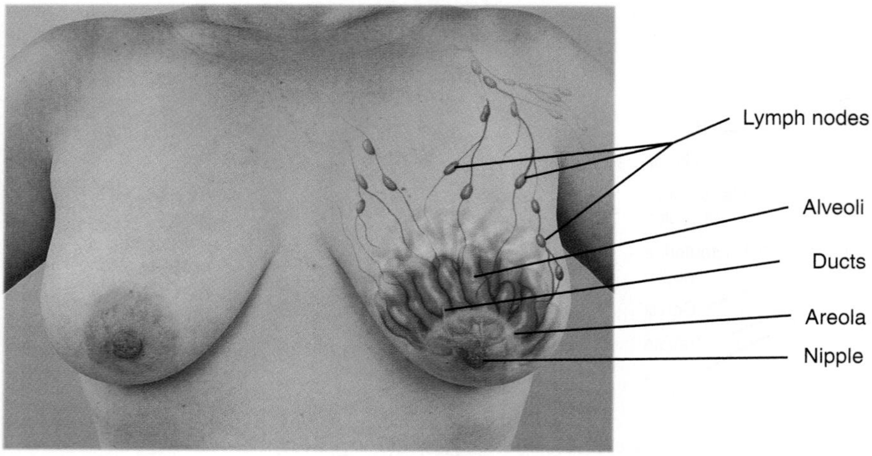

FIGURE 6.10 Anatomy of the breasts.

Hall, 2001). Together, secretion of estrogen and LH and follicular growth continue until one follicle achieves full maturation. At that time, the other follicles begin to atrophy. Secretion of LH increases, stimulating the secretion of progesterone in larger quantities than of estrogen.

Ovulation is rupture of the mature follicle and release of its ovum. It occurs as estrogen secretion diminishes and progesterone secretion increases, usually at approximately day 14 of the menstrual cycle. Sexual intercourse within 72 hours of ovulation has the potential

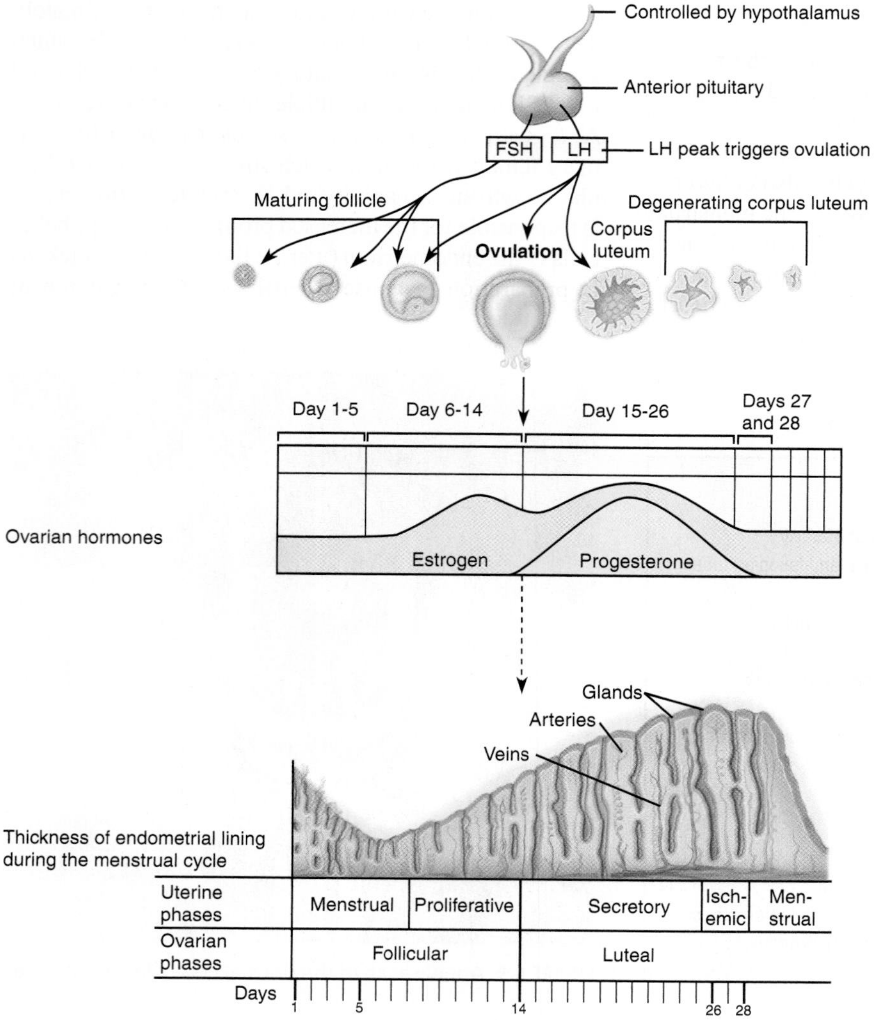

FIGURE 6.11 The 28-day (average) menstrual cycle.

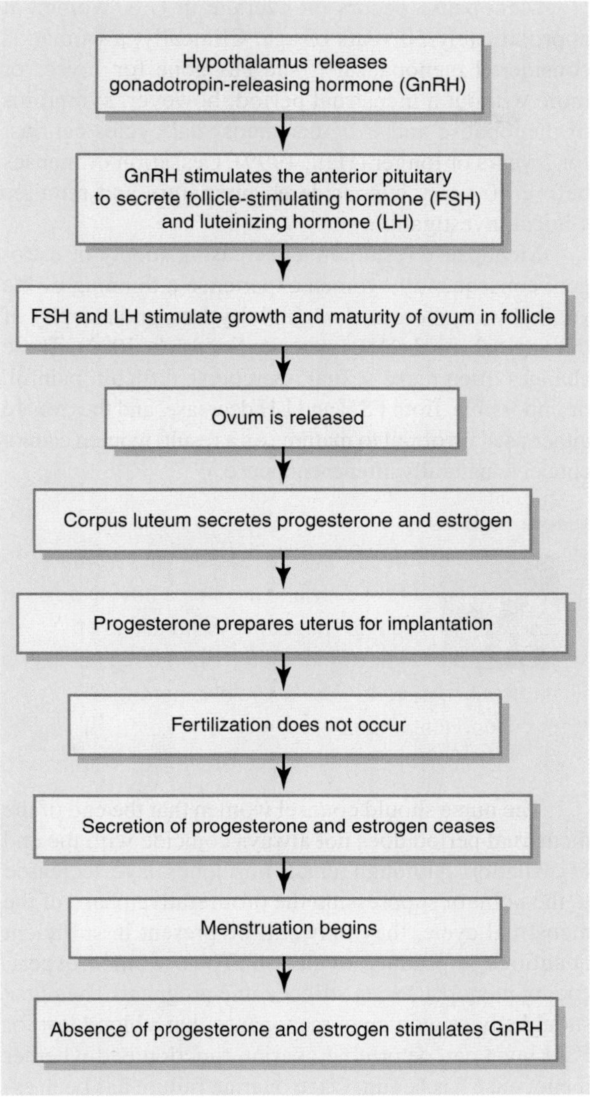
Hypothalamus releases gonadotropin-releasing hormone (GnRH)
GnRH stimulates the anterior pituitary to secrete follicle-stimulating hormone (FSH) and luteinizing hormone (LH)
FSH and LH stimulate growth and maturity of ovum in follicle
Ovum is released
Corpus luteum secretes progesterone and estrogen
Progesterone prepares uterus for implantation
Fertilization does not occur
Secretion of progesterone and estrogen ceases
Menstruation begins
Absence of progesterone and estrogen stimulates GnRH

FIGURE 6.12 Summary of female reproductive hormones.

to result in pregnancy. Methods of contraception (see Chap. 8) and fertility testing in cases of difficulty conceiving (see Chap. 10) are related to identifying ovulation and avoiding or having intercourse at this time, depending on desired outcomes.

The **secretory phase** (progesterone phase) is under the control of progesterone and lasts from approximately day 15 to day 28 of the menstrual cycle. Shortly after ovulation, the ruptured follicle remains. Granulation cells surround the empty follicle and fill with fluid (luteinize) to form a mass called the **corpus luteum.** The corpus luteum secretes a large amount of progesterone and a smaller amount of estrogen. Progesterone increases blood supply to the endometrium and adds nourishing and secretory glycoprotein and lipid deposits to the endometrial lining, making it receptive to implantation (Critchley et al., 2001).

If a sperm does not fertilize the ovum during ovulation, the **menstrual phase** occurs on day 1 of the new cycle and lasts until approximately day 4. The plush endometrial lining that developed in anticipation of a fertilized ovum is sloughed off as a bloody discharge through the vaginal canal. The withdrawal of progesterone and estrogen acts as a positive feedback mechanism to the hypothalamus to secrete GnRH. Secretion of GnRH begins the proliferative phase, reinitiating the menstrual cycle.

Recent studies show that the withdrawal of progesterone is responsible for uterine desquamation and repair; it also activates the inflammatory process of vasoconstriction, white blood cell invasion, and the complement cascade (Critchley et al., 2001). Activation of these processes would explain some of the discomfort that some women experience during menstruation.

Adulthood

Experts in sexual behavior have categorized phases of sexual arousal and orgasm. Identifying and using categorical phases enable sexual behaviorists to describe normal function and disorders. Most attempts at establishing these phases are adaptations of the original sexual response cycle studies conducted by Masters and Johnson in 1966 (Levin, 2002).

Male Sexual Response

The physiology of the male sexual response consists of penile erection, lubrication, ejaculation of semen through the internal urethra, and resolution:

- Both psychogenic stimulation from the brain and physical stimulation of the glans penis can result in erection of the penis.
- Upon sustained stimulation of the penis through intercourse or other mechanisms, the internal urethra ejects a fluid that lubricates the receptacle and further heightens sexual arousal.
- Ejaculation of semen occurs at the climax (orgasm) in spasms that originate in the sympathetic nervous system. The impulses travel from the reflex arc located at L1 and L2 to the genital organs (Guyton & Hall, 2001).
- Resolution occurs after ejaculation as the penis returns to normal size and sexual excitement disappears. Unlike in women, who are capable of multiple orgasms within a short period, vasocongestion returns to baseline much faster in men; therefore, men have limited capacity for multiple orgasm (Mah & Binik, 2001).

Female Sexual Response

The sexual response phases discussed earlier for males (desire, excitement, plateau, orgasm, and resolution) also are appropriate classifications for female sexual response. Because of male and female anatomic differences, however, females are capable of having sexual intercourse without experiencing the sexual response phases.

The female sexual response can be described from an anatomic and physiologic perspective. Stimulation of the external genitalia, specifically the labia majora, labia minora, and clitoris, can cause sexual arousal. Once aroused, genital vasocongestion results from stimulation of the reflex arc located at S1 and S2. Lubricating fluid allows vigorous penetration of the vagina without pain; tenting of the anterior vaginal wall and elevation of the cervix also occur, but the etiology for these changes is not known. Rapid firing of nerve impulses exceeds the threshold, resulting in orgasm (Levin, 2002). Presently, no scientific evidence can explain orgasm, but it is known that vaginal and uterine contractions characterize orgasm and that degrees of intensity vary by person and with each occurrence (Levin, 2002).

Researchers have not been able to identify the reason for vaginal tenting and cervical elevation during female sexual arousal. Two possible explanations include the following:

- Tenting and elevation enlarge the vaginal canal, reducing friction around the penis, delaying ejaculation, and giving the female (who achieves orgasm more slowly than the male) more time.
- Tenting and elevation create a reservoir under the cervix for storing ejaculate, providing time for the ejaculate to be decoagulated and liquefied, thus freeing sperm to be capacitated to fertilize the ovum (Levin, 2002).

During resolution, sexual excitement decreases, and the neurons return to the normal state. Women have a longer resolution phase than men. For this reason, women can have a second orgasm (or more) if stimulation continues.

Relationship Between Timing and Fertility

Conception is more likely in the absence of female orgasm because sperm require 10 to 15 minutes after ejaculation to decoagulate and achieve the motility required to travel the length of the female uterus and fallopian tubes (Levin, 2002). Widely accepted research has shown, however, that conception is likely when intercourse occurs within 72 hours of ovulation, and that there is no evidence that age of sperm in the ejaculate affects its viability or that the timing of intercourse affects the sex of the offspring (Wilcox, Weinberg, & Baird, 1995).

Middle and Older Adulthood

"My husband and I found that our sex life improved once I reached menopause. The act became solely a question of pleasure and enjoyment, without worries over contraception or pregnancy. And with the children grown and out of the house, concerns about privacy and being quiet no longer mattered. Without these stresses, I was able to enjoy sex again in a way I hadn't for almost 30 years!"

A 58-year-old woman who has been menopausal for 7 years.

Menopause occurs on average in U.S. women at approximately 50 years of age. Clinically, a woman is considered menopausal if she has gone for 1 year or more without a menstrual period; however, symptoms of menopause and irregular menstrual cycles can last for 2 years or longer (Hall, 1999). Cessation of menses before 40 years is considered premature and requires clinical investigation.

Menopause results in a decreasing supply of estrogen; consequently, women experience a thinning of the vaginal wall, increased vaginal dryness, and atrophy of the vaginal canal (DeLamater & Friedrich, 2002). These changes often make sexual intercourse difficult, painful, or impossible. Both FSH and LH decrease, and the ova are either used up or fail to mature. As a result, women cannot conceive naturally after menopause.

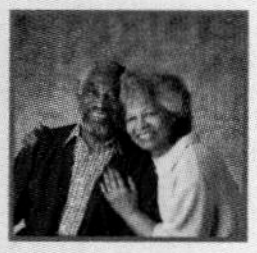

Recall Patti, the 54-year-old woman who describes problems having sex with her husband. What areas of assessment would the nurse likely focus on relative to Patti's age and potential physiologic changes?

The nurse should counsel women that the end of the menstrual period does not always coincide with the end of ovulation. Although female hormones have decreased to the point of suppressing the proliferative phase of the menstrual cycle, they may still be present in sufficient quantities to produce ovulation. Thus, women experiencing menopause can still become pregnant. The nurse should advise women in menopause that a blood test for FSH level can determine ovarian function and whether menopause has begun. Once ovarian failure has been established, the woman has reached menopause, and pregnancy is not a possibility.

Similarly, **andropause** (decreased production of androgens in men), also known as *male menopause,* occurs as early as 40 years as a result of decreased testosterone that accompanies aging. Because of decreased testosterone, aging men experience delays in achieving erections (DeLamater & Friedrich, 2002). With less testosterone, they produce less sperm. The testes become less firm, ejaculation is less forceful, pubic hair thins, and scalp hair thins or is lost. Unlike women, who no longer can reproduce naturally when menopause is established fully, men never stop producing sperm and can reproduce for a lifetime.

In the past, society tended to assume that older people did not engage in sexual activity. More recent research, however, has shown that sex continues well past menopause and andropause. Both men and women are known to be satisfactorily engaged in active sex lives well into their 80s and beyond (DeLamater & Friedrich, 2002; Shelton, 1997; Steinke, 1994; Zeis & Kasl-Godley, 2001). Maintenance of sexuality in older adulthood is an integral part of mental and physical health, self-esteem, and self-worth.

Sexual health histories on older clients should be done routinely along with providing health information and teaching about protective sex and risky sexual behavior. A thorough sexual history helps identify problems in sexual relationships. Examples include **dyspareunia** (painful sexual intercourse) related to decreased estrogen levels and resulting vaginal dryness in women, erectile dysfunction in men, and psychological problems such as feelings of rejection when the spouse or partner no longer desires sexual intercourse. See Nursing Care Plan 6.2.

As people age, sexual expression needs to be adapted to reflect physical limitations and capabilities. As men age, the force and frequency of penile erections often decrease, the time to achieve effective erection increases, and the erection does not last as long. Nurses can explain these normal phenomena and suggest ways of adaptation.

Medications prescribed to treat illnesses can cause sexual dysfunction. Examples include antihypertensive drugs, insulin, and some antidepressants. Often men will not take these medications because of actual or feared sexual dysfunction. Nurses can assist by explaining the side effects to clients and their partners and enlisting their cooperation and assistance in following the drug regimen. The nurse needs to communicate openly, provide accurate information, and listen actively to be effective in stressing the importance of compliance with the medication regimen.

CULTURAL PERSPECTIVES

To facilitate the most optimal sexual expression among clients, it is important that the nurse be aware of cultural perspectives related to sexual choices and behaviors, including culturally influenced attitudes, behaviors, and beliefs related to sex and reproduction. It is of equal importance for the nurse to always avoid treating clients based on cultural stereotypes and to plan care for each person based on individualized needs, values, and issues.

White (Caucasian) North Americans

White North Americans, particularly those of Northern European origin, exhibit few overtly specific cultural practices related to sex and reproduction. They routinely celebrate neither menarche nor male nocturnal emission. They deal with the various physical and emotional symptoms of menopause by accessing traditional as well as complementary/alternative therapies and look to health providers for relief. Until 2003, a common treatment for menopause was hormone replacement therapy (HRT), the most common form of which combined progesterone and estrogen. The use of estrogen alone for menopausal symptoms had demonstrated decreased low-density lipoprotein (LDL) blood levels. Another reason for the widespread use of HRT was decreased incidence of postmenopausal osteoporosis. Despite these benefits, results of the Women's Health Initiative study published in the *Journal of the American Medical Association* showed that combination HRT for relief of menopausal symptoms had life-threatening adverse effects (Kuller & Women's Health Initiative, 2003). The risks that the use of HRT posed for stroke and thrombosis were so dangerous that the researchers halted the study and issued new guidelines. Current evidence suggests that clinicians should carefully consider HRT for women based on risks versus benefits, duration of therapy and other individualized factors.

Asian North Americans

According to Okazaki (2002), Asians are more reserved than whites in their sexual values and attitudes. They emphasize conservative moral and social conduct and consider sex outside marriage inappropriate and harmful to the honor of the family (Okazaki, 2002). In comparison to white, Asian North Americans expect to have their first sexual intercourse later, children later, and fewer sexual partners over their lifetimes (Okazaki, 2002).

This conservatism extends to sex education and health screening. These women are less likely to engage in women's health screening and risk prevention than are women of other cultures (Okazaki, 2002). They are less likely to have discussed birth control, pregnancy, and other sexually oriented topics in their homes (Okazaki, 2002). Nurses should keep these considerations in mind when working with Asian Americans, particularly when explaining the importance of routine screening tests (such as for breast and cervical cancer).

Hispanic North Americans

U.S. Hispanic women have a risk for HIV that is 7 times the risk for white American women, a disparity that is thought to be the result of socioeconomic factors, cultural influences, and perceptions of invulnerability (Faulkner & Mansfield, 2002). Hispanic culture expects Hispanic women to see themselves as asexual, similar to the Virgin Mary, and to not discuss or enjoy sex. Women are supposed to depend on their husbands (considered to be oversexed) to teach them about sex (Faulkner & Mansfield, 2002). Because Hispanic women tend not to discuss sex, they may miss opportunities to learn how to protect themselves from HIV, other STIs, and unwanted pregnancies. The focus of behavior change for Hispanic women is to encourage communication about sex with their sexual partner and the consequences of unprotected intercourse.

NURSING CARE PLAN 6.2

The Client With Pain During Intercourse

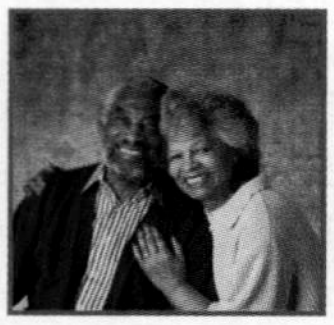

The nurse asks Patti how sexual problems have affected her marital relationship. Patti states that her husband has been patient, but the lack of intimacy is causing a strain. She also says that her husband thinks it is his fault. "He thinks I no longer find him attractive. That isn't true. It just hurt so much the last few times we had sex, that I'm afraid to do it anymore."

Assessment of Patti's sexual history reveals that she went through menopause approximately 2 years ago and that the problems with sex started around the same time. During discussion of sexual activity, Patti mentions that she wishes her husband would spend more time on foreplay, but that she's embarrassed to talk about this with him. "I don't want him to feel criticized. He's such a good man, and I know he wants me to be happy."

NURSING DIAGNOSIS

Sexual Dysfunction related to physiologic or psychologic issues

EXPECTED OUTCOMES

1. The client will understand the cause of the sexual dysfunction and take measures to treat it.
2. The client will resume a satisfying sexual relationship and adapt to altered function (if necessary).

INTERVENTIONS	RATIONALES
Refer the client for a comprehensive physical evaluation.	Health care professionals must look for physical causes of pain during intercourse and make sure that there is not an underlying problem that needs to be addressed.
Explain the age-related changes associated with menopause, including vaginal atrophy and resulting irritability and dyspareunia.	Understanding normal changes in aging may help the client realize that her experience is not uncommon or necessarily a reflection of her marital sexual relationship. Her knowledge also can assist her to communicate effectively about the problems with her husband.
Discuss possible treatment modalities with the client. Include information about estrogen tablets or creams, as well as over-the-counter moisturizers and lubricants.	Such modalities can provide the lubrication and protection against irritation needed to ensure a pleasurable sexual experience.
Discuss alternative methods for sexual expression. Explore personal values and cultural beliefs about sexual activity, and suggest methods for sexual gratification that are consistent with the client's beliefs.	The client can engage in activity other than vaginal intercourse with her spouse. Both partners may achieve orgasm through methods such as mutual masturbation or oral-genital stimulation.

Continued

NURSING CARE PLAN 6.2 ● The Client With Pain During Intercourse

INTERVENTIONS	RATIONALES
Instruct the client on techniques of clear and honest communication. Encourage her to express her feelings to her spouse. Model effective listening and how to elicit feedback.	Improved communication abilities will foster greater emotional intimacy and help prevent misunderstandings and resentment.
Encourage the client to engage in cuddling and caressing with her husband.	Physical and emotional intimacy can strengthen their overall relationship.

EVALUATION

1. The client verbalizes understanding possible causes of the pain during sex and takes steps to treat it.
2. The client reports beginning to engage in pleasurable sexual behaviors again with her husband.

African Americans

As reported previously, African American adolescents are significantly more likely to have sexual intercourse before 13 years of age than are Hispanic and white Americans (Grunbaum et al., 2002). African American girls are socialized to value traditionally masculine traits of independence and assertiveness as well as traditionally feminine traits of expressiveness and nurturance (Belgrave et al., 2000). This socialization may permit girls to feel more self-confident in sexual matters, promoting riskier behavior. On the positive side, African American teen girls are known to have greater self-esteem and a more positive body image than white American girls of the same age (Belgrave et al., 2000).

Little research has been conducted on the experience of African American women in menopause. Older African American women have respect from and are accorded positions of power in their communities, which are organized to provide support to members (Rousseau & McCool, 1997). This strong support network is most likely instrumental in assisting women through midlife crises. Physiologically, African American women have an increased risk for postmenopausal breast cancer but a decreased risk for fractures because they experience slower bone loss than white women (Rousseau & McCool, 1997). Nurses and health professionals need to focus specifically on teaching breast self-examination to these clients.

POSITIVE AND NEGATIVE ASPECTS OF SEXUAL PRACTICES AND BEHAVIORS

The Centers for Disease Control and Prevention (CDC, 2002) define exposure categories for contracting HIV/AIDS and uses them to track incidence of these STIs. By creating such categories, health professionals can better pinpoint the groups at greatest risk for exposure to not

● COMPLEMENTARY/ALTERNATIVE MEDICINE 6.1

Alternatives to Hormone Replacement Therapy

With the risks associated with hormone replacement therapy, many women are turning to over-the-counter, botanical, and complementary products to ease the menopausal transition. Examples of products used to relieve menopausal symptoms are black cohosh, ginseng, and soy protein–based isoflavones (not soy alone). Women in the Middle East, China, Japan, and Italy have used some of these products for many years to treat problems related to menopause. Although few clinical trials show proper dose, most of these products are considered safe with a degree of effectiveness based on the severity of the symptoms, purity of the product, and dose taken (Gass & Taylor, 2003).

only HIV/AIDS but also several other STIs, including hepatitis. Data from the CDC show that the following groups are at highest risk for exposure to HIV/AIDS:

- Men who have sex with men
- Men who are injecting drug users
- Men who have sex with men and are injecting drug users
- Women whose male sexual partners engage in sex with men
- Women who are injecting drug users

Sexual behaviors, including those above, can pose risks for contracting STIs, including HIV/AIDS, and for having unplanned pregnancies. Table 6.1 shows negative aspects of risky sexual practices and associated outcomes. The key to avoiding negative or undesired outcomes is the practice of safer sex. Safer sex is called "safer" rather than safe because no method is 100% safe, other than total abstinence. Teaching Tips 6.2 provides information on safer sex options for physical intimacy.

One major risk factor for sexual health problems is having multiple sexual partners. Health care professionals should encourage clients to maintain monogamous sexual relationships to reduce their risks for health problems. They should advise clients to screen sexual partners for disease by asking about previous relationships and the possibility of having acquired a past STI. It is important to note that both heterosexual women and lesbians should be screened because lesbians may have had heterosexual experiences themselves or have had partners who have had heterosexual experiences. The desired outcomes are to reduce the risk for HIV/AIDS to the client and the client's contacts and to reduce the risk for other STIs (see Chap. 4). Reducing risk means that clients should avoid having unprotected sex and should minimize their number of partners.

Unwanted pregnancies are another potential negative outcome of unprotected vaginal intercourse. They can lead to difficult psychological and social choices about whether to end or continue the pregnancy. The number of abortions in the United States peaked in 1990 and has been declining since (Finer & Henshaw, 2003). The reason for the decline is thought to be increased education about contraception and a decreased number of physicians willing to perform abortion. In addition, some youth have embraced the concept of abstinence. The health care provider should not overlook abstinence as an option in providing counseling about birth control and avoiding unwanted pregnancies (see Chaps. 8 and 9).

TABLE 6.1 Negative Aspects of Sexual Practices and Potential Outcomes

SEXUAL PRACTICE	NEGATIVE OUTCOMES
Unprotected anal sex	Sexually transmitted infections HIV/AIDS Hepatitis A, B, and C Anal fissures and abscesses Colitis, enteritis, gastrointestinal disturbances Scabies, pubic lice
Unprotected vaginal sex	Sexually transmitted infections HIV/AIDS Hepatitis A, B, and C Unplanned pregnancy Scabies, pubic lice
Unprotected oral sex	Sexually transmitted infections Urethritis HIV/AIDS Hepatitis A, B, and C

SEXUAL ORIENTATION AND RELATED ISSUES

Several theories exist about the etiology of homosexuality and bisexuality. Researchers believe that a combination of biologic, social, and environmental events determine sexual orientation. Research studies by Hamer, Hu, Magnuson, Hu, and Pattatucci in 1993 and Turner in 1995 suggest the involvement of a chromosomal marker in sexual orientation. Sequencing and mapping of the human genome have been completed only recently, with findings still being evaluated. Many causal relationships for several elements of human experience may soon be discovered, including the genetic components of sexual orientation.

Gay Identity Development

QUOTE 6-1

"Homosexuality . . . is nothing to be ashamed of . . . it cannot be classified as an illness. . . . We consider it to be a variation of the sexual function . . . It is a great injustice to persecute homosexuality . . . and a cruelty, too."

Sigmund Freud in a letter dated April 9, 1935, to a woman requesting treatment for her son. The Letters of Sigmund Freud *(1961).*

Parents, peers, friends, and relatives attempt to socialize children into their respective societally accepted biologic roles from birth. This socialization extends to the realm of sexuality as well. Parents tend to naturally expect that their children will begin to show interest in members of the opposite sex, particularly as adolescence approaches.

Parents may feel some apprehension about their child's sexual orientation if their son seems indifferent to girls or their daughter maintains tomboyish traits into the teen years. Gay identities usually begin to develop in the prepubertal stage. Often the gay child feels or is noticed as being "different." Some hide their gay identity or reveal it late in life because of perceived pressure to follow heterosexual expectations.

● TEACHING TIPS 6.2 Safer Sex Options for Physical Intimacy

TEACHING POINTS

A common nursing role is educating clients in a variety of health care settings (community groups, clinics, hospitals) about the prevention of sexually transmitted infections (STIs). The following is a listing of guidelines for safer sex that the nurse may wish to share with clients.

SAFER SEXUAL ACTIVITIES

- Massage
- Masturbation
- Hugging
- Hand-to-genital touching (hand job)
- Mutual masturbation
- Body rubbing
- Erotic books and movies
- Dry kissing
- All sexual activities when both partners are monogamous, trustworthy, and known by testing to be free of HIV

POSSIBLY SAFER SEXUAL ACTIVITIES

- Wet kissing with no broken skin, cracked lips, or damaged mouth tissue
- Vaginal or rectal intercourse using latex or synthetic condom correctly
- Oral sex on a man using latex or synthetic condom
- Oral sex on a woman using a latex or synthetic barrier such as a female condom, dental dam, or modified male condom, especially if she does not have her period or a vaginal infection with discharge
- All sexual activities when both partners are in a long-term monogamous relationship and trust each other

UNSAFE SEXUAL ACTIVITIES IN THE ABSENCE OF HIV TESTING, TRUST, AND MONOGAMY

- Any vaginal or rectal intercourse without a latex or synthetic condom
- Oral sex on a man without a latex or synthetic condom
- Oral sex on a woman without a latex or synthetic barrier such as a female condom, dental dam, or modified male condom, especially if she is having her period or has a vaginal infection with discharge
- Semen in the mouth
- Oral–anal contact
- Sharing sex toys or douching equipment
- Blood contact of any kind, including menstrual blood, or any sex that causes tissue damage or bleeding

From Mohr, W. K. (2006). *Psychiatric–mental health nursing* (6th ed.). Philadelphia: Lippincott Williams & Wilkins.

Stages

Table 6.2 shows the stages of developing a gay identity. Women move through the stages at slightly different rates than do men. The stages do not represent every homosexual person: many gay and lesbian people move through the stages faster or slower, or appear to skip a stage. As society becomes more accepting of a wider variety of sexual orientations, acceptance of gay and lesbian identities is likely to occur earlier (Perrin, 2002).

Sensitization. This stage typically represents preadolescence. Girls with a lesbian sexual orientation report being more interested in sports than are same-sex peers; boys with gay sexual orientation report not being interested in sports, preferring solitary activities, such as reading and music (Perrin, 2002). Both boys and girls may be attracted vaguely to members of the same sex, but usually preadolescents do not label the attraction as sexual.

Identity Confusion. During this stage, many gay and lesbian people begin to recognize their vague same-sex attraction as potentially homosexual. Because they have identified up to now with the heterosexual community, confusion or cognitive dissonance emerges about identity. Self-recognition of homosexuality has been happening earlier, with the average age now being 17 years for gay males and 18 years for lesbians (Perrin, 2002).

Social stigma related to homosexuality often prevents rapid self-acceptance of the **minority sexual orientation.** This lack of self-acceptance often leads to denial, attempts to eliminate the same-sex attraction (repair), or avoidance of recognition of these feelings. In some cases, the person may redefine himself or herself as **bisexual** (having an attraction to or sexual relationships with members of the same sex and the opposite sex).

Identity Assumption. In this stage, the person accepts the gay or lesbian identity, associates with others who are gay, and begins homosexual experimentation. If the gay or lesbian person does not achieve self-acceptance, he or she may be isolated from both heterosexual and homosexual societies, and a life of secrecy and fear of discovery begins (Perrin, 2002). To elaborate, if a gay or lesbian person denies homosexuality and joins the heterosexual community, a secret life of "passing" as heterosexual begins. During "passing," the gay or lesbian person does not quite "fit in" with the heterosexual community. People notice that he or she lacks interest in heterosexual relationships; the absence of a "partner" automatically eliminates the person from some heterosexual circles. One might think

TABLE 6.2 Stages in the Formation of a Gay Identity

STAGE	APPROXIMATE AGE	CHARACTERISTICS
Sensitization	Before puberty	Has gender neutrality or cross-gender interests Feels "different" from same-sex peers
Identity confusion	Early adolescence	Has same sex arousal, activity, or both Has inner turmoil and confusion Inadequate coping mechanisms include attempts to justify behavior or avoidance of similar situations May become socially isolated to hide behavior or become heavily involved in heterosexual activity
Identity assumption	Adolescence	Accepts same sex behavior, same sex friends, and activities Explores sexual minority culture and activities Inadequate coping behavior includes keeping lifestyle secret or, alternatively, flaunting gay status
Commitment	Adulthood	Accepts and discloses gay identity Develops same-sex intimacy and joins the gay community Inadequate coping includes keeping gay identity secret, becoming socially isolated, and sometimes turning to alcohol and drugs

Adapted from Troiden, R. R. (1988). Homosexual identity development. *Journal of Adolescent Health Care, 9*(2), 105–113.

that this experience is similar to living as a single heterosexual person; however, this assumption is incorrect. A heterosexual single person maintains his or her true sexual orientation and builds a network of friends, both male and female, who accept the person as straight. The single heterosexual person always has the potential for an intimate relationship. A "passing" homosexual person does not live this way because he or she has not declared a sexual orientation. Therefore, he or she cannot form consensual relationships based on trust and loses the potential for intimate relationships. By the same token, the homosexual person "passing" as a heterosexual person cannot form consensual relationships in the gay community either. Relationships he or she establishes will be superficial and different from those that he or she would develop if trying to join the gay community as a gay person. Elements of truth and trust are missing from the relationships of a person who is "passing." He or she is living a lie; the result is social isolation, "self-hatred, and despair" (Perrin, 2002, p. 77).

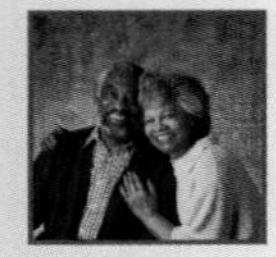

Recall Patti, the woman who reports that she is having pain during intercourse. What if, instead, Patti had reported that she secretly had always been attracted to other women and no longer wanted to pretend with her husband? How would the nurse have changed her approach to the client's problem?

Commitment. In the last stage, *commitment,* the gay or lesbian accepts the homosexual identity, maintains intimate relationships, and takes an active role in the homosexual community (Perrin, 2002). At this stage, the homosexual is openly gay or lesbian and does not wish to be heterosexual.

Disclosure (Coming Out)

Much has been written about the lack of parental, peer, and community support for homosexuals, especially gay and lesbian adolescents. In addition, physical and psychological abuse of sexual minorities is common in societies with a heterosexual majority. Acceptance by family, peers, and community plays an important role in the ability of sexual minority youths to reach the stage of commitment and maintain acceptance of self and lifestyle.

Disclosure of homosexual orientation is the equivalent of "coming out." Disclosure usually occurs first with a close friend who is also gay or lesbian, then with role models such as teachers and community leaders, who are also gay or lesbian (Perrin, 2002). Gay and lesbian adolescents often need assistance from professionals in disclosing to parents when it appears that parental support is not available (Cant, 2006).

Psychosocial and Cultural Issues

Homosexuals are at risk for psychosocial problems because of societal stigma against their sexual orientations. Exactly when they most need social support, homosexual youths are dealing with nonacceptance. Nonacceptance occurs in many forms. Many youths report being harassed, ignored, physically assaulted, and verbally abused (Perrin, 2002). In addition, studies have shown that youths with a minority sexual orientation, such as homosexuality, are more likely than heterosexual youths to attempt suicide (McAndrew & Warne, 2004; Savin-Williams, 2001). Other alterations in coping include depression, isolation, and substance abuse.

To better understand the social implications of being a minority of any kind, nurses should consider the concept of stigma. Various sources define **stigma,** an undesirable attribute, as being in a reduced form compared with the usual person (Drury & Louis, 2002). A stigmatized person has some attribute that the general population considers unusual, different, and undesirable. This stigmatization involves more frequent monitoring of the person from the minority background, as well as interpreting his or her behavior according to stereotypes about that minority. Consider, for example, past experiences in classrooms in which people with disabilities are pupils. Attention is drawn immediately to the person with a disability, who stands out in a crowd and becomes an object of continuous scrutiny and monitoring by the "normal" population.

The openly gay or lesbian person, as a result of his or her minority status, is a visible subject of frequent monitoring by the general population (the majority). Others judge the stigmatized gay or lesbian person based on stereotypes. As stigmatized people, gays and lesbians feel compelled to "hide," "pass as straight," or "come out" and face the full effects of that choice, regardless of whether they are fully ready to do so. Once the gay or lesbian person has "come out," his or her relationships with all segments of society change. Because society tends to assume that all people have a heterosexual orientation, gay and lesbian people face judgment on two planes: as a person and as a homosexual person. Many gays and lesbians have extreme difficulty integrating the homosexual self into overall self because they are viewing themselves through the eyes of the heterosexual community.

One strategy that some heterosexuals use in an attempt to show acceptance of homosexual people, ironically, has the opposite effect. In some cases, heterosexuals act as though there is nothing different about the gay or lesbian person, or they avoid the issue altogether. The strategy of accepting the homosexual person without acknowledging his or her sexual orientation is paramount to setting up a power base to control the issue. To further explain, if a heterosexual person decides to ignore a friend's homosexuality and to not relate to the friend as homosexual, the heterosexual person has, in essence, placed a restriction of silence on the relationship. The lack of discussion permits denial of the friend's homosexual status, causing the friend to "pass." Thus, seeming blindness to sexual orientation (as well as to ethnicity, race, age, disability, or gender) does not equate with acceptance and lack of prejudice.

COLLABORATIVE CARE: ALTERNATIVE SEXUAL ORIENTATION

Nurses and other health care professionals need to address differences in sexual orientation to identify medical and other problems specific to the person. It is important for nurses to view sexual orientation as part of the client's psychosocial and biologic makeup. Each person presents with unique and individual needs as a result of homosexuality, bisexuality, or heterosexuality. For example, the nurse should approach the collaborative care of clients with alternative sexual orientations with an appreciation and respect for each client's worth and dignity with a nonjudgmental attitude (Kirton et al., 2001). Health care professionals can provide enormous support to clients by assisting them through periods of disclosure to others and simply making them feel accepted and valued as they are.

Assessment

The nurse should complete a sexual history on all clients. Because sex is a sensitive issue for many, the nurse may begin by asking the client to agree to answer the questions in the sexual history. Privacy and confidentiality are essential. The health professional should convey to the client the importance of the sexual history in identifying risks and planning care. The nurse should ask questions professionally and with concern. See Assessment Tool 6.1 for appropriate questions to ask in a sexual, nonreproductive history in any setting. When a person discloses that he or she has an alternative sexual orientation, the nurse can include the questions presented in Assessment Tool 6.2.

The nurse can use the assessment in evaluating risks to sexual health, as well as overall physical, psychological, and social consequences of such risks. Along with the client, the nurse can integrate the findings in developing appropriate client-centered interventions.

Select Potential Nursing Diagnoses

When a client has a minority sexual orientation, nursing diagnoses frequently involve psychosocial issues. Some potential nursing diagnoses are as follows.

- **Ineffective Sexuality Patterns** related to possible transmission of disease
- **Deficient Knowledge** about sexual orientation and lack of information about protection from STIs
- **Anticipatory Grieving** related to loss of psychosocial well-being
- **Ineffective Health Maintenance** related to lack of information about acquisition and transmission of disease
- **Ineffective Sexuality Patterns** related to fear of acquiring an STI and impaired relationship with significant other

● ASSESSMENT TOOL 6.1 Appropriate Questions in a Sexual (Nonreproductive) History

- Are you in now or have you been in a sexual relationship?
- Is your relationship with a person of the same sex or opposite sex?
- Are you having sexual intercourse in this relationship?
- Is the sexual intercourse vaginal-penile, anal, oral, or manual?
- Do you prefer relationships with men, women, or both?
- Are you worried about sexually transmitted infections (STIs) such as HIV?
- Have you ever had an STI?
- Does your partner have an STI? Has your partner had an STI in the past?
- Have you had multiple sexual partners?
- How many partners have you had in the past year?
- Do you use contraception? If so, what kind?
- Do you use condoms or other protection during sex?
- Does your partner use protection or contraception?
- Does your partner have multiple sex partners?
- Are you happy with your sexuality?
- Have you been sexually abused?

- **Impaired Social Interaction** related to sociocultural dissonance
- **Sexual Dysfunction** related to ineffective or absent role model and conflicting values
- **Risk for Powerlessness** related to low self-esteem
- **Risk for Infection** related to high-risk behavior and lack of knowledge about safer sex methods
- **Risk for Situational Low Self-Esteem** related to decreased power and control over environment
- **Risk for Suicide** related to low self-esteem, isolation, fear, and powerlessness
- **Risk for Delayed Psychosocial Adjustment** related to denial of sexual orientation (not NANDA)

Planning/Intervention

Many of the above nursing diagnoses are indirectly or directly related to Deficient Knowledge related to lack of exposure to information. When assisting a client to deal with issues of sexual orientation, as well as other matters related to sexuality, the nurse should tailor planning, interventions, and goals to the client's specific circumstances. NIC/NOC Box 6.1 provides some common interventions and outcomes related to the issue of sexual orientation.

Related nursing interventions for clients with minority sexual orientation focus on the following strategies:

- Determine the client's stage of sexual orientation identity development.
- Teach the client the stages of sexual orientation identity development.
- Assist the client to accept his or her homosexual orientation.
- Determine high-risk behaviors for health problems; discuss findings with the client.
- Provide safer sex education.

● ASSESSMENT TOOL 6.2 Sexual Assessment of Clients with Minority Sexual Orientation

The following are questions the nurse can ask when taking a history from a homosexual or bisexual client:

- Do you consider yourself homosexual or bisexual? How long have you been "out" to yourself about your orientation? Do you wish to have, or have you had, any same-sex sexual experiences?
- What are your thoughts or feelings about your orientation? If you have positive feelings about being homosexual or bisexual, how do you feel you developed this outlook? If you have negative feelings about being homosexual or bisexual, how do you cope with these feelings? Do you feel you have accepted your homosexuality or bisexuality?
- Are you "out" in your life (at work or school)? Of your family and friends who know, how do they feel about your orientation?
- Whom do you consider as your support system? Do they know you are homosexual or bisexual? Do you have homosexual or bisexual friends? Has being "out" or "closeted" about your orientation caused any problems in your family, place of work, church, or social relationships? How do you deal with these problems?
- Do you have a lover or life partner? Do you and your partner have any unresolved issues that need to be addressed? How have AIDS and other sexually transmitted infections affected your sex life and relationship? Do your family and friends know the nature of your relationship? Are they supportive?

Adapted from Smith, B. S. (1992). Nursing care challenges: Homosexual psychiatric patients. *Journal of Psychosocial Nursing, 30*(12), 15–21.

NIC/NOC Box 6.1 Sexual Orientation

NIC

- Complex Relationship Building
- Coping Enhancement
- Counseling
- Decision-Making Support
- Emotional Support
- Grief Work Facilitation
- Health Education
- Infection Protection
- Risk Identification
- Self-Awareness Enhancement
- Self-Esteem Enhancement
- Self-Responsibility Facilitation
- Support Group
- Support System Enhancement
- Teaching: Disease Process
- Teaching: Safer Sex
- Teaching: Sexuality

NOC

- Coping
- Decision Making
- Grief Resolution
- Knowledge: Health Behaviors
- Knowledge: Sexual Functioning
- Psychosocial Adjustment: Life Change
- Risk Control: Sexually Transmitted Diseases
- Self-Direction of Care
- Self-Esteem Enhancement
- Sexual Identity: Acceptance

- Encourage monogamous relationships; explain the dangers and risks associated with multiple sexual partners.
- Provide information about community resources and support groups geared toward clients with minority sexual orientations.
- Refer the client to a counselor if appropriate.
- Offer support if the client is facing family issues related to his or her sexual orientation.
- Encourage the client to discuss episodes of being a target of homophobic jokes.
- Provide referrals for spiritual counseling if desired.
- Screen the client for suicidal thoughts.
- Refer the client for appropriate medical screening and laboratory tests for STIs.

Evaluation

The nurse evaluates the effectiveness of interventions for specific goals based on each client's particular concern. Possible desired outcomes for the client dealing with issues related to sexual orientation include the following:

- The client verbalizes behavior considered "high risk" for STIs, the types of STIs that can result from high-risk behavior, and understanding of how STIs are acquired and transmitted.
- The client verbalizes strategies for safer sex.
- The client identifies positive and negative aspects of sexual orientation and designs a plan to manage threats to psychological well-being.
- The client develops a plan to disclose sexual orientation to family and close friends.
- The client verbalizes names and phone numbers of relevant support groups.
- The client identifies a role model of the same sexual orientation.
- The client identifies positive aspects of sexual orientation and specific individual talents and abilities that contribute to the improvement of the community to which he or she belongs.
- The client verbalizes no suicidal ideation.

SEXUAL AND REPRODUCTIVE RITES OF PASSAGE

The concept of **cultural identity** includes "religion, rites of passage, language, dietary habits, and leisure activities" (Bhugra et al., 1999, p. 245). **Rites of passage** are traditions, often ceremonious, that mark specific points or milestones in a human life. They have the positive function of demonstrating that the culture has accepted a person as part of the community; thus, they are associated with a strong sense of belonging. Rites of passage go beyond celebrations. For example, a baby shower is a celebration. It is not a rite of passage, however, because it does not signify a transformation, is not a tradition embraced by one culture, has not been passed down for generations, is not associated with standard symbolic dress or ritual, and is not required for acceptance into a culture.

The Vision Quest is a rite of passage for some Native American tribes. A medicine man takes an adolescent male into a sweat chamber fired by burning cedars and assists the teen with his prayers (Delaney, 1995). Then, he takes the boy to an isolated spot where the teen prays and fasts for 4 to 5 days until a vision comes to him about how he will spend the rest of his life (Delaney, 1995). Symbolism, tradition, ritual, assistance from elders, and cultural acceptance guide and transform the male from teen to adult.

It has been proposed that certain cultures have modified rites of passage that relate more to modern times (Delaney, 1995). Because of the enslavement of African Americans in the United States, many feel that their rites of passages were taken from them (Fleming, 1996). Consequently, some African American groups are developing programs geared to re-establishing rites of passage for events including birth, adulthood, eldership, and death (Fleming, 1996). The purpose of the National Rites of Passage Institute (www.ritesofpassage.org) is to return roots to African American youth and to socialize them into becoming productive citizens.

Female Circumcision

Some cultures support female circumcision because of profound religious beliefs. They conduct the rituals as part of religious ceremonies. Contrary to popular assumptions, many women consider the procedure more than a rite of passage: they associate the practice with cultural cleanliness, respect, loyalty, religious piety, and proof of virginity, which brings honor to the family. In these cultures, uncircumcised females are stigmatized as unworthy of marriage, and their children are ostracized because they have been born to uncircumcised women (Vissandjee et al., 2003; Wright, 1996). Those who support female circumcision and emigrate to countries that ban or oppose the practice sometimes change their perceptions after leaving their countries of origin. Many immigrants to the West still believe in female circumcision, however, and return their females to their home countries for the procedure (Vissandjee et al., 2003).

Female circumcision can take three different forms. The first and most traditional procedure is *Sunna circumcision* (surgical removal of the tip of the clitoris). The second is *clitoridectomy,* or removal of the entire clitoris. The third, *infibulation,* is removal of the entire clitoris, labia minora, and sometimes labia majora, with closure of the vaginal canal: a ridge for the urinary meatus and a small hole for menstruation are constructed (Wright, 1996; Young, 2002). With infibulation, the closed vaginal canal often requires cutting for intercourse and restitching after childbirth.

Cultures that practice female circumcision posit several rationales for the procedure. Examples include that it:

- Reduces sexual pleasure for the woman, thus preventing her promiscuity
- Reduces gender ambiguity
- Increases chances for marriage (because of increased sexual pleasure for the man as a result of the decreased size of the vaginal opening)
- Preserves virginity and proof of it

Lay midwives and other people who perform female circumcision (eg, male barbers) may use nonsterile tools such as knives and razors and no analgesia to perform the procedure (Wright, 1996). In 1998, the World Health Organization (WHO) estimated that 135 million young women had undergone some form of female circumcision and that 2 million girls and women undergo this procedure annually (Moshovis, 2002). Infection, hemorrhage, shock, and death are immediate postprocedural complications. Long-term problems include dysmenorrhea, urinary tract infection, incontinence, urinary retention, and reproductive tract infections.

Recently, concern has arisen among Western health care professionals about female circumcision. U.S. and Canadian health professionals are being sought to assist with procedures in people migrating from countries where female circumcision is common. This development puts physicians in the position of considering the procedure from an ethical decision-making model. Opponents deplore the practice, believing that it decreases women's power and ensures male domination over them. Some physicians feel conflicted, believing that at least if they performed the procedure, regardless of whether they agreed with it, the client would suffer fewer complications.

Male Circumcision

Male circumcision originated with native West African tribes more than 5,000 years ago (Chessler, 1997). The four types of male circumcision are *simple* (removal of the prepuce or foreskin), *subincision* (simple circumcision followed by slitting of the penis to expose the glans), *salkh* (cutting a strip of skin from the navel to the lower thigh), and *superincision* (cutting the preputium from the upper surface to the pubic area) (Chessler, 1997).

Male circumcision is a rite of passage in some cultures. The Jewish faith requires the circumcision of all healthy males on the eighth day after birth. The Jewish procedure is done by a *mohel,* a ritual expert, outside the hospital during a celebration (the *bris*) with many relatives and friends.

In the Muslim faith, circumcision is a religious obligation; however, the ritual differs greatly from that practiced by Jews. Muslim boys are required to be circumcised sometime before adulthood, and the ceremonies often are held for a group of boys circumcised at one time (Miller, 2002). Eight days of celebration precede the circumcisions; after the ceremony, the boys' foreskins are buried in the ground (Miller, 2002).

In the United States, nonreligious male circumcision is a medical procedure unrelated to religion or culture. In 1977, circumcision was the most common surgical procedure performed on males in the United States; it is still performed on 60% of U.S. boys (Miller, 2002), but is neither supplied nor rejected by the ASAP. See Chapter 20 for more discussion of preoperative, intraoperative, and postoperative care.

The U.S. cultural norm of male circumcision results partly from the influence of Jewish and Muslim populations (Miller, 2002). In some cases, families base the decision about circumcising their sons on issues of social acceptance and "normality." Until recent years, the commonality of circumcision often caused men with uncircumcised penises to experience a sense of socially undesirability or "differentness." They experienced (and in some cases may still undergo) stigmatization as effeminate, deformed, and even unclean. Other families want circumcision for their male child because they believe it will cause him less confusion if his male genitalia share the same appearance as those of the father and other male relatives.

Medical rationales for circumcision have been that it promotes cleanliness and prevents smegma (whitish collection of dead cells) from accumulating under the foreskin (Miller, 2002). Other medical rationales for circumcision include prevention of HIV, penile cancer, cervical cancer in women, urinary tract infections, and masturbation. These rationales have been challenged. Complications include ". . . meatal ulceration, hemorrhage, infection, retention of the plastic bell ring, concealed penis, urethral fistula, urinary retention, glans necrosis, injury and loss of glans, excessive skin loss, skin bridge, and preputial cysts" (Chessler, 1997, p. 561). The glans covered by a foreskin has a natural moist lubrication thought to have a beneficial effect to women during sexual intercourse by providing a moist gliding action that lubricates the vagina and prevents dyspareunia (painful intercourse). The penis with an uncovered glans is dry because the foreskin serves to keep the glans moist, which is the normal state.

Questions to Ponder

1. A 6-year-old boy undergoes surgery for a ruptured appendix. During the operation, surgeons discover that the boy has two functional ovaries. Because the boy has had male external genitalia from birth (except for smaller than usual testes), the parents have raised the child as a boy. Health care professionals refer the family to a psychologist for counseling.
   - What are some gender issues that the family will have to consider?
   - Should a sex assignment as female be made and surgery to construct a vagina be planned? If so, why? If not, why?
2. You are working as a nurse in a combined labor, delivery, and nursery unit on the day shift. An obstetrician rushes up to you at 10:00 AM and shouts, "Prepare the Lewis baby and the Marcus baby for circumcision right now. I have to be in the operating room with a client having a cesarean section at 10:45 AM. I will be back in 5 minutes." As you are strapping the two infant boys to the circumcision board, you are worrying that you have not had time to adequately premedicate the infants and that the infants will suffer pain.
   - What strategies can you implement at the moment?
   - What strategies can you use to prevent this problem in the future?

SUMMARY

- Development of the sexual self is an important part of a person's identity, integrated sense of self, ability to reproduce, and ability to fulfill role functions.
- The human germ cell goes through three stages before birth: pre-embryonic (gestational days 1 to 14), embryonic (gestational day 15 through gestational week 8), and fetal (end of gestational week 8 to birth).
- The internal sex organs determine the infant's gender; however, in some cases, gender is ambiguous. Gender assignment usually is based on the internal organs, except in cases of late discovery, in which gender is assigned based on the felt identity of the child.
- Hermaphroditism and female and male pseudohermaphroditism are examples of variations in normal sexual development.
- Gender constancy does not occur in children until approximately 7 years.
- Origins of sex role behavior can be traced to historical, cultural, social, and religious influences.
- During fertilization, the man ejaculates approximately 120 million sperm cells in a fluid from his penis, but only one sperm fertilizes the female ovum in a single birth.
- The male hormone testosterone is responsible for the development of male sex characteristics, development and maintenance of muscle mass, and bone density.
- The menstrual cycle depends on the female hormones of gonadotropin, luteinizing hormone, follicle-stimulating hormone, estrogen, and progesterone.
- The menstrual cycle is divided into three phases: proliferative, secretory, and menstrual. Ovulation occurs between the proliferative and secretory phases.
- Conception is more likely when sexual intercourse occurs within 72 hours of ovulation.
- Female menopause is established after 1 year of no menstrual bleeding. Menopause is associated with the inability to conceive.
- Men and women remain sexually active until old age.
- Sexual intercourse and unwanted pregnancies are community health concerns in the United States.
- Nurses encourage parents, families, and friends to accept their gay and lesbian children. Likewise, the community needs to recognize and accept the gay and lesbian population.
- Gay and lesbian people go through developmental stages until making a commitment to the gay and lesbian identity.
- Because the sexual self is an integral part of the self, the nurse conducts a sexual history on all clients who seek or need care irrespective of disease process, sexual orientation, and age (from puberty to death).
- Female circumcision of women younger than 18 years is illegal in the United States.

REVIEW QUESTIONS

1. Molly is a 3-year-old girl who frequently plays with Michael, a 3-year-old boy who lives next door. One day, Michael brings his toy trucks and railroad cars to Molly's house for Molly to see. While Michael is there, Molly intently plays with Michael's dump truck. She pretends that she is driving and hauling dirt. Molly's mother, Jill, sees this and is concerned that Molly seems so interested in playing with the trucks, because this is a "boy's" activity. Which of the following is the probable rationale for Jill's concern?
   A. Jill is afraid that Molly will get hurt playing with toys that boys like.
   B. Jill is worried that Molly will try to keep the trucks and Michael will be upset.
   C. Jill is worried that Molly will lose interest in all her other toys.
   D. Jill is concerned that Molly is showing early signs of lesbian traits.
2. The nurse discusses with Jill her concerns about her 3-year-old daughter Molly and Molly's interest in trucks. Which of the following is the most appropriate advice for the nurse to offer?
   A. Jill should continue to watch for more signs of male gender–specific behavior.
   B. Jill should not worry because behavior is not gender specific until school age.
   C. Jill should take Molly to a child psychologist as soon as possible.
   D. Jill should quietly put Michael's toys out of sight.
3. A mother of a newborn girl, who is visiting the United States from Nigeria for 1 year, has asked a nurse to investigate circumcision for her baby girl. In her religion, circumcision for baby girls is a long-held religious belief signifying piety and purity. Which of the following is the best response to the new mother?
   A. "Female circumcision is absolutely immoral, and I cannot help you with that."
   B. "In the United States, female circumcision is a reportable crime."
   C. "In the United States, the law prohibits female circumcision until age 18 years."
   D. "I will arrange a consult for you with a physician qualified for this surgery."
4. The nurse is working with a group of children of various ages. Which of the following children would the nurse expect to show the most androgyny?
   A. A 3-year-old boy
   B. A 4-year-old girl
   C. A 6-year-old boy
   D. A 7-year-old girl
5. Mary, 50 years old, has not had a menstrual period for 14 months. She asks the nurse if she is considered menopausal. Which response from the nurse would most accurately describe Mary's sexual reproduction status?
   A. Mary has reached menopause and cannot conceive.
   B. Mary has not reached menopause and may still conceive.
   C. Mary has reached menopause, but may still conceive.
   D. Mary has not reached menopause, but she can no longer conceive.
6. The nurse is working with a client who has been found to have premature testosterone production and secretion. Which of the following would the nurse expect to find in the client's history and medical record?
   A. Learning disabilities
   B. Aggressive behavior in school
   C. Short stature
   D. Feminization
7. During a routine examination, a client mentions recently experiencing erectile dysfunction frequently, even though he has no previous history of this problem. Which of the following responses from the nurse would be most appropriate?
   A. "Have you recently begun taking any new medications?"
   B. "How does your partner feel about this problem?"
   C. "How much exercise have you been doing lately?"
   D. "Have you tried engaging in any new sexual practices?"
8. A nurse educator is teaching a group of nurses the best approaches for educating families with teenagers about sexual issues. Which of the following interventions would the nurse be most likely to advocate?
   A. Teach all families the necessity of providing their teens with birth control.
   B. Discuss high-risk behaviors that can lead to sexually transmitted infections.
   C. Reassure teens with possible minority sexual orientation that they are too young to know.
   D. Inform parents that they must discuss sexual issues even if teens are embarrassed.

REFERENCES

American Academy of Pediatrics. (2001). Sexual education of children and adolescents. *Pediatrics, 108*(2), 498–501.

American Academy of Pediatrics. (1999). Circumcision policy statement. *Pediatrics, 103*(2), 686–693.

American Nurses Association. (2001). *Code of ethics for nurses with interpretive statements.* Washington, DC: American Nurses Publishing.

American Psychiatric Association. (2000). *Fact sheet: Gay, lesbian, and bisexual issues.* Washington, DC: American Psychiatric Publishing, Inc.

Baker, R. (1996). *Sperm wars: The science of sex.* New York: Basic Books.

Baker, R., Bellis, M. A., & Baker, R. R. (1995). *Human sperm competition: Copulation, masturbation and infertility.* Georgetown, TX: Landes Bioscience.

Belgrave, F. Z., Van Oss Marin, B., & Chambers, D. (2000). Cultural, contextual, and intrapersonal predictors of risky sexual attitudes among urban African American girls in early adolescence. *Cultural Diversity and Ethnic Minority Psychology, 6*(3), 309–322.

Berger, K. S. (2004). *The developing person through the life span* (6th ed.). New York: Worth Publishing.

Berman, J. (2005). Physiology of female sexual function and dysfunction. *International Journal of Impotence Research, 17,* S44–S51.

Bhugra, D., Bhui, K., Mallett, R., Desai, M., Singh, J., & Leff, J. (1999). Cultural identity and its measurement: A questionnaire for Asians. *International Review of Psychiatry, 11,* 244–249.

Bickley, L. S. (2006). *Bates' guide to physical examination and history taking* (9th ed.). Philadelphia: Lippincott Williams & Wilkins.

Byrd, J. E., Hyde, J. S., DeLamater, J. D., & Plant, E. A. (1998). Sexuality during pregnancy and the year postpartum. *Journal of Family Practice, 47*(4), 305–308.

Cant, B. (2006). Exploring the implications for health professionals of men coming out as gay in healthcare settings. *Health and Social Care in the Community, 14*(9), 9–16.

Centers for Disease Control and Prevention. (2002). Update: AIDS—United States, 2000. *Morbidity and Mortality Weekly Report, 51*(27), 592–595.

Chessler, A. J. (1997). *Justifying the unjustifiable: Rite v. wrong. Buffalo Law Review, 45,* 555–613.

Chrisler, J. C., & Zittel, C. B. (1998). Menarche stories: Reminiscences of college students from Lithuania, Malaysia, Sudan and the United States. *Health Care for Women International, 19*(4), 303–304.

Critchley, H. O., Kelly, R. W., Brenner, R. M., & Baird, D. T. (2001). The endocrinology of menstruation: A role for the immune system. *Clinical Endocrinology, 55,* 701–710.

Davis, D. S. (2001). Male and female genital alteration: A collision course with the law? *Health Matrix Cleveland, 11*(2), 487–570.

DeJudicibus, M. A., & McCabe, M. P. (2002). Psychological factors and the sexuality of pregnant and postpartum women. *Journal of Sex Research, 39*(2), 94–103.

DeLamater, J., & Friedrich, W. N. (2002). Human sexual development. *Journal of Sex Research, 39*(1), 10–14.

Delaney, C. H. (1995). Rites of passage in adolescence. *Adolescence, 30*(120), 891–898.

Drury, C. A., & Louis, M. (2002). Exploring the association between body weight, stigma of obesity, and health care avoidance. *Journal of the American Academy of Nurse Practitioners, 14*(12), 554–561.

Egan, S. K., & Perry, D. G. (2001). Gender identity: A multidimensional analysis with implications for psychosocial adjustment. *Developmental Psychology, 37*(4), 451–463.

Faulkner, S. L., & Mansfield, P. K. (2002). Reconciling messages: The process of sexual talk for Latinas. *Qualitative Health Research, 12*(3), 310–328.

Finer, L. B., & Henshaw, S. K. (2003). Abortion incidence and services in the United States in 2000. *Perspectives on Sexual and Reproductive Health, 35*(1), 6–15.

Fleming, M. (1996). Rites of passage. *Essence, 26*(12), 118–119.

Gass, M. L., & Taylor, M. B. (2003). Alternatives for women through menopause. *American Journal of Obstetrics and Gynecology, 185*(2), S47–S56.

Grunbaum, J. A., Kann, L., Kinchen, S. A., Williams, B., Ross, J. G., Lowry, R., & Kolbe, L. (2002). Youth risk behavior surveillance—United States, 2001. *Journal of School Health, 72*(8), 313–328.

Guyton, A., & Hall, J. (2001). *Textbook of medical physiology* (10th ed.). Philadelphia: W. B. Saunders.

Hall, L. L. (1999). Taking charge of menopause. *FDA Consumer, 33*(6), 16–21.

Hamer, D. H., Hu, S., Magnuson, V. L., Hu, N., & Pattatucci, A. M. (1993). A linkage between DNA markers on the X chromosome and male sexual orientation. *Science, 261*(5119), 321–327.

Kirton, C., Talotta, D., & Zwolski, K. (2001). *Handbook of HIV/AIDS nursing.* St. Louis: Mosby.

Kriplani, A., Abbi, M., Kriplani, A. K., Bal, S., Ammini, A. C., & Kucheria, K. (1999). Laparoscopic removal of gonadal tumors in male pseudohermaphrodites. *Journal of Gynecologic Surgery, 99*(15), 49–54.

Krone, N., Wachter, I., Stefanidou, M., Roscher, A. A., & Schwarz, H. P. (2000). Mothers with congenital adrenal hyperplasia and their children: Outcome of pregnancy, birth, and childhood. *Clinical Endocrinology, 55,* 523–529.

Kuller, L. H., & Women's Health Initiative. (2003). Hormone replacement therapy and risk of cardiovascular disease: Implications of the results of the Women's Health Initiative. *Journal of the American Heart Association,* 23(1), 11–16.

Lean, W. L., Deshpande, A., Huston, J., & Grover, S. R. (2005). Cosmetic and anatomic outcomes after feminizing surgery for ambiguous genitalia. *Journal of Pediatric Surgery, 40*(12), 1856–1860.

Levin, R. J. (2002). The physiology of sexual arousal in the human female: A recreational and procreational synthesis. *Archives of Sexual Behavior, 31*(5), 405–411.

Lobel, T. E., Gruber, R., Govrin, N., & Mashraki-Pedhatzur, S. (2001). Children's gender-related inferences and judgments: A cross-cultural study. *Developmental Psychology, 37*(6), 839–846.

Mah, K., & Binik, Y. M. (2001). The nature of human orgasm: A critical review of major trends. *Clinical Psychology Review, 21*(6), 823–856.

Masters, W. H., & Johnson, V. E. (1966). *Human sexual response.* Philadelphia: Lippincott Williams & Wilkins.

Mazza, V., DiMonte, I., Ceccarelli, P. L., Rivasi, F., Falcinelli, C., Forabosco, A., & Volpe, A. (2002). Prenatal diagnosis of female pseudohermaphroditism associated with bilateral luteoma of pregnancy: Case report. *Human Reproduction, 17*(3), 821–824.

McAndrew, S., & Warne, T. (2004). Ignoring the evidence dictating the practice: Sexual orientation, suicidality and the dichotomy of the mental health nurse. *Journal of Psychiatric and Mental Health Nursing, 11*(4), 428–434.

McTaggart S. J., Algar, E., Chow, C. W., Powell, H. R., & Jones, C. L. (2001). Clinical spectrum of Denys-Drash and Frasier syndrome. *Pediatric Nephrology, 16,* 335–339.

Michailidis, G. D., Papageorgiou, P., Morris, R. W., & Economides, D. L. (2003). The use of three-dimensional ultrasound for fetal gender determination in the first trimester. *British Journal of Radiology, 76*(907), 448–451.

Miller, G. P. (2002). Circumcision: Cultural-legal analysis. *Virginia Journal of Social Policy & the Law, 9,* 497–585.

Moshovis, P. P. (2002). When cultures are wrong. *Journal of the American Medical Association, 288*(9), 1181–1182.

Murray, R. B., & Zentner, J. P. (2001). *Health promotion strategies through the lifespan* (7th ed.). Upper Saddle River, NJ: Prentice Hall.

Okazaki, S. (2002). The influences of culture on Asian Americans' sexuality. *Journal of Sex Research, 39*(1), 34.

Perrin, E. (2002). *Sexual orientation in child and adolescent health care.* New York: Kluwer Academic/Plenum Publishers.

Pinyerd, B., & Zipf, W. B. (2005). Puberty—timing is everything! *Journal of Pediatric Nursing, 20*(2), 75–82.

Rosenblum, K., & Travis, T. (2002). *The meaning of difference: American constructions of race, sex and gender, social class, and sexual orientation.* Boston: McGraw-Hill.

Rousseau, M. E., & McCool, W. F. (1997). The menopausal experience of African American women: Overview and suggestions for research. *Health Care for Women International, 18*(3), 233.

Sadler, T. W. (2004). *Langman's medical embryology* (9th ed.). Baltimore: Lippincott Williams & Wilkins.

Savin-Williams, R. C. (2001). Suicide attempts among sexual-minority youths: Populations and measurement issues. *Journal of Consulting and Clinical Psychology, 69*(6), 983–999.

Shelton, D. (1997). You are never too old. *Natural Way for Better Health, 2*(6), 1–3.

Souzo, P. (1996). Book reviews. *Scientific American, 274*(1), 102–103.

Steinke, E. E. (1994). Knowledge and attitudes of older adults about sexuality in aging: A comparison of two studies. *Journal of Advanced Nursing 19,* 477–485.

Tenore, J. L. (2003). Methods for cervical ripening and induction of labor. *American Family Physician, 67*(10), 2123–2128.

Turner, W. J. (1995). Homosexuality, type 1: An Xq28 phenomenon. *Archives of Sexual Behavior, 24*(2), 109–134.

Van der Kamp, H. J., Noordam, K., Elvers, B., Van Baarle, M., Otten, B. J., & Verkerk, P. H. (2001). Newborn screening for congenital adrenal hyperplasia in the Netherlands. *Pediatrics, 108*(6), 1320–1324.

Vissandjee, B., Kantiebo, M., Levine, A., & N'Dejuru, R. (2003). The cultural context of gender identity: Female genital excision and infibulation. *Health Care for Women International, 24,* 115–124.

Wang, N. J., Song, H. R., Schanen, N. C., Litman, N. L., & Frasier, S. D. (2005). Frasier syndrome comes full circle: Genetic studies performed in an original patient. *Journal of Pediatrics, 146*(6), 843–844.
Wiederman, M. (1998). A new perspective on the old battle of the sexes. *Journal of Sex Research, 35*(1), 120–123.
Wilcox, A. J., Weinberg, C. R., & Baird, D. D. (1995). Timing of sexual intercourse in relation to ovulation: Effects on the probability of conception, survival of the pregnancy, and sex of the baby. *New England Journal of Medicine, 333*(23), 1517–1521.
Woelfle, J., Hoepffner, W., Sippel, W. G., Branswig, J. H., Heidemann, P., Deiss, D., et al. (2002). Complete virilization in congenital adrenal hyperplasia: Clinical course, medical management, and disease-related complications. *Clinical Endocrinology, 58,* 231–238.
Wright, J. (1996). Female genital mutilation: An overview. *Journal of Advanced Nursing, 24,* 251–259.
Young, J. S. (2002). Female genital mutilation. *Journal of the American Medical Association, 288*(9), 1130.
Yunger, J. L., Carver, P. R., & Perry, D. G. (2004). Does gender identity influence children's psychological well-being? *Developmental Psychology, 40*(4), 572–582.
Zeiss, A., & Kasl-Godley, J. (2001). Sexuality in older adults' relationships. *Generations, 25*(2), 18–25.

CHAPTER 7

Family Formation

Rebecca Cahill and Thelma Sword

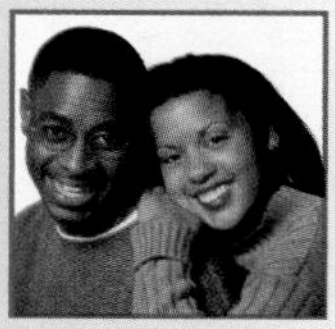

Olivia and her husband Tyler have been married for 3 years. They have shared many activities together, such as skiing, camping, and traveling. The couple has just found out that they are going to have their first child. Olivia and Tyler are excited about the baby. During a regular prenatal visit to the health clinic, Olivia confides to the nurse, "I'm feeling a bit overwhelmed by the pregnancy. And Tyler seems happy about the baby coming, but lately, he seems a bit distant from me."

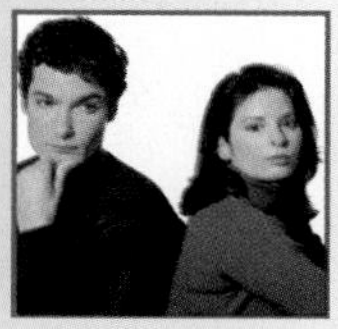

Jacob and Rachel, a Jewish couple who have undergone 5 years of unsuccessful infertility treatments, have arranged for a private adoption of a female baby born to a young single Jewish girl. They have been in contact with the biological mother almost daily during the pregnancy. When the biological mother goes into labor, she calls Jacob and Rachel to attend the birth of their new daughter. Rachel chooses to be present in the delivery room; Jacob goes to the health care facility but remains outside in the waiting room.

You will learn more about these families later in this chapter. Nurses working with these clients and others like them need to understand the content of this chapter to manage care and address issues appropriately. Before beginning, consider the following points related to the above scenarios:

- Does anything about either case present any issues of immediate concern or worry? Explain your answer.
- Which type of family structure or arrangement is depicted for each couple? How are these structures similar? Different?
- What areas would the nurse need to assess with Olivia and Tyler? With Rachel and Jacob?

LEARNING OBJECTIVES

On completion of this chapter, the reader should be able to:

- Compare and contrast the family theories of Bowen, Satir, and Friedman.
- Explain how nurses can use the family theories presented in this chapter when assessing and communicating with families.
- Recognize common family forms in the contemporary United States and Canada.
- Identify ways in which the nurse develops the nursing care plan based on the family's culture and specific family form.
- Describe the processes of domestic and international adoption and implications related to the differing family forms.
- Apply the nursing process to families in formation.

KEY TERMS

agency adoptions
blended family
closed adoption
cultural competence
cultural relativism
differentiation of self
ecomap
extended family
extended kin network
family
genogram
international adoption
open adoption
private adoption
single-parent family
system
traditional nuclear family
triangles
two-parent family

The **family** represents the unit of interrelationships from which a person functions in society. Definitions of family and current family structures have evolved to include new varieties and configurations not seen in the past. Every area of nursing care needs to recognize and address the issues that today's families face. This is especially true in maternity and women's health care because the family as a whole is the target of health care delivery.

This chapter presents theories of family that apply directly to the nursing care of women and their families. The focus is on various forms of the family in the 21st century. The chapter includes various sociocultural perspectives. Adoption issues are addressed from both the domestic and international perspective; additionally, personal experiences with adoption are presented. The chapter closes with a section on collaborative care when working with families.

DEFINITIONS OF FAMILY

Several definitions of family exist. Some basic definitions include the following:

- Two or more people living together related by blood, marriage, or adoption (Fields, 2003a)
- The primary unit of socialization and the basic structural unit of the community
- An institution of society that preserves and transmits culture (Chen & Ratkin, 2002)
- Who they say they are (Wright & Leahey, 2006)

Additional perspectives on defining the family are found in Box 7.1.

Families Viewed as Systems

Families can be viewed as a microcosm of our world (Satir, 1988). Changes in U.S. and Canadian demographics in

BOX 7.1 Perspectives on the Family

- "The family is the factory where a person is made, and adults are the people-makers" (Satir, 1972).
- "Family refers to two or more persons who are joined together by bonds of sharing and emotional closeness and who identify themselves as being part of a family" (Freidman, 1992, p. 9).
- "Family is an open and developing system of interacting personalities with a structure and a process enacted in relationships among the individual members, regulated by resources and stressors and existing within the larger community" (Cooley, 2000, p. 240).

recent years have had a major influence on families and the roles of their members (Tiedje & Darling-Fisher, 2003). Nurses need a basic understanding of some theoretical foundations of family dynamics to provide direction to nursing care.

The first concept is that the family can be viewed as a system (Von Bertalanffy, 1968). In this context, **system** means a unit in which the whole is greater than the sum of its parts. The following basic principles of systems apply to families:

- Systems have boundaries.
- Boundaries may be open or closed.
- Systems need rules to function.
- Interrelationships occur with interchangeable causes and effects.
- Communication feedback must occur within the system.

Systems operate within the larger environment, and whatever affects the system as a whole affects each of its parts. For example, when one member of the family has an alteration of health, each family member, as well as the family as a unit, is affected (Fig. 7.1).

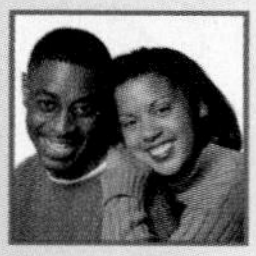

Consider the family system of Olivia and Tyler, who are expecting their first child. Obviously the family unit will change with the birth of the baby. How might the family system already be changing during the pregnancy?

At their foundation, theories of families as systems assume that "human behavior is regulated by the same natural processes that regulate the behavior of all other living things" (Kerr & Bowen, 1988, p. 3). Murray Bowen (1978) and Virginia Satir (1974) are two theorists who have developed systems frameworks for understanding

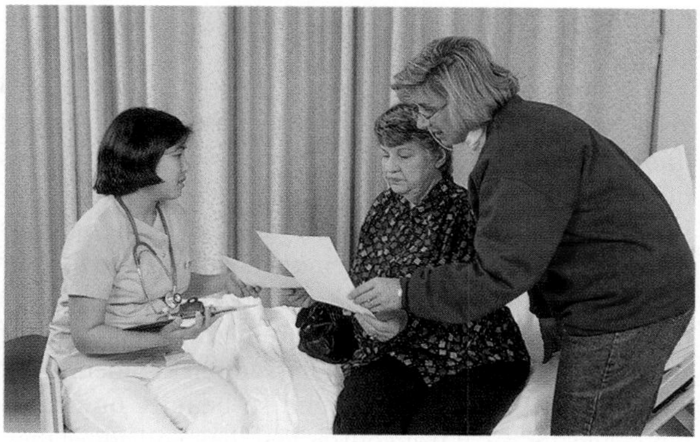

FIGURE 7.1 Health alterations can affect the entire family unit, whether the ill person is an older parent, a sibling, or another relative. Nurses must strive to work with families to help them through such times of adjustment. (Photo © B. Proud.)

the activity within the family. Another theorist, Marilyn Friedman (1992), who addresses nursing specifically, challenged nurses to view families as units and to provide appropriate assessments of the family as a whole. Although these theoretical perspectives were developed decades ago, they remain applicable to families today. Nursing can integrate the concepts associated with these theories to guide nursing practice in the care of families.

Bowen's Theory

Bowen based his family systems theory on his earlier work with families dealing with schizophrenia. Observations of clients with schizophrenia when alone and then later with their families demonstrated the existence of key factors in these relationships. When the clients made contact with relatives, the emotional effects of these interactions were observable in the clients. Bowen distinguished the family relationship system from the family emotional system. The *relationship system* described what happened, whereas the *emotional system* explained why. Bowen (1978) noted these factors and found that they repeated themselves with clients who did not have schizophrenia and their families.

Bowen presented concepts that provided a greater understanding of the person within a system called the family. His theory emphasizes the need for balance within the emotional system. Bowen identified three concepts—(1) differentiation of self, (2) triangles, and (3) anxiety—as key to gaining insight into the meaning of activities within the family system.

Differentiation of Self. Differentiation of self, according to Bowen, means how much a person can separate himself or herself from other family members. It involves the ability to separate emotions from thoughts. Differentiation of self represents individuality and separateness among family members. It is thought to form the basis of how people cope with life challenges (Murdock & Gore, 2004).

As newborns develop, they instinctively begin to grow emotionally separate from their parents and siblings: thinking, feeling, and acting for themselves. The process of differentiation of self involves a combination of learning to be an individual and learning to separate emotions from thinking (Fig. 7.2). The more differentiated the self becomes, the less automatic emotional reactions the person will display. Without learning differentiation of self, children simply function in reaction to others (Kerr & Bowen, 1988). They depend so heavily on acceptance and approval from others that they will adjust their thoughts, words, and actions to please others and will dogmatically adhere to established behaviors and ideas without thinking critically about them.

Triangles. The concept of communication within triangles is important. Initially, communication occurs between two people. Often, two-person interactions are emotional, tense, or unstable (Cooley, 2000). The two-person interaction provides no outlet for the inevitable conflicts that arise when two people have opposite views, feelings, or reactions to issues of importance to both parties. "When emotional tension in a two-person system exceeds a certain level, it triangles a third person, permitting the tension to shift about within the triangle" (Bowen, 1978, p. 174). A **triangle** is a three-person system and is the smallest system available to form a stable relationship system. Triangles develop naturally with time as two people reach out and form relationships with others. A triangle can handle much more tension than two-person communication because it allows tension to shift among three relationships. Shifting tension, however, may not mean that anything is satisfactorily resolved.

Triangles are constantly fluctuating. In the triangle, each of the three sides represents the different people in the communication process. Family members may be positioned on any side in any given situation. The dynamics of the triangle are changing constantly. In situations of moderate tension, one side of the triangle is considered the "close" (or supportive) side, whereas the other side is considered "distant." The side of closeness is preferred in calm periods within the family, whereas the distant side is desired during periods of anxiety.

Triangles create situations of "odd person out," with one of the three parties always left outnumbered, outvoted, or excluded in some way (Fig. 7.3). For example, when a father takes his daughter's side in an argument, the mother feels left out; when parents present a "united front" against a misbehaving child, the child feels left out. Being the "odd person out" is difficult to tolerate and generates anxiety.

Anxiety. Significant in Bowen's theory is the concept of anxiety. *Anxiety* is defined traditionally as response to a real or imagined threat (see Chap. 5). Within the context of Bowen's theory, as anxiety increases, the likelihood that people will respond with automatic rather than thoughtful actions also increases (Mauer & Smith, 2005). The varying level of anxiety within the family as a whole and experienced by individual members over time affects the communication within triangles as well as each person's ability to achieve differentiation of self. Additionally, the amount of anxiety within a family system directly affects the emotional reactivity of its members.

When increased anxiety is present, people tend to respond in automatic ways rather than with thoughtful responses and actions. Families with members with poor differentiation of self have more relationship-dependent and relationship-prescribed interactions, which result in increased anxiety (Kerr & Bowen, 1988). The amount and level of anxiety affect emotional closeness or distance within the family (Charles, 2001).

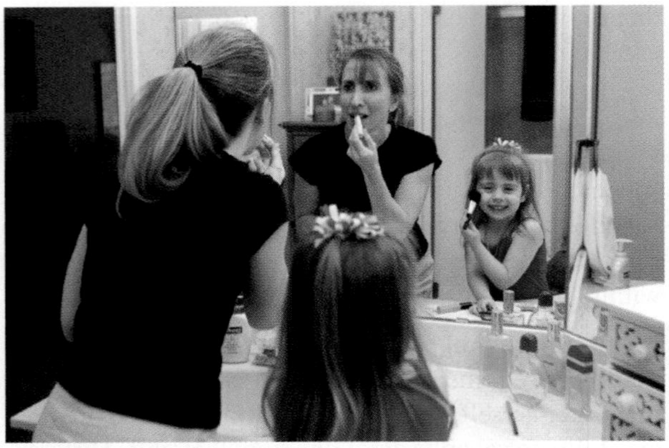

FIGURE 7.2 Young children base their self-perceptions on the opinions of those close to them, especially their parents. They often engage in imitative behaviors as a way to gain parental approval.

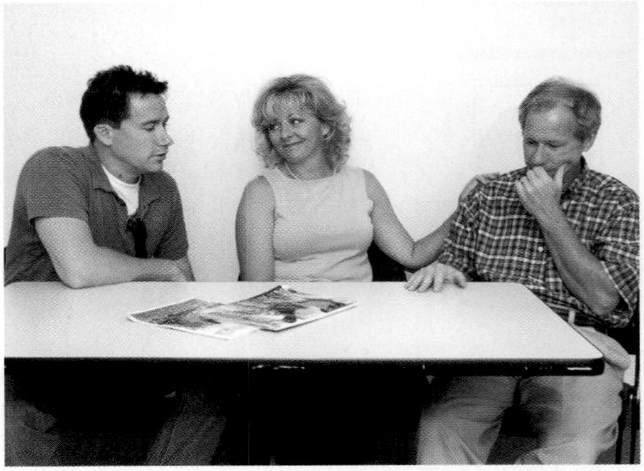

FIGURE 7.3 Triangles can have varying outcomes. They often leave one person in the triangle feeling excluded or outnumbered. Such feelings can contribute to anxiety and family tension.

QUOTE 7-1

"When I was growing up, it always seemed like my sister and father would have the same points of view and 'gang up' on me and my mother in discussions and arguments. Now that I have my own children, I can see how difficult it can be to navigate discussions and make everyone feel like their voice is heard and that no one is taking sides."

From a mother with three children

Application to Nursing. When interacting with families, nurses may be drawn into the family triangle. The nurse needs to possess awareness of these communication dynamics and therapeutic communication techniques to maintain a neutral position in interactions (Table 7.1). Understanding the role of anxiety in the family system can assist nurses as they care for clients in stressful, anxiety-provoking health care situations. The nurse needs to work against becoming involved in family conflicts and concentrate on helping relatives communicate with one another. See Nursing Care Plan 7.1.

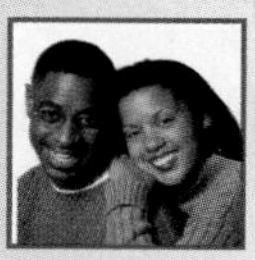

Consider Olivia and Tyler. Imagine that Olivia's anxiety continues to increase, causing her to lean more heavily on Tyler. At the same time, Tyler reacts to Olivia's "neediness" critically. He further distances himself, leaving Olivia feeling isolated. Applying Bowen's theory, how might the birth of the newborn cause a triangle in this situation?

TABLE 7.1 Therapeutic Communication Techniques

TECHNIQUE	PURPOSE	EXAMPLE
Giving broad openings	Communicates a desire to begin a meaningful interaction Allows the client to define the problem or issue	"What would you like to discuss today?" "Tell me about how you have been doing."
Paraphrasing	Reflects the meaning of the client's message in the nurse's words Allows for clarification Lets the client know that the nurse has understood the message	"So you're saying that your husband is unwilling to work on the marriage any more."
Offering general leads	Encourages client to continue elaborating Communicates the nurse's interest in listening	"I see." "Uh-huh."
Reflecting feelings	Reflects the emotion underlying the client's message Conveys empathy	"It sounds like you're feeling hopeless about the situation."
Focusing	Encourages the client to expand upon one part of a statement Concentrates on a single issue Useful technique with clients who are confused or overwhelmed by many issues at the same time	"Can you give me an example of how that typically happens for you?" "Let's go back to ___ because I'm not sure I follow you." "What is it about ___ that bothers you?"
Voicing doubt	Gentle way of challenging the client's perceptions Encourages reconsideration	"Really?" "Are you sure that your parents will never accept your decision?"
Clarifying	Makes clear that which is vague or not meaningful May help clients clarify their own understanding	"I'm not sure what you mean by ___."
Placing events in time sequence	Allows the client to organize thoughts Provides clues to recurring patterns Helps the nurse follow the client's train of thought and understand what is happening	"So how did this start?" "What happened next?"
Giving information	Allows for teaching and clarification	"Several halfway houses have work programs."
Encouraging formulation of a plan	Encourages client to think about solutions without the nurse giving advice Helps the client problem-solve	"What do you think you should do about this problem?" "What are your options, as you see them?"
Testing discrepancies	Helps the client become aware of inconsistencies in statements versus behaviors Allows for gentle confrontation	"You say that you want to participate in this group, but I notice that you have missed the past three meetings."

NURSING CARE PLAN 7.1

The Family in Transition

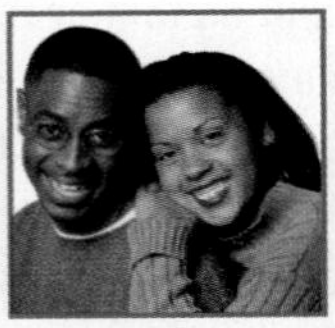

Recall Olivia and Tyler from the beginning of the chapter. The nurse prompts Olivia to provide more information about her feelings of being overwhelmed and that her husband is becoming "distant" since she became pregnant. Olivia states, "Sometimes I feel like such a wimp. I find myself asking Tyler for help with things that I never would have before I was pregnant. He's really not used to this. Sometimes, he ignores me and says I'm behaving like a child. He tells me he wonders what will happen when a real baby is around. I'm not sure what's happening. What kind of mother will I be?"

NURSING DIAGNOSIS

Anxiety related to changes in responsibilities, roles, relationships, and family structure secondary to pregnancy

EXPECTED OUTCOMES

1. The couple will identify problem issues and areas of concern.
2. The client will state areas in which she needs assistance.

INTERVENTIONS	RATIONALES
Assess the client's level of understanding about pregnancy and changes.	Assessment provides a baseline to identify specific client needs and to develop an individualized plan.
Discuss with the client her concerns, feelings, and perceptions related to pregnancy and its possible effects.	Discussion provides opportunities to emphasize positive aspects of the current situation; verbalization of concerns aids in establishing sources of stress and problem areas that need to be addressed.
Communicate accurate facts; answer questions honestly.	Open and honest communication promotes trust and helps correct any misconceptions or misinformation.
Discuss the physiologic and psychological changes of pregnancy (see Chap. 12), including their basis and measures to cope with them.	Adequate knowledge of possible changes and measures to cope with them helps to alleviate concerns related to the unknown.
Include the client's partner in the discussion about pregnancy, both partner's needs, and necessary adaptations.	The participation of both partners increases feelings of control over the situation and promotes support and sharing.
Encourage the couple to communicate clearly and openly about events, issues, or concerns.	Clear communication is essential for sharing information.
Provide the couple with information about support groups, Web sites, and other sources of appropriate information.	Shared experiences and knowledge of similar situations can aid in preparing the couple for what to expect.
Investigate sources of available support, such as extended family, friends, and community; encourage the couple to use these sources.	Additional sources of support are helpful in alleviating anxiety and stress.
Continue to assess the client's and partner's adaptation and functioning at subsequent visits.	Continued assessment aids in monitoring progress of the situation and provides opportunities to address concerns that may arise as the pregnancy progresses.

Continued

NURSING CARE PLAN 7.1 ● The Family in Transition

EVALUATION

1. The couple identifies realistic measures to cope with the demands of pregnancy and the family.
2. The couple develops a workable plan that promotes healthy functioning of both partners, the fetus/newborn, and overall family.

Satir's Theory

Virginia Satir was a pioneer in family therapy who described aspects of family processes that she observed during her work with families. In Satir's (1972) work *Peoplemaking,* she viewed the family as the environment where people are created. Understanding some of Satir's concepts is helpful in gaining insight into working with families. "All the ingredients in a family that count are changeable and correctable: individual self-worth, communication, system, and rules" (Satir, 1972, p. xii).

Self-Worth. Self-worth is a basic human need and part of Maslow's hierarchy of needs. Self-esteem or self-worth includes a person's subjective appraisal of himself or herself as having both positive and negative aspects (Sedikides et al., 2004). Developing a sense of self and self-worth assists people with coping and the development of healthy relationships in their lives (Clark, 2003). As a child develops within the family, he or she develops ideas and feelings about self. According to Satir, the daily ongoing interactions with family members can foster or discourage these ideas and feelings. These interactions commonly are called the "communication within the family" and involve verbal and nonverbal behaviors to convey messages.

Communication. Communication includes verbal and nonverbal messages sent and received as family members make contact with one another. Communication includes talking and listening. "Communication is the largest single factor determining what kinds of relationships [one] makes with others and what happens to each in the world" (Satir, 1988, p. 51). It is through this communication that the family rules are developed.

Rules. Rules are part of every family and provide the structure for the family's system of operation. All families need rules, which provide structure for the family system. Rules include how family members should feel and act (Satir, 1988). Rules are the guidelines used within the family to set standards about what is considered acceptable or unacceptable (Hitchcock et al., 2003). There are rules about behavior, communication, and relationships. For example, families have rules about what is acceptable behavior at the dinner table, rules about how anger is expressed, and rules about sharing.

Systems. Family systems can be closed or open based on how the family reacts to change from inside and outside the family. Closed systems are rigidly connected or disconnected with little exchange of information; open systems are interconnected, responsive, and sensitive to one another with free-flowing information (Satir, 1988). The open, healthy family system finds its connection to people and organizations outside the family. Communication within this open family system becomes:

- A tool for helping children learn
- A way to communicate the rules of the family
- A means of conflict resolution within the family
- The method for nurturing the self-esteem of individual family members (Satir, 1988)

An open family system encourages greater interpersonal development of the people within the family. Nevertheless, closed systems may be an expression of cultural beliefs and are not necessarily unhealthy.

Individuals learn feelings of worth within the family system, providing a means by which members can express how they feel to improve communication and foster self-worth. Satir (1972) proposes a simple, straightforward means for family members to communicate how they are feeling about their own self-esteem or self-worth. By using the example of an old black pot that is either full (high pot: feelings of high self-esteem) or empty (low pot: feelings of shame or guilt, low self-esteem), families can learn to communicate their feelings to one another. Children with a "high pot" can succeed even with failure in school and among peers, whereas children with a "low pot" can experience success yet continue to doubt their self-worth (Satir, 1988).

Application to Nursing. Nurses can apply Satir's theory to families in many different circumstances. For example, with the knowledge that communication is learned, nurses can encourage new parents to use effective communication tools to develop a foundation of healthy family communication for the new baby. Communication provides the means for the infant to learn everything about the world and to develop feelings of worth. Through healthy communication, parents can provide the growing child with a foundation of nurturing.

Assessing communication among family members and within the family as a whole helps the nurse understand the unique dynamics involved. In certain situations, nurses may need to facilitate family meetings to identify family goals, foster mutually acceptable interventions, and clarify misunderstandings.

Friedman's Theory

Friedman's (1992) systems theory focuses on family nursing. It stresses a key interrelational characteristic of the family system—the whole is greater than the sum of its parts. Friedman identifies specific activities or functions of the family as the basis for wholeness. Family function is the family's purpose with respect to individual, family, other social systems, and society (Hanson, 2006). The major functions of families described by Friedman (1992, 2003) include affective, socialization, reproductive, economic, and health care functions. Families carry out these functions through different roles within a wide range of cultural settings, as discussed next and in Table 7.2.

Affective Function. The affective function represents a vital activity for the family. In a rapidly changing 21st-century society, the person depends on the family to meet the affection and emotional needs of the members. With families in poverty and experiencing significant stress, risks are increased that the affection needs of members will be displaced for the more basic function of meeting physical needs (Friedman, 1992).

Socialization Function. It is within the structure of the family that socialization of its members begins. For children, an important foundation for successful maturation occurs with the activities of socialization. Appropriate use of language, behavior, and communication skills and core family values are part of the socialization that occurs within the family. The child's many learning experiences build up as this lifelong process of "internalizing the appropriate set of norms and values" (Friedman, 1992, p. 76) continues for all family members (Fig. 7.4).

Reproductive Function. Families always have been the traditional structure for procreation. The myriad family forms in today's society still support the family's reproductive function as a prerequisite to the continuation of our society. Nevertheless, this function now takes on many forms, including adoption, artificial insemination, and surrogate mothering (see Chap. 10). In addition, the roles and influence of extended family members are changing, with many family members often providing child care and support.

The reproductive function of the family is also facing current challenges. Concerns over rampant population growth and teen pregnancy affect undeveloped and industrialized countries alike. Annually, many U.S. adolescent pregnancies end in abortion or miscarriage. The resultant grief, with its own physical, emotional, social, and cognitive responses, poses additional health concerns for women and families (Wheeler & Austin, 2001).

Economic Function. The economic function of the family is vital for obtaining adequate financial resources to meet material needs (Friedman, 1992). Historically, the family head supported the family, providing the financial resources needed. In today's society, the head of the family varies greatly. Additionally, the community resources available to provide help to families with financial obligations are wide ranging (Hitchcock et al., 2003).

The economic function of the family has changed in this new century. In today's society, many women work outside the home. Two-income families are common and often necessary for economic stability. Although children in the United States and Canada typically do not work to provide economic support of the family, their employment as they become teenagers may be a factor in allowing them to enjoy luxuries and "extras." Families have taken on the role and function of consumers of goods and services (Geistfeld, 2005).

Health Care Function. Providing the essentials to keep the family healthy is the health care function. Such essentials include food, clothing, and shelter, as well as health care itself. Health care practices of families are diverse. Use of home remedies or healers, for example, may be culturally based. In addition, the family may or may not be aware of community health prevention activities. Despite such diversity, families support the health and wellbeing of their members.

Application to Nursing. Nurses working with families need to understand each family's health beliefs, decision-making activities, and knowledge about health to provide the most appropriate care. When family rituals are interrupted or functions are jeopardized, the nurse should serve to help fix the problems and limit disruptions.

In maternal, newborn, and women's health care, nurses need to respond to the increasing diversity represented in today's families. Understanding existing theories and seeking new models for family assessment can equip nurses to address the various needs families present. Nurses will "encounter families from diverse and interconnected world economies where culture, ethnicity, and race are predicted to become increasingly blended throughout the next 50 years" (Denham, 2003, p. 151).

● **TABLE 7.2 Friedman's Family Functions**

FUNCTION	DESCRIPTION	IMAGE
Affective	Support and respect with affirmation occurs within the family.	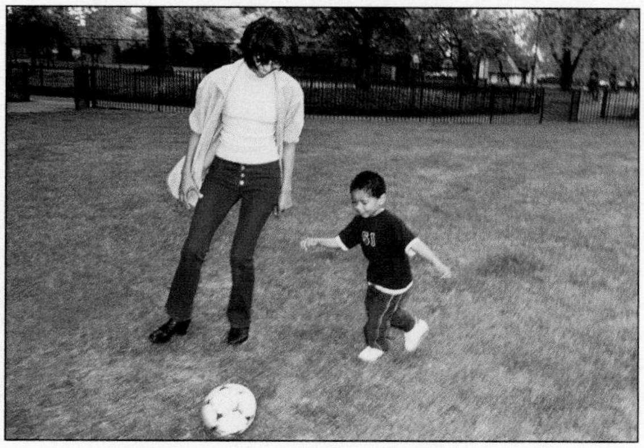
Socialization	The shared culture and values of the family members are articulated and learned.	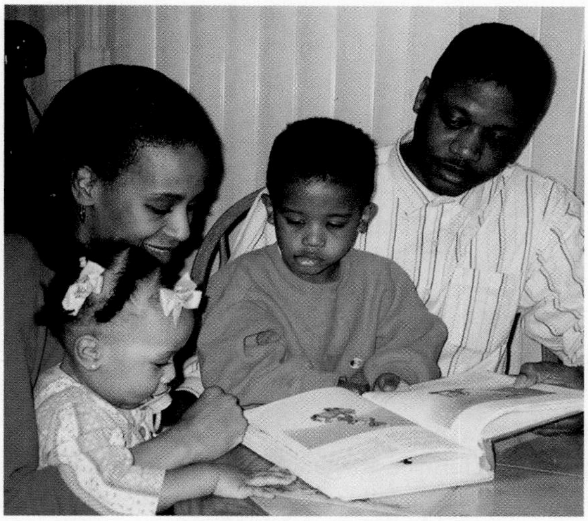
Reproductive	Choices regarding procreation are made within the family.	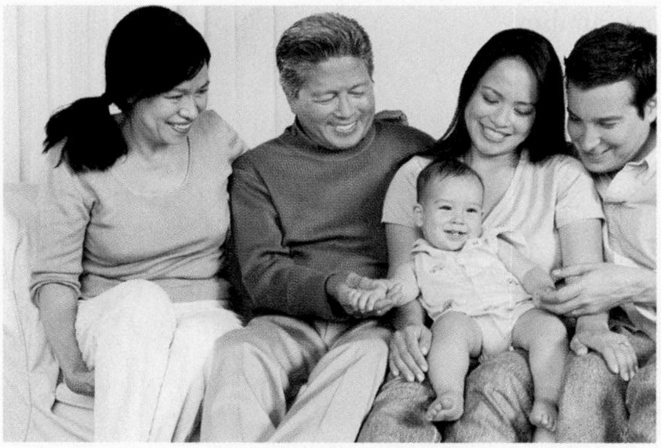

Continued

TABLE 7.2 Friedman's Family Functions *(Continued)*

FUNCTION	DESCRIPTION	IMAGE
Economic	Financial resources hold the family together.	
Health care	Provisions for the physical necessities of life are made.	

Nonsystem Views of Family

Regardless of form or structure, family processes are similar in some ways for all families. Roles, values, decision making, and life cycle are elements of family processes that have the potential to play out uniquely within individual families.

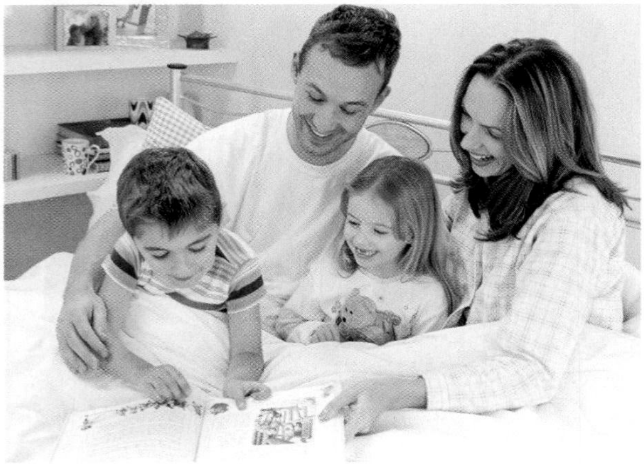

FIGURE 7.4 A main function of families is to socialize and educate children.

Family Roles

A role can be considered a consistent behavior in a particular situation (Wright & Leahey, 2006). Family members assume various roles to enhance the functioning of the family as a unit. Roles may vary based on a family's cultural expectations. Roles are not constant but are influenced by each person's interactions with other family members. Role flexibility is essential as a dimension of how the family copes and adapts to change (Friedman et al., 2003).

Women's roles have changed in the past decade, with more individualized defining of the woman's behavior in the family. Men's roles have also expanded. Men are more active in the fathering role than in the past (Fig. 7.5). Tiedje and Darling-Fisher (2003) reported "approximately 17% of preschool children are cared for by their fathers while mothers work" (p. 350). As mothers' roles in the family change, fathers' roles have responded with increased participation in the care of children. Nurses' responses to these changes need to include "awareness on the behalf of the providers, and intentional inclusion of a standard father-friendly format" (Tiedje & Darling, 2003, p. 353) in the interactions with fathers.

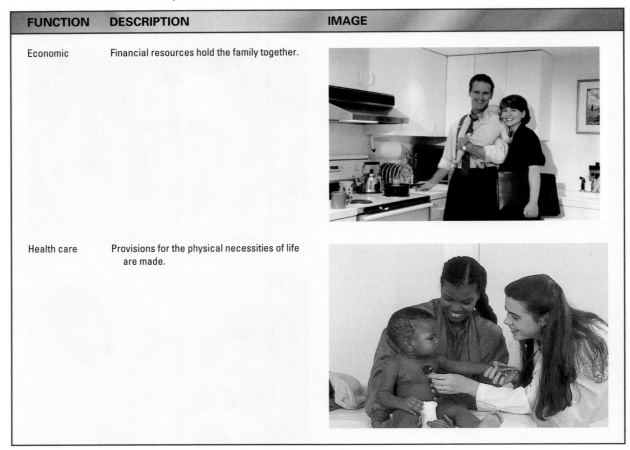

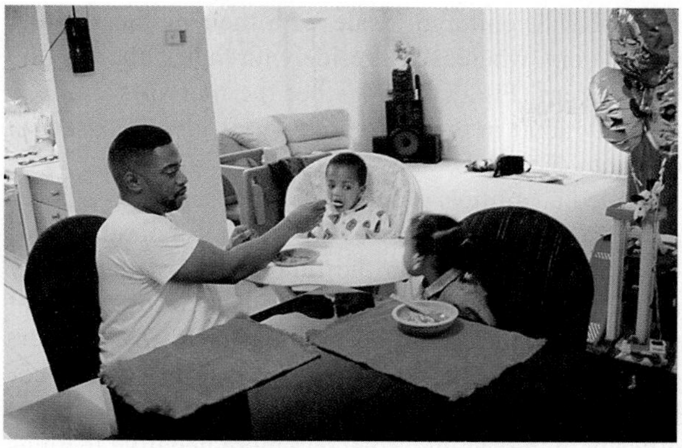

FIGURE 7.5 Many of today's fathers are taking active roles in child care, with some dads providing the predominant child care while mothers work outside the home.

Other roles emerge, as grandparents need care within the family. Alternatively, if parents become ill, children assume roles and responsibilities normally assigned to the parents. Zey (2005) discussed the *longevity revolution,* or the fact that average life expectancy has increased during the past century. Longevity may influence the roles within marriage and families. "Multigenerative families could become more common as families live longer" (Zey, 2005, p. 20). Roles remain fluid and changing within families to meet the needs as they arise.

QUOTE 7-2

"My husband never ceases to amaze me in terms of how well he has embraced his role as parent. When we decided that he would stay home to take care of Harry while I worked, I worried that my husband would be bored or would feel weird about not having outside employment. But both of them are thriving, and frankly I think my husband is innately more nurturing and patient than I'll ever be."

A woman whose husband is staying home to be the primary caregiver of their young son

Family Values

Hanson (2006) explained family values as the family's own unique system of ideas, attitudes, and beliefs about commonalities that unite the family. Cultural perspectives enhance these common ideas. Family dynamics have the potential for constant change. The basic values of the family anchor the family in society. "As families grow and change over time, so, too, do their values" (Hitchcock et al., 2003, p. 631).

Family Decision Making

One essential task of the family is decision making, which combines the use of power and communication. Good communication within the family lays the foundation for effective decision-making strategies. Traditionally, parents take on the role of the decision makers. Allocating power on a daily basis between parents effectively distributes decision-making responsibilities. Families with open and honest communication strategies within the family can foster greater joint problem solving among family members (Friedman et al., 2003). Cultural values and beliefs are foundational elements for how decision making will be handled within any given family. Often, even the communication of the decision is overshadowed by the cultural framework of the family.

Family Life Cycle

Much has been written about the predicted stages with the life cycle of families. Friedman, Bowden, and Jones (2003) labeled the life events that signify a change as family stage markers (p. 108). Duvall's classic work on the eight stages of the life cycle of traditional families provides a framework for the recognition of the stages through which families progress:

- Stage 1: Beginning families
- Stage 2: Childbearing families
- Stage 3: Families with preschool children
- Stage 4: Families with school-aged children
- Stage 5: Families with teenagers
- Stage 6: Families launching young adults
- Stage 7: Middle-aged parents
- Stage 8: Family in retirement (Duvall, as cited in Friedman et al., 2003).

When considering life cycles and developmental stages of families, the change that precipitated the stage must be considered. Adjustments, such as birth of a child, geographic relocations, or a youngest child leaving home to attend college, affect the functioning of the family. During each phase, the family achieves certain tasks. Completion of each task makes the transition to the next phase smoother for each member of the family and the family as a whole. Anything that hinders or delays the family's progression through the stages may pose additional difficulties for the family in the next phase of the life cycle.

FAMILY ARRANGEMENTS AND STRUCTURES

Although the view of the family has changed drastically over the years, the concept of a family made up of a mother, father, children, house, car, and pets frequently persists. Currently in the United States and Canada, however, no one "norm" exists for a family. Family forms have various structures, arrangements, and configurations. Nurses should remember that families come in all shapes, sizes, and varieties. Nurses avoid quick assumptions about a client and what his or her family unit may be. Careful assessment, including asking questions about the family system and the family resources, as opposed to relying on assumptions or stereotypes, is crucial when planning care for families. Some of the more common forms are discussed next.

Traditional Nuclear and Two-Parent Families

In a report for the U.S. Census Bureau, Fields (2001) defined the **traditional nuclear family** as married parents with biological children and no other people living in the household (Fig. 7.6). According to this report, 56% of U.S. children lived in a nuclear family, an increase of 5% from 1991. Across various ethnic groups, the differences in percentages were noticeable. For example, the percentage of white non-Hispanic children living in nuclear families was the highest at 65%. The next highest group, at 58%, was Asian and Pacific Islanders, followed by Hispanics at 48%, and African Americans at 29%.

Interestingly, a 2003 report by Fields derived from 2002 data no longer included the concept of the nuclear family. The 2003 report focused on the **two-parent family,** defined as a child "living with a parent who is married with his or her spouse present" (Fields, 2003a, p. 3). The second parent could have had a biological, step, or adoptive relationship with the child. Using this definition, 69% of children younger than 18 years lived in a two-parent family in 2002 (Federal Interagency Forum on Child and Family Statistics [FIFCFS], 2003).

Single-Parent Families

This chapter defines a **single-parent family** as a family headed by an adult not currently living with a spouse. This structure includes, but is not limited to men or women who are separated, divorced, or widowed. Later in the chapter, families headed by partners with same-sex unions are discussed.

The single-parent family presented in Fields' (2003a) report does not always refer to a single adult alone in a household. Subsequently, the report's information has been difficult to interpret. The clearest data show that 23% of U.S. children reside with their mothers as the only parent, whereas 5% reside with their fathers as the only parent (Fig. 7.7). Whether the man or woman is the only adult in the household varies greatly based on ethnicity (Fig. 7.8).

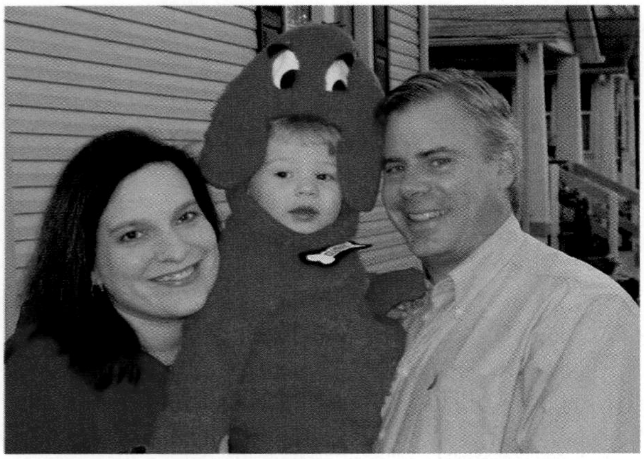

FIGURE 7.6 The traditional nuclear family consists of a married couple with their biological child or children.

Media, political groups, and other segments of society have raised concerns for many years about the influence of cohabitation on the functioning of the family unit. According to Kalil (2002), evidence suggests that the quality of the cohabiting relationship differs from the quality of the marital relationship. In Kalil's study, cohabiting parents experienced more depression, decreased efficacy in the parental role, and more negative feelings toward children. Moreover, Kalil mentions that children born into a cohabiting relationship are less likely to see their fathers after the relationship terminates, as compared with children born into a marriage that ends in divorce.

Review of the latest data from the Centers for Disease Control and Prevention shows that birth rates to unmarried women younger than 20 years declined from 1994 to 2001; however, birth rates to unmarried women 20 to 24 and 40 to 44 years old increased. In 2001, 34% of U.S. births were to unmarried women (FIFCFS, 2003) (Fig. 7.9). These data are significant because children born to single mothers are thought to be at increased risk for long-term adverse health consequences resulting from their family's potentially limited financial, emotional, and social resources (FIFCFS, 2003).

Nurses should note that even though an abundance of information exists on the hardships of the single-parent family experience, the quality of the experience that children have in the home is equally important. Fraenkel (2004) summarized qualities of the home environment that promote all children's well-being to include the following:

- Role models of appropriate behaviors
- Fair and respectful discipline
- Supervision
- Affection
- Responsiveness
- Encouragement

Regardless of the structure or form of the family, an environment in which the child is safe and in which his or her needs are consistently met is the most important component of that child's overall well-being.

Families With Same-Sex Parents

Most available information about families in which the sex of the parents is the same focuses on families headed by female partners (Fig. 7.10). According to the Urban Institute (2003):

> *Ninety percent of all U.S. counties have at least one same-sex couple with children under 18 in the*

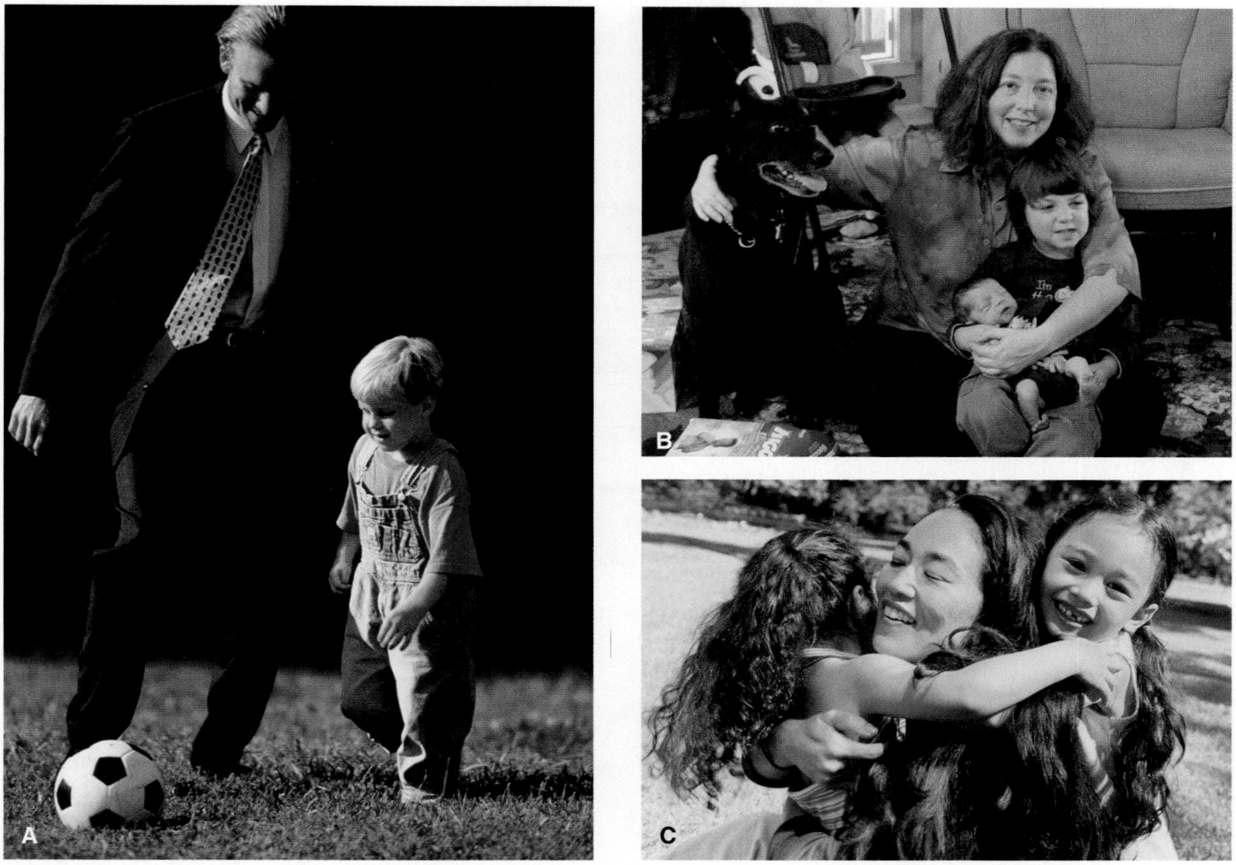

FIGURE 7.7 Single-parent families are led by adults who are not currently living with a spouse. The head of the household can be the father (**A**) or the mother (**B**) and (**C**).

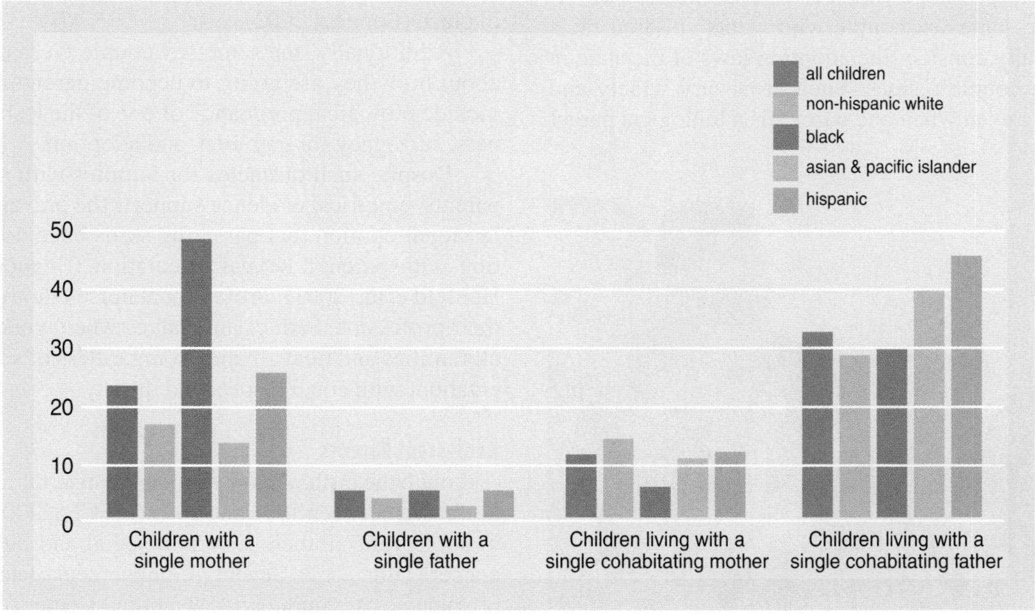

FIGURE 7.8 Children with single parents and proportion with cohabiting single parents.

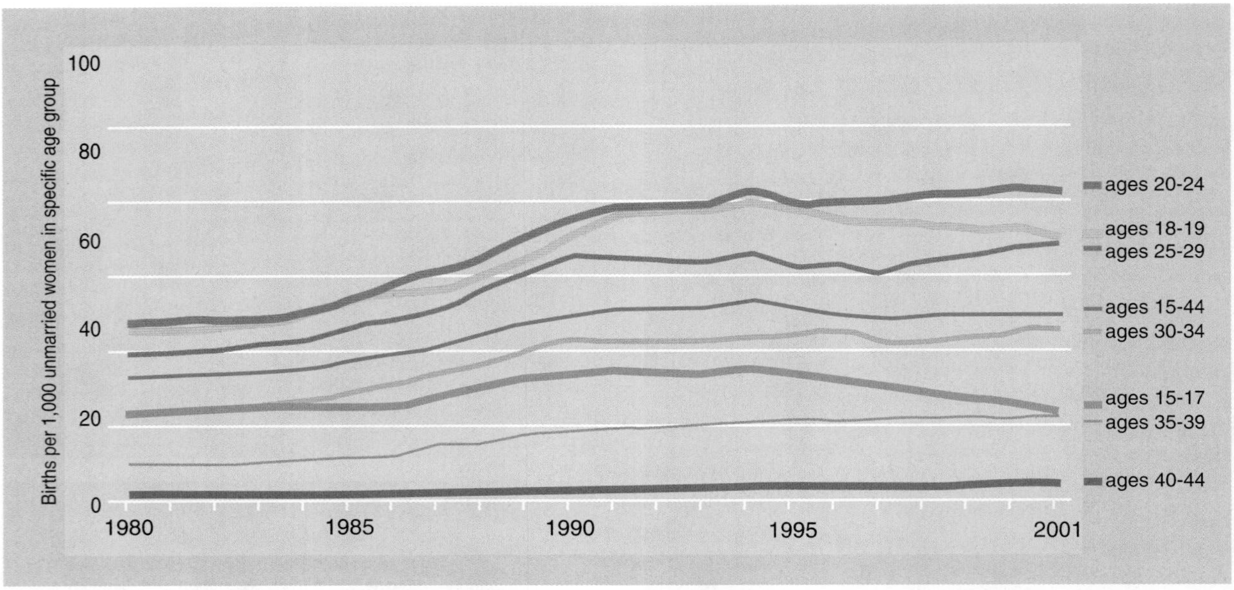

FIGURE 7.9 Birth rates for unmarried women by age of mother, 1980–2001.

> *household. . . . Only ten states have laws supportive of gay and lesbian couple adoption. More than a third of all U.S. counties (1082) have a higher proportion of same-sex couples with children than the national average of two per thousand.*

Couples of the same sex who decide to incorporate children into their family face issues not shared by heterosexuals. In most states, same-sex couples do not have the legal opportunity to marry and thus gain certain protections and privileges open to heterosexuals. For example, the same-sex couple who wants children must automatically consider the adoption laws of the state in which the couple resides. Such laws vary widely and often apply even when one partner is a biological parent to the child (referred to as *second parent adoption*). Problems can arise when a child with same-sex parents does not have a legal relationship with both parents. Examples include denial of health care coverage from a nonadoptive parent's health insurance policy, denial of emergency medical treatment, and custody or financial support issues should the biological parental relationship end through separation or death. In the case of death, a child may be denied Social Security benefits if the nonadoptive parent dies before the child is 18 years old; inheritance of the nonadoptive parent's estate may be denied without a will in place (Bennett, 2002).

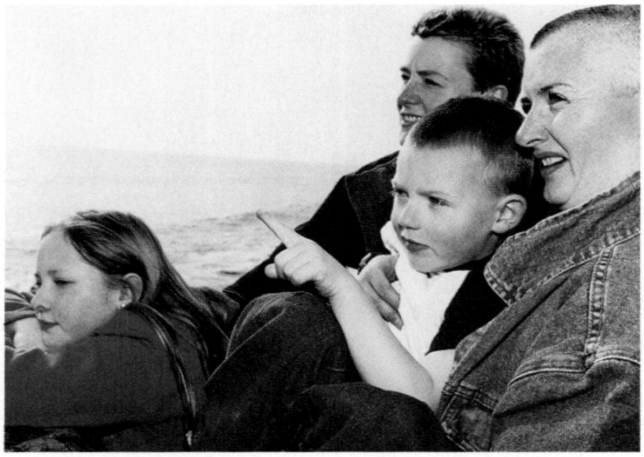

FIGURE 7.10 A family headed by lesbian parents.

Additionally, the same-sex couple faces decisions about how they are going to become parents. Options include biological pregnancy of one of the lesbian partners, surrogacy for gay men, and adoption.

Despite such obstacles for families with same-sex parents, empirical evidence supports the prevailing professional opinion that parenting skills have no correlation with parental sexual orientation (Bennett, 2002; Hunfeld et al., 2001). Professional nurses should uphold their professional ethics and values when working with all families and treat all clients, regardless of sexual orientation, with equal respect and dignity.

Adolescent Parents

Although the birth rate for women younger than 20 years decreased between 1994 and 2001 (FIFCFS, 2003), births to adolescent mothers remain a social and health care concern (Fig. 7.11). Seventy-eight percent of adolescent pregnancies are unintended (National Center for Health Statistics [NCHS], 2002). Teens who become pregnant

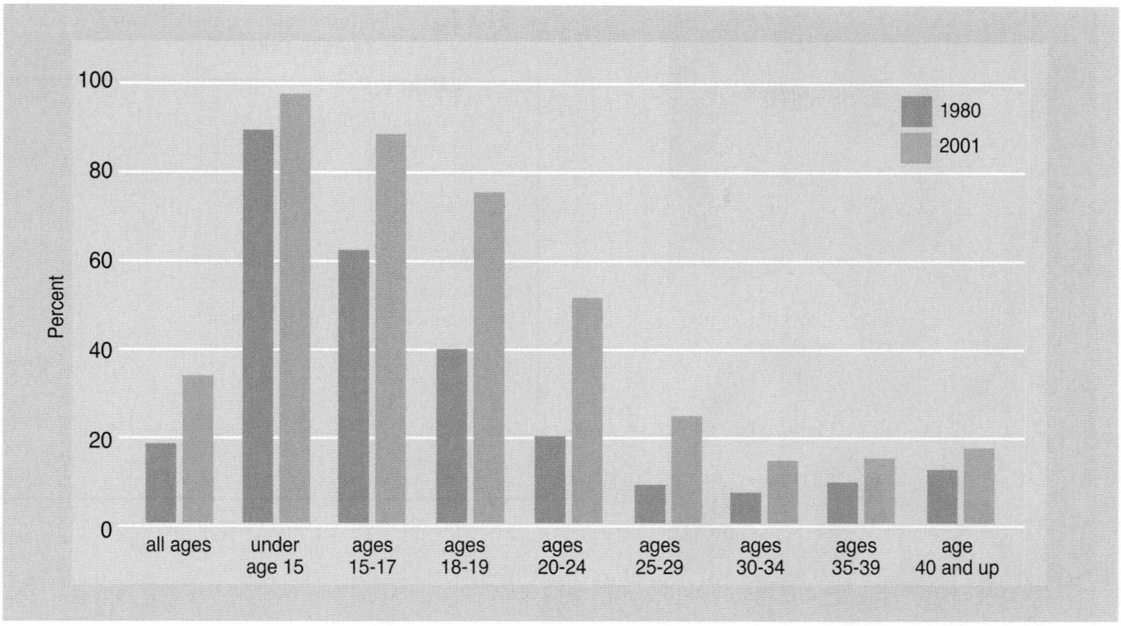

FIGURE 7.11 Percentages of all births that are to unmarried women by age of mother in 1980 and 2001.

usually have not completed their education; findings show that they are at increased likelihood of needing public assistance, have fewer employment opportunities, and are likely to experience marital instability when compared with their peers overall (NCHS, 2002). Infants born to adolescent mothers also are at increased risk for low birth weight, infant mortality, and infant morbidity. They may require assistance to meet developmental milestones (NCHS, 2002).

A recent summary of the available literature related to the experiences of adolescent motherhood found common themes (Clemmens, 2003). Teenage mothers reported stressors related to facing the reality of responsibilities presented with motherhood and difficulty balancing their adolescent needs and their mothering responsibilities. Although stressors exist, the teenage mothers also reported that motherhood was a positively transforming experience in their lives. Additionally, the teenage mothers found the infant to be a stabilizing force. Many of the teenage mothers identified having a child to be a turning point toward a positive future.

Nurses working with pregnant teens should try to address issues of health promotion. It is essential to try to make expectant teen mothers understand that maternal health directly affects fetal health. Such instruction can be challenging during the teen years, when many young women are struggling with issues related to body image. Nevertheless, the nurse should strive to work with adolescents to initiate or to maintain healthy behaviors not only for the pregnancy outcome, but also in the hopes that such behaviors will persist throughout the young woman's life (Montgomery, 2003a).

Working with adolescent parents requires nurses to be aware of this group's growth and development issues. Nurses should consider resources available to help promote the health of the adolescent family. Adolescents often prefer peer support in educational offerings. Therefore, community or clinic-based offerings with role-playing or demonstration may be more effective than one-on-one teaching strategies. Some teaching priorities important for the developing adolescent family include infection protection, nutrition, infant feeding, substance abuse, mental health, and goal setting for the future (Montgomery, 2003b).

Blended Families

In a **blended family,** children from a previous marriage are brought into a family of a married couple. This structure also may be referred to as *stepfamilies, remarried families,* or *reconstituted families* (Clark, 2003). Additional children may result from the new marriage, blending all the individuals into one cohesive family structure (Fig. 7.12).

Myths and stereotypes about stepparents have influenced society's acceptance of blended families and, indeed, may contribute to the dynamics of family relationships themselves. For example, a child who is aware of the myth of the "wicked stepmother" may interpret neutral actions or language as negative. Or a stepfather may be reluctant to set valid rules for behavior in his own house out of a fear of overstepping his boundaries. Research by Ganong and Coleman (2004) indicates the success of the blended family may be directly related to the stepparent–stepchild relationship. Blended families need to acknowledge their new kinship ties and work

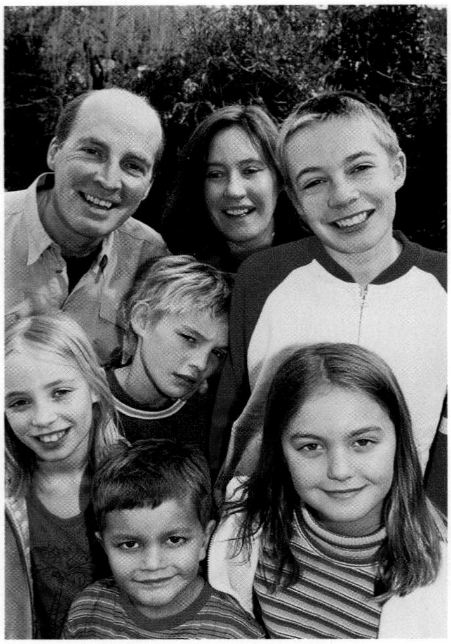

FIGURE 7.12 The blended family consists of a married couple with children from previous marriages, and possibly their own biological children. In this family, three of the children are the biological offspring of the father, one of the children is the biological offspring of the mother, and the youngest child is the biological child of both parents.

BOX 7.2 Physiologic Risks for Pregnant Woman 35 Years or Older

- Decreased fertility (starting in early 30s)
- Increased risk for naturally occurring twins
- Increased risk for chronic health problems complicating pregnancy (eg, diabetes, hypertension)
- Increased risk for bearing a child with chromosomal disorder (especially Down syndrome)
- Increased risk for miscarriage
- Increased risk for placenta previa
- Increased risk for low-birth-weight newborn or premature birth
- Increased risk for ectopic pregnancy
- Higher incidence of fetal distress and prolonged labor
- Increased rate of cesarean births

From March of Dimes. (2002). Pregnancy after 35. *Quick reference: Fact sheets for professionals & researchers.* White Plains, NY: Author.

to stabilize the potential for problematic relationships. Jones (2003) offers the advice that the family should abandon any attempts to view the situation as a traditional nuclear family; instead, they should strive to create a unique stepfamily story.

The legal status of stepparents is somewhat complex. Public policy does not adequately recognize the influence or rights of the stepparent. For example, stepparents typically have no legal status in relationship to the child and no legal authority to discipline or give medical treatment authorization (Jones, 2003).

Families of Mothers Older Than 35

The term *older parent* usually implies that a pregnant woman is 35 years or older. The age of 35 as a benchmark has resulted from research suggesting women this age or older face unique physiologic risks based on age alone (March of Dimes, 2002).

What does it mean to form a family, by any means, when one or both of the parents are older? In 1997, Stark compared the psychosocial adjustment of women 35 years or older during pregnancy with those of 32 years or younger to determine the conflicts faced in adjusting to pregnancy and upcoming parenthood. Results demonstrated that the older group had significantly less fear of loss of control in labor and decreased fear of helplessness. The study also showed, however, that the older women faced more role confusion and conflict with new motherhood relative to their established careers.

Many women turn to their mothers for support during pregnancy. Older women forming families may be caring for their own aged or sick mothers; their mothers may be deceased. In such cases, support from the baby's grandmother may be lacking and leave a sufficient void in the older mother's life. Also, having friends experiencing childbearing or childrearing simultaneously can be a support for many families. This support from friends may be more difficult to find for older parents, whose friends may be past the childbearing and childrearing stage.

Stark addressed life experience and confidence in skills and knowledge gained through it as positive in the transition to motherhood and found older mothers to have better education, higher incomes, and earlier prenatal care than younger women. A 2002 exploratory study by Viau and colleagues examined the health concerns and health-promoting behaviors of 50 pregnant women older than 35 years. Findings showed that these women were proactive about health care, freely asked questions, sought out information related to health care, and interviewed health care providers to make sure the "fit" was good between their and their providers' expectations. This study also noted that 86% of participants had adopted or had enhanced their health promotion behaviors before or during pregnancy. Although this study addressed the limitations of the sample (which consisted predominately of married, well-educated, insured, and economically stable women), the overall U.S. demographic trend of increasing births in this age group correlates with the sample reflected (Viau et al., 2002). Stein and Susser (2000) have suggested that children of older parents do better in school and usually experience a better socioeconomic situation; additionally, life experience of the parents provides some resiliency for dealing with the stressors of parenting.

Extended Families

An **extended family** is one in which a child lives with at least one parent and at least one other person who is not a part of the nuclear family. Often, extended families consist of a multigenerational mix of relatives, nonrelatives, or both. According to Fields (2001), 14% of all U.S. children live in extended families (Fields, 2001). The extended family form can be found most often as a temporary arrangement because of illness, divorce, teenage pregnancy, and older family members who need assistance. It also is more common among working class and recent immigrant families (Friedman et al., 2003).

A variation of the extended family is the **extended kin network** family. In this form, two or more households in close proximity to each other share social support, responsibility, goods, and services. The extended kin network family is most common among Hispanic groups (Friedman et al., 2003).

Grandparents as Primary Caregivers

In some situations, grandparents have primary parenting responsibilities for their grandchildren (Fig. 7.13). Frequent factors that precipitate the need for grandparents to parent their grandchildren include drug abuse by biological parents, divorce, child abuse, incarceration, teenage pregnancy, or death of biological parents. Because these events are major stressors, children in these families may be at risk for increased mental or physical health needs.

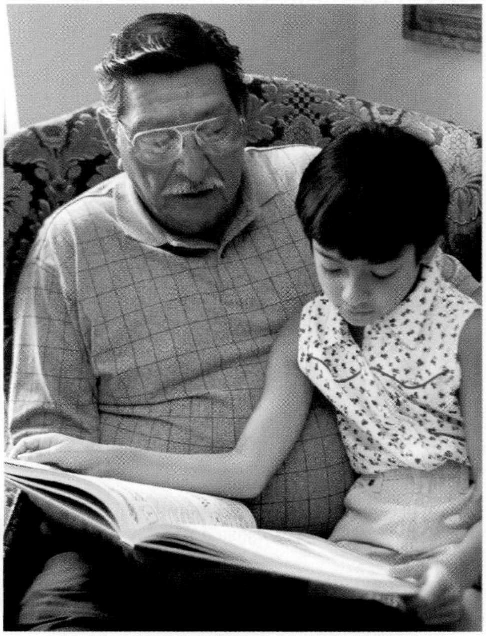

FIGURE 7.13 This grandfather is the primary caregiver of his granddaughter.

Grandparents with primary parenting responsibilities face unique challenges. As a group, they also have more physical and mental health challenges than their noncaregiving peers (Hayslip & Kaminski, 2005). Additionally, among households in which grandparents raise children without the children's parents, 30% are below the poverty level, and 36% do not have health insurance for the children (Fields, 2003b).

Despite the challenges of this family form, benefits have been noted (Hayslip & Kaminski, 2005). Specifically, grandparents themselves report that the experience gives them a feeling of contribution and having a "second chance" at parenting. Children raised by grandparents have been found to have fewer behavioral problems in school than their peers. Ninety percent of grandparents surveyed in a small study reported they would choose to take primary responsibility for their grandchildren if they had to make the decision a second time. Nurses working with families headed by grandparents need to assess for needs in the areas of parenting skills, social support system, economic issues, and legal custody issues (Hayslip & Kaminski, 2005).

CULTURAL PERSPECTIVES

Nurses must be culturally sensitive and competent as they provide care to women and families. **Cultural competence** includes attaining cultural knowledge, having an open attitude, and implementing appropriate clinical skills (Callister, 2001). With this combination, the nurse is prepared to "provide holistic care that addresses the needs of diverse populations" (American Association of Colleges of Nursing, 1998, p. 15). The influence of culture on family dynamics cannot be overlooked or ignored.

Understanding different cultures from the perspective of **cultural relativism** will guide nursing interactions and perceptions during caregiving. Purnell and Paulanka (2003) define cultural relativism as "the belief that the behaviors and practices of people should be judged only from the context of their cultural system" (p. 352). A difficulty arises because the nurse is responsible for some knowledge of the client's cultural beliefs. When communication is smooth, some of this understanding develops during assessment. The best source of information regarding specific cultural practices is the client. Nurses also need adequate knowledge about the widely represented cultures that they may encounter.

Although it remains important for nurses to have general knowledge about the cultures with which they frequently work, it is paramount to avoid stereotyping clients based on their ethnic or religious cultural groups. Many clients follow only some or few of the typical customs of their cultural groups. For example, some people of Jewish descent follow kosher dietary laws, whereas others do not.

The U.S. Bureau of the Census (2001) indicates some 32.5 million foreign-born people within the population. This figure represents 11.5% of the U.S. population. The breakdown of the region of birth is as follows:

- Latin America, 52.2%
- Asia, 25.5%
- Europe, 14%
- Other regions, 8.3%

When these figures are combined with the many second- and third-generation American-born citizens, the ever-increasing need for culturally competent nursing care is evident. Providing culturally competent care is required of all nurses. With each opportunity to learn from the literature and from clients and families, nurses become increasingly knowledgeable about various cultural groups. Learning to view the behaviors of others from an understanding of the client's cultural background is an important initial step in gaining cultural expertise.

Remembering always to include cultural components in a client assessment offers additional opportunities for focusing on the client's culture. Boyle (2003) suggests including the following areas in a cultural assessment:

- Family/kin system
- Social life
- Language and traditions
- Value orientation and cultural norms
- Religion
- Health beliefs and practices
- Political systems

The literature and the Internet can provide vast resources for increasing cultural knowledge and competence. See Table 7.3.

Hispanic Culture

People with origins in Latin America, Central America, and South America represent members of the Hispanic community. The Hispanic cultural group represents the fastest growing segment of the U.S. population (Purnell & Paulanka, 2003). The typical family pattern is patriarchal, with the male viewed as having wisdom, strength, and self-confidence (*machismo*). Some movement toward more democratic roles for women is seen in second- and third-generation Hispanic families (D'Avanzo & Geissler, 2003; Purnell & Paulanka, 2003).

The mother's role within the family is to care for the home and the children. Hispanic women are typically in charge of health matters in the family. The mother is a position of honor. The father tends to make decisions made on behalf of the family in matters outside the home (Purnell & Paulanka, 2003).

Most Hispanic families highly value children and large families. Children represent the continuation of the family structure and extension of cultural values (Purnell & Paulanka, 2003). Callister and Birkhead (2002) found the support of the maternal grandmother to be a powerful influence. Family and extended family needs are strong components of the Hispanic value system.

Health care practices may include the use of home or folk remedies and lay healers. It is common in Hispanic culture to turn to the family for advice and care at the initial onset of an illness. Although the family is an important source of information and support regarding health

TABLE 7.3 Helpful Web Sites for Cultural Information

WEB SITE NAME	CONTENTS	WEB ADDRESS
U.S. Department of Health and Human Services Health Resources and Services Administration	Links to federal health resource information	www.askhrsa.org
Maternal and Child Health Bureau	Information and additional links to topics about maternal and child health	http://mchb.hrsa.gov
La Leche League International	Information to promote and educate mothers about breastfeeding	www.laleche.org
Bright Futures	Sponsored by the American Academy of Pediatrics with information and links to provide prevention and health promotion for infants, children, adolescents, and their families	http://brightfutures.aap.org
National Head Start Association	Private nonprofit organization for meeting the needs of Head Start children and families	www.nhsa.org
Family Voices	National clearinghouse for information and education concerning the health care of children with special health needs	www.familyvoices.org

matters, many Hispanics also seek guidance and care from health care providers for illness.

One barrier to Hispanic women seeking prenatal care is that Hispanic cultures tend to seek health care only for illness. A notable exception is the Cuban culture, which tends to value preventive health care, leading to high participation in prenatal care and other wellness-focused health care services (Purnell & Paulanka, 2003).

When working with traditional Hispanic families, nurses should incorporate an understanding of the strong family network by (1) recognizing the male as head of the household, (2) including family members in assessment and planning interventions, and (3) using the family meeting to promote successful health care interventions (Purnell & Paulanka, 2003) (Research Highlight 7.1). Some specific examples of providing culturally sensitive care for Hispanics in the clinical setting include addressing the man if present with his wife, allowing for extended family involvement in care of the new family, and allowing time and space for family communication.

Asian Culture

The term *Asian* is used collectively for people or groups from China, Korea, the Philippines, Japan, and Southeast Asia. According to the 2000 U.S. Census, 3.6% of the American population is of Asian heritage.

Strong loyalty to the family is a traditional Asian value. The family system is the core of relationships. In Asian cultures, individuals may subordinate personal interests to those of the family. Harmony and honor are important concepts for relationships (Purnell & Paulanka, 2003).

A patriarchal family style tends to influence authority and communication within Asian families. Family members are expected to care for one another. Traditional marriage, the nuclear family, and involvement of extended families are important. The male as head of the household assumes major responsibility for the family (Munoz & Luckmann, 2005; Purnell & Paulanka, 2003). Among Asian groups, extended family members have a sense of obligation to provide care and help to relatives. Older adults are held in high honor and esteem.

The mother–child relationship in Asian families tends to be strong. Frequently, mothers are quite protective of their children from birth onward, and emphasis on fostering independence may be minimized. Respect for authority and listening to one's elders are emphasized (Purnell & Paulanka, 2003).

Some Asian Americans combine complementary modalities with Western health care practices. Traditional Asian health care practices include maintaining a balance between the forces of yang and yin (Purnell & Paulanka, 2003). Many Asian practices of healing are finding their way into Western health care systems. Examples include acupuncture, Tai chi, and herbal therapy. Nurses need to inquire about remedies used at home and what seems to be helpful. Family members may be present to provide personal care at the hospital, and when possible and appropriate, opinions of family members are an important part of the plan of care (Purnell & Paulanka, 2003).

Jewish Culture

Belonging to the Jewish culture means identifying with and being part of a people, a religion, and potentially many varied subcultures (Selekman, 2003). Three main Jewish denominations are found within the faith component. These are the orthodox, conservative, and reform traditions (Munoz & Luckmann, 2005). Each denomination has a different understanding of what beliefs a Jewish person should hold and how he or she should live. Despite such doctrinal variations, an overall consistency about what it means to be Jewish remains among the different segments.

Family life depends greatly on the individuals involved and is influenced by the branch of Judaism fol-

● RESEARCH HIGHLIGHT 7.1 Paternal Influences on the Timing of Prenatal Care Among Hispanics

PURPOSE: To explore and better understand the influences of the expectant father on when Hispanic women begin prenatal care.

DESIGN: Researchers surveyed 300 pregnant Hispanic women recruited from clinics that gave services to low income and medically needy clients. These women sought prenatal care on or before 35 weeks' gestation. The survey focused on their own pregnancy intentions and those of their male partners.

RESULTS: Findings showed that the father's pregnancy intention had a protective effect on early prenatal care. In pregnancies intended by the father but not intended by the mother, the women were less likely to delay care, as compared with those pregnancies unintended by both partners.

NURSING IMPLICATIONS: When working with Hispanic clients, involvement of the male partners in family planning, prenatal care, and childbirth education can be critical to success, in addition to being culturally appropriate.

Sangi-Haghpeykar, H., Mehta, M., Posner, S., & Poindexter, A. N. 3rd (2005). *Maternal and Child Health Journal, 9*(2), 159–163.

lowed, the geographical regions from which ancestors originated, and other factors. Each family varies in terms of who acts as the key decision-maker and which responsibilities women and men hold related to the home and children. Although actual roles and duties vary widely, Jewish mothers and fathers generally tend to share parental responsibilities equitably. Both men and women can play active roles in supporting the home and raising the children, with specific duties varying according to each family's dynamics (Munoz & Luckmann, 2005).

Children are considered a blessing in Jewish families, who frequently value education highly, both in terms of academics and faith traditions. When a child is ill, nurses should appreciate the value placed on children, which may foster great concern from parents over care received and outcomes.

Special ceremonies for children include the recognition of adulthood through a *bar mitzvah* for 13-year-old boys and a *bat* or *bas mitzvah* for 12- or 13-year old girls (Figure 7.14). It is only in the last century that girls also were recognized in this manner, and some orthodox Jews do not have bat mitzvah ceremonies (Selekman, 2003). Other Orthodox families celebrate different types of "rite of passage" ceremonies.

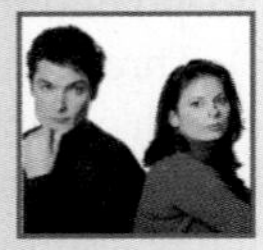

Think back to Jacob and Rachel, the couple choosing private adoption. How might the value that the Jewish culture places on children have influenced their decision to continue fertility treatments for 5 years before choosing to adopt?

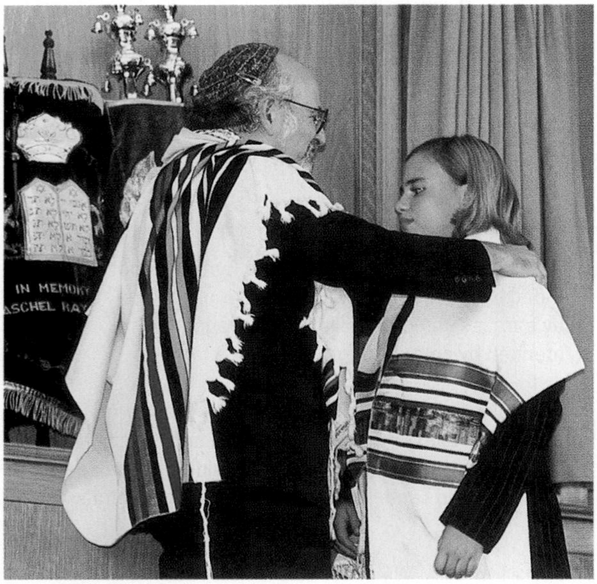

FIGURE 7.14 The bat mitzvah is a rite of passage for many Jewish girls.

Some Jewish families maintain traditional adherence to strict dietary customs known as kosher, which outlines specific guidelines for the processing, preparation, and consumption of food. Kosher practices involve abstaining from birds/beasts of prey and seafood and not mixing meat and dairy products (which could necessitate cooking an animal in its mother's milk). Such measures help to ensure that Jewish people eat food that has been prepared and come from sources that are not associated with spiritual "negatives," such as sickness, pain, uncleanliness, or abuse. Nurses should be cognizant of kosher practices and include careful assessment of dietary habits when obtaining the health history of Jewish clients.

Another unique component of Jewish custom is the practice of separation that dictates the male's avoidance of the female during times of vaginal bleeding (Selekman, 2003). For this reason, some Jewish men may attend childbirth but not touch their wives during this time. Nurses who are aware of this belief can honor the participation of husbands within the Jewish belief system.

Native American Culture

According to the Bureau of Indian Affairs (n.d.), 562 American Indian tribes are federally recognized with the United States. Every tribe has distinct customs and practices. Navajo Indians represent the largest tribe; for this reason, the following discussion focuses on this group.

The family and the tribe are greatly valued among Navajos. Navajo families traditionally are based on a matriarchal structure. The family is an extended network with many relatives living in close proximity. When couples marry, the husband joins the wife's relatives. The grandmother and mothers are the center of Navajo social networks. Extended families often provide considerable care of children and newborns, with women being the verbal health care decision makers (Still & Hodgins, 2003).

Navajo men care for livestock and the farm, whereas Navajo women care for home and family. These women tend to function with great independence. A male leader may arise in the extended family to offer some direction to the group (Still & Hodgins, 2003).

Children are highly valued and welcomed into the extended family. Children learn to respect and honor traditional native wisdom. Many celebrations focus on stages of growth and development. One custom is to name the child at birth, but not reveal the name until the "first laugh celebration" (when the child expresses its first laugh). This custom is believed to protect the child's soul and self-identity. Navajo children are encouraged to help their parents and are allowed considerable freedom in their own decision making (Still & Hodgins, 2003).

Health care practices attempt to align a sense of harmony with environment and family (Leininger, 1991). There is a strong link with traditional supernatural forces, religion, and healing influenced by the use of native healers. Native healers can typically be grouped into one of three categories, based on the spiritual forces they work with: good, evil, or both (Still & Hodgins, 2003).

Increasingly, the Indian Health Services Agency has been focusing on encouraging the integration of traditional native healing practices with the megaculture's health care services. The prevalence of many pregnancy-related ceremonies, taboos, and herbal medicines has posed problems for Native Americans seeking birth in hospital settings (Still & Hodgins, 2003). Culturally appropriate and competent care for these clients may necessitate accommodations for traditional American Indian birthing practices within a hospital environment.

Nurses should involve the appropriate elderly woman who is the family decision maker as needed. Nurses also should recognize that many members of this extended family may be present at the health care facility when a client is ill or has given birth (Hanley, 2004). When planning teaching about a newborn, the nurse should assess who will provide primary care to the child so that he or she can be included in educational sessions. Nurses caring for Navajo children may be concerned with the heightened decision making allowed the children by their parents, such as refusing medication. For the expectant Navajo woman, the nurse should include specific assessment questions that will honor and respect traditional healing beliefs.

African American Culture

Historically, African Americans have faced vast challenges and experienced many struggles related to race. Despite the scope and breadth of this group, many African Americans feel a sense of solidarity with one another, possibly because of common experiences of racism or marginalization (Munoz & Luckmann, 2005).

The family structure in African American families is frequently matriarchal, with much emphasis on extended family. Unlike many other cultures, the single female head of household role is not stigmatized in African American culture. Grandmothers are often the most revered member of the family unit (Fig. 7.15). It is not unusual for African Americans to emphasize privacy regarding family and health-related matters (Glanville, 2003).

Glanville (2003) has identified three common themes in the African American culture: the prevalence of danger and evil in the world, the vulnerability of the individual to external forces, and the need for outside assistance because of a sense of helplessness. These ideas can influence health-seeking behaviors. Illness is typically associated with pain; thus, African Americans are more likely to pursue treatment for conditions that elicit pain than for conditions without pain, such as hypertension. Folk medicine practices are common (Glanville, 2003).

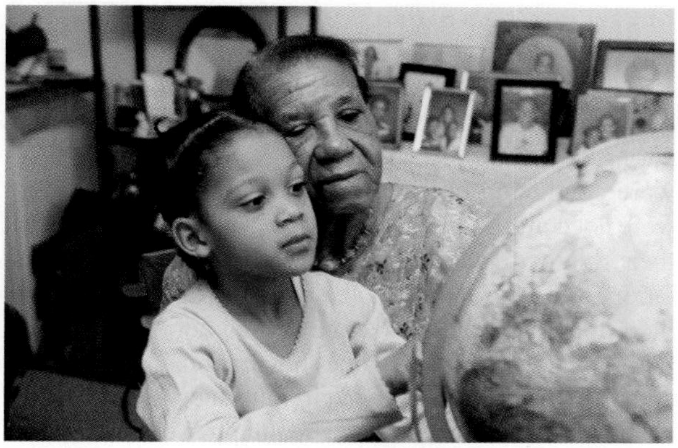

FIGURE 7.15 African American grandmothers often are the most respected members of their families.

Muslim Culture

People of Arab descent represent various subcultures. This section focuses on common themes found in people with ancestry in the many countries of the Arabian Peninsula. Although this group represents various behaviors, thoughts, and religious attitudes, Islam is the most common religion of the group. People who practice Islam are called Muslims.

Muslim family structures are patriarchal, with women having subordinate roles to men. Age is another determinant of status, with young people subordinate to their older counterparts. Typical gender roles include women having responsibility for child care and the success of marriage. Men are considered breadwinners, decision makers, and protectors of the family. In public, women may show submissive behaviors to men, but within the marriage, the wife may strongly influence decisions made for the family. Children are important in Muslim and Arab families; cooperation and respect are key themes in childrearing (Kulwicki, 2003).

Women are typically modest. As a form of protection in situations that involve contact with men, some Muslim women wear garments that show only the face and hands. Because of a strong sense of female modesty, some Muslims typically view childbirth as an activity involving women only. The preference for female birth attendants is strong (Kulwicki, 2003).

Family status and reputation are important aspects of Muslim culture. Fertility is encouraged; giving birth is considered important to promoting family status. Pregnancy is viewed as a natural process, although certain practices are restricted during pregnancy: attending funerals, cutting hair, stealing, gossiping, and having sexual intercourse (Bahar et al., 2005).

FAMILIES GROWING THROUGH ADOPTION

The process of adoption has undergone many changes during the past 30 years. Before the 1970s, many adoptions were conducted in secrecy. Often, biological mothers were not comfortable stating publicly that they had placed their child with adoptive services, fearing shame, humiliation, or both. Many adopted children were unaware of their nonbiological connection to their adoptive parents. Although these circumstances have not changed entirely and in all cases, attitudes and circumstances are evolving. Health care providers, mental health providers, adoption workers, and the general public are becoming more educated about and amenable to discussing adoption openly. The vast secrecy that once accompanied adoption is becoming less common (Pavao, 2005). **Open adoptions** (adoptions in which the biological parents, adoptee, and adoptive parents have an ongoing association, ranging from picture or letter sharing to open visitation) are becoming more frequent.

To help promote positive approaches to adoption, nurses working with both birth and adoptive parents should be sensitive to the language used when discussing this topic. Table 7.4 suggests positive adoption language that nurses may want to add to their vocabulary when working in these circumstances.

Birth or Biological Parents

The decision whether to place a child for adoption is difficult and, in many cases, agonizing. Birth parents have to sort through many realities as they make this choice. They must consider available resources and supports should they decide to raise or to continue to raise a child. They also need to evaluate the possibility of single parenthood, finances, their own emotional pain and suffering, and the child's best interests. Sometimes, family and friends provide guidance, but in many cases, birth parents cannot count on objective support from such people. When considering their options, many birth parents seek help from unbiased, trained professionals such as social workers, therapists, or counselors to assist with the complex decision making involved. Most reputable adoption agencies or hospitals have access to such professionals to assist birth parents with the issues. Because relinquishment of a child for adoption is a decision with lifelong and permanent ramifications, it is important that birth parents make their choice objectively while considering emotional aspects of the situation (Pavao, 2005).

Pre-Adoptive Parents

Pre-adoptive parents also have special needs to consider. Sometimes, adoption is the first choice for people to add children to their families. Other couples decide to adopt after being diagnosed with infertility (see Chap. 10). Some couples have endured years of infertility treatments without success. Others decide to pursue adoption once they receive a diagnosis of infertility and choose not to pursue fertility treatments. Some couples with infertility or people close to them may view the decision to adopt as a "second choice" to having a biological child. Issues surrounding infertility involve loss that requires griev-

TABLE 7.4 Positive Adoption Language

NEGATIVE LANGUAGE	POSITIVE REPLACEMENT
Real parents	Birth parents
Natural parent	Biological parents
Own child	Birth child
Adopted child	My child
Illegitimate	Born to unmarried parents
Give up	Terminate parental rights
Give away	Make an adoption plan
Keep	Parent
Adoptable child; available child	Waiting child
Begetter	Biological father
Reunion	Making contact with
Adoptive parent	Parent
Foreign adoption	International adoption
Adoption triangle	Adoption triad
Disclosure	Permission to sign a release
Track down	Search
An unwanted child	Child placed for adoption
Child taken away	Court terminated
Handicapped child	Child with special needs
Foreign child	Child from abroad
Is adopted	Was adopted

ing. Some parents believe that finally achieving parenthood will help resolve issues of loss related to infertility.

Because of the highly charged and complex issues involved, it is important that all pre-adoptive parents are psychologically and emotionally ready for the challenges they will face both during the adoption process and from society, their relatives, and their other support systems. Enlisting the help of a social worker, therapist, or counselor who is trained in adoption-related issues is crucial to ensuring that these parents are ready for the road ahead (Pavao, 2005).

Once parents have chosen to adopt, they face a multitude of decisions, many of which they may feel unprepared to make. Many pre-adoptive parents dream of adopting an infant similar to themselves in terms of race, ethnicity, health status, and other parameters. The reality is that most pre-adoptive parents are white and the number of white infants overall and available for adoption is decreasing. Therefore, pre-adoptive parents need to consider the benefits and risks of domestic versus international adoption, adopting a child of a different race, adopting an older child, and using a public agency, private agency, or private attorney. Many pre-adoptive parents who are not properly educated on the pros and cons of different options make choices based on anecdotal information from peers or stories they have heard through the media. Advice from a knowledgeable social worker, therapist, or counselor can be helpful in these circumstances (Pavao, 2005).

The shortest line to obtain a child is not always the best line. As Pavao (2005) points out, "Adoption is about finding families for children, not about finding children for families" (p. 24). See Figure 7.16 for a model that parents can use to help consider the aspects necessary in the decision-making process.

Types of Adoption

In general, there are three basic types of adoption: agency domestic, private domestic, and international. Adoption laws vary tremendously from state to state. Limiting the discussion to the three basic types provides a general overview of the process. After reviewing the differences, this section discusses some specific considerations, such as transracial and special needs adoption.

Domestic Agency Adoptions

Agency adoptions occur through a licensed organization that does all necessary legal, administrative, and social work to ensure processes are handled efficiently and in children's best interests. They can be facilitated by either public or private adoption agencies. This section focuses on the similarities between public and private agencies but also notes cases with extensive differences.

Agency adoptions are legal in every American state. The most notable difference between a public and a private agency are the fees. For a public agency, fees range from free to $2500; with a private agency, fees range from $4000 to more than $30,000 (National Adoption Information Clearinghouse [NAIC], 2003a). Some programs can provide financial assistance for pre-adoptive parents: federal tax credits, state tax credits, some special adoption subsidies, employer benefits, and adoptions loans (NAIC, 2002d).

An advantage to agency adoption is that social workers advised by attorneys guide both birth and pre-adoptive parents through every step of the process. Another advantage is that the fee is set, so even if one birth mother changes her mind, the fee covers costs until the agency finds another available child. Pre-adoptive parents need to find an agency that meets their individual needs. Investigating and seeking references are key. Pre-adoptive parents should check the agency's record of placing children in families, check with their state to see if it has an adoption regulatory agency to inquire about complaints, and check references from former clients (NAIC, 2003c). Drawbacks to agency adoption include that the wait for a child can be long. Often, bureaucracy is difficult to manage.

QUOTE 7-3

"I think the agency could have done more to make the adopting families feel better connected . . . to the process during the long time it took to actually receive a child. It was 'no news is no news.' "

An adoptive mother's recollection of her experience with agency adoption

Domestic Private Adoptions

In a **private adoption,** arrangements are made without involvement from a licensed agency. Initial contacts may be between the pre-adoptive parents and a pregnant woman or between a pregnant woman and an attorney depending on state laws. Because laws vary drastically in each state, it is prudent for potential adoptive parents to seek advice from an attorney who is knowledgeable about adoption law in their state of residence and any states where they may consider seeking an adopted child (NAIC, 2003d). The cost of private adoption can range from $8000 to more than $30,000 (NAIC, 2003a).

Private adoptions have both positive and negative aspects. The wait for a child is usually shorter than with an agency; criteria for placement are typically less rigid. Some people who do not qualify as adoptive parents with agencies can sometimes succeed with private adoption. Risks are greater, however, because the validity of a private adoption is more likely to be challenged than it would be with an agency. Also, with the close contact that usually occurs between pre-adoptive and birth parents, **closed adoption** (adoption with no contact between birth and adoptive parents) is usually not an option. Finally, the emotional and financial costs cannot be regained if a private adoption does not go through (NAIC, 2003d).

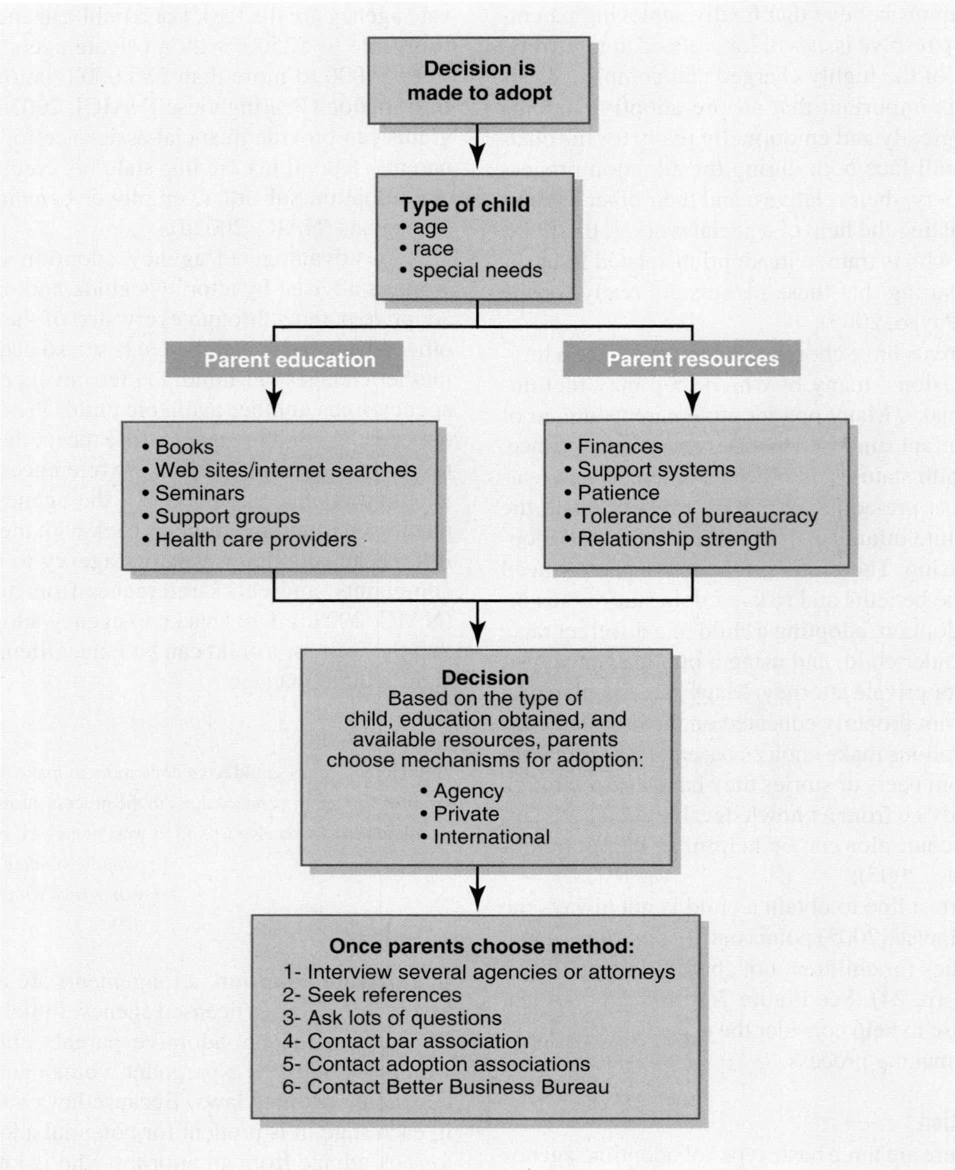

FIGURE 7.16 Decision tree for adoption.

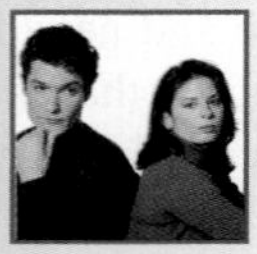

Recall Jacob and Rachel, the couple involved in a private adoption. In their state, the child will not require outside foster care. The birth mother will initially relinquish her rights and assign guardianship to Jacob and Rachel 48 hours after birth.

After giving birth, the biological mother asks to briefly see the baby girl. After she touches the newborn and tears run down her cheek, she then hands the baby to Rachel and tells her to love her daughter.

Imagine if the birth mother asks to see the baby again. How should the nurse respond?

International Adoptions

International adoptions are those in which the adoptive parent or parents and child are from two different countries; they can be handled through an agency or a private attorney. Although complex, international adoptions are gaining popularity as newborns available for adoption in the United States and Canada continue to decrease. International adoptions are usually the most costly. In addition to the costs of the adoption itself, the pre-adoptive parents have to pay for other items, such as international travel and lodging. Often, adoptive parents pay to reimburse for foster care provided to the adoptive child (NAIC, 2003a). Some means for reimbursement of international adoption costs are available, such as the federal tax credits, potential employer benefits, and adoption loans. In addition, some airlines and hotels offer discounts for parents traveling to adopt (NAIC, 2002d).

Some pre-adoptive parents prefer international adoption because they view future custody issues with birth parents as unlikely. The process requires either an attorney or agency skilled in this type of adoption because the process is complex (U.S. State Department, 2002).

International adoption is not an option in all countries. Prospective adoptive parents must carefully consider possibilities, including the child's culture of origin and whether travel to that region is viable for them. Table 7.5 shows the number of adoptions from the top five countries for international adoption from 1993 to 2002.

QUOTE 7-4

"Our children couldn't look more different. Our oldest is blonde with blue eyes, while our youngest is Asian, with black hair and dark eyes. The girls are very close and have been since they first met. . . . Completing the adoption was quite an adventure, but it was well worth it!"

A woman talking about her family, which consists of parents, a biological child, and a child adopted from China

Special Circumstances With Adoption

Sometimes, circumstances make the adoption process complex and cumbersome. Some children with various conditions are labeled as "special needs" and are particularly hard to place. Examples include children with physical or health problems; children older than 5 years; minority children; children with a history of abuse, neglect, or emotional problems; sibling groups, children who are HIV positive, and children with documented conditions that can lead to future problems (NAIC, 2003b).

Funding may be available to assist parents who choose to adopt special needs children. Ongoing assistance may be available for long-term medical conditions. Pre-adoptive parents need to fully investigate the resources required to properly care for such a child to make sure that their family is capable of meeting the child's needs (NAIC, 2002d, 2003a).

Transracial or transcultural adoption also may be an option. Parents should examine their beliefs and attitudes about race and ethnicity and their current lifestyle for multicultural aspects. They also may wish to consider adopting siblings of the same race. Once parents have adopted transracially, it is important for them to tolerate no racially or ethnically biased remarks in their home, surround themselves with supportive family and friends, celebrate the uniqueness of all cultures, expose the child to a variety of experiences, take the child to places where he or she can be with people from their ethnic group, and keep the dialogue open regarding race and culture (NAIC, 2002b).

COLLABORATIVE CARE: WORKING WITH FAMILIES

Assessment

Assessment of the family requires a broad approach because it includes assessment of the family as a whole as well as assessment of the individual members. Key components of a family assessment include the following:

- Family structure and function
- Roles, tasks, and responsibilities of each member
- Family developmental stage
- Family dynamics, power, and decision making
- Family support systems
- Health beliefs and practices
- Culturally related issues
- Community interactions

Family assessment data typically reveal strengths, weaknesses, and stressors. Learning about the family's established support systems and past successful coping mechanisms provides valuable information for planning care. Additionally, although families already may have some knowledge of available community resources, the nurse may be able to recommend further sources of support based on the assessment process.

TABLE 7.5 Number of Children Adopted From Top Five Countries for International Adoptions, 1993–2002

2002	2001	2000	1999	1998	1997	1996	1995	1994	1993
China, 5053	China, 4681	China, 5053	Russia, 4348	Russia, 4491	Russia, 3816	China, 3333	China, 2130	Korea, 1795	Korea, 1775
Russia, 4939	Russia, 4279	Russia, 4269	China, 4101	China, 4206	China, 3597	Russia, 2454	Russia, 1896	Russia, 1530	Russia, 746
Guatemala, 2219	S, Korea, 1870	S. Korea, 1794	S. Korea, 2008	S. Korea, 1829	S. Korea, 1654	Korea, 1516	Korea, 1666	China, 787	Guatemala, 512
S. Korea, 1779	Guatemala, 1609	Guatemala, 1518	Guatemala, 1002	Guatemala, 911	Guatemala, 788	Guatemala, 427	Guatemala, 449	Paraguay, 483	Colombia, 426
Ukraine, 1106	Ukraine, 1246	Romania, 1122	Romania, 895	Vietnam, 603	Romania, 621	Romania, 555	India, 371	Guatemala, 436	Paraguay, 412

Data from U.S. State Department: *Immigrant Visas issued to orphans coming to the U.S. Retrieved May 1, 2006, from http://travel.state.gov/Family/adoption/stats/stats_451.html.*

Structure and Function

Ideally, the nurse completes a family assessment using a tool that provides cues about the family's specific details and needs. Skills in interviewing and observation assist the nurse with family data collection. The Friedman Family Assessment Model and the Calgary Family Assessment Model are two widely used assessment tools. Friedman's model assesses family strategies within the dimensions of system maintenance, coherence, system change, and individualization (Denham, 2003). It has a short and a long form. Sections of the short form are as follows:

- Identifying data
- Developmental stage of the family
- Environmental data
- Family structure
- Family functions
- Family stress, coping, and adaptation (Friedman et al., 2003)

The Calgary Model includes structural, developmental, and functional categories for assessment (Assessment Tool 7.1). It emphasizes the identification of strengths and resources. Repeated use of a family assessment tool assists nurses to refine their skills.

Nurses also can use assessment tools to organize data about a family visually and to map relationships. Examples include genograms and family maps. The **genogram** (Assessment Tool 7.2) uses visual links and other symbols to represent family relationships. In essence, it depicts a family tree (Diem & Moyer, 2005). Most genograms cover the parents, siblings, and children over three generations. They can depict structural and functional patterns, relationships, and significant life events.

Ecomaps are family maps (Assessment Tool 7.3). Whereas the genogram illustrates relationships within the family, the ecomap depicts the family's relationship to the larger community (Diem & Moyer, 2005). After the assessment is completed, the nurse can refer to the ecomap while evaluating the family's external support systems.

Roles and Tasks

As discussed earlier, family roles can be informal or formal as members perform tasks with a given situation within the family. Formal roles are expected roles; for example, father as income earner, mother as homemaker. Informal roles hold a significant place in the family dynamics. Examples may include encourager, harmonizer, blocker, follower, martyr, scapegoat, or go-between (Clark, 2003). The nurse should note the presence of these formal and informal roles as part of the assessment process.

Gathering information about the family's place in the life cycle also assists the nurse with assessing roles and tasks. Sometimes, during completion of a genogram, information about family tasks and roles flows naturally

● ASSESSMENT TOOL 7.1 Components of the Calgary Family Assessment Model

STRUCTURAL ASSESSMENT

Internal

- Family composition
- Gender
- Sexual orientation
- Rank order or birth order of children
- Subsystems in the family
- Boundaries

External

- Extended family
- School
- Church
- Health care systems

Context

- Ethnicity
- Race
- Social class
- Religion
- Environment

DEVELOPMENTAL ASSESSMENT

- Stages of the family
- Associated tasks

FUNCTIONAL ASSESSMENT

Instrumental

- Activities of daily family living

Expressive

- Communication patterns
- Problem solving
- Roles of family members
- Influence and power of different members over other members
- Family beliefs
- Alliances

● ASSESSMENT TOOL 7.2 Sample Genogram

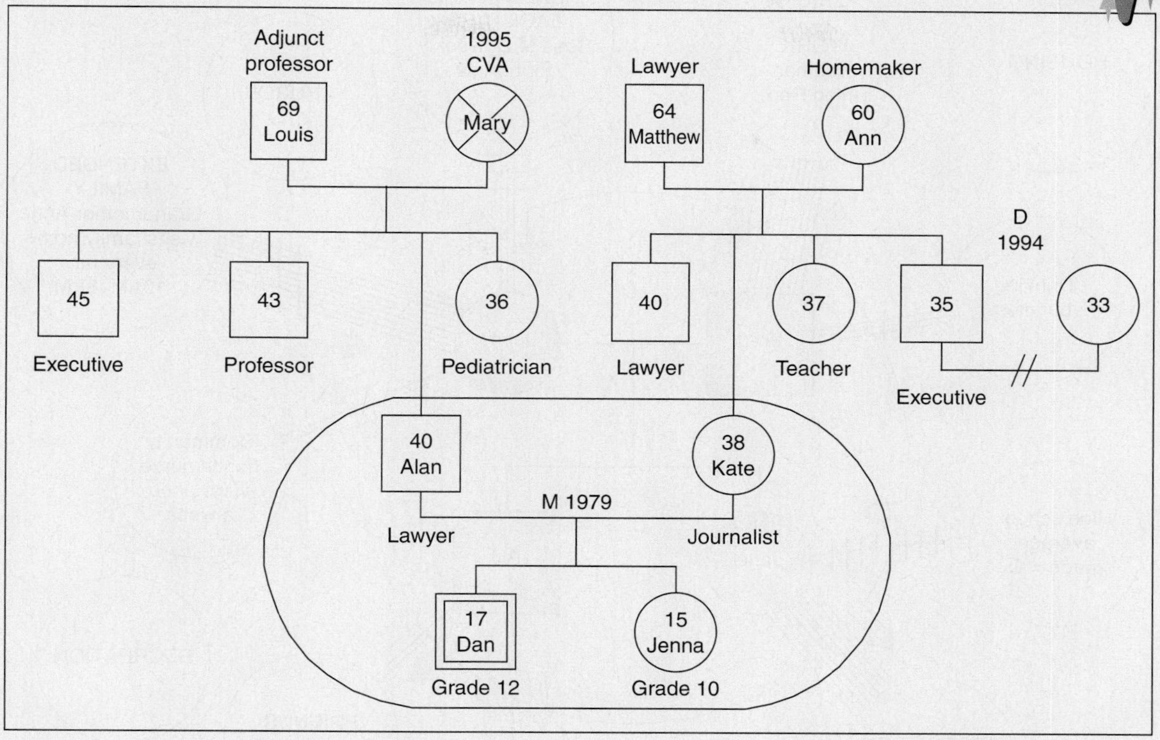

from the discussion. The nurse's understanding of systems and developmental theories provides a framework for seeking information about family roles and tasks as part of the interviewing process of the assessment. With the birth of a child, the family may be required to reassign roles and tasks.

Dynamics and Communication Patterns

Communication patterns and level of anxiety are core elements in assessing family dynamics. Communication has many levels, and family members naturally develop their own way of interacting. Verbal and nonverbal communication patterns within the family should be considered, "as should the listening ability of the family members" (Clark, 2003, p. 301). Keeping in mind Satir's (1988) information about self-esteem and family interactions and Bowen's (1978) systems theory and discussion of anxiety, the nurse should assess family dynamics in interaction with family members. Assessing communication style is one of the first steps in assessing family dynamics (Maurer & Smith, 2005). What is the family style?

- Receptive (open to suggestions)
- Distancing (has difficulty connecting to resources)
- Resistive (denies or disagrees with suggestions)
- Rigid (has fixed way of dealing with problems)
- Ordered (clearly spells out roles and communication)
- Dependent (prefers to look to others for direction) (Cooley, as cited in Maurer & Smith, 2005).

In the course of this assessment, the level of anxiety within the family should become clear. If anxiety is high, future assessment may need to focus on family coping. All these assessments will produce more data if a family meeting can be part of the entire process.

Family as Part of the Community

Assessing the family within the community is best accomplished with a home visit. Home visits can include an assessment of the home environment for safety issues that need to be addressed. When a home visit is not possible, the detailed information from the ecomap can provide a basic assessment of the family's role within the community. The nurse should remember that some families who belong to a resource-rich community still have difficulty accessing and connecting with the needed resources and should do whatever is possible to assist them to do so.

Family Culture

Additionally, the nurse should complete a family cultural assessment to have full information about the family's

ASSESSMENT TOOL 7.3 Sample Ecomap

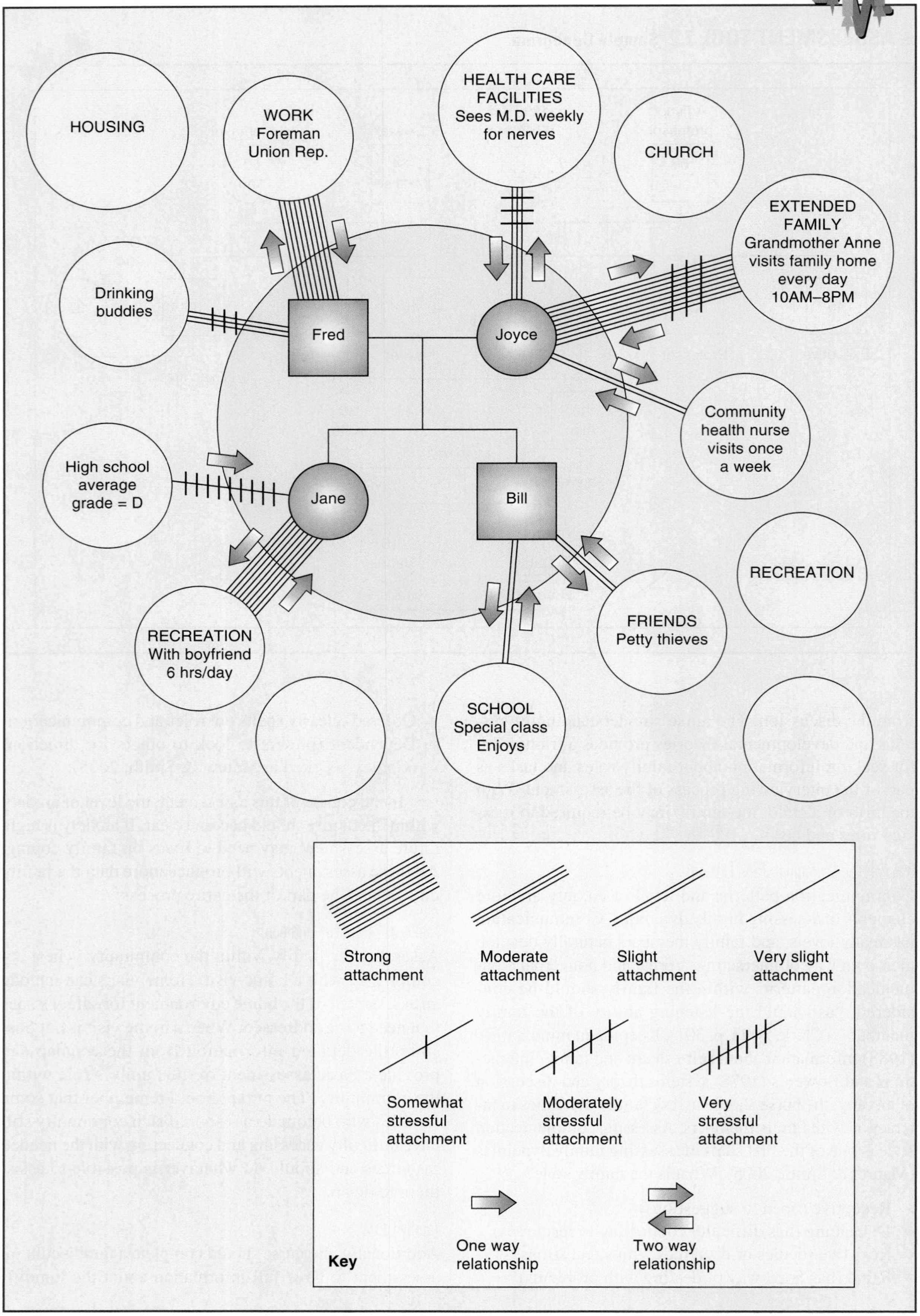
HOUSING
WORK
Foreman
Union Rep.
HEALTH CARE FACILITIES
Sees M.D. weekly for nerves
CHURCH
EXTENDED FAMILY
Grandmother Anne visits family home every day 10AM–8PM
Drinking buddies
Fred
Joyce
Community health nurse visits once a week
High school average grade = D
Jane
Bill
RECREATION
RECREATION
With boyfriend 6 hrs/day
FRIENDS
Petty thieves
SCHOOL
Special class
Enjoys
Strong attachment
Moderate attachment
Slight attachment
Very slight attachment
Somewhat stressful attachment
Moderately stressful attachment
Very stressful attachment
Key
One way relationship
Two way relationship

norms, beliefs, and culturally related health care practices. Gaining insight into culturally influenced perspectives on health care is a valuable component of understanding the family dynamics in any given situation (Rozzano, 2003).

Select Potential Nursing Diagnoses

Determining a family diagnosis may be new to some nurses who are more familiar with arriving at diagnoses for individual clients. Some commonly applicable family diagnoses include the following:

- **Deficient Knowledge**
- **Impaired Verbal Communication**
- **Risk for Impaired Parent/Infant/Child Attachment**
- **Risk for Caregiver Role Strain**
- **Compromised Family Coping**
- **Disabled Family Coping**
- **Health-Seeking Behaviors**
- **Interrupted Family Processes**
- **Readiness for Enhanced Family Processes**
- **Impaired Home Maintenance Management**
- **Impaired Parenting**
- **Ineffective Family Therapeutic Regimen Management**
- **Parental Role Conflict**

Although the nurse is responsible for determining appropriate family diagnoses based on the specific assessment data, he or she should confirm with the family members that this diagnosis correctly addresses the problems identified.

Planning/Intervention

Planning involves forming the desired outcomes (goals) and choosing interventions to help meet them. Outcomes need to be realistic, specific, and measurable. NIC/NOC Box 7.1 summarizes interventions and outcomes commonly applicable to family situations.

When planning care and intervening, the nurse should work in partnership with family members. Together, they can establish a plan to address the family's observed and verbalized needs (Nursing Care Plan 7.2). Planning is also a time for the nurse to empower family members to become part of the solution to their own problems. The

NIC/NOC Box 7.1 Family Care

Common NIC Labels

- Abuse Protection Support: Child
- Abuse Protection Support: Domestic Partner
- Abuse Protection Support: Elder
- Caregiver Role Strain
- Childbirth Preparation
- Complex-Relationship Building
- Conflict Mediation
- Culture Brokerage
- Development Enhancement: Child
- Family Involvement Promotion
- Family Therapy
- Grief Work Facilitation: Perinatal Death
- Home Maintenance Assistance
- Parenting Promotion
- Postpartal Care
- Prenatal Care
- Respite Care
- Risk Identification
- Risk Identification: Childbearing Family
- Role Enhancement
- Sibling Support
- Support System Enhancement
- Teaching: Infant Nutrition
- Teaching: Infant Safety
- Teaching: Infant Stimulation
- Teaching: Toddler Nutrition
- Teaching: Toddler Safety

Common NOC Labels

- Abuse Cessation
- Abuse Protection
- Caregiver Home Care Readiness
- Caregiver Stressors
- Caregiver Well-Being
- Caregiver-Patient Relationship
- Child Adaptation to Hospitalization
- Child Development
- Family Coping
- Family Functioning
- Family Health Status
- Family Integrity
- Family Normalization
- Family Participation in Professional Care
- Family Physical Environment
- Family Resiliency
- Family Social Climate
- Family Support During Treatment
- Knowledge: Child Physical Safety
- Knowledge: Fertility Promotion
- Knowledge: Parenting
- Knowledge: Pregnancy
- Knowledge: Preconception Maternal Health
- Knowledge: Postpartum Maternal Health
- Parent–Infant Attachment
- Parenting
- Parenting Performance
- Role Performance

NURSING CARE PLAN 7.2

A Family Growing Through Adoption

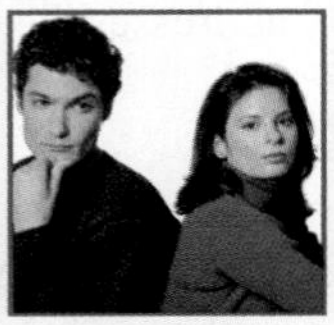

Think back to Jacob and Rachel, the Jewish couple at the beginning of the chapter who are adopting a baby girl. The birth mother has relinquished the baby to the couple. Jacob and Rachel are holding their daughter closely, pointing out some of her features. They state, "She is so beautiful, really a dream come true. We have to learn so much about caring for her."

Six hours after the birth, you check on the birth mother who tearfully states that she knows she is making a good decision but would like to hold the baby for awhile to say goodbye. After informing Jacob and Rachel of this request, they agree to honor it. They state, "Do you think she has changed her mind?"

NURSING DIAGNOSIS

Readiness for Enhanced Parenting related to new role as parents and limited knowledge of newborn care

EXPECTED OUTCOMES

1. The couple will identify areas of needed information about newborn care.
2. The couple will identify basic newborn care measures.

INTERVENTIONS	RATIONALES
Assess the parents' level of understanding about newborn care.	Assessment provides a baseline to identify specific client needs and to develop an individualized teaching plan.
Explore the couple's exposure to newborn care; correct any misconceptions or myths; allow time for questions.	Information about exposure provides additional foundation for teaching and provides opportunities to clarify or correct misinformation and teach new information.
Provide the parents with teaching materials related to newborn care in various forms, such as in writing or via videos.	Teaching materials in various formats enhances learning; written materials can be used as a reference at home.
Demonstrate newborn care measures; allow parents to participate in care, offering anticipatory guidance and suggestions; have parents return demonstrate care measures, such as bathing, feeding, and diapering (see Chap. 20).	Participation enhances learning; return demonstration allows for evaluation of that learning.
Encourage the use of en face positioning and close cuddling during feeding; instruct parents in newborn's cues and appropriate responses.	Proper positioning during feeding and appropriately responding to cues promotes the development of trust in newborn.
Investigate availability of community resources for support; if necessary, arrange for a home health care follow-up.	The birth of a newborn brings about many changes in the family unit. Community resources and follow-up provide additional support and assistance if needed.

Continued

NURSING CARE PLAN 7.2 ● A Family Growing Through Adoption

EVALUATION

1. Parents demonstrate beginning independence with newborn care.
2. Parents exhibit ability to identify and respond to newborn cues.

NURSING DIAGNOSIS

Fear related to possible change in birth mother's decision

EXPECTED OUTCOMES

1. The couple will state an understanding of the rationale for the birth mother's request.
2. The couple will report decreased fear that birth mother may change her mind.

INTERVENTIONS	RATIONALES
Explain the underlying reason for the birth mother's request.	Explanation aids in providing factual, concrete information to allay misconceptions and fears.
Inform the couple that the birth mother's request is part of the grieving process.	Grieving requires knowledge of the person. Allowing the birth mother to know the newborn as a person facilitates this process.
Gently remind the couple that the birth mother can still change her mind.	Legally, the birth mother has a specified time in which to make her decision. Knowledge of this by all parties is crucial.
Ensure open, honest communication.	Such communication promotes trust and enhances the nurse–client relationship.
Provide emotional support to the couple as they cope with the situation; enlist the aid of other relatives if appropriate.	Additional support promotes positive coping.

EVALUATION

1. The couple states that their fears about a change in decision are decreased.
2. The couple demonstrates behaviors that indicate incorporating the newborn into their family unit.

nurse should ascertain specific initial priorities to ensure the family's enhanced compliance with any plan that might be devised (Fig. 7.17).

While working with the family, the nurse should make them aware of various community resources available. Although communities vary in the availability and provision of such resources, the nurse can collaborate with a social worker to connect families to local supports.

In choosing interventions necessary to meet desired outcomes, the nurse should consider both the actions and the supports needed to implement the actions. Priorities should be clear if the nurse remains focused on the desired outcome. The nurse can involve the family by providing choices of possible interventions that would meet the desired outcome and explaining the pros and cons of potential interventions.

Evaluation

Evaluation of the outcomes of the planned interventions is necessary to determine the success of the plan. Whenever possible, family members should participate in the follow-up evaluation. Doing so with the nurse will provide additional learning about what worked for the family and what did not seem helpful.

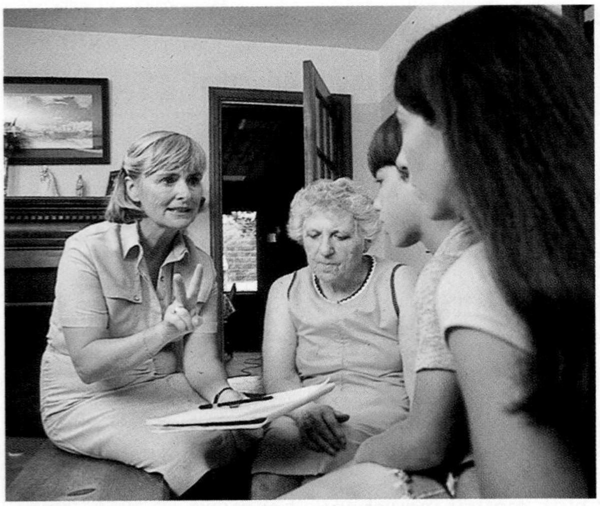

FIGURE 7.17 The nurse working with families needs to regularly monitor compliance of the members with established plans and interventions.

Questions to Ponder

1. Think about your experiences in the clinical setting in working with families. What experiences do you have in which you worked well with a family? Can you identify factors that positively influenced that situation?
2. Think of an experience in which working with a family was difficult. Have you learned anything new that you could apply to that situation?
3. Think of a personal situation in which your family had contact with the health care system. In your personal situation, assess the use and effectiveness of the nursing process.
4. What is your family like? Think about all the cultural groups with whom you personally identify. How have your personal experiences with family and culture influenced your view of other families?

SUMMARY

- Many definitions of family are found in the literature, but nurses need to acknowledge that families are individually defined.
- System theory views families as greater than the sum of its members.
- Families have roles and tasks, values, methods of decision making, patterns of communication, and unique cultural aspects.
- Culture strongly influences families during the childbearing and childrearing stages. Although some general information about ethnic groups is available, nurses need to ask each client and family about their specific cultural beliefs and practices.
- Using the nursing process of assessment, planning and intervention, and evaluation, nurses can provide family-centered care.

REVIEW QUESTIONS

1. Understanding that the health status of one family member affects the other family members is reflected in
   A. communication theory.
   B. systems theory.
   C. family functional theory.
   D. cultural theory.
2. The nurse is working with a married couple who has two biological children, one child from the father's previous marriage, and one child from the mother's previous relationship. The nurse identifies the family structure as a/an:
   A. nontraditional family.
   B. compound family.
   C. blended family.
   D. extended family.
3. In assessing family dynamics, the nurse should collect information about the family processes. Which of the following questions might best provide data about family processes?
   A. "Who makes the decisions in the family?"
   B. "Tell me about your family illnesses."
   C. "Describe how the children are disciplined."
   D. "What recreational activities do you do as a family?"
4. Which of the following examples illustrates healthy family communication?
   A. Verbal messages go through a third party for interpretation.
   B. Family members freely discuss problems with each other.
   C. Family members seldom share thoughts and feelings with each other.
   D. Expressed verbal messages rarely match internal feelings.
5. According to Bowen's Family System Theory, the level of differentiation involves
   A. tensions within a two-person system.
   B. separation of emotions and thoughts.
   C. observed triangles within the family.
   D. communication that facilitates family cooperation.
6. An appropriate approach for the nurse to implement when confronted with triangling is
   A. ask questions to assess the situation.
   B. support the logical position observed in the communication.
   C. suggest possible solutions.
   D. leave and allow the family to solve the problem alone.

7. A couple dealing with infertility asks the nurse to explain the difference between an open and a closed adoption. Which of the following responses, if made by the nurse, is most correct?
   A. In an open adoption, the birth mother retains the right to visit the child.
   B. In a closed adoption, the adopted child never knows identity of the biological parents.
   C. In an open adoption, parental satisfaction is higher for both biological and adoptive parents.
   D. In a closed adoption, the birth parents and adoptive parents do not exchange identifying information.
8. All of the following adoptive children would be considered "special needs" except
   A. a white infant born with a severe heart defect.
   B. a group of triplets.
   C. a child 6 years of age.
   D. a 6-month-old.

REFERENCES

American Association of Colleges of Nursing. (1998). *The essentials of baccalaureate education for professional nursing practice.* Washington, DC: Author.

Bahar, Z., Okcay, H., Ozbicakci, S., Beser, A., Ustun, B., & Ozturk, M. (2005). The effects of Islam and traditional practices on women's health and reproduction. *Nursing Ethics, 12*(6), 557–570.

Bennett, L. (2002). *The state of the family: Laws and legislation affecting gay, lesbian, bisexual and transgender families.* Washington, DC: Human Rights Campaign Foundation.

Bowen, M. (1978). *Family therapy in clinical practice.* New York: Jason Aronson.

Boyle, J. S. (2003). Culture, family and community. In M. M. Andrews & J. S. Boyle (Eds.), *Transcultural concepts in nursing care* (4th ed., pp. 315–360). Philadelphia: Lippincott Williams & Wilkins.

Callister, L. C. (2001). Culturally competent care of women and newborns: Knowledge, attitude and skills. *Journal of Obstetric, Gynecologic, & Neonatal Nursing (JOGNN), 30*(2), 209–215.

Callister, L. C., & Birkhead, A. (2002). Acculturation and perinatal outcomes in Mexican immigrant childbearing women: An integrative view. *Journal of Perinatal and Neonatal Nursing, 16*(3), 22–38.

Charles, R. (2001). Is there any empirical support for Bowen's concepts of differentiation of self, triangulation and fusion? *American Journal of Family Therapy, 29,* 279–292.

Clark, M. J. (2003). *Community health nursing* (4th ed.). Upper Saddle River, NJ: Prentice Hall.

Clemmens, D. (2003). Adolescent motherhood: A meta-synthesis of qualitative studies. *American Journal of Maternal/Child Nursing, 28*(2), 93–99.

Cooley, M. (2000). A family perspective in community health nursing. In C. Smith & F. Maurer (Eds.), *Community health nursing* (pp. 237–255). Philadelphia: W. B. Saunders.

D'Avanzo, C. E., & Geissler, E. M. (2003). *Mosby's cultural health assessment* (3rd ed.). St. Louis: Mosby.

Denham, S. A. (2003). Familial research reveals new practice model. *Holistic Nursing Practice, 17*(3), 143–151.

Diem, E., & Moyer, A. (2005). *Community health nursing projects: Making a difference.* Philadelphia: Lippincott Williams & Williams.

Federal Interagency Forum on Child and Family Statistics. (2003). *America's children: Key national indicators of well-being 2003.* Washington DC: Author.

Fields, J. (2001). *Living arrangements of children: Fall 1996,* (P70-74). Washington, DC: U.S. Census Bureau.

Fields, J. (2003a). *America's families and living arrangements: 2003* (P20-553). Washington, DC: U.S. Census Bureau.

Fields, J. (2003b). *Children's living arrangements and characteristics: March 2002* (P20-547). Washington, DC: U.S. Census Bureau.

Fraenkel, P. (2004). The many meanings of family and the role of fathers. NYU School of Medicine: Child Study Center. Retrieved December 28, 2005, from http://www.aboutourkids.org.

Friedman, M. M. (1992). *Family nursing: Theory and practice* (3rd ed.). Norwalk, CT: Appleton & Lange.

Friedman, M. M., Bowden, V. R., & Jones, E. G. (2003). *Family nursing: Research, theory, and practice* (5th ed.). Upper Saddle River, NJ: Prentice Hall.

Ganong, L. H., & Coleman, M. (2004). *Stepfamily relationships: Development, dynamics, and interventions.* New York: Kluwer Academic/Plenum Publishers.

Geistfeld, L. V. (2005). Consumer economics and family economics: The charge, the response. *Journal of Consumer Affairs, 39*(2), 409–413.

Glanville, C. (2003). People of African American heritage. In L. D. Purnell & B. J. Paulanka (Eds.), *Transcultural health care: A culturally competent approach* (2nd ed., pp. 40–53). Philadelphia: F. A. Davis.

Hanley, C. E. (2004). Navajos. In J. N. Giger & R. E. Davidhizar (Eds.), *Transcultural nursing: Assessment & intervention* (4th ed., pp. 255–277). St. Louis: Mosby.

Hanson, S. M. H. (2006). *Family health care nursing: Theory, practice, and research* (3rd ed.). Philadelphia: F. A. Davis.

Hayslip, B., & Kaminski, P. L. (2005). Grandparents raising their grandchildren: A review of the literature and suggestions for practice. *Gerontologist, 45*(2), 262–269.

Hitchcock, J. E., Schubert, P. E., & Thomas, S. A. (2003). *Community health nursing: Caring in action* (2nd ed.). Clifton Park, NY: Delmar Learning.

Hunfeld, J. A., Fauser, B. C., deBeaufort, I. D., & Passchier, J. (2001). Child development and quality of parenting in lesbian families: No psychosocial indications for a-priori withholding of infertility treatment. A systematic review. *Human Reproduction Update, 7*(1), 579–590.

Jones, A. C. (2003). Reconstructing the stepfamily: Old myths, new stories. *Social Work, 48*(2), 228–236.

Kalil, L. A. (2002). Cohabitation and child development. In A. Booth & A. C. Crouter (Eds.), *Just living together: Implications of cohabitation on families, children, and social policy* (pp. 153–159). Mahwah, NJ: Lawrence Erlbaum Associates, Inc., Publishers.

Kerr, M. E., & Bowen, M. (1988). *Family evaluation.* New York: W. W. Norton.

Kulwicki, A. D. (2003). People of Arab heritage. In L. D. Purnell & B. J. Paulanka (Eds.), *Transcultural health care: A culturally competent approach* (2nd ed., pp. 90–105). Philadelphia: F. A. Davis.

Leininger, M. M. (1991). Selected culture care findings of diverse cultures using culture care theory and ethnomethods. In M. M. Leininger (Ed.), *Culture care diversity & universality: A theory of nursing* (pp. 345–371). New York: National League for Nursing Press.

Luetschwager, J. A. (2000). Adoption: Comparison of state statutes, analysis of barriers, and the role of nursing. *Journal of Nursing Law, 7,* 31–48.

March of Dimes. (2002). Pregnancy after 35. *Quick reference: Fact sheets for professionals & researchers.* White Plains, NY: March of Dimes.

Mauer, F. A., & Smith, C. M. (2005). *Community/public health nursing practice: Health for families and populations.* St. Louis: Elsevier.

Montgomery, K. S. (2003a). Health promotion for pregnant adolescents: Nurses can help improve outcomes during this opportune time. *AWHONN Lifelines, 7*(5), 432–444.

Montgomery, K. S. (2003b). Nursing care for pregnant adolescents. *Journal of Obstetric, Gynecologic, and Neonatal Nursing, 32*(2), 249–257.

Monoz, C., & Lockmann, J. (2005). *Transcultural Communication in nursing* (2nd ed.). Albany, NY: Thomson Delmar Learning.

Murdock, N. L., & Gore, P. A. (2004). Stress, coping, and differentiation of self: A test of Bowen theory. *Contemporary Family Therapy, 26*(3), 319–335.

National Adoption Information Clearinghouse. (2002a, Nov. 13). The adoption home study process. Retrieved April 19, 2006, from http://naic.acf.hhs.gov/pubs/f_homstu.cfm.

National Adoption Information Clearinghouse. (2002b, Nov. 13). Transracial and transcultural adoption. Retrieved April 19, 2006, from http://naic.acf.hhs.gov/pubs/f_trans.cfm.

National Adoption Information Clearinghouse. (2002c, Nov. 13). Intercountry adoption. Retrieved April 19, 2006, from http://naic.acf.hhs.gov/pubs/f_inter/index.cfm.

National Adoption Information Clearinghouse. (2002d, Nov. 15). Resources to help defray adoption cost. Retrieved April 19, 2006, from http://naic.acf.hhs.gov/pubs/f_inter/index.cfm.

National Adoption Information Clearinghouse. (2003a, Jan. 28). Cost of adopting. Retrieved April 19, 2006, from http://naic.acf.hhs.gov/pubs/f_adoptoption.cfm.

National Adoption Information Clearinghouse. (2003b, Jan. 14). Adopting a child with special needs. Retrieved April 19, 2006, from http://naic.acf.hhs.gov/pubs/f_specne/index.cfm.

National Adoption Information Clearinghouse. (2003c, July). Adoption: Where do I start? Retrieved April 19, 2006, from http://naic.acf.hhs.gov/index.cfm.

National Adoption Information Clearinghouse. (2003d, May 20). Legal issues of independent adoption. Retrieved April 19, 2006, from http://naic.acf.hhs.gov/index.cfm.

National Center for Health Statistics. (2002, Feb.). Births: Final data for 2000. *National Vital Statistics Report, 50*(5).

Paulson, R. J., Boostanfar, R., Saadat, P., Mor, E., Tourgeman, D. E., Slater, C. C., Francis, M. M., & Jain, J. K. (2002). Pregnancy in the sixth decade of life: Obstetric outcomes in women of advanced reproductive age. *Journal of the American Medical Association, 288,* 2320–2323.

Pavao, J. M. (2005). *The family of adoption.* Boston: Beacon Press.

Purnell, L. D. & Paulanka, B. J. (2003). *Transcultural health care: A culturally competent approach* (2nd ed.). Philadelphia: F. A. Davis.

Rozzano, L. (2003). Culture perspective. *Holistic Nursing Practice, 17*(1), 8–10.

Satir, V. (1972). *Peoplemaking.* Palo Alto, CA: Science and Behavior Books.

Satir, V. (1988). *The new peoplemaking.* Mountain View, CA: Science and Behavior Books.

Schmidley, D. (2003, Feb.). *Current population reports: The foreign-born population in the United States: March 2002.* U.S. Census Bureau.

Sedikides, C., Gregg, A., Rudich, E., Kumashiro, M, & Rusbult, C. (2004). Are normal narcissists psychologically healthy? Self-esteem matters. *Journal of Personality & Social Psychology, 87*(3), 400–416.

Selekman, J. (2003). People of Jewish heritage. In L. D. Purnell & B. J. Paulanka (Eds.), *Transcultural health care: A culturally competent approach* (2nd ed., pp. 234–248). Philadelphia: F. A. Davis.

Smith, C. M., & Mauer, F. A. (2000). *Community health nursing.* Philadelphia: W. B. Saunders.

Stark, M. A. (1997). Psychosocial adjustment during pregnancy: The experience of mature gravidas. *Journal of Obstetric, Gynecologic, & Neonatal Nursing, 26,* 206–211.

Stein, Z., & Susser, M. (2000). The risk of having children in later life: Social advantage may make up for biological disadvantage. *British Medical Journal, 320,* 1681–1682.

Still, O., & Hodgins, D. (2003). Navano Indians. In L. D. Purnell & B. J. Paulanka, *Transcultural health care: A culturally competent approach* (2nd ed. pp. 279–293). Philadelphia: F. A. Davis.

Urban Institute (2003). Gay and lesbian families in the census: Couples with children. *Checkpoints: Data releases on economic and social issues.* Washington, DC: Office of Public Affairs—The Urban Institute.

Tiedje, L. B., & Darling-Fisher, C. (2003). Promoting father-friendly healthcare. *The American Journal of Maternal/Child Nursing, 28*(6), 350–357.

U.S. Bureau of Census. (2001, May). *Overview of race and Hispanic origin.* Retrieved September 24, 2003, from http://eire.census.gov/popest/data/national/asro.php.

U.S. State Department. (2000). *Fact sheet: Child Citizenship Act of 2000.* Retrieved August 23, 2003, from http://travel.state.gov/chilcitfaq.html.

U.S. State Department. (2002). *International adoptions* [Brochure]. Retrieved October 25, 2003, from http://travel.state.gov/int'ladoption.html.

U.S. State Department. (2006). *International adoption.* Retrieved January 3, 2006, from http://travel.state.gov/family/adoption.

Von Bertalanffy, L. (1968). *General system theory.* New York: George Braziller.

Viau, P. A., Padula, C. A., & Eddy, B. (2002). An exploration of health concerns & health-promotion behaviors in pregnant women over age 35. *American Journal of Maternal/Child Nursing, 27,* 328–334.

Wendlan, C. L., Byrn, F., & Hill, C. (1996). Donor insemination: A comparison of lesbian couples, heterosexual couples and single women. *Fertility and Sterility, 65*(4), 764–770.

Wheeler, S. R., & Austin, J. K. (2001). The impact of early pregnancy loss on adolescents. *American Journal of Maternal/Child Nursing, 26*(3), 154–159.

Wright, L. M., & Leahey, M. (2006). *Nurses and families: A guide to family assessment and intervention* (4th ed.). Philadelphia: F. A. Davis.

Zey, M. G. (2005, Nov.–Dec.). The super-longevity revolution: How it will change our lives. *Futurist,* 16–21.

SPECIAL REPRODUCTIVE AND HEALTH CONCERNS

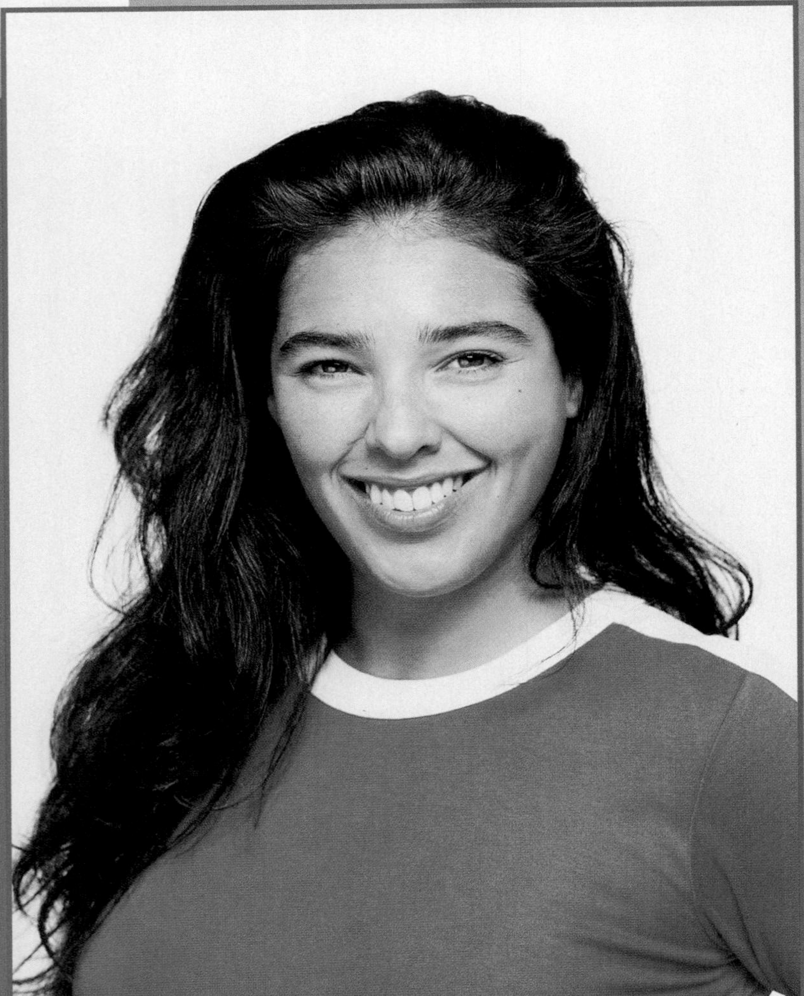

UNIT 2

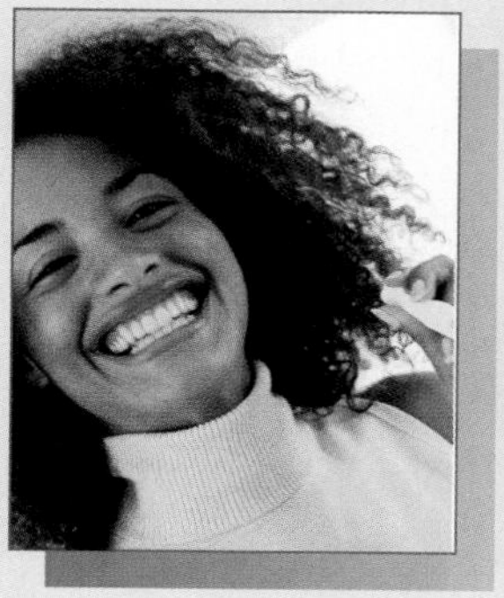
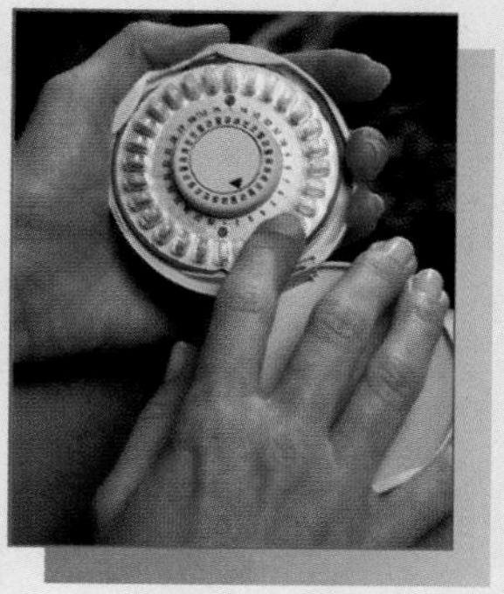
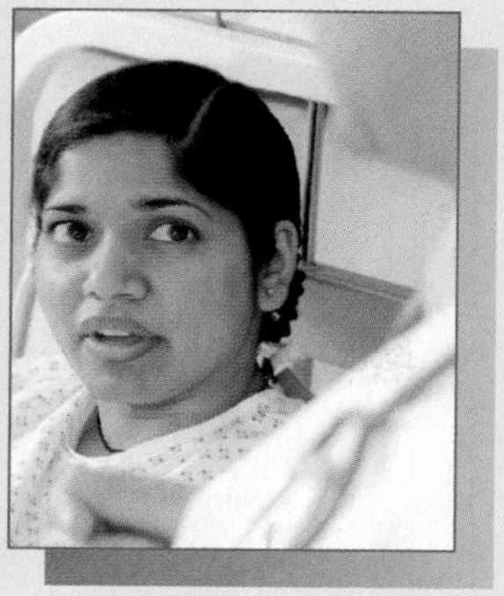
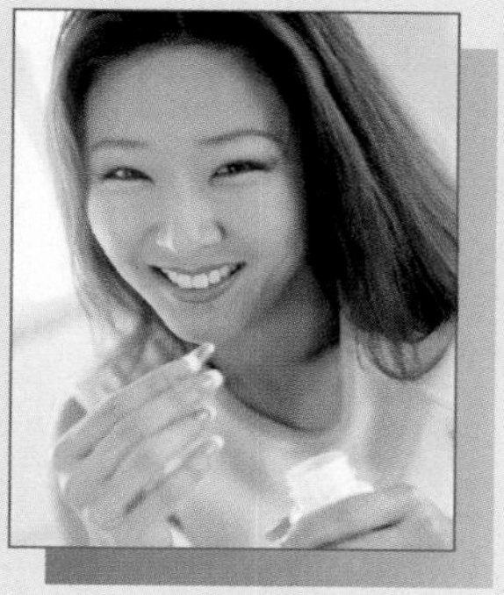

Unit 2 explores important topics associated with reproductive health, although not specifically tied to the process and act of childbearing itself. It describes those issues and concerns that contribute to an environment in which women feel empowered to control the timing and circumstances that best promote healthy gestation. It also discusses ways for health care providers to assist clients with effectively preventing, responding to, and managing the consequences of unexpected reproductive outcomes. Examples of topics covered in this unit include contraception, abstinence, voluntary pregnancy termination, infertility, and alternative childbearing arrangements. The section also contains detailed explorations of genetics and embryonic/fetal development, focusing on problems that can develop or manifest during these phases and associated contributing factors. It reviews significant preventive and diagnostic screening tests and interventions that prospective parents can take to optimize family health.

CHAPTER 8

Fertility Control and Contraception

Eileen Scaringi

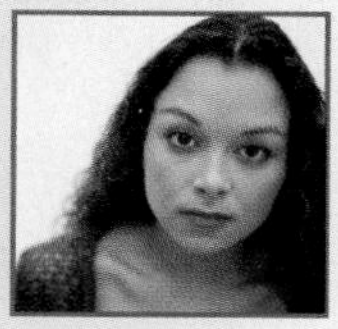

Veena, 26 years old, comes to the clinic for information about contraception. She reports that she's been having sexual intercourse occasionally for 4 years and has used condoms in the past. She wants to explore options other than condoms so that she can feel "more in control over avoiding pregnancy."

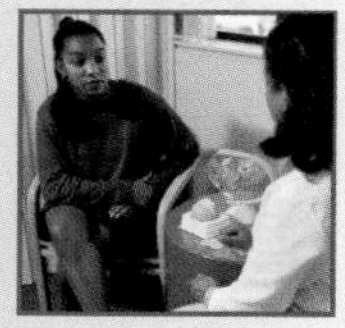

During a scheduled health maintenance visit, Kenya, 19 years old, mentions that she will be married in 4 months to Darrell. The client says that she and her fiancé are both virgins and are planning to wait until their wedding night to have sexual intercourse. The couple follows strict religious beliefs that do not permit contraception. "We'd like to have children someday, but I really would like to avoid pregnancy until I finish college," Kenya reports. She mentions that she has heard about natural family planning and wonders if the nurse can provide more information.

You will learn more about Veena's and Kenya's stories later in this chapter. Nurses working with such clients need to understand the material in this chapter to manage care and address issues appropriately. Before beginning this chapter, consider the following points related to the above scenarios:

- Does anything about either case present any issues of immediate concern? Are there areas for which the nurse must obtain more information? Explain your answers.
- How might the ages of the clients involved influence the nurse's approach to care?
- What health-related areas should the nurse investigate with Veena? What about with Kenya?
- What measures can the nurse take to approach the clients with sensitivity and adequate information? How can the nurse ensure understanding of concepts taught?

LEARNING OBJECTIVES

On completion of this chapter, the reader should be able to:

- Describe a brief history of contraception and social forces that have helped to shape its development and availability.
- Explain the mechanism of action, effectiveness, contraindications, correct usage, side effects, and danger signs for specific contraceptive methods.
- Identify appropriate teaching for women about emergency contraception.
- Discuss natural family planning methods.
- Describe surgical methods of limiting fertility.
- Elicit a thorough health history for clients seeking contraception, taking into consideration sexual orientation and cultural beliefs.
- Identify appropriate counseling measures for barrier, hormonal, and intrauterine methods of contraception.

KEY TERMS

abstinence
bilateral tubal ligation
cervical cap
combined oral contraceptives (COCs)
contraception
contraceptive sponge
diaphragm
female condom
fertility awareness methods
intrauterine device (IUD)
lactational amenorrhea method
male condom
natural family planning
pelvic inflammatory disease (PID)
sexually transmitted infections (STIs)/ sexually transmitted diseases (STDs)
typical use failure rate
vasectomy
withdrawal

Since ancient times, women and men have sought to control their fertility (Box 8.1). **Contraception** means any method used to prevent pregnancy. The introduction of the oral contraceptive in 1960 ushered in a new era of fertility control and contributed to an increased sense of sexual freedom for women, who had new opportunities to determine when, how often, and with whom they would become pregnant. Birth control methods continue to evolve; examples of recently developed devices include the contraceptive patch and the vaginal contraceptive ring.

Society traditionally has placed contraceptive responsibility, along with child nurturing, on women. Except for the male condom, withdrawal, and vasectomy, all currently available contraceptive methods are female focused. Although research into male methods continues, obstacles to development and use include the undesired side effects of infertility and interference with sexual performance (Lyttle & Kopf, 2003; Waites, 2003). Continued political pressure is necessary to promote the development of these options.

Hindrances that impede contraceptive development include the organization of and resources available for research, current federal regulations, product liability issues, and the attitudes of the U.S. public (Kaeser, 1990; Lyttle & Kopf, 2003; Reaves, 2002). Neither the government nor pharmaceutical companies have demonstrated a commitment to the research and development of new contraceptive methods (Kreinin, 2002).

This chapter provides a historical and social context for fertility control. The chapter explores various methods of fertility control, including barrier, hormonal, intrauterine, behavioral, and surgical methods. It describes collaborative care measures for the client seeking information about contraception and family planning. Nurses need to be prepared to provide teaching and assistance to

BOX 8.1 Brief History of Contraception

2000–1000 BCE. Ancient Egyptian writings discuss vaginal pessaries and mixtures to insert into the vagina to prevent conception.
500–600 BCE. Biblical writings discuss withdrawal.
500 BCE. Aristotle suggests covering the cervix with cedar oil to prevent pregnancy.
100–200 CE. The Talmud describes the insertion of sponges soaked with vinegar or wine to prevent pregnancy.
150 CE. Roman mythology describes the use of a goat bladder as a condom.
300–400 CE. St. Augustine prohibits contraception.
1100–1200 CE. Islamic writings discuss withdrawal.
1200–1300 CE. The Roman Catholic church approves only "natural methods" of contraception.
1583 CE. The writings of Fallopius describe linen "sheath" or condom.
1725–1798 CE. Casanova writes about condoms made from animal intestines and cervical caps made from lemons.
1800–1900 CE. Rubber condoms are introduced, along with the cervical cap, diaphragm, and sponges with spermicide.
1882. The first birth control clinic, located in Holland, opens.
1909. The IUD is introduced.
1916. Margaret Sanger opens the first birth control clinic in the United States.
1960. The oral contraceptive is marketed in the United States.
1965. The U.S. Supreme Court removes the final legal obstacles to distribution of contraceptive information.
1992. Depo-Provera is introduced in the United States.
2000. The FDA approves Mirena and Lunelle.
2001. The FDA approves NuvaRing and Ortho Evra.

women seeking a method best suited to their needs and lifestyles while ensuring adequate understanding of the abilities, mechanisms, benefits, and risks of different methods.

HISTORICAL PERSPECTIVES

In ancient times, options for limiting pregnancy were few and included prolonged lactation, ingested and inserted plant extracts (Green, 1971) and, in some cultures, infanticide. Withdrawal of the penis before ejaculation was another widely used method; some cultures today continue to rely on it as a primary mechanism of birth control. Magical rites, formulas, and potions also were common methods, along with douching, positioning, and moving the body violently (Bullough & Bullough, 1994; Schenker & Fabenou, 1993).

Early Egyptian writings discuss vaginal insertion of a mixture of crocodile dung, honey, and gum-like substances for the prevention of pregnancy. These writings also describe an occlusive vaginal pessary, a forerunner to the modern diaphragm. Aristotle recommended covering the cervix and vagina with cedar oil. The Bible describes withdrawal (*coitus interruptus*), and Hippocrates mentions an intrauterine device in his writings. The Hebrew Talmud details the insertion into the vagina of a sponge soaked in vinegar or wine, while the Romans may have used goat intestines as a barrier in their efforts to prevent pregnancy (Bullough & Bullough, 1994; Himes, 1970).

In 1583, Gabriele Fallopius, an Italian anatomist for whom the fallopian tubes are named, first described a linen "sheath" or condom. During this time, the primary use of the condom was not as a contraceptive, but as a way to combat syphilis. In the 18th century, Casanova described the use of a lemon half as a cervical cap and also wrote about condoms made from animal intestines. Such condoms, however, were expensive and had to be washed for reuse. In the 19th century, mass-produced rubber condoms became available, as did a cervical cap, diaphragm, and sponge with spermicide.

Organized religion often has shaped social policies toward contraception. Jewish and Christian religions have interpreted the Biblical narrative describing withdrawal as a prohibition against wasting semen. In the 13th century, the Roman Catholic Church put forth its policy of only "natural methods" of fertility control (ie, sex only during a "safe" period and intercourse without ejaculation); this doctrine remains in force. The Protestant tradition followed similar prohibitions against contraception, which were manifested as vigorous legislation against "obscenity." In 1873, the Comstock Laws made the advertisement of information on abortion and contraception illegal.

Religious and political policies severely limited public awareness of birth control until two seemingly disparate political groups sought to promote contraception: the social radicals, who saw childbirth as destructive to women and large families as a major contributor to poverty, and the eugenicists, who desired to stop the poor from "breeding." Aletta Jacobs opened the first birth control clinic in Holland in 1882. Zealous U.S. legislation and law enforcement quickly shut down the first clinic opened by Margaret Sanger in Brooklyn in 1916. A militant socialist who coined the phrase "birth control," Sanger had been distributing pamphlets on fertility control and had to flee to Europe to avoid prosecution. She continued a lifelong crusade to increase the availability of contraception, and her American Birth Control League was the forerunner of today's Planned Parenthood.

In 1909, the IUD was introduced. The rhythm method was first described in 1932. Charles Knowlton's *The Fruits of Physiology,* published in 1933, recommended douches made of sodium bicarbonate, alum, zinc phosphate, sodium chloride, vinegar, rose leaves, or raspberry leaves or roots to prevent pregnancy. Although it was postulated in 1919 that ingestion of progesterone would prevent pregnancy, it was not until the 1940s that Russell Marker overcame the difficulty of the large quantity of hormone needed by synthesizing the steroid from Mexican yams.

Mass-market oral contraception was introduced in 1960. "The pill" has been credited with initiating a sexual revolution. Oral contraceptives provided highly effective protection. The first trials for oral contraception with progesterone were done in Puerto Rico. After discovering that estrogen acted as a "contaminant," it was removed from the pill. When pregnancy rates subsequently increased, 150 μg of estrogen was re-added. Subsequently, the dose of estrogen has been decreased with each new generation of oral contraceptives, which currently contain as little as 20 μg. Progesterone-only formulations are available today as well.

In 1965, the U.S. Supreme Court removed the last legal obstacles restricting the dissemination of contraception information. Since then, various hormonal methods have become available. The U.S. Food and Drug Administration (FDA) approved depot medroxyprogesterone acetate (DMPA) in 1982 and the levonorgestrel implant, Norplant, in 1990. Most recently, the FDA approved the combined injectable (Lunelle) in 2000 and the transdermal contraceptive (Ortho-Evra) and vaginal contraceptive ring (NuvaRing) in 2001. Additional research is currently underway to expand contraceptive choices.

TYPES OF CONTRACEPTIVE METHODS

Table 8.1 provides an overview of the various methods of contraception discussed in this chapter. These methods can be subclassified as follows: barrier, hormonal, intrauterine, behavioral, and surgical.

Barrier Methods

Barrier methods rely on mechanical devices to prevent sperm from entering the female reproductive tract. Some of them also provide protection against **sexually transmitted infections (STIs),** also called **sexually transmitted diseases (STDs).** Barrier methods include male and female condoms, diaphragms, and cervical caps.

Male Condom

Until the early 1900s, the **male condom** was one of the few widely available methods of contraception. Today, male condoms are available in latex, natural membrane (usually sheep intestine), and polyurethane forms. They come in various sizes and colors, with or without lubricants or spermicides, and with or without a reservoir tip (Fig. 8.1). Condoms are also available textured and flavored. No prescription for condoms is needed.

Latex and polyurethane condoms protect against the transmission of STIs, including HIV. Natural membrane condoms do not protect against virus transmission (ie, HIV and human papillomavirus [HPV]); however, some clients prefer them because they facilitate increased male sensitivity during intercourse.

Mechanism of Action and Effectiveness. Condoms work by containing ejaculate and its estimated 300 million sperm, preventing them from entering the female reproductive tract and, subsequently, conception. **Typical use failure rates** (rate at which the method fails to prevent pregnancy, factoring in incorrect and inconsistent use, as well as failure despite correct application and use with every act of intercourse) range from 7% to 15% (Hatcher et al., 2004; Walsh et al., 2003). Condoms used with spermicide (see next section) decrease the likelihood of pregnancy, especially in the event of slippage or breakage of the condom. Evidence to suggest that condoms marketed as lubricated with spermicide are more effective than condoms not lubricated with spermicide is insufficient (Hatcher et al., 2004).

Contraindications and Side Effects. An allergy to latex in either partner is the only contraindication for use of latex condoms. Primary symptoms of latex allergy include genital irritation or burning. Clients with latex allergy remain candidates for natural membrane or polyurethane condoms, as well as other contraceptive options discussed in this chapter.

Client Teaching and Collaborative Interventions. Some clients may not understand correct placement or use of condoms. One method by which nurses can educate them is to demonstrate correct use with a model of a penis or a similarly shaped object. The nurse also can ask the client for a return demonstration on the model to validate understanding, provided the client is comfortable doing so. If a model penis is unavailable, the nurse can use a banana instead.

As discussed earlier, latex and polyurethane condoms protect against STIs, but natural membrane condoms contain microscopic holes through which virus particles may pass. Thus, clients seeking use of condoms for STI prevention require instruction about ensuring that they are using latex or polyurethane types.

Before use of condoms, the client, partner, or both should check them for date of expiration and to be sure that the packaging is intact. To be used correctly, the condom must be placed over the erect penis before any genital contact is made with the partner (Fig. 8.2). Application of the condom before the man enters the partner is critical because the man may release a few drops of semen before ejaculation, even if he is unaware that this has happened. Although this ejaculate consists mostly of semen from the Cowper's and prostate glands, it also contains some sperm, making this fluid potentially fertile. The fluid also could contain virus particles.

The client or partner should place the correct side of the condom on the glans (tip) of the penis and unroll the

(text continues on page 282)

TABLE 8.1 Summary of Contraceptive Methods

METHOD	MECHANISM OF ACTION	TYPICAL USE FAILURE RATE	BEST CANDIDATES	NONCONTRACEPTIVE BENEFITS AND ADVANTAGES	SIDE EFFECTS AND DISADVANTAGES	CONTRAINDICATIONS
Barrier Methods						
Male condom	Encases the penis to hold ejaculate and prevent sperm from entering female reproductive tract	15%	Those looking for an over-the-counter product Cooperative male partners	Latex and polyurethane forms protect against STIs	May be perceived as interruptive of sex	Latex allergy (may use natural membrane or polyurethane)
Female condom	Provides a barrier between the penis and female reproductive tract	21%	Women willing to accept 21% failure rate	Controlled by woman Protects against STIs	Difficult to insert	Severe vaginal prolapse
Diaphragm (with spermicide)	Covers the cervix to prevent sperm from entering; spermicide kills sperm	16%	Women comfortable inserting device into vagina	May be inserted 6 hours before sex Protects against some STIs	Needs to be professionally fitted	Frequent UTIs Allergy to spermicide
Cervical cap (with spermicide)	Covers the cervix to prevent sperm from entering; spermicide kills sperm	16–32%	Women comfortable inserting device into vagina	May be inserted 6 hours before intercourse and left in for 48 hours	Needs to be professionally fitted No STI protection	Latex allergy Cervical infection
Contraceptive sponge	Blocks cervix from sperm, traps sperm; releases spermicide to kill sperm	17–24%	Women comfortable inserting device into vagina; those looking for an over-the-counter product controlled by the woman	May be inserted up to 24 hours before intercourse Does not need reinsertion or replacement within 24-hour period for subsequent acts of intercourse	No STI protection	Allergy to spermicide
Spermicide	Reduces mobility of sperm and blocks penetration into cervix	29% (Varies depending on use with or without other methods)	Women at low risk for HIV Women comfortable inserting spermicide into vagina	Foam immediately effective	May have unpleasant taste Film and suppositories require 15 minutes to become effective No STI protection	Spermicidal allergy
Hormonal Methods						
Combined oral contraceptives	Prevent ovulation and sperm penetration at cervix	8%	Women who can remember to take each day	Lower risk for ovarian and endometrial cancer Decreased acne and dysmenorrhea	Nausea Headaches BTB No STI protection	History of breast cancer or DVT Migraines with focal/neurologic changes CAD Smokers older than 35 years

Continued

TABLE 8.1 Summary of Contraceptive Methods *(Continued)*

METHOD	MECHANISM OF ACTION	TYPICAL USE FAILURE RATE	BEST CANDIDATES	NONCONTRACEPTIVE BENEFITS AND ADVANTAGES	SIDE EFFECTS AND DISADVANTAGES	CONTRAINDICATIONS
Contraceptive patch	Prevents ovulation and sperm penetration at cervix	8%	Teenagers who cannot remember a pill each day	Patch is changed once a week	Breast tenderness Nausea Headaches BTB No STI protection	Same as COCs
Vaginal contraceptive ring	Prevents ovulation	8%	Women who cannot remember a pill each day	Removed in 21 days; new ring inserted 7 days later	Vaginitis Vaginal discharge Other COC SEs; No STI protection	Same as COCs
Progestin-only pills	Prevents sperm penetration at cervix	8%	Women who cannot take estrogen (breastfeeding women)	No estrogen-related side effects	BTB Amenorrhea Ovarian cysts Headaches	Breast cancer Liver disease Impaired absorption Certain medications
DMPA	Suppresses ovulation Prevents sperm penetration at cervix	3%	Women who cannot take estrogen	Decreased risk for endometrial cancer, PID, and ectopic pregnancy May decrease seizures Reduces sickle cell crises	Irregular bleeding Amenorrhea Slow return to fertility Weight gain No STI protection Clinic visits every 70–90 days	History of breast cancer, MI, or stroke Liver disease
Progestin-only implant (Implanon)	Prevents sperm penetration at cervix Suppresses ovulation Thins endometrium	<1%	Available 2006: Women who cannot take estrogen	Decreased dysmenorrhea	Irregular bleeding Headaches No STI protection	Breast cancer Liver disease Certain medications
Intrauterine Methods						
Copper IUD	Inhibits sperm motility Destroys sperm	<1%	Women at low risk for STIs Women who cannot take hormones	Cost effective Decreased risk for ectopic pregnancy	Heavier bleeding, dysmenorrhea No STI protection	Women at risk for STIs Allergy to copper Cervicitis

Continued

Levonorgestrel IUD (Mirena)	Prevents sperm penetration at cervix Thins endometrium Suppresses ovulation	<1%	Women who desire a long-acting, highly effective method	Decreased menstrual flow and dysmenorrhea Decreased risk for ectopic pregnancy	Irregular bleeding Amenorrhea No STI protection Ovarian cysts	Women at risk for STIs Breast cancer Liver disease
Behavioral Methods						
Abstinence	Not having sexual intercourse	Not available	Those who wish to refrain from sexual intercourse	Guarantees avoidance of pregnancy and STIs	Difficult to maintain	None
Natural family planning/fertility awareness method	Abstaining or using a barrier method or withdrawal during fertile period	25%	Those who cannot use other methods Women with regular cycles	Woman more aware of her cycle	Must be committed to abstain or use other methods during fertile time No STI protection Requires training	Women with irregular cycles
Withdrawal	Prevents deposit of sperm into vagina	27%	Women willing to accept an increased risk for pregnancy	Method readily available	Requires great self-control No STI protection	Men who cannot withdraw before ejaculating
Lactational amenorrhea method (LAM)	Lactation inhibits ovulation	1%–2%	Mothers who are exclusively breastfeeding and have not had a menses	Facilitates postpartum weight loss Decreases risk for breast cancer	No STI protection	Infant older than 6 months old Return of menses Women with blood-borne disease or taking drugs contraindicated in breastfeeding
Surgical Methods						
Surgical sterilization	Female: occludes fallopian tubes Male: occludes vas deferens	<1%	Those wishing to have no (or no more) children	Female: decreased risk for ovarian cancer Male: easier, less expensive, and more effective than female	Surgical risks (greater for female) Possible regret No STI protection	Those unsure of a permanent method

BTB, breakthrough bleeding; CAD, coronary artery disease; COC, combined oral contraceptives; DMPA, depot medroxyprogesterone acetate; PID, pelvic inflammatory disease; STI, sexually transmitted infection.

Adapted from Hatcher, R. A., Trussell, J., Stewart, F., Cates, W., Stewart G., Guest, F., & Kowal, D. (2004). *Contraceptive technology* (18th ed.). New York: Artent Media.

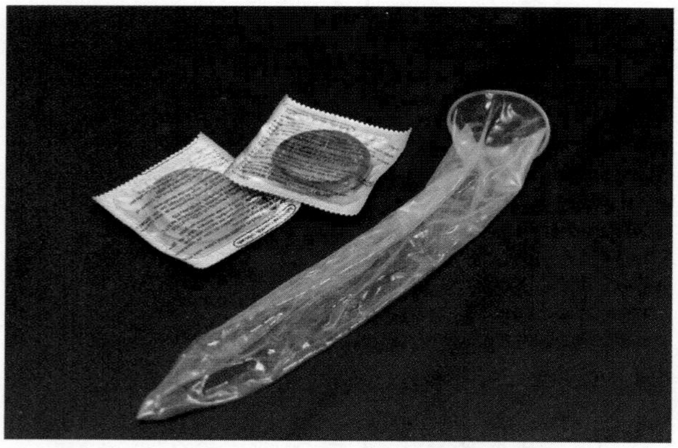

FIGURE 8.1 Male condoms are available in various colors, textures, and sizes.

condom down the shaft while holding onto the tip of the condom, to provide a reservoir for the ejaculate. If the condom is placed inside out, the couple should discard and replace it with a new one. If the condom-covered penis is placed into the partner's mouth or anus, a new condom should be applied before vaginal intercourse to ensure that it is intact and free of bacteria. For extra protection, clients may choose to wear two condoms.

After ejaculation, the man should hold the condom in place while removing the penis from the vagina or other orifice. He should pull down on the tip of the condom while sliding the condom down the shaft, to prevent spillage of the ejaculate. Each act of intercourse requires a new condom.

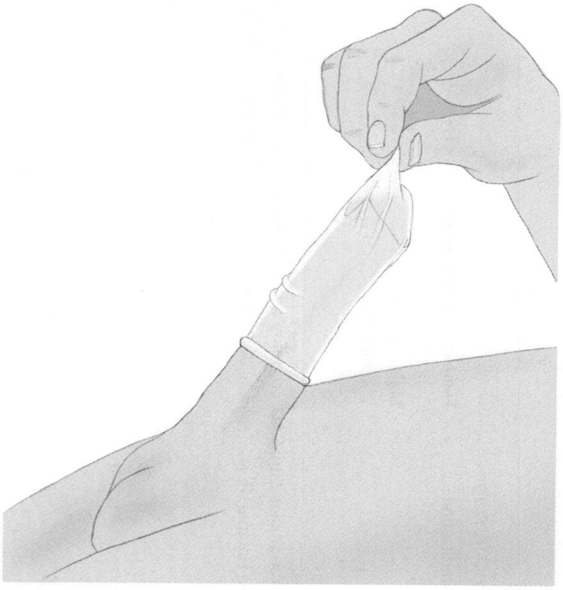

FIGURE 8.2 The client places the condom over the erect penis before making any genital contact with the partner. Some space should be left at the tip of the condom to contain the ejaculate.

Clients should not use petroleum- or oil-based products with latex condoms because these substances can weaken the latex and increase the risk for breakage. Use of a water-based lubricant (eg, KY Jelly, Astroglide, water, saliva) with condoms is acceptable.

Female Condom

The **female condom,** introduced in 1993, consists of a barrier of polyurethane inserted into the vagina and an outer ring that extends to cover the labia (Fig. 8.3). The composition of the female condom may provide protection from and for the labial tissues, which are a common site for herpes simplex virus (HSV) and HPV infections. Female condoms also protect against other STIs, including HIV (Hatcher et al., 2004). They are available without a prescription.

Mechanism of Action and Effectiveness. Like male condoms, female condoms work by containing ejaculate during sexual intercourse. The smaller of the two polyurethane rings in the closed end of the condom should be inserted as deep as possible into the vagina, leaving the larger ring at the open end outside the vagina.

The female condom can be inserted up to 8 hours before intercourse; it must be left in place until after intercourse is completed. Reuse of the female condom is not recommended. The typical use failure rate is 21% (Hatcher et al., 2004).

Contraindications and Side Effects. The only contraindication to use of the female condom is difficulty with insertion, which may result from a woman's discomfort with touching herself or an inability to follow the instructions. Female condoms may produce noise during intercourse, which some clients find distracting or undesirable. They protect against STIs only with correct use. Some clients find the appearance of the female condom unusual; its use may be problematic for male partners who are not used to the appearance of this device.

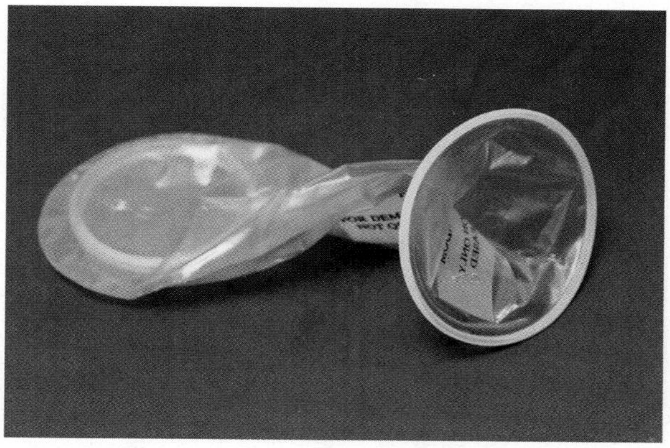

FIGURE 8.3 The female condom.

Client Teaching and Collaborative Interventions. Clients who choose the female condom need instruction about insertion, which can be challenging. The woman should compress and guide the condom into the vagina with the inner, small ring, until the outer ring rests against the vulva (Fig. 8.4). To avoid inserting the penis outside the condom, one partner should manually insert the penis into the vagina during sexual intercourse. Also, one partner should hold the outer ring in place during intercourse to prevent the condom from slipping into the vagina. The nurse should advise clients not to reuse female condoms. He or she also should instruct clients not to use male and female condoms together because the resultant friction may cause slippage.

Diaphragm

The **diaphragm** consists of a dome and flexible ring, which is sized from 50 to 100 mm (Fig. 8.5). Although most diaphragm domes are made of latex, one silicone model is available. Available types of rings include arching, flat spring, and coil spring, which are designed to fit variations in pelvic anatomies. Diaphragms are available only with a prescription. They must be used with spermicidal cream or jelly.

Mechanism of Action and Effectiveness. The diaphragm is placed into the vagina to cover the cervix so that sperm cannot enter there for fertilization. Use of spermicidal foam and jelly increases effectiveness. The typical use failure rate for diaphragms with spermicide ranges from 16% to 20% (Hatcher et al., 2004). Diaphragms may provide limited protection against STIs (Minnis & Padian, 2005).

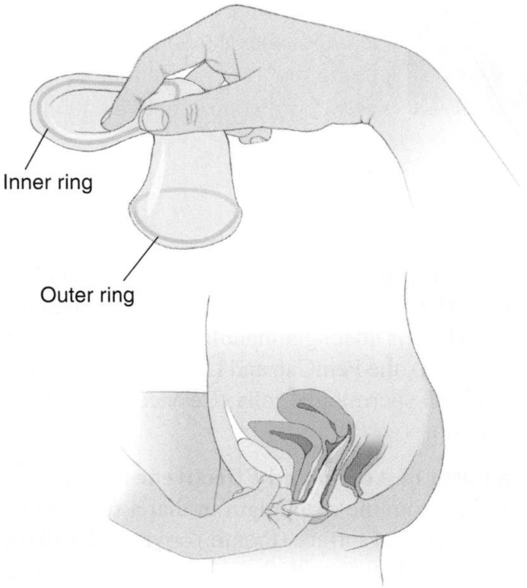

FIGURE 8.4 The client should compress and guide the inner ring of the female condom into the vagina, with the outer ring resting against the vulva.

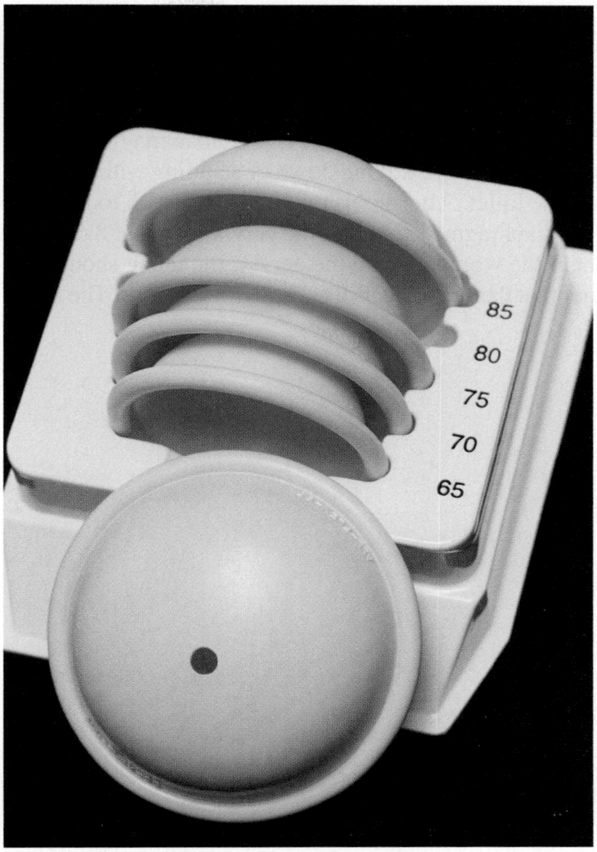

FIGURE 8.5 The diaphragm covers the cervix to prevent sperm from entering the female reproductive tract.

Contraindications and Side Effects. Women with a history of frequent urinary tract infections (UTIs) are not good candidates for diaphragms because their use increases risk for UTIs (Information from your family doctor, 2004). The increased risk may be related to compression of the diaphragm on the urethra or increased vaginal bacteria. Other contraindications include spermicidal allergy, latex allergy, and inability to insert and remove the device from the vagina. Clients should not use a diaphragm during menstruation; doing so increases the risk for toxic shock syndrome (Youngkin & Davis, 2004). Clients with latex allergy who wish to use a diaphragm may be candidates for a silicone diaphragm.

Client Teaching and Collaborative Interventions. Clients who choose diaphragms must be fitted for them by a health care provider to determine appropriate type and size. Before use, the client should hold the diaphragm dome side down while placing a tablespoon of spermicidal cream or jelly in the dome. She also should place additional spermicide around the ring. To correctly insert a diaphragm, the client should hold the diaphragm dome side down between the thumb and middle finger, squeeze the edges together, and place the diaphragm into the vagina (Fig. 8.6A). The diaphragm should fit snugly between the symphysis pubis and beneath the cervix, while covering the cervix and touching the lateral vaginal walls (Youngkin & Davis, 2004). The woman may find insertion easier if she is lying down or standing with one foot on the toilet. After insertion, she must check to feel that the diaphragm is covering the cervix (see Fig. 8.6B). To help the woman locate the cervix, the nurse should tell her that the cervix feels like the tip of the nose. The nurse should allow the client private time to practice inserting and removing the diaphragm.

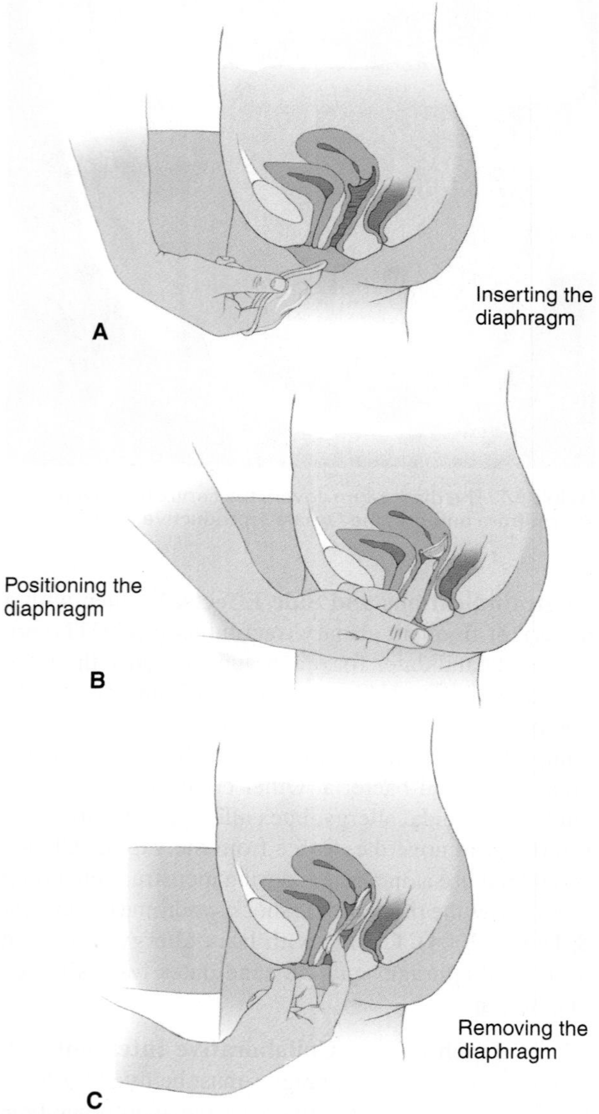

FIGURE 8.6 (**A**) To insert the diaphragm, the client holds the dome side down between thumb and middle finger. She squeezes together the edges and places the device into the vagina. (**B**) To check for correct insertion, the client reaches inside her vagina to feel for the cervix and make sure that the diaphragm is covering it. (**C**) For removal, the client hooks her finger above the diaphragm's ring and pulls it out.

The diaphragm should remain in place 6 to 8 hours after intercourse. The nurse should instruct the client not to douche after use and to wait 3 hours after removal for any douching. If intercourse is repeated, the woman should leave the diaphragm in place and insert additional spermicide into the vagina.

To remove the diaphragm, the client should hook a finger above the ring and pull it out (see Fig. 8.6C). After removal, the client should wash the diaphragm with mild soap and water only, dry it, and store it in the case. The nurse should advise against the use of any powders or oil-based lubricants with a diaphragm because these substances may weaken the integrity of the latex dome (Speroff & Darney, 2001).

Before each use, the client should verify that the diaphragm is intact by filling the dome with water and inspecting for leaks. Any leaks indicate the need for replacement of the diaphragm and use of an alternate method of contraception until the new diaphragm is ready and fitted. Regardless of whether the diaphragm is leaking, the client should replace the device every 2 years (Hatcher et al., 2004), and she should visit a health care provider for assessment of the fit of the diaphragm annually (Speroff & Darney, 2001). Additionally, after pregnancy or a weight change of 20% or more, the client needs to be refitted for proper size (Hatcher et al., 2004). Although weight change may not necessitate a new diaphragm size, such changes can contribute to alterations of the vaginal shape (Hatcher et al., 2004; Speroff & Darney, 2001).

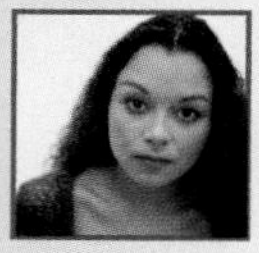

Veena described wanting to feel "more in control over avoiding pregnancy." Would a diaphragm be an appropriate contraceptive option for the nurse to suggest?

Cervical Cap

The **cervical cap** consists of a firm rubber cap with a rim sized to fit over the cervix (Fig. 8.7). Types include the Prentif (which is no longer manufactured but may still be in circulation), the FemCap and Lea's Shield. They must be used with spermicidal jelly. Cervical caps require a prescription.

Mechanism of Action and Effectiveness. The cervical cap differs from the diaphragm in that a seal forms between the cervical surface (Prentif) or vaginal wall (FemCap or Lea's Shield), with the rim of the cap holding the mechanism in place. The FemCap and Lea's Shield have a strap to assist with removal. Typical use failure rates range from 16% to 20% for nulliparous women and from

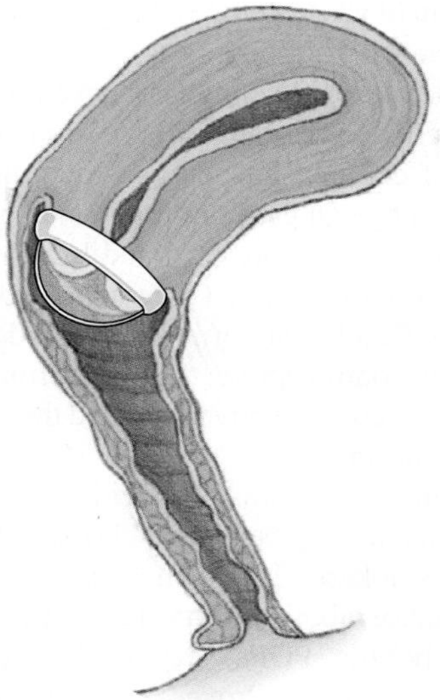

FIGURE 8.7 The rim-sized cervical cap fits over the cervix. It requires concomitant use of spermicide.

32% to 40% for multiparous women (Hatcher et al., 2004). The reason for such a high failure rate in multiparas is because pregnancy and childbirth cause the cervix to become softer and more pliable. This renders the cervical cap less capable of remaining in place.

Contraindications and Side Effects. Latex allergies (for Prentif and FemCap) and spermicide allergies, as well as an unevenly shaped cervix, are contraindications. Women who are uncomfortable with touching their bodies would not be good candidates for the cervical cap, which requires insertion and removal directly into and from the vagina.

Client Teaching and Collaborative Interventions. The prescription-only cervical cap must be fitted by a health care provider. For use of the Prentif cap, the client must fill one third of the Prentif cap with spermicidal jelly or cream. She then should insert the cap into the vagina over the cervix. After insertion, the client should gently try to dislodge the Prentif cap to ensure that the suction is intact; she should do this again after 1 minute.

With the FemCap, the client should place ¼ tsp of spermicide in the bowl, spread a thin layer of spermicide over the brim (except for where the finger and thumb are holding the brim), and put an additional ½ tsp of spermicide on the outside of the dome. She then should insert the cap into the vagina over the cervix. For repeated intercourse, the FemCap should remain in place, but additional spermicide should be added.

Before inserting the Lea's Shield, the bowl of the device is filled with spermicidal jelly, and the device is inserted into the vagina, strap down. No additional spermicide is necessary for repeated acts of intercourse.

Regardless of type, clients should not use the cap with any petroleum-based products in the vagina, which may weaken the device's structural integrity. The client should leave the cervical cap in place at least 6 hours (8 hours for the Lea's Shield) but no longer than 48 hours after intercourse. She should not use it during menstruation. Removal is by applying firm, pulling pressure on the rim or strap to break the suction. Following removal, the client should clean the cap with mild soap and water and dry it. The cervical cap does not protect against STIs. The FDA recommends that the woman have a follow-up Pap test after 3 months of use, then return to normal yearly screening (Hatcher et al., 2004).

Contraceptive Sponge

The **contraceptive sponge** fits over the woman's cervix and releases spermicide to prevent fertilization. This soft and concave over-the-counter device was reintroduced to the U.S. market in 2005 after several years' absence resulting from manufacturer malfunction. The previous problems have been fixed with the current device.

Mechanism of Action and Effectiveness. The sponge itself acts as a physical barrier between the cervix and sperm trying to penetrate it. It is made of polyurethane, which traps and absorbs semen. Finally, the sponge regularly releases spermicide built into the product over 24 hours. The typical use failure rate ranges from 14% to 28%, although these results are based primarily on the previously available sponge in the 1980s and early 1990s (Hatcher et al., 2004).

Contraindications and Side Effects. Women who are uncomfortable with touching their bodies are not good candidates for the sponge. The device may cause irritation or allergic reactions to spermicide. Finally, all users must be cautioned not to leave the device in place for more than 30 hours because doing so can increase the risk for toxic shock syndrome.

Client Teaching and Collaborative Interventions. The client can insert the sponge up to 24 hours before intercourse. She does not need to remove or replace it to engage in more than one act of intercourse. The client needs to wait 6 hours after the last act of intercourse before removing the sponge, but she should not leave the sponge in place for more than 30 hours.

To insert the sponge, the client should hold the unpackaged device in one hand with the "dimple" side up and make sure that the loop is dangling under the sponge. Then, the client needs to wet the sponge thoroughly with clean water, which will activate the spermicide. The client should squeeze the wet sponge gently until it becomes sudsy, but stop before she squeezes it dry. Next, the client should fold the sides upward until the sudsy sponge looks narrow and long, with the loop beneath dangling from one end of the fold to the other. The client should then point the folded end of the sponge toward the vagina for insertion, sliding the sponge into the vaginal opening as far as she can. Once the sponge is in place, the client should check to make sure that her cervix is not exposed and that she can still feel the string loop.

To remove the sponge, the client should wait at least 6 hours after the last act of intercourse. She should reach into the vagina with her finger to find the string loop. Then, the client should bear down and push the sponge toward the vaginal opening, while hooking the finger around the string loop or grasping the sponge between her thumb and forefinger.

Spermicidal Products

Spermicidal foam, cream, film, suppositories, and jelly are available over the counter. As already discussed, they are frequently used in conjunction with other barrier devices; diaphragms and cervical caps require their use for optimal effectiveness. The active ingredient in most spermicides is Nonoxynol-9.

Spermicides act as a barrier at the cervix and decrease sperm motility on contact. The typical use failure rate of spermicide alone is 29% (Hatcher et al., 2004). When used with other barrier contraceptive devices, effectiveness increases. Alone, spermicide does not protect against STIs.

Spermicide allergy is a contraindication for use. Symptoms may include genital irritation or burning. Clients may perceive the drainage of the foam or suppository from the vagina as messy or unappealing. When used during oral sex, partners may report an unpleasant taste.

The World Health Organization (WHO, 2006) recommends that women at high risk for contracting HIV not use spermicides, either alone or as part of another method, because spermicide has been found to increase transmission (Centers for Disease Control and Prevention, 2002; D'Cruz & Uckun, 2004; Stephenson, 2000). Studies also have shown that spermicide does not protect against gonorrhea or chlamydia (Roddy et al., 2002). Research is ongoing to develop effective *microbicides* to help protect against STIs, but to date no effective microbicide is available (WHO, 2006).

To allow enough time for the spermicide to dissolve and to coat the vagina, the client should insert film and suppositories at least 15 minutes, but not longer than 1 hour, before intercourse. Spermicidal foam is effective immediately after placement in the vagina. The couple should complete intercourse within 60 minutes of spermicidal insertion. For repeated acts of intercourse, they should use additional spermicide. The nurse instructs women using spermicide not to douche or bathe for at least 6 hours after intercourse.

Hormonal Methods

Hormonal methods of contraception have two variations. Combined methods use both estrogen and progestin (a synthetic form of progesterone). Progestin-only methods do not include any estrogen.

Combined hormonal methods have multiple mechanisms of action, including suppression of ovulation, thickening of cervical mucus, and thinning of the endometrium. They can cause multiple side effects; however, they also have short-term and long-term benefits unrelated to contraception (Freeman, 2002; Rager & Omar, 2005). Combined hormonal methods include the combined oral contraceptive, the transdermal contraceptive, the vaginal contraceptive ring, and the combined injectable contraceptive.

Progestin-only methods provide highly effective contraception and may be a good choice for breastfeeding women, smokers older than 35 years, and those at risk for thromboembolic events. These methods include progestin-only pills (POPs), depomedroxyprogesterone acetate (DMPA or Depo-Provera), and levonorgestrel injectables (the Norplant system). Mirena is an intrauterine system that combines the mechanisms of progestin with an intrauterine device (see Intrauterine Methods).

Combined Oral Contraceptives

QUOTE 8-1

"Can we imagine how well women would take their pills if they could use them to control when (and if) they menstruated? I think today would be a good day to find out."

Anita L. Nelson, "The Pill at 40—A New Look at a Familiar Method," Family Planning Perspectives, March 2000.

Combined oral contraceptives (COCs) rely on administration of estrogen and progestin to control fertility. Progestin provides the main mechanism for contraception (Speroff, Glass, & Kase, 1999), whereas estrogen stabilizes the endometrium to decrease breakthrough bleeding. Estrogen also increases the risk for thromboembolic events such as deep vein thrombosis (DVT), myocardial infarction (MI), and stroke (Speroff & Darney, 2001). For this reason, the estrogen content of COCs has dropped dramatically since their introduction. Whereas early oral contraceptives contained 100 to 150 μg of ethinyl estradiol, available brands today contain 20 to 50 μg.

Types. Various COCs are available by prescription, including triphasic (dosages of estrogen or progestin vary) and monophasic (dosages are constant). COCs come in 28-day packs, which include 21 active pills and 7 placebos, and 21-day packs, which contain only active pills (Fig. 8.8). Mircette provides 21 days of combined hormones, 2 days of placebos, and 5 days of 10-μg ethinyl estradiol.

A recently developed system combines ethinyl estradiol and levonorgestrel (*Seasonale*). This approach relies on 84 active pills and 7 placebo pills (Hatcher et al., 2004) for a 91-day treatment cycle, resulting in only four menstrual periods a year. Another mechanism by

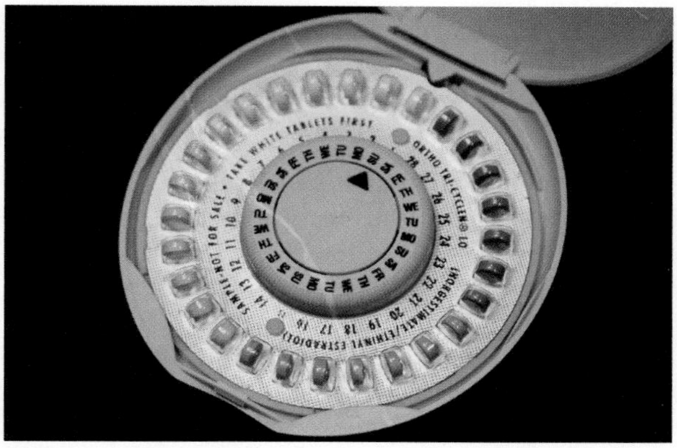

FIGURE 8.8 A sample pack of combined oral contraceptives.

which menstruation can be minimized to 4 times a year is for the health care provider to place the client on continuous COCs by instructing her to take three monophasic packs in a row without taking the placebo week, and then taking the active pills and the placebo pills of the fourth pack.

Mechanism of Action and Effectiveness. COCs prevent pregnancy primarily by suppressing ovulation, thickening cervical mucus, decreasing tubal motility, and thinning the endometrium. Suppression of the hypothalamus-pituitary-ovarian axis prevents ovulation because the exogenous hormones in COCs provide negative feedback to the hypothalamus' secretion of gonadotropin-releasing hormone (GnRH). This in turn suppresses pituitary secretion of follicle-stimulating hormone (FSH) and luteinizing hormone (LH). Without proper circulating levels of FSH and LH, the ovaries will not develop a follicle and release an egg.

Without follicular development and its accompanying surge in estrogen production, the cervical mucus fails to thin as normal before ovulation. As a result, penetration of the mucus by the sperm becomes difficult. Without normal FSH or LH stimulation, the thinner endometrial lining decreases the ability of a fertilized egg to implant. The thinner lining also leads to decreased menstrual flow for most women.

Combined oral contraceptives have a typical user failure rate ranging from 1% to 8% (Hatcher et al., 2004).

Contraindications and Side Effects. Women who wish to use COCs must be carefully screened for several contraindications, listed in Box 8.2. Users should not be pregnant, less than 3 weeks postpartum, or breastfeeding. Women older than 35 years who smoke are at increased risk for a thromboembolic event and therefore should not take COCs. A family history of DVT or clotting disorders also may present an increased risk for a thromboembolic event COCs (Hatcher et al., 2004).

In addition to an increased risk for DVT, stroke, and MI, users of COCs also incur a higher risk for cholelithiasis and hypertension (Hatcher et al., 2004). Women taking COCs with a family history of breast cancer have not been found to have an additional risk for breast cancer (Burkman et al., 2004; Collaborative Group on Hormonal Factors in Breast Cancer, 1996). Women with renal, kidney, or adrenal disease should not take Yasmin, a COC that contains a progestin derived from spironolactone (Archer, 2001). Spironolactone has antimineralocorticoid properties that may help clients with premenstrual symptoms, hypertension, and weight gain (Foidart, 2005; Krattenmacher, 2000).

BOX 8.2 Contraindications to Use of Combined Oral Contraceptives

- Migraines with neurologic symptoms
- Coronary artery disease or cerebral vascular disease
- Severe diabetes
- Hypertension
- Liver disease
- Breast or endometrial cancer
- Deep vein thrombosis
- Unexplained vaginal bleeding

Less serious side effects of COCs include breakthrough bleeding, breast tenderness, headaches, and nausea. Often, these side effects decrease after 1 to 2 months of use. Taking the pill in the evening or with food may help alleviate nausea. Some women gain weight while taking COCs, but average weight gain is no different from women taking placebos (Hatcher et al., 2004). There has been no demonstrated infertility following any length of COC use.

Potentially beneficial side effects include decreased acne; lighter and shorter menstrual flow, and thus a decreased risk for anemia; and decreased dysmenorrhea (Burkman et al., 2004). A reduced risk for endometrial and ovarian cancer has been documented in women taking COCs (Burkman et al., 2004; Grimes, 2001). In addition, women who use COCs are at lower risk for colorectal cancer (Beral et al., 1999), ovarian cysts, and benign breast disease (Hatcher et al., 2004).

Client Teaching and Collaborative Interventions. The nurse should instruct the client to start the COCs as prescribed, on either the first day of her menstrual period or the first Sunday within her menstrual period. The client should use a backup method of contraception for the first week. If the woman has been instructed to take COCs continuously (monophasic only), she will skip the placebo pills and start a new pack. Otherwise, she may expect a menstrual period during the placebo week. The nurse should encourage women to take the placebos to maintain the scheduled dosing and as a reminder to start a new package. Occasionally, women do not have a menstrual flow, which would indicate a test for pregnancy if they have missed or taken late any pills during that pack.

The client needs to take the pill at the same time each day, within 2 to 3 hours. Otherwise, she may experience breakthrough bleeding or pregnancy. For one missed or late pill, the nurse should instruct the client to take the pill as soon as she remembers and to use backup contraception for 7 days thereafter. If the missed pill was at the beginning of the pack, the health care provider may offer her emergency contraception (Hatcher et al., 2004) (discussed later in this chapter). The client may choose to take missed pills 12 hours apart to avoid nausea. For two missed pills, the woman should take a pill every 12 hours until her regimen is caught up, and be offered emergency contraception, again using a backup method for 1 week.

With three or more missed pills, the nurse should instruct the woman to contact her primary health care provider. She may be offered emergency contraception and counseled to use a backup method of contraception until her next menses, when she would start a new pack of pills. As with any restart, a week of backup contraception is advised.

Some antibiotics (tetracyclines) may decrease levels of circulating hormones. Thus, the nurse should advise the client using COCs who must take antibiotics to use a backup method of contraception during her antibiotic regimen and for 7 days after. Herbal preparations containing St. John's wort also may lead to decreased effectiveness (Redmond & Self, 2002) and require backup contraception with concomitant use.

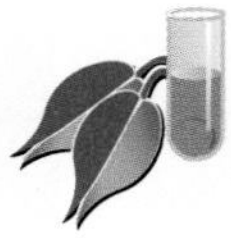

The nurse instructs women to monitor for dangerous side effects. A helpful pneumonic is ACHES (Box 8.3).

Women just starting or restarting COCs will be given 3 months of the pills and instructed to return to their health care providers before refills are needed for assessment of blood pressure and evaluation for side effects. See Teaching Tips 8.1.

Transdermal Contraceptive Patch

The transdermal contraceptive patch (Ortho Evra), introduced in 2002, provides an alternative delivery system of estrogen and progestin (Fig. 8.9). The woman applies the patch once a week; over those 7 days, 6 mg of progestin and 0.75 mg of ethinyl estradiol are released in a consistent amount each day. The patch may be placed on the buttocks, abdomen, or upper outer arm, but not on the breasts.

Mechanism of Action and Effectiveness. The mechanisms of action and effectiveness of the transdermal contraceptive are the same as for COCs. Data are currently unavailable on typical failure rates, but one study showed a lower failure rate with the patch than with COCs (Audet et al., 2001). Patch users have significantly better compliance (correct and consistent use) than pill users (Hatcher et al., 2004). Studies also have shown a slightly higher failure rate in women who weigh more than 198 lbs (Zieman et al., 2001). Although it is not understood why heavier women have more of a risk for pregnancy, theories include decreased absorption or decreased hormone levels resulting from increased blood volume (Does weight play a role, 2002).

Contraindications and Side Effects. Contraindications and side effects of COCs also apply to users of the transdermal contraceptive. In addition, users of the patch may experience skin reactions at the application site. Rotation of the application site is encouraged.

Client Teaching and Collaborative Interventions. Ortho Evra is prescribed in boxes of three transdermal patches. The nurse should instruct the client to start the patch on either the first day of the next menstrual period or the first Sunday within the next menstrual period. If she applies the patch within 5 days of the onset of menses, the woman needs no backup contraception. One week from the day of original application, the client should remove the patch and apply a new one. She will not apply a patch on the fourth week and will experience withdrawal bleeding (have a menstrual period). If the primary care provider prescribes a continuous patch regimen (9 weeks of continual dosing), she will start a new box every 3 weeks.

Studies have shown effective adhesiveness of the patch with showering and even daily swimming (Zacur et al., 2002). To promote adhesion, the nurse should instruct the client to press the patch firmly if it seems to be releasing from the skin. If the patch will not adhere, the client should remove the current patch and apply a new patch for the rest of that week.

If the woman applies the patch 1 to 2 days late, it remains effective. If she is more than 2 days late in applying a new patch, the nurse should instruct her to start a new package when her menstrual flow begins or the first Sunday within her next menstrual flow. The client should use backup contraception until she has applied the new patch, if used within the first 5 days of menses.

BOX 8.3 ACHES

- **A**bdominal pain (may indicate gallbladder disease)
- **C**hest pain (possibly indicating myocardial infarction)
- **H**eadaches that are severe (may indicate a stroke)
- **E**ye problems, such as blurred vision or changes in vision (possibly indicating a stroke)
- **S**evere leg pain (may indicate deep vein thrombosis)

TEACHING TIPS 8.1 Starting Oral Contraceptives

For a woman starting oral contraceptives for the first time, the nurse should review the following information carefully:

- *How to start:* Depending on the prescription, the woman may begin taking the first active hormone pill on the first day of menses or on the Sunday after menses begins. She may request to start on a Sunday because then her menstrual flow would occur only on weekdays. It is important for her to understand to start on the first Sunday of her menses (she may still be bleeding), not to wait for the Sunday after menses ends. Have a sample pack available so that the woman can see how to remove the pill from the packaging. Allow time for questions. Advise the client to use a backup method of contraception for the first week. Discuss alternatives for backup method; advise her to always have her choice available.
- *How to take the pill:* The woman needs to take the pill at the same time each day (within 2 to 3 hours). Ask her when she thinks she will take it: does she wake up or go to bed at a consistent time? If not, she may want to set a watch timer at, for example, noon to remind her. To help her remember to take the pill, she might choose to put the pack next to her toothbrush or something else that she uses every day (eg, deodorant). Counsel her regarding common side effects: nausea, breakthrough bleeding, and breast tenderness. If she experiences nausea, she can take the pill with food or at a different time of day (switching from morning to evening would constitute a late pill and necessitate backup for 7 days). Breakthrough bleeding is worse in smokers, which gives an additional incentive to quit smoking.
- *What to do if she misses pills:* For one missed or late pill, the client should take the pill as soon as she remembers and use backup contraception for 7 days thereafter. If the missed pill was at the beginning of the pack, the health care provider may offer her emergency contraception (Hatcher et al., 2004). The client may choose to take missed pills 12 hours apart to avoid nausea. For two missed pills, the woman should take a pill every 12 hours until she is caught up, and be offered emergency contraception, again using a backup method for 1 week. With three or more missed pills, the woman should contact her primary health care provider.
- Danger signs include abdominal pain, chest pain, headaches, eye problems (blurred or lost vision), and severe leg pain.

The nurse should counsel the client to monitor for ACHES (see Box 8.3). Women just starting or restarting use of the transdermal contraceptive should return to their health care provider after 3 months for assessment of blood pressure and evaluation for side effects.

The client should be careful not to apply the patch to any area on which she uses lotions, makeup, moisturizers, or creams. She also should avoid application to any red or irritated skin area, as well as to sites with open sores, abrasions, or cuts. If the skin at the application site becomes mildly irritated (a normal side effect), the client can remove the current application and apply a new patch to a new location.

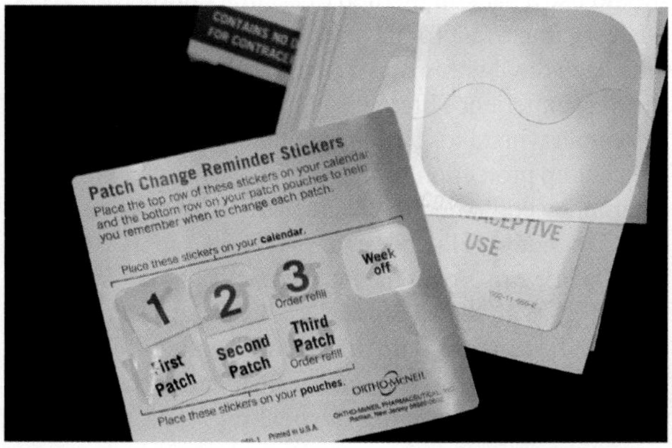

FIGURE 8.9 The client changes the transdermal contraceptive patch weekly. She can apply it to the arms, trunk, or buttocks, but not the breasts.

If a patch becomes loose, the client should remove it and replace it with a new one. She does not need additional contraception if she is certain that the patch has been detached for 24 hours or fewer. If the patch has been loose for more than 24 hours or if the client is unsure of how long it was detached from the skin, she should remove it and apply a new one. She also will need to begin a new 4-week cycle, with a new day 1 and a new day for changing the patch. For the first week of the new cycle, the woman needs to use backup contraception, such as a condom with spermicide.

A client who wants to discontinue use of the patch as part of her plans for conception should first discuss this situation with her health care provider. The provider should be able to guide the client in decision making involving the best timing for attempting pregnancy. He or she may recommend that the woman use nonhormonal contraception until her natural menstrual cycles are regularly established to better facilitate the dating of any pregnancy that ensues.

Vaginal Contraceptive Ring

The vaginal contraceptive ring (NuvaRing) was released in 2002. This 2-inch flexible ring contains estrogen and progestin, which are released slowly over 21 days (Fig. 8.10). The mechanism of action is suppression of ovulation. Effectiveness is similar to that of COCs (Stewart & Barnhart, 2002).

Contraindications for the vaginal contraceptive ring are the same as those for COCs (Hatcher et al., 2004). Some users may experience vaginitis or vaginal discharge (Veres et al., 2004). Women also may experience headache, nausea, weight gain, or breast pain. This device may not be acceptable to users who are not comfortable inserting and removing the ring from the vagina.

The nurse should instruct the client to compress the ring between two fingers and insert the ring up into the vagina. Clients may find insertion easier while standing with one leg up, squatting, or lying down. The woman should insert the ring during the first 5 days of her menstrual period. The nurse should teach her to use a backup method of contraception for the first 7 days. The woman should remove the ring after 3 weeks, which will result in withdrawal bleeding. After 7 ring-free days, the client should insert a new ring.

If the client leaves in a ring up to 35 days, she may remove it and insert a new ring after 7 days without concern for pregnancy. The nurse should advise that if the client leaves a ring in place for longer than 35 days, the client should use a backup method of contraception until she has a menses, when she may reinsert a new ring. She also should use a backup method for the first 7 days.

The nurse should advise the user not to remove the ring for intercourse; however, she can remove the ring for up to 3 hours without decreasing contraceptive efficacy. The nurse also should advise clients not to douche. The client may use any necessary vaginal medications.

In rare cases, the ring may be expelled spontaneously, related to intercourse, tampon removal, or constipation. An essential teaching item is for the nurse to remind the woman that she should always have an extra ring available in case the ring is lost. The woman and partner usually cannot feel the ring during intercourse. One study showed that the ring does not hinder sexual comfort for women or their partners (Novak et al., 2003).

The nurse should remind the woman using the vaginal contraceptive ring to monitor for ACHES (see Box 8.3). Women just starting or restarting the vaginal contraceptive ring require assessment of blood pressure and evaluation for side effects after 3 months of use (Hatcher et al., 2004).

FIGURE 8.10 The vaginal contraceptive ring releases estrogen and progestin slowly over 21 days to suppress ovulation.

Progestin-Only Pills

Progestin-only pills (POPs; also known as minipills) provide a continuous dose of progestin (no placebo pills). They prevent pregnancy primarily by thickening the cervical mucus; however, they also help prevent ovulation. Additionally, they inhibit implantation by thinning the endometrium. The typical use failure rate for POPs is 8%, but effectiveness approaches 100% in women who are exclusively breastfeeding infants (Hatcher et al., 2004).

Contraindications to POPs include unexplained vaginal bleeding, pregnancy, history of breast cancer, and liver disease. Gastrointestinal disease that interferes with absorption (active colitis), as well as use of certain medications (ie, rifampin, certain anticonvulsants, St. John's Wort, griseofulvin), also are contraindications because they increase hepatic clearance. It is unclear whether there is an interaction with orlistat (Xenical), a prescription weight-loss medication (Hatcher et al., 2004). Breakthrough bleeding is a common side effect in women taking POPs, as are amenorrhea, ovarian cysts, and headaches.

The nurse should instruct the client to begin her POPs as prescribed, on the first 5 days of menses, immediately postpartum, or after the 6-week postpartum examination if she has not resumed sexual relations. She should use a backup method of contraception for 7 days. It is very important for the user to take the pill at the same time each day, within 2 to 3 hours. If she takes a pill late, she may experience breakthrough bleeding or pregnancy. A woman who takes a pill more than 3 hours late should use backup protection for 2 days. She also may be offered emergency contraception if she has had intercourse in the past 3 to 5 days (Hatcher et al., 2004).

Debate exists over the interference of broad-spectrum antibiotics with the effectiveness of POPs (Hatcher et al., 2004). The nurse should advise women taking POPs to monitor for new or worsening headaches, changes in vision, or trouble moving or speaking.

Depo-Medroxyprogesterone Acetate (DMPA or Depo-Provera)

DMPA had been available internationally for 25 years; it was introduced in the United States in 1992. This in-

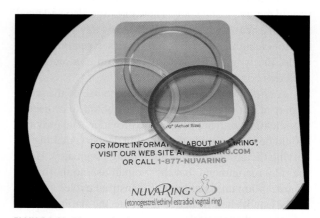

jectable progestin is given intramuscularly into the deltoid or gluteus maximus muscle every 11 to 13 weeks.

DMPA prevents pregnancy by suppressing ovulation, thickening the cervical mucus, thinning the endometrium, and slowing tubal motility. It has a typical use failure rate of 3% (Hatcher et al., 2004). Contraindications for use include pregnancy; unexplained vaginal bleeding; history of breast cancer, myocardial infarction, or stroke; current DVT; liver disease; and sensitivity to DMPA. A common side effect of DMPA is irregular bleeding; users also experience weight gain at an average of 5.4 lbs in the first year and 16.5 lbs after 5 years (Hatcher et al., 2004). Other side effects include amenorrhea, breast tenderness, headaches, tenderness at the injection site, hair loss, depression, and decreased libido (Hatcher et al., 2004). Additionally, women may experience amenorrhea for many months and nonovulatory cycles for more than 1 year after cessation of DMPA, with an average return to fertility 10 months after the last injection (Hatcher et al., 2004).

Women begin DMPA during the first 5 days of a menstrual period or immediately postpartum. Breastfeeding women may choose to wait 6 weeks until the milk supply is established because high doses of exogenous progesterone may interfere with the stimulus for milk synthesis (Hatcher et al., 2004). Women starting DMPA should use backup contraception for the first 7 days. The nurse should counsel women to expect irregular menstrual bleeding for the first year of use. The nurse should explain that amenorrhea is also likely and is not harmful, but that women should monitor for symptoms of pregnancy.

Women should return for their next injection in 11 to 13 weeks. It is helpful for the nurse to provide a calendar that lists the next visit (Freeman, 2004). If the next injection is scheduled at 12 weeks, this would provide a 1-week "grace period" if the woman misses her appointment. If a woman is more than 90 days past the last injection, the nurse may counsel her to return during her next menses to receive her next injection. Because of the length of time it may take for menses to resume, clinicians may choose to give an injection without a menses if they are certain the woman is not pregnant.

Long-term effects of DMPA on bone mineralization are uncertain; therefore, the nurse should advise the client to take appropriate levels of calcium (1,000 mg for women 18 years to menopause). Regular exercise will assist in maintaining bone density and preventing weight gain (see Chap. 2). The nurse also should offer DMPA users advice on healthy nutrition. To monitor for allergic reactions, the nurse may ask women to wait in the office for 20 minutes after injection. Women who experience heavy bleeding require screening for cervical infection, cancer, pregnancy, and anemia. Clinicians may advise the use of ibuprofen, 800 mg three times a day for 3 days, estrogen daily for 5 days, or the addition of COCs for 1 to 2 months to control bleeding (Hatcher et al., 2004). A woman considering pregnancy within 1 year may not be an ideal candidate for Depo-Provera because there is an average 10-month delay in return to fertility.

Progestin-only Implants

The levonorgestrel system (Norplant) is no longer marketed in the United States, and the etonogestrel system (Implanon) is to be released in 2006. Implanon is a single implant inserted under the skin on the medial aspect of the upper arm. The implant releases a continual dosage of the progestin, which is effective for 3 years. The mechanisms of actions include thickening cervical mucus, preventing ovulation and thinning the endometrium.

Contraindications are the same as for progestin-only pills, and side effects include menstrual changes (irregular bleeding and amenorrhea), headaches and acne. Advantages include use for women who have contraindications to estrogen use, and decreased menstrual pain. The typical use failure rate is less than 1% (Hatcher et al., 2005).

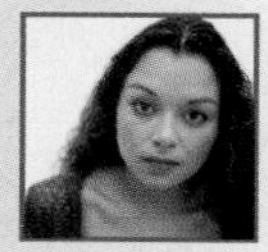

Veena, the 22-year-old woman seeking contraceptive options, verbalizes an interest in combined hormonal contraceptive methods, but states, "I'm terrible with remembering to take pills." What alternatives could the nurse suggest?

Intrauterine Methods

Intrauterine devices (IUDs) are plastic T-shaped objects inserted into the uterus for contraception (Fig. 8.11). Several models of IUDs were available in the 1970s until studies showed that certain types, including the Dalcon Shield, increased risks for uterine perforation and **pelvic inflammatory disease (PID).** Currently, two intrauterine contraceptives are available in the United States: the Paraguard T380A (the Copper T), which was first marketed in 1988; and the levonorgestrel intrauterine system (Mirena), which was introduced in 2000.

A physician, midwife, or nurse practitioner inserts the IUD during the woman's menses, midcycle, or immediately postpartum. Expulsion is least likely if insertion occurs at midcycle. The health care provider performs a bimanual examination and with a speculum in place (see Chap. 2). He or she then places the IUD contained inside an insertion tube into the uterine cavity and then withdraws the tube and the cuts the string to approximately 1 inch. The client may feel some discomfort or cramping during the procedure.

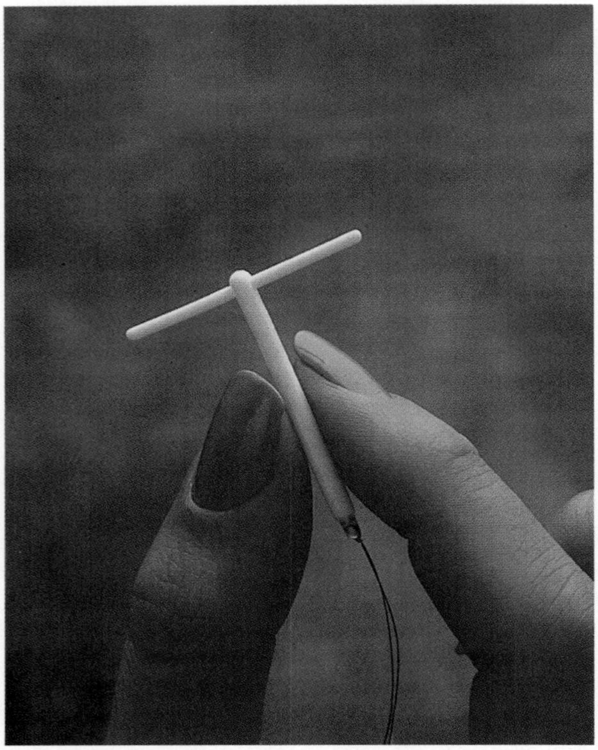

FIGURE 8.11 Intrauterine devices (IUDs) are inserted by a health care provider directly into the uterus.

Use of IUDs is not advised in nulliparous women. Management of pregnancy with an IUD in place varies depending on the circumstances.

Women should monitor for serious side effects with IUDs, using the pneumonic PAINS:

- **P**eriod late or abnormal spotting (indicating a possible pregnancy)
- **A**bdominal pain or pain with intercourse (indicating a possible infection)
- **I**nfection exposure (to any STI) or abnormal vaginal discharge (any new discharge or change in discharge)
- **N**ot feeling well, fever, chills
- **S**tring missing, longer or shorter

Women should check to ensure that the string is still in place after each menses. They also should check after insertion for any problems, because these devices come with a 3-month warranty. If the woman changes sexual partners, she should consider using latex condoms to protect against STIs.

Copper IUD

The copper IUD prevents fertilization by creating a hostile uterine environment in which copper ions inhibit sperm motility and an inflammatory endometrial process phagocytosizes the sperm. It provides 10 years of contraception with a 0.8% typical use failure rate (Hatcher et al., 2004). Use is appropriate for breastfeeding women.

Contraindications to the copper IUD include women who are not in a monogamous relationship (at risk for STIs), are HIV positive, are pregnant, or have undiagnosed vaginal bleeding, cervicitis, pelvic infection, recent endometritis, suspected uterine or cervical cancer, or an allergy to copper. Side effects of the copper IUD include increased menstrual flow and dysmenorrhea, anemia, risk for uterine perforation, and a vasovagal reaction with insertion or expulsion. For these reasons, women who normally experience heavy menstrual flow and dysmenorrhea are not good candidates for the copper IUD.

In most countries, the copper IUD is the most popular IUD. Its very low failure rate makes its effectiveness comparable to that of surgical sterilization.

Advantages to use of the copper IUD generally outweigh the risks for women who have never given birth and are younger than 20 years of age. These devices can be safely inserted at any point in the menstrual cycle, as long as the provider feels reasonably confident that the client is not pregnant.

Mirena

Mirena thickens the cervical mucus, impairs sperm migration, and alters the endometrium to prevent implantation. It also inhibits ovulation. Mirena provides 5 years of contraception and has a 0.1% typical use failure rate (Hatcher et al., 2004). Contraindications for the Mirena IUD are the same as for with the copper IUD (except allergy to copper), breast cancer, undiagnosed vaginal bleeding, and liver disease. Mirena users may experience irregular bleeding or amenorrhea, expulsion, uterine perforation (rare), ovarian cysts, headaches, or breast tenderness. They are at decreased risk for ectopic pregnancy and often have decreased flow and decreased dysmenorrhea. Mirena also may be used in the treatment of endometriosis, menorrhagia, or uterine fibroids.

Behavioral Methods

Some women, for personal or religious reasons, choose not to use devices or hormonal methods for contraception, but still wish to avoid pregnancy. Health care providers may instruct such clients about behavioral methods of controlling their pregnancy status.

Abstinence

Abstinence means not engaging in vaginal intercourse. Some people also include refraining from anal and oral sex as part of abstinence. Abstaining from vaginal intercourse is the most reliable method of contraception because it provides no opportunity for sperm to enter the woman's reproductive tract to fertilize an ovum. It also can help control the spread of many STIs.

Those who follow abstinence do so for various reasons. For some people, it coincides with religious or ethical beliefs. Others simply wish to take no chances of becoming pregnant. Abstinent clients may participate in other forms of sexual behavior that they consider "safe" or "acceptable." Examples include kissing, masturbation, sexual fantasy, and oral sex.

Fertility Awareness and Natural Family Planning

Fertility awareness methods (FAMs) of contraception focus on determining a woman's time of ovulation. Some FAMs rely on the use of barrier devices if a couple engages in vaginal intercourse during the fertile period. **Natural family planning** (NFP) relies on sex only during nonfertile periods and abstinence during the determined period of fertility. For both FAMs and NFP, clients may choose to follow the rhythm (calendar) method, the cervical mucus ovulation detection method, the symptothermal method, or the Standard Days method. All have a typical use failure rate of 25%.

Clients who choose NFP must be highly motivated to abstain from intercourse during the fertile days. They also must be capable of understanding the concept of fertile days and of tracking daily temperature. If using the cervical mucus ovulation detection or symptothermal method, the client must be comfortable with checking her cervical mucus. Breastfeeding, recent childbirth, or pregnancy loss may affect signs of fertility and thus make these methods harder to use. There are no side effects to FAMs (Fig. 8.12).

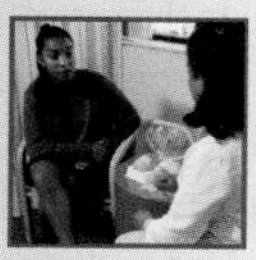

At the start of the chapter, you met Kenya, a 19-year-old seeking information about NFP. What assessment data are critical to ascertain when developing her teaching plan?

Rhythm (Calendar) Method. The rhythm or (calendar) method calls on the client to track the length of her menstrual cycles. The nurse should explain that ovulation takes place 12 to 16 days before the start of the next menstrual flow. The first day of the fertile time cannot be predicted with perfect accuracy but may be estimated by tracking six menstrual cycles and subtracting 18 from the shortest cycle (day 1 or first day of menses to day 1 or first day of next menses). The last day of the fertile period would be the longest cycle length minus 11. To prevent conception, the nurse should advise the client to use a barrier method or to abstain from intercourse on the first day of fertility through the last day of the fertile period. Thus, a woman with a longest cycle of 35 days

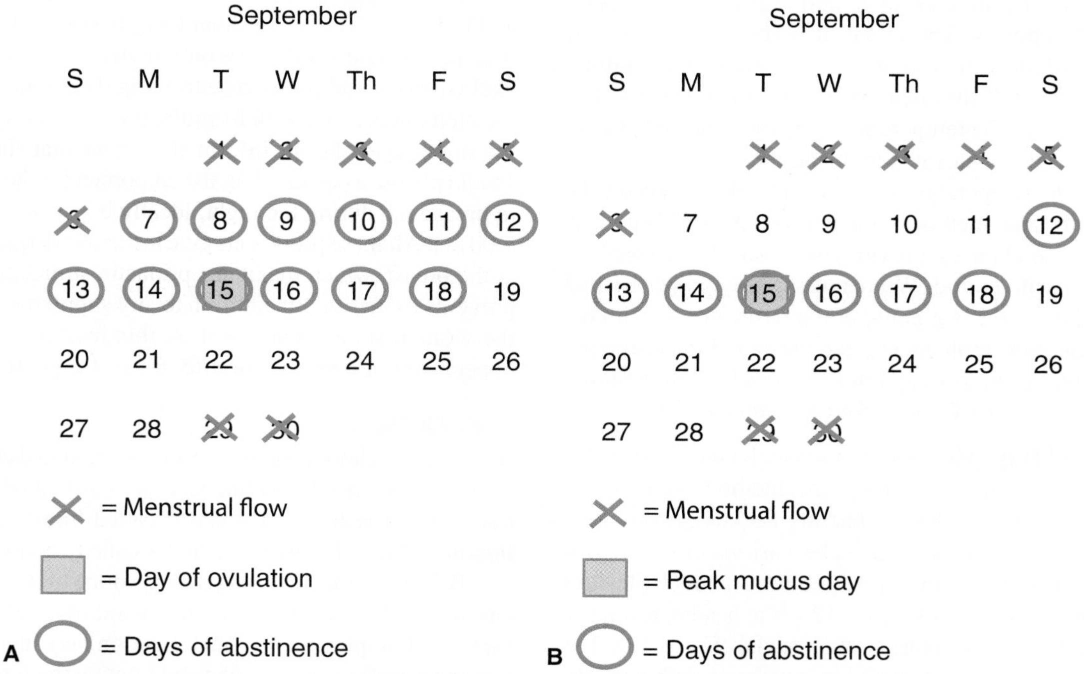

FIGURE 8.12 Sample logs kept by clients using (**A**) the calendar method and (**B**) the cervical mucus ovulation detection method. For both methods, the days circled in red indicate times when the client should abstain from intercourse or use a barrier method if engaging in intercourse to minimize chances of conception.

and a shortest cycle of 30 days would use a barrier method or abstain from day 12 (30 minus 18) to day 24 (35 minus 11). Women with irregular cycles cannot accurately predict ovulation; therefore, they are not good candidates for the calendar method.

Cervical Mucus Ovulation Detection Method. The nurse should teach clients who want to use this method about the changes in cervical mucus that occur around ovulation. At this time, a woman's vaginal discharge may become clear and stretchy (indicating fertile mucus). The nurse should teach the client to check at the introitus with her fingers or tissue paper for the appearance and character of mucus each morning for several months. Women must have abstained for 24 hours to make the test interpretable. To prevent pregnancy, clients should use a barrier method or abstain from intercourse at the first appearance of fertile mucus through the third day after the last appearance of fertile mucus.

Basal Body and Symptothermal Methods. The basal body temperature (BBT) method is based on the woman's temperature changes around the time of ovulation, with an approximate 0.5°F decrease before ovulation and a 0.4° to 0.8°F increase with ovulation. The client needs to take her temperature every day at approximately the same time, usually when she first awakens, and definitely before getting out of bed or eating, which may alter the temperature. Use of a digital or basal body thermometer is advisable. A basal body thermometer is specially calibrated with a smaller range and thus larger and easy-to-read numbers. The client also should document if she overslept or was ill, which may affect temperature. If tracking BBT, the client should abstain or use a barrier method when the temperature drops and through 3 consecutive days of elevated temperature.

As the temperature drop may not always occur, the symptothermal method, which combines BBT with cervical mucus changes, provides more accuracy in predicting the fertile period. Women using the symptothermal method mark the beginning of the fertile period with the appearance of fertile mucus and the end of the fertile period with the fourth day after an elevated temperature. See Nursing Care Plan 8.1 for more information.

Standard Days Method. Women with menstrual cycles that last 26 to 32 days can use this method, which relies on the use of cycle beads (fertility necklace) consisting of different colored beads. The various colors represent the first day of the cycle (red bead), nonfertile days (6 brown beads), fertile days (12 white beads), and more nonfertile days (13 more brown beads) (Fig. 8.13). The client moves a band forward by one bead each day, abstaining during the white beads, and moving the band to the red bead on the first day of the next menses (Arevalo, Jennings, & Sinai, 2002).

Withdrawal

Withdrawal, or *coitus interruptus,* is the removal of the penis from the vagina before ejaculation to prevent the introduction of sperm into the vagina. With a typical use failure rate of 27%, it has no contraindications or side effects (Hatcher et al., 2004). Nevertheless, the man must be able to predict ejaculation and to control the urge to remain in the vagina. Before intercourse, the man should urinate to remove any sperm that may be present from a previous ejaculation; before insertion, he should wipe the penis clean of any pre-ejaculatory fluid.

Lactational Amenorrhea Method (LAM)

The **lactational amenorrhea method** (LAM) is appropriate for breastfeeding mothers in the first 6 months after childbirth, provided that these women have no menstrual periods and that their infants are breastfeeding exclusively (see Chap. 21). The only contraindications other than the appearance of menses or supplementation with formula feeding include taking medications not recommended in breastfeeding and blood-borne infections that could be passed to the infant (eg, HIV).

LAM has no side effects; studies have shown that breastfeeding reduces the risk for breast cancer (Collaborative Group on Hormonal Factors in Breast Cancer, 2002) and facilitates postpartum weight loss (Hatcher et al., 2004). The typical use failure rate is 2% (Hatcher et al., 2004).

LAM suppresses ovulation because breastfeeding continually releases prolactin, which inhibits the FSH and LH cycle. The nurse should emphasize to the client that this method is effective only if she is breastfeeding exclusively. In addition to instructing the woman not to supplement nursing with formula, juice, water, or food, the nurse also should inform the client that the baby should not use a pacifier. It is also important for the mother to breastfeed during the night, ideally between 2:00 and 4:00 AM. All these provisions give the baby adequate time at the breast, which maintains prolactin stimulation and prevents ovulation. In addition to any supplementation, the woman should not count on this method after the appearance of a menses or after 6 months postpartum.

Surgical Methods

If a client has chosen not to have any or additional children, he or she may choose a permanent surgical method of contraception. The female method is called **bilateral tubal ligation** (BTL). The male method is called **vasectomy.**

Bilateral tubal ligation (BTL) is done under general anesthesia that, through one of several methods, interrupts the fallopian tubes. Tubal ligation may involve removing a section of each tube and ligating the remaining ends through clips, bands, or cautery (Fig. 8.14). A new approach involves the placement under hysteroscopy of a device consisting of two concentric metal coils into the

NURSING CARE PLAN 8.1

The Client Interested in Natural Family Planning

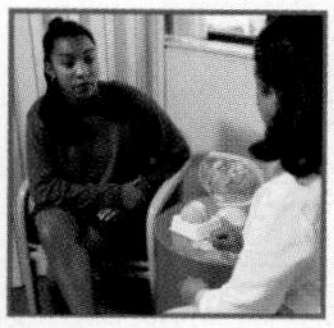

Recall Kenya from the beginning of this chapter. Assessment reveals menarche at age 12 years, with menstrual cycles every 30 to 31 days and lasting an average of 4 to 5 days. Kenya states, "Sometimes I get mild cramps on the first day, but then they disappear." She describes her flow as moderate with some small clots occasionally. "Darrell and I are hoping that we can use natural family planning. But neither of us is too sure what it involves."

NURSING DIAGNOSIS

Deficient Knowledge related to natural family planning (NFP) methods and their use

EXPECTED OUTCOMES

1. The client will identify methods for NFP.
2. The client will choose a contraceptive method of NFP that is realistic for her.

INTERVENTIONS	RATIONALES
Assess the client's level of understanding about NFP.	Assessment provides a baseline to identify specific client needs and to develop an individualized teaching plan.
Explore the client's exposure to NFP methods; correct any related misconceptions or myths; allow time for questions.	Information about exposure provides additional foundation for teaching and gives opportunities to clarify or correct misinformation.
Discuss with the client whether religious beliefs allow the use of a barrier method of contraception.	Further knowledge of religious beliefs helps guide appropriate suggestions for the couple. Fertility awareness methods may involve use of a barrier method.
Assess the client's level of comfort with touching her sexual organs and ability to do so.	Some NFP methods require obtaining a sample of cervical mucus from the vaginal area to determine fertility. Discomfort with doing so may prohibit use of such methods.
Teach the client about the various methods, including the mechanism of action, degree of effectiveness, advantages and disadvantages, and steps of use for each.	Information about each method provides a foundation from which the client can make an informed decision.
Encourage the client to bring her partner to the next visit to continue discussion of methods.	Participation from the client's partner provides support and enhances the chances for a successful experience.
Review menstrual cycle and ovulation; instruct client and partner in how to determine fertile period.	NFP methods rely on determining ovulation and fertile periods.
Assess the client's and partner's degree of motivation for abstaining from sexual intercourse during fertile days.	Couples choosing NFP methods must be highly motivated to abstain from intercourse during fertile periods.

Continued

NURSING CARE PLAN 8.1 ● The Client Interested in Natural Family Planning *(Continued)*

INTERVENTIONS	RATIONALES
Teach the client and partner how to use method correctly; have couple return demonstrate/verbalize steps; provide reinforcement and reinstruction as necessary.	Correct use of method enhances success.

EVALUATION

1. The client states the rationale for her choice of NFP method.
2. The client and partner verbalize steps for correct use of method chosen.
3. The client and partner state that they are comfortable with the method chosen.

fallopian tubes (Westhoff & Schnare, 2003). Failure rates vary from 0.8% to 3.7%, with younger women experiencing higher failure rates (Hatcher et al., 2004).

The client must sign a consent form 30 days before BTL. The procedure is not readily reversible; therefore, it is important to ascertain that the woman is sure in her decision. One study has shown regret after 14 years in 40% of women younger than 30 years having tubal sterilization (Hatcher et al., 2004). Research has shown that women who have had a BTL are at lower risk for ovarian cancer (Hankinson et al., 2002). The nurse also should counsel the woman regarding potential complications, including possible wound infection, bladder or vessel damage, hemorrhage, and death. Medicaid will not pay for BTL in women younger than 21 years.

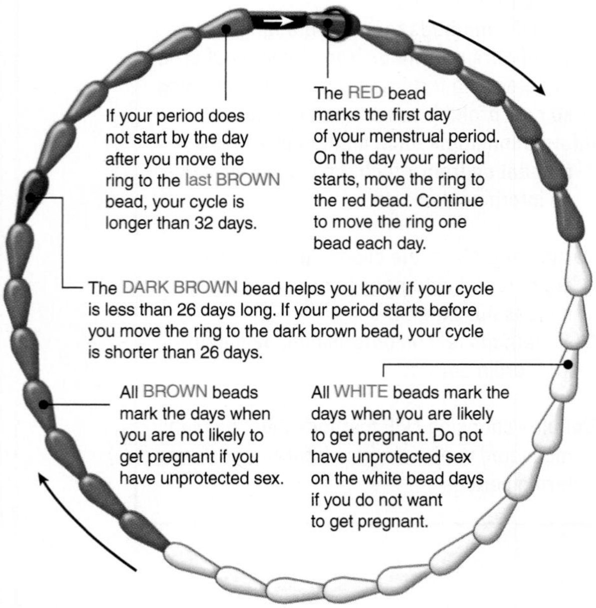

FIGURE 8.13 Fertility (cycle) beads can be used with the Standard Days method of fertility awareness.

Male sterilization, or vasectomy, involves ligation or cauterization of the vas deferens, which thus prevents delivery of sperm (Fig. 8.15). This procedure is safer than BTL and provides a typical use failure rate of 0.15% (Hatcher et al., 2004). Possible side effects include hematoma, bruising, wound infection, or adverse reaction to local anesthesia. The nurse should counsel men that vasectomy has not been shown to interfere with sexual function. Men should also return for two sperm counts of zero before depending on the vasectomy for contraception.

Both vasectomy and BTL are considered permanent. Even though vasectomy reversal is possible, the nurse should counsel men and their partners to consider this option carefully to prevent regret.

Emergency Contraception

Nurses should counsel all women at risk for unplanned pregnancy regarding *emergency contraception* in the event of rape or contraceptive failure (eg, condom breakage, missed pills, failure to use method). Previously called the "morning-after pill," this method has been renamed emergency contraception to reflect its effectiveness up to 72 hours after intercourse and the in-

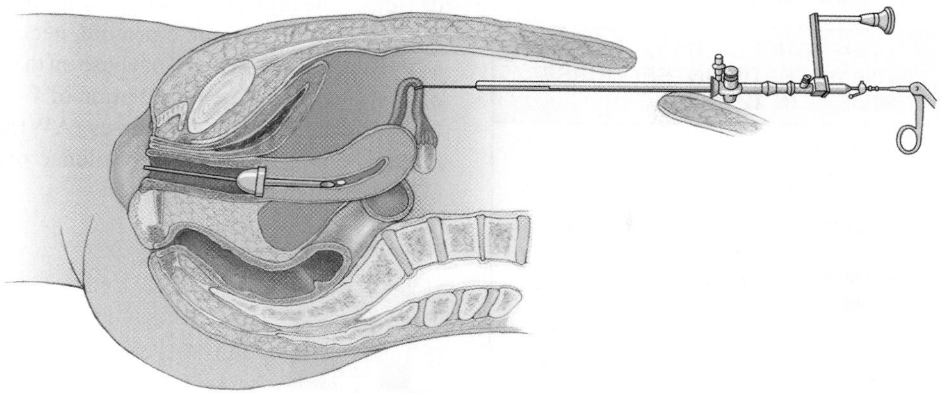

FIGURE 8.14 In tubal ligation, a section of each fallopian tube is removed, and the remaining ends are clipped, banded, or cauterized.

clusion of the copper IUD, which can be inserted up to 5 days after intercourse.

Emergency contraception prevents pregnancy through hormones that delay ovulation and may prevent implantation or thicken cervical mucus. Alternately, the mechanism of action by insertion of the copper IUD is prevention of implantation. Emergency contraception does not abort an established pregnancy. Emergency contraception with POPs or Plan B failed in only 1.1% of 967 women, whereas COCs have been found to have a 2% to 3% failure rate (Hatcher et al., 2004). Rates improve if the method is given in the first 24 hours after intercourse.

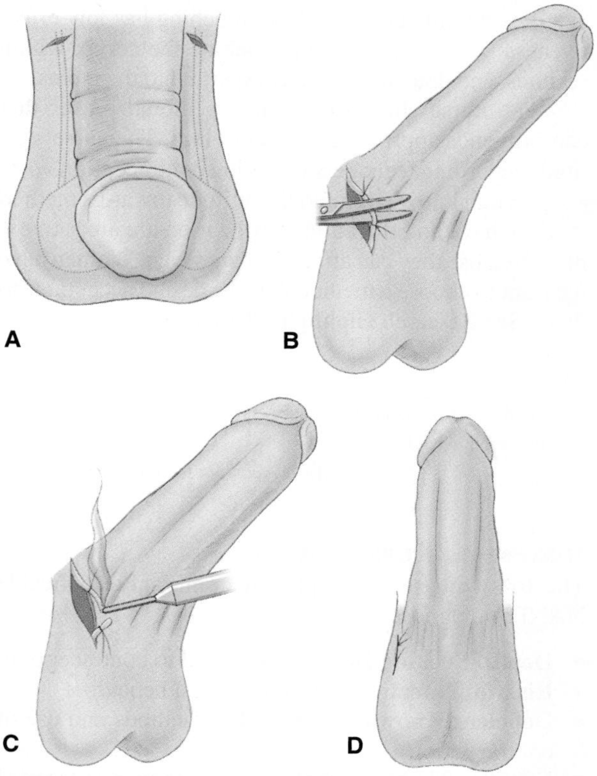

FIGURE 8.15 (**A**) Vasectomy involves ligation or cauterization of the vas deferens to prevent delivery of sperm. (**B**) The surgeon cuts through the vas deferens. (**C**) The ends of the vas deferens are cauterized and (**D**) sutured.

The only contraindication to use of emergency contraception with POPs or Plan B is a previously established pregnancy or undiagnosed vaginal bleeding. Also, women who should not use COCs for emergency contraception include those who have an acute migraine or have a history of deep venous thrombosis or pulmonary embolism. Side effects to the use of COCs include nausea and vomiting. Nausea and vomiting also may occur with POP or Plan B use. For side effects of the copper IUD, see Intrauterine Methods.

Women should be aware that emergency contraception is effective up to 72 hours after unprotected intercourse. The sooner it is provided, the more effective it is at preventing pregnancy. Some clinicians may choose to provide a prescription in advance in the event that it is needed; in some states, pharmacists are allowed to dispense Plan B.

After it is established that the woman is not pregnant through determination of recent menses or negative pregnancy test, the copper IUD may be inserted in appropriate candidates. Alternately, they should take both Plan B tablets (Hatcher et al., 2005), or the first dose of certain COCs or POPs (Table 8.2). The dose of COCs or POPs is repeated in 12 hours.

The nurse should counsel women to continue to use a method of contraception until their next menses. They may experience an early or delayed menses from delayed ovulation; counsel them to obtain a pregnancy test if no menses occurs in 2 to 3 weeks. Emergency contraception is not suitable as a continuous method of

● TABLE 8.2 Dosages of Emergency Contraception

BRAND	DOSE: TAKE UP TO 72 H AFTER UNPROTECTED INTERCOURSE, REPEAT IN 12 H
Plan B	1 white pill
Ovrette	20 yellow pills
PREVEN	2 light blue pills
Ovral	2 white pills
Lo/Ovral	4 white pills
Nordette	4 light orange pills
Tri-Levlen, Triphasil	4 light yellow pills

contraception; thus, counsel women on the use of other methods.

COLLABORATIVE CARE: THE CLIENT SEEKING FERTILITY CONTROL

Nurses who provide care about fertility control, family planning, and contraception to clients have an opportunity to teach important information and to assist with decision making. They are responsible for taking a detailed history, listening to each client's needs and concerns, and providing the detailed education and follow-up necessary for making practical choices and successfully using selected methods (Freeman, 2004).

Assessment

Assessment Tool 8.1 presents questions that can guide health history taking necessary for education about fertility control. Before initiating any teaching, the nurse should obtain the client's full medical and sexual history, as well as family history. Ascertaining the client's sexual orientation, desire for pregnancy or its prevention, and any beliefs that may influence decisions guides the encounter. The need for protection against STIs is an indication for use of condoms, perhaps in addition to other methods focusing primarily on avoiding pregnancy. The client also may choose abstinence or FAM/NFP, and nurses should be familiar with these methods.

Because of the intimate nature of the questions asked, it is imperative for nurses to provide a nonjudgmental atmosphere in which clients feel free to share. It helps to begin questioning with less threatening questions, including past medical history or menstrual history, and to normalize the situation by letting clients know that the nurse asks all women these questions (Fig. 8.16).

The nurse should not assume that a client is or is not sexually active, or that she has had freedom in her relationships to implement preferred contraceptive methods. For example, in some cases, sexual abuse precludes a woman from having control over the ability to use devices. Questions regarding history of abuse and current abuse help the nurse provide necessary referrals, as well as assess the effects of abuse on the chosen method of contraception. The Association of Women's Health, Obstetrical and Neonatal Nurses (AWHONN) advises that screening for domestic violence occur with each client encounter (see Chap. 5).

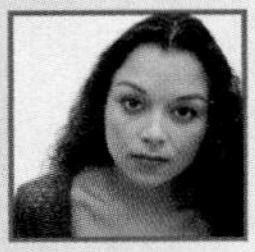

Think back to Veena, the 22-year-old from the beginning of the chapter who wants to explore options for contraception. What areas should the nurse address during assessment to assist Veena in making an informed choice?

Given that 49% of U.S. pregnancies are unintended (Henshaw, 1998), it is imperative that the nurse provides the information needed for successful use of the chosen method. The nurse must take time to listen to the woman and to ask questions about how she feels and what she knows about contraception. It is important to clear up any misinformation and misperceptions she may have received from the media, peers, or others. For example, one urban legend is that douching with Coca-Cola after intercourse can prevent pregnancy. In fact, douching has low effectiveness because sperm can penetrate the cervix within seconds, and douching can push sperm into the uterus.

The nurse should recognize personal biases that can influence approaches to counseling. The nurse's attitude regarding teenagers receiving contraception without parental knowledge and the attitude toward a method that can have an effect after fertilization are areas to explore because they can affect the care given. Women have the right to choose a method that is safe and acceptable to them. See Research Highlights 8.1 and 8.2.

QUOTE 8-2

"It is hard to know what to choose. Everyone seems to have a different view about what is best."

An 18-year-old sexually active woman.

Select Potential Nursing Diagnoses

The following are examples of commonly applicable NANDA diagnoses:

- **Health-Seeking Behaviors** related to contraception
- **Risk for Infection** related to sexual behaviors
- **Deficient Knowledge** related to methods and use of contraception
- **Effective Therapeutic Regimen Management** related to method of contraception
- **Ineffective Therapeutic Regimen Management** related to noncompliance, inability to use method of contraception, or side effects of method

ASSESSMENT TOOL 8.1 Fertility Control and Planning

MENSTRUAL HISTORY

- How old were you when you had your first period?
- What day did your last menstrual period start?
- Was it a normal period?
- What was the first day of your previous menstrual period?
- How often do you have a menstrual period?
- How many days are there from the first day of one menstrual period to the first day of the next period?
- How many days do you bleed?
- Do you have cramping with your periods? If so, what do you take for them?

FAMILY, MEDICAL, AND OBSTETRIC HISTORY

- Has anyone in your family ever had a heart attack or stroke? If so, at what age?
- Has anyone in your family ever had breast cancer?
- Has anyone in your family ever had a blood clot or clotting disorder?
- Have you ever had the following:
  - A blood clot?
  - A heart attack?
  - A stroke?
  - High blood pressure?
  - Migraine headaches? If so, do you have any visual changes (blurred vision, seeing spots) or changes in sensation (numbness or tingling in your hands or feet) with these headaches?
- Have you ever had cancer? Where?
- Have you had any unexplained vaginal bleeding?
- Do you have a clotting disorder?
- Do you have varicose veins?
- Have you ever had a urinary tract infection? If so, how many have you had?
- Are you allergic to any medications? To latex? To spermicides?
- Have you ever had a sexually transmitted infection (STI)?
  - Gonorrhea
  - Chlamydia
  - Syphilis
  - Herpes
  - Genital warts
  - Trichomoniasis
- Have you ever had pelvic inflammatory disease (PID?)
- Have you ever been pregnant? If so, what were the outcomes (live birth, abortion, miscarriage)?
- Do you have plans to become pregnant? If so, when?

SEXUAL HISTORY

- Have you ever had sexual intercourse? (vaginal/anal/oral)
- What do you do to protect yourself from HIV or other infections? What do you do that may be putting you at risk for HIV or other infections?
- How many partners have you had in your lifetime?
- How many partners do you have now? How many have you had in the last 3 to 6 months?
- Are your partners male or female or both?
- Do you ever use alcohol or drugs in connection with sexual activity? Do you ever exchange sex for drugs, shelter, or money?
- Have you ever been forced to have sex?
- Do you enjoy sex? Do you have orgasms? Do you or your partner have any questions or concerns about sex?
- When was the last time you had vaginal intercourse?
- (If partner is male):
  - Did you use anything to prevent pregnancy?
  - Are you seeking to become pregnant at this time?
  - How often do you have vaginal intercourse?

ABUSE SCREEN

- Are you afraid of your partner or someone important to you?
- Within the last year, have you been hit, slapped, kicked, or otherwise physically hurt by anyone? By whom? How often?
- Are you in a relationship where you are treated badly?
- Have you been forced to engage in sexual activities? If yes, by whom? How many times?

SOCIAL/CONTRACEPTIVE HISTORY

- Do you smoke or chew tobacco?
- Do you have any cultural or religious beliefs that influence your view of birth control (eg, a belief that prohibits any contraception except abstinence, or a belief that prohibits use of contraception with a mechanism that prevents implantation of the fertilized egg).
- What birth control methods (e.g., birth control pill, Depo-Provera, condoms), if any, have you used before? Did you like or dislike the methods (if any)? Did you have any problems with those methods?
- What methods of birth control are you considering?
- What is important to you in a birth control method?
- Do you have any concerns or questions about birth control?

Planning and Intervention

Methods of planning and intervention relate directly to the method chosen. Specific measures are discussed under Client Teaching and Collaborative Interventions for each contraceptive choice. NIC/NOC Box 8.1 outlines common interventions and desired outcomes when working with clients on issues related to fertility control and contraception.

After obtaining a client history, the nurse can present available methods and proceed to focus counseling on ap-

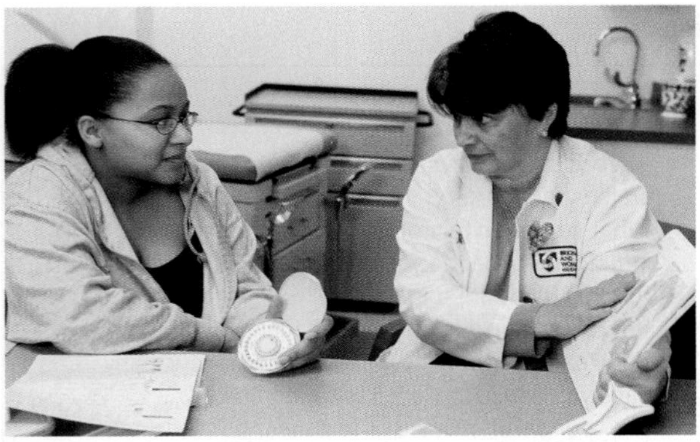

FIGURE 8.16 As with all issues related to sexuality, the nurse shows sensitivity and shapes the interaction according to the client's comfort level and responses when discussing family planning, contraception, and prevention of sexually transmitted infections.

propriate or desired methods. Factors that influence method choice include medical contraindications, cost, tolerability of side effects, ability to use method, partner involvement, individual values, cultural background, and plans for future fertility (Hatcher et al., 2004; Youngkin & Davis, 2004). For example, partner involvement is integral for the use of the male condom and for NFP.

After offering the woman the methods of contraception that she desires and that are safe for her, the nurse should clarify proper use of the methods. It also is suggested that the nurse counsel the woman regarding emergency contraception and ensure that the woman has decided on a backup method of contraception. Written information is valuable to reinforce teaching, much of which may be new to the woman. It also helps to have a sample of the method, such as a condom, diaphragm, or pill pack. See Nursing Care Plan 8.2 for more information.

Evaluation

The woman should be able to call the nurse for information in the event of a question or problem. After the woman has used a method for 3 months, it is helpful to schedule a follow-up appointment to assess for side effects and danger signs, and provide further teaching if necessary. The nurse should verify correct use at each follow-up visit as well. If side effects are present, the nurse provides teaching on how to deal with side effects. If the side effects are dangerous, the nurse alerts the clinician immediately.

Questions to Ponder

1. A 16-year-old female client presents for an annual examination. She is currently sexually active with male partners and uses no method of contraception, but states that she is not interested in pregnancy at this time. After you discuss the available methods of contraception, she is unsure if she wants to use any method because she does not want to experience any potential side effects.
   - Why do you think this teenager may be hesitant about using contraception?
   - What attitudes on your part could interfere with providing care to this woman?
   - How could you assist this teenager to make a good decision?

● RESEARCH HIGHLIGHT 8.1 Nurses' Description and Evaluation of Reproductive Health Counseling for Adolescent Females.

PURPOSE: The goal was to identify ways for nurses to provide useful counseling about reproductive health to teenage females.

DESIGN: Researchers interviewed five nurses with expertise in family planning with adolescents.

RESULTS: The nurses supported the appropriateness of adult reproductive health counseling for teens and expressed frustration regarding the unused potential of expert nurses in this area. Strategies to improve care for adolescent females include fostering critical thinking because teens are concrete thinkers who have difficulty with future-oriented thinking; including the significant other in the reproductive health care visit; and monitoring for cues that may suggest a nonconsensual nature of sexual activity. To maximize the effectiveness of this type of care, the expert nurses stressed the importance of allowing adequate time for a comprehensive assessment, especially given the high incidence of sexual abuse and vulnerability to STIs for this age group. They also indicated the value of taking time to listen to teens not only to obtain information but also to promote self-esteem, which is critical to reducing risky behavior. They emphasized strategies to reduce risks for STIs, including discussions of abstinence.

Other plans identified to improve care include consistency of caregiver to develop the client's trust and self-esteem, the creation of clinics designed specifically for adolescents, the presentation of alternatives to sexual intercourse, and problem-solving in stressful situations, as well as literature and videos to reinforce new behaviors.

Lambke, M. R., & Kavenaugh, K. (1999). Nurses' description and evaluation of reproductive health counseling for adolescent females. *Health Care for Women International, 20*(2), 147–162.

● RESEARCH HIGHLIGHT 8.2 Why Are Teens Still Getting Pregnant Despite Contraceptive Options?

PURPOSE: The goal was to heighten knowledge about trends in teen pregnancy and to better target pregnancy prevention programs.

DESIGN: Fourteen focus groups consisting of 65 male and female students were convened at schools and community agencies in both rural and urban areas.

RESULTS: Teens cited peer pressure, pressure from male partners, and the desire to fit in as reasons for having sex. They noted the influential role that older siblings and the media play in legitimizing sexual activity. Other identified themes included difficulty communicating with adults and accessing programs. Teens named clinics as their first choice for information. They expressed a desire for more information on how to practice safer sex, as well as prevention counseling and treatment.

These teens felt that confidentiality from health care professionals is essential, including within the clinic, as well as in terms of parents, partners, and school administrators. They also voiced a desire for dialogues about choices, not lectures on abstinence. They listed low-cost or free services as important, in addition to the availability of peer counselors working in the clinic. These findings provide suggestions for contraceptive care, including the importance of providing information nonjudgmentally and respectfully, carefully guarding confidentiality, and seeking ways to make care more accessible. They also suggest that any programs addressing teen sexuality should involve teens themselves in their planning and implementation.

Kendig, S., & Omvig, K. (2001). Why are teens still getting pregnant despite contraceptive options? *Contemporary Nurse Practitioner, Spring/Summer*, 10–13, 16–20.

2. A 24-year-old woman states that although she desires to prevent transmission of STIs, her male partner will not agree to use a condom. He claims that he "does not have a disease."
   - How can you support the client in her situation?
   - What are some suggestions you can give her to negotiate the use of condoms?
   - What are her alternatives to prevent STIs?

NIC/NOC Box 8.1 Contraceptive Education

Common NIC Labels
- Anticipatory Guidance
- Behavior Management: Sexual
- Behavior Modification
- Family Planning: Contraception
- Health Education
- Health Screening
- Impulse Control Training
- Learning Facilitation
- Self-Responsibility Facilitation
- Sexual Counseling
- Teaching: Safe Sex
- Teaching: Sexuality
- Values Clarification

Common NOC Labels
- Decision Making
- Knowledge: Conception Prevention
- Knowledge: Sexual Functioning
- Risk Control: Sexually Transmitted Diseases
- Risk Control: Unintended Pregnancy
- Self-Esteem
- Sexual Functioning

SUMMARY

- Throughout history, humans have sought to control fertility. Options have increased with time; several devices have emerged since the first oral hormonal contraceptive in 1960.
- Most contraceptive methods depend on and are controlled by the female. Additional male-oriented contraceptive devices are undergoing research, but political and social forces limit interest in and funding for further development.
- Barrier devices of contraception include male and female condoms, diaphragm, cervical cap, contraceptive sponge, and spermicide. These mechanisms work by providing physical blocks between sperm and the woman's reproductive tract. Male and female condoms have the additional benefit of helping to prevent STIs.
- Hormonal methods of contraception can be based on medications that combine delivery of progestin and estrogen, or that use progestin only. The various types of medications work to suppress ovulation, thin the endometrium, and thicken cervical mucus to create an environment inhospitable for fertilization.
- Combined methods of hormonal contraception include combined oral contraceptives, the transdermal contraceptive patch, the combined injectable contraceptive (Lunelle), and the vaginal ring.
- Progestin-only methods of hormonal contraception include progestin-only pills, Depo-Provera injections, and Norplant.
- Intrauterine devices are inserted into the woman's uterus by a primary care provider. They release copper or hormones that create an environment hostile to sperm and fertilization.

NURSING CARE PLAN 8.2

A Client Seeking Information About Contraceptives

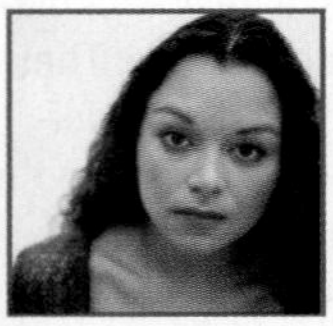

Recall Veena, 26 years old, who is exploring options for contraception. Veena's health history indicates no major medical problems, including no STIs. Her weight is appropriate for her height, and her menstrual cycle is normal (every 29 days), with occasional cramping.

NURSING DIAGNOSIS

Health-Seeking Behaviors related to contraceptive alternatives

EXPECTED OUTCOME

The client will verbalize that she understands various contraceptive alternatives, how they work, and their benefits and risks.

INTERVENTIONS	RATIONALES
Take measures to protect the client's privacy and to facilitate a relaxed atmosphere of trust. Close the door or curtain to the examination area. Minimize distractions. Assure the client that information provided will be kept confidential.	A client who feels comfortable and accepted and that the nurse is maintaining privacy is more likely to be frank about concerns related to sexuality and reproduction.
Discuss the mechanisms of action, use, reliability, costs, and side effects of different contraceptive methods.	Accurate information facilitates the client's decision making about the best choice for her needs.

EVALUATION

1. The client expresses understanding of the methods discussed.
2. The client verbalizes interest in three methods discussed with the nurse.

NURSING DIAGNOSIS

Decisional Conflict related to contraceptive alternatives

EXPECTED OUTCOME

The client will choose one of the methods identified by the follow-up appointment in 4 weeks.

INTERVENTIONS	RATIONALES
Discuss the client's lifestyle and how the three possibilities she identified interact with her circumstances.	Assessing the client's circumstances may help the nurse and client further narrow the choices. For example, if the client has a poor memory or a very busy schedule, oral

Continued

NURSING CARE PLAN 8.2 ● A Client Seeking Information About Contraceptives

INTERVENTIONS	RATIONALES
	contraceptives (which she needs to take at the same time every day for maximum effectiveness) may not be the best choice. If she is uncomfortable touching herself, a diaphragm may be unsuitable.
Continue to discuss the mechanisms of action, use, reliability, costs, and any side effects of the three potential options. Explore those factors that seem most important to the client (eg, finances, possible physical effects).	Additional information should help the client further narrow her options. Understanding her priorities may give clues about which factors are most important in determining the best choice.
Provide brochures and other information about the three options for the client to read at home.	The client may feel less pressured to decide and may be able to think more clearly with additional time; having backup information available at home can assist her as she chooses.
Review and discuss the ongoing need for safer sex practices (see Chap. 6).	The client is making a contraceptive choice based on a desire to avoid pregnancy; however, many contraceptives do not protect against STIs. The client still will need to use condoms to protect against STIs.
Reinforce the necessity of ongoing follow-up care, regardless of the actual method chosen.	Ongoing health maintenance will be essential to evaluate the client's compliance and satisfaction with the chosen method. It also will be necessary to protect against any related problems or complications.

EVALUATION

1. The client verbalizes that she will think about and read the information provided in the next few weeks.
2. The client schedules a follow-up appointment.
3. The client chooses to use a diaphragm and returns to the clinic at the follow-up appointment for appropriate instruction and related care.

- Behavioral methods include abstinence, fertility awareness, withdrawal, and lactational amenorrhea. These approaches require different types of behavior control and abilities on the part of users to prevent pregnancy.
- Surgical methods include bilateral tubal ligation for women and vasectomy for men. These permanent forms of sterilization are appropriate only for those clients who are definite about their decisions to have no or no more children.
- Emergency contraception is available for women up to 72 hours after unprotected intercourse. Options include POPs, COCs, and the insertion of an IUD. All women at risk for unintended pregnancy should be counseled on emergency contraception and how to obtain it if needed.
- Nurses providing teaching and interventions for fertility control and contraception should obtain the client's complete health history, including past medical history, family history, menstrual history, and sexual history to provide appropriate assistance.
- For each contraceptive device or approach, the nurse should understand and be familiar with its mechanism of action, advantages, disadvantages, side effects, contraindications, and effectiveness to provide adequate guidance for clients.

REVIEW QUESTIONS

1. A 28-year-old client comes to the physician's office to explore various methods of birth control. Upon reviewing the client's history, which of the following should the nurse identify as a contraindication for COCs?
   A. Fibrocystic breast changes
   B. Deep vein thrombosis
   C. Smoking
   D. Irritable bowel syndrome
2. A client calls the clinic and says that she had sex without birth control recently and wants to use emergency contraception. In preparing a response, the nurse should include that the latest time emergency contraception can be used effectively is
   A. 12 hours after unprotected intercourse.
   B. 24 hours after unprotected intercourse.
   C. 48 hours after unprotected intercourse.
   D. 72 hours after unprotected intercourse.
3. The nurse is teaching a client who has begun using COCs about problems to report immediately and advises the client to remember the acronym ACHES. The nurse knows that teaching has been effective when the client reports that ACHES stands for
   A. Abnormal periods, Chest pain, Headaches—severe, Eye problems—blurred or changes in vision, Severe leg pain.
   B. Abnormal periods, Clotting with periods, Headaches—severe, Eye problems—blurred or changes in vision, Severe leg pain.
   C. Abdominal pain, Chest pain, Hair loss, Eye problems—blurred or changes in vision, Severe leg pain.
   D. Abdominal pain, Chest pain, Headaches—severe, Eye problems—blurred or changes in vision, Severe leg pain.
4. The nurse is teaching a couple about correct condom use. Which of the following statements if made by the man indicates that he needs more instruction?
   A. "I'll be sure to put on the condom before making any contact with my partner's genitals."
   B. "I will make sure that when I am wearing the condom, it is tight against the glans of my penis."
   C. "To remove the condom, I'll slide it down while holding the top and pulling the tip, with my penis still erect."
   D. "I will make sure that we use a brand new condom every time we engage in sexual activity."
5. The nurse is caring for a client who reports using spermicide as her regular method of contraception. Which statement, if made by the client, should indicate to the nurse that further education is needed?
   A. "Spermicides protect against HIV."
   B. "Spermicide is a method the woman controls."
   C. "Spermicide can be inserted 15 minutes before sex."
   D. "Spermicides are available without a prescription."
6. The nurse is preparing a teaching plan on noncontraceptive benefits of COCs. Which of the following should not be included in the teaching plan?
   A. Protection against breast cancer
   B. Decreased acne
   C. Prevention of HIV
   D. Decreased dysmenorrhea
7. A client is just starting Depo-Provera injections. The nurse is preparing to schedule a follow-up appointment for her. The most optimal appointment time would be in
   A. 3 months.
   B. 4 months.
   C. 6 months.
   D. 12 months.
8. A client in her last trimester of pregnancy who intends to breastfeed her baby asks the nurse which contraceptive options will be available to her. Which of the following responses from the nurse is most correct?
   A. Lactational amenorrhea method, progestin-only pills, Depo-Provera
   B. Combined oral contraceptives, copper IUD, progestin-only pills
   C. Copper IUD, vaginal contraceptive ring, diaphragm
   D. Condoms, spermicides, contraceptive patch
9. When teaching a client about the correct use of a diaphragm for contraception, the nurse should make the following statement:
   A. "You must remember to remove the diaphragm immediately after intercourse."
   B. "You should not use your diaphragm while you are menstruating."
   C. "Remove the diaphragm to add spermicide when you have sex more than once at a time."
   D. "You will need to replace your diaphragm every 5 years."
10. The nurse is assisting a client with placement of the transdermal contraceptive. Which alternative sites can the nurse and client choose for placement?
    A. On the client's abdomen or buttocks
    B. On the client's abdomen, buttocks, or upper arm
    C. On the client's abdomen, buttocks, or upper torso
    D. On the client's buttocks only

REFERENCES

Archer, D. (2001). Evaluation of a new oral contraceptive progestogen, drospirenone with ethinyl estradiol (Yasmin). *Contraceptive Technology Update, 22*(Suppl. 9), 1–4.

Arevalo, M., Jennings, V., & Sinai, I. (2002). The Standard Days method: A new method of family planning (research notes). *Sexual Health Exchange, 2002*(2), 6–8.

Audet, M. C., Moreau, M., Koltun, W. D., Waldbaum, A. S., Shangold, G., Fisher, A. C., Creasy, G. W., for the Ortho Evra/Evra 004

Study Group. (2001). Evaluation of contraceptive efficacy and cycle control of a transdermal contraceptive patch vs. an oral contraceptive: A randomized control trial. *Journal of the American Medical Association, 285*(18), 2347–2354.

Beral, V., Hermon, C., Kay, C., Hannaford, P., Darby, S., & Reeves, G. (1999). Mortality associated with oral contraceptive use: 25 Year follow-up cohort of 46,000 women from Royal College of General Practitioners' oral contraceptive study. *British Medical Journal, 318*(7176), 96–100.

Bullough, V. L., & Bullough, B. (1994). A brief history of population control and contraception (Symposium: Overpopulation & Contraception). *Free Inquiry, 14*(2), 16–23.

Burkman, R., Schlesselman, J. J., & Zieman, M. (2004). Safety concerns and health benefits associated with oral contraception. *American Journal of Obstetrics and Gynecology, 190*(S4), S5–S22.

Centers for Disease Control and Prevention. (2002). Nonoxynol-9 spermicide contraception use: United States, 1999. *Journal of the American Medical Association, 287*(9), 2938–2940.

Collaborative Group on Hormonal Factors in Breast Cancer. (1996). Breast cancer and hormonal contraceptives: Collaborative reanalysis of individual data on 53,297 women with breast cancer and 100,239 women without breast cancer from epidemiological studies. *Lancet, 347*(9017), 1713–1727.

Collaborative Group on Hormonal Factors in Breast Cancer, & Beral, V. (2002). Breast cancer and breastfeeding: Collaborative reanalysis of individual data from 47 epidemiological studies in 30 countries, including 50,302 women with breast cancer and 96,973 women without the disease. *Lancet, 360*(9328), 187–195.

Dailard, Cynthia. (2003). Understanding 'Abstinence': Implications for Individuals, Programs and Policies. *The Guttmacher Report on Public Policy, 6*(5), 4–6.

D'Cruz, O. J., & Uckun, F. M. (2004). Clinical development of microbicides for the prevention of HIV infection. *Current Pharmaceutical Design, 10*(3), 315–336.

Does weight play a role in effectiveness (of Ortho Evra contraceptive patch)? (2002). *Contraceptive Technology Update, 23*(7), 81–83.

Foidart, J. M. (2005). Added benefits of drospirenone for compliance. *Climacteric, 8*(S3), 28–34.

Freeman, S. (2002). The continuing evolution of oral contraceptives. *Women's Health Care: A Practical Journal for Nurse Practitioners, 1*(5), 8–15.

Freeman, S. (2004). Nondaily hormonal contraception: Considerations in contraceptive choice and patient counseling. *Journal of the American Academy of Nurse Practitioners, 16*(6), 226–238.

Green, S. (1971). *The curious history of contraception.* New York: St. Martin's Press.

Grimes, D. A. (2001). Health benefits of oral contraception: Update on endometrial cancer prevention. *Contraception Report, 12*(3), 4–7.

Grimes, D. A., & Wallach, M. (Eds.) (1997). Modern contraception updates from The Contraception Report. NJ: Emron.

Hankinson, S. E., Hunter, D. J., Colditz, G. A., Willett, W. C., Stampfer, M. J., Rosner, B., et al. (2002). *A pocket guide for managing contraception.* GA: Bridging the Gap Foundation.

Hatcher, R. A., Trussell, J., Stewart, F., Cates, W., Stewart, G., Guest, F., & Kowal, D. (2004). *Contraceptive technology* (18th ed.). New York: Artent Media.

Hatcher, R. A., Zieman, M. et al. (2005). *A Pocket Guide to Managing Contraception.* Tiger, Georgia: Bridging the Gap Foundation.

Hennekens, C. H., & Speizer, F. E. (1993). Tubal ligation, hysterectomy and risk of ovarian cancer: A prospective study. *Journal of the American Medical Association, 270*(23), 2813–2818.

Henshaw, S. (1998). Unintended pregnancy in the United States. *Family Planning Perspectives, 30*(1), 24–29.

Himes, N. E. (1970). *Medical history of contraception.* New York: Schocker Books.

Hutti, M. (2003). New & emerging contraceptive methods. *AWHONN Lifelines, 7*(1), 33–39.

Information from your family doctor. Birth control using a diaphragm. (2004). *American Family Physician, 69*(1), 103.

Kaeser, L. (1990). Contraceptive development: Why the snail's pace? *Family Planning Perspectives, 22*(3), 131–133.

Kaunitz, A. M., Garceau, R. J., Cromie, M. A., & the Lunelle Study Group. (1999). Comparative safety, efficacy & cycle control of Lunelle™ monthly contraceptive injection (medroxyprogesterone acetate/estradiol expionate injectable suspension) and Ortho Novum 777 oral contraceptive (norethindrone/ethinyl estradiol triphasic). *Contraception, 60*(4), 179–187.

Kendig, S., & Omvig, K. (2001). Why are teens still getting pregnant despite contraceptive options? *Contemporary Nurse Practitioner, Spring/Summer,* 10–13, 16–20.

Krattenmach, R. (2000). Drospirenone: Pharmacology and pharmacokinetics of a unique progestogen. *Contraception, 62*(1), 29–38.

Kreinin, T. (2002). New approaches to contraception are needed (from the President). *SEICUS Report, 31*(2), 3.

Lambke, M. R., & Kavenaugh, K. (1999). Nurses' description and evaluation of reproductive health counseling for adolescent females. *Health Care for Women International, 20*(2), 147–162.

Lyttle, C. R., & Kopf, G. S. (2003). Status and future direction of male contraceptive development. *Current Opinion in Pharmacology, 3*(6), 667–671.

Minnis, A. M., & Padian, N. S. (2005). Effectiveness of female controlled barrier methods in preventing sexually transmitted infections and HIV: Current evidence and future research directions. *Sexually Transmitted Infections, 81*(3), 193–200.

Nelson, A. L. (2000). The pill at 40: A new look at a familiar method. *Family Planning Perspectives, 32*(2), 89–90.

Novak, A., de la Logeb, C., Abtezc, L., & van der Muelen, E. (2003). The combined contraceptive vaginal ring, NuvaRing®: An international study of user acceptability. *Contraception, 67*(3), 187–194.

Rager, K. M., & Omar, H. A. (2005). Hormonal contraception: Noncontraceptive benefits and medical contraindications. *Adolescent Medical Clinics, 16*(3), 539–551.

Rahimy, M., Cromie, M., Hopkins, N., & Tong, D. (1999). Lunelle monthly contraceptive injection (medroxyprogesterone acetate and estradiol cypionate injectable suspension): Effects of body weight and injection site on pharmacokinetics. *Contraception, 60*(4), 201–208.

Reaves, N. D. (2002). Unresolved issues in contraceptive health policy. *Health Care of Women International, 23*(8), 854–860.

Redmond, A., & Self, T. (2002). Oral contraceptives and drugs that compromise their efficacy. *Journal of Critical Illness, 17*(8), 306–308.

Roddy, R., Zekang, L., Ryan L., Tamoufe, U., & Tweedy, K. (2002). Effect of nonoxynol-9 gel on urogenital gonorrhea and chlamydia infection: A randomized control trial. *Journal of the American Medical Association, 287*(9), 1117–1121.

Schenker, J., & Fabenou, V. (1993). Family planning: Cultural and religious perspectives. *Human Reproduction, 8*(6), 969–976.

Speroff, L., & Darney, P. (2001). *A clinical guide for contraception.* Philadelphia: Lippincott Williams & Wilkins.

Speroff, L., Glass, R. H., & Kase, N. G. (1999). *Clinical gynecologic endocrinology and infertility* (6th ed.). Philadelphia: Lippincott Williams & Wilkins.

Stephenson, J. (2000). Widely used spermicide may increase, not decrease, risk of HIV transmission. *Journal of the American Medical Association, 284*(8), 949.

Stewart, F. H., & Barnhart, K. T. (2002). The vaginal contraceptive ring: Efficacy, cautions and frustrations. *Contraceptive Technology Reports, 23*(2), SSSI–SSS9.

Veres, S., Miller, L., & Burington, B. (2004). A comparison between the vaginal ring and oral contraceptives. *Obstetrics and Gynecology, 104*(3), 555–563.

Waites, G. M. (2003). Development of methods of male contraception: Impact of the World Health Organization Task Force. *Fertility and Sterility, 80*(1), 1–15.

Walsh, T. L., Frezieres, R. G., Peacock, K., Nelson, A. L., Clark, V. A., Bernstein, L., & Westoff, C., & Schnare, S. M. (2003). Male and female sterilization: An update. *Dialogues in Contraception, 7*(8), 5–7.

World Health Organization. (2006). Microbicides. Retrieved February 21, 2006, from http://www.who.int/hiv/topics/microbicides/microbicides/en/.

Wraxall, B. G. (2004). Effectiveness of the male latex condom: Combined results for three popular condom brands used as controls in randomized clinical trials. *Contraception, 70*(5), 407–413.

Youngkin, E. Q., & Davis, M. S. (2004). *Women's health: A primary care clinical guide* (3rd ed.). Stamford, CT: Appleton & Lange.

Zacur, H., Hedon, B., Mansour, D., Shangold, G., Fisher, A., & Creasy, G. (2002) Integrated summary of Ortho Evra™/Evra™ contraceptive patch adhesion in varied climates and conditions. *Fertility and Sterility, 77*(2), 32–35.

Zieman, M., Guillebaud, J., Weisberg, E., Shangold, G. A., Fisher A. C., & Creasy, G. W. (2001). Integrated summary of contraceptive efficacy with the Ortho Evra transdermal system. *Fertility and Sterility, 76*(3), S19.

RESOURCES

www.contraceptiononline.org/contrareport
www.managingcontraception.com
www.ippf.org
www.plannedparenthood.org
www.arhp.org (Association of Reproductive Health Professionals)
www.4women.gov (National Women's Health Information Center)
www.sexualityandu.ca
www.seicus.org (Education)
www.not-2-late.com (Emergency contraception information and providers)
www.advocatesforyouth.org (Adolescent Reproductive health)
www.familyplanning.net (NFP)
www.ccli.org (NFP)
California Association of Natural Family Planning
1217 Tyler St.
Salinas, CA 93906
(877) 332-2637
www.canfp.org (Natural Family Planning)
National Center for Women's Health, Pope Paul VI Institute
6901 Mercy Road
Omaha, NE 68104-2604
(402) 390-6600
www.popepaulvi.com (Natural Family Planning)

CHAPTER 9

Voluntary Pregnancy Termination

Judith Lewis

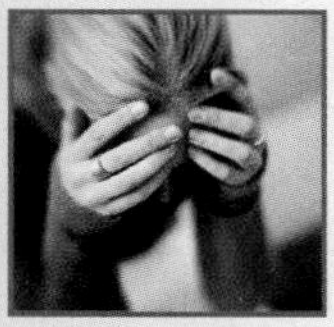

Patti, a single 24-year-old client with a 3-year-old daughter, comes to the physician's office for a checkup. She says that she's been very tired, nauseous, and just "not feeling herself." Examination reveals that Patti is 9 weeks pregnant. The client is shocked by the news and cries inconsolably. She states, "Another baby? What will I do?"

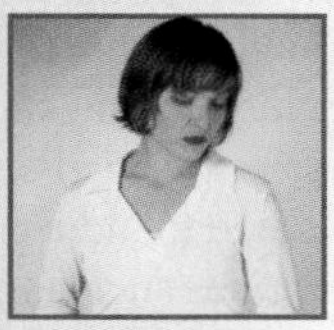

Gina, 44 years old, is recovering from an abortion she underwent after an amniocentesis at 16 weeks' gestation revealed severe congenital abnormalities in the fetus. During a follow-up discussion with the nurse, Gina, visibly exhausted, states, "This is the hardest decision I ever had to make."

You will learn more about Patti's and Gina's stories later in this chapter. Nurses working with such clients need to understand the material in this chapter to manage care and address issues appropriately. Before beginning, consider the following points related to the above scenarios:

- What is your initial reaction to the circumstances presented in each case? Do you have different responses to each client for any reason? Explain your answer.
- How might each client's particular situation influence the nurse's approach to care?
- How are the clients similar? Different?
- What other details should the nurse investigate with Patti? What about with Gina?
- What measures can the nurse take to approach the topics involved with sensitivity and adequate information?

LEARNING OBJECTIVES

On completion of this chapter, the reader should be able to:

- Discuss the historical perspective of pregnancy termination.
- Describe the current legal and social context of voluntary pregnancy termination in the United States and Canada.
- Identify religious, ethical, and social considerations related to elective abortion.
- Explain various procedures used in abortion.
- Outline nursing care considerations for clients who have terminated their pregnancies.

KEY TERMS

abortion
laminaria tents
viability

Abortion may be defined as the termination of pregnancy before the fetus reaches the age of **viability,** or the point at which vital organs are able to support life independently outside the uterus. In most cases, the age of viability is considered the end of the second trimester, or 24 weeks' gestation. Viability is a medical, not a legal, term; the point of viability varies for each pregnancy and is determined by physicians on a case-by-case basis. Pregnancy terminations that occur spontaneously are discussed in Chapters 13 and 16. This chapter focuses on voluntary termination of pregnancy.

Nurses often are in positions to provide information to pregnant women about options available to them, and to inform them of appropriate resources. Understanding the health-related, social, and legal issues associated with pregnancy termination will help nurses provide suitable care for their clients.

HISTORICAL PERSPECTIVES

Evidence has shown that human beings have attempted to control family size throughout history (Riddle, 1992). During some periods and in various locations, people desired large families with many children. During others, the preferred family size was smaller. Ways of controlling family size included abstinence, primitive contraception (see Chap. 8), and voluntary abortion. Although abortion has been practiced for centuries, it has been used considerably less frequently than contraception in limiting family size. Throughout history, preventing pregnancy has been more socially desirable than terminating pregnancy (Riddle, 1992).

Ancient Times

Abortion has been available and used to control childbirth since the earliest days of recorded history. It is mentioned in the Hippocratic Oath (Box 9.1). Scholars disagree about the actual intent of the statement in the Oath (Riddle, 1992). There also is considerable evidence that the proscription was not practiced widely.

In ancient times, women who wanted to induce abortion tried to do so by performing exercises such as carrying heavy loads, jumping, walking, and horseback riding. They also ingested diuretics and laxatives and took sitz baths with poultices containing various materials (eg, old olive oil, iris oil, ox bile, linseed). Another means of inducing abortion included inserting vaginal suppositories composed of agents such as myrtle and wallflower.

Middle Ages and Beyond

During the Middle Ages, knowledge of antifertility measures existed in classical texts, but it is unclear how much of this information the average citizen would have known or been able to obtain. Church fathers spoke against the use of contraception and abortion. The dearth of information about abortion and contraception in medieval sources leads one to believe that these topics were not safe to discuss. Medieval writings contain a great deal of material about herbal remedies but usually do not mention their abortifacient qualities.

During the 17th and 18th centuries, traditional knowledge regarding abortion continued to decline. The passage of the Ellenborough Act of 1803 made abortion illegal for subjects of the British Crown. This development marked the beginning of the criminalization of

BOX 9.1 The Hippocratic Oath

I swear by Apollo Physician and Asclepius and Hygieia and Panaceia and all the gods and goddesses, making them my witnesses, that I will fulfill according to my ability and judgment this oath and this covenant:

To hold him who has taught me this art as equal to my parents and to live my life in partnership with him, and if he is in need of money to give him a share of mine, and to regard his offspring as equal to my brothers in male lineage and to teach them this art—if they desire to learn it—without fee and covenant; to give a share of precepts and oral instruction and all the other learning to my sons and to the sons of him who has instructed me and to pupils who have signed the covenant and have taken an oath according to the medical law, but to no one else.

I will apply dietetic measures for the benefit of the sick according to my ability and judgment; I will keep them from harm and injustice.

I will neither give a deadly drug to anybody if asked for it, nor will I make a suggestion to this effect. Similarly I will not give to a woman an abortive remedy. In purity and holiness I will guard my life and my art.

I will not use the knife, not even on sufferers from stone, but will withdraw in favor of such men as are engaged in this work.

Whatever houses I may visit, I will come for the benefit of the sick, remaining free of all intentional injustice, of all mischief and in particular of sexual relations with both female and male persons, be they free or slaves.

What I may see or hear in the course of the treatment or even outside of the treatment in regard to the life of men, which on no account one must spread abroad, I will keep to myself holding such things shameful to be spoken about.

If I fulfill this oath and do not violate it, may it be granted to me to enjoy life and art, being honored with fame among all men for all time to come; if I transgress it and swear falsely, may the opposite of all this be my lot.

(Edelstein, 1967)

From Edelstein, L. (1967). The Hippocratic Oath: Text, translation and interpretation. In: O. Temkin & C. L. Temkin (Eds.), *Ancient Medicine: Selected papers of Ludwig Edelstein* (pp. 3–64). Baltimore: Johns Hopkins University Press.

abortion. Dr. Pascoe of Cornwall, England, was convicted in 1852 for administering oil of savin to a woman who had aborted. Such convictions made physicians reluctant to become involved with matters concerning abortion.

Modern Changes

In the 1960s, the women's movement and the availability of oral contraceptives encouraged many women to expect and to demand control over their reproductive capacity. Although abortion was an option in the 1960s, a woman first had to have a three-physician panel certify that continuing the pregnancy was detrimental to her physical or emotional health. As a result, access to such services varied widely. Often those women who lacked financial or personal resources were denied needed procedures, whereas affluent or "well-connected" women had little difficulty obtaining access to abortion services.

Many women without access to safe, aseptic, physician-performed abortions resorted to contacting people who performed abortions in unclean and unsafe conditions. Women who sought so-called back-alley abortions or attempted to self-induce abortions often experienced significant morbidity and mortality resulting from infection, hemorrhage, or other complications (Boston Women's Health Book Collective, 2005). Many of these procedures injured women so greatly as to jeopardize or ruin their future reproductive capacity. There are anecdotal accounts of these activities, but as a result of the shame and secrecy surrounding these procedures, reliable data do not exist. *If These Walls Could Talk* (1996), a video depicting the struggles faced by women experiencing unintended pregnancies in 1952, 1974, and 1996, presents a powerful portrayal of the dangers that women seeking to terminate their pregnancies faced before abortion services became legal.

RELIGIOUS PERSPECTIVES

In 1869, Pope Pius IX put forth the position of the Roman Catholic Church on *ensoulment,* or the moment at which a soul takes on the characteristics of personhood. Pius IX asserted that ensoulment occurs at the moment of conception and that any termination of pregnancy was not permitted. In the Catholic view, the conceptus has the same moral standing as any other soul; therefore, the fetus's right to life is equal to the mother's. There is no concept of being able to select the well-being of one soul over another. Catholics believe that the Pope's word is considered absolute because he is God's emissary on earth. Church doctrine specifies that followers cannot question a Papal decree.

Other Christian religions have roots in Catholicism but differ from it in many ways, including the acceptance of Papal decree on the view of abortion. There are a wide variety of perspectives on the acceptability of abortion among Protestant denominations. Generally speaking, fundamentalist denominations are more vociferous in their objections to abortion than are other Christian faiths.

QUOTE 9-1

"I believe abortion is a sad and undesirable choice. But I also question the morality of bringing children into this world that won't be supported, taken care of, or loved in the way they need to be to thrive. And I also don't feel comfortable judging another woman's actions in those circumstances."

A 34-year-old Catholic woman struggling with her views on abortion

Judaism regards the conceptus as water up to 40 days after conception. Jews view the fetus as part of the woman's body from 40 days' after conception until the point that the presenting part is delivered. Lewis (2003a; 2003b) discusses the status of abortion in Jewish law. Although Judaism has a strong pro-life bias, the life and health of the woman are of prime importance. This religion permits, or even encourages, abortion when continuing a pregnancy would endanger the woman's life or affect her physical or emotional health adversely (Schenker, 2000). Abortion on demand would be acceptable for the first 40 days of pregnancy; after that, Jews would treat the fetus as any other part of a woman's body. Judaism believes that the human body is to be treated with great respect, so would not be in favor of damaging or mutilating a healthy body part. Therefore, Judaism would not be in favor of abortion on demand after 40 days gestation, although the concept of adversely affecting a woman's physical or emotional health is often interpreted quite liberally.

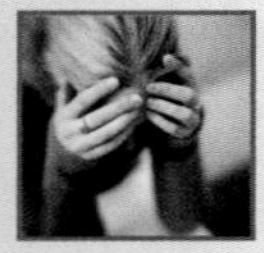

Remember Patti, the client from the beginning of the chapter who just found out she is at 9 weeks' gestation with an unplanned pregnancy. Suppose Patti's history reveals that she is Jewish. How might this influence the nurse's approach with her?

In Islam, abortion is permitted under special circumstances only (Atighetchi, 1994; Schenker, 2000).

CURRENT LEGAL AND POLITICAL CLIMATE

The United States

Abortion has been an issue of considerable political debate in the United States for the last third of the 20th century. The landmark 1973 decision by the US Supreme Court on Roe v. Wade was a watershed. Roe v. Wade affirmed that a woman has a basic right to privacy and autonomy that permits first-trimester abortion on demand. The court left decisions about second-trimester abortions to the discretion of the states and strongly discouraged third-trimester abortions. This decision has been argued for the past 30 years, and efforts to diminish its jurisdiction have been numerous. The current status of abortion and reproductive rights on a state-by-state basis can be reviewed at http://www.naral.org. The information changes with each state's legislative session, so the reader is encouraged to check the Internet for the current status in a particular jurisdiction.

Many arguments against abortion assert that the fetus, as well as the mother, has certain rights. Annas (1998) notes that the fetus is not a person under the Constitution and asserts that states cannot make abortion a crime for either client or physician before the fetus is viable. States can outlaw abortion after viability only if there is an exception that permits abortion to protect the life or health of the woman. States can impose restrictions on abortion before viability only if those restrictions do not create a substantial obstacle to a woman's obtaining an abortion. Roe v. Wade ensured that women have the constitutional right to privacy, and that this privacy is broad and fundamental enough to encompass her decision to terminate her pregnancy.

Approximately 50% of all pregnancies are unintended, and approximately 50% of those unintended pregnancies end in abortion (Kaiser Family Foundation, 2002). Excluding miscarriages, approximately 24% of all pregnancies end in abortion (Finer & Henshaw, 2005). Abortion rates have continued to decline over the past several years; in 2002, the US abortion rate was 16 per 1000 women 15 to 44 years old (Strauss et al., 2005). According to Henshaw (1998), more than 30 million women had an abortion from 1973 to 1998. Even though rates continue to decline, abortion remains one of the most common surgical procedures in the United States today.

Who has abortions? Approximately 18% of women having abortions are teenagers, 33% are between the ages of 20 and 24 years, and 49% are 25 years or older (Strauss et al., 2005). More than 80% are unmarried, and approximately 55% are white (Strauss et al., 2005). Approximately 60% of women having abortions have given birth previously. More than 50% of all abortions occur within the first 8 weeks of pregnancy, and almost 90% are performed during the first trimester (Strauss et al., 2005). Only 1% of abortions are performed at 21 weeks' gestation or later (Henshaw, 1998; Strauss et al., 2005). Most commonly, these abortions are for severe fetal abnormalities diagnosed late in gestation or for conditions that put the mother's life in jeopardy.

Canada

The term *abortion* in Canada refers to any pregnancy terminated up until 20 weeks' gestation. Although abortion was a criminal offense in Canada for many years, it was decriminalized in 1988. Canada does not have any specific legislation related to abortion. The government views it as a medical procedure and regulates it the same way as all other medical procedures. Abortion may be performed on request, and there is no requirement that the woman provide documentation other than the fact that she does not want the pregnancy.

NURSING PERSPECTIVES, ROLES, AND RESPONSIBILITIES

For most people, their feelings and beliefs about abortion are intensely private and based on personal ethical systems rather than simply scientific evidence. These beliefs span the entire range of possibilities, from abortion on demand from conception until the onset of labor, to a total ban on abortion from the moment of conception, regardless of the rationale. Each person is entitled to his or her beliefs. The controversy for many arises when personal beliefs conflict with the legally protected rights of individual women (Marek, 2004).

QUOTE 9-2

"I want to provide the best care possible to my clients, but how can I support them in a decision with which I disagree?"

A pro-life nursing student struggling with abortion-related concerns for clients

Although personal beliefs are appropriate guides to personal decision making, they are inappropriate guides to professional practice. Each person, whether client or nurse, has a right to uphold personal beliefs and to act on them to the extent protected by the Constitution. As professionals, nurses are obligated to present to clients the gamut of options available in a fashion respectful of all possible choices and in a way that does not inherently bias the client (Assessment Tool 9.1).

The first step in being able to provide such an objective perspective is becoming aware of personal beliefs and biases. If a nurse believes that abortion is the best alternative for a client carrying a fetus with a genetic abnormality, he or she needs to be aware that this is a *personal* perspective (Marek, 2004). If a nurse thinks that abortion is never appropriate under any circumstances, he or she needs to be conscious of this belief because he or she may, consciously or unconsciously, show that bias in presenting information to a client facing an unwanted pregnancy (Cignacco, 2002).

The decision to terminate a pregnancy is never easy (Hess, 2004) (Research Highlight 9.1). Clearly, the client making this decision may wish she never had to make such a choice. Those who reach this conclusion come to it for various reasons (Finer et al., 2005). It is appropriate to provide clients with information about options. It is *never* appropriate to make it evident that one option is more acceptable to the nurse than any other. If a client asks the nurse, "What would you do if you were facing this decision?" the only appropriate response is something like, "What I would do is not relevant; what is important is ensuring that you have the information you need to make this choice, because you, and not me, are the one who has to decide what to do." Clients make many decisions that are different than the nurse may make under the same circumstances. The nurse's responsibility with clients deciding on the outcome of a pregnancy is the same as would exist with a client's decision to have a surgical procedure, adhere to a medication regimen, or make any other health-related decision. NIC/NOC Box 9.1 highlights some applicable nursing interventions and outcomes for a client experiencing an abortion.

Decision-Making Process

Clients elect to terminate pregnancies for reasons such as concerns about maternal health, genetic conditions

● ASSESSMENT TOOL 9.1 Decision Tree of Pregnancy Options

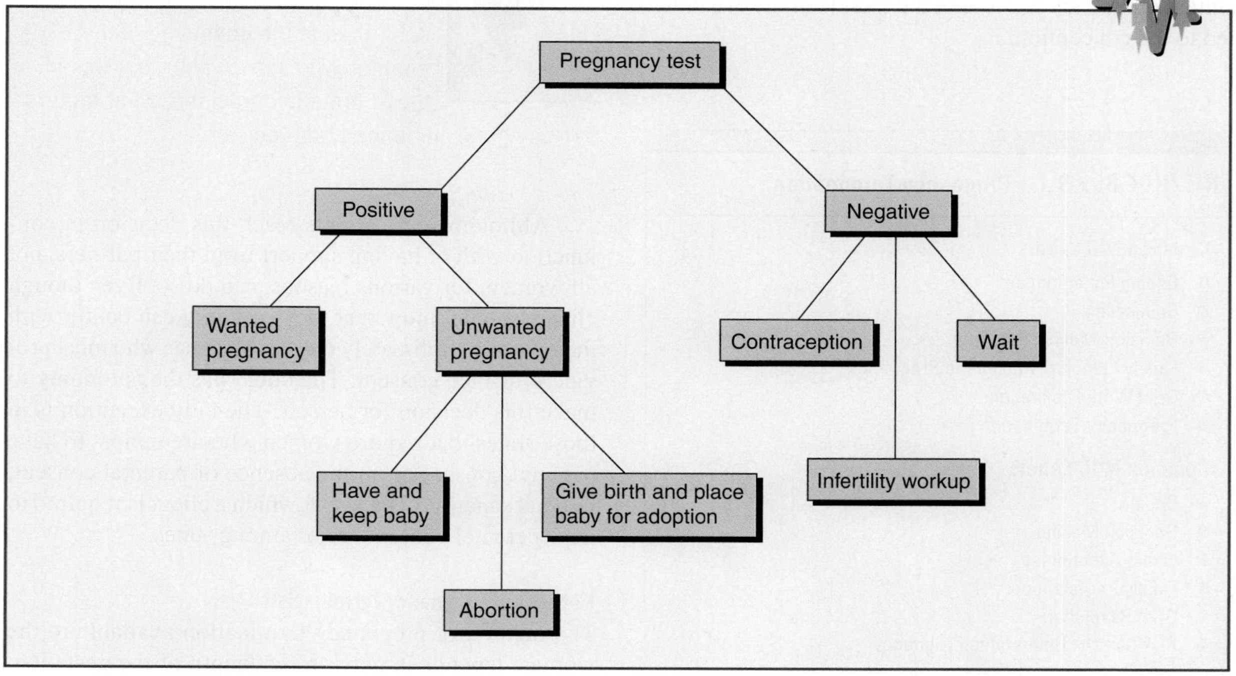

● RESEARCH HIGHLIGHT 9.1 Dimensions of Women's Long-Term Postabortion Experience

PURPOSE: To describe and explore the experience of women 5 years or more after a first-trimester voluntary abortion.

METHODS: The researcher constructed a phenomenologic study of audio-recorded semistructured interviews with 17 women. Clients were of various ethnicities, religions, socioeconomic backgrounds, ages, and marital statuses.

RESULTS: Five themes were common among the women's experiences: making the decision, coping with memories, gaining perspective, seeking help, and recognizing worth. Most participants integrated and found meaning in the experience of abortion. The women had both positive and negative consequences of having decided to abort a pregnancy.

NURSING IMPLICATIONS: This study supports the importance of avoiding unwanted pregnancy through abstinence and contraception. Nursing counseling and assistance throughout the abortion decision-making process needs to be sensitive and acknowledge spiritual and emotional issues.

Hess, R. F. (2004). *MCN—The American Journal of Maternal and Child Nursing, 29*(3), 193–198.

affecting the fetus, rape, incest, and personal circumstances (Finer et al., 2005). The reasons may be intensely personal and as varied as women themselves. For some clients with chronic medical conditions, a contraceptive failure that resulted in pregnancy may place their own lives in jeopardy. Clients in abusive relationships who become pregnant may elect abortion so that they do not have permanent ties to the male partner with whom they would share offspring (Copelon et al., 2005; Leung et al., 2002). Those who know that they or their partners are carriers of genetic conditions may seek prenatal genetic diagnosis with the goal of terminating those pregnancies that would bear severely affected children (see Chap. 11). Victims of rape or incest may wish to terminate any resultant pregnancy because of the trauma of the event that led to the conception.

NIC/NOC Box 9.1 Pregnancy Termination

Common NIC Labels

- Coping Enhancement
- Counseling
- Decision-Making Support
- Family Planning: Unplanned Pregnancy
- Grief Work Facilitation
- Pregnancy Termination Care

Common NOC Labels

- Coping
- Decision Making
- Family Functioning
- Family Participation
- Grief Resolution
- Risk Control: Unintended Pregnancy

The nurse's role should be to assess the client's condition; to provide factual, nondirective teaching about the types of abortion available and other possible alternatives, including keeping the child or surrendering the child for adoption after birth (see Chap. 7); and to ensure that the client makes decisions with adequate knowledge and sufficient autonomy. The client needs to decide and feel comfortable and confident that the choice is the best possible alternative, given the circumstances surrounding the pregnancy. Nursing Care Plan 9.1 highlights the care of a client considering pregnancy termination.

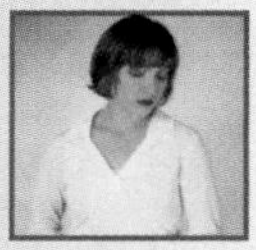

Consider Gina, the 44-year-old woman described at the beginning of the chapter who had an abortion. Based on the information provided, what factors may have influenced her decision?

Although some clients reach this decision in conjunction with or having support from their partners, not all women, for various reasons, can do so. Even though clients should know that they certainly can confer with their partners, ultimately they are the ones who must provide informed consent. The client has the autonomy to make this decision for herself. The only exception is in those states that require women who are minors to have parental consent or, in the absence of parental consent, judicial sanction. The age at which a client is required to have parental consent varies among states.

Methods of Pregnancy Termination

The method of pregnancy termination available to the woman depends largely on the length of the gestation.

NURSING CARE PLAN 9.1

The Client Considering an Abortion

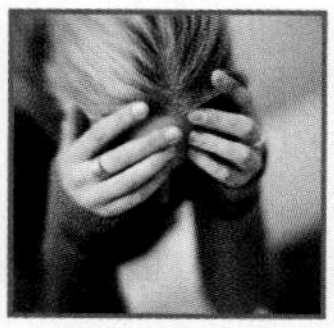

Recall Patti from the beginning of this chapter. She states, "There is no way I can have another baby. I can't afford it. My daughter can't be put through this. I broke up with her father a month ago, and he'll never support me through another pregnancy. He'll just say it's my fault and that he's glad to be rid of me." She sobs. "I never thought I'd have to consider an abortion. How am I going to make it through?"

NURSING DIAGNOSES

- **Decisional Conflict** related to uncertainty about abortion and lack of available support
- **Ineffective Coping** related to anxiety about abortion, situational crisis, and inadequate social support

EXPECTED OUTCOMES

1. The client will make an informed decision about the abortion by the next visit.
2. The client will identify areas of stress related to her current situation.
3. The client will demonstrate beginning positive coping mechanisms.

INTERVENTIONS	RATIONALES
Assess the client's level of understanding about abortion and options available.	Assessment provides a baseline to identify specific client needs and to develop an individualized plan of care.
Communicate accurate facts and answer questions; clarify any misconceptions or misinformation.	Clear communication helps provide accurate information to aid in alleviating fears and clarifying misinformation.
Provide the client with a chance to discuss any concerns, fears, or worries about her situation; encourage the client to share her feelings.	Communication can reveal sources of stress and any problematic areas that need to be addressed; sharing of feelings aids in promoting positive coping.
Ask the client about available support systems (eg, family, friends).	Identifying such supports helps to establish sources of assistance when the client needs help from other people.
Assist the client to identify possible areas for support. Provide her with information about support groups, Web sites, and other avenues for education and assistance.	Shared experiences and knowledge of similar situations for others can help the client prepare for what to expect and to realize that she is not alone.
Ask the client about measures used to cope with previous stressful situations; determine which measures were successful. Reinforce use of successful strategies; instruct the client in simple relaxation techniques, as appropriate.	Identifying previous coping strategies helps to determine effective strategies for use in this situation. Simple relaxation techniques provide one means of positive coping.

Continued

NURSING CARE PLAN 9.1 ● The Client Considering an Abortion *(Continued)*

INTERVENTIONS	RATIONALES
Provide the client with information (including brochures and pamphlets) related to viable options and choices nonjudgmentally; encourage the client to review material before the next visit. Encourage her to actively participate in decision making related to options; focus on one aspect at a time.	Nurses are obligated to provide the client with all possible options without personal bias. Active participation promotes feelings of control; focusing on one aspect reduces the risk for feeling overwhelmed.
Assist the client with scheduling a return visit in 1 week.	Follow-up is necessary to determine the client's decision.

EVALUATION

1. The client states she is comfortable with her decision.
2. The client exhibits behaviors congruent with her decision.
3. The client verbalizes areas of concern related to her situation.
4. The client reports using relaxation techniques for times when she feels stressed.

Although most abortions performed in North America are surgical, a small but growing number of women are electing medical terminations (Scott et al., 2003; Strauss et al., 2005).

First-Trimester Methods

Vacuum Aspiration. Most first-trimester abortions are performed by vacuum aspiration (Strauss et al., 2005) (Fig. 9.1). Usually, the client visits the clinic or doctor's office the day before the procedure for insertion of laminaria tents. Laminaria tents are small cones of dried seaweed that, when exposed to moisture, expand, thus painlessly dilating the cervix. The clinician inserts the laminaria during examination with a speculum. The client then wears a tampon to hold the tents in place. Alternatively, the clinician may apply prostaglandin gel to the cervix to soften it.

Just before the procedure, the client may elect to take a mild sedative. Local anesthesia in the form of a lidocaine paracervical block is common. The clinician performs a bimanual examination to document the size of the uterus. He or she cleanses the cervix, which is held by a *tenaculum* (a surgical instrument used to grasp and stabilize the cervix). The clinician inserts a thin plastic catheter through the cervix; this catheter is connected to a vacuum aspirator or syringe. The aspirator or syringe then evacuates the contents of the uterus. During the procedure, the nurse should support the woman, letting her know that she may experience mild to moderate cramping.

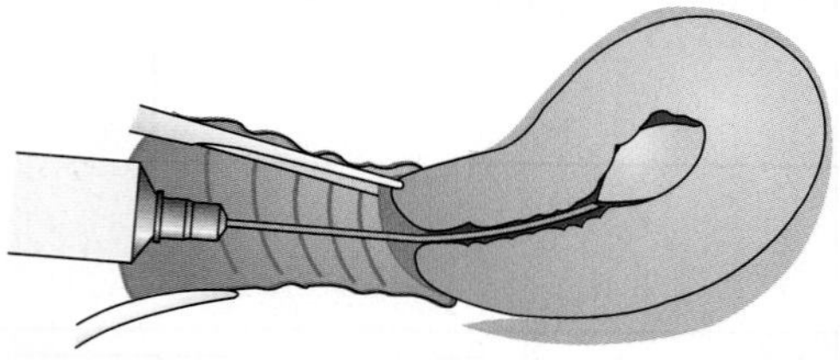

FIGURE 9.1 Vacuum extraction.

After the aspiration, the clinician ensures that the uterine contents have been removed completely. Health care providers should monitor the client for 1 to 2 hours to ensure that her vital signs are stable and that she is not experiencing excessive blood loss. They should instruct her to expect bleeding similar to that of a heavy menstrual period in duration and intensity. They should teach her to avoid the use of tampons while she is actively bleeding, as well as sexual activity until bleeding ceases. Other teaching measures include instructing the client to contact a clinician if she has an elevated temperature, excessive cramping or tenderness, or excessive bleeding, and to expect resumption of menses 4 to 6 weeks after the procedure.

Some health care providers request a return visit, at which time they perform a pelvic examination and pregnancy test to ensure that the pregnancy has been terminated successfully (Scott et al., 2003). As appropriate, they also may offer instruction about and prescription for contraceptives.

Methotrexate and Misoprostol. Methotrexate is cytotoxic and has been used as a chemotherapeutic agent for many years. It also is used to treat unruptured ectopic pregnancies, rheumatoid arthritis, choriocarcinoma, and psoriasis. It is lethal to proliferating trophoblastic tissues and leads to abortion by blocking folic acid in fetal cells, preventing them from dividing. Misoprostol is a prostaglandin-based drug that is used for cervical ripening and abortion. Used together, methotrexate and misoprostol have a 95% success rate in early pregnancy termination (Hatcher et al., 2004).

Treatment regimens vary, but they all require at least two visits to the health care provider. Typically, at the initial visit, the client receives an injection of methotrexate into the gluteal muscle. Researchers disagree about the optimal timing for insertion of misoprostol, which can be dispensed in either suppository or pill form. When a suppository is used, the provider should give the woman 800 μg of misoprostol and instruct her to insert this into the vagina 3 to 7 days after the methotrexate injection. When pills are used, the provider should teach the client to use a tampon to hold them in place in the vagina for 12 hours or until active vaginal bleeding begins. As opposed to self-administration of the suppository or pill form, some providers prefer for the client to return to the office or clinic for the provider to insert the substance. Regardless of form used or type of insertion, providers should give all women undergoing this procedure an acetaminophen-codeine preparation for discomfort. See Teaching Tips 9.1 for more information.

All clients are required to return to the clinic 3 to 7 days after administration of misoprostol to ensure that the abortion has been complete. Some cases require a second administration of misoprostol. Some clients require a surgical abortion by vacuum aspiration if the medical procedure is not effective in terminating the pregnancy (see later discussion).

Mifepristone and Misoprostol. Mifepristone, or RU486, acts as a progesterone antagonist (Pharmacology Box 9.1). It is used as emergency contraception, as well as for early abortion, in many countries throughout the world, including France, Sweden, and China. Supplementing it with misoprostol enhances its efficacy. Side effects are more pronounced in women whose pregnancies are more advanced (Scott et al., 2003). Clients using mifepristone report abortion experiences similar to those who experience spontaneous abortion, with cramping and bleeding (Hatcher et al., 2004).

Acetaminophen can control most discomfort; some providers add codeine to acetaminophen. Blood loss is proportional to the length of gestation, but typically less than 100 mL. Contraindications include suspected ectopic pregnancy, renal failure, and concurrent use of steroids or anticoagulant therapy.

For most clients, this combination requires a minimum of three visits to the clinician. On the first visit, the client takes 600 mg of mifepristone. Although some women expel the pregnancy with just this intervention, most need to return to the clinic 2 days later for oral administration of 400 mcg of misoprostol. After administration of the misoprostol, providers should observe the client for a minimum of 4 hours; most women experience abortion during this time. Two weeks later, the client again returns to the clinic for an examination to ensure that the abortion is complete. Because the procedure is not done frequently in the United States, most clinicians have less experience with this regimen than with the others, so routines may vary considerably.

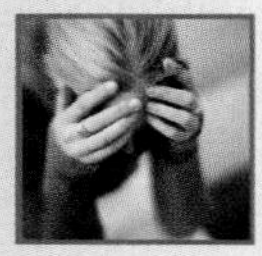

Think back to Patti, the single woman who has just found out that she is 9 weeks pregnant. Patti makes an informed decision to have an abortion, which is scheduled for next week. Which options would be available for her?

Second-Trimester Methods

Solution Infusions. Infusions of hypertonic solutions such as saline or urea often are used to terminate second-trimester pregnancies (Fig. 9.2). Typically, the clinician inserts laminaria tents the day before or just before the

TEACHING TIPS 9.1 Self-Insertion of Misoprostol

The provider instructs the client as follows:

- Insert the medication at bedtime or some other time when you can rest.
- Eat sparingly because of the possibility of nausea.
- Drink sufficient fluids to maintain hydration and avoid postural hypotension.
- Insert the medication deep into the vagina with clean hands; remain supine for at least 30 minutes.
- Expect cramping and bleeding to begin within 12 hours.
- Take acetaminophen and codeine every 4 hours as needed for cramping; notify the health care provider if the bleeding is heavy enough to soak through four sanitary napkins in less than 2 hours.
- Do not take folate or vitamins containing folate for 1 week after methotrexate administration.

● PHARMACOLOGY 9.1 Mifepristone (Mifegyne)

CLASSIFICATION: Abortifacient

ACTION: A progesterone antagonist that stimulates uterine contractions and sloughing of endometrium, causing an implanted trophoblast to loosen from the placental wall (can be used up to 49 days' gestational age)

PREGNANCY CATEGORY: X

DOSAGE: One-time dose of 600 mg PO

POSSIBLE ADVERSE EFFECTS:
Headache, vomiting, diarrhea, heavy uterine bleeding

NURSING INTERVENTIONS

- Drug can cause such nausea that client may appreciate being premedicated with an antiemetic.
- Drug is usually followed within 48 hours with a prostaglandin for greater effect.
- Client may need a uterine dilatation and curettage (D&C) if heavy bleeding does not resolve.
- Client needs to be counseled regarding effective birth control measures to avoid having to take mifepristone again in the future.

procedure. He or she asks the woman to empty her bladder before the procedure begins to avoid inadvertent injury to that organ. Then, the client undergoes an amniocentesis, in which amniotic fluid is withdrawn and a similar amount of hypertonic solution is infused. Alternatively, the clinician may insert prostaglandins vaginally. The goal of the infusion or insertion is to stimulate uterine contractions and expulsion of the uterine contents. In some cases, intravenous oxytocin is used to facilitate contractions and to shorten the time between medication administration and abortion.

Abortion by infusion and insertion methods is expensive and costly. For this reason, these procedures are used infrequently today (Hatcher et al., 2004).

Dilatation and Evacuation (D&E). This procedure is similar to a first-trimester vacuum aspiration but requires greater cervical dilatation because of the increased volume of uterine contents (Fig. 9.3). It also is more uncomfortable. Thus, it is more common for the client to request sedation before beginning. Many providers use this procedure through 20 or more weeks' gestation, although some prefer to do the procedure before 16 weeks' gestation. For some women who undergo diagnostic amniocenteses for genetic abnormalities, however, results are not definitive before 16 weeks.

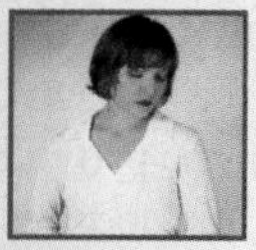

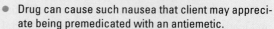

Remember Gina, the 44-year-old woman who had an abortion for severe fetal physical and congenital abnormalities. Which type of abortion procedure was most likely performed?

Aftercare

The earlier in the pregnancy an abortion is performed, the safer the procedure. Medical complications of abortion are small when compared with the medical risk of pregnancy and childbirth (Scott et al., 2003); they include problems such as hemorrhage, infection, and incomplete abortion. Many providers encourage return visits to ensure that no complications exist.

Nursing implications include the following:

- Ensure that women who are Rh negative receive RhoGAM (see Chap. 18).
- Teach women to recognize and report warning signs:
  - Fever
  - Chills

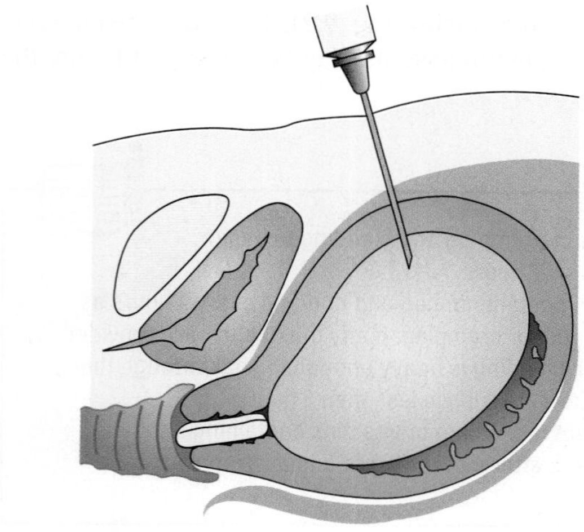

FIGURE 9.2 Saline induction.

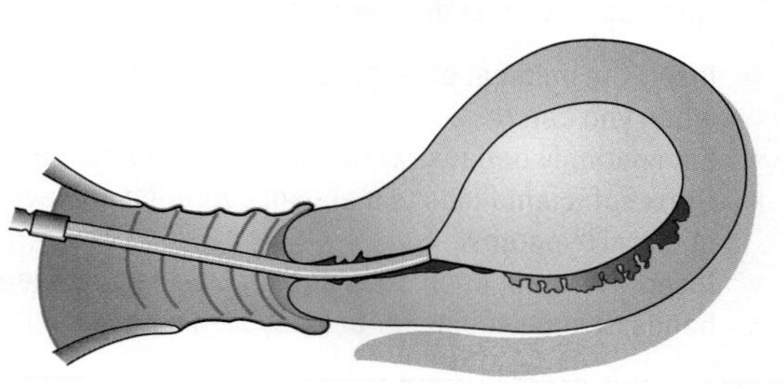

FIGURE 9.3 Dilatation and extraction (D&E).

- Abdominal pain
- Abdominal tenderness
- Excessive or prolonged bleeding
- Foul-smelling vaginal discharge
- Lack of menses by 6 weeks after the procedure (Hatcher et al., 2004)

For some clients experiencing mid to late second-trimester abortion, there is the possibility of lactation. Nurses should prepare women for this possibility and encourage them to have a tight-fitting bra and nursing pads available. When lactation occurs, some clients find it especially distressing. Nurses can help by providing anticipatory guidance so that the client is not surprised or frightened if she begins to lactate.

No evidence has shown that first-trimester abortions affect future fertility or pregnancy risks. Although some women experience sadness and show signs of stress during and after the procedure, others report relief. Psychological and emotional sequelae largely will vary with the client (Broen et al., 2005). Nursing Care Plan 9.2 highlights the care of a client after an abortion.

The client may be fertile almost immediately after undergoing an abortion. The nurse should offer the client information about contraception as appropriate (see Chap. 8). She can begin almost any method of contraception immediately; insertion of an intrauterine device may be performed as soon as termination of the pregnancy is confirmed. Because some contraceptive methods take time to become effective, the nurse may suggest a backup method of contraception as a supplement until the woman has had her first postabortion menses.

CONCLUSION

From a health perspective, abortion as performed in the United States and Canada today is safe and effective. Although some states have introduced mandatory waiting periods and the need for minors to have parental consent, and some health insurance plans do not cover elective abortion, Roe v. Wade (1973) guarantees the right of a woman to determine whether she will terminate her pregnancy.

The decision to terminate a pregnancy is never easy. It certainly is preferable to avoid an unintended pregnancy. For some, who are the victims of rape or incest, the choice to avoid the pregnancy is not possible. For others, who are at risk for producing children with genetic abnormalities, the option of prenatal genetic diagnosis followed by termination of affected fetuses allows them the possibility of having a biologic child not affected by the condition of concern.

Women have been having abortions for as long as people have been having sex. For the past 30 years in the United States, they have had the option of having these abortions under conditions that do not compromise their lives or future reproductive capacity. If abortion is once again made illegal, many women who elect to terminate their pregnancies once again will turn to self-induced or black-market abortions that can lead to increased maternal morbidity and mortality.

Questions to Ponder

1. Iona, 27 years old, comes to the clinic for confirmation of a positive home pregnancy test. She is afraid that her husband of 5 years will become physically abusive if she has another baby. She states that they cannot afford to support the children they already have and that he has threatened to "kill her" if she ever gets pregnant again.
   - What is your reaction to this scenario?
   - What options are available to the client?
2. John and Mary have just received the results of prenatal genetic testing, which reveals that their 18-week fetus has Tay-Sachs disease (see Chap. 4). One previous child with Tay-Sachs died at 35 months old after a long period of suffering. John and Mary have a 3-year-old unaffected child at present. They state that watching another child suffer from this genetic condition is more than they could bear.
   - What are your feelings about these circumstances?

SUMMARY

- Women have sought ways to control family size since the beginning of recorded history.
- It is preferable to control conception, but women with unintended pregnancy may elect to terminate the pregnancy for a variety of reasons.
- Religion, culture, and legal access to safe abortion services all affect women's utilization of abortion services.
- Clients with unintended pregnancy who do not have access to safe abortion services often seek less safe ways to terminate unwanted pregnancies. This adversely affects women's health.
- People have strong feelings about abortion that are based as much in faith traditions as they are in scientific knowledge.
- Medical and surgical procedures are available for both first- and second-trimester abortions.

REVIEW QUESTIONS

1. A nurse who believes abortion is unacceptable under all circumstances should
   A. share her beliefs with clients.
   B. share beliefs with clients if asked.
   C. keep her personal beliefs to herself.
   D. never work in women's health.
2. Which of the following is an example of a surgical abortion?

NURSING CARE PLAN 9.2

The Client Recovering from Abortion

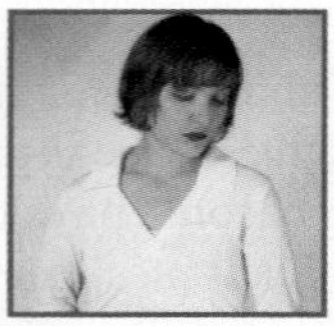

Gina, the 44-year-old woman from the beginning of the chapter, has undergone a dilatation and evacuation procedure. She is awake, alert, and able to tolerate food and fluids. Her vital signs are within acceptable parameters. She has moderate vaginal bleeding and is complaining of only mild cramping at present. She states, "I feel like it was the right choice for me, my husband, and my family. But it's hard not to consider what might have been."

NURSING DIAGNOSIS

Anticipatory Grieving related to the loss of the fetus and an unknown future

EXPECTED OUTCOMES

1. The client will verbalize feelings about the loss.
2. The client will demonstrate acceptance of the loss.
3. The client will begin the grief process.

INTERVENTIONS	RATIONALES
Explore with the client the meaning of the loss of the fetus to her and to her family; encourage her to openly verbalize her feelings and concerns.	Exploration and encouraging verbalization of feelings provide the client with a safe outlet.
Assess the client for possible feelings of guilt associated with her decision to abort.	Guilt may affect her ability to progress through the grieving process.
Review the client's reasons for her decisions.	Such review helps to minimize any misconceptions and questions related to her decision and aids in lessening any feelings of guilt.
Assist the client to identify personal past coping strategies that have been successful.	Doing so helps to determine effective strategies for use in this situation.
Reassure the client that her feelings are common; encourage participation in support groups as appropriate.	Reassurance helps reduce anxiety and fear. Support groups promote sharing of feelings with others who have had similar experiences.
Encourage the client to include spouse and other family members in visits and discussion of feelings.	Participation of other relatives promotes sharing and provides support for one another. Sharing of feelings promotes positive coping.
Provide the client and family with information about the grieving process and stages of grief.	Information about grieving provides a basis for the client and her family to understand what is happening to them.
Allow the client (and family members) time to cry; use appropriate methods to help them express feelings comfortably (eg, role-playing, activity, drawing).	Expression of feelings is essential to progress through the grief process.
Arrange for a follow-up visit with the client.	A follow-up visit allows time to reassess and evaluate the client's progress.

EVALUATION

1. The client continues to state that she made the correct decision.
2. The client demonstrates positive methods of coping.
3. The client demonstrates acceptance of decision and of the loss.

A. Dilatation and evacuation
B. Plan B
C. RU486
D. Methotrexate

3. When counseling clients of the Jewish faith about abortion, which of the following would the nurse need to consider?
   A. The fetus is considered to have a soul immediately after being conceived.
   B. Four months need to pass before abortion would be viewed as taking a life.
   C. The religion permits abortion when pregnancy threatens the woman's health.
   D. The fetus has rights equal to those of the mother from the moment of conception.
4. When providing care to a client considering an abortion, which of the following should the nurse do first?
   A. Identify personal beliefs and biases related to abortion rights.
   B. Present information on what the nurse believes the client needs.
   C. Provide teaching about Constitutional rights related to abortion.
   D. Share decision-making responsibilities with the client.
5. After teaching a client who is scheduled to undergo a vacuum aspiration, which client statement indicates the nurse's teaching has been successful?
   A. "The physician will give me an injection into my buttocks and a suppository several days later."
   B. "I'll get some pills from the physician one day and then come back to the clinic in about 2 days for some more pills."
   C. "I'll get a local anesthetic and then the physician will use a small catheter to remove what's in my uterus."
   D. "The physician will do an amniocentesis, take out some fluid, and replace it with a strong salt solution."
6. Which of the following would the nurse include in the discharge teaching plan for a client undergoing a dilatation and evacuation?
   A. Using tampons for any vaginal bleeding
   B. Resuming sexual activity in 24 hours
   C. Notifying the care provider for temperature elevations
   D. Using a moderately strong narcotic analgesic for pain
7. A woman who has had an abortion is Rh negative. Which of the following would the nurse expect to administer?
   A. Prostaglandin
   B. Laminaria
   C. Methotrexate
   D. RhoGAM

REFERENCES

Annas, G. J. (1998). Partial-birth abortion, Congress, and the Constitution. *New England Journal of Medicine, 339*(4), 279–283.

Atighetchi, D. (1994). The position of Islamic tradition on contraception. *Medicine and the Law, 13*(7–8), 717–725.

Boston Women's Health Book Collective. (2005). *Our bodies, ourselves: A new edition for a new era.* New York: Touchstone.

Broen, A. N., Moum, T., Bodtker, A. S., & Ekeberg, O. (2005). The course of mental health after miscarriage and induced abortion: A longitudinal, five-year follow-up study. *BMC Medicine, 3,* 18.

Centers for Disease Control and Prevention. (2002). Abortion surveillance—United States, 1998. *Morbidity and Mortality Weekly Report, 51*(SS03), 1–32.

Cignacco, E. (2002). Between professional duty and ethical confusion: Midwives and selective termination of pregnancy. *Nursing Ethics, 9*(2), 179–191.

Copelon, R., Zampas, C., Bruise, E., & Devore, J. (2005). Human rights begin at birth: International law and the claim of fetal rights. *Reproductive Health Matters, 13*(26), 120–129.

Edelstein, L. (1967). The Hippocratic Oath: Text, translation and interpretation. In O. Temkin & C. L. Temkin (Eds.): *Ancient medicine: Selected papers of Ludwig Edelstein* (pp. 3–64). Baltimore: Johns Hopkins University Press.

Finer, L. B., & Henshaw, S. K. (2005). Estimates of U.S. abortion incidence in 2001 and 2002. Retrieved March 23, 2006, from http://www.guttmacher.org/pubs/2005/05/18/ab_incidence.pdf.

Finer, L. B., Frohwirth, L. F., Dauphinee, L. A., Singh, S., & Moore, A. M. (2005). Reasons U.S. women have abortions: Quantitative and qualitative perspectives. *Perspectives in Sexual and Reproductive Health, 37*(3), 110–118.

Hatcher, R. A., Trussell, J., Stewart, F., Nelson, A. L., Cates, W., Guest, F., Kowal, D. (2004). *Contraceptive technology* (18th rev. ed.). New York: Ardent Media.

Henshaw, S. K. (1998). Abortion incidence and services in the United States, 1995–1996. *Family Planning Perspectives, 30*(6), 263–270.

Hess, R. F. (2004). Dimensions of women's long-term postabortion experience. *MCN—The American Journal of Maternal and Child Nursing, 29*(3), 193–198.

If these walls could talk. (1996). Home Box Office.

Jones, R. K., et al. (2002). Patterns in the socioeconomic characteristics of women obtaining abortions in 2000–2001. *Perspectives on Sexual and Reproductive Health, 34,* 226–235.

Kaiser Family Foundation. (2002). *Abortion in the United States.* Menlo Park, CA: Author.

Lewis, J. A. (2003a). The Jewish perspective. In M. L. Moore (Ed.), *Cultural perspectives in childbearing* (pp. 78–91). New York: March of Dimes.

Lewis, J. A. (2003b). Jewish perspectives on pregnancy and childbearing. *MCN—The American Journal of Maternal/Child Nursing, 28*(5), 306–312.

Leung, T. W., Leung, W. C., Chan, P. L., & Ho, P. C. (2002). A comparison of the prevalence of domestic violence between patients seeking termination of pregnancy and other general gynecology patients. *International Journal of Gynaecology and Obstetrics, 77*(1), 47–54.

Marek, M. J. (2004). Nurses' attitudes toward pregnancy termination in the labor and delivery setting. *Journal of Obstetrical, Gynecological, and Neonatal Nursing, 33*(4), 472–479.

Riddle, J. M. (1992). *Contraception and abortion from the ancient world to the Renaissance.* Cambridge, MA: Harvard University Press.

Roe v. Wade. (1973). 410 US 113.

Schenker, J. G. (2000). Women's reproductive health: Monotheistic religious perspectives. *International Journal of Gynaecology and Obstetrics, 70*(1), 77–86.

Scott, J. R., Gibbs, R. S., Karlan, B. Y., & Haney, A. F. (2003). *Danforth's obstetrics and gynecology* (9th ed.). Philadelphia: Lippincott Williams & Wilkins.

Strauss, L. T., Herndon, J., Chang, J., Parker, W. Y., Bowens, S. V., & Berg, C. J. (2005). Abortion surveillance—United States, 2002. *Morbidity and Mortality Weekly Report Surveillance Summaries, 54*(7), 1–31.

CHAPTER 10

Fertility Challenges

Judith A. Lewis and Jennifer J. Black

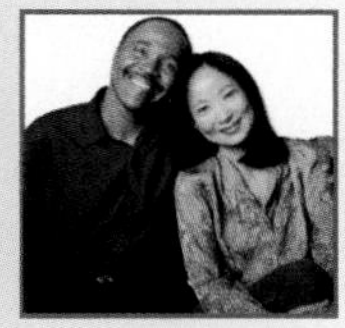

Ted and Joan have been undergoing preliminary evaluation for infertility. The couple has been married for 5 years; they have been trying to get pregnant for the past 2 years. Ted is 39, and Joan is 37. For both partners, their medical histories are negative for any major medical problems.

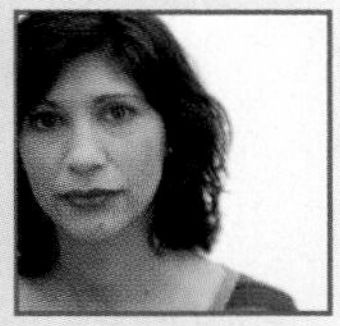

Stacy, 42 years old, was married for the second time 1 year ago. She is visiting the examiner for a routine reproductive examination. Before they begin, Stacy asks if there is something that she can discuss. "My husband and I have been trying to get pregnant for several months now. It's not happening." Her voice begins to shake. "My ex-husband and I tried to have a baby for years and it never came to be, even though the doctors couldn't find anything wrong. It's one of the reasons my first marriage did not work out. I am so afraid the same thing will happen again."

Nurses working with such clients need to understand the material in this chapter to manage care effectively and address each issue appropriately. Before beginning this chapter, consider the following points related to the above scenarios:

- What additional information does the nurse require from each client?
- How would you suggest the nurse balance the physical needs of each client with the emotional, psychosocial, and spiritual challenges that infertility may impose?
- What measures should the nurse consider for involving the male partners in these scenarios?
- What next steps would you expect for Ted and Joan? For Stacy?

LEARNING OBJECTIVES

On completion of this chapter, the reader should be able to:

- Define infertility.
- Identify populations affected by infertility.
- Identify religious and ethical considerations concerning infertility.
- List common causes of infertility.
- Describe methods of diagnosis and options for treatment of infertility.
- Identify collaborative interventions to help people cope with infertility.
- Describe alternatives to infertility treatment.

KEY TERMS

assisted hatching
assisted reproductive technologies
cervical stenosis
endometriosis
gamete intrafallopian transfer (GIFT)
impaired fecundity
infertility
intracytoplasmic sperm injection (ICSI)
in vitro fertilization (IVF)
polycystic ovarian syndrome
premature ovarian failure
primary infertility
secondary infertility
zygote intrafallopian transfer (ZIFT)

Infertility, a medical diagnosis of the reproductive system, is defined as the inability to achieve pregnancy after 1 year of frequent, unprotected intercourse (DeMasters, 2004). Women older than 35 years having difficulty conceiving may receive a diagnosis of infertility before a full 12 months. **Primary infertility** applies to a man or woman who has never been able to conceive. **Secondary infertility** applies to an inability to conceive after one or both partners have conceived previously. **Impaired fecundity** is the term used when a couple can achieve pregnancy, but the woman cannot carry the pregnancy to a viable birth. A diagnosis of impaired fecundity usually is given after a woman has had two miscarriages.

Infertility affects approximately 10% to 15% of U.S. couples (Centers for Disease Control and Prevention [CDC], 2003). Both women and men may experience conditions that contribute to infertility. Although many people tend to think of infertility as a problem affecting heterosexual couples desiring to have children, infertility may be a problem for single women, single men, and gay and lesbian couples. People in many kinds of situations may seek services to treat infertility.

For most women, family planning involves taking measures to ensure that they can avoid unintended pregnancy, and then taking steps to conceive a child when they are ready to have children. These women have control of their fertility. These choices and control over human reproduction are not available to women with infertility. Loss of these alternatives can be devastating, placing stress on relationships and leading to decreased self-esteem and depression (Bernstein, Lewis, & Seibel, 1994; Brucker & McKenry, 2004; Olshanky, 2003).

HISTORICAL PERSPECTIVES

Infertility has likely existed as long as humans have—instances of it are recorded in the Hebrew Bible. Sarah and Abraham, Rebecca and Isaac, and Rachel and Jacob all were frustrated in their attempts to bear children. Other Old Testament women who experienced infertility include Michal, the wife of King David, and Hannah, the wife of Elkanah (Gold, 1988).

Historical accounts of kings disposing of wives because of their inability to bear children are numerous. It seems that, because the woman bore the pregnancy, the inability to achieve the pregnancy was always thought to be her fault. In many parts of the world, this myth still persists.

RELIGIOUS AND CULTURAL PERSPECTIVES

Most religions and cultures view children as a blessing. Some cultures place a value on children of a specific gender. For example, couples whose ancestry can be traced to India often express a strong preference for male children (Malhi, 1995).

Jewish Perspectives

In the Bible, God commands humans to "be fruitful and multiply" (Genesis 1:28). Dorff (1998) notes that Judaism considers childbearing both an obligation and a commandment (*mitzvah*). Thus, observant Jews highly desire the ability to procreate, and the Jewish faith considers seeking medical intervention to treat infertility acceptable. Lewis (2003) notes that because people cannot be commanded to do something of which they are incapable, the commandment to reproduce would not be an obligation for the infertile couple. Although sexual relations within marriage are seen as a part of fulfilling the commandment of procreation, Judaism has no requirement that the sole purpose of intercourse is the creation of offspring. Sex that is not for the purpose of procreation is acceptable. The *ketubah,* or marriage contract, obligates the man to provide for the woman in all manners, including physical intimacy.

There are few situations in which sex is prohibited in Judaism, such as on the Day of Atonement (Yom Kippur) and during the immediate mourning period for a parent, sibling, or child. Orthodox Jewish families may follow the rules of *niddah,* or family purity, which considers women ritually impure during and immediately following menstruation. At this time, these women must refrain from any physical contact with men, including sexual intercourse, until they visit the *mikveh,* or ritual bath for immersion after 7 days with no vaginal bleeding have passed. These proscriptions may affect the timing of diagnostic and therapeutic interventions. Health care providers should encourage couples with these dilemmas to confer with their Rabbi.

Because sex outside heterosexual marriage is not in keeping with religious traditions, Judaism does not deal with issues of infertility among single women or lesbians.

Muslim Perspectives

Muslims look to the Qur'an for guidance regarding infertility. They generally accept assistive reproductive techniques when the husband's sperm and wife's eggs are used. Self-masturbation generally is forbidden, but it is acceptable for the wife to help with the collection of sperm. Use of donor gametes or surrogates is thought to produce an illegitimate child and is discouraged. In Islamic countries, polygamy (multiple wives) is an acceptable practice that allows a man to take a second wife if the first cannot bear children. In all cases, couples are encouraged to look to Allah for guidance before making any reproductive decisions (Islam and Infertility, n.d.).

Catholic Perspectives

Observant Catholics rely on rulings from the Vatican to determine permissible activities. Catholic doctrine prohibits sexual activity outside of marriage, frowns upon masturbation, and permits no form of artificial contraception. Couples may find that the only acceptable way of collecting a semen specimen is through the use of a condom with a hole in it, so that the act of sex still carries the possibility of conception. Many assisted reproductive technologies may be unacceptable to Catholic women and men. Again, clients should seek specific guidance from the Church and the parish priest.

MYTHS, FACTS, AND RESOURCES

As discussed previously, the belief that the female partner is primarily responsible for unwanted infertility is but one common myth associated with infertility. Table 10.1 lists other myths, as well as facts that refute them. Perhaps the most pervasive myth suggests that if couples adopt, they will become pregnant. Although pregnancy has followed an adoption in some cases, the thousands of couples who adopt and do not have a subsequent pregnancy are ignored. Although infertile women benefit from correct information, well-meaning but ill-informed advice from friends and colleagues can be more hurtful than helpful.

Valid sources of information are available for infertile men and women. Box 10.1 provides a sample of a wide variety of reliable Internet resources. Some sites listed are for women with specific concerns and perspectives, whereas others are geared toward health care professionals. A good starting point when looking for client-centered material is the Resolve Web site (www.resolve.org). A nurse named Barbara Eck Menning founded this national, not-for-profit organization, which has many local chapters that provide support and information. Many infertile women have found Resolve's meetings and group support invaluable. Their Web site contains much educational and referral material as well.

For health care providers, the Nurses in Reproductive Medicine section of the American Society for Reproductive Medicine (ASRM) Web site (www.asrm.org) provides information, standards of practice, and connections to other nurses working in infertility and reproductive endocrinology settings.

A search using the word "infertility" on www.google.com yielded 1.59 million hits. Although many sources contain accurate information, several are vague

(text continues on page 326)

● **TABLE 10.1 Infertility Myths and Facts**

MYTH	FACT
Infertility is a woman's problem.	Male factors account for 30% of cases of infertility. Of the remainder, female factors account for 35%, combined factors account for 20%, and unexplained factors are responsible for 15%.
Infertility is rare.	Estimates are that 1 in 6 people experience infertility at some point. Approximately 4.5 million couples experience infertility each year. Fewer than 2 million infertile couples actually seek medical help. It is a common health problem.
Infertility is all in your head. If you relax and stop thinking about it, you will get pregnant.	Infertility causes stress; stress doesn't cause infertility. Infertility is a medical problem and disorder of the reproductive system.
If you adopt a baby, you will get pregnant.	The pregnancy rate after adopting is the same as for those who do not adopt.
People who can't have babies do not know proper sex techniques.	Infertility is not a sexual disorder. It is a medical condition.
Sex every day will increase your chances of getting pregnant.	Sex every 36 to 48 hours around the time of ovulation optimizes sperm concentration and increases the chances of conception.
For some couples, getting pregnant just takes time.	Couples in which the female partner trying to achieve pregnancy is younger than 35 years should seek consultation after 12 months of unprotected intercourse and no conception. Couples in which the female partner trying to achieve pregnancy is 35 years or older should seek consultation after 6 months of unprotected intercourse without conception.
Infertility happens only to couples who have never had a child before.	Secondary infertility (infertility after successful past pregnancies) is possible.
Maybe this is God's way of telling you that you aren't meant to be parents.	Such a statement is painful for anyone to hear and can be very discouraging. Infertility is a medical condition.
My spouse or partner might leave me if we can't conceive a child.	Although infertility can put stress on any relationship, most couples survive infertility crises with their relationship intact. Many couples find that the process of learning new ways of relating to each other during the experience of infertility brings them closer together.
Painful menstruation causes infertility.	Painful menstruation alone does not affect fertility. Progressively worsening menstrual pain may indicate endometriosis, a condition that may affect fertility. The pain escalates with each menstrual cycle and over time as scarring and adhesions form.
Blood group "incompatibility" between husband and wife can cause infertility.	There is no relationship between blood groups and fertility.
I'm not getting pregnant because most of the sperm leaks out after intercourse.	Loss of seminal fluid after intercourse is perfectly normal, and most women notice some discharge immediately after sex. This discharge is not a cause of infertility.
If you work at it and want it enough, you'll get pregnant.	Unlike many aspects of life, infertility may be beyond your control.
A man can judge his fertility by the thickness and volume of his semen.	Semen consists mainly of seminal fluid, secreted by the seminal vesicles and prostate. Volume and consistency of semen are not related to potential for fertility, which depends on sperm count. Microscopic examination is necessary for assessment of sperm count.
Infertility is hereditary.	If your mother, grandmother, or sister had difficulty becoming pregnant, this does not mean you will have the same problem. Most infertility problems are not hereditary. The exception is if a family had a genetic problem that interfered with fertility.
A retroverted (tipped) uterus causes infertility because the semen cannot swim into the cervix.	Approximately 20% of women have a retroverted uterus. If the retroverted uterus is freely mobile, this normal physiologic variation will not cause infertility.
A woman ovulates from the left ovary one month and the right ovary the next month.	It is true that only one ovary ovulates each month. The pattern, however, is not necessarily regular from side to side.
Placing pillows under the woman's hips during and after intercourse enhances fertility.	Sperm are already swimming in cervical mucus as sexual intercourse is completed. They will continue to travel up the cervix to the fallopian tube for the next 48 to 72 hours. Hip position really does not matter.
Menstrual cycles shorter or longer than every 28 days are irregular.	The length of a woman's menstrual cycle often varies. As long as a woman can count on having her period at a regular interval each month, the number of days in her particular cycle is normal.

Continued

TABLE 10.1 Infertility Myths and Facts

MYTH	FACT
A man's sperm count will be the same each time it is examined.	Sperm counts vary, based on the time between ejaculations, illness, and medications.
I have no problems having sex. Because I am virile, my sperm count must be normal.	There is no correlation between male fertility and virility. Men with totally normal sex drives may have no sperm at all.
Azoospermia (no sperm) results from excessive masturbation in childhood.	Masturbation is normal, and most boys and men indulge in it. It does not affect sperm count. Men do not "run out" of sperm because the testes constantly produce sperm.
Women who have had voluntary abortions are at risk for infertility when they want to become pregnant.	Precautions are taken with elective abortions to prevent subsequent infertility. Antibiotics are given both during and after the procedure to prevent infection and possible scarring and adhesions. The risk for perforation of the uterus or its arteries is minimal.

From ASRM. (2006). *Frequently asked questions about infertility.* Retrieved February 9, 2006, http://www.asrm.org/Patients/faqs.html.

BOX 10.1 Internet Resources for Infertility

General Information Sites

www.ihr.com/infertility. The site for Internet Health Resources (IHR) provides extensive information about in vitro fertilization, ICSI, infertility clinics, donor egg and surrogacy services (eg, surrogate mothers), natural infertility treatment, male infertility services, sperm banks, pharmacies, infertility books and videotapes, sperm testing, infertility support, and drugs and medications (eg, Metrodin, Pergonal, Clomid).

www.inciid.org. The InterNational Council on Infertility Information Dissemination, Inc. Web site includes comprehensive, consumer-targeted coverage of cutting-edge technologies and treatments. It has a good glossary, basic and advanced articles about specific topics, and excellent bulletin boards.

www.fertilitext.org. This site integrates the combined knowledge of professionals and practitioners in the reproductive health and fertility treatment communities. Its information is enhanced through collaborations with a growing network of participating organizations, fertility specialists, and visitors.

www.americaninfertility.org. This site acts as a lifetime resource for men and women needing reproductive information and support, and to forward the causes of adoption and reproductive health through advocacy, education, awareness building, and research funding. Membership is required for some services.

www.infertilitynetwork.org. Infertility Network is a registered Canadian charity providing information and support to those who have difficulty conceiving or carrying a pregnancy to term, to help them make informed choices.

www.resolve.org. The National Infertility Association, Resolve's Helpline, Medical Call-In Hour, Physician Referral Services, Member-to-Member Contact System, and Family Building Magazine focus on supporting couples navigating the maze of infertility.

www.ferti.net. The Worldwide Fertility Network disseminates infertility information among professional workers, researchers, and clients.

www.members.optushome.com.au/. Since 1993, the Donor Conception Support Group of Australia, Inc. is a self-funding organization run by volunteers. It now has a membership of approximately 600 adults and 300 children around the world.

www.ein.org. The Electronic Infertility Network shares information about infertility and the work of infertility support associations, within Europe and the rest of the world.

www.reproductivescience.com. IntegraMed America is a national network of fertility centers dedicated to helping women achieve pregnancy. Their Web site allows users to contact fertility centers, apply for loans online, and more.

http://members.aol.com/ladenwaitn/index.html. The Ladies in Waiting Infertility Support Web site is for married Christian women dealing with infertility.

Sites for Particular Medical Conditions

http://endo-online.org. The Endometriosis Association is a nonprofit, self-help organization dedicated to providing information and support, educating the public and medical community, and conducting and promoting research about endometriosis.

www.pcosupport.org. The Polycystic Ovarian Syndrome Association is a voluntary organization dedicated to promoting research and understanding of polycystic ovarian syndrome (PCOS).

Sites for Miscarriage Support

www.growthhouse.org/natal.html. Growth House, Inc. provides end-of-life support, including for grief related to pregnancy and infant death.

www.hannah.org. Hannah's prayer is a Christian infertility and pregnancy loss support network.

Continued

BOX 10.1 Internet Resources for Infertility *(Continued)*

www.hern.org/~hand/. Houston's Aid in Neonatal Death is a Houston-based pregnancy and infant loss support group.

www.sandsvic.org.au. SANDS is a support group for parents who experience miscarriage, stillbirth, or neonatal death.

Sites for Medical Specialists and Clinical Research

www.asrm.com. The American Society of Reproductive Medicine is committed to supporting and sponsoring educational activities for the lay public and continuing medical education activities for professionals engaged in the practice and research of reproductive medicine.

www.smru.org. This site for the Society for Male Reproduction and Urology (SMRU) contains information about male reproduction and urology physicians.

www.socrei.org. This professional Web site for the Society for Reproductive Endocrinology and Infertility (SREI) contains a search function for finding Reproductive Endocrinologists.

www.reprodsurgery.org. This site for the Society of Reproductive Surgeons (SRS) contains information about reproductive surgeons.

Surrogacy Sites

www.opts.com. The Organization of Parents Through Surrogacy (OPTS) Web site provides mutual support and surrogate parenting information.

www.surromomsonline.com. Surrogate Mothers Online provides information, support, and friendship to actual and potential surrogate mothers as well as parents and prospective parents.

www.surrogacy.com. The American Surrogacy Center, Inc. (TASC) promotes the exchange of information on medical infertility treatments, surrogacy alternatives, current legal status, and practitioners.

Sites About Adoption

www.Adoption.com. This site contains extensive adoption information, including Usenet Newsgroups, Mailing Lists, E-mail help, and search capabilities.

www.netexpress.com/users/adoptez/infertl.htm. The Adoption Made Easy Web site provides assistance in guiding couples through the infertility and adoption process by developing unique and confidential infertility/adoption plans.

www.adoptionstogether.org. Adoptions Together, Inc is an adoption agency.

www.bethany.org. The Bethany Adoption Services site contains extensive adoption information.

www.Adopting.org. This site contains extensive adoption information.

www.adopt.org. This site for the National Adoption Center has a photo listing and other adoption information.

and misleading. Others focus on personal stories with suggestions that do not apply to all women. Because of the intensely personal nature of infertility, many women are incredibly vulnerable. Nurses can assist women to critically analyze information from the Internet so that they do not become victims of unscrupulous people and practices.

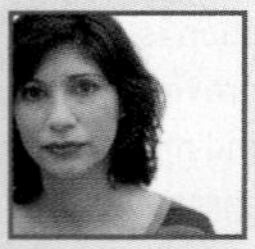

Remember Stacy, the 42-year-old woman undergoing a routine examination, who voices concerns about her ability to get pregnant. What if Stacy states, "Maybe this is God's way of telling me I wasn't supposed to be a mother." What nursing responses would be most appropriate?

CAUSES OF INFERTILITY

Box 10.2 categorizes the major causes of infertility. Generally, causes tend to be biologic, environmental, related to lifestyle, or physical in nature. The physical factors can be grouped further as female factor, male factor, or combined.

Biologic Factors

Advancing Age

"I spent much of my 20s and 30s taking steps to avoid becoming pregnant. I never thought that when I was finally ready to have a child, the option might not be open to me."

A 42-year-old woman undergoing fertility treatments

Chief among biologic factors in infertility is age. In general, a woman's fertility begins at menarche, peaks during her 20s, and then declines gradually until menopause, when it ends. Because women increasingly are electing to become established in their careers before they have children, they often delay attempting pregnancy until after their peak years of fertility. Women who delay pregnancy until later in life may find that their biologic clock has moved more quickly than anticipated. The quality and number of ova, as well as the quality of sperm, decline with age (Lane, 2006; Swanton & Child, 2005). The timing of the hormonal changes associated with menopause varies in women, which may pose challenges for some older women who have delayed pregnancy to a point at which they also are perimenopausal.

Sexually Transmitted Infections

Women who have multiple sexual partners, or who have sex with partners who have had multiple partners, are at

BOX 10.2 Causes of Infertility

Biologic
Age
Genetics
Sexually transmitted infections

Environmental/occupational
Heat
Chemicals
Radiation
Environmental toxins

Lifestyle
Smoking
Alcohol use
Substance/drug use
Delaying pregnancy
Decreased frequency of coitus
Obesity

Physical

Female Factors
Cervical factors
Uterine factors
Tubal factors
Hormonal factors
Ovulatory factors
Coital factors
Endometriosis

Male Factors
Sperm production
Sperm transport
Ejaculatory problems
Coital factors
Genetic factors

Combined Factor
Sperm antibodies
Coital difficulties

Unknown Cause

increased risk for acquiring sexually transmitted infections (STIs) (Niccolai et al., 2004; Santelli et al., 1998). Some infections, such as chlamydia, are associated closely with decreased fertility (Idahl et al., 2004). Women with untreated or chronic pelvic infections are at risk for having narrowed or blocked fallopian tubes, which decreases the possibility of fertilization, increases the risk for ectopic pregnancy, or both (Mardh, 2004).

Genetic Conditions

The cause of infertility may be genetic. For example, Turner's syndrome is a condition in which one of the two sex chromosomes is completely or partially absent, resulting in a phenotypic female with gonadal dysgenesis in 90% of cases (Beers & Berckow, 2004). Those with Turner's syndrome have markedly compromised or completely absent fertility. Men with cystic fibrosis, another genetic condition, almost always are infertile because of a congenital bilateral absence of the vas deferens. Many men with mild cystic fibrosis are diagnosed with the condition only when they seek counseling and treatment for infertility (Kolettis & Sandlow, 2002; Sharlip et al., 2002). Clients with infertility related to genetic conditions require counseling about their chances of passing the same conditions to offspring, should they be able to achieve pregnancy, carry a fetus to viability, or both.

Environmental Factors

Many environmental toxins can affect fertility. As women gain increasing access to employment opportunities, they become exposed to workplace hazards from which they were once shielded. Environmental hazards include toxic chemicals, excessive heat, air pollution, and noise. For example, until gas-scavenging systems were required in operating rooms, women working in operating rooms were at increased risk for spontaneous abortions (Panni & Corn, 2002).

Lifestyle Factors

Many lifestyle choices can affect fertility adversely. Cigarette smoking negatively affects both male and female fertility (Practice Committee of the ASRM, 2004; Windham et al., 2005). Heavy alcohol consumption negatively influences fertility and has adverse affects on the developing fetus (Klonoff-Cohen, Lam-Kruglick, & Gonzalez, 2003). Use of illegal substances can interfere with the hypothalamic-pituitary feedback loop and the production of gonadotropins (Farah, 2000). Dual-career couples with heavy job demands may find themselves with decreased opportunities for sexual activity at the optimal time for conception.

Obesity can affect fertility (Linne, 2004). Fat cells convert adrenal hormones into estrogens. A steady supply of estrogen from this peripheral source ultimately will interfere with the ovarian production of estrogen, disrupting ovulation and causing infertility.

Several of the lifestyle factors affecting fertility are modifiable. Nurses should encourage clients to decrease behaviors that may compromise their fertility. They should promote healthy lifestyles that include abstention from cigarettes, recreational drugs, and excessive alcohol consumption. Exercise, healthy diet, and stress management are essential (see Chap. 2). Clients also should be counseled on safe sexual practices and be made aware of potential environmental hazards that may affect fertility. See Teaching Tips 10.1 for more information.

TEACHING TIPS 10.1 Methods to Enhance Fertility

The nurse should counsel the client or couple as follows:

- Reduce stress, particularly stress related to the issue of becoming pregnant. Discuss your desires and frustrations with your partner, particularly if sex starts to become a "chore."
- Avoid use of douches and lubricants before, during, and after intercourse. These substances can interfere with sperm motility and alter the chemical balance of cervical mucus.
- After engaging in intercourse, the woman trying to become pregnant should remain flat in bed. This position can help sperm flow more steadily to the cervix. The woman should not rise from this position for 20 to 30 minutes.
- The best timing for sexual intercourse is every 36 to 48 hours while the woman is ovulating. Discuss methods for predicting ovulation and planning intercourse to achieve pregnancy directly with your health care provider.
- Maintain good nutrition.
- Get regular exercise.
- Avoid tobacco, alcohol, and recreational drugs.

Physical Factors and Classification

Approximately one third of infertility problems are attributable to female-factor infertility; slightly less than one third are tied to male-factor infertility (ASRM, 2006). Approximately 20% of problems result from combined male and female factors (ASRM, 2006). In approximately 15% of cases, infertility cannot be classified as attributable to any one party or cause (ASRM, 2006).

Female Factor Infertility

Hormonal Problems. In women, infertility can result from alterations in hormonal activity of the hypothalamus, pituitary gland, thyroid gland, adrenal glands, or ovaries. Each organ has an important role in secreting hormones necessary for a normal menstrual cycle (Fig. 10.1).

Hypothalamus. Alterations in the hypothalamus cause changes in levels of estrogen and gonadotropin-releasing hormone (GnRH). Such alterations may result from stress, eating disorders, or intensive exercise (eg, gymnastics). Conditions in which body fat and total body weight are decreased markedly may lead to anovulation. If a cause for the hypothalamic disturbance can be identified, the condition may be easily reversible. Treatment is more difficult if the etiology of the disturbance is unknown (Star, Lommel & Shannon, 2004).

Pituitary Gland. The pituitary gland secretes follicle-stimulating hormone (FSH) and luteinizing hormone (LH), both of which are key regulators of ovulation. FSH is responsible for the events that trigger the development of the ovarian follicle, and LH level surges with ovulation. The pituitary gland also is responsible for the production of prolactin, which normally emerges after childbirth to promote lactation. Elevated prolactin levels in the non-breastfeeding woman can cause anovulatory cycles and resultant infertility. Although a common cause of elevated prolactin levels is a tumor called a pituitary adenoma, certain medications can lead to this problem, as can hypothyroidism (Star et al., 2004).

Thyroid Gland. Alterations in thyroid hormones also may be related to infertility. In the hypothyroid state, a woman may experience increased frequency of menstruation. The unopposed thyroid-releasing hormone (because the thyroid is not producing enough thyroid hormones) from the hypothalamus stimulates the pitu-

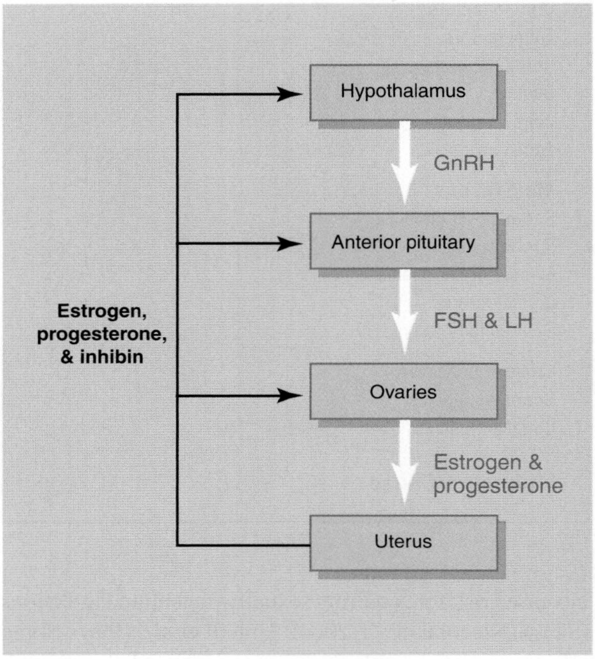

FIGURE 10.1 Role of hormones in fertility. Gonadotropin-releasing hormone (GnRH) released from the hypothalamus regulates production of luteinizing hormone (LH) and follicle-stimulating hormone (FSH) in the anterior pituitary. LH stimulates the release of estrogen and progesterone from the ovaries. FSH stimulates maturation of the ovarian follicle. Estrogen, a hormone produced by the ovaries, is responsible for secondary sex characteristics and cyclic changes in the lining of the uterus and vagina. Progesterone, another hormone produced by the ovaries, prepares the uterus for the development of the fertilized ovum and maintains the uterus throughout pregnancy.

itary gland to make excess prolactin. In turn, this situation interferes with the pituitary feedback cycle and may affect production of LH and FSH.

In the hyperthyroid state, the woman may experience decreased or absent menses. Hyperthyroid conditions are often autoimmune in nature and coexist with autoimmune ovarian problems, in which antibodies are directed at the ovaries and prevent them from participating in menses (Becks & Burrow, 2000).

Hyperthyroidism and hypothyroidism in men can alter spermatogenesis by interfering with the hypothalamic-pituitary feedback loop (Shaban, 2003).

Adrenal Gland. Adrenal dysfunction can lead to male and female infertility. The adrenal glands produce androgens in men and women (in women, estrogen and progesterone usually counter these androgens). In some conditions, such as adrenal hyperplasia and adrenal tumors, excess androgen is produced. Secondary to this excess steroid production, women may experience ovulatory failure; men may experience azoospermia (Beers & Berckow, 2004).

Ovaries. The ovaries also secrete hormones, and alterations in ovarian function may be related to infertility. **Polycystic ovarian syndrome** (PCOS) is a common cause of ovarian dysfunction (Lane, 2006). Manifestations of PCOS include the following symptoms in any combination: obesity, hirsutism, amenorrhea or irregular menses, and subsequent infertility. The condition is associated with a hypothalamic-pituitary-ovarian imbalance that results in elevated levels of estrogen, testosterone, and LH. There is also associated hyperinsulinemia and impaired glucose tolerance. The condition also is linked with the adverse health outcomes of cardiovascular disease, type 2 diabetes mellitus, and endometrial carcinoma (Farah, 2000).

Treatment depends on the symptoms most bothersome to the client. The health care provider may prescribe oral contraceptives to regulate menstruation and decrease levels of LH and testosterone (decreasing hirsutism). If the client desires pregnancy, the health care provider may prescribe clomiphene (Clomid) to correct the hormone imbalance and induce ovulation. He or she also may prescribe metformin to treat impaired glucose tolerance. Metformin reduces glucose produced in the liver and increases the cellular uptake of glucose. Another drug class that may be prescribed is the glitazones to increase insulin sensitivity in the muscles and adipose tissue and to inhibit hepatic glucose production.

Another common condition is **premature ovarian failure.** All the eggs that a woman ever will produce develop in a rudimentary fashion while she is still in utero (see Chap. 11). Her number of eggs decreases steadily until menopause (Swanton & Child, 2005). In some women, however, this process is accelerated markedly, so that they begin to experience symptoms of menopause 10 or more years earlier than would normally be expected (Swanton & Child, 2005). Causes include genetic conditions with chromosomal abnormalities, autoimmune disease, surgical removal of the ovaries, or damage to the ovaries by virus, chemotherapy, or radiation. Women with premature ovarian failure may not be able to become pregnant with their own eggs. Symptoms of menopause (eg, hot flashes, vaginal dryness, decreased libido) can be treated with hormone replacement. Clients with this condition need to take preventive measures against osteoporosis and heart disease (see Chap. 2).

Tubal Problems. In some women, the cause of infertility is tubal. Fallopian tubes can become narrowed or scarred from ascending pelvic infection, inflammation from an intrauterine device [IUD], surgical adhesions, or previous ectopic pregnancy. Pelvic adhesions from conditions such as endometriosis (see later discussion) can prevent free movement of the fallopian tubes, making them less able to capture extruded eggs. Tubal problems can result in the inability of egg and sperm to meet or of the fertilized ovum to reach the uterus. In some women, previous sterilization surgery may be reversed successfully; in others, the tubes may be reanastomosed successfully, but these women still cannot achieve fertility.

Cervical Problems. The reason for infertility may be a problem in the uterine cervix. Examples include cervical stenosis and suboptimal cervical mucus.

Cervical stenosis is the narrowing or closing of the cervical os. It may be congenital or the result of previous surgery from improper healing or scarring. This closing of the cervical opening can impair or prevent the ability of sperm to enter the uterus for fertilization of an egg.

Cervical mucus provides nutrients for sperm as they move toward the egg. This mucus also can either facilitate or prevent the passage of sperm into the uterus. The structure of cervical mucus acts as a filter for abnormally formed sperm and sperm with antibodies attached. Cyclic influences of hormones on mucus also make it more or less navigable by sperm. Near ovulation, estrogens cause the mucus to become watery and penetrable by sperm so that the sperm can swim easily toward the egg awaiting fertilization. Progesterone causes the mucus to become viscous and impenetrable by sperm.

Uterine Problems. Some women have anatomic alterations of the uterus that compromise fertility. For example, fibroid tumors can mechanically obstruct the cervix, endometrial cavity, or fallopian tubes, preventing union of egg and sperm. They also can distort the endometrial cavity and interfere with proper implantation of a fertilized egg. A tumor may impede blood flow to the developing embryo because the tumor requires vasculature to support it. This often is found to be the cause of infertility in women who have had multiple miscarriages (Marchionni et al., 2004).

Diethylstilbestrol [DES] is a synthetic estrogen that was used from the 1950s to the 1970s to reduce incidence of early pregnancy loss, intrauterine fetal demise, and preterm delivery. It was later determined that DES actually may have increased rates of spontaneous abortion, preterm delivery, and perinatal death; its use was banned in 1971 (Goldberg & Falcone, 1999). Unfortunately, the effects of DES were not limited to the women who took it themselves. Women whose mothers took DES during their pregnancies may have congenital abnormalities that compromise fertility. DES is believed to interfere in mullerian development with subsequent reproductive structure abnormalities. A "DES daughter" may have vaginal abnormalities (eg, adenosis), cervical abnormalities (eg, collars, hoods, septae), and uterine malformations (eg, T-shaped uterus, constriction bands) (Goldberg & Falcone, 1999). In addition to structural reproductive abnormalities, DES also may cause poor cervical mucus, endometriosis, and irregular menses, which can all contribute to infertility (Goldberg & Falcone, 1999). Men with in utero exposure to DES may have sperm and semen abnormalities that do not affect their fertility (Schrager & Potter, 2004).

Endometrial Problems. Endometriosis is a condition in which bits of the endometrial lining, normally attached to the inner lining of the uterus, become part of the abdominal cavity (Fig. 10.2). This misplaced endometrial tissue undergoes the same cyclic changes as intrauterine endometrium. Resulting cyclic stimulation and bleeding of the endometrial tissue cause local inflammation, scarring, and adhesions. These problems, in turn, can lead to anatomic distortions that preclude normal functioning and, subsequently, to infertility. In addition, the woman with endometriosis can experience dyspareunia (severe discomfort with intercourse), which may cause her to avoid or to limit coitus.

Male Factor Infertility

Sperm Problems. Male infertility can result from problems with sperm production or transport (Table 10.2). Normal semen contains at least 20 million sperm per milliliter, of which 50% demonstrate normal forward progression and 30% or more have normal morphology (Mayo Clinic, 2004). The normal ejaculate is at least 2 mL in volume (Mayo Clinic, 2004). Decreased volume may result from retrograde ejaculation, a condition in which the sphincter between the urethra and bladder relaxes. As a result, some ejaculate enters the bladder rather than being expelled through the penis into the vagina of the female partner. A low sperm count may result from increased scrotal temperature, infection, or chronic illness. Trauma or infection may lead to decreased sperm motility. High numbers of sperm with abnormal morphology may result from environmental toxins or testicular cancer (Star et al., 2004).

Sperm transport problems are often anatomic in nature. Hydroceles, spermatoceles, or varicoceles are abnormalities that cause increased vascularity, raising the temperature in the scrotum and diminishing the viability of sperm (Mayo Clinic, 2004). Congenital bilateral absence of the vas deferens causes total obstruction of the transport system. In this condition, sperm are

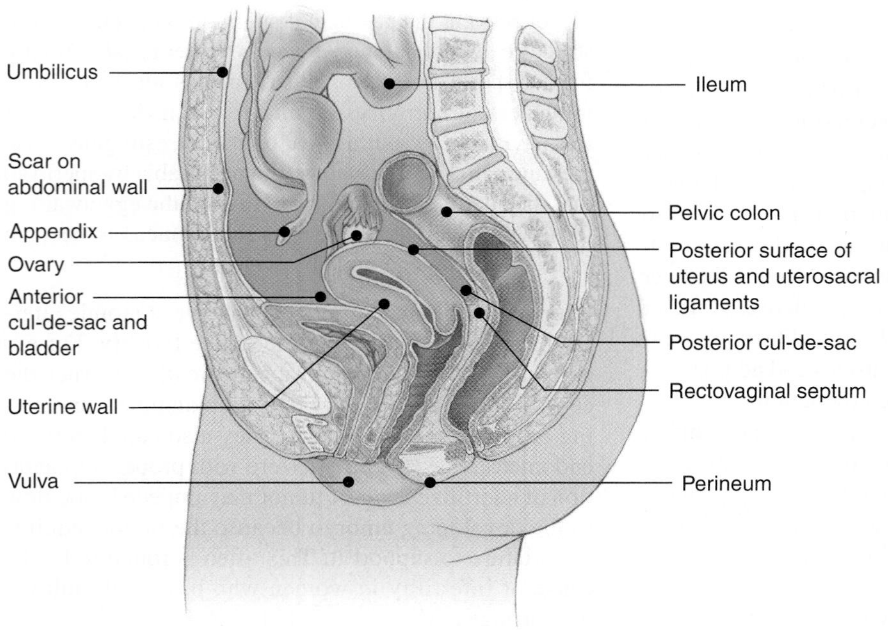

FIGURE 10.2 Common sites of endometriosis.

TABLE 10.2 Normal Values for Semen Analysis

Volume	2–5 mL
Liquefaction	Complete in 20–30 min
Count	>20 million per mL
Motility	>60% mobile after 1 h
	>50% mobile after 2 h
Morphology	<40% of total
White blood cells	None
Bacteria	None to few

manufactured in normal quantities and of normal quality, but their ability to traverse the tubules is impaired. Men with cystic fibrosis almost always have congenital bilateral absence of the vas deferens, causing absolute infertility.

Erectile and Ejaculatory Problems. The penis must introduce sperm into the vagina for successful transfer of sperm through the cervix and into the uterus and fallopian tubes. Some men have difficulty achieving and maintaining an erection, making successful completion of intercourse impossible. Other men can achieve an erection, but suffer from premature ejaculation, in which they ejaculate before sperm are introduced into the vagina, thereby eliminating the chance for fertilization of an egg. Men with spinal cord injury or neuropathies may fail to ejaculate or have retrograde ejaculation, in which case semen is delivered to the man's bladder instead of to the woman's vagina.

Hypospadias. Still other men have hypospadias, a condition in which the urethral opening is on the underside of the penis rather than at its tip (Fig. 10.3). In some cases, the urethral opening is at the juncture of the penis and the scrotum. A man with hypospadias may be able to have sexual intercourse, but the ejaculate is not delivered deep into the vagina, making it less likely that sperm will reach the outer third of the fallopian tube. A man with severe hypospadias may deliver his ejaculate totally on his partner's external genitalia.

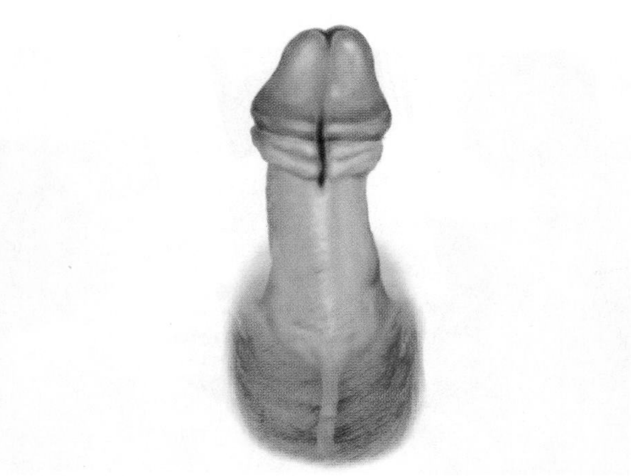

FIGURE 10.3 Hypospadias may be a male physical factor contributing to infertility.

Other Causes of Infertility

Some couples have *combined factor infertility,* in which the woman makes antibodies to her partner's sperm. These people may not have impaired fertility alone; however, as a couple, the antisperm antibodies in the female's cervical mucus cause the sperm to become immobile before they can traverse the cervix.

Other couples have difficulty with sexual intercourse because of anatomic factors. Examples include obesity and confusion or limited knowledge about coital technique. Environmental factors such as inadequate privacy may lead to hasty coital episodes that end prematurely.

Infertility of Unknown Cause

"The most difficult parts of dealing with infertility for us have been the uncertainty and the lack of closure. No one has been able to explain why we can't get pregnant. Every time we make love, I wonder if maybe this time we'll be lucky. The ongoing disappointments are sometimes unbearable."

A man who has been trying with his wife for pregnancy for more than 3 years

Infertility for which a definitive cause cannot be identified accounts for 15% of all cases (ASRM, 2006). This situation can be especially frustrating for clients, particularly because they never know whether their situation is modifiable or unchangeable. They may feel guilt if they decide to give up trying; alternatively, they may feel increasing frustration for continuing their quest to have a biologic child without results. These clients may need additional counseling and resources to handle the especially challenging physical and psychological effects of this situation.

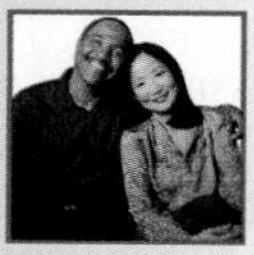

Ted and Joan, the couple described at the beginning of the chapter, have decided to pursue further testing for infertility. During a visit, Ted states, "What if they can't find anything wrong?" How should the nurse respond?

COLLABORATIVE CARE: INFERTILITY

The realization that a couple has a problem with infertility can generate stress and negative emotions. Societal and cultural messages exalt sexual prowess and performance. Couples who cannot successfully achieve pregnancy may feel inadequate and that they do not measure up to societal standards (Brucker & McKenry, 2004).

ASSESSMENT TOOL 10.1 Infertility Questionnaire

SELF-IMAGE

1. I feel bad about my body because of our inability to have a child.
2. Since our infertility, I feel I can do anything as well as I used to.
3. I feel as attractive as before our infertility.
4. I feel less masculine/feminine because of our inability to have a child.
5. Compared with others, I feel I am a worthwhile person.
6. Lately, I feel I am sexually attractive to my wife/husband.
7. I feel I will be incomplete as a man/woman if we cannot have a child.
8. Having an infertility problem makes me feel physically incompetent.

GUILT/BLAME

1. I feel guilty about somehow causing our infertility.
2. I wonder if our infertility problem is due to something I did in the past.
3. My spouse makes me feel guilty about our problem.
4. There are times when I blame my spouse for our infertility.
5. I feel I am being punished because of our infertility.

SEXUALITY

1. Lately I feel I am able to respond to my spouse sexually.
2. I feel sex is a duty, not a pleasure.
3. Since our infertility problem, I enjoy sexual relations with my spouse.
4. We have sexual relations for the purpose of trying to conceive.
5. Sometimes I feel like a "sex machine," programmed to have sex during the fertile period.
6. Impaired fertility has helped our sexual relationship.
7. Our inability to have a child has increased my desire for sexual relations.
8. Our inability to have a child has decreased my desire for sexual relations.

Note: The questionnaire is scored on a Likert scale, with responses ranging from "strongly agree" to "strongly disagree." Each question is scored separately, and the mean score is determined for each section (Self-image, Guilt/Blame, and Sexuality). The total mean score is then divided by 3. A final mean score of greater than 3 indicates distress.

From AWHONN. Bernstein, J., Potts, N., and Mattox, J. H. (1985). Assessment of psychological dysfunction association with infertility. *Journal of Obstetric, Gynecologic, and Neonatal Nursing, 14*(Suppl.), 64S, Table 1. Washington, DC: Author.

Couples who seek fertility treatment find themselves talking about the most intimate details and activities with complete strangers. Some couples disagree about the acceptability of doing so, thereby placing stress on a relationship that already may be strained. Sometimes women seek consultation during their annual gynecologic examinations and wish to have diagnostic assessment alone because their male partners are unwilling to discuss the issue.

Assessment

For some couples, the expense of the assessment process is a barrier. As of 2006, only eight states mandate insurance coverage for fertility treatment (International Council on Infertility Information Dissemination, Inc., 2004). Still other couples delay assessment and diagnosis because of the schedule necessary to complete the workup. Diagnostic tests are scheduled at specific times during a woman's cycle, often necessitating that she miss work. These absences can lead to further loss of income at a time when the cost of the infertility evaluation is increasing expenses.

Nurses caring for those experiencing infertility should be aware of the tremendous emotional stress that this condition can place on individuals, couples, and those who care for them (Assessment Tool 10.1). Sensitivity and support from nurses may make a tremendous difference in the ability of clients to maintain self-esteem and control during a difficult time. Nurses can remind couples that other options, such as adoption and child-free living, exist. If clients or couples express interest in such alternatives, nurses can act as advocates and supply resources and information. In all cases, the nurse works to ensure that clients understand that they themselves maintain control over options they wish to pursue and when they want to cease treatment (Fig. 10.4).

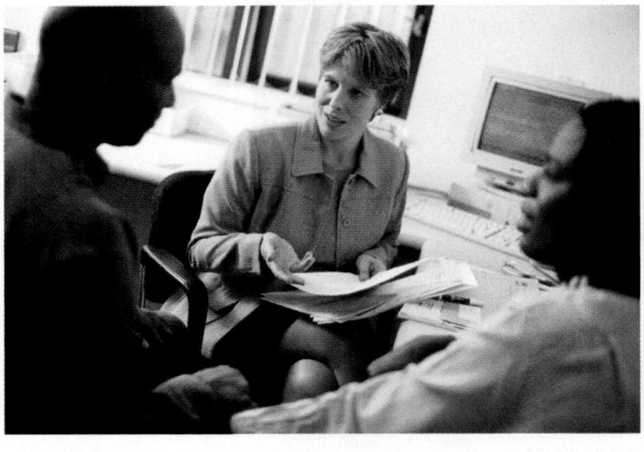

FIGURE 10.4 The nurse works as an advocate for clients and ensures that all decisions related to fertility rest with the woman or the woman and her partner.

Assessment of the Man

Assessment of the male partner should be completed early in the diagnostic process because it involves fewer invasive procedures and is less costly than is the process for women. Although some reproductive endocrinologists evaluate both men and women, a urologist usually completes the workup of the male partner.

Health History

The first step is gathering a complete health history, which should include the following information:

- Whether the man has ever achieved pregnancy with this or any other partner
- Exposure to environmental agents, such as chemicals or other toxins
- Exposure to heat, including the use of steam baths or wearing tight underwear or trousers
- Smoking, alcohol, or recreational drug use
- History of STIs
- History of postpubertal mumps or orchitis (which cause testicular atrophy), or genital trauma
- Family history, including whether his mother took DES during her pregnancy with him
- Family history of cystic fibrosis (congenital absence of vas deferens)
- Use of prescription or over-the-counter medications, or use of chemotherapeutic drugs
- Dietary adequacy

Assessment Tool 10.2 provides a sample Medical History Form to evaluate for male-factor infertility.

● ASSESSMENT TOOL 10.2 Infertility History Form for Men

Name:
Address:
Occupation: Age:
Employer:
Bus. Tel.:
Referred by:
Birth Place:
Birth Date:

Date:
Tel.:
Religion:
Ins.:
Cert. No.:
Gr. No.:
Name Rel./Friend:
Address:

All previous occupations:

List all states or countries in which you have lived:

Education: Please encircle the last grade you completed — Grade 5 6 7 8 — High School 1 2 3 4 — College 1 2 3 4 — Post Grad. ________ yrs. Degrees

CHIEF COMPLAINTS
Please list all symptoms you have NOW.
1. ______________
2. ______________
3. ______________
Routine checkup—no symptoms [ ]

P.I. Please do not write in this space.

Family History		Age	If Living Health	Age at Death	If Deceased Cause
Father					
Mother					
Brother or sister	1.				
	2.				
	3.				
	4.				
	5.				
Husband or wife					
Son or daughter	1.				
	2.				
	3.				
	4.				
	5.				
	6.				
	7.				

Please Encircle Has any blood relative had			Who
Cancer	no	yes	
Tuberculosis	no	yes	
Diabetes	no	yes	
Heart trouble	no	yes	
High blood pressure	no	yes	
Stroke	no	yes	
Epilepsy	no	yes	
Mental illness	no	yes	
Suicide	no	yes	
Congenital deformities	no	yes	

NOTE:
This is a confidential record of your medical history and will be kept in this office. Information contained here will not be released to any person except when you have authorized us to do so.

Continued

● ASSESSMENT TOOL 10.2 Infertility History Form for Men *(Continued)*

PERSONAL HISTORY
ILLNESS: Have you had
(Please Encircle all Answers no or yes)

Measles or German measles .... no yes	Gonorrhea or syphilis .... no yes	Mycins or other antibiotics .... no yes
Chickenpox or mumps .... no yes	Anemia or jaundice .... no yes	Merthiolate or mercurochrome ... no yes
Whooping cough .... no yes	Epilepsy .... no yes	Any other drug .... no yes
Scarlet fever or scarlatina .... no yes	Migraine headaches .... no yes	Any foods .... no yes
Pneumonia or pleurisy .... no yes	Tuberculosis .... no yes	Adhesive tape .... no yes
Diphtheria or smallpox .... no yes	Diabetes or cancer .... no yes	Nail polish or other cosmetics .... no yes
Influenza .... no yes	High or low blood pressure .... no yes	Tetanus antitoxin or serums ...... no yes
Rheumatic fever or heart disease ..... no yes	Nervous breakdown .... no yes	INJURIES: Have you had any
Arthritis or rheumatism .... no yes	Food, chemical or drug poisoning ... no yes	Broken bones .... no yes
Any bone or joint disease .... no yes	Hay fever or asthma .... no yes	Sprains or dislocations .... no yes
Neuritis or neuralgia .... no yes	Hives or eczema .... no yes	Lacerations (extensive) .... no yes
Bursitis, sciatica or lumbago ...... no yes	Frequent colds or sore throat ...... no yes	Concussion or head injury .... no yes
Polio or meningitis .... no yes	Frequent infections or boils .... no yes	Ever been knocked out .... no yes
Bright's disease or kidney infection ... no yes	Any other disease .... no yes	TRANSFUSIONS: Have you ever had
	ALLERGIES: Are you allergic to	Blood or plasma transfusion ...... no yes
	Penicillin or sulfa .... no yes	Weight: now ________ one year ago ________
	Aspirin, codeine or morphine .... no yes	Max ________ when ________ Height ________

Please review the section you have just completed and wherever you answered "yes" fill in the year (guess if necessary) and also where there is more than one illness to a line encircle the ones you have had. Example: Chickenpox or mumps.................... 1961....................... no (yes)

SURGERY: Have you had
Tonsillectomy .... no yes
Appendectomy .... no yes
Any other operation (give details) ... no yes

Give DETAILS below of all hospitalizations for surgery or illness including name and address of Doctor and Hospital ....

Have you ever been advised to have any surgical operation which has not been done? [1] no [2] yes what...........

Systems: Please check those you have had.
Eye disease [ ], Eye injury [ ], Impaired sight [ ], Ear disease [ ], Ear injury [ ], Impaired hearing [ ],
Trouble with: Nose [ ], Sinuses [ ], Mouth [ ], Throat [ ], Have you checked any in this group?.............................. no yes
Fainting spells [ ], Loss of consciousness [ ], Convulsions [ ], Paralysis [ ], Frequent or severe headaches [ ],
Dizziness [ ], Depression or anxiety [ ], Hallucinations [ ], Have you checked any in this group? .... no yes
Enlarged glands [ ], Goiter or enlarged thyroid [ ], Skin disease [ ], Have you checked any in this group? .... no yes
Chronic or frequent cough [ ], Chest pain or angina pectoris [ ], Spitting up of blood [ ], Night sweats [ ],
Shortness of breath [ ], Palpitation or fluttering heart [ ], Swelling of hands, feet, or ankles [ ],
Varicose veins [ ], Extreme tiredness or weakness [ ], Have you checked any in this group? .... no yes
Kidney disease or stones [ ], Bladder disease [ ], Albumin, sugar, pus, etc. in urine [ ], Difficulty in
urinating [ ], Awake to urinate nightly [ ], Have you checked any in this group?.. no yes
Stomach trouble or ulcers [ ], Indigestion [ ], Liver or gallbladder disease [ ], Colitis or other bowel disease [ ]
Appendicitis [ ], Hemorrhoids or rectal bleeding [ ], Constipation or diarrhea [ ], Recent change in bowel
action or stools [ ], Recent change in appetite or eating habits [ ], Have you checked any in this group? .... no yes

HABITS: Do you
Sleep well? .... no yes
Use alcoholic beverages .... no yes
Every day? .... no yes
Smoke? .... no yes
How much?..............
Exercise enough .... no yes
Is your diet well balanced? .. no yes

List any drugs or medications you take regularly or frequently:
____
____
____
____
____
____
____
____

Continued

● ASSESSMENT TOOL 10.2 Infertility History Form for Men

MARITAL HISTORY

Prior marriage?.. When? (Dates) ....

Was pregnancy achieved?.. Any other proof of fertility? ....

....

....

Is sex entirely satisfactory?.. Estimated frequency of coitus (intercourse) per month: ......

Reaction of wife: .... Remarks: ....

....

....

....

INFERTILITY STUDIES

	Result	Date	Where Done
Semen analysis:	....	....	....
Thyroid tests:	....	....	....
Hormone tests:	....	....	....
Medicines given:	....	....	....
Other tests:	....	....	....

....

....

(Courtesy of Division of Human Reproduction, Hospital of the University of Pennsylvania, Philadelphia, PA)

Physical Examination

The physical examination focuses on secondary sex characteristics, as well as the structure and function of the male reproductive organs.

Laboratory and Diagnostic Testing

Laboratory testing is done to ensure general well-being and may include assessment of serum FSH and testosterone levels (Sharlip et al., 2002). Depending on results of these tests, LH, free testosterone, and prolactin levels may be tested (Speroff & Fritz, 2004). See Table 10.3 for a complete summary of male hormone levels that may be examined.

Conditions such as diabetes should be ruled out. Diabetes in men can cause bladder neck dysfunction and result in retrograde ejaculation. A complete semen analysis

● TABLE 10.3 Male Hormone Levels

HORMONE TO TEST	NORMAL VALUES	WHAT VALUE MEANS
Testosterone	270–1100 ng/dL	Testosterone production is stimulated by Leydig cells in the testicles. Low levels of testosterone combined with low FSH and LH are diagnostic of hypogonadotropic hypogonadism.
Free testosterone	0.95–4.3 ng/dL	
% Free testosterone	0.3%–5%	A normal male has about 2% free, unbound testosterone.
Follicle-stimulating hormone (FSH)	1–18 mIU/mL	Basic hormone testing for males often only includes FSH and testosterone.
Prolactin	<20 ng/mL	A level two or three times that of normal may indicate a pituitary tumor, such as a prolactinoma, which may lead to decreased sperm production. Elevations can be treated with bromocriptine.
Luteinizing hormone (LH)	2–18 mIU/mL	LH stimulates Leydig cells and production of testosterone. A problem with LH levels alone is rarely seen, so testing is only needed if testosterone level is abnormal.
Estradiol (E2)	10–60 pg/mL	
Progesterone (P4)	0.3–1.2 ng/mL	

Available at: http://www.fertilityplus.org/faq/hormonelevels.html

should be performed on a specimen collected after 2 to 3 days of abstinence from intercourse. During a semen analysis, the examiner evaluates the volume of ejaculate, the percentage of motile sperm, the percentage of sperm with normal morphology, the total sperm count, liquefaction (semen should become liquefied within 60 minutes), and the number of white blood cells (indicates possible inflammation). The specimen usually is collected by masturbation. It is acceptable for the man to collect the specimen at home or in another private setting and deliver it to the laboratory within a specified period. If the specimen requires transport to the laboratory, the man should carry the specimen in an inner pocket so that it remains at body temperature until it can be analyzed.

Some men cannot produce a specimen by masturbating or have religious or other personal reservations about masturbating. Collecting the specimen in an unlubricated condom that does not contain any spermicides and is used during intercourse is possible. For the couple whose religion prohibits both masturbation and the use of condoms, poking a small hole in the condom before applying it may satisfy those concerns.

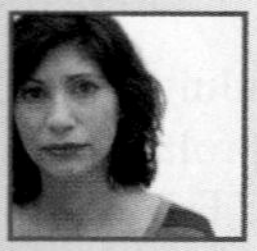

Stacy, the 42-year-old woman from the beginning of the chapter, reports that in her previous marriage, the health care providers couldn't find anything wrong. What questions would be important for the nurse to ask when assessing Stacy's situation?

Assessment of the Woman

Health History

Assessment of the woman also includes a detailed health history. The health care provider asks about genetic conditions like sickle cell anemia, β-thalassemia, or Tay-Sachs disease; a history of DES use by the woman's mother; previous pregnancies with this or another partner; surgery or trauma; infectious diseases; substance abuse; chronic illness; and dietary adequacy. He or she also elicits use of drugs, cigarettes, and alcohol; and family history of unexplained mental retardation, birth defects, perinatal or neonatal deaths, and chronic or early-onset health problems (Farah, 2000). Assessment Tool 10.3 provides a sample form used to evaluate for female factor infertility.

Physical Examination

The physical examination focuses on secondary sex characteristics, structure and function of the reproductive organs, and general well-being.

Laboratory and Diagnostic Testing

Laboratory tests to evaluate for infertility in the woman include routine analyses, evaluation of hormonal levels (serum progesterone, FSH, LH, and prolactin), Pap testing, and testing for chlamydia. See Table 10.4 for a complete summary of female hormone levels that may be examined.

Early in the workup, the health care team must document the status of the woman's immunity to rubella so that those clients without an appropriate titer can receive immunization in a timely fashion. Also, the health care provider should ensure that the woman is taking a folic acid supplement, as is recommended for all women of childbearing age, to reduce the risk for having a pregnancy in which the fetus has a neural tube defect.

Monitoring of Basal Body Temperature

This technique is used to predict the time of ovulation based on the thermogenic properties of serum progesterone. Body temperature should increase by 0.4° to 0.8°F when progesterone levels are highest, just after ovulation (Speroff & Fritz, 2004). The health care provider will ask the woman to keep a chart for several months monitoring her basal body temperature. Each morning, the client records her temperature immediately upon awakening (at rest) using the same thermometer. She plots the temperatures on a chart so that a pattern develops; subsequently, she can establish the time of ovulation, which precedes the increase in temperature. The woman also records her menses, any events that would alter her temperature (eg, infections, insomnia), and when she has intercourse. She also can record any symptoms, such as twinges during ovulation and the nature and character of her cervical mucus.

The nurse should evaluate the chart with the couple, helping to determine whether ovulation is occurring (just before the increase in body temperature) and, if cycles are regular, when to time intercourse to maximize chances of conception. A sample temperature chart is provided in Figure 10.5.

Postcoital Testing

Another test performed early in the workup is a *postcoital test.* It may be scheduled on or just before the expected date of ovulation, if a recurrent pattern can be determined from the basal body temperature chart. The health care provider instructs the woman to have intercourse 6 to 8 hours before her scheduled appointment and to avoid showering or douching between having sexual relations and arriving for the test. After a pelvic examination, the clinician removes and microscopically examines the woman's cervical mucus to determine its quality and character, as well as the number and motility of sperm (Fig. 10.6).

Many couples find this test stressful, viewing it as a quantitative assessment of sexual functioning. Because of this pressure, they often cannot complete intercourse at the prescribed time. Providers should warn them of

(text continues on page 340)

● ASSESSMENT TOOL 10.3 Infertility History Form for Women

Name:
(Nee):
Address: Age:
Occupation:
Employer:
Bus. Tel.:
Referred by:
Birth Place:
Birth Date:

Date:
Tel.:
Ins.:
Cert. No.:
Gr. No.:
Name Rel./Friend:
Address:

Unit No.:
Husb.:
Occupation: Age:
Employer
Bus. Address:
Bus. Tel.:
Religion: Husband: Wife:
[ ] Single [ ] Divorced
[ ] Married [ ] Widow (er)

All previous occupations:

List all states or countries in which you have lived:

Education: Please encircle the last grade you completed — Grade 5 6 7 8; High School 1 2 3 4; College 1 2 3 4; Post Grad. ________ yrs. Degrees

Date of last physical exam.
Chief Complaints: Please list all symptoms you have NOW.
1. ____________
2. ____________
3. ____________
Routine checkup—no symptoms [ ]

P.I. Please do not write in this space.

Family History		Age	If Living Health	Age at Death	If Deceased Cause
Father					
Mother					
Brother or sister	1.				
	2.				
	3.				
	4.				
	5.				
Husband or wife					
Son or daughter	1.				
	2.				
	3.				
	4.				
	5.				
	6.				

Please Encircle Has any blood relative had			Who
Cancer	no	yes	
Tuberculosis	no	yes	
Diabetes	no	yes	
Heart trouble	no	yes	
High blood pressure	no	yes	
Stroke	no	yes	
Epilepsy	no	yes	
Mental illness	no	yes	
Suicide	no	yes	
Congenital deformities	no	yes	

NOTE: This is a confidential record of your medical history and will be kept in this office. Information contained here will not be released to any person except when you have authorized us to do so.

PERSONAL HISTORY
ILLNESS: Have you had
(Please Encircle all Answers no or yes)

- Measles or German measles . . . no yes
- Chickenpox or mumps . . . no yes
- Whooping cough . . . no yes
- Scarlet fever or scarlatina . . . no yes
- Pneumonia or pleurisy . . . no yes
- Diphtheria or smallpox . . . no yes
- Influenza . . . no yes
- Rheumatic fever or heart disease . . . no yes
- Arthritis or rheumatism . . . no yes
- Any bone or joint disease . . . no yes
- Neuritis or neuralgia . . . no yes
- Bursitis, sciatica or lumbago . . . no yes
- Polio or meningitis . . . no yes
- Bright's disease or kidney infection . . . no yes
- Gonorrhea or syphilis . . . no yes
- Anemia or jaundice . . . no yes
- Epilepsy . . . no yes
- Migraine headaches . . . no yes
- Tuberculosis . . . no yes
- Diabetes or cancer . . . no yes
- High or low blood pressure . . . no yes
- Nervous breakdown . . . no yes
- Food, chemical or drug poisoning . . . no yes
- Hay fever or asthma . . . no yes
- Hives or eczema . . . no yes
- Frequent colds or sore throat . . . no yes
- Frequent infections or boils . . . no yes
- Any other disease . . . no yes

ALLERGIES: Are you allergic to

- Penicillin or sulfa . . . no yes
- Aspirin, codeine or morphine . . . no yes
- Mycins or other antibiotics . . . no yes
- Merthiolate or mercurochrome . . . no yes
- Any other drug . . . no yes
- Any foods . . . no yes
- Adhesive tape . . . no yes
- Nail polish or other cosmetics . . . no yes
- Tetanus antitoxin or serums . . . no yes

INJURIES: Have you had any

- Broken bones . . . no yes
- Sprains or dislocations . . . no yes
- Lacerations (extensive) . . . no yes
- Concussion or head injury . . . no yes
- Ever been knocked out . . . no yes

TRANSFUSIONS: Have you ever had

- Blood or plasma transfusion . . . no yes

Weight: now ________ one year ago ________
Max ________ when ________ Height ________

Please review the section you have just completed and wherever you answered "yes" fill in the year (guess if necessary) and also where there is more than one illness to a line encircle the ones you have had. Example: Chickenpox or mumps . . . 1961 . . . no (yes)

Continued

● ASSESSMENT TOOL 10.3 Infertility History Form for Women *(Continued)*

SURGERY: Have you had
Tonsillectomy .... no yes
Appendectomy .... no yes
Any other operation (give details) .... no yes

Give DETAILS below of all hospitalizations for surgery or illness including name and address of Doctor and Hospital....

Have you ever been advised to have any surgical operation which has not been done? [1] no [2] yes what............

Systems: Please check those you have had.
Eye disease [ ], Eye injury [ ], Impaired sight [ ], Ear disease [ ], Ear injury [ ], Impaired hearing [ ],
Trouble with: Nose [ ], Sinuses [ ], Mouth [ ], Throat [ ], Have you checked any in this group? .... no yes
Fainting spells [ ], Loss of consciousness [ ], Convulsions [ ], Paralysis [ ], Frequent or severe headaches [ ],
Dizziness [ ], Depression or anxiety [ ], Hallucinations [ ], Have you checked any in this group? .... no yes
Enlarged glands [ ], Goiter or enlarged thyroid [ ], Skin disease [ ], Have you checked any in this group? .... no yes
Chronic or frequent cough [ ], Chest pain or angina pectoris [ ], Spitting up of blood [ ], Night sweats [ ],
Shortness of breath [ ], Palpitation or fluttering heart [ ], Swelling of hands, feet, or ankles [ ],
Varicose veins [ ], Extreme tiredness or weakness [ ], Have you checked any in this group? .... no yes
Kidney disease or stones [ ], Bladder disease [ ], Albumin, sugar, pus, etc. in urine [ ], Difficulty in
urinating [ ], Awake to urinate nightly [ ], Have you checked any in this group? .... no yes
Stomach trouble or ulcers [ ], Indigestion [ ], Liver or gallbladder disease [ ], Colitis or other bowel disease [ ]
Appendicitis [ ], Hemorrhoids or rectal bleeding [ ], Constipation or diarrhea [ ], Recent change in bowel
action or stools [ ], Recent change in appetite or eating habits [ ], Have you checked any in this group? .... no yes

HABITS: Do you

Sleep well? .... no yes
Use alcoholic beverages..... no yes
Every day?............... no yes
Smoke?.................... no yes
How much?.............
Exercise enough............ no yes
Is your diet well balanced?... no yes

List any drugs or medications you take regularly or frequently:

______
______
______
______
______
______

OBSTETRICAL-GYNECOLOGICAL REVIEW

Age at first menstruation ______ Age at first coital experience ___ Number of living children (at present) ___
Number of pregnancies ______
Number of live births ______ Number of multiple pregnancies ______
Number of stillbirths (more than 20 weeks) ______
Number of abortions, miscarriages (20 weeks or less) ___
Number of children dead ___ Age of oldest child ___
Number of births with deformities ______

GYNECOLOGICAL HISTORY

Are menstrual cycles regular?........ Are your periods similar?........
Interval between periods ....
Length of flow .... Date of last menstrual cycle ....
Amount of flow .... [1] Light [2] Moderate [3] Heavy
Was the quality, quantity, and duration of flow for this last cycle similar in comparison with previous cycles?.................................
[1] No (specify how it differed) ....
.... [2] Yes
Has there been any bleeding in between periods? ....
[1] No [2] Yes (specify) ....
Were any medications taken during cycle? ....
[1] No [2] Yes (specify)
Dysmenorrhea (menstrual discomfort) ....
[1] None [2] Intermittent [3] Constant
Type of menstrual discomfort experienced
[1] None [3] Dull [5] Cramp
[2] Sharp [4] Ache [6] Backache

PREMENSTRUAL SYMPTOMS

Bloating.............................. no yes
Breast tenderness..................... no yes
Pelvic pain .... no yes
Backache .... no yes
Headache .... no yes
Irritability.......................... no yes
Edema .... no yes
Acne .... no yes

INTERMENSTRUAL DISCHARGE

Type [1] None [3] Yellow [5] White
[2] Tan [4] Bloody [6] Other (specify)
Amount .... Scant Heavy
Itching .... no yes
Odorless .... no yes
Frequent .... no yes
Regular pattern .... no yes

Continued

ASSESSMENT TOOL 10.3 Infertility History Form for Women

MARITAL HISTORY

Prior marriage?.......... When? (Dates) .... Was pregnancy achieved? ....

Is sex entirely satisfactory? .... Dyspareunia (discomfort during coitus): no ....yes ....

Estimated frequency of coitus .... Does coitus occur during menses? Yes .... No ....

(sexual intercourse) per month:..........

Reaction of husband:.......... On which days of flow? ....

Remarks: .... Is this consistent? ....

....

....

INDICATE THE INFORMATION FOR ANY OF THE FOLLOWING STUDIES WHICH YOU HAVE HAD

	Date	Result	Doctor
Basal body temperature record:			
Biopsy test:			
Thyroid test:			
Gas (Rubin) test:			
X-ray of uterus and tubes:			
Postcoital test: (survival of seed in your secretions)			
Cautery of cervix:			
Hormone test:			
Inseminations:			
Medicines given:			
Other:			

(Courtesy of Division of Human Reproduction, Hospital of the University of Pennsylvania, Philadelphia, PA)

TABLE 10.4 Female Hormone Levels

HORMONE TO TEST	TIME TO TEST	NORMAL VALUES	WHAT VALUE MEANS
Follicle-stimulating hormone (FSH)	Day 3	3–20 mIU/mL	FSH is often used as a gauge of ovarian reserve. In general, under 6 is excellent, 6–9 is good, 9–10 fair, 10–13 diminished reserve, 13+ very hard to stimulate. In PCOS testing, the LH:FSH ratio may be used in the diagnosis. The ratio is usually close to 1:1, but if the LH is higher, it is one possible indication of PCOS.
Estradiol (E2)	Day 3	25–75 pg/mL	Levels on the lower end tend to be better for stimulating. Abnormally high levels on day 3 may indicate existence of a functional cyst or diminished ovarian reserve.
Estradiol (E2)	Day 4–5 of meds	100+ pg/mL or 2× day 3	There are no charts showing E2 levels stimulation because there is a wide variation depending on how many follicles are being produced and their size. Most doctors will consider any increase in E2 a positive sign, but others use a formula of either 100 pg/mL after 4 days of stims, or a doubling in E2 from the level taken on cycle day 3.
Estradiol (E2)	Surge/hCG day	200+ pg/mL	The levels should be 200–600 per mature (18 mm) follicle. These levels are sometimes lower in overweight women.
Luteinizing hormone (LH)	Day 3	<7 mIU/mL	A normal LH level is similar to FSH. An LH that is higher than FSH is one indication of PCOS.
Luteinizing hormone (LH)	Surge day	>20 mIU/mL	The LH surge leads to ovulation within 48 hours.

Continued

● **TABLE 10.4 Female Hormone Levels *(Continued)***

HORMONE TO TEST	TIME TO TEST	NORMAL VALUE	WHAT VALUE MEANS
Prolactin	Day 3	<24 ng/mL	Increased prolactin levels can interfere with ovulation. They may also indicate further testing (MRI) should be done to check for a pituitary tumor. Some women with PCOS also have hyperprolactinemia.
Progesterone (P4)	Day 3	<1.5 ng/mL	Often called the follicular phase level. An elevated level may indicate a lower pregnancy rate.
Progesterone (P4)	7 dpo	>15 ng/mL	A progesterone test is done to confirm ovulation. When a follicle releases its egg, it becomes what is called a corpus luteum and produces progesterone. A level over 5 probably indicates some form of ovulation, but most doctors want to see a level over 10 on a natural cycle, and a level over 15 on a medicated cycle. There is no midluteal level that predicts pregnancy. Some say the test may be more accurate if done first thing in the morning after fasting.
Thyroid-stimulating hormone (TSH)	Day 3	0.4–4 uIU/mL	Midrange normal in most labs is about 1.7. A high level of TSH combined with a low or normal T_4 level generally indicates hypothyroidism, which can have an effect on fertility.
Free triiodothyronine (T_3)	Day 3	1.4–4.4 pg/ml	Sometimes the diseased thyroid gland will start producing very high levels of T_3 but still produce normal levels of T_4. Therefore, measurement of both hormones provides an even more accurate evaluation of thyroid function.
Free thyroxine (T_4)	Day 3	0.8–2 ng/dL	A low level may indicate a diseased thyroid gland or may indicate a nonfunctioning pituitary gland that is not stimulating the thyroid to produce T_4. If the T_4 is low and the TSH is normal, that is more likely to indicate a problem with the pituitary.
Total testosterone	Day 3	6–86 ng/dL	Testosterone is secreted from the adrenal gland and the ovaries. Most would consider a level above 50 to be somewhat elevated.
Free testosterone	Day 3	0.7–3.6 pg/mL	
Dehydroepiandrosterone sulfate (DHEAS)	Day 3	35–430 µg/dL	An elevated DHEAS level may be improved through use of dexamethasone, prednisone, or insulin-sensitizing medications.
Androstenedione	Day 3	0.7–3.1 ng/mL	
Sex hormone–binding globulin (SHBG)	Day 3	18–114 nmol/L	Increased androgen production often leads to lower SHBG
17-Hydroxyprogesterone	Day 3	20–100 ng/dL	Midcycle peak would be 100–250 ng/dL; luteal phase, 100–500 ng/dL
Fasting insulin	8–16 hours fasting	<30 mIU/mL	The normal range here doesn't give all the information. A fasting insulin of 10–13 generally indicates some insulin resistance, and levels above 13 indicate greater insulin resistance.

MRI, magnetic resonance imaging; PCOS, polycystic ovary syndrome; dpo, days post ovulation.
Available at: http://www.fertilityplus.org/faq/hormonelevels.html.

this development ahead of time and reassure them that it is common. Some health care facilities do not schedule the appointment ahead of time but have a clinician available for walk-in appointments, so that the woman can call to schedule the appointment after completing intercourse. Other couples agree for the woman to not let her partner know which specific day the test is scheduled, thus decreasing performance anxiety that may affect the male partner.

Endometrial Biopsy

An *endometrial biopsy,* performed during the second phase of a woman's menstrual cycle, provides information about hormonal influences on the adequacy of the endometrial lining and its ability to support a fertilized egg (Fig. 10.7). It is relatively noninvasive but gives basically the same information as serum progesterone levels or the basal body temperature (ie, that the client is ovulating). For this reason, it is not used unless the

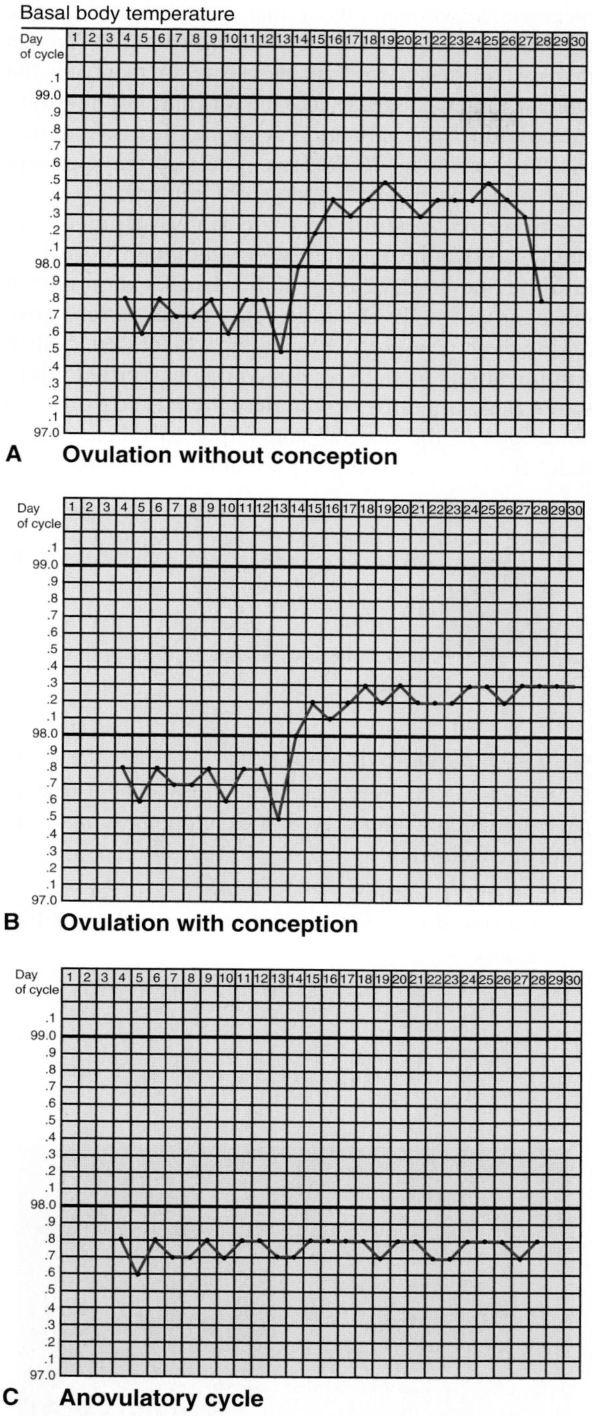

FIGURE 10.5 Sample basal body temperature chart recordings.

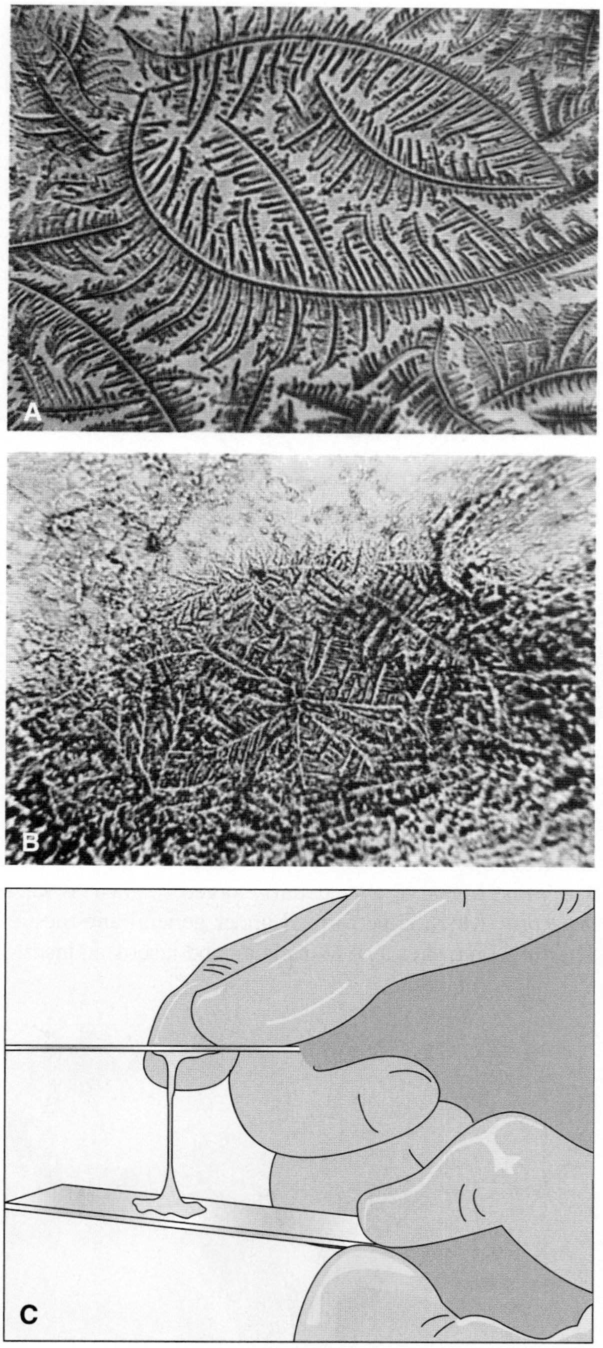

FIGURE 10.6 During assessment of cervical mucus, examiners will look for a ferning pattern to the mucus under the microscope. (**A**) shows ferning; (**B**) shows incomplete ferning. Another quality they will evaluate for is spinnbarkeit (the ability to stretch a distance before breaking), shown in part (**C**).

diagnostician also wishes to rule in or out endometrial hypertrophy.

Hysteroscopy and Hysterosalpingogram

A *hysteroscopy* or *hysterosalpingogram* may be performed to view the uterine cavity and determine tubal patency. These tests often are performed immediately after menses, when the woman is unlikely to be pregnant and the chance of disrupting a spontaneous pregnancy is minimal. Dye may be injected through the cervix under fluoroscopy (Fig. 10.8). The examiner then notes whether the dye traverses the uterus and fallopian tubes into the

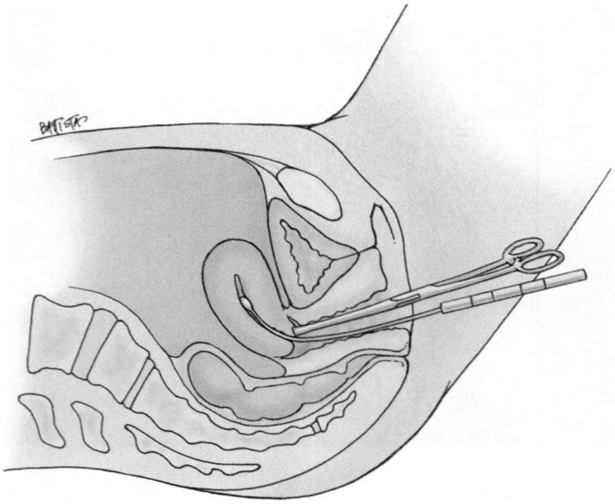

FIGURE 10.7 During endometrial biopsy, the examiner takes samples from the uterine lining to assess the hormonal levels of the endometrial tissue.

abdominal cavity. This test also can help determine the shape of the uterine cavity. Congenital defects of the uterine cavity (eg, septate uterus) or endometrial polyps or fibroids may be interfering with implantation or embryonic development. The hysterosalpingogram will show uterine or fallopian abnormalities but will not differentiate the cause. Laparoscopy is used to pinpoint the cause.

Laparoscopy

The most invasive test, usually saved for last, is *laparoscopy,* which is performed under general anesthesia. The surgeon makes a small incision and inserts an instrument into the woman's abdominal cavity to introduce gas, which is used to extend the abdominal cavity. The surgeon then inserts the laparoscope. He or she can then view the woman's internal organs, looking for causes of infertility such as adhesions, structural abnormalities, or endometrial implants (Fig. 10.9). He or she also may perform some minor ablation of endometrial implants.

Some physicians forego the hysterosalpingogram and insert dye through the cervix, looking for spillage into the abdominal cavity under direct vision during the laparoscopy. In rare occasions, complications arise during the procedure, necessitating a laparotomy. Such complications include bleeding and inadvertent injury to internal structures, which may include scarring and adhesions of the ovaries and fallopian tubes, potentially further compromising a woman's fertility.

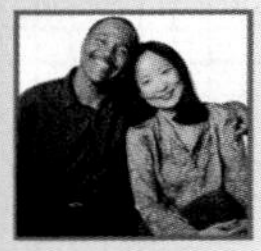

Joan, described at the beginning of the chapter, is scheduled to undergo a laparoscopy. She asks, "How will this test help us?" What teaching should the nurse provide?

Select Potential Nursing Diagnoses

Many nursing diagnoses can apply to the client or couple experiencing infertility. Some common examples include the following:

- **Ineffective Coping**
- **Situational Low Self-Esteem** related to the inability to conceive

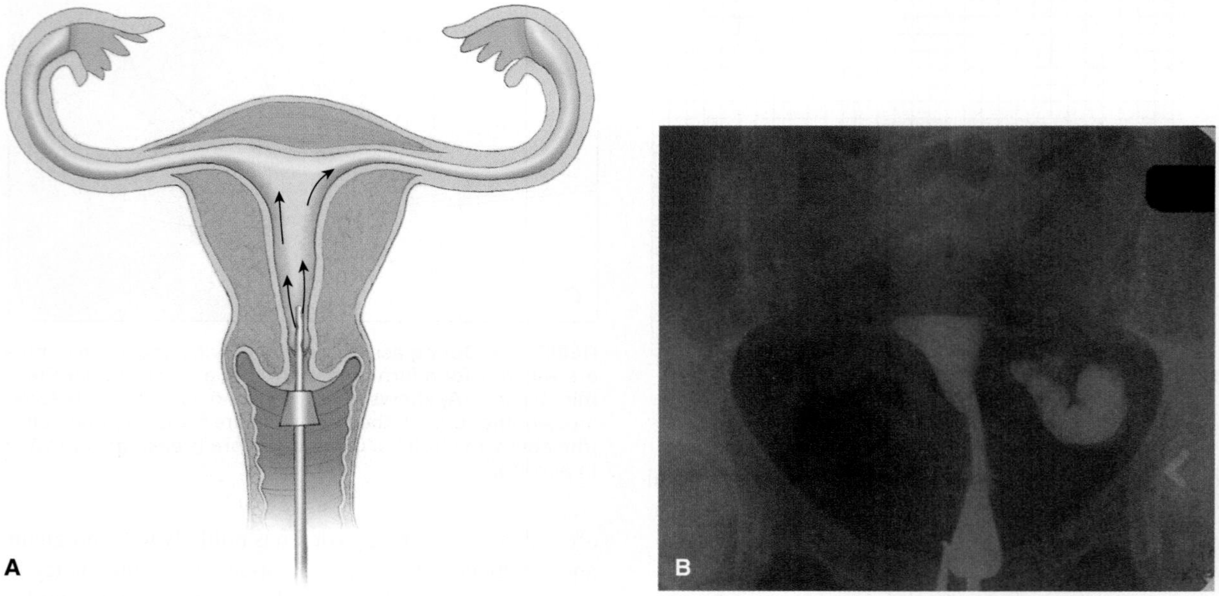

FIGURE 10.8 (**A**) During a hysterosalpingogram, examiners inject a dye into the woman's uterus. The dye outlines the uterus and fallopian tubes during radiography for evaluation of patency. (**B**) This image shows blockage of the right fallopian tube (*left* on image). The area remains dark and difficult to discern, indicating the inability of contrast medium to pass through.

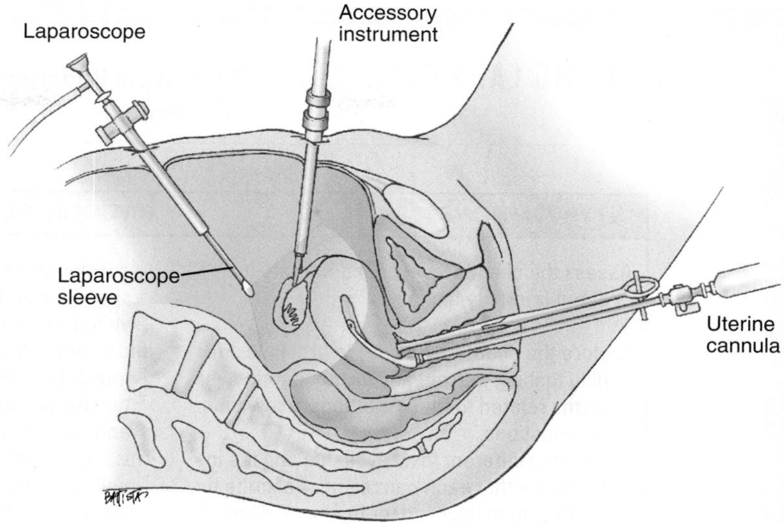

FIGURE 10.9 Diagnostic laparoscopy, the most invasive test for infertility, is used to visualize the internal pelvic organs directly, as well as to check for tubal patency.

- **Anxiety** related to diagnostic procedures, treatments, and outcomes
- **Deficient Knowledge** related to effects of lifestyle on fertility
- **Powerlessness** related to inability to control aspects of the situation
- **Grieving** related to actual or perceived losses

Planning and Intervention

Expected outcomes are individualized based on the client's particular circumstances (Nursing Care Plans 10.1 and 10.2). Some expected outcomes common to most clients might be as follows:

- The client (couple) will verbalize a realistic understanding of their circumstances and knowledge about any identified causes, as well as possible options.
- The client (couple) will discuss emotions related to the situation.

NIC/NOC Box 10.1 provides an overview of common intervention and outcome labels applied to infertility and its treatment.

(text continues on page 346)

NURSING CARE PLAN 10.1

The Couple Undergoing Examination of Infertility

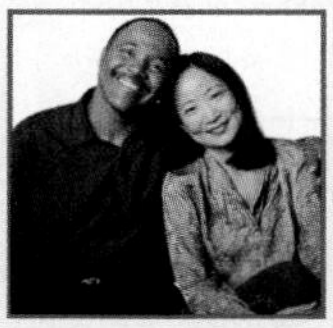

Recall Ted and Joan from the beginning of this chapter. Health history taking indicates that Joan's menstrual cycle is regular. Baseline vital signs and laboratory test results are normal. While discussing their situation, Joan says, "I know that Ted and I have to have some tests, but it sounds like there are so many. What are all these tests? This whole situation is so overwhelming. And, forget privacy. That's a thing of the past."

NURSING DIAGNOSIS

Deficient Knowledge related to infertility testing procedures and their indications

EXPECTED OUTCOMES

1. The client will identify the reasons for different testing procedures.
2. The client will state the implications of the results of testing.

Continued

NURSING CARE PLAN 10.1 ● The Couple Undergoing Examination of Infertility *(Continued)*

INTERVENTIONS	RATIONALES
Assess the client's level of understanding about infertility testing.	Assessment provides a baseline to identify specific client needs and to develop an individualized teaching plan.
Explore the client's exposure to previous infertility testing; correct any misconceptions or myths related to these methods; allow time for questions.	Information about exposure provides additional foundation for teaching and provides opportunities to clarify or correct misinformation and teach new information.
Explain the different tests available and the information that each can reveal. Describe the various methods used for testing and indications for each; include the client's husband in the discussion.	This information will help alleviate anxiety about unknown aspects of the process. Infertility testing involves testing of the male and female client. Involving the client's husband aids in preparing him for the tests.
Obtain a health history and physical examination of client and her husband.	Health history and physical examination aid in revealing possible factors contributing to infertility.
Inform the client's husband about blood tests and semen analysis; instruct husband how to collect semen sample and transport it to the laboratory properly.	Blood testing reveals information about hormonal levels; semen analysis provides information about the adequacy of the husband's sperm. Proper timely transport to the laboratory of the semen specimen is necessary for accurate results.
Instruct the client how to monitor basal body temperature, explaining that ovulation usually precedes the increase in temperature. Also encourage the woman to record additional information such as menses, times of intercourse, and events such as insomnia or infection.	Basal body temperature is used as a measure to determine ovulation. Documentation of additional information provides information about possible factors affecting temperature readings.
Teach client about postcoital testing, endometrial biopsy, hysteroscopy and hysterosalpingogram, and laparoscopy as appropriate.	Additional testing with these procedures may be indicated to determine possible causes of infertility.
Review the results of testing, explaining the findings in terms the couple can understand.	Knowledge of test results aids in couple's understanding of the underlying cause of infertility and proposed methods for treatment.
Offer support and guidance throughout the testing period.	Infertility testing can be a source of anxiety and frustration.

EVALUATION

1. The client explains the rationale for specific testing procedures.
2. The couple demonstrates understanding the tests and results.

NURSING DIAGNOSIS

Powerlessness related to lack of privacy involving sexual activity secondary to infertility testing

EXPECTED OUTCOMES

1. The couple will state that they feel some control over their sexual activity.
2. The couple will verbalize feelings of being less overwhelmed with testing.

Continued

NURSING CARE PLAN 10.1 ● The Couple Undergoing Examination of Infertility

INTERVENTIONS	RATIONALES
Assess the couple's concerns and feelings related to testing.	Assessment provides a baseline from which to develop an individualized plan of care.
Allow the couple to verbalize their feelings related to lack of privacy and feelings of sexual functioning on demand; encourage couple to role-play situations.	Verbalization of feelings allows for sharing and offering of support; role-playing provides an outlet for concerns and provides opportunities for teaching and support.
Reassure couple that their feelings are common; encourage them to participate in support groups.	Reassurance that feelings are common reduces anxiety and fear; participation in support groups promotes sharing of feelings with others who have similar experiences.
Encourage couple to actively participate in decision making related to testing as appropriate, such as which tests to complete first; advise the couple to focus on one aspect of testing at a time.	Active participation promotes feelings of control; focusing on one aspect minimizes feelings of being overwhelmed.
Remind couple about their reason for undergoing infertility testing, the ultimate outcome of having a child.	Reminding the couple helps to reinforce their commitment and desire for the ultimate outcome.

EVALUATION

1. The couple states they feel some control over their current situation.
2. The couple participates in infertility testing with minimal anxiety.

NURSING CARE PLAN 10.2 ● The Client Contemplating Fertility Testing

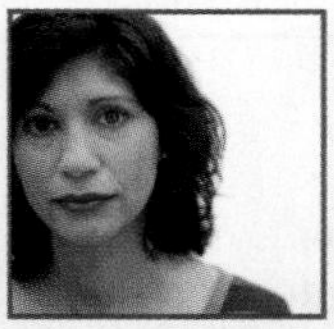

Remember Stacy, the 42-year-old woman from the beginning of the chapter. During her visit she openly talks about her situation. "As much as I want to know if we can hold out hope for having a baby, I'm afraid to learn the results. What if I am the one with the problem? I don't want to rob my husband of his chance to have a family."

NURSING DIAGNOSES

- **Situational Low Self-Esteem** related to feelings of failure secondary to concerns about inability to conceive a child
- **Anxiety** related to uncertainty of fertility status

EXPECTED OUTCOMES

1. The client will verbalize positive feelings about self and her relationship with her husband.
2. The client will state reduced anxiety about her fertility status.
3. The client and husband will verbalize feelings about their relationship and effect of infertility and its treatments on their relationship.

Continued

NURSING CARE PLAN 10.2 ● The Client Contemplating Fertility Testing *(Continued)*

INTERVENTIONS	RATIONALES
Assess the client's beliefs about her reproductive function, self-esteem, and body image. Explore her current understanding about fertility and its effect on her self-esteem and body image.	Assessment provides a baseline from which to develop appropriate strategies for teaching and care.
Communicate accurate facts and answer questions; clarify any misconceptions or misinformation.	Clear communication helps to provide accurate information to aid in alleviating fears and clarifying misinformation.
Explain the different tests available and the information that each can reveal.	This information will help alleviate anxiety about unknown aspects of the process.
Ask the client about measures used to cope with previous stressful situations; determine which measures were successful.	Identifying previous coping strategies helps to determine effective strategies for use in this situation.
Encourage client to include husband in visits.	Participation of client and husband promotes sharing.
Provide the couple with a chance to discuss any concerns, fears, or worries about their situation; encourage client and husband to share feelings.	Communication can reveal sources of stress and any problematic areas that need to be addressed; sharing of feelings aids in promoting positive coping.
Ask the couple about available support systems (eg, family, friends).	Identifying available support systems helps to help establish sources of assistance when one or both partners need help from other people.
Provide the couple with information about support groups, Web sites, and other avenues for education and assistance.	Shared experiences and knowledge of similar situations for others can help the couple prepare for what to expect and to realize that they are not alone.
Work with the client and her husband to establish measures to deal with infertility testing; role-play situations involving possible outcomes.	Establishing measures and role-playing helps clients be prepared for situations to promote adequate coping.
Assess client and partner for behaviors indicative of maladaptation or difficulty coping.	Early identification of problems fosters prompt treatment and can help prevent a crisis from escalating.

EVALUATION

1. The client demonstrates positive coping strategies related to infertility status.
2. The client and her husband identify helpful supports to deal with stresses related to infertility and its treatment.
3. The couple verbalize support and a firm commitment to each other regardless of the outcome.
4. The couple verbalize a realistic plan to handle their feelings about the situation and to address matters appropriately once they know more information.

Treatment options depend on the diagnosis. For some couples, financial concerns contribute to choices about which treatment options to pursue and how long to continue them. All options require strict adherence to complex regimens that involve expensive medications, scheduled sex, and repeated visits to the health care facility to monitor the woman's cycle and to plan treatment. The stress of the process can strain the couple's relationship and finances (Schneider & Forthofer, 2005). When working with clients considering treatments, the

NIC/NOC Box 10.1 Infertility Management

NIC

- Anxiety Reduction
- Calming Technique
- Coping Enhancement
- Counseling
- Decision-Making Support
- Emotional Support
- Family Planning: Infertility
- Fertility Preservation
- Genetic Counseling
- Preconception Counseling
- Reproductive Technology Management
- Specimen Management
- Support System Enhancement
- Teaching: Procedure/Treatment

NOC

- Anxiety Control
- Coping
- Decision Making
- Family Coping
- Knowledge: Fertility Promotion
- Knowledge: Treatment Procedures

nurse should emphasize that the decision whether to have treatment, which options to try, and when to say "enough" are theirs and theirs alone.

Many couples spend tens or hundreds of thousands of dollars pursuing the dream of a biologic child. Because of the emotional and financial investments involved, the nurse should counsel clients to ensure that the clinic with which they are working has experience and reasonable success in the modality of treatment most appropriate for the particular fertility problem. Clinics report their success rates to the ASRM; these are available from the CDC. Data are complex and difficult to interpret. A strong objective source for assistance in deciphering data is Resolve. This referral service can help clients determine whether the data they are reviewing are appropriate to their particular situation.

Costs and success rates for various treatments vary. Some women have insurance coverage for some options, but not for others. Health care providers may advise some couples to try options for different durations depending on their diagnosis, age, and personal preferences. See Box 10.3 for a summary of progressive treatment options for infertility.

"I got married last year and we tried to reverse my husband's vasectomy, but we couldn't. The only way I am going to get pregnant is through artificial insemination. But my insurance company will pay for my fertility treatment only if I have been married for at least 2 years to a man who is fertile. Who comes up with these rules?"

BOX 10.3 Progressive Treatment Options for Infertility

Male Infertility

Intrauterine insemination
Therapeutic donor insemination

Female Infertility

Ovulation induction
Assisted reproductive therapy
- In vitro fertilization
- Gamete intrafallopian transfer or zygote intrafallopian transfer
- In vitro fertilization with donor oocytes
- Intracytoplasmic sperm injection
- Gestational carrier

Artificial Insemination

Artificial insemination involves the use of a thin, flexible catheter to insert sperm directly into the vagina or directly into the uterus (Fig. 10.10). This procedure reduces the distance that sperm have to travel and can be effective in maximizing the chances of conception if the male partner's sperm count is relatively low. The semen sample is obtained by masturbation. After liquefaction, the specimen is centrifuged to separate the sperm from the seminal fluid. The sperm pellet is then resuspended in a nutritive medium and inserted into the uterus through a thin flexible catheter. The seminal fluid is removed because prostaglandins in the fluid could cause an anaphylactic reaction if delivered directly into the uterus. This procedure can be effective if the woman's cervical mucus contains antisperm antibodies by bypassing the vagina and cervix and delivering the sperm directly into the uterus. It also might be inserted into the vagina (unwashed sperm). The male partner who has a neurologic deficit rendering him incapable of erection and ejaculation can undergo electrical stimulation for ejaculation and delivery of the sperm into the vagina.

Donor Sperm

In cases in which the male partner has a genetic condition that the couple does not want to risk transmitting, the male is totally azospermic, or there is no male partner, a frozen specimen from an anonymous donor can be used. Sperm donor agencies generally adhere to donor screening guidelines but are self-regulated (Speroff & Fritz, 2004). Sperm donors should be screened for any transmittable problematic conditions before they donate. Speroff and Fritz (2004) recommend that there be repeat screenings (at each donation) for syphilis, gonorrhea, chlamydia, hepatitis B and C, cytomegalovirus, and HIV. The specimens should be frozen and quarantined for 6 months, at which time the donor should return for additional HIV testing. If the donor is found to be HIV negative, then the sample (whose sperm must be viable

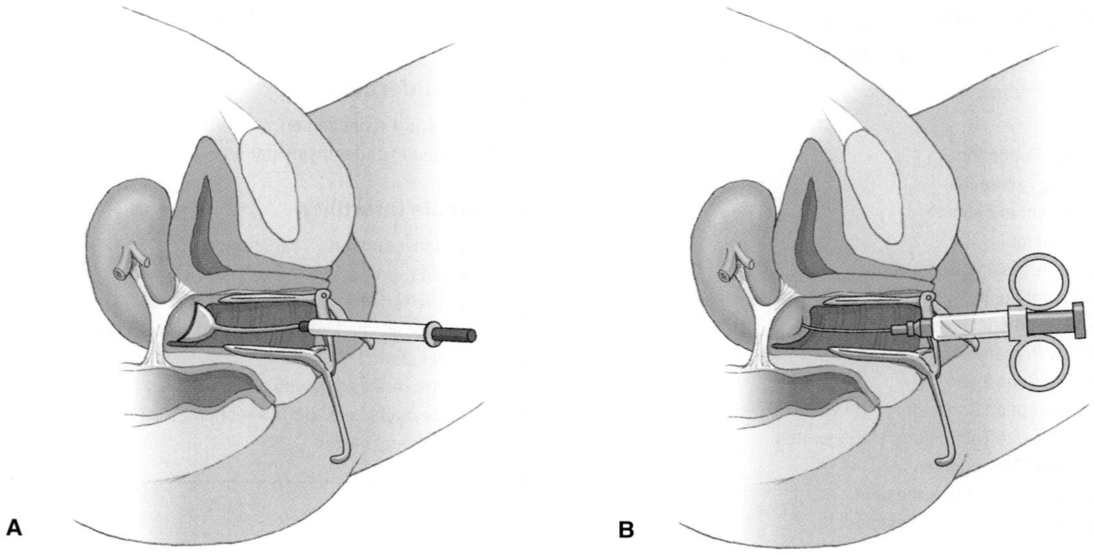

FIGURE 10.10 Procedure for artificial insemination. (**A**) A cervical capping device is used to place semen directly in contact with the cervix. (**B**) Semen is injected directly into the uterine cavity.

and motile after freezing) is released for use. Genetic screening should be included to determine carrier status of conditions like cystic fibrosis. Family and personal history and physical examination also are conducted to ensure the donor's general health. Couples can match sperm donors for any number of characteristics, depending on their personal preferences. Lesbians and single women who desire pregnancy may prefer the term *alternative insemination* to describe the process.

Ovarian Induction (Fertility Drugs)

Women who have alterations in ovulation may be treated with ovulation-inducing drugs (eg, clomiphene citrate [Clomid]) (Table 10.5). Medication regimens may take several months to achieve a satisfactory response, and the medications carry significant side effects. The risk for ovarian hyperstimulation is significant. In this condition, because of high levels of circulating hormones (serum estradiol and exogenous gonadotropins), the ovaries become enlarged. In extreme cases, intravascular fluid volume can shift into the peritoneal space, with resultant hypovolemia, oliguria, hemoconcentration, and massive ascites, which can result in death (Beers & Berckow, 2004). Thus, health care providers must monitor the woman's cycles to prevent this condition. If hyperstimulation does occur, the provider should instruct the woman to stop medication, avoid intercourse, and reduce the level of medication during a subsequent cycle.

Use of fertility drugs increases the chance of multiple gestation, which poses several risks to mother and fetus (see Chap. 13). Parents may face the prospect of reducing the number of fetuses for the safety of the mother and other fetuses. Often, one medication is used to mature and develop several follicles at once, and another is used to suppress the release of the follicles. With some medications, especially in combination, titrating the dose to provide the desired response and minimize untoward responses can be difficult. The level of risk depends on the medications and should be considered when planning treatment.

Women undergoing ovulation induction may engage in sexual intercourse or artificial insemination, depending on the availability of a male partner and the presence of male factor infertility.

Assisted Reproductive Technologies

For some couples, artificial insemination, use of donor sperm, or administration of fertility drugs does not produce pregnancy. They then must decide whether to pursue **assisted reproductive technologies** (ARTs). The CDC (2005) defines ART as all fertility treatments in which both eggs and sperm are handled. In general, these procedures involve surgically removing eggs from a woman's ovaries, combining them with sperm in the laboratory, and returning them to the woman's body or donating them to another woman. These procedures are expensive and considerably invasive. Success rates vary widely and depend on the specific procedure, the experience of the clinician, the age of the woman, the quality of the sperm, and the quality of the eggs. Many of the procedures involve similar steps, but some techniques may be more acceptable to couples than others, based on religious and personal beliefs.

In Vitro Fertilization

In vitro fertilization (IVF) was the first ART procedure developed (Fig. 10.11). The woman takes ovulation-inducing medications so that multiple follicles develop

TABLE 10.5 Commonly Used Fertility Drugs

CATEGORY	ACTION	DOSE	EXAMPLE
Selective estrogen receptor modulator (SERM)	Stimulates ovulation by causing the hypothalamus to produce GnRH, which causes the pituitary to produce more FSH and LH, which stimulates the ovary to release an egg	Tablets, start with 50 mg/day for 5 days; may increase to 200 mg/day	Clomid or Serophene (clomiphene citrate)
Follitropins (gonadotropins)	Similar to body's FSH; stimulates growth and maturation of ovarian follicle	75 IU/day	Fertinex (urofollitropin)
Menotropins (gonadotropins)	Promotes growth and maturation of ovarian follicle	Intramuscular regimens vary	Pergonal (FSH and LH from urine)
Human chorionic gonadotropin (hCG)	Induces ovulation by stimulating release of egg from mature follicle	2,000–10,000 units IM	Pregnyl (hCG extracted from urine)
GnRH agonists	Suppress production of LH and FSH, preventing premature LH surge and development of only one dominant follicle	Lupron—depot 375 mg every 28 days for 6 months; Synarel—200 μg intranasally twice daily for 6 months	Lupron (leuprolide acetate) Synarel (nafarelin acetate)
GnRH antagonists	Inhibits release of LH from pituitary to prevent premature LH surge	250 μg/day injected under the skin	Antagon (ganirelix acetate)
Progesterone	Prepares uterus for implantation of fertilized egg and maintain pregnancy	Vaginal suppositories, 25–50 mg twice daily or 50 mg each night; rectal suppositories, 12.25 mg every 12 hours; capsule, 100 mg orally 3 times day	Progesterone suppository, troche, or gel
Ergot alkaloid	Interrupts prolactin feedback to pituitary, allows for release of LH and FSH	Oral dose of 5–7.5 mg/day	Bromocriptine (Parlodel)

FSH, follicle-stimulating hormone; GnRH, gonadotropin-releasing hormone; LH, luteinizing hormone.

and mature. Serial ultrasounds are used to monitor the follicles. When the lead follicle reaches the appropriate size, the woman or her partner administers an intramuscular injection of a drug such as human chorionic gonadotropin. The purpose of the injection is so that the timing of ovulation can be determined accurately, and an egg retrieval procedure can be scheduled just before the expected ovulation. The retrieval is done under conscious sedation and with ultrasound guidance.

After the eggs are retrieved, they are fertilized with sperm from the male partner or a donor. An endocrinologist performs the fertilization in the laboratory. Several

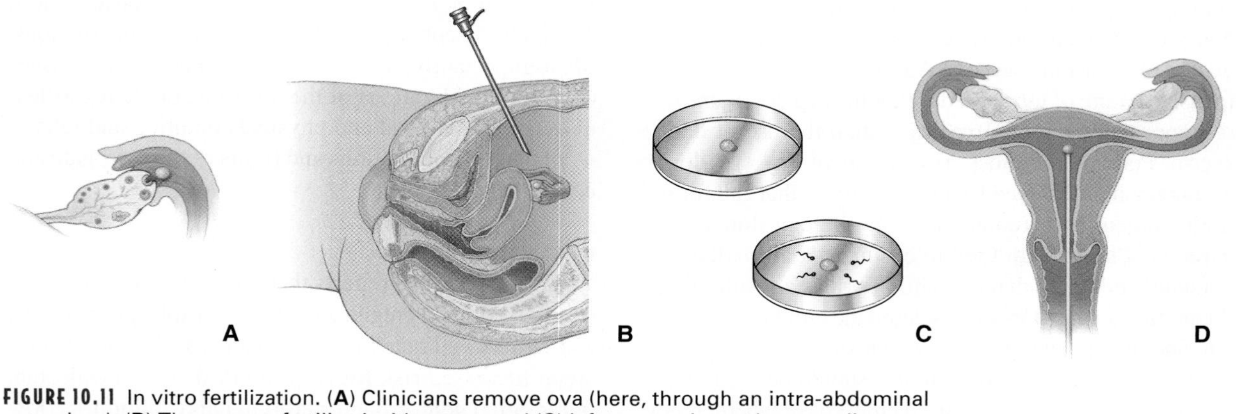

FIGURE 10.11 In vitro fertilization. (**A**) Clinicians remove ova (here, through an intra-abdominal procedure). (**B**) The ova are fertilized with sperm and (**C**) left to grow in a culture medium. (**D**) The fertilized ova are inserted into the woman's uterus for potential implantation.

days later, the woman returns to the physician's office for transfer of a set number of embryos into her uterus through the cervix. Any excess embryos can be cryopreserved for future use or destroyed.

Gamete Intrafallopian Transfer

Another ART is called **gamete intrafallopian transfer (GIFT).** In this procedure, the eggs are retrieved as described previously, but then the eggs and sperm are deposited directly into the woman's fallopian tube. Fertilization takes place in vivo. For some couples, this procedure satisfies religious prohibitions against artificial fertilization because any fertilization takes place within the woman and no embryos are left for cryopreservation.

Zygote Intrafallopian Transfer

Zygote intrafallopian transfer (ZIFT) involves egg retrieval, fertilization in the laboratory, and transfer of the zygotes directly to the fallopian tube. This is done at an earlier stage of development than for those embryos inserted into the uterus during IVF.

In Vitro Fertilization With Donor Eggs

Women who do not ovulate or who are of advanced age (ie, older than 35 years) may wish to use donor eggs. These may come from family members or anonymous donors. With donor eggs, ovulation-inducing medications are used to synchronize the cycles of the egg donor and the recipient. Eggs are then retrieved and fertilized with sperm obtained from the male partner or a donor. The embryos are then transferred to the recipient as in IVF. The use of donor eggs is a relatively new development, with several donor egg programs found throughout the country. The ASRM also has a set of guidelines for donor screening, but again, donor agencies are self-regulated and should be researched. Because of the necessity for synchronization of the cycles of both the egg donor and egg recipient, and because until recently unfertilized eggs could not be preserved, women wishing to undergo IVF with donor eggs must travel to the location of the participating clinic, often staying there for several weeks until transfer can be accomplished and appropriate diagnostic tests can be conducted to determine success. Additionally, because of the invasive nature of the procedure for the egg donor, the use of donor eggs is more expensive than the use of donor sperm. Perhaps the most critical part of any egg donor arrangement is the need for legal contracts that call for relinquishment of parental rights by the egg donor. The agreement must be drafted to ensure that all parties understand and agree that any child born as a result of egg donation is indisputably considered the child of the recipient and that the egg donor has no responsibility for rearing and caring for the child. It also should be established who has the rights to any unused embryos or whether they are to be destroyed or donated to other infertile couples.

Intracytoplasmic Sperm Injection

If the male partner's sperm count is very low, chances of success may increase with direct injection of a single sperm into the egg, a process called **intracytoplasmic sperm injection (ICSI).** The procedure is similar to IVF, except that the sperm are introduced directly into the cytoplasm of the egg. If the eggs are from a woman of advanced maternal age, microscopic holes may be drilled in the zona pellucida, a procedure referred to as **assisted hatching.**

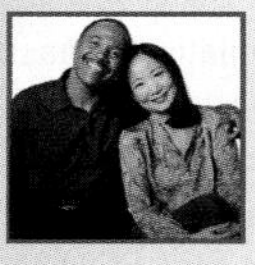

Ted and Joan from the beginning of the chapter have undergone fertility testing and decide to pursue ART. Their religious beliefs, however, forbid artificial fertilization. Which method would be most appropriate for them to choose?

Surrogate or Gestational Carriers

Some women cannot carry a pregnancy to term because of an absent or malformed uterus. In such cases, the client may choose to employ a surrogate or gestational carrier to produce a baby genetically related to the mother, father, or both. In this case, a procedure similar to IVF is performed, and then the resultant embryos are placed in the surrogate's uterus. After the child's birth, the surrogate surrenders him or her to the party or parties who legally adopt the child.

There have been several highly publicized cases in which, after birth, the surrogate declines to relinquish the child. For this reason, this procedure involves extensive preconception contracts to adequately protect against future legal problems. In such contracts, the surrogate, who often is a married woman who has completed her family, agrees to certain conditions, including refraining from sexual activity with her own partner, so that there is no possibility of spontaneous conception. She also agrees to abstain from activities that may put the fetus at risk (eg, smoking, alcohol or illegal drug consumption) and agrees to comply with the obstetrician's instructions. Most importantly, the contract should cover such issues as parental obligations of the infertile couple regardless of the child's mental and physical condition and release of all parental obligations and rights of the surrogate and her partner.

Multifetal Reduction

The ASRM (2001) reports that "preterm birth occurs in over 50% of twin pregnancies, 90% of triplet pregnancies, and virtually all quadruplet pregnancies." Preterm babies are at increased risk for respiratory distress syndrome, intracranial hemorrhage, cerebral palsy, blindness, low birth weight, and neonatal morbidity and mortality (see

Chap. 22). Mothers also experience more cases of gestational hypertension, gestational diabetes, anemia, and polyhydramnios with multiple gestations (ASRM, 2001). If more than one or two embryos implant and begin development, by use of fertility medication or by ART, reduction of the number of viable fetuses may be necessary. Fetal reduction may increase the chance of the mother having one or two healthy babies instead of a miscarriage or premature birth of three or more babies who are more likely to die or to suffer from long-term disability. This situation can be stressful for a couple who has spent limitless time and energy trying to become pregnant. The possibility should be discussed and a plan decided before treatment begins. Nurses can facilitate this conversation and help the client or couple to develop a plan before they are faced with the decision to reduce the number of fetuses.

Evaluation

The couple should have a reasonable expectation of the probability of success of any treatment. Infertility practices vary widely in the experience of the clinicians and the success rates of their protocols. Statistics can be difficult to interpret because "success" rates may be reported in terms that are not comparable. For example, definitions of what is considered a pregnancy, demographics and risk factors of the client populations served, and variability among clinicians are all variables that may change across practice settings.

Although women undergo infertility treatment in hopes of achieving a pregnancy, those who do become pregnant face additional challenges. Bernstein, Lewis, and Seibel (1994) studied women who became pregnant after a history of infertility. They found that differences exist in the way that these women process their pregnancy, as well as subtle differences in maternal–fetal attachment, self-concept, and coping during pregnancy. Although the woman may have achieved a pregnancy, the pregnancy has not "cured" the infertility. The infertility diagnosis remains and for the woman seems like a chronic condition. There is some speculation that women who have infertility may have differences in how they act as parents. There is concern that parents may treat these highly desired, long-hoped-for children differently by being more intense or overprotective as a consequence of the incredible risks and investments involved in conceiving.

Women dealing with secondary infertility also may not receive the support they need. Because they have successfully had at least one child, others may dismiss their feelings of loss and desperation. Nurses sensitive to the issues raised by infertility and its related emotional costs can better support parents and help them cope effectively with the normal stresses of parenthood.

Questions to Ponder

1. A woman whose husband has azoospermia tells the nurse that she plans to become pregnant using donor sperm without her husband's knowledge. She is afraid that he will not approve of this but is confident that once she gives birth he will love the child on first sight.
   - What are your personal feelings about her decision?
   - What obligations do you have to share her plans with her husband?
   - What resources are available to you?
2. A couple who is attempting pregnancy through the use of ART is debating whether they will tell friends, relatives, or the resultant offspring about circumstances surrounding the conception.
   - What are the benefits and risks of secrecy?
   - What resources are available to the couple?

SUMMARY

- Infertility, or the inability to achieve pregnancy after 1 year of regular, unprotected intercourse, affects approximately 10% to 15% of U.S. couples.
- Causes of infertility include biologic, chemical, environmental, and lifestyle factors. Male and female factors, as well as combined factors, account for most cases. For some couples, no identifiable cause can be ascertained.
- Diagnostic assessment includes evaluating both partners. Assessment of the male partner should be completed early in the diagnostic process.
- Treatment options depend on the diagnosis and can cause significant financial and practical burdens. Nurses can help couples understand the reasonable expectation of probability of success and refer clients to sources for support, such as Resolve.
- Religious, ethnic, cultural, and personal values may play important roles in couples' responses to diagnosis and may influence their acceptance of various options.

REVIEW QUESTIONS

1. The nurse is providing anticipatory guidance to a couple about to undergo an infertility workup. Which of the following components for the male partner should the nurse share will be evaluated initially?
   A. ejaculatory response
   B. serum prolactin levels
   C. serum testosterone level
   D. history and physical examination
2. A nurse is reviewing the potential findings that fertility testing may reveal. One partner says, "It will be such a relief to find out what the problem is so we

can fix it." Which of the following responses from the nurse would be most appropriate?
A. "I'm sure it will be a great relief, but testing can be very stressful, so be prepared."
B. "Because of the time involved in testing, you may feel discouraged and want to give up. Don't."
C. "It is important for you to review each test carefully before we start so you know exactly what to expect."
D. "Although testing often identifies the cause of infertility, some cases of infertility remain unexplained even after testing."

3. A nurse is reviewing the laboratory test results of a client's cervical mucus. Which of these findings indicates that the client's cervical mucus is conducive to conception?
A. pH of 5
B. ferning
C. no spinnbarkeit
D. rectal temperature of 97.4°F

4. The nurse instructs a male client about the proper technique for collecting a semen specimen for analysis. Which of these statements, if made by the client, would indicate that he understands the instructions?
A. "I will ejaculate into a sterile container."
B. "I will deliver the ejaculate to the laboratory within 30 minutes."
C. "I will place ice around the container in which I am transporting the ejaculate."
D. "I will not ejaculate for 3 days before providing you with the specimen."

5. The nurse should include which of the following statements when teaching a woman about monitoring her basal body temperature?
A. "Look for an increase in body temperature of approximately 3 degrees."
B. "Look for a decrease in your temperature followed by a sharp increase."
C. "Look for periodic dips in your temperature over 24 hours about 1 week before your period is due."
D. "Look for an increase in your temperature for 2 days, followed by a return to your baseline temperature."

6. A client who is experiencing difficulty becoming pregnant asks the nurse if her infertility is the result of an induced abortion she had several years ago. The nurse's response should be based on the understanding that
A. spontaneous abortions are related to infertility.
B. infertility is generally independent of a history of induced abortions.
C. there is a direct relationship between induced abortions and subsequent infertility.
D. infertility may be related to guilt and remorse women feel following abortions.

7. The 40-year-old male partner of an infertile couple shares all the following information with the nurse during his health history. Which piece of data indicates the need for health education to improve the chances of achieving a pregnancy?
A. The man is moderately obese.
B. The man is a writer who works out of his home.
C. The man smokes one-half a pack of cigarettes per day.
D. The man drinks 1 to 2 alcoholic beverages per day.

8. The nurse is reviewing the chart of a 32-year-old client who has been diagnosed with impaired fecundity. Which of these data support the diagnosis?
A. The woman has a history of first-trimester spontaneous abortion.
B. The woman's sexual partner's semen analysis revealed a low sperm count.
C. The woman has not become pregnant after 1 year of unprotected intercourse.
D. The woman had two induced abortions during her late teens and early twenties.

9. The 34-year-old female partner of an infertile couple shares all the following information with the nurse during the health history. Which piece of data indicates the need for health education to improve the chances of achieving a pregnancy?
A. The woman is moderately obese.
B. The woman works as a massage therapist in a health spa.
C. The woman drinks approximately three alcoholic beverages per week.
D. The couple have had unprotected intercourse every other day during the middle of her menstrual cycle for 6 months.

10. The nurse is discussing the use of infertility medications with an infertile couple. Which of these statements, if made by one or another of the partners, would suggest that additional information is needed?
A. "A number of different medications may be needed during each cycle."
B. "We will both take medication at different times of my wife's menstrual cycle."
C. "Depending on the medication, you will be teaching my husband how to give me a daily injection."
D. "The risk for having a multiple gestation is related to the length of time that we will be needing the medication."

REFERENCES

American Society for Reproductive Medicine. (2006). *Frequently asked questions about infertility.* Retrieved February 9, 2006, from: http://www.asrm.org/Patients/faqs.html.

American Society for Reproductive Medicine. (2001). *Patient's fact sheet: Complications of multiple gestation.* Retrieved September 18, 2004, from http://www.asrm.org/Patients/FactSheets/complications-multi.pdf.

Becks, G., & Burrow, G. (2000). Thyroid disorders and pregnancy. Retrieved September 18, 2004 from http://www.thyroid.ca/articles/EngE11A.html.

Beers, M., & Berckow, R. (2004). *The Merck manual of diagnosis and therapy* (17th ed.). Retrieved February 9, 2006, from http://www.merck.com/mrkshared/mmanual/home.jsp.

Bernstein, J., Lewis, J., & Seibel, M. (1994). Effect of previous infertility on maternal–fetal attachment, coping styles, and self-concept during pregnancy. *Journal of Women's Health, 3*(2), 125–133.

Brucker, P. S., & McKenry, P. C. (2004). Support from health care providers and the psychological adjustment of individuals experiencing infertility. *Journal of Obstetric, Gynecologic, and Neonatal Nursing, 33*(5), 597–603.

Centers for Disease Control and Prevention. (2003). *2001 Assisted reproductive technology success rates: National summary and fertility clinic reports.* Retrieved September 10, 2004, from http://www.cdc.gov/reproductivehealth/art.htm.

Centers for Disease Control and Prevention. (2005). *Assisted reproductive technology.* Retrieved February 9, 2006, from http://www.cdc.gov/ART/index.htm.

DeMasters, J. (2004). Male infertility. *Advance for Nurses, 6*(1), 19–25.

Dorff, E. N. (1998). *Matters of life and death: A Jewish approach to modern medical ethics.* Philadelphia: Jewish Publication Society.

Farah, L. (2000). *Infertility: Etiology and evaluation.* Retrieved September 10, 2004, from http://www.dcmsonline.org/jax-medicine/2000journals/may2000/infertility.htm.

Gold, M. (1988). *And Hannah wept.* Philadelphia: Jewish Publication Society.

Goldberg, J., & Falcone, T. (1999). Effect of diethylstilbestrol on reproductive function. *Fertility and Sterility, 72*(1), 1–7.

Idahl, A., Boman, J., Kumlin, U., & Olofsson, J. (2004). Demonstration of *Chlamydia trachomatis* IgG antibodies in the male partner of the infertile couple is correlated with a reduced likelihood of achieving pregnancy. *Human Reproduction, 19*(5), 1121–1126.

International Council on Infertility Information Dissemination, Inc. (2004). States mandating insurance coverage for infertility and pregnancy loss. Retrieved February 9, 2006, from http://www.inciid.org/article.php?cat=insurance101&id=15&pagenumber=2.

Islam and Infertility (n.d.). Retrieved September 15, 2004, from http://www.angelfire.com/la/IslamicView.

Jarzabek, K., Zbucka, M., Pepinski, W. Szamatowicz, J., Domitrz, J., Janica, J., et al. (2004). Cystic fibrosis as a cause of infertility. *Reproductive Biology, 4,* 119–129.

Klonoof-Cohen, H., Lam-Kruglick, P., & Gonzalez, C. (2003). Effects of maternal and paternal alcohol consumption on the success rates of in vitro fertilization and gamete intrafallopian transfer. *Fertility and Sterility, 79*(2), 330–339.

Kolettis, P., & Sandlow, J. (2002). Clinical and genetic features of patients with unilateral absence of the vas deferens. *Urology, 60,* 1073–1076.

Lane, D. E. (2006). Polycystic ovary syndrome and its differential diagnosis. *Obstetrics and Gynecology Survey, 61*(2), 125–135.

Lewis, J. A. (2003). Jewish perspectives on pregnancy and childbearing. *MCN—The American Journal of Maternal Child Nursing, 28*(5), 306–312.

Linne, Y. (2004). Effects of obesity on women's reproduction and complications during pregnancy. *Obesity Review, 5*(3), 137–143.

Malhi, P. (1995). Influence of gender preference for children on fertility behavior: A comparative study of men and women in Haryana. *Journal of Family Welfare, 41*(2), 53–60.

Marchionni, M., Fambrini, M., Zambelli, V., Scarsselli, G., & Susini, T. (2004). Reproductive performance before and after abdominal myomectomy: A retrospective analysis. *Fertility and Sterility, 82*(1), 154–159.

Mardh, P. (2004). Tubal factor infertility, with special regard to chlamydial salpingitis. *Current Opinion in Infectious Diseases, 17,* 49–52.

Mayo Clinic. (2004). *Sperm smarts: Optimizing fertility.* Retrieved February 9, 2006, from http://www.mayoclinic.com/health/fertility/MC00023.

Niccolai, L., Ethier, K., Kershaw, T., Lewis, J., Meade, C., & Ickovics, J. (2004). New sex partner acquisition and sexually transmitted disease risk among adolescent females. *Journal of Adolescent Health, 34,* 216–223.

Olshanky, E. (2003). A theoretical explanation for previously infertile mothers' vulnerability to depression. *Journal of Nursing Scholarship, 35,* 263–269.

Panni, M., & Corn, S. (2002). The use of a uniquely designed anesthetic scavenging hood to reduce operating room anesthetic gas contamination during general anesthesia. *Anesthesia & Analgesia, 95*(3), 656–660.

Practice Committee of the ASRM. (2004). Smoking and infertility. *Fertility and Sterility, 81*(4), 1181–1186.

Pritts, E. (2001). Fibroids and infertility: A systematic review of the evidence. *Obstetrical & Gynecological Survey, 56*(8), 483–491.

Santelli, J., Brener, N., Lowry, R., Bhatt, A., & Zabin, L. (1998). Multiple sexual partners among U.S. adolescents and young adults. *Family Planning Perspectives, 30,* 271–275.

Schneider, M. G., & Forthofer, M. S. (2005). Associations of psychosocial factors with the stress of infertility treatment. *Health Social Work, 30*(3), 183–191.

Schrager, S., & Potter, B. (2004). Diethylstilbestrol exposure. *American Family Physician, 69*(10), 2395–2400.

Shaban, S. (2003). Male infertility overview: Assessment, diagnosis, and treatment. Retrieved September 18, 2004, from http://www.ivf.com/shaban.html.

Sharlip, I., Jarow, J., Belker, A., Lipshultz, L., Sigman, M., Thomas, A., et al. (2002). Best practice policies for male infertility. *Fertility and Sterility, 77*(5), 873–882.

Speroff, L., & Fritz, M. (2004). *Clinical gynecologic endocrinology and infertility* (7th ed.). Philadelphia: Lippincott Williams & Williams.

Star, W. L., Lommel, L. L., & Shannon, M. T. (2004). *Women's primary health care: Protocols for practice* (2nd ed.). San Francisco: UCSF Nursing Press.

Swanton, A., & Child, T. (2005). Reproduction and ovarian ageing. *Journal of the British Menopause Society, 11*(4), 126–131.

Windham, G. C., Mitchell, P., Anderson, M., & Lasley, B. L. (2005). Cigarette smoking and effects on hormone function in premenopausal women. *Environmental Health Perspectives, 113*(10), 1285–1290.

CHAPTER 11

Genetics, Embryology, and Preconceptual/Prenatal Assessment and Screening

Shirley Jones

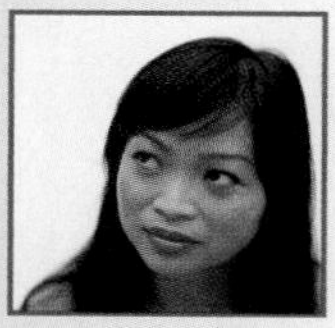

Carmen, 22 years old and recently married, comes to the health care facility to discuss preconception health screening. During her interview, Carmen states, "My spouse and I would like to start trying for a baby right away. But my mother mentioned a genetic problem a distant cousin had years ago. Several of my relatives have diabetes, heart disease, and other chronic conditions. I'm afraid that if my baby had a problem, it would be my fault."

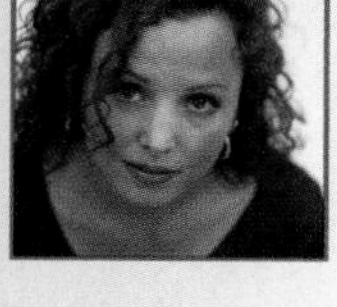

April, 36 years old, and her husband Alex, 37 years old, come to the prenatal clinic. April is at 13 weeks' gestation. She gave birth to their first child, a healthy daughter, 4 years ago. With this pregnancy, the couple attempted to conceive for 2 years. During this appointment, April states, "According to the Internet, I'm now considered of 'advanced maternal age.' The risk of having a child with genetic problems has increased so much! Should I be worried about Down syndrome?"

Nurses working with such clients need to understand the material in this chapter to manage care and address issues appropriately. You will read more about these clients later. Before beginning, consider the following points:

- How should the nurse tailor care to best suit the needs of these clients and their families?
- What aspects of teaching do these clients require?
- What issues are similar for the women? What issues are different?
- What factors might affect April's pregnancy adversely?
- Which types of screening and diagnostic testing would the nurse expect April to undergo? Carmen?
- How would the nurse intervene to enhance each client's health, well-being, and comfort?

LEARNING OBJECTIVES

On completion of this chapter, the reader should be able to:

- Summarize gametogenesis, embryogenesis, and fetal growth and development.
- Identify the etiology of risk factors that can affect conception, gestation, and embryonic/fetal growth and development adversely.
- Discuss preconception health risk assessment and counseling from the view of health care providers, sociocultural communities, and clients seeking these services.
- Describe the effects of advances in human genetics on informed decision making and consent.
- Discuss strategies to enhance the health, well-being, and comfort of clients seeking preconception or prenatal health risk assessment and counseling.
- Describe the scope of preconception, prenatal, and postnatal screening and diagnostic procedures available to clients.

KEY TERMS

allele
association
blastomere
chromosome
chronic sorrow
deformation
disruption
dizygotic twins
dominant
dysmorphology
gametogenesis
genes
genetic counseling
genetics
genotype
informed decision making and consent
malformation
meiosis
mitosis
monozygotic twins
morula
multifactorial disorder
mutations
nucleotide
oocyte
phenotype
recessive
sequence
sex linked
spermatid
syndrome
teratogen
variation
zygote

One of every 33 U.S. babies is born with a birth defect (Centers for Disease Control and Prevention [CDC], 2004). The risk for conceiving a child with a birth defect is increased for some people with medical, genetic, or parental age factors. This chapter provides the reader with awareness and understanding of the many preconception and prenatal development issues that await clients in their journey to have a healthy biologic child. The material found here serves to provide health care professionals with the knowledge and resources needed to identify reproductive risks and to present information about alternatives to clients. The foundation for this knowledge is built through a review of basic genetics, embryology, and fetal development. The chapter continues with discussions of appropriate preconception screening and assessment techniques. It also explores in detail prenatal screening and evaluation techniques and associated collaborative care interventions.

GENETICS AND CELL BIOLOGY

Variation is the life cycle outcome of each person's unique response to nature (genetic code) and nurture (environment), beginning before conception and ending with death. It is ever changing and ever present throughout a person's biopsychosocial growth and development. **Genetics** is the field of study that investigates variations within the human genome.

The breadth and diversity of genetic characteristics are remarkable given that each person is 99.9% the same as any other human being. The importance and potential influence of the seemingly small level of variation become self-evident when one considers that the human genome consists of 3 billion base pairs, each solely or jointly responsible for the myriad of human characteristics. Thus, a 0.1% difference accounts for the possibility of 3 million variations in an infinite number of combinations from one person to the next (Guttmacher & Collins, 2002).

Chromosomes, Genes, and DNA

Somatic cells are the basic biologic foundation of every human organ and system. They help maintain the growth, development, and well-being of each person. *Germ cells* are the reproductive cells located in the *gonads* (ovaries, testes). The sole function of germ cells is to preserve the human species through replication. Both somatic and germ cells consist of a nucleus surrounded by cytoplasm (Fig. 11.1). The nucleus contains 46 chromosomes (two copies of each of 23 different chromosomes) that together compose the entire human genome. **Chromosomes** are threadlike strands that carry genes and transmit hereditary information. Within the cytoplasm are multiple organelles, including ribosomes and mitochondria.

Each chromosome consists of deoxyribonucleic acid (DNA), proteins, and a small amount of ribonucleic acid (RNA). DNA is made up of sugar (deoxyribose), a phosphate group, and a nitrogenous base (purine or pyrimidine). Together, these substances form a **nucleotide** that joins with other nucleotides to create a strandlike chain. DNA is responsible for the genetic code required for the synthesis of all amino acids. First described by Watson and Crick (1953), the double helix structure of DNA is the product of two strands of DNA held together by hydrogen bonds formed from the complementary pairing of nitrogen bases: adenine with thymine (purine bases) and cytosine with guanine (pyrimidine bases). The molecular structure is similar to a ladder twisted into a spiral staircase, with the strands of DNA forming the sides and the base pairs forming the rungs. The specific one-to-one pairing of the nitrogenous bases is the foundation of DNA's ability to perfectly and intrinsically replicate itself. This process leads to separation of the two strands and the use of each as a template for two new DNA molecules. When mistakes in this process occur, the cell attempts to mediate and repair these errors (Friedberg, 2003). Not all **mutations** are repaired, however, and those that remain become part of the new DNA molecule and all future replications of that DNA strand.

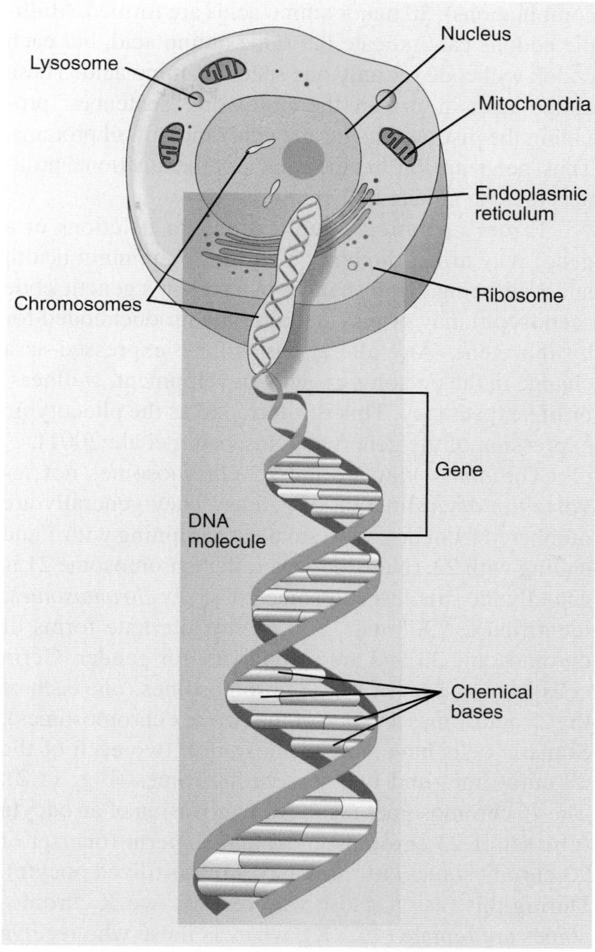

FIGURE 11.1 Schematic drawing of the contents of a cell and the physical structure of DNA. Note that each chemical base only pairs with its reciprocal chemical base.

RNA also is composed of a sugar (ribose), a phosphate group, and a nitrogenous base (purine or pyrimidine). Unlike DNA, RNA is single stranded and uses the pyrimidine uracil instead of thymine. All three types of RNA (messenger, ribosomal, and transfer) are necessary for translation of the genetic code into the synthesis of polypeptides (protein) (Alberts, 2003). This process is associated with the ribosomes found in the cellular cytoplasm. The unidirectional flow of genetic information from DNA to RNA to protein is the central principle of molecular genetics.

Genes, the basic units of heredity, are located along the DNA of each chromosome. The number of different genes per chromosome depends on the sizes of both gene and chromosome. Each gene is a unique sequence (both number and order) formed from the nucleotides along the DNA strands. The four nitrogenous bases (**A** = adenine, **T** = thymine, **C** = cytosine, **G** = guanine) of DNA form three-letter "words" referred to as *codons.* From the 64 possible codons (four unique letters in three-letter combinations), 20 major amino acids are formed. Multiple codons can indicate the same amino acid, but each codon will code for only one specific amino acid. These amino acids in turn are the multiword "sentences" providing the instructions for the generation of all proteins. Thus, genes are the "recipe book" for the functional products that the human body requires.

Errors (mutations, duplications, or deletions of a gene) may affect the body's ability to maintain health and well-being. Such changes in a person's genetic code (**genotype**) may or may not alter the product coded for by that gene. Any alterations will be expressed as a change in the person's growth, development, wellness, or life expectancy. This is referred to as the phenotypic expression of the genotype (Nussbaum et al., 2001).

The *autosomes* are the 22 chromosomes not involved in determination of gender. They generally are numbered from largest to smallest beginning with 1 and ending with 22. (Note, however, that chromosome 21 is actually the smallest autosome.) The *sex chromosomes,* identified as "X" and "Y," are the alternate forms of chromosome 23 and are responsible for gender. Germ cells have one set of the 23 chromosomes (one each of the 22 autosomes and one of the two sex chromosomes). Somatic cells have 46 chromosomes, two each of the 22 autosomes and two sex chromosomes (Fig. 11.2). The 46 chromosomes result from the fusion of an **oocyte** (one set of 23 chromosomes) and a sperm (one set of 23 chromosomes) to form a **zygote** (fertilized oocyte). During this fusion, those who receive two X chromosomes are female (46,XX), whereas those who receive one X and one Y chromosome are male (46,XY). Because females may give only an X to their children but males may give either an X or a Y, the chromosome complement of each sperm determines the zygote's gender.

Mitosis and Meiosis

All cells (somatic and germ) undergo a life cycle of birth, maturation, replication, and death. The process undertaken by somatic cells is called **mitosis** (Fig. 11.3). The process used by germ cells is called **meiosis;** it leads to the formation of gametes (Fig. 11.4). The similarities and differences between the two processes may be summarized as replication *with* (meiosis) or *without* (mitosis) a reduction in total chromosome count (diploid cell = 2n, or 2 × 23 = 46 chromosomes). Both mitosis and meiosis are critical to the accurate and consistent transmission of genetic information from parent to all descendant cells.

Mitosis

Mitosis is the cellular process that enables an embryo to become a fetus, a fetus to become a child, and a child to become an adult. It is the body's natural process of growth and development performed in association with cellular repair and replacement.

The five phases of mitosis are interphase, prophase, metaphase, anaphase, and telophase:

- During *interphase,* the cell "rests" from mitotic division but performs metabolic functions, depending on the type of cell (eg, nerve, skin, muscle, brain, blood). The cell also prepares for mitotic replication and division by gathering the additional RNA, amino acids, and nucleotides it will need at the end of this phase. The replicated sides of each chromosome (*sister chromatids*) are joined together at the *centromere.*
- *Prophase* is the beginning of cellular division. This phase is identified microscopically by visualization of

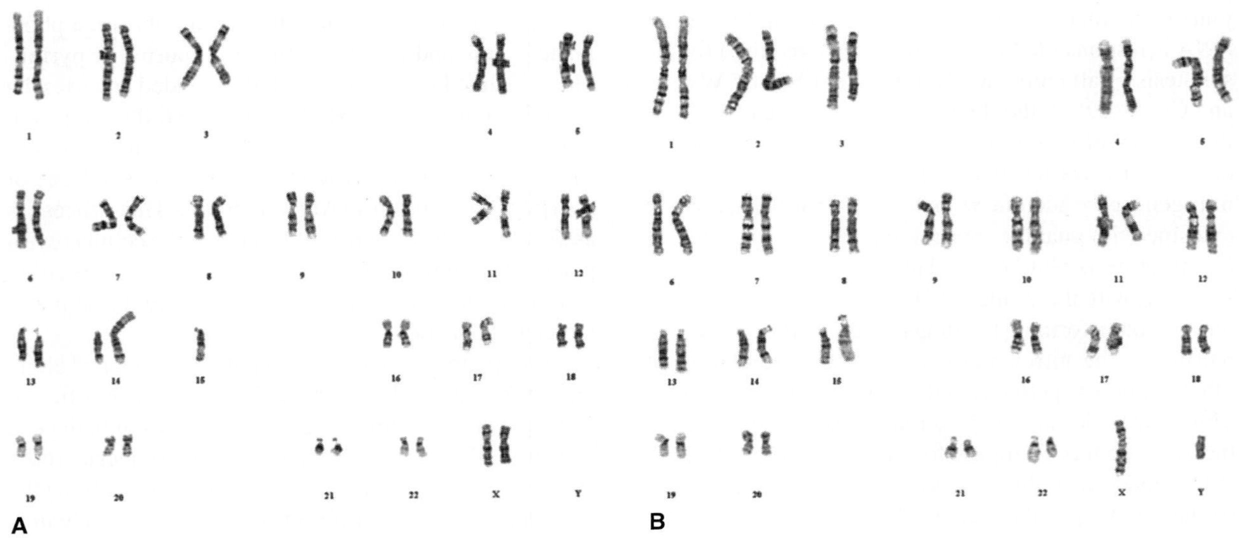

FIGURE 11.2 (**A**) Normal female karyotype (46,XX). (**B**) Normal male karyotype (46,XY). (Courtesy of A. Donnenfeld, Genzyme Genetics, Santa Fe, NM.)

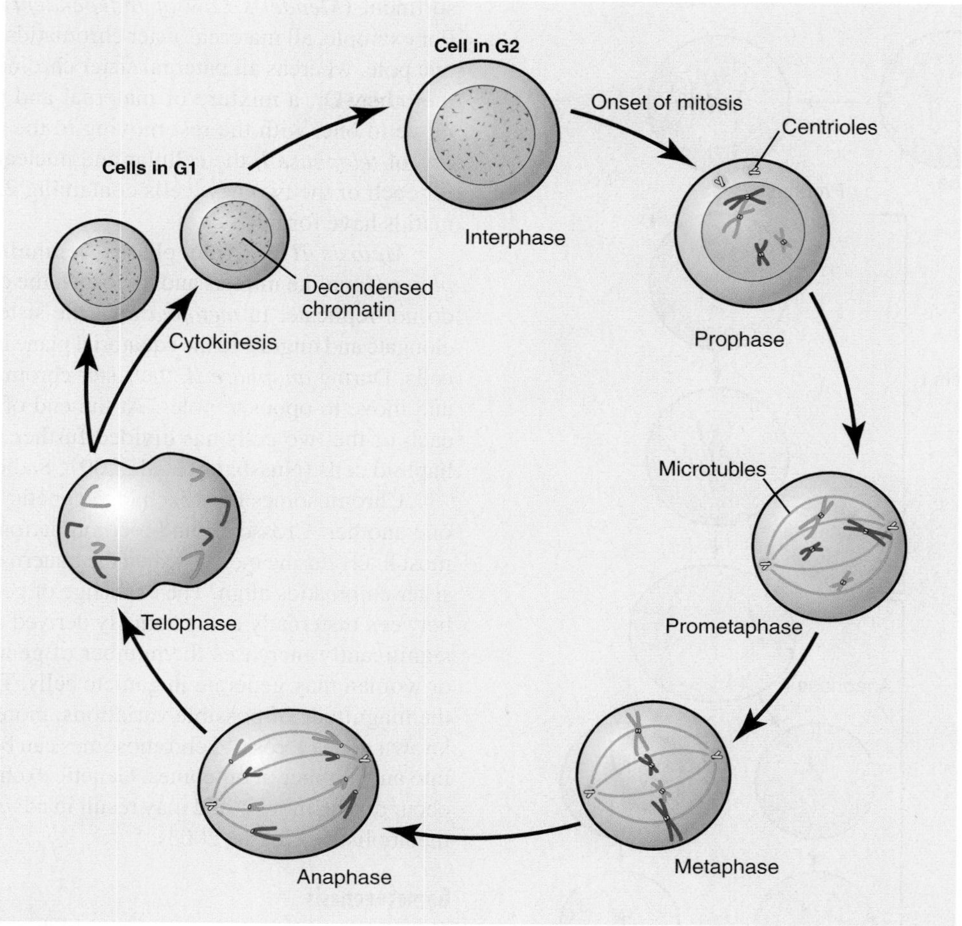

FIGURE 11.3 Mitosis. Diagrammatic representation using only two chromosome pairs. *Purple* represents maternal chromosomes; *coral* represents the paternal chromosomes. During metaphase, each chromosome lines up along the equatorial plane. In total, 46 chromosomes compose each cell.

the condensed chromosomes and migration of the duplicated centrioles to opposite poles of the cytoplasm. Once the chromosomes have reached their highest density, they begin to migrate to the cell's equatorial plane. The spindle fibers also form.

- The key aspects of *metaphase* are complete migration of the chromosomes and linkage by the spindle fibers of the centrioles to the centromeres of each chromosome. At this point, the chromosome appears microscopically in the traditional notation of either an "X" or inverted "U."
- *Anaphase* is marked by splitting of the centromeres as the two sets of spindle fibers pull them to opposite cellular poles. The result is separation of the sister chromatids and formation of new daughter chromosomes. As the daughter chromosomes reach their respective poles, an indentation begins to form in the cell membrane.
- During the last stage of *telophase,* two new cellular membranes form through the furrowed region of the original cell, and two new daughter cells appear. The chromosomes within each uncoil and become less dense. The nuclear membrane surrounding the chromosomes reforms in each daughter cell (see Fig. 11.13) (Lashley, 1998; Nussbaum et al., 2001).

Meiosis

As mentioned earlier, the process of meiosis enables the diploid germ cells to divide and produce haploid gamete cells (n = 23 chromosomes). Meiosis is marked by two separate reductions in the number of chromosomes after completion of their initial replication during interphase. The outcome of meiosis is four new haploid cells rather than two diploid cells.

Meiosis I includes prophase I, metaphase I, anaphase I, and telophase I. The hallmark of meiosis I is the pairing of homologous chromosomes during *metaphase I* so that the maternal and paternal sister chromatids for each of the 23 distinct chromosomes lie next to each other along the cell's equatorial plane (see Fig. 11.4).

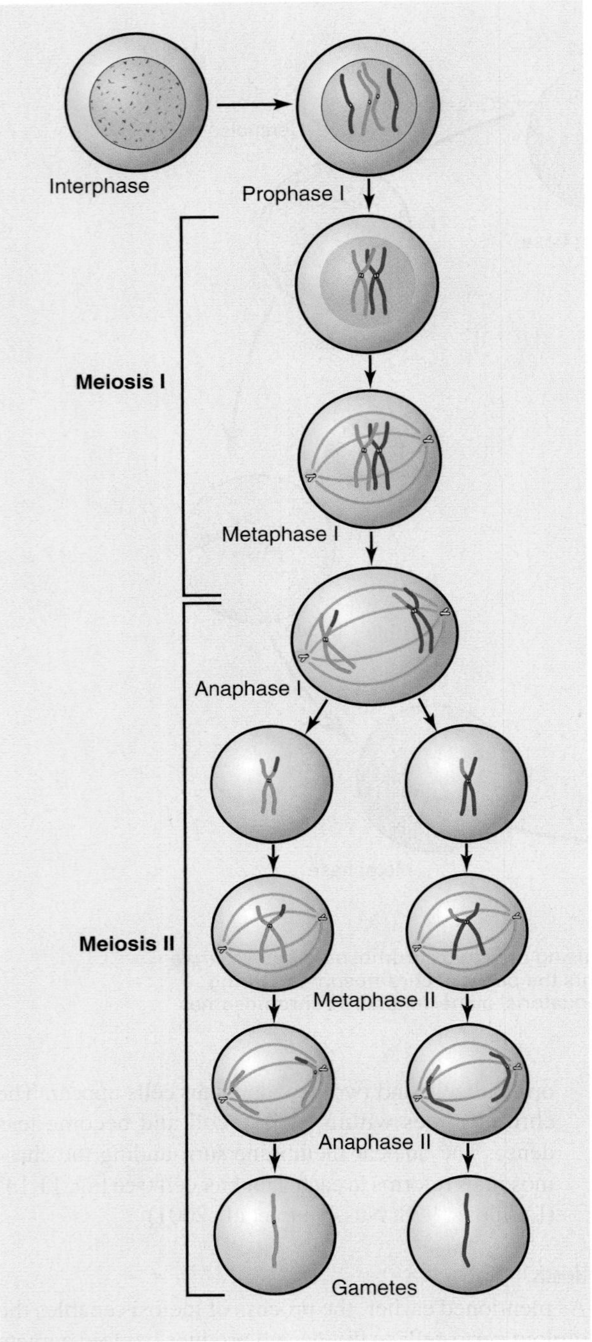

FIGURE 11.4 Meiosis. Diagrammatic representation using two homologous pairs of chromosomes. The 23 homologous pairs line up along the equatorial plane during metaphase I. This permits the potential for exchange of pieces of sister chromatids during metaphase I pairing.

(In mitosis, homologous sister chromatids do not pair with each other.) In *anaphase I,* the homologous pairs separate, with each sister chromatid moving toward opposite poles (*Mendel's Law of Segregation*). Furthermore, the movement to opposite poles is in a random assortment (*Mendel's Law of Independent Assortment*). For example, all maternal sister chromatids may move to one pole, whereas all paternal sister chromatids move to the other. Or, a mixture of maternal and paternal may move to one, with the rest moving to the other. By the end of *telophase I,* the cellular and nuclear membranes for each of the two new cells containing 23 sister chromatids have formed.

Meiosis II has four phases beginning with *prophase II;* unlike mitosis and meiosis I, the chromosomes do not replicate. In *metaphase II,* the sister chromatids elongate and migrate to the equatorial plane in the two new cells. During *anaphase II,* the sister chromatids separate and move to opposite poles. At the end of *telophase II,* each of the two cells has divided further into two new haploid cells (Nussbaum et al., 2001; Sadler, 1995).

Chromosomes may exchange genetic material with one another. Crossover and recombination of DNA are most likely during meiosis when the maternal and paternal sister chromatids align. The exchange of genetic material between maternally and paternally derived chromosomes significantly increases the number of genotypes a man or woman may generate in gamete cells. To underscore the magnitude of possible variations, more than 30,000 known genes across 46 chromosomes can be recombined into any number of outcomes. Genetic exchange also can occur during mitosis and may result in adverse effects on metabolism (Alberts, 2003).

Gametogenesis

Gametogenesis is the process by which primordial germ cells yield gametes (oocytes and **spermatids**) to help maintain continuity of the human species. The cells that give rise to gametes are formed by the 3rd week of gestation and join with somatic cells to form primitive gonads by the 5th week of gestation (Sadler, 2005). Male primordial germ cells remain dormant in the testes until puberty. Female primordial germ cells, however, begin to differentiate after formation of the primitive ovary in the embryo. Development of germ cells is by mitotic division. Mature oocytes and spermatids form through meiosis.

Spermatogenesis and Spermiogenesis

Each testis is composed primarily of 70 cm of tightly coiled seminiferous tubules, in which *spermatogenesis* occurs (Speroff et al., 1999). At puberty, the male germ cells form two types of cells: spermatogonia A and spermatogonia B. A continuous supply of sperm stem cells forms through the ongoing mitotic division of spermatogonia A. Throughout the adult male's reproductive life, selected spermatogonia A cells go on to form spermatogonia B cells. Spermatogonia B cells in turn give rise to primary spermatocytes, which in turn produce spermatids through meiotic division. This process requires approximately 50 days.

The final maturation of spermatids occurs over the next 12 to 26 days (Speroff et al., 1999). This process is called *spermiogenesis* and consists of four critical components that provide sperm with progressive motility and the ability to fertilize oocytes (Sadler, 1995). Step 1 is condensation of the spermatid nucleus. Step 2 is shedding of most of the spermatid cytoplasm. Step 3 is formation of the acrosome cap, which covers the nuclear surface of the spermatid and contains the enzymes necessary to penetrate the outer layers of the oocyte. This penetration permits transfer of the sperm nucleus with its chromosomes into the cytoplasm of the oocyte. Step 4, the final step, is formation of the neck, midpiece, and tail of the sperm, which facilitates its movement through the female cervix and uterus to the fallopian tubes in preparation for fertilization of the oocyte (Fig. 11.5). The seminiferous tubules transport sperm to the epididymis, where full motility is reached in preparation for ejaculation through the vas deferens and movement through the female reproductive tract. The life cycle of a sperm is approximately 75 to 90 days (Speroff et al., 1999).

Oogenesis

Approximately 46 days after fertilization (Nussbaum et al., 2001), the primitive gonads complete differentiation and become the testes or ovaries. In the female embryo, oogenesis begins at this point, as opposed to initiation of spermatogenesis at the onset of puberty in the male.

The genetic female's primordial germ cells become oogonia. Each oogonium replicates many times through mitotic division to increase in overall number and form clusters surrounded by epithelial (somatic) cells from the ovarian surface. From 3 to 5 months' gestation, the oogonia begin to differentiate into primary oocytes. Epithelial cells from the ovarian cortex encase each oocyte and eventually form the primordial follicle. Once a primary oocyte forms, DNA replication is complete, and the cell enters meiosis I. It remains suspended in this phase throughout childhood. Starting with menarche and continuing with each subsequent menstrual cycle over the next 35 to 40 years of a woman's reproductive life, one or more oocytes "awaken" and continue maturation by completing meiosis II (Nussbaum et al., 2001; Sadler, 1995; Speroff et al., 1999).

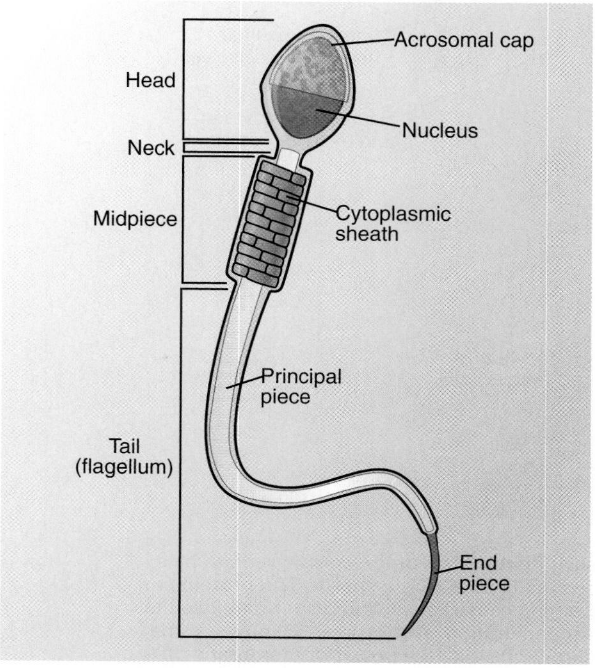

FIGURE 11.5 Normal sperm morphology.

By the 5th month of gestation, the number of oogonia reaches a lifetime maximum of approximately 6 to 7 million. Over the next 4 months, that number decreases to 1 to 2 million. This magnitude of rapid depletion, however, slows. By puberty, the number of primary oocytes has diminished to 200,000 to 400,000 (Speroff et al., 1999). Given that the reproductive female will have approximately 500 menstrual cycles in her lifetime, the surviving primary oocytes provide ample potential for conception. Remember that a primary oocyte may be in meiosis I for 50 years or more before completing the meiotic cycle and maturing into a secondary oocyte available for sperm penetration and fusion (Speroff et al., 1999).

With each menstrual cycle, 5 to 15 primordial follicles begin to mature in response to follicle-stimulating hormone (FSH), although as many as 1,000 attempt maturation (Sadler, 1995; Speroff et al., 1999). (See Chap. 6 for discussion of the endometrial cycle.) The primary oocyte within the primordial follicle also responds and begins to complete meiosis I. Usually one primordial follicle matures faster than the others and becomes the primary or "lead" follicle. In response to luteinizing hormone (LH), the primary oocyte completes meiosis I and forms a secondary oocyte and first polar body. During meiosis, the oocyte replicates its DNA and transfers 23 sister chromatids to each new daughter cell, but it does not equally divide the cell's cytoplasm between the two new cells. The primary oocyte receives nearly all the cytoplasm. This process repeats when the secondary oocyte and second polar body are formed. Each receives 23 chromatids, but the secondary oocyte receives the largest portion of the cytoplasm. Therefore, oogenesis results in one mature secondary oocyte from a single oogonium, whereas spermatogenesis results in four secondary spermatocytes from a single spermatogonium.

With the formation of the secondary oocyte, the graafian (mature) follicle releases the developing oocyte from the ovary (ovulation), and the fimbriae brush the oocyte into the fallopian tube. The oocyte enters meiosis II as it travels down the fallopian tube. Fertilization of the oocyte by a sperm occurs in the fallopian tube. If fertilization does not occur, the oocyte dies and is reabsorbed. The secondary oocyte completes meiosis II only if a sperm fertilizes it. At completion of meiosis II, a zygote (fertilized oocyte) and second polar body have formed.

Fertilization and Implantation

Each menstrual cycle provides a narrow window of opportunity for fertilization. The ovulated oocyte remains capable of fusing with a sperm for only 24 hours. Sperm survive in the female reproductive tract for no more than 72 hours. In addition to these short lifespans, multiple sperm must encounter the secondary oocyte and use the cumulative enzymes within their acrosome caps to assist a single sperm to penetrate and fuse with the secondary oocyte. Although the normal ejaculate has 200,000,000 to 300,000,000 sperm, only 300 to 500 actually reach the oocyte, further decreasing the odds of conception (Speroff et al., 1999).

Before sperm encounter the secondary oocyte, they must undergo capacitation in the female reproductive tract. This process lasts approximately 7 hours and results in the removal of the protective protein covering the acrosome cap. It must happen for sperm to penetrate the cells (corona radiata) that surround the oocyte (Fig. 11.6).

After entry of the sperm, the oocyte continues with the final steps of meiosis II, forming the second polar body and the mature oocyte with its pronucleus containing 23 chromosomes. The head of the sperm contains its pronucleus with 23 chromosomes; the sperm sheds its neck and tail. The two pronuclei come to lie next to each other and begin to replicate their DNA. At the conclusion of fertilization, the normal diploid number is returned to the developing cell, the gender is determined, and cleavage of the zygote by mitotic division is initiated (Sadler, 2005).

As the developing zygote travels down the fallopian tubes to the uterine cavity, it repeats mitotic cell division,

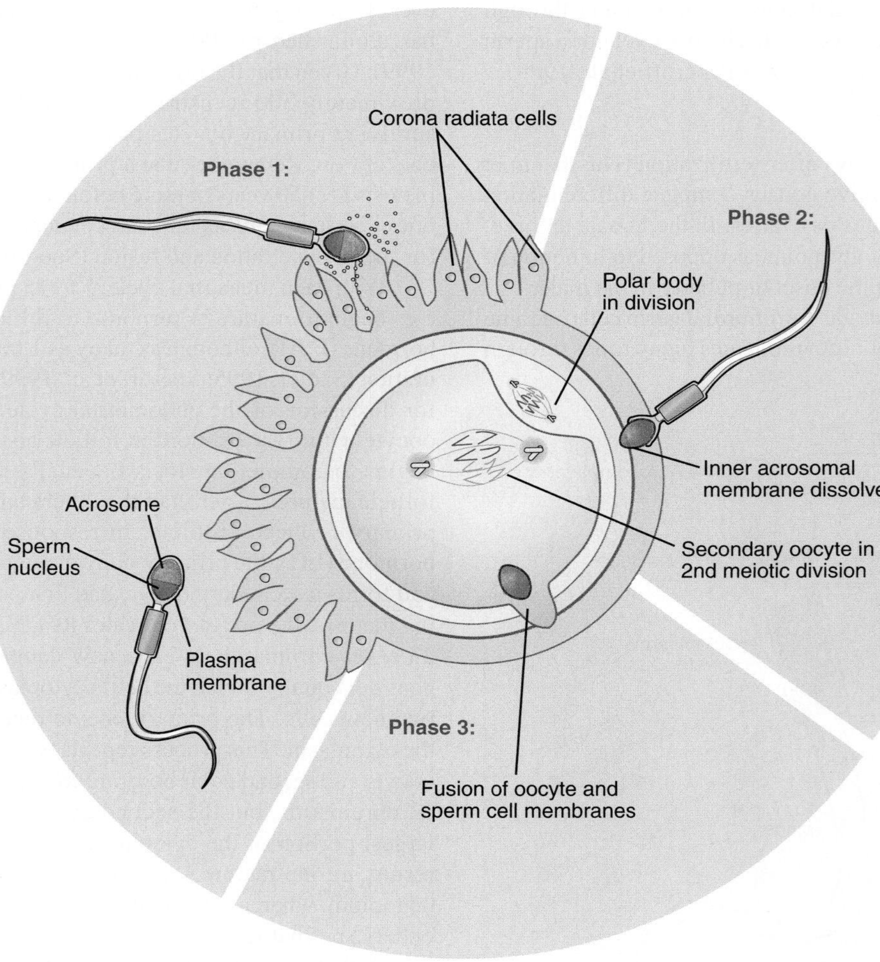

FIGURE 11.6 The three phases of fertilization. Phase 1: Penetration of the corona radiata by several sperm. Phase 2: Penetration of the zona pellucida by a single sperm. The proteins on the zona pellucida bind sperm to its surface. This binding causes capacitated sperm to lose the plasma membrane and release enzymes required for penetration. This process is known as the *acrosome reaction.* Phase 3: Fusion of the oocyte membrane with the posterior membrane of the sperm head. Upon fusion of the membranes, chemical changes in the zona pellucida prevent any other sperm from entering the oocyte's cytoplasm. (Adapted from Sadler, T. W. [1995]. *Langman's medical embryology* [7th ed.]. Philadelphia: Lippincott Williams & Wilkins.)

forming new cells (**blastomeres**) enclosed within the zona pellucida of the former oocyte. Each new blastomere is smaller than the parent cells. Approximately 5 days after fertilization, the **morula** (dividing embryo that contains 16 or more blastomeres) enters the uterine cavity. Fluid enters the intercellular spaces, and the blastomeres differentiate. Some blastomeres flatten along the circumference of the former oocyte to form the trophoblast, whereas others migrate to one pole to form the embryoblast. The space left by this segregation of the two cell masses is the blastocele. At this point, the zona pellucida is dissolved and lost, allowing the cells of the developing embryoblast to embed into the uterine mucosa. Full implantation is complete approximately 7 days after fertilization if the endometrium has responded appropriately to the proliferative and secretory phases of the menstrual cycle (Sadler, 2005).

EMBRYOLOGY AND FETAL DEVELOPMENT

Human gestation lasts 40 weeks (10 lunar months). The first 2 weeks correlate with development of the oocyte and endometrial lining. The field of embryology uses 38 weeks as the total length of gestation, beginning from the day of oocyte fertilization and zygote formation rather than from the first day of the last menstrual period (LMP) (Sadler, 2005). The embryonic calculation more accurately reflects the duration of human gestation because the proliferative phase of the menstrual cycle may last from days to weeks (Speroff et al., 1999). *The following discussion of embryology uses the standard of 38 weeks' gestation. Unless otherwise stated, all other references to gestation in this chapter use the obstetrical standard of 40 weeks.*

The 1st and 2nd weeks of gestation are known as the *pre-embryonic period,* which begins with fertilization and ends with the appearance of the fetal pole within the blastocyst. The *embryonic period* extends from the 3rd to 8th week of gestation and is marked by differentiation of the embryonic tissue into the multiple and specialized tissue cells of the human body. The *fetal period* lasts from the 9th to the 38th week of gestation and is characterized by the growth and development of fetal organs and tissues. See Table 11.1 for a summary of pre-embryonic, embryonic, and fetal development.

Pre-embryonic Development

As described earlier, the zygote has the normal diploid number of 46 chromosomes. This single cell enters into a series of rapid mitotic divisions, which continue as the zygote travels down the fallopian tube to the uterine cavity. Once the zygote begins mitotic cellular division, it is referred to as an embryo. The number of cells visible on microscopic examination is used to describe the stage of embryo development (eg, 2-cell embryo, 5-cell embryo, 10-cell embryo).

Before the blastocyst forms approximately 5 to 7 days after fertilization, each blastomere (cell) within the embryo can differentiate into any type of tissue. This law of biology is referred to as *totipotency* (Sadler, 1995; Speroff et al., 1999). For this reason, one or more blastomeres may die or be removed without harm to the developing embryo. Totipotency permits the formation of multiple gestations and survival of the embryo after preimplantation biopsy. Once differentiation occurs at approximately the 3rd week, cellular totipotency is lost.

By the beginning of the 2nd week, the blastocyst has embedded partially into the endometrium. At this time, it consists of the outer cells (trophoblast), the inner cell mass (embryoblast), and the blastocele cavity. The embryoblast appears flat and is known as the bilaminar germ disk with two layers: hypoblast and epiblast. The amniotic cavity and membrane (amnion) begin to form within the epiblast. Growth of the germ disc is slow during this period. Endometrial changes as a result of implantation lead to a decidual reaction that appears as a halo around the gestational sac (Fig. 11.7).

Normally, the blastocyst implants in the main uterine body on either the anterior or posterior wall. This permits the placenta to develop embedded within tissue prepared for the invasive fusion of the trophoblast and the growth of the fetus to full term. If the blastocyst implants near or over the internal os, a partial or complete placenta previa occurs (see Chap. 13). With careful monitoring, this abnormality of implantation can result in a normal birth. Implantation also can occur outside the uterus (extrauterine or ectopic pregnancy) (American College of Obstetricians and Gynecologists, 1989). It may occur in the ampullary (90%) or isthmic portion of the fallopian tube (8%) (Fig. 11.8). The remaining 2% of ectopic pregnancies develop in the interstitial tissue of the abdominal cavity or the cornea of the uterus.

Membranes and Placenta

Structural Development. Differentiation of the trophoblast during the pre-embryonic phase begins the formation of the placenta and fetal membranes (amnion and chorion) (Figs. 11.9A–C). Vacuoles appear in the syncytiotrophoblast (syncytium) and form lacunae (see Fig. 11.9A). The lacunar (intervillous) spaces form an intercommunicating network; the expanding syncytiotrophoblast carries these spaces into the endometrial lining. This expansion causes erosion of maternal capillaries, which become distended with increased maternal blood to the endometrium. The lacunae merge with the capillaries to establish the flow of maternal blood to the trophoblast layer of the blastocyst (see Fig. 11.9B). By the end of the 2nd week, the cytotrophoblast develops villous structures that penetrate the syncytiotrophoblast. The syncytium surrounds the cytotrophoblast columns, but the two tissues do not fuse. This side-by-side interstitial proximity of the lacunae and primary villi is the beginning of uteroplacental circulation.

TABLE 11.1 Embryonic and Fetal Development

Week 3

Beginning development of brain, spinal cord, and heart
Beginning development of the gastrointestinal tract
Neural tube forms, which later becomes the spinal cord
Leg and arm buds appear and grow out from body

Week 4

Brain differentiates
Limb buds grow and develop more

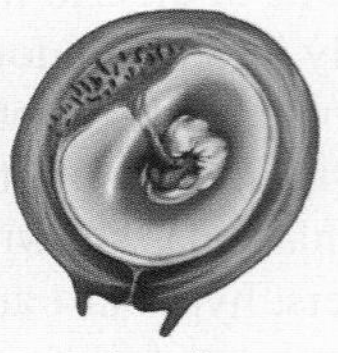

4 weeks

Week 5

Heart now beats at a regular rhythm
Beginning structures of eyes and ears
Some cranial nerves are visible
Muscles innervated

Week 6

Beginning formation of lungs
Fetal circulation established
Liver produces RBCs
Further development of the brain
Primitive skeleton forms
Central nervous system forms
Brain waves detectable

Week 7

Straightening of trunk
Nipples and hair follicles form
Elbows and toes visible
Arms and legs move
Diaphragm formed
Mouth with lips and early tooth buds

Week 8

Rotation of intestines
Facial features continue to develop
Heart development complete
Resembles a human being

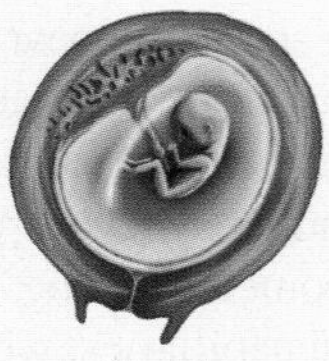

8 weeks

Weeks 9–12

Sexual differentiation continues
Buds for all 20 temporary teeth laid down
Digestive system shows activity
Head comprises nearly half the fetus size
Face and neck are well formed
Urogenital tract completes development
Red blood cells are produced in the liver
Urine begins to be produced and excreted
Fetal gender can be determined by week 12
Limbs are long and thin; digits are well formed

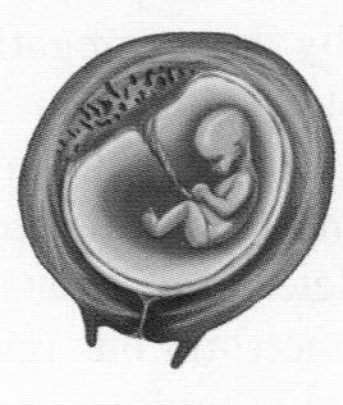

12 weeks

Weeks 13–16

A fine hair develops on the head called *lanugo*
Fetal skin is almost transparent
Bones become harder
Fetus makes active movement
Sucking motions are made with the mouth
Amniotic fluid is swallowed
Fingernails and toenails present
Weight quadruples
Fetal movement (also known as *quickening*) detected by mother

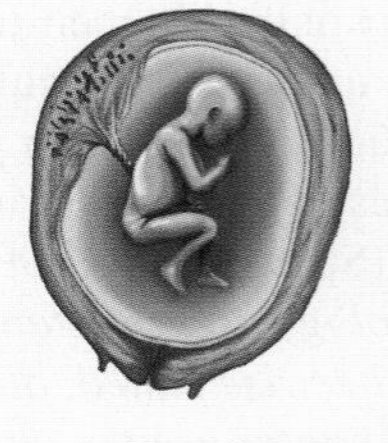

16 weeks

Weeks 17–20

Rapid brain growth occurs
Fetal heart tones can be heard with stethoscope
Kidneys continue to secret urine into amniotic fluid
Vernix caseosa, a white greasy film, covers the fetus
Eyebrows and head hair appear
Brown fat deposited to help maintain temperature
Nails are present on both fingers and toes
Muscles are well developed

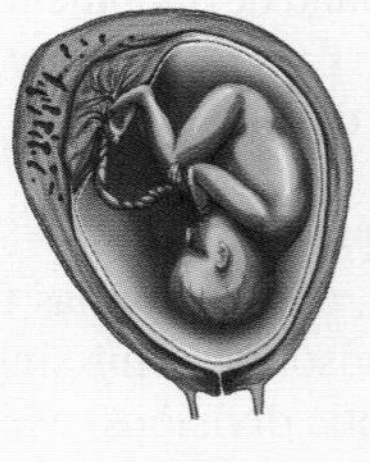

20 weeks

Continued

TABLE 11.1 Embryonic and Fetal Development

Weeks 21–24

Eyebrows and eyelashes are well formed
Fetus has a hand grasp and startle reflex
Alveoli forming in lungs
Skin is translucent and red
Lungs begin to produce *surfactant*

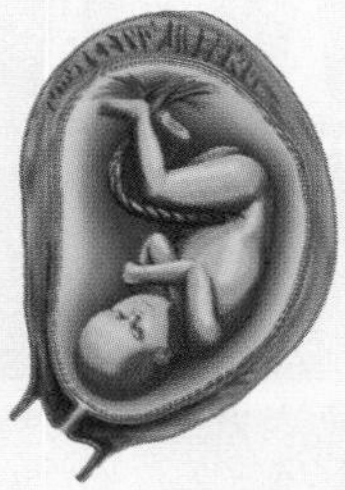

25 weeks

Weeks 25–28

Fetus reaches a length of 15 inches
Rapid brain development
Eyelids open and close
Nervous system controls some functions
Fingerprints are set
Blood formation shifts from spleen to bone marrow
Fetus usually assumes head-down position

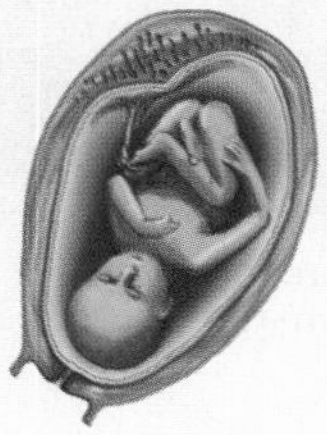

28 weeks

Weeks 29–32

Rapid increase in the amount of body fat
Increased central nervous system control over body functions
Rhythmic breathing movements occur
Lungs are not fully mature
Fetus stores iron, calcium, and phosphorus

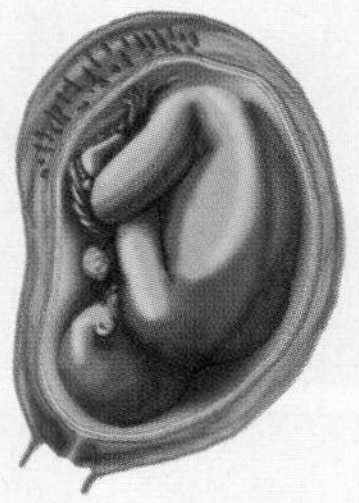

32 weeks

Weeks 33–38

Testes are in scrotum of male fetus
Lanugo begins to disappear
Increase in body fat
Fingernails reach the end of fingertips
Small breast buds are present on both sexes
Mother supplies fetus with antibodies against disease
Fetus is considered full term at 38 weeks
Fetus fills uterus

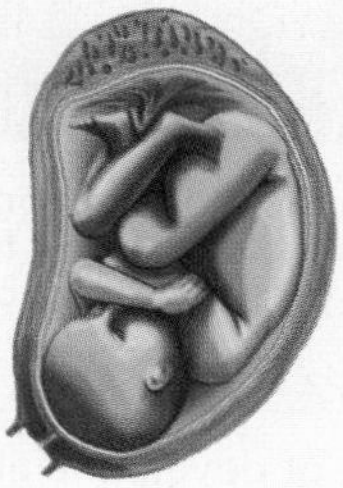

37 weeks

During the 3rd week of development, the villi at the embryonic pole further differentiate into two types of structures used to (1) anchor the chorionic sac to the maternal decidua and (2) exchange nutrients and other products with the mother (see Fig. 11.9C).

Concurrent with development of the villi, cells from the hypoblast form the exocoelomic cavity at the pole opposite the embryoblast (abembryonic). (*Note: Embryologists use spherical geography to describe the location of structures within an embryo, eg, pole, equator, or circumference.*) This cavity is the primitive yolk sac. Cells from the primitive yolk sac begin to form the extraembryonic mesoderm, a connective tissue that fills the space between the trophoblast and amnion. This mesoderm gives rise to the extraembryonic coelom (chorionic cavity) that surrounds the yolk sac and amniotic cavity.

On about day 13, cells from the hypoblast form the secondary yolk sac, which nourishes the developing embryo until the placenta fully forms. The connecting stalk attaches the embryoblast within the amniotic cavity to the trophoblast; the amniotic membrane does not cross this stalk (see Fig. 11.9C). The stalk develops blood vessels and surrounds the allantois by the 5th week of development. It fuses with the elongating secondary yolk sac (vitelline duct) and vitelline vessels to become the primitive umbilical cord by 10 weeks' gestation. By 12 weeks, the allantois, vitelline duct, and vitelline vessels regress, leaving the umbilical vessels (two arteries and one vein) encased within Wharton's jelly. Wharton's jelly serves as a protective surface barrier for the otherwise exposed umbilical vessels. At term, the umbilical cord is approximately 50 to 60 cm long and 2 cm in diameter.

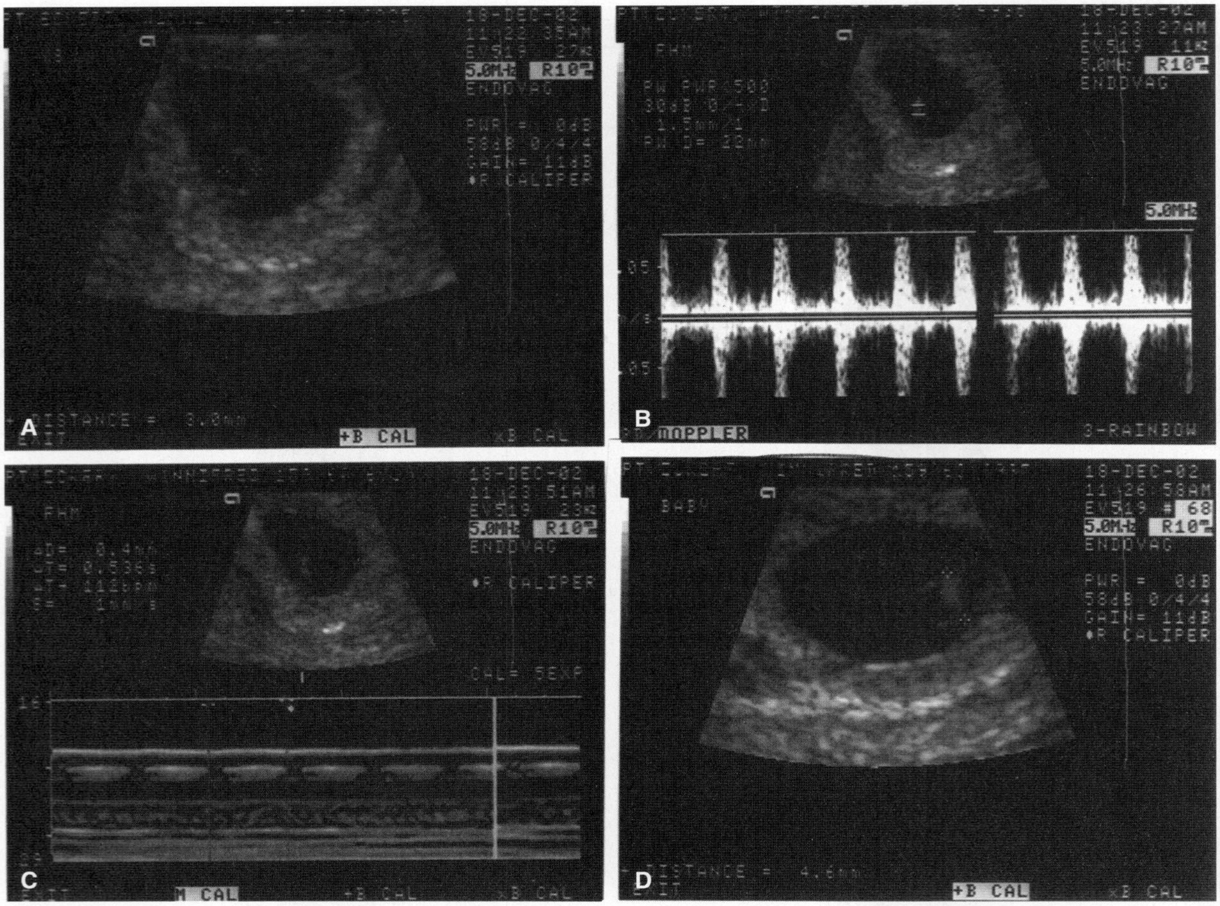

FIGURE 11.7 Five-week obstetrical sonographic evaluation. (**A**) Yolk sac. (**B**) Doppler recording of fetal heart tones. (**C**) Measurement of fetal heart rate of 112 beats/minute. (**D**) Crown–rump measurement of fetal pole. (Courtesy of M. Munch, The Fertility Center, York, PA.)

By the 8th week of development, the small villous projections cover the entire surface of the gestational sac. Initially, these villi are attached loosely to the trophoblast and are aspirated easily during chorionic villus sampling (CVS; discussed later in this chapter). Over the next 4 weeks, the villi over the embryonic pole continue to grow (forming the bushy chorion frondosum), while the villi at the abembryonic pole degenerate, creating the smooth chorion laeve. Similarly, the uterine decidua in proximity to the abembryonic pole thins and disintegrates as the gestational sac increases. The exposed chorion laeve expands with growth of the sac and fuses with the surfaces of the uterine cavity opposite the embryonic pole. This fusion creates a temporary closure of the uterine opening, which remains in place until gestation ends. Conversely, the decidual plate proliferates over the surface of the chorionic plate of the chorion frondosum. Within the gestational sac, the amnion also expands and obliterates the chorionic cavity. With this loss of space between the amnion and chorion, the two membranes fuse to form the "bag of waters," the amniochorionic membrane (bag) that surrounds the developing fetus.

The area between the chorionic and decidual plates contains the intervillous spaces (lakes) filled with maternal blood. It is into these intervillous lakes that the villi grow. By the 4th month, the chorion frondosum has developed 15 to 20 large villus trunks. The decidua basalis forms septa that grow between each villus trunk and surrounds the free villi branches. The septa do not descend to the chorionic plate, permitting the villus trees to remain connected to each other and the chorionic plate. Importantly, syncytial cells cover the outer layer of the septa, which together create the critical placental membrane barrier between the maternal blood in the intervillous spaces and the vessels of the embryonic villi. Growth of the septa segregates the villus trunks into compartmental structures known as *cotyledons.* These structures are visible on the maternal side of the placenta and appear as rugated liver. The fetal side of the placenta is smooth with evidence of large arteries and veins that converge toward the insertion site of the umbilical cord (Fig. 11.10). At the end of 38 weeks' gestation, the placenta covers approximately 15% to 30% of the internal uterine surface. It is approximately 15 to 20 cm in diameter, 3 cm deep, and 500 to 600 g. This

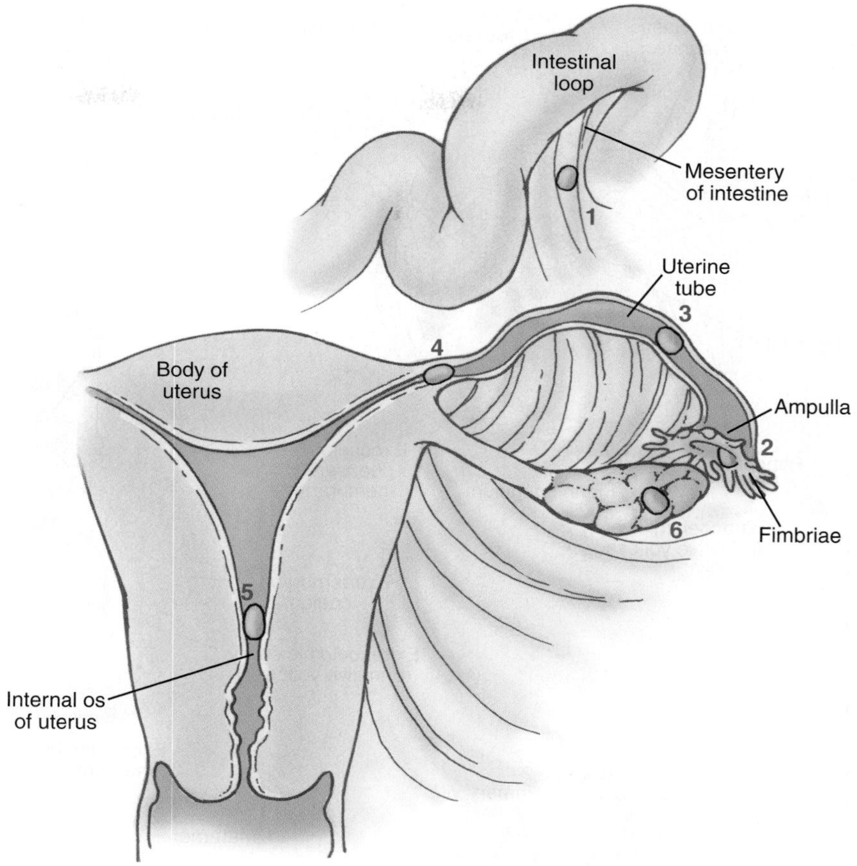

FIGURE 11.8 Diagrammatic representation of abnormal implantation sites. (Adapted from Sadler, T. W. [1995]. *Langman's medical embryology* [7th ed.]. Philadelphia: Lippincott Williams & Wilkins.)

growth is the result of the continued proliferation of the existing villus trunks (Sadler, 1995, 2005).

Spiral arteries (80 to 100) traverse the decidual plate to enter the intervillous lakes and provide maternal blood to the cotyledons. Endometrial veins return the blood to the maternal circulation. The differences in the pressure gradients between the maternal and fetal circulations force maternal blood into and out of the intervillous lakes in cycle with maternal blood pressure changes. The spiral arteries have a pressure of 70 mm Hg, the intervillous spaces have a pressure of 10 mm Hg, and the closed vascular system of the fetus maintains a fairly constant pressure of 30 mm Hg (Tuchmann-Duplessis et al., 1975). Placental circulation of 150 mL of blood occurs 3 to 4 times per minute. Further differentiation of the tissues between the chorionic and decidual plates during the 4th and 5th months of development enhance this process, bringing the syncytial membrane of the intervillous lakes into close proximity with the endothelial lining of the fetal vessels. Given the approximate 4 to 14 m^2 of villi surface area, this rate of exchange is achieved easily. Monitoring the pregnancy for placental function is necessary, however, given that the placenta begins to undergo changes suggesting a diminishing exchange between maternal and fetal circulations. Possible changes in the villi and fetal capillaries may reduce their permeability. Occasionally, these changes result in the infarction of an intervillous lake or an entire cotyledon. If changes are substantial, they affect the exchange of metabolic and gaseous products, harming the unborn fetus (Scott et al., 1999).

Function of the Placenta. The placenta serves two primary functions: exchange of metabolic and gaseous products between the fetal and maternal circulatory systems and production of hormones necessary for fetal development and continuation of the pregnancy (Table 11.2). The exchange of metabolic and gaseous products across the placental membrane occurs by three mechanisms:

- *Simple diffusion:* the passive movement of molecules from a higher concentration to a lower concentration. Substances exchanged across the placenta by simple diffusion include oxygen, carbon dioxide, water, hormones, electrolytes, and many drugs.
- *Facilitated or active transport:* the energy-consuming movement of molecules against an electrochemical gradient. Amino acids, free fatty acids, carbohydrates, and vitamins pass through the placenta by active transport.
- *Pinocytosis:* protrusion of the cell surface membrane to engulf a molecule. Albumin and maternal antibodies require pinocytosis for placental transport.

Transfer of maternal antibodies to the fetus confers acquired passive immunity on the newborn for several

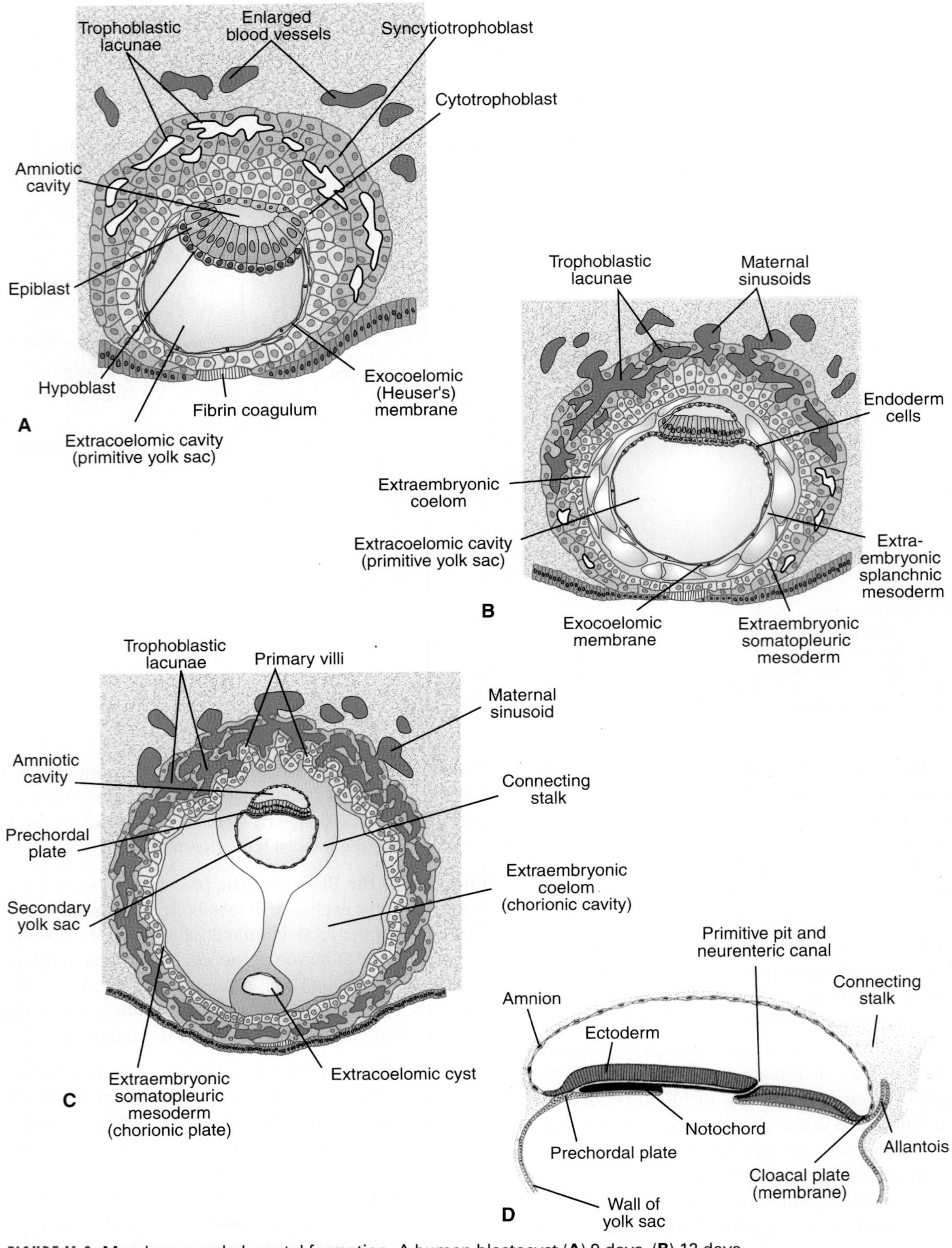

FIGURE 11.9 Membrane and placental formation. A human blastocyst (**A**) 9 days, (**B**) 12 days, (**C**) 13 days after fertilization, and (**D**) trilaminar germ disc forms during 3rd week after fertilization. (Adapted from Sadler, T. W. [1995]. *Langman's medical embryology* [7th ed.]. Philadelphia: Lippincott Williams & Wilkins.)

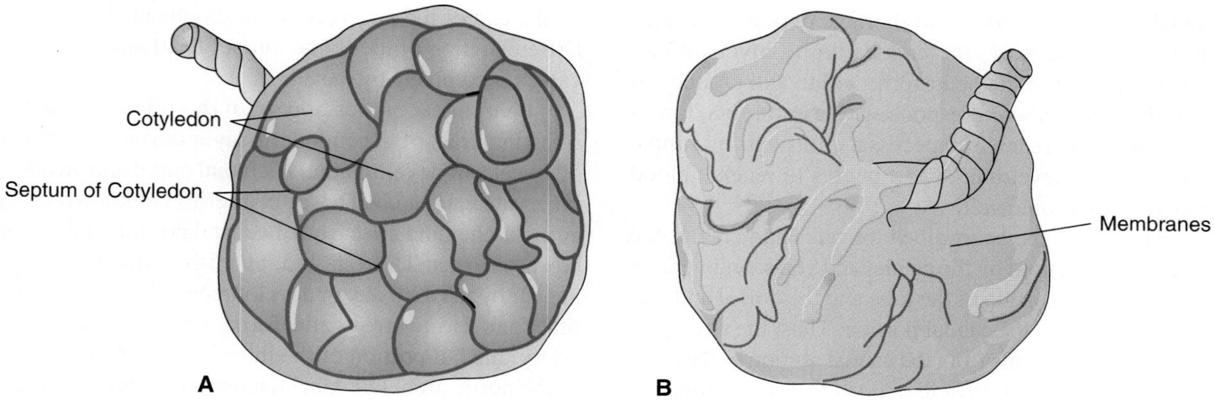

FIGURE 11.10 Placenta. (**A**) Maternal side. (**B**) Fetal side.

months after birth. The placenta produces the hormones progesterone, estriol, human chorionic gonadotropin (hCG), and somatomammotropin. Progesterone helps maintain the pregnancy. Estriol (estrogen) stimulates uterine growth and development of the maternal mammary glands. The hCG indicates the presence and health of a gestation. Somatomammotropin, a growth hormone, preferentially provides the fetus with glucose from the maternal circulatory system (Scott et al., 1999).

Function of the Amniotic Fluid. Amniotic fluid fills the amniotic cavity and protects the developing fetus. This clear fluid increases from 30 mL at 10 weeks' gestation to approximately 900 mL by 37 weeks. It is produced primarily by substances from the maternal blood supply and cells of the amniotic cavity. The fetus begins to swallow amniotic fluid and void at approximately 5 months' gestation. Fetal urine, however, largely consists of water, given that the placenta, not the fetal kidneys, filters fetal waste products to the maternal circulation.

The amniotic fluid is replaced every 3 hours and serves several key functions:

- Prevents injury to the fetus by providing a shock-absorbing cushion
- Separates the embryo from the other placental membranes
- Provides for movement early and throughout gestation, which is critical to fetal growth

Without an adequate volume of amniotic fluid, fetal malformations develop.

Circulation

The cardiovascular system begins to develop midway through the 3rd week of gestation (Sadler, 2005). The heart, blood vessels, and blood cells form from the mesoderm layer of the trilaminar embryo. In response to embryologic changes in the endoderm, the splanchnic mesoderm produces angioblasts that form clusters of angiocysts on the lateral sides of the disk-shaped embryo. These clusters migrate toward the cephalic pole, where they merge and form a horseshoe-shaped structure of small blood vessels. The anterior central segment of this structure becomes the cardiogenic area and, later, part of the heart tube. A second set of angiogenic cells appears on each side of the cardiogenic area. These bilateral cell clusters form the two dorsal aortae. Closure of the neural tube, followed by rapid brain development, causes the germ disk to fold cephalocaudally as well as laterally. This dual folding brings the caudal ends of the two dorsal aortae together, and they merge. The very distal ends of each tube, however, remain open. Later in development, these openings merge through the aortic arches with the cardiogenic area to form the heart tube. This folding also causes the cardiogenic area to move

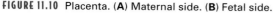

TABLE 11.2 Substances That Traverse the Placental Membrane

SUBSTANCES LEAVING MATERNAL CIRCULATION	SUBSTANCES LEAVING FETAL CIRCULATION
Oxygen	Carbon dioxide
Water	Water
Electrolytes	Urea
Carbohydrates	Waste products
Lipids	Hormones
Proteins	
Hormones	
Antibodies	
Viruses*	
Drugs*	

*Most viruses and many drugs (prescribed, over-the-counter, and recreational) cross the placenta from the maternal to fetal circulation and may adversely affect the fetus.

From Scott, J. R., DiSaia, P. J., Hammond, C. B., & Spellacy, W. N. (1999). *Danforth's obstetrics and gynecology* (8th ed.). Philadelphia: Lippincott Williams & Wilkins.

caudally from the cervical to thoracic region of the embryo. Simultaneously, the endocardium, myocardium, and epicardium of the heart form within and around the primitive heart tube. In response to the embryo's diminishing ability to receive all necessary nutrients by simple diffusion, the developing heart begins to receive blood from the embryonic veins.

By day 28, the heart tube elongates and creates the cardiac loop, caused by the caudal and ventral movement of the cephalic portion of the tube and the dorsal and cranial movement of the caudal portion. Thus, the atrial portion of the heart forms from the caudal section of the heart tube, whereas the ventricular portion forms from the cephalic portion. The major septa of the heart have formed by the end of the 5th week of development (Fig. 11.11). Differentiation of the four-chamber heart and associated valves is complete by the 8th week.

Pharyngeal arches appear in the primitive gastrointestinal tract of the endoderm layer during the 4th and 5th weeks of development. A cranial nerve and an artery innervate each arch. These six arteries are known as the aortic arches and arise from the distal portion of the truncus arteriosus. The 1st, 2nd, and 5th aortic arches disappear by the 29th day of development. The 3rd, 4th, and 6th continue to grow and form the common carotid artery, medial portion of the internal carotid artery, part of the aortic arch, left subclavian arteries, proximal segment of the right subclavian artery, proximal portion of

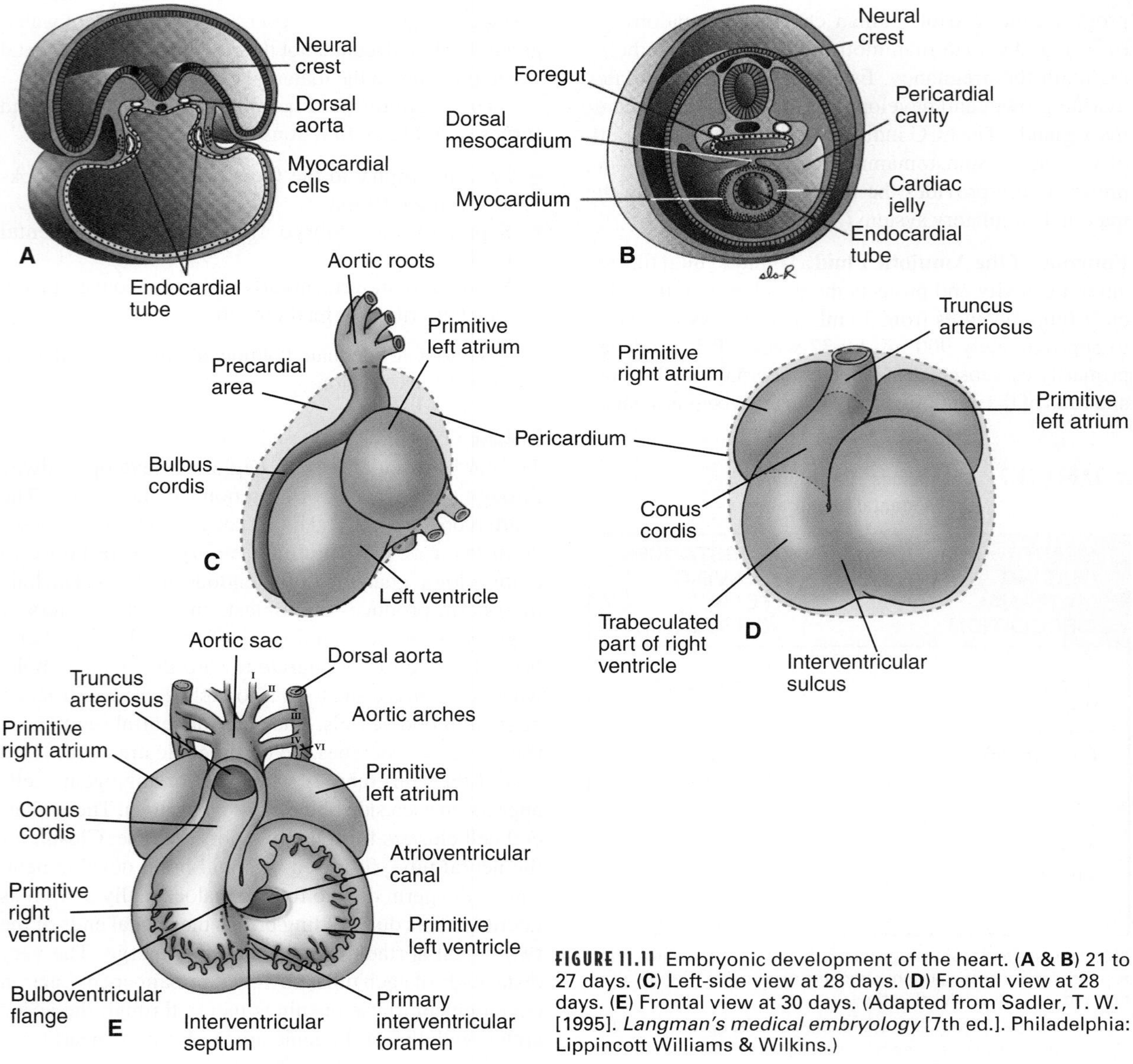

FIGURE 11.11 Embryonic development of the heart. (**A & B**) 21 to 27 days. (**C**) Left-side view at 28 days. (**D**) Frontal view at 28 days. (**E**) Frontal view at 30 days. (Adapted from Sadler, T. W. [1995]. *Langman's medical embryology* [7th ed.]. Philadelphia: Lippincott Williams & Wilkins.)

the right pulmonary artery, and ductus arteriosus. During this time, the vitelline and umbilical arteries form. The vitelline arteries initially supply the yolk sac; in the adult, they fuse to form the celiac, superior mesenteric, and inferior mesenteric arteries that nourish the gastrointestinal tract. The umbilical arteries form as paired branches of the dorsal aorta, travel alongside the allantois, and fuse with the connecting stalk to become the umbilical cord. The proximal portions of these arteries form the internal iliac and superior vesical arteries, whereas the distal segments form the medial umbilical ligaments after birth.

Concurrent with the development of the fetal arterial system, the venous system is established with the appearance of the vitelline, umbilical, and cardinal veins by the end of the 5th week of development. In later embryonic development, the vitelline veins give rise to the portal system (hepatocardiac portion of the inferior vena cava, portal vein, and superior mesenteric vein). The main drainage system of the early embryo consists of the cardinal veins. Later, these veins will form the caval system. Only one of the umbilical veins is sustained beyond the early embryonic period. As placental circulation increases, the left umbilical vein enlarges to form a primary communication with the ductus venosus and secondary branches with the hepatic sinusoids. At birth, the umbilical vein and ductus venosus lose their lumens and, respectively, become the ligamentum teres hepatic and ligamentum venosum.

The placenta is the main source of fetal nourishment and oxygen–carbon dioxide balance. The fetal respiratory and gastrointestinal systems do not have primary responsibility for these functions until after birth. The umbilical vein captures the maternal oxygen (80% saturation) crossing the placenta and transports it to the ductus venosus, where it continues through the inferior vena cava to the right and left atria. From there, the increasingly desaturated blood empties into the descending aorta and travels back to the placenta through the two umbilical arteries (58% saturation upon return to the placental membrane) (Sadler, 2005; Tuchmann-Duplessis et al., 1975).

With cessation of placental blood at birth and pressure changes in the heart and lungs that accompany postnatal circulation and spontaneous respiration, four major changes occur in the infant vascular system (Sadler, 2005). The closure of the umbilical vein, umbilical arteries, and ductus venosus are the result of the constriction caused by the umbilical cord clamp. The increased pressure in the right atrium closes the oval foramen (foramen ovale) between the left and right atria. Spontaneous respiration results in the release of bradykinin, which signals the smooth muscle surrounding the ductus arteriosus to contract and force closure of this structure (Sadler, 2005). Figure 11.12 compares human circulation before and after birth. Chapter 20 discusses fetal-to-newborn transitions in more detail.

Embryonic Development

As mentioned earlier, the embryonic phase lasts from the 3rd to 8th week of development (see Table 11.1). The 3rd week is critical to further development because it is when *gastrulation* occurs. Gastrulation is the process by which the primitive streak begins to form on the surface of the epiblast and in turn initiates formation of the trilaminar germ disk composed of ectoderm, mesoderm, and endoderm. By day 15 or 16, the primitive streak that begins at the caudal pole of the germ disk migrates toward the prechordal plate at the cephalic pole. The primitive node is a raised area encompassing the cephalic end of the pit that forms within the primitive streak. Through the process of invagination, epiblast cells selectively journey to the primitive streak, separate from the epiblast, and then migrate beneath it to lie between the epiblast and hypoblast layers. These cells differentiate into the endoderm and mesoderm. The remaining epiblast becomes the ectoderm. This migration continues until the cells move beyond the boundaries of the germ disk to join with the yolk sac and amnion; they travel bilaterally around the prechordal plate to meet, fuse, and form the cardiogenic plate (Sadler, 2005; Scott et al., 1999).

Through the same process of invagination, prenotochordal cells punctuate the hypoblast to create two layers along the midline of the embryo from the primitive pit to the prechordal plate. The notochord forms when cells of the notochordal plate propagate and detach in response to the developing endoderm around the primitive streak. The notochord develops cranially to caudally as the primitive streak moves toward the caudal pole. It lies beneath the neural tube and becomes the source of the axial skeleton. Throughout these two processes of invagination, the germ disk changes shape from nearly round to an elongated teardrop, with the cephalic end broader than the caudal pole. This change results from the significant migration of cells to the cephalic region, which continues through the 4th week. The primitive streak begins to disappear at the cephalic pole by the end of the 4th week, while it remains functional at the caudal pole through the 5th week before disappearing entirely. This process of cephalic (first) to caudal (last) development is constant throughout the embryonic phase (Fig. 11.13) (Sadler, 2005; Scott et al., 1999).

Organogenesis

Organogenesis begins on day 19 with formation of the neural plate, the foundation of the central nervous system (Table 11.3). The neural plate develops from the thickening of the ectoderm lying atop the notochord. It

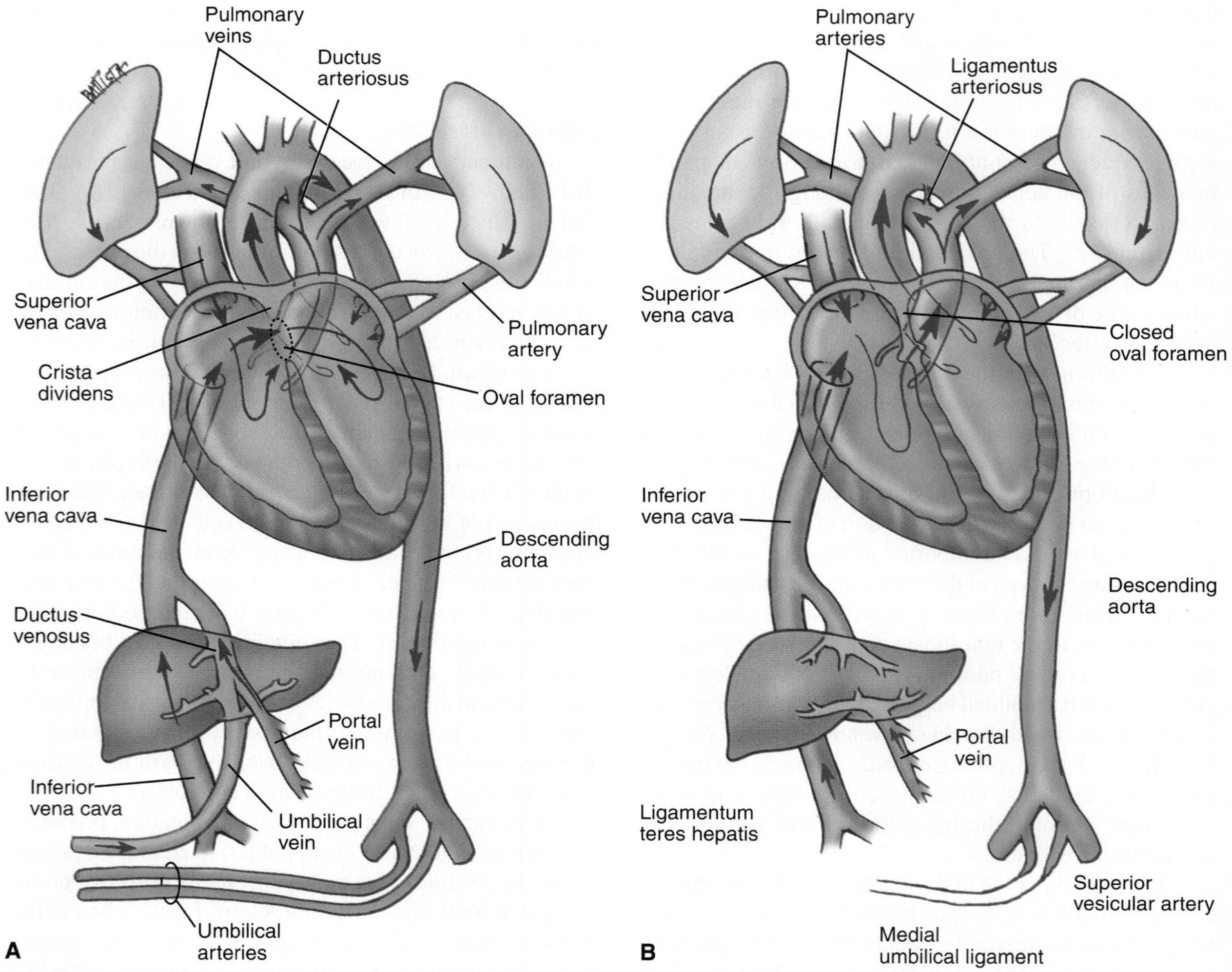

FIGURE 11.12 Human circulation (**A**) before birth and (**B**) after birth. (Adapted from Sadler, T. W. [1995]. *Langman's medical embryology* [7th ed.]. Philadelphia: Lippincott Williams & Wilkins.)

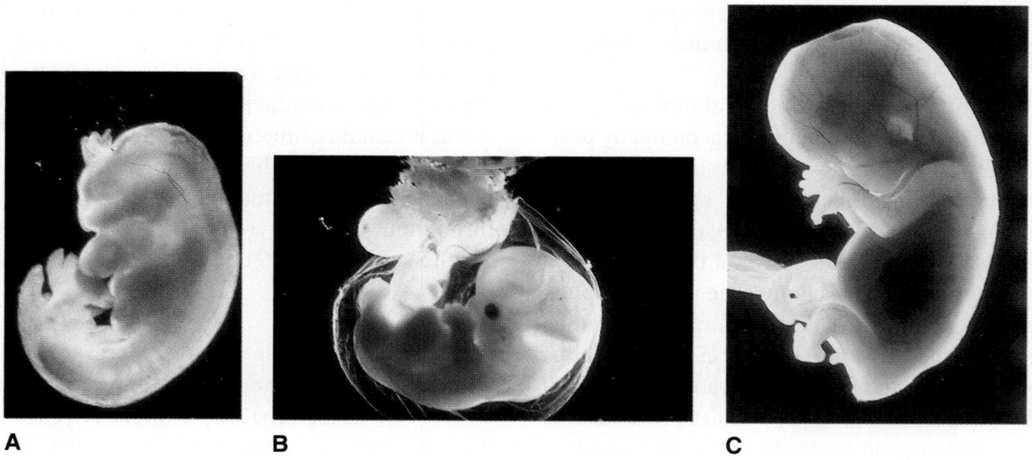

FIGURE 11.13 (**A**) Four-week embryo. (**B**) Five-week embryo. (**C**) Six-week embryo.

TABLE 11.3 Timing of Organogenesis by Embryonic Layer

LAYER	TISSUE FORMED	EMBRYONIC WEEK DEVELOPMENT BEGINS	ASSOCIATED DEVELOPMENTAL DEFECTS
Ectoderm			
	Central nervous system	3	Encephalocele Exencephaly Holoprosencephaly Hydrocephalus Neural tube defects
	Eye	4	Coloboma iridis Congenital cataracts Cyclopia Microphthalmia
	Peripheral nervous system	4	Meningomyelocele Myeloschisis
	Tooth enamel	6	Natal teeth
	Mammary and sweat glands	7	Polymastia Polythelia
	Ear (external)	8	Preauricular appendages Preauricular pits
	Pituitary	8	Pharyngeal hypophysis
	Skin and nails	8	Ichthyosis Nail hypoplasia
	Hair	12	Hypertrichosis
Mesoderm			
Parietal (somatic)	Parietal layer of serous membranes of peritoneal, pleural, and pericardial cavities	3 to 4	Cleft sternum Diaphragmatic hernia Gastroschisis
Visceral (splanchnic)	Cardiac muscle (myocardium)	3	Atrial and ventricular septal defects Tetralogy of Fallot Transposition of the great vessels
	Visceral layer of serous membranes covering abdominal organs, lungs, and heart	3 to 4	
	Smooth muscle of arteries, veins, lymph vessels, and blood and lymph cells	4 to 5	Coarctation of the aorta Cystic hygroma Patent ductus arteriosus
	Stromal and muscular wall of gastrointestinal tract	4 to 5	Congenital hiatal hernia Duodenal atresia Esophageal stenosis Extrahepatic biliary atresia Imperforate anus Omphalocele Pyloric stenosis Rectoanal atresia
Paraxial → somitomeres and somites	Cartilage, bone	4	Achondroplasia Amelia Cleft palate Clubfoot Cranioschisis → anencephaly Craniosynostosis Mandibulofacial dysostosis Osteogenesis imperfecta Polydactyly

Continued

● **TABLE 11.3 Timing of Organogenesis by Embryonic Layer *(Continued)***

LAYER	TISSUE FORMED	EMBRYONIC WEEK DEVELOPMENT BEGINS	ASSOCIATED DEVELOPMENTAL DEFECTS
	Subcutaneous tissue	4	
	Skeletal muscle	4 to 5	No pectoralis major muscle Prune belly syndrome
Intermediate	Kidneys, ducts, cortex of adrenal glands	4	Congenital adrenal hyperplasia Horseshoe kidney Pelvic kidney Polycystic kidney disease Renal agenesis → oligohydramnios
	Gonads, ducts, uterus	6 to 7	Cryptorchism Gonadal dysgenesis Hydrocele Hypospadias Inguinal hernia Testicular feminization Uterine bicornis Uterine didelphys
Endoderm			
	Respiratory tract epithelium	4	Esophageal atresia → polyhydramnios Tracheoesophageal fistula
	Gastrointestinal tract epithelium, including stomach, liver, gallbladder, and pancreas	4 to 5	Hirschsprung's disease Meckel's diverticulum Meconium ileus
	Urinary bladder epithelium	6	Exstrophy of the bladder
	Parenchyma of thyroid, parathyroids, liver, and pancreas	6 to 7	Hepatic tumor Thyroglossal cyst
	Tympanic cavity and eustachian tube	6 to 7	Deafness

Data from Sadler, T. W. (1995). *Langman's medical embryology* (7th ed.). Philadelphia: Lippincott Williams & Wilkins; Sanders, R. C. (2002). *Structural fetal abnormalities: The total picture.* St. Louis: Mosby.

grows toward the primitive streak while the bilateral edges become more prominent and form the neural folds. These folds proliferate until they join and fuse medially in the midsection to form the beginning of the neural tube. The neural folds of the cephalic pole close by day 25 and grow rapidly to form the vesicles of the brain. The caudal neural folds seal to form the spinal cord by day 27. Over the next 5 weeks, the ectoderm gives rise to the peripheral nervous system; sensory epithelium of the nose, eye, and ear; epidermis; subcutaneous, mammary, and pituitary glands; and tooth enamel.

The mesoderm further differentiates into three layers: paraxial, intermediate, and lateral (parietal and visceral). The paraxial mesoderm gives rise to somites, which develop cephalocaudally from days 20 to 35, creating a maximum 42 to 44 pairs. Six to eight of these pairs are lost, leaving 3 occipital, 7 cervical, 12 thoracic, 5 lumbar, 5 sacral, and 3 to 5 coccygeal pairs. Each somite produces sclerotome (cartilage and bone surrounding the notochord and spinal cord), myotome (striated and smooth muscle), and dermatome (skin) cells. The nephrogenic cord is formed by intermediate mesoderm and gives rise to the excretory components of the urinary and reproductive systems. Parietal mesoderm and ectoderm adhere to form the lateral and ventral body wall. The serous membranes of the peritoneal, parietal, and pericardial cavities and the spleen, blood vessels, and blood are all derivatives of visceral mesoderm (Sadler, 2005).

The rapid growth of the central nervous system and somites precipitates cephalocaudal and lateral folding of the embryo, respectively. This positional change profoundly affects development of the gastrointestinal tract, the primary organ system formed by endoderm. As the embryo becomes crescent shaped, the layer of endoderm forms a continuous tube from the cephalic to caudal ends of the embryo and passively changes its orientation in response to cephalocaudal bending. As a result, the yolk sac is pulled inside the body of the embryo and is constricted to form the vitelline duct. The endoderm also generates the parenchyma of the thyroid, parathyroids, liver, and pancreas; the epithelial lining of the respiratory tract, urinary bladder, urethra, tympanic cavity, and auditory tube; the tonsils; and the thymus gland (Sadler, 2005; Scott et al., 1999).

Appearance

The appearance of the embryo changes significantly from the 3rd to the 8th week. Initially, the embryo looks like a flattened spherical disk. By the end of this phase, eyes, ears, fingers, and toes are readily identifiable. Embryo size during this period is determined by measuring the distance from vertex of the cranium to the midpoint between the apices of the buttocks (crown–rump length, or CRL) (Table 11.4) (Callen, 1994; Sadler, 2005).

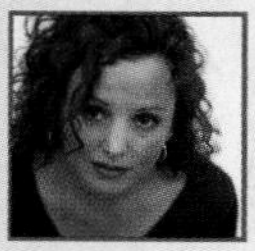

Recall April, described at the beginning of the chapter. Her pregnancy is of 13 weeks' gestation. Suppose April asks, "How much does my baby weigh now?" How would the nurse respond?

Teratology

The embryonic phase consists of 6 weeks of rapid growth and development. Alterations may develop from the genotype determined at conception, a spontaneous (de novo) change in maturation, or an adverse gestational environment. These changes are referred to as *congenital malformations, congenital anomalies,* or *birth defects.* Once the oocyte has been fertilized, the first two causes of congenital malformations are unalterable. The last is preventable. Nurses should remember, however, that most women are not aware they are pregnant until they are 6 to 8 weeks' obstetrical age, which correlates with the 4th to 6th week of embryonic development. This period is significant in its level of organogenesis (see Table 11.3) (Lewis, 2001). Thus, the effects of an adverse gestational environment may already be present before confirmation of pregnancy and initiation of prenatal care.

Teratology is the field of study that investigates and evaluates the causes of structural or functional damage to the developing embryo or fetus. The outcome for the embryo or fetus exposed to a **teratogen** may include any of the following (Lashley, 1998):

- No apparent effect
- Congenital anomalies
- Prenatal or perinatal death
- Altered growth
- Postnatal functional or behavioral deficits or aberrations
- Carcinogenesis

The principles of teratology describe the factors considered when evaluating probable cause for any alteration in normal embryonic and fetal development. Fundamental to these principles is the gestational age when intrauterine exposure occurs, dose and length of contact with the suspected teratogen, and genotype of the fetus (Lashley, 1998; Sadler, 2005). Table 11.5 presents agents associated with human malformations.

TABLE 11.4 Embryo and Fetal Size by Gestational Age

GESTATIONAL AGE (WEEKS*)	CRL LENGTH	WEIGHT (GM)	BIPARIETAL DIAMETER† (CM)	FEMUR LENGTH† (CM)
2	0.2 mm			
3	2–3 mm			
4	4–6 mm			
5	5–8 mm			
6	10–14 mm			
7	17–22 mm			
8	28–30 mm			
9–12	5–8 cm	10–45	2.5–3.0	1.0–1.7
13–16	9–14 cm	60–200	3.1–4.5	1.8–2.7
17–20	15–19 cm	250–450	4.6–5.5	2.8–3.8
21–24	20–23 cm	500–820	5.6–6.6	3.9–4.8
25–28	24–27 cm	900–1300	6.7–7.4	4.9–5.7
29–32	28–30 cm	1,400–2,100	7.5–8.4	5.8–6.6
33–36	31–34 cm	2,200–2,900	8.5–9.2	6.7–7.4
37–38	35–36 cm	3,000–3,400	9.2–9.7	7.5–7.9

*Weeks listed are based on embryology standard of 38 weeks' gestation. Add 2 weeks to each gestational age to correlate with the obstetrical standard of 40 weeks' gestation.

†BPD and femur are typically not measured until 12 weeks gestation.

Data from Sadler (1995), Sadler (2005), and Callen, 1994.

TABLE 11.5 Selected Agents Associated With Human Malformations

CATEGORY	AGENT	CONGENITAL MALFORMATION
Chemical	ACE inhibitors	Growth retardation, fetal death
	Alcohol	Fetal alcohol syndrome characterized by short palpebral fissures, maxillary hypoplasia, heart defects, mental retardation
	Amphetamines	Cleft lip, cleft palate, heart defects
	Aminopterin	Anencephaly, hydrocephaly, cleft lip, cleft palate
	Cocaine	Growth retardation, microcephaly, behavioral abnormalities, gastroschisis
	Diphenyl-hydantoin	Fetal hydantoin syndrome characterized by facial defects, mental retardation
	Formaldehyde	Growth retardation
	Iodine	Hypothyroidism, goiter
	Isotretinoin	Vitamin A embryopathy characterized by small, abnormally shaped ears, mandibular hypoplasia, cleft palate, heart defects
	Lead	Growth retardation, neurologic disorders
	Lithium	Heart malformations
	LSD	Limb defects, central nervous system defects
	Methotrexate	Limb defects, central nervous system defects
	Organic mercury	Multiple neurologic symptoms similar to cerebral palsy
	PCB	Growth retardation, gum hyperplasia, skull anomalies, developmental retardation
	Quinine	Deafness, limb anomalies, visceral defects, visual problems
	Streptomycin	Eighth cranial nerve damage (ear)
	Tetracycline	Discoloration and hypoplasia of tooth enamel
	Thalidomide	Limb defects, heart malformations
	Trimethadione	Cleft palate, heart defects, urogenital and skeletal abnormalities
	Valproic acid	Neural tube defects, heart, craniofacial and limb anomalies
	Warfarin	Chondrodysplasia, microcephaly
Hormones	Androgens	Masculinization of female genitalia
	Diethylstilbestrol (DES)	Malformations of the uterus, fallopian tubes, upper vagina, uterine cancer, malformed testes
	Maternal diabetes	Heart and neural tube defects
Infectious	Cytomegalovirus	Microcephaly, blindness, mental retardation
	Hepatitis virus	Biliary atresia, hepatic damage
	Herpes simplex virus	Microphthalmia, microcephaly, retinal dysplasia
	HIV	Microcephaly, growth retardation, HIV
	Parvovirus B19	Growth retardation
	Rubella virus	Cataracts, glaucoma, heart defects, deafness
	Syphilis	Mental retardation, deafness
	Toxoplasmosis	Hydrocephalus, cerebral calcifications, microphthalmia
	Varicella virus	Limb hypoplasia, mental retardation, muscle atrophy
Physical	Radiation (x-ray)	Microcephaly, spina bifida, cleft palate, limb defects
	Smelter emissions	Growth retardation, Wilms' tumor, multiple system anomalies
	Hyperthermia	Anencephaly

Note: This is a selected list of teratogenic agents. Absence of an agent from this list does not imply safe use during pregnancy. Not all fetuses will develop the congenital malformations described above.

ACE, angiotensin-converting enzyme; LSD, lysergic acid diethylamide; PCB, polychlorinated biphenyls.

Data from Harper (2001), Lashley (1998), and Sadler (1995).

Incidence of major structural congenital anomalies at birth is 2% to 3% and rises to 4% to 6% by 5 years, when additional findings are identified upon a child's admittance to school (CDC, 2004; Lashley, 1998). Minor congenital anomalies may be benign or associated with other birth defects that together significantly affect the newborn's health or well-being. The probability of an associated major defect increases with the number of minor anomalies found. There is a 3% chance of a major defect if one minor anomaly is present, a 10% chance with two minor anomalies, and a 20% chance with three or more (Sadler, 1995).

Anomalies are classified as malformations, disruptions, or deformations and may occur as part of a syndrome, association, or sequence event:

- A **malformation** is the complete or partial absence of a fetal structure.
- A **disruption** is a change in the morphology of a structure after its formation (eg, bowel atresia, amniotic bands).
- A **deformation** is the result of a mechanical event that abnormally molds an otherwise healthy tissue; it is often reversible after birth (eg, clubfeet).
- A **syndrome** is a clustering of multiple anomalies known to be primary outcomes of a single event.
- A **sequence** is a number of secondary alterations that develop from a major defect.
- An **association** is the presentation of a cluster of anomalies known not to be associated with either a syndrome or sequence event (Nussbaum et al., 2001).

Multiple Gestations

The number of multiple gestations has risen sharply over the past two decades (American Society for Reproductive Medicine, 2000). The U.S. incidence of twin births rose from approximately 2% (18.9 per 1,000 births) in 1980 to 3% (29.3 per 1,000 births) in 2000 (Martin et al., 2002). The most common form of multiple gestations is twins (Zhang et al., 2002), the two types of which are **monozygotic** (MZ) **twins** and **dizygotic** (DZ) **twins.** Traditionally, MZ twins are called "identical," and DZ twins are called "fraternal." Triplets and all other high-order multiple gestations may be MZ, DZ, or both.

MZ twins share the same genotype, although exposure to different environmental factors throughout their individual lives may result in the expression of different **phenotypes.** The natural incidence of MZ twins is 3 to 4 per 1,000 births (Sadler, 2005). These gestations result from an alteration in zygote development. Early in this process, the single cell mass becomes two or more independent structures, each capable of developing into a normal fetus (Fig. 11.14). The timing of the separation determines whether MZ babies share the same chorion, placenta, amnion, or all these. If the early embryo divides into two separate and distinct structures before the trophoblast has formed, they will not share the same chorion, placenta, or amnion. These MZ twins are noted to be dichorionic-diamniotic and may be identified initially as DZ. Their relationship requires genetic studies to determine that they are MZ infants. The most common incidence of MZ twins occurs 5 to 7 days after fertilization and results from the splitting of the inner cell mass of the blastocyst before formation of the amnion. These MZ twins have one placenta and one chorion, but two amnions (monochorionic-diamniotic). A rare form of MZ twinning is division of the bilaminar germ disk just before the primitive streak develops approximately 8 to 10 days after fertilization. This type creates a monochorionic-monoamniotic gestation. Conjoined (Siamese) twins are the result of the incomplete separation of the bilaminar germ disk. These twins may be joined at the chest-abdomen (thoracopagus), spine (pygopagus), or cranium (craniopagus). Some conjoined twins have been successfully separated (Sadler, 2005).

DZ twins represent more than two thirds of twin births and are reported to have a natural incidence of 7 to 11 per 1000 births (Sadler, 2005). Their occurrence is known to be influenced by the mother's ethnicity, age, parity, nutrition, and family history. Africans are more likely to give birth to twins than whites, and whites have a higher incidence of twin births than Asians. Incidence also increases with advancing maternal age and parity, good nutrition, and presence of twins in the maternal family history (Bortolus et al., 1999). DZ or multizygotic gestations result when separate sperm independently fertilize two or more oocytes within a single menstrual cycle. The placenta and chorion of each gestation may fuse together if the implantation sites for each embryo are in close proximity. This may result in the identification of a DZ twin gestation as MZ. DZ and multizygotic siblings share the same genetic relationship as any siblings born to the same genetic mother and father, whether birth occurs on the same day or years apart.

Fetal Development

The 9th to 38th weeks of development are called the fetal phase and are characterized by the exponential growth and maturation of the organs and systems developed during the embryonic phase. By the end of the 12th week, the fetus is 2.5 million times bigger than the zygote (Fig. 11.15). The exception to this rapid growth is the fetal head, which at 12 weeks makes up 50% of the CRL and by 20 weeks represents only 35% of the total crown–heel length (CHL). This ratio further decreases over the next 20 weeks; at birth, the head is 25% of the CHL (Callen, 1994; Sadler, 2005). The probability of malformations decreases during the fetal phase, although the central nervous system remains sensitive to teratogens. Deformations also may continue if the uterus, volume of amniotic fluid, and fetus do not develop in synchrony (Scott et al., 1999).

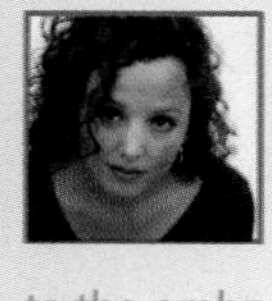

Think back to April, the 37 year old who is pregnant for the second time. Which period of gestational development is her pregnancy experiencing according to the embryologic standard?

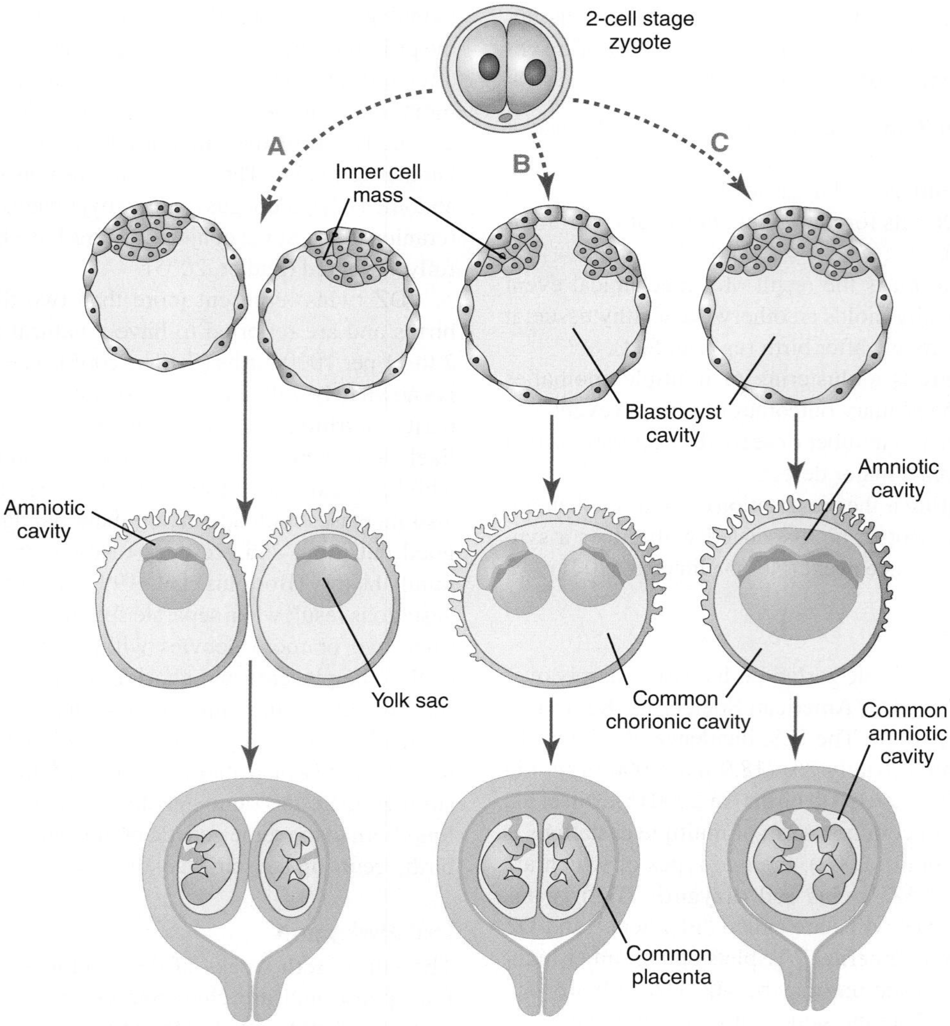

FIGURE 11.14 Diagrammatic representation of three types of monozygotic twins. (**A**) Separation occurs at the two-cell stage; twins are dichorionic-diamniotic. (**B**) Complete separation of the inner cell mass; twins are monochorionic-diamniotic. (**C**) Late separation of the inner cell mass; twins are monochorionic-monoamniotic. (Adapted from Sadler, T. W. [1995]. *Langman's medical embryology* [7th ed.]. Philadelphia: Lippincott Williams & Wilkins.)

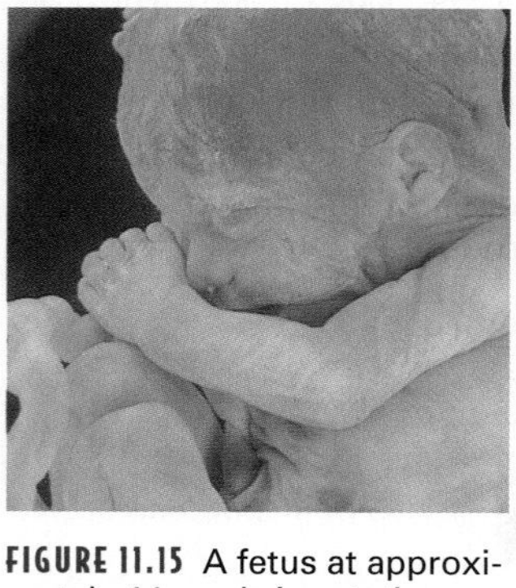

FIGURE 11.15 A fetus at approximately 14 weeks' gestation.

At the end of the 12th week, the eyes are in their medial location, the ears are rotated upward and outward, the limbs are proportional to the fetal trunk, the external sex is differentiated, and primary ossification centers are evident in the skull and long bones. Fetal movement is visible on ultrasound, but the mother typically is not aware of this activity.

At the end of the 20th week, the fetus has grown to 50% of its expected CHL at birth; however, fetal weight increases little from weeks 9 to 20 (see Table 11.4). Fine hair called *lanugo* covers the fetus; scalp hair and eyebrows are evident by the end of the 5th month. Importantly, the mother begins to experience fetal movement between the 16th and 20th weeks.

During the 7th and 8th month of fetal development, the fetus gains 50% of its birth weight. Deposits of subcutaneous tissue are laid down during this period in preparation for newborn metabolic functions and fluctuations in temperature in the postnatal environment. Chances of extrauterine survival before the 7th month are much lower than after the 7th month because the central nervous and respiratory systems undergo vast maturation during these last months of gestation. Critical physiologic processes associated with these systems must be completed during the last 2 months to enhance the neonate's survival (see Chap. 22).

By 38 weeks, the normally developed fetus has the anatomic structures and physiologic functions necessary for extrauterine life. The CHL is 48 to 58 cm. Weight is 3,000 to 3,400 g, and gender is readily identifiable by the well-defined external genitalia (Sadler, 2005).

PRECONCEPTION HEALTH ASSESSMENT AND SCREENING

Health assessment, screening, and counseling are vital behaviors for clients (see Chap. 2). Throughout the 20th century, scientific evidence mounted supporting health promotion and risk assessment to enhance the odds of the conception, gestation, and birth of a healthy child. The advent of modern medical genetics in the 1950s and the initiation of the Human Genome Project (HGP) in 1990 further supported the important role of health promotion and risk screening in positive reproductive outcomes.

Despite many years of public education by the U.S. Public Health Service and the March of Dimes Foundation about the importance of preconception health, preparation for and timing of most conceptions remain unplanned (Moos, 2004). Lack of reproductive planning can postpone health promotion behaviors until after the first prenatal appointment, usually at 8 weeks' gestation (Moos, 2003). The significance of this delay becomes clear when one remembers that the embryonic development of most organs and body systems is nearly complete by 9 to 10 weeks' gestation.

The scope of preconception health assessment, screening, and counseling continues to advance with knowledge identified through the ongoing HGP. Health care is moving broadly from an orientation of disease management to one of risk identification and prevention to promote lifelong health and wellness (Collins et al., 2003). This paradigm shift is especially important for clients who wish to optimize not only their own health but also the long-term well-being of their children.

Many clients who seek preconception health assessment are aware of a positive history for a risk factor. Examples include prior spontaneous loss of one or more pregnancies, inability to conceive, prior fetal anomaly, or a known genetic disorder within the reproductive family. Among women who seek preconception counseling because they will be 35 years or older when they give birth, many are identified to have non–age-related risk factors that would not have been addressed had they not sought counseling because of advanced maternal age. Such risk factors are not exclusive to clients of advanced maternal age and encompass chronic conditions (eg, hypertension, diabetes, cardiovascular disease, renal disease) and adult genetic disorders (eg, sickle cell anemia, Marfan syndrome) (see Chap. 4). These two groups, however, make up only a small portion of those women who conceive each year (Cefalo & Moos, 1995).

To eliminate gaps in service, many programs and agencies continuously attempt to increase public awareness of preconception health assessment. Examples include the federal government through the Public Health Service; state governments through Public Health Departments; the March of Dimes through national, regional, and local educational programs; and the media through public service campaigns. Despite such efforts, to date the CDC reports limited downward change in the incidence of the 21 congenital anomalies monitored (Martin et al., 2002).

Nurses in various health care settings should be prepared to either provide information about or perform preconception screening and counseling (Lea et al., 2000). One opportunity to disseminate such information is during annual gynecologic examinations; however, many women of childbearing age fail to seek this service. Examples of other settings in which nurses may share preconceptual health information are Planned Parenthood, pediatric offices, employee health services, school health services, and any health care encounter that includes a discussion of implications for reproduction (ie, diagnosis of a chronic disease).

Genetic Services

People who seek genetic services may be concerned about their own risk for a genetic disorder, a genetic disorder in their child, the risk for transmission of a genetic disorder to their child, or the effects of adverse environmental exposure on their health or that of their child. Most clients do not express concern for possible genetic risk until they approach conception and birth. Other people seek genetic services only when they or their child are suspected to have a genetic disorder, and further evaluation is recommended (Harper, 2001; Lashley, 1998).

Providing Genetic Counseling

Genetic counseling is the framework that guides the performance of genetic screening, diagnosis, evaluation, and intervention (Fig. 11.16). It is a process of information gathering, clinical and laboratory evaluation, and information sharing about the occurrence of or risk for a genetic disorder within a family. The goal is to provide appropriate and accurate information in a nondirective manner so that the client can make an informed decision about personal or family health and health care (Harper, 2001).

Nurses routinely provide counseling to clients about genetic concerns. Genetics nurses, genetic counselors, medical geneticists, clinical geneticists, and other health professionals with advanced training in human genetics provide genetic counseling, evaluation, diagnosis, and therapy (International Society of Nurses in Genetics and American Nurses Association, 1998). Collaboration

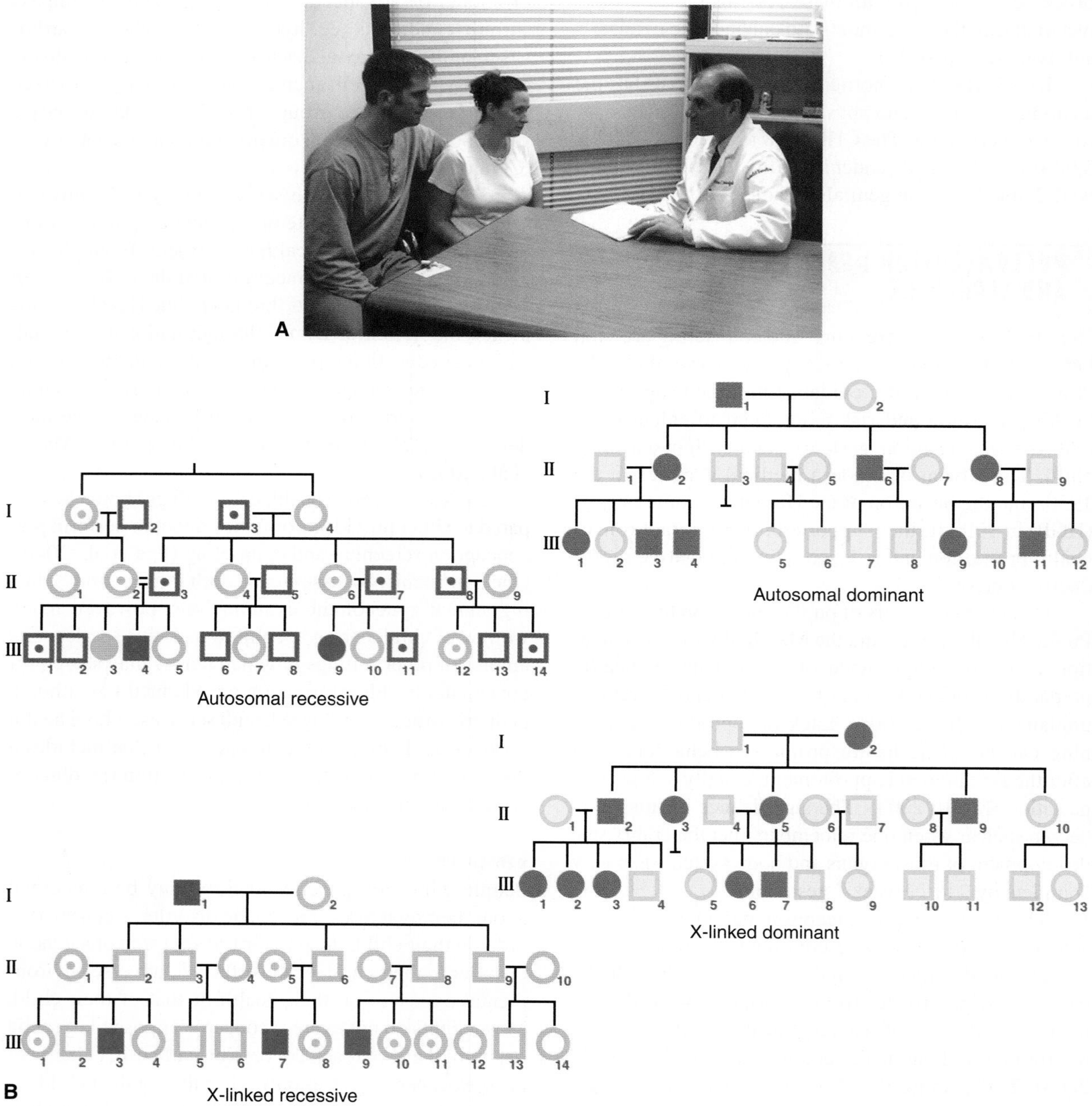

FIGURE 11.16 A couple receives genetic counseling. The provider uses teaching aids to assist the couple to understand genetic principles. See Assessment Tool 11-3 for explanations of the pedigrees. (Courtesy of Society Hill Genetics, Philadelphia.)

between the nurse and the genetics specialist is integral to the provision of preconception and prenatal health assessment and care. The nurse should integrate knowledge of genetics and associated health care implications to engage in the dialogue inherent within this collaborative relationship (Lashley, 1997). Importantly, the nurse needs to assimilate and synthesize this knowledge to provide comprehensive and appropriate care to each client (Lea et al., 2000).

Understanding Basic Genetic Principles

To provide appropriate client care and give accurate information, nurses need awareness of certain fundamental genetic principles: Mendelian patterns of inheritance, expression, penetrance, imprinting, anticipation, and polygenic and multifactorial inheritance (Lewis, 2001).

Mendelian Patterns of Inheritance. Mendelian patterns of inheritance are based on the fundamental biologic principle that each human gene has two copies: one on the maternal chromosome and one on the paternal chromosome (Nussbaum et al., 2001). Genes are categorized based on their location on a specific chromosome (loci). They are described as autosomal (chromosomes 1 to 22) or **sex linked** (X or Y chromosome). As a result of human genetic evolution, many genes have one or more alternate forms known as **alleles.** If both the maternal and paternal alleles for a specific locus are the same, then the person is said to be *homozygous* for that gene. Conversely, if the maternal and paternal alleles for a specific locus are different, then the person is said to be *heterozygous.* Because more than 30,000 genes are in the human genome, all humans are heterogenic as a result of genetic evolution. In addition, some genetic traits require only one copy of an allele to be expressed (**dominant** trait), whereas others require two copies of the same allele to be expressed (**recessive** trait). If a trait is caused by an autosomal dominant, autosomal recessive, X-linked dominant, or X-linked recessive gene, a specific pattern of inheritance is found within families, which is identified easily with the construction of a pedigree. See Table 11.6 for more information.

People with one dominant allele and one recessive allele for a given loci that requires two recessive alleles for expression are considered "carriers" of the recessive allele. Because they are not homozygous for the recessive allele, they do not express the associated phenotype; however, they can pass the recessive allele to any children. If the child subsequently receives two copies of the recessive allele (one from each parent), he or she will be homozygous for the recessive trait and will express its effects. For example, a father has brown eyes and a mother has blue eyes. The expression of brown eyes requires only one copy of the dominant allele (brown) for eye color. The expression of blue eyes requires two copies of the recessive form (blue). If the brown-eyed parent is homozygous, then all children of this couple will have brown eyes because the father can transmit only the dominant allele. If, however, he is heterozygous with one dominant allele (brown) and one recessive allele (blue), then each child has a 50% chance to be a brown-eyed heterozygote like the father and a 50% chance to be a homozygous blue-eyed child like the mother (Lashley, 1998; Lewis, 2001).

An inheritable permanent change in the DNA of a gene is known as a *mutation.* Some mutations have a benign or no effect; others result in an adverse alteration. Typically, such changes affect growth, development, and wellness. As with all other human traits, disorders caused by a single copy of an altered gene follow dominant patterns of inheritance, whereas disorders that require two copies of the altered gene follow recessive patterns of inheritance. More than 3,000 autosomal dominant disorders, 1,500 autosomal recessive disorders, and 300 X-linked disorders have been identified (National Center for Biotechnology Information, 2003).

TABLE 11.6 Characteristics of Single-Gene Disorders

CHARACTERISTIC	AUTOSOMAL RECESSIVE	AUTOSOMAL DOMINANT	SEX-LINKED RECESSIVE	SEX-LINKED DOMINANT
Gender bias	None	None	Males only	Higher percentage in females
Transmission	Horizontal	Vertical	Vertical	Sporadic
Risk for occurrence	25% affected; 50% carriers	50% affected	50% affected males; 50% carrier females	50% children of affected females; 100% daughters of affected males
Unique characteristics	Consanguinity	Male-to-male transmission	Unequal X-inactivation results in affected daughters	X-inactivation modifies effect on daughters

Some dominant disorders (eg, Huntington's disease, or HD) do not appear until adulthood and are referred to as *adult-onset disorders.* In some cases, an altered dominant gene confers a 100% chance of expression, but clinical features have not yet developed; this is considered a *presymptomatic disorder.* The term *predisposition* describes clients who have an altered gene, but do not have a 100% chance of expressing its clinical manifestations unless another concurrent biologic event occurs (Lashley, 1998; Nussbaum et al., 2001).

Several recessive disorders have increased frequencies among specific ethnic groups. This is the result of generations of people consistently establishing reproductive relationships within and among their same ethnic group, causing repeated transmission of carrier status from parent to child. See Tables 11.7 to 11.10.

TABLE 11.7 Selected Genetic Disorders by Population or Ethnic Group

POPULATION OR ETHNIC GROUP	GENETIC DISORDER	PATTERN OF INHERITANCE
Acadian (Nova Scotia)	Niemann-Pick disease, type D	AR
Afrikaner	Porphyria variegata	AR
Åland Islanders	Ocular albinism (Forsius-Erikson type)	XR
Amish	Ellis-van Creveld	AR
	Hemophilia B	XR
	Limb-girdle muscular dystrophy	AR
	Pyruvate kinase deficiency hemolytic anemia	PG/MF
Armenians	Familial Mediterranean fever	AR
	Familial paroxysmal polyserositis	AR
Asians	Dubin-Johnson syndrome (Iranian Jews, Japan)	AR
	Reduced penetrance in females	
	G6PD deficiency, Mediterranean type	XR
	Ichthyosis vulgaris (Iraq, India)	AD
	Metachromatic leukodystrophy (Habbanite Jews, Saudi Arabia)	AR
	Phenylketonuria (Yemen)	AR
	Werdnig-Hoffman disease (spinal muscular atrophy infantile type I; Karaite Jews)	AR
Blacks (African)	β-Thalassemia	AR
	G6PD deficiency, African type	AR
	Hemoglobin C disease	AR
	Hereditary persistence of hemoglobin F	AR
	Lactase deficiency (adult)	AR
	Sickle cell disease	AR
Burmese	Hemoglobin E disease	AR
Chinese	α-Thalassemia	AR
	Lactase deficiency (adult)	AR
	G6PD, Chinese type	AR
	Werdnig-Hoffman disease (spinal muscular atrophy infantile type I)	AR
Costa Ricans	Malignant osteopetrosis	AR
Druze	Alkaptonuria	AR
English	Cystic fibrosis	AR
	Hemachromatosis type I	AR
	Hereditary amyloidosis type III (spinocerebellar atrophy)	AR
	Werdnig-Hoffman disease (spinal muscular atrophy infantile type I)	AR
French Canadians	Morquio's syndrome	AR
	Tay-Sachs disease	AR
	Tyrosinemia	AR
Finns	Aspartylglycosaminuria	AR
	Congenital nephrosis	AR
	Diastrophic dwarfism	AR
	Generalized amyloidosis syndrome V	AD
	Polycystic liver disease	AD
	Retinoschisis	XR

Continued

TABLE 11.7 Selected Genetic Disorders by Population or Ethnic Group

POPULATION OR ETHNIC GROUP	GENETIC DISORDER	PATTERN OF INHERITANCE
Filipino	Torsion dystonia type 7	XR
Gypsies (Czech)	Congenital glaucoma	AR
Hopi Indians	Tyrosinase-positive albinism	AR
Hungarians	Werdnig-Hoffman disease (spinal muscular atrophy infantile type I)	AR
Icelanders	Phenylketonuria	AR
Inuit Eskimos	Amyloidosis	AR
	Congenital adrenal hyperplasia	AR
	Methemoglobinemia	AR
	Pseudocholinesterase deficiency	AR
Irish	Neural tube defects	PG/MF
	Phenylketonuria	AR
Japanese	Acatalasemia	AR
	Cleft lip/palate	PG/MF
	Oguchi's disease	AR
Jews (Ashkenazi)	Bloom's syndrome	AR
	Canavan's disease	AR
	Cystic fibrosis	AR
	Factor XI (PTA) deficiency	AR
	Familial dysautonomia (Riley-Day syndrome)	AR
	Fanconi anemia (group C)	AR
	Gaucher disease type III (adult)	AR
	Niemann-Pick disease (infantile)	AR
	Tay-Sachs disease	AR
	Torsion dystonia (adult)	AR
Jews (Sephardic)	Ataxia-telangiectasia (Morocco)	AR
	Cystinuria (Libya)	AR
	Glycogen storage disease type III (Morocco)	AR
Lapps	Congenital dislocation of hip	PG/MF
Lebanese	Dyggve-Melchior-Clausen syndrome	XR
Mediterranean (Italians, Greeks)	β-Thalassemia	AR
	Familial Mediterranean fever	AR
	G6PD deficiency, Mediterranean type	XR
Navaho Indians	Ear anomalies	PG/MF
Polynesians	Clubfoot	PG/MF
Polish	Phenylketonuria	AR
Portuguese	Joseph's disease	AD
Scandinavians (Danes, Swedes, Norwegians)	α-Antitrypsin deficiency	AR
	Cholestasis-lymphedema (Norwegians)	AR & AD
	Dupuytren's disease	AD & MF/PG
	Krabbe's disease	AR
	Lecithin cholesterol acyltransferase (LCAT) deficiency	AR
	Phenylketonuria	AR
	Sjögren-Larsson syndrome (Swedes)	AR
Scots	Cystic fibrosis	AR
	Hereditary amyloidosis, type III	AD
	Phenylketonuria	AR
	Werdnig-Hoffman disease (spinal muscular atrophy infantile type I)	AR
Thailanders	Hemoglobin E disease	AR
	Lactase deficiency, adult	AR
Zuni People	Tyrosinase positive albinism	AR

AD, autosomal dominant; AR, autosomal recessive; G6PD, glucose-6-phosphate dehydrogenase; MF, multifocal; PG, polygenetic; XR, X-linked recessive.

From Burrow & Farris (1988), Lashley (1998), and Online Mendelian Inheritance in Man (2003), http://www.ncbi.nlm.nih.gov/.

TABLE 11.8 Eastern European Jewish Carrier Screening

DISEASE	DISEASE INCIDENCE	JEWISH CARRIER FREQUENCY	DETECTION RATE	TESTING METHOD	NON-JEWISH CARRIER FREQUENCY	NON-JEWISH CARRIER DETECTION RATE
Tay-Sachs	1/3,000	1/30	98% by Hex A enzyme 94% by DNA-based test	Enzyme-leukocyte* DNA-based test	1/30 French Canadians, Cajuns; 1/250 other populations	98% by Hex A enzyme
Cystic fibrosis	1/2,500–3,000	1/26–29	97%	DNA	See Table 11.9	See Table 11.9
Canavan's disease	1/6,400	1/40	98%	DNA	Unknown	Unknown†
Niemann-Pick disease (type A)	1/32,000	1/89	95%	DNA	Unknown	Unknown†
Fanconi's anemia (group C)	1/32,000	1/90	99%	DNA	Unknown	Unknown†
Bloom's syndrome	1/40,000	1/100	95%–97%	DNA	Unknown	Unknown†
Gaucher's disease	1/900	1/15	95%	DNA	Unknown	Unknown†
Dysautonomia	1/3,600	1/32	99%	DNA	Unknown	Unknown†

Note: For DNA-based testing, 10 mL should be obtained in yellow-top ACD-A or lavender-top EDTA tubes. For enzyme testing, specimen requirements may vary between laboratories; call laboratory for instructions. Numbers may not be exact; for clinical comparison only.

*Tay-Sachs carrier testing by enzyme on pregnant women and those on oral contraceptives must be done through leukocytes.

†Unless familial mutation is known, DNA testing in the non-Jewish population will have a lower detection rate than in the Jewish population.

From Genetic Pocket Screening Facts. (2001). March of Dimes Birth Defects Foundation (09-1618-01). Reprinted with permission.

● **TABLE 11.9 Cystic Fibrosis DNA Testing**

ETHNICITY	DISEASE INCIDENCE	CARRIER FREQUENCY	CARRIER DETECTION RATE* (%)	AT-RISK COUPLE† DETECTION RATE (%)
Northern European	1/2,500	1/25–29	85–90	80
Southern European	1/2,500	1/25–29	70	50
Ashkenazi Jewish	1/2,800	1/26–29	97	95
Hispanic	1/8,100	1/46	57	32
African American	1/14,500	1/60–65	72	50
Asian	1/32,000	1/90	30	10
Other populations	Extremely variable	Extremely variable	70, generally	50

Note: For DNA-based testing, 10 mL should be obtained in yellow-top ACD-A or lavender-top EDTA tubes. Numbers may vary between laboratories.

*Carrier detection rates are dependent on the number of mutations screened by the laboratory

†At-risk couple—couple in which both members are found to be carriers and thus have a 25% chance of having a baby with cystic fibrosis.

From March of Dimes Birth Defects Foundation. (2001). *Genetic screening pocket facts.* Publication No. 09-1618-01, White Plains. NY: Author. Reprinted with permission.

Penetrance and Expression. Some variations that occur between genotype and phenotype are explained through the principles of *penetrance* (the percentage of people with the gene who manifest the associated characteristics) and *expression* (the degree to which the characteristics of a gene are manifest within the person). These two biologic processes account for the prior inability to classify some congenital disorders according to Mendelian principles. Such conditions did not appear to follow any of the four standard patterns of inheritance, although they consistently recurred within extended families (Harper, 2001; Lashley, 1998). The relationship between penetrance and expression for those at risk for transmission of an adverse genetic trait is profound. For example, some people with the autosomal dominant form of osteogenesis imperfecta express the disorder by having blue sclera and no other problems; others experience recurrent skeletal fractures even with mild trauma. In addition, within the same family, parent and child may express the disorder to different degrees. An example is seen in families with a history of tuberous sclerosis, a disorder characterized by epilepsy, learning difficulties,

● **TABLE 11.10 Hemoglobinopathies**

ETHNICITY	β-THAL TRAIT	α-THAL TRAIT*	SICKLE CELL TRAIT*	HEMOGLOBIN C TRAIT†	OTHER HEMOGLOBIN VARIANTS
Mediterranean	1/20–30	1/30–50 trans§	1/30–50	Rare	D, G, Lepore
African American	1/75	1/30 trans§	1/12	1/50	0, D
Non-Hispanic Caribbean, West Indian	1/50–75	1/30 trans§	1/12	1/30	0, D
West African	1/50	1/30 trans§	1/6	1/20–30	0, D
Hispanic Caribbean	1/75	Variable	1/30	Rare	Variable
Hispanic Mexican, Central American	1/30–50	Variable	1/30–200	Rare	J, E
Asian	1/50	1/20 cis§	Rare	Rare	E
Southeast Asian	1/30	>1/20 cis§	Rare	Rare	E
Asian Subcontinent (Indian, Pakistani)	1/30–50	Variable	1/50–100	Rare	D, 0, E
Middle Eastern	1/50	Variable	1/50–100	Rare	D, 0, E, J

†Sickle cell prep or dex is not an appropriate screening tool for hemoglobinopathies.

‡CBC and hemoglobin electrophoresis are adequate screens for all ethnic backgrounds.

*α-Thalassemia is an exclusion diagnosis unless DNA analysis is utilized.

^Numbers may not be exact; for clinical comparison only.

§Cis α-thal trait (mutations carried on the same chromosome) has more clinical significance than trans α-thal trait (each mutation is carried on opposite chromosomes of a homologous pair).

From March of Dimes Birth Defects Foundation. (2001). *Genetic screening pocket facts.* Publication No. 09-1618-01. White Plains, NY: Author. Reprinted with permission.

behavioral problems, and skin lesions. Although a highly penetrant gene, some people have no disorder-related problems, even though they have both a parent and a child with clinical manifestations (National Center for Biotechnology Information, 2003).

Imprinting and Anticipation. Imprinting and anticipation further explain the variability in findings among people with Mendelian single-gene disorders (Harper, 2001; Wilkins-Haug, 1993). *Imprinting* means that an allele demonstrates a different phenotypic effect depending on whether the child received the allele from mother or father. For example, a child will show characteristics of Beckwith-Wiedemann syndrome (eg, exomphalos, macroglossia, gigantism) if the mother transmits the allele for this disorder located on the "p" arm of chromosome 11. Conversely, the child will not express symptoms if the father transmits the same allele (Harper, 2001). Another example involves Prader-Willi syndrome (PWS) and Angelman syndrome (AS). PWS is characterized by obesity, muscular hypotonia, mental retardation, short stature, and hypogonadotropic hypogonadism. AS is characterized by severe retardation, ataxia, hypotonia, epilepsy, absence of speech, and unusual facies. It is now understood that the same gene on chromosome 15 causes both PWS and AS, but expression depends on the parent of origin. PWS is the outcome of maternal transmission, whereas AS is the outcome of paternal transmission (Lashley, 1998; National Center for Biotechnology Information, 2003).

In most cases, the amount of DNA within a gene is stable and does not change from one generation to the next. Nevertheless, among certain autosomal dominant disorders, this biologic principle is false. Myotonic dystrophy, fragile X syndrome, and HD are known to increase in severity with subsequent generations (Crawford et al., 2001; Harper, 2001). The cause is an expansion in the number of trinucleotides within the gene. This increased repetition of trinucleotides occurs during meiotic division and does not follow any established pattern; that is, a change may or may not occur in any or all subsequent generations of successive meioses. This is the biologic principle of *anticipation.*

Multifactorial Inheritance. *Multifactorial inheritance* means that multiple genes and their interactions with environmental factors regulate the expression of a phenotypic trait. It is the most common form of inheritance in the general population (Box 11.1). The presence or absence of a critical mass of interacting factors mediates expression of the disorder. Using the threshold model (Fig. 11.17), if the threshold is reached, then the person manifests signs of the disorder. Unlike Mendelian inheritance, the risk for a **multifactorial disorder** in a first-degree relative is disorder specific and depends on *heritability* (historical frequency of the disorder when manifested within an extended family) and incidence within the overall population. Generally, the risk for recurrence is equal to the square root of the population incidence. Thus, if a couple has given birth to one child with spina bifida (general population frequency, 1:1,000), the specific risk for recurrence in a subsequent pregnancy is approximately 1:32 (Harper, 2001). The risk for occurrence within a nuclear family increases if the woman and her reproductive partner are related genetically (Bennett et al., 2002). Estimates are that first cousins share the same alleles for approximately one eighth of all their genes (Nussbaum et al., 2001). This significantly increases the likelihood of transmission of a Mendelian or multifactorial disorder to a child conceived with their gametes.

BOX 11.1 Common Multifactorial Disorders

Congenital Anomalies

- Anencephaly
- Cleft lip with/without cleft palate
- Cleft palate
- Clubfoot
- Dislocation of the hip
- Heart defects
- Hypospadias
- Pyloric stenosis
- Spina bifida

Childhood and Adult Disorders

- Asthma
- Cancers
- Crohn's disease
- Diabetes (type 1)
- Hypertension
- Multiple sclerosis
- Peptic ulcer
- Psoriasis
- Systematic lupus erythematosus

Data from Lashley, F. R. (1998). Clinical genetics in nursing practice (2nd ed.). New York: Springer, and National Center for Biotechnology Information (2003). Online Mendelian inheritance in man. Available at: http://www.ncbi.nlm.nih.gov.

In addition to the genes contained on the chromosomes within the nucleus of every cell, the mitochondria found in the cytoplasm of the cell contain at least 60 unique genes (National Center for Biotechnology Information, 2003). The mutation rate among mitochondrial genes is higher than for the genes found on the chromosomes. Mitochondrial disorders are relatively rare and typically affect the brain, skeletal, and heart muscle (Lashley, 1998; Tinkle & Castora, 2002). Importantly, these disorders are transmitted maternally. Sons and daughters are affected equally, but fathers do not transmit the disorder to any children.

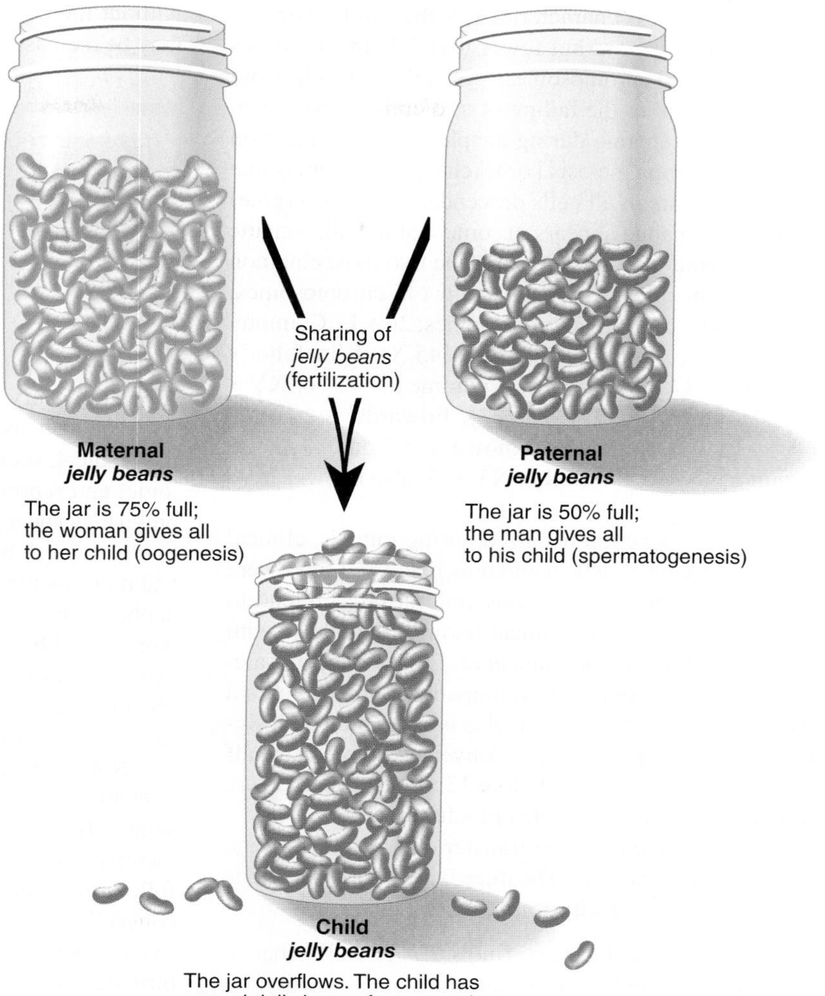
Sharing of
jelly beans
(fertilization)
Maternal
jelly beans
The jar is 75% full;
the woman gives all
to her child (oogenesis)
Paternal
jelly beans
The jar is 50% full;
the man gives all
to his child (spermatogenesis)
Child
jelly beans
The jar overflows. The child has
enough jelly beans for one and one
half jars. Also, the jar should be shrunk
a bit from environmental wear and tear.

FIGURE 11.17 Jelly bean jar threshold model.

Duplications, Deletions, and Translocations. Structural changes in chromosomes result from deletions, duplications, or translocations. These problems account for 3% to 7% of spontaneous gestational losses (Lashley, 1998).

A *deletion* is the breakage and removal of a portion of a chromosome. It may occur on either distal end or within the chromosome itself (broken middle sections reattach to form a single structure). The best-known deletion syndrome is *cri-du-chat,* which results from the absence of the "p" arm of chromosome 5. Infants with cri-du-chat have an abnormal cry that sounds like a cat. DiGeorge's syndrome results from absence of a small portion of the "q" arm of chromosome 22 (Sanders, 2002).

A *duplication* is insertion of additional DNA within a chromosome, which may or may not have adverse phenotypic effects. Charcot-Marie-Tooth syndrome, a peripheral neuropathy, results from a replicated segment on the "p" arm of chromosome 17.

Disorders also may result from deletions or duplications of one or more entire chromosomes. Such changes either increase or decrease the amount of genetic material found in that person's genome. They are categorized as alterations in either number or structure. *Euploidy* is the correct complement of 46 chromosomes (diploid, 2n = 46 chromosomes). *Polyploidy* is a change in the total number of chromosomes. Examples include multiple haploid sets (n = 23 chromosomes) such as triploidy (3n = 69 chromosomes) and tetraploidy (4n = 92 chromosomes). Triploidy most frequently results from the simultaneous fertilization of the oocyte by two separate sperm. A failure in meiotic division of the diploid oocyte or sperm also can produce a triploid zygote. Failure of the first mitotic division of the zygote causes tetraploidy. Approximately 25% of spontaneously aborted fetuses are found to have either triploidy or tetraploidy, neither of which is compatible with life beyond the neonatal period (Lashley, 1998).

Aneuploidy is characterized by the addition or deletion of one or more but fewer than 23 chromosomes ($2n \pm 1$ or 2 or 3 chromosomes). Aneuploidy results from *nondisjunction,* or the failure of two homologous chromosomes to separate during anaphase. Nondisjunction may occur during meiosis I or II (change in chromosome number appears in all cells descended from the zygote) or mitosis (change appears in some, but not all, somatic cells; referred to as mosaicism). The two most common forms of aneuploidy are *monosomy* (45 chromosomes; $2n - 1$) and *trisomy* (47 chromosomes; $2n + 1$). Common examples are Turner's syndrome (45,X), Klinefelter's syndrome (47,XXY), Down syndrome (47,XX or XY + 21, also known as trisomy 21), Edwards' syndrome (47,XX or XY + 18; also known as trisomy 18), and Patau's syndrome (47,XX or XY +13; also known as trisomy 13) (Fig. 11.18).

If nondisjunction occurred during mitosis, clinical findings depend on which and how many cell lines were affected. People with chromosomal mosaicism tend to have fewer and milder clinical findings than those with other aneuploidy (Nussbaum et al., 2001). Each mosaicism mentioned previously is compatible with life beyond the neonatal period, but each also is associated with significant phenotypic findings. Conversely, more than half of spontaneous abortions before 12 weeks' gestation are found to have one of the aneuploidies (Harper, 2001).

A *translocation* is the transfer of a segment of one chromosome to another. The three types of translocations are reciprocal, nonreciprocal, and Robertsonian.

- Reciprocal translocation is the breakage and exchange of segments between two chromosomes; usually, no genetic material is lost.
- Nonreciprocal translocation is the breakage of a single segment from one chromosome with attachment to another. Each translocation may be balanced (all genetic material is retained) or unbalanced (genetic material increases or decreases). The incidence of balanced translocations in the general population is 1 in 625; affected individuals generally have a normal phenotypic appearance.
- Robertsonian translocations involve only chromosomes 13, 14, 15, 21, and 22. They are referred to as acrocentric because the "p" arm is replaced by short satellite projections. The long arms of two of these chromosomes fuse at the centromere, and the genetic material contained within the satellite projections is lost. This rearrangement is found in approximately 1 in 900 people, typically without a phenotypic effect (Lashley, 1998).

Importantly, all translocations profoundly affect gametogenesis. It is necessary for the gametes of a balanced or Robertsonian translocation carrier to segregate and divide during meiosis to maintain the integrity of the proper genetic complement. If not, a zygote is produced without the correct amount of genetic material, which may be the basis for recurrent loss of pregnancy.

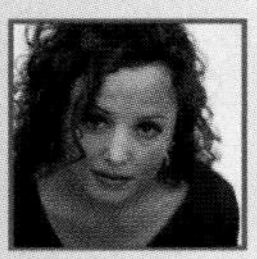

April mentioned concern over an increased risk for Down syndrome during her recent examination with the nurse. How does this type of genetic disorder occur?

Health History Assessment

A health history can identify reproductive and perinatal risk factors. This assessment includes information about the medical, social, environmental, nutritional, gynecologic, and reproductive history of the woman desiring pregnancy and assessment of the history of her reproductive partner. A health history also contains the medical and reproductive history of the parents, siblings, nieces, nephews, aunts, uncles, cousins, and grandparents of the woman and her partner, which the health care provider assesses for risk factors. To ensure that all information is obtained, the client may complete a prepared health history form (Assessment Tool 11.1).

Nurses should use the information obtained to provide appropriate preconception or prenatal health counseling. They also should use the assessment findings to identify risk factors that require further investigation and follow-up. Nurses may initiate a referral for genetic counseling if findings indicate that the client, reproductive partner, or both are at risk for having a child with a birth defect or genetic disorder (Lea et al., 2000).

A preconception health assessment may reveal information that clients perceive as sensitive, private, and highly confidential (Scanlon & Fibison, 1995). Such assessment has the profound potential to alter a client's self-image and relationships. Many clients fear that insurers, employers, and social communities will use genetic information to discriminate against them and their family. Legislation is pending to protect genetic information against insurance or employment discrimination; however, abilities to regulate or prevent discrimination by social communities are limited. Therefore, each nurse in every health care setting must consider and address the following questions carefully (International Society of Nurses in Genetics, 2001):

- Where is the appropriate place to record genetic information?
- What constitutes appropriate informed consent for genetic testing and evaluation?
- What is the nurse's responsibility to provide genetic information to clients?
- What is the nurse's responsibility to the client and family confronted with genetic information?

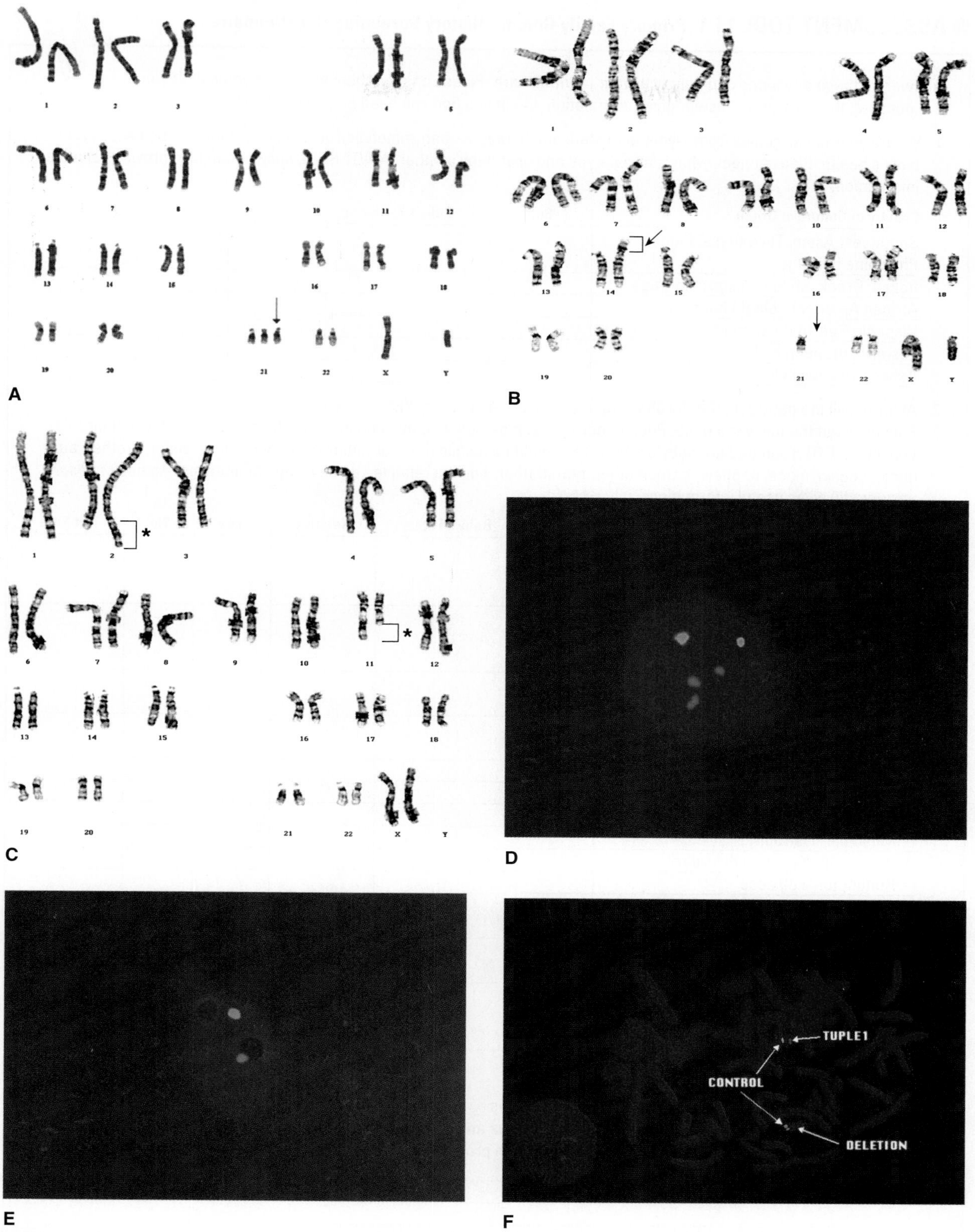

FIGURE 11.18 Karyotypes of abnormal and normal chromosome complements. (**A**) Male with trisomy 21. (**B**) Robertsonian translocation of chromosomes 14 and 21. Note that missing chromosome 21 is attached to chromosome 14. (**C**) Translocation of distal portion of chromosome 11 to chromosome 2. (**D**) Female with trisomy 21. (**E**) Normal male. (**F**) Normal for DiGeorge's syndrome probe. (Courtesy of A. Donnenfeld, Genzyme Genetics, Santa Fe, NM.)

● ASSESSMENT TOOL 11.1 Primary Family Genetic History Screening Questionnaire

Answering these questions can help with your prenatal care. Please answer them as well as you can. If you are not sure, the "not sure" answer gives information, too. If you find you need help, please just ask.

1. Where your family comes from—your ancestors and heritage—can sometimes give important information about your baby's health. Please check what is true for you and your baby's father. A NOT SURE answer can also provide valuable information.

Country or Culture of Origin	**Self**	**Baby's Father**	**Yes**	**No**	**Not Sure**
Southwest Asian, Taiwanese, Chinese, Philippine heritage					
Italian, Greek, Middle Eastern heritage					
African American (black) heritage					
Hispanic/Puerto Rican heritage					
Eastern European heritage					
Ashkenazi Jewish heritage					

2. At birth, will the baby's mother be 35 years or older (circle one) YES NO
3. Please fill out the following table. Put a check for each person who has one of the problems listed and give their relationship to BOTH you and the baby's father. This could be a child (born or unborn), mother, father, sister, brother; aunt, uncle, cousin, niece, nephew, grandmother, grandfather, *and* the relative can be living of deceased. Again, a *not sure* answer still gives useful information.

Condition	**Self**	**Baby's Father**	**Relative**	**Yes**	**No**	**Not Sure**
Has anyone ever had a baby with an opening in its back or spine (called spina bifida)?						
Has anyone ever had a baby with an opening in its head (called anencephaly)?						
Has any family member ever been diagnosed as mentally retarded?						
Has anyone ever had a baby, live-born or not, with Down syndrome (trisomy 21)?						
Has anyone ever been diagnosed with:						
Cystic fibrosis?						
Fragile X syndrome?						
Muscular dystrophy?						
Hemophilia/bleeding disorder?						
Huntington's disease						
Was anyone ever born with a heart defect?						
Was anyone ever born with a cleft lip/palate?						
Has anyone ever given birth to a baby with another kind of birth defect? Name, if known.						

(Please check one)	**Yes**	**No**	**Not Sure**
4. Has a woman in either family had 2 or more miscarriages			
5. Has a woman in either family had 1 or more miscarriages **and** a stillbirth?			

6. Has anyone in either family inherited a disease or health problem?__________
If so, what? __________
Name of condition__________

From Practice Based Genetics Curriculum for Nurse Educators. (2000). Foundation for Blood Research with funding from NIH, NHGRI, Grant #R25 HG0-1686. Reprinted with permission.

Continued

● ASSESSMENT TOOL 11.1 Primary Family Genetic History Screening Questionnaire

FOR PREGNANT WOMEN

(Please check one)	Yes	No	Not Sure
7. Have you ever been treated for PKU? (also called phenylketonuria)			
8. Are you on insulin?			
9. Are you on any other prescribed medication?			

10. If you are on any other prescribed medication, please name it (*this could include lithium for depression (Eskalith, Lithobid, Lithonate) or seizure medication (Dilantin, valproic acid, Depakene, Tegretol, Altretol, Mysoline, Tridione) or acne medication (Accutane isotretinoin)*):

____
____
____
____

Are there medication problems, issues, or questions that are of concern to you? If the answer is "yes," please tell the nurse.

Patient's Name ____________________ **DOB** ____________________

Nurse's Name ____________________ **Date** ____________________

- Is the level of confidentiality required by genetic information different from other medical information?

These questions are critical for appropriate management of genetic information and the process of informed decision making. Informed decision making, which integrates the ethical principles of autonomy, justice, and beneficence (Rothstein & Anderlik, 2001; Scanlon & Fibison, 1995), is the hallmark of preconception health assessment. Its goals are as follows:

1. Methodical, organized, and complete identification of personal risk factors
2. Provision of individualized, nondirective, nonjudgmental education and counseling
3. Timely access to complementary services, such as genetic and nutritional counseling and behavioral modification programs (Moos, 2003).

If these goals are met, then the client can approach reproductive issues with the knowledge necessary to make informed choices.

Screening Process

Preconception health assessment provides the opportunity for clients to initiate health behaviors known to be beneficial to the conception, development, and birth of children. Going through this process tends to engender positive feelings among those who do so because they feel empowered to optimize the health and well-being of future children. Conversely, this process also may cause feelings of anger, guilt, and anxiety as clients learn and share information. Therefore, nurses should protect the right of clients *to choose* or *to choose not* to seek preconception health screening and counseling (i.e., "right to know" versus "right not to know"). To that end, nurses should precede each step of the health assessment with (1) an explanation of the process, information that may or may not be learned, and possible implications of that knowledge; and (2) an opportunity for dialogue. As touched on earlier, this is the foundation of the process of informed decision making (Box 11.2) (Scanlon & Fibison, 1995). It is part of the informed consent process

● BOX 11.2 Components of Informed Decision Making and Consent for Genetic Testing or Evaluation

The process of informed decision making and consent includes, but is not limited to, the presentation of the following information before the performance of a genetic test or evaluation:

- The purpose of the screening or diagnostic test
- The nature of the disorder in question
- Reasons for completing the testing or evaluation
- Benefits of the testing or evaluation
- Risks of the testing or evaluation, including physical, psychological, social
- Alternative procedures
- Available interventions or treatments, including the lack of such interventions
- Subsequent decisions that will be likely after results are disclosed
- Available counseling services
- Implications of results for family members
- Institutional confidentiality standards
- Sensitivity and specificity of the test
- Unexpected results

From Jones, S. L. (2000). Reproductive genetic technologies: Exploring ethical and policy implications. *Lifelines, 4,* 33–36.

(the process of assessing and documenting consent after informed decision making). It is *not* a component of implied consent (consent by acceptance of an intervention without shared dialogue) (Shuster, 1997).

Using Standardized Risk Assessment Forms

To ensure *methodical, organized, and complete identification of personal risk factors,* the woman and her reproductive partner should complete a standardized health risk assessment form (see Assessment Tool 11.1). Health care providers may identify and add questions as needed (Lashley, 1998; Moos, 2004).

In some cases, the woman's partner is not involved in this process, either by choice or circumstance. Although the full complement of risks will not be available in such cases, it is still helpful for the woman to go through this screening to identify potential maternal risk factors.

Examples of other areas appropriate to address are as follows:

- Social history—exposure to or use of alcohol, cigarettes, drugs, radiation, or toxic chemicals
- Nutrition history—required or chosen dietary restrictions, any eating disorders, use of dietary supplements
- Medical history—any systemic condition (eg, thyroid, kidney, cardiovascular disease)
- Infectious disease history—occurrence of or exposure to any infectious disease or blood-borne pathogen such as herpes simplex, hepatitis, or HIV
- Reproductive history—any male or female reproductive organ anomalies such as congenital bilateral absence of the vas deferens, gonadal dysgenesis, or bicornuate uterus
- Ethnic background—any disorder known to occur more frequently in a specific population

Common Areas of Concern

QUOTE 11-1

"We waited so long to get pregnant . . . and now I fear I may be too old!"

In response to preconception counseling for a woman older than 35 years

Parental Age. As maternal age advances, so does the rate of aneuploidy (Nussbaum et al., 2001). The result is increased rates of pregnancy loss and birth of infants with chromosomal anomalies (Nussbaum et al., 2001). Most women and men are aware that advanced maternal age (older than 35 years) may affect a pregnancy adversely. This awareness is the direct outcome of (1) the adoption of practice standards that obligate obstetricians, gynecologists, and women's health nurses to appropriately disseminate this information; and (2) the considerable media exposure about this issue through public service campaigns, news programs, and storylines in popular entertainment.

Conversely, the general public and some health care providers are less aware that advanced paternal age (older than 45 years at conception) unfavorably affects fetal growth and development (American College of Medical Genetics, 1996a; Astolfi et al., 2004; Kazaura et al., 2004; Klonoff-Cohen & Natarajan, 2004). As discussed earlier, spermatogenesis begins at puberty and continues throughout the rest of the man's life. Estimates are that one new gene mutates each time spermatogonia replicate before spermatocyte meiosis. Most of these mutations are benign or lethal to embryo development; however, approximately 1 in 10 spermatocytes carries a new deleterious gene mutation (Nussbaum et al., 2001). Natural selection through programmed cell death (apoptosis) eliminates many of these anomalous spermatocytes from the pool of viable sperm. Nevertheless, apoptosis declines as paternal age advances (Singh et al., 2002) and correlates with decreased male fertility and increased incidence of fetuses with single gene disorders of paternal origin.

Many clients seeking preconception counseling because one or both partners are of advanced reproductive age have limited knowledge of the biologic mechanisms that adversely alter their probability of giving birth to a healthy child. The nurse should identify their current level of knowledge and preconception counseling expectations. The nurse should encourage the completion of a Preconception Health Screening questionnaire (see Assessment Tool 11.1) to fully identify and assess all related reproductive issues. Collection of the information necessary to respond accurately to the questionnaire facilitates recognition by clients of the importance of preconception health risk assessment and counseling.

People of advanced reproductive age require information about the possible outcomes for a child conceived with their genetic gametes. The nurse should offer education and counseling using incidence tables for chromosome anomalies associated with advanced maternal age (Table 11.11) and review characteristics of disorders that may occur through paternal transmission of a spontaneous new mutation as a result of advanced paternal age (Table 11.12). Examples of normal and anomalous karyotypes (see Figs. 11.2 and 11.18) illustrate possible outcomes of chromosome nondisjunction. The nurse should present and discuss the scope of reproductive options available (Assessment Tool 11.2). A review of the full range of prenatal diagnostic procedures, including preimplantation genetic diagnosis (Munne et al., 2002), is integral to preconception counseling for advanced reproductive age. The nurse also should discuss the benefits and risks of donor gametes from people younger than 35 years. This option reduces, but does not eliminate, the incidence of chromosomal anomalies and spontaneous new mutations per pregnancy conceived (see Chap. 10).

Presentation and discussion of reproductive alternatives assist clients to make an informed choice as to which reproductive option aligns best with their beliefs

TABLE 11.11 Risk for Having a Liveborn Child or Fetus With a Chromosome Abnormality

	INCIDENCE		
MATERNAL AGE	All Chromosome Anomalies at Birth	Down Syndrome at Birth	Down Syndrome at Amniocentesis*
20–24	1 in 500	1 in 1,400	
25–29	1 in 435	1 in 1,100	
30	1 in 384	1 in 900	
31		1 in 900	
32	1 in 323	1 in 750	
33		1 in 625	1 in 420
34	1 in 238	1 in 500	1 in 333
35	1 in 192	1 in 385	1 in 250
36	1 in 156	1 in 300	1 in 200
37	1 in 127	1 in 225	1 in 150
38	1 in 102	1 in 175	1 in 115
39	1 in 83	1 in 140	1 in 90
40	1 in 66	1 in 100	1 in 70
41	1 in 53	1 in 80	1 in 50
42	1 in 42	1 in 65	1 in 40
43	1 in 33	1 in 50	1 in 30
44	1 in 26	1 in 40	1 in 25
45+	1 in 8 to 1 in 21	1 in 25	1 in 20

*The incidence of Down syndrome is slightly higher at time of chorionic villus sampling (performed at 9 to 12 weeks' gestation) than at amniocentesis (performed at 16 weeks' gestation) as a result of ongoing spontaneous loss of these fetuses from 12 to 16 weeks' gestation.

Adapted from risk tables published in Harper, P. S. (2001). *Practical genetic counseling* (5th ed.). New York: Oxford University Press, and Beers, M. H., & Berkow, R. (2003). *The Merck manual of diagnosis and therapy* (17th ed.). Available at: http://www.merckmedicus.com.

TABLE 11.12 Selected Examples of Disorders Associated With Advanced Paternal Age

DISORDER	MENDELIAN PATTERN OF INHERITANCE
Achondroplasia	Autosomal dominant
Acrodysostosis	Autosomal dominant
Apert's syndrome	Autosomal dominant
Basal cell nevus syndrome	Autosomal dominant
Crouzon's craniofacial dysostosis	Autosomal dominant
Duchenne's muscular dystrophy	X-linked recessive*
Hemophilia A	X-linked recessive*
Marfan syndrome	Autosomal dominant
Neurofibromatosis	Autosomal dominant
Oculodentodigital dysplasia	Autosomal dominant
Progeria	Autosomal dominant†
Treacher Collins syndrome	Autosomal dominant
Waardenburg syndrome	Autosomal dominant

*Spontaneous mutation would occur in the maternal grandfather of the child conceived within a family with no prior history of hemophilia A or Duchenne's muscular dystrophy.

†Progeria has also been reported to be an autosomal recessive disorder.

Adapted from Lashley, F. R. (1998). *Clinical genetics in nursing practice* (2nd ed.). New York: Springer.

and values. Social communities (family, friends, work, and culture) and religious doctrine often influence or dictate viable and nonviable reproductive services to consider. Some people choose to realize their goal (addition of a child to the family unit) by pursuing alternatives that violate the beliefs of their community. These people require assistance from health care providers to access specialized services confidentially and privately to minimize the risk for social discrimination.

Reproductive History. The reproductive history of both the woman and her partner can identify potential risk factors as they pursue the desire for a biologic child. If both people previously have achieved the birth of a child (together or with different partners), it is highly probable that this couple will conceive and give birth. Numerous clinical studies provide evidence of multiple risk factors that together result in the poor monthly fecundity rate (20%) found among females (Evers, 2002). Absence of a prior conception and birth alone is not sufficient evidence to warrant a reproductive evaluation, but additional questioning can help eliminate or identify potential risks that together indicate potential reproductive failure.

To ensure a comprehensive review, the nurse should identify and assess reproductive history for potential risk factors and provide education about the implications of findings. Congenital or acquired reproductive malformations (eg, congenital absence of the vas deferens, septate

● ASSESSMENT TOOL 11.2 Preconception Decision Making: Reproductive Options for Individuals at Risk for the Transmission of a Genetic Disorder

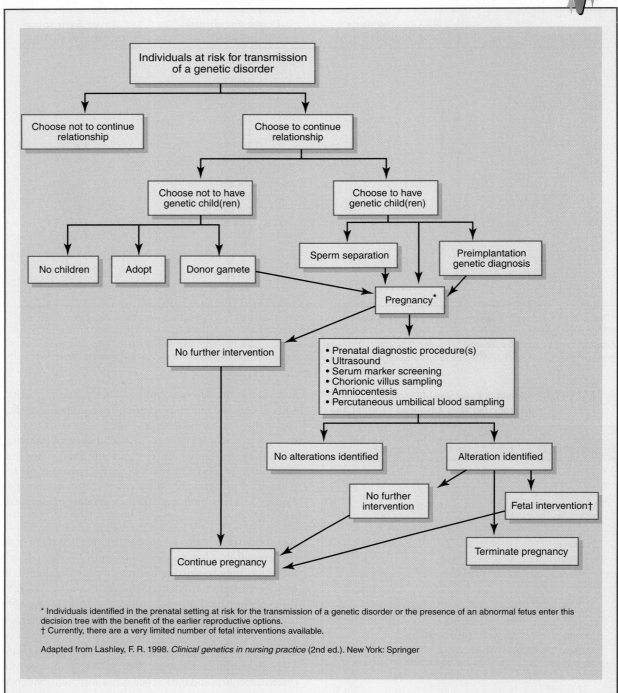

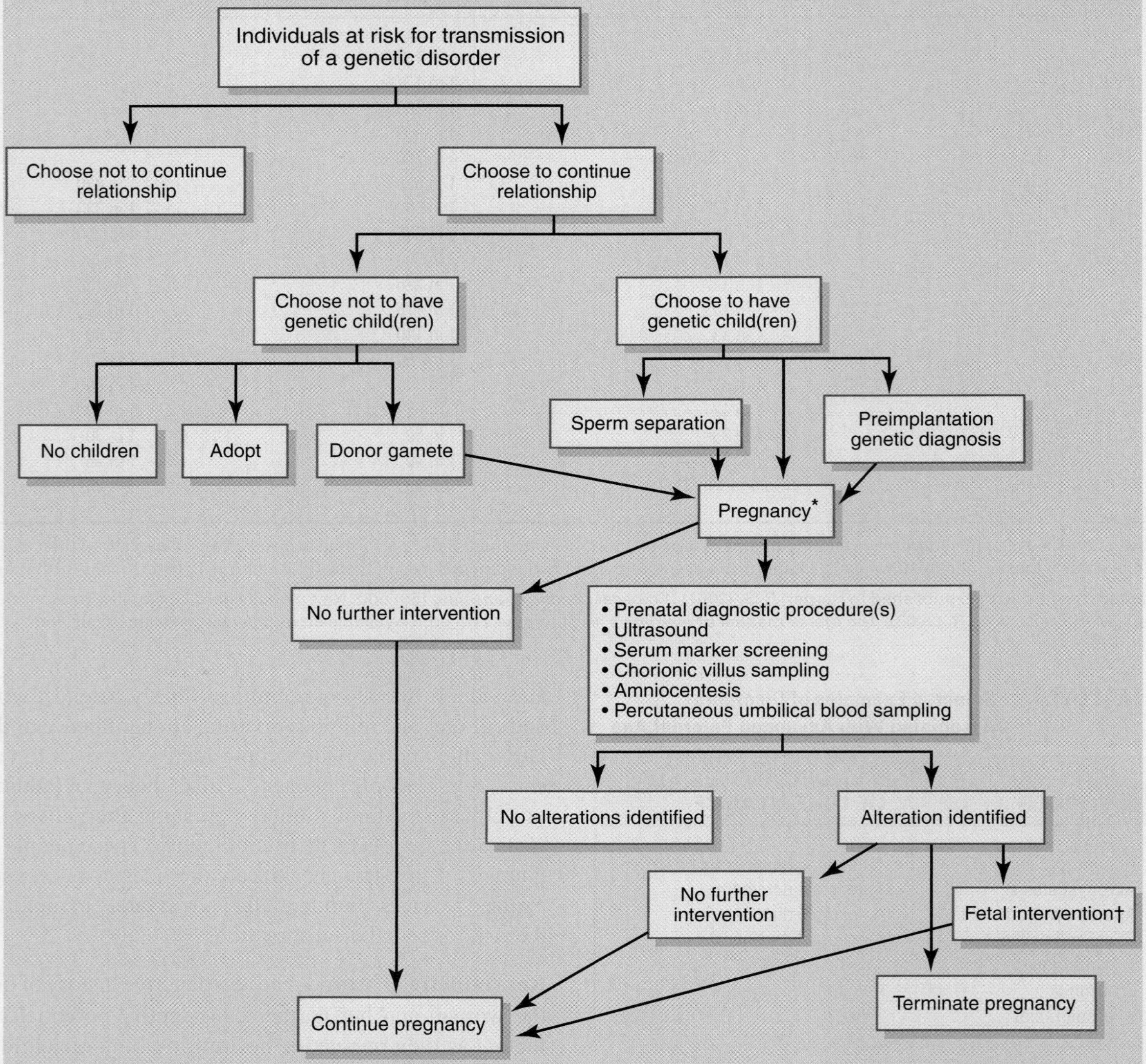

* Individuals identified in the prenatal setting at risk for the transmission of a genetic disorder or the presence of an abnormal fetus enter this decision tree with the benefit of the earlier reproductive options.
† Currently, there are a very limited number of fetal interventions available.

Adapted from Lashley, F. R. 1998. *Clinical genetics in nursing practice* (2nd ed.). New York: Springer

uterus); loss of ovarian or testicular reserve (ie, no oocytes or spermatocytes); irregular menstrual cycles (eg, premature ovarian failure); infections; autoimmune disorders; and hormonal imbalances (eg, hyperprolactinemia, thyroid disorders, insulin resistance) may lead to an inability to conceive or carry a pregnancy to term (see Chap. 10). Chromosomal rearrangements in the fetus from an inherited unbalanced translocation or microdeletion may result in spontaneous pregnancy loss during the first trimester.

Recurrent miscarriage, also called *recurrent pregnancy loss (RPL),* is the loss of three or more pregnancies before 20 weeks' gestation (Carp et al., 2001). Analyses performed on the products of conception from sporadic miscarriages suggest a strong correlation between chromosomal anomalies and pregnancy loss (more than half of cases show chromosomal rearrangements). Most of these losses result from nondisjunctions rather than from parental transmissions of unbalanced translocations. Among those couples experiencing RPL, less than 10% have a parental chromosomal rearrangement (Lashley, 1998; Nussbaum et al., 2001). In fact, the incidence of abnormal parental karyotypes correlates inversely with the number of previous spontaneous losses (Ogasawara et al., 2000). That is, a chromosomal rearrangement in the client's cells is less likely to be identified as the cause as the frequency of RPL increases.

The complexity of establishing the probable cause of a suspected conception failure or history of RPL is increased by the potential need for the client to be evaluated by both reproductive endocrinology (infertility) and genetics specialists. Many of the diagnostic tests required for these specialty evaluations may be completed within the primary care setting. The nurse should coordinate the completion of requisite tests (serum hormone levels, physical examinations, chromosome analysis) and review results before referral of the client to one or more specialists. The results of the initial evaluation may lead to elimination or redirection of a planned referral. The nurse should counsel the client about the importance of and method for obtaining a fetal karyotype if pregnancy loss recurs.

If an irreversible cause (eg, parental chromosomal anomaly, malformation of reproductive organs, sterility) of reproductive failure is identified, the nurse should teach the client about the scope of reproductive options available. The nurse also should encourage and assist clients as they evaluate and reflect on their feelings and beliefs about these alternatives. Referral for counseling is appropriate if the woman, partner, or both express displeasure with themselves or each other or discomfort with suggested alternatives.

Family History and Ethnicity. Screening and diagnostic tests within the preconception health risk assessment process identify and eliminate potential concerns for clients proactively seeking a healthy pregnancy outcome. Allele form analysis for a single gene may be indicated. This type of screening test is used in preconception and prenatal settings to identify healthy people at risk for transmitting an altered allele to their child. Its use is indicated when there is a family history of an adult-onset disorder not yet apparent in the at-risk reproductive partner. Depending on the disorder, this form of testing is known as presymptomatic (eg, HD) or predisposition (eg, breast cancer). Carrier screening is also appropriate if the family history or ethnic group of either reproductive partner suggests the potential transmission of a single copy of an altered recessive allele.

If both the woman *and* her partner have the same altered recessive allele, then each pregnancy has a 25% chance of resulting in the birth of a child with a genetic disorder. Likewise, each pregnancy has a 25% chance of the birth of a healthy child without an altered allele. There is a 50% chance that each pregnancy produces a child who is a healthy carrier of one copy of the altered allele just like the parents (Lea & Williams, 2002).

If a woman *or* her partner is at risk for transmitting a dominant altered allele to the fetus, then each pregnancy has a 50% chance of resulting in the birth of a child with the same presymptomatic or predisposition risk as the at-risk parent. Similarly, each pregnancy has a 50% chance of ending with a child without the altered allele and its associated phenotypic risk.

One of the most basic preconception screening tools is the question, "What is your ethnic group?" (see Tables 11.7 to 11.10.). This information initiates and directs one aspect of assessment of risk factors for a specific client. For example, if a woman is white and of French Canadian ancestry, her carrier risk is increased for cystic fibrosis and Tay-Sachs disease. Likewise, if her reproductive partner is white and of Icelandic ancestry, his carrier risk is increased for cystic fibrosis and phenylketonuria.

Completion of a pedigree assists with identification of family members who have or are at risk for other single-gene disorders not necessarily specific to any ethnic or population group. Advances in molecular, biochemical, and cytogenetic testing permit determination of individual risk (present, absent, probable) for many known genetic disorders. Professional practice standards form the basis of protocols for recommended genetic screening tests (American College of Obstetricians and Gynecologists & American College of Medical Genetics, 2001; Genetic testing for cystic fibrosis, 1997). Current clinical protocols include a basic scope of preconception or prenatal tests.

The nurse should be prepared that inquiry into a client's ethnic or population background may elicit fears of racial bias or other discrimination, resulting in the client's conscious decision not to provide requested data. Although a clinical protocol may dictate performance of one or more genetic screening tests, the principles of **informed decision making and consent** require the nurse to educate and counsel before doing so (Burke, 2002; Tinkle, 2002). Typically, an explanation of the science and basis of the protocol eliminates client resistance. The nurse should work with clients to ensure that they understand the rationale for testing. He or she is obligated to (1) assist with the process of informed decision making, (2) document that process, and (3) support the decision, whether the client elects to pursue or not to pursue genetic testing.

If a family history of a dominant or recessive genetic disorder is suspected or positive, the nurse, based on his or her own knowledge and scope of practice, should provide education and counseling or referral for genetic counseling specific to that disorder. The need for dissemination of information and dialogue about common genetic disorders (eg, cystic fibrosis, sickle cell anemia) in primary care settings is growing. Multiple resources are available to learn about and prepare materials for use when discussing such disorders with clients (American Sickle Cell Anemia Association, 2003; Brown & Schwind, 1999; Cystic Fibrosis Foundation, 2003; Richards et al., 2002). The nurse should coordinate all referral services and provide supportive counseling throughout the process.

Environmental Influences. A preconception screening assessment can identify environmental influences that may affect pregnancy outcome. Health care providers assess paternal health during a cycle of spermatogenesis, maternal health before conception as well as throughout gestation, and the ecological environment in which the woman and partner reside and work. Men exposed to toxic substances such as heat, radiation, viruses, bacteria, alcohol, and prescription and recreational drugs are more likely to have decreased morphologically and genetically normal sperm in a single ejaculate. This results in reproductive failure preconception and postfertilization (Speroff et al., 1999). Women exposed to similar toxic agents experience diminished ovarian reserve, poor endometrial lining development, and abnormal fetal development (see Table 11.5). Likewise, chronic and acute diseases decrease fecundity and increase fetal wastage (Evers, 2002; Speroff et al., 1999).

Men and women alike require proper nutrition and normal endocrine function to sustain gametogenesis and, for the woman, gestation and normal fetal development. Abnormal levels of prolactin, thyroid-stimulating hormone (TSH), gonadotropin-releasing hormone (GnRH), FSH, testosterone, estrogen, and progesterone interfere with normal gametogenesis and embryo implantation (see Chap. 10). Women specifically require additional vitamins and minerals to support fetal growth and development (see Chap. 3). Especially important is additional folic acid to reduce the risk for neural tube defects (March of Dimes Foundation, 1999).

The nurse should evaluate the client's health and exposure to toxic substances. Ideally, each reproductive partner completes a medical health history and preconception screening questionnaire. The nurse should review the responses and clarify any ambiguities. This aspect of preconception health risk assessment addresses the following areas of concern (Lashley, 1998; Scott et al., 1999):

1. Lack of natural or acquired immunity to common infectious diseases: rubella, rubeola, hepatitis B, varicella, mumps
2. Any severe or uncontrolled chronic disorders: diabetes, hypertension, thyroid disorders, systemic lupus erythematosus, kidney disease, epilepsy
3. Use of or exposure to radiation or hormonal, chemical, or biologic agents detrimental to fetal development: alcohol, radioactive materials, oral contraceptives, prescribed or recreational drugs, toxoplasmosis
4. Any maternal genetic disorder that affects normal fetal development (eg, phenylketonuria, factor V Leiden) (Kupferminc et al., 1999)
5. Lack of proper diet or supplemental vitamins and minerals sufficient to assist with proper fetal development

Many environmental factors that adversely affect conception, growth, and fetal development are reversible, controllable, or both. The nurse should identify reversible health risks and educate clients about actions required to confirm and subsequently eliminate those risks. Recommended standards for some risk factors are available from professional organizations; the nurse can use them during discussion. For example, AWHONN (2003) recommends that all women begin taking 400 μg of synthetic folic acid daily at least 1 month before conception and continue that intake throughout the first 3 months of pregnancy.

The nurse should assess immune levels for diseases known to have available vaccines. He or she should coordinate appropriate laboratory testing and subsequent recommendations for vaccination. Internists, endocrinologists, or nephrologists refer women with chronic or uncontrolled diseases for evaluation based on the specific diagnosis. The nurse should coordinate the referral services and gather summary reports for each completed referral.

The nurse should educate and counsel clients about social or work environment activities that affect fetal development. He or she should provide support for people who require assistance to eliminate a risk factor from the environment or refer them to the appropriate non–health care agency. Examples include Human Resources at their employment site, the Department of Occupational Health and Safety, and Alcoholics Anonymous.

A special situation exists for women with a chronic disease (eg, diabetes) or genetic disorder (eg, phenylketonuria). They can take steps to optimize the gestational environment (eg, control of glucose and insulin levels, reduction in circulating phenylalanine), but they cannot reduce the risk to the level experienced by those without phenylketonuria or diabetes. The nurse should provide them with education and counseling about alternative reproductive options (see Chap. 10).

Constructing Pedigrees

To assist with summarizing and analyzing information obtained from the questionnaire, the health care provider may construct a pedigree (genogram). Assessment Tool 11.3 presents guidelines for pedigree completion, with symbols

● ASSESSMENT TOOL 11.3 Guidelines for Pedigree (Genogram) Completion

1. Complete pedigree using a pencil and 6-inch ruler.
2. Begin the pedigree by placing the consultand (the person giving the history) on the appropriate line.
3. Move from the proband (the first individual diagnosed with an alteration of their genes) out, completing each generation.
4. Generations appear on the pedigree from the top to the bottom of the page, oldest to youngest.
5. Number generations from top to bottom using Roman numerals.
6. Fathers appear to the left of mothers.
7. Siblings appear in the order of birth from left to right.
8. Group like siblings who are without symptoms in one symbol.
9. Number siblings and cousins from left to right using "1, 2, 3. . . ".
10. Identify the age of the individual or age at death under the symbol.
11. Create a legend allowing for multiple findings.

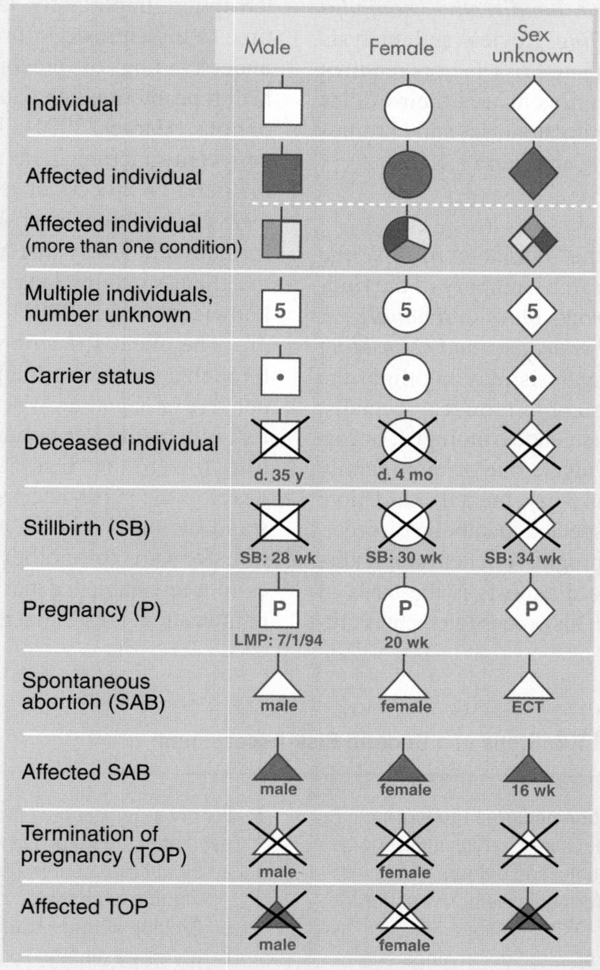

From Jones, S. L. (1999a). Genetically transmitted diseases: Identification and counseling. In *Management of genetic information: Implications for nursing practice* (32nd Annual Postgraduate Course Syllabus). Birmingham, AL: American Society of Reproductive Medicine. Reprinted with permission.

commonly used (Bennett et al., 1995). After drawing the pedigree, the health care provider reviews it with the client for accuracy and completeness. It is not unusual for this review to elicit additional and important information that the client forgot when responding to questions "about the family" rather than "about the individual family member." This careful review of individual family members tends also to identify symptoms, characteristics, or diagnoses that need further investigation before completion of assessment of the information (Spahis, 2002). A family member may alter or fail to provide information to protect privacy and prevent discrimination. These "family secrets" often must be uncovered to obtain vital facts for correct interpretation of information provided.

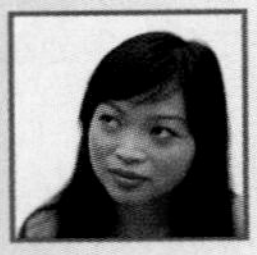

Remember Carmen, the recently married client who wants to begin having children. Carmen is concerned about the possibility of disease transmission to her fetus. Would completing a pedigree be helpful in this situation? Why or why not?

Assessment Tool 11.4 outlines a genetic risk assessment. The nurse should complete this assessment before *the provision of individualized, nondirective, nonjudgmental education and counseling.* Review and analysis of the pedigree to identify potential risk factors requires nurses to be familiar with teratogens and their effects (see Table 11.5), as well as mitochondrial and chromosomal disorders. See Nursing Care Plan 11.1.

Information Sharing

After carefully reviewing the available results, the health care provider should draft a summary of the findings in preparation for the *provision of individualized, nondirective, nonjudgmental education and counseling* with the client. This initial analysis may highlight the need for additional information or referral to a specialist such as a geneticist, neurologist, endocrinologist, or cardiologist. The necessity to evaluate one or more family members with a developmental delay, mental retardation, musculoskeletal anomaly, suspected metabolic disorder, congenital malformation, or progressive neurologic disorder to establish a definitive diagnosis is the basis of such a referral (Spahis, 2002). This process element is critical to the accurate delineation of preconception risk for some clients.

To ensure the appropriate provision of information, nurses should identify the full scope of reproductive options available to the client based on specific preconception risk. Concurrently, nurses should carefully identify and seek to understand their values and beliefs as well as their accompanying inherent biases. This self-assessment is critical to providing *individualized, nondirective, nonjudgmental education and counseling.*

The setting chosen for preconception health counseling should be quiet, private, and free of frequent interruption. Importantly, the nurse should allot sufficient time to disseminate information and assess the client's understanding of preconception risk, recommended health promotion behaviors, and available reproductive options (Harper, 2001). The nurse should identify and correct misinterpretations and misunderstandings through the iterative process of reflective questioning (Lashley, 1998). In addition, he or she should prepare and share information in a way that aligns with and accommodates the client's culture, language, education level, and prior knowledge (Weil, 2001).

The client's reaction to the information identified through a preconception health risk assessment may be positive or negative. When an unexpected or anticipated risk is presented, the client may express anger and hostility toward the "bearer of bad news." Nurses need to develop the skills necessary to assist clients to understand the basis of such a response and be prepared to transfer care to another health care provider if they cannot re-establish a therapeutic relationship. This level of interaction is essential if clients are to achieve increased

● ASSESSMENT TOOL 11.4 Steps of a Genetic Risk Assessment

1. Complete a three-generation pedigree (genogram).
   a. Identify and speak about every person individually.
   b. Use standardized symbols (see below).
   c. Follow the guidelines for pedigree construction (see Assessment Tool 11.3).
2. Review the pedigree for repeated occurrence of a medical or genetic disorder.
   a. All health issues should be identified.
   b. All health issues should be verified, not assumed.
3. Review the pedigree for isolated occurrence of a medical or genetic disorder.
   a. Lack of phenotypic expression does not eliminate genotypic risk.
   b. Confirm paternity.
4. Identify the ethnicity of the genetic parents.
   a. Identify genetic risks associated with ethnicity.
   b. Confirm paternity.
5. Follow organizational protocol for further evaluation and/or referral
   a. Establish a center specific protocol for preconception evaluation.
   b. Provide written information about genetic tests.
   c. Identify a genetic specialist(s) to whom referrals can be made.
6. Review findings and therapeutic options with the consultand.

From Jones, S. L. (1999a). Genetically transmitted diseases: Identification and counseling. In *Management of genetic information: Implications for nursing practice* (32nd Annual Postgraduate Course Syllabus). Birmingham, AL: American Society of Reproductive Medicine. Reprinted with permission.

NURSING CARE PLAN 11.1

The Client Seeking Preconception Health Screening

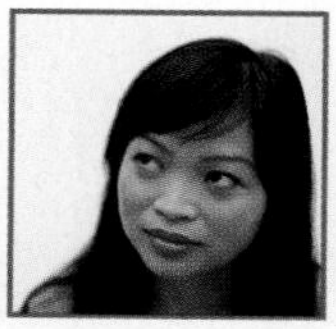

Remember Carmen, the 22-year-old who desires pregnancy but is concerned about transmitting genetic or other disorders to her baby. Further assessment of Carmen reveals the following: history of seasonal allergies with use of over-the-counter decongestants; weight appropriate for height; and vital signs within acceptable parameters.

Further discussion of family history reveals that twins run in Carmen's family. "What if I have twins?" she says. "I'm not sure I could handle that!"

NURSING DIAGNOSIS

Anxiety related to uncertainty about fetal health secondary to family history

EXPECTED OUTCOMES

1. The client will identify specific areas causing her concern.
2. The client will state measures to minimize anxiety.
3. The client will report a decrease in anxiety levels.

INTERVENTIONS	RATIONALES
Assess the client's level of understanding about pregnancy and fetal health.	Assessment provides a baseline to identify specific client needs and develop an individualized plan.
Discuss with the client her concerns, feelings, and perceptions related to pregnancy and fetal health and possible effects on current family situation.	Discussion provides opportunities to emphasize positive aspects; verbalization of concerns aids in establishing sources of stress and problem areas to address.
Communicate accurate facts and answer questions honestly. Reinforce facts. Encourage the client not to blame herself if problems are found.	Open and honest communication promotes trust and helps to correct misperceptions or misinformation. Facts help dispel unfounded fears, myths, and guilt.
Evaluate which past coping strategies have been most effective.	Use of appropriate coping strategies aids in reducing anxiety.
Emphasize that the client can use this time to make health or lifestyle changes.	Health promotion behaviors can help reduce risks in pregnancy.
Obtain an assessment risk and complete a client pedigree.	Assessment risk and pedigree aid in determining possible areas that may pose threats to fetal health.
Review with the client measures used throughout pregnancy to monitor fetal well-being; include appropriate screening and diagnostic testing that may be done.	Knowledge of ongoing surveillance techniques aids in alleviating stress related to the unknown.
Encourage the client to include her husband in follow-up visits.	Participation of the client's partner promotes sharing, provides support, and enhances the chances for success.
Question the client about available support systems, such as family, friends, and community.	Additional sources of support are helpful in alleviating anxiety.
Provide client with information about support groups, Web sites, and other sources of information related to pregnancy and fetal health.	These resources can help the client to prepare for what to expect.

Continued

NURSING CARE PLAN 11.1 ● The Client Seeking Preconception Health Screening *(Continued)*

EVALUATION

1. The client openly verbalizes concerns about pregnancy and fetal health.
2. The client demonstrates positive methods of coping.
3. The client reports that her anxiety level has diminished.

NURSING DIAGNOSIS

Deficient Knowledge related to pregnancy and factors affecting fetal health

EXPECTED OUTCOMES

1. The client will verbalize accurate information about pregnancy and ways to ensure fetal health.
2. The client will identify possible screening and diagnostic tests needed to ensure fetal health.

INTERVENTIONS	RATIONALES
Assess the client's knowledge about her body and typical changes in pregnancy.	This information establishes a baseline from which to develop appropriate teaching strategies.
Describe fetal growth and development and factors that may affect fetal health, including exposure to teratogens.	An accurate description of fetal growth and development is essential to understanding risk factors.
Encourage the client to avoid exposure to possible teratogens; urge her to contact her primary health care provider about the use of an over-the-counter decongestant during pregnancy.	Exposure to teratogens can result in fetal malformations, disruptions, and deformations.
Explain the basic principles of genetics, including inheritance of disorders; review the client's pedigree and correlate information with explanation.	Information about genetics provides an understanding about the need for possible screening and testing.
Discuss multiple gestation, including factors that increase the risk; review the client's pedigree for possible risks associated with twin births.	A maternal family history of twin births increases the client's risk for twins.
Instruct the client about possible screening and testing based on history, risk assessment, and pedigree.	Information about possible upcoming testing helps to prepare the client and minimize anxiety and fear of the unknown.
Provide client with written material about healthy behaviors and testing.	Written material provides additional means of teaching and provides opportunities for review and reinforcement.

EVALUATION

1. The client demonstrates healthy behaviors related to pregnancy and fetal health.
2. The client verbalizes an understanding of the rationale for screening and diagnostic testing.

knowledge and understanding about the importance of (1) good maternal health and health care before and during pregnancy; (2) implementation of health promotion behaviors; (3) identification and reduction of perinatal risk factors; (4) elimination of toxic exposures; (5) stabilization of maternal disorders; and (6) informed dialogue and shared decision making.

Anticipatory Care

The results of preconception health risk assessment may reveal the need for multiple health care, community, or family services. Clients may be unaware of the breadth, availability, and accessibility of such services. The nurse's knowledge and skills align well with the role of care coordinator and frequently can help clients to identify and navigate the diverse forms of assistance they seek or need (Lea et al., 2000). A key aspect of anticipatory care is *timely access to complementary services, such as genetic and nutritional counseling and behavioral modification programs.*

Through anticipatory care, nurses can assist clients to respond to the recommendations from the preconception health risk assessment. Nursing interventions (Lea et al., 2000) include the following:

- Establishment of institutional protocols and policies for the completion of a referral
- Timely initiation of appropriate referrals
- Reduction or elimination of barriers to services (Suther & Goodson, 2003), such as geographic location (use of teleconferencing), cost (insurance benefits appeal, public health funds), knowledge (education of professional and administrative staff), or time (coordination of services to limit total number of visits required)
- Management of genetic information (Scanlon & Fibison, 1995)
- Protection of confidentiality and privacy
- Written summary of the findings and recommendations appropriate for the client's knowledge level
- Bidirectional dialogue that is iterative over time
- Development of materials sensitive to the client's culture whether defined as geographic, ethnic, sexual orientation, social, disability, or language (Weil, 2001)
- Dissemination of information to other individuals, family members, or health care providers (if requested by the client)

The nurse also should use the skills, knowledge, and interventions integral to the completion of a comprehensive preconception health risk assessment after a pregnancy is established or a child with a suspected or known genetic disorder is born. The information gleaned can help clients anticipate concerns for the current situation as well as future pregnancy considerations. As the HGP further advances knowledge of human genome variation and the molecular basis of disease, such knowledge and skills will be requisite for nurses in all health care settings.

PRENATAL SCREENING AND DIAGNOSTIC PROCEDURES

As with preconception screening and counseling, the goal of prenatal screening and diagnosis is to provide individualized, nondirective, nonjudgmental education and counseling after a methodical, organized, and complete identification of prenatal risk factors. Based on the assessment, education, and counseling performed, providers identify and recommend prenatal screening or diagnostic tests for the client. The process of informed decision making and consent is the framework directing this aspect of prenatal care (see Box 11.2). Clients must understand that prenatal screening and diagnosis do not usually result in identification, treatment, and cure. Rather, the process leads to identification of a fetus with an anomaly and the need for the client to decide whether to continue the pregnancy. The simple analogy is the story of Pandora's box. Once the box is opened and the knowledge inside is shared, the information cannot be put back into the box and forgotten.

Health care providers should apprise clients who seek prenatal counseling of the benefits and limitations of prenatal screening and diagnosis before such clients give procedural consent. This includes discussion of the following key points (Harper, 2001; Nussbaum et al., 2001):

- What is the risk the fetus will be affected?
- What are the nature and probable consequences of the disorder of concern?
- Are appropriate postnatal treatments available for the disorder of concern?
- What are the risks, benefits, and limitations of the available and disorder-appropriate procedures?
- How long will it take to receive the results of the screening or diagnostic procedures?
- What is the frequency and possible need for a repeat procedure?
- Is the risk of the procedure perceived to be outweighed by the information to be learned?

This dialogue may lead to the discovery of sensitive information (eg, nonpaternity) with social implications. It also may cause *iatrogenic worry,* which is emotional discomfort solely resulting from the information learned (Kenen et al., 2000). Importantly, most women who seek prenatal screening and diagnosis receive reassuring information after the performance of one or more such procedures. All women also must understand that seeking this service does not imply an obligation to terminate a pregnancy found to have a fetus with an anomaly. The primary goal of prenatal diagnosis is to identify whether a fetus has an anomaly. It is the sole decision of the woman and her reproductive partner to determine how to use that information, including termination of the pregnancy or preparation through knowledge acquisition for the birth and parenting of a child with a specific disorder.

Screening and diagnostic tests are different, although both are used within the prenatal setting. Screening tests typically are used when large populations (eg, the entire U.S. prenatal population) are to be assessed to identify the smaller group of people appropriate for referral to more complex and costly services. Examples in the prenatal population are maternal serum alpha-fetoprotein (MSAFP) screening tests for neural tube defects and chromosomal anomalies or level 1 ultrasound screenings for gestation dates and number of fetuses. Diagnostic tests generally are used to confirm or to eliminate suspected anomalies among the smaller group of at-risk people. Examples include three-dimensional ultrasound to assess for structural anomalies and amniocentesis for analysis of chromosome complement. Sometimes, the outcome of a diagnostic test is inconclusive. Diagnostic testing does not guarantee the definitive identification or nonexistence of a fetal anomaly. Table 11.13 compares the multiple prenatal screening and diagnostic procedures.

Four methods are used to perform a genetic test (Lea & Williams, 2002; Nussbaum et al., 2001). *Direct molecular analysis* of the DNA or RNA of a sequenced gene is performed by polymerase chain reaction (PCR) amplification and gel electrophoresis. *Linkage analysis* uses PCR amplification and gel electrophoresis to detect alleles (DNA marker alleles) known to be located close to and likely to segregate with the altered allele of concern that has not yet been sequenced. *Biochemical assays* assess the absence or presence (and at what level) of an enzyme or protein product from the gene of concern through traditional radioimmune assays and biochemical tests. *Cytogenetic analysis* is the microscopic examination of metaphase chromosomes after the cell is stained with Giemsa (G-banding) to create the light and dark bands specific to the individual chromosomes. A picture of the stained chromosomes is taken, and a karyotype is prepared (see Fig. 11.18).

The methodologic confluence of molecular genetics and cytogenetics permits the rapid examination of one or more specific DNA (gene) sequences or the number and structural arrangement of chromosomes or chromosomal regions within a cell. This merger of technologies is fluorescence in situ hybridization (FISH). Metaphase chromosomes are denatured on laboratory slides (that is, "in situ") to expose the strands of DNA comprising each chromosome. A complementary fluorescently labeled strand of nucleic acid molecules attempts to bond (hybridization) to a specific DNA sequence that may or may not be available in the specimen under analysis. Under microscopic examination, the results of the application of FISH are evaluated (Nussbaum et al., 2001). The fluorescent staining of large portions or whole chromosomes is known as chromosome painting. FISH technology is progressing to permit comparative genome hybridization (examination of the total amount of a specific DNA sequence within a cell, especially useful in tumor evaluation) and spectral karyotyping (painting of the entire chromosome complement within a cell). Importantly, results are available rapidly because cells do not have to be cultured before analysis.

There are multiple indications for referral to and completion of prenatal genetic counseling, whether screening, diagnostic, or both. These risk factors are identified through the completion of a prenatal health assessment form by the woman and her reproductive partner. Typically the same form prepared and used in the preconception health care setting is used for prenatal evaluation of risk (see Assessment Tool 11.1). Seven standards of care and one sociocultural indication warrant referral of the woman and her partner to prenatal genetic services:

1. Advanced maternal (older than 35 years) or paternal (older than 45 years) age
2. Birth of previous child with a chromosome anomaly
3. A chromosomal rearrangement in one of the genetic parents
4. Known or suspected family history of a genetic disorder
5. Family history of an X-linked disorder for which no disorder-specific test is available
6. First- or second-degree relative with a neural tube defect
7. An anomaly found on ultrasound or abnormal serum marker screening test
8. Increased parental anxiety (people who know or provide care to those with genetic disorders; recipients of donor gametes)

Prenatal screening and testing are not limited to the first and second trimesters of pregnancy or solely to the diagnosis of fetal anomalies. They also are performed during the third trimester to assess fetal maturity (lung), fetal anemia, and uteroplacental function.

Nursing Care Plan 11.2 describes a scenario in which a couple must face decision making related to prenatal screening and diagnostic procedures. It describes the difficulties that clients can face when trying to determine how much information they want to know in the early stages of pregnancy. NIC/NOC Box 11.1 presents some general interventions and outcomes relative to prenatal screening procedures and counseling.

Maternal Serum Marker Screening

Maternal serum marker screening first became available in prenatal care settings in the late 1980s. MSAFP was the first biochemical marker to be analyzed. Elevated levels of MSAFP are associated with pregnancies found

(text continues on page 406)

TABLE 11.13 Comparison of Prenatal Screening and Diagnostic Procedures

	MATERNAL SERUM MARKER SCREENING	ULTRASOUND EVALUATION	CHORIONIC VILLUS SAMPLING (CVS)	AMNIOCENTESIS	PERCUTANEOUS UMBILICAL BLOOD SAMPLING (PUBS)	PREIMPLANTATION GENETIC DIAGNOSIS (PGD)	PLACENTAL FUNCTION (NST OR OCT)
Typical Reason for Procedure	Screening test for neural tube defects and chromosome anomalies	Screening test for genetic disorders; diagnostic procedure for structural anomalies	Diagnostic procedure for chromosome anomalies and genetic disorders*	Diagnostic procedure for chromosome anomalies, neural tube defects, abdominal wall defects, genetic disorders,* and lung maturity†	Diagnostic procedure for fetal disorders that require analysis of fetal blood serum levels‡	Diagnostic procedure for select chromosome anomalies and genetic disorders*	Screening procedure to assess uteroplacental insufficiency
Timing of Procedure§	15–20 weeks ‖	4–40 weeks	10–12 weeks	15–20 weeks; though may be performed thru 40th week†	19–40 weeks (typically performed at 19–21 weeks)	Days 3–5 after fertilization (at about 2.5 weeks)	Typically initiated by 32nd to 34th week
Length of Time for Results	3–7 days	Immediate	7–14 days**	7–14 days	1–5 days	24 hours	Immediate
Sampling Method (Quantity of Specimen Required for Analysis)	Maternal venous blood sample (7–10 mL)	Abdominal or vaginal ultrasound (one or more scans)	Transabdominal needle*** or transcervical catheter ultrasound-guided aspiration of chorionic villi (15–35 mg)	Transabdominal ultrasound guided needle aspiration of amniotic fluid (20–30 mL)***	Transabdominal ultrasound-guided needle aspiration of fetal blood from the umbilical cord (1 mL for a CBC; 3 mL for a karyotype)	Mechanical or laser biopsy of blastomeres from the day 3 to day 5 embryo (1–2 blastomeres per embryo)	External monitoring of fetal heart accelerations or late decelerations (in response to oxytocin) (One or more assessments)
Adverse Events	Bruising at needle insertion site	None known	Spontaneous loss of pregnancy; infection with or without loss of pregnancy; premature rupture of membranes; spotting or bleeding	Spontaneous loss of pregnancy; infection with or without loss of pregnancy; premature rupture of membranes; puncture of fetus or placenta	Spontaneous loss of pregnancy; infection with or without loss of pregnancy; premature rupture of membranes; puncture of fetus or placenta	Destruction of the embryo; loss of microscopic blastomere during transfer to test tube; inconclusive test results	Induction of labor in response to oxytocin

Continued

TABLE 11.13 Comparison of Prenatal Screening and Diagnostic Procedures *(Continued)*

	MATERNAL SERUM MARKER SCREENING	ULTRASOUND EVALUATION	CHORIONIC VILLUS SAMPLING (CVS)	AMNIOCENTESIS	PERCUTANEOUS UMBILICAL BLOOD SAMPLING (PUBS)	PREIMPLANTATION GENETIC DIAGNOSIS (PGD)	PLACENTAL FUNCTION (NST OR OCT)
Risks and Disadvantages	False-positive and false-negative results; potential for additional testing where no anomaly exists	Identification of structural anomalies with an unknown prognosis or no known treatment	0.5%–2% loss rate; 2% ambiguous results; if done before 9 weeks, increased incidence of limb reduction defects	0.5%–1.0% loss rate; potential for second-trimester termination of pregnancy	2%–5% loss; potential for second-trimester termination of pregnancy	No embryo transfer for 20%–30% of PGD cycles; high cost	Equivocal results requiring repeat testing
Benefits	Noninvasive primary screening test	Noninvasive broad screening test with rapidly advancing technology (3D images)	Permits a first-trimester termination of pregnancy	Permits assessment of multiple genetic risks from a single sample; broadly available; largest provider experience	Direct access to fetal blood	Assessment of embryo before implantation, allowing women to choose or not choose to transfer the embryo to the uterus	Noninvasive assessment of uteroplacental function

*Diagnosis is limited to those genetic disorders for which the genetic sequence of the altered gene has been identified.

†Fetal lung maturity may be assessed by measuring the lecithin-to-sphingomyelin (L/S) ratio in amniotic fluid.

‡Examples are fetal anemia secondary to Rh isoimmunization and fetal drug levels of antiarrhythmic agents.

§Based on 40 weeks' gestation calculated from first day of last menstrual period (LMP).

||First-trimester assessment of free β-hCG and PAPP-A done in conjunction with ultrasound evaluation of the fetal nuchal translucency (under clinical investigation).

**For cytogenetic or PCR molecular analysis. Fluorescent in situ hybridization results may be available in 1–2 days, but current technology provides limited information.

***An 18, 20, or 22 gauge needle (such as a spinal needle) is used.

NST, nonstress test; OCT, oxytocin challenge test.

Data from Harper (2001), Jones & Headrick (1992), and Scott, DiSaia, Hammond & Spellacy (1999).

NURSING CARE PLAN 11.2

The Client Facing Prenatal Diagnosis Options

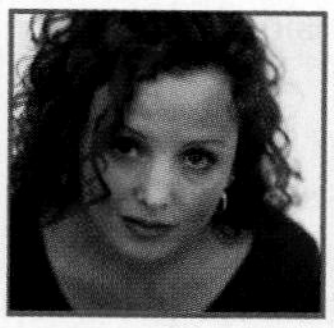

As discussed at the beginning of the chapter, April and Alex have conceived after 2 years. During the interview, the nurse notes that April is concerned about her increased risk for chromosomal anomalies given her "advanced maternal age." April states, "I read that our chance of having a child with Down syndrome has risen to the point that invasive testing is the lesser of the two risks. If we have such testing, what if I am one of the women who miscarries a healthy fetus after an amniocentesis? I could never forgive myself. But if I give birth to a child with Down syndrome, I just don't know how I'll handle it. . . ."

NURSING DIAGNOSES

- **Decisional Conflict** related to personal values and beliefs secondary to lack of knowledge
- **Anxiety** related to increased risks for genetic abnormalities and potential complications associated with prenatal screening and testing

EXPECTED OUTCOMES

1. The couple will identify the advantages and disadvantages of the prenatal diagnosis options.
2. The couple will express concerns about age-related risk and the scope of prenatal testing options.
3. The couple will describe the resources and support needed to make an informed decision.
4. The couple will make a timely and informed decision.

INTERVENTIONS	RATIONALES
Take measures to protect privacy and to facilitate a relaxed atmosphere of trust.	Clients who feel comfortable and accepted and that the nurse is maintaining privacy are more likely to be frank about concerns related to prenatal screening and testing.
Include both partners in the discussion; encourage them to work together in the informed decision-making process.	Disturbances in self-esteem, body image, and personal relationships are more likely if clients do not support each other.
Provide education and counseling about the identified risk factors and available diagnostic options.	Lack of information causes stress; in turn, stress fosters the inability to make an informed decision.
Explore the couple's exposure to prenatal screening and testing; assist them to identify and list their fears and concerns; correct any misunderstandings related to these methods; allow time for questions.	Such information provides an additional foundation for teaching and opportunities to clarify or correct misinformation. Unrecognized fears can lead to indecision from not understanding fully the basis of the anxiety.
Review possible options for screening and testing, including risks and benefits of each; provide the couple with written information about the various methods; suggest other sources of information, such as couples who have undergone testing and local community agencies.	Increased knowledge promotes informed decision making. Use of written material allows opportunities for review and discussion. Talking with others who have had similar experiences allows the couple to share feelings and to feel that they are not alone.

Continued

NURSING CARE PLAN 11.2 ● The Client Facing Prenatal Diagnosis Options *(Continued)*

Encourage the couple to discuss concerns, fears, and beliefs with each other.	Sharing of feelings promotes mutual decision making.
Explore the risks of not deciding.	Prenatal diagnosis has a limited window of opportunity. It requires a timely decision before options become unavailable.
Assure the couple that it is solely their choice about whether to undergo prenatal diagnosis.	The client needs support in a potential decision to ***not*** pursue prenatal diagnosis.
Explore the couple's ethical and spiritual beliefs; arrange for a possible referral to a spiritual leader or encourage them to speak with a spiritual leader of their choice.	Prenatal diagnosis may include voluntary interruption of pregnancy as one potential outcome. Ethics and values affect the decision whether to terminate a pregnancy. A spiritual leader may assist the couple to understand personal ethics and values in the context of prenatal choice.
Arrange for a follow-up visit with the client and her husband in 2 to 3 weeks.	Follow-up is necessary to determine the couple's progress to a decision and provides opportunities for additional teaching, support, and guidance.

EVALUATION

1. The couple states appropriate information related to prenatal testing and diagnosis.
2. The couple identifies the risks and benefits of prenatal testing.
3. The couple makes an informed choice to participate or not participate in prenatal counseling and diagnosis by the mid second trimester.
4. The couple states that they are comfortable with their decision.

NIC/NOC Box 11.1 Prenatal Screening and Counseling

NIC

- Active Listening
- Anxiety Reduction
- Coping Enhancement
- Counseling
- Decision-Making Support
- Emotional Support
- Genetic Counseling
- Mutual Goal Setting
- Support System Enhancement
- Values Clarification

NOC

- Anxiety Control
- Decision Making
- Fear Control
- Information Processing
- Participation: Health Care Decisions

to have fetuses with anencephaly and open or closed neural tube defects (Fig. 11.19). As a sole biochemical marker, MSAFP identifies 95% of fetuses with anencephaly, 80% of fetuses with open spina bifida, and 5% of fetuses with closed spina bifida (Scott et al., 1999). To correctly interpret MSAFP levels, the laboratory needs confirmation of gestational age, fetal viability, single or multiple gestation, maternal weight, race, and presence or absence of maternal diabetes (Nussbaum et al., 2001).

A result is provided as "multiples of the median" (MoM) for a specific population incidence of neural tube defects (NTDs). The U.S. incidence of NTDs is approximately 1 in 1,000 to 2,000, with the highest level in the Appalachian region. Each laboratory establishes specific standards for positive or negative findings per MoM; however, most laboratories use 2.5 MoM as the upper range of normal (Scott et al., 1999).

The addition of maternal serum unconjugated estriol (uE3) and hCG to the MSAFP analysis (referred to as "triple screen") and age-related risk assessment permits screening for the risk for trisomy 21 (Down syndrome) and trisomy 18 (Edwards' syndrome). The MoMs for

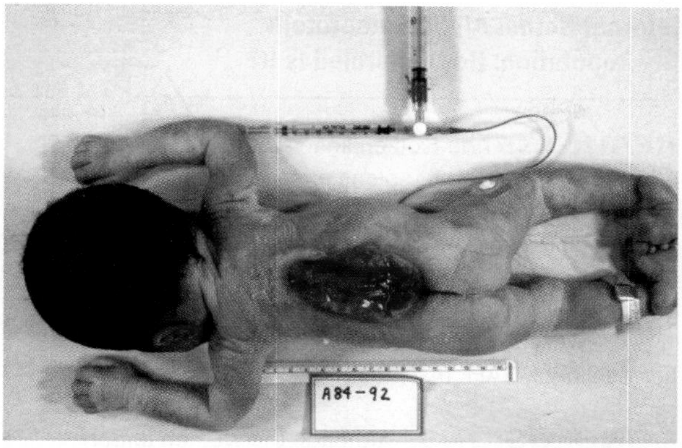

FIGURE 11.19 Stillborn infant with neural tube defect. (Courtesy of A. Donnenfeld, Society Hill Genetics, Philadelphia.)

MSAFP and uE3 are usually less than 1 and typically less than 0.72 and 0.73, respectively, whereas the hCG level is significantly elevated above 2 MoMs for pregnancies found to have a fetus with Down syndrome. In contrast, pregnancies found to have a fetus with Edwards' syndrome have MSAFP, uE3, and hCG with lower MoMs. The sensitivity of the trimarker assays for Edwards' syndrome is greater than 80%, whereas the sensitivity for Down syndrome is 60% (Nussbaum et al., 2001).

Multiple other biochemical markers have been investigated in an effort to increase the sensitivity of maternal serum screening in the second trimester. Inhibin-A (INH-A) was found to vary less with gestational age than other biochemical markers (Benn, 2002a). INH-A is linked closely with hCG levels and is elevated in fetuses with trisomy 21. The addition of INH-A to the panel of MSAFP, uE3, and hCG resulted in the recognition of the "quad test" as a replacement for the triple screen (Benn, 2003). There are, however, little prospective data given the interest of researchers in first-trimester testing (Benn, 2002a).

The ability to perform first-trimester maternal serum screening for Down syndrome and Edwards' syndrome is being investigated. Pregnancy-associated placental protein (PAPP-A) and free β-hCG are the biochemical markers used in association with assessment of the nuchal translucency (enlarged subcutaneous fluid-filled space at the back of the fetal neck) (Benn, 2002b; Spencer, 2000). PAPP-A is typically low and β-hCG significantly elevated in a pregnancy found to have a fetus with trisomy 21; the nuchal translucency (NT) is of concern if it measures greater than 3 mm (Benn, 2002b). Of concern is the significant potential variability from one ultrasonographer to another performing the NT measurement (Wapner et al., 2003). The multicentered First Trimester Maternal Serum Biochemistry and Fetal Nuchal Translucency Screening Study Group reported an 85% detection rate for trisomy 21 and a 91% detection rate for trisomy 18 within a study population of 8,500 singleton pregnancies (Wapner et al., 2003).

COLLABORATIVE CARE: MATERNAL SERUM MARKER SCREENING

Assessment

Most women progress through prenatal care with limited understanding of the various assessments and tests that providers perform. Most first encounters with prenatal genetic screening are the request to perform the maternal serum triple screen at 15 to 20 weeks' gestation. The nurse should be prepared to provide education and support for clients before obtaining their consent for testing. To conduct the test, a venous blood sample is obtained from the woman and analyzed for MSAFP, uE3, and hCG.

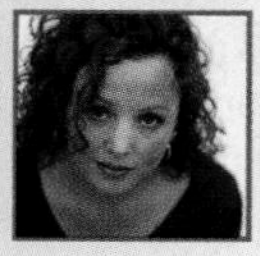

April is 37 years old. This is her second pregnancy. Would she be a suitable candidate for maternal serum marker screening?

Select Potential Nursing Diagnoses

The following are examples of potentially applicable NANDA diagnoses:

- **Risk for Ineffective Role Performance** related to uncertainty about prenatal screening
- **Risk for Anxiety** related to false-positive test results
- **Deficient Knowledge** related to risks and benefits of screening tests

Planning/Intervention

The adherence to the principles of informed decision making and consent for maternal serum triple screen testing is fundamental to the performance of this standard of practice (American College of Medical Genetics, 1996b) (Research Highlight 11.1). The client must understand the purpose, benefits, risks, limitations, and follow-up care associated with this screening test (see Table 11.13). It is especially important for her to understand that this screening test can have false-negative (misidentification of a fetus as free of a neural tube defect or chromosome anomaly when one exists) and false-positive (misidentification of a fetus as at-risk for a neural tube defect or chromosome anomaly when one does not exist) results. The nurse should assist the client to understand this important limitation of a screening test.

When an abnormal result is presented to the client, the nurse should provide supportive counseling and reiterate the difference between a screening and diagnostic test. Depending on the level of MoM abnormality, the nurse should reassure the client that the fetus is more likely to not have than to have an NTD or chromosome anomaly. The nurse should clarify the diagnostic tests recommended for confirmation or elimination of risk for an NTD or chromosome anomaly. Typically, this includes performance of a diagnostic ultrasound and amniocentesis for assessment of amniotic fluid AFP and fetal chromosomes

● RESEARCH HIGHLIGHT 11.1 Informed Consent for Maternal Serum Alpha-Fetoprotein Screening in an Inner City Population: How Informed Is It?

OBJECTIVE: Nurses are frequently the health care professionals who seek informed consent from clients for complex procedures. The standard that they should use to measure client understanding of complicated protocols has not been defined clearly. The purpose of this study was to determine whether women who received information from a provider and viewed a videotape about maternal serum alpha-fetoprotein (MSAFP) screening gained knowledge sufficient to meet the criteria to participate in voluntary shared decision making (informed consent).

DESIGN: The researchers recruited 53 inner-city pregnant women (58% Hispanic, 39% African American, 3% white) 15 to 19 weeks pregnant from a northeastern Women's Health Center to participate in this prospective qualitative study. They prepared 12 open-ended questions to assess the women's level of knowledge after interacting with the provider and viewing the videotape. The researchers conducted audiotaped personal interviews with each woman who verbally responded to the identified questions. They performed content analysis on the interviews to identify the level of understanding about MSAFP screening among the women.

RESULTS: Two women answered all questions correctly, but no one answered all questions incorrectly. As the content of the questions became more complex, fewer women answered them correctly. Sixty-two percent of the women answered the first question "What is MSAFP?" correctly, whereas only 18% answered correctly the question, "What does a positive low MSAFP test mean?"

CONCLUSIONS: Although the women understood that the test was voluntary, they did not demonstrate consistent knowledge about it or the meaning of positive results. This did not deter 80% of women from immediately signing the informed consent document and proceeding with the MSAFP test. The remaining 20% requested additional information. This study did not answer the question of how to measure comprehension and the level necessary and sufficient to consider a woman "informed." The researchers support the method of interactive dialogue to evaluate comprehension.

Freda, M. C., DeVore, N., Valentine-Adams, N., Bombard, A., & Merkatz, I. R. (1998). *Journal of Obstetric, Gynecologic, and Neonatal Nursing, 27*(1), 99–106.

(Nussbaum et al., 2001). The nurse should provide emotional and care support for this phase of informed decision making and consent, which includes referral to genetic services if diagnostic ultrasound or amniocentesis is not available in the primary obstetrical care setting.

Evaluation

Evaluation varies according to the individualized plan and interventions. It is vital for the nurse to assess the process of informed decision making and consent undertaken by the client. Sometimes, health care providers perceive and label decisions to *not* proceed with screening or diagnostic testing as noncompliant behavior. If the nurse perceives that a decision to not proceed is made after appropriate education and counseling and that the client understands the benefits and risks of the procedure, then the nurse supports the decision and advocates on the client's behalf if questioned by other health care professionals.

Ultrasound Evaluation

QUOTE 11-2

"In a level 2 ultrasound setting, the patients come expecting the worst. With preliminary screening, these patients don't."

A sonographer in response to a routine ultrasound with an adverse outcome

Introduced in the 1970s, ultrasound is the most widely known prenatal screening and diagnostic procedure. As a result of advances in this technology, the general public expects a child's first picture to be an ultrasound snapshot taken during the second trimester. This parental expectation is the result of news and marketing campaigns that demonstrate the clear depiction of the fetus' individual physical features through the use of three-dimensional sonographic imaging. This noninvasive technology creates an aura of wonder among those who witness the ability to look into the world of the developing fetus.

Ultrasound is performed with a transabdominal or transvaginal handheld device called a *transducer.* Sound waves pass through the transducer and abdominal or vaginal wall to bounce off the fetus. The transducer captures a moving ("real-time") or still image of the fetus and sends it back to the ultrasound machine. The image appears as a two- or three-dimensional volume snapshot of the fetus. Three-dimensional imaging requires sophisticated computer processor technology to transform sound waves into sculpture-like fetal images (Kurjak et al., 2002).

Ultrasound is used as both a screening and diagnostic test (Raynor, 2003). As a screening instrument, it is used to identify gestational age, number of fetuses, and fetal viability. It also is used as an adjunct to correct interpretation of maternal serum marker screening, identification of pregnancies at higher-than-age-appropriate risk for chromosomal anomalies, and performance of invasive tests (Nussbaum et al., 2001). As a diagnostic tool, ultrasound imaging is used to identify and evaluate specific structural anomalies associated with genetic disorders and isolated birth defects.

Ultrasound is a safe, noninvasive tool with no known teratogenic risks to mother or fetus (Raynor, 2003). The perceived lack of harm and the availability of routine visualization of the fetus increase the likelihood that a prenatal ultrasound scan will be performed. Nevertheless, the general public often neglects to understand the limitations of ultrasound and the potential for no available prognostic information if an anomaly is identified (Goldberg, 2004). This may lead to parental iatrogenic worry and possible interruption in prenatal parent–fetus bonding (Kohut et al., 2002). Ultrasound requires the dissemination of information about the potential for unanticipated findings and associated consequences, whether it is used for screening, diagnosis, or social information (eg, baby book picture, gender identification).

COLLABORATIVE CARE: ULTRASOUND

Assessment

Informed decision making and consent have *not* been a traditional component of the performance of ultrasound for screening or diagnosis. The nurse should assess the client's understanding of the scope of potential benefits, risks, and limitations of sonographic imaging before performance of the procedure. Informed consent before screening or diagnostic ultrasound is highly desirable and assists with preparation for any subsequent need to disclose unexpected findings. In addition, real-time two- and three-dimensional volume imaging allows the client to visualize fetal movement before she may experience physical perception. The nurse should educate and counsel the client referred for ultrasound to rule out a suspected disorder about her ability (and the acceptability) to choose or choose not to observe the ultrasound scan.

Early gestation (less than 12 weeks') is visualized using a transvaginal approach (provider preferred for best visualization) or transabdominal approach (requires the woman's bladder to be full to assist with transmission of the sound waves to the fetus). Some clients will not agree to the use of a transvaginal probe for social or cultural reasons. The nurse should identify and counsel them to determine whether transvaginal sonography would be a viable alternative if the woman inserted the transducer probe herself. If this option is not acceptable, then the nurse should inform the person performing the scan of the client's preference.

Ultrasound imaging of the second- and third-trimester fetus generally is accomplished using transabdominal ultrasound. The available volume of amniotic fluid precludes the need for a full bladder during these scans.

Select Potential Nursing Diagnoses

The following are examples of potentially applicable NANDA diagnoses:

- **Risk for Impaired Parent/Fetal Attachment** related to identification of fetal anomalies
- **Risk for Powerlessness** related to parental perception of inability to alter fetal outcome
- **Deficient Knowledge** related to advantages and disadvantages of fetal sonographic evaluation

Planning/Intervention

Screening during the first trimester includes assessment of gestational age, viability (cardiac activity), number of embryos, size of gestational and yolk sacs, and growth (see Fig. 11.7). In addition to these components of a level 1 (basic) scan, skilled sonographers and physicians can evaluate the normality of the fetal NT. This structure lies between the skin and soft tissue atop the cervical spine and is evident during 10 to 14 weeks' gestation. An NT above 2.1 mm at 11 weeks or 3.0 mm at 14 weeks correlates highly with an increased risk for fetal chromosome aneuploidy (Bindra et al., 2002). It also may indicate a cardiac anomaly or other genetic syndrome not associated with a chromosomal anomaly (Box 11.3). The nurse should counsel and educate the client about the implications of NT assessment and the recommendation for confirmation or elimination of risk through the use of amniocentesis and fetal chromosome analysis. This dialogue includes information about the client's ability to thoughtfully consider whether to proceed with an amniocentesis after the outcome of NT assessment is known.

Assessment of the fetal nasal bone currently is being investigated as an additional ultrasound screening marker. Absence of the nasal bone has been found to be indicative of Down syndrome in fetuses scanned during either the first or second trimester (Vintzileous et al., 2003).

Physicians use ultrasound to assist with the safe performance of amniocentesis and CVS (see Table 11.13). The nurse should educate and counsel the client about each procedure and the benefit of adjunct sonography in the reduction of fetal risk. He or she should share the importance of understanding the scope of identifiable findings in this nondiagnostic use of sonography with the client to ensure informed decision making and consent.

Throughout gestation, ultrasound is used to diagnose and evaluate fetal structural anomalies (Sanders, 2002) (Box 11.4). The nurse should educate and counsel the woman about this technology (Figs. 11.20 and 11.21). It is especially important for the client to understand that the presence of a structural anomaly is a

BOX 11.3 The Importance of Nuchal Translucency Screening

Case History

A woman presented for chorionic villous sampling at 11 weeks' gestation indicated by (1) advanced maternal age (39 years), and (2) abnormal nuchal fold measuring 4.9 mm. The chromosome analysis following chorionic villus sampling (CVS) was a normal 46,XY. Because a skilled sonographer performed the nuchal fold measurement and recorded a finding of nearly 5 mm (the highest acceptable measurement for a fetus of any age), the woman was counseled that the fetus was at significant risk for other anomalies. At 18.5 weeks, the woman returned for diagnostic ultrasound. The fetus was found to have bilateral bowed femurs and forearms, lower sacral protrusion, developing "lemon sign" of the frontal skull, bilateral hydronephrosis, and bilateral edema of the feet (see below). Definitive diagnosis could not be made, but given the anomalies, the woman was counseled that the fetus was expected to have a poor postnatal prognosis.

Upon birth of the fetus, examination suggested the autosomal dominant disorder camptomelic dysplasia. This case highlights the importance of performing diagnostic ultrasound in conjunction with CVS.

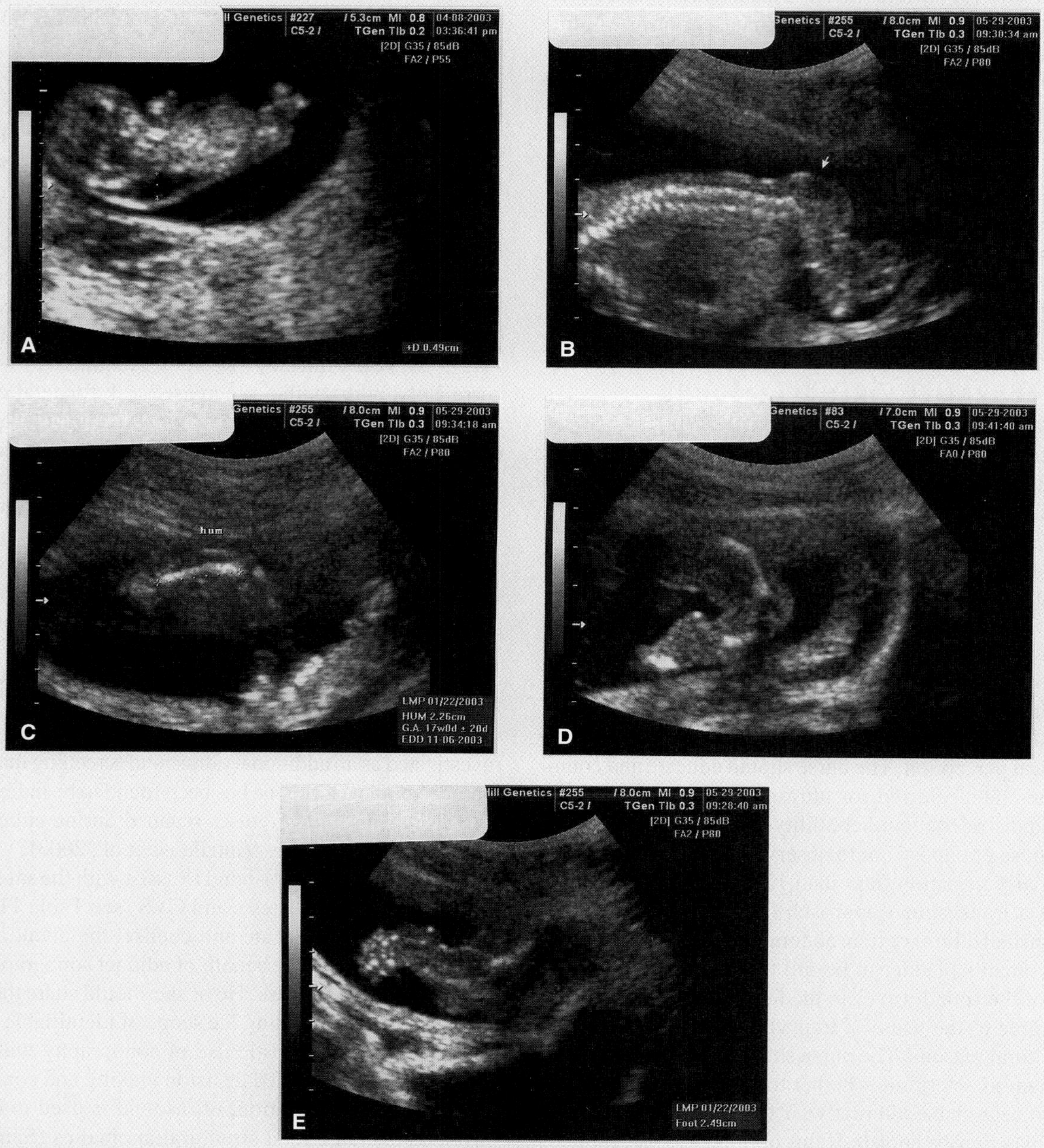

(A) 11-week-old fetus; nuchal fold of 4.9 mm. **(B)** 18.5-week-old fetus; sacral protrusion. **(C)** Bowed humerus. **(D)** Bowed femur. **(E)** Edema of foot. (Courtesy of S. Majewski, Society Hill Genetics, Philadelphia.)

BOX 11.4 Selected Examples of Structural Defects That Ultrasound Imaging Can Confirm

Agenesis of the corpus callosum
Anencephaly
Cardiac malformations
Cerebellar hypoplasia
Cleft lip
Cleft palate
Clubfoot
Conjoined twins
Cystic hygroma
Diaphragmatic hernia
Duodenal atresia
Encephalocele
Exomphalos
Genital anomalies
Holoprosencephaly
Hydrocephalus
Neural tube defects
Nuchal edema
Nonimmune hydrops
Obstructive uropathy
Omphalocele
Polycystic kidney disease
Polydactyly
Radial ray defects

confirmatory diagnosis. The absence of a structural anomaly, however, is not absolute. The procedure may fail to reveal an anomaly as a result of fetal position or limited skill of the person performing the ultrasound scan. The sensitivity and specificity of diagnostic ultrasound continue to advance with ongoing improvement of three-dimensional volume imaging and yield a declining incidence of false-negative scans (Fig. 11.22).

Evaluation

Evaluation of the knowledge and expectations of the client who seeks or is referred for gestation ultrasound are of significant importance to the process of informed decision making, the client's comfort and well-being, and the preservation without disruption of the growing bond between parent and fetus. Evaluation of the client's knowledge and understanding of possible follow-up interventions also is required.

Invasive Diagnostic Tests

Three methods are available to evaluate fetal chromosomes, genes, or blood chemistry: amniocentesis, CVS, and percutaneous umbilical cord sampling. Each is performed to obtain a fetal specimen for analysis and evaluation. Given their invasive nature, none is performed unless there is a clinical indication (see Table 11.13).

Amniocentesis

Amniocentesis (often referred to simply as "amnio") became available in the clinical setting in the 1960s, following closely the confirmation of the correct number of chromosomes in the human genome. The establishment of the positive correlation between advanced maternal age and increased risk for birth of a child with a chromosomal anomaly provided further impetus for the adoption and integration of this technology as a standard of care within the prenatal setting (see Table 11.11) (Nussbaum et al., 2001). Amniocentesis for prenatal genetic assessment typically is performed between 15 and 20 weeks' gestation.

With amniocentesis, a needle is inserted through the maternal abdominal and uterine walls to place the needle tip within the amniotic sac in a space filled with amniotic fluid and free of fetal parts (Fig. 11.23). Ultrasound is used to identify an appropriate site and to guide the needle to that area safely. Approximately 20 to 30 mL of amniotic fluid is withdrawn, which represents approximately 10% of the total volume available at 15 to 20 weeks' gestation. The developing skin of the fetus sheds cells into the amniotic fluid. These cells are separated from the amniotic fluid, grown in laboratory culture dishes, and analyzed for chromosomal (method: cytogenetic analysis) or single gene (method: molecular genetic analysis) disorders. The amniotic fluid is used to determine the level of MSAFP. A third-trimester amniocentesis is performed to assess the lecithin-to-sphingomyelin (L/S) ratio to evaluate fetal lung maturity in the gestation at risk for preterm delivery.

Chorionic Villus Sampling

Chorionic villus sampling (CVS), available in the United States since the 1980s, typically is performed between 10 and 12 weeks' gestation, but sometimes is offered up to 14 weeks (Jenkins & Wapner, 1999). Before the differentiation of chorionic tissue into the well-organized structure of the placenta, villi cover the entire surface of the chorionic sac (see earlier discussion). These villi are easily detached for laboratory analysis of the fetus' genetic health.

Performance of CVS is completed by applying gentle syringe suction through a needle (transabdominal approach) or catheter (transvaginal approach) to detach villi from the chorionic sac (Fig. 11.24). Similar to amniocentesis, cytogenetic and molecular genetic testing is performed on the villi. Because amniotic fluid is not obtained, MSAFP analysis is not completed. An MSAFP screen and ultrasound evaluation at 15 to 16 weeks' gestation is the appropriate adjunct to CVS. CVS originally was offered beginning with the 8th week of gestation. In the 1990s, reports surfaced raising concern about a possible association between CVS and infants born with limb reduction defects. Careful review of the international CVS

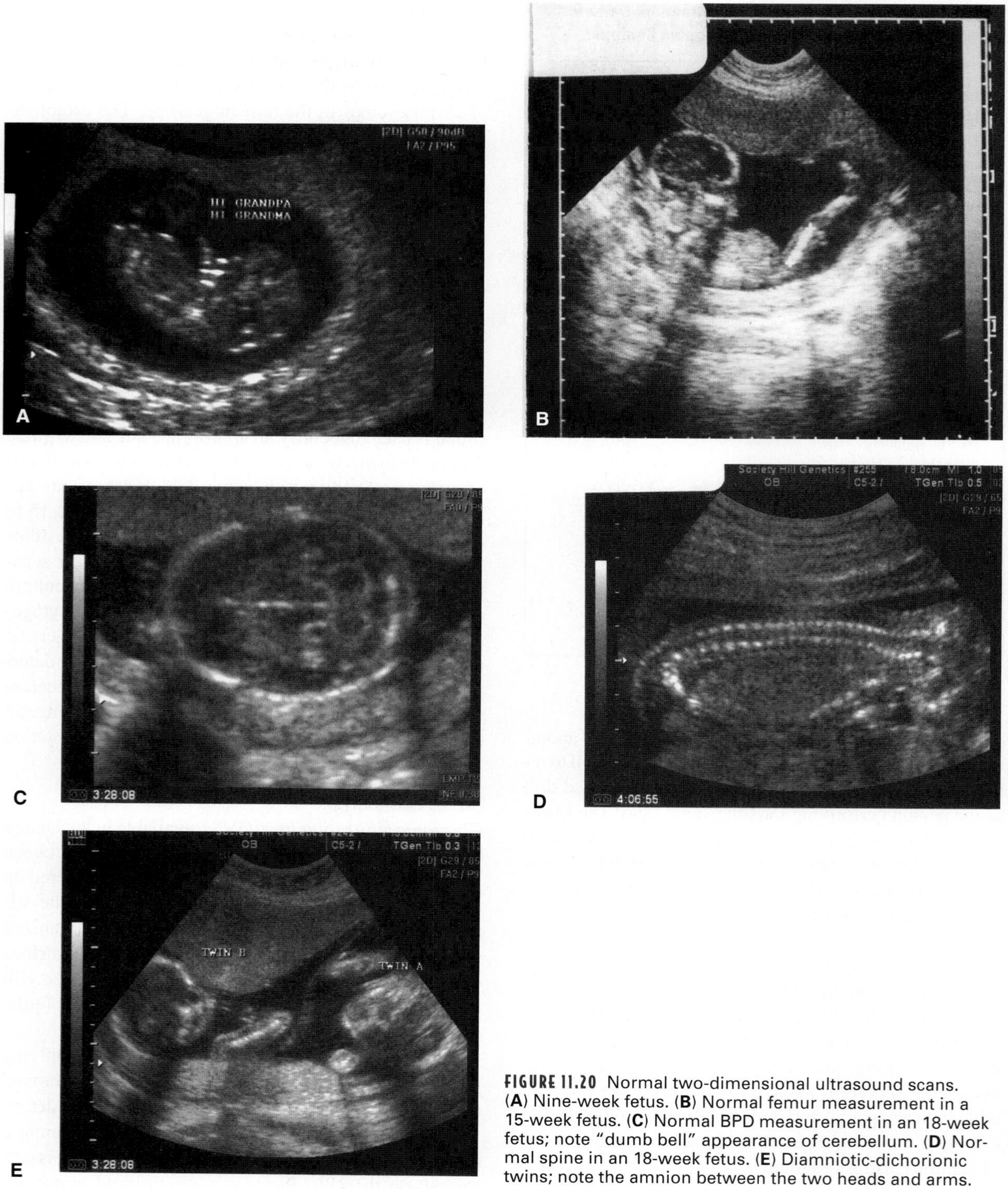

FIGURE 11.20 Normal two-dimensional ultrasound scans. (**A**) Nine-week fetus. (**B**) Normal femur measurement in a 15-week fetus. (**C**) Normal BPD measurement in an 18-week fetus; note "dumb bell" appearance of cerebellum. (**D**) Normal spine in an 18-week fetus. (**E**) Diamniotic-dichorionic twins; note the amnion between the two heads and arms.

registry identified a probable correlation if the procedure is performed during 8 or 9 weeks' gestation. Conversely, this correlation is not found among infants born after CVS performed between 10 and 14 weeks' gestation (Froster & Jackson, 1996; Nussbaum et al., 2001).

Percutaneous Umbilical Blood Sampling

Percutaneous umbilical blood sampling (PUBS) is performed when direct access to fetal blood is required for evaluation of the health and well-being of the fetus. PUBS is performed under ultrasound guidance (Fig. 11.25).

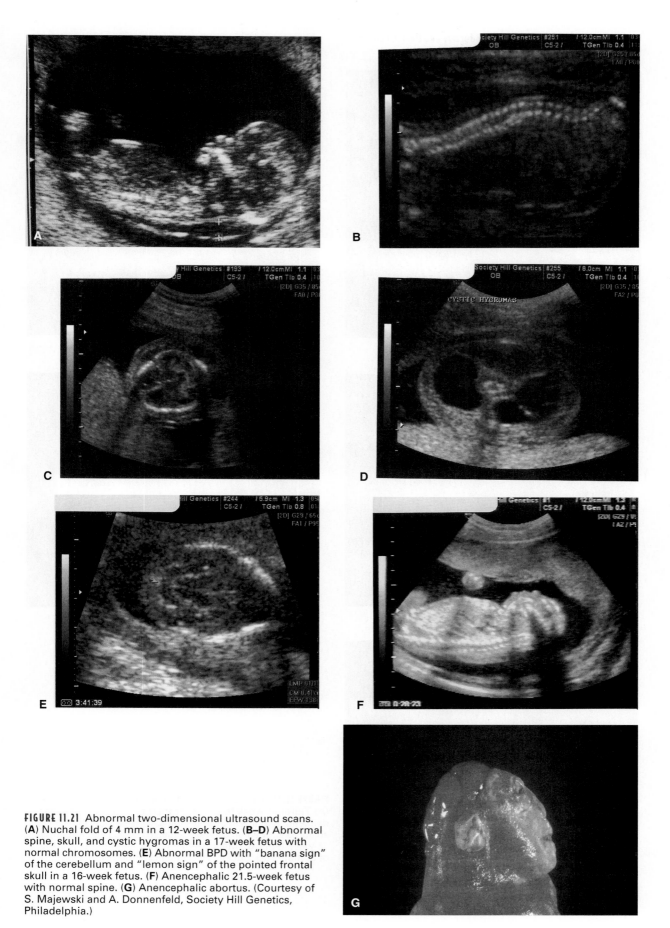

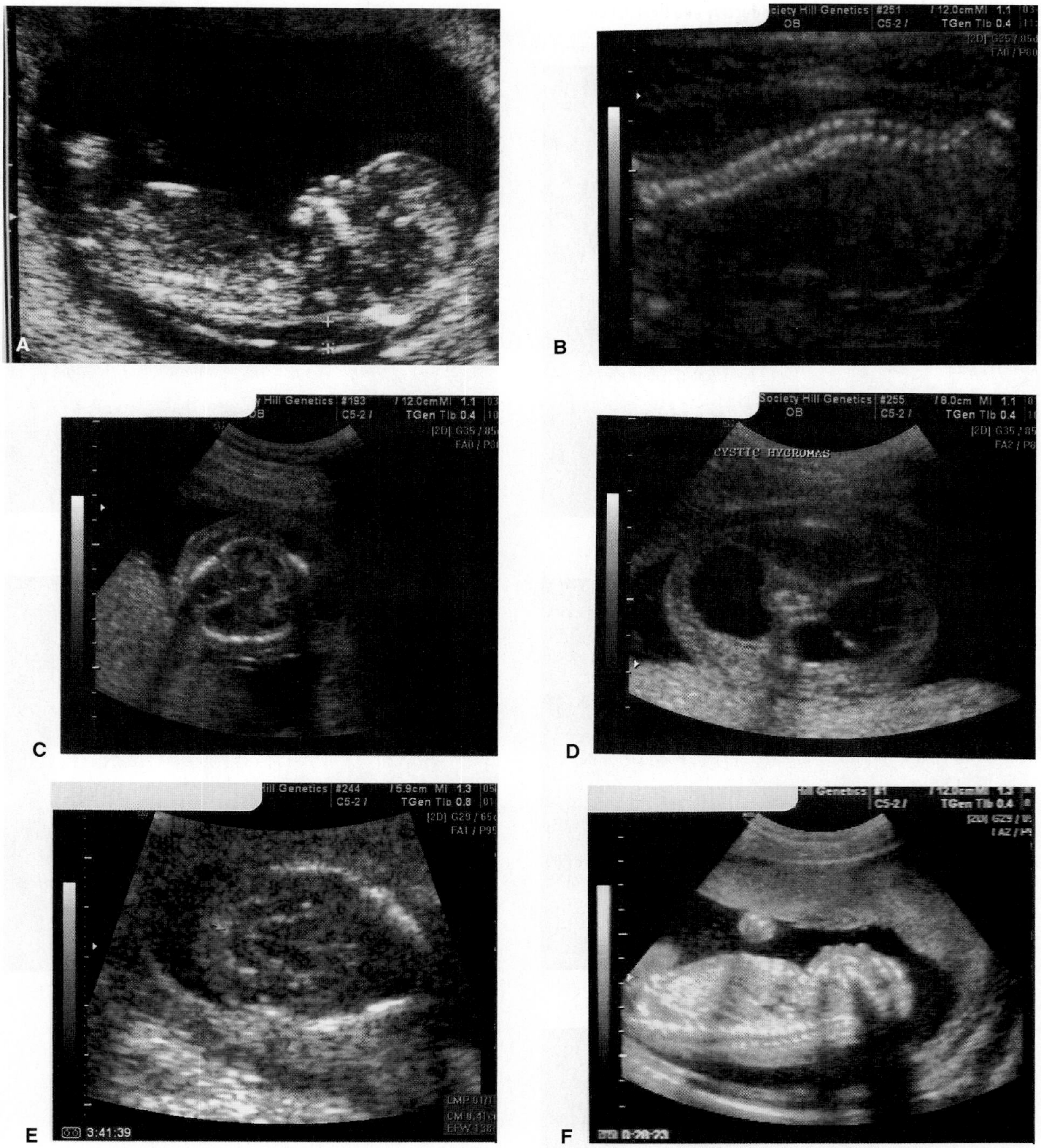

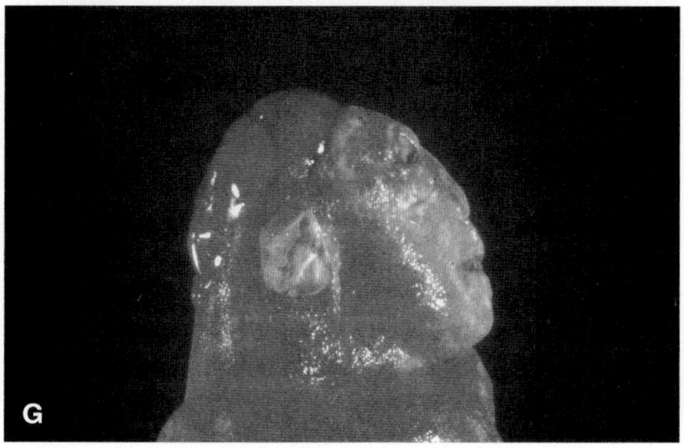

FIGURE 11.21 Abnormal two-dimensional ultrasound scans. (**A**) Nuchal fold of 4 mm in a 12-week fetus. (**B–D**) Abnormal spine, skull, and cystic hygromas in a 17-week fetus with normal chromosomes. (**E**) Abnormal BPD with "banana sign" of the cerebellum and "lemon sign" of the pointed frontal skull in a 16-week fetus. (**F**) Anencephalic 21.5-week fetus with normal spine. (**G**) Anencephalic abortus. (Courtesy of S. Majewski and A. Donnenfeld, Society Hill Genetics, Philadelphia.)

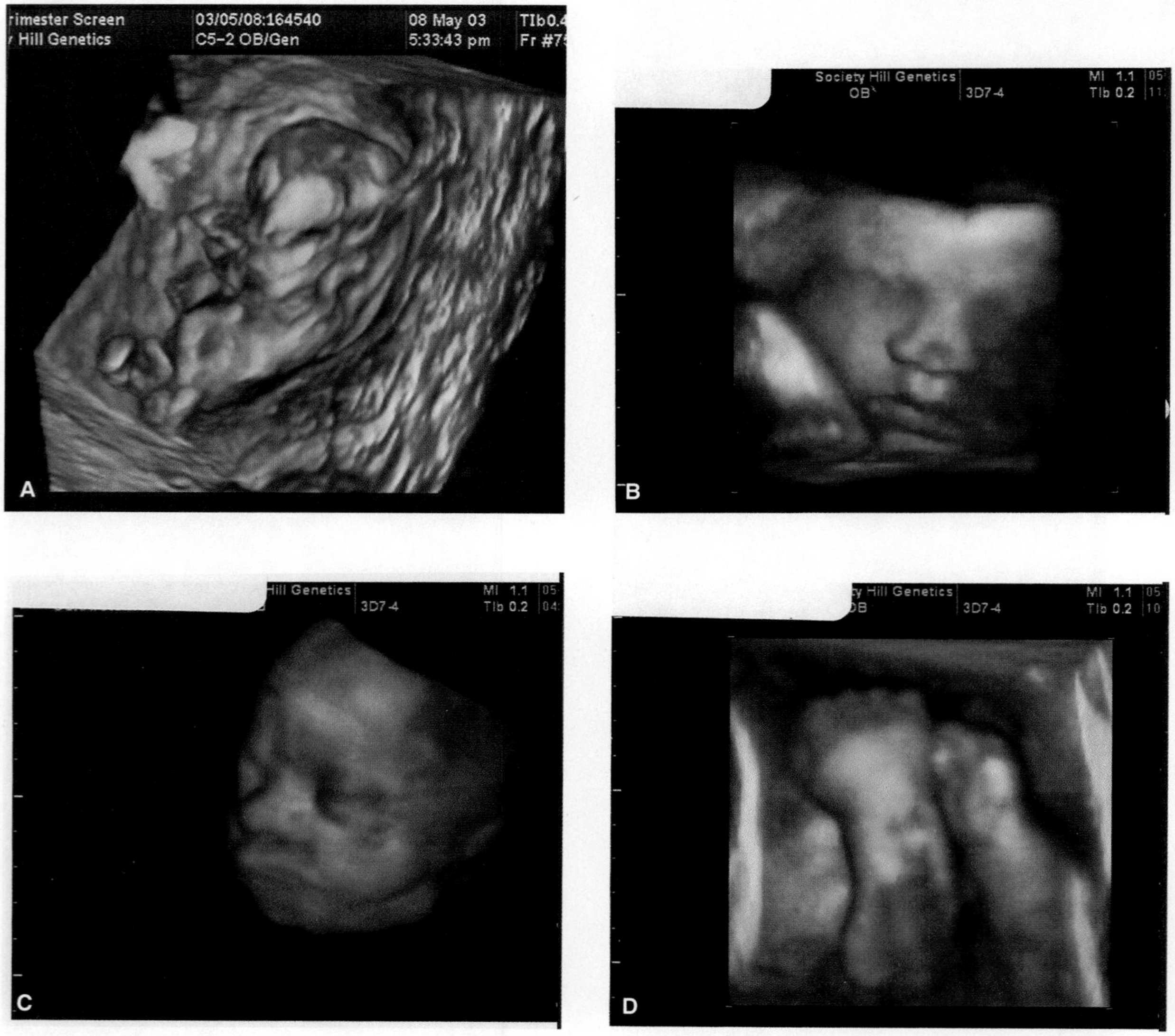

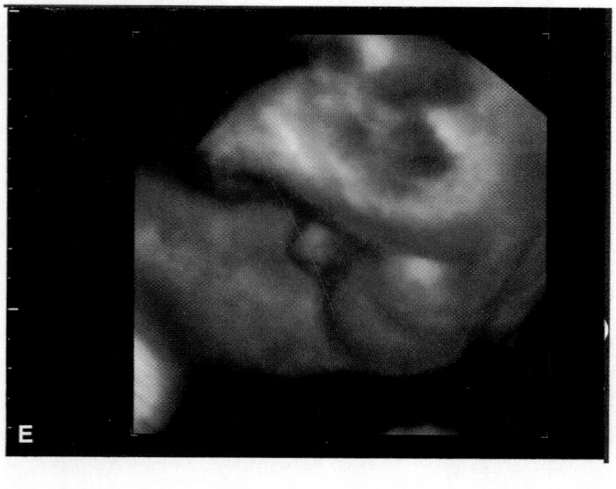

FIGURE 11.22 Normal three-dimensional ultrasound scans. (**A**) Thirteen-week fetus. (**B**) Frontal face view; note clear delineation of lips in 36-week fetus. (**C**) Side view of face; note ability to view ear in 35-week fetus. (**D**) Hands and forearms of 36-week fetus. (**E**) Male genitalia of 29-week fetus. (Courtesy of S. Majewski, Society Hill Genetics, Philadelphia.)

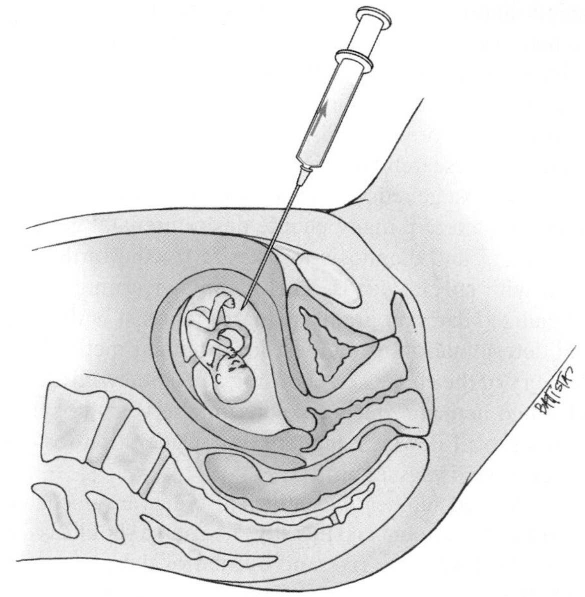

FIGURE 11.23 Amniocentesis.

A fine needle is inserted through the abdominal and uterine walls into the umbilical vein. The indications for PUBS have diminished with advances in molecular genetic disorder identification. Examples of disorders that continue to be evaluated by PUBS are anemia secondary to Rh isoimmunization and fetal drug levels secondary to receiving antidysrhythmic agents. The technique used to perform PUBS also provides a method for fetal transfusion of blood or administration of drugs (Scott et al., 1999).

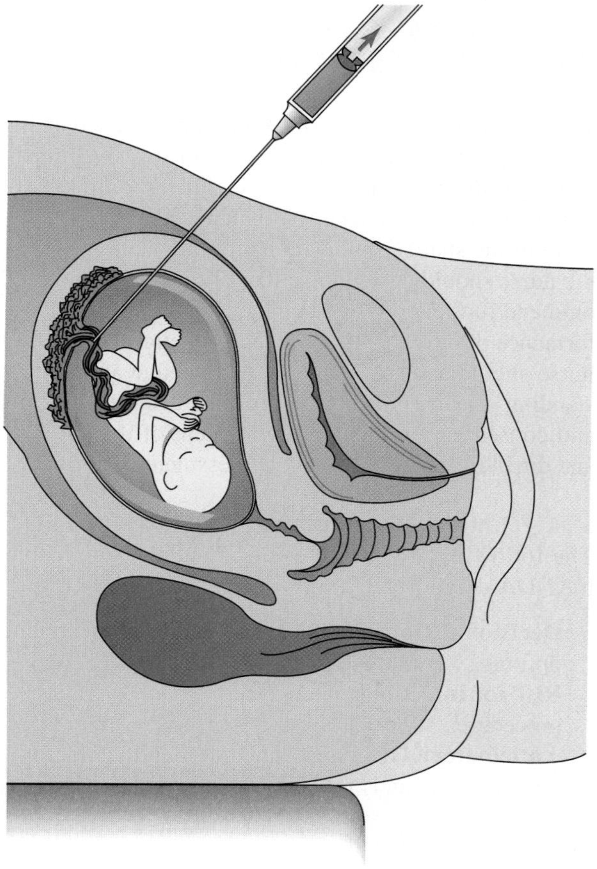

FIGURE 11.25 Percutaneous umbilical blood sampling.

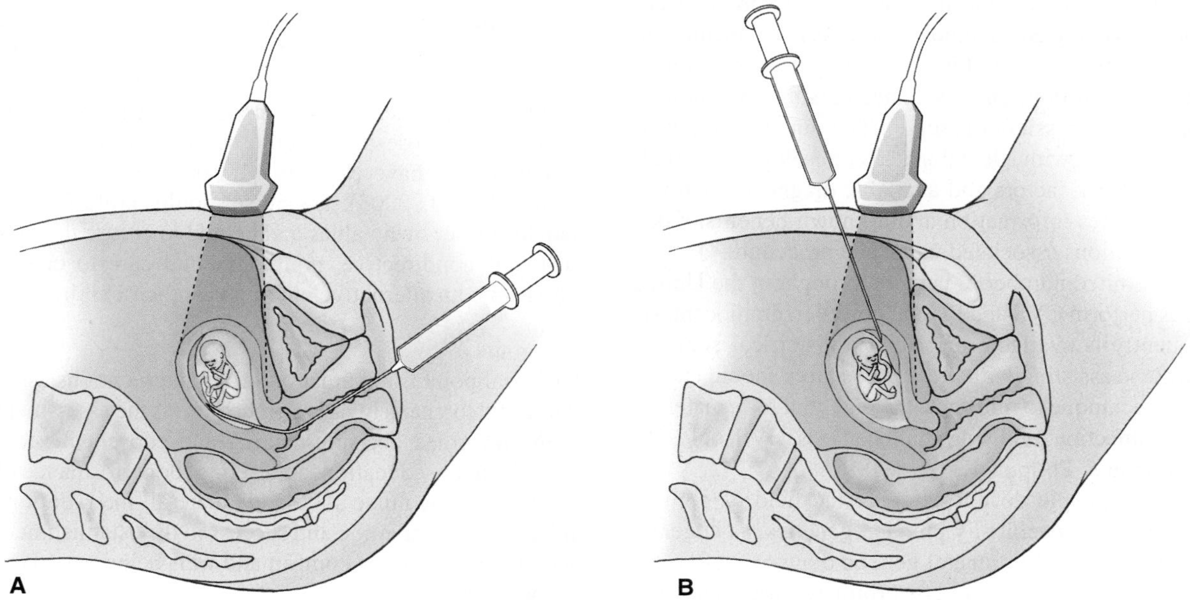

A B

FIGURE 11.24 Chorionic villus sampling. (**A**) Transvaginal sampling. (**B**) Transabdominal sampling.

COLLABORATIVE CARE: INVASIVE DIAGNOSTIC TESTS

Assessment

The completion and assessment of a prenatal screening questionnaire can reveal indications for invasive prenatal diagnostic procedures (see Assessment Tool 11.1). If review of the completed questionnaires identifies one or more of the standard indications for prenatal diagnosis, the nurse should advise the client of this result and recommend further counseling and evaluation. Before performance of or referral for prenatal genetic services, the nurse should assess the client's knowledge and understanding of each procedure. Informed decision making and consent are an integral component of this process and direct the type and level of assessment performed.

Select Potential Nursing Diagnoses

The following are examples of potentially applicable NANDA diagnoses:

- **Decisional Conflict** related to scope of treatment options
- **Risk for Infection** related to performance of invasive procedures
- **Anticipatory Grieving** related to identification of a fetal anomaly and "loss" of expected healthy child

Planning/Intervention

QUOTE 11-3

"We wanted this pregnancy so much . . . why me?"

In response to an abnormal result after a prenatal diagnostic procedure

As knowledge of genetics advances, the ability to provide appropriate and disorder-specific prenatal genetic counseling and diagnosis increases. It is incumbent on nurses to integrate this developing body of clinical genetics knowledge and associated nursing care implications into professional practice. The nurse should provide the client with education and counseling about their identified risk factors and available diagnostic options. This includes information about known benefits, risks, and limitations associated with each procedure.

A limited number of centers throughout the United States perform CVS and PUBS; however, amniocentesis frequently is available in primary obstetrical settings. The nurse assisting with these procedures should ensure sterile technique to minimize the potential for a maternal or fetal infection following amniocentesis, CVS, or PUBS (Workman & Philpott-Howard, 1997).

Most people do not perceive the field of clinical genetics, and specifically prenatal genetics, as eugenic. Clients opposed to prenatal genetic diagnosis often assume that they are required to terminate a pregnancy if a genetic anomaly is identified (Chen & Schiffman, 2000). Sometimes, family, social, cultural, or religious communities impose such perceptions. The nurse should provide supportive counseling and teaching to assist clients to make an informed decision about services they wish to pursue (Research Highlight 11.2). Although the prognosis for most genetic disorders or congenital anomalies cannot be altered, many people desire prenatal genetic counseling and diagnosis to prepare for the birth of a child with special needs. This includes learning about specialized care, programs available to assist with care, and determination of the best location and method for delivery of the child (i.e., choosing a hospital with an established neonatal intensive care unit versus a hospital with a level I newborn nursery or consideration for cesarean versus vaginal birth).

A limited number of identified disorders are amenable to prenatal treatment and therapy. The nurse should assist clients to assess the risk and burden of the prenatally untreated disorder in comparison to the risk and benefit of prenatal treatment. If clients and health care providers perceive the long-term benefit to the fetus who is a candidate for prenatal treatment to outweigh the immediate risk, then the nurse should assist by coordinating referral services for this highly specialized prenatal health care. An example is the fetus identified with urinary bladder outlet obstruction. It is critical for the fetus to void in utero to ensure the necessary volume of amniotic fluid for proper musculoskeletal development, as well as reduction of kidney damage subsequent to the blockage of urinary explosion. Prenatal treatment is the placement of a vesicoamniotic shunt performed under ultrasound guidance (Donnenfeld et al., 2002).

Nurses expect that clients who seek prenatal genetic counseling and diagnosis desire the birth of a child without genetic disorders or congenital anomalies. The nurse should assess expectations to ensure a collective understanding of viewpoints by client and partner, as well as health care providers. For example, researchers describe the preferential desire of some people within the deaf community to have children with hearing impairment (Martinez et al., 2003). The nurse should carefully evaluate his or her own values and beliefs to ensure the provision of nondirective, nonjudgmental care to clients who desire an alternative outcome for their child.

Evaluation

The focal point for evaluation of the interventions associated with prenatal invasive procedures is the assessment of the informed decision-making and consent process requisite to the education, counseling, or performance of these tests. The nurse should evaluate all interventions initiated for completion and success in the establishment or maintenance of the comfort and well-being perceived by the client.

RESEARCH HIGHLIGHT 11.2 One Day You're Pregnant and One Day You're Not: Pregnancy Interruption for Fetal Anomalies

OBJECTIVE: The prevalent use of prenatal diagnosis by ultrasound, maternal serum screening, chorionic villus sampling, and amniocentesis results in the identification of fetal anomalies. The purpose of the pilot study was to investigate the processes operating within the experience of women electing the option of second-trimester pregnancy interruption.

DESIGN: The researchers used the inductive and descriptive research method of phenomenology to carry out the study and analyze the 75- to 90-minute audiotaped unstructured interviews with three women who had voluntarily interrupted a pregnancy for fetal anomalies 4 to 6 weeks before the interview. The women were recruited from a convenience sample drawn from a private perinatal practice providing prenatal diagnosis at an urban tertiary care center in the Pacific Northwest.

RESULTS: "One day you're pregnant and one day you're not" is the common theme that describes the experience of women experiencing second-trimester pregnancy interruption. Intertwined processes characterize this transition period. "The hardest thing we ever did" is further described by four phases: beginning the nightmare, making the decision, finding meaning, and redefining normal. "Saying hello and goodbye" was found to have three stages: fighting love, doing the right thing, and reconnecting.

CONCLUSIONS: Clinical implications for the care of women experiencing the life-altering event of second-trimester pregnancy interruption are identified and presented.

Bryar, S. H. (1997). *Journal of Obstetric, Gynecologic, and Neonatal Nursing, 26*(5), 559–566.

Preimplantation Genetic Diagnosis and Related Technologies

Maternal serum marker screening, diagnostic ultrasound, CVS, and amniocentesis are recognized and readily available methods of prenatal diagnosis. All these procedures share one common disadvantage: each is performed after the fetus is well established within the uterus. If prenatal diagnostic testing identifies a fetal anomaly, options available to the client are limited. Historically, clients known to be at risk for transmission of a genetic disorder to their child before conception have had five reproductive options: adopting, choosing to have no children, using donor gametes, chancing the conception and birth of a child free of the genetic disorder, and undergoing prenatal diagnosis with prenatal choice about whether to continue a pregnancy found to have a genetic disorder. For some people, none of these reproductive alternatives is acceptable within the context of their social, cultural, or religious community. For others, selection is the least harmful choice in a group of emotional land mines.

Together, the development of in vitro fertilization (IVF) (see Chap. 10) and advances in molecular genetics provide a sixth reproductive alternative. *Preimplantation genetic diagnosis* (PGD) is genetic evaluation of the embryo created through IVF. First described in 1990, PGD may be performed by biopsy of the polar body, blastomere, or blastocyst. Each method has distinct advantages and disadvantages (Verlinsky & Kuliev, 1998) (Table 11.14). Most PGD programs preferentially use the method of blastomere biopsy.

COLLABORATIVE CARE: PREIMPLANTATION GENETIC DIAGNOSIS

Assessment

PGD provides a reproductive alternative for those opposed to clinical interruption of a pregnancy. Clients identified through preconception assessment screening to be at risk for transmission of a genetic disorder may elect to avail themselves of this earliest possible form of "prenatal diagnosis." This decision should occur through informed decision making about the scope of reproductive options available. The nurse should assist the client to make this assessment by providing information and counseling about each alternative (see Table 11.14).

Disorders that may be evaluated through PGD currently are limited to a small percentage of the total genetic disorders described. Because the analysis generally is performed on only one or two cells, each PGD program must carefully and extensively validate the success of each test within its laboratory setting. Selected examples of disorders for which PGD is offered include chromosomal rearrangements, chromosomal aneuploidy (for advanced maternal age), HD, myotonic dystrophy, spinal muscular atrophy, cystic fibrosis, sickle cell anemia, Fanconi's anemia, and gender identification in X-linked genetic disorders (Pickering et al., 2003). This list expands continuously; the nurse should help the client by investigating the applicability of PGD to the specific disorder of concern.

For those women considering PGD because of risk for transmission of an X-linked genetic disorder, the

TABLE 11.14 Comparison of Preimplantation Genetic Diagnosis Methods

	POLAR BODY BIOPSY	BLASTOMERE BIOPSY	BLASTOCYST BIOPSY
Embryologic Timing of Procedure	Extrusion of first polar body just before fertilization or extrusion of second polar body immediately after fertilization	Second or third day after oocyte fertilization	Fifth or sixth day after oocyte fertilization
Length of Time for Results	1–2 days	1–2 days	1–2 days
Sampling Method	Mechanical or laser opening of the zona pellucida of the oocyte or zygote; gentle aspiration of the polar body	Mechanical or laser opening of the zona pellucida of the embryo; gentle aspiration of 1–2 blastomeres	Mechanical or laser opening of the zona pellucida of the blastocyst; gentle aspiration of trophoblast cells
Adverse Events	Destruction of oocyte/zygote; mechanical loss of microscopic material; failure of oocyte to fertilize; failure of zygote to cleave	Destruction of embryo; mechanical loss of blastomeres; failure of embryo to progress	Destruction of blastocyst; mechanical loss of trophoblast cells; failure of blastocyst to implant when transferred
Advantages	May be performed on the unfertilized oocyte or the pre-embryo zygote	High probability of accurate diagnosis; ability to test for affect of maternal and paternal alleles; ability to identify gender*	Provides 10 to 30 trophectoderm cells for analysis; ability to test for effect of maternal and paternal alleles; ability to identify gender*
Disadvantages	Applicable to only single gene disorders; cannot identify gender*; higher probability of misdiagnosis	Results dependent on the analysis of only 1 to 2 cells; inability to diagnose genetic mosaicism	Inability to grow most embryos to blastocyst stage; high blastocyst loss after biopsy procedure

*At present, many X-linked disorders are not detectable by direct analysis of the altered gene sequence. Because each male embryo has a 50% chance of having the altered allele, female embryos are preferentially chosen for implantation.

Data from Verlinsky, Y., & Kuliev, A. (1998). Preimplantation genetic diagnosis. In A. Milunsky (Ed.), *Genetic disorders in the fetus: Diagnosis, prevention & treatment* (4th ed.). Baltimore: Johns Hopkins University Press, and Jones, S. L., & Fallon, L. A. (2002). Reproductive options for individuals at risk for transmission of a genetic disorder. *Journal of Obstetric, Gynecologic, and Neonatal Nursing, 31*(2), 193–199.

nurse also may provide information about sperm separation technology. This process enriches the ejaculate used to inseminate the IVF oocyte with sperm carrying the chromosome complement of the desired gender. In cases of X-linked disorders, the desired gender is female, given that males have a 50% chance of being affected by the disorder, whereas females have a 50% chance of being carriers like their mothers. Two different processes have been used to separate sperm. The passage of a prepared ejaculate through an albumin gradient separates X-bearing from Y-bearing sperm (Beernink et al., 1993; Rose & Wong, 1998). This method of sperm sorting (Ericsson method) is used primarily for people seeking gender selection for social reasons. Sperm separation also may be performed by passing sperm through a flow cytometric cell sorter that recognizes the 2.8% total DNA content difference between X- and Y-bearing sperm (Vidal et al., 1998). This technology (MicroSort™) has a high success rate associated with the conception and birth of female children (Genetics and IVF Institute, 2003).

Select Potential Nursing Diagnoses

The following are examples of potentially applicable NANDA diagnoses:

- **Spiritual Distress** related to perceived status of the human embryo
- **Dysfunctional Grieving** related to desire for a "healthy" child
- **Ineffective Sexuality Patterns** related to fear of conception and transmission of genetic risk to a biologic child

Planning/Intervention

Dissemination of information and discussion about PGD must occur before conception for it to be considered a reproductive option. Once a pregnancy is confirmed, PGD is no longer a viable alternative. The nurse in the preconception setting should provide this information to the client. If a client presents after conceiving, the nurse should identify an appropriate time to apprise her of this reproductive alternative for consideration before any future conceptions. Important to this dialogue is information about the cost of PGD and the limited insurance benefit coverage.

Typically, people who seek PGD know they have the altered gene of concern. In contrast, many people at risk for transmission of HD do not wish to know whether they have the HD gene (Richards, 2003). Usually, they do not want to know if they have the HD gene because they then know for sure that at some point they will develop this adult-onset degenerative neuromuscular disorder. Like most people desiring children, they strongly hope to have a healthy child free of the HD risk. The nurse should share with these people information about the option to use PGD technology to eliminate transmission of the HD gene to their offspring and not learn their own HD status (Stern et al., 2002). Through the process of informed decision making, these people can choose to *not* be informed of the genetic status of the biopsied embryos or the status of the at-risk parent. They agree that only unaffected embryos are transferred after biopsy and analysis. The nurse should explain the advantage of achieving a pregnancy unaffected by HD, whereas the at-risk parent does not learn his or her own genetic status and reviews the disadvantages of cost and unnecessary treatment if the at-risk parent does not in fact have the HD gene (Jones & Fallon, 2002).

The nurse should provide anticipatory care to clients to support them as they seek PGD services (Jones & Krysa, 1998; Willie et al., 2004). The depth and scope of this intervention are determined by the comfort level of the "fertile" reproductive woman receiving this specialized service alongside "infertile" women, given IVF technology is the clinical component of a PGD program (see Chap. 10). Frequently, the "fertile" woman expresses feelings of guilt that she strives to have *a healthy child* as opposed to the infertile woman who desires *a child.* It is imperative that the nurse support the woman and assure her that seeking this service is appropriate and not a selfish act.

Flow cytometric separation of sperm is currently in clinical trial (Genetics and IVF Institute, 2003). The nurse should provide information to the client about the technology, requirements for participating in a clinical trial, and implications of that participation. The principles of informed decision making and consent are fundamental to a clinical trial protocol.

Evaluation

Evaluation varies according to the individualized plan of care and related interventions. This is especially true for the client who receives information about newer technologies that permit the performance of PGD, nondisclosing PGD, or sperm separation. The nurse should assess the client's response to the information and interventions and provide additional education, counseling, and support as indicated.

Evaluation of the Placenta and Fetal Well-Being

Antepartum testing is a specialized form of prenatal screening and diagnosis generally performed during the third trimester. The goals are to identify any fetal episodes of distress to prevent permanent injury or death and to evaluate whether the fetus is healthy so that invasive procedures are not implemented unnecessarily (Scott et al., 1999). Fetal hypoxia or asphyxia secondary to uteroplacental insufficiency is the primary concern.

The placenta is an organ with a limited life cycle and built-in obsolescence. Although the placenta generally functions appropriately throughout gestational weeks 38 to 42, embryonic and in utero events can alter its efficiency and duration, which may have long-term effects. Examples include abnormal development or number of cotyledons, placenta infarction, and premature (partial) placental separation from the uterine wall. The procedures available for testing the placenta and fetal well-being are discussed in extensive detail in Chapter 12.

POSTNATAL SCREENING AND DIAGNOSTIC PROCEDURES

For most clients, the birth of a child is a special and memorable event. They anxiously await confirmation from their obstetrical and pediatric care providers of the child's gender and health. The obstetrical care providers initially assess newborns in the delivery room; other health care providers complete more comprehensive evaluations after transfer of the baby to the newborn nursery or, if necessary, the neonatal intensive care unit (see Chaps. 20 and 22). Initial assessment focuses on clinical markers included in the Apgar score (color, respiratory effort, muscle tone, heart rate, and reflex irritability) and physical appearance. Comprehensive evaluation includes a head-to-toe assessment of all body systems.

Two facets of newborn assessment require knowledge of genetic principles and their associated clinical implications: newborn screening for inherited metabolic and hearing disorders and evaluation of the newborn with one or more dysmorphic features. If an abnormality is identified, the family unit typically is referred for follow-up with a genetics specialist.

Parents of a newborn identified to have an anomaly associated with adverse implications for health and well-being experience psychological sequela typically associated with the death of a family member or close friend. Parental reactions follow a sequential process of shock, denial, sadness, and anger; adaptation; and reorganization (Krafft & Krafft, 1998; Lowes & Lyne, 2000). The sequence often is interrupted and restarted as the child enters each new chronologic age and meets difficulty or inability to accomplish age-appropriate tasks of daily living. This leads to the parental experience of **chronic**

sorrow, a continuous reliving of the initial interaction that confirmed the child's genetic or congenital disorder.

Newborn Screening Programs

Newborn screening is the oldest population genetics screening program in the United States. It is the outgrowth of a state-based screening program for phenylketonuria begun by Robert Guthrie and Robert MacCready in 1962. All 50 states and the District of Columbia have state-mandated newborn screening programs. The original and primary purpose is to identify genetic disorders (typically resulting in altered biochemical function) and to institute treatment before the onset of clinical symptoms (Lloyd-Puryear & Forsman, 2002). In addition to screening for metabolic disorders, more than 30 states require assessment for hearing loss (Newborn Screening Task Force, 2000). Likewise, several states have added screening for cystic fibrosis (CF), perceiving the importance of initiating treatment for the associated pancreatic insufficiency before significant onset of symptoms. Controversy exists as to whether CF meets the criteria of "treatable disorder" described in the key elements of a newborn screening program (Nussbaum et al., 2001).

Because newborn screening programs are regulated and managed at the state level, national consistency is limited as related to the disorders included in individual screening programs and funding available. Some states mandate screening for as few as 4 disorders; others screen for 36. Most states screen for 8 or fewer disorders and usually do not require parental consent before performance (Table 11.15) (Government Accounting Office, 2003). The laboratory method used to analyze the newborn blood specimen also varies across state programs. In contrast, the principles that guide the development, establishment, and continuation of a newborn screening program are universal and well established (Box 11.5).

The Newborn Screening Task Force (2000) convened by the American Academy of Pediatrics and the Health Resources and Services Administration in 1999 published recommendations for standardization of tests

TABLE 11.15 Genetic Disorders Most Commonly Included in State Newborn Screening Programs*

DISORDER	NUMBER OF STATES THAT MANDATE SCREENING OF THIS DISORDER	NATIONAL INCIDENCE†	POTENTIAL OUTCOMES IF DISORDER IS UNTREATED	TREATMENT
Phenylketonuria (PKU)	51	1 in 13,947‡	Mental retardation, seizures	Low-phenylalanine diet
Congenital hypothyroidism	51	1 in 3,044§	Mental retardation, stunted growth	Thyroid hormone
Galactosemia	50	1 in 53,261‖	Brain damage, liver damage, cataracts, death	Galactose-free diet
Sickle cell diseases	44	1 in 3,721** 1 in 7,386***	Organ damage, delayed growth, stroke	Penicillin, vaccinations
Congenital adrenal hyperplasia (CAH)	32	1, 18,987	Death due to salt loss, reproductive and growth difficulties	Hormone and salt replacement
Biotinidase deficiency	24	1 in 61,319	Mental retardation, developmental delay, seizures, hearing loss	Biotin supplements
Maple syrup urine disease (MSUD)	24	1 in 230,028	Mental retardation, seizures, coma, death	Dietary management and supplements
Homocystinuria	17	1 in 343,650	Mental retardation, eye problems, skeletal abnormalities, stroke	Dietary management and vitamin supplements

*Data are as of December 2002; more than 4 million births occur each year; includes all 50 states and the District of Columbia.

†Incidence rates are based on data from 1990 to 1999.

‡Includes classic phenylketonuria and clinically significant phenylketonuria variant.

§Includes only primary congenital hypothyroidism.

‖Includes only classic galactosemia.

**Incidence of sickle cell anemia.

***Incidence of hemoglobin sickle C disease.

Adapted from Government Accounting Office. (2003). Newborn screening: Characteristics of state programs. A Report to Congressional Requesters. Available at: http://www.gao.gov.

BOX 11.5 Key Elements of a Newborn Screening Program

1. Treatment is available.
2. Early intervention prevents morbidity and mortality.
3. A test is required to identify the disorder in a timely manner.
4. The test is highly sensitive (no false-negative results) and reasonably specific (limited false-positive results).
5. Frequency and severity of the disorder warrant identification.
6. Available infrastructure includes:
   a. Parental education (and consent if required)
   b. Timing screening
   c. Follow-up programs
   d. Referral resources
   e. Accurate data collection systems
   f. Access to interventions and treatment
   g. Policies to protect confidentiality and privacy

performed and methods used. Professional organizations such as the Association of Women's Health, Obstetric, and Neonatal Nurses (2002) have published position papers that affirm the importance of this standardization. Chapter 20 discusses newborn screening in more detail.

Dysmorphology Assessment

Dysmorphology, the branch of clinical genetics that specializes in birth defects, combines knowledge of genetic principles, developmental mechanisms, and the natural history of a wide variety of congenital anomalies (Nussbaum et al., 2001). It is the most rapidly growing area within clinical genetics as a result of advances in molecular DNA analysis that permit identification of the genotypes of many disorders previously categorized solely according to phenotype expression. A dysmorphologic assessment is used to evaluate stillborn infants, newborns, children, and adults with disorders thought to result from a malformation, deformation, or disruption in development caused by altered genes, chromosomal rearrangements, or in utero teratogen exposure.

COLLABORATIVE CARE: DYSMORPHOLOGY ASSESSMENT

A dysmorphic feature is an abnormality of shape, size, or structure. Each finding traditionally is classified as minor or major. Among normal newborns, more than 13% have at least one minor anomaly, whereas only 1% have two or more minor anomalies (Lashley, 1998). If an infant is found to have two minor dysmorphic features, the health care provider should carefully assess for one or more major anomalies that may not be readily apparent. This is especially important if three or more minor anomalies are identified. A cluster of dysmorphologic features may be categorized as a syndrome, sequence, or association (see Embryonic Development).

Assessment

The nurse should determine whether a comprehensive family, medical, and reproductive history was completed in the preconception or prenatal setting. If the parent acknowledges this assessment and evaluation, the nurse should assist in procuring this information. If it does not exist, then the nurse should request that the woman and reproductive partner complete a health assessment questionnaire. The construction and review of a three- or four-generation pedigree is especially important.

A careful review of the pregnancy history specific to the conception and birth of the person under evaluation is critical to the differential diagnosis in cases of a suspected genetic or environmental cause for dysmorphic findings (Harper, 2001). For example, infants with fetal alcohol syndrome can have cardiac malformations (eg, ventricular septal defect), central nervous system anomalies (eg, microcephaly), facial abnormalities (eg, micrognathia), truncal and skeletal anomalies (eg, diaphragmatic hernia), and genitourinary malformations (eg, hypoplastic external genitalia). Similarly, DiGeorge's syndrome (velocardiofacial syndrome) is characterized by conotruncal abnormalities (eg, tetralogy of Fallot), facial abnormalities (eg, micrognathia), renal obstruction, thymic disorders (absent), and diaphragmatic hernia. Fetal alcohol syndrome results from the ingestion of alcohol by the woman during her pregnancy and has a 0% recurrence risk if the same woman does not consume alcohol in any future pregnancy. DiGeorge's syndrome results from a microdeletion of the "q" arm of chromosome 22 and has a 50% recurrence if the microdeletion also is identified in the parents (Sanders, 2002).

Physical examination is the primary tool of a dysmorphologic evaluation. The nurse should precisely measure height, weight, head, neck, face, eyes, limbs, hands, feet, and trunk (Fig. 11.26). He or she should record information about the appearance of the skin, nails, teeth, genitalia, and cry. This permits accurate analysis of serial observations of these findings. Photography in conjunction with precise measurements provides the most accurate documentation of the findings. The nurse should educate, counsel, and reassure the woman, child, or man of the importance of this method of documentation, although highly sensitive and personal. In addition, radiography is used to assess bone density and structure (to rule out disorders such as lethal bone dysplasias and osteogenesis imperfecta); cytogenetic, biochemical, and DNA analyses (to confirm or rule out a genetic basis) are performed as part of the dysmorphologic assessment. It is particularly important to perform an autopsy on a stillborn

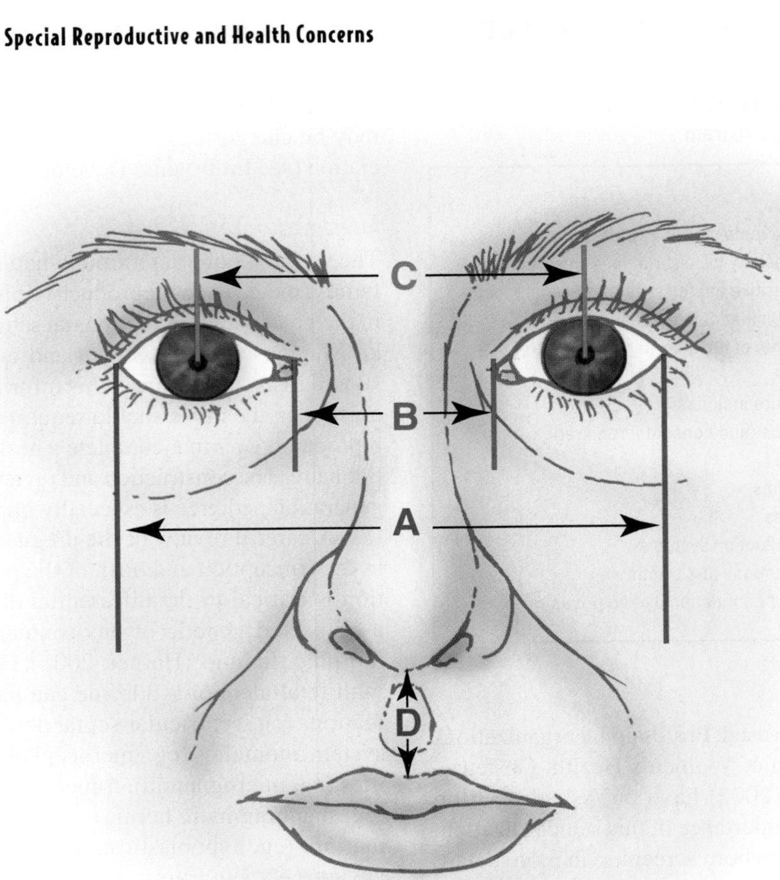

FIGURE 11.26 Facial measurements in a dysmorphologic evaluation. (Reprinted with permission from the March of Dimes, White Plains, NY.)

infant to evaluate the structure and formation of internal organs, the site of many major malformations.

Select Potential Nursing Diagnoses

The following are examples of potentially applicable NANDA diagnoses:

- **Chronic Sorrow** related to the recurring sadness
- **Caregiver Role Strain** related to overwhelming daily needs of infant
- **Social Isolation** related to uncertainty that others will accept the infant

Planning/Intervention

Some obstetrical and pediatric providers believe that the completion of a dysmorphologic evaluation does not contribute to the child's welfare and provides only an academic research opportunity for the dysmorphologist. In fact, dysmorphologic evaluations are important to provide if multiple minor or major anomalies are identified, including for deceased or stillborn infants. The correct diagnosis permits dissemination of appropriate and accurate information about recurrence risk for a future pregnancy. It also reduces the likelihood of a child being labeled with an incorrect diagnosis, leading to potential life-threatening or life-restricting events. For example, the person diagnosed with fetal alcohol syndrome has mental retardation, whereas the person with DiGeorge's syndrome does not. A reversal of these diagnoses can profoundly affect long-term well-being.

The parents of children diagnosed with genetic or congenital disorders experience chronic sorrow. The nurse should assist these clients to identify community resources to assist with daily care, health requirements, and educational needs. He or she should provide information about parent support groups, respite care, school programs, and public health services. Given that resources provided or mandated vary widely among states, the nurse should become familiar with his or her state program to assist the family with the identification of, navigation through, and coordination of services. The nurse also should assist the family by aligning services with the language, social, cultural, and religious beliefs of the identified community.

Evaluation

Evaluation is based on the individualized plan of care for each woman, man, or child. Evaluation of the perceived success of the available resources and programs within the community is essential. Ongoing evaluation of the family unit is central to this process to ensure that members are accessing the appropriate services.

Questions to Ponder

1. A woman and her reproductive partner come for preconception counseling. The nurse performs a preconception health risk assessment and evaluation. The results show both people to carry the ΔF508 mutation of the *CFTR* gene associated with CF. The couple does not wish to have a child with CF. They request information about the scope of available reproductive options but are concerned that their family and religious community will not support any choice they make.
   - What information should the nurse be aware of before responding to the couple about their reproductive options?
   - What support might help the couple as they process the information and choose an appropriate reproductive alternative?
   - What are your personal feelings about prenatal diagnosis and choice (therapeutic interruption of a pregnancy)?
2. A young couple, both 28 years old, report a paternal family history of HD. The mother of the young man, diagnosed with HD at 45 years old, is now in an assisted living facility because of the severity of her neuromuscular degeneration. The young man's two older siblings had DNA analysis performed, and both have received the HD gene, although neither is currently symptomatic. This couple very much wants to have a child without the HD gene and prefers that they both are the genetic parents of the child. The young man does not want to know his HD status; he currently has no manifestations of HD. They have heard about nondisclosing PGD as a way to achieve these dual goals. They state they want preliminary information from a primary care provider before seeking out a PGD program.
   - What are your personal feelings about facilitating someone to have PGD when there is a reasonable likelihood that embryos found to have the HD gene will be disposed of and not transferred to the woman's uterus?
   - Do you believe that someone can make an informed choice not to be informed?
   - What information do you need to know before responding to the couple?
   - Can someone give consent not to be informed?

SUMMARY

- Variation is the life-cycle outcome of each person's unique response to nature and nurture beginning before conception and ending with death.
- *Somatic cells* make up every organ and system and maintain growth, development, and well-being. *Germ cells* are the reproductive cells of the ovary and testis; their function is preservation through replication of the human species.
- Each chromosome consists of DNA, proteins, and a small amount of RNA. Genes, the basic units of heredity, are located along the DNA of each chromosome. Each gene is a unique sequence formed from the nucleotides along the DNA strands.
- A change in the genetic code may or may not alter the product coded for by that gene. An alteration will be expressed as a change in growth, development, wellness, life expectancy, or all these factors.
- *Mitosis* is the body's natural process of growth and development performed in association with cellular repair and replacement. *Meiosis* is the unique cell division that occurs in the diploid germ cells to produce gamete cells containing only 23 chromosomes.
- Male germ cells remain dormant in the testes until puberty. Then, the life cycle of each sperm is approximately 75 to 90 days. Female embryos begin differentiation of the germ cells after the primitive ovary forms. Oogonia remain suspended until puberty; over the next 40 years, oocytes develop as part of the menstrual cycle.
- The oocyte can fuse with sperm for only 24 hours after ovulation. Sperm survive no more than 72 hours after they are deposited in the female reproductive tract.
- Once the zygote begins to cleave (mitotic cellular division), it is referred to as an embryo. The number of cells visible microscopically is used to describe the stage of embryo development.
- Before formation of the blastocyst (5 to 7 days after fertilization), each blastomere can differentiate into any type of tissue (totipotency). With differentiation, totipotency is lost.
- Normally, the blastocyst implants on either the anterior or posterior wall of the main uterine body. The placenta thus develops embedded within tissue prepared for the invasive fusion of the trophoblast and fetal growth to full term.
- The two primary functions of the placenta are exchange of metabolic and gaseous products between

the fetal and maternal circulatory systems and production of hormones necessary for fetal development and continuation of gestation.

- Amniotic fluid surrounds and protects the developing fetus. It separates the fetus from other placental membranes, providing for the movement critical to normal fetal growth and development. Without adequate amniotic fluid, fetal malformations occur.
- Differentiation of the four-chamber heart and associated valves is complete by the 8th embryologic week.
- The *ectoderm* gives rise to the peripheral nervous system; sensory epithelium of the nose, eye, and ear; epidermis; subcutaneous, mammary, and pituitary glands; and tooth enamel. The *mesoderm* gives rise to cartilage and bone; striated and smooth muscles; skin cells; excretory components of the urinary and reproductive systems; serous membranes of the peritoneal, parietal, and pericardial cavities; spleen; blood vessels; and blood. The *endoderm* gives rise to the gastrointestinal tract; parenchyma of the thyroid, parathyroids, liver, and pancreas; epithelial lining of the respiratory tract, urinary bladder, urethra, tympanic cavity, and auditory tube; tonsils; and thymus gland.
- The incidence of major structural congenital anomalies at birth is 2% to 3% and rises to 4% to 6% by 5 years of age, when additional findings are identified upon admittance to school. Anomalies are classified as malformations, disruptions, or deformations and may be part of a syndrome, association, or sequence event.
- Multiple gestations have risen sharply over the past 2 decades. Monozygotic gestations result from altered zygote development. They share the same genotype, although exposure to different environmental factors throughout their lives may result in different phenotypes. Dizygotic gestations share the same genetic relationship as any siblings born to the same genetic mother and father.
- The goal of genetic counseling is to provide appropriate, accurate, and nondirective information so that clients can make informed decisions about their own and their children's health and health care.
- Preconception health assessment may elicit sensitive, private, and highly confidential information. It has the profound potential to alter a client's self-image and relationships.
- Informed decision making links the goals of preconception screening and counseling with the principles of autonomy, justice, and beneficence to ensure appropriate management of genetic information.
- Each step of the health assessment should be preceded by an explanation of the process, information that may be learned, and possible implications of that knowledge; and the opportunity for dialogue between client and health care provider.
- Multifactorial inheritance is the expression of a phenotypic trait regulated by multiple genes and their interaction with environmental factors. It is the most common form of inheritance in the general population.
- Chromosomal rearrangements are categorized as alterations in either number or structure.
- Aneuploidy increases as maternal age advances. This results in a higher rate of pregnancy loss and birth of infants with chromosome anomalies.
- Advanced paternal age is associated with increased incidence of spontaneous new mutations in the fetus.
- Congenital or acquired malformations of the reproductive organs, loss of ovarian or testicular reserve, irregular menstrual cycle, infections, autoimmune disorders, and hormonal imbalances may result in the inability to conceive, carry a pregnancy to term, or both.
- Recurrent miscarriage is the loss of three or more pregnancies before 20 weeks' gestation.
- *Screening tests* typically are used to assess large populations to identify those appropriate for referral to more complex and costly services. *Diagnostic tests* generally are used to confirm or eliminate suspected anomalies among at-risk clients.
- The four methods available to evaluate fetal chromosomes, genes, or blood chemistry are CVS, amniocentesis, percutaneous umbilical cord sampling, and preimplantation genetic diagnosis.
- Antepartum testing is performed during the third trimester to identify fetuses experiencing distress so that interventions may be implemented to prevent permanent injury or death.
- The primary purpose of newborn screening is to identify genetic disorders and institute treatment in the newborn before the onset of clinical symptoms.
- A dysmorphologic assessment can evaluate stillborns, infants, children, and adults with disorders thought to result from a malformation, deformation, or disruption in development from altered genes, chromosomal rearrangements, or in utero teratogen exposure.

REVIEW QUESTIONS

1. A client presents with a clinical diagnosis of tuberous sclerosis. To determine his or her phenotype, which method of assessment would the nurse expect to be used?
   A. Construction and review of a pedigree
   B. Chromosome analysis
   C. Direct DNA analysis
   D. Physical examination and evaluation
2. A woman gives birth to twins. The provider informs the woman that the children are dizygotic. This information is best determined by
   A. identification of one distinct placenta and one bag of water.

B. identification of one distinct placenta and two separate bags of water.
C. identification of two distinct placentas and two separate bags of water.
D. same gender for both infants.

3. Parents of monozygotic twins ask if the children will experience identical growth and development. To best answer the parents, the nurse should explain
A. each infant shares the same genotype and phenotype; thus, growth and development can be expected to be identical.
B. each infant shares the same genotype, but the environment will alter phenotype; thus, growth and development may vary.
C. each infant has a different genotype, but the same phenotype; thus, growth and development will not vary.
D. each infant is the same as any other two siblings and will have variable growth and development.

4. The placenta functions to
A. prevent passage of antibodies from mother to child.
B. provide a direct exchange of blood between mother and child.
C. provide an exchange of metabolic and gaseous products between mother and child.
D. prevent passage of teratogenic agents from mother to child.

5. A 32-year-old woman comes to the clinic and reports a history of three losses of pregnancy before 12 weeks' gestation. She would like to become pregnant again, but is anxious that she may spontaneously abort. To determine an appropriate plan for this woman, the nurse should next
A. ask whether chromosome analysis was performed on any of the abortuses.
B. construct a family pedigree.
C. obtain a peripheral blood sample for chromosome analysis.
D. obtain a peripheral blood sample for serum hormone analysis.

6. A 28-year-old woman comes for counseling after receiving abnormal results on her MSAFP at 15 weeks' gestation. To determine an appropriate plan for this woman, the nurse should next
A. confirm gestational age and viability.
B. refer the woman for genetic counseling.
C. refer the woman for amniocentesis.
D. obtain a new specimen and repeat the analysis.

7. A Caucasian woman comes for prenatal care. Her family history is negative for any known incidence of a genetic disorder. Her immediate plan of care should include
A. collection of a blood sample for cystic fibrosis mutation screening.
B. construction of a pedigree.
C. education about her risk to be a carrier for CF and the availability of a screening test.
D. no further education about genetic risk factors.

8. A 37-year-old woman presents for prenatal care at 7 weeks' gestation. She requests information about CVS and wants to know when this procedure is best performed. The nurse correctly shares that CVS is performed at
A. 6 to 8 weeks of gestation.
B. 8 to 9 weeks of gestation.
C. 10 to 12 weeks of gestation.
D. 15 to 16 weeks of gestation.

9. A woman, 36 weeks' pregnant, is undergoing a nonstress test. Her obstetrical provider did not explain the purpose of the test but informed her that it needed to be done in the next 2 days. The client is anxious and concerned. The nurse supports the woman by explaining the purpose of the test is
A. to identify whether the fetus is at risk for uteroplacental insufficiency and whether delivery should be initiated.
B. to identify whether the fetus is at risk for uteroplacental insufficiency and whether alteration of maternal nutrition and exercise is required.
C. to identify whether the fetus has sufficient amniotic fluid.
D. to identify whether the mother has gestational diabetes.

10. A nurse is performing a home visit for a new mother and baby. After assessing health and breastfeeding ability, the most important inquiry the nurse should make is
A. how much support the woman is receiving from family and friends.
B. if a blood sample was obtained from the infant for newborn screening.
C. if the infant is being supplemented with formula.
D. if the mother can sleep when the infant sleeps.

RESOURCES

Continuing Education

Williams, J. K., & Lea, D. H. (2002). *Genetic issues for perinatal nurses* (2nd ed.). White Plains, NY: March of Dimes Birth Defects Foundation.

Online Resources

American Society of Human Genetics (ASHG): Professional society for genetics healthcare specialists. Available at: http://www.ashg.org.

Centers for Disease Control and Prevention: Updates and publishes aggregate incidence of birth defects. Available at: http://www.cdc.gov.

Gene Tests: Catalog and description of genetic tests currently available. Available at: http://www.genetests.org.

Genetic Alliance: Organization dedicated to the establishment of partnerships among professionals, consumers and industry to promote healthy lives for everyone affected by genetics. Available at: http://www.geneticalliance.org.

International Society of Nurses in Genetics (ISONG): Professional society for genetic nurses. Available at: http://www.isong.org.

March of Dimes (MOD): Organization committed to the prevention of birth defects through education and research. Available at: http://www.marchofdimes.com.

National Center for Biotechnology Information (NCBI): Maintains the database that catalogs Mendelian inheritance in man. Available at: http://www.ncbi.nlm.nih.gov.

National Human Genome Research Institute (NHGRI): The branch of the National Institutes of Health (NIH) charged with management and coordination of the national Human Genome Project. Available at: http://www.genome.gov.

National Society of Genetic Counselors (NSGC): Professional society for genetic counselors. Available at: http://www.nsgc.org.

Office of Genomics and Disease Prevention: Branch of the Centers for Disease Control charged with the collation and dissemination of genetic information to healthcare providers and recipients. Available at: http://www.cdc.gov.

REFERENCES

Alberts, B. (2003). DNA replication and recombination. *Nature, 421*(6921), 431–435.

American College of Medical Genetics. (1996a). Statement on guidance for genetic counseling in advanced paternal age. *American College of Medical Genetics Newsletter, 6,* 13.

American College of Medical Genetics. (1996b). Statement on multiple marker screening in pregnant women. *American College of Medical Genetics Newsletter, 6,* 14.

American College of Obstetricians and Gynecologists & American College of Medical Genetics. (2001). *Preconception and prenatal carrier screening for cystic fibrosis.* Washington, DC: Author.

American College of Obstetricians and Gynecologists. (1989). *Ectopic pregnancy* (Number 126). Washington, DC: Author.

American Sickle Cell Anemia Association. (2003). FAQ's: Sickle cell anemia. Available at: http://www.ascaa.org.

American Society for Reproductive Medicine. (2000). *Multiple pregnancy associated with infertility therapy.* Practice Committee Report. Available at: http://www.asrm.org.

Association of Women's Health, Obstetric and Neonatal Nurses. (2003). *Preconceptional use of folic acid. Clinical position statement.* Available at: http://www.awhonn.org.

Association of Women's Health, Obstetric and Neonatal Nurses. (2002). *National standards for newborn screening. Policy position statement.* Available at: http://www.awhonn.org.

Astolfi, P., Pasquale, A., & Zonta, L. A. (2004). Late paternity and stillbirth risk. *Human Reproduction, 19*(11), 2497–2501.

Beernink, F. J., Dmowski, W. P., & Ericsson, R. J. (1993). Sex preselection through albumin separation of sperm. *Fertility and Sterility, 59*(2), 382–386.

Beers, M. H., & Berkow, R. (2003). *The Merck manual of diagnosis and therapy* (17th ed.). Available at: http://www.merckmedicus.com.

Benn, P. A. (2002a). Advances in prenatal screening for Down syndrome. I. General principles and second trimester testing. *Clinica Chimica Acta, 323*(1–2), 1–16.

Benn, P. A. (2002b). Advances in prenatal screening for Down syndrome. II. First trimester testing, integrated testing, and future directions. *Clinica Chimica Acta, 324*(1–2), 1–11.

Benn, P. A. (2003). Improved antenatal screening for Down's syndrome. *Lancet, 361*(9360), 794–795.

Bennett, R. L., Motulsky, A. G., Bittles, A., Hudgins, L., Uhrich, S., Doyle, D. L., Silvey, K., Scott, C. R., Cheng, E., McGillivray, B., Steiner, R. D., & Olson, D. (2002). Genetic counseling and screening of consanguineous couples and their offspring: Recommendations of the National Society of Genetic Counselors. *Journal of Genetic Counseling, 11*(2), 97–119.

Bennett, R. L., Steinhaus, K. A., Uhrich, B., O'Sullivan, C. K., Resta, R. G., Lochner-Doyle, D., Markel, D. S., Vincent, V., & Hamanishi, J. (1995). Recommendations for standardized human pedigree nomenclature. *Journal of Genetic Counseling, 4*(4), 267–279.

Bindra, R., Heath, V., & Nicolaides, K. H. (2002). Screening for chromosomal defects by fetal nuchal translucency at 11 to 14 weeks. *Clinical Obstetrics and Gynecology, 45*(3), 661–670; discussion, 730–732.

Bortolus, R., Parazzini, F., Chatenoud, L., Benzi, G., Bianchi, M. M., & Marini, A. (1999). The epidemiology of multiple births. *Human Reproduction Update, 5*(2), 179–187.

Brown, T., & Schwind, E. L. (1999). Update and review: Cystic fibrosis. *Journal of Genetic Counseling, 8*(3), 137–162.

Bryar, S. H. (1997). One day you're pregnant and one day you're not: Pregnancy interruption for fetal anomalies. *Journal of Obstetric, Gynecologic and Neonatal Nursing, 26*(5), 559–566.

Burke, W. (2002). Genetic testing. *New England Journal of Medicine, 347*(23), 1867–1875.

Burrow, G. N., & Ferris, T. F. (1988). *Medical complications during pregnancy* (3rd ed.). Philadelphia: W. B. Saunders.

Callen, P. W. (1994). *Ultrasonography in obstetrics and gynecology* (3rd ed.). Philadelphia: W. B. Saunders.

Carp, H., Toder, V., Aviram, A., Daniely, M., Mashlach, S., & Barkai, G. (2001). Karyotype of the abortus in recurrent miscarriage. *Fertility and Sterility, 75*(4), 678–682.

Cefalo, R. C., & Moos, M. K. (1995). *Preconceptional health care* (2nd ed.). St. Louis: Mosby.

Center for Disease Control. (2004). Birth defects: Frequently asked questions. Available at: http://www.cdc.gov.

Chen, E. A., & Schiffman, J. F. (2000). Attitudes toward genetic counseling and prenatal diagnosis among a group of individuals with physical disabilities. *Journal of Genetic Counseling, 9*(2), 137–152.

Collins, F. S., Green, E. D., Guttmacher, A. E., & Guyer, M. S. (2003). A vision for the future of genomics research: A blueprint for the genomic era. *Nature, 422*(6934), 835–847, insert.

Crawford, D. C., Acuna, J. M., & Sherman, S. L. (2001). FMR1 and the fragile X syndrome: Human genome epidemiology review. *Genetics in Medicine, 3*(5), 359–371.

Cystic Fibrosis Foundation. (2003). Living with CF. Available at: http://www.cff.org.

Donnenfeld, A. E., Lockwood, D., Custer, T., & Lamb, A. N. (2002). Prenatal diagnosis from fetal urine in bladder outlet obstruction: Success rates for traditional cytogenetic evaluation and interphase fluorescence in situ hybridization. *Genetics in Medicine, 4*(6), 444–447.

Evers, J. L. H. (2002). Female subfertility. *Lancet, 360,* 151–159.

Freda, M. C., DeVore, N., Valentine-Adams, N., Bombard, A., & Merkatz, I. R. (1998). Informed consent for maternal serum alpha-fetoprotein screening in an inner city population: How informed is it? *Journal of Obstetric, Gynecologic and Neonatal Nursing, 27*(1), 99–106.

Friedberg, E. C. (2003). DNA damage and repair. *Nature, 421*(6921), 436–440.

Froster, U. G., & Jackson, L. (1996). Limb defects and chorionic villus sampling: Results from an international registry, 1992–1994. *Lancet, 347*(9000), 489–494; editorial discussion, 484–485.

Genetics and IVF Institute. (2003). MicroSort®: Current clinical trial results. Available at: http://www.microsort.com.

Genetic testing for cystic fibrosis. (1997, April 14–16). *NIH Consensus Statement, 15*(4), 1–37.

Goldberg, J. D. (2004). Routine screening for fetal anomalies: Expectations. *Obstetrics and Gynecology Clinics of North America, 31*(1), 35–50.

Government Accounting Office. (2003). Newborn screening: Characteristics of state programs. Available at: http://www.gao.gov.

Guttmacher, A. E., & Collins, F. S. (2002). Genomic medicine: A primer. *New England Journal of Medicine, 347*(19), 1512–1520.

Harper, P. S. (2001). *Practical genetic counseling* (5th ed.). New York: Oxford University Press.

International Society of Nurses in Genetics and American Nurses Association. (1998). *Statement on the scope and standards of genetics in clinical nursing practice.* Washington, DC: American Nurses Publishing.

International Society of Nurses in Genetics. (2001). Privacy and confidentiality of genetic information: The role of the nurse. A Position Statement. Available at: http://www.globalreferrals.com.

Jenkins, T. M., & Wapner, R. J. (1999). First trimester prenatal diagnosis: Chorionic villus sampling. *Seminars in Perinatology, 23*(5), 403–413.

Jones, S. L. (1999a). Genetically transmitted diseases: Identification and counseling. In *Management of genetic information: Implications for nursing practice* (32nd Annual Postgraduate Course Syllabus). Birmingham, AL: American Society of Reproductive Medicine.

Jones, S. L. (1999b). Legislative initiatives, genetic diagnosis and treatment: Clinical ramifications. In *Management of genetic information: Implications for nursing practice* (32nd Annual Postgraduate Course Syllabus). Birmingham, AL: American Society of Reproductive Medicine.

Jones, S. L. (2000). Reproductive genetic technologies. *AWHONN Lifelines, 4*(5), 33–36.

Jones, S. L., & Fallon, L. A. (2002). Reproductive options for individuals at risk for transmission of a genetic disorder. *Journal of Obstetric, Gynecologic, and Neonatal Nursing, 31*(2), 193–199.

Jones, S. L., & Headrick, E. G. (1992). Integration of clinical genetics into assisted reproductive technologies: Implications for nursing practice. *NAACOG's Clinical Issues in Perinatal and Women's Health Nursing, 3*(2), 301–312.

Jones, S. L., & Krysa, L. W. (1998). Comfort care interventions in a preimplantation genetic testing program. *Holistic Nursing Practice, 12*(3), 20–29.

Kazaura, M., Lie, R. T., & Skjaerven, R. (2004). Paternal age and the risk of birth defects in Norway. *Annals of Epidemiology, 14*(8), 566–570.

Kenen, R., Smith, A. C. M., Watkins, C., & Zuber-Pittore, C. (2000). To use or not to use: The prenatal genetic technology/worry conundrum. *Journal of Genetic Counseling, 9*(3), 203–217.

Klonoff-Cohen, H. S., & Natarajan, L. (2004). The effect of advancing paternal age on pregnancy and live birth rates in couples undergoing in vitro fertilization or gamete intrafallopian transfer. *American Journal of Obstetrics and Gynecology, 191*(2), 507–514.

Kohut, R. J., Dewey, D., & Love, E. J. (2002). Women's knowledge of prenatal ultrasound and informed choice. *Journal of Genetic Counseling, 11*(4), 265–276.

Krafft, S. K., & Krafft, L. J. (1998). Chronic sorrow: Parents' lived experience. *Holistic Nursing Practice, 13*(1), 59–67.

Kupferminc, M. J., Eldor, A., Steinman, N., Many, A., Bar-Am, A., Jaffa, A., Fait, G., & Lessing, J. B. (1999). Increased frequency of genetic thrombophilia in women in complications of pregnancy. *New England Journal of Medicine, 340*(1), 9–13.

Kurjak, A., Kupesic, S., & Kos, M. (2002). Three-dimensional sonography for assessment of morphology and vascularization of the fetus and placenta. *Journal of Society of Gynecologic Investigation, 9*(4), 186–202.

Lashley, F. R. (1997). *The genetics revolution: Implications for nursing.* Washington, DC: American Academy of Nursing.

Lashley, F. R. (1998). *Clinical genetics in nursing practice* (2nd ed.). New York: Springer.

Lea, D. H., & Williams, J. K. (2002). Genetic testing and screening: Use them as a part of routine nursing practice. *American Journal of Nursing, 102*(7), 36–43.

Lea, D. H., Williams, J. K., Jenkins, J., Jones, S. L., & Calzone, K. (2000). Genetic health care: Creating interdisciplinary partnerships with nursing in clinical practice. *National Academies of Practice Forum, 2*(3), 177–186.

Lewis, J. A. (2001). *Genetics and the perinatal and women's health nurse.* Washington, DC: Association of Women's Health, Obstetric and Neonatal Nurses.

Lloyd-Puryear, M. A., & Forsman, I. (2002). Newborn screening and genetic testing. *Journal of Obstetric, Gynecologic & Neonatal Nursing, 31*(2), 200–207.

Lowes, L., & Lyne, P. (2000). Chronic sorrow in parents of children with newly diagnosed diabetes: A review of the literature and discussion of the implications for nursing practice. *Journal of Advanced Nursing, 32*(1), 41–48.

March of Dimes Birth Defects Foundation. (1999). Folic acid. Available at: http://www.marchofdimes.com.

March of Dimes Birth Defects Foundation. (2001). *Genetic screening pocketfacts.* Publication No. 09-1618-01. White Plains, NY: Author.

Martin, J. A., Hamilton, B. E., Venture, S. J., Menacker, F., & Park, M. M. (2002). Births: Final data for 2000. National vital statistic reports, 50(5). Hyattsville, MD: National Center for Health Statistics. Available at: http://www.cdc.gov.

Martinez, A., Linden, J., Schimmenti, L. A., & Palmer, C. G. S. (2003). Attitudes of the broader hearing, deaf, and hard-of-hearing community toward genetic testing for deafness. *Genetics in Medicine, 5*(2), 106–112.

Moos, M. K. (1998). Truth or consequences? *Obstetrical and Gynecological Survey, 53*(12), 731.

Moos, M. K. (2003). *Preconception health promotion: A focus for women's wellness* (2nd ed.). White Plains, NY: March of Dimes.

Moos, M. K. (2004). Preconceptional health promotion: Progress in changing a prevention paradigm. *Journal of Perinatal & Neonatal Nursing, 18*(1), 2–13.

Munne, S., Cohen, J., & Sable, D. (2002). Preimplantation genetic diagnosis for advanced maternal age and other indications. *Fertility and Sterility, 75*(2), 234–236.

National Center for Biotechnology Information. (2003). Online Mendelian inheritance in man. Available at: http://www.ncbi.nlm.nih.gov.

Newborn Screening Task Force. (2000). Serving the family from birth to the medical home: A report from the Newborn Screening Task Force. *Pediatrics, 106*(2), S383–S427.

Nussbaum, R. I., McInnes, R. R., & Willard, H. F. (2001) *Thompson and Thompson genetics in medicine* (6th ed.). Philadelphia: W. B. Saunders.

Ogasawara, M., Aoki, K., Okada, S., & Suzumori, K. (2000). Embryonic karyotype of abortuses in relation to the number of previous miscarriages. *Fertility and Sterility, 73*(2), 300–304.

Pickering, S., Polidoropoulos, N., Caller, J., Scriven, P., Ogilvie, C. M., Braude, P., & the PGD Study Group. (2003). Strategies and outcomes of the first 100 cycles of preimplantation genetic diagnosis at the Guy's and St. Thomas' Center. *Fertility and Sterility, 79*(1), 81–90.

Raynor, B. D. (2003). Routine ultrasound in pregnancy. *Clinical Obstetrics and Gynecology, 46*(4), 882–889.

Richards, C. S., Bradley, L. A., Amos, J., Allitto, B., Grody, W. W., Maddalena, A., McGinnis, M. J., Prior, T. W., Popovich, B. W., & Watson, M. S. (2002). Standards and guidelines for CFTR mutation testing. *Genetics in Medicine, 4*(5), 379–391.

Richards, F. (2003). Couples' experiences of predictive testing and living with the risk or reality of Huntington disease: A qualitative study. *American Journal of Medical Genetics, 126*(A), 170–182.

Rose, G. A., & Wong, A. (1998). Experiences in Hong Kong with the theory and practice of the albumin column method of sperm separation for sex selection. *Human Reproduction, 13*(1), 146–149.

Rothstein, M. A., & Anderlik, M. R. (2001). What is genetic discrimination, and when and how can it be prevented? *Genetics in Medicine, 3*(5), 354–358.

Sadler, T. W. (1995). *Langman's medical embryology* (7th ed.). Philadelphia: Lippincott Williams & Wilkins.

Sadler, T. W. (2005). *Langman's essential medical embryology.* Philadelphia, PA: Lippincott Williams & Wilkins.

Sanders, R. C. (2002). *Structural fetal abnormalities: The total picture.* St. Louis: Mosby.

Scanlon, C., & Fibison, W. (1995). *Managing genetic information: Implications for nursing practice.* Washington, DC: American Nurses Publishing.

Scott, J. R., DiSaia, P. J., Hammond, C. B., & Spellacy, W. N. (1999). *Danforth's obstetrics and gynecology* (8th ed.). Philadelphia: Lippincott Williams & Wilkins.

Shuster, E. (1997). Fifty years later: The significance of the Nuremberg Code. *New England Journal of Medicine, 337*(20), 1436–1440.

Singh, N. P., Muller, C. H., & Berger, R. E. (2002). DNA double strand breaks and apoptosis in human sperm: Effects of donor age. *Fertility & Sterility, 78*(3), S69–S70.

Spahis, J. (2002). Human genetics: Constructing a family pedigree. *American Journal of Nursing, 102*(7), 44–49.

Spencer, K. (2000). Screening for trisomy 21 in twin pregnancies in the first trimester using free β-hCG and PAPP-A, combined with fetal nuchal translucency thickness. *Prenatal Diagnosis, 20,* 91–95.

Speroff, L., Glass, R. H., & Kase, N. G. (1999). *Clinical gynecologic endocrinology and infertility* (6th ed.). Philadelphia: Lippincott Williams & Wilkins.

Stern, H. J., Harton, G. L., Sisson, M. E., Jones, S. L., Fallon, L. A., Thorsell, L. P., Getlinger, M. E., Black, S. H., & Schulman, J. D. (2002). Non-disclosing preimplantation genetic diagnosis for Huntington disease. *Prenatal Diagnosis, 22,* 503–507.

Suther, S., & Goodson, P. (2003). Barriers to the provision of genetic services by primary care physicians: A systematic review of the literature. *Genetics in Medicine, 5*(2), 70–76.

Tinkle, M. B. (2002). Cystic fibrosis: Are nurses ready to be on the front line? *AWHONN Lifelines, 6*(2), 134–139.

Tinkle, M. B., & Castora, F. (2002). Mitochondrial disorders: A clinician's primer. *MEDSURG Nursing, 11*(1), 25–29.

Tuchmann-Duplessis, H., David, G., & Haegel, P. (1975). *Illustrated human embryology, Volume 1*. New York: Springer Verlag.

Verlinsky, Y., & Kuliev, A. (1998). Preimplantation genetic diagnosis. In A. Milunsky (Ed.), *Genetic disorders in the fetus: Diagnosis, prevention & treatment* (4th ed.). Baltimore: Johns Hopkins University Press.

Vidal, F., Fugger, E. R., Blanco, J., Keyanfar, K., Catala, V., Norton, M., Hazelrigg, W. B., Black, S. H., Levinson, G., Egozcue, J., & Schulman, J. D. (1998). Efficiency of MicroSort flow cytometry for producing sperm populations enriched in X- or Y-chromosome haplotypes: A blind trial assessed by double and triple colour fluorescent in-situ hybridization. *Human Reproduction, 13*, 308–312.

Vintzileous, A., Walters, C., & Yeo, L. (2003). Absent nasal bone in the prenatal detection of fetuses with trisomy 21 in a high risk population. *Obstetrics & Gynecology, 101*(5), 905–908.

Wapner, R., Thom, E., Simpson, J. L., Pergament, E., Silver, R., Filkins, K., et al. (2003). First-trimester screening for trisomies 21 and 18. *New England Journal of Medicine, 349*(15), 1405–1413.

Watson, J. D., & Crick, F. H. C. (1953). Molecular structure of nucleic acids. *Nature, 171*(4356), 737–738.

Weil, J. (2001). Multicultural education and genetic counseling. *Clinical Genetics, 59*(3), 143–146.

Willie, M. D., Weitz, B., Kerper, P., & Frazier, S. (2004). Advances in preconception genetic counseling. *Journal of Perinatal & Neonatal Nursing, 18*(1), 28–40.

Wilkins-Haug, L. (1993). The emerging genetic theories of unstable DNA, uniparental disomy, and imprinting. *Current Opinion in Obstetrics and Gynecology, 5*, 179–185.

Workman, M. R., & Philpott-Howard, J. (1997). Risk of fetal infection from invasive procedures. *Journal of Hospital Infections, 35*, 169–174.

Zhang, J., Meikle, S., Grainger, D. A., & Trumble, A. (2002). Multifetal pregnancy in older women and perinatal outcomes. *Fertility and Sterility, 78*(3), 562–568.

PREGNANCY

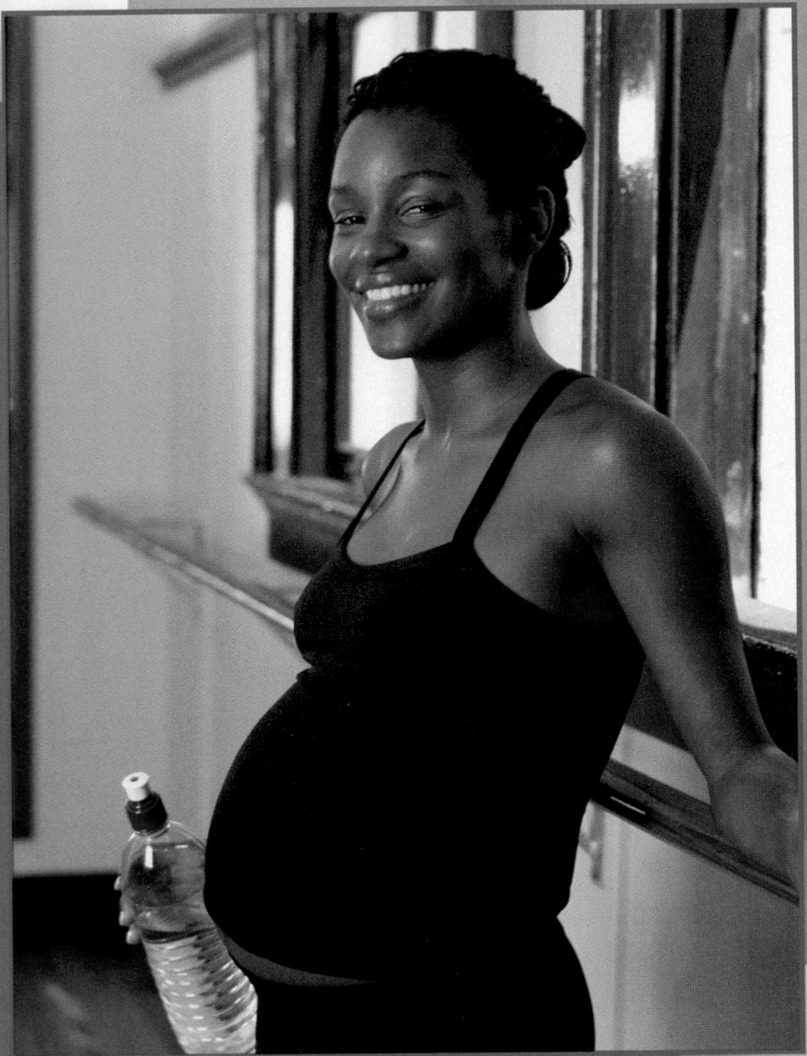

UNIT 3

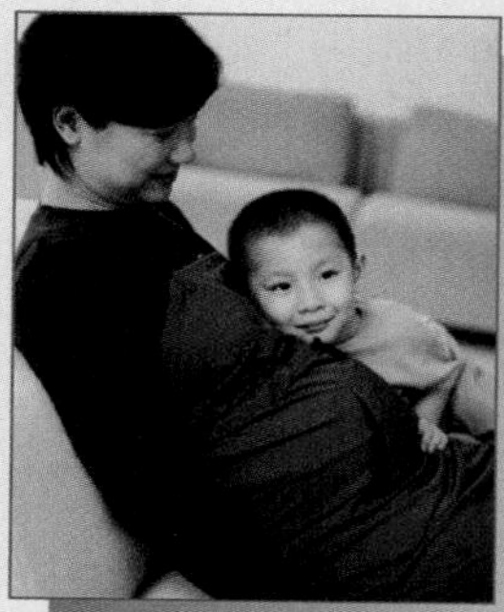 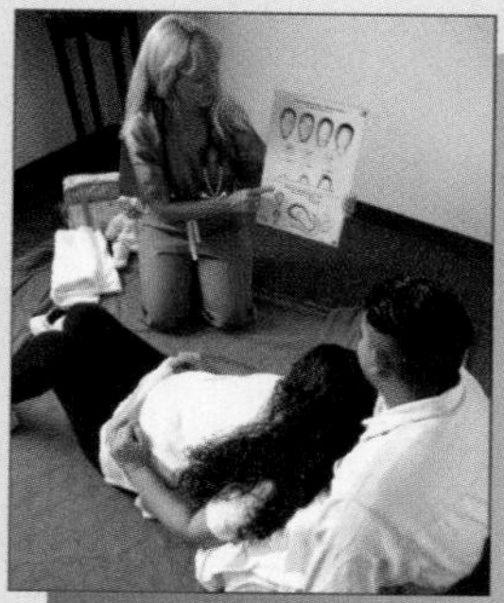 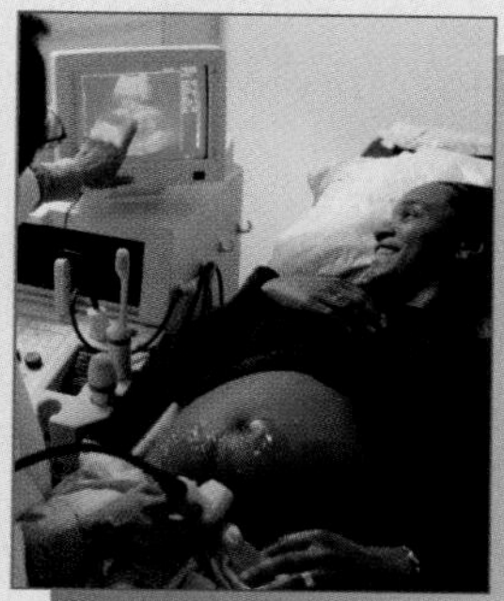 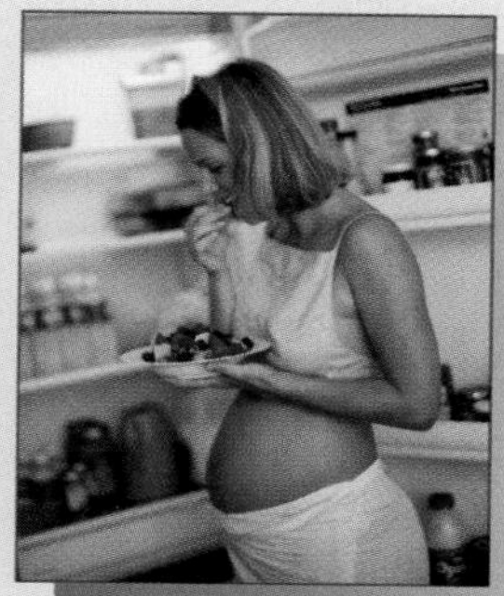

Few life events are as wonderful, ambivalent, memorable, and defining as pregnancy. While the process of gestation has many common threads and themes for all women, each mother's experience is unique. Furthermore, the same woman may experience pregnancy differently each time that she goes through it. The changes that the expectant woman undergoes involve not only her physical, psychological, spiritual, emotional, interpersonal, and social dimensions. Providing appropriate support for the pregnant client, as well as her partner, significant others, and extended family and friends, is one of the most important crucial aspects of quality collaborative health care.

This unit describes the process of normal pregnancy, expected changes in each trimester, and associated management approaches for the normal discomforts and adjustments that accompany this life event. It also discusses those conditions and circumstances that render a pregnancy as high risk, with measures that health care providers should take to protect the health of mother and fetus. The unit explores different methods of preparing for pregnancy, childbirth, and parenthood, emphasizing the role that educational programs can play in improving outcomes not only for individual clients, but also for families and the overall public.

CHAPTER 12

Process of Pregnancy

Robin Evans

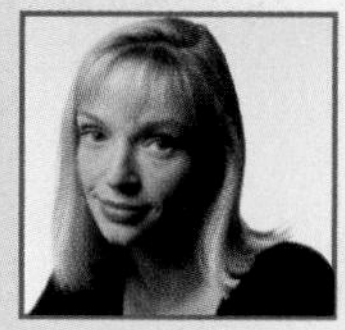

Millie, 38 years old, G3P2002, has just learned she is at 12 weeks' gestation with an unplanned pregnancy. Although she expresses excitement, Millie also verbalizes apprehension. "I thought I was done forever with diapers and night feedings. I also forgot how tired and nauseous you feel during the first trimester." She says she is concerned about fetal well-being because she is older than when she went through her previous pregnancies. She also wonders how she'll have enough time for the rest of her family once the new baby arrives.

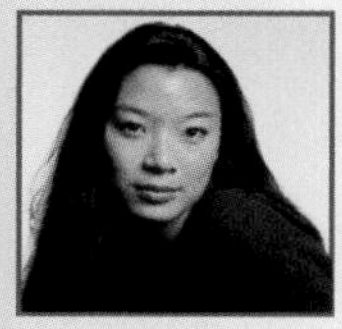

Kathy, 26 years old, G1P0, comes to the prenatal clinic for a regular visit at 32 weeks' gestation. While the nurse is collecting assessment data, Kathy relates that her feet have been swollen and that she has been constipated. She states "I never expected pregnancy to have so many physical effects. I'm worried about my feet. Do you think something is wrong with the pregnancy?"

You will learn more about Millie's and Kathy's stories later in this chapter. Nurses working with these clients and others like them need to understand the material in this chapter to manage care and address issues appropriately. Before beginning, consider the following points related to the above scenarios:

- How can the nurse reassure both clients, while appropriately addressing any problems for each that might exist?
- What differences might these clients experience based on their ages, previous pregnancy histories, and other circumstances?
- What topics and assessment questions might the nurse focus on next for each woman?
- How can the nurse effectively integrate each client's physical, psychological, and sociocultural pregnancy-related concerns?

LEARNING OBJECTIVES

On completion of this chapter, the reader should be able to:

- Discuss variations in pregnancy, including those based on age, sociocultural considerations, and religion.
- Describe common physical and psychological changes in pregnancy.
- Identify the presumptive, probable, and positive signs of pregnancy.
- Summarize the components of an assessment for pregnant women, focused on appropriate history taking, physical examination, and laboratory evaluation.
- Summarize the components of the assessment of fetal activity and well-being.
- Discuss strategies to enhance women's health and comfort during pregnancy.
- Discuss substances that may have teratogenic effects on the fetus.

KEY TERMS

amenorrhea
Braxton-Hicks contractions
cephalopelvic disproportion
Chadwick's sign
chloasma
diastasis
fundus
Goodell's sign
Hegar's sign
Leopold's maneuvers
leukorrhea
lightening
linea nigra
Montgomery's tubercles
morning sickness
multigravida
Naegele's rule
oligohydramnios
operculum
para
primigravida
quickening
striae gravidarum
supine postural hypotension syndrome
teratogen

Pregnancy is one of life's most profound experiences. During the early part of the 20th century, women spent a considerable portion of their reproductive years pregnant, producing large families. The advent of birth control provided options previously not available to limit family size (see Chap. 8). In the latter part of the 20th century, some countries actually began to limit the number of children people could have, enforcing deterrents to producing more than one child.

This chapter addresses the components of appropriate care of pregnant women, examining the process of pregnancy from several perspectives. A common and incorrect assumption is that all women experience pregnancy the same way. Many factors, however, contribute to clients' responses. Knowledge and understanding of these variations allow nurses to give anticipatory health education, as well as to provide care specific to the client's and family's actual needs. The chapter explores physical and psychological changes during pregnancy, including their etiology. It describes appropriate assessments necessary to identify any potential or actual challenges to the well-being of woman, fetus, or both. Maintenance of maternal and fetal well-being helps ensure a positive outcome of the pregnancy. The chapter discusses strategies that may enhance the health and comfort of pregnant clients. This knowledge provides nurses an opportunity to assist clients to improve self-image and self-care.

VARIATIONS IN RESPONSES TO PREGNANCY

The way the client and family experience pregnancy is influenced by such things as age, sociologic and cultural background, and religion. Viewing all women of the same age, ethnic origin, race, culture, sexual orientation, economic status, or religious beliefs as the same, however, will not lead to sensitive and appropriate health care provision. The nurse needs to see each individual as just that—an individual who may or may not subscribe to stereotypes or generalizations. For example, although women may be of a particular culture or ethnic origin, the extent to which they follow traditional customs varies. The nurse should view each woman within the context of her environment, including cultural, historical, political, and economic factors, while remembering that the client is unique and requires individualized, pertinent, and specific care (Callister, 2005).

Age-Related Variations

A woman's potential to become pregnant may cover a span from early adolescence to the late 40s. The average age of U.S. mothers has been increasing steadily during the past 30 years, with relatively fewer mothers younger than 20 years and more mothers 35 years or older (U.S. Department of Health and Human Services [USDHHS], 2005). The average age of mothers at the time of birth increased from 24.6 in 1970 to 27.2 in 2000, whereas the median age (the middle point if the ages of all mothers were arranged from highest to lowest) of mothers having their first baby increased from 22.1 in 1970 to 24.6 in 2000 (Matthews & Hamilton, 2002).

Pregnancy in Adolescence

In 2000, the U.S. teenage pregnancy rate was 48.5 births for every 1000 women 15 to 19 years of age (Matthews & Hamilton, 2002). In 2003, the birth rate for teenagers declined to its lowest rate in more than 6 decades and an average of 34% lower than the peak teenage birth rate in 1991 (USDHHS, 2005). In 2002, Canada's rate of teen pregnancy was 33.9 for every 1000 women aged 15 to 19 years (Statistics Canada, 2005). Teen mothers bring unique perspectives to pregnancy that may not always be consistent with how society views them (Fig. 12.1). They often are portrayed as young women who have made poor choices, adding significant costs to society, both in financial terms and in terms of their parental suitability (Geronimus, 2003). Because often they have not completed schooling, their ability to provide adequate support for themselves and their children is viewed as compromised. They are seen as not yet having had time to accomplish their own tasks of adolescence, leading to increased risk for negative consequences (SmithBattle, 2000b). Attitudes have begun to shift during the past decade. Researchers are attempting to understand from various perspectives the choices and experiences of these young women (Hanna, 2001; Seamark & Lings, 2004; SmithBattle, 2000a, 2000b), rather than only focusing on the more traditional view of immature, inexperienced, irresponsible "children raising children" (SmithBattle, 2000b), whose lack of parenting skills may put children at risk. For example, Hanna (2001) and SmithBattle (2000a) identified that teen mothers viewed raising a child as a way to demonstrate responsibility, in contrast to the more common public discourse. A metasynthesis by Clemmens (2003) revealed that although parenthood was challenging for them, teen mothers also saw motherhood as a positively transforming and stabilizing influence, as well as a turning point for the future.

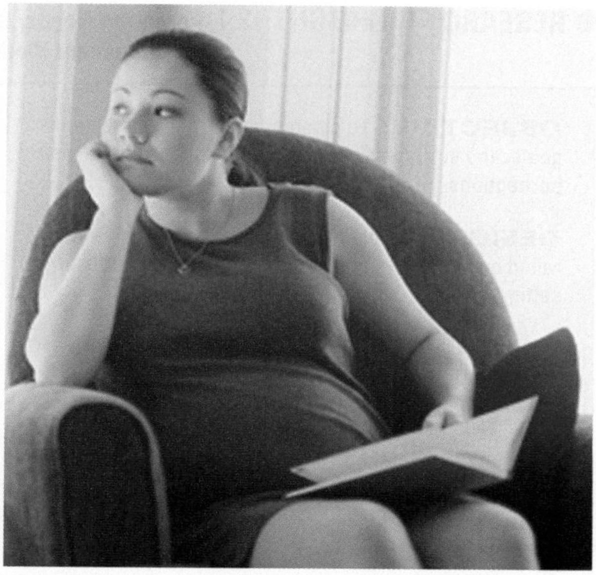

FIGURE 12.1 Although pregnancy in adolescence poses unique challenges, expectant teens may see parenthood as a demonstration of responsibility, a transformative experience, a source of stability, and a life turning point.

Nevertheless, teen mothers do have challenges. They often are less likely to complete school and are more likely to earn less income than those women who delay childbearing until after 20 years old, a fact probably related more to socioeconomic disadvantage than to becoming a teen mother (Geronimus, 2003; SmithBattle, 2000b). Adolescents are less likely to have regular access to health care than younger children and older persons (Centers for Disease Control and Prevention [CDC], 2005). Contributing factors include an inability to pay for services, lack of insurance coverage, coverage limits, transportation issues, and concerns about confidentiality (CDC, 2005).

Teen mothers have differing levels of support from family or partners, a concept that may be somewhat culturally determined. African American and Latina teens appear to have more support from family members than do white teens, although this may be changing (Geronimus, 2003; SmithBattle, 2000b). For the families of teen mothers, the transition to parenthood and grandparenthood can be abrupt and complicated (Dallas, 2004). Teens themselves tend to emphasize the need for support and knowledge to be successful in their new role of parenting (Stiles, 2005). See Research Highlight 12.1.

● RESEARCH HIGHLIGHT 12.1 Parenting Needs, Goals, and Strategies of Adolescent Mothers

OBJECTIVE: To pinpoint and organize the needs, goals, and strategies of teen mothers according to their perceptions.

DESIGN: This microethnographic qualitative study relied on interviews and focus groups in a naturalistic setting.

PARTICIPANTS AND SETTING: Five unmarried 18-year-old mothers from a Southern U.S. urban secondary school participated. The researchers analyzed data using a clustering technique and a modified multistage method.

RESULTS: The adolescent mothers emphasized a need for knowledge and support. They identified as goals career, happiness, and independence; they targeted the strategies of support groups, life skills and formal education, and employment.

CONCLUSIONS: The findings can assist nurses to develop programs and activities that emphasize and include peer support and education. Chances for success are increased if nursing interventions focus on needs for both teens and children; are multidisciplinary, flexible, accepting, and supportive; occur in a comfortable environment; and include the adolescents' children and other family members.

Stiles, A. S. (2005). *MCN—The American Journal of Maternal and Child Nursing, 30*(5), 327–333.

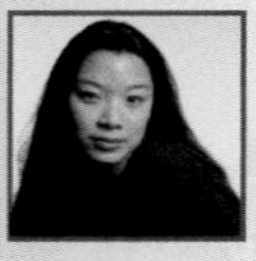

Remember Kathy, the 26-year-old at the beginning of the chapter who is in her 32nd week of gestation. Imagine that Kathy were 16 years old and single. What areas would be especially important for the nurse to assess?

Pregnancy After 35

In 2003, U.S. women 40 to 44 years had a birth rate of 8.7 births for every 1000 women, reflective of the steady rise in pregnancy in older women since 1980, when the rate was 3.9 births for every 1000 women (USDHHS, 2005). Women older than 35 years have an increased incidence of subfertility and inability to conceive (see Chap. 10) (Beckmann et al., 2002; Fong & McGovern, 2004). They often believe that it is "now or never" (Bondas & Eriksson, 2001; Dobrzykowski & Stern, 2003), which may contribute to anxiety about conceiving. When women older than 35 years are pregnant, they tend to be more highly educated, proactively seek information, and have fewer peers with whom to share the pregnancy experience (Neumann & Graf, 2003). Many pregnant women older than 35 years, however, experience challenges that may affect pregnancy, including obesity, preexisting hypertension, depression, and socioeconomic disadvantages (Carolan, 2003; Neumann & Graf, 2003). Some studies have shown women older than 35 years to be at increased risk for cesarean birth (Cunningham et al., 2005; Kozinsky et al., 2002; Ziadeh & Yahaya, 2001). They may experience increased anxiety as concern about potential outcomes for both self and baby become more prominent, although little evidence indicates that such worry affects pregnancy detrimentally. It is unclear whether the pregnant woman 35 years or older is at increased risk because of the pregnancy itself or because other health-related risks increase with age (Neumann & Graf, 2003). Fortunately, most pregnancies to women older than 35 years are normal and result in healthy maternal and newborn outcomes (Neumann & Graf, 2003). (See Nursing Care Plan 12.1.)

Pregnancy from 20 to 35 Years

Traditionally, the age span of 20 to 35 years has been considered the opportune time for pregnancy. Mothers within this range usually have completed their high school education. Number of years of completed education has been correlated positively with birth weight and decreased perinatal morbidity and mortality (Barron, 2001). Although women in this age group have fewer risk factors associated with pregnancy and birth, socioeconomic factors unrelated to age may continue to play a role in the outcome of the pregnancy. For example, women in lower socioeconomic groups may be unable to access adequate prenatal care because a "disproportionate number of women of childbearing age are uninsured or underinsured" (Barron, 2001, p. 133). They may be at increased risk for preterm labor related to their occupation if it requires long periods of standing or heavy work.

Sociocultural Variations

Many nurses and health care professionals assume that all women and their significant others experience pregnancy and its associated rites of passage similarly. Pregnancy and parenthood, however, have different meanings and rituals for each woman. These experiences are influenced

NURSING CARE PLAN 12.1

The Client in Early Pregnancy

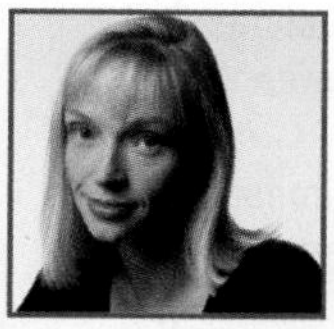

Recall Millie from the beginning of this chapter. Review of her pregnancy history reveals that both previous pregnancies were normal and resulted in vaginal births at 38 and 39 weeks, respectively. Her oldest child weighed 7 lb, 2 oz at birth; her second child weighed 6 lb, 14 oz. In addition to problems with "morning sickness," Millie also reports constipation and hemorrhoids. She states, "My children are very active in after-school activities and sports. And I'm the one who drives them back and forth. Sometimes I feel like a chauffeur. My husband helps when he can, but he usually has to go out of town for a few days each month for business. I'm just worried that I won't be able to keep up with everything."

NURSING DIAGNOSIS

Anxiety related to client's age and the increased physical and psychological demands associated with current pregnancy and current family lifestyle

EXPECTED OUTCOMES

1. The client will verbalize concerns related to pregnancy.
2. The client will identify areas in which she needs assistance.

INTERVENTIONS	RATIONALES
Assess the client's level of understanding about age and pregnancy.	This information serves as a baseline for specific client needs and an individualized plan.
Discuss with the client her concerns, feelings, and perceptions related to pregnancy and age and possible effects on current family situation.	Discussion provides opportunities to emphasize positive aspects; verbalization of concerns helps establish sources of stress and areas that need to be addressed.
Communicate accurate facts and answer questions honestly.	Open, honest communication promotes trust and helps correct any misinformation.
Review the client's previous pregnancy history.	This information gives clues to potential problems and aids in identifying the client's reactions and coping abilities.
Discuss possible effects of increased age on pregnancy and measures to reduce risks.	Adequate knowledge of possible effects and risk-reduction measures helps alleviate concerns related to the unknown.
Ask the client to describe her typical daily schedule and activities; review with her areas that might be problematic.	Knowledge of a typical routine offers a baseline; identifying potential problem areas facilitates teaching and anticipatory guidance.
Investigate sources of available support, such as family, friends, and community; encourage the client to use them.	Additional sources of support are helpful in alleviating anxiety and stress.
Encourage the client to obtain adequate rest and nutrition; discuss ways to accomplish them within her current situation.	Adequate rest and nutrition are essential to promote a positive pregnancy outcome.

Continued

NURSING CARE PLAN 12.1 ● The Client in Early Pregnancy *(Continued)*

INTERVENTIONS	RATIONALES
Include the client, partner, and children in discussion about the pregnancy, client needs, and necessary adaptations.	Client and family participation increases feelings of control over the situation and promotes support and sharing.
Provide the family with information about support groups, Web sites, and other sources of appropriate information.	Shared experiences and knowledge of similar situations can aid in preparing the client and family for what to expect.
Continue to assess the family's adaptation and functioning at subsequent visits.	Continued assessment aids in monitoring progress of the situation and provides opportunities to address concerns that may arise as the pregnancy progresses.

EVALUATION

1. The client identifies realistic measures to cope with the demands of pregnancy and family.
2. The client and family develop a workable schedule that promotes maternal, fetal, and family health.
3. The client demonstrates use of appropriate support services.
4. The client reports a decrease in anxiety at next visit.

by language and cultural differences, ethnicity, sexual orientation, and socioeconomic status (Box 12.1).

Cultural, Racial, and Ethnic Influences

Variations among people within a culture exist and influence how much a client follows culturally related beliefs (Callister, 2001a). Some may see cultural traditions and beliefs about childbirth as "old wives tales" (Lauderdale, 2003). Women from a certain race may have no affiliation with the culture of that race. An important part of cultural assessment and sensitivity, therefore, is learning the client's degree of affiliation with her cultural group; the cultural beliefs and practices that she follows; her patterns of decision making, language, and communication; the family's parenting style and role; dietary practices; and culturally influenced expectations of the health care system (Callister, 2001b).

Sociocultural beliefs can influence a woman's experience of pregnancy and her beliefs about and practices during gestation. For example, some cultures commonly implicate prenatal thoughts, dreams, and behaviors as explanations for negative effects on the developing fetus (Callister, 2001a). Some African and Hispanic Americans believe that the pregnant woman should not raise her arms above the head because doing so can lead to nuchal cord (Lauderdale, 2003). The amount of support and involvement from extended family in pregnancy, birth, and childrearing is another area with cultural, ethnic, and racial determinants (Callister, 2001b; Cesario, 2001; Lagana, 2003; Lemon, 2002; Liu & Moore, 2000; Raines & Morgan, 2000). For example, some people of West Indian and Chinese heritage consider it inappropriate for men to be present at birth (Callister, 2001b; Lauderdale, 2003). In such cases, it would be most appropriate for a woman's health care providers to be female.

Although belief in the concepts of "hot" and "cold" is common to several cultures, how each culture expresses that belief differs. For example, women from southeast Asia (Callister, 2001b; Raines & Morgan, 2000) and Latinas (Lemon, 2002) believe that balance should be maintained between hot and cold: during pregnancy (considered to be a hot condition), women eat cold foods; following birth (believed to deplete the woman's body of the hot element), they eat hot foods to balance the cold state. The designation of foods as hot or cold is unrelated to the temperature of the food; rather, it refers to the effect that the food has on the body.

Latina custom may result in women requesting to take the placenta home, so that they can bury it deeply to prevent animals from eating it (believed to result in an inability to bear any more children) and to decrease the woman's pain (Lemon, 2002). These women usually

BOX 12.1 Cultural Influences on Pregnancy

The following are some generalities about common findings in various ethnic groups. The nurse should remember that each client's circumstances require unique assessment and care.

African Americans

- Have extensive networks of extended families, friends, and neighbors who participate in childrearing and may be present during labor and birth to "be there," not to provide care
- Highly respect their elders and value children
- Often are demonstrative and comfortable with touch and physical contact
- May believe that all animate and inanimate objects have good or evil spirits
- May rely on family healers or spiritualists
- May practice *pica* (ingestion of nonfood items, such as clay or starch)
- May be expressive of pain
- May wear garlic, amulets, and copper or silver bracelets
- Do not want baby's head or hands touched without first asking permission, from a belief that doing so can transmit "bad vibes" and germs
- Believe raising arms above the head may cause the cord to wrap around the baby's neck

Haitians

- Carry a "spit" cup during pregnancy from a belief that they should not swallow saliva
- Bathe for first 3 days postpartum in a special water boiled with herbs; for next 3 days bathe in water in which leaves have been soaked and warmed by the sun
- Take cold baths 1 month after birth to tighten muscles and bones believed to have been loosened during childbirth
- Wear a piece of linen or a belt tightly around the waist postpartum to prevent gas from entering the body
- Avoid eating white foods such as milk, lobster, and white beans postpartum to prevent vaginal discharge and hemorrhage

West Indians (Jamaica, Trinidad, and Barbados)

- Do not allow father of baby to visit during labor or birth
- Rely exclusively on breastfeeding

Chinese

- Believe events are predestined
- Strive for spirituality
- Believe in Yin and Yang: balance that should be maintained between hot and cold
- Eat "cold" foods such as chicken, fish, vegetables, and fruit during pregnancy (considered a hot condition) because eating "hot" foods is believed to cause abortion or premature labor
- May not want to take prenatal vitamins, which they consider a hot medication
- Believe that exposure of the genital area is inappropriate
- Value humility and modesty; may find an open gown and vaginal examinations embarrassing
- Believe it is inappropriate for any man to view the woman's body, and thus desire female health care providers
- Consume "hot" foods to balance the "cold" postpartal state for 40 days after birth
- Value pericare and hygiene, but refrain from showering for up to 2 to 4 weeks postpartum
- Rear children within the extended family
- Are distressed when others touch the newborn's head, which parents consider sacred
- Assume an upright or squatting position for birth
- Believe newborn should be swaddled for first few days to prevent exposure to winds

Hispanics and Latinas

- Have large, cohesive family groups with a family decision-making process and extensive physical and emotional support
- Consult husband or significant others about major health decisions
- Frequently use folk medicine
- View motherhood as most important role; pregnancy is an important family event
- Have a sense of present, so may not realize effects of behavior on future of pregnancy and baby—they may be late or absent from prenatal visits
- Believe that fate or God controls their destiny
- Follow folk traditions thought to prevent birth defects (eg, wear a safety pin attached to an undergarment to protect the fetus from cleft lip or palate)
- Believe raising hands above head while pregnant may cause knots in baby's umbilical cord
- May believe that defects or injury to fetus are related to unsatisfied cravings
- May avoid vitamins or iron during pregnancy because of the belief that they are harmful
- Believe in hot and cold theory of disease prevention and health promotion
- Believe that walking during labor makes birth occur more quickly
- Fear cesarean birth, which they view as life threatening for the mother
- Avoid showers for several days postpartum
- May place black onyx on or near the newborn to ward off the evil eye
- May view colostrum as "bad" or "old" milk and avoid breastfeeding during the first few postpartal days

Mexican Americans

- Take no illicit drugs, alcohol, tobacco, or over-the-counter medications for fear of hurting the baby
- Refrain from becoming angry, believing that doing so harms the fetus
- Walk daily and avoid naps to promote fetal activity

Continued

BOX 12.1 Cultural Influences on Pregnancy *(Continued)*

- Dress warmly, covering head and feet, based on a belief that exposure to cold can lead to illness
- Believe that one ultrasound is acceptable but repeated ultrasounds might hurt the baby
- Want to be near their kin
- Believe that food cravings are to be satisfied to prevent fetal harm
- Sleep flat on the back to protect the baby
- Avoid cold air during pregnancy

Native American Tribes

- Value oral traditions passed on from previous generations
- Allow elders to play a dominant role in decision making
- Allow traditional healers to use feathers, cornmeal, grasses, rocks, or medicine bags in rituals (These should not be disturbed if left at bedside or on crib or bassinette.)
- May avoid eye contact and limit touch
- Prefer watching and listening as methods of learning
- Often do not see the past as related to present problems, making assessment challenging
- Believe in nonaggressive harmony
- Believe if woman becomes angry or mad or argues, the child also will behave that way
- View childbearing as part of normal life cycle
- Focus on pregnancy during time woman is pregnant, not on what will follow
- Believe that swimming or bathing in cold water every day will toughen mother's and baby's system
- Remain active during pregnancy to aid baby's circulation (Crow)
- Do not tie knots or braid or allow the baby's father to do so to avoid causing difficult labor (Navaho)
- Avoid traditional ceremonies like Yei or Squaw dances to prevent spirits from harming the baby (Navaho)

Whites

- Highly value involvement of partners
- View technology as beneficial and necessary to ensure safe delivery and a healthy baby
- May desire little medical interference, home birth, or water birth
- Value early prenatal care and education

Data from Andrews & Hanson, 2003; Berry, 1999; Callister, 2001b; Cesario, 2001; Lagana, 2003; Lauderdale, 2003; Lemon, 2002; Page, 2004; Raines & Morgan, 2000

consult their husband, significant others, and important family members about major health decisions (Callister, 2001b). Mexican American women become more conscientious about eating a healthy diet, avoiding alcohol, remaining calm for fear of hurting the baby, and increasing their activity to encourage regular walking while discouraging lifting, bending, or standing a prolonged time or rigorous exercise (Lagana, 2003). Although support of families in the Mexican American culture is well recognized (Page, 2004), geographic separation of families may fragment this support (Lagana, 2003). See Research Highlight 12.2.

Traditional Native American culture is built on a strong spiritual foundation with an orientation focused on the circular medicine wheel. Living in complete harmony with nature is important. People who follow this culture value listening and the role of elders. They may avoid eye contact, which they view as disrespectful (Cesario, 2001).

Lesbian Pregnancy

Artificial insemination, in vitro fertilization, surrogacy, and adoption have enabled people who have struggled with fertility issues to achieve pregnancy and childbirth (see Chap. 10); these methods also have facilitated parenthood for gay and lesbian parents (Lauderdale, 2003) (Fig. 12.2). Although lesbian and heterosexual mothers generally share most of the basic components of the transition to parenthood, lesbian clients also face several challenges that can compromise the integrity of their perinatal mental health (Ross, 2005). For example, lesbians may be at increased risk for a lack of social support, particularly from their families of origin (Ross, 2005). They may be exposed to stress from homophobic discrimination, as well as insurance and resources issues if their health care coverage for fertility and other procedures is limited because of their sexual orientation. Attitudes of health care personnel also may compromise health care provided (McManus et al., 2006). Nevertheless, lesbian pregnancies are more likely to be planned, and lesbian families generally have a more equitable distribution of child care, which may provide some protective effects on mental health (Ross, 2005). Studies have shown that lesbian couples primarily want to receive an attitude of respect for and understanding of their choices (Lauderdale, 2003).

Influence of Poverty

Poverty creates problems for all pregnant women, regardless of age, race, ethnicity, or sexual orientation. Limited resources compromise the ability of poor clients to provide adequate housing and food for themselves and any children they may have. Lack of money leads to problems accessing reliable transportation and child care, both of which are frequent causes of lack of prenatal care (CDC, 2005). The racial gap in access to ad-

● RESEARCH HIGHLIGHT 12.2 Come Bien, Camina y No Se Preocupe—Eat Right, Walk, and Do Not Worry: Selective Biculturalism During Pregnancy in a Mexican American Community

OBJECTIVE: To describe the pregnancy experiences of Mexican American women living in a small, predominantly Mexican American town and to examine the influence of acculturation on those experiences.

DESIGN: Focused ethnographic study using semi-structured, formal interviews and content analysis. Participants were recruited using snowball technique and purposeful sampling to draw approximately equal numbers of U.S.-born and Mexico-born women.

PARTICIPANTS AND SETTING: Twenty-nine Mexican American women were interviewed about their pregnancy experience and also completed the Acculturation Rating Scale for Mexican Americans (ARSMA). Inclusion criteria included motherhood, ability to speak Spanish or English, and reported Mexican cultural heritage. Interviews were conducted at a setting of participant's choice and in their preferred language. Additional data about the pregnancy experience were collected from prenatal care provider interviews, participant observation, event analysis, and review of public records, including birth statistics, population census, and historical records from the area.

RESULTS: Study findings verified the persistence of many Mexican American culture pregnancy beliefs described in the 1970s and 1980s. What had changed was that women had taken on broader societal roles outside of the home. Women reported that during pregnancy, they tried to adhere to more traditional Mexican cultural beliefs.

Lagana, K. (2003). *Journal of Transcultural Nursing, 14,* 117–124.

equate prenatal care has narrowed during the past 15 to 20 years, although it is actually widening between white and African American mothers 17 years and younger (Health Resources and Services Administration, 2002; Shiao et al., 2005). Women enrolled in a program that provides extra food may share the food with other impoverished family members. Attitudes of health care workers may influence the mother's perceptions of herself and her environment. For example, community workers who visit the mother in her home can contribute to decreased self-respect by unconsciously making inconsiderate remarks about the home environment (Allender & Spradley, 2005).

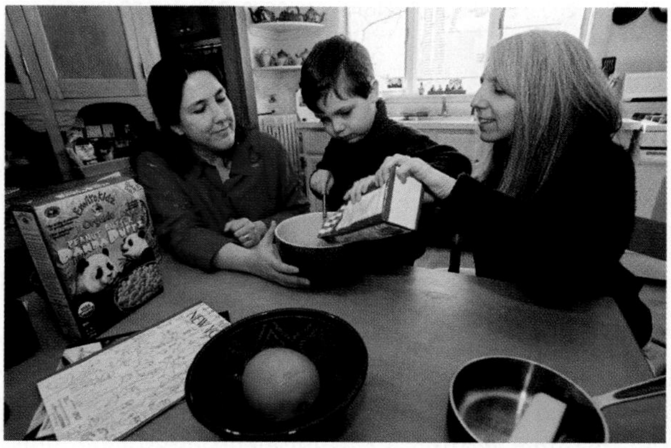

FIGURE 12.2 Families with lesbian parents are growing in U.S. and Canadian societies. Pregnant lesbians benefit from health care provision that is sensitive, respectful, and supportive.

Religious Variations

Religion may play a factor in the pregnant woman's life and response to pregnancy (Box 12.2). Just as with culture, assessing each client and family individually is essential because the degree to which they adhere to religious beliefs and teachings may vary. As well, some religions are divided into orthodox and nonorthodox sects, with even more variation in the views and laws to which members adhere. The following sections review some common religious issues related to pregnancy and childbirth that nurses should be aware of when working with clients.

Islam

Some Muslim women prefer cold foods, believing that pregnancy causes the body to become hot (Bradshaw, 2000). The Muslim Sabbath begins Thursday at sundown and ends Friday at sundown, so women may not schedule prenatal appointments during this time (Bradshaw, 2000; Roberts, 2002). During Ramadan, the Islamic holy month, most Muslims limit food and water intake to the night hours. As a result, nutrition may be compromised during this time. Muslim women also may refrain from medical attention during Ramadan (Bradshaw, 2000).

Buddhism

Buddhist traditions include meditating, chanting, burning incense, and lighting candles. Pregnant Buddhist clients may prefer a peaceful birth environment conducive to a meditative state (Northcott, 2002). Orthodox Buddhists may follow a vegan diet and refuse food after midday unless for medical reasons. Buddhists may refuse opiates,

BOX 12.2 Religious Influences on Pregnancy

Muslims

- Eat cold food to counter the belief that pregnancy causes the body to become hot
- Avoid scheduling appointments on Friday, which is their Sabbath
- Perform ritual circumcision of males during childhood
- Fast from sunrise to sunset during the month of Ramadan; they also may avoid medical attention during this period
- Eat and use no pork, pork products, or alcoholic beverages
- Prefer female caregivers
- Practice a ritual cleansing at the end of each menstrual period

Buddhists

- May meditate, chant, burn incense, and light candles
- Prefer a peaceful birth environment
- May follow vegan diet and refuse food after midday
- May refuse opiates, sedatives, or tranquilizers

Hindus

- Prohibit consumption of all meats

Jews

- Follow the kosher laws that mandate consumption of only select animals and fish (eg, animals with a cleft hoof who chew cud, only fish with fins and scales); ritual slaughtering of allowed animals to ensure minimal suffering; prohibition of mixing of dairy and meat dishes at the same meal
- Perform circumcision on all male children on the 8th day of life (conducted by a specially educated individual called a mohel, who may or may not be a physician)
- Observe Sabbath from Friday at sundown to Saturday at sundown
- In Orthodox clients, avoid physical contact with husband from appearance of the mucus plug or other vaginal blood, when regular contractions have been established, and/or the cervix is fully dilated (ends at either 6 weeks or 3 months postpartum)
- Practice a ritual cleansing 7 days after completion of menstruation and at end of period of separation identified above following childbirth

Mormons

- Prohibit alcohol, tobacco, coffee, and tea
- Prohibit pork, certain seafood (including shellfish), and fermented beverages
- May follow a vegetarian diet
- May request husband to lay hands on woman's head and give a blessing for strength, comfort, and well-being as she labors and gives birth

Jehovah's Witnesses

- Accept no blood or blood products
- Accept blood volume expanders as long as not derived from blood products
- Forbid therapeutic abortion, sterilization, and artificial insemination

Roman Catholics

- Accept only natural methods of birth control (abstinence, rhythm method, temperature method, or ovulation method) (see Chap. 8)
- View abortion as morally wrong
- Accept the Sacrament of the Sick and Eucharist (Communion) for those who are ill
- Ill infants may be baptized in an emergency

Protestant Denominations (Includes Lutherans, Anglicans, Presbyterians, Episcopalians, Baptists, Congregationalists, Adventists, and Churches of Christ)

- Beliefs and practices are diverse and vary among denominations

Data from Andrews & Hanson, 2003; Bennett et al., 2005; Bradshaw, 2000; Collins, 2002; Lewis, 2003; Northcott, 2002; Roberts, 2002

sedatives, and tranquilizers, because of their effects on awareness and consciousness (Northcott, 2002). For pregnant clients in labor, the health care team may need to be prepared to assist with nonpharmacologic pain management techniques (see Chap. 14).

Judaism

People of the Jewish faith may belong to different affiliations that reflect varying levels of adherence to Jewish Law. Orthodox Jews strictly follow the Law, whereas Conservative, Reconstruction, and Reform Jews are more liberal (Lewis, 2003). Orthodox Jewish women may feel more comfortable with female providers. Once her membranes rupture, the Orthodox Jewish pregnant woman will abstain from any physical (including sexual) contact with her husband for approximately 12 days (Collins, 2002). This teaching does not prohibit the man's presence in the room with her, however. Certain activities are forbidden during the Sabbath, which begins at sunset Friday and continues until nightfall on Saturday (25 hours). For example, Jews may not do anything considered "work." Examples include driving, cooking, bathing, writing, or using electricity or the telephone (including the call bell). If a cesarean birth is necessary during this time, the Orthodox couple may provide verbal consent only.

Jehovah's Witnesses

Jehovah's Witnesses do not accept blood or blood products. Thus, if a pregnant Jehovah's Witness develops anemia or postpartum hemorrhage, she will not accept blood transfusions (Bennett et al., 2005). Blood volume expanders are acceptable as long as they are not derived from blood products (Andrews & Hanson, 2003). Amniocentesis is acceptable, but therapeutic abortions and artificial insemination are forbidden (Andrews & Hanson, 2003).

Roman Catholicism

Roman Catholicism views only abstinence and natural family planning as acceptable methods of contraception (Andrews & Hanson, 2003) (see Chap. 8). Voluntary abortion is considered morally wrong (see Chap. 9). When a pregnant Catholic is ill, she may be given the Sacrament of the Sick, Eucharist, or both (Andrews & Hanson, 2003). Ill newborns may be baptized in an emergency, rather than waiting for the traditional baptism, which normally occurs after a few weeks or months of the baby's birth.

Protestantism

Protestantism is an umbrella term for several non-Catholic denominations of Christianity, including Lutherans, Anglicans, Presbyterians, Baptists, Congregationalists, Adventists, and Church of Christ. Religious beliefs and practices within and among these denominations are diverse and varied (Andrews & Hanson, 2003). These and all clients, regardless of religious affiliation, require individualized assessment to determine appropriate adaptations to care.

PHYSIOLOGIC CHANGES IN PREGNANCY

During pregnancy, several changes occur within the body (Table 12.1). Some are obvious, whereas others are less noticeable.

Weight

Average weight gain during a singleton pregnancy is approximately 25 to 35 lb for women with a normal pre-pregnancy body mass index (BMI) (Institute of Medicine [IOM], 1990). An average 25 lb is distributed among the fetus, amniotic fluid, and placenta (11 lb); uterus and breasts (2 lb); increased blood volume (4 lb); extracellular fluid (about 3 lb); and maternal stores (5 lb) (Luppi, 2001). During the first several days following birth, the woman excretes the additional fluid in urine once she loses the placenta's fluid-retaining hormones. See Chapter 3 for more detailed discussion of recommendations for weight gain depending on the woman's pre-pregnancy weight and BMI.

The recommended weight gain for multiple births is higher, at least 40 lb for a twin pregnancy (IOM, 1990). Most of this weight gain occurs in the last two trimesters.

Cardiovascular System

Major changes occur within the woman's cardiovascular system during pregnancy. These changes are necessary for adequate placental and fetal circulation.

Because of increasing uterine size, the maternal heart shifts upward and to a more transverse position, causing it to appear enlarged on radiographic examination. Blood pressure remains unchanged despite the increased blood volume; it actually decreases slightly during the second trimester (approximately 5 to 10 mm Hg for both systolic and diastolic pressures), returning to pre-pregnancy values by the third trimester. These changes to blood pressure may result from increased production of prostaglandins or altered vascular resistance (Cunningham et al., 2005; Luppi, 2001).

Maternal blood volume begins to rise in the first trimester, increases most significantly during the second trimester, and then increases at a slower rate in the third trimester, eventually stabilizing in the last weeks of pregnancy. In the late stages of pregnancy, approximately 500 mL of blood flows through the maternal circulation to the placenta each minute, and blood volume at birth is increased approximately 45% above pre-pregnancy values to approximately 1500 mL (Cunningham et al., 2005). Increased levels of aldosterone and estrogen are primarily responsible; these hormones cause the kidneys to retain more fluid. The increased blood volume provides adequate circulation to the placenta to ensure appropriate oxygen and nutrients for the developing fetus. It also helps to compensate for the blood loss experienced during childbirth, which usually ranges from 500 to 600 mL with a vaginal birth and up to 1000 mL with a cesarean birth (Bridges et al., 2003).

Because of the increased blood volume and basal metabolic rate (BMR), maternal cardiac output increases 30% to 40% to 5 to 7 L/min, usually by approximately 27 weeks' gestation, when it plateaus until term (Luppi, 2001). Stroke volume increases approximately 50% (Luppi, 2001). The woman's pulse increases approximately 10 beats/minute, primarily in the second trimester, with minimal change during the third trimester (Guyton & Hall, 2006).

When the pregnant woman lies supine, especially in the third trimester when the fetus experiences its greatest growth spurt, she may experience what is referred to as **supine postural hypotension syndrome.** Characteristics of this syndrome include lightheadedness, faintness, and palpitations. This develops from the pressure of the gravid uterus pushing the vena cava against the vertebrae. Occlusion of the vena cava decreases blood flow

● **TABLE 12.1 Physiologic Changes in Pregnancy and Expected Time Frames**

TRIMESTER	WEEK	PHYSIOLOGIC CHANGES
First	1–2	Implantation of blastocyst
		Human chorionic gonadotropin secreted
	6	Nausea and vomiting
	8	Fetal outline visible on ultrasound
	10–12	Fetal heart audible by Doppler
	16	Changes in skin pigmentation
		Possible expression of colostrum
Second	18–20	Quickening
		Fetal heart audible on fetoscope
	20	Fetal outline palpable through abdominal wall
		Human placental lactogen secreted
Third	27	Increased blood volume, cardiac output, and pulse
		Uterine enlargement, leading to supine postural hypotension, shortness of breath, edema, hemorrhoids, and lordosis
	38	Lightening

from the extremities, causing decreased cardiac output and hypotension. Maternal hypotension is potentially dangerous because it leads to decreased placental circulation and subsequent decreased oxygen to the fetus. A preventive measure for supine postural hypotension is to tell the woman early in pregnancy to refrain from lying on her back, and instead to lie on her side or to sit upright. A corrective measure is for the woman to lie laterally, preferably on the left side, or to put a wedge under her right hip (Fig. 12.3).

Edema in the lower extremities may result from impeded venous return caused by pressure of the growing fetus on the pelvic and femoral areas (Cunningham et al., 2005). Edema worsens with dependency, especially prolonged standing or sitting. Decreased venous return also predisposes the woman to varicosities, including hemorrhoids, which the vascular relaxation resulting from circulating progesterone may exacerbate.

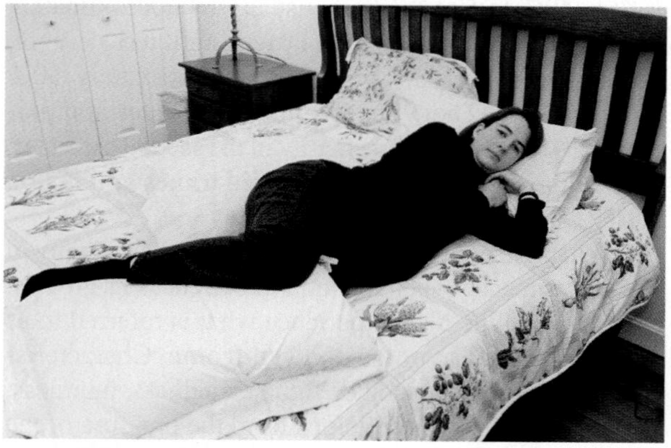

FIGURE 12.3 To avoid supine postural hypotension and to provide relief to her back, the client should lie on her side.

Hematologic System

Plasma volume increases approximately 45% to 50% by term to 1200 to 1300 mL. Erythropoiesis results from increased estrogen and progesterone and accompanies this increased fluid, resulting in an increased red blood cell (RBC) mass as the RBC volume increases 20% to 30% to 250 to 450 mL (Luppi, 2001). As the increase in RBC volume is relatively less than the increase in plasma, hemodilution results, which often is referred to as *physiologic anemia of pregnancy* (Cunningham et al., 2005, Luppi, 2001). This occurs most frequently during the second trimester; in the third trimester, plasma volume decreases, whereas the RBC mass continues to increase (Cunningham et al., 2005). For this reason, anemia is defined as less than 11 g/dL (110 g/L) in the first and third trimesters and less than 10 g/dL (100 g/L) during the second.

Most pregnant women require some iron supplementation. Women may enter pregnancy with relatively low iron stores because of the depletion that occurs during monthly menses. The fetus requires approximately 300 mg/day of iron (Beckmann et al., 2002); the woman needs an additional 500 mg/day of iron, especially in the second trimester, because of the increased circulating RBC mass (Scholl, 2005). Compounding this increased need for iron is the fact that decreased gastric acidity may impair iron absorption. Thus, many primary care providers prescribe iron supplementation during pregnancy to prevent anemia (Scholl, 2005).

The need for folic acid also increases during pregnancy to prevent maternal megaloblastic anemia (large nonfunctioning RBCs), which has been linked to an increased risk for neural tube defects (Findlay, 2000; Viteri & Berger, 2005). Because folic acid helps synthesize the DNA necessary for rapid cell growth, ideally women should begin increasing their intake at least 3 months before becoming pregnant (Health Canada, 2003). It is recommended that all women of childbearing age who could become pregnant consume 400 μg/day (0.4 mg/day) of folic acid (Health Canada, 2003; March of Dimes, 2003) (see Chap. 3). Extra folic acid also helps the woman produce additional RBCs and supports placental and fetal growth. It also may help decrease other birth defects such as cleft palate, cleft lip, and some heart defects (Findlay, 2000; van Rooij, 2004).

Respiratory System

Pregnancy affects the respiratory system most notably in the later stages. As a result of increased oxygen demands of the fetal and maternal tissues, the amount of oxygen the woman uses increases by approximately 20% by the end of pregnancy (Luppi, 2001). A corresponding amount of carbon dioxide also forms. The effect of these changes, thought to be caused by progesterone, is increased respiratory effort, occasional dyspnea, and $PaCO_2$ decreased to slightly below normal (Cunningham et al., 2005; Luppi, 2001).

The growing fetus puts pressure on and displaces the diaphragm upward (Fig. 12.4). This crowding causes a distinct feeling of shortness of breath, especially during the late stages. Once **lightening** (movement of the fetal head into the pelvis) occurs, the woman experiences relief from dyspnea and again can breathe easily.

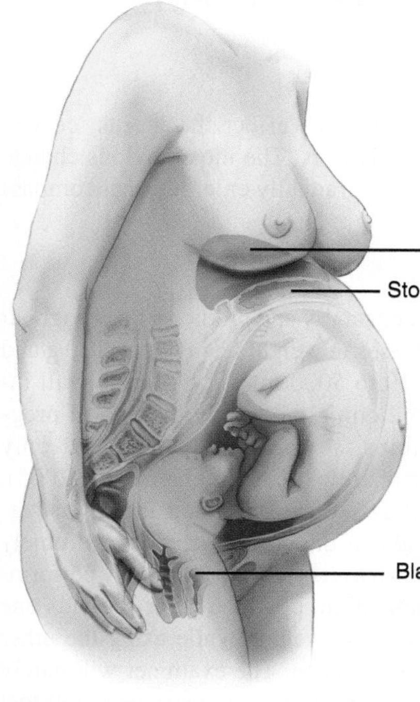

FIGURE 12.4 The growing uterus and fetus push up the liver, compress the stomach and bladder, and displace the diaphragm upward.

Gastrointestinal System

In early pregnancy, many women experience nausea and vomiting. Although researchers have hypothesized that the cause may be increased levels of human chorionic gonadotropin (hCG) and estrogen, they have not established a clear etiology. Nausea and vomiting commonly are referred to as "morning sickness" because many women experience it when first rising in the morning. Morning sickness actually is a misnomer, however, because it can occur any time of day. It usually subsides by the third month of pregnancy.

Hyperemesis gravidarum, a more severe form of nausea and vomiting, may be diagnosed in women with nausea and vomiting that lasts beyond 3 months or that imposes dangerous health effects. Examples of such effects include weight loss, dehydration, electrolyte imbalance, ketonuria, and ketonemia. Clients with this condition may require hospitalization with fluid and electrolyte replacement. Any underlying pathophysiology must be ruled out. See Chapter 13 for more discussion.

Many gastrointestinal system changes occur predominantly in the second and third trimesters. Women may experience heartburn as the growing fetus displaces the stomach. Relaxation of the cardioesophageal sphincter, resulting from effects of progesterone, also may cause reflux of gastric contents into the esophagus, adding to heartburn (Beckmann et al., 2002). Decreased intestinal motility results from pressure of the growing fetus on the intestine and the effects of progesterone, leading to constipation. The gallbladder tends to become sluggish, possibly because of the effects of progesterone on smooth muscle. Subsequent stasis of bile and the increased cholesterol levels in pregnancy may predispose women to gallstones (Lindseth & Bird-Baker, 2004).

Integumentary System

Extra pigmentation often appears, caused by increased melanocyte-stimulating hormone secreted by the pituitary and the melanocyte-stimulating effects of estrogen and progesterone (Cunningham et al., 2005; Luppi, 2001). A dark line (**linea nigra**) may be visible from just under the sternum to the pubis, separating the abdomen vertically into two hemispheres (Fig. 12.5). Darkened areas also may appear on the face, primarily over the nose and cheeks (**chloasma**). Chloasma also is referred to as the "mask of pregnancy." Once melanocyte-stimulating hormones decrease in the postpartum period, the increased pigmentation also usually disappears (Cunningham et al., 2005). Pigmentation may again appear with oral contraceptive use (Luppi, 2001).

As pregnancy advances, the abdominal skin becomes stretched. This results in small ruptures in the connective layer of the skin, leading to what are commonly referred to as "stretch marks" or **striae gravidarum.** These marks

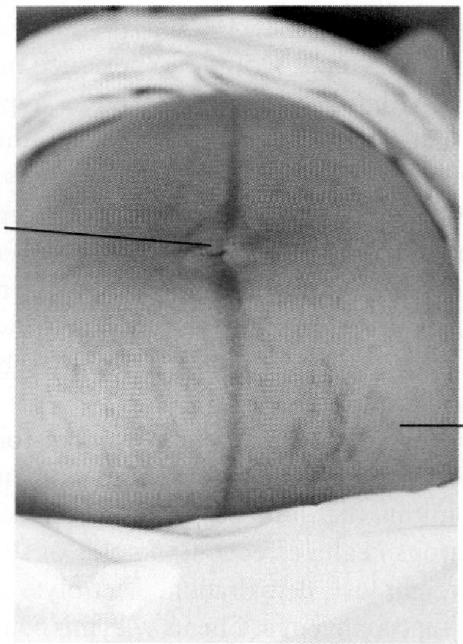

FIGURE 12.5 Skin changes in pregnancy include linea nigra and striae gravidarum.

tend to fade following birth of the baby, becoming more silver or white, although they never completely disappear (see Fig. 12.5). Striae also may appear on the breasts as they enlarge and on any other body parts with large weight gain. Some women use moisturizers, including cocoa butter, in an attempt to decrease these body changes. Some women also believe that the massage that accompanies application of these products is beneficial in preventing or decreasing skin changes.

With the progression of pregnancy, the rectus muscle may stretch to the point that it actually separates. This is known as **diastasis.** If it occurs, a pyramid shape may appear in the lower abdomen when the woman raises her head from a flat surface, as the underlying muscles protrude through the separation. If a diastasis does occur, the client should refrain from doing sit-ups until 1 to 2 weeks postpartum and avoid lifting anything heavy, both of which may exacerbate the separation or lead to development of a hernia.

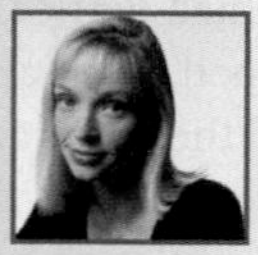

Remember Millie, the 38-year-old woman from the beginning of the chapter who just found out that she was pregnant with her third child. When performing her physical assessment, would you expect to find striae gravidarum? Why or why not?

Endocrine System

The biggest change to the endocrine system is caused by the placenta, which produces several hormones, including large amounts of estrogen and progesterone, hCG, human chorionic somatomammotropin or human placental lactogen (hPL), relaxin, and prostaglandins (Guyton & Hall, 2006).

- Estrogen causes breast and uterine enlargement.
- Progesterone helps maintain the endometrium, inhibits uterine contractility, and aids in breast development.
- The trophoblast cells of the placenta secrete hCG early in pregnancy; hCG stimulates progesterone and estrogen, which help maintain the pregnancy until the placenta can assume this function at approximately 7 weeks' gestation.
- The placenta secretes hPL at approximately 20 weeks' gestation; hPL acts as an insulin antagonist, freeing up fatty acids for energy so that glucose is available for fetal growth.
- Relaxin is responsible for softening the collagen in joints and the cervix; it also plays a role in inhibition of uterine contractions.
- Prostaglandins affect the contractibility of smooth muscle, to such an extent that some researchers theorize that a decrease in them may trigger labor (Guyton & Hall, 2006).

The thyroid gland increases up to 50% during pregnancy, causing increased release of thyroxin. Increased secretion of adrenocortical hormones, together with increased thyroxin, leads to an increased BMR (Guyton & Hall, 2006). Consequently, the pregnant woman frequently has sensations of overheating, which also is related to increased blood volume. The parathyroid gland also enlarges slightly, causing increased use of calcium and vitamin D.

Reproductive System

Pregnancy-related changes affect the uterus, cervix, ovaries, vagina, and breasts. The most obvious change is in the uterus, which gradually enlarges to encompass the growing fetus.

Uterus

The uterus grows constantly and predictably throughout pregnancy. It increases in weight from 50 to 1100 g and in capacity from 10 to 5000 mL. The uterine wall increases from 1 to 2 cm, although by the end of pregnancy the wall thins, so that it is supple and only approximately 1.5 cm thick (Cunningham et al., 2005).

At approximately 6 weeks' gestation, the lower uterine segment just above the cervix becomes extremely soft. The provider can assess for this finding by performing bimanual examination, in which he or she puts one finger of one hand in the vagina while using the other hand to palpate the abdomen. The examiner will barely be able to feel the lower uterine segment, or it will feel extremely thin. The uterus flexes easily over the cervix. This softening is referred to as **Hegar's sign** (Fig. 12.6).

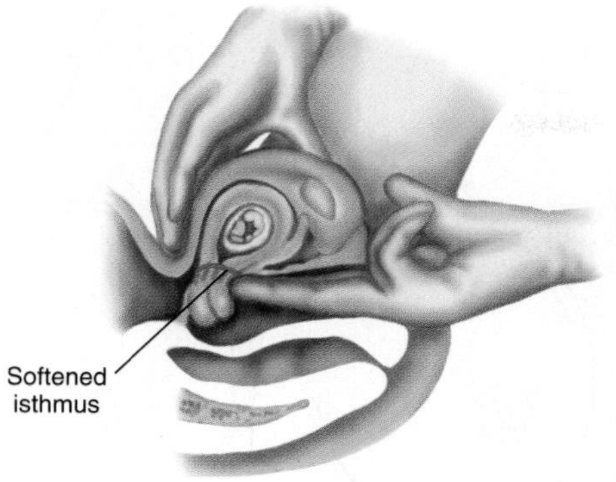

FIGURE 12.6 Hegar's sign in pregnancy is a softening of the lower uterine segment just above the cervix. Upon palpation, the area becomes difficult to feel or feels extremely thin; additionally, the uterus flexes easily over the cervix.

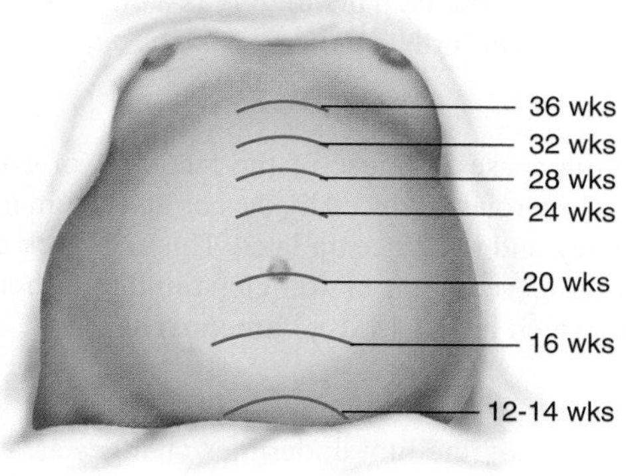

FIGURE 12.7 Fundal height corresponds to the week of gestation.

Uterine contractions begin at approximately 12 weeks' gestation and last for the duration of gestation; their strength increases as pregnancy advances. The woman may begin to feel these **Braxton-Hicks contractions,** which contribute to increased placental perfusion, as waves across the uterus in the early part of the third trimester. They are palpable and visible on monitor strips. During the last month of pregnancy, Braxton-Hicks contractions may increase so much that the client mistakes them for labor contractions. Most clients are taught about Braxton-Hicks contractions, with the expectation that they will be able to distinguish between them and true labor contractions. Research suggests, however, that teaching about Braxton-Hicks contractions before 37 weeks' gestation leads to confusion (Poole et al., 2001). Whenever the woman learns about Braxton-Hicks contractions, it is essential for nurses also to provide comprehensive education about the signs of premature labor (see Chap. 16).

By 20 to 24 weeks, the uterine wall becomes thin enough to allow a skilled examiner to palpate the fetal outline. This palpation, termed **Leopold's maneuvers,** assists providers to determine the position of the fetus. It also facilitates auscultation of the fetal heart. Both of these assessments are presented later in this chapter.

The height of the **fundus** (the top of the uterus) should correspond with the week of gestation (Fig. 12.7). For example, at 28 weeks' gestation, the distance from the pubis to the fundus should be approximately 28 cm. At 34 weeks' gestation, it should be 34 cm. At approximately 38 weeks in the primigravida, uterine height decreases to the level of its height at 36 weeks. This phenomenon, termed *lightening,* occurs as the fetal head settles into the pelvis in preparation for birth.

Health care providers can measure symphysis–fundal height in one of two ways (Fig. 12.8). Using the first method, the nurse places one end of a tape measure at the client's symphysis pubis and extends the tape up to and over the curve of the fundus. When using the second method, the nurse again places one end of the tape measure at the symphysis pubis of the woman. He or she then extends the tape up to the curve of the fundus, but stops before going over the curve. Either method is acceptable; however, all practitioners should consistently use the same method to prevent discrepancies in measurements.

Cervix

The cervix becomes more vascular and edematous in response to increased circulating estrogen from the placenta (Cunningham et al., 2005). Increased vascularity causes the cervix to become dark violet rather than pale pink. Increased fluid between the cells causes the cervix to soften; this softening, **Goodell's sign,** is significant. The consistency of the nonpregnant cervix is similar to the tip of the nose, whereas the consistency of the pregnant cervix is like that of the ear lobe. Just before labor, the cervix further softens until it can be compared to the

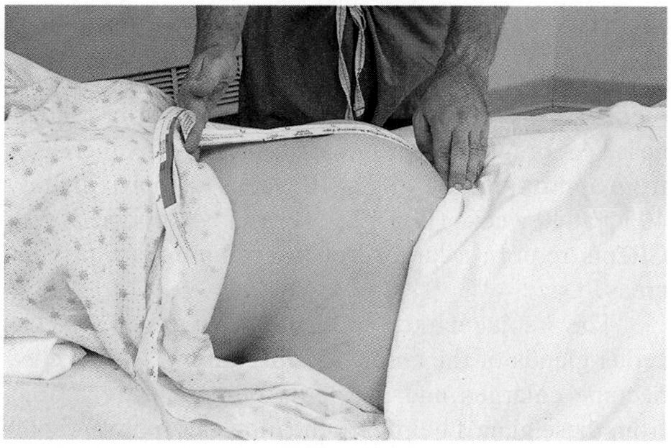

FIGURE 12.8 The nurse assesses symphysis–fundal height with a tape measure.

consistency of butter. This finding is a characteristic of being "ripe" for birth.

Ovaries

Ovulation ceases because of the feedback of estrogen and progesterone produced by the corpus luteum in early pregnancy and the placenta later. This feedback causes cessation of secretion of follicle-stimulating hormone (FSH), which in turn leads to **amenorrhea.**

Vagina

The vaginal epithelium undergoes changes as a result of circulating estrogen. Increased vascularity changes the color of the vaginal wall from the pre-pregnant pink to deep violet (**Chadwick's sign**). Increased estrogen also affects the vaginal epithelium and underlying tissue, causing them to become hypertrophic and enriched with glycogen. As the endocervical glands hypertrophy and increase, they form a tenacious coating of mucus, or **operculum.** This mucus plug serves as a barrier to prevent bacteria from entering the vagina, thus preventing infection in the fetus and membranes.

The pH of vaginal secretions changes from an alkaline value above 7 to an acidic value of 4 or 5. The primary cause is the bacteria *Lactobacillus acidophilus,* which grows in the glycogen-enriched environment (Cunningham et al., 2005). This pH change has favorable effects because it helps prevent bacterial invasion of the vagina during the pregnancy. It also, however, has unfavorable effects because it provides an environment that encourages the growth of *Candida albicans,* a yeast infection that causes itching, burning, and a white, cheesy discharge. Although treatment of *C. albicans* primarily aims to promote comfort, it is also necessary to prevent transmission to the newborn as he or she passes through the vaginal canal at birth. Treatment may include miconazole (Monistat), clotrimazole (Gyne-Lotrimin), or nystatin (Cunningham et al., 2005).

Breasts

Breast changes result from high levels of circulating estrogen and progesterone and increased blood flow (Murray, 2003). During the first trimester, women may report such symptoms as tingling, fullness, or tenderness. As pregnancy progresses, breast size increases from approximately 45 g at 10 weeks to approximately 405 g at 40 weeks (Fig. 12.9) (Fraser & Cooper, 2003). Clients require a larger bra to accommodate this increased size.

The areolae darken and increase in size. The sebaceous glands of the areola (**Montgomery's tubercles**) become enlarged and may be protuberant. Secretions from these glands help keep the nipples supple and prevent drying and cracking during lactation. Blue veins may become prominent over the breasts as vascularity to the area increases. By 16 weeks, the nipples may begin to express *colostrum,* the thin, watery, high-protein fluid that is the precursor to breast milk (see Chap. 21).

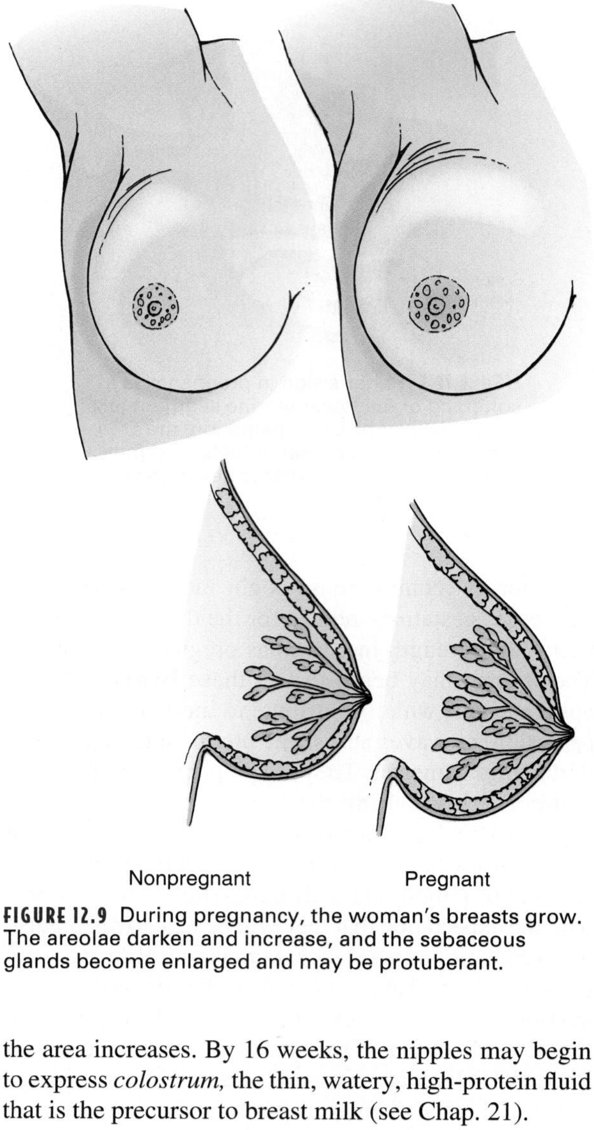

FIGURE 12.9 During pregnancy, the woman's breasts grow. The areolae darken and increase, and the sebaceous glands become enlarged and may be protuberant.

Urinary System

During the first trimester, the pregnant woman may experience urinary frequency until the uterus rises out of the pelvis and relieves pressure on the bladder. Such frequency returns in the later stages of pregnancy as lightening occurs and the fetal head again puts pressure on the bladder (Fig. 12.10).

Total body water increases by approximately 6.5 L by the end of pregnancy (Cunningham et al., 2005). During pregnancy, the woman's kidneys must filter not only the maternal but also the fetal waste products. The kidneys also must be able to handle the increased renal blood flow. Kidney size increases approximately 1.5 cm (Luppi, 2001). Glomerular filtration rate (GFR) and renal plasma flow begin to increase in early pregnancy to meet the increased need of the circulatory system. By the beginning of the second trimester, the GFR has in-

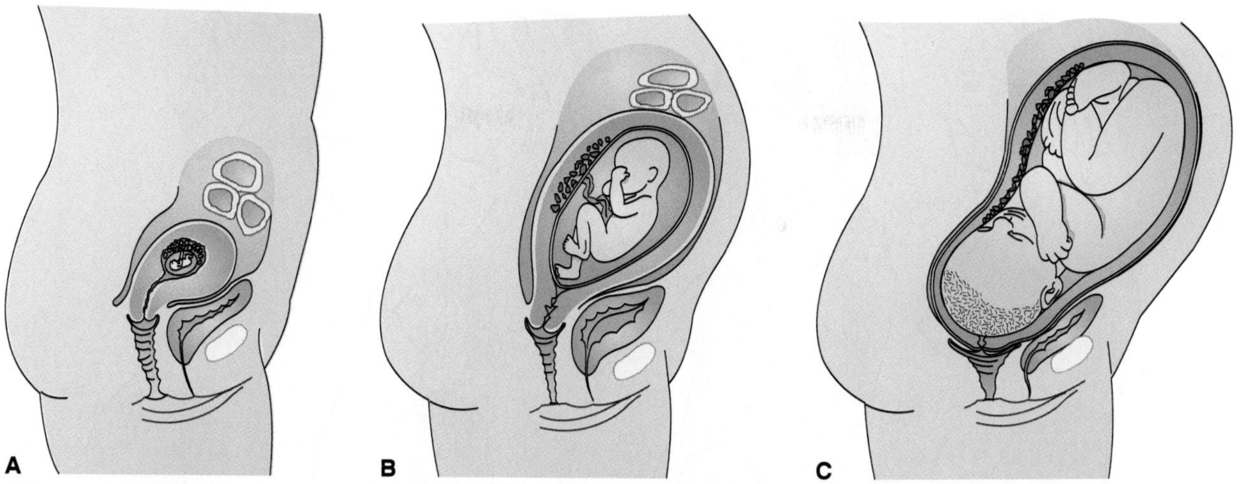

FIGURE 12.10 Urinary frequency in pregnancy is related to the changing position of the uterus as the fetus grows. (**A**) In early pregnancy, pressure of the uterus against the bladder leads to increased urinary frequency. (**B**) In the second trimester, the uterine position changes so that bladder pressure is relieved. (**C**) Toward the end of pregnancy, the uterus once again is pressing on the bladder, leading to increased frequency.

creased approximately 50% and will remain at this level for the rest of the pregnancy (Cunningham et al., 2005; Luppi, 2001). The renal plasma flow increases by 30% to 60% at the same time but will decrease during late pregnancy to term, where it will be approximately 50% above that of the nonpregnant woman (Cunningham et al., 2005; Luppi, 2001). As a result of these increases, blood urea nitrogen (BUN) and serum creatinine levels decrease. Amino acids and water-soluble vitamins are lost in greater amounts in the urine.

The increased GFR, antidiuretic hormone (ADH), prostaglandins, and progesterone and decreased vascular resistance cause the woman to excrete sodium. The body increases its sodium reabsorption in the tubules to aid in maintenance of osmolarity. Progesterone causes an increased response of the renin-angiotensin-aldosterone system, which leads to increased aldosterone production, which in turn aids sodium resorption. Estrogen and cortisol also have an effect on increasing sodium absorption (Cunningham et al., 2005; Luppi, 2001).

The higher GFR leads to increased filtration of glucose into the renal tubules. Because resorption of glucose by the tubule cells occurs at a fixed rate, some glucose will accidentally spill into the urine during pregnancy. As well, glucose is spilled into the urine at lower levels of serum glucose.

The ureters increase in diameter because of the increased progesterone level. Ureteral compression from the enlarging uterus and ovarian vein plexus and pressure of the ureters against the pelvic brim may lead to hydronephrosis and hydroureter (Cunningham et al., 2005). Pressure on the urethra may lead to poor bladder emptying and subsequent bladder infection. During later gestation, the enlarging uterus may cause pressure on the bladder that may lead to urinary stasis and pyelonephritis if not relieved. These infections are significant because each increases the risk for preterm labor (Maloni, 2000).

Musculoskeletal System

Calcium and magnesium needs increase because the fetal bones are forming and plasma levels are low. Calcium intake should be 1300 mg/day in pregnant women 18 years or younger and 1000 mg/day in pregnant women older than 18 years (National Institutes of Health [NIH], 2003). Magnesium intake should be 400 mg/day in pregnant women 18 years and younger and 350 mg/day in women older than 18 years (NIH, 2003). Calcium supplements have been shown to protect infants against low birth weight (Merialdi et al., 2003). Some studies have shown calcium supplementation as effective in reducing the incidence of pre-eclampsia (Merialdi et al., 2003), whereas others have found no effect (Roberts et al., 2003).

As pregnancy progresses, the pelvic joints become more pliable under the influence of relaxin. This increased flexibility facilitates delivery of the fetus but also may cause discomfort to the woman. Sometimes the symphysis pubis separates up to 3 to 4 mm, leading to difficulty walking.

The increasing weight of the fetus and protrusion of the belly cause lordosis, an abnormal forward curvature of the spine in the lumbar region, as the woman attempts to maintain a center of gravity (Fig. 12.11). She may subsequently experience a chronic backache.

Physiologic Differences Related to Age and Race/Ethnicity

Many physiologic changes during pregnancy are common to all women regardless of age, race, or ethnicity.

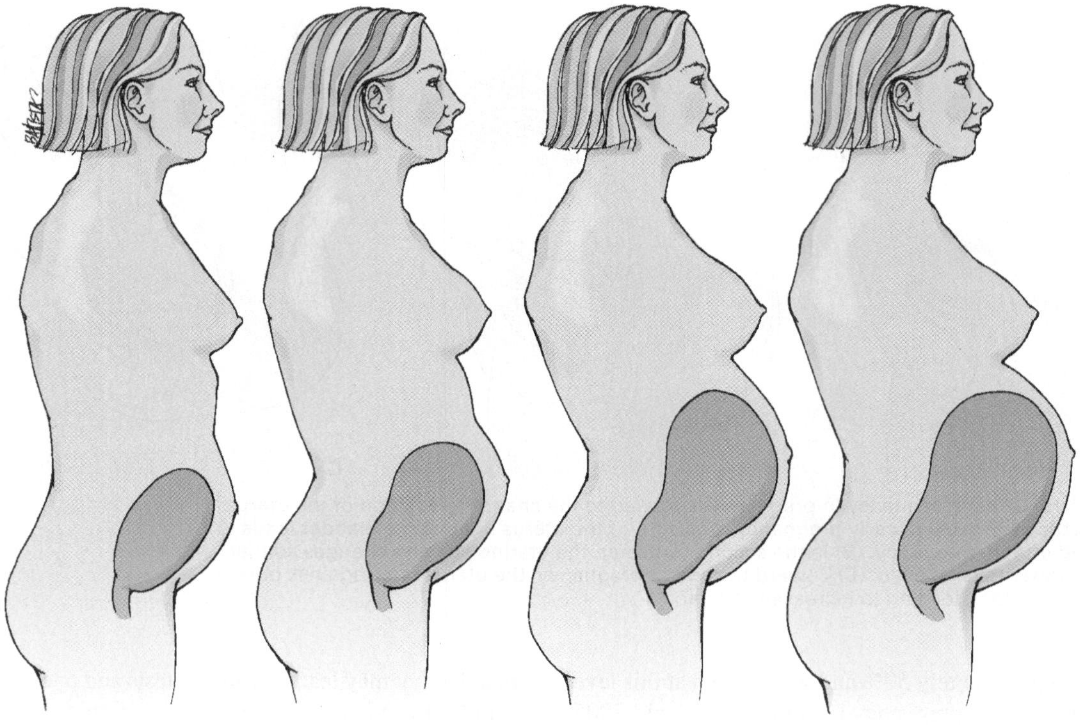

FIGURE 12.11 Progressive maternal postural changes in pregnancy.

Some differences, however, are unique to certain age groups or to people of specific race or ethnicity.

Adolescent mothers who have not yet completed their own growth may be at increased risk for related complications, including **cephalopelvic disproportion** (CPD), which increases the risk for cesarean birth. They are at increased risk for low-birth-weight babies, preterm labor, and pregnancy-induced hypertension (PIH), although some studies suggest that the risk for PIH is more related to parity than age (Barron, 2001; Stevens-Simon et al., 2002). These risks are increased with younger adolescents, especially those who conceive within 2 years of menarche (Stevens-Simon et al., 2002). Risks such as inadequate nutrition, poor health, and those related to poverty also may have negative effects on a pregnancy (Stevens-Simon et al., 2002).

Women older than 35 years have higher incidences of preexisting conditions, such as diabetes and hypertension (Ozalp et al., 2003). Preexisting hypertension increases the risk for developing abruptio placentae and pregnancy-induced hypertension, which may lead to low-birth-weight infants (Poole et al., 2001). The risk for cesarean birth is increased for these women (Kozinsky et al., 2002). Questions have been raised about whether the increased rate of preterm and cesarean birth is related to a higher incidence of maternal complications or simply age (Kozinsky et al., 2002; Tough et al., 2002).

Little research exists that identifies differences among minority groups or the prevalence of alterations among women of childbearing age within these groups. Mexican American women usually give birth to infants with higher birth weights than African American and European American women with similar risk factors (Berry, 1999). Low-birth-weight infants born to Mexican American women, however, have a higher mortality rate than either of the other two groups. One study (Braveman et al., 2001) found that African American women were three times more likely and Asian American women twice as likely to give birth to a low-birth-weight infant than European American women, regardless of age, parity, education, or poverty level.

Several diseases or alterations that may affect pregnancy seem to be prevalent in women of childbearing age from different ethnic or racial backgrounds. The incidence of diabetes is increased in American Indian and African American women. Tuberculosis is more prevalent in American Indian and Asian women. Preexisting hypertension is more frequent in African American women, as is sickle cell anemia. Tay-Sachs disease is more common in the Ashkenazi Jewish population. Thalassemia is most common in those from the Mediterranean, Middle East, and Southeast Asia (Callister, 2001b). See Chapter 4 for more discussion.

African American women have a higher risk for dying from pregnancy-related causes such as hemorrhage, pregnancy-induced hypertension, and pulmonary embolism than do white women (Anachebe & Sutton, 2003). Some reasons that have been hypothesized for this difference include differences in access to care and the quality and content of that care (Anachebe & Sutton, 2003). African American women and women of other ethnic minorities have a higher rate of infant mortality than do white women.

PSYCHOLOGICAL AND EMOTIONAL CHANGES IN PREGNANCY

Many psychological changes for the client and her significant others are common throughout pregnancy. Even if a pregnancy is planned, many women are surprised to find themselves actually pregnant. They may feel somewhat ambivalent, questioning whether the timing is right or how they should modify career plans. A client may experience fears about the pregnancy, labor, and birth. If the pregnancy is unintended, these feelings may be more pronounced. Such clients may consider the possibility of abortion or other alternatives in the early months of the unwanted pregnancy (Finer et al., 2005). Still other clients are overjoyed to learn that they are pregnant, particularly if they experienced problems conceiving or waited a long time to try.

QUOTE 12-1

"I keep vacillating between being incredibly excited and happy to being terrified about the responsibility of being a parent."

A woman who has just found out she is expecting

Reactions of Woman and Partner

During the first trimester, the pregnancy may not seem real to the pregnant woman. She may have little evidence other than amenorrhea and confirmation of a positive pregnancy test from her caregiver that she is actually pregnant. As a consequence, she may become conscious of any body changes that lend additional support to validate the pregnancy. Both the woman and her partner may feel somewhat overwhelmed by the mood swings the woman may experience (Driscoll, 2001).

The second trimester of pregnancy often is more idyllic than the first. Problems with morning sickness usually have passed, the threat of spontaneous abortion is decreased, and the woman frequently will have seen the outline of the fetus on an ultrasound to confirm that there actually is a pregnancy. Women, particularly primigravidas, may choose to wear maternity clothes before truly needing them as outward confirmation of the pregnancy. Alternatively, some women experience feelings of grief at the loss of usual body shape and size. One highlight of the second trimester is quickening, which usually occurs at approximately 20 weeks' gestation. This provides proof to the woman that there is an actual baby and promotes bonding with him or her (Driscoll, 2001). The nurse needs to be sure that he or she is not projecting onto the woman and her significant others how they should feel. Sometimes, ambivalence remains, or expected feelings do not occur. This is also a time when the partner can be more involved in the pregnancy. Feeling the baby's movements and hearing the fetal heart during visits to the care provider help to increase the partner's involvement.

During the third trimester, the woman often experiences mounting apprehension about what is to come (Driscoll, 2001). Physical discomforts return as the baby grows. The mother begins to prepare for the birth of the baby. Both parents are more involved in planning for labor and birth. This may be when they attend prenatal classes together. The partner may feel increased concern for the woman as she becomes more uncomfortable and the end of the pregnancy nears. Near the end of the pregnancy, the woman often experiences a surge of energy (Pillitteri, 2007). She may use this increased energy to clean and organize the home. The nurse should inform the mother about this phenomenon and encourage her to resist the temptation to work, resting instead to save her energy for the stress of the labor ahead. In the weeks leading up to her due date, she may want to consider preparing meals ahead of time and freezing them to be used in the early days after her return home postpartum.

Reactions of Grandparents-to-Be

The parents of the pregnant woman (and her partner) also must accept the reality of the pregnancy and the coming grandchild. They often provide support and may become closer to their children, especially the pregnant woman. Nevertheless, grandparents also have adaptations to make for themselves. They may be unsure about the level of involvement that is expected during the pregnancy, birth, and after (Pillitteri, 2007). They may have issues of their own that influence their interest in and involvement with the expectant parents and the experience. They may live a considerable distance away from the expectant family, which curtails their involvement. Younger grandparents-to-be often continue to work and to be involved in other activities that may limit their available time and interest. They also may have some adjustments to make in accepting the pregnancy and the fact that they will be grandparents, feeling that they are too young for the role. Other issues such as retirement, death of friends, or menopause of the grandmother may influence reactions and subsequent involvement with the pregnancy and child. Nurses should remain sensitive to any cultural patterns of communication or interaction that may influence the plan of care.

Reactions of Other Children

The idea of a younger sibling coming into the family may present challenges for other children. There is no "best" time to accomplish this; however, the introduction of the coming addition of the sibling should be based on the age, developmental level, and experience of the other children. Parents should tell the child about the coming baby before or when they tell other family members to decrease any risk that they will hear the news accidentally or from someone else. Depending on the child's age, it may be most appropriate to begin actions to minimize potential sibling rivalry early in the pregnancy. Children who are very young may experience anxiety and frustration when the expectant mother is more fatigued. The child may feel deprived of attention. Young children need consistency. They need to know that familiar places, people, and things will continue once the new baby arrives. If planning for the new arrival involves moving children from a crib to another bed, parents should do so at a minimum of several weeks before the baby's birth.

Young toddlers frequently show regressive behavior, reverting to thumb sucking, wanting to drink from a bottle, or wetting or soiling after toilet training. One possible reason is because the toddler sees the new baby getting attention for doing these things (Pillitteri, 2007). If the new parents are aware of this possibility, they are much less frustrated if it occurs.

Families should include school-aged children in the pregnancy as it progresses. They should provide information in a quantity and at a level appropriate for the child's developmental stage and interest. Feeling fetal movements, listening to the fetal heart, and attending sibling preparation classes help children to feel that they are part of the pregnancy (Fig. 12.12).

Older children and adolescents may appear to be knowledgeable but have many misconceptions. They may feel uncomfortable with the evidence of their parents' sexuality or may worry about changes to the family structure. They may be concerned that they will be expected to shoulder additional responsibilities. Parents should provide the older child or adolescent the opportunity to voice their concerns. They should create opportunities for them to be involved in the preparation for the new child.

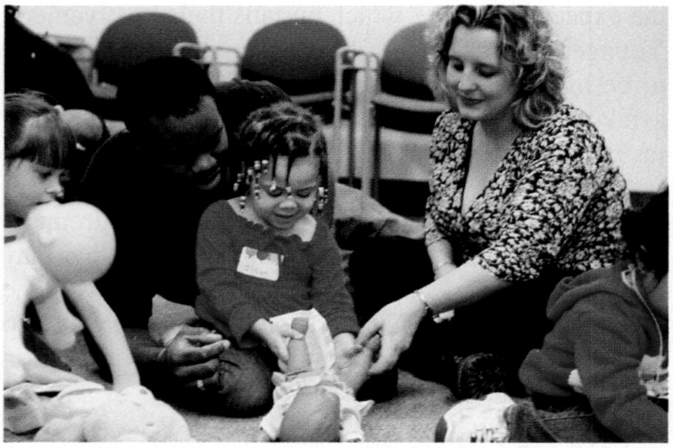

FIGURE 12.12 Sibling preparation classes can help children adjust to the changes in their family and make them feel like they are part of the experience.

Changing attitudes and facility policies frequently allow children to be present at the child's birth. This changing practice facilitates involvement of siblings in the birth and feeling a part of the process. Children often attend classes that prepare them to be present at the birth. In addition to the positive aspects of involving the children, however, negative aspects also may arise. Children may become frightened or upset at seeing their mother in pain. A specific person should be designated to provide support to the children during the labor and birth. If the children cannot continue to be present, this person should provide support and care to them. Following the birth, parents need to continue to focus on assisting children to feel that they are part of the family.

SIGNS OF PREGNANCY

Several changes that women experience are used to diagnose pregnancy. These include *presumptive* or subjective signs, *probable* or objective signs, and *positive* or diagnostic signs.

Presumptive Signs

Presumptive signs of pregnancy are those subjective changes the woman herself experiences. They do not confirm a pregnancy because other factors also may cause them. In conjunction with other signs, however, they can be diagnostic.

The first sign that women generally experience is amenorrhea. In a woman with regular cycles, one or two missed menstrual periods suggest pregnancy. Another presumptive sign is **"morning sickness,"** nausea and vomiting that often occurs in the morning and fades during the day. Women actually may experience variations in nausea and vomiting, however, which range from distaste of certain foods or odors, vomiting throughout the day, or vomiting at night. Nausea and vomiting usually appear 6 weeks after the first day of the last menstrual period and last for approximately 6 to 12 weeks, ending with the beginning of the second trimester. Occasionally, nausea and vomiting are prolonged beyond this time frame.

Excessive fatigue may begin within a few weeks after the first day of the last menstrual period and may be present during the entire first trimester. Women in the first trimester also may experience urinary frequency, which develops as the enlarging uterus exerts pressure on the bladder. This will diminish as the uterus rises in the abdomen, returning again near the end of pregnancy.

QUOTE 12-2

"I was prepared to feel nauseous, but that wasn't a big problem for me. Instead, I felt completely exhausted all the time for the first 4 months!"

A client recounting her pregnancy experience

The woman may notice breast changes, including enlargement, tingling sensations, and tenderness, during the first few weeks of pregnancy. Pigmentation of the nipples and areolae also may change, along with increased visibility of the veins, especially in those women with fair skin, occurring after the second month.

The woman may experience **quickening,** the first perception of fetal movement. Clients often describe quickening as a fluttering in the abdomen that increases in frequency and duration until the movements become perceptible as distinct fetal movements that will continue throughout the pregnancy. Quickening usually occurs between 16 and 20 weeks' gestation (Cunningham et al., 2005).

Probable Signs

Probable signs of pregnancy are those objective changes assessed by the examiner. Even though they are more diagnostic than presumptive signs, they are not a definitive diagnosis—again, probable signs may result from other factors.

Changes to the uterus and vagina are the only probable signs detectable in the first trimester. They include softening of the cervix (Goodell's sign); the dark violet coloration of the cervix, vagina, and vulva (Chadwick's sign); and the softening of the lower part of the uterus between the cervix and the body (Hegar's sign). Increased circulation to the area and circulating estrogen cause these changes, which usually are evident by 6 to 8 weeks' gestation.

Progressive uterine enlargement, especially accompanied by continuing amenorrhea, is usually evidence of pregnancy. This enlargement may be more pronounced in multigravidas, whose abdominal musculature has lost some tone from previous pregnancies. The fundus of the uterus is palpable just above the symphysis pubis at 10 to 12 weeks' gestation and at the level of the umbilicus at 20 to 22 weeks. The examiner may use Leopold's maneuvers to feel the fetal outline beginning at approximately 24 weeks' gestation. Abdominal palpation may reveal Braxton-Hicks contractions at approximately the 28th week.

The hCG appears in the serum of pregnant women shortly after implantation of the fertilized oocyte, reaching measurable levels 8 to 9 days after ovulation (Guyton & Hall, 2006). The hCG level peaks between 60 to 70 days' gestation and then declines until about 100 to 130 days when the level reaches its lowest point (Cunningham et al., 2005). Pregnancy tests are based on maternal blood or urine tests assessing for hCG. Blood serum tests are used more frequently than urine tests because hCG is detected earlier in serum and therefore results can be obtained earlier. One of two techniques is generally used to detect hCG levels: radioimmunoassay (RIA) or enzyme-linked immunosorbent assay (ELISA) (Table 12.2). Findings of these tests are considered probable rather than positive because luteinizing hormone, secreted by the pituitary, is similar to hCG and can sometimes cause a false-positive result. As well, conditions other than pregnancy can cause increased hCG.

Several different over-the-counter home pregnancy kits are available that manufacturers indicate are up to 97% accurate if used exactly according to directions. Varying degrees of accuracy, however, have been reported (Consumer Reports, 2003). These tests are based on recognition of hCG in the urine (Wilcox et al., 2001). The woman dips the reagent strip into her urine stream or into a container containing her urine. If she detects a color change on the strip or a line appears, the result is

TABLE 12.2 Pregnancy Tests

TEST	COMPONENTS	RESULTS
RIA (radioimmunoassay test)	This assay is usually done in a laboratory setting. Radioactively labeled markers bind with AB against hCG. The test is dependent on competition between this radiolabeled AB and nonradiolabeled hCG in the blood sample tested. "Free" and "bound" are then separated and the unbound radioactivity is assayed.	Standard curves predict how much hCG will be present at varying times in the pregnancy. The results of the RIA are compared with these standard curves.
ELISA (enzyme-linked immunosorbent assay test)	Uses a monoclonal AB bound to a solid-phase support (usually plastic), which binds the hCG in the test sample. A second AB is added to "sandwich" the test sample hCG. It is the second AB to which an enzyme, such as alkaline phosphatase, is linked. When substrate for this enzyme is added, a blue color develops.	The intensity of the blue color is proportional to the amount of enzyme and thus to the amount of second AB bound and the amount of hCG in the test sample.

AB, antibody; hCG, human chorionic gonadotropin.

From Cunningham, F. G., Gant, N. F., Leveno, K. J., Bloom, S. L., Hauth, J. C., Gillstrap, L. C. III, & Wenstrom, K. D. (2005). *Williams obstetrics* (22nd ed.). New York: McGraw-Hill.

positive (Cunningham et al., 2005). The indicated time frame of the test is 3 to 5 minutes.

Most manufacturers suggest the woman wait until the day of her missed menstrual period to test; if done too early, results are unreliable. Some pregnancy tests on the market suggest that they can detect hCG at lower levels and thus test for pregnancy as early as 6 to 8 days after conception (see http://www.at-home-pregnancy-tests.com/pregnancytests.html and http://www.early-pregnancy-tests.com/pregnancytests.html). It may be difficult to accurately predict, however, when conception has actually occurred. Implantation does not always occur before the expected onset of menses, nor is the hCG level produced this early in sufficient amounts for home pregnancy kits to detect. Even using a pregnancy test approximately 100 times more sensitive than home pregnancy tests in detecting for hCG, Wilcox and colleagues (2001) found that not all pregnancies resulted in a positive pregnancy test by the first day of the missed period.

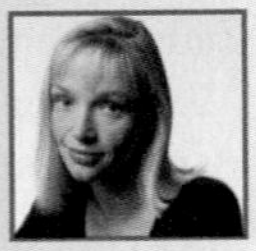

Millie has just found out that she is 12 weeks pregnant. What probable signs would you expect Millie to have exhibited that suggest pregnancy?

Before the advent of home pregnancy kits, women had to visit their health care provider to find out if they were pregnant. Because it is now possible for women to do pregnancy tests at home, they may delay accessing prenatal care. The nurse should encourage early and regular prenatal care once a client has identified probable signs of pregnancy. He or she should instruct the client that a positive pregnancy test result confirms only that trophoblastic tissue has secreted hCG. The test does not provide positive confirmation of either pregnancy or its location. For example, gestational trophoblastic neoplasia (an uncommon but serious cancer that secretes hCG) results in a positive pregnancy test with no accompanying pregnancy. An ectopic pregnancy also may produce a positive result and may be missed if the woman does not seek early prenatal care. The client should discontinue use of oral contraceptives at least 5 days before the test to prevent false-positive results.

Because of the possibility of false-negative results with home pregnancy tests, a provider must further evaluate any negative test result when the woman continues to show other signs of pregnancy.

Evaluation should focus on the response of the client and her significant others. The nurse should recognize that a range of responses is possible. Whether the pregnancy is intended or not, reactions vary widely. Clients may experience joy, excitement, ambivalence, apprehension, or fear, even if a pregnancy was intended. Reactions may depend on past experiences with pregnancy, stories relayed by others, and anticipation. The nurse and client should plan further care based on this evaluation.

If a pregnancy is unintended or unwanted, the woman may consider abortion as an option in the early months (see Chap. 9). If the pregnancy is unwanted and therapeutic abortion is not an option, the woman may consider adoption as an alternative. The nurse should provide consultations with other health care workers, including social workers, to enable the woman to obtain additional information about the options available and to make preliminary plans.

Positive Signs

Positive signs are those signs that absolutely confirm pregnancy: a fetal heart, fetal movements that the examiner can feel, and visualization of the fetus on ultrasound. Positive signs are completely objective and cannot result from any other cause or pathology. They usually are undetectable until the third month at the earliest.

An examiner may hear the fetal heart or see it on ultrasound (Fig. 12.13). The fetal heart is detectable by ultrasound Doppler as early as 8 to 12 weeks' gestation (Cunningham et al., 2005). It can be detected by 17 to 19 weeks on auscultation with a stethoscope or fetoscope (Cunningham et al., 2005). Normal at a rate of 120 to

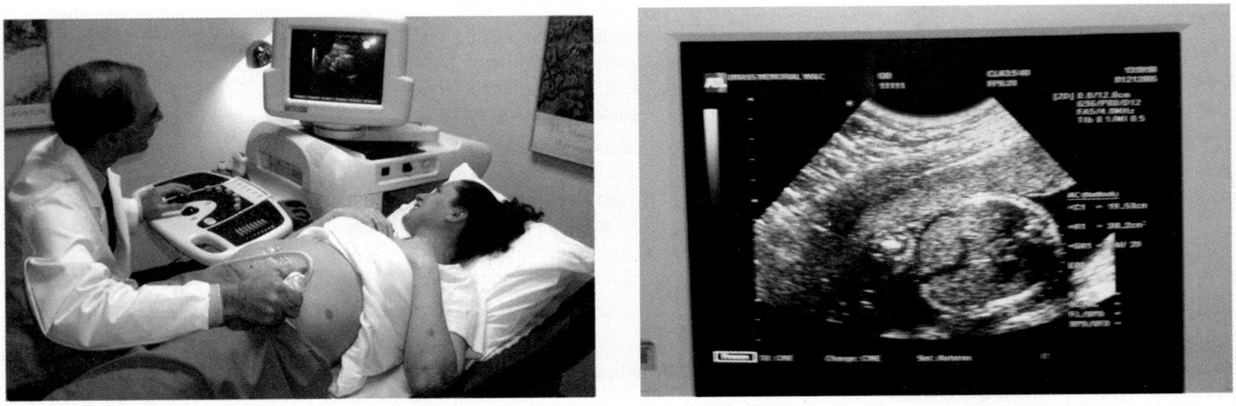

FIGURE 12.13 The appearance of the fetal heart on ultrasound is a positive sign of pregnancy.

160 beats/minute, it is best heard over the fetus's back. Movement of the fetal heart first occurs at approximately the fourth week and can be detected by echocardiography as early as 48 days after the first day of the last normal menses or by transvaginal sonography (see Chap. 11) by the fifth week (Cunningham et al., 2005).

Auscultation of the abdomen over the uterus may reveal the uterine soufflé. This soft swooshing sound results from the flow of the increased blood volume and vascularity of the uterus and placenta. Because the rate of the uterine soufflé matches the maternal pulse, the examiner should palpate the radial pulse of the mother simultaneously with auscultation of the abdomen. If it is the uterine soufflé that is heard, the beats of the soufflé will match the palpated maternal pulse beats. If the beats that are heard do not match the palpated maternal pulse beats, the examiner can be confident that he or she is hearing the fetal heart tones. This assessment is essential because fetal heart rate (FHR) may be diminished in periods of fetal distress.

An examiner usually can feel fetal movements after 20 weeks' gestation (Cunningham et al., 2005), although maternal obesity may interfere until later in the pregnancy when the fetus is larger. If ultrasound is done at 4 to 6 weeks, a gestational sac may be seen, which confirms the pregnancy.

ANTEPARTAL HEALTH ASSESSMENT

Health care providers offer information about assessment findings and their meanings to the pregnant client and her designated significant others. They use information gathered during assessments to plan individualized care throughout the pregnancy and for labor and birth. Nurses also provide information about anticipated changes to assist the client and family to plan interventions related to such changes.

Assessment of maternal health is an extremely important part of care, both at the initial prenatal visit and throughout pregnancy. Any alterations in maternal health pose concerns for the woman's well-being and can also potentially hinder fetal growth, development, and well-being, thus requiring close monitoring. Nurses and other health care providers can identify risk factors that may pose problems for the woman, fetus, or both during pregnancy, labor, and birth. They can then plan care to decrease such risks. Continuing prenatal care can identify additional risk factors that may not exist or manifest themselves at the first visit and assist the health care team to ensure healthy pregnancy outcomes.

Initial Prenatal Maternal Health Assessment

Once a client identifies herself to a health care practitioner as believing she is pregnant, the provider should perform an assessment to confirm the pregnancy. Nurses and other health care providers should conduct a thorough assessment (history taking and physical examination) of the pregnant client at the first prenatal visit. The health history should cover a complete menstrual, sexual, and pregnancy history; family history of the woman to determine whether any familial or genetic disorders may affect maternal or fetal health (see Chap. 11); history of any previous pregnancies and births; and past illnesses. The physical examination should be comprehensive, with accompanying laboratory and diagnostic evaluations.

If pregnancy is not confirmed, the provider should assess for alternative causes of the identified symptoms (Table 12.3). The nurse should educate the pregnant client about relief measures for symptoms to promote comfort as much as possible.

Health History

During the first prenatal visit, a comprehensive health history provides a wealth of information that nurses and other health care providers use to assess risks associated with the pregnancy, plan appropriate care, and help ensure positive outcomes. The woman's physical and emotional health before pregnancy is as important as her physical and emotional health during gestation. Assessment Tool 12.1 provides a suggested organization for a thorough health history, along with rationales and recommended questions.

Menstrual History. The nurse should obtain the client's menstrual history, which includes age at onset of menarche; frequency, regularity, duration, and amount of blood loss with normal menstrual periods; any history of dysmenorrhea; and date of the first day of the last normal menstrual period. This portion of the history helps identify any irregularities in the client's normal menses that may affect calculation of the estimated date of delivery (EDD). Irregular menstrual periods often correspond with irregular ovulation; in such cases, the EDD may be less reliable. It is also important to identify that the last menstrual period was normal. Some clients experience bleeding with implantation and may misinterpret this event as a menstrual period.

Sexual and Sexually Transmitted Infection (STI) History. An appropriate sexual history includes type of birth control used and when the woman discontinued it. Recent use of hormonal contraception (eg, oral contraceptives) may delay ovulation, which may affect calculation of the EDD. Use of an intrauterine device (IUD), if still in place, may threaten the integrity of the pregnancy and increases the risk for spontaneous abortion, sepsis, and preterm birth (Cunningham et al., 2005). Failure to use a latex condom may, depending on the situation, increase risks for HIV and other STIs. A pregnancy that occurs despite use of contraception may necessitate discussion of the desirability of the pregnancy.

The nurse should identify any history of STIs, which may be transmitted through sexual intercourse or sexual

● **TABLE 12.3 Signs of Pregnancy and Possible Alternative Explanations**

SIGNS OF PREGNANCY	POSSIBLE ALTERNATIVE EXPLANATIONS
Presumptive Signs	
Amenorrhea	Endocrine disorder Lactation Malnutrition, including anorexia nervosa or bulimia Excessive exercise Emotional stress Early menopause
Nausea and vomiting	Gastrointestinal disorders Emotional stress Acute infection
Fatigue	Lack of sleep Overexertion Anemia Other illnesses
Urinary frequency	Urinary tract infection Cystocele Emotional stress
Breast changes	Premenstrual changes Chronic cystic mastitis Breast cysts
Quickening	Increased peristalsis Flatus Abdominal muscle contractions
Probable Signs	
Goodell's sign	Estrogen–progesterone contraceptive pill
Chadwick's sign	Increased vascular congestion
Hegar's sign	Other hormonal influences Anatomically soft walls of nonpregnant uterus
Enlarged uterus	Uterine tumor Uterine fibroids
Braxton-Hicks contractions	Hematomas Soft myoma
Changes in pigmentation	Contraceptives
Positive pregnancy test results	Luteinizing hormone secreted by pituitary Gestational trophoblastic neoplasia Ectopic pregnancy

contact with the genitals, rectum, or mouth. STIs also may be transmitted in other ways. These STIs include gonorrhea; syphilis; HIV; human papillomavirus (HPV), which commonly manifests as genital warts; herpes simplex virus (HSV), which causes genital herpes; chlamydia; hepatitis B and C; and vaginitis, which may be caused by organisms such as trichomonas and *C. albicans*. Identification of a history of STIs is important because it may affect care planned during pregnancy and delivery.

Along with the risks for cervical and other cancers, chronic hepatitis, cirrhosis, and other complications common for all women, pregnant women have additional consequences that may arise from STIs, which may be apparent at birth or appear at a later date. Pregnancies complicated by STIs have an increased risk for stillbirth, preterm labor, low birth weight, conjunctivitis, pneumonia, neonatal sepsis, neurologic damage, congenital abnormalities, and meningitis (CDC, 2004; Cunningham et al., 2005). Congenital abnormalities may include blindness, deafness, or other organ damage.

Mothers can transmit STIs to newborns before, during, or after birth. For example, syphilis can cross the placenta and infect the fetus, causing congenital syphilis (Carey, 2003). Gonorrhea, chlamydia, and genital herpes are transmitted as the infant passes through the birth canal during delivery (Dapaah & Dapaah, 2003).

HIV can cross the placental barrier and infect the fetus. Medication is available to help decrease fetal

ASSESSMENT TOOL 12.1 Prenatal Health Assessment Form

MENSTRUAL HISTORY

RATIONALE *Identify irregularities in normal menstrual cycle that may affect calculation of estimated date of delivery (EDD).*

Suggested questions:

- Tell me about your normal menstrual cycle.
- Tell me about your last menstrual period. When did it occur? Was it the same as or different from your normal periods?
- When did you begin to menstruate?
- How frequently do you get your menstrual period?
- Do your cycles stay the same or change from month to month? Is there any variation between cycles?
- How many days does your period normally last?
- How many pads/tampons do you saturate each day?

SEXUAL HISTORY

RATIONALE *Recent use of birth control pills may delay ovulation. An IUD in place increases risk for spontaneous abortion or ectopic pregnancy. Early identification of sexually transmitted infections will prevent prolonged fetal exposure to effects of infection and will facilitate planning of appropriate care.*

Suggested questions:

- Tell me about what type of birth control you have been using.
- When did you discontinue using it?
- Tell me about any sexually transmitted infections you may have had.
- Have you ever had gonorrhea (clap), syphilis, HIV, genital warts, genital herpes, chlamydia, or hepatitis? If you have, describe when and how you were treated.
- Has your partner ever had any of these infections? If so, describe when and how your partner was treated.
- Have you ever had a vaginal infection? If you have, tell me about what it was like and how it was treated.
- How many sexual partners have you had?
- Have you ever had unprotected sex? If you have, tell me when this happened.

PAST PREGNANCY HISTORY

RATIONALE *A history of past pregnancies helps identify potential complications in the current pregnancy. A history of past labors and births will assist in planning for the current pregnancy.*

Suggested questions:

- Tell me about any other pregnancies you have had.
- How many other pregnancies have you had?
- What dates were your children born?
- Have you had any babies that were premature or born earlier than they were supposed to be?
- How early were they born?
- Have you had any miscarriages or abortions? If you had a therapeutic abortion, how was it done and were there any complications?
- How far along were you in your pregnancy when you had any miscarriage or abortion?
- How is the current health of your other children?
- Did you have any problems with any of your other pregnancies such as bleeding, high blood pressure, headaches, blurring of your vision or spots before your eyes, pain, or diabetes? If you have, describe when the problems occurred and how they were treated.
- How much did each of your children weigh at birth?
- What gender was each of your children?
- What type of birth did you have with each of your children?
- Did you have any problems with other births? If you did, can you describe what happened?
- Did you have any babies that were born other than head first?
- Were you given any medicine to start your labor?
- Did you have any complications from your other births?
- Was the placenta delivered on its own?
- Did you have anything to help with pain during your previous labor(s)?

CURRENT PREGNANCY HISTORY

RATIONALE *A history of the current pregnancy will provide baseline information that will guide planning for future evaluation and health promotion activities.*

Suggested questions:

- Was this pregnancy planned or unplanned?
- Did you become pregnant on your own or did you use some intervention? If so, what intervention did you use?
- Have you had any problems with this pregnancy such as nausea or vomiting, bleeding, pain, or headache? If so, please elaborate.

PAST MEDICAL AND SURGICAL HISTORY

RATIONALE *Some illnesses or conditions may predispose the woman to increased risk during the pregnancy.*

Suggested questions:

- Tell me about any past illnesses or surgeries.
- Have you had any problems with your heart such as rheumatic fever or hypertension?

Continued

ASSESSMENT TOOL 12.1 Prenatal Health Assessment Form *(Continued)*

- Has anyone ever told you that you had diabetes?
- Have you had any lung problems such as difficulty breathing, asthma, or tuberculosis?
- Have you ever had seizures or been told you have epilepsy?
- Have you ever had problems with your kidneys or urinary infections?
- Have you ever had surgery before? If so, why did you have surgery?
- What kind of anesthetic did you have? Did you have any problems with the anesthetic?
- Have you ever had a blood transfusion? If so, why did you have it and when? Did you have any problems with it?
- What kinds of illnesses did you have when you were a child?
- What kinds of vaccinations have you had?
- Have you ever had any problems with feelings of anxiety, sadness, depression, fatigue, or had difficulty getting up?
- Have you experienced any major changes such as moving, a change in or loss of a relationship, job (your or family member)? What happens when such things occur? How do you react?

FAMILY HISTORY

RATIONALE ***Some conditions may be hereditary or familial.***

Suggested questions:

- Tell me about any illnesses in your family or the baby's father's family.
- Has anyone in your family had heart trouble, lung problems, diabetes, tuberculosis, or asthma?
- Has anyone in the baby's father's family had any of these problems?
- Has anyone in either family been diagnosed with cancer? If so, what kind?
- Has anyone in either family been born with any birth defects?
- Has anyone in either family been born with any inherited disease, blood disorders, mental retardation, or any other problems?
- Have there been twins or triplets born in either family?
- Has anyone in your family delivered a baby before the ninth month of pregnancy?

SOCIAL/CULTURAL HISTORY

RATIONALE ***Information may increase knowledge about potential risks to mother or fetus. Information about cultural history may influence plan of care.***

Suggested questions:

- Tell me about your habits and anything that I should know to assist you to incorporate your culture into your pregnancy experience.
- Do you smoke cigarettes? If so, how much do you smoke?
- Do you drink alcohol? How much alcohol do you drink each day? What kind of alcohol do you drink?
- Do you use any street drugs such as cocaine, speed, marijuana, or anything else? If you do, what kind of drugs do you use and how often do you use them?
- Do you use any prescription or over-the-counter drugs?
- Does any of your family or friends consider your habits to be a problem?
- Do any of your habits interfere with your daily living?
- Are there any special practices that you or your partner want to incorporate from your culture into your plan for this pregnancy? Is there anything that we can assist you with to accomplish this?
- If you needed help (such as someone to baby sit, lend you money, listen when you are upset), whom would you ask?

HISTORY OF ABUSE

RATIONALE ***Intimate partner abuse affects a significant number of women and frequently escalates during pregnancy. Physical, emotional, and sexual abuse crosses race, culture, ethnicity, social class, and gender. Therefore, all women may be at potential risk. Abuse may have serious consequences for both the mother and fetus.***

Suggested questions:

- Have you been hit, slapped, kicked, or otherwise physically hurt by someone within the last year?
- If yes, by whom and how many times?
- Have you been hit, slapped, kicked, or otherwise physically hurt by someone since you've been pregnant?
- If yes, by whom and how many times?
- Has anyone forced you to have sexual activities within the last year?
- If yes, by whom and how many times?
- Are you afraid of your partner or anyone else?
- Have you had negative comments made about you or your sexual performance within the last year?
- If yes, by whom and how many times?
- Can you freely access your family's money?

susceptibility to HIV; it is often initiated early in the pregnancy and continued until birth. Some studies have found, however, that transmission can be significantly reduced, even if medication is started in the third trimester (Patchen & Beal, 2001). HIV also can be transmitted during birth and, unlike other STIs, can be transmitted postpartally in breast milk (Dapaah & Dapaah, 2003).

Past Pregnancies. The nurse should obtain a history of past pregnancies, including whether they were planned. Complications arising in previous pregnancies may predispose the woman to a higher risk for the same complications in the present pregnancy. Information about the course of past labors and births may be useful in planning the course of this pregnancy.

A woman who has never been pregnant is called a nulligravida. If this is the client's first pregnancy, she is referred to as a **primigravida.** If this is a second or subsequent pregnancy, the term **multigravida** is used. The term **para** sometimes is used to denote the number of births after the 20th week of gestation. Because this term provides less clarity and health care providers sometimes interpret it inconsistently, a system that provides more comprehensive data about the status of past pregnancies and births is used frequently. Providers often use the acronym GTPAL to determine these more comprehensive data:

- G—the total number of pregnancies that the woman has had, including the current one
- T—the number of infants born at term (at 37 or more weeks' gestation)
- P—the number of infants born prematurely (after 20 weeks' gestation but before completion of 37 weeks' gestation)
- A—the number of pregnancies that ended in either therapeutic or spontaneous abortion (before 20 weeks' gestation)
- L—the number of children currently alive to whom the woman has given birth

Thus, a woman currently pregnant for the fifth time, with three children currently alive (delivered at 38 weeks, 40 weeks, and 32 weeks), and who had a spontaneous abortion at 14 weeks will have a GTPAL recorded as 5-2-1-1-3. A woman currently pregnant for the third time who gave birth to twins at 35 weeks and a single baby at 42 weeks, all of whom are currently alive, will have a GTPAL of 3-1-2-0-3. After delivering her baby at 39 weeks, her GTPAL will change to 3-2-2-0-4.

The nurse should assess past pregnancies for their duration. If a woman has had multiple lost pregnancies before 20 weeks' (the legal age of fetal viability), it may suggest an incompetent cervix (see Chap. 13). The nurse also should assess for complications in previous pregnancies that may have significance or implications for this pregnancy. Examples include bleeding, hypertension, headaches, blurred vision, pain, and gestational diabetes. Bleeding in a past pregnancy may have implications for the current pregnancy, based on the cause and outcome. For example, if the bleeding resulted in a spontaneous abortion, the risk for recurrence may be increased (Cunningham et al., 2005). Hypertension, headaches, blurred vision, or pain may have been indicative of pregnancy-induced hypertension. If pregnancy-induced hypertension or gestational diabetes complicated a previous pregnancy, risk for recurrence in this pregnancy will be increased (Kendrick, 2001; Poole, 2001).

The nurse should identify the birth weight of previous children. If any were classified as small for gestational age (SGA), intrauterine growth restriction (IUGR) may have complicated the pregnancies. If so, risk for recurrence in the current pregnancy may be increased. If children from previous pregnancies were large for gestational age (LGA), risk for development of gestational diabetes in the current pregnancy may be increased (Kendrick, 2001). The risk for an LGA infant in the current pregnancy is also increased if a previous pregnancy produced an LGA infant (Cunningham et al., 2005). Women whose infants are LGA are at increased risk for cephalopelvic disproportion (CPD) or shoulder dystocia (Cunningham et al., 2005). Regardless of whether a previous pregnancy resulted in an SGA or LGA infant, the nurse always should closely monitor the rate of fetal growth in the current pregnancy.

The nurse should identify the types of previous births, including any that were through cesarean section, required instruments such as forceps or vacuum extractors, or were complicated by a presentation other than vertex (head first). He or she should identify the reasons for any previous cesarean births. Indications may have no influence on this birth or may continue to be significant. For example, cesarean birth because of breech presentation will have fewer implications unless it recurs in this pregnancy (Cunningham et al., 2005). If cesarean birth occurred because of dystocia (failure to progress), chances are increased that this will continue to present indications for cesarean birth in this pregnancy.

Assessment should include a review of any complications of previous pregnancies, including retained placenta or postpartum hemorrhage. The risk for these recurring increases in subsequent pregnancies (James, 2001), so it is useful to have this information to monitor the birth and postpartum period more closely.

The nurse should document any labor analgesia or anesthesia used during previous births. This information will be useful in assessing the woman's tolerance to pain and planning care for labor and childbirth.

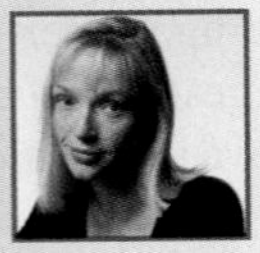

Consider Millie, described at the beginning of the chapter and in Nursing Care Plan 12.1. Based on her history, how would you document her history of past pregnancies using the GTPAL method? Imagine that Millie had also had a spontaneous abortion at age 22 and that her 11-year-old was born at 34 weeks' gestation instead of 39 weeks. What would her GTPAL be now?

Past Medical and Surgical History. The nurse should elicit information about the woman's past medical and surgical history. He or she should review cardiovascular or bleeding disorders; respiratory illnesses including asthma and tuberculosis; renal illnesses including urinary tract infections (UTIs); hypertension; diabetes; epilepsy; past surgeries; anesthetic problems; transfusions; allergies; childhood illnesses; and emotional alterations.

Cardiovascular disorders may predispose the client to increased risk because pregnancy generates increased blood volume and BMR and subsequent increased cardiac output (see Chap. 13). Bleeding disorders may predispose the woman to thrombophlebitis, episodes of bleeding, and postpartum hemorrhage.

Respiratory illnesses have implications for both maternal and fetal well-being. Women with asthma may have decreased respiratory capacity, which may be further compromised by fetal enlargement and subsequent pressure on the diaphragm. This decreased respiratory capacity also may affect the fetus because decreased oxygen in the maternal circulation decreases oxygen to the placenta and subsequent diffusion to the fetus. Active tuberculosis may spread from mother to fetus either across the placenta or, more commonly, following birth (Laibl & Sheffield, 2005).

Women who have had a previous UTI may be at increased risk for developing subsequent infections. A UTI in pregnancy can lead to increased risk for preterm labor (Morgan, 2004).

Women with a history of hypertension are at increased risk for developing pregnancy-induced hypertension (Cunningham et al., 2005). Knowledge of preexisting hypertension, then, should lead to increased surveillance during pregnancy. Women with preexisting diabetes are at increased risk during pregnancy. See Chapter 13 for further information on these conditions.

Women with epilepsy often have little or no difficulty during pregnancy; however, in some instances, seizure activity may be exacerbated (Cunningham et al., 2005). The plan of care for these women includes close follow-up to ensure maintenance of appropriate medication. Medication must be balanced to provide the antiseizure characteristics the mother requires without posing a risk for congenital anomalies to the fetus, which may be caused by some anticonvulsants (Cunningham et al., 2005).

The nurse should use information about past surgeries and anesthesia to anticipate care that may be needed should cesarean birth be required. Additionally, past surgery, depending on its nature, may have implications for the plan of care during pregnancy. The nurse should use information about past transfusions to plan further assessment that may be needed to determine the woman's hepatitis B and C status.

Information about childhood illnesses is a valuable resource about immunity that the client probably has acquired, although occasionally immunity is not achieved after exposure to an illness. The nurse should obtain the client's vaccination history, if known. See Box 12.3 for vaccination safety during pregnancy. Using both information about childhood illnesses and the vaccination history to ascertain the client's immunity status, the nurse may provide information about appropriate avoid-

BOX 12.3 Vaccination Safety during Pregnancy

Live Virus Vaccines

- MMR (measles, mumps, rubella): Contraindicated during pregnancy because it can cause congenital malformations including blindness, heart defects, and deafness
- Varicella zoster: Contraindicated during pregnancy
- Polio (Sabin type): Contraindicated during pregnancy, because of potential virus transmission to fetus

Live Bacterial Vaccines

- Typhoid: Risks vs. benefits should be evaluated for individual situation
- Yellow fever: Give in high-risk areas only

Inactivated Virus Vaccines

- Influenza: Can be given on request after the first trimester
- Rabies: No contraindication related to pregnancy
- Hepatitis A and B: No contraindication related to pregnancy
- Japanese encephalitis: Risks vs. benefits should be evaluated for individual situation

Inactivated Bacterial Vaccines

- Pneumococcus: No contraindication related to pregnancy
- Meningococcus: No contraindication related to pregnancy
- Haemophilus: No contraindication related to pregnancy
- Cholera: Risks vs. benefits should be evaluated for individual situation

Toxoids

- Tetanus–Diphtheria: No contraindication related to pregnancy

Sources: Clemen-Stone, et al, 2002; Cunningham, et al., 2005.

ance of exposure to others who may be ill. Exposure to rubella and chickenpox in the nonimmune woman can result in congenital anomalies.

Family History. The nurse should assess the family background of the mother and, if known, the father for any known conditions or alterations relating to the cardiovascular and respiratory systems, kidney disease, and bleeding disorders. He or she should identify any history of diabetes, congenital or fetal anomalies, epilepsy or seizures, emotional problems, cancer, HIV, or hepatitis. A history of any of these variations from normal may provide important information in identifying potential risks to the pregnant woman or unborn child. Identification of multiple births, especially fraternal, in the family may indicate ovulation twice in 1 month, which may predispose the woman to multiple births.

Habit History. Assessment includes the use of cigarettes, alcohol, and illicit, prescribed, and over-the-counter drugs, including amounts and types consumed. Smoking increases the risk for problems related to birth weight, placental abnormalities, and sudden infant death syndrome (Anderson et al., 2005; Magee et al., 2004; Zdravkovic et al., 2005). Alcohol increases the risk for fetal alcohol syndrome and fetal alcohol effects (Floyd et al., 2005). The use of drugs like cocaine and narcotics during pregnancy is associated with congenital anomalies, SGA, risk for placenta abruption, and neonatal abstinence syndrome (Askin, 2001; Cunningham et al., 2005).

Nutrition History. A review of the pregnant woman's dietary habits, preferences, and knowledge is critical. Chapter 3 discusses nutritional assessment and pregnancy-related needs and adjustments in thorough detail.

History of Abuse. Intimate partner abuse affects approximately 21% to 30% of U.S. women (Anderson, 2002). Acts of abuse frequently escalate during pregnancy (Anderson et al., 2002), although the exact prevalence is unknown. Factors that may be associated with an increased risk for abuse include younger age, substance abuse of both the woman and her partner, and unintended pregnancy (Espinosa & Osborne, 2002). Women who have been abused tend to have more episodes of depression and anxiety and fewer sources of support; they also tend to begin prenatal care later (Espinosa & Osborne, 2002). Serious consequences of abuse during pregnancy include placenta abruption, premature rupture of the membranes, low birth weight, and death of the mother, fetus, or both (Boy & Salihu, 2004; Plichta, 2004). Abuse may be physical, emotional, or sexual.

Because the woman may have only one prenatal visit or be afraid to disclose abuse until a trusting relationship is established, health care providers should ask questions at every visit (Anderson, 2002). Because abuse crosses race, culture, religion, social status, and gender, they should do this assessment with all pregnant women. Women who are not in abusive situations generally do not express offense at being asked such questions, perhaps because domestic violence is so prevalent that many women know someone who has been in that situation (Renker & Tonkin, 2006). The nurse should ask questions in privacy, away from the partner, other family members, or significant others (Stenson et al., 2005). Because she may be slow to respond, the woman needs adequate time to answer.

Assessment findings that may suggest abuse include infrequent prenatal visits that begin late in the pregnancy, poor weight gain, signs of possessiveness or jealousy in the woman's partner, apparent fear of her partner, or lack of eye contact or conversation (Anderson, 2002). Although the nurse may believe that the woman should leave the situation, he or she must understand that the woman may not be at a stage where this is seen as a viable option (Lutz, 2005).

Physical Examination

A complete physical examination should be performed. Vital signs and an initial weight need to be established as baseline data (Fig. 12.14). If the pre-pregnancy weight is known, the nurse should include it. Nurses and other providers can then use these baseline data to compare with changes that occur throughout pregnancy and to identify potential problems identified.

Expected Date of Delivery. Providers calculate the EDD. This date was formerly known as expected date of confinement (EDC). Because childbirth is no longer seen as a "confinement," the terminology has changed to expected date of delivery (EDD) or expected date of birth (EDB).

The most common way to calculate the EDD is to use **Naegele's rule.** The woman identifies the first day of her last normal menstrual period; Naegele's rule subtracts

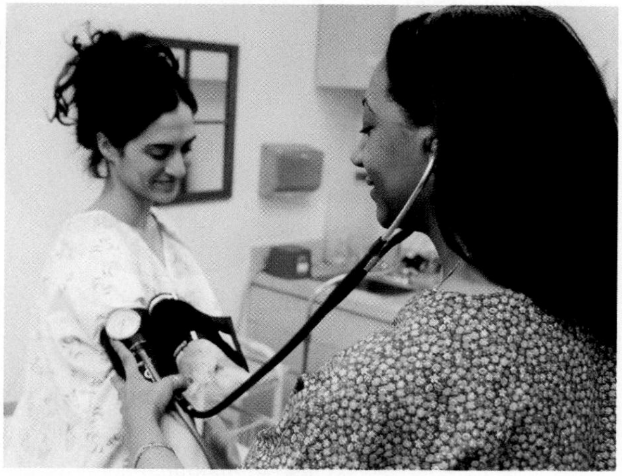

FIGURE 12.14 The nurse takes the client's blood pressure during the first prenatal visit and at all subsequent appointments.

3 months and adds 7 days to this date to give an EDD. For example, the first day of a client's last normal menstrual period was May 6. Subtracting 3 months would be February; adding 7 days would be 13. Therefore, the EDD is February 13 of the following year. Providers also can use the EDD wheel (Fig. 12.15) to calculate the EDD. To do so, providers match the line indicating the day of the last period with the appropriate date. The date on the outside wheel that falls on the line indicating 40 weeks is the EDD.

Some women have irregular periods or bleed throughout their cycle, which makes the use of Naegele's rule or the EDD wheel less reliable. As well, some women are simply not sure of the date of their last menstrual period, especially in the case of an unplanned pregnancy or when the woman pays little attention to the frequency of her periods. In these cases, providers use alternative methods to determine EDD. One such method to date pregnancy is ultrasound to visualize the gestational sac and regular measurements of the embryo/fetus (see Chap. 11). The most common measurements include biparietal diameter (distance from side to side) of the fetal head, head circumference, crown–rump length, abdominal circumference, and femoral length. Standard measurements have been established at different gestations, facilitating estimation of the pregnancy (Cunningham et al., 2005).

Ultrasound has been shown to have little effect on embryogenesis or fetal growth (Hershkovitz et al., 2002). The 2000 safety statement of the International Society for Ultrasound in Obstetrics and Gynecology, which was reconfirmed in 2002, indicates that "routine clinical scanning of every woman during pregnancy . . . is not contraindicated" (Abramowicz et al., 2002, p. 105), but that technicians should keep exposure time to the lowest levels that will permit obtaining diagnostic information. The use of the Doppler ultrasound is not recommended during the first trimester of pregnancy unless in exceptional cases after approval of the local ethical committee because of the high temperatures that may be produced (Abramowicz et al., 2002; Hershkovitz et al., 2002).

Providers also can use the EDD wheel to determine the weeks of gestation of the pregnancy. They match up the line indicating the EDD with the appropriate date and then find the current date on the outside wheel. Following that line toward the inner circle will provide the gestation in weeks and days.

General Survey. The nurse should assess physiologic changes that the woman has been experiencing. This includes both presumptive and probable signs of pregnancy. Although these help to confirm the pregnancy, the nurse also uses the information to develop a plan of care to identify anticipated changes to the woman to

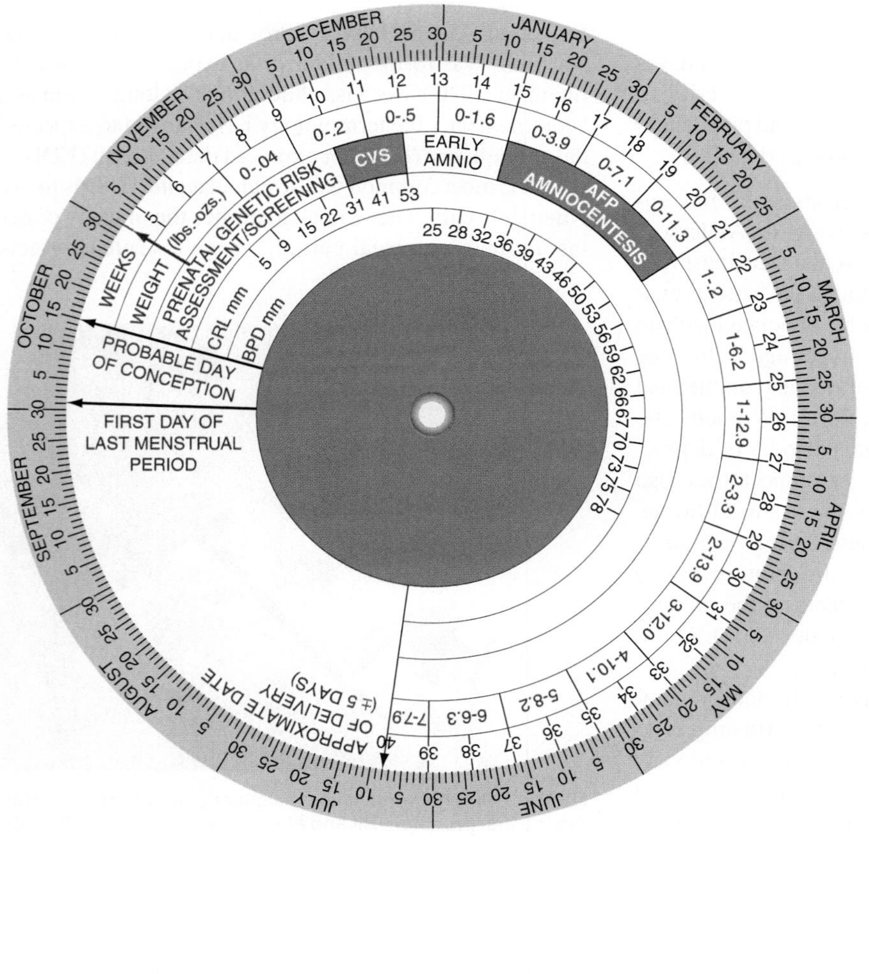

FIGURE 12.15 The EDD wheel helps health care providers estimate a client's due date. This client's last menstrual period (LMP) was October 1. Her due date according to the wheel is July 8 of the following year. (Used with permission. Copyright March of Dimes, 2003.)

decrease anxiety and to assist the woman to prevent or decrease the symptoms.

An organized approach, often according to body systems, usually is easiest to follow to complete the physical examination. The initial assessment includes a general survey of the woman and her state of nourishment, grooming, posture, mood, affect, and general appearance. Poor grooming and posture and a flat affect may suggest some mental health issues, including depression. A woman appearing poorly nourished with poor grooming may have decreased resources and may benefit from a social services consultation.

Skin. Assessment of the skin includes evaluation of any scars. These may be from a previous cesarean section or tracks caused by intravenous drug use. In combination with bruising, scars may suggest physical abuse. Skin variations may include chloasma, linea nigra, and striae.

Breasts. The client should undergo a clinical breast examination (see Chap. 2). The pregnant breasts may appear enlarged, perhaps with striae (Fig. 12.16). The areolae and nipples also may appear enlarged and with darker pigmentation. Montgomery's tubercles may be visible on the areola; the nipples may begin to express colostrum during the last trimester.

Heart and Lungs. When assessing the heart and lungs, the nurse may hear a functional, soft, blowing systolic murmur from the increased cardiac volume (Fig. 12.17). The nurse should note any other murmur and refer the finding to appropriate health care team members. The increased blood volume and resulting increased cardiac output add significantly to the workload of the heart.

Abdomen. The nurse should palpate and inspect the abdomen. Striae and linea nigra may be present. Depending on the gestation of the pregnancy, the nurse may assess symphysis–fundal height.

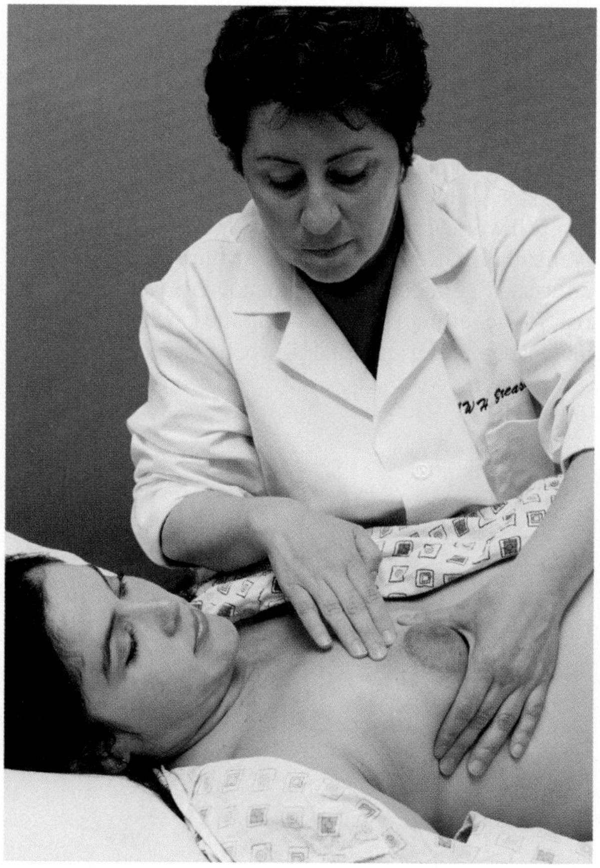

FIGURE 12.16 The nurse examines the pregnant client's breasts.

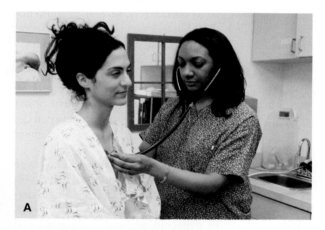

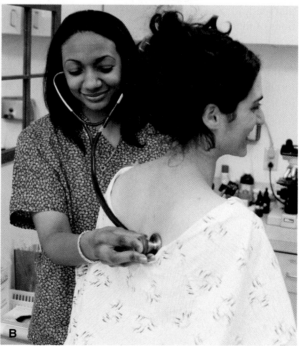

FIGURE 12.17 The nurse assesses the client's (**A**) heart and (**B**) lungs. A soft, blowing systolic murmur from the increased cardiac volume is a normal finding.

Genitalia. The examination includes assessment for cervical and vaginal changes as part of assessment of the probable signs of pregnancy, including Chadwick's, Hegar's, and Goodell's signs. A Pap smear and vaginal cultures are necessary to provide baseline data.

Pelvimetry. The pelvis may be assessed later in pregnancy if engagement of the presenting part has not occurred (Viccars, 2003). Assessment includes the pubic arch, inclination, and curve of the side walls; the prominence of the ischial spines; and the shape of the sacrum.

The pelvic bones are assessed for size and shape to determine the adequacy of the pelvis for vaginal birth. The two most important measurements are the *diagonal conjugate* and the *bi-ischial diameter*. The diagonal conjugate indicates the anteroposterior diameter of the pelvic inlet. It is measured by pointing the second and third fingers, when placed within the vagina, toward the sacral promontory (Fig. 12.18A). The distance of the fingers is then measured to estimate the diagonal conjugate. The measurement ideally is at least 11.5 cm.

To measure the bi-ischial diameter, the examiner forms his or her hand into a closed fist, which he or she then places across the woman's perineum between the ischial tuberosities (Fig. 12.18B). This measurement ideally is at least 8 cm.

There are four classifications of pelves. Each type has a characteristic shape, although individual pelves will have some variations and may have characteristics of several types (Cunningham et al., 2005). These four classifications include the gynecoid, android, anthropoid, and platypelloid. See Box 12.4 for depictions and explanations of these types.

Laboratory Evaluation and Disease Screening

Laboratory evaluation should be done to identify the mother's ABO blood type and Rh, as well as any antibodies. If the mother's Rh is negative, the father's blood type should be identified, if possible. This is useful in determining any potential for Rh incompatibility (see Chap. 16). A rubella titer should be done to identify immunity, indicated by a value of 1:32 or greater. If the pregnant woman is nonimmune, she should avoid exposure to rubella during her pregnancy, because of the associated risk for spontaneous abortion and congenital anomalies. Once she has delivered the baby, she should be given an MMR (measles, mumps, rubella) vaccination to increase her immunity. She should not become pregnant within 1 month of receiving the vaccine; it is believed to be safe if she is breastfeeding.

The woman should have a baseline hemoglobin and urinalysis. The urinalysis will indicate any asymptomatic bacteriuria, which is common in pregnancy. If this is not treated, it may lead to acute symptomatic UTI, which occurs in approximately 25% of affected women (Cunningham et al., 2005). Bacteria in the urine, combined with urinary stasis that occurs in pregnancy, put the woman at increased risk for pyelonephritis. Bacteriuria or pyelonephritis increases the risk for preterm labor (Cunningham et al., 2005).

The hemoglobin is done as a baseline on which to evaluate future values. Hemoglobin normally decreases during pregnancy because iron is actively transferred to the fetus and the red blood cell mass of the mother increases. Continued evaluation is essential to ensure that hemoglobin values are maintained within safe ranges. Abnormal values, especially in late pregnancy (considered to be less than 11.0 g/dL or 110 g/L), are usually the result of iron deficiency and indicate the need for additional exogenous iron (Cunningham et al., 2005).

All women should be offered HIV testing at the first prenatal visit. Repeat testing in the third trimester before 36 weeks' gestation is recommended for women at high risk for acquiring HIV, including those who have multiple sex partners, use illicit drugs, or have a partner infected

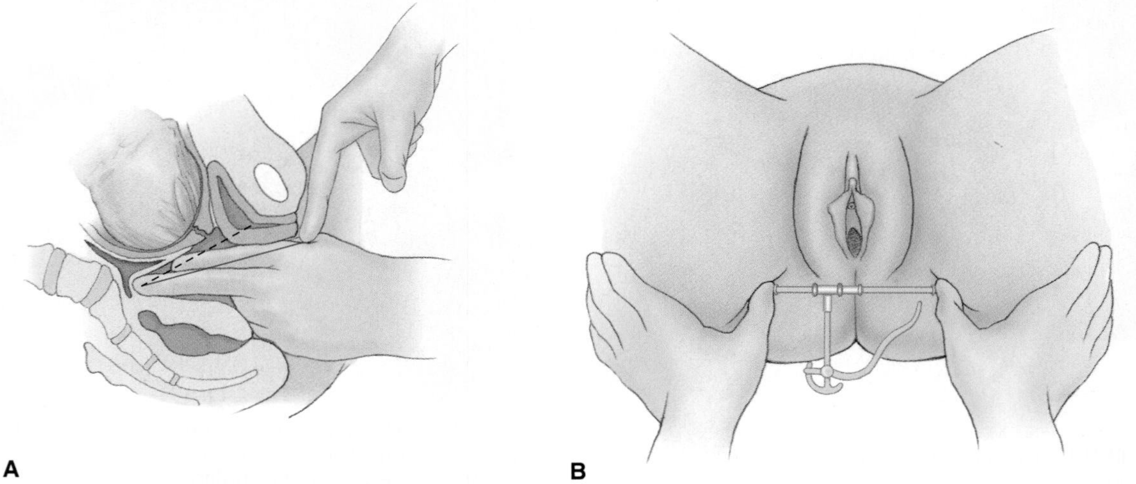

FIGURE 12.18 (**A**) Diagonal conjugate (*solid line*). (**B**) Ischial diameter.

BOX 12.4 Types of Pelves

Gynecoid

- Inlet is round or oval.
- Pubic arch is wide, at least 90 degrees.
- Ischial spines are not prominent.
- Side walls are straight and parallel.
- Posterior pelvis is round and wide.
- Anteroposterior diameter is only slightly less than the transverse diameter.
- Distance between promontory of sacrum and symphysis pubis (obstetrical conjugate) is 11 cm or more.
- Distance between promontory of sacrum and lower edge of symphysis pubis (diagonal conjugate) is 12–13 cm.
- Distance between ischial spines (interspinous) is 10 cm.
- Transverse diameter of inlet is 13.5 cm.
- Transverse diameter of outlet is 10–11 cm.
- Anteroposterior diameter between the lower margin of the symphysis pubis and the tip of the sacrum is 9.5–11.5 cm.

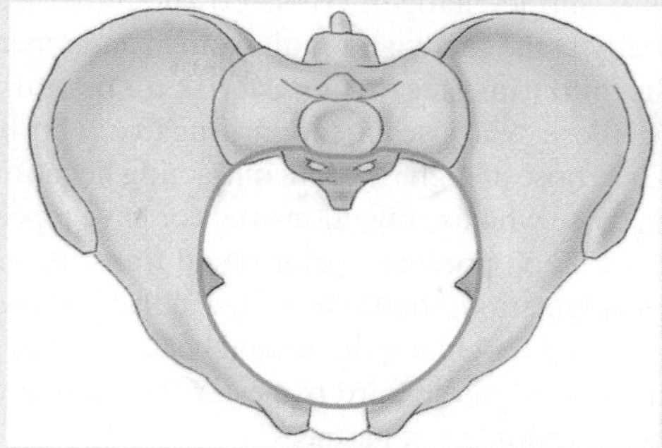

Android

- Inlet is heart shaped.
- Anterior of pelvis is narrow and triangular.
- Pubic arch is narrow, less than 90 degrees.
- Sacrum is straight and usually forward.
- Ischial spines are prominent.
- Side walls are straight and parallel.
- Posterior pelvis is shallow.
- Anteroposterior and transverse diameters are adequate, but posterior sagittal diameter is decreased.

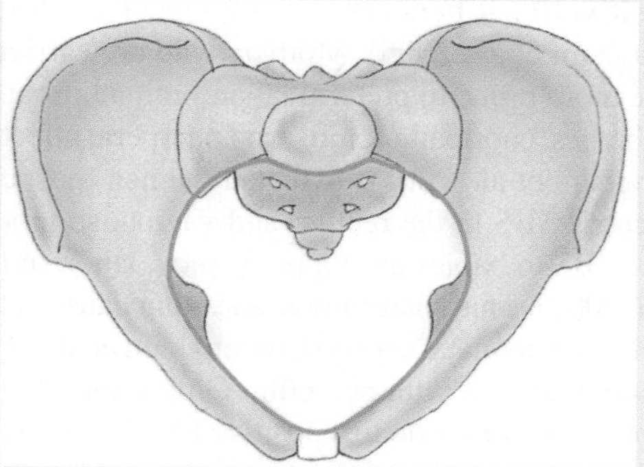

Anthropoid

- Inlet is oval shaped.
- Pubic arch is slightly narrowed from 90 degrees.
- Sacrum longer and usually straight.
- Ischial spines are somewhat prominent but pose little problem because of the size of the posterior segment.
- Side walls are straight.
- Posterior pelvis is somewhat large.
- Anteroposterior diameter is long with a short (although adequate) transverse diameter.

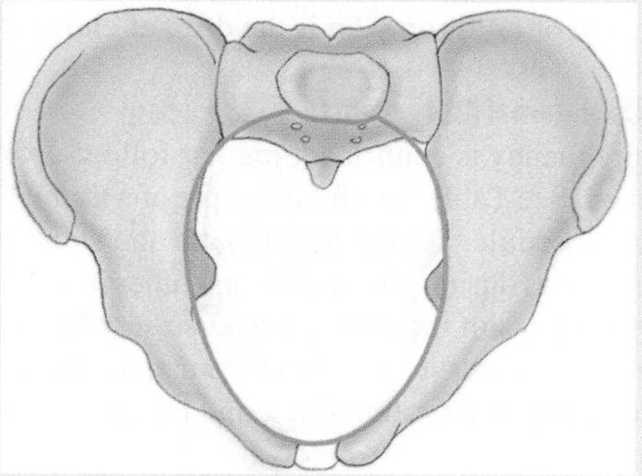

Platypelloid

- Inlet is flattened and oval shaped.
- Pubic arch is wide.
- Sacrum is short, quite curved, and inclines backward.
- Ischial spines are somewhat prominent but are insignificant because of the width of the interspinous diameter.
- Anteroposterior diameter is short with a wide transverse diameter.
- Angle of anterior pelvis is wide.
- Pelvis is quite shallow.

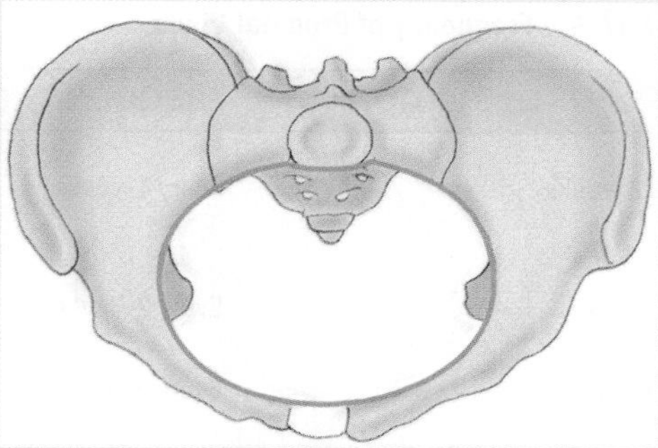

with HIV. A syphilis test should be done on all women at the first prenatal visit and for anyone who has a stillbirth. Hepatitis B surface antigen (HbsAG) should be tested serologically at the first visit for all women and repeated during the third trimester for those at risk for hepatitis B, including those who use injection drugs or who have other STIs. Those at high risk for contracting hepatitis C, including those who use injection drugs or have repeated exposure to blood products, prior blood transfusion, or organ transplantation, should be tested at the first prenatal visit. Testing for chlamydia should be done at the first visit and repeated in the third trimester for women who have new or multiple sex partners.

The American College of Obstetricians and Gynecologists (ACOG, 2002) recommends screening of all pregnant women for group B streptococci (GBS), rather than the risk-based screening that was previously recommended. It is common for pregnant women to be asymptomatic carriers of GBS; 15% to 20% have a culture positive for it between 23 to 26 weeks' gestation (Cunningham et al., 2005). Mothers who are carriers of GBS are more prone to preterm labor, premature rupture of membranes, chorioamnionitis, and puerperal infections (Cunningham et al., 2005). Affected women most commonly carry GBS in the rectum and vagina, so mothers can pass GBS to babies during pregnancy, labor, or birth (ACOG, 2002). This bacterium is a leading cause of fetal infections and neonatal sepsis (Cunningham et al., 2005). Antibiotic treatment with penicillin G or ampicillin during labor for women who test positive for GBS is recommended to assist in preventing transmission (Cunningham et al., 2005). For women who are allergic to penicillin, clindamycin or erythromycin is the drug of choice.

Follow-Up Maternal Assessments

Once a pregnancy is confirmed, regular follow-up visits are planned. See Table 12.4 for a sample of a normal prenatal visit schedule. During the prenatal and subsequent visits, as well as during phone calls and other interactions that may occur with the client, the nurse should provide anticipatory guidance to assist the woman to understand expected changes, their timelines, and potential comfort measures.

Continuing prenatal assessments during each subsequent visit include vital signs and weight, FHR when audible, symphysis fundal height, position of the fetus when palpable, edema, discomforts of pregnancy, any risk factors, and any concerns that the woman may have. The examiner may palpate the fetal outline using Leopold's maneuvers and auscultate and assess the fetal heart. See Nursing Procedures 12.1 and 12.2.

Continued regular prenatal care is essential for the remainder of the pregnancy to monitor maternal well-being and fetal growth and well-being. Once the pregnancy is confirmed positively and the client can see or hear evidence of the fetus, it may be the first time she realizes that she is truly pregnant. It provides positive proof to her that a baby really is growing inside her. This may be the first time that she feels confident enough to begin to plan for the arrival. The nurse should continue to provide support and anticipatory guidance to the pregnant woman and her significant others in continuing prenatal care. He or she should give information about prenatal classes as well as other support services that may be available in the woman's community.

Assessment of Fetal Activity and Well-Being

Assessment of fetal activity and well-being throughout the pregnancy is vital to ensuring a favorable outcome. Health care providers use several methods and tools to accomplish this assessment. These include assessment of fetal activity, the biophysical profile, modified biophysical profile, contraction stress test, and umbilical artery Doppler velocimetry.

Fetal Activity

The nurse can establish assessment of fetal activity by having the mother keep a journal. An example of such a tool is a record of daily kick count. Beginning at 32 to 34 weeks (26 to 28 weeks for those women at high risk for antepartum fetal death), the mother rests on her left side with her hand on her abdomen at the same time each day. She counts the time it takes to feel 10 fetal movements, which should occur in less than 2 hours (Barron, 2001; Cunningham et al., 2005). If she does

TABLE 12.4 Frequency of Prenatal Visits

WEEKS OF GESTATION	FREQUENCY OF VISITS	SPECIAL INVESTIGATIONS
Up to 28 weeks	Every 4 weeks	15–20 weeks: Alpha fetoprotein 20 weeks: Level 2 diagnostic ultrasound 24–28 weeks: Gestational diabetes
28–36 weeks	Every 2–3 weeks	28 weeks: Anti-D antibodies if mother is Rh negative. If none present, give anti-D immune globulin.
36+ weeks	Every week	

NURSING PROCEDURE 12.1

Performing Leopold's Maneuvers

PURPOSE

To determine fetal presentation, position, and attitude

ASSESSMENT AND PLANNING

- Assess the client's knowledge of and previous experience with the procedure.
- Review the client's medical record to determine estimated date of delivery (EDD) and week of gestation.
- Gather necessary equipment
  - Warmed, clean hands

IMPLEMENTATION

1. Explain the procedure to the client *to help alleviate anxiety.*
2. Have the client empty her bladder *to promote client comfort and minimize uterine distention from interfering with palpation.*
3. Perform hand hygiene.
4. Assist the client to the supine position with her knees slightly flexed *to help relax abdominal muscles;* place a small pillow under one side *to prevent supine hypotension syndrome.*
5. Expose the abdominal area and inspect the abdomen *to identify any bulging prominences, asymmetry, and indentations.*
6. Position yourself at the side of the bed, facing the client. Place both hands on the uterine fundus and palpate for its contents *to identify the fetal body part occupying the fundus.* Identify the fetal body part palpated by consistency, shape, and mobility. *A soft irregular object that does not move freely suggests the buttocks; a smooth, firm, regular object that moves independently suggests the head (breech presentation).*
7. Then move your hands to the sides of the maternal abdomen, placing the palmar surface one hand on each side of the abdomen. Gently palpate one side of the abdomen while using the opposite hand to support the abdomen and *uterus to locate the fetal back and extremities.* Repeat using the opposite action. *The fetal back will feel hard and smooth; the extremities will feel irregular and nodular.*

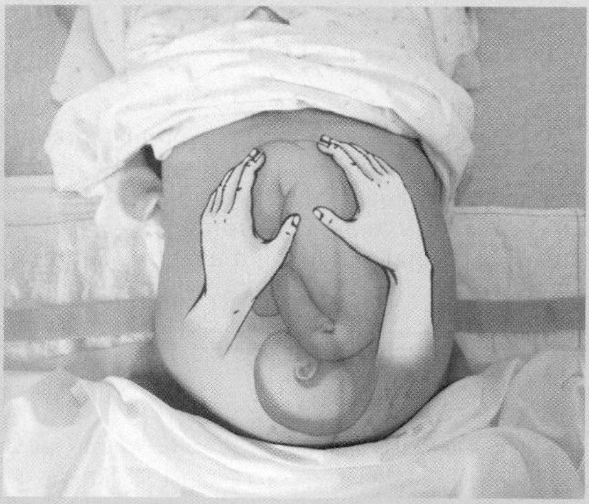

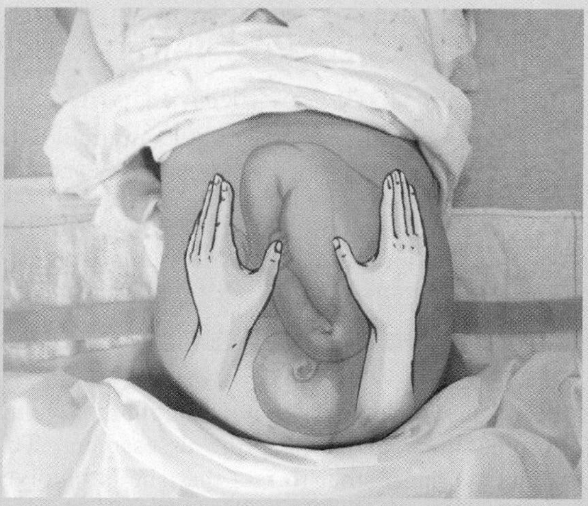

Continued

NURSING PROCEDURE 12.1 CONTINUED

Performing Leopold's Maneuvers

8. Place one hand just above the symphysis pubis and, using your thumb and fingers, attempt to grasp the presenting part of the fetus. Feel for a hard, round object *to identify the head as the presenting part* or a soft irregularly shaped object *to identify breech presentation.* While palpating, attempt to move the object *to determine possible engagement of the head. Free movement denotes that the presenting part is not engaged.*
9. Turn and face the client's feet. Using the first three fingers of each hand, begin to palpate in a downward fashion moving toward the symphysis pubis, along both sides of the abdomen, *to identify the degree of fetal flexion.* Feel for a hard bony area. If this area is on the opposite side of where the fetal back was palpated, then the fetus is in an attitude of flexion; if the area is on the same side as the fetal back, the fetus is in an attitude of extension.
10. Assist the woman to a comfortable position.
11. Document the findings in the client's medical record.

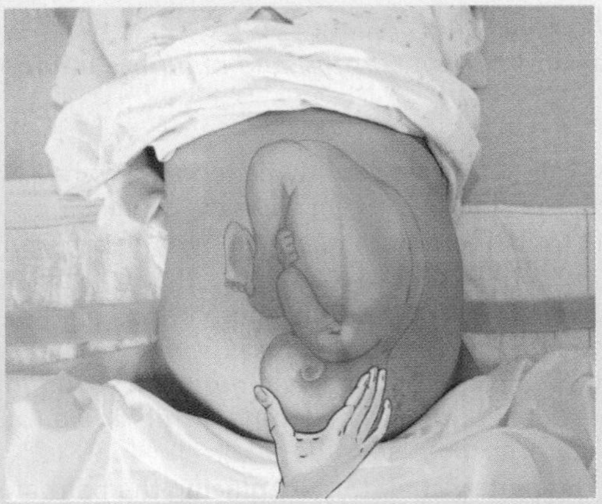

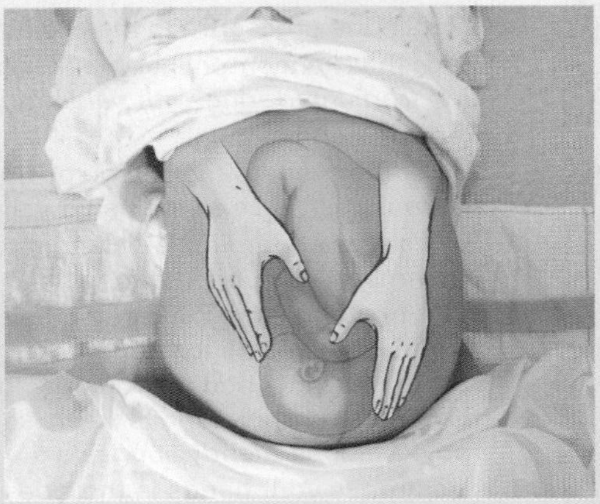

EVALUATION

- The client tolerated the procedure without difficulty.
- The fetal position, presentation, and attitude were within normal parameters.

AREAS FOR CONSIDERATION AND ADAPTATION

Perinatal Considerations

- Remember that Leopold's maneuvers can be performed throughout a woman's pregnancy.
- Use Leopold's maneuvers to assist in determining where best to auscultate fetal heart tones.
- If the woman is in labor, perform these maneuvers in between contractions.
- Place a pillow under the client's shoulders if necessary to promote comfort.
- Do not perform the fourth maneuver (palpating for fetal attitude) if the fetus is in the breech position.

not feel 10 movements in 2 hours, the mother should drink some juice and repeat the assessment. This record assists the mother to feel that she is involved in care. The record provides information for the care provider about fetal well-being. The nurse is responsible for teaching the mother how to perform these assessments and evaluating each assessment for signs of fetal well-being.

QUOTE 12-3

"I feel lucky that this baby is very active. With my daughter, there were times when I'd get worried when I didn't feel the kicking for a few hours. This baby kicks constantly. Of course, I wish he'd settle down at 4:00 AM sometimes!"

A woman comparing her experiences of fetal activity in two pregnancies

(text continues on page 472)

NURSING PROCEDURE 12.2

Assessing Fetal Heart Rate

PURPOSE

To evaluate fetal well-being

ASSESSMENT AND PLANNING

- Assess the client's knowledge of and previous experience with the procedure.
- Determine the client's estimated date of delivery (EDD) and number of weeks' gestation.
- Check the client's medical record for baseline information related to fetal heart rates.
- Review the client's medical record for information related to any previous pregnancies and outcomes.
- Gather equipment
    - Ultrasonic Doppler device

    Or

    - Fetoscope
    - Water-soluble conductive gel (for ultrasonic Doppler device)
    - Washcloth or tissue

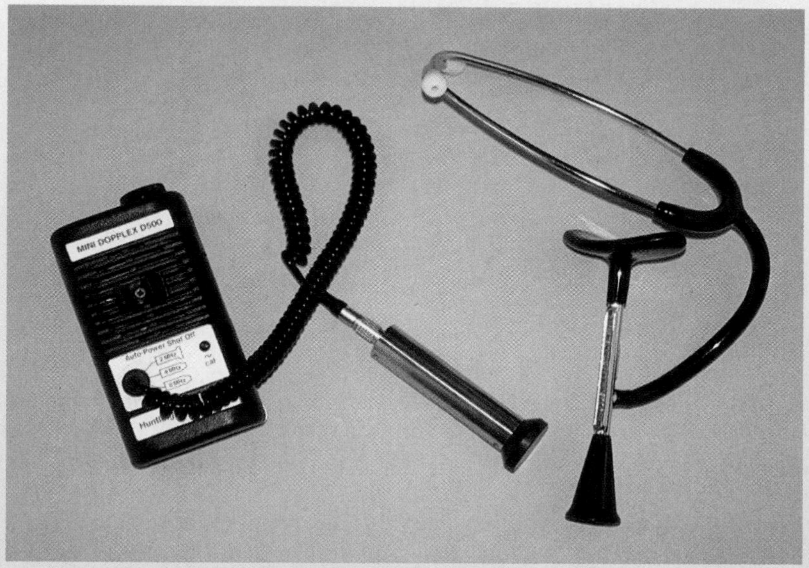

Doptone (*left*) and fetoscope (*right*).

IMPLEMENTATION

1. Explain the procedure to the client and answer any questions that she may have *to help allay any fears and anxieties.*
2. Assist the woman to the supine position *to allow for easy access to the abdominal area.* Provide privacy.
3. Perform hand hygiene.
4. Expose the client's abdomen and perform Leopold's maneuvers *to identify fetal back and best location to hear fetal heart tones.* (See Nursing Procedure 12.1.)
5. Apply water-soluble gel to client's abdomen in the area of the fetal back or to the device *to ensure adequate contact of the device to the client's skin and enhance sound transmission.*
6. If the ultrasonic device has ear pieces, place them into the ears; then turn on the device.

Continued

NURSING PROCEDURE 12.2 CONTINUED

Assessing Fetal Heart Rate

7. Position the device on the client's abdomen at the location of the fetal back *to hear the heart sounds;* alternatively, place the device beginning at the midline, midway between the umbilicus and symphysis pubis; if necessary, slowly move the device laterally *to hear the heart sounds;* move the device slowly and slightly until you hear the sounds the loudest.

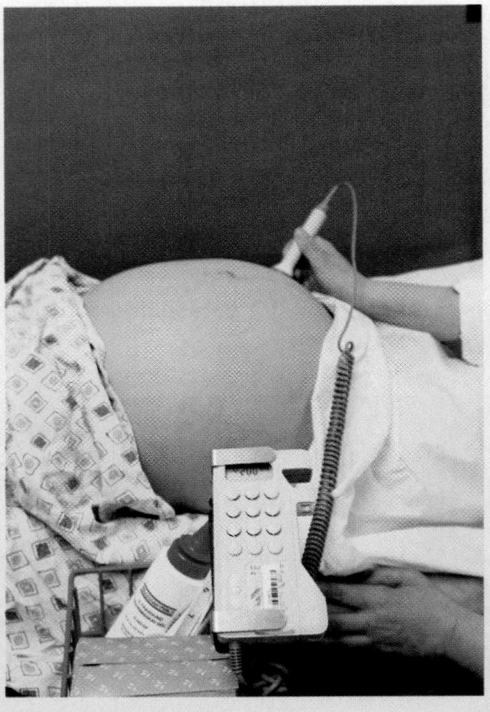

Step 7. The examiner applies the Doppler ultrasound device.

8. Count the client's pulse rate *to determine that what is heard is the fetal heart rate and not the maternal heart rate.* If the rates are the same, reposition the device and count again.
9. Once you have confirmed the fetal heart rate, count it for one full minute; also note the rhythm.
10. Remove the device and wipe the client's abdomen with a washcloth or tissue *to remove water-soluble gel;* provide the client with information about fetal well-being based on fetal heart rate.
11. Wipe the device *to remove the gel;* perform hand hygiene.
12. Document the fetal heart rate and rhythm and location of fetal heart sounds.

EVALUATION

- The fetal heart rate was within the normal range of 120 to 160 beats/minute.
- The client tolerated the procedure without difficulty.

AREAS FOR CONSIDERATION AND ADAPTATION

Perinatal Considerations

- If this is the client's first prenatal visit, assess the client for presumptive, probable, and positive signs of pregnancy.

Continued

NURSING PROCEDURE 12.2

Assessing Fetal Heart Rate

- Keep in mind that fetal heart rate assessment is performed at every prenatal visit.
- If using a fetoscope, do the following:
    - Do not apply water-soluble gel.
    - Place the ear pieces in the ears and attach the fetoscope to your head, positioning the instrument centrally.
    - Gently place the bell of the fetoscope onto the woman's abdomen, depressing the client's abdomen approximately ½ inch.

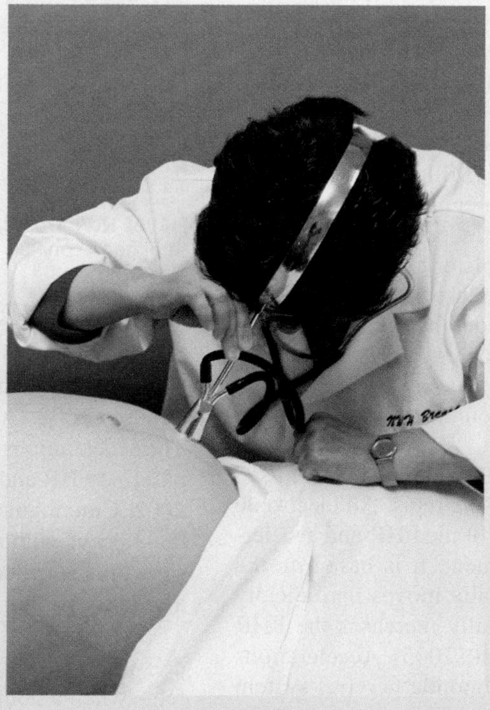

The examiner positions the fetoscope.

- Move the scope slowly from side to side on the client's abdomen until you hear the heart sounds clearly and loudly.
- At the same time, assess the client's pulse rate for 15 to 30 seconds *to ensure that what you are hearing is not the mother's heart rate.*
- If both rates are the same, reposition the scope and repeat the previous step.
- Once the rates are different, then count the fetal heart rate for 1 full minute.

- During labor, monitor fetal heart rate intermittently or continuously as per the facility's policy, using a fetoscope, ultrasonic Doppler device, or external or internal electronic fetal monitoring.
- When using electronic fetal monitoring during labor, evaluate fetal heart rate and rhythm in light of uterine contractions. (See Chapter 15 for more information.)

Community-Based Considerations

- Expect to assess fetal heart rate at every home visit.
- Notify the client's primary care provider about changes in fetal heart rate outside the normal range of 120 to 160 beats/minute.

Biophysical Profile

The biophysical profile (BPP) is also being used increasingly as a tool to assess fetal well-being. It is used to evaluate the "probability of a given fetus having or not having sufficient delivery of oxygen to select primary and secondary target organs, including the fetal brain, kidney and to a lesser extent lung, so as to maintain normal function" (Manning, 2002, p. 975). The BPP comprises both a nonstress test (NST; using electronic fetal monitoring) and ultrasound evaluation. The NST is done to determine FHR reactivity; obstetrical ultrasound assesses fetal breathing movements, gross fetal body movements, fetal tone, and the volume of amniotic fluid (Barron, 2001). Because the BPP provides a more comprehensive examination of fetal well-being than does evaluation of FHR alone, the false-negative rate is often comparable or superior when compared with any single test (contraction stress test or NST) used to predict the fetus at risk for poor outcome (Miller, 2002; Sprong, 2003). Examples may include pregnancies complicated by maternal hypertension, diabetes, premature rupture of the membranes, postmaturity, history of previous fetal death, or maternal reports of decreased fetal movements. Although the information provided by the BPP may be useful in identifying a fetus in jeopardy at a specific point and the fetal condition during the past several weeks (Manning, 2002), it cannot be definitively used as a predictor of future well-being.

The NST is a part of the BPP but also may be used alone to assess the condition of the fetus. An electronic fetal monitor provides a tracing of the FHR and accelerations of the FHR with movement. It is based on the knowledge that the fetus normally moves periodically and that fetal movement normally increases the FHR (Barron, 2001; Cunningham et al., 2005). Accelerations imply an intact central and autonomic nervous system not affected by uterine hypoxia (Cunningham et al., 2005; Preboth, 2000).

The NST is relatively simple, quick, and noninvasive. It can be done on an outpatient basis and interpreted with relative ease. Nevertheless, the fetus may be in a sleep cycle during the 20 to 30 minutes that the test takes, making it difficult to obtain a suitable tracing or requiring the test to take longer (Andres, 2002).

The woman should be in bed in a semi-Fowler's position. There is no requirement for any dietary restriction; however, she should not have smoked recently. Each of two transducers is held in place with soft fabric belts snugly fastened. The tocodynamometer transducer (which measures uterine activity) is placed over the fundus of the uterus. The Doppler FHR transducer (which measures FHR) is covered with transducer gel and placed over the position where the FHR is most readily heard (usually over the fetal back, ascertained by using Leopold's maneuvers) (Fig. 12.19). The woman remains in bed for a minimum of 20 minutes.

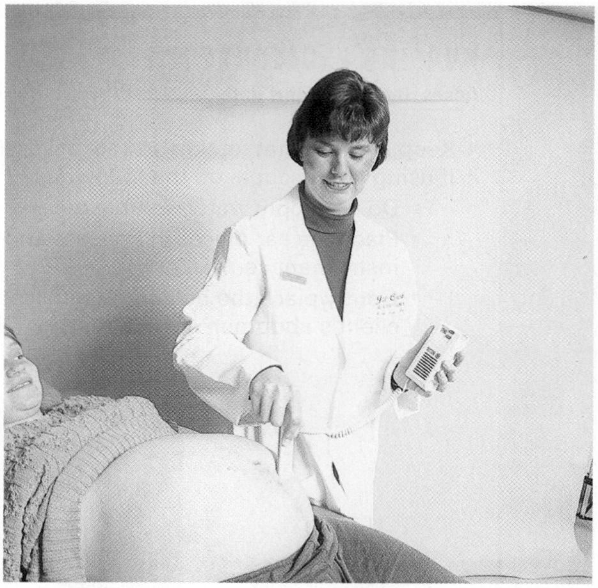

FIGURE 12.19 Doppler ultrasound can be used to check for fetal heart tones.

Results of the NST should show what is termed a reactive tracing. This means that the tracing shows two or more accelerations in association with fetal movements (Andres, 2002; Cunningham et al., 2005; Preboth, 2000). The accelerations must be at least 15 beats/minute above baseline FHR and must last at least 15 seconds (Andres, 2002, Cunningham et al., 2005). The two accelerations must occur within 20 minutes. A tracing that does not show this is called a nonreactive strip and may indicate a need for further evaluation.

Vibroacoustic stimulation (VAS) may be used to deliver both vibratory and acoustic stimulation to the fetus when a nonreactive strip is obtained or to shorten the time needed to obtain a reactive strip (Andres, 2002; Miller, 2002; Sprong, 2003). An artificial larynx is positioned on the abdomen over the fetus and a stimulus lasting 1 second is applied. The fetus responds to this stimulation with a startle that results in acceleration of the FHR. If there is no response to this stimulation, it may be repeated up to three times for progressively longer periods (up to 2 to 3 seconds) with 1 minute between each period of stimulation (Andres, 2002; Cunningham et al., 2005).

A second component of the BPP is fetal breathing movements that are visible on ultrasound. These movements differ from those in neonates (Cunningham et al., 2005). In the fetus, the chest wall collapses paradoxically during inspiration, and the abdomen protrudes; in the neonate, the opposite occurs. Gasps, sighs, and rapid irregular bursts of breathing have been identified in the fetus (Cunningham et al., 2005). At least one episode of breathing movements that lasts at least 30 seconds over 30 minutes is considered normal for the BPP.

Fetal body movements comprising at least three separate and distinct episodes of body or limb movements in 30 minutes are considered normal (Andres, 2002; Cunningham et al., 2005). Simultaneous movements of the limbs or trunks are counted as one movement. The nurse must distinguish periods of rest in the fetus from a lack of activity because of a compromised uterine environment.

The fetus begins to flex and stretch its arms and legs by about 13 weeks' gestation (Cunningham et al., 2005). At least one episode of both extension and flexion of fetal extremities or the opening or closing of a hand within 30 minutes indicates normal body tone (Barron, 2001; Cunningham et al., 2005).

Amniotic fluid volume is an important component of the BPP. The kidneys and lungs are the principal sources of amniotic fluid. The production of fetal urine falls with hypoxemia or acidemia (Manning, 2002). It takes approximately 15 days for amniotic fluid to progress from a normal volume to a barely abnormal volume, and approximately 23 days to reach severe **oligohydramnios** (Manning, 2002). Therefore, amniotic fluid volume may be the most obvious sign of chronic fetal hypoxemia or acidemia. Abnormal amniotic fluid volumes also may indicate congenital anatomic anomalies or fetal growth restrictions (Schrimmer & Moore, 2002). At least one pocket of amniotic fluid that measures at least 2 cm in vertical diameter should be visible on ultrasound to be considered normal (Barron, 2001; Cunningham et al., 2005).

Table 12.5 indicates the interpretation of the variables, each of which is assigned a score of 2 or 0. A score of 1 is not an option. A score of 10 or 8, with a normal amount of amniotic fluid, indicates a normal, nonasphyxiated fetus. A score of 8 with oligohydramnios suggests that there may be chronic fetal asphyxia present and the fetus should be delivered. A score of 6 is indicative of possible fetal asphyxia. If the amniotic fluid volume is abnormal, the fetus should be delivered. If the amniotic fluid volume is normal, the test is considered questionable and warrants additional investigation. A score of 4 or less is considered to be probably fetal asphyxia; the test should be repeated again the same day and if the score is 6 or less, the fetus should be delivered (Cunningham et al., 2005).

Modified Biophysical Profile

The modified BPP combines the NST with the amniotic fluid index (AFI). Advantages of the modified BPP include the decreased time needed to complete the test and relative ease of completion of the test with the added benefit that it appears to be as predictive of fetal status as other approaches (Barron, 2001; Cunningham et al., 2005). The AFI measures the sum of the deepest amniotic fluid pocket in each of the four quadrants of the uterus (Miller, 2002). Each pocket must be free of umbilical cord or fetal extremities. The AFI is considered indicative of the long-term function of the placenta. An AFI greater than 5 cm represents an adequate volume of amniotic fluid (Cunningham et al., 2005; Sprong, 2003). A modified BPP is considered abnormal if the AFI is less than 5 cm, regardless of reactivity of the NST (Sprong, 2003).

Contraction Stress Test

A contraction stress test (CST) may be used to evaluate function of the placenta. This test previously was called an oxytocin contraction test (OCT), a term now used infrequently. It indicates response of the FHR, and thus the placenta, to uterine contractions. Because the uteroplacental circulation is compromised during a contraction (as a result of decreased blood flow to the intervillous space by the contracting uterus), there is transient decreased fetal oxygenation during the contraction (Huddleston, 2002). If there is reasonable uteroplacental function, the

TABLE 12.5 Biophysical Profile

VARIABLE	NORMAL (SCORE = 2)	ABNORMAL (SCORE = 0)
Fetal breathing movements	At least one episode of breathing movements lasting at least 30 seconds in a 30-minute period	Absent respirations or no episode of breathing movements lasting at least 30 seconds in a 30-minute period
Gross body movements	At least three separate and distinct episodes of body or limb movements in 30 minutes	Two or fewer episodes of body or limb movements in 30 minutes
Fetal tone	At least one episode of extension and flexion of fetal extremities or the spine	Slow extension with return to partial flexion or movement of limb in full extension only or no movement
Amniotic fluid volume	At least one pocket of amniotic fluid measuring at least 2 cm in vertical diameter	Either pocket of fluid is less than 2 cm in vertical diameter or no pocket
Fetal heart reactivity	Two or more accelerations of the fetal heart of at least 15 beats/min above baseline and lasting at least 15 seconds associated with fetal movement within 20 minutes	Less than two accelerations or acceleration less than 15 beats/min in a 20-minute period

fetus will have adequate basal oxygenation (the level when there is no uterine contraction) and will be able to cope with the temporary decrease in circulation during a contraction (Huddleston, 2002). If there is a deterioration of the uteroplacental function leading to marginal basal oxygenation, any decrease in uteroplacental circulation (such as with a contraction) will cause late FHR decelerations (see Chap. 15) (Cunningham et al., 2005; Huddleston, 2002). Recurrent late decelerations indicate fetal hypoxemia. The variable decelerations that accompany contractions also may result from fetal umbilical cord compression, which may be associated with oligohydramnios (Beckmann et al., 2002).

The CST should not be performed when uterine activity is undesirable, such as with placenta previa or a previous vertical uterine scar (Huddleston, 2002). The CST also should be avoided when risk for preterm labor and delivery is increased, including multiple gestation, incompetent cervix, previous preterm delivery, or hydramnios (Huddleston, 2002).

For the CST, the woman is positioned in bed in a semi-Fowler's position or with a wedge or pillow under one hip (preferably the right) to prevent occlusion of the aorta, which may reduce uterine blood flow to such a degree that late decelerations of the FHR occur and produce false-positive results (Huddleston, 2002). Each of two transducers is held in place with a soft fabric belt that is snugly fastened. The tocodynamometer transducer (which measures uterine activity) is placed over the fundus of the uterus. The Doppler FHR transducer (which measures FHR) is covered with transducer gel and placed over the position where the FHR is most readily heard (usually over the fetal back, ascertained by using Leopold's maneuvers). The test may take between 20 and 90 minutes (Cunningham et al., 2005; Huddleston, 2002), during which time the woman remains in bed.

An initial 20-minute NST provides a baseline recording. In 10% to 15% of procedures, spontaneous uterine activity seen during the NST is adequate and further stimulation of contractions is not needed (Huddleston, 2002). Adequate uterine activity for a CST is defined as three uterine contractions that each last 40 to 60 seconds within 10 minutes (Cunningham et al., 2005; Huddleston, 2002). If spontaneous uterine activity is not adequate but late decelerations occur, further stimulation of uterine activity is contraindicated (Fig. 12.20).

If there is no, or inadequate, spontaneous uterine activity and no late decelerations have occurred, contractions are stimulated using either nipple self-stimulation or, rarely, an oxytocin infusion. Nipple stimulation is used most frequently, primarily because of cost and time savings as well as decreased discomfort to the woman

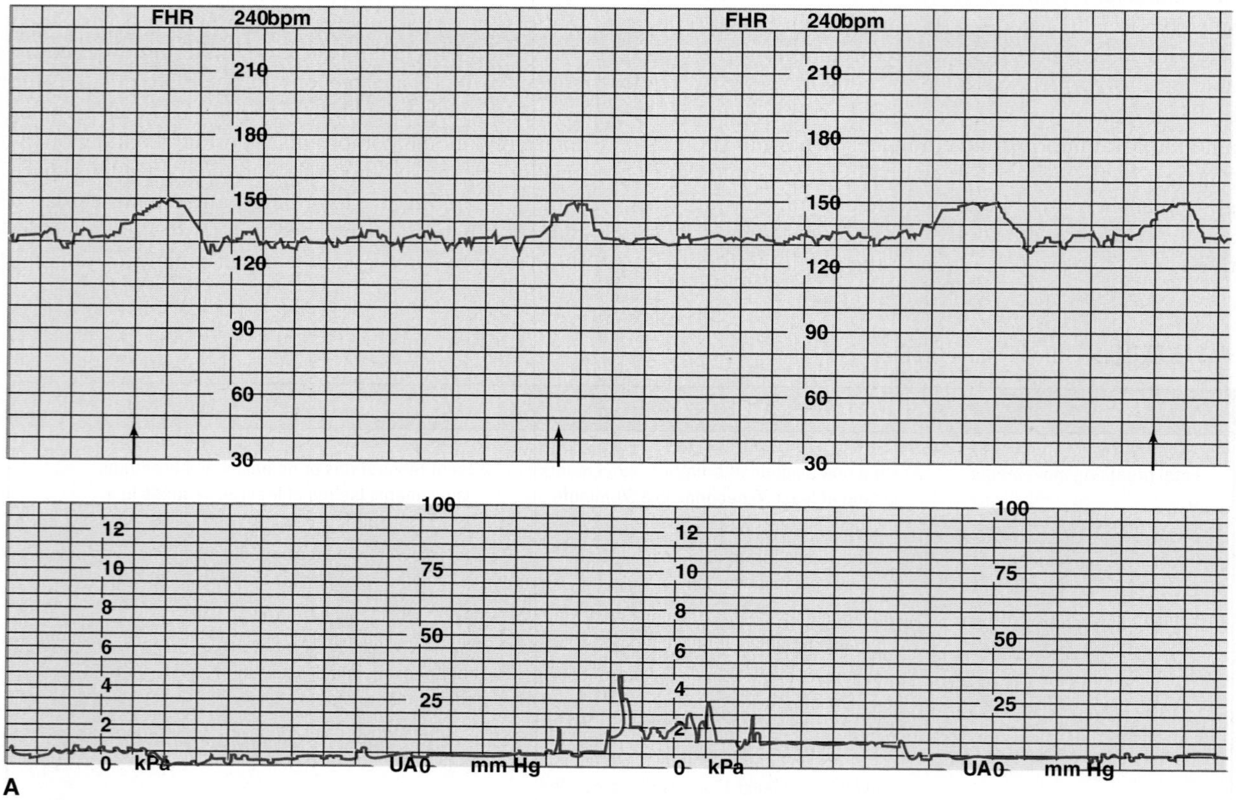

FIGURE 12.20 (**A**) A rhythm strip. The upper portion is the fetal heart rate (FHR), and the lower portion is uterine activity. *Arrows* represent fetal movement.

Continued

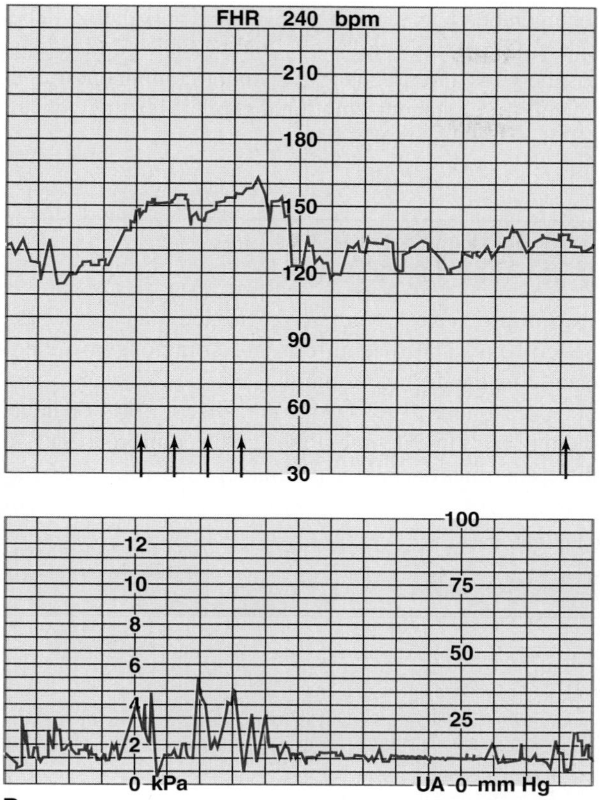

B

FIGURE 12.20 *(Continued)* (**B**) Baseline FHR is 130 to 131 beats/min. The strip shows FHR accelerations in response to fetal movement (*arrows*).

(Huddleston, 2002). With nipple self-stimulation, the woman rapidly but gently rubs one nipple through light clothing with her fingertips in a to-and-fro motion for 2 minutes (Cunningham et al., 2005; Huddleston, 2002). She then stops the stimulation for 5 minutes. During this time, uterine activity is monitored both with the monitor and manually (Huddleston, 2002). If there are no adequate contractions after 5 minutes, the woman again stimulates her nipple for 2 minutes and rests for 5 minutes. Stimulation is stopped immediately if a contraction begins. Two cycles or less than 4 minutes have been found to result in adequate uterine contraction in approximately 75% of women (Huddleston, 2002). Stimulation of contractions using nipple self-stimulation has resulted in tests of shorter duration than those using oxytocin infusion (Huddleston, 2002).

Previous guidelines for nipple self-stimulation suggested that continuous stimulation of both bared nipples was appropriate (Huddleston, 2002). The ACOG is endorsing self-stimulation of only one nipple through light clothing, however, because of its acceptability to women and because it is less likely to cause uterine hyperstimulation (Huddleston, 2002).

Although now used rarely to stimulate contractions (Huddleston, 2002), if oxytocin infusion is administered, it is delivered as a low-dose infusion piggyback by pump at an initial rate of 0.5 mU/min. The rate is increased slowly until adequate uterine contractions are achieved.

The CST is said to be negative if no late decelerations are seen with any contraction (Cunningham et al., 2005; Huddleston, 2002). It is said to be positive if late decelerations accompany 50% or more of the contractions, regardless of the number of contractions (Cunningham et al., 2005; Huddleston, 2002). If these late decelerations occur before the achievement of adequate contractions, the test should be discontinued (Huddleston, 2002). The test is considered equivocal-suspicious if there are intermittent late decelerations or significant variable decelerations (Cunningham et al., 2005). The test is considered equivocal-hyperstimulatory if the decelerations occur with contractions lasting longer than 90 seconds or more frequently than every 2 minutes (Cunningham et al., 2005). If there are fewer than 3 contractions in 10 minutes or the tracing is not interpretable, the test is considered unsatisfactory (Cunningham et al., 2005).

Umbilical Artery Doppler Velocimetry

Umbilical artery Doppler velocimetry is the newest technique to assess fetal well-being. The test is based on the belief that the shape of uterine artery velocity waveform is unique and differs in the fetus with normal growth and the fetus with growth restriction. The waveform is characterized by "high end-diastolic velocities with continuous forward blood flow throughout diastole" (Divon & Ferber, 2002, p. 1015). As the pregnancy progresses, the degree of end-diastolic flow shows a typical increase. When end-diastolic flow is decreased, intrauterine growth restriction occurs (Cunningham et al., 2005; Divon & Ferber, 2002). This is thought to result in part from poorly vascularized placenta villi (Cunningham et al., 2005; Divon & Ferber, 2002). With extreme cases of placental dysfunction, the end-diastolic flow may be absent or reversed (Cunningham et al., 2005; Divon & Ferber, 2002). Absent or reversed end-diastolic flow is considered an ominous sign indicating fetal compromise that may precede fetal death (Cunningham et al., 2005; Divon & Ferber, 2002). Perinatal mortality in reversed end-diastolic flow has been reported to be approximately 33%, whereas mortality in absent end-diastolic flow has been 10% (Cunningham et al., 2005).

Although abnormal Doppler studies have been associated with lower arterial and venous pH values, increased intrapartum fetal distress, and a higher incidence of neonatal respiratory distress syndrome (Divon & Ferber, 2002), Doppler is currently recommended only for the diagnosis of fetal growth restrictions (Cunningham et al., 2005; Divon & Ferber, 2002; Sprong, 2003). The blood flow in other fetal vessels has been evaluated, but at this time, only assessment of the umbilical artery has proved to be a reliable predictor of perinatal outcome (Cunningham et al., 2005; Divon & Ferber, 2002).

Collaborative Management

The nurse should examine the findings from each assessment of fetal well-being to anticipate the appropriate plan of care. For example, if the fetus displays normal activity, the NST is reactive, the BPP score is 10, the CST is negative (no late decelerations), and the end-diastolic flow is satisfactory, these findings suggest no compromise of the fetus and satisfactory uteroplacental perfusion. Any or all of the tests may be repeated depending on risk factors associated with the pregnancy and the clinical condition that prompted the testing. If assessment findings are abnormal, either alone or in combination, the nurse should anticipate further evaluation. Subsequent management depends on the results of this further evaluation, gestational age, degree of oligohydramnios (if assessed), and maternal condition. It is important for nurses to remember that the mother and significant others will be concerned about the test results and possible implications for the fetus and pregnancy. A major component of the nurse's care includes emotional support for the woman and her significant others.

ANTICIPATORY GUIDANCE RELATED TO PREGNANCY

During pregnancy, women experience many changes. Several physical discomforts are common; however, each client will have a unique experience. Therefore, not everyone will experience all discomforts or have them to the same degree. Physical discomforts occur at different times during the pregnancy. See Table 12.6 for

TABLE 12.6 Common Discomforts of Pregnancy, Etiology, and Relief Measures

DISCOMFORT	ETIOLOGY	RELIEF MEASURES
First Trimester		
Urinary frequency	Pressure of growing uterus on bladder	Decrease fluid intake at night. Maintain fluid intake during day. Void when feel the urge.
Fatigue	Possibly, increased metabolic requirements or nocturia	Rest frequently. Go to bed earlier.
Sleep difficulties	Often related to other signs and symptoms (eg, nocturia, palpitations)	Rest frequently. Decrease fluid intake at night.
Breast enlargement and sensitivity	Effect of hormones, especially estrogen and progesterone	Wear a good supporting bra with wide shoulder straps. Assess for other conditions.
Nasal stuffiness and epistaxis	Elevated estrogen levels	Avoid decongestants. Use humidifiers, cool mist vaporizers, and normal saline drops.
Ptyalism (excessive salivation)	Unknown	Perform frequent mouth care. Chew gum or suck hard candies.
Nausea and vomiting	Unknown	Avoid food or smells that exacerbate condition. Eat dry crackers or toast before rising in morning. Eat small, frequent meals.
Second and Third Trimesters		
Urinary frequency	After lightening, pressure of fetal head on bladder	Void when feel the urge. Decrease fluid intake at night. Maintain fluid intake during day.
Shortness of breath	Growing fetus, which puts pressure on diaphragm	Use extra pillows at night to keep more upright. Limit activity during day.
Heartburn	Displacement of stomach by growing fetus Relaxation of cardioesophageal sphincter	Eat small, more frequent meals. Use antacids. Avoid overeating and spicy foods.
Dependent edema	Impeded venous return from pressure of fetus on pelvic area	Avoid standing for long periods. Elevate legs when laying or sitting. Avoid tight stockings.
Varicosities	Weight of uterus, which causes pooling and engorgement of veins in lower extremities Heredity, age, obesity	Rest in Sims' position. Elevate legs regularly. Avoid crossing legs. Avoid tight stockings. Avoid long periods of standing.

Continued

TABLE 12.6 Common Discomforts of Pregnancy, Etiology, and Relief Measures

DISCOMFORT	ETIOLOGY	RELIEF MEASURES
Hemorrhoids	Constipation Pressure of enlarging uterus on pelvic and rectal veins	Maintain regular bowel habits. Use prescribed stool softeners. Apply witch hazel compresses and topical or anesthetic ointments to area.
Constipation	Pressure of growing fetus on intestine, causing decreased peristalsis Possibly, ingestion of iron	Maintain regular bowel habits. Increase roughage in diet. Increase fluids. Find iron preparation that is least constipating.
Leukorrhea	Response to increased estrogen levels	Take a daily bath or shower. Do not douche or use tampons. Wear cotton underwear.
Backache	Lumbar lordosis that develops to maintain balance in later pregnancy	Wear shoes with low heels. Walk with pelvis tilted forward. Use firmer mattress. Perform pelvic rocking or tilting.
Leg cramps	Decreased serum calcium level Increased serum phosphorus level Interference with circulation	Extend affected leg and dorsiflex the foot. Elevate lower legs frequently. Apply heat to muscles. Evaluate diet.
Balance alterations	Growing uterus, which throws off the woman's center of gravity	Wear shoes with low heels. Walk with pelvis tilted forward.
Round ligament pain	Tension on round ligament from enlarging uterus	Rise slowly from sitting to standing or lying to sitting. Apply a warm heating pad to abdomen or take a warm (not hot) bath. Bring knees up toward abdomen.
Flatulence	Decreased gastric motility Pressure of growing uterus on large intestine	Avoid gas-forming foods. Chew food thoroughly. Engage in regular daily exercise. Maintain regular bowel routine.
Carpal tunnel syndrome	Compression of medial nerve in carpal tunnel of wrist; weight gain and edema may contribute	Avoid aggravating hand movements. Elevate affected arm. Wear splint.
Faintness	Pooling of blood in lower extremities Anemia	Rise slowly from sitting to standing. Evaluate hemoglobin and hematocrit. Avoid hot stuffy environments.
Mood swings	Hormonal influences	The woman and her partner need information about these mood swings to understand that they are normal. This assists them to cope with them.

a summary of common discomforts, their etiologies, and suggested relief measures.

After providing anticipatory guidance, the nurse should remember to evaluate the effectiveness of interventions used to assist with the discomforts of pregnancy. If implemented measures have been ineffective, the nurse may need to investigate further to ensure there is not an alternative reason for the problems. Symptoms that continue to increase with associated metabolic or psychological complications may need treatment. For example, the client with uncontrolled nausea and vomiting that leads to dehydration and significant weight loss may need intravenous fluids for hydration and nourishment. See Nursing Care Plan 12.2 and NIC/NOC Box 12.1.

Urinary Frequency

Early in pregnancy, clients experience urinary frequency from the growing uterus compressing the bladder. Although little can be done to solve this problem, the nurse should advise clients who experience it to consider decreasing fluid intake in the evening before going to bed. Doing so assists in decreasing urine production, which may limit the number of times a client has to get up during the night to void. The nurse should advise clients not to reduce their fluid intake during the day because appropriate fluids are important to maintain hydration and to increase blood volume. The nurse should counsel clients to void whenever they feel the urge. Urine that stays in the bladder for an extended time increases the risk

NURSING CARE PLAN 12.2

A Client With Common Discomforts of Pregnancy

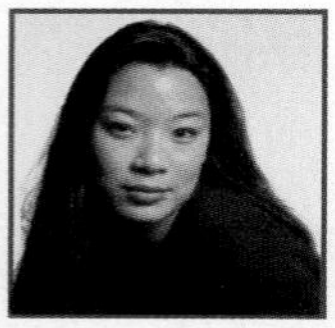

Consider Kathy from the beginning of the chapter. Assessment of her feet reveals pitting edema. On further questioning, Kathy says that she is employed as a cashier at the local supermarket. Once she finishes work for the day, she usually goes home, makes supper, and does some housework. She goes to bed about 10:00 PM, having gotten up at 6:30 AM. She has been decreasing her fluid intake in the evening because she occasionally still has urinary frequency. She does not like to eat vegetables.

NURSING DIAGNOSIS

Constipation related to decreased peristalsis secondary to pregnancy

EXPECTED OUTCOMES

1. The client will verbalize the underlying etiology of constipation.
2. The client will identify two strategies to decrease constipation.

INTERVENTIONS	RATIONALES
Use both oral and written materials to teach the client about the pressure that the growing fetus places on the intestine, which causes decreased peristalsis.	Assisting the client to understand the reasons for constipation will help her choose effective strategies to decrease the problem. Understanding the etiology will help decrease anxiety.
Assist the client to choose vegetables and fruit that she likes in her diet.	Dietary roughage helps the stool retain fluid and decreases constipation.
Assist the client to plan increased fluid intake throughout the day.	Doing so will facilitate softer stool. Planning the increase during the day will assist the client with the urinary frequency she experiences at night.
At her next visit to the prenatal clinic, ask the client if she has experienced any changes in her stools. Assess for any further discomforts.	Doing so will reveal if the actions have been successful or if further planning is needed. The client will be less anxious if she has achieved success.

EVALUATION

1. The client verbalizes understanding of the reasons for constipation.
2. The client reports improvements in her stool pattern.
3. The client lists specific vegetables and fruit that she now includes in her diet.
4. The client reports that increased fluid has been successful in treating her constipation and avoiding urinary frequency at night.

NURSING DIAGNOSIS

Health-Seeking Behaviors related to discomforts of pregnancy

EXPECTED OUTCOMES

1. The client will verbalize the underlying etiology of dependent edema.
2. The client will take measures to control swelling and to avoid overexertion.

Continued

NURSING CARE PLAN 12.2 ● A Client With Common Discomforts of Pregnancy

INTERVENTIONS	RATIONALES
Using oral and written material, instruct the client about the impeded venous return from the fetal pressure on the pelvic area.	Assisting the client to understand the reasons for the edema will assist her to choose effective strategies to decrease the problem. Understanding the etiology will help decrease her anxiety.
Assist the client to identify ways that she can decrease the time that she stands.	Doing so will assist with venous return and should decrease the edema. Having the client identify the strategies assists both client and nurse to plan realistic interventions. The client will be more likely to continue to use suggestions if she has had more control.
Assist the client to identify appropriate clothing that will prevent further occlusion of the venous return.	Avoiding tight stockings will assist with prevention.
At the client's next visit to the clinic, assess the edema.	Doing so facilitates further planning and interventions if these are not successful.

EVALUATION

1. The client identifies two strategies to decrease dependent edema.
2. The client verbalizes understanding of the causes of edema and repeats material taught.
3. The client reports more frequent rest periods and going into work 30 minutes later each day.

NIC/NOC Box 12.1 Pregnancy and Related Care

Common NIC Labels

- Anticipatory Guidance
- Childbirth Preparation
- Constipation/Impaction Management
- Family Integrity Promotion: Childbearing Family
- Family Planning: Unplanned Pregnancy
- Learning Facilitation
- Nutritional Counseling
- Prenatal Care
- Surveillance: Late Pregnancy
- Ultrasonography: Limited Obstetric

Common NOC Labels

- Coping
- Decision Making
- Family Coping
- Fetal Status: Antepartum
- Knowledge: Maternal–Child Health
- Knowledge: Pregnancy
- Maternal Status: Antepartum

for UTI (Mittal & Wing, 2005). The nurse also should teach that urinary frequency will be alleviated when the uterus rises into the abdominal cavity, although it will return with lightening in the third trimester.

Fatigue and Sleep Problems

Pregnant women often are fatigued because of nocturia and increased metabolic requirements. They experience frequent sleep difficulties related to other signs and symptoms, such as palpitations. Suggestions to manage fatigue and sleep difficulties include getting more frequent rest periods, going to bed earlier, and resting in a modified Sims' position to reposition some fetal weight onto the bed. The nurse also may advise the client to use pillows under the abdomen and between the legs for support.

Breast Sensitivity and Other Discomforts

The breasts enlarge and become more sensitive from the effects of circulating hormones, especially estrogen and progesterone. The nurse should recommend wearing a supportive bra with wide shoulder straps that decrease pressure on the shoulders and avoiding any stimulus that seems to exacerbate breast sensitivity.

Increased estrogen levels may cause nasal stuffiness and epistaxis (nosebleeds) (Youngkin & Davis, 2004). Suggestions to manage nasal stuffiness include humidification of the room air and saline drops or spray. These suggestions also may help control epistaxis. Additional suggestions for epistaxis include local application of a moisturizer such as petroleum jelly, avoidance of forceful blowing of the nose, and avoidance of excessive overexertion or heating that may exacerbate epistaxis.

Ptyalism (excessive salivation) may occur for unknown reasons. Frequent mouth care and chewing gum or sucking hard candy may assist with ptyalism (Cunningham et al., 2005).

Gastrointestinal Problems

One of the most frequent discomforts of early pregnancy is nausea and vomiting, the cause of which is unknown. Hormonal and emotional factors have been investigated with inconsistent results. Because clients with nausea and vomiting often experience it as morning sickness, the nurse may recommend that they eat dry crackers or toast before rising. The nurse should counsel clients to avoid foods or smells that exacerbate nausea. Small, frequent meals also may assist to control nausea.

During the second and third trimesters, pregnant clients may experience heartburn as the cardioesophageal sphincter relaxes and the growing fetus displaces the stomach upward, leading to gastroesophageal reflux. Small, frequent meals may assist with heartburn, along with avoiding overeating and spicy foods. Limiting food and fluids before bed and sleeping in a semi-Fowler's position may help. Antacids also may be useful. The most consistent relief is provided by the use of liquid forms of antacids and histamine-2 receptor inhibitors (Katz, 2003). Women should be told that antacids containing aluminum may cause constipation; those containing magnesium may cause diarrhea. The client should discuss antacids with her primary care provider before using them.

The pressure of the enlarging uterus on the pelvic and rectal veins may lead to hemorrhoids. Adding to the development of hemorrhoids and the resulting discomfort, pregnant women are prone to constipation as the pressure of the growing fetus on the intestine decreases peristalsis. The use of iron supplements may exacerbate constipation. Women may experience flatulence from decreased gastric motility and the pressure of the growing uterus on the large intestine.

The nurse should encourage regular bowel habits to decrease constipation, hemorrhoids, and flatulence. Increasing roughage and fluids in the diet, avoiding or reducing constipating foods such as cheese, and increasing fluid intake may all assist with constipation. After consultation with her primary care provider to ensure that there are no contraindications, the client may find a regular program of mild exercise helpful. Stool softeners may assist with constipation and hemorrhoids. Witch hazel compresses, topical analgesics, or anesthetic ointments also may help if the constipation is related to hemorrhoids. The client can decrease flatulence by avoiding gas-forming foods and chewing food thoroughly.

Vascular Problems

Dependent edema, especially of the ankles and feet, results from the impeded venous return caused by the pressure of the growing fetus on the pelvic area. The pooling and engorgement of the veins in the lower extremities also leads to varicose veins, which can be exacerbated by heredity, age, or obesity. Leg cramps may develop from decreased serum calcium level, increased serum phosphorus level, and interference with circulation of the extremities.

The nurse should advise the client to avoid long periods of standing and to elevate the legs while sitting, which may help decrease dependent edema, varicosities, and leg cramps (Fig. 12.21). If the client develops a leg cramp, she should extend the affected leg and dorsiflex the foot. Application of heat to the muscle also may be helpful. Clients should avoid crossing their legs and wearing tight stockings to prevent varicosities. They also should avoid massaging the calf muscle.

Dyspnea

Dyspnea arises from the crowding caused by the growing fetus on the diaphragm, the increased oxygen the client uses, and the resulting carbon dioxide that forms. Use of extra pillows at night to prop the client in bed into a more semi-sitting position may assist with shortness of breath. If shortness of breath occurs during the day as well, the client may need to limit her activities.

Leukorrhea and Vaginal Problems

Leukorrhea (increased vaginal secretions) often results in response to increased estrogen levels. A daily bath or shower, along with the use of cotton underwear and panty liners, will increase comfort and decrease risk for

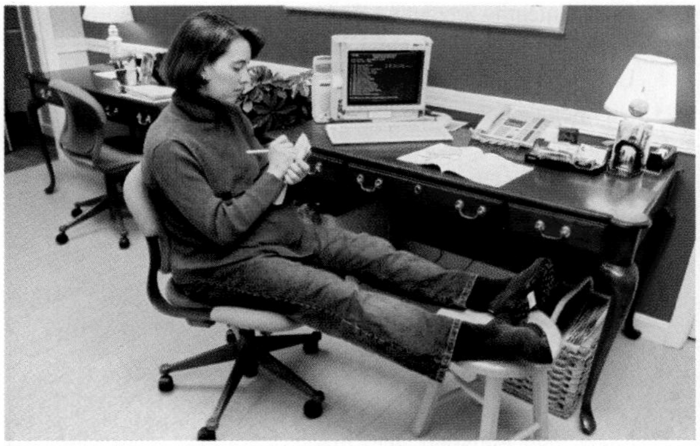

FIGURE 12.21 Leg elevation can prevent or decrease edema, varicosities, and leg cramps during pregnancy.

infection. The woman should avoid douching because of the risk for vaginal infection.

Round Ligament Pain

As the uterus enlarges, tension is put on the round ligament, often resulting in pain. Rising slowly from a sitting to standing position or from a lying to sitting position may decrease this pain. Bringing the knees up to the abdomen also may help decrease some of the pain. Assuming a position on the hands and knees and lowering the head to the floor, while keeping the buttocks in the air, may alleviate unremitting ligament pain.

Carpal Tunnel Syndrome

Weight gain, edema, and traction on the median nerve from postural changes resulting in median nerve compression may contribute to the development of carpal tunnel syndrome, a condition that causes tingling, numbness, and burning in the fingers and hands (Bahrami et al., 2006; Cunningham et al., 2005). The nurse should advise the client that gentle range of motion of the affected hand every 4 hours may assist with mild symptoms. If symptoms are more severe, the client may need a soft wrist splint to avoid pressure on the median nerve in the mid-palm area. The nurse should counsel the client to avoid repetitive wrist motion, flexion, or extension and encourage her to alternate and take frequent breaks from activities.

Supine Hypotension Syndrome

Clients in the later stages of pregnancy may be at increased risk for faintness as blood pools in the lower extremities. If the client lies on her back, pressure from the gravid uterus compresses the vena cava, causing supine hypotensive syndrome. This results in hypotension with diaphoresis and possible syncope. The client can avoid supine hypotensive syndrome by maintaining a side-lying position during pregnancy, especially resting on the left side, which increases placental circulation and oxygenation. Slowly rising from sitting to standing and avoiding hot humid environments also will help prevent postural hypotension.

Backache

The growing uterus disrupts the pregnant client's center of gravity, compromising her balance (Fig. 12.22). Backache and lordosis can develop in late pregnancy as the client tries to maintain her balance. The client can relieve backache by wearing shoes with lower heels, performing pelvic rocking or tilting exercises, and walking with the pelvis tilted backward. Warm (not hot) baths that do not exceed 30 minutes may be helpful. Use of a firmer mattress also may provide relief. The client also should practice good body mechanics by bending both knees when lifting, holding objects close to her body, lifting with her leg muscles, and avoiding heavy lifting. Regular exercise (after consultation with the primary care provider) also may assist with strengthening back and abdominal muscles and thus decreasing backache.

Bathing

Tub bathing is acceptable during pregnancy as long as the woman's membranes are intact. Bathing with ruptured membranes is contraindicated because of the risk

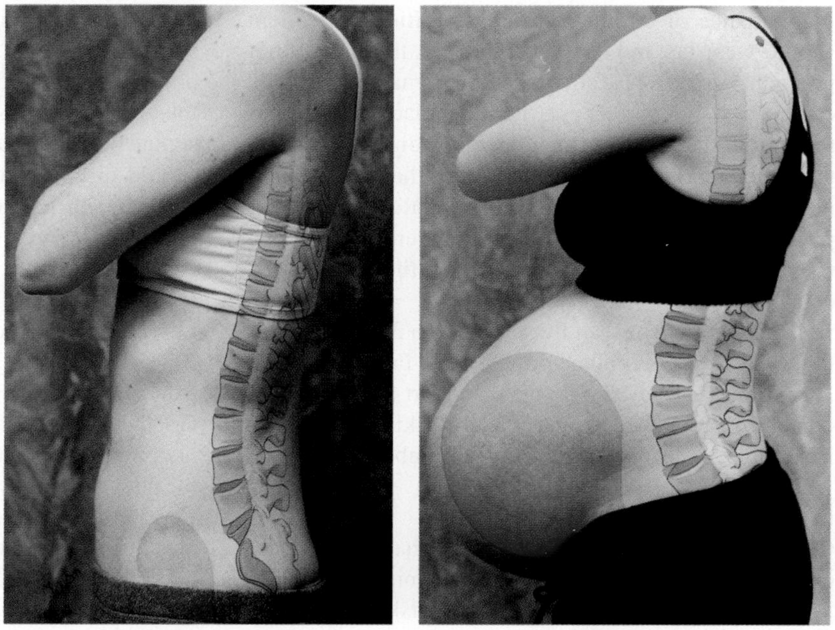

FIGURE 12.22 The postural changes from the first trimester (**A**) to the third trimester (**B**) disrupt the pregnant client's center of gravity and sense of balance.

A. Early pregnancy **B.** Late pregnancy

for infection. Because of the problems with balance in the last trimester, showers at the end of pregnancy may be preferable. The temperature of the water should not exceed 39°C (102°F) to avoid raising the core body temperature, which may lead to postural hypotension. The use of saunas and whirlpool baths is not recommended because of the intense heat.

Working

Working during pregnancy generally is not contraindicated, although there may be individualized instances in which it is not recommended. If the client works in a high-risk area (ie, an occupation that is physically or emotionally hazardous), additional precautions may be necessary, or she may need to transfer to another area. Pregnant clients who continue to work should take the opportunity to rest periodically throughout the day whenever possible. Those whose work requires prolonged standing should be especially conscious of sitting frequently; prolonged standing has been found to increase the risk for preterm labor (McCulloch, 2002).

Travel

There is no contraindication to travel for pregnant women, unless they have medical or obstetrical complications. Travel may be contraindicated for clients with cardiovascular conditions complicated by pregnancy, congenital or acquired heart disease, multiple gestations after 22 weeks, or incompetent cervix. Long-distance travel may not be advisable when pregnancy is complicated by threatened abortion, vaginal bleeding, history of preterm labor, or other obstetrical complications.

Travel by car is often tiring, especially late in pregnancy. Frequent rest stops are necessary to assist with maintenance of circulation to extremities. The client should wear lap and shoulder seatbelts throughout her pregnancy to decrease any risk for maternal injury (Beck et al., 2005). For correct use, the client places the lap portion of the seatbelt over the upper portion of her thighs, under her abdomen. She then positions the shoulder harness between the breasts. Both belts should be snugly applied. Seatbelts also will decrease exaggerated flexion of the woman's torso, which may lessen the risk for placental separation (Fig. 12.23).

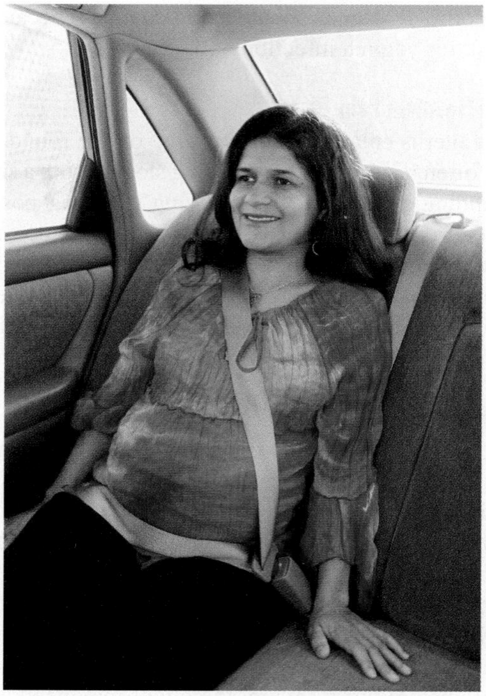

FIGURE 12.23 The pregnant client should wear a seatbelt as shown.

Pregnant clients can fly safely up to 36 weeks' gestation (ACOG Committee on Obstetric Practice, 2002). During flights, they should wear support hose and periodically exercise the legs and ankles, walking in the aisles if possible, to decrease the risk for thrombophlebitis.

Exercise

Generally, the pregnant client does not have to limit exercise. She should, however, avoid becoming excessively fatigued or doing any activity that may risk injury to herself or her fetus. Clients who have been accustomed to aerobic exercise before pregnancy should be allowed to continue; however, they should not begin new activity or increase their level or intensity (Fig. 12.24). Clients who have continued their pre-pregnancy exercise routine during pregnancy have been found to have shorter active labors, fewer cesarean births, and less fetal distress in labor (Cunningham et al., 2005). Women who have been sedentary before pregnancy should not take part in aerobic exercise that is any more strenuous than walking (Cunningham et al., 2005) and should consult with their primary care provider before starting. All pregnant clients must avoid exercise that involves extended time in the supine position in the second and third trimesters. They should discontinue exercise if they have any signs of oxygen deprivation such as extreme fatigue, dizziness, or extreme shortness of breath. They should not exercise if exercise might adversely affect any obstetrical or medical condition, such as incompetent cervix, risk factors for preterm labor, or pregnancy-induced hypertension.

Dental Care

Good dental care during pregnancy is important. Studies have suggested that active periodontal disease increases the client's risk for pre-eclampsia (Cockney, 2003; Contreras et al., 2006). The client should schedule a dental checkup in early pregnancy and inform the dentist about her pregnancy to assist in avoiding teratogenic substances. Dental x-rays may be taken if a lead apron fully covers the abdomen (Katz, 2003). There is no evidence

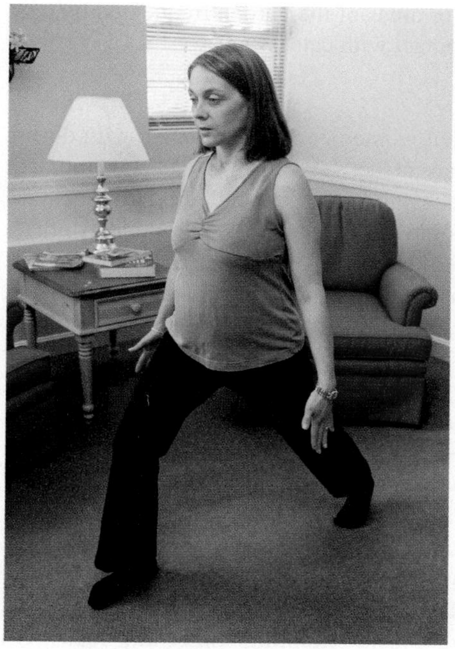

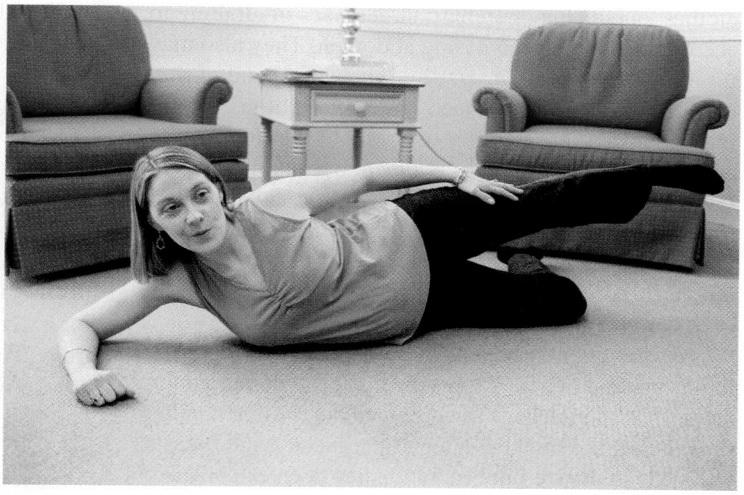

FIGURE 12.24 The pregnant client can continue her normal exercise routine, which may strengthen the abdominal and back muscles. She should not start new routines during this time, however.

that suggests that pregnancy aggravates dental caries (Cunningham et al., 2005).

Sexual Concerns

Both the client and her partner may express concerns about sexuality and intercourse during pregnancy. Although there is no reason why the healthy woman need abstain from intercourse or orgasm during pregnancy, some sources suggest that women should avoid coitus and orgasm in the last 4 weeks of pregnancy (Cunningham et al., 2005). Regardless of suggestions, studies have found that the frequency of coitus decreases as pregnancy progresses (Sayle et al., 2003). Clients may engage in intercourse less frequently because of decreased desire or fear of causing harm in the pregnancy.

Intercourse or orgasm is contraindicated in cases of known placenta previa, or ruptured membranes (Cunningham et al., 2005; Katz, 2003). The amniotic sac provides protection from infection; once it has ruptured, the risk for infection increases (Freda, 2002). Nipple stimulation, vaginal penetration, or orgasm may cause uterine contractions secondary to the release of prostaglandins and oxytocin (Katz, 2003). Therefore, women who are predisposed to preterm labor or threatened abortion may choose to avoid intercourse (Katz, 2003).

It is normal for desire for sexual intercourse to decrease or increase during pregnancy (Freda, 2002). Sometimes, the cause is discomforts of pregnancy, such as nausea or vomiting. Discussing these changes with the client's partner helps decrease misunderstandings and feelings of inadequacy in either partner. Other changes that may influence sexual desire or activity include the normally increased amount and odor of vaginal secretions and increased breast sensitivity, especially in the first trimester, that may be exacerbated by touching of breasts or positions that increase the pressure put on them.

In later stages, once the abdomen is significantly enlarged, alternate positions may be more comfortable for some women. Examples of positions that may increase comfort include the woman in the superior position or a side-by-side position. If the woman experiences discomfort from vaginal penetration, the couple may find alternative methods of sexual expression, such as cuddling, masturbation, or oral sex. It is important for the partner to refrain from blowing into the pregnant woman's vagina because doing so may cause an air embolism, which has been shown to be fatal (Cunningham et al., 2005; Freda, 2002).

Some women report increased sexual desire during pregnancy. Possible reasons for this increase include not having to worry about birth control, as well as the increased blood flow to the pelvic region that increases libido and sexual satisfaction. Decreased desire may result from those times when the woman is not feeling well. Occasionally, concerns may develop about potential changes in the woman's body and the couple's relationship. The nurse should provide the opportunity for each to verbalize their concerns and correct any misinformation or myths. The nurse also should encourage the couple to initiate and maintain an open dialogue.

Clothing

As the client's abdomen enlarges, the need for different clothing becomes apparent. Before buying maternity clothes, clients may purchase larger sizes of clothing to accommodate their increasing abdomen. They also may insert elastic or cloth inserts into the waist band of regular clothing until they need maternity clothes. Clothing should be loose fitting to promote comfort and to accommodate the growing abdomen. Because new clothing can be expensive and is worn for a relatively short time, suggestions to economize include sharing clothes with friends and family, sewing one's own clothing, and buying used clothing. Recently, stores that sell lightly used clothing at reduced prices have emerged.

As the client's breasts increase, she will require a larger bra and benefit from bras that provide maximum support. Although some recommend purchasing nursing bras during the last trimester of pregnancy, the breasts will change in size once lactation has been established. Thus, purchasing nursing bras while pregnant may not be helpful.

Nutrition

Nutrition is important because the client must ensure that both she and the fetus receive the calories and nutrients they require. Chapter 3 provides extensive discussion of nutritional needs and adaptations required during pregnancy.

Pets

Pets provide companionship, especially to clients who may be home more than usual during pregnancy. They may present additional challenges, however, to expectant mothers and their significant others. Pets may demonstrate jealousy of the new baby, similar to sibling rivalry, when they have held a central position in the family. It might be helpful for the expectant client to pretend to carry a baby around the house. Additionally, many pregnant women give additional time and affection to their pets, in anticipation of their having less time to do so once the baby is born. Rather than helping the pet, however, this may increase the animal's feelings of jealousy because it emphasizes the differences in attention that they are receiving once the baby is part of the family. Books and other resources are available that will provide assistance to the family in dealing with this.

The protozoan *Toxoplasma gondii* causes toxoplasmosis, an illness that presents few problems to adults but can produce profound effects on the fetus, including spontaneous abortion and congenital toxoplasmosis, if contracted during pregnancy. The likelihood of fetal infection increases with gestation (Minkoff & Gibbs, 2003). Eating undercooked meat, drinking unpasteurized milk, or having contact with the feces of infected cats facilitates contact with *T. gondii* (Cunningham et al., 2005). Fecal oocytes are spread through the air and can cause infection through inhalation. The nurse should counsel the pregnant woman to avoid contact with the cat litter box or areas of the garden frequented by cats. Otherwise, contact with cats is safe.

Teratogens

Substances that women come into contact with during pregnancy may affect fetal growth and development adversely. Such substances are called **teratogens** (see Chap. 11). Some teratogens are legal, whereas others are illegal. Some effects of teratogens are evident at birth, whereas others are not detected until years later. For example, female children of women who took the drug diethylstilbestrol (DES) during pregnancy did not show any adverse effects until years later when those who had been exposed in utero developed vaginal and cervical cancer in adolescence. Structural abnormalities of the reproductive tract in female children led to infertility and increased risk for ectopic pregnancy, spontaneous abortions, and preterm labor (Cunningham et al., 2005). Exposed male children had increased risk for epididymal cysts, microphallus, cryptorchidism, and testicular hypoplasia (Cunningham et al., 2005). On the other hand, babies demonstrated the adverse effects of thalidomide (shortened limbs) as soon as they were born.

Many substances can be teratogens or have teratogenic effects, including x-rays and pesticides. Medications are the most frequently recognized and researched teratogens. Other examples include rubella, alcohol, syphilis, and toxoplasmosis.

COLLABORATIVE CARE: TERATOGENS

Assessment

Maternal use of teratogenic substances may be known or unknown during pregnancy, either to the woman herself or to health care providers. Assessment should focus primarily on determining any substances that the woman may come into contact with. The nurse also should discuss with the client the frequencies and amounts of such contact (eg, how often and the amount of alcohol ingested).

Select Potential Nursing Diagnoses

The following are examples of commonly applicable NANDA diagnoses:

- **Risk for Fetal Injury** related to prenatal exposure to drugs
- **Deficient Knowledge** related to substances that adversely affect fetal development

Planning/Intervention

During pregnancy, the client needs information about substances that may have teratogenic effects on the fetus and what those effects may be. The nurse can provide such discussion and answer questions as needed.

Medications, including both over-the-counter and prescription drugs, are the most well-documented teratogens. Although women may be aware of the hazards of prescription drugs during pregnancy, such awareness does not always extend to over-the-counter medications (Werler et al., 2005). The greatest danger to the fetus is during the organogenesis of the first trimester (see Chap. 11). Maternal exposure to medications may occur before a woman knows that she is pregnant. Therefore, if possible, the nurse should suggest that the client begin avoiding medications once she makes the decision to become pregnant.

Caffeine has not been directly implicated as a teratogen; however, excessive intake may be implicated in spontaneous abortion (Cunningham et al., 2005; Katz, 2003). Caffeine also interferes with the absorption of iron (Lloyd, 2003). The commonly accepted recommendation is for women to try to limit their intake of caffeine during pregnancy.

Nicotine has been demonstrated to cause decreased birth weight in neonates (Bernstein et al., 2005). It also has been associated with an increased risk for placenta abruptio, preterm birth, and perinatal death (Cunningham et al., 2005). Babies born to mothers who smoke during pregnancy have an increased incidence of sudden infant death syndrome and lower respiratory tract infections (Gaffney, 2001; Lannero et al., 2006; Viccars, 2003). The nurse should give information to clients about the risks. If it is difficult for a client to quit smoking, the nurse should inform her that any decrease is beneficial. If significant others around the client smoke, rather than the woman herself, the nurse should suggest that they smoke in places other than around the client.

Infants of mothers who ingest alcohol are at increased risk for fetal alcohol syndrome (FAS) and fetal alcohol effects (FAE) (see Chap. 22). No level of alcohol has been determined safe during pregnancy, so the nurse should caution women to avoid all alcohol during pregnancy. Alcohol can pass through the placental barrier, resulting in an alcohol content in the fetal blood equivalent to the maternal alcohol content.

The use of cocaine during pregnancy increases the risk for placenta abruptio, stillbirth, low birth weight, neonatal addiction and subsequent withdrawal, and some birth defects (Barron, 2001; Beckmann et al., 2002; Cunningham et al., 2005). Marijuana has not been proved to be a teratogen (Yankowitz, 2003); however, it may be used in combination with other drugs that may be teratogens (Pillitteri, 2007). Therefore, the health care provider should assess the client for use of marijuana. Because the use of marijuana is more acceptable in society today, women may admit to using it while denying other drug use.

Pollution also may be a teratogen. The nurse should caution pregnant women to limit their exposure outside on days when pollution levels are significant.

Evaluation

Health care providers should continue to evaluate the client's behaviors. They may determine that additional teaching and support are necessary. Referral to support groups may be appropriate. Providers should closely monitor newborns who were exposed to teratogenic substances in utero.

COMMUNITY AND HOME CONCERNS

The role of the community in a client's pregnancy varies, often related to cultural practices. For example, clients and families from Latino cultures may be more likely to have significant support from the community and extended family (McGlade et al., 2004). Other clients may have little knowledge of community programs and resources. Many clients, however, are interested in prenatal classes and may access these from public health offices, private groups, or other organizations. The nurse should be aware of the availability of these classes within the community and provide accurate information to clients and support people.

Many families today face difficult issues, such as poverty, homelessness, unemployment, chemical dependency, family and neighborhood violence, and lack of support systems. Early recognition of any of these problems may assist the nurse to provide referrals to appropriate resources. Examples include social workers, food and nutrition supplement programs (including Women, Infants, and Children Special Supplemental Food Program), and social services.

Questions to Ponder

During an appointment with the prenatal clinic, a woman's partner tells the nurse that the woman has been using cocaine throughout her pregnancy and continues to do so. He says that he is concerned about the health of the fetus and wants something done to prevent her from continuing to use drugs.

1. Discuss your personal feelings about a pregnant woman who knowingly continues to use drugs that she has been repeatedly told will cause serious harm to the baby.
2. Explore your personal feelings about the partner wanting to have something done to prevent her from continuing to use drugs.

3. Identify the additional information might be helpful for the nurse to have before responding.
4. Clarify the legal and ethical considerations that need to be considered.

SUMMARY

- Women experience pregnancy in various ways. In addition to age, ethnicity, race, culture, sexual orientation, economic status, and religion also have effects. Each woman is unique. Nurses should not make assumptions that a particular client fits into any one stereotype. For example, although a woman may be from a particular culture, the extent to which she follows traditional customs may vary. The nurse must view each woman within the context of her environment.
- Women who present with pregnancy may range in age from younger than 15 to older than 45 years. Each age group faces unique challenges with pregnancy.
- Blood volume at delivery increases approximately 30%. Cardiac output increases by 30% to 40%. Pulse increases approximately 10 beats/minute.
- Supine postural hypotension syndrome may present problems of lightheadedness and faintness as the pressure of the gravid uterus compresses the vena cava if the woman lies on her back.
- Impeded venous return to the legs and pelvis may result in edema of the lower extremities, varicosities, and hemorrhoids.
- As the fetus grows, it pushes the diaphragm up so that the woman experiences shortness of breath in the latter stages of pregnancy. As it exerts pressure on other abdominal organs, it causes constipation, flatus, and heartburn.
- Changes to the integumentary system include pigmentation changes of the face and abdomen and the development of striae.
- Hormones that are increased in pregnancy, including estrogen, progesterone, human chorionic gonadotropin, human placental lactogen, relaxin, and prostaglandins, cause breast enlargement and tingling, leukorrhea, and mood swings.
- The glomerular filtration rate and the renal plasma flow increase in the kidneys.
- As the woman's abdomen grows, she develops a lordosis in an attempt to maintain her balance with her shifting center of gravity. This may lead to chronic backache.
- Women experience a number of psychological changes as they move through pregnancy, including surprise, fear, excitement, and apprehension. Changes are also experienced by partners, grandparents, and siblings.
- Presumptive signs are the subjective signs that the mother experiences. They include amenorrhea, morning sickness, excessive fatigue, urinary frequency, changes in the breasts, and quickening. Probable signs are those objective signs that the examiner assesses. They include Goodell's sign, Chadwick's sign, Hegar's sign, enlargement of the uterus, Braxton-Hicks contractions, skin pigmentation changes, and pregnancy tests. Positive signs absolutely confirm pregnancy. They include the presence of a fetal heart, fetal movements that can be felt by the examiner, and visualization of the fetus on ultrasound.
- The health history of the pregnant woman should include a menstrual history, sexual history, history of sexually transmitted infections, history of past pregnancies, past medical and surgical history, history of abuse, childhood illnesses, family background of the mother and father, and the use of drugs, alcohol, and tobacco.
- Physical examination of the pregnant woman should include the estimated date of delivery, physiologic changes the woman has been experiencing, and a complete physical examination of all body systems. A pelvic examination should include assessment of the pelvis. The mother's ABO and Rh, rubella titer, hemoglobin, and urinalysis should be assessed.
- Fetal well-being can be evaluated through maternal assessment of activity, the biophysical profile, the modified biophysical profile, the nonstress test, the contraction stress test, and the umbilical artery Doppler velocimetry. Each of these alone provides relatively limited information; in combination, however, greater confidence in care decisions will be achieved.
- Women will not be able to solve the common problems associated with pregnancy, but they may be able to manage the symptoms sufficiently to be comfortable for most of the pregnancy. Strategies include decreasing fluid intake in the evening, taking frequent rest periods, wearing a supportive bra, avoiding foods that are bothersome, eating small and frequent meals, elevating legs regularly, increasing roughage in the diet, and rising slowly from sitting to standing.
- Several substances are teratogenic to the developing fetus. Examples include prescription and over-the-counter medications, nicotine, alcohol, cocaine, and pollution.

REVIEW QUESTIONS

1. During a prenatal visit, a 38-year-old woman, G1P0, who is at 28 weeks' gestation, expresses increased concerns about the pregnancy. Which of the following would the nurse recognize as the most likely potential cause for anxiety?
   A. Fear of the unknown
   B. Fear of losing the pregnancy
   C. Ambivalence about the pregnancy
   D. Changes in the woman's mental health

2. A woman comes to a prenatal clinic seeking care. She is new to the area, having recently arrived from Bangladesh. She identifies herself as a Muslim. Which intervention would be most important to consider when planning her care?
   A. Ensure an interpreter is available.
   B. Question her about what traditions of the Muslim faith she follows.
   C. Ensure no appointments are scheduled on Fridays.
   D. Assign her to a provider with a small workload so that more time can be spent with her.
3. A woman who is at 26 weeks' gestation calls the office nurse and shares that she has been experiencing all the following symptoms. Which symptom would suggest to the nurse that additional information is needed?
   A. Nasal stuffiness
   B. Urinary frequency
   C. Tingling in the breasts
   D. Darkened spots on the nose and cheeks
4. A woman, G2P0010, who is at 14 weeks' gestation says that she isn't sure she is pregnant. She believes that her symptoms may indicate something is wrong with her. Which of these statements would it be best for the nurse to use to reassure the woman?
   A. "Once you feel the baby move you will feel better about being pregnant."
   B. "Many women feel this way early in pregnancy, so you are not alone."
   C. "Your pregnancy test came back positive, so you don't need to worry."
   D. "An ultrasound will provide the best assurance that you are pregnant."
5. During a health assessment of a woman who is pregnant for the fourth time, she indicates that she has 5-year-old twin boys who were born at 32 weeks and a 3-year-old daughter born at 41 weeks. She relates that she miscarried last year. All her children are currently healthy. What is the appropriate way to record her gravida and para status?
   A. 4-2-1-1-3
   B. 4-1-2-1-3
   C. 4-1-1-1-3
   D. 3-1-1-1-3
6. A young woman attends the prenatal clinic for her first visit. She indicates that the first day of her last normal menstrual period was December 2. Using Naegele's rule, her expected date of delivery (EDD) is September
   A. 2.
   B. 5.
   C. 9.
   D. 12.
7. The nurse is preparing a teaching plan in anticipation of meeting with a client who is at 34 weeks' gestation, G3P2011, and is concerned about the development of varicose veins in both legs. The nurse should include all the following information in the teaching plan *except:*
   A. Shoes should have flat or minimal heels.
   B. Massage both legs daily.
   C. Plan exercise focusing on the lower extremities.
   D. Reassure the client that they will disappear after birth.
8. A client, G2P1001, who is 33 weeks pregnant, comes to the nurse-midwifery office for a routine visit. She shares with the nurse that she has been experiencing difficulty getting to sleep, backaches, swelling of her ankles, and shortness of breath. Which of these statements would it be best for the nurse to make?
   A. "Tell me more about each of these."
   B. "These are normal changes of pregnancy."
   C. "They will go away in another few weeks."
   D. "Share with me your concerns about these symptoms."
9. During a prenatal assessment, a woman indicates that she has several cats and dogs at home. Which of the following information should the nurse share with the woman?
   A. No changes are necessary to the woman's routines.
   B. The client should avoid emptying the cats' litter box.
   C. Someone else should feed the animals.
   D. The client should avoid cleaning up the dog's waste.
10. A woman, G4P2103, who is at 38 weeks' gestation has had a biophysical profile. Results show a pocket of amniotic fluid measuring 2 cm in vertical diameter and that the fetus is stretching and flexing its arms and legs and has moved discretely three times in 30 minutes. The fetal heart rate is 132 beats/minute with three increases to 160 beats/minute accompanying movements. The ultrasound showed breathing movements lasting 45 seconds. Based on these findings, the nurse should conclude that the fetus is
    A. healthy.
    B. sleeping.
    C. in need of immediate birth.
    D. in need of repeat testing in 4 to 6 hours.

REFERENCES

Abramowicz, J. S., Kossoff, G., Marsal, K., & Ter Haar, G. (2002). Safety statement, 2000 (reconfirmed 2002). *Ultrasound Obstetrical Gynecology, 19,* 105.

Allender, J. A., & Spradley, B. W. (2005). *Community health nursing concepts and practices* (6th ed.). Philadelphia: Lippincott.

American College of Obstetricians and Gynecologists (ACOG). (2002). ACOG Committee Opinion: Number 279, December 2002. Prevention of early-onset group B streptococcal disease in newborns. *Obstetrics & Gynecology, 100*(6), 1405–1412.

American College of Obstetricians and Gynecologists (ACOG) Committee on Obstetric Practice. (2002). ACOG committee opinion.

Air travel during pregnancy. *International Journal of Gynaecology and Obstetrics, 76*(3), 338–339.

Anachebe, N. F., & Sutton, M. V. (2003). Racial disparities in reproductive health outcomes. *American Journal of Obstetrics & Gynecology, 188,* S37–S42.

Anderson, B. A., Marshak, H. H., & Hebbeler, D. L. (2002). Identifying intimate partner violence at entry to prenatal care: Clustering routine clinical information. *Journal of Midwifery & Women's Health, 47,* 353–359.

Anderson, C. (2002). Battered and pregnant: A nursing challenge. *AWHONN Lifelines, 6,* 95–99.

Anderson, M. E., Johnson, D. C., & Batal, H. A. (2005). Sudden infant death syndrome and prenatal maternal smoking: Rising attributed risk in the Back to Sleep era. *BMC Medicine, 3*(1), 4.

Andres, J. G. (2002). Intrauterine growth restriction: Perinatal issues and management. In E. J. Martin (Ed.), *Intrapartum management modules* (3rd ed., pp. 399–437). Philadelphia: Lippincott Williams & Wilkins.

Andrews, M. M., & Hanson, P. A. (2003). Religion, culture and nursing. In M. M. Andrews & J. S. Boyle (Eds.), *Transcultural concepts in nursing care* (4th ed., pp. 432–502). Philadelphia: Lippincott Williams & Wilkins.

Askin, D. F. (2001). Newborn adaptation to extrauterine life. In K. R. Simpson & P. A. Creehan (Eds.), *AWHONN's perinatal nursing* (2nd ed., pp. 494–512). Philadelphia: Lippincott Williams & Wilkins.

Bahrami, M. H., Rayegani, S. M., Fereidouni, M., & Baghbani, M. (2005). Prevalence and severity of carpal tunnel syndrome (CTS) during pregnancy. *Electromyography and Clinical Neurophysiology, 45*(2), 123–125.

Barron, M. L. (2001). Antenatal care. In K. R. Simpson & P. A. Creehan (Eds.), *AWHONN's perinatal nursing* (2nd ed., pp. 125–172). Philadelphia: Lippincott Williams & Wilkins.

Beck, L. F., Gilbert, B. C., & Shults, R. A. (2005). Prevalence of seat belt use among reproductive-aged women and prenatal counselling to wear seat belts. *American Journal of Obstetrics and Gynecology, 192*(2), 580–585.

Beckmann, C. R. B., Ling, F. W., Laube, D. W., Smith, R. P., Barzansky, B. M., & Herbert, W. N. P. (2002). *Obstetrics and gynecology* (4th ed.). Philadelphia: Lippincott Williams & Wilkins.

Bennett, M., Macri, C. J., & Bathgate, S. L. (2005). Erythropoietin use in a pregnant Jehovah's Witness with anemia and beta-thalassemia: A case report. *Journal of Reproductive Medicine, 50*(2), 135–137.

Bernstein, I. M., Mongeon, J. A., Badger, G. J., Solomon, L., Heil, S. H., & Higgins, S. T. (2005). Maternal smoking and its association with birth weight. *Obstetrics and Gynecology, 106*(5 Pt. 1), 986–991.

Berry, A. (1999). Mexican American women's expressions of the meaning of culturally congruent prenatal care. *Journal of Transcultural Nursing, 10,* 203–212.

Bondas, T., & Eriksson, K. (2001). Women's lived experiences of pregnancy: A tapestry of joy and suffering. *Qualitative Health Research, 11,* 824–840.

Boy, A., & Salihu, H. M. (2004). Intimate partner violence and birth outcomes: A systematic review. *International Journal of Fertility and Women's Medicine, 49*(4), 159–164.

Bradshaw, J. (2000). The impact of maternity on the Muslim family. *Midwifery Today—International Midwife, Summer*(54), 58–60.

Braveman, P., Cubbin, C., Marchi, K., Egerter, S., & Chavez, G. (2001). Measuring socioeconomic status/position in studies of racial/ethnic disparities: Maternal and infant health. *Public Health Reports, 116,* 449–463.

Bridges, E. J., Womble, S., Wallace, M., & McCartney, J. (2003). Hemodynamic monitoring in high-risk obstetrics patients: Expected hemodynamic changes in pregnancy. *Critical Care Nurse, 23,* 53–63.

Callister, L. C. (2005). What has the literature taught us about culturally competent care of women and children? *MCN—The American Journal of Maternal and Child Nursing, 30*(6), 380–388.

Callister, L. C. (2001a). Culturally competent care of women and newborns: Knowledge, attitude, and skills. *Journal of Obstetrics, Gynecology and Neonatal Nursing, 30,* 209–215.

Callister, L. C. (2001b). Integrating cultural beliefs and practices into the care of childbearing women. In K. R. Simpson & P. A. Creehan (Eds.), *AWHONN's perinatal nursing* (2nd ed., pp. 68–93). Philadelphia: Lippincott Williams & Wilkins.

Carey, J. C. (2003). Congenital syphilis in the 21st century. *Current Women's Health Report, 3*(4), 229–302.

Carolan, M. (2003). The graying of the obstetric population: Implications for the older mother. *Journal of Obstetrics, Gynecology and Neonatal Nursing, 32,* 19–27.

Centers for Disease Control and Prevention (CDC). (2005). Unintended and teen pregnancy prevention: Teen pregnancy. Retrieved March 7, 2006, from http://www.cdc.gov/reproductivehealth/UnintendedPregnancy/Teen.htm.

Centers for Disease Control and Prevention (CDC). (2004). STDs and pregnancy. Retrieved March 9, 2006, from http://www.cdc.gov/std/STDFact-STDs&Pregnancy.htm#affect.

Cesario, S. K. (2001). Care of the Native American woman: Strategies for practice, education and research. *Journal of Obstetrics, Gynecology and Neonatal Nursing, 30,* 13–19.

Clemmens, D. (2003). Adolescent motherhood: A meta-synthesis of qualitative studies. *MCN—The American Journal of Maternal and Child Nursing, 28*(2), 93–99.

Cockney, C. D. (2003). On the edge: Periodontal disease linked to preeclampsia risk. *AWHONN Lifelines, 7,* 211.

Collins, A. (2002). Nursing with dignity. 1. Judaism. *Nursing Times, 98,* 34–35.

Consumer Reports. (2003). When the test really counts. *Consumer Reports, 68,* 45–47.

Contreras, A., Herrera, J. A., Soto, J. E., Arce, R. M., Jaramillo, A., & Botero, J. E. (2006). Periodontitis is associated with preeclampsia in pregnant women. *Journal of Peridontology, 77*(2), 182–188.

Cunningham, F. G., Gant, N. F., Leveno, K. J., Bloom, S. L., Hauth, J. C., Gillstrap, L. C., III, & Wenstrom, K. D. (2005). *Williams obstetrics* (22nd ed). New York: McGraw-Hill.

Dallas, C. (2004). Family matters: How mothers of adolescent parents experience adolescent pregnancy and parenting. *Public Health Nursing, 21*(4), 347–353.

Divon, M. Y., & Ferber, A. (2002). Doppler evaluation of the fetus. *Clinical Obstetrics and Gynecology, 45,* 1015–1025.

Dobrzykowski, T. M., & Stern, P. N. (2003). Out of sync: A generation of first-time mothers over 30. *Health Care for Women International, 24,* 242–253.

Driscoll, J. W. (2001). Psychosocial adaptation to pregnancy and postpartum. In K. R. Simpson & P. A. Creehan (Eds.), *AWHONN's perinatal nursing* (2nd ed., pp. 115–124). Philadelphia: Lippincott Williams & Wilkins.

Espinosa, L., & Osborne, K. (2002). Domestic violence during pregnancy: Implications for practice. *Journal of Midwifery & Women's Health, 47,* 305–317.

Findlay, M. (2000). Folic acid: Helping to prevent birth defects. *Alabama Nurse,* 27, 16–17.

Finer, L. B., Frohwirth, L. F., Dauphinee, L. A., Singh, S., & Moore, A. M. (2005). Reasons U.S. women have abortions: Quantitative and qualitative perspectives. *Perspectives in Sexual and Reproductive Health, 37*(3), 110–118.

Floyd, R. L., O'Connor, M. J., Sokol, R. J., Bertrand, J., & Cordero, J. F. (2005). Recognition and prevention of fetal alcohol syndrome. *Obstetrics & Gynecology, 106*(5 Pt. 1), 1059–1064.

Fong, S., & McGovern, P. (2004). How does age affect fertility? *Contemporary OB/GYN, 49*(4), 37–46.

Freda, M. C. (2002). *Perinatal patient education.* Philadelphia: Lippincott Williams & Wilkins.

Gaffney, K. F. (2001). Infant exposure to environmental tobacco smoke. *Journal of Nursing Scholarship, 33,* 343–348.

Geronimus, A. T. (2003). Damned if you do: Culture, identity, privilege, and teenage childbearing in the United States. *Social Science & Medicine, 57,* 881–893.

Guyton A., & Hall, J. (2006). *Textbook of medical physiology* (11th ed). Philadelphia: W. B. Saunders.

Hanna, B. (2001). Negotiating motherhood: The struggles of teenage mothers. *Journal of Advanced Nursing, 34,* 456–464.

Health Canada. (2003). *Folic acid.* Retrieved March 9, 2006, from http://www.hc-sc.ca/English/folicacid/.

Health Resources and Services Administration. (2002). HRSA study finds narrowing racial gap in women's use of prenatal care. Retrieved March 9, 2006, from http://newsroom.hrsa.gov/releases/2002releases/prenatal.htm.

Hershkovitz, R., Sheiner, E., & Mazor, M. (2002). Ultrasound in obstetrics: A review of safety. *European Journal of Obstetrics & Gynecology and Reproductive Biology, 101,* 15–18.

Huddleston, J. F. (2002). Continued utility of the contraction stress test? *Clinical Obstetrics and Gynecology, 45,* 1005–1014.

Institute of Medicine. (1990). *Nutrition during pregnancy. I. Weight gain.* Washington, DC: Author.

James, D. C. (2001). Postpartum care. In K. R. Simpson & P. A. Creehan (Eds.), *AWHONN's perinatal nursing* (2nd ed., pp. 446–475). Philadelphia: Lippincott Williams & Wilkins.

Katz, V. L. (2003). Prenatal care. In J. R. Scott, R. S. Gibbs, B. Y. Karlan, & A. F. Haney (Eds.), *Danforth's obstetrics and gynecology* (9th ed., pp. 1–34). Philadelphia: Lippincott Williams & Wilkins.

Kendrick, J. M. (2001). High risk pregnancy—diabetes. In K. R. Simpson & P. A. Creehan (Eds.), *AWHONN's perinatal nursing* (2nd ed., pp. 219–235). Philadelphia: Lippincott Williams & Wilkins.

Kozinsky, Z., Orvos, H., Katona, M., Zoboki, T., Pal, A., & Kovacs, L. (2001). Perinatal outcome of induced and spontaneous pregnancies of primiparous women aged 35 or over. *International Journal of Gynecology & Obstetrics, 76,* 23–26.

Kozinsky, Z., Orvos, H., Zoboki, T., Katona, M., Wayda, K., Pal, A., & Kovacs, L. (2002). Risk factors for cesarean section of primiparous women aged over 35 years. *Acta Obstetric Gynecology Scandinavian, 81,* 313–316.

Lagana, K. (2003). Come bien, camina y no se preocupe—eat right, walk, and do not worry: Selective biculturalism during pregnancy in a Mexican American community. *Journal of Transcultural Nursing, 14,* 117–124.

Laibl, V. R., & Sheffield, J. S. (2005). Tuberculosis in pregnancy. *Clinical Perinatology, 32*(3), 739–747.

Lannero, E., Wickman, M., Pershagen, G., & Nordvall, L. (2006). Maternal smoking during pregnancy increases the risk of recurrent wheezing during the first years of life (BAMSE). *Respiratory Research, 5*(7), 3.

Lauderdale, J. (2003). Transcultural perspectives in childbearing. In M. M. Andrews & J. S. Boyle (Eds.), *Transcultural concepts in nursing care* (4th ed., pp. 95–131). Philadelphia: Lippincott Williams & Wilkins.

Lemon, B. S. (2002). Exploring Latino rituals in birthing. *AWHONN Lifelines, 6,* 443–445.

Lewis, J. A. (2003). Jewish perspectives on pregnancy and childbearing. *MCN—The American Journal of Maternal and Child Nursing, 28*(5), 306–312.

Lindseth, G., & Bird-Baker, M. Y. (2004). Risk factors for cholelithiasis in pregnancy. *Research in Nursing Health, 27*(6), 382–391.

Liu, J., & Moore, J. (2000). Perinatal care: Cultural and technical differences between China and the United States. *Journal of Transcultural Nursing, 11,* 47–54.

Lloyd, C. (2003). Common medical disorders associated with pregnancy. In D. M. Fraser & M. S. Cooper (Eds.), *Myles textbook for midwives* (14th ed., pp. 321–356). Philadelphia: Elsevier Science.

Luppi, C. J. (2001). Physiologic changes of pregnancy. In K. R. Simpson & P. A. Creehan (Eds.), *AWHONN's perinatal nursing* (2nd ed., pp. 96–114). Philadelphia: Lippincott Williams & Wilkins.

Lutz, K. F. (2005). Abused pregnant women's interactions with health care providers during the childbearing year. *Journal of Obstetric, Gynecologic, and Neonatal Nursing, 34*(2), 151–162.

Magee, B. D., Hattis, D., & Kivel, N. M. (2004). Role of smoking in low birth weight. *Journal of Reproductive Medicine, 49*(1), 23–27.

Maloni, J. (2000). Preventing preterm birth: Evidence-based interventions shift toward prevention. *AWHONN Lifelines, 4,* 26–33.

Manning, F. A. (2002). Fetal biophysical profile: A critical appraisal. *Clinical Obstetrics and Gynecology, 43*(4), 975–985.

March of Dimes. (2003). March of Dimes resources for professionals. Retrieved March 9, 2006, from http://www.marchofdimes.com/professionals/690_4089.asp.

Martin, J. J. (2002). Maternal and fetal response to labor. In E. J. Martin (Ed.), *Intrapartum management modules* (3rd ed., pp. 19–60). Philadelphia: Lippincott Williams & Wilkins.

Matthews, T. J., & Hamilton, B. E. (2002). Mean age of mother, 1970–2000. *National Vital Statistics Reports, 51*(1), 1–16.

McCulloch, J. (2002). Health risks associated with prolonged standing. *Work, 19*(2), 201–205.

McGlade, M. S., Saha, S., & Dahlstrom, M. E. (2004). The Latina paradox: An opportunity for restructuring prenatal care delivery. *American Journal of Public Health, 94*(12), 2062–2065.

McManus, A. J., Hunter, L. P., & Renn, H. (2006). Lesbian experiences and needs during childbirth: Guidance for health care providers. *Journal of Obstetric, Gynecologic, and Neonatal Nursing, 35*(1), 13–23.

Merialdi, M., Barroli, G., Villar, J., Abalos, E., Gulmezoglu, A. M., Kulier, R., & de Onis, M. (2003). Nutritional interventions during pregnancy for the prevention or treatment of impaired fetal growth: An overview of randomized controlled trials. *Journal of Nutrition, 133,* 1626S–1631S.

Miller, D. A. (2002). Outpatient antepartum testing. In W. C. Hill (Ed.), *Ambulatory obstetrics* (pp. 221–232). Philadelphia: Lippincott Williams & Wilkins.

Minkoff, H. L., & Gibbs, R. S. (2003). Obstetric and perinatal infections. In J. R. Scott, R. S. Gibbs, B. Y. Karlan, & A. F. Haney (Eds.), *Danforth's obstetrics and gynecology* (9th ed., pp. 339–364). Philadelphia: Lippincott Williams & Wilkins.

Mittal, P., & Wing, D. A. (2005). Urinary tract infections in pregnancy. *Clinical Perinatology, 32*(3), 749–764.

Morgan, K. L. (2004). Management of UTIs during pregnancy. *MCN—The American Journal of Maternal and Child Nursing, 29*(4), 254–258.

National Center for Health Statistics. (2002). *National vital statistics report, 50.* Retrieved March 9, 2006, from http://www.cdc.gov/nchs/fastats/pdf/nvsr50_05t3.pdf.

National Institute of Health. (2003). *Dietary reference intakes. Elements.* Retrieved March 9, 2006, from http://www4.nationalacademies.orb/iorn/iornhome.nsf/Wfiles/Webtableminerals.pdf.

Neumann, M., & Graf, C. (2003). Pregnancy after age 35. *AWHONN Lifelines, 7,* 423–430.

Northcott, N. (2002). Nursing with dignity. 2. Buddhism. *Nursing Times, 98,* 36–38.

Ozalp, S., Tanir, H. M., Sener, T., Yazan, S., & Keskin, A. E. (2003). Health risks for early (< or = 19) and late (> or = 35) childbearing. *Archives of Gynecology and Obstetrics, 268*(3), 172–174.

Patchen, L., & Beal, M. W. (2001). Preventing perinatal transmission of HIV: An evidence-based update for midwives. *Journal of Midwifery & Women's Health, 46,* 354–365.

Pillitteri, A. (2007). *Maternal & child health nursing* (5th ed.). Philadelphia: Lippincott Williams & Wilkins.

Plichta, S. B. (2004). Intimate partner violence and physical health consequences: Policy and practice implications. *Journal of Interpersonal Violence, 19*(11), 1296–1323.

Poole, J. H. (2001). High risk pregnancy: Hypertensive disorders. In K. R. Simpson & P. A. Creehan (Eds.), *AWHONN's perinatal nursing* (2nd ed., pp. 173–190). Philadelphia: Lippincott Williams & Wilkins.

Preboth, M. (2000). ACOG guidelines on antepartum fetal surveillance. *American Family Physician, 62,* 1184–1188.

Raines, D. A., & Morgan, Z. (2000). Culturally sensitive care during childbirth. *Applied Nursing Research, 13,* 167–172.

Renker, P. R., & Tonkin, P. (2006). Women's views of prenatal violence screening: Acceptability and confidentiality issues. *Obstetrics & Gynecology, 107*(2 Pt. 1), 348–354.

Roberts, J. M., Balk, J. L., Bodnar, L. M., Belizan, J. M., Bergel, E., & Martinez, A. (2003). Nutrient involvement in preeclampsia. *Journal of Nutrition, 133,* 1684S–1692S.

Roberts, K. S. (2002). Providing culturally sensitive care to the childbearing Islamic family. *Advances in Neonatal Care, 2*(4), 222–228.

Ross, L. E. (2005). Perinatal mental health in lesbian mothers: A review of potential risk and protective factors. *Women Health, 41*(3), 113–128.

Sayle, A. E., Savitz, D. A., & Williams, J. F. (2003). Accuracy of reporting of sexual activity during late pregnancy. *Paediatric and Perinatal Epidemiology, 17*(2), 143–147.

Scholl, T. O. (2005). Iron status during pregnancy: Setting the stage for mother and infant. *American Journal of Clinical Nutrition, 81*(5), 1218–1222.

Schrimmer, D. B., & Moore, T. R. (2002). Sonographic evaluation of amniotic fluid volume. *Clinical Obstetrics and Gynecology, 45,* 1026–1038.

Seamark, C. J., & Lings, P. (2004). Positive experiences of teenage motherhood: A qualitative study. *British Journal of General Practice, 54*(508), 813–818.

Shiao, S. Y., Andrews, C. M., & Helmreich, R. J. (2005). Maternal race/ethnicity and predictors of pregnancy and infant outcomes. *Biological Research for Nursing, 7*(1), 55–66.

SmithBattle, L. (2000a). Developing a caregiving tradition in opposition to one's past: Lessons from a longitudinal study of teenage mothers. *Public Health Nursing, 17,* 85–93.

SmithBattle, L. (2000b). The vulnerabilities of teenage mothers: Challenging prevailing assumptions. *Advances in Nursing Science, 23,* 29–40.

Sprong, C. Y. (2003). Fetal monitoring. In J. R. Scott, R. S. Gibbs, B. Y. Karlan, & A. F. Haney (Eds.), *Danforth's obstetrics and gynecology* (9th ed., pp. 159–172). Philadelphia: Lippincott Williams & Wilkins.

Statistics Canada. (2005). Pregnancy outcomes by age group. Retrieved March 7, 2006, from http://www40.statcan.ca/l01/cst01/hlth65a.htm.

Stenson, K., Sidenvall, B., & Heimer, G. (2005). Midwives' experiences of routine antenatal questioning relating to men's violence against women. *Midwifery, 21*(4), 311–321.

Stevens-Simon, C., Beach, R. K., & McGregor, J. A. (2002). Does incomplete growth and development predispose teenagers to preterm deliver? A template for research. *Journal of Perinatology, 22,* 315–323.

Stiles, A. S. (2005). Parenting needs, goals, and strategies of adolescent mothers. *MCN—The American Journal of Maternal and Child Nursing, 30*(5), 327–333.

Tough, S., Newburn-Cook, C., Johnston, D., Svenson, L., Rose, S., & Belick, J. (2002). Delayed childbearing and its impact on population rate changes in lower birth weight, multiple birth and preterm delivery. *Pediatrics, 109,* 399–403.

U.S. Department of Health and Human Services (USDHHS). (2005). *National Center for Health Statistics, health, United States 2005, with chartbook on trends in the health of Americans.* Hyattsville, MD: Author.

Van Rooij, I. A., Ocke, M. C., Straatman, H., Zielhuis, G. A., Merkus, H. M., & Steegers-Theunissen, R. P. (2004). Periconceptional folate intake by supplement and food reduces the risk of nonsyndromic cleft lip with or without cleft palate. *Preventive Medicine, 39*(4), 689–694.

Viccars, A. (2003). Antenatal care. In D. M. Fraser & M. S. Cooper (Eds.), *Myles textbook for midwives* (14th ed., pp. 251–274). Philadelphia: Elsevier Science.

Viteri, F. E., & Berger, J. (2005). Importance of pre-pregnancy and pregnancy iron status: Can long-term weekly preventive iron and folic acid supplementation achieve desirable and safe status? *Nutrition Review, 63*(12 Pt. 2), S65–76.

Werler, M. M., Mitchell, A. A., Hernandez-Diaz, S., & Honein, M. A. (2005). Use of over-the-counter medications during pregnancy. *American Journal of Obstetrics and Gynecology, 193*(3 Pt. 1), 771–777.

Wilcox, A. J., Baird, D. D., Dunson, D., McChesney, R., & Weinberg, C. R. (2001). Natural limits of pregnancy testing in relation to the expected menstrual period. *Journal of the American Medical Association, 286,* 1759–1761.

Yankowitz, J. (2003). Ultrasound in obstetrics. In J. R. Scott, R. S. Gibbs, B. Y. Karlan, & A. F. Haney (Eds.), *Danforth's obstetrics and gynecology* (9th ed., pp. 129–142). Philadelphia: Lippincott Williams & Wilkins.

Youngkin, E. Q., & Davis, M. S. (2004). *Women's health: A primary care clinical guide.* Upper Saddle River, NJ: Prentice Hall.

Zdravkovic, T., Genbacev, O., McMaster, M. T., & Fisher, S. J. (2005). The adverse effects of maternal smoking on the human placenta: A review. *Placenta, 26*(Suppl. A), S81–86.

Ziadeh, S., & Yahaya, A. (2001). Pregnancy outcome at age 40 and older. *Archives of Gynecology and Obstetrics, 265,* 30–33.

CHAPTER 13

High-Risk Pregnancy

Nancy Watts

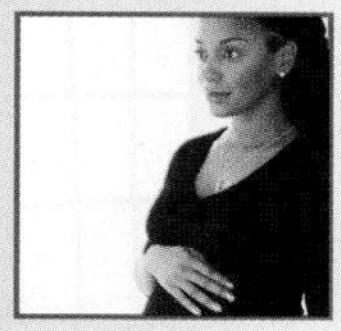

Selena, a 39-year-old African American woman, comes to the clinic at 27 weeks' gestation with her second pregnancy. During this routine prenatal visit, she will undergo screening for diabetes. Her blood glucose level remained normal throughout her first pregnancy, which ended with the vaginal birth of a healthy 9 lb, 10 oz son. Selena states, "My mother found out 2 years ago that she has diabetes. Am I now at risk?"

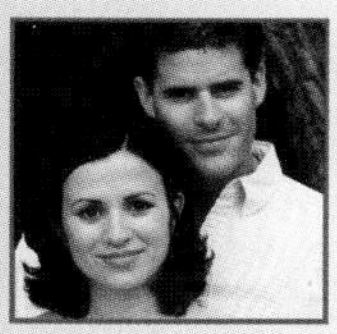

Harriet, a 33-year-old client at 28 weeks' gestation with her fourth pregnancy, is being evaluated in the health care provider's office. During her second and third pregnancies, Harriet developed pregnancy-induced hypertension (PIH) managed with bedrest at home for several weeks. Her obstetric history (GTPAL) is documented as 41203. "My last two babies were born at 34 and 33 weeks because of my blood pressure problems," she reports. Her children are 2, 4, and 7 years old.

You will learn more about Selena's and Harriet's stories later. Nurses working with these and similar clients need to understand this chapter's content to manage care and address issues appropriately. Before beginning, consider the following points:

- Does anything about either scenario above present issues of immediate concern? Explain.
- Would you consider each client's pregnancy to be high risk? Why or why not?
- How are Selena and Harriet similar? How are they different?
- What details does the nurse need to investigate with Selena? What about Harriet?
- What areas of concern and teaching would the nurse need to address with each client?

LEARNING OBJECTIVES

Upon completion of this chapter, the reader should be able to:

- Explain what is meant by the term *high-risk pregnancy.*
- Identify the role of risk assessment in pregnancy, as well as areas of focus in performing such evaluation.
- Outline a comprehensive approach to the care of the pregnant woman with asthma.
- Describe factors that may contribute to pregnancy outcomes in pregnant women with cardiovascular disease and appropriate management strategies for various types of clients.
- Discuss common signs and symptoms associated with anemia during pregnancy and their management.
- Identify the major problem related to concurrent pregnancy and systemic lupus erythematosus.
- Describe appropriate screening and treatment measures for various infections that pose dangerous risks to mother, fetus, or both during pregnancy.
- Compare several renal and urinary problems that can develop in the expectant woman and associated levels of care.
- Outline key interventions for the pregnant woman with diabetes.
- Discuss why psychosocial disorders may be more prevalent in pregnant women and management strategies within the context of gestational and fetal growth.
- Understand reasons for universal screening of all pregnant women for abuse.
- Identify potential indicators that suggest abuse in a pregnant client.
- Explain why screening for smoking, alcohol use, and other substance abuse in pregnancy is so essential.
- Define the criteria for a diagnosis of hyperemesis gravidarum.
- List the various classifications of hypertension in pregnancy.
- Outline general treatment strategies and interventions for women with hypertension in pregnancy.
- Describe what is meant by acute HELLP syndrome and measures for evaluating successful treatment.
- Explain the usual management of pPROM.
- Identify why pregnant women are at increased risk for disseminated intravascular coagulation.
- Compare and contrast various placental problems in pregnancy that can pose risks to maternal and fetal health.
- Name complications commonly associated with pregnancy in adolescence.
- List ideal outcomes in cases of multiple gestation.
- Explain the difference between miscarriage and stillbirth.
- Compare and contrast ectopic pregnancy with gestational trophoblastic disease.

KEY TERMS

cerclage
cervical insufficiency
disseminated intravascular coagulopathy
eclampsia
ectopic pregnancy
gestational diabetes
gestational trophoblastic disease
high-risk pregnancy
hyperemesis gravidarum
incompetent cervix
miscarriage
multiple pregnancy
obesity
peripartum cardiomyopathy
placenta previa
placental abruption
pre-eclampsia
stillbirth

A **high-risk pregnancy** may be defined as "one in which the life or health of the mother or fetus is made vulnerable because of a medical or obstetric condition" (Cannon et al., 2000, p. 435). Approximately 25% of pregnancies are considered high risk based on this definition (Youngkin & Davis, 2004). Health problems that predispose the mother, fetus, or both to complications frequently exist before the pregnancy, although sometimes they develop or show manifestations for the first time with gestation. Examples of common health problems in pregnancy may include cardiac disease, autoimmune disorders, and diabetes. Obstetric complications involve those conditions directly related to gestation itself (Gilbert & Harmon, 2003). Examples include placental abnormalities and premature rupture of membranes. In addition, some pregnancies are considered high risk because of specific circumstances related to the mother's lifestyle, environment, or situation. Examples include adolescent pregnancy, violence, poverty, mental illness, substance use, lack of access to prenatal care, and trauma.

This chapter reviews medical, obstetric, and other factors that may compromise pregnancy and general measures taken to monitor and manage gestational complications. Discussions of conditions that pose special or increased risks in labor and birth and their management are found in Chapter 16.

PREGNANCY RISK ASSESSMENT

Many pregnant clients with chronic preexisting health conditions can anticipate close monitoring of their gestation and may not associate a need for hospitalization or home care as a crisis or emergency. Their ability to accommodate a preexisting health problem may correlate with their adaptation to a high-risk pregnancy (Gupton et al., 2001). Clients who develop unexpected complications, however, may experience great stress, anger, and anxiety and feel unprepared to deal with the threat to themselves and to their fetuses. They may need more time to adjust to the situation and to express feelings to supportive others (Gilbert & Harmon, 2003).

Regardless of when a problem posing risk developed, high-risk pregnancy is stressful for any family anticipating a baby's birth. The major reason for risk assessment is to guide rational planning for appropriate care, including the need for ongoing consultation and site of birth. Such planning is extremely important in geographic areas lacking intensive or special care facilities. In such cases, special modifications may be necessary, such as increased prenatal visits to a family physician; more aggressive involvement from a midwife or obstetrician; ongoing home care; monitoring in an institutional setting; or admission to a tertiary-level facility in advance of labor and birth.

Variables such as anxiety, stress, social support, and self-esteem influence a client's risk status. Women may view their risk status differently from the health care provider. The client's personal perceptions and understandings are important to consider when care providers assess pregnancy and plan care (Gupton et al., 2001). Assessment Tool 13.1 gives guidelines for areas of the health history and physical examination to focus on when evaluating a pregnancy's risk.

Psychosocial Risk Factors

For some clients, pregnancy is unplanned, unwanted, or both. At times, women face concomitant challenges during pregnancy, such as job changes, unemployment, relocation, unstable relationships, death of a significant person, or onset or worsening of a medical condition. Unchecked stress related to these developments may intensify or be the risk factor leading to psychological problems. Hormonal changes associated with reproduction also increase the possibility of psychiatric diagnoses.

Psychosocial stressors associated with high-risk pregnancy include the following:

- Lack of control
- Concern or anxiety over fetal well-being
- Boredom
- Feelings of helplessness and powerlessness
- Sense of isolation, confinement, and being a prisoner
- Missing out on normal activities
- Separation from home and family
- Physical discomforts
- Medication side effects
- Timelessness
- Changing self-image
- Sick role
- Concerns about children
- Role reversal
- Difficulties in relationship with partner
- Lack of privacy (if hospitalized)
- Incompatible roommates (if hospitalized)

Antenatal psychosocial health assessment is a critical component of prenatal care. Completion of the Antenatal Psychosocial Health Assessment (ALPHA) document (Assessment Tool 13.2) at 20 weeks' gestation can assist care providers to screen for the above problems, in addition to poor parenting skills, substance abuse, and mood disorders (Comley & Mousmanis, 2003).

Economic Risk Factors

Low-income women may struggle to gain access to and pay for health care. Lack of prenatal care is associated with adverse perinatal outcomes (Cannon et al., 2000). Many women with low-paying jobs are not educated for other positions or must take whatever work they can find

● ASSESSMENT TOOL 13.1 Common Risk Factors in Pregnancy

BIOPHYSICAL FACTORS

- Genetic disease
- Cardiovascular disease
- Hypertension
- Diabetes
- Autoimmune disorder
- Adolescent pregnancy
- Late-life pregnancy
- Uterine, cervical, or placental abnormalities
- Infections (including sexually transmitted infections)
- Asthma
- Poor nutrition
- Underweight or overweight
- Multiple gestation

PSYCHOSOCIAL FACTORS

- Mood disorders
- Anxiety disorders
- Eating disorders
- Stress
- Substance use
- Domestic violence

SOCIAL FACTORS

- Poverty
- Lack of social support
- Decreased or absent access to health care
- Family problems (eg, divorce, illness, relocation)

because of family responsibilities. Single women who are the heads of their households make up approximately 20% of U.S. families, a structure that studies show to be economically disadvantaged (Youngkin & Davis, 2004).

Single poor women and their families are the largest group of Americans at the bottom of the economic structure (Keating-Lefler & Wilson, 2004). Butterworth (2004) describes an association between single-parent status and increased risk for mental illness. Single mothers also report sexual abuse in childhood, anxiety, and depression more frequently (Butterworth, 2004). In the midst of poverty and inadequate resources, these women must juggle work and responsibility for their family's well-being. The health status of those with high poverty rates is compromised; in the United States, this group consists largely of single women and their families (Keating-Lefler & Wilson, 2004). Single mothers also experience great stress from physical, emotional, and psychological challenges. They are at risk for significant losses in pregnancy because they may be isolated from friends, male partners, family, themselves (their "old self"), and their dreams (Keating-Lefler & Wilson, 2004).

Most clients who develop a high-risk pregnancy and can no longer work experience economic stress; such problems are compounded when a woman is single and must provide economically for herself and others. Nurses working in occupational health are in a strategic position to assist such women to continue to support themselves and their dependents. Advocacy for childbearing women to have flexible work hours, to coordinate prenatal visits within working hours, to obtain information on various health and wellness topics associated with pregnancy, and to facilitate rest periods throughout the day can enable them to continue working. Assessment for occupational teratogens is also important; substances to look for include lead, mercury, medications, and extremely high temperatures (Cannon et al., 2000).

Nurses working with single women need to help identify potential sources of support (including forming new groups of pregnant single women), encourage dreams and visions for the future, and assist with practical financial assistance. Strategies that also enhance personal capacity and resources may have the most potential for success (Fig. 13.1).

Nutrition-Related Risk Factors

Overall, poor nutrition can compromise maternal weight gain, resulting in a low-birth-weight infant. In 1999, 7.6% of U.S. infants were small for gestational age; 11.8% were premature (Fowles, 2002) (see Chap. 22). Deficiencies in iron, iodine, and calcium affect a woman's ability to maintain a healthy pregnancy. One significant nutritional risk

● ASSESSMENT TOOL 13.2 ALPHA (Antenatal Psychosocial Health Assessment)

- How do you and your partner solve arguments?
- Do you ever feel frightened by what your partner says or does?
- Have you ever been hit, pushed, shoved, or slapped by your partner?
- Has your partner ever humiliated or psychologically abused you?
- Have you ever been forced to have sex against your will?

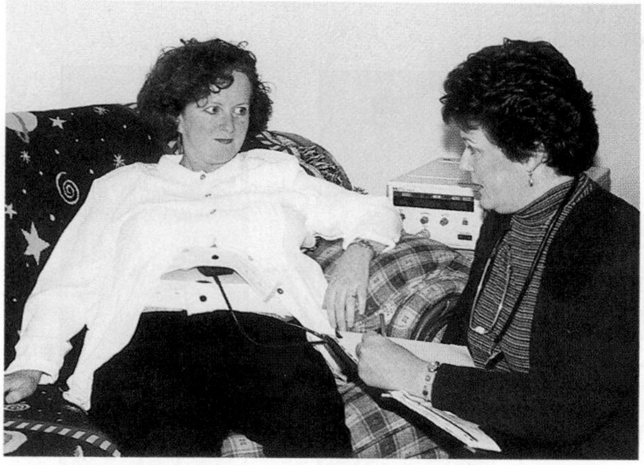

FIGURE 13.1 Single pregnant women, especially those with other risk factors in pregnancy, need additional systems of support and help with obtaining resources. (Photo by Melissa Olson, with permission of Health Home Coming, Inc., Bensalem, PA.)

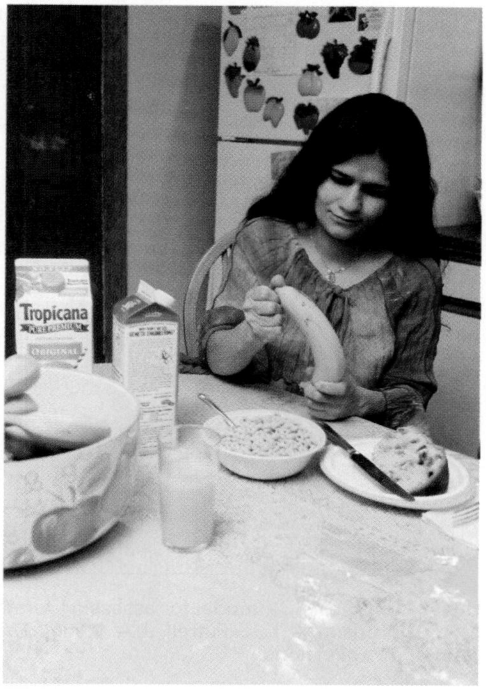

FIGURE 13.2 Ensuring adequate and appropriate nutritional choices in pregnancy is a significant area of nursing focus in all clients and one area requiring ongoing monitoring for risk.

to fetal development is deficiency of folic acid, specifically in the first trimester. At least 50% of neural tube defects can be prevented with folic acid supplementation that begins before conception and continues in the first trimester (Comley & Mousmanis, 2003) (see Chaps. 3, 11, and 22).

Poor nutrition can result from inadequate financial resources to obtain food, poor appetite, lifestyle choices such as smoking or alcohol use, or ongoing nausea and vomiting associated with pregnancy (Luke, 2005). Slowed fetal weight gain has been linked to preterm labor (Luke, 2005). This risk is increased if the mother herself was born with low birth weight (twofold increase in giving birth to a low-birth-weight infant and doing so prematurely) (Luke, 2005).

Counseling with a dietitian and referral to appropriate community resources may help ensure maternal and fetal health. Pattern of weight gain is more important than total number of pounds to ensure optimal birth outcomes (Fowles, 2002). Adequate intake of both water and milk is critical. Women taking prenatal vitamins within the first 3 gestational months are twice less likely to have low-birth-weight babies than women who do not use such supplements (Fowles, 2002). The nurse should offer nutritional information throughout the pregnancy, assessing types of foods as well as numbers of servings and emphasizing the importance of increased intake of fruits and vegetables (Fig. 13.2). If the client and nurse have a cultural or language barrier, an interpreter can assist as necessary to ensure that the client understands nutritional needs and practices and to offer culturally integrated suggestions (Fowles, 2002).

Family-Related Considerations

Researchers and theorists have described pregnancy and childbirth as a crucial period in which the steady state of the family is disrupted, requiring its members to use coping mechanisms for adaptation. When coping skills are strong, growth or change results (Zwelling & Phillips, 2001). If coping abilities are insufficient to meet the challenges, crisis occurs (see Chap. 7). High-risk pregnancy poses even greater challenges than usual. The ABCX model of family response to stress illustrates this adaptation and the potential for crisis (Fig. 13.3). Support for the entire family unit as well as each person within it is a critical enhancement to inherent coping abilities and strategies.

Family-centered care, with its emphasis on the family unit and collaboration, can promote positive coping with high-risk pregnancy. Knowledge can empower families; information about specific conditions, treatments, and overall plans of care can help them deal with expected and unexpected developments. Sensitivity and integration of unique customs is respectful and fosters collaboration (Zwelling & Phillips, 2001).

A high-risk pregnancy carries the potential for separation of the client from her newborn, other family members, or both. This threat increases the chance for family crisis and the need for support from health care providers. Encouragement of family-centered practices, policies, and collaboration in health care facilities can strengthen the family unit and prepare relatives for this transitional period.

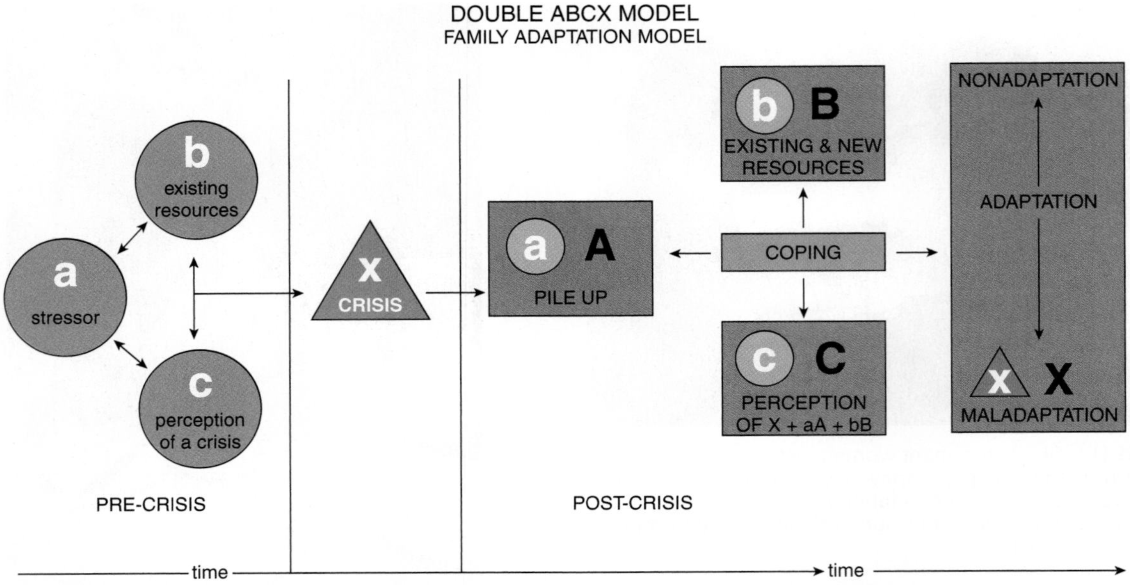

FIGURE 13.3 The ABCX model for assessing family dynamics. (From McCubbin, H. I., Thompson, E. A., Thompson, A. L., & Futrell, J. A. [2000]. *The dynamics of resilient families.* Thousand Oaks, CA: Sage Publications.)

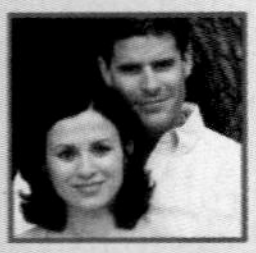

Consider Harriet, the 33-year-old woman pregnant with her fourth child described at the beginning of the chapter. During her previous two pregnancies, she was placed on bedrest at home. If bedrest is necessary with this pregnancy, how might this affect the family unit?

COMMON INTERVENTIONS IN HIGH-RISK PREGNANCY

Certain interventions are common in high-risk pregnancy, regardless of the presenting problem. This section focuses on some common methods of monitoring and preserving maternal and fetal health in cases of high-risk pregnancy. NIC/NOC Box 13.1 highlights common general nursing interventions and outcomes associated with high-risk pregnancy.

Fetal Health Surveillance

Fetal surveillance is critical to the management of high-risk pregnancy. Regular fetal monitoring allows health care providers to assess perfusion and oxygenation, as well as the potential for hypoxia or acidosis (Armour, 2004). As discussed in detail in Chapter 12, fetal surveillance methods include fetal movement counting, nonstress testing (NST), Doppler studies, and biophysical profiles. Together, these methods can minimize the chances of fetal morbidity and mortality (Malcus, 2004). Evaluations of fetal circulation, neurology, and heart rate also can give crucial information throughout the antenatal period (Malcus, 2004).

Bedrest

Bedrest for the mother, whether in a health care facility or at home, may be prescribed in cases of high-risk pregnancy (Fig. 13.4). Bedrest restricts movement and can isolate the woman from family and friends. Hospitaliza-

NIC/NOC Box 13.1 High-Risk Pregnancy

Common NIC Labels

- Electronic Fetal Monitoring: Antepartum
- Family Integrity Promotion: Childbearing Family
- Health Education
- High-Risk Pregnancy Care
- Labor Suppression
- Prenatal Care
- Risk Identification
- Surveillance
- Ultrasonography: Limited Obstetric

Common NOC Labels

- Fetal Status: Antepartum
- Knowledge: Pregnancy
- Maternal Status: Antepartum
- Prenatal Health Behavior
- Risk Control
- Risk Detection

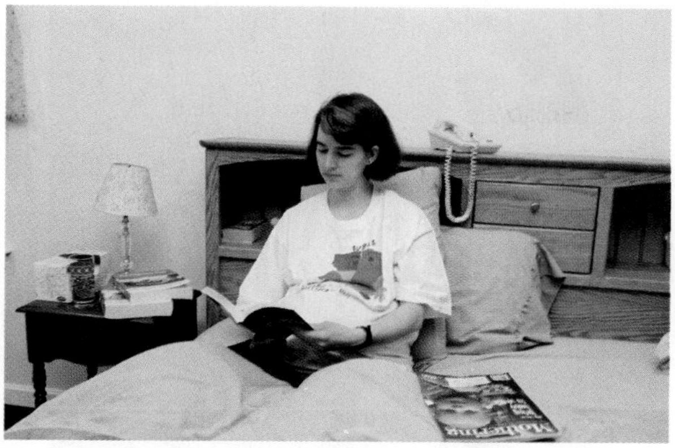

FIGURE 13.4 Bedrest is a common intervention employed in high-risk pregnancies to prevent preterm labor. Sources of activity (eg, reading) and interaction (eg, telephone) are important for women requiring bedrest to help prevent loneliness, isolation, and depression.

tion usually is necessary if the client lives far from family or other support people, or if she, the fetus, or both require increased medical attention. This treatment carries its own risks, such as decreased muscle tone, constipation, fatigue, fear, and depression (Cunningham, 2001). Weight gain during bedrest has been linked to decreased muscle mass, intracellular and extracellular fluid loss, and calcium loss. Additional problems may include sleep disturbances, fatigue, and auditory changes related to fluid shifts to the head while supine (Cunningham, 2001). Regardless of the setting for bedrest, clients may experience negative emotions. Social isolation can have a negative effect because contact with family and friends may be vital to maternal psychosocial well-being. Increased anxiety and emotional lability over weeks or months of bedrest can strain relationships and alter family dynamics. Absence from the home or decreased involvement in daily routines also can be hard on children or those caring for them (Maloni et al., 2001). Financial costs can be extensive. The woman may be required to leave her job, other children may need care from paid providers, or the family may need to pay for transportation back and forth to the facility giving care.

Women asked about bedrest therapy in the hospital described their experience as "feeling like a prisoner" (Cunningham, 2001). Stress-related symptoms included mood swings, boredom, isolation, and loneliness. Some women, however, described feeling safer as a result of the reassurance provided by frequent fetal assessments. See Research Highlight 13.1.

HEALTH COMPLICATIONS IN PREGNANCY

Health complications in pregnancy can pose significant challenges for the woman, fetus, family, and health care team. Ideally, clients whose problem existed before gestation were prepared for the pregnancy and received appropriate preconception counseling and care (see Chap. 11). Referral to an obstetrician specializing in maternal and fetal medicine or a medical specialist, genetic counselor, or both may have been completed before pregnancy. Beginning this care and continuing to assess this woman and family up through the postpartum period is extremely important for healthy outcomes.

● RESEARCH HIGHLIGHT 13.1 Impact of Prescribed Activity Restriction During Pregnancy on Women and Families

OBJECTIVES: Examination of the lived experience of women and their families with prescribed activity restriction during pregnancy for treatment of preterm labor.

SAMPLE: The sample included 58 women, 42 partners, and 27 health care providers. Women were drawn from an intensive care center, community hospital, and private physician practices. Participants had to be at least 18 years old, able to read and understand English, and sign an informed consent.

METHOD: Multiple interviews were held with women on activity restrictions because of threatened preterm labor at 2-week intervals until birth occurred.

RESULTS: "Doing the best we can" was a dominant theme identified by women and their partners. Their main goal was to protect the high-risk pregnancy; although the restrictions were stressful, the families attempted to balance them with their needs. Some families described themselves as "on the edge" as they tried to juggle the demands of their other children, loss of income, and daily stresses. After their infants' births, families spoke little about the restriction experience. Most related information involved postpartum weakness and difficulty regaining strength.

CONCLUSIONS: Assisting women to cope with activity restriction for preterm labor involves individual assessment of their circumstances and supports. Whether in the hospital or at home, women should be helped to find community resources for their families' needs. Teaching should include realistic expectations of postpartum maternal physical abilities if they have been on restricted activity programs during pregnancy.

May, K. (2001). *Health Care for Women International*, 22, 29–41.

Some conditions (eg, asthma) may improve during pregnancy; others (eg, diabetes) may shift continually with other physiologic adjustments that naturally accompany the various gestational stages. Part of admission for a woman in labor includes review of significant components of her health history such as current conditions, previous surgeries, psychiatric disorders, substance use, and medications taken during pregnancy.

ASTHMA

Asthma, the most common obstructive pulmonary disorder in pregnant women, is a concurrent factor in 4% to 8% of pregnancies (Blaiss, 2004; Kwon et al., 2004). Morbidity and mortality from asthma during pregnancy are increasing. The most common exacerbation period is from 24 to 36 weeks' gestation, with the most infrequent and usually mildest incidents in the last month (Blaiss, 2004). Risk for prenatal asthma exacerbation is related directly to asthma severity, which increases in approximately 30% of pregnant women, decreases in 30%, and stays stable in the remaining 40% (Schatz, 2003). Asthma is more common and severe in African American women and in women of all races with lower socioeconomic status. Beckmann (2002) describes the physical effects of asthma in pregnancy as decreased exercise, walking outside, climbing stairs, and even performing housework because of shortness of breath, coughing, wheezing, and increased upper respiratory infections. Low birth weight may result from ongoing chronic asthmatic changes.

Pregnant clients with asthma should receive care from a team of asthma specialists and an obstetrician or nurse-midwife. Members should perform frequent pulmonary function tests because abnormalities in pulmonary gas exchange produced by worsening asthma can lead to fetal hypoxia. Pregnant clients can participate in self-care by using a peak expiratory flow (PEF) meter to determine their lung volume and capacity 3 times a day, recording findings to review with health care providers (Beckmann, 2002) (Fig. 13.5). Monthly assessment of such findings is beneficial, as is spirometry (National Institutes of Health [NIH] & National Asthma Prevention Program Working Group, 2004).

Prenatal asthma treatment is based on a stepwise approach focused on maintaining adequate control (Fig. 13.6). Evidence of such control includes minimal or no chronic symptoms day or night, minimal exacerbations, no activity limitations, maintenance of pulmonary function, minimal use of short-acting inhaled β_2 agonists, and minimal or no adverse effects from medications (NIH & National Asthma Prevention Program Working Group, 2004). Clients may be prescribed corticosteroids, which may decrease birth weight and increase the risk for pregnancy-induced hypertension. The team should review concerns regarding fetal weight gain and well-being. They also may need to revise the plan if concerns increase over time.

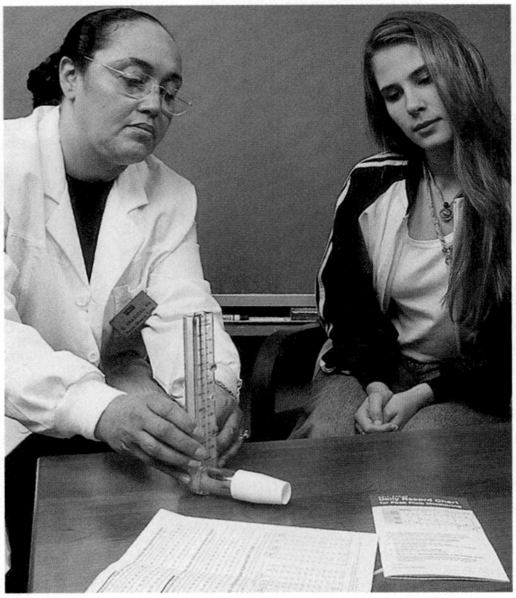

FIGURE 13.5 The nurse teaches the pregnant client with asthma how to use the peak flow monitor.

During labor, initial maternal assessments focus on vital signs (especially respiratory rate and temperature), coping ability, and pain management preferences. Because stress may cause or trigger an asthma attack, continual monitoring for any signs or symptoms is essential. Positive findings include shortness of breath, increased respiratory rate (above 12 to 24 breaths/min), and increased inspiratory or expiratory effort. An oxygen saturation monitor may be attached to the client's finger; a level less than 95% indicates a need for increased oxygenation. The health care team should assess the client's progress depending on any presenting symptoms. The laboring client also may require intravenous (IV) fluids for hydration, arterial blood gas evaluations, radiographic studies, and an electrocardiogram (ECG) (Boyle, 2002). Medications taken throughout pregnancy (eg, inhalers) should remain available. The nurse should stay with the client and provide continuous support because a consistent nursing presence can decrease anxiety and increase security.

The team should avoid administering pain medications such as meperidine (Demerol) or morphine because of their associated histamine release. Prostaglandin E preparations should not be used in clients with asthma undergoing labor augmentation or induction because they may contribute to bronchospasm. In such cases, oxytocin (Syntocinon) is the medication of choice. The team must review the risks and benefits of any procedure or test before beginning.

Classify severity: clinical features before treatment or adequate control	symptoms/day / symptoms/night	PEF or FEV_1 / PEF variability	**Medications** required to maintain long-term control: Daily medications
4 Severe persistent	Continual / Frequent	60% / >30%	Preferred treatment: • High dose inhaled corticosteroid AND • Long-acting inhaled $beta_2$-agonist AND, if needed • Corticosteroid tablets or syrup long term (2 mg/kg/day, generally not to exceed 60 mg/day). (Make repeat attempts to reduce systemic corticosteroid and maintain control with high-dose.) Alternative treatment: • High dose inhaled corticosteroid* AND • Sustained-release theophylline to serum concentration of 5-12 mcg/ml
3 Moderate persistent	Daily / >1 night/week	>60% - <80% / >30%	Preferred treatment: EITHER • Low-dose inhaled corticosteroid* and long-acting inhaled $beta_2$-agonist OR • Medium-dose inhaled corticosteroid* IF Needed (particularly in patients with recurring severe exacerbations): • Medium-dose inhaled corticosteroid* and long-acting inhaled $beta_2$-agonist Alternative treatment: • Low-dose inhaled corticosteroid* and either theophylline or leukotriene receptor antagonist† IF Needed • Medium-dose inhaled corticosteroid* and either theophylline or leukotriene receptor antagonist†
2 Mild persistent	>2 days/week but <daily / >2 nights/month	>80% / 20% - 30%	Preferred treatment: • Low-dose inhaled corticosteroid* Alternative treatment (listed alphabetically): •Cromolyn, leukotriene receptor antagonist†, OR sustained-release theophylline to serum concentration of 5-12 mcg/ml
1 Mild intermittent	2 days/week / 2 nights/month	80% / <20%	• No daily medication needed • Severe exacerbations may occur, separated by long periods of normal lung function and no symptoms. A course of systemic corticosteriods is recommended.

Quick relief

All patients

- Short-acting bronchodilator: 2-4 puffs short-acting inhaled $beta_2$-agonist‡ as needed for symptoms.
- Intensity of treatment will depend on severity of exacerbation; up to 3 treatments at 20-minute intervals or a single nebulizer treatment as needed. Course of systemic corticosteroid may be needed.
- Use of short-acting inhaled $beta_2$-agonist‡ >2 times a week in intermittent asthma (daily, or increasing use in persistent asthma) may indicate the need to initiate (increase) long-term-control therapy.

Step down

Review treatment every 1-6 months; a gradual stepwise reduction in treatment may be possible.

Step up

If control is not maintained, consider step up. First, review patient medication technique, adherence, and environmental control.

Goals of therapy: asthma control

- Minimal or no chronic symptoms day or night
- Minimal or no exacerbations
- No limitations on activities; no school/work missed
- Maintain (near) normal pulmonary function
- Minimal use of short-acting inhaled $beta_2$-agonist‡
- Minimal or no adverse effects from medications

Notes

- The stepwise approach is meant to assist, not replace, the clinical decision making required to meet individual patient needs.
- Classify severity: assign patient to most severe step in which any feature occurs (PEF is percent of personal best; FEV_1 is percent predicted).
- Gain control as quickly as possible (consider a short course of systemic corticosteroid), then step down to the least medication necessary to maintain control.
- Minimize use of short-acting inhaled $beta_2$-agonist‡ (e.g., use of approximately one canister a month even if not using it every day indicates inadequate control of asthma and the need to initiate or intensify long-term control therapy).
- Provide education on self-management and controlling environmental factors that make asthma worse (e.g., allergens, irritants).
- Refer to an asthma specialist if there are difficulties controlling asthma or if in Step 4 care is required. Referral may be considered if Step 3 care is required.

* There are more data on using budesonide during pregnancy than on using other equal inhaled corticosteroids.
† There are minimal data on using leukotriene receptor antagonists in humans during pregnancy, although there are reassuring animal data submitted to FDA.
‡ There are more data on using albuterol during pregnancy than on using other short-acting inhaled $beta_2$-agonists.

FIGURE 13.6 Stepwise approach to asthma management in pregnancy and lactation. (From U.S. Department of Health and Human Services. [2005]. *NAEPP working group report on managing asthma during pregnancy: Recommendations for pharmacological treatment.* 2004 Update. Rockville, MD: Author.)

Assessment of fetal health during pregnancy varies according to the severity of maternal asthma, maternal respiratory rate, and other individual circumstances. If no fetal risk factors exist when a client is in labor, fetal health may be evaluated by auscultation as long as the fetal heart rate remains within the institution's normal range. If any change in fetal heart rate is concerning (eg, decelerations) or maternal asthma worsens, electronic fetal monitoring may be required. Reassuring findings include variability of 6 to 25 beats per minute (bpm), with a baseline rate of 110 to 160 bpm and no decelerations (Association of Women's Health, Obstetric and Neonatal Nurses [AWHONN], 2003).

Adequate respiratory function, ability to cope with labor and birth, presence of support person as per the client's wishes, and verbalized understanding of all aspects of care and fetal well-being are desired outcomes. Documentation, which demonstrates consistency of care, would include identification of all triggers, medications, appropriate therapies, and monitoring.

CYSTIC FIBROSIS

Cystic fibrosis (CF) is a genetic disorder affecting multiple organs (see Chap. 4). In the past, clients with CF often did not live to adulthood. Recently, however, advances in treatment have prolonged the lifespan of these clients. Some women with CF are becoming pregnant.

Normal pregnancy causes decreased residual volume. Some women with CF cannot maintain the vital capacity or increased cardiac output of pregnancy, which increases risk for premature birth (Barak et al., 2005) (see Chap. 22). In pregnant clients with CF, nurses should observe for signs of malabsorption and monitor maternal weight and pancreatic enzymes during each visit. The nurse should administer oral supplements or nasogastric feedings as ordered. During the intrapartal period, the nurse should monitor the client's fluid and electrolyte balance and frequently assess results of laboratory testing and vital signs. Adequate oxygenation is essential. The nurse should monitor the results of pulse oximetry and, if problems arise, administer oxygen as ordered. Generally, local or epidural anesthesia is preferred for clients with CF ready to give birth. Breastfeeding is permitted once sodium content has been determined; if the sodium content of the mother's milk is high, breastfeeding is contraindicated (Lawrence & Lawrence, 2005).

CARDIOVASCULAR DISEASE

Cardiovascular complications occur in approximately 1% to 3% of U.S. pregnancies (Arafeh & Baird, 2006). The two most common subdivisions are acquired and congenital disorders. Acquired disorders are decreasing in Western countries (largely as a result of the decline of rheumatic fever) but remain a concern in developing areas. The number of women of childbearing age with congenital heart disease is increasing because advances in both diagnosis and intervention have improved survival rates and health, facilitating the ability of these clients to achieve and to maintain pregnancy (Arafeh & Baird, 2006; Kuczkowski, 2004).

Twenty percent of pregnant women with cardiac disease give birth to newborns who are preterm, small for gestational age, or both (see Chap. 22) (Siu et al., 2001). These neonatal complications are associated with maternal risk factors of poor functional class or cyanosis, left heart obstruction, anticoagulation, smoking, and multiple gestation (Siu et al., 2001).

Etiology and Pathophysiology

Physiologic adaptations in pregnancy pose significant risks for women with cardiovascular disease (Ramsey et al., 2001). Blood volume and cardiac output increase as early as the first trimester. With some conditions (eg, Marfan syndrome), the additional volume may increase the risk for congestive heart failure, aneurysm, or both. Toward the end of pregnancy, the increased uterine size encroaches on the inferior vena cava, decreasing venous return and lowering cardiac output when in the supine position (Ramsey et al., 2001). Risks for women who have cardiovascular problems are further increased because of the hypercoagulable state normal to pregnancy. Pregnant women with artificial valves and atrial fibrillation are at increased risk for arterial thrombosis (Arafeh & Baird, 2006). Any type of therapeutic anticoagulation increases the risk for hemorrhage. Electrocardiographic changes also are common in pregnancy, including sinus tachycardia, shift in the QRS axis, and atrial and ventricular dysrhythmias (Ramsey et al., 2001).

Certain risk factors can help predict which clients are at highest risk for morbidity and mortality: (1) history of a prior cardiac event or dysrhythmia, (2) prepregnancy heart disease greater than or equal to class III on the New York Heart Association (NYHA) system, and (3) ejection fraction less than 40% (Martin & Foley, 2003). Smoking, multiple gestation, and use of heparin or warfarin also are linked to a greater potential for neonatal complications (Martin & Foley, 2003).

Types

Manifestations depend on the specific cardiac problem (Gilbert & Harmon, 2003). Maternal functional status is based on the following NYHA (2006) classification:

- Class I: asymptomatic at all activity levels, uncompromised
- Class II: symptomatic with increased activity, slightly compromised

- Class III: symptomatic with ordinary activity, markedly compromised
- Class IV: symptomatic when resting, incapacitated

Generally, pregnant clients with class I or II heart disease have a favorable prognosis, although their functional status may worsen. For example, 44% of women with cardiac disease develop congestive heart failure and pulmonary edema in the third trimester (Ramsey et al., 2001).

Newborns of clients with congenital heart disease have a 2% to 5% risk for congenital heart malformations (Lupton et al., 2002; Ramsey et al., 2001). The health care team must review the functional status associated with the condition together with the potential risk for congenital heart disease in the newborn.

Mitral Stenosis

Mitral stenosis is the most common rheumatic valvular lesion in pregnant clients; approximately 25% of women become symptomatic for the first time while pregnant (Arafeh & Baird, 2006). Mitral stenosis decreases left atrial outflow as well as left ventricular diastolic filling, resulting in a fixed cardiac output. These clients need adequate diastolic filling time to complete cardiac output. Any increase in heart rate shortens the diastolic period more than the systolic, decreasing time for blood to flow across the mitral valve. The increased heart rate and blood volume inherent in pregnancy contribute to the potential for symptoms in the latter half of gestation, particularly during labor and birth. Treatment may include activity restriction to prevent tachycardia, β blockers to control heart rate, and carefully monitored diuretic therapy to treat pulmonary edema (Martin & Foley, 2003).

Mitral Valve Prolapse

Mitral valve prolapse, the most common congenital heart lesion, occurs in 17% of women of childbearing age (Ramsey et al., 2001). It can be asymptomatic or cause palpitations, chest pain, or both. The increased blood volume and decreased systemic vascular resistance of pregnancy actually improve mitral valve function, allowing women with mitral valve prolapse to tolerate pregnancy well (Martin & Foley, 2003). Auscultation may reveal a midsystolic click and murmur, which may decrease with advancing pregnancy because of increased peripheral vasodilation.

Peripartum Cardiomyopathy

Peripartum cardiomyopathy (PPCM) is the term used for heart failure in the last month of pregnancy or within 5 months of childbirth without previous heart disease or identifiable cause (Martin & Foley, 2003). Approximately 1 in 3000 women develop PPCM, which has a mortality rate as high as 56% (Martin & Foley, 2003). Risk factors include multiparity, multiple gestation, gestational hypertension, advanced maternal age, and African American race (Martin & Foley, 2003). Signs and symptoms include nocturnal dyspnea, chest pain, cough, increasing fatigue, peripheral edema, and, on physical examination, rales and murmurs (Ramsey et al., 2001). This problem is discussed in more detail in Chapter 19.

Atrial Septal Defects

Atrial septal defects are commonly seen during pregnancy and are usually asymptomatic (Ramsey et al., 2001). The increased plasma volume of pregnancy can cause dysrhythmias as gestation progresses, but generally this condition is well tolerated.

Collaborative Management: Pregnancy

The most important factors to consider in pregnant clients with cardiac disease are the specific cardiac lesion and whether it has been corrected surgically (Table 13.1). Preconception is the best time to provide the necessary information regarding maternal and fetal risks related to the specific problem (see Chaps. 4 and 11). Once pregnancy is established, fetal echocardiography is critical to prenatal diagnosis of congenital heart disease and important to include in care of women with a history of congenital cardiac disease. Generally, the management of pregnant clients with serious cardiac disease should occur in health care facilities with the capacity and resources for intensive maternal, fetal, and neonatal care (Ramsey et al., 2001).

All pregnant clients require thorough and ongoing physical examination (see Chap. 12). Clients with cardiovascular problems need particular attention paid to heart sounds and pulse rate, as well as questions regarding childhood illnesses, exercise, episodes of dyspnea, and surgery. Symptoms of fatigue, difficulty breathing, palpitations, and lower-extremity edema can be attributed to pregnancy or worsening cardiac disease, so it is important to attempt to differentiate the cause (Martin & Foley, 2003). Clients should be asked about heart murmurs before pregnancy, any activity limitations, chest pain, cyanosis, or previous rheumatic fever (Mason & Bobrowski, 1998). Clients with positive responses should be suspected of having cardiac disease; appropriate classification and diagnosis are important to their ongoing care.

Antepartal blood volume progressively increases, peaking at 28 to 32 weeks' gestation. This period is a critical time to observe the status of the pregnant client with a cardiac condition (Arafeh & Baird, 2006). Beginning at 28 weeks, her visits to the health care provider may need to occur weekly to protect her health during this pivotal time.

Diagnostic studies include chest x-ray, electrocardiogram, arterial blood gas analysis, and echocardiogram. Consultation with a cardiologist is usual during

● **TABLE 13.1 Selected Heart Conditions in Pregnancy**

PROBLEM	EXPLANATION	TREATMENT/MANAGEMENT
Aortic stenosis	A narrowed opening of the aortic valve results in obstructed left ventricular ejection.	Confirmation of diagnosis by echocardiography Antiarrhythmic drugs, β blockers, or both to reduce the risk for other cardiac problems Bedrest, activity restrictions, and close maternal and fetal monitoring
Atrial septal defect	Congenital opening between the atria, with left-to-right shunting of blood and greater left-sided pressure	Atrioventricular nodal–blocking agents Electrical cardioversion Rest and activity limitations
Mitral valve prolapse	Prolapse of the leaflets of the mitral valve into the left atrium during ventricular contraction	Usually, no special precautions needed during pregnancy
Mitral valve stenosis	Obstructed blood flow from atria to ventricle, with possible resultant pulmonary hypertension and edema, as well as right ventricular failure	Diuretics, anticoagulants, and β blockers to treat symptoms In severe cases, bedrest and activity restriction
Peripartum cardiomyopathy	Heart failure of unknown etiology in the last month of gestation to 5 months postpartum in women with no preexisting heart disease	Diuretic therapy Vasodilators Inotropic agents
Ventricular septal defect	Opening in the ventricular septum	Rest and activity limitations

initial diagnosis and for ongoing care and follow-up. The team providing care should decide the appropriate facility for labor and birth, timing of birth, additional needed supplies (eg, hemodynamic monitoring, endocarditis prophylaxis), preferred method of anesthesia, anticoagulant therapy, and needs for early admission (Arafeh & Baird, 2006).

General treatment measures include careful use of antepartum activity restriction, bedrest, or both based on the specific cardiac lesion and functional class; avoidance of anemia by regular laboratory testing and iron supplementation; and intensive maternal and fetal monitoring for potential complications (Ramsey et al., 2001). Frequent rest throughout the day is necessary to meet the increased demands that pregnancy imposes on the cardiac system. Assisting with diet counseling helps ensure appropriate weight gain based on the client's prepregnancy body mass index. A fetal echocardiogram at 18 to 22 weeks' gestation, as well as ongoing monitoring of growth and development, provides clues to fetal well-being.

Collaborative Management: Labor and Birth

Assessment during labor includes careful history taking to pinpoint medications and their dosages, explanations about the effects of cardiac disease during pregnancy and labor, and physical examination, including vital signs. The team needs to understand the client's support for labor, plan for birth, initial labor stage, cervical dilation, effacement, and fetal well-being. Signs and symptoms of complications include fatigue, difficulty breathing or shortness of breath, palpitations, and increasing edema of the feet and ankles (Martin & Foley, 2003).

During labor, demands on the cardiovascular system increase by as much as 50% (Ramsey et al., 2001). Uterine contractions cause fluctuating levels in venous return and sympathetic tone. Placental separation and uterine involution cause physiologic autotransfusion of approximately 500 mL of blood, increasing risks for pulmonary edema and cardiogenic shock (Ramsey et al., 2001). Care at this time focuses on reducing maternal cardiac workload, specifically from tachycardia. Epidural analgesia is beneficial in decreasing intrapartum fluctuations in cardiac output, maternal blood pressure, and pulse (see Chap. 17).

Vaginal birth after 36 weeks' gestation is the goal of care because it poses fewer hemodynamic changes than does cesarean birth. Each case is considered individually, however, depending on the severity of the maternal lesion, symptoms associated with pregnancy, and results of completed tests for fetal lung maturity (Gilbert & Harmon, 2003). Changes in the labor plan are based on maternal and fetal well-being. The client and her family need to be kept informed of her progress throughout pregnancy and labor and of any required changes in care.

Monitoring of a laboring woman with cardiac disease may include readings of central venous pressure, pulmonary wedge pressure, and oxygen saturation. Intake and output should be monitored accurately; specific assessments for individualized care (eg, anticoagulant therapy) are necessary (Gilbert & Harmon, 2003). Depending on severity of the condition, continuous maternal ECG monitoring may be required. Vital signs are assessed every 15 to 60 minutes, with auscultation of the lung fields every 1 to 4 hours. During insertion of monitoring lines, the nurse looks for changes in waveforms or dysrhythmias, which may signify a need for repositioning. Measuring urine output to ensure at least 30 mL/hour is essential for adequate circulating volume. Oxygen therapy and use of the left lateral recumbent position may help. Staff from the intensive care nursery should be on hand to ensure adequate newborn care.

Most institutions would consider maternal cardiac disease a risk factor necessitating continuous electronic fetal monitoring during labor. External monitoring may be adequate; in some cases, internal monitoring with an intrauterine pressure catheter (IUPC) and a fetal scalp electrode (FSE) is used so that data about contraction intensity and fetal heart rate patterns are consistent. Nonreassuring patterns (eg, late decelerations), together with labor progress and potentially a fetal scalp pH sample, need to be evaluated.

Balancing this client's risk and care with the anticipation of birth as a joyous occasion is important. If the mother must be separated from her newborn for any period, facilitating postpartum visitation as soon as possible is vital. Encouraging breastfeeding per the woman's choice also must begin as soon as possible (Arafeh & Baird, 2006).

ANEMIA

Anemia, which affects approximately 50% of pregnant clients, occurs when the quantity or quality of circulatory red blood cells (RBCs) decreases (Casanova et al., 2005). Problems with quantity occur when RBCs are destroyed or lost earlier than their 120-day life cycle. Problems related to quality include microcytic (too small), macrocytic (too large), hypochromic (hemoglobin concentration too low), or hyperchromic (hemoglobin concentration too high) RBCs. Regardless of type, all anemias cause similar signs and symptoms: fatigue, palpitations, chest pain, and shortness of breath with exercise.

Iron-Deficiency Anemia

The iron requirement in pregnancy is 3 to 4 mg/day and increases with gestation as the woman's body works to build the maternal RBC mass, expand plasma volume, and facilitate placental growth (Scholl, 2005). This requirement is challenging to meet with a typical Western diet (Bodnar et al., 2005), and current researchers believe that 50% of women do not have adequate iron stores for pregnancy (Scholl, 2005). Risks for iron-deficiency anemia are increased in black women, clients using antacids or tetracyclines, low-income women, and clients with a concurrent zinc deficiency (Bodnar et al., 2005).

Signs and symptoms of iron-deficiency anemia include fatigue, decreased endurance, and compromised work efficiency. Cognitive deficits and mood swings also are possible, including problems with short-term memory, verbal learning, and depression. Accompanying reduced immune function poses additional health risks (Bodnar et al., 2005). Iron-deficiency anemia also has been associated with preterm birth and low birth weight (Kirkham et al., 2005).

To assess for iron-deficiency anemia, hemoglobin and hematocrit values should be tested in all pregnant clients as part of initial prenatal care. Preferably, these studies are done in the first trimester to separate true anemia from physiologic changes associated with pregnancy. Other evaluations include serum ferritin, transferrin saturation, and free erythrocyte protoporphyrin (Bodnar et al., 2005). A dietary review, possibly with a nutritionist or dietitian, may be appropriate. The client may be prescribed prenatal vitamins with supplemental iron. Discussion of finances may be appropriate to ensure that the client can afford the foods and supplements needed to provide adequate iron or to offer assistance through a social worker, nutritionist, community program, or other avenue. Client teaching focuses on the importance of iron for energy, weight gain, and fetal well-being.

Sickle Cell Anemia

Sickle cell anemia, the most common genetic disorder in the United States, occurs predominantly in African Americans (see Chap. 4). This homozygous recessive illness is characterized by chronic hemolytic anemia. A woman with sickle cell anemia normally has a decreased hemoglobin level (7 to 8 g/dL), as well as a decreased oxygen-carrying capability, to which she likely has adjusted (Blackburn, 2003). Pregnancy, however, may pose new or added problems as the increased blood volume also increases her anemia. Assisting the client to achieve or maintain healthy hemoglobin levels without acute episodes of vascular occlusion is the goal. Careful monitoring involves ongoing blood work and fetal assessment.

Clients with sickle cell anemia may experience chronic hemolytic anemia, acute episodes of vascular occlusion (sickle cell crises), or both. Those with chronic anemia may appear jaundiced and suffer from gallstones, splenomegaly, and slow-healing ulcers. Pyelonephritis and pneumonia are also common. Clients with acute crises may describe pain resulting from sickled cells clustering together in the microvasculature, particularly in the bones and chest. Occlusions in the brain increase the risk for stroke. The heart, liver, and spleen may be affected. Sickle cell crises may increase in frequency and severity with gestation (Blackburn, 2003). Placental infarction and fetal hypoxia can occur during one or more episodes of acute vascular occlusion, with the potential adverse effects of preterm labor, intrauterine growth restriction (IUGR), and stillbirth.

Assessment of the pregnant woman with sickle cell anemia should include a complete health history and physical examination. Laboratory testing should involve a complete blood count, differential, reticulocyte count, blood urea nitrogen, glucose, direct bilirubin, and urinalysis. Questions about previous episodes should include type, amount, and location of pain as well as any helpful treatment. Understanding potential triggers and any precipitating factors (eg, infection) is also helpful. Hydroxyurea (Droxia, Hydrea) may be ordered to reduce acute crises. Folic acid supplements may be beneficial and usually are tolerated well. For the client with sickle cell crisis, fluids and analgesics are appropriate. See Chapter 4 as well.

AUTOIMMUNE DISEASES

Autoimmune diseases affect women of childbearing age more than any other group. Research findings suggest a link with these disorders and increased levels of estrogen and other steroids, the naturally enhanced immunity resulting from pregnancy, or a combination of these factors. Chapter 4 discusses various autoimmune problems common to women; the following paragraphs explore two of the most significant of these illnesses in relation to pregnancy.

Systemic Lupus Erythematosus

Systemic lupus erythematosus (SLE) is a complex, chronic, inflammatory autoimmune disease that can affect numerous organs. Deposits of antigen–antibody complexes in capillaries and various visceral structures are characteristic (Sibai, 2003). SLE often begins or worsens during the childbearing years (Zhang & Chen, 2003); incidence may be as high as 1:1000 in women 20 to 50 years old (Gilbert & Harmon, 2003). The disease is marked by intermittent remissions and exacerbations (see Chap. 4). Clients are prone to clotting problems, with increased rates of pulmonary emboli, deep vein thromboses, and cerebrovascular accidents.

Fertility in women with SLE usually is normal. Pregnancy-related risk factors include IUGR, prematurity, stillbirth, and miscarriage, in addition to maternal hypertension, proteinuria, or both. One factor cited as related to pregnancy outcomes for clients with SLE is the duration of remission of the illness before pregnancy. Zhang & Chen (2003) report that 80% of those in remission for at least 1 year before conceiving were free from exacerbations of SLE during pregnancy. In that same study, those at risk for problems had remission for less than 6 months before conceiving. Extensive preconception counseling should include a discussion of risks and benefits as well as planning for the best time to conceive for both maternal and fetal health.

The major difficulty in pregnancy for women with SLE involves the placenta, which can have various abnormalities and forms of compromise. The inflammatory autoimmune response inherent with this disease leads to placental vasculopathy, with subsequent fibrin deposition and areas of infarction. As a result, placental circulation can be decreased, and the fetus may suffer from malnutrition and its dangerous consequences (Zhang & Chen, 2003). In pregnant women with SLE, placental weight tends to be smaller, and the placental villi are thinner and slimmer.

Nurses, obstetricians, rheumatologists, and social workers are team members likely to have significant roles in evaluating the health of the pregnant client with SLE. Visits to the primary care provider should occur every 2 weeks during the first two trimesters and then weekly during the third trimester. Evaluations of renal function, blood pressure, and fetal growth are critical to locate any changes that might suggest maternal or fetal compromise. Corticosteroid therapy has been shown to improve outcomes in pregnancies involving mothers with SLE (Zhang & Chen, 2003). Glucocorticosteroids are the drug class of choice. The smallest therapeutic dose should be prescribed, with the primary care provider increasing the amount during times of stress (eg, labor).

Preterm birth, IUGR, and gestational hypertension are potential risks. Teaching about the signs and symptoms of preterm labor, scheduling fetal monitoring, and communicating with the client about findings throughout the pregnancy are therapeutic and supportive nursing interventions (see Chap. 16). Discussing the need for close follow-up, child care, and transportation assistance may help ensure the client's compliance with appointments and interventions.

Collaborative planning for labor and birth is necessary before admission. Once the client arrives at the birthing area, she needs individualized attention to her care needs. Initial assessment includes routine blood tests, evaluation of blood pressure, monitoring for signs of edema or proteinuria, and checks of creatinine clearance and urine output. Evaluation of cardiac function by ECG and invasive monitoring may be necessary. Auscultation of breath and lung sounds helps determine pulmonary function. The team must check for signs of disseminated intravascular coagulation by evaluating complete blood count, platelet count, prothrombin time, and International Normalized Ratio (INR); additionally, maternal blood may be needed for group and crossmatch. Physical examination focuses on labor's progress; a vaginal examination is performed unless contraindicated. The client may be administered antihypertensive drugs and high-dose prednisone. Continuous fetal monitoring and ongoing communication can decrease maternal anxiety about fetal well-being as labor continues. Cesarean birth may be determined safest depending on the specific risks and benefits to both mother and fetus. Expected outcomes include a normal fetal heart rate, normal labor progress, pain management per the woman's wishes, and birth without coagulopathy.

Antiphospholipid Syndrome

Antiphospholipid syndrome (APS) is an autoimmune disorder characterized by the presence of circulating antiphospholipids. The two most common types are lupus anticoagulants and anticardiolipin antibodies. Low levels of antiphospholipids may be found in 2% to 4% of all women; however, 0.2% have levels associated with pregnancy complications. The rate of pregnancy loss in women with untreated APS is as high as 90% (Silver & Branch, 1997). Up to 30% of pregnancies in women with APS are marked by abnormal fetal growth, gestational hypertension, and placental abnormalities (Silver & Branch, 1997). Thrombosis is the most serious risk associated with APS, with occlusions occurring in various locations.

Laboratory testing for antiphospholipids should be done when the maternal health history reveals recurrent spontaneous abortions, unexplained pregnancy loss in the second or third trimester, venous thrombosis, arterial thrombosis, stroke, SLE, autoimmune thrombocytopenia, or prolonged clotting assay. The client with APS requires treatment from a team including social workers, nurses, obstetricians, hematologists, and pharmacists. Communication among members and with the client and family ensures collaborative care and desired outcomes. Fetal growth and development should be assessed weekly from 28 weeks' gestation onward through NST, biophysical profiles, Doppler studies, or all these methods. Monitoring of maternal blood pressure and renal function also is essential.

One potential treatment for the pregnant client with APS is a combination of prednisone (40 mg/day) with low-dose aspirin (80 mg/day). Although effective, it increases the risks for preterm birth and gestational hypertension. Another potential treatment is low-molecular-weight heparin; this drug poses risks for abnormal bleeding and fractures but has been successful in decreasing occlusion. Individual factors need to be considered to determine the most effective therapy.

INFECTIONS

Routine prenatal care for all pregnant clients includes obtaining a detailed medical history, testing for sexually transmitted infections (STIs), and offering laboratory testing for human immunodeficiency virus (HIV). Intrapartum infections require knowledge and skill from health care providers to decrease the risk for vertical transmission from mother to fetus. Such transmission may occur through ascending infection in the birth canal, blood exchange, or direct contact with vaginal or cervical secretions.

HIV

As discussed in Chapter 4, clients may not develop symptoms of HIV for 10 years or longer. As of December 2002, approximately 19.2 million women worldwide were living with HIV (Burdge et al., 2003). Improvements in treatment are extending the lives of many of these women; some such clients are choosing to become pregnant.

Most pediatric transmissions of HIV are acquired perinatally (Burdge et al., 2003). The transmission rate from infected mother to fetus without treatment is 25% (Gilbert & Harmon, 2003). Maternal HIV status should be determined during pregnancy with appropriate consent and testing, maternal treatment initiated before birth, and subsequent infant treatment at birth. Nurses should encourage all women to consent to an HIV test early in pregnancy to facilitate prompt diagnosis and treatment for their fetus or newborn. Treatment during pregnancy significantly reduces the risk of the infant acquiring the disease.

Collaborative interventions focus on teaching about the risks and benefits of all aspects of care in relation to the infection. A multidisciplinary team involves nurses, obstetricians, HIV specialists, social workers, dietitians, and pharmacists. All care providers should use universal precautions at all times (standard of care for all women), including wearing goggles during birth.

The nurse should use open-ended questions to determine the client's knowledge about her infection and plans for newborn care. Some women choose not to share information about their health with family members, partners, or both; therefore, nurses must be careful to ask initial questions about HIV status of the woman alone. Assessment also should include evaluations of the client's emotional state and coping ability. The nurse should review and document community resources the client already is using when planning care during pregnancy and after the baby's birth.

An estimated 50% to 80% of perinatal transmissions of HIV occur during labor and birth (Katz, 2004). Treatment goals during labor are to provide individualized care to the client based on the clinical and immunologic stage of her disease and to prevent perinatal HIV transmission (Katz, 2004). Antiretroviral therapy, most commonly oral zidovudine (ZVD), may have been started during pregnancy and will be given intravenously during childbirth (Pharmacology Box 13.1). The goal is to reduce the maternal viral load, thus decreasing the chances of disease transmission. Medical interventions such as rupturing the membranes or using a fetal scalp clip (internal monitoring) are avoided. Vaginal examinations should be minimized. Prolonged ruptured membranes increase the risk for HIV transmission; thus, care should be taken to decrease exposure of the fetus or newborn to maternal body fluids (Katz, 2004). Antibiotic therapy should be considered at least 4 hours before birth. Cesarean birth is an option being studied as a way to decrease perinatal HIV transmission.

Some HIV-positive women also are injection drug users. They may be ambivalent about their pregnancies

● PHARMACOLOGY 13.1 Zidovudine (ZVD)

ACTION: Inhibits retroviral replication, including HIV; helps block maternal–fetal transmission of HIV

PREGNANCY CATEGORY: C

DOSAGE: 100 mg 5 times a day from gestational week 14 to labor's onset

POSSIBLE ADVERSE EFFECTS: Nausea and vomiting, headache, skin rash, fatigue, paresthesias

NURSING CONSIDERATIONS

- Ensure that the client schedules and attends regular appointments for monitoring of blood tests.
- Emphasize to the client that she must follow strictly the dosage and administration instructions given to her with the medication.
- Assist the client to manage any nausea that may accompany use of the drug.
- Teach the client that use of zidovudine does not protect against transmitting HIV to others through sexual contact or contaminated blood.

From Karch, A. M. (2005). *2005 Lippincott's nursing drug guide.* Philadelphia: Lippincott Williams & Wilkins.

or worried about fetal health (Katz, 2004). Emotional support involves being nonjudgmental during care provision. Describing interventions and involving the client in choices for labor support (eg, music, pain management) are important. Depression also has been associated with an HIV diagnosis; thus, encouraging the client's resourcefulness and coping skills can contribute to increasing her health behaviors (Boonpongmanee et al., 2003).

Postpartum discussions should focus on obtaining the client's feedback about care received during labor and birth, giving her opportunities to discuss her memories and perceptions of the experience. Testing for HIV in the newborn and, if necessary, providing ongoing medical treatment for him or her are extensions of the care started during pregnancy. See Chapter 22 for more information on care of the newborn with HIV.

Sexually Transmitted Infections

More than 56 million U.S. adolescents and adults have STIs other than HIV (Thomas, 2001). As discussed in detail in Chapter 4, STIs are most common during the reproductive years. Women have more frequent and more serious complications from STIs than do men (Youngkin & Davis, 2004). Viral STIs are often difficult to treat; the person may have the virus for the rest of his or her life.

As part of prenatal care, nurses should ask every woman questions about sexual activity, previous STIs, and risk factors for STIs (eg, number of partners). Reviewing the sexual history of a pregnant woman with an STI also is important to help determine any requirements for reporting in her geographic area. Physical examination should include thorough assessment of the perineal area for any warts, malodorous or unusual vaginal discharge, redness, or bleeding.

Treatment of bacterial STIs is tailored to the pregnant woman's situation; follow-up should be implemented during prenatal care. Treatment of viral STIs may not remove the virus; the nurse may need to educate the woman about ongoing safety and preventive health measures.

Planning for screening, treatment, and follow-up for STIs is important during pregnancy. Collaboration with the woman is key to ensuring that she continues to complete preventive measures, treatments, or both. See Table 13.2.

Group B Streptococcus

Incidence of group B streptococcus (GBS) sepsis is 1.8 per 1000 births, and GBS is a major cause of neonatal morbidity and mortality (CDC, 2005a). In pregnant women, GBS usually is asymptomatic but can cause urinary tract infections (UTIs), amnionitis, endometritis, and wound infection (Chandran et al., 2001). Newborn infection results from vertical transmission, making maternal colonization an identifiable risk factor. Other risk factors include preterm labor, birth of a previous infant colonized with GBS, and membranes ruptured longer than 18 hours.

Current recommendations for prenatal care before labor include taking a swab at 35 to 37 weeks' gestation from the vaginal introitus and anorectum of all pregnant women so that results are available during labor (Chandran et al., 2001). The client who tests positive for GBS and her family should receive information about the need for intrapartal antibiotics at least 4 hours before birth. Penicillin G, 5 million units IV initially, with 2.5 million units IV every 4 hours until birth, is the preferred treatment. If no swab has been taken or the results of testing are unavailable, treatment is based on risk factors during labor: temperature above 100°F, rupture of membranes greater than 18 hours, or preterm labor.

Further education is necessary postpartum. Although the risk for transmission of GBS is highest in the first 24 hours, it persists for up to 7 days following birth. Thus, the nurse should review signs and symptoms of infection with the family before discharge.

TABLE 13.2 Infections in Pregnancy and Potential Fetal Effects

INFECTION	POTENTIAL FETAL EFFECTS	COLLABORATIVE CARE CONSIDERATIONS
Toxoplasmosis	Neurodevelopmental disabilities related to damage of the central nervous system: cranial deformity, microcephaly, hydrocephaly	Conduct routine antepartal screening to detect this virtually asymptomatic protozoan infection; promptly treat. Caution pregnant women to avoid emptying cat litter boxes or working in soil contaminated with cat feces. Remind women to cook all meats thoroughly. Consider use of pyrimethamine after first trimester (this drug reduces folic acid levels, which are necessary to protect against neural tube defects before the second trimester). Monitor newborn for hyperbilirubinemia if sulfonamides are prescribed.
Rubella	Teratogenic, particularly to fetal eyes, ears, heart, and brain, resulting in congenital cataracts, deafness, cardiac anomalies, mental and motor deficits, congenital cleft lip and cleft palate, intrauterine growth restriction	Remind all pregnant women to avoid contact with children who have rashes; reinfection is possible in women with rubella antibodies. Review results of antepartal rubella titer; provide counseling about results and possible implications. Assess fetal biophysical profile and ultrasound findings. Give postpartal vaccination to women who do not demonstrate immunity to rubella with cautions to avoid conception within 1 month of vaccination. Take specimens for culture from newborn's nose and throat. Isolate newborn from other newborns in the nursery. Assess for evidence of congenital anomalies. Provide supportive and restorative care measures. Teach specialized feeding techniques for cleft lip and palate. Promote attachment and bonding.
Syphilis	Possible fetal demise; if infection persists beyond 18 weeks' gestation, cognitive deficits and orthopedic deformities (osteochondritis) Congenital syphilis	Perform VDRL on initial antepartal visit with immediate antibiotic therapy if indicated. Give instructions regarding safe sex practices. Monitor newborn for rash, obstructed nasal breathing, and excessive nasal secretions. Give immediate antibiotic therapy and follow-up care to newborn.
Cytomegalovirus (CMV)	Severe disability; damage to cranial nerves leading to blindness; deafness and hepatic dysfunction from transplacental exposure; exposure during vaginal birth or from contaminated breast milk serious only in very low-birth-weight newborns	Detect maternal infection (asymptomatic) with CMV-IgG and IgM by ELISA testing. Routine testing for CMV in newborns is not performed, although antibodies may be isolated in maternal or newborn serum for diagnosis. Provide antepartal teaching to avoid exposure. Perform meticulous handwashing before meals and avoid contact with young children in crowds such as nursery schools or daycare settings (to reduce risk for droplet transmission).
Herpes simplex virus type 2 (HSV-2)	Congenital herpesvirus infection from transplacental inoculation with vesicles at birth or infection during birth when vulvar lesion present Infection leading to encephalitis, convulsions, shock, and death Neurologic damage in newborn survivors	Plan for cesarean rather than vaginal birth if woman has active herpes lesions. Assess newborn for oral ulcerations and skin lesions (pinpoint clustered vesicles surrounded by erythema). Monitor for onset of birth-acquired infection, such as poor feeding, fever, and lethargy preceding eruption of skin lesions. Administer prescribed antiviral agent, acyclovir (Zovirax). Restrict newborn handling or feeding if active lesions present. Restrict health care providers with fever blisters or cold sores from nursery because of the severity of infection and the high risk for neurologic sequelae in the newborn.

Continued

● **TABLE 13.2 Infections in Pregnancy and Potential Fetal Effects *(Continued)***

INFECTION	POTENTIAL FETAL EFFECTS	COLLABORATIVE CARE CONSIDERATIONS
Gonorrhea	Severe eye infection resulting from conjunctival inoculation of *Neisseria gonorrhoeae* during vaginal birth (ophthalmia neonatorum) Blindness (if untreated) from corneal damage	Ensure early antepartal diagnosis; treat with penicillin or ceftriaxone (Rocephin). Give neonatal eye prophylaxis at birth. Assess newborns born outside the hospital for fiery red conjunctiva and thick yellow crusting exudate from the eyes; treat with IV antibiotics and topical antibiotic ointment. Use sterile normal saline eye irrigations for thick suppuration.
Hepatitis B virus (HBV)	Hepatitis B infection with potential for becoming a chronic carrier	Promptly wipe contaminated blood and secretions from the newborn after birth. Bathe baby as soon as possible in an open isolette with a radiant warmer to prevent cold stress. Perform gentle nasal and oropharyngeal suction to avoid a break in mucous membranes, which could provide the entry route for inoculation of the virus. Give HBV vaccine at birth to prevent future HBV infection. Give immune serum globulin to infants of mothers testing positive for HBV. Do not give injections before the first bath because HBV skin surface contamination can invade the newborn when the needle pierces the skin. Do not begin breastfeeding until after the administration of immune serum globulin (provides passive immunity) because virus is found in breast milk.
Chlamydia	Eye infection from conjunctival inoculation during vaginal birth	Administer bilateral eye prophylaxis at birth with erythromycin ophthalmic ointment. Assess newborns born outside the hospital for edema and erythema of the eyelids and purulent exudates. Give systemic antibiotic therapy as prescribed for the newborn, mother, and mother's sexual contacts.
Candidiasis	Thrush (oral *Monilia*)	Assess newborn for white-coated tongue resembling milk curds; scrape from the tongue to reveal red, raw patches. Observe for poor feeding or signs of oral pain when suckling. Give prompt and aggressive topical antifungal therapy with nystatin to prevent systemic infection; application to lesions of the oral mucosa, the buccal space, or the tongue; ensuring contact with the lesion rather than allowing the infant to suck and swallow directly from the dropper. Give antifungal treatment to mother and her sexual contacts to prevent reinfection.
Human immunodeficiency virus (HIV)	Possible HIV infection resulting from placental transmission, perinatal exposure, or breast milk	Give antepartal zidovudine therapy to reduce placental transfer of virus to fetus. Counsel mother not to risk exposure through breastfeeding. Reassure mother that because of transfer of antibodies through the placenta, all newborns will test positive for HIV, but this does not mean that the disease is present. Treat toddlers who remain positive after 18 months old with long-term strategies to support nutrition and prevent opportunistic illness.
Group B streptococcus (GBS)	**Early onset** (day of birth): rapidly progressing pneumonia and respiratory distress **Late onset** (2–4 wks): meningitis, intracranial pressure, bulging fontanels; neurologic deficits in survivors	Ensure health care providers practice strict handwashing between caring for newborns. Administer IV antibiotic therapy (penicillin) during labor 4 or more hours before birth. Monitor newborn blood cultures following prolonged rupture of membranes, if no prophylaxis. Give antibiotic therapy to newborns of mothers who are GBS positive, if symptomatic and no prophylaxis.

Rubella

Today, rubella (German or "three-day") measles is rare in the United States and Canada; in 2002, 82 total U.S. cases were reported (CDC, 2005b). A population-based immunization strategy in both countries has effectively decreased the risk for rubella infection during pregnancy. The largest risk to the developing fetus occurs in the first trimester, when congenital rubella syndrome (CRS) may result. Approximately 25% of affected newborns have tremors, increased irritability, small head size, and hypotonia at birth (Comley & Mousmanis, 2003). By the end of the first year, these children may have psychomotor retardation, progressive hearing loss, or visual deficits with new impairments emerging with development (Comley & Mousmanis, 2003).

Symptoms of rubella infection include a rash that may or may not be itchy beginning on the face and progressing to the trunk. Transmission is by droplet and may occur up to 7 days before and 7 days after the rash (CDC, 2005b). In adults, lymph node edema, joint pain, and mild fever may accompany the rash.

Screening for rubella immunity is normally part of blood testing completed at the first antenatal visit. Evidence of immunity is determined by the amount of maternal immunoglobulin G (IgG) antibodies. A client with no or less than adequate evidence of immunity should be told about her status and offered postpartum immunization. She also should be educated about this disease and alerted to take preventive measures for the first 3 months of gestation so that she may avoid groups of children who may not be immunized.

Toxoplasmosis

Toxoplasma gondii, a protozoan parasite, infects up to one third of the world's population through ingestion or handling undercooked meat (pork and lamb) or handling cat feces (Montoya & Liesenfeld, 2004). In clients infected for the first time while pregnant, the parasite can enter the fetal circulation through the placenta. Positive maternal status before pregnancy poses little or no fetal risks unless the infection happens a few months before conception. Early maternal infection tends to result in severe congenital toxoplasmosis, usually leading to spontaneous abortion. With late maternal exposure, the newborn appears normal but may have a subclinical infection (Montoya & Liesenfeld, 2004). Congenital toxoplasmosis ranges from 1 to 10 per 10,000 births (Montoya & Liesenfeld, 2004).

Detection of IgG antibodies to *T. gondii* should be assessed in early pregnancy; their absence would identify clients at risk for toxoplasmosis. Cautions about cooking meat thoroughly, avoiding the handling of cat feces, and using gloves while gardening outdoors should be individualized for those at risk, although these guidelines are important for all pregnant women (Montoya & Liesenfeld, 2004). Treatment with spiramycin should be initiated as quickly as possible if diagnosis of recently acquired maternal infection is found, as should information and education for the woman and family.

Cytomegalovirus

Cytomegalovirus (CMV) is the most common cause of congenital infection leading to neurologic impairment (Damato & Winnen, 2002). The illness acquired during gestation can result in stillbirth or miscarriage, IUGR, congenital anomalies, or other infections. In some cases, affected infants appear asymptomatic at birth but develop progressive sensorineural problems, including hearing impairment. The greatest risks to the pregnant woman include contact with infected children in daycare centers or health care settings. Frequent handwashing is encouraged in these environments. No treatment exists for CMV; thus, nurses should encourage women to practice sound hygiene while pregnant. Another nursing role may be to provide supportive counseling to clients if ultrasound or other diagnostic testing reveals sequelae of congenital CMV infection.

Parvovirus

Parvovirus B19 is the smallest DNA-containing virus that infects mammalian cells (White, 2003). Infection with parvovirus B19 (fifth disease or erythema infectiosum) is common among young children, particularly from March to May (Fig. 13.7). Transmission occurs by inhaled particles, hand-to-mouth contact, and contaminated blood. Symptoms include headache, fever, malaise, gastrointestinal upset, sore throat, and cough. The distinctive rash described as "slapped cheek" has a red appearance against relatively pale skin, usually appearing on the face before spreading to the trunk and limbs and fading in color. Approximately 50% of adults are immune from

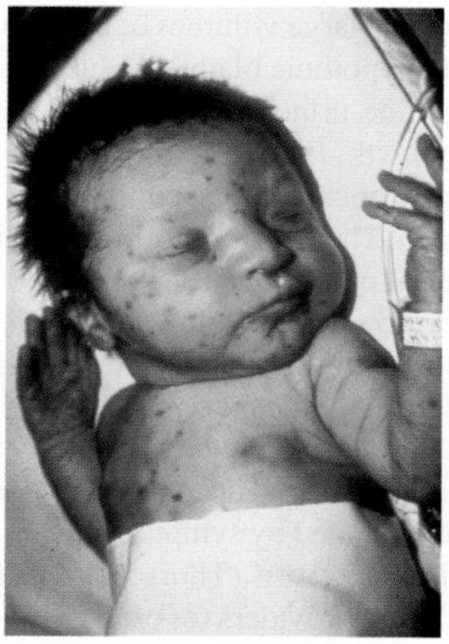

FIGURE 13.7 An infant born with congenital rubella.

prior infection; therefore, incidence in pregnancy is decreased (White, 2003). Adults who contract the disease may describe joint pain, particularly in the hand and wrist.

Pregnant women who contract this infection transmit it to their fetuses in up to 30% of cases (Goff, 2005; White, 2003). Complications can include spontaneous abortion, fetal anemia, fetal nonimmune hydrops, and miscarriage (Goff, 2005). Clients with symptoms or history of exposure should have blood work that includes serology, IgG, and IgM (enzyme-linked immunosorbent assay [ELISA] and indirect fluorescent antibody [IFA]). Serial ultrasounds may assist in a diagnosis of hydrops; if so, the pregnant woman should be referred to an obstetrician and a tertiary care center for management of this high-risk fetus (White, 2003).

RENAL AND URINARY PROBLEMS

During pregnancy, kidney volume, weight, and size increase, as does dilation of the ureters and renal calyces as a result of hormonal influences and obstruction by the enlarging uterus. The obstructive effect along with urinary stasis predisposes pregnant women to UTIs, pyelonephritis, and symptomatic infections from vesicoureteral reflux. It is also possible for bacteria from the gastrointestinal area to contaminate the perineal area.

Renal blood flow increases during gestation 70% to 85% (Thorsen & Poole, 2002). Other renal adaptations in pregnancy include changes in protein excretion, tubular function, acid–base regulation, and osmoregulation. These developments are reflected in laboratory test results; for example, protein excretion can reach an upper limit of 300 mg/day (the usual normal limit is 150 mg/day). Awareness of such pregnancy-related variations is vital to be able to quickly recognize and address abnormalities (see Chap. 12).

UTIs and Pyelonephritis

During pregnancy, large volumes of urine may remain in the ureters and hypotonic bladder. Glucose, protein, and amino acids in the urine provide an ideal environment for bacterial growth. Edema and hyperemia of the bladder mucosa also increase susceptibility to infection in pregnant women. The static column of urine in the ureters leads to bacterial migration (Blackburn, 2003). Asymptomatic bacteriuria develops in 2% to 10% of pregnant women. Although this number is similar to rates in nonpregnant women, significant complications can develop during pregnancy such as preterm birth, low birth weight, hypertension, and maternal anemia. A further 3% of pregnancies are complicated by symptomatic UTIs, including pyelonephritis and cystitis (Thorsen & Poole, 2002).

All health care providers for pregnant women should be alert to the possibility of asymptomatic and symptomatic UTIs. Describing symptoms to be aware of (eg, urinary burning and frequency) to pregnant women during the first prenatal visit can help them recognize differences between UTI and normal pregnancy changes. Testing urine at every prenatal visit is crucial. The most common method of assessment is urinalysis by dipstick (Thorsen & Poole, 2002). The one exception may be the client with hypertension who should have a dipstick test, followed by 24-hour urine collection if the urinary protein level is greater than 1+. A woman with underlying renal disease should have a baseline 24-hour urine collection that may be continued with serial 24-hour tests to determine renal involvement. Diagnosis of asymptomatic bacteriuria is based on a midstream urine collection that reveals at least 100,000 colonies/mL of a single organism. The most common bacterium isolated is *Escherichia coli.*

Treatment of UTIs in pregnant women may include ampicillin if *E. coli* is identified as the causative organism. High-dose antibiotics usually are required because of the increased excretion that stems from increased renal blood flow (Gilbert & Harmon, 2003). Reculturing at the end of therapy is important to ensure that the infection has cleared. If necessary, treatment can be reinitiated up to 2 more times. An antimicrobial agent (eg, nitrofurantoin) may be prescribed if ampicillin is unsuccessful. Discussion of hygiene that includes wiping from front to back after urination and sexual intercourse, extra fluid intake, and cotton underwear is important.

The most common symptoms of pyelonephritis include costovertebral angle tenderness, high fever, chills, myalgia, nausea, and vomiting. Maternal temperature typically "spikes" and then falls to normal or even hypothermic levels. These symptoms should prompt a urinalysis that typically shows numerous leukocytes and bacteria. A complete blood count usually shows a significantly increased leukocyte count with a left shift. Treatment includes admitting the client to the health care facility and beginning generalized IV antibiotic therapy until results from culture and sensitivity are available. Once results are known, drug therapy is individualized to the client's illness. If there is no response within 24 hours of therapy, blood cultures should be drawn to ensure that sepsis has not developed. IV therapy should continue until 24 to 48 hours after temperature is normal and right-sided tenderness has resolved. Oral antibiotics can then continue for 10 to 14 days as ordered (Thorsen & Poole, 2002). Ongoing assessment of urine by urinalysis, dipstick, or both throughout the rest of pregnancy is essential to prevent recurrences.

Acute Renal Failure

In 1999, the rate of live births to women of all races and ages with a history of renal disease was 7 per 1000 (Thorsen & Poole, 2002). Acute renal failure (ARF) may occur in clients with a prepregnancy diagnosis of renal disease, from a pregnancy-associated event such as gestational hypertension, or from a non–pregnancy-associated problem such as trauma (Thorsen & Poole, 2002). Clients who experience ARF have a sudden decrease in renal function with an increased serum creatinine level and oliguria.

Management of the pregnant client with ARF requires a collaborative approach to protect maternal health and fetal well-being. Determining the ability of the health care facility to manage this woman's care and to transfer her appropriately as needed is vital. A thorough health history and physical examination are important. Decreased intake (eg, hyperemesis gravidarum, laxative use with eating disorders) or diarrhea can lead to volume depletion and increase risk for ARF. Hypertension and concealed hemorrhage also are risk factors. Assessment of vital signs is critical to evaluate maternal well-being. For example, increased blood pressure readings may indicate fluid overload. Increased pulse and respiratory rate may precede pulmonary edema. Maternal pulse oximetry is appropriate as indicated by the woman's clinical condition. Fatigue, malaise, irritation, and disorientation may be seen. Laboratory testing may include complete blood count, coagulation profile, and electrolytes. A 24-hour urine collection should be started. Evaluation of hemoglobin is necessary to ensure that the client does not develop anemia from decreased erythropoietin production. Awareness of symptoms of anemia (ie, shortness of breath, easy fatigue, impaired fetal growth) can help monitor for this condition.

Fetal monitoring through NST and fetal movement counts also is mandatory. Ultrasound imaging of the kidneys may be required to assist with a diagnosis. If diuretics are used as treatment, monitoring of electrolyte levels is extremely important (Gilbert & Harmon, 2003).

DIABETES MELLITUS

As discussed in Chapter 4, various types of diabetes mellitus affect women. In type 1 (10% to 20% of cases), pancreatic β cells are destroyed gradually or suddenly, and the client requires administration of insulin to stay alive (Kozak, 2002). In type 2 (80% to 90% of cases), the client has abnormal insulin secretion as well as insulin resistance. Hereditary and environmental factors are involved in the development of both conditions.

Women with type 1 or type 2 diabetes who become pregnant require adaptations to manage their condition and their pregnancy successfully. Ideally, these clients plan their pregnancy carefully with health care team members at a high-risk pregnancy clinic. The goal is to maintain or achieve "ideal" blood glucose control to decrease the risk for congenital anomalies, fetal macrosomia, and spontaneous abortion (see Chaps. 16 and 22). A woman with type 1 or 2 diabetes may need to alter her treatment during pregnancy to reflect changes in insulin requirements, assessment for retinal and renal disease, and glucose monitoring. Careful follow-up by a multidisciplinary team throughout pregnancy in preparation for labor and birth is essential.

In **gestational diabetes,** a woman develops or recognizes carbohydrate intolerance for the first time during pregnancy. Approximately 4% of pregnant women experience gestational diabetes, which varies in severity for each client (Kozak, 2002). Risk factors include previous history of gestational diabetes, previous birth of a large for gestational age infant, history of stillbirth or spontaneous abortion, family history of type 2 diabetes, obesity, advancing maternal age, glucosuria, and hypertension. High-risk ethnic groups include African Americans, Hispanics, Native North Americans, Pacific Islanders, and South or East Asian Americans (Kozak, 2002).

Current recommendations are for pregnant women to undergo screening for gestational diabetes between 24 and 28 weeks' gestation; women with risk factors should be screened earlier (Fig. 13.8). This screening is done with a 1-hour plasma glucose measurement following a 50-g glucose load given at any time of the day. A result greater than 10.3 mmol/L confirms gestational diabetes. A result between 7.8 and 10.2 mmol/L is an indication for the woman to undergo a 75-g oral glucose tolerance test.

Regardless of the type of diabetes involved, the risk for congenital anomalies in infants born to mothers with diabetes is higher than in the general population (4% to 11% vs. 2% to 3%) (Kozak, 2002). Maintaining strict glucose control throughout pregnancy decreases this risk. During labor and birth, diabetes increases both maternal and fetal risks, including gestational hypertension, shoulder dystocia, and need for cesarean or operative birth (see Chap. 16).

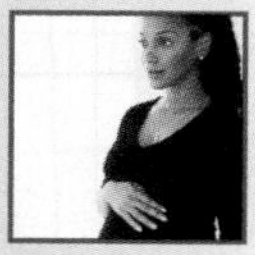

Think back to Selena, the 39-year-old client pregnant for the second time. What risk factors would the nurse identify as placing Selena at increased risk for gestational diabetes?

COLLABORATIVE CARE: DIABETES IN PREGNANCY

Pregnant women with diabetes may develop complications. A team approach is necessary to involve them and their families in management of the condition, promotion of health, prevention of hospitalization, and control of any complications. Balancing pregnancy and diabetes is stressful. The woman may have financial concerns related to the supplies required for monitoring. Learning

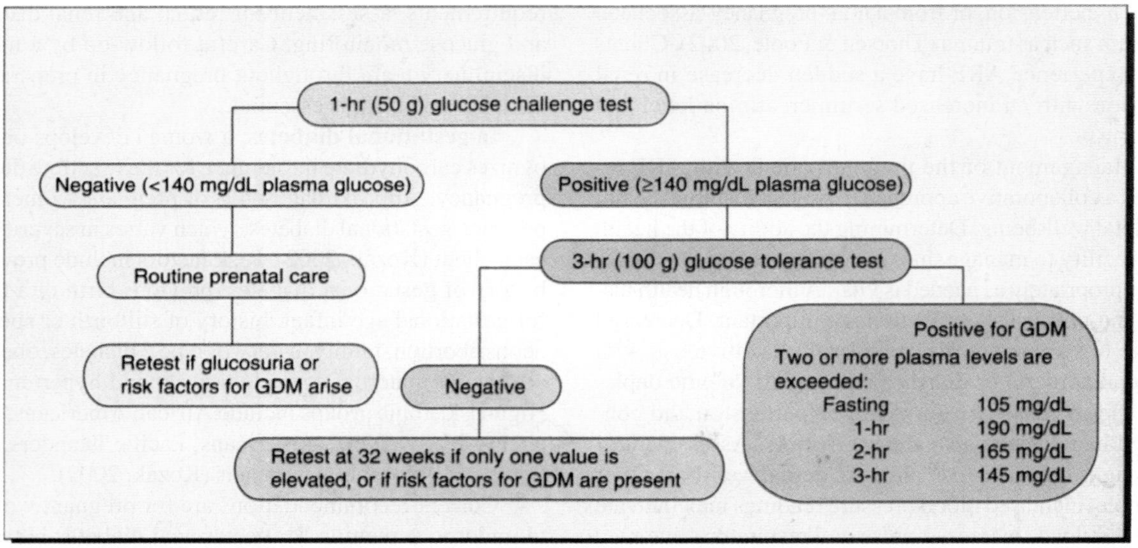

FIGURE 13.8 Screening guidelines for gestational diabetes mellitus (GDM).

about diabetes, planning meals, and testing blood glucose levels can be emotionally and physically taxing. Risks for other problems, such as gestational hypertension, polyhydramnios, UTIs, intrapartal trauma, and retinopathy, are increased. Health care providers need to be aware of such complications and constantly monitor for them (Kozak, 2002).

Treatment during pregnancy should include dietary counseling and review, glucose monitoring instruction, and insulin therapy. Normally, an endocrinologist and obstetrician are members of the client's team. Others involved may include social workers, community nutrition and diabetic clinic staff, and public health nurses. NIC/NOC Box 13.2 highlights some common nursing interventions and outcomes for pregnant women with diabetes.

In some cases, fetal size leads to a decision to induce labor (see Chap 16). Such a choice is based on indicators of fetal well-being as monitored through assessment of fetal lung maturity and NST. Care in labor and birth must be ongoing; including the client and family in activities such as self-monitoring glucose during labor or consulting an endocrinologist can facilitate involvement and continuity. Level of care required during labor and birth depends on whether the client was taking insulin before labor and her blood glucose levels during labor.

NIC/NOC Box 13.2 Pregnancy and Diabetes

Common NIC Labels

- High-Risk Pregnancy Care
- Medication Administration: Subcutaneous
- Prenatal Care
- Teaching: Disease Process
- Teaching: Prescribed Diet
- Teaching: Prescribed Medication

Common NOC Labels

- Fetal Status: Antepartum
- Knowledge: Diabetes Management
- Knowledge: Diet
- Knowledge: Pregnancy
- Knowledge: Treatment Regimen
- Maternal Status: Antepartum

Assessment

Assessment of the pregnant client with preexisting diabetes should include type, onset, duration, and treatment. The nurse should review a history of any complications such as retinopathy, neuropathy, or cardiovascular disease. He or she should explore the client's support systems, dietary understanding, stress levels, motivation, and coping methods. The woman should undergo a glycosylated hemoglobin test (HbA1c) to reveal her glucose control over the previous 3 months. Additional tests include serum creatinine and urinalysis for microalbumin.

The client diagnosed with gestational diabetes who is 24 to 28 weeks' pregnant requires immediate intervention from a diabetic care team. Their assessment includes reviewing support systems, nutrition and diet, coping strategies, family history, lifestyle, and genetics.

For cases of both preexisting and gestational diabetes, careful nursing assessment on admission to the birthing unit includes review of pregnancy history, diabetes management, support systems, cultural differences (which may give clues about stress and anxiety levels), and results of screening tests (eg, urine, blood glucose levels). Recording her insulin therapy during pregnancy and last dose, if appropriate, would be important, as would her last oral intake.

Evaluation every hour for hypoglycemia should be ongoing during labor and birth. Signs and symptoms include shakiness, dizziness, sweating, clumsy or jerky movements, hunger, headache, pale skin color, and confusion. Assessment of fetal well-being depends on institutional policy but usually includes intermittent auscultation or continuous electronic fetal monitoring depending on the severity of the diabetes and risk to the fetus.

Select Potential Nursing Diagnosis

The following are examples of commonly applicable NANDA diagnoses in cases of diabetes in pregnancy:

- **Anxiety** related to maternal and fetal health with diabetes and pregnancy
- **Deficient Knowledge** related to new medical diagnosis
- **Risk for Ineffective Health Maintenance** related to a new diagnosis of diabetes or previous diagnosis together with pregnancy
- **Imbalanced Nutrition: Risk for More Than Body Requirements** related to an inability to assess diet in initial stages of diet planning
- **Ineffective Coping** related to stress of managing pregnancy and diabetes

Planning/Intervention

Reviewing Blood Glucose Self-Monitoring

During pregnancy, the nurse should assist the client to review or to learn techniques of blood glucose monitoring (Fig. 13.9). The client needs to self-assess her blood glucose level four times a day (prandial and preprandial) using an accurate monitor; she needs to record results on a written log that allows for easy tracking of patterns. Risk for nocturnal hypoglycemia is increased, so testing during the night may be required. The nurse should provide guidelines for findings that mandate communication with the diabetic team. Nursing Care Plan 13.1 highlights some key aspects of nursing care.

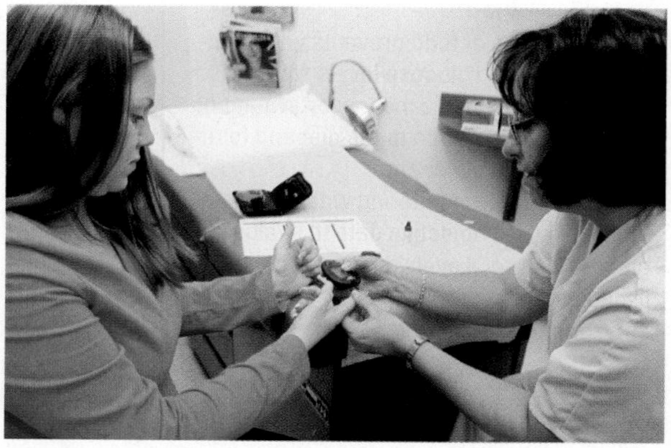

FIGURE 13.9 This client with gestational diabetes is learning techniques for self-monitoring of blood glucose levels.

Promoting Diet Management

Dietary management is extremely important when pregnancy and diabetes coexist. A dietitian can assist with individualizing meals to ensure tight blood glucose control, appropriate weight gain, and adequate nutrition. Together, the nurse and dietitian should consider the client's cultural and socioeconomic status when assisting her to plan meals. A diet with 2000 to 2500 cal/day spaced over three meals and three snacks meets the needs of most women in their second and third trimesters. The care team generally tries to structure maternal weight gain to be approximately 2.2 to 6.6 lb (1 to 3 kg) in the first trimester and 0.4 lb/week (0.18 kg/week) for the remainder of gestation (Kozak, 2002).

Encouraging Activity and Exercise

A physiotherapist may help to assess this woman's history of exercise and tailor a program to meet her needs for energy balance. Walking, swimming, riding a bicycle, and housecleaning should be encouraged. Good posture, positioning, and body mechanics for lifting and decreasing stress on joints (eg, the pelvic area) are important (Kozak, 2002).

Administering Insulin

Women with type 1, type 2, or gestational diabetes may require insulin during pregnancy. Some clients just starting insulin find injecting themselves difficult and require support and encouragement. The nurse should review equipment, type of insulin, and injection tool (pen, needle) with the client and then go over the details a second time for the client to practice.

Clients who take insulin need to be aware of their risk for hypoglycemia (abnormally low blood glucose), why it happens, when it can occur, how to prevent it, and how to treat it. They may need to have glucagon with them at all times in case of a hypoglycemic episode.

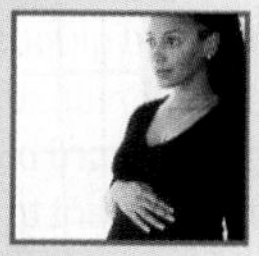

Screening tests indicate that Selena has gestational diabetes. As part of the treatment plan, she is to perform blood glucose self-monitoring four times a day. She says, "My mother only tests her blood twice a day. Why do I have to do it four times a day?" How should the nurse respond?

(text continues on page 516)

NURSING CARE PLAN 13.1

The Client With Gestational Diabetes

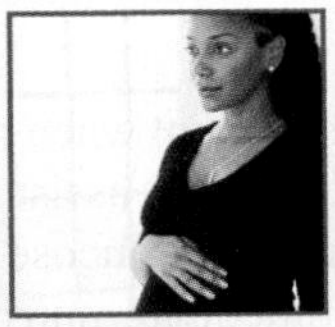

The results of Selena's screening test for gestational diabetes are positive. Her primary care provider prescribes a special diet and blood glucose self-monitoring. Selena states, "I'm in shock. How will this affect my baby? And what if I need shots?"

NURSING DIAGNOSES

- **Deficient Knowledge** related to disease process, treatment, and effects on pregnancy and fetus
- **Anxiety** related to uncertainty about insulin therapy and possible effects on fetal outcome

EXPECTED OUTCOMES

1. The client will demonstrate an understanding of gestational diabetes and treatment.
2. The client will verbalize effects of diabetes on pregnancy and fetus.
3. The client will report less anxiety related to the condition and pregnancy.

INTERVENTIONS	RATIONALES
Assess the client's knowledge of gestational diabetes and associated risks.	Assessment provides a baseline from which to develop an individualized teaching plan.
Explore the client's exposure to diabetes, including gestational diabetes; correct any misconceptions; allow time for questions.	Information provides an additional foundation for teaching and opportunities to clarify misinformation.
Review the client's history for risk factors, such as previous birth of an LGA infant and family history of type 2 diabetes.	Identification provides a basis for developing appropriate measures to reduce the risk associated with these factors.
Review the physiologic mechanisms underlying gestational diabetes; teach the client about various treatment options.	Education promotes understanding.
Work with the client to develop an appropriate plan for activity and exercise, based on her preferences and ability.	Activity and exercise assist glucose control. A client-tailored program enhances the chances for compliance. Collaboration fosters cooperation and feelings of control.
Review the client's dietary program, including the need for evenly spaced meals and snacks throughout the day. Monitor weight at each visit.	Well-timed intake of food prevents wide fluctuations in blood glucose levels. Weight monitoring provides a means for evaluating the client's adherence to the diet and fetal growth and development.
Teach the client how to perform blood glucose self-monitoring; have her return-demonstrate the skill. Urge her to check and to record blood glucose levels as ordered. Tell the client to notify the health care provider promptly if levels are outside established parameters.	Blood glucose self-monitoring with documentation provides objective data to evaluate glucose control. Levels outside of established parameters may indicate the need for adjustments to the regimen.

Continued

NURSING CARE PLAN 13.1 ● The Client With Gestational Diabetes

INTERVENTIONS	RATIONALES
Teach the signs and symptoms of hypoglycemia, including factors contributing to its development and measures to treat it. Instruct the client to check blood glucose levels if she develops any signs and symptoms.	Early identification and prompt intervention for hypoglycemia reduce the risk for injury to the client and her fetus.
Evaluate the client's past coping strategies to determine which have been most effective.	Use of appropriate coping strategies aids in reducing anxiety.
Encourage the client to include her partner in follow-up visits.	Participation of the client's partner promotes sharing, provides support to the client, and enhances the chances for a successful experience.
Question the client about available support systems, such as family, friends, and community resources. Enlist the aid of social services as necessary to assist with possible stressors such as financial concerns and child care.	Stress can upset blood glucose control. Additional sources of support are helpful in alleviating anxiety.
Provide information about support groups, Web sites, and other resources related to gestational diabetes, pregnancy, and fetal health.	Shared experiences and knowledge of similar situations can prepare the client for what to expect.

EVALUATION

1. The client describes gestational diabetes and its effect on pregnancy.
2. The client identifies the role of measures used to control gestational diabetes.
3. The client demonstrates a beginning ability to perform blood glucose self-monitoring.
4. The client shows use of positive coping measures to reduce anxiety level.

NURSING DIAGNOSIS

Risk for Injury (maternal and fetal) related to effects of diabetes on pregnancy

EXPECTED OUTCOMES

1. The client will verbalize the need for glucose control during pregnancy.
2. The client will maintain blood glucose levels within acceptable parameters.
3. The client will demonstrate progression of pregnancy with fetal growth and development appropriate for gestational age.

INTERVENTIONS	RATIONALES
Assess maternal status at each visit; monitor vital signs, including blood pressure. Reinforce the need for more frequent follow-up during pregnancy.	Ongoing assessment is essential for early identification of potential problems. Gestational diabetes increases risks for gestational hypertension. Frequent follow-up provides multiple opportunities to assess maternal and fetal well-being.

Continued

NURSING CARE PLAN 13.1 ● The Client With Gestational Diabetes *(Continued)*

INTERVENTIONS	RATIONALES
Measure fundal height at each visit; prepare the client for diagnostic and laboratory testing. Monitor fetal heart rate.	Fundal height provides an estimation of fetal growth. Diagnostic and laboratory testing provides information about maternal and fetal well-being. Fetal heart rate is an indicator of fetal well-being.
Review blood glucose levels for fluctuations. Expect to include insulin administration if blood glucose levels are outside established parameters. Instruct the client in administration and related care.	Strict blood glucose control is necessary to prevent congenital anomalies and fetal macrosomia. Insulin may be necessary to maintain blood glucose control.
Assess for signs and symptoms of hypoglycemia, especially if insulin is necessary. Instruct the client in measures to control hypoglycemia.	Untreated hypoglycemia poses a danger to the mother and fetus.
Prepare the client for necessary fetal surveillance, such as biophysical profiles and nonstress testing, especially during the third trimester. Teach her how to perform fetal count kicks.	Fetal surveillance provides information about fetal well-being, aids in early detection of possible complications, and promptly enables any necessary intervention.
Discuss care that may be required during labor and birth.	Discussion helps the client prepare for labor and birth and provides a baseline for additional teaching once labor starts.
Reinforce the need for client adherence to the treatment regimen and follow-up.	Adherence and follow-up enhance the chances for a successful outcome.

EVALUATION

1. The client demonstrates understanding of glucose control measures.
2. The client exhibits acceptable blood glucose levels.
3. The client progresses through pregnancy without complications.
4. The fetus demonstrates gestational age–appropriate growth and development.

Monitoring the Fetus

Intensive fetal monitoring begins toward the end of pregnancy (third trimester) with fetal movement counting, biophysical profiles, and NST. These evaluations all are done to reduce the risk for trauma, stillbirth, or both.

Providing Care During Labor and Birth

The woman who comes to the birthing unit with preterm labor and receives corticosteroids to enhance fetal lung maturity (usually 12 to 24 hours between doses) requires increased insulin for those 2 days. An explanation of this treatment as well as the interaction between corticosteroids and diabetes should be provided.

During labor, the goal of insulin therapy is to maintain blood glucose concentrations of 60 to 80 mg/dL to decrease the risk for neonatal hypoglycemia (Gilbert & Harmon, 2003). Insulin needs commonly decrease at the beginning of labor and fall to zero during the active phase. Maternal glucose requirements are 2.5 mg/kg/min. Her blood glucose levels should be monitored hourly. IV insulin should be administered as 25 units of regular insulin in 250 mL of NS, with the line flushed with 25 mL to decrease the insulin-binding capacity to plastic surfaces (Gilbert & Harmon, 2003). The insulin solution should be maintained on an infusion pump while piggybacked to a main IV line to ensure the woman's safety.

Areas that require careful monitoring include the progress of labor (increased risk for prolonged labor from fetal macrosomia), maternal temperature every 1 to 4 hours, vital signs hourly, and continuous fetal health surveillance by electronic monitoring depending on institutional policy. Urine should be assessed for ketones at every void or every 4 hours if the woman has an indwelling catheter. Intake and output should be evaluated hourly (Gilbert & Harmon, 2003). Assessment for hypoglycemia during labor and birth should be ongoing.

Evaluation

Any type of diabetes in pregnancy increases maternal and fetal risks. Ongoing involvement from a team of specialists is essential to ensure maximum maternal and fetal health. The goals are fetal and maternal well-being throughout pregnancy, labor, and birth as evidenced by consistently normal blood glucose levels, normal fetal monitoring results as per institutional policy, and coordinated multidisciplinary care.

PSYCHOSOCIAL DISORDERS AND PROBLEMS

Chapter 5 discusses mental health and mental illness during the adolescent and adult years in detail. The following sections explore the effects of some common psychiatric problems when they develop or coincide with pregnancy. Postpartum psychiatric illnesses are explored in detail in Chapter 19.

Depression in Pregnancy

The most common U.S. illness is major depression, particularly affecting women of childbearing age (Dietch & Bunney, 2002). Major depression is a cluster of signs and symptoms that include at least five or more of the following for at least 2 weeks:

- Mood changes, usually sadness, anxiety, or irritability
- Negative changes in sleep patterns (eg, insomnia)
- Appetite changes
- Weight changes
- Change in activity levels
- Fatigue
- Decreased motivation
- Decreased interest in other things, life in general, or both
- Decreased libido
- Decreased ability to concentrate, usually with a shortened attention span
- Feelings of helplessness and worthlessness
- Thoughts of dying (American Psychiatric Association [APA], 2000)

Depression is associated more commonly with the postpartum period (see Chap. 19); however, women can experience depression anytime in life, including pregnancy. A milder form of depression, dysthymia, is described as a loss of enthusiasm or joy and ongoing fatigue (Dietch & Bunney, 2002). See Chapter 5.

All women of childbearing age should be made aware of the signs and symptoms of depression. For pregnant women, open-ended questions to ask, particularly during the first prenatal visit, include the following:

- What changes have you noticed about how you feel lately?
- What changes have you noticed about how you have been behaving lately?
- How are these changes affecting you personally? Your family?
- How do these changes make you feel? (Dietch & Bunney, 2002)

These questions may lead to a discussion of particular signs and symptoms, especially changes in appetite, eating, sleeping, and mood.

A careful history both of the pregnancy and factors causing stress or low self-esteem is important for individualizing the care plan. Counseling, whether individual or group, is crucial to assist with review of symptoms, build on maternal strengths, and assist in developing self-esteem and interpersonal relationships (Dietch & Bunney, 2002). Behavioral therapy also may be an option; it involves completing a series of tasks to facilitate changes, enhance self-esteem, and improve problem-solving skills.

Pharmacology may include tricyclic antidepressants, monoamine oxidase inhibitors (MAOIs), or selective serotonin reuptake inhibitors (SSRIs). Side effects include decreased appetite, nausea, decreased deep sleep, and drowsiness (Dietch & Bunney, 2002). The nurse should review these side effects during client teaching if pharmacology is part of the treatment plan. The nurse also should discuss with the client and her family the risks versus benefits of using pharmacologic treatment for depression in pregnancy. Collaborative approaches should explore such options as counseling and increased prenatal visits. Assisting the client to evaluate areas of stress and offering counseling to her partner and family also may be appropriate.

Bipolar Disorder

Bipolar disorder affects 0.5% to 1.5% of people in the United States. Clients usually are in their teens or early adulthood at onset of bipolar illness, putting them at risk during their reproductive years. Rapid cycling and depressive characteristics are more common in women than in men with this problem (Yonkers et al., 2004).

Review of health history of the pregnant woman with bipolar illness should include her prior response to various medications, the severity of her illness, the duration of normal mood with and without medications, the time between episodes when she has discontinued medications, and recovery with pharmacotherapy (Yonkers et al., 2004). A client with a stable condition may be able to stop taking medications for some time before conception and during the first trimester, to decrease the risk for teratogenic effects. Discontinuation of maintenance pharmacologic treatment, however, may lead to relapse, particularly if withdrawal is abrupt and not tapered (Yonkers et al., 2004). Before conception, the client and health care provider may test the stability of the woman's condition by tapering medication slowly and closely monitoring for symptoms. Should symptoms manifest quickly, the client and provider may decide that remaining on medication during pregnancy is the best plan.

Ongoing pharmacotherapy may be necessary if the client has a tendency to self-harm, protracted recovery time, impaired insight, or lack of sufficient support systems (Yonkers et al., 2004). The risk for fetal malformations depends on the properties of the specific medication involved and when in gestation the drugs are taken. In planning treatment, it is critical to minimize risks to both mother and fetus while also limiting maternal morbidity from an active phase of bipolar disorder. An informed choice, together with prenatal care given by both an obstetrician and psychiatric specialist, is important.

For the woman who continues to take medications during pregnancy, the lowest effective dose must be used, with consideration given to those drugs that have the least teratogenic potential (Yonkers et al., 2004). Older agents with case and cohort data (research evidence for use during pregnancy) should be tried and evaluated first. Fetal screening and assessment should be part of this client's care plan. Lithium, valproate, or olanzapine may be used during pregnancy.

Domestic Violence

Abuse is defined as "someone using power over another person to try to harm that person, or to exert control that will harm that person either immediately, or eventually if repeated over time" (Health Canada, 1999). Abuse may be physical, emotional, verbal, financial, or sexual. Clients who report the highest rates of abuse are typically in their childbearing years (15 to 45 years old) (Watts, 2004). Domestic violence is a term used to represent an ongoing pattern of control that includes physical or sexual abuse or threats, emotional abuse, stalking, economic control, and control of social contacts.

Abuse may begin or increase during pregnancy. Jasinski (2004) describes both maternal and fetal consequences of pregnancy-related violence. These include delayed or absent prenatal care, low birth weight, premature labor, unhealthy maternal behaviors (eg, substance abuse), fetal trauma, recurrent UTIs, postpartum depression, and social isolation. In other cases, pregnancy is the woman's first entry into the health care system and her first contact with a helping profession. Those who care for pregnant women frequently are in a unique position to screen for and to treat cases of abuse. Evidence also suggests that women want health care providers to ask direct and nonthreatening questions about violence (Jasinski, 2004).

COLLABORATIVE CARE: THE PREGNANT CLIENT WHO IS ABUSED

Assessment

All health care facilities should screen all women for abuse routinely. Care providers should be alert for suggestive indicators such as chronic pain; insomnia; irritable bowel syndrome; migraines; arthritis; UTIs; injuries to the face, breasts, abdomen, and buttocks; anxiety; depression; fractures; unexplained bruises; areas of redness consistent with slaps; lacerations; and multiple injuries in various stages of healing. Any type of screening must be done with the woman privately. A nonthreatening and nonjudgmental approach may include a general statement about the prevalence of abuse in society. For example:

"In the United States, approximately 10% to 20% of women have been abused at some time in their lives. Out of concern for all the women to whom I provide care, I ask whether you have ever been hit, kicked, or punched in your current intimate relationship. Also, do you feel personally safe in your home? Have you ever been hurt or frightened in your home?"

The "SOS" is a screening tool that may be used with pregnant women in a clinic setting. The letters SOS describe the process of **S**creen, **O**ffer options, and **S**afety. The nurse should first tell the woman that "We're concerned about the health effects of partner abuse so we ask a few questions of all of our clients." Then, he or she can ask the following questions:

- Do you ever feel unsafe at home?
- Has anyone at home hit you or tried to injure you in any way?
- Have you ever felt afraid of a partner? (Watts, 2004 quoting Mian, 2000, p. 232)

The woman who responds positively to having been abused either currently or in the past needs to know that she did not deserve this, that help can be provided, and that her situation may threaten the course of labor and birth.

For clients in labor, accurate, confidential assessment is critical. Antenatal documentation may provide information that questions regarding abuse have been asked previously. Abuse screening should take place again privately in the labor assessment area, with responses documented.

Labor and birth sometimes trigger memories of childhood sexual abuse as women experience their bodies in new and different ways. Potential triggers during this time include expressions of pain, strangers in the room, vaginal examinations, pushing efforts, perineal pain, and even breastfeeding (Hobbins, 2004). Private discussion with the woman who has described past experiences of abuse would be helpful in knowing how to assist her to cope during labor and birth (Fig. 13.10).

Select Potential Nursing Diagnoses

The following are examples of commonly applicable NANDA diagnoses for the client who has experienced abuse:

- **Fear** related to possible injury or ongoing abuse
- **Anxiety** related to maternal and fetal health and well-being
- **Chronic Pain** related to ongoing or beginning abuse
- **Deficient Knowledge** related to safety and support
- **Pain** related to labor and birth and increased anxiety caused by abuse or memories of abuse
- **Impaired Parenting** related to abuse or past abuse

Planning/Intervention

If a woman responds positively about abuse during screening, nurses and other care providers must make resources available and assist her to form an emergency safety plan. Inclusion of any children in this plan is important to ensure their safety. Every effort must be made to protect this woman; therefore, charting and all information given must remain confidential. Clients entering prenatal care must be treated with respect and dignity, regardless of their stories.

Ensuring one-to-one nursing care throughout labor can facilitate the client's trust. Encouraging her choices relative to pain medications and comfort measures would be important to giving the client a feeling of control. Providing her with information regarding her care may promote her participation in and acceptance of labor and birth. Ensuring that she receives information to make a safety plan that she can implement at any time if needed would be critical to postpartum follow-up. Assisting her to verbalize concerns and questions privately also would be important. Culturally sensitive care would ensure the presence of a translator other than a family member and asking open-ended questions.

Evaluation

The goal of care for all women is to screen for abuse and, depending on answers, provide encouragement and support. For women dealing with abuse issues, information about community resources and shelters is a measure by which to provide needed assistance.

Confidentiality and privacy of both the woman's records and conversations are essential. Ensuring safety and well-being is also crucial. Safety of the fetus or newborn also must be considered; measures to promote family bonding need to be enacted, even in what might be a painful and emotional atmosphere.

Substance Use

Many substances can have negative consequences on maternal and fetal health during pregnancy. Antenatally, the nurse should ask all women about their use of tobacco,

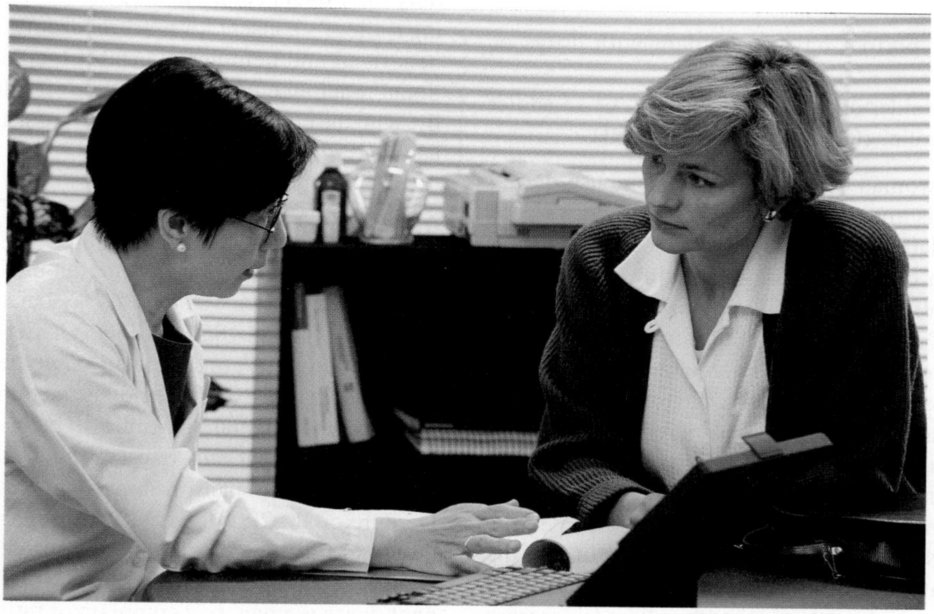

FIGURE 13.10 Well before labor begins, the nurse should try to discuss sensitive issues, such as past abuse, with the client to help prepare her for emotions and feelings she may experience during childbirth.

marijuana, cocaine, alcohol, and other recreational or prescription drugs.

Alcohol use in pregnancy contributes to birth defects and developmental delays. Heavy or binge drinking has been linked to fetal alcohol syndrome (FAS); low levels of alcohol use may cause low birth weight (see Chap. 22). Facial anomalies as well as learning deficits may be partly the result of alcohol use in pregnancy. Fetal alcohol spectrum disorder is a new term describing the various problems that can accompany maternal alcohol use. A safe level of alcohol use during pregnancy has not been determined (Comley & Mousmanis, 2003).

Women who smoke during pregnancy are at increased risk for preterm labor and IUGR. Other problems associated with maternal tobacco use include miscarriage and tubal pregnancy (Comley & Mousmanis, 2003).

Most women who use substances in pregnancy use more than one drug (Table 13.3). It may be difficult to separate the effects of one from the other. Other factors such as poverty, lack of family support, and inadequate education may be equal risk factors in this woman's pregnancy.

Effective care for women who use substances and their fetuses is multifaceted and involves cooperation and collaboration from the woman and her family, social workers, physicians, midwives, community health workers, and family and children's services. One tool that has been developed to begin the discussion about substance abuse is the four Ps:

- Have you ever used drugs or alcohol during this **p**regnancy?
- Have you had a problem with drugs or alcohol in the **p**ast?
- Does your **p**artner have a problem with drugs or alcohol?
- Do you consider one of your **p**arents to be an addict or an alcoholic? (Gilbert & Harmon, 2003)

When a woman describes substance abuse during pregnancy, it is important for the health care provider to respond in relation to the effects of her behavior on her health and on that of her fetus. Remaining nonthreatening but assessing her motivation to taper use or quit is essential. Discussing family and social supports also is important to the success of intervention.

If the substance involved is heroin or opioids, a treatment plan that includes methadone may need to be considered with a gradual tapering that allows the woman to not suffer from obstetrical complications or withdrawal. Frequent monitoring and hospitalization for some time would be most beneficial if available, depending on the treatment plan. Adapting a plan of care depending on the substance involved that assists the client to decrease or quit without complications to her pregnancy is the goal. Encouragement, praise, and self-esteem are important to include as additional goals in treatment.

Eating Disorders

Western society's fascination with thinness has contributed to many young women working hard to attain a body image smaller than normal. For some clients, the natural weight gain that accompanies pregnancy is difficult. Women may struggle with prenatal visits that require objective checks of weight.

In the past 30 years, reported cases of bulimia nervosa and anorexia nervosa have increased (see Chap. 5) (Mitchell-Gieleghem et al., 2002). Currently, 5% to 10% of women have bulimia or anorexia; 90% of these women are in the childbearing years (Little & Lowkes, 2000). Pregnancies complicated by anorexia or bulimia are at high risk for gestational hypertension, small-for-gestational-age newborns, breech presentation, miscarriage, vaginal bleeding, and cesarean birth (Little & Lowkes, 2000).

The client with an eating disorder who presents for prenatal care needs a careful health history. Many women attempt to deny an eating disorder. If the client has been slow to gain weight, seems unwilling to talk about her weight, or has a body mass index lower than 19, an eating disorder should be suspected. For women who admit to having an eating disorder, important blood tests include serum electrolytes, thyroid function, blood urea nitrogen, and serum creatinine. Requesting her permission or consent to have a social worker visit her or referral to community services is important.

Little and Lowkes (2000) report that eating disorders frequently increase in intensity in the first postpartum year; some clients attempt to control the weight of their infants as well. Assisting women with eating disorders to find help immediately postpartum may protect not only their own health but also that of their baby. Seeking a client's consent for nutritional consultation can be beneficial and help her to establish appropriate nutritional requirements during her recovery. Involving family, with the client's permission, may assist her to achieve her goals.

OBESITY

Obesity is becoming more common in North America. The U.S. prevalence of obesity associated with pregnancy ranges from 18.5% to 35% (Galtier-Dereure et al., 2000). Increased consumption of processed and fast foods, decreased exercise, and fascination with computers and other sedentary pastimes all increase the chances of excessive weight gain. Excess weight before pregnancy increases risks for many maternal complications (Galtier-Dereure et al., 2000). Obesity in pregnancy poses the potential for hypertension, vascular disease, diabetes, and need for cesarean birth (Cesario, 2003). The pregnant obese woman may complain of fatigue, backache, pelvic pain, or UTI. All these common complaints in pregnancy are increased for obese women because of the additional musculoskeletal strain, cardiac workload, and

TABLE 13.3 Maternal Substance Abuse

SUBSTANCE	EFFECTS	MANAGEMENT GUIDELINES
Alcohol	Fetal alcohol syndrome Spontaneous abortion Low birth weight Low Apgar scores	Identify and confirm cases of alcohol abuse. Educate women regarding danger to fetus: permanent cognitive impairment, facial deformity, microcephaly, growth deficiencies, and behavioral problems. Refer woman to alcohol treatment facility. Use supportive network and follow-up to reduce alcohol intake.
Cocaine	Congenital anomalies of the brain, kidneys, and urogenital tract Small for gestational age (SGA), intrauterine growth restriction (IUGR) Prematurity Birth asphyxia secondary to placental abruption Brain infarcts Neurobehavioral abnormalities	For newborns, perform massage therapy to soothe, calm, and reduce behavioral disorganization: stroke the prone newborn over each area of the body systematically, moving from trunk outward to extremities. Talk soothingly in low tones to calm baby. If newborn is unstable or preterm, use gentle palmar touch to head and abdomen at several intervals each day (Mainous, 2002). Ensure adequate non-nutritive sucking; swaddle newborn snugly. Reduce environmental stimuli. Administer sedation as ordered.
Smoking or exposure to secondhand tobacco smoke	Spontaneous abortion SGA Low birth weight Increased risk for sudden infant death syndrome (SIDS) Increased incidence of abruptio placentae and placenta previa Birth defects including congenital urinary tract anomalies	Educate women about dangers to fetus and self. Evaluate woman's desire and ability to quit. If woman cannot or is unwilling to quit, form a contract to ration or limit cigarettes per day. Give support and positive reinforcement. Provide information about alternative methods of stress relief. Encourage partner/family to support client's efforts to decrease smoking.
Heroin	IUGR SGA Increased incidence of SIDS Newborn withdrawal Poor feeding in the newborn Dehydration and electrolyte imbalance related to vomiting and diarrhea	Begin maternal methadone therapy to reduce risk for spontaneous abortion or possible fetal demise (after 32 to 34 weeks' gestation) secondary to heroin withdrawal. Administer sedatives and methadone to newborn. Swaddle newborn for comfort; give gentle persistence and stimulation for feeding. Use soft preemie nipples to reduce energy expenditure associated with feeding. Conduct massage and give gentle human touch to help decrease restlessness and improve habitation. Decrease noise, noxious stimuli, and light.
Marijuana	Preterm birth Decreased birth weight and length Possible delays in growth and development in preschooler	Assess for concurrent use of other harmful substances: alcohol, cocaine, methamphetamines. Educate women about drug's potential long-term effects on the child's language, memory, and development. Give psychological support if drug use is a form of self-medicating to avoid an unpleasant or abusive home environment. Provide social service referrals as needed.

chance for infection their extra weight imposes. These clients also need to be assessed regularly for any signs of labor depending on gestation because many symptoms they experience also can be indications of preterm labor. Chapter 16 discusses in detail specific issues related to obesity and the labor and birth process.

COMMON GESTATIONAL COMPLICATIONS

Major complications specifically related to gestation and pregnancy are relatively few. Nevertheless, they can pose significant risks to mother, fetus, or both. This section discusses those problems of gestation inherently related to the state of pregnancy itself. In addition, it explores two common types of special risk: adolescent pregnancy and multiple gestation. The section concludes with those conditions leading to pregnancy loss and care for the grieving family.

HYPEREMESIS GRAVIDARUM

Most women experience mild to moderate nausea and vomiting during pregnancy, which usually begins by 4 to 6 weeks' gestation, increases in severity by 8 to 12 weeks, and commonly resolves by 20 weeks (von Dadelszen, 2000). Women with **hyperemesis gravidarum** have severe nausea and vomiting, a weight loss of 5% or more from their prepregnancy value, dehydration, and electrolyte imbalances (Youngkin & Davis, 2004). Hyperemesis gravidarum is a high-risk problem because it increases chances for pregnancy loss, IUGR, maternal activity restriction, fatigue, and depression.

Many risk factors are associated with severe nausea and vomiting in pregnancy (NVP), including younger maternal age, nulliparity, low socioeconomic status, unplanned pregnancy, passive smoking, previous pregnancy with NVP, increased body mass index, eating disorders, ethnicity, and fetal female gender (suggesting an immune mechanism). One etiologic theory is that NVP results from an olfactory response with specific trigger odors in some women; another is that the problem stems from motion hypersensitivity (von Dadelszen, 2000). Dysregulation of gastric rhythms also has been proposed as a cause. Gestational hormones, particularly human chorionic gonadotropin (hCG), have been investigated for their role, particularly because rising levels of hCG are correlated with increased NVP in the first trimester. No etiology has been proven as of this writing. A deficiency of vitamin B_6 is associated with NVP, but it is uncertain whether this occurs before or after NVP.

Some researchers have linked hyperemesis gravidarum to psychosocial conflicts inherent in pregnancy: fear and anxiety regarding changing or new roles, possible adverse socioeconomic repercussions of childbirth, and whether the pregnancy was planned. Symptoms decrease with hospitalization, leading researchers to think that some women may view the hospital as a "safe place," potentially pointing to emotional and psychological contributors to NVP (Deuchar, 2000).

NVP can negatively affect family relationships and the pregnant client's ability to work: 75% of employed women with NVP reported time lost from their jobs, and 50% felt that NVP adversely compromised their relationship with their partner (Mazzotta et al., 2000). NVP has been compared with the severity of nausea experienced by clients undergoing chemotherapy (Society of Obstetricians and Gynaecologists of Canada [SOGC], 2002). Hospitalized women with hyperemesis gravidarum have described social alienation and withdrawal to cope with the embarrassment and pervasiveness of the problem. They describe loneliness, being overwhelmed, and hopelessness, particularly when faced with little understanding from family, friends, and health care providers (O'Brien et al., 2002). See Research Highlight 13.2.

Assessment Findings

It may be a challenge for some women to find a health care provider while experiencing hyperemesis gravidarum, which usually begins during the first 10 weeks of pregnancy. Access to help may depend on whether the client already has a family doctor, has had medical confirmation of her pregnancy, and is well enough to attend appointments. Potentially, this client may present at the emergency department for assistance.

A thorough history is necessary. Frequency, severity, and duration of episodes are important to ascertain. Triggers or precipitating factors (eg, odors, times of day, specific foods) also would be helpful to know. The nurse should ask about strategies that the woman may have tried such as dietary modifications or herbal medications (eg, black cohosh). Information from family and friends may provide insight about how the client is coping.

Physical examination is essential to rule out other diagnoses and to confirm the pregnancy. Routine procedures include urinalysis (protein, ketones, and glucose) as well as current weight. Blood work may include a complete blood count, electrolytes, liver enzymes, and thyroid and bilirubin levels.

Collaborative Management

Several clients with hyperemesis gravidarum have one or more admissions to a health care facility (as many as 14 per 1000 births) (SOGC, 2002). Hospitalization may be necessary if assessment reveals dehydration and a need for IV therapy to correct electrolyte imbalances. Initially, the client's status will be nothing by mouth (NPO) during IV hydration. Fluids should not be taken again until the client has gone 48 hours without vomiting.

During hospitalization, nursing care involves monitoring intake and output, including emesis; assessing urine for ketones and protein; taking daily weights; and providing nutritional counseling as needed. Mouth care while the client is NPO and a quiet environment with attention to minimizing odors (to try and prevent this potential cause of nausea) may decrease the severity of symptoms. Medical care may include pharmacologic therapy (Pharmacology Box 13.2).

Critical to this woman's emotional needs is support provided by health care providers combined with the recognition of her need for isolation when she is feeling nauseous. Demonstrated understanding about the severity and reality of this syndrome is essential (O'Brien et al., 2002). Women experiencing NVP have identified an in-

● RESEARCH HIGHLIGHT 13.2 Isolation from "Being Alive": Coping with Severe Nausea and Vomiting of Pregnancy

OBJECTIVE: To understand how pregnant women cope with severe nausea and vomiting.

SAMPLE: Twenty-four pregnant women admitted for nausea and vomiting to a Canadian hospital participated. They ranged in age from 18 to 41 years, came from various cultural backgrounds, and had different levels of education. Eight women were pregnant for the first time; 15 were having their second pregnancy, and 1 woman was expecting for the third time.

METHOD: This descriptive-exploratory study relied on semistructured interviews. Data analysis was concurrent with information collection. Researchers reviewed emerging results with a focus group for comment, confirmation, and clarification to ensure that participants recognized their own experience in the presented description.

RESULTS: Women identified increasing loneliness and isolation beginning early in pregnancy and continuing for the duration of their symptoms. Although the women themselves recognized that the symptoms were not minor and that strategies to deal with them were not working, their support people did not appreciate their difficulties. They also emphasized that health care professionals did not understand the extent and debilitating nature of the problem. Participants described nausea and vomiting as "taking over their lives," eventually feeling as if they had no life of their own. For many, symptoms subsided by 22 weeks' gestation. Two participants elected to have abortions, and two continued to have severe nausea and vomiting up until birth.

NURSING IMPLICATIONS: Nurses providing care to pregnant women hospitalized because of nausea and vomiting need to understand the emotional effects of this problem. Assisting clients to reduce predisposing and coexisting factors that exacerbate nausea and vomiting may help.

O'Brien, B., Evans, M., & White-McDonald, E. (2002). *Nursing Research, 51,* 302–308.

ability to communicate to others the pervasiveness of their symptoms as a concern. The nurse who provides care should assist the client and her family to discuss the experience, identify interventions that may be helpful, and communicate openly.

Depending on the severity of symptoms, total parenteral nutrition (TPN) also may be started in the hospital and continued at home. The home care nurse would focus on evaluating the results of hydration and IV therapy; he or she also would explore the client's coping strategies and support systems. Teaching parameters may include eating smaller and more frequent meals, taking fluids between meals, decreasing cooking odors, eating whatever the woman can tolerate, and using complementary therapies such as ginger or vitamin B_6 supplements (SOGC, 2002). Indications of improving health include increased fluid intake, weight gain, adequate hydration, and successful employment of coping strategies.

HYPERTENSIVE PROBLEMS

Hypertension is an absolute blood pressure (BP) value equal to or greater than 140/90 mm Hg, a diastolic BP value greater than or equal to 90 mm Hg, or both. Most pregnant women have an internal "clock" that regulates BP, showing an increase during the day, a peak during the early evening, and a decrease between midnight and 4 AM. Hypertensive disorders occur in 10% of pregnant women

● PHARMACOLOGY 13.2 Promethazine (Phenergan)

ACTION: Blocks cholinergic receptors in the vomiting center of the brain, thus mediating nausea and vomiting in cases of hyperemesis gravidarum

PREGNANCY CATEGORY: C

DOSAGE: 25 mg orally; repeat doses of 12.5 to 25 mg as needed every 4 to 6 hours. Drug can be given parenterally or rectally if client cannot tolerate oral administration. IM or IV dosages are 12.5 to 25 mg, not to be repeated more frequently than every 4 hours.

POSSIBLE ADVERSE EFFECTS: Confusion, dizziness, restlessness, epigastric distress, urinary frequency, dysuria

NURSING CONSIDERATIONS

- Implement safety precautions to protect the client against injury secondary to the drug's sedative effects.
- Emphasize to the client to try to maintain an adequate fluid intake.

From Karch, A. M. (2005). *2005 Lippincott's nursing drug guide.* Philadelphia: Lippincott Williams & Wilkins.

and are a major cause of maternal mortality (Gilbert & Harmon, 2003). They develop most often in primiparas, particularly those who are obese; are younger than 18 years or older than 35 years; have diabetes, APS, or both; are of low socioeconomic status; or fail to receive prenatal care (Poole, 1997). Multiparas are also at risk, particularly those with a new partner in this pregnancy, preexisting hypertension, renal disease, diabetes, or multiple gestation (SOGC, 2000).

Hypertension in pregnancy is classified as follows:

- Gestational hypertension with or without proteinuria: this category is used for hypertension first noted after 20 weeks' gestation
- Preexisting hypertension (chronic): hypertension that exists before pregnancy, past 42 days postpartum, or both (Bridges et al., 2003)
- Preexisting hypertension with superimposed gestational hypertension (combination)

Proteinuria is considered to be greater than 1+ on a dipstick or greater than 300 mg/L with a 24-hour urine collection (should be considered if dipstick indicates greater than 1+). Edema is not considered part of the diagnosis for gestational or chronic hypertension. U.S. guidelines on high BP follow the above descriptions and include a further definition: *transient hypertension.* This retrospective diagnosis is given to a client whose BP returns to normal by 12 weeks postpartum; however, increased BP may recur in future pregnancy and predict future primary hypertension (Chobanian et al., 2003).

Pre-eclampsia refers specifically to hypertension after 20 weeks' gestation with proteinuria. It is more common in multiparas, women carrying multiple fetuses, women with hypertension for 4 years or more, clients with a family history of pre-eclampsia or hypertension in a previous pregnancy, and clients with renal disease (Chobanian et al., 2003). Pre-eclampsia can progress to life-threatening **eclampsia,** a medical emergency, at any time in pregnancy, labor, or early postpartum. Signs of eclampsia include convulsive facial twitching and tonic–clonic contractions (Youngkin & Davis, 2004). These developments usually are preceded by an acute increase in BP and worsening signs of multiorgan development, such as increased liver enzymes, proteinuria, blurred vision, and hyperreflexia.

In women who develop gestational hypertension, BP begins to increase during the second half of pregnancy; they may not experience the pregnancy-related decrease in BP at night. Normal fluctuations in BP during pregnancy are the reason for two evaluations at least 6 hours apart for hypertension in pregnant women. Vasospasm, which causes poor perfusion, is thought to be the mechanism for increased BP and total peripheral resistance in pregnancy. Vasospasm decreases blood flow and changes the function of many organs and systems. Intra-arterial lesions caused by vasospasm initiate the coagulation cascade, resulting in endothelial damage. Decreased placental perfusion is an important pathophysiologic change that accompanies hypertension in pregnancy. A direct fetal effect can be IUGR from decreased placental circulation. As hypertension progresses, the woman also may develop an increased sensitivity to vasopressors, reduced plasma volume, altered proximal renal tubular function, and activation of the coagulation cascade (Patrick & Roberts, 1999).

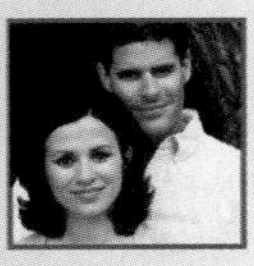

Consider Harriet, the woman pregnant with her fourth child described at the beginning of the chapter. What risk factors might predispose Harriet to pre-eclampsia?

COLLABORATIVE CARE: THE PREGNANT CLIENT WITH HYPERTENSION

When a client is pregnant, her health care providers need to be alert for any signs or symptoms of hypertension. Ongoing assessments of proteinuria, BP, and fetal health are critical components of each prenatal visit. Any increase in BP requires follow-up questions about headache, epigastric pain, and visual disturbance. Those providing care should collaborate in their assessment and planning. If hypertension is diagnosed, team members may include an obstetrician and home care nurses to adequately provide the treatment that this woman and fetus require. Antenatal admission to the hospital may be considered based on the distance of the woman's residence from the facility; signs of increasing blood pressure, proteinuria, or both; and the woman's specific requirements for care.

Treatment of the client with symptoms of multiorgan involvement and hypertension during labor involves assessment of signs and symptoms, laboratory testing, monitoring of fetal well-being, and review of the prenatal history. Multiorgan involvement and subsequent symptoms can result from vascular constriction or vasospasm and movement of fluid intracellularly (Fig. 13.11). The effects of hypertension and vasospasm on the placenta and fetus are always a primary concern. Vasospasm and endothelial damage can lead to reduced placental perfusion, which can decrease fetal development, leading to IUGR.

Multiorgan involvement with hypertension that develops early in pregnancy is considered an obstetric emergency (SOGC, 2000). This situation demands involvement from a hematologist, neonatologist, obstetrician, internal medicine specialist, neonatal nurses, maternity nurses, social workers, and pharmacists.

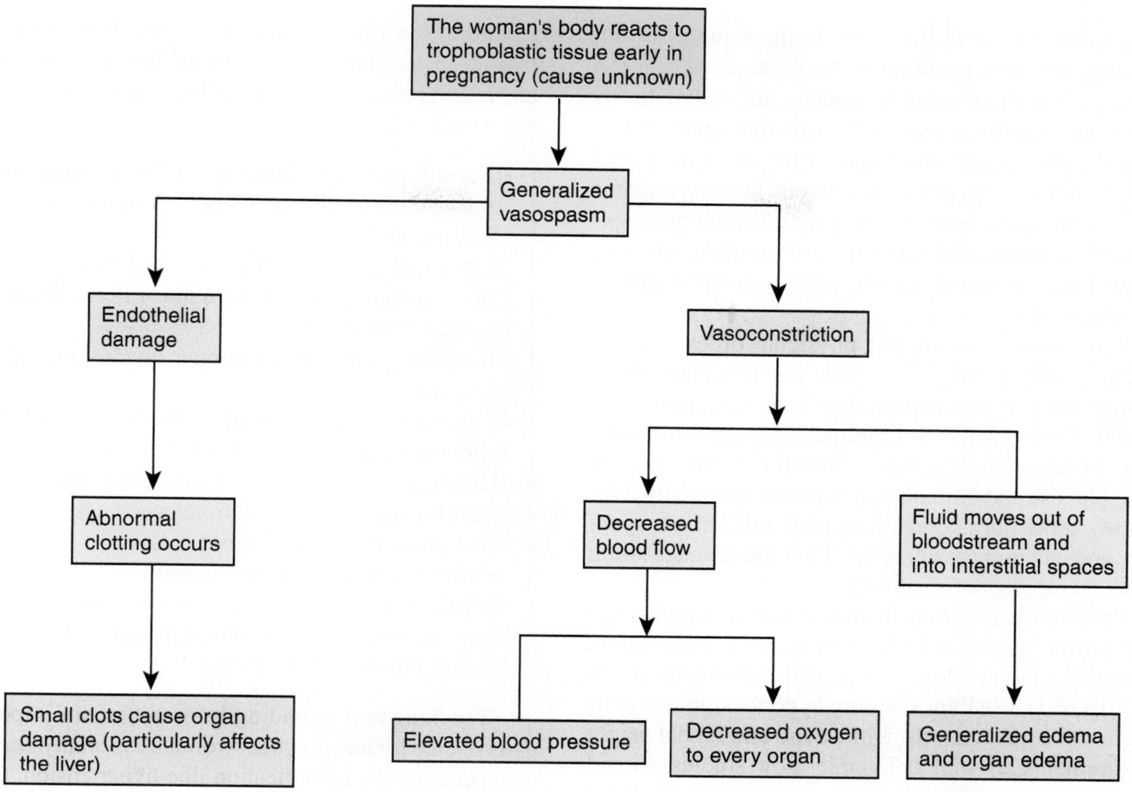

FIGURE 13.11 Pregnancy-induced hypertension can cause a cascade of problems.

Assessment

Prompt recognition of hypertension in pregnancy is based on comprehensive knowledge that includes understanding of anatomy and physiology, application of clinical skills, and awareness of possible complications (eg, abruptio placenta, acute renal failure, pulmonary edema, cerebral hemorrhage). Assessment begins with taking the woman's BP, evaluating urine for output and protein, and checking neurologic signs. Careful monitoring of vital signs, neurologic status, renal function, and hematologic values is important (Chobanian et al., 2003; Patrick & Roberts, 1999).

A thorough medical and family history must focus on any underlying cardiovascular disease, diabetes, pulmonary disease, migraine headaches, or seizure disorder. Questions about the woman's perinatal history should emphasize presence of increasing BP throughout the pregnancy, fetal demise or IUGR in a previous pregnancy, and prepregnancy BP. Other assessment parameters include amniotic fluid volume, fetal growth, and current fetal status (Poole, 1997).

The nurse always should take BP with the client sitting and her arm at heart level (Fig. 13.12). The cuff must be of the appropriate size, with an accurate sphygmomanometer and Korotkoff sounds I and IV recorded. The nurse should take the woman's BP in both arms initially to assess for differences that may be caused by anatomy, position, or other factors.

A head-to-toe assessment of the client with diagnosed hypertension would include taking BP with the client in the lateral position. Repeat BPs should be taken

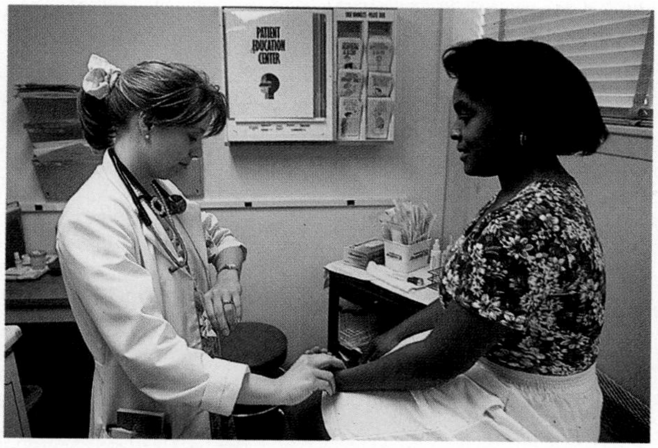

FIGURE 13.12 Although ongoing evaluations of blood pressure for all pregnant clients are essential, they are of special importance in women with a history of hypertensive problems. (© Bob Kramer.)

in the same arm, with the client in the same position, and using the same machine for consistency. The nurse should ask the client about headaches, any visual disturbances (eg, blurring, scotomata), irritability, and tremors. He or she also should investigate if the client has experienced any bleeding, petechiae, or both. Other symptoms to investigate include any right upper quadrant pain, epigastric pain, nausea and vomiting, urine output and color, and swelling. Asking about fetal activity and movements also is important.

Laboratory tests are per physician orders. Likely studies include hemoglobin, platelets, complete blood count, fibrinogen, partial thromboplastin time, prothrombin time (INR), alanine transaminase, aspartate transaminase, lactate dehydrogenase, bilirubin (liver function tests), glucose and ammonia (to rule out acute fatty liver disease), proteinuria, creatinine, urea, uric acid, magnesium, and calcium (baseline level in case of magnesium sulfate therapy) (SOGC, 2000).

Fetal assessment may include continuous fetal monitoring if the woman is in labor or an NST if she is not, ultrasound, Doppler flow studies, and amniotic fluid volume. IUGR is a risk for ongoing hypertension and antihypertensive medications. Ultrasound and fundal height measurements, as well as Doppler flow studies, should be used to monitor fetal growth and development (Sibai & Chames, 2003).

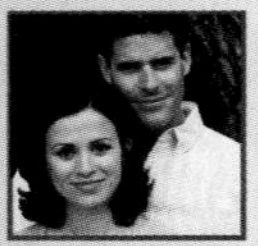

Remember Harriet, the woman at 28 weeks' gestation with a history of gestational hypertension. Imagine that she is diagnosed with gestational hypertension in this pregnancy. For what complications are she and her fetus at risk?

Select Potential Nursing Diagnoses

The following are examples of commonly applicable NANDA diagnoses in a pregnant client with hypertension:

- **Anxiety** related to pregnancy and fetal growth and development with gestational hypertension
- **Ineffective Health Maintenance** related to gestational hypertension
- **Pain** related to specific symptoms of gestational hypertension
- **Risk for Compromised Family Coping** related to diagnosis of or required treatment for gestational hypertension
- **Social Isolation** related to potential bedrest therapy

Planning/Intervention

The plan of care for a woman with gestational hypertension may occur at home or in a health care facility, depending on the distance of her residence from the institution, available resources, and her access to monitoring equipment (Fig. 13.13). Ongoing monitoring may include the following:

- BP readings every 4 hours while the woman is awake
- Assessments for any facial or abdominal edema
- Daily weights
- Neurologic symptoms (eg, hyperreflexia, clonus)
- Checks for any persistent occipital or frontal headaches or visual disturbances
- Monitoring for any right upper quadrant or epigastric pain
- Evaluation for any proteinuria by dipstick daily to be followed by a 24-hour collection if greater than 1+
- Hematocrit and platelet counts twice a week
- Liver function tests 1 to 2 times per week
- Fetal movement counts twice a day
- Nonstress test 2 to 3 times a week
- Biophysical profile once to twice a week
- Doppler studies to determine placental blood flow weekly (Barton et al., 1999)

Teaching and providing information are important parts of care for any pregnant woman, especially one who is experiencing a complication like hypertension. Common concerns and questions these clients may have include the following:

- Why did this happen to me?
- Why did I not hear of this condition before I became ill?
- Why did I not feel ill?
- Will it happen again in my next pregnancy?
- Why do I feel like I have failed?
- Will this have long-term effects on my health?
- Does gestational hypertension run in families? (Cheyne & McQueen, 1999)

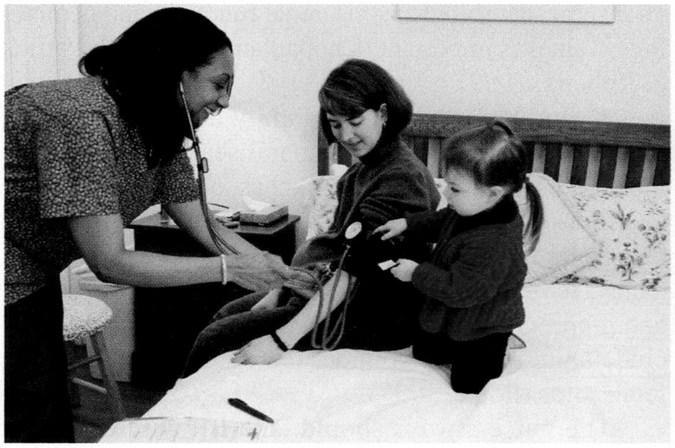

FIGURE 13.13 Depending on her condition and distance from a health care facility, the expectant client with hypertension may receive ongoing blood pressure monitoring at home.

Pharmacologic treatments may be necessary, including those drugs that a woman with preexisting hypertension was taking before becoming pregnant (Table 13.4). Oral β blockers are the preferred medication because they minimize the severity of hypertension and the need for additional antihypertensive drugs (Montan, 2004). Atenolol, metoprolol, and pindolol are common agents prescribed during pregnancy. Side effects may include a small-for-gestational-age baby (see Chap. 22). See Nursing Care Plan 13.2 for additional information.

Current research is focusing on the use of calcium during pregnancy to decrease the development of hypertension. Further studies are needed, but women at high risk may benefit. Low-dose aspirin (75 mg) also may decrease gestational hypertensive effects in high-risk women (Montan, 2004).

Indications that birth should occur quickly include the following:

- Persistent increase in maternal BP to severe hypertension
- Development of severe or persistent cerebral symptoms
- Persistent right upper quadrant or epigastric pain
- Progressive thrombocytopenia
- Abnormal liver enzymes with hemolysis
- Onset of labor, rupture of membranes, or bleeding
- Severe growth retardation shown on ultrasound or Doppler studies
- Nonreactive NST with abnormal biophysical profile
- Decreased amniotic fluid volume (oligohydramnios)
- Gestational age of 38 to 40 weeks

A woman's BP is not a reliable indicator of her risk for seizures. The central nervous system involvement in gestational hypertension can progress to headaches and visual disturbances, decreased level of mentation, seizure, or eclampsia. Magnesium sulfate is the agent of choice

TABLE 13.4 Hypertensive Drugs Used in High-Risk Pregnancy

DRUG	ACTION	DOSAGE	ADVERSE EFFECTS	SPECIAL CONSIDERATIONS
Furosemide (Lasix)	Inhibits resorption of sodium and chloride	Slow IV bolus of 10 to 40 mg over 1 to 2 minutes	Anorexia, dizziness, electrolyte imbalances, muscle cramps and spasms, orthostatic hypotension, vertigo, vomiting	Assess the client's urine output hourly.
Hydralazine hydrochloride (Apresoline)	Relaxes the vascular smooth muscle, improving blood perfusion	Slow IV bolus of 5 to 10 mg every 20 minutes	Anorexia, diarrhea, headache, nausea and vomiting, tachycardia	Be sure to withdraw this drug gradually to prevent rebound hypertension.
Labetalol hydrochloride (Normodyne)	α_1 and β blocker	Bolus dose of 10 to 20 mg, with IV infusion of 2 mg/min until desired blood pressure is reached	Constipation, dizziness, fatigue, flatulence, gastric pain, vertigo	Regularly assess the client for development of any adverse effects; help to manage those that may arise.
Magnesium sulfate	Blocks neuromuscular transmission; assists with vasodilation	IV loading dose of 4 to 6 g over 30 minutes; maintenance infusion of 2 to 4 g/hr as ordered	Toxicity: cardiac and central nervous depression, flushing, hypotension, sweating	Be sure to monitor the client's serum magnesium levels carefully to prevent toxicity. Check deep tendon reflexes and ankle clonus. Ensure that calcium gluconate 10% is readily available as an antidote.
Nifedipine (Procardia)	Calcium channel blocker	10 mg orally for three doses; then every 4 to 8 hours	Angina, cough, diarrhea, dizziness, nasal congestion, peripheral edema	Regularly assess the client for development of any adverse effects; help to manage those that may arise.
Sodium nitroprusside	Arterial and venous vasodilator	IV infusion, with dose titrated according to blood pressure values	Abdominal pain, apprehension, diaphoresis, palpitations, restlessness, retrosternal pressure	Protect medication from effects of light by wrapping drug container in foil or other opaque material.

From Karch, A. M. (2005). *2005 Lippincott's nursing drug guide.* Philadelphia: Lippincott Williams & Wilkins.

NURSING CARE PLAN 13.2

The Client With Gestational Hypertension

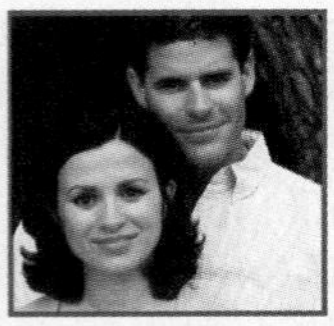

During this prenatal visit, Harriet's urine test for protein is 2+. Her blood pressure is 150/98 mm Hg. Harriet is asked to return to the office the next morning to have her blood pressure checked again. On her return visit, her urine is 2+ for protein, and her blood pressure is 158/96 mm Hg. She is diagnosed with gestational hypertension.

NURSING DIAGNOSIS

Risk for Injury (maternal and fetal) related to elevated blood pressure and resultant effects on maternal and fetal status

EXPECTED OUTCOMES

1. The client will demonstrate a blood pressure less than 140/90 mm Hg.
2. The client will remain free of signs and symptoms of eclampsia.
3. The fetus will demonstrate gestational age–appropriate growth and development.

INTERVENTIONS	RATIONALES
Assess the client's blood pressure at each visit; compare readings in each arm. Also assess fetal heart rate.	These assessments provide objective information about maternal and fetal status and aid in detecting trends that may signify a developing problem.
Question the client about any central nervous system complaints such as headaches, visual disturbances, irritability, or tremors.	Central nervous system disturbances may indicate possible progression to eclampsia.
Continue to assess urine by dipstick for protein; prepare client for 24-hour urine collection.	A 24-hour urine collection helps confirm proteinuria and evaluates renal function.
Administer antihypertensive agents as prescribed. Instruct the client in medication therapy.	Antihypertensive agents aid in controlling blood pressure.
Obtain fundal height measurements at each visit; assist with scheduling the client for follow-up ultrasounds.	Fundal height measurements help estimate fetal growth and development. Ultrasounds provide information about the intrauterine environment and fetal well-being.
Monitor the client's weight and assess for edema, especially of the hands and face.	Weight is a reliable indicator of fluid status. Edema of the hands and face may suggest fluid overload.
Arrange for laboratory testing such as CBC, coagulation studies, renal and hepatic function tests, and serum magnesium and calcium levels.	Gestational hypertension can affect multiple organs. Laboratory testing provides a baseline for future comparison and continued monitoring. Serum calcium and magnesium levels provide a baseline should magnesium sulfate therapy be necessary.
Teach the client how to monitor fetal activity and movement.	Fetal activity and movement indicate fetal well-being.

Continued

NURSING CARE PLAN 13.2 ● The Client With Gestational Hypertension

INTERVENTIONS	RATIONALES
Assist with arranging for fetal assessment studies such as nonstress test, ultrasound, Doppler flow studies, and amniotic fluid volume.	Gestational hypertension can affect placental functioning, which can interfere with fetal well-being. Fetal assessment studies aid in determining fetal status.
Teach about danger signs and symptoms to report immediately, such as severe persistent headaches or visual disturbances, right upper quadrant or epigastric pain, and change in fetal activity or movement.	These signs may indicate continued elevation of blood pressure that may progress to eclampsia.
Arrange for continued follow-up of client at home; initiate referral for home care as appropriate.	Continued follow-up provides further opportunities for assessment, teaching, and support.

EVALUATION

1. The client maintains a blood pressure below 140/90 mm Hg.
2. The client exhibits no signs and symptoms of preeclampsia progressing to eclampsia.
3. The fetus demonstrates gestational age–appropriate growth and development.
4. The client gives birth to a healthy newborn at term without complications.

in cases of hypertension and proteinuria with risk factors for eclampsia. The dosage initially is 4 g IV, followed by 1 to 2 g/hour IV. Side effects are weakness, paralysis, decreased respirations, and decreased urinary output. The client's reflexes should be checked regularly while she is receiving magnesium sulfate and the antidote, IV calcium gluconate 10% over 3 minutes, should be available if needed. Patellar–tendon response is the most common reflex assessed because of its ease of access (Fig. 13.14). Absence of deep tendon reflex is often the first sign of magnesium toxicity. Frequent blood work to assess for the therapeutic level of magnesium should be completed every 4 to 6 hours or per institutional policy. Other blood work to monitor the woman's condition, such as a complete blood count and liver function tests, would be done at the same time to minimize the number of venipunctures.

Close monitoring is required to prevent seizure activity, cerebral vascular accident, and intracranial pressure. Supplies kept at the client's bedside for acute episodes include diazepam, calcium gluconate 10%, ephedrine, epinephrine, hydralazine, magnesium sulfate 50%, phenytoin, and IV solutions such as sodium chloride (saline) and sterile water. Various needles, IV supplies, reflex hammer, tourniquet, blood collection tubes, and airways also are important. These could be kept together in a box taken to the bedside if a client with hypertension presents in an acute episode.

An opportunity to "debrief" after the woman has given birth would be extremely helpful in answering her questions and concerns. Reviewing information provided 1 to 2 weeks later is ideal. A public health nurse may be the best health care provider to accomplish this task.

Evaluation

Care for the woman with hypertension in pregnancy includes assessment, monitoring of both the woman and her fetus, and provision of the safest environment for both. Prolonging the pregnancy if the fetus is growing is preferred to a preterm birth and its associated complications. Use of low-dose aspirin and other medications may assist in avoiding the acute episodes that must be treated with advanced fetal and maternal monitoring and interventions including birth.

HELLP SYNDROME

The acronym HELLP is used to indicate a syndrome involving hemolysis (microangiopathic hemolytic anemia),

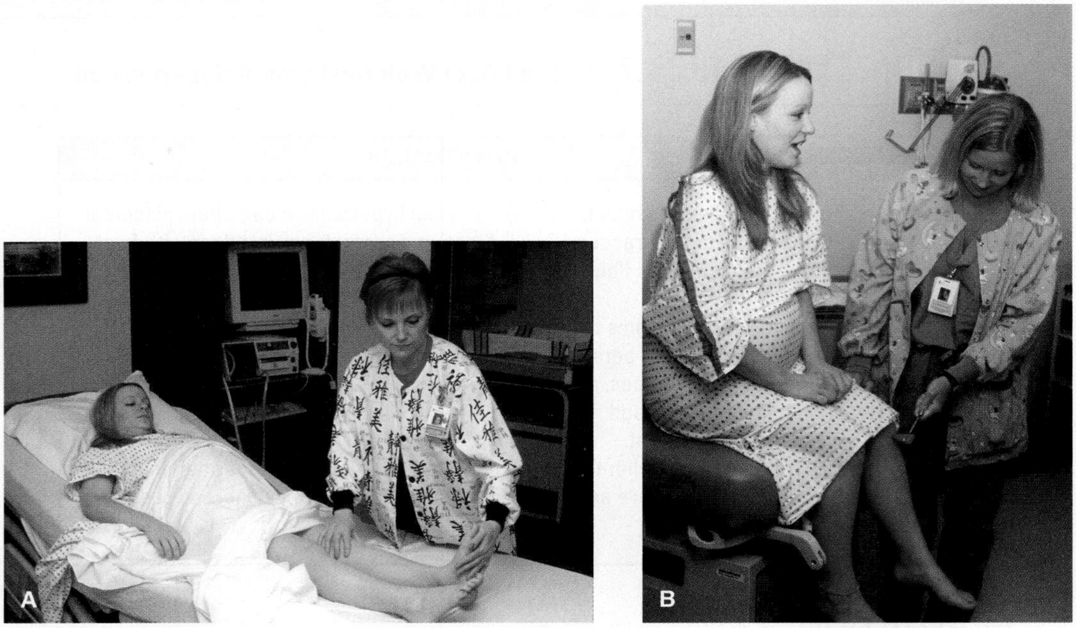

FIGURE 13.14 Monitoring for pre-eclampsia includes evaluations for nervous system irritability. (**A**) To assess for *ankle clonus,* the nurse should dorsiflex and then release the woman's foot on both sides. Movements should be smooth. Jerky and rapid movements may indicate worsening hypertensive problems. (**B**) The nurse can assess the client's *patellar reflexes* by using a reflex hammer to strike the woman's patellar tendon quickly and firmly. A patellar reflex occurs when the leg and foot move (documented as 2+). An absent reflex in either leg may be a sign of developing pre-eclampsia.

elevated liver enzymes, and a low platelet count (Barton & Sibai, 2004). HELLP syndrome complicates 0.1% to 0.4% of all pregnancies (Kidner & Flanders-Stepans, 2004). It can occur independently or along with gestational hypertension (Padden, 1999). Pregnant women may develop symptoms of HELLP syndrome as early as 17 weeks' gestation or as late as 7 days postpartum. Approximately 66% of clients develop HELLP antenatally, whereas 33% develop it after giving birth (Magann & Martin, 1999). Maternal hypertension can involve multiple organs and require immediate decisions about care. Complications include liver hematoma or rupture, stroke, cardiac arrest, seizure, disseminated intravascular coagulation, and renal damage (Kidner & Flanders-Stepans, 2004). Maternal mortality rates are as high as 24%; fetal mortality rates range from 30% to 40% (Magann & Martin, 1999).

Endothelial dysfunction is the underlying pathology in HELLP syndrome. It begins at implantation, causing incomplete maternal spiral artery transformation and activation of intravascular coagulation. This in turn causes vascular ischemia and fibrin deposits with vasospasm and clotting cascade activation (Kidner & Flanders-Stepans, 2004).

Assessment Findings

HELLP syndrome frequently results from mismanagement or misdiagnosis because of the various vague symptoms the woman may include in the initial complaint (Kidner & Flanders-Stepans, 2004). Early presentations of nausea and vomiting may be associated with gallbladder dysfunction or gastrointestinal disturbance before HELLP syndrome is investigated (Baskett, 1999). The client may describe epigastric or right upper quadrant pain or nonspecific virus-like symptoms (Barton & Sibai, 2004). The pain is likely to result from obstructed blood flow in the hepatic sinusoids blocked by fibrin deposition. Any pregnant woman who presents with malaise or a viral-type illness in the third trimester needs a complete blood count and liver function testing for HELLP (Padden, 1999). Significant weight gain with generalized edema usually is associated with HELLP syndrome (Barton & Sibai, 2004).

Diagnosis is based on laboratory evidence of hemolytic anemia, hepatic dysfunction, and thrombocytopenia (Magann & Martin, 1999). A peripheral blood smear shows evidence of damaged erythrocytes (burr cells, schistocytes, and helmet cells) caused by vasoconstriction, vasospasm, and damaged endothelial cells (microvascular injury). Decreased prothrombin time and platelet count occur later because of a decreased lifespan of the circulating platelets (3 to 5 days rather than the normal 8 to 10 days) as well as increased platelet aggregation from decreased resistance to platelet activating factor (Magann & Martin, 1999).

Ongoing monitoring of a critically ill woman with HELLP syndrome should include visual assessments, reflexes, strict intake and output, BP, and fetal heart rate. The nurse should ensure that the client is not experiencing epigastric pain or headache.

Collaborative Management

HELLP syndrome is something of a unique gestational experience because fear of death may be prominent for the mother. Loneliness, anxiety, powerlessness, and depression are emotions commonly described by hospitalized women with high-risk pregnancies. The speed with which treatment decisions must be made when a woman has HELLP syndrome and the information provided to her, however, may heighten a sense of doom and anxiety. Some clients have described a premonition even before HELLP was diagnosed that "things were not right with this pregnancy" (Kidner & Flanders-Stepans, 2004).

A team approach is vital to providing the best care. Frequently, internists as well as obstetricians, nutritionists, physiotherapists, and pharmacists are part of treatment planning. Management approaches are based on estimated gestational age, maternal health, and fetal status (Padden, 1999). Ongoing evaluations of maternal platelet count and lactate dehydrogenase level are critical for prediction of worsening symptoms. Complaints of severe right upper quadrant, shoulder, or neck pain require evaluation through liver imaging to assess for subcapsular hematoma or hepatic rupture (Padden, 1999). Blood should be cross-matched continually and reserved for labor and birth. Ongoing fetal assessments include daily fetal movement counts, NSTs, biophysical profiles, and Doppler studies.

If gestational age is estimated as 32 weeks or less, therapy may include corticosteroid administration for fetal lung maturation, transfer to a tertiary care facility, bedrest, fluid replacement, and fetal assessment (Barton & Sibai, 2004). If gestation is more than 32 weeks but less than 34 weeks, corticosteroids may still be given along with conservative measures to prolong the pregnancy as long as is safe for both mother and fetus. Consultation with a health care team member can assist the family to prepare for birth regardless of gestation (Padden, 1999).

Antihypertensive therapy should be initiated if maternal BP is greater than 160/110 mm Hg. Magnesium sulfate may be used to prevent seizures. The initial bolus is 4 to 6 g followed by an infusion of 2 g/hour measured by infusion pump and assessed together with magnesium blood levels and urine output. Toxicity can be treated with 10 to 20 ml of 10% IV calcium gluconate (Padden, 1999). Hydralazine (Apresoline) or labetalol (Normodyne) may be given to decrease the risk for maternal cerebral hemorrhage, and placental abruption.

Up to 25% of women with HELLP syndrome develop serious complications such as DIC, placental abruption, adult respiratory distress syndrome, hepatorenal failure, pulmonary edema, and hepatic rupture. Many require blood products. Infant morbidity and mortality range from 10% to 60% depending on severity of the maternal disease. These infants are at increased risk for IUGR and respiratory distress syndrome (see Chap. 22) (Padden, 1999).

Postpartum counseling should focus on the client's risk for recurrence of HELLP syndrome (19% to 27%) and gestational hypertension (43%) in future pregnancies. Screening for antiphospholipid antibodies may be done before another pregnancy (Padden, 1999).

PRETERM PREMATURE RUPTURE OF MEMBRANES

Premature rupture of the fetal membranes (PROM) is a complication in approximately 8% of pregnancies (Mercer, 2004). Preterm PROM (pPROM) occurs before 37 weeks' gestation, is responsible for 30% of all cases of PROM (Mercer, 2004), and leads to 30% to 40% of all preterm births (see Chap. 22). In many cases, women have a short time (often up to 1 week) following pPROM before they experience labor and childbirth. With advances in health care technology, the period of latency may increase in the future (Weitz, 1999).

Risk factors for pPROM include maternal nutritional deficiencies, tobacco use, and poor maternal weight gain (Weitz, 1999). Maternal connective disorders also have been linked to pPROM. Infections with group B streptococci, chlamydia, gonorrhea, and bacterial vaginosis have been shown to reduce fetal membrane strength and elasticity (Weitz, 1999). Prior preterm birth or contractions in the current pregnancy are also risk factors (Mercer, 2004).

Chorioamnionitis occurs in approximately 20% to 25% of women with pPROM and is a more significant problem with earlier gestations, as well as positive gonorrhea or GBS status (Weitz, 1999). Intrauterine death occurs in 1% of cases from cord accident, oligohydramnios, cord compression, or abruptio placentae. *Amniotic band syndrome,* which is the adherence of tough bands derived from the fetal membranes, may constrict fetal parts, leading to deformities and, in severe cases, potential amputation of a fetal limb. Increased incidence of fetal anomalies is associated with pPROM (Weitz, 1999). A small number of women can have spontaneous resealing of the membranes and restoration of a normal amniotic fluid volume, particularly with pPROM following amniocentesis (Mercer, 2004).

COLLABORATIVE CARE: pPROM AND PROM

During pregnancy, the nurse should be aware of a client's risk factors for pPROM. He or she also should discuss with the client smoking cessation, nutritional counseling, and signs and symptoms of preterm labor in routine prenatal care (see Chaps. 12 and 16).

Fetal fibronectin, a protein produced by the fetal membranes and normally found in the cervicovaginal fluid until approximately 20 weeks' gestation, can be tested as a predictor of pPROM, preterm labor, or both. Fetal fibronectin found between 24 and 34 weeks' gestation in the cervicovaginal fluid in a woman with intact fetal membranes may indicate an increased risk for preterm birth. Collection is done by placing a sterile cotton swab in the posterior fornix of the external cervical os for a minimum of 10 seconds and then preserving it in a tube for analysis.

Assessment

Women may describe pPROM as a "gush of fluid," a "pop," or "leaking." In such instances, the nurse should discuss with the client the timing and date of the event. Questions about fluid color, amount, and consistency are important, as are fetal movements, contractions, vaginal bleeding, and fever (Weitz, 1999). Questions about frequency and burning associated with urination as well as sexual activity and douching practices are needed to rule out a urinary tract infection and other causes of discharge.

Objective assessments should include maternal vital signs, fetal heart rate, abdominal palpation for contractions, and uterine tenderness. The nurse should inspect the perineal area for fluid, odor, endocervical mucus, or bloody discharge. A sterile speculum examination may be required to determine fluid leaking from the os. Such examination also would permit visualization for cord prolapse, presenting part, and any vaginal bleeding, as well as swabs for culture and sensitivity for *Chlamydia trachomatis* and *Neisseria gonorrhoeae* (Mercer, 2004). A rectal or vaginal swab for GBS should be obtained at this time if not done within the past 6 weeks (Mercer, 2004). Digital examination should be avoided to decrease the immediate risk for infection (Weitz, 1999).

Nitrazine and fern tests aid in the diagnosis of pPROM. The Nitrazine test involves application of vaginal fluid secretions to sterile pH paper. Vaginal pH is normally 4.5 to 6.0 and does not change the yellow color of the paper, whereas amniotic fluid is alkaline and changes the paper to dark blue. The fern test is performed by gathering vaginal secretions onto a microscopic slide (sterile swab). The fern pattern that appears microscopically is determined by the high salt content of amniotic fluid and strongly indicates pPROM.

If a client's findings indicate a need for bedrest, hospitalization, or both, individual assessment of her support systems and ability to communicate with them is vital when making plans for provision of care.

Select Potential Nursing Diagnoses

The following are examples of commonly applicable NANDA diagnoses:

- **Risk for Infection** related to pPROM
- **Risk for Maternal/Fetal Injury** related to pPROM (eg, oligohydramnios causing a cord accident, maternal infection, or both)
- **Risk for Deficient Fluid Volume**
- **Constipation** related to bedrest therapy
- **Anxiety** related to fetal and maternal risks for injury and preterm birth
- **Fatigue** related to hospital environment for care provision

Planning/Intervention

The most common treatment for pPROM is bedrest with ongoing assessment for fever, chills, and change in amniotic fluid (color, odor) that would indicate chorioamnionitis. Temperature assessment every 8 hours together with a white blood cell count as part of a complete blood count every other day assists with assessing for chorioamnionitis (Mercer, 2004). Uterine tenderness and tachycardia also suggest chorioamnionitis. Uterine contractions and fetal heart rate assessments should be done daily. Antenatal corticosteroids are ordered if the pregnancy is less than 34 weeks but viable (at least 23 to 24 weeks) (Mercer, 2004). If gestation is 32 to 36 weeks, amniotic fluid may be collected for fetal lung maturity testing. Amniotic fluid assessed for lecithin-to-sphingomyelin (L/S) ratio can predict fetal lung maturity if the client goes into labor.

A diagnosis of pPROM may necessitate hospitalization. Nursing interventions for the hospitalized client focus on helping her communicate with family from whom she may be separated. She also may need assistance with obtaining financial aid to help support her household while she is away. Common assistive measures include ensuring her access to a telephone, computer, and letter-writing materials; additionally, the facility should promote a liberal visiting policy. Assisting the client with passive and stretching exercises performed in bed would help to pass time. Consultation with a physiotherapist is appropriate. A nutritionist can help ensure adequate weight gain and access to preferred foods and portion sizes. Other activities are for neonatal staff visit to assist the client in understanding care that the fetus will receive if born prematurely, show prenatal videos, and provide other educational materials focusing on preparation for labor and birth.

Evaluation

Prolonging pregnancy to allow for further fetal growth and development without maternal infection is the goal for this woman and fetus. Constant fetal and maternal assessment is required to ensure that appropriate interventions are initiated to ensure safety.

CERVICAL INSUFFICIENCY/INCOMPETENCE

Incompetent cervix, or painless cervical dilation, can progress to pPROM and preterm birth and is the cause of 10% to 25% of second-trimester fetal losses (Terkildsen et al., 2003). The term cervical incompetence carries a negative connotation that may increase the emotions and physical burdens associated with recurrent pregnancy losses to women and families. **Cervical insufficiency**

is therefore a more sensitive term, suggesting that the cervix is a dynamic structure with compliance and length unique to each woman (Williams & Iams, 2004). The sequence of events involved in insufficiency may or may not repeat itself in future pregnancies. Affected clients can therefore be placed into three groups: those with a history of two or more second-trimester pregnancy losses without labor, those with ultrasound findings during pregnancy showing a shortened cervix, and those with evidence of advanced dilation and effacement but no evidence of regular contractions (Williams & Iams, 2004). Composition of cervical tissue and maternal stress may lead to premature cervical dilation. An inverse relationship between cervical length and preterm birth is well established (Belej-Rak et al., 2003).

Risk factors for premature cervical dilation include excessive cervical dilation for curettage or biopsy, history of previous cervical lacerations during childbirth, and cervical or uterine anomalies (see Chap. 4). A history of short labors, losses at early gestations, or both also may contribute.

Transvaginal ultrasound is used to assess cervical length, effacement, and dilation. Cervical length remains fairly stable throughout pregnancy until the third trimester, when it progressively shortens. The median length is 35 to 40 mm from 14 to 22 weeks and 30 mm after 32 weeks. Effacement begins at the internal cervical os and proceeds distally through a process called *funneling* (Williams & Iams, 2004). The discovery of cervical thinning and dilation in a woman is a stronger predictor of insufficiency in a nullipara than in a multipara.

Cerclage (suturing) early in the second trimester has the potential to decrease fetal morbidity and mortality in cases of cervical insufficiency (Williams & Iams, 2004) (Fig. 13.15). The suturing helps prevent cervical relaxation and dilation. A cerclage may be prophylactically placed at 13 to 14 weeks' gestation for clients with a history of cervical insufficiency leading to previous loss. Emergency cerclage may be performed at 20 to 23 weeks' gestation, but risks include pPROM, chorionitis, and preterm birth. Placement at 22 weeks' gestation may help the pregnancy to proceed to at least 28 weeks, promoting the chances for a better fetal outcome. The client is advised to limit her activity (potentially bedrest at home or in the hospital) and to avoid long periods of standing (more than 90 minutes) and intercourse.

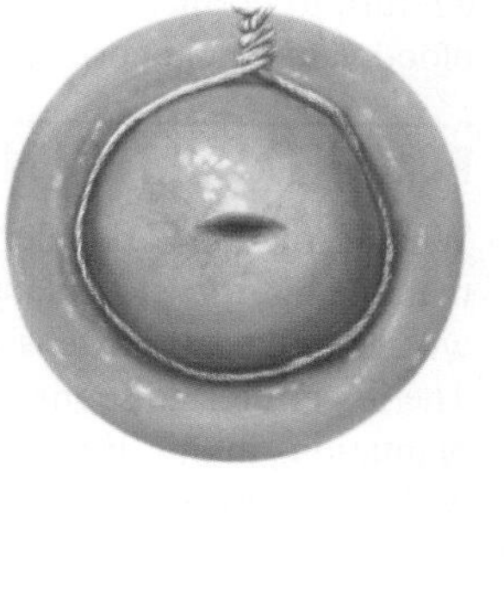

FIGURE 13.15 Cervical cerclage may be used in cases of cervical insufficiency.

If cerclage successfully maintains the pregnancy, the suture is removed in the physician's office at 37 weeks' gestation (term) to encourage normal labor. If the health care team determines that an earlier cesarean birth would be best for the woman and family, the cerclage is removed at the same time.

Wherever this woman is receiving care, she requires support to cope with the ongoing stress associated with her condition. Encouraging her to communicate with other mothers at home with restricted activity would be helpful, as would contact with community supports such as public health nurses, occupational therapists, and physical therapists.

Effectiveness of treatment is indicated by a pregnancy that reaches term without premature labor. Ensuring that the woman and her family have coped with decreased mobility and limitations related to avoiding labor is an integral part of successful therapy as well.

DISSEMINATED INTRAVASCULAR COAGULOPATHY

Disseminated intravascular coagulopathy (DIC) is a complex coagulation disorder caused by activation of both the clotting and fibrinolytic systems (Lurie et al., 2000) (Fig. 13.16). *Coagulo* refers to clotting, and *pathy* means "disease of," so DIC simply means a disorder with multiple defects in the coagulation cascade that cause inappropriate clotting throughout the vascular system (Geiter, 2003). During pregnancy, a woman's blood is hypercoagulable. Events unique to pregnancy can trigger DIC: abruptio placentae, intrauterine fetal demise, and gestational hypertension. Release of placental tissue factor may activate the prothrombinase complex that causes DIC. Sepsis can also be a trigger.

The presentation of DIC can be acute, chronic, or low grade. Low-grade presentation occurs when coagulation activity increases for a short time and then is restored to normal or if the body can compensate for a short time with the consumption of coagulation factors (Geiter, 2003). With the heightened coagulation of pregnancy, it is important to be aware of the chronic presentation of DIC and test for it as appropriate.

Assessment Findings

Signs and symptoms of DIC can be subtle or obvious, as with hemorrhage:

- Oozing or bleeding from IV sites, previous incisions, mucous membranes, patchy cyanosis, gangrene
- Altered level of consciousness, subarachnoid bleeding, cerebrovascular accident
- Hemoptysis, pulmonary embolus, acute respiratory distress syndrome

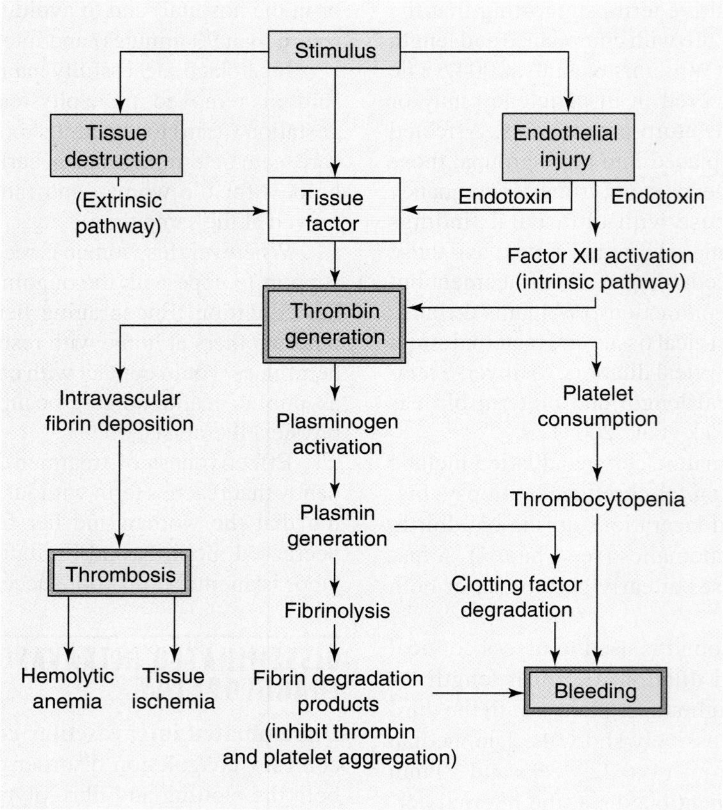

FIGURE 13.16 Pathways in normal blood coagulation and fibrinolysis versus in disseminated intravascular coagulation.

- Gastrointestinal bleed, abdominal distention, bowel infarction, constipation, diarrhea
- Hematuria, oliguria, renal insufficiency or failure (Geiter, 2003)

Diagnostic tests include a complete blood count (platelet count that decreases by 50% or more from baseline would be indicative), prothrombin time, activated partial thromboplastin time, fibrinogen, fibrin degradation products and D-dimer (fibrin degradation products that only increase with rapid clot dissolution).

Collaborative Management

Health care providers should be aware of potential triggers for DIC, which may develop suddenly in an obstetric client. A hematologist may be part of the multidisciplinary team. In cases of confirmed DIC, important measures include looking for the cause, rapidly infusing blood and IV fluids as needed, giving continuous oxygen, and assisting with organ perfusion (Baskett, 1999). Once the cause has been identified, therapy specific to it (eg, antibiotics to treat gram-negative sepsis) should be initiated. Adequate tissue perfusion prevents ischemia, necrosis, or both. Increasing or initiating IV therapy as well as the delivery of packed red blood cells can be instrumental in treating hemorrhage. Closely monitoring vital signs, particularly oxygen saturation, blood pressure, and pulse, is critical to ensuring the woman's recovery (Geiter, 2003). Heparin therapy may slow coagulation, particularly in situations such as incomplete abortion. Whole blood does not contain clotting factors, so a ratio of four units of blood to one unit of fresh frozen plasma should be considered. Cryoprecipitate and platelets also may be considered. The goal is to keep the hematocrit above 30% (hemoglobin at 100 or greater). Each unit of blood is expected to raise the hemoglobin by 1.5 g/dL.

Communicating to the client and her family members about care, what is being done, and why is essential so that they understand what is happening. Being honest while remaining supportive and competent is extremely important at this time. Ensuring that the client is receiving appropriate care in a facility that can ensure a safe birth is a primary goal. Effective treatment would be determined by a return to normal clotting time, maintenance of normal blood values, and normal level of consciousness.

PLACENTAL ALTERATIONS

When growth and development of a pregnancy are normal, the blastocyst implants in the upper uterine portion, which has the most extensive blood supply (see Chap. 11). The lower uterine segment is thinner, and placental implantations in this area put the placenta in direct contact with the myometrium.

Placenta Previa

Placenta previa is a condition in which the blastocyst implants in the lower uterine segment, over or very close to the internal os (Fig. 13.17). This condition occurs in 0.4% to 0.9% of all pregnancies after 20 weeks' gestation and is the major cause of bleeding in the third trimester (Usta et al., 2005). Approximately 90% of placentas that initially implant low migrate upward. A possible explanation for this migration is that as the lower uterine segment grows, the placenta moves away from the os; alternatively, chorionic villi may develop in one area but remain dormant in another (Gilbert & Harmon, 2003). The degree to which the placenta covers the cervical os determines the diagnosis of total, partial, or marginal.

Placenta previa is classified as major or minor degree and further categorized as type I, II, III, or IV. Approximately 50% of all cases are minor, and 50% are major.

Minor degree includes the following:

- Type I (lateral or low-lying) implantation: includes the lower uterine segment but not the internal os
- Type II (marginal) implantation: includes the lower edge of the placenta extending to but not covering the internal os

Major degree includes the following:

- Type III (partial): the placenta partially covers the dilated internal os
- Type IV (complete or central): the placenta completely covers the internal os, even when fully dilated (Baskett, 1999)

Etiology and Pathophysiology

Early in the second trimester, the unformed lower uterine segment extends only 0.5 cm from the internal cervical os. Ultrasounds performed during this time show 5% of all placentas as low-lying and close to the internal os (Baskett, 1999). As the lower uterine segment develops over the last 12 weeks, the upper uterine segment and attached placenta appear to move up and away from the cervix (placental migration). By term, only 1 in 250 placentas remain low lying (placenta previa). Ultrasound at term is a highly accurate method of placental localization (<2% false negative or positive) (Baskett, 1999). Operative interventions on the uterus that cause damage to and scar tissue formation in the endometrium increase the risk for low implantation. Such problems may decrease the possibility for the natural expansion that facilitates placental migration away from the cervical os.

Risk Factors

Risk factors for placenta previa include previous cesarean birth, previous placenta previa, previous pregnancy termination, multiparity, maternal age older than 35 years, smoking, and use of cocaine (Usta et al., 2005). Other possible contributing factors include uterine anomalies (eg, bicornuate or septate uterus), a short interval between pregnancies, living at a high altitude, and Asian ethnicity (an 86% higher incidence of placenta previa than the general population).

Complications

Associated complications include coagulopathy, postpartum hemorrhage (because the lower segment contracts poorly and lacerates easily), uterine rupture, and vasa previa. Other placental abnormalities are possible because of poor development at the implantation site.

Assessment Findings

The most common signs and symptoms of placenta previa are antepartum hemorrhage and fetal malpresentation in late pregnancy because of displacement by the low occupying placenta. Near term, the lower uterine segment is formed and stretched. The edge of a placenta implanted in this area may separate from the uterine wall, causing

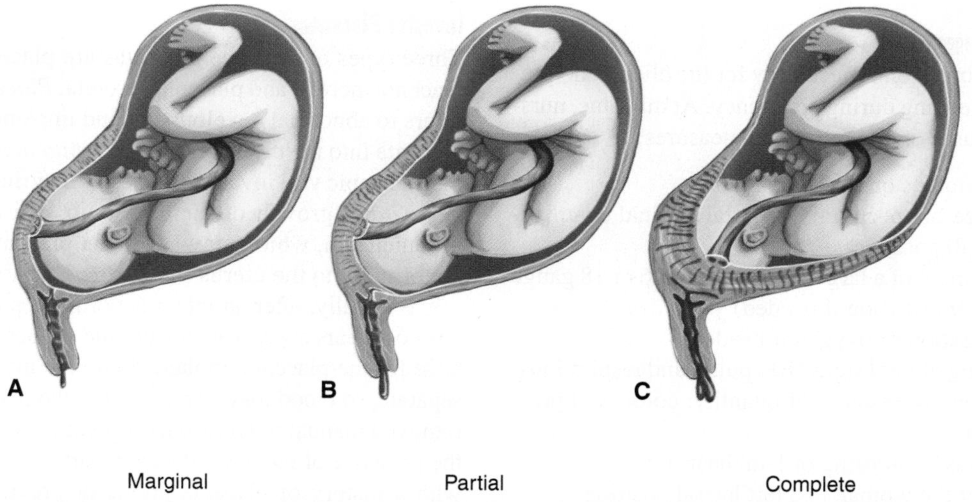

FIGURE 13.17 (**A**) Marginal placenta previa. (**B**) Partial placenta previa. (**C**) Complete placenta previa.

bleeding that is normally painless. Generally, the first bleeding episode associated with placenta previa is rarely fatal, with maternal death occurring in 0.03% of all cases (Baskett, 1999). Major degrees of placenta previa bleed earlier, more often, and more heavily than minor degrees. Bleeding generally does not cause retention or contractions; 10% of women do not begin bleeding until labor starts (Alexander & Schneider, 2000).

Other presenting symptoms include the following:

- A uterus felt to be "soft" on palpation
- Fetal heart present with a normal rate
- Shock and anemia (corresponding with the amount of blood lost)
- Increased risk for postpartum hemorrhage (lower uterine segment has less contractility)
- Abnormalities of the placenta and cord insertion (Baskett, 1999)

Any bleeding after 20 weeks' gestation warrants investigation by transabdominal or transvaginal ultrasound to determine the placental location. A sterile speculum examination can help determine other causes of bleeding such as cervicitis. An asymptomatic placenta previa identified before the last half of the third trimester has a 90% chance of moving to the normal location; therefore, serial ultrasounds should be performed every 2 to 3 weeks to determine whether placenta previa still exists (Gilbert & Harmon, 2003). Bleeding usually stops but may resume at a later date.

With more women undergoing ultrasound examination early in the second trimester, more low-lying placentas are being noted and documented, with additional ultrasounds performed closer to term to monitor the condition's progress. If a woman is diagnosed with placenta previa, careful individualized plans are developed to include a cesarean birth at 37 to 38 weeks, ensuring that blood for transfusion is available to minimize risks to the woman and fetus.

Collaborative Management

Antenatal admission is necessary for the client who presents with bleeding during pregnancy. At this time, nursing care focuses on the following measures:

- Clotting studies on a blood sample
- Avoidance of speculum or digital vaginal examination if at all possible
- Establishment of a large-bore IV line (16 or 18 gauge for blood transfusion if needed)
- Administration of oxygen if needed
- Monitoring of vital signs (BP, pulse, and respirations)
- If bleeding, assessment of quantity, color, and presence of clots
- Continuous monitoring of fetal heart rate
- Caring for the woman in a left lateral position
- Anticipation of cesarean birth and monitoring closely for postpartum hemorrhage (general anesthesia would be considered if the woman is hypovolemic, still bleeding, or both; spinal anesthesia would be considered if bleeding stops and volume status is within normal limits)

The nurse should speak calmly to the woman and support persons, explaining interventions and their purposes. He or she should identify the roles of various care providers and document care, teaching, and outcomes.

Signs of improved tissue perfusion include blood clotting, vital signs within normal limits, and decreased blood loss. Evidence of the woman's ability to cope with the situation includes decreased maternal tension and verbalized understanding of interventions. Signs of significant blood loss are shock (hypotension, pale, clammy skin), measured vaginal bleeding (soaked pads), and labored breathing.

Bedrest may initially be part of the plan until bleeding has stopped for at least 3 days, at which time the woman may be discharged to home care. Blood for transfusion must be available at all times; any anemia should be treated. The woman who is Rh negative needs to receive Rh immune globulin (see Chap. 22). Diagnostic ultrasound is used to determine the exact placental location.

Team members collaborate with the woman regarding where she will receive ongoing care, depending on her distance from an appropriate health care facility. Options for home care depend on the degree of placenta previa, point of gestation, and safety concerns. The woman who is less than 34 weeks needs corticosteroids as per institutional policy to increase fetal lung maturity. Many women with placenta previa give birth before 35 weeks' gestation. See Chapter 16 for discussions of cesarean birth and for considerations when placenta previa is first noted in a laboring client.

Invasive Placentas

Three types of invasive placentas are placenta accreta, placenta increta, and placenta percreta. *Placenta accreta* refers to abnormal development and implantation of the placenta into the myometrium. *Placenta increta* is when the chorionic villi invade into the myometrium. *Placenta percreta* is growth of the chorionic villi through the myometrium, which may allow the placenta to adhere abnormally to the uterus (Gilbert & Harmon, 2003).

Normally, after an infant is born, the placenta separates or shears away from the uterine surface. It is impossible for the placenta implanted into the myometrium to separate, so blood loss increases until the placenta can be removed manually. Ultrasound is necessary to determine the presence of invasive placenta, particularly in women with a history of placenta previa or previous cesarean birth. Both these conditions significantly increase the risk for invasive placenta (Gilbert & Harmon, 2003). For example, the risk for placenta accreta is 8 times greater with one cesarean birth and 4 times greater still with a history of two or more cesarean births (Usta et al., 2005).

Decision making regarding this woman's location of care is important and based on many factors such as amount of bleeding, fetal health status, and maternal status. Various assessments are used to evaluate fetal health, including fetal movement counts, auscultation of the fetal heart rate, NST, biophysical profiles, and Doppler studies.

The usual treatment for clients at 24 to 36 weeks' gestation is simply to monitor for any signs of a developing problem, provided that the client is not bleeding. If hemorrhage is severe, however, cesarean birth may be scheduled even for an immature fetus. Steroids may be administered to accelerate fetal lung maturation in gestations less than 34 weeks. An IV line (18 gauge to allow for blood transfusion as required), with blood cross-matched at all times should be part of the nursing care of the hospitalized client. Currently, in some geographic areas, women diagnosed with placental problems are hospitalized and prescribed bedrest awaiting fetal maturation. In other areas, antenatal care is conducted at home to allow women to remain with their families while being monitored for signs of labor.

Circumvallate Placenta

With a *circumvallate placenta,* the edges roll under the placenta during development, and a membrane forms around the entire outside edge (Alexander & Schneider, 2000). Causes include deep uterine implantation and bleeding early in gestation. Circumvallate placenta occurs in approximately 1% of pregnancies (Alexander & Schneider, 2000). Bleeding can occur if the membranous edge separates. If bleeding is absent or controlled, the client can receive care similar to that used for women with minor placenta previa. If bleeding persists or increases, cesarean birth is necessary (Alexander & Schneider, 2000). See Chapter 16.

Placental Abruption

Placental abruption (abruptio placentae) is the premature separation of a normally implanted placenta from the uterine wall (Fig. 13.18). This serious complication is the most common cause of intrapartal fetal death (Usta et al., 2005).

Etiology

The cause of placental abruption is unknown. Risk factors include advanced maternal age, cigarette smoking, hypertension, cocaine and alcohol use, unusually short cord, trauma, polyhydramnios, pPROM, gestational hypertension, and diabetes. Poor nutrition, increased parity, multiple gestation, and male fetal gender also are associated. Women with a previous abruption have a 10-fold risk of recurrence in another pregnancy (Carter, 1999).

Placental abruption can result from bleeding followed by hematoma formation and then rebleeding. This cycle can continue, causing ongoing separation of the placenta from the uterine wall. The displaced portion of the placenta is no longer perfused, interrupting the maternal–fetal circulation. Fetal death can result, as can maternal DIC.

Classification

Placental abruption normally is classified as mild, moderate, or severe. Approximately 90% of cases are mild to moderate and do not lead to any fetal concerns, maternal hypotension, or coagulopathy (Palmer, 2002). Further classifications are as follows:

- *Marginal or apparent:* separation is near the edge of the placenta; blood can escape

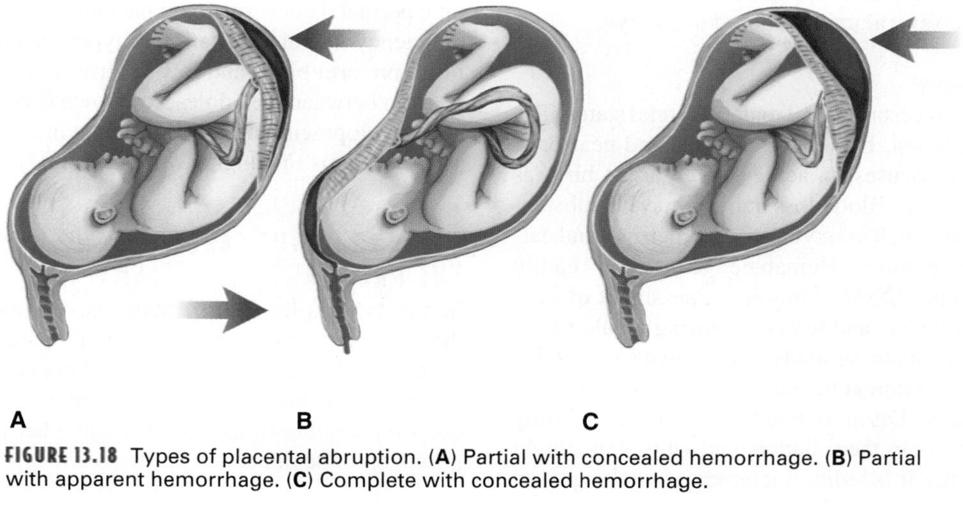

FIGURE 13.18 Types of placental abruption. (**A**) Partial with concealed hemorrhage. (**B**) Partial with apparent hemorrhage. (**C**) Complete with concealed hemorrhage.

- *Central or concealed:* separation is in the center of the placenta; blood is trapped in a pocket of the placenta
- *Mixed or combined:* part of the separation is near the edge; part is concealed in the center (Gilbert & Harmon, 2003)

Assessment Findings

Presenting symptoms depend on the degree and type of detachment. Onset may be sudden. The goal of care is to recognize and to treat the cause of any visible bleeding as quickly as possible. Visible vaginal blood loss can be misleading because the "true" maternal blood loss may be concealed behind the placenta (Palmer, 2002).

The nurse should assess for the color and amount of vaginal bleeding, as well as for uterine tenderness and rigidity. Pain in the abdomen or back may be sudden, sharp, and severe. Concealed blood causes uterine pressure and myometrial contractions, which result in abdominal tenderness and pain. If the woman is undergoing epidural anesthesia, palpation may reveal continuous abdominal rigidity.

Because of the pregnant state, the vital signs of a woman experiencing placental abruption may not indicate accurately her degree of blood loss or shock. Symptoms of shock usually do not occur until hemorrhage is significant. They may include hypotension, tachycardia, decreased urinary output, shallow and irregular respirations, pallor, and thirst.

The fetal heart should be monitored continuously in the case of suspected placental abruption; indicators include increased or absent resting tone in the tocodynometer and repetitive late or variable decelerations.

Ongoing blood loss can result in coagulopathy and progress in a few cases to DIC. It is critical for health care providers to work together to continually evaluate through laboratory testing, physical examination, and fetal monitoring to ensure ongoing health and safety. Laboratory testing includes a complete blood count, hemoglobin and hematocrit, platelet count, fibrinogen and fibrin-split products, and type and cross-match. It also is critical to hold several units of blood in reserve.

Collaborative Management

Care depends on gestation and maternal–fetal status. The goal is stabilization. If the fetus is alive and near or at term, the team focuses on achieving cesarean birth as quickly as possible. Blood loss at birth may be substantial; medications such as oxytocin, ergometrine, and carboprost tromethamine (Hemabate) should be readily available (Palmer, 2002). Ongoing assessment of vital signs, pain, bleeding, and fetal monitoring would be essential components of all plans of care. See Chapter 16.

If the fetus is immature and blood loss is slow, birth can be postponed. Discussion with this client and family is necessary to help them understand why plans might change suddenly if bleeding increases or vital signs indicate hemorrhage. Interventions must include measures for evaluating blood test results and reassessing the condition. Ultrasound to check for "concealed" bleeding may be required.

In cases of severe abruption, the fetus may die in utero. In such cases, the decision for a vaginal or cesarean delivery is based on risks for hemorrhage or other complications related to optimizing maternal health.

ADOLESCENT PREGNANCY

In recent years, the pregnancy rate among adolescents has decreased; nevertheless, this issue continues to have serious societal implications in both Canada and the United States (Rentschler, 2003). One million U.S. teen pregnancies occur annually; approximately 2% to 4% of these young women place their child with adoptive services, and 41% terminate their pregnancies (American Academy of Pediatrics [AAP] & American College of Obstetricians and Gynecologists [ACOG], 2002). Of those younger than 18 years who give birth, 80% are unmarried (AAP & ACOG, 2002).

In most cases, teen pregnancy is unplanned. Developmentally, adolescents tend to be in the "concrete thinking" phase, in which use of contraception, particularly condoms, as part of future planning and avoidance of adverse consequences does not enter into decision making. The young woman (and her partner) may think that pregnancy will never happen to them and that they are somehow protected from risky behavior (Feroli & Burstein, 2003). In some cases, teens may intentionally try to become pregnant without appreciating the responsibilities and risks inherent in assuming the parental role. Risk factors for teen pregnancy include high rates of sexual activity, sexual or physical violence in the home, and cultural values and norms that accept adolescent parenting (Neinstein & Farmer, 2004).

If a pregnant teen chooses to continue with the gestation, she is at greater risk for perinatal complications than a pregnant woman between 20 to 35 years old. Specific perinatal concerns for expectant teens include iron-deficiency anemia, gestational hypertension, operative birth, preterm birth, and low-birth-weight infant. Competition between the adolescent's own needs for growth and development and fetal demands may contribute to such problems (Youngkin & Davis, 2004).

COLLABORATIVE CARE: THE PREGNANT ADOLESCENT

Some states in the United States have laws mandating the involvement of a pregnant teen's parents (AAP & ACOG, 2002). In other states and Canada, the pregnant adolescent is considered an independent client: it is her decision whether to inform or involve her parent in the provision of health care.

Assessment

Assessment parameters for pregnant teens are similar to those for any pregnant woman (see Chap. 12). For clients of this developmental stage, assessment of social support systems is especially critical. Encouraging teens to involve helpful family members and friends when making decisions may be beneficial.

Select Potential Nursing Diagnoses

The following are examples of NANDA diagnoses commonly applicable to pregnant adolescents:

- **Risk for Ineffective Health Maintenance** related to inadequate prenatal care and nutrition
- **Risk for Imbalanced Nutrition: Less Than Body Requirements**
- **Risk for Delayed Growth and Development**
- **Fatigue**
- **Deficient Knowledge**
- **Risk for Situational Low Self-Esteem**

Planning/Intervention

At the first prenatal appointment, providing information about the teen's options is important. Generally, the choices are to continue with the pregnancy and raise the baby, to continue with the pregnancy and place the child with adoptive services, or to terminate the pregnancy. Educating the client about procedures, processes, and the risks and benefits involved with each choice is critical to her decision-making. It also is important to ensure that the teen asks questions and verbalizes understanding of information she is given.

If the client decides to terminate her pregnancy, advice, instructions, or both should be given in a straightforward, nonthreatening manner (see Chap. 9). If she chooses to continue the pregnancy, scheduling follow-up appointments to review information as well as to perform the necessary examinations is important. Additional interventions may include referrals to community nursing, social services, or both for extra support (AAP & ACOG, 2002). Monitoring the teen's psychosocial needs throughout the gestation and attempting to find resources and ways to meet them is an integral part of client advocacy (Fig. 13.19). See Research Highlight 13.3.

Evaluation

Giving the pregnant teen a chance to collaborate with health care providers when formulating plans of care is critical. Desired outcomes are for the adolescent to understand her alternatives and to identify people she wants involved in her care. If the client elects to continue the pregnancy, desired outcomes are for care providers to develop a good working relationship with her, encourage her attendance at prenatal visits, and provide ongoing care as needed for her specific circumstances.

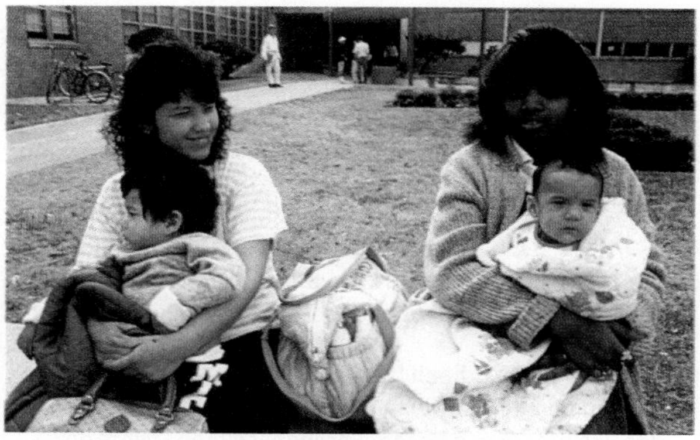

FIGURE 13.19 Adolescents may benefit socially from school-sponsored programs that continue after pregnancy to facilitate interactions with other young mothers and their children.

MULTIPLE PREGNANCY

Multiple pregnancy (gestation with two or more fetuses) is considered high risk because it has an increased potential for fetal abnormalities, prematurity, discordant fetal growth, and fetal growth restriction (Malcus, 2004). Other associated risks include gestational hypertension, anemia (maternal blood volume is 500 mL or more than in single pregnancy), and increased discomforts such as constipation (Watson-Blasioli, 2001). Prenatal health care providers should be alert for these complications.

Incidence of multiple pregnancy is increasing for many reasons: older maternal ages, frequent use of reproductive-assisted technology, and hereditary factors (Watson-Blasioli, 2001; Zach & Pramanik, 2004). Between 1980 and 1994, the U.S. twin birth rate increased by 30%, whereas the triplet birth rate quadrupled (Zach & Pramanik, 2004). In Canada, the number of twins increased by 35% and triplets by 58% (Healy & Gaddipati, 2005). See Chapter 11 for details on developmental processes that lead to multiple gestation and the different types.

Care of clients with multiple gestation is challenging throughout pregnancy, labor, and birth. Mothers are at risk for preterm labor, hypertension, anemia, placental dysfunction, and cord abnormalities (Ellings et al., 1998). Ongoing assessment of fetal well-being is important. Twin studies have shown that fetal heart rate accelerations are simultaneous 52% of the time and that both fetuses have synchronous behavior patterns 95% of the time (sleep or awake state) (Hayward, 2003). Thus, NSTs for women with multiple gestation should be done with fetal monitors that can simultaneously record two or more fetal heart rates. Frequent review of the results is necessary to protect the health of all fetuses being assessed.

The frequency of ultrasound evaluation in multiple gestation depends on the preferences of the primary care

RESEARCH HIGHLIGHT 13.3 Pregnant Adolescents' Perspectives of Pregnancy

OBJECTIVE: The purpose of this qualitative study was to obtain a clearer understanding of teens' perspectives on pregnancy and parenting.

SAMPLE: Twenty unmarried teens pregnant for the first time and planning to keep the child were interviewed during the second or third trimester.

METHOD: Each teen participated in a 60- to 90-minute interview with questions such as "What was life like before you became pregnant?" and "What do you think it will be like being a mother?" The researchers grouped data into themes using grounded theory and the constant comparative method.

RESULTS: These young women described three major themes. "The Pregnant Me—Unexpected Changes" involved surprise that pregnancy-related changes included new emotions, lifestyle choices, and future plans, as well as the many unexpected physical manifestations of gestation. "Transformed Relationships" referred to responses from others including peers, partners, and significant adults. The final theme, "Envisioning Motherhood," included the responses of fear, awe, and desire to be a "good mother."

CONCLUSION: The teens in this small sample size described positive feelings about pregnancy and the hope of being good parents. They communicated a wish to protect their fetuses through lifestyle changes, such as decreasing smoking and improving eating habits.

NURSING IMPLICATIONS: Community nurses, particularly those working with teens (eg, school nurses) need to build on positive responses and give opportunities for pregnant adolescents to support one another. Assisting teens to become more aware of the process of pregnancy can help them anticipate changes, which may improve their coping. Support groups that begin during and continue after pregnancy might promote ongoing lifestyle improvements as well as enhancing parenting skills.

Rentschler, D. (2003). *Journal of Maternal–Child Nursing, 28,* 378–382.

provider and other risk factors. As with singleton pregnancy, ultrasound is used to determine gestation, fetal growth, and amniotic fluid volume. In multiple gestation, ultrasound also is necessary to determine chorionicity, one of the most important determinants of outcome. Twin–twin transfusion syndrome complicates approximately 15% of monochorionic multiple gestations and is associated with a mortality rate of 30% to 50% (Kumar & O'Brien, 2004). Risk factors for this problem include a single monochorionic placenta, polyhydramnios, oligohydramnios, and same-sex fetuses. Positive findings include a chronically distended bladder in one fetus, fetal growth discordance, and evidence of fetal cardiac dysfunction (Gilbert & Harmon, 2003). In cases of twin–twin transfusion syndrome, the family needs care from a facility that can provide individualized evaluation and counseling to mother and fetuses (Kumar & O'Brien, 2004). Because of the risks of this syndrome, the SOGC (2000) recommends that, if possible, clinicians check chorionicity as soon as multiple pregnancy is diagnosed. It can be determined as early as 10 to 14 weeks' gestation.

Monochorionic, monoamniotic placentation is a rare condition of multiple gestation associated with a mortality rate as high as 50% from cord entanglement, knots, congenital anomalies, and prematurity (SOGC, 2000). Cord entanglement occurs in almost all monoamniotic twins. Other sonographic features of a monoamniotic pregnancy include the following:

- No dividing amniotic membrane
- A single placenta
- Same-sex fetuses
- Adequate amniotic fluid surrounding each fetus
- Fetuses moving freely within the uterine cavity (SOGC, 2000)

COLLABORATIVE CARE: MULTIPLE PREGNANCIES

Care for the client with a multiple gestation mainly involves educating the client and family about their many options for care. Plans must be flexible enough to accommodate emergency interventions (eg, cesarean birth) as necessary while facilitating the woman's participation in decision making (eg, feeding choices, support people, early comfort measures depending on gestation and fetal positions). Team members should give realistic information as pregnancy progresses to dispel myths. They should encourage the client to discuss fears and worries openly (Ellings et al., 1998). The following paragraphs focus on care during pregnancy of the woman carrying more than one fetus. Chapter 16 presents special considerations relative to labor and birth in multiple gestation.

Assessment

Ongoing prenatal assessment of cervical length may help predict the chances of preterm birth. Restricted activity may be recommended or simply initiated as a practical necessity because of the mobility limitations imposed by the increased fetal weight. Planning for this possibility can decrease the client's social isolation and increase her ability to cope. Upper-body exercises and physiotherapy also may be helpful for clients who must remain on bedrest (Mariano & Hickey, 1998). Restricted activity and leaving employment early in the pregnancy, however, have not been shown to decrease the likelihood of preterm birth (SOGC, 2000).

Assessment of maternal weight gain is critical. Although specific recommendations must be tailored to each woman's prepregnant body mass index (see Chap. 12), a general guideline is that a woman expecting twins should gain 24 lbs by 24 weeks and approximately 1 lb/week thereafter. A woman expecting triplets should gain 36 lbs by 24 weeks and 1 lb/week thereafter (Mariano & Hickey, 1998). When discussing nutrition, the care provider should emphasize quality and variety while ensuring that the woman is eating adequate servings of all food groups (Mariano & Hickey, 1998). Other discussion topics to cover include ways to manage constipation, consume sufficient nutrients, and deal with nausea and vomiting; problems in these areas may necessitate referral to a dietitian.

Ongoing ultrasounds during pregnancy provide information on fetal growth and development and help detect any anomalies, rates of which are 40% higher in multiples (SOGC, 2000). For each fetus in a multiple pregnancy, growth is similar to that found in a single pregnancy until approximately 32 to 35 weeks' gestation, when the rate for the multiples slows.

During each prenatal visit, the primary care provider checks the lie and presentation of each fetus, which will be critical determining factors relative to the type of birth (vaginal or cesarean). Ultrasound as well as abdominal palpation should be used to confirm the fetal positions.

Select Potential Nursing Diagnoses

The following are examples of commonly applicable NANDA diagnoses in cases of multiple gestation:

- **Anxiety** related to maternal and fetal health concerns
- **Fear** related to labor, birth, and the health of the mother and fetuses
- **Constipation** related to decreased gastrointestinal functioning
- **Risk for Imbalanced Nutrition** related to the demands of multiple pregnancy
- **Risk for Ineffective Health Maintenance** related to multiple pregnancy care requirements
- **Deficient Knowledge** related to specialized care for multiple pregnancy
- **Risk for Compromised Family Coping** related to the increased demands of multiple newborns

Planning/Intervention

Maternal–fetal attachment has been studied mainly in terms of single pregnancies. Damato (2000) concluded that nurses should ask nonjudgmental questions regarding a woman's emotional adjustment to a multifetal pregnancy. Differing feelings for each fetus may not be unusual, and parents should understand that such attitudes are valid. Parents may need time to process the circumstances related to their high-risk pregnancy and the potential for preterm birth. If labor happens early, interrupted antepartal attachment may compromise perinatal bonding. If the woman's partner is involved, nurses should include him or her as much as possible in prenatal care and encourage his or her support. They also should refer the client and her support people to associations or clubs that encourage the sharing of hopes and fears in cases of multiple gestation.

Multifetal pregnancies are associated with many financial, personal, and social costs for the families involved. Nurses should provide anticipatory information to these families to prepare them for the increased emotional, financial, and practical stresses they are likely to experience. Participation in organizations such as the Parents of Multiples Birth Association (POMBA) before birth helps establish a source for support and networking. Community nurses are ideally placed to visit families during the prenatal periods to prepare them. Referral to a social worker, counseling services, family support programs, or all of these may be appropriate.

Ongoing discussion with this woman and family regarding social support and preparation for infant care after birth is necessary. Parents of multiples are at increased risk for divorce, child abuse, and postpartum depression related to increased emotional and financial stress (Mariano & Hickey, 1998). Assistance in coping skills and anticipation of the need for increased social support can be extremely valuable.

Because of the risk for preterm labor associated with a multiple pregnancy, the nurse should teach the client the signs and symptoms of this problem. The mean weekly frequency of uterine contractions is higher than in a singleton pregnancy; additionally, contractions gradually increase with gestation (Mariano & Hickey, 1998).

Evaluation

In cases of multiple pregnancy, ideal outcomes are for the woman to reach 36 to 37 weeks' gestation with all fetuses growing and developing normally, with progress toward the birth of all healthy infants while maintaining the health of the mother. Close fetal monitoring through movement counts, Doppler studies (as appropriate), biophysical profiles, and NST are measures by which to monitor progress. Verbalization from family members that they are prepared for their postpartal circumstances is equally important. See Chapter 16 for more information.

PERINATAL LOSS

From the earliest moments of learning about a pregnancy, parents envision their infant's future, with expectations and hopes for their life together (Michon et al., 2003). Regardless of the point of gestation at which it happens, a lost pregnancy can be difficult for the family involved. Parents who experience perinatal loss move through the stages of shock and numbness, searching and yearning, disorganization and depression, and reorganization. They adjust to the loss at varying paces depending on support systems, individual coping strategies, strengths, and other stressors. Generally, the bereavement process lasts 6 to 24 months. According to Michon and colleagues (2003), the grief experienced by mothers is usually of greater intensity than that of fathers.

Societal changes have contributed to increased parental grieving over perinatal loss. The lower infant mortality rate and scientific advances have fostered expectations for pregnancies to continue without disruption, which encourages women to bond early with their fetuses. Methods of reproductive control may increase a woman's motivation to plan pregnancy for a specific time or point in her life. When a pregnancy is lost under such conditions, sadness and mourning are likely to be greater.

Early Pregnancy Loss

Most pregnancy losses occur within the first trimester (Abboud & Liamputtong, 2003). **Miscarriage** is the term used for a pregnancy lost before 20 weeks' gestation. Some states include no signs of life and weight below 350 g in the definition; in Canada, the weight is less than 500 g. If the fetal weight is greater than 500 g, gestation is longer than 20 weeks, or both, funeral arrangements are needed.

The medical term for pregnancy loss before 20 weeks' gestation is *abortion,* regardless of whether the event is elective or spontaneous (Table 13.5). Nurses should be sensitive to the terminology they use when discussing a pregnancy loss with clients and their families, however, because some people may view the term "abortion" as unkind, judgmental, or inappropriate.

When a client experiences a miscarriage, feelings may vary from relief (if the pregnancy was unwanted) to extreme sadness and despair (Gilbert & Harmon, 2003). The woman may feel like a failure or want acknowledgement of the loss from everyone to whom she announced the pregnancy. Usually, few interventions can prevent a miscarriage; however, the client may blame herself or be blamed by others (Abboud & Liamputtong, 2003). A second-trimester loss may be especially difficult because the client and family are likely to have experienced objective validations of the pregnancy's existence, such as seeing the fetus through ultrasound, hearing the fetal heartbeat, or feeling fetal movements. Because most pregnancy losses occur before 12 weeks' gestation, a second-trimester miscarriage may be harder because it is less expected.

Common causes of early pregnancy loss include genetic abnormalities, uterine or cervical problems, infections, substance abuse, and maternal medical conditions (eg, diabetes, hypothyroidism). Two other common problems related to early pregnancy loss are ectopic pregnancy and gestational trophoblastic disease.

Ectopic Pregnancy

Ectopic pregnancy, a life-threatening condition, occurs when the products of conception implant anywhere other than the uterus (Fig. 13.20). It happens in approximately 1.5% of pregnancies (Royal College of Obstetricians and Gynaecologists [RCOG], 2002). Most ectopic implanta-

TABLE 13.5 Classifications of Abortion

TYPE	DEFINITION	MANAGEMENT
Complete abortion	Passage of all products of conception, revealed by ultrasound showing an empty uterus	Follow-up care to discuss related issues, family planning needs, psychosocial concerns
Habitual abortion	Three or more consecutive spontaneous abortions	Identification and treatment of underlying cause (if possible) If related to cervical insufficiency, cerclage in future pregnancies to promote successful outcome
Incomplete abortion	Passage of some of the products of conception, revealed by ultrasound showing retained material in the uterus	Dilation and curettage (D&C) or administration of prostaglandin analog to evacuate the uterus
Inevitable abortion	Pregnancy loss that cannot be prevented	If products of conception are not passed spontaneously, vacuum curettage or administration of prostaglandin analog to evacuate the uterus
Missed abortion	Retained nonviable embryo for 6 weeks or more	Uterine evacuation by suction curettage or D&C, depending on the stage of the pregnancy Induction of labor as a nonsurgical option
Threatened abortion	Vaginal bleeding early in gestation, with no passage of embryonic or fetal tissue	Possibly, mild activity restriction

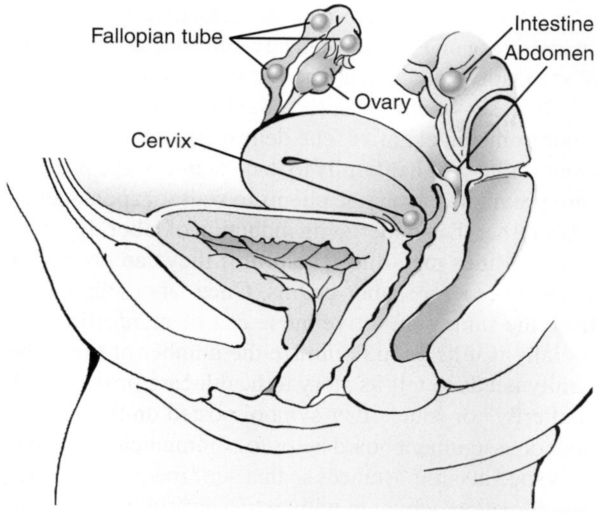

FIGURE 13.20 Sites for implantation of an ectopic pregnancy may include the fallopian tubes, ovary, intestines, abdomen, and cervix.

tions involve the fallopian tubes; as gestation continues, bleeding and pain develop. If untreated, the tube can rupture, causing severe hemorrhage that may lead to maternal collapse and death (Abbott, 2004).

Causes and risk factors for ectopic pregnancy include blocked or narrowed fallopian tubes that prevent ova from reaching the uterus; previous pelvic infection; history of chlamydia infection; previous appendicitis; history of infertility or cesarean birth; age older than 35 years; and smoking (Abbott, 2004).

Presenting symptoms may include a positive pregnancy test, vaginal bleeding, and abdominal pain, which usually is one sided but not necessarily on the side of the ectopic implantation. Bleeding may range from spotting to severe hemorrhage. A classic sign of a ruptured ectopic pregnancy is shoulder tip pain caused by internal bleeding irritating the diaphragm. Bladder pain may accompany urination, and the client may feel pressure in the bowels. Dizziness, pallor, and nausea may precede collapse. Up to 75% of affected clients present with subacute systems (Abbott, 2004). Transvaginal ultrasound can confirm the diagnosis from 4 weeks' gestation onward.

Treatment may involve drugs (eg, methotrexate) or laparoscopic surgery. The emergency surgery and reality of the lost pregnancy can pose challenges to the client's psychological health and relationships. Women who have experienced ectopic pregnancy describe it as "a termination without consent" (Abbott, 2004, p. 33). Initial feelings may include pain, fear for personal safety, and concern for future fertility. The linkage with past STIs as a risk factor may heighten a woman's emotions over this experience. Providing supportive care and expressing sympathy are important interventions; the nurse also should give information about community resources.

Gestational Trophoblastic Disease

Gestational trophoblastic disease (GTD) means abnormal proliferation and degeneration of the trophoblastic villi. When GTD occurs, gestational tissue exists, but the pregnancy is not viable. As the gestational cells degenerate, they fill with fluid (Fig. 13.21). In addition to the typical early indicators of pregnancy (ie, amenorrhea, fatigue, breast tenderness), signs and symptoms of molar pregnancy include brownish vaginal bleeding, anemia, hyperemesis gravidarum, edema, disparity between uterine size and gestational age, elevated hCG levels, absent fetal heart sounds, and a characteristic molar pattern on ultrasound.

Two types of GTD are complete and partial hydatidiform moles. With a complete molar pregnancy, all the villi swell and form cysts. This problem has an accompanying risk for *choriocarcinoma,* a dangerous and rapidly spreading malignancy. With a partial molar pregnancy, some villi form normally. Partial moles rarely lead to choriocarcinoma. Regardless of type, the uterine contents must be immediately evacuated by dilation and curettage and tested for any evidence of malignancy. If no malignancy is found, the client must undergo follow-up tests of hCG levels for the next 12 months to ensure that any remaining tissue does not turn malignant. Chemotherapy may be used prophylactically or as treatment (see Chap. 4). Because of the risks for cancer, the client must be careful to avoid pregnancy for 1 year following GTD.

Late Pregnancy Loss

Stillbirth is the term used when a pregnancy of more than 20 weeks' gestation ends in fetal death. Stillbirth happens in approximately 1 in 43 U.S. births (Chichester, 2005). Causes include cord accident, extreme prematurity, and congenital abnormalities (Gilbert & Harmon, 2003). Another type of stillbirth is when one fetus in a multiple

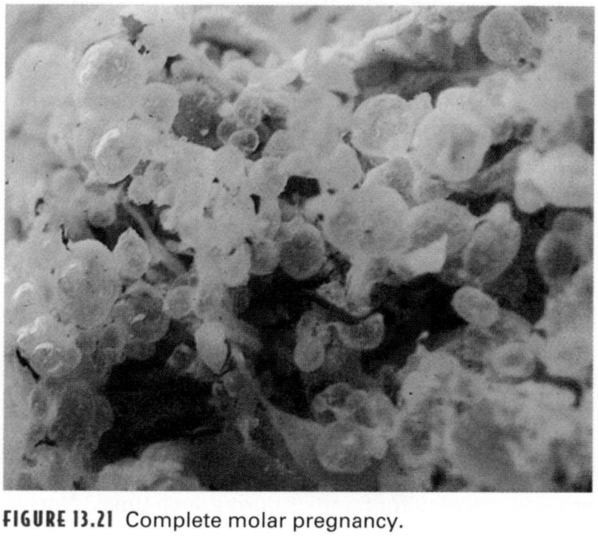

FIGURE 13.21 Complete molar pregnancy.

gestation dies before or during labor and birth. In this event, the family may struggle with the ambivalence of celebrating the birth of the living baby or babies, while grieving for the one who has died

COLLABORATIVE CARE: PREGNANCY LOSS

When a family has lost a pregnancy, health care providers must provide sensitive collaborative interventions that focus on information, understanding, and physical care. The team may involve physicians, midwives, nurses, public health nurses, and social workers. Ongoing communication about each professional's role and the care given can help ensure that the needs of the client and family are met. In some cases, families must deal with both birth and death within a short time and need extra support during this transition period (Chichester, 2005).

Assessment

Depending on when a gestation is lost, a client may come to the labor and delivery area describing decreased or no fetal movements over an extended period. Fear, anxiety, and a desire for reassurance are common emotions at such times. The nurse should assess the fetal heart rate; if he or she cannot reassure the parents quickly, the nurse should notify the client's primary care provider immediately to move forward with additional evaluations. The next step would involve biophysical profiling or a real-time scan, the results of which would indicate fetal health or confirm fetal demise.

Select Potential Nursing Diagnoses

The following NANDA diagnoses are commonly applicable in cases of perinatal loss:

- **Chronic Sorrow**
- **Risk for Dysfunctional Grieving**
- **Social Isolation** related to the grief process
- **Interrupted Family Processes** related to grief

Planning/Intervention

Once a gestation has been confirmed as lost, parents may feel shocked, confused, fearful that they may have contributed to the event, or angry. Commonly, women and their partners search for an answer about what went wrong. Nurses should understand that such questioning is normal while trying to learn whether a desire to blame someone or something for the loss is at the root of the concern (Abboud & Liamputtong, 2003). Giving short and simple explanations, allowing parents to be together (if the woman has come alone, she should be asked about her preferences for someone to be with her), and providing a quiet place for grieving are helpful immediate interventions. Many facilities have a "quiet" room that provides privacy for families during such times. Nurses who cry at this event should feel reassured that this response is not unusual and can be a comforting expression of sympathy to the client and her significant others.

In cases of stillbirth, the client may not experience labor immediately after fetal demise, which may be difficult for her and her family to understand. Some primary care providers encourage clients to wait for spontaneous labor rather than undergoing induction of labor. In either case, families may find it helpful if they can grieve for some time before labor begins. Once labor starts, care from the same supportive nurse can be comforting, especially if it helps to minimize the number of times the family needs to tell its story to health care providers. A "butterfly" or some other symbol posted on the client's door or assignment board helps to communicate the family's special circumstances so that staff members are prepared to approach them with extra sensitivity. Assisting the client to make decisions about pain relief methods and comfort measures may facilitate positive feelings about this time. Giving information about emotions and reactions that they may experience also can be helpful. Describing in simple terms the legal aspects necessary for an autopsy and a funeral is important.

Encouraging families to decide how much time to spend with their baby after delivery is over and whether they want keepsakes such as pictures, a lock of hair, or footprints may result in better memories of the experience (Gilbert & Harmon, 2003). Alexander and Schnieder (2000) write that respectful and compassionate pictures for parents to keep can assist in their mourning. Photos of the baby's foot or hand in a parent's or sibling's hand may be powerful and treasured remembrances. Some cultures, such as Old Order Amish, view photographs as "graven images," however, and would not appreciate this approach.

Various cultures mourn and grieve losses differently. To provide culturally sensitive care, nurses must first identify their own values to facilitate respect for the wide-ranging emotions, customs, and wishes that others may bring to this experience (Chichester, 2005). Religion also may influence preferences for care. Some families may desire the presence of a support person from their faith or immediate baptism of the stillborn infant. Asking clients about such wishes helps to ensure the provision of culturally sensitive care (Chichester, 2005).

Parents who have experienced perinatal loss have described the following interventions as helpful (Gilbert & Harmon, 2003):

- Support from a significant person during the experience
- Seeing the fetal tissue
- Holding the baby
- Saving mementos
- Being given time to grieve
- Being allowed choices (decision making)

- Having sensitive caregivers
- Hearing words or phrases such as "I don't know what to say," "I am sorry, I can't imagine what this must be like for you," and "What is this like for you?" (Unhelpful statements such as "You can have another one" or "Time heals all wounds" are not comforting at this time [Jonas-Simpson & McMahon, 2005]).

Health care providers need to acknowledge the client's physical and emotional pain (Abboud & Liamputtong, 2003). The mother requires immediate support and must be discouraged from focusing on self-blame. She needs to be able to request care or counseling later if she requires it. Encouraging fathers to discuss their feelings either with their partners, in individual counseling, or in support groups might be appropriate. Each member of the couple may not have legitimate means of expressing his or her own loss while supporting the other person. For the sake of their relationship, each person should be encouraged to assist the other to grieve at an individual pace and to use referrals as necessary (Abboud & Liamputtong, 2003).

Evaluation

Ensuring that family members feel that their wishes for care, privacy, comfort, and information were met is key. Facilitating a smooth discharge from the health care facility is critical. Nurses also must do what they can to ensure that such families do not receive surveys from the facility about their experience or donation requests.

Questions to Ponder

1. Ms. C (G3, TPAL 1102) has just been diagnosed with an anterior placenta previa. Her plan of care includes bedrest, biweekly biophysical and nonstress testing, vital signs every 12 hours, and fetal movement counting bid. Ms. C's two children are 5 and 3 years old, her husband is a shift worker at an automotive plant, and her parents live 300 miles away. Describe how you would assess Ms. C's support system and teaching regarding her need for hospitalization at present.
2. Ms. C. has had no further episodes of bleeding, and the decision has been made to send her home on Home Care with weekly fetal monitoring at home, daily fetal movement counts, and instructions to return weekly for an ultrasound to monitor the baby's growth and development. Describe the teaching that you would do before Ms. C's discharge.

SUMMARY

- High-risk pregnancies involve conditions or complications that can endanger the safety of the mother, fetus, or both. The situation may involve the need for monitoring to prevent a maternal or fetal problem such as with maternal obesity, substance use, or adolescent pregnancy; a significant health problem that existed before or developed during the pregnancy; or a health problem directly related to the gestation.
- A high-risk pregnancy is a stressor that requires risk assessment to guide planning for appropriate care, including the need for ongoing consultation and place of birth. Assessment of possible psychosocial, economic, nutritional, and family-related stressors is essential.
- The pregnant woman with asthma requires a stepwise approach to care to maintain adequate control of her symptoms during pregnancy. Use of corticosteroids may lead to decreased birth weight and increased risk for gestational hypertension.
- The New York Heart Association's classification is used to determine the functional status of a pregnant woman with heart disease. Women with class I or II heart disease have a favorable prognosis, but their functional status may worsen with the physiologic changes of pregnancy. Gestational weeks 28 to 32 are a critical time for the pregnant woman with heart disease because the increased blood volume peaks at this time.
- Fatigue, palpitations, and potentially chest pain or shortness of breath with exercise are common signs and symptoms associated with anemia during pregnancy. Iron-deficiency anemia is associated with preterm birth and low birth weight.
- The major problem related to pregnancy and systemic lupus erythematosus involves the placenta with inflammatory responses that include infarctions, fibrin deposits, and small placental size. As a result, decreased placental circulation and fetal malnutrition can occur.
- Planning for screening, treatment, and follow-up for STIs is important during pregnancy. Collaboration with the woman is key to ensuring that she continues to complete preventive measures, treatments, or both. Testing for group B streptococcus (via swab obtained from the vaginal introitus and anorectum) is recommended for all pregnant women at 35 to 37 weeks' gestation so that the results of testing are available when the woman enters labor.
- The most common cause of asymptomatic bacteriuria is *Escherichia coli.* Costovertebral angle tenderness, high fever, chills, myalgia, nausea, and vomiting are common signs and symptoms of pyelonephritis. The pregnant woman with acute renal failure requires immediate therapy that includes frequent assessments of vital signs, breath sounds, fluid intake, and urine output as well as fetal monitoring such as nonstress testing and fetal movement counts.

- Key interventions for the pregnant woman with diabetes include blood glucose self-monitoring; diet management; activity and exercise; insulin administration (if required); and fetal monitoring.
- Although depression is associated more commonly with the postpartum period, women can experience depression anytime in life, including pregnancy. Women are at risk for developing bipolar disorder during their reproductive years.
- Health care providers need to be alert for indicators that may suggest that a woman is a victim of abuse; these include chronic pain and insomnia; irritable bowel syndrome; migraine headaches; arthritis; UTIs; injuries to the face, breasts, abdomen, and buttocks; anxiety; depression; fractures; unexplained bruises; areas of redness consistent with slap injuries; lacerations; and multiple injuries consistent with stages of healing.
- Alcohol abuse in pregnancy is a causative factor in birth defects and developmental delays; heavy or binge drinking has been linked to fetal alcohol syndrome. A safe level of alcohol use during pregnancy has not been identified. Smoking during pregnancy is linked to preterm labor and intrauterine growth restriction.
- Hyperemesis gravidarum, which usually begins during the first 10 weeks of pregnancy, is manifested by nausea and vomiting, a greater than 5% weight loss, dehydration, and electrolyte imbalance.
- Hypertension in pregnancy is classified as gestational hypertension with or without proteinuria (typically first noted after 20 weeks' gestation); preexisting hypertension (chronic); and preexisting hypertension with superimposed gestational hypertension. Pre-eclampsia refers to hypertension after 20 weeks' gestation with proteinuria; it can progress to eclampsia (seizures).
- Decreased placental perfusion is a key pathophysiologic change with hypertension in pregnancy. Magnesium sulfate is the drug of choice for treating hypertension and proteinuria with risk factors for eclampsia. Close monitoring is necessary to prevent magnesium toxicity.
- Acute HELLP syndrome in a pregnant woman requires immediate and careful attention to both the mother and fetus. Successful treatment involves a balance between antenatal treatment and birth of a viable infant in the safest location for the family. Lung maturation is commonly used to determine the best time for the fetus to be born.
- The most common treatment for pPROM is bedrest with ongoing assessment for fever, chills, and change in amniotic fluid (color and odor) that would indicate chorioamnionitis.
- During pregnancy, a woman's blood is hypercoagulable, and events unique to pregnancy, such as abruptio placentae, intrauterine fetal demise, and gestational hypertension, can trigger disseminated intravascular coagulation.
- Placenta previa, a condition in which the placenta covers the cervical os to varying degrees, is the major cause of bleeding in the third trimester and commonly manifested by painless vaginal bleeding. Placental abruption, the premature separation of a normally implanted placenta from the abdominal wall, is manifested by vaginal bleeding, uterine tenderness, and rigidity. It is the most common cause of intrapartal fetal death.
- A pregnant adolescent is at greater risk for perinatal complications; adolescence is a risk factor for iron-deficiency anemia, gestational hypertension, operative birth, preterm birth, and low birth weight infant.
- With a multiple pregnancy, the ideal outcomes are for the woman and family to reach 36 to 37 weeks' gestation with all fetuses growing and developing normally, culminating in the birth of all healthy infants and preservation of the mother's health. Close monitoring of fetal health through movement counts, Doppler studies, biophysical profiles, and nonstress testing are useful in monitoring the status of the pregnancy.
- Parents experiencing perinatal loss move through bereavement and adjust to their loss at their own pace depending on their support systems, individual coping strategies, strengths, and other stressors. This process averages about 6 to 24 months.
- Miscarriage is the term used to denote a pregnancy loss before 20 weeks' gestation. The medical term for a pregnancy loss before 20 weeks is abortion, regardless of whether it is elective or spontaneous. Stillbirth is the term used to denote a pregnancy that has lasted more than 19 weeks' gestation and ends without signs of life.
- Most ectopic pregnancies occur in the fallopian tube. The woman usually complains of pain on one side with some bleeding ranging in amount and character. Shoulder tip pain caused by irritation to the diaphragm is a classic sign of a ruptured ectopic pregnancy.
- Gestational trophoblastic disease occurs as one of two types: complete molar pregnancy in which all the villi swell and form cysts; and partial mole in which some villi form normally. A complete molar pregnancy increases the woman's risk for developing choriocarcinoma, whereas partial moles rarely lead to this malignancy.

REVIEW QUESTIONS

1. When assessing a pregnant woman with asthma, the nurse would be most alert for exacerbation of asthmatic symptoms during which gestational weeks?
   A. 6–12
   B. 12–24
   C. 24–36
   D. 36 to 40

2. A pregnant woman with sickle cell anemia develops chronic hemolytic anemia. Which findings should the nurse least likely assess?
   A. Severe bone pain
   B. Jaundice
   C. Splenomegaly
   D. Cholelithiasis
3. Which of the following should the nurse include when describing the care that will be required during labor to a pregnant client with HIV?
   A. Artificial rupturing of membranes
   B. Internal electronic fetal monitoring
   C. Expected cesarean birth
   D. Antibiotic therapy before birth
4. After teaching a group of students about the effects of parvovirus infection on the fetus, which effect if stated by the group indicates the need for additional teaching?
   A. Fetal death
   B. Hypotonia
   C. Anemia
   D. Nonimmune hydrops
5. A pregnant woman comes to the clinic complaining of a high fever, chills, and flank pain. Assessment reveals costovertebral angle tenderness. She states, "My temperature will go up high and then go back to normal, sometimes even a little below normal." Which of the following should the nurse suspect?
   A. Pyelonephritis
   B. Acute renal failure
   C. Gestational hypertension
   D. Hypoglycemia
6. The nurse teaches a pregnant client with gestational diabetes how to perform blood glucose self-monitoring. Which statement, if made by the client, indicates effective teaching?
   A. "I'll test my blood every morning before breakfast."
   B. "I'll make sure to eat a light snack before testing my blood."
   C. "I'll keep a log for each result with my 4 times a day testing."
   D. "I'll give myself the insulin and then test my blood."
7. The nurse determines that a pregnant woman who has come to the clinic is a victim of abuse. Which of the following would be least important when providing nursing care to this client at this time?
   A. Maintaining confidentiality
   B. Ensuring client and fetus safety
   C. Making a referral to a local shelter
   D. Establishing a one-to-one relationship
8. A client, admitted to the hospital with hyperemesis gravidarum resulting in dehydration and electrolyte imbalance, is NPO. When should the nurse expect that the client will be allowed to start taking oral fluids again?
   A. When the client's bowel sounds return
   B. After 6 hours of receiving intravenous fluids
   C. When the client reports that she feels hungry
   D. After the client has not vomited for 48 hours.
9. A client with pre-eclampsia is receiving magnesium sulfate intravenously. Which assessment finding would lead the nurse to suspect that the client is experiencing magnesium toxicity?
   A. Muscle weakness
   B. Absent patellar reflex
   C. Seizures
   D. Respiratory rate of 18 breaths/minute
10. A client with a complete molar pregnancy comes to the clinic for follow-up after dilation and curettage. Which statement should indicate to the nurse that the client needs additional teaching about her condition?
   A. "I need to make appointments to have my hormone levels checked for the next year."
   B. "I know that this condition has put me at risk for a dangerous type of cancer."
   C. "I hope to get pregnant again, but I know that I need to wait for at least a year."
   D. "I know that the umbilical cord wrapped around my baby's neck, causing problems."

REFERENCES

Abbott, L. (2004). Ectopic pregnancy: Symptoms, diagnosis and management. *Nursing Times, 100,* 32–33.

Abboud, L. N., & Liamputtong, P. (2003). Pregnancy loss: What it means to women who miscarry and their partners. *Social Work in Health Care, 36,* 37–62.

Alexander, J., & Schneider, F. (2000). Vaginal bleeding associated with pregnancy. *Primary Care, 27,* 137–150.

American Academy of Pediatrics and the American College of Obstetricians and Gynecologists. (2002). *Guidelines for perinatal care* (5th ed.). Washington: Authors.

American Psychiatric Association. (2000). *Diagnostic and statistical manual of mental disorders* (4th ed., text revision). Washington: Author.

Andrist, L. (2003). Media images, body dissatisfaction, and disordered eating in adolescent women. *Journal of Maternal Child Nursing, 28,* 119–123.

Arafeh, J., & Baird, S. (2006). Cardiac disease in pregnancy. *Critical Care Nursing Quarterly, 29*(1), 32–52.

Armour, K. (2004). Antepartum maternal–fetal surveillance: Using surveillance to improve maternal and fetal outcomes. *AWHONN Lifelines, 8,* 233–240.

Association of Women's Health, Obstetric and Neonatal Nurses (AWHONN). (2003). *Fetal heart monitoring: Principles and practices* (3rd ed.). Dubuque: Kendall/Hunt Publishing Co.

Barak, A., Dulitzki, M., Efrati, O., Augarten, A., Szeinberg, A., Reichert, N., et al. (2005). Pregnancies and outcome in women with cystic fibrosis. *Israel Medical Association Journal, 7*(2), 95–98.

Barton, J., & Sibai, B. (2004). Diagnosis and management of hemolysis, elevated liver enzymes, and low platelets syndrome. *Clinics in Perinatology, 31*(4), 807–833.

Barton, J., Witlin, A., & Sibai, B. (1999). Management of mild pre-eclampsia. *Clinical Obstetrics and Gynecology, 42,* 455–469.

Baskett, T. (1999). *Essential management of obstetric emergencies* (3rd ed.). Bristol: Clinical Press Ltd.

Beckmann, C. (2002). A descriptive study of women's perceptions of their asthma during pregnancy. *Journal of Maternal–Child Nursing, 27*(2), 98–102.

Belej-Rak, T., Okun, N., Windrim, R., Ross, S., & Hannah, M. E. (2003). Effectiveness of cervical cerclage for a sonographically shortened cervix: A systematic review and meta analysis. *American Journal of Obstetrics and Gynecology, 189*(6), 1679–1687.

Blackburn, S. T. (2003). *Maternal, fetal and neonatal physiology: A clinical perspective* (2nd ed.). St. Louis: Saunders.

Blaiss, M. (2004). Managing asthma during pregnancy: The whys and hows of aggressive control. *Postgraduate Medicine, 115*(5), 55–65.

Bodnar, L., Cogswell, M., & McDonald, T. (2005). Have we forgotten the significance of postpartum iron deficiency? *American Journal of Obstetrics and Gynecology, 193,* 36–44.

Boonpongmanee, C., Zauszniewski, J. A., & Morris, D. L. (2003). Resourcefulness and self-care in pregnant women with HIV. *Western Journal of Nursing Research, 25*(1), 75–92.

Bridges, E., Womble, S., Wallace, M., & McCartney, J. (2003). Hemodynamic monitoring in high-risk obstetrics patients. II. Pregnancy-induced hypertension and preeclampsia. *Critical Care Nurse, 23,* 52–56.

Burdge, D. R., Money, D. M., Forbes, J. C., Walmsley, S. L., Smaill, F. M., Boucher, M., et al. (2003). Canadian consensus guidelines for the management of pregnancy, labour and delivery and for postpartum care in HIV-positive pregnant women and their offspring (summary of 2002 guidelines). *Canadian Medical Association Journal, 168*(13), 1671–1674.

Butterworth, P. (2004). Lone mothers' experience of physical and sexual violence: Association with psychiatric disorders. *British Journal of Psychiatry, 184,* 21–27.

Cannon, R., Schmidt, J., Cambardella, B., & Browne, S. (2000). High-risk pregnancy in the workplace: Influencing positive outcomes. *American Association of Occupational Health Nursing, 48,* 435–446.

Carter, S. (1999). Overview of common obstetric bleeding disorders. *Nurse Practitioner, 24,* 50–73.

Casanova, B., Sammel, M., & Macones, G. (2005). Development of a clinical prediction rule for iron deficiency anemia in pregnancy. *American Journal of Obstetrics and Gynecology 193,* 460–466.

Centers for Disease Control and Prevention. (2005a). Early-onset and late-onset neonatal group B streptococcal disease—United States, 1996–2004. *MMWR: Morbidity and Mortality Weekly Report, 54*(47), 1205–1208.

Centers for Disease Control and Prevention. (2005b). Rubella. Retrieved April 6, 2006, from http://www.cdc.org.

Cesario, S. K. (2003). Obesity in pregnancy: What every nurse needs to know. *AWHONN Lifelines, 7*(2), 118–125.

Chandran, L., Navaie-Waliser, M., Zulqarni, N. J., Batra, S., Bavir, H., Shah, M., & Lincoln, P. P. (2001). Compliance with group B streptococcal disease prevention guidelines. *MCN—American Journal of Maternal Child Nursing, 26*(6), 313–319.

Cheyne, H., & McQueen, J. (1999). Care of the woman with hypertension in pregnancy: The viewpoint of the midwife. *Bailliere's Clinical Obstetrics and Gynaecology, 13,* 107–113.

Chichester, M. (2005). Multicultural issues in perinatal loss. *AWHONN Lifelines, 9*(4), 312–320.

Chobanian, A., Bakris, G., Black, H., Cushman, W., Green, L., Izzo, J., et al. (2003). Seventh report of the Joint National Committee on Prevention, Evaluation and Treatment of High Blood Pressure. *Hypertension, 42,* 1206.

Comley, L., & Mousmanis, P. (2003). *Improving the odds: Healthy child development.* Toronto: Ontario College of Family Physicians.

Cunningham, E. (2001). Coping with bed rest: Moving toward research-based nursing interventions. *AWHONN Lifelines, 5,* 51–55.

Damato, E. (2000). Maternal–fetal attachment in twin pregnancies. *Journal of Obstetric, Gynecologic, and Neonatal Nursing, 29,* 598–605.

Damato, E. G., & Winnen, C. W. (2002). Cytomegalovirus infection: Perinatal implications. *Journal of Obstetric, Gynecologic, and Neonatal Nursing, 31*(1), 86–92.

Deuchar, N. (2000). The psychological and social aspects of nausea and vomiting of pregnancy. In G. Koren & R. Bishai (Eds.), *Nausea and vomiting of pregnancy: State of the art 2000* (pp. 10–14). Toronto: Motherisk, Hospital for Sick Children.

Dietch, K., & Bunney, B. (2002). The "silent" disease: Diagnosing and treating depression in women. *AWHONN Lifelines, 6,* 140–145.

Ellings, J., Newman, R., & Bowers, N. (1998). Intrapartum care for women with multiple pregnancy. *Journal of Obstetrical and Neonatal Nursing, 27*(4), 466–472.

Fowles, E. (2002). Comparing pregnant women's nutritional knowledge to their actual dietary intake. *Journal of Maternal–Child Nursing, 27,* 171–177.

Galtier-Dereure, F., Boegner, C. & Bringer, J. (2000). Obesity and pregnancy: Complications and cost. *American Journal of Clinical Nutrition, 71*(5), 1242S–1248S.

Geiter, H. (2003). Disseminated intravascular coagulopathy. *Dimensions of Critical Care Nursing, 22,* 108–114.

Gilbert, E., & Harmon, J. (2003). *Manual of high-risk pregnancy and delivery* (3rd ed.). St. Louis: Mosby.

Goff, M. (2005). Parvovirus B19 in pregnancy. *Journal of Midwifery and Women's Health, 50*(6), 536–538.

Gupton, A., Heaman, M., & Cheung, L. (2001). Complicated and uncomplicated pregnancies: Women's perception of risk. *Journal of Obstetric, Gynecologic, and Neonatal Nursing, 30,* 192–201.

Hayward, K. (2003). Cobedding of twins: A natural extension of the socialization process. *Journal of Maternal–Child Nursing, 28,* 260–263.

Health Canada. (1999). *A handbook for health and social service professionals responding to abuse during pregnancy.* Retrieved March 3, 2003, from http://www.hc-sc.gc.ca/hppb/familyviolence/html/femexpose_e.html.

Healy, A. J., & Gaddipati, S. (2005). Intrapartum management of twins: Truths and controversies. *Clinics in Perinatology, 32*(2), 455–473.

Hobbins, D. (2004). Survivors of childhood sexual abuse: Implications for perinatal nursing care. *Journal of Obstetric, Gynecologic, and Neonatal Nursing, 33*(4), 485–497.

Jasinski, J. (2004). Pregnancy and domestic violence: A review of the literature. *Trauma, Violence and Abuse, 5,* 47–64.

Jonas-Simpson, C., & McMahon, E. (2005). The language of loss. When a baby dies prior to birth: Cocreating human experience. *Nursing Science Quarterly, 18*(2), 124–130.

Katz, A. (2004). Neonatal HIV infection. *Neonatal Network, 23*(1), 15–20.

Keating-Lefler, R., & Wilson, M. (2004). The experience of becoming a mother for single, unpartnered, Medicaid-eligible, first-time mothers. *Journal of Nursing Scholarship, 36,* 23–29.

Kidner, M. C., & Flanders-Stepans, M. B. (2004). A model for the HELLP syndrome: The maternal experience. *Journal of Obstetric, Gynecologic, and Neonatal Nursing, 33,* 44–53.

Kirkham, C., Harris, S., & Grzybowski, S. (2005). Evidence-based prenatal care. I. General prenatal care and counseling. *American Family Physician, 71*(7), 1307–1316.

Kozak, S. (2002). *Diabetes: Antepartum, intrapartum, postpartum and newborn nursing care. A self-directed learning module.* Vancouver, BC: Women's Hospital.

Kwon, H., Belanger, K., & Bracken, M. (2004). Effect of pregnancy and stage of pregnancy on asthma severity: A systematic review. *American Journal of Obstetrics and Gynecology, 190,* 1201–1210.

Kuczkowski, K. M. (2004). Labor analgesia for the parturient with cardiac disease: What does the obstetrician need to know? *Acta Obstetricia et Gynecologica Scandinavica, 83,* 223–233.

Kumar, S., & O'Brien, A. (2004). Recent developments in fetal medicine. *British Medical Journal, 328,* 1002–1006.

Lawrence, R. A., & Lawrence, R. M. (2005). *Breast-feeding: A guide for the medical profession* (6th ed.). St. Louis: Mosby.

Little, L., & Lowkes, E. (2000). Critical issues in the care of pregnant women with eating disorders and the impact on their children. *Journal of Midwifery and Women's Health, 45*(4), 301–307.

Luke, B. (2005). The evidence linking maternal nutrition and prematurity. *Journal of Perinatal Medicine, 33,* 500–505.

Lupton, M., Oteng-Ntim, E., Ayida, G., & Steer, P. (2002). Cardiac disease in pregnancy. *Current Opinion in Obstetrics and Gynecology, 14,* 137–143.

Lurie, S., Feinstein, M., & Mamet, Y. (2000). Disseminated intravascular coagulopathy in pregnancy: Thorough comprehension of etiology and management reduces obstetricians' stress. *Archives of Gynecology and Obstetrics, 263*(3), 126–130.

Magann, E., & Martin, J. (1999). Twelve steps to optimal management of HELLP syndrome. *Clinical Obstetrics and Gynecology, 42,* 532–550.

Malcus, P. (2004). Antenatal fetal surveillance. *Current Opinion in Obstetrics and Gynecology, 16,* 123–128.

Maloni, J., Brezinski-Tomasi, J., & Johnson, L. (2001). Antepartum bed rest: Effect upon the family. *Journal of Obstetric, Gynecologic, and Neonatal Nursing, 30,* 165–173.

Mariano, C., & Hickey, R. (1998). Multiple pregnancy, multiple needs. *Canadian Nurse, 94*(9):26–30.

Martin, S., & Foley, M. (2003). Adult-onset heart disease in pregnancy. *Patient Care for the Nurse Practitioner, 2,* 1–16.

Mason, B., & Bobrowski, R. (1998). High risk pregnancy. *Contemporary Ob/Gyn.* Retrieved August 11, 2003, from http: 80-obgyn. pdr.net.proxy.lib.uwo.ca: 2048.

Mazzotta, P., Magee, L., Maltepe, C., Lifshitz, A., Navioz, Y., & Koran G. (2000). The perception of teratogenic risk by women with nausea and vomiting of pregnancy. In G. Koren & R. Bishai (Eds.), *Nausea and vomiting of pregnancy: State of the art 2000* (pp. 157–172). Toronto: Motherisk, Hospital for Sick Children.

Mercer, B. (2004). Preterm premature rupture of the membranes: Diagnosis and management. *Clinics in Perinatology, 31,* 765–782.

Mian, P. (2000). The role of the clinical nurse specialist in the development of a domestic violence program. *Clinical Nurse Specialist, 14,* 229–234.

Michon, B., Balkou, S., Hivon, R., & Cyr, C. (2003). Death of a child: Parental perception of grief intensity—end of life and bereavement care. *Pediatric Child Health Journal, 8,* 363–366.

Mitchell-Gieleghem, A., Mittelstaedt, M. E., & Bulik, C. M. (2002). Eating disorders and childbearing: Concealment and consequences. *Birth, 29*(3), 182–191.

Montan, S. (2004). Drugs used in hypertensive diseases in pregnancy. *Current Opinion in Obstetrics and Gynecology, 16*(2), 111–115.

Montoya, J., & Liesenfeld, O. (2004). Toxoplasmosis. *Lancet, 363,* 1965–1976.

National Institute of Health and National Asthma Education and Prevention Program Working Group. (2004). Managing asthma during pregnancy: Recommendations for pharmacologic treatment. Retrieved March 1, 2006, from http://www.nhlbi.nih.gov/health/prof/lung/asthma/astpreg/astpreg_qr.pdf.

Neinstein, L., & Farmer, M. (2004). Teenage pregnancy. In L. Neinstein (Ed.), *Adolescent health care: A practical guide* (4th ed.). Philadelphia: Lippincott Williams & Wilkins.

O'Brien, B., Evans, M., & White-McDonald, E. (2002). Isolation from "being alive": Coping with severe nausea and vomiting of pregnancy. *Nursing Research, 51,* 302–308.

Padden, M. O. (1999). HELLP syndrome: Recognition and perinatal management. *American Family Physician.* Retrieved March 3, 2004, from http://www.aafp.org/afp/990901ap/829.html.

Palmer, C. (2002). Obstetric emergencies and anesthetic management. *Current Reviews for Perianesthesia Nurses, 24,* 121–132.

Patrick, T., & Roberts, J. (1999). Current concepts in preeclampsia. *Journal of Maternal–Child Nursing, 24,* 193–201.

Poole, J. (1997). Aggressive management of HELLP syndrome and eclampsia. *American Association of Critical-Care Nurses Clinical Issues, 8,* 524–538.

Ramsey, P., Kirk, D., & Ramin, S. (2001). Cardiac disease in pregnancy. *American Journal of Perinatology, 18,* 245–265.

Rentschler, D. (2003). Pregnant adolescents' perspectives of pregnancy. *Journal of Maternal–Child Nursing, 28,* 378–382.

Royal College of Obstetricians and Gynaecologists. (2002). *Clinical guidelines for tubal pregnancies.* London: Author.

Schatz, M., Dambrowski, M. Wise, R., Thom, E., Landon, M., Mabie, W., et al. (2003). Asthma morbidity during pregnancy can be predicted by severity classification. *Journal of Allergy and Clinical Immunology, 112*(2), 283–288.

Scholl, T. (2005). Iron status during pregnancy: Setting the stage for mother and infant. *American Journal of Clinical Nutrition, 8,* 1218S–1222S.

Sibai, B. & Chames, M. (2003). Hypertension in pregnancy: Tailoring treatment to risk. *OBG Management, 15*(7).

Silver, R., & Branch, D. (1997). Autoimmune disease in pregnancy: Systemic lupus erythematosus and antiphospholipid syndrome. *Clinics in Perinatology, 24,* 291–320.

Siu, S., Sermer, M., Colman, J., Alvarez, A., Mercier, L., Morton, B., et al. (2001). Prospective multicenter study of pregnancy outcomes in women with heart disease. *Circulation, 104,* 515–521.

Society of Obstetricians and Gynaecologists of Canada (SOGC). (2000). Management of twin pregnancies (Parts I & II). *Journal of Obstetricians and Gynecologists of Canada, 91,* 519–526, 607–610.

Society of Obstetricians and Gynaecologists of Canada (SOGC). (2002). The management of nausea and vomiting of pregnancy. *Journal of Obstetricians and Gynecologists in Canada, 24,* 817–823.

Terkildsen, M., Parilla, B., Kumar, P., & Grobman, W. (2003). Factors associated with success of emergent second-trimester cerclage. *Obstetrics and Gynecology, 101,* 565–569.

Thomas, D. (2001). Sexually transmitted viral infections: Epidemiology and treatment. *Journal of Obstetric, Gynecologic, and Neonatal Nursing, 30,* 316–323.

Thorsen, M., & Poole, J. (2002). Renal disease in pregnancy. *Journal of Perinatal and Neonatal Nursing, 15,* 13–29.

Usta, I., Hobeika, E., Musa, A., Gabriel, G., & Nassar, A. (2005). Placenta previa-accreta: Risk factors and complications. *American Journal of Obstetrics and Gynecology, 193,* 1045–1049.

Von Dadelszen, P. (2000). The etiology of nausea and vomiting of pregnancy. In G. Koren & R. Bishai (Eds.), *Nausea and vomiting of pregnancy: State of the art 2000* (pp. 5–9). Toronto: Motherisk, Hospital for Sick Children.

Watson-Blasioli, J. (2001). Double-take: Defining the need for specialized prenatal care for women expecting twins: A Canadian perspective. *AWHONN Lifelines, 5,* 34–42.

Watts, N. (2004). Screening for domestic violence: A team approach for maternal/newborn nurses. *AWHONN Lifelines, 8,* 210–219.

Weitz, B. (1999). Premature rupture of the fetal membranes: An update for advanced practice nurses. *Journal of Maternal–Child Nursing, 26,* 86–92.

White, A. (2003). Parvovirus B19 infection in pregnancy. *Perinatal Outreach Program of Southwestern Ontario, 25.*

Williams, M., & Iams, J. (2004). Cervical length measurement and cervical cerclage to prevent preterm birth. *Clinical Obstetrics and Gynecology, 47*(4), 775–783.

Yonkers, K., Wisner, K., Stowe, Z., Leibenluft, E., Cohen, L., Miller, L., et al. (2004). Management of bipolar disorder during pregnancy and the postpartum period. *American Journal of Psychiatry, 161,* 608–620.

Youngkin, E., & Davis, M. (2004). *Women's health: A primary care clinical guide* (3rd ed.). Upper Saddle River, NJ: Pearson Education.

Zach, T., & Pramanik, A. (2004). Multiple births. *eMedicine.* [On-line]. Available at: http://www.emedicine.com.

Zhang, W., & Chen, S. (2003). An overview on systemic lupus erythematosus pregnancy. *Modern Rheumatology, 13,* 293–300.

Zwelling, E., & Phillips, C. (2001). Family-centered maternity care in the new millennium: Is it real or is it imagined? *Journal of Perinatal and Neonatal Nursing, 15,* 1–12.

CHAPTER 14

Educational Preparation for Pregnancy, Childbirth, and Parenthood

Barbara Hotelling

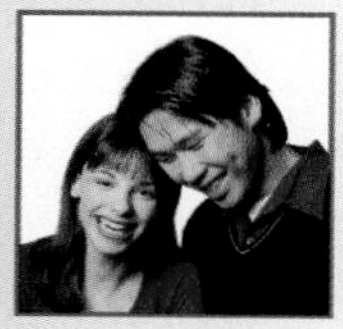

Belinda, 29 years old, comes to the community health center for a prenatal visit at 14 weeks' gestation with her first pregnancy. She mentions that she and her husband have been talking about labor and birth. Belinda states, "He thinks we should have 'natural childbirth,' but I might want an epidural. I don't want to be in pain. People are constantly telling me horror stories about labor."

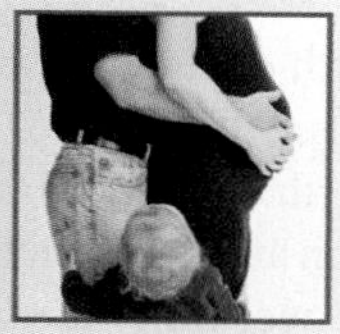

Clarice, now at 22 weeks' gestation, comes to the clinic for a prenatal visit. Her partner of 7 years, Joel, accompanies her. During the visit, Clarice and Joel mention that their 3-year-old son has been acting out lately. "This all started right after we told him we were expecting another baby," they report.

You will learn more about these stories later in this chapter. Nurses working with such clients need to understand the content here to manage care and address issues appropriately. Before beginning, consider the following points related to the above scenarios:

- What areas related to childbirth education need to be considered for each client? What types of teaching programs might be helpful for Belinda? For Clarice?
- How might each client's circumstances influence the nurse's approach to care?
- How are the scenarios similar? How are they different?
- What details will the nurse need to investigate with Belinda? What about Clarice?
- What methods of follow-up evaluation might the nurse want to consider for each client?

LEARNING OBJECTIVES

Upon completion of this chapter, the reader should be able to:

- Describe the relationship between childbirth preparation and health promotion for women, infants, children, and general society.
- Summarize the evolution of childbirth education from past women's networks to today's formal classes.
- Explore different theoretical approaches to childbirth preparation.
- Identify specific types of childbirth preparation classes and their areas of focus and emphasis.
- Describe the influences fear, pain, and control can have over a client's preferences for labor and birth preferences.
- Explain collaborative care approaches to educating parents throughout the childbearing cycle.

KEY TERMS

certified nurse-midwife (CNM)	Mother-Friendly Childbirth Initiative
doula	psychoprophylaxis
hypnobirthing	twilight sleep
midwife	holistic
normal birth	

Childbirth education is an important vehicle of health promotion for women, infants, and families. The pendulum has swung over a period of approximately 300 years from information about pregnancy, birth, parenting, and breastfeeding being supplied woman-to-woman, to being given by physicians to women in an authoritative, "medicalized" fashion, to today's environment that combines aspects of both models. The pendulum also has swung between women's desire for natural birth and anesthetized birth.

Is birth a pathologic event or normal physiology? Does childbirth education provide parents with the information they need to make careful choices about how they give birth, or is it merely preparation for a medicalized labor? Who controls decisions about how a woman gives birth—the mother herself, her health care attendants, or other people? Answers to these questions vary depending on the provider of childbirth education, the client's previous pregnancy experiences, and the information a society sends about pain during labor. Control in birth is an issue with significant ramifications because research has shown a significant relationship between a woman's perception of such control during labor and her ongoing ability to integrate the birth experience and assume care for her newborn (Simkin, 1991, 1996).

This chapter explores childbirth education. It considers the history of such preparation and the evolution of different methods and approaches over time. It explains the importance and roles of various types of classes and common themes encountered. The chapter also explores the role of nurses and other health care providers and ways they can best assist clients and families with instruction, decision making, and role adjustments.

CHILDBIRTH EDUCATION

Childbirth education has been a consistent, powerful health promotion tool for women, children, and families since the earliest classes in maternal hygiene, nutrition, and baby care (Nichols & Humenick, 2000). Pregnancy, for many parents, is a teachable moment. For example, as an expectant mother bonds with her fetus, she may be willing to change risky behaviors for the sake of her future child. She may become more careful about her diet and try harder to choose foods and beverages that optimize fetal growth and health, even if these selections are not her usual preferences (Fig. 14.1). She may consult her health care provider before taking any over-the-counter medications. She may quit smoking. Exercise may become part of her daily routine, or she may begin to develop networks with others who want to discuss childbirth. Such lifestyle changes may be beyond and better than what she normally would do if she were concerned only with her own welfare.

Extending health promotion improvements to more pregnant women and across many sociocultural groups is an important consideration for health care providers, particularly within the context of recent data from the National Center for Health Statistics (NCHS). Current findings show U.S. life expectancy to be longer than ever before; however, the infant mortality rate increased from 6.8 deaths per 1000 live births in 2001 to 7 deaths per 1000 live births in 2002 (NCHS, 2005). This increase in infant fatalities is the first time since 1958 that this rate did not decline or remain unchanged (NCHS, 2005). Although many factors may have contributed to the higher incidence of infant deaths, a concern exists that pregnant women are not doing enough to preserve and promote their own as well as fetal health. As stated in *Healthy People 2010,* "the health of mothers, infants, and children is of critical importance, both as a reflection of the current health status of a large segment of the U.S. population and as a predictor of the health of the next generation" (U.S. Department of Health and Human Services [U.S. DHHS], 2000).

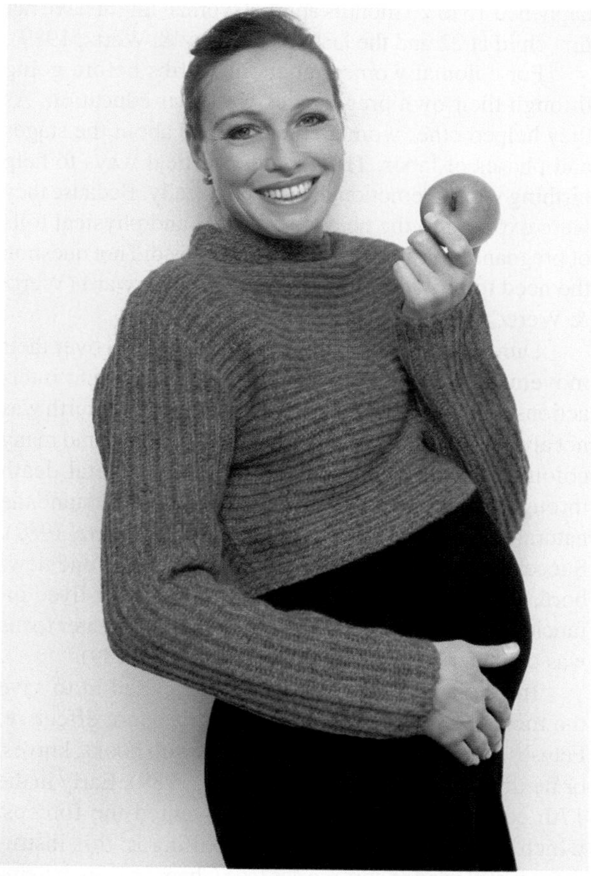

FIGURE 14.1 Pregnancy has been called a "teachable" moment. Many women are motivated to make healthier choices when they are expecting because of the direct effects of their decisions on their fetus.

Childbirth education can contribute significantly to the promotion of healthy lifestyles. People who take prenatal classes receive extensive information about nutritional and fluid needs during pregnancy, exercise suited to lifestyle and preferences, smoking cessation, stress management, dangerous medications and street drugs, ways to foster healthy relationships, and the importance of avoiding alcohol. Expectant parents who begin classes as early as the first trimester can initiate health-promoting behaviors sooner and improve their chances of giving birth to a full-term, adequately nourished infant who experiences minimal fetal stress.

The prevention of preterm birth is currently a major focus of many health-oriented organizations and programs, such as the March of Dimes (Table 14.1). From 1993 to 2003, the U.S. rate of preterm birth increased nearly 12% (March of Dimes, 2005). Lifestyle and environmental factors that increase the risk for preterm labor and birth include receiving late or no prenatal care, smoking, drinking alcohol, using illegal drugs, being exposed to diethylstilbestrol (DES), experiencing domestic violence (including physical, sexual, or emotional abuse), lacking social support, being under excessive stress, and working long hours with long periods of standing (March of Dimes, 2005). Animal studies have shown the adverse effects of stress on pregnancy outcomes. Stressed animals have a higher incidence of preterm birth and low infant birth weight. In humans, stress contributes to increased risky behaviors such as smoking, drinking alcohol, and using drugs (Wirth, 2001). Childbirth education provides women and their families with the information they need to motivate them toward healthier lifestyles and provides a supportive environment that encourages positive lifestyle changes.

QUOTE 14-1

"One of the best things that happened when I became pregnant was that it forced me to really think about the choices I was making relative to health, diet, and exercise. I adopted so many behaviors that were easy to ignore when I was thinking only of myself."

From an expectant parent

Ideally, the decision to become a parent is made consciously and within an environment that incorporates holistic, health-promoting, and empowering childbirth education. Additionally, such education is rooted in collaborative communication and targeted toward relevant

● **TABLE 14.1 Statistical Analysis of Preterm and Low-Birth-Weight Outcomes in the United States**

UNITED STATES STATISTICS	1993	2003	HEALTHY PEOPLE 2010 OBJECTIVES
Preterm	11.0%	12.3%	7.6%
Low birth weight	7.2%	7.9%	5.0%

From March of Dimes. (2005). Born too soon and too small in the United States. March of Dimes Birth Defects Foundation. Retrieved November 1, 2005, from http://www.marchofdimes.com/peristats.

times during conception, pregnancy, birth, and postpartum. An example would be information about nutrition during these different stages. For the woman seeking conception, midwives or nurses counseling her would focus teaching on ensuring that nutrient intake optimizes a healthy fetal environment and maintains or improves maternal health. They would emphasize the importance of folic acid supplementation, which can prevent fetal neural tube defects (Charles et al., 2005). During pregnancy, nutrition teaching likely would emphasize dietary measures to combat nausea, boost the immune system, and protect maternal iron stores. For women who plan to breastfeed, education also would focus on measures to promote an optimal milk supply. In the postpartum period, teaching would center on the chosen newborn feeding method, nutritional strategies to help the woman's body adjust to the nonpregnant state, and ways to obtain extra energy and nutrients needed for the demanding requirements of childrearing. At each phase, health care providers and other educators should communicate with one another to ensure that information is coordinated, accurate, and consistent. A unified approach assists clients to internalize health-promoting behaviors that can benefit families for a lifetime.

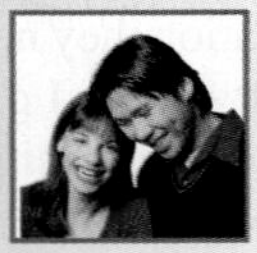

Recall Belinda, the woman at 14 weeks' gestation described at the beginning of the chapter. What specific areas would the nurse need to address to help guide Belinda and her husband in their decisions about childbirth?

Historical Perspectives

Women have a tradition lasting for centuries of educating one another about pregnancy and methods of participation in labor and birth. Sheila Kitzinger describes it as "the women's network" (Nolan, 1997), by which women learn about birth and baby care from their mothers, sisters, and female relatives. The following paragraphs explore the evolution of childbirth education in the United States from colonial times to the present.

Colonial America

English settlers brought "social birth" to colonial America (Wertz & Wertz, 1989). Birth was the exclusive province of women, who aided one another during labor and throughout the postpartum *lying-in* period of 3 to 4 weeks. Female relatives and friends provided continuous emotional and physical support to mother and newborn, whereas midwives provided skilled care. The lying-in period gave the mother time to rest, regain strength, and successfully nurse and care for her baby without interruption. Extended childbearing was the norm. Births usually happened 15 to 20 months apart; a woman might have her first child at 22 and the last at 40 (Wertz & Wertz, 1989).

For colonial women, attending births before going through their own pregnancies was their education. As they helped other women, they learned about the stages and phases of labor. They found practical ways to help birthing women emotionally and physically. Because they were exposed to the heavy emotional and physical tolls of pregnancy, birth, and childrearing, they did not question the need to provide support for weeks afterward (Wertz & Wertz, 1989).

During labor, colonial women had control over their movement, nutrition, hydration, positioning, and interactions with their newborns. Nevertheless, childbirth was not always joyful. Antibiotics were unavailable, and many colonial mothers anticipated their own or fetal death throughout pregnancy. They did not fully understand the natural processes of birth and pain (Wertz & Wertz, 1989). Successful childbirth meant survival of mother and newborn. Many stillbirths, miscarriages, and short-lived infancies went unrecorded, suggesting that the greater focus was on maternal survival (Wertz & Wertz, 1989).

In England, surgeons were being called in to save the mother's life when vaginal birth was not effective. Fetuses were extracted from the uterus with hooks, knives, or flexible materials (Wertz & Wertz, 1989). Early in the 17th century, Peter Chamberlen invented the forceps, which removed the fetus without killing it; this instrument is still used in some cases (see Chap. 16). Such items were the possession of the creator and not necessarily shared. For example, the Chamberlens kept forceps exclusively within their own family for more than 100 years.

Colonial physicians lacked prestige and authority, and midwives attended most births. Nevertheless, men who had received medical training in Europe came back to the colonies with new talents and knowledge to help laboring women and were eager to use these skills to enhance their importance within the community. For example, during the 1700s and 1800s, Parisian surgeons and midwives worked together in hospital-schools to understand birth and learn how best to assist difficult labors. They trained colonial physicians in what was called *male midwifery.* When these physicians returned to the colonies with advanced empiric knowledge, women began choosing them over existing midwives (Wertz & Wertz, 1989).

1800s to Early 1900s

Throughout the 18th and 19th centuries, social birth began to fade, making emotional and physical support for laboring women less available. The change to medicalized physician-led birth also was a product of a shift in childbirth setting from home to hospital. Before the 1800s, hospitals mainly cared for poor, homeless, or working-class married women giving birth (Wertz & Wertz, 1989). Those who labored in hospitals were commonly exposed to infections. Oliver Wendell Holmes was the first U.S. physician to identify puerperal fever as an infection transmitted by doctors. He published his findings in 1843, asking "doctors to cease practice when they or their patients became ill" (Wertz & Wertz, 1989, p. 121). Not until the mid-1880s did Dr. Ignaz Philipp Semmelweiss, a Hungarian doctor, demonstrate statistically that puerperal fever was contagious and could be prevented through antiseptic means (Wertz & Wertz, 1989). As a result, hospitals became safer, and laboring women of all classes began going to them.

In 1900, approximately 90% of births occurred at home. By 1979, 99% of births took place in hospitals (Zwelling, 1996). Physicians had assumed much control over information about birth. Friends and relatives were not primary sources of information; they could no longer regularly provide support for laboring and birthing women. With the shift toward hospitalized birth, childbirth education all but disappeared. It was kept alive by the relatively small number of women who could not afford birth in the hospital and were attended by other women at home.

Anesthesia for Childbirth

Women began choosing anesthesia to deal with the painful, lonely hospital birth experience. The first U.S. administration of obstetric ether was in 1847. That same year James Young Simpson, Chair of Midwifery at the University of Edinburgh's School of Medicine, administered diethyl ether to a laboring patient. This use of anesthesia in birth received much criticism. Medical authorities recognized the potency of ether and feared its effects on both mother and newborn. "Childbirth," they said, "is a physiologic process best managed with the least possible interference" (Caton et al., 2002, p. S25). Physicians who used ether or chloroform found these anesthetics difficult to administer and time-consuming (Caton et al., 2002). Slowly, anesthetics that were easier to administer emerged.

The Twilight Sleep Movement

In 1902, a method of amnesic-analgesia called *Dammerschlaf* combined scopolamine and morphine and was delivered through the recently developed hypodermic syringe (Pitcock & Clark, 1992). Women were kept in darkened rooms with quiet nurses protecting their amnesic state. The goal was for the mother to remember nothing of labor's physical discomforts. This popular method came to be known in the United States as **twilight sleep.**

Feminists contributed to the demand for wider availability of twilight sleep. Many women were eager to embrace any method that modern medicine could employ to protect them against the pain and dangers they associated with labor and childbirth (Bing, 2000). Rallies of the Twilight Sleep Association in major cities were successful in forcing physicians to provide this form of analgesia (Pitcock & Clark, 1992). Use of this method began to dwindle, however, with reports of dangerous delays in newborn respirations associated with this method. The final blow to twilight sleep came from the sudden death of one of its most visible advocates, Frances X. Carmody, in a twilight sleep birth (Pitcock & Clark, 1992). Despite the disappearance of twilight sleep, messages persisted that women did not have to suffer in childbirth and that freedom from labor pain was healthy. "American and English feminists included better obstetric care and anesthesia as part of their campaign for women's rights" (Caton et al., 2002).

Modern Approaches to Childbirth

After World War II, women began to seek consciousness, control, dignity, and companionship in birth. Natural birth activists in England, Russia, and France were conducting research to demonstrate the concept that pain could be deconditioned and a new response to it could be created (Nichols & Humenick, 2000). Theories that began at this time are still in vogue today and form the basis of many childbirth education programs used internationally.

Dick-Read

In the 1940s, Grantley Dick-Read, an English obstetrician, was attending a birth and offered the mother chloroform as the fetal head began to crown. The mother rejected the medication. When Dick-Read asked her later about the refusal, she replied, "It didn't hurt. It wasn't meant to, was it, doctor?" (Rothman, 1991). In 1944, Dick-Read published *Childbirth Without Fear,* addressing the **holistic** nature of childbirth, in which the mind and body are connected. Dick-Read posited that the basic cause of labor pain was fear that produced tension. By educating pregnant women in physical exercise, relaxation, and breathing, Dick-Read believed that the fear–tension–pain cycle could be broken. Creating healthy bodies and attitudes in advance would prepare laboring women to deal with the strong physical sensations of childbirth (Nichols & Humenick, 2002).

Psychoprophylaxis

In Russia, Erofeeva based research loosely on Pavlov's experiments showing the mind–body connection in response to pain. Velvosky's trial-and-error experiments emphasized prevention of pain through psychological strategies rather than chemicals. This stimulated Nikolayev to name the training method **psychoprophylaxis** (Ondeck, 2000). He emphasized controlled breathing, abdominal stroking, and applying pressure points on the hip and back to manage pain without pharmacology.

In 1959, Elisabeth Bing and Marjorie Karmel began providing psychoprophylactic classes to other women. Together, they started the first childbirth education organization, the American Society for Psychoprophylaxis in Obstetrics (ASPO) (Bing, 2000). This group sought to bring together noninterventionist obstetricians interested in reducing the use of analgesia and anesthesia during childbirth, parents who wanted more control over labor, and educators who wanted to make psychoprophylaxis accessible. At the same time, the Maternity Center Association convened local consumer groups for the purposes of "parents and professionals working together to provide parents with the knowledge of alternatives to make an informed choice" (Nichols & Humenick, 2000).

Lamaze

Fernand Lamaze visited Nikolayev's clinic in 1951 and brought the psychoprophylactic method of childbirth to Western Europe. It was in the Parisian Lamaze clinic that Marjorie Karmel (see earlier discussion) learned about psychoprophylaxis and used it successfully with her first childbirth. When she and her husband returned to the United States, she sought a physician who would help her have the same satisfying and safe experience she had had with Lamaze. With great difficulty, she managed to have another fulfilling birth, using medication only as requested (Karmel, 1981).

In 1908, the American Red Cross launched prenatal classes that focused on maternal hygiene, nutrition, and baby care (Ondeck, 2000). These classes were the mainstay of childbirth education until the 1960s, with the founding of ASPO/Lamaze and the International Childbirth Education Association (ICEA). As discussed, ASPO/Lamaze was an organization of parents, professionals, and providers, whereas the ICEA began as a federation of local groups focused on creating a consumer-based organization to improve maternity services (Ondeck, 2000). Subsequent childbirth education organizations focused on reform and alternatives to medicalized practices. In the 1970s, the National Association of Parents and Professionals for Safe Alternatives in Childbirth (NAPSAC) promoted the demedicalization of childbirth. Robert Bradley, a Denver obstetrician, promoted nonmedicated birth and the need for fathers to serve as active coaches for laboring and birthing women (Ondeck, 2000).

COMMON THEMES IN CHILDBIRTH EDUCATION AND PREPARATION

When women and their families are getting ready for childbirth, themes of fear, concern over pain, and desire for control are common and tend to recur. This has been true throughout history. As discussed, early preparation for birth was not formalized but consisted of the passing of information from one woman to another (Zwelling, 1996). First-hand education occurred by women attending other births. Nevertheless, the absence of antibiotics and appropriate measures of infection control resulted directly in legitimate and widespread fears of maternal or fetal demise. "References to feelings of joy and ecstasy in giving birth are absent from women's diaries throughout the colonial period. A woman who bore and reared seven or eight children, several of whom were likely to die, while carrying on the tasks of farm life, perhaps found the word 'joy' inappropriate even for an easy birth" (Wertz & Wertz, 1989, p. 20). By the 20th century, research into the physiology and psychology of pain grew to include inquiry into the relationships between pain perception and culture, spirituality, satisfaction in childbirth, expectations, stress, personal control, parity, social class, education, and maternity services.

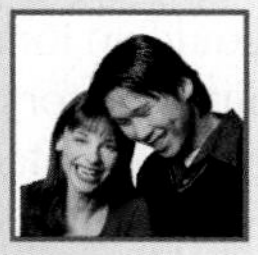

Think back to Belinda, the pregnant woman from the beginning of the chapter who wants to make decisions relative to labor pain management. How does what Belinda currently knows or believes reflect some of the historical influences associated with childbirth education?

Walsh (2001) comments on the strong influence culture can have on a woman's experience of birth pain. Regardless of whether a relief measure is nonpharmacologic or pharmacologic, if it conflicts with the client's belief systems, her perception of the experience and transition to her maternal role may be negatively compromised (Walsh, 2001). Areas in which culture may influence choices include the authority figure in the birthing process, site of birth, level of activity during birth, beliefs about body parts, and reaction to interventions (Walsh, 2001).

Simkin (1991, 1992) found that women remember many details of their birth experiences and that their long-term satisfaction is heavily influenced by their sense of control over what happened, participation in care-related decisions, treatment by attending professionals, sense of accomplishment, and self-esteem. The clinical features of labor, pain, and interventions may be less crucial to the client's satisfaction than are her ability to control the experience, make choices, and be supported by others.

Pain Assessment

In a study of Jordanian women, Abushaikha and Oweis (2005) found a discrepancy between women's experiences of labor pain intensity and the assessment of such pain by their caregivers. Baker and colleagues (2001) found a similar discrepancy in their analysis of Australian mothers' and midwives' pain scores throughout 13 labors and births. This study showed a high correlation between the midwives' and mothers' scores in mild to moderate pain but low correlation relative to severe pain. The researchers concluded that although nonverbal cues are appropriate for pain assessment, interventions may be better mediated by verbal cues. These findings indicate a need for health care providers to focus on both verbal and nonverbal cues to provide a positive childbirth experience (Baker et al., 2001).

In 1997, a joint effort by the University of Wisconsin–Madison Medical School and the Joint Commission on Accreditation of Healthcare Organizations (JCAHO) led to the integration of pain assessment and management into JCAHO standards (Crosby et al., 2002). These standards were developed to recognize each client's right to the assessment and treatment of pain, to monitor the management of pain within each health care organization, and to educate staff and clients about the importance of effective pain management (U.S. Department of Veterans Affairs, 2006). JCAHO required compliance starting 2001 by hospitals, home care agencies, long-term care facilities, behavioral health facilities, outpatient clinics, and health plans to assess pain in all clients, record the results in a way that facilitates regular follow-up, educate relevant providers in pain assessment and management, and establish policies and procedures that support appropriate delivery of pain medications (Crosby et al., 2002). Additionally, the JCAHO standards mandated nurses to assess pain experienced by clients with arthritis, victims of trauma, and laboring women using the same measurement tool. They also required nurses to perform evaluations with supporting documentation at each assessment.

One purpose of the JCAHO standards was to help achieve decreased levels of pain in laboring women. Nevertheless, the existing standards have some basic flaws. Interventions to reduce pain in a trauma victim would not necessarily be effective in reducing pain in a laboring mother. The trauma victim would benefit from rapid pharmacologic treatment, whereas the laboring mother would benefit from nonpharmacologic management that enhances endogenous release of endorphins. For this reason, two nurse birth educators, Amis and Green (2005), developed a tool based on JCAHO recommendations to make pain assessment relevant for laboring women. Using *Assessment of Effective Coping During Labor,* nurses can identify a client's preferences for labor pain management and provide suggestions for nonpharmacologic interventions based on her reported level of pain. See Assessment Tool 14.1.

Research Investigations

In 2002, the results of the first U.S. survey of women's childbearing experiences (*Listening to Mothers)* were released. According to its findings, epidural anesthesia (used by 63% of participants) was rated highest in pain relief of both pharmacologic and nonpharmacologic methods. The next four highest-rated methods included immersion in a pool or tub, showers, and "birth balls" (Fig. 14.2). Four of the five lowest-rated methods included narcotics and breathing techniques (Declercq et al., 2002). Interestingly, the study showed that although many women knew that epidurals provide highly effective pain relief, most remained uninformed about the potential side effects (see Chap. 17). Researchers continue to investigate the most effective method of pain relief causing the fewest complications. A question not frequently addressed is whether labor pain should be eliminated in the first place.

Does labor pain serve a useful purpose? Leap and Anderson (2004) conducted a qualitative study on midwives' attitudes toward pain in childbirth and identified rationales for working with pain rather than fighting or fleeing it:

- Considering the task of the human body in moving the baby from inside to outside, the physiology of pain is normal.
- Pain stops women and allows them to find a place of safety for giving birth.
- The enormity of this transformational occasion requires an unusual behavior pattern for the woman.
- During this time of transition, the physical and emotional characteristics of pain help a woman summon her support systems.
- Pain triggers the mother's altruistic behaviors toward babies.
- The woman experiences pain and joy together in the transition from being pregnant and growing a baby to becoming a mother.

ASSESSMENT TOOL 14.1 Assessment of Effective Coping During Labor

Upon admission, ask the laboring woman about her preferences:
Which of the following best describes your plan for pain management during labor?

_____(a) I would like to have an unmedicated birth. Please do not offer me any type of pain medication. If I decide that I want medication for pain, I will ask for it.
_____(b) I want to see how it goes. I would like to try nonpharmacologic (nondrug) pain management strategies, but I may decide to use pain medications too.
_____(c) I would like to have a small dose of pain medication (narcotic) by injection ("shot") or put into my IV (if I have an IV.)
_____(d) I would like to have epidural analgesia.

During labor, ask the laboring woman how well she feels she is coping with her contractions. Give her a scale of 0 (coping well) to 10 (not coping at all).

Coping Rating	Suggested Nonpharmacologic Nursing Comfort Strategies
0–3 She is coping well.	Encourage her—tell her how well she is doing. Reassure her that labor is going normally; provide reassuring touch to shoulder or hand. Offer to stay with the laboring woman if her labor partner needs a short break. Inform her of options available such as a tub and/or shower.
4–7 She is struggling with her contractions.	If possible, provide continuous support; provide reassuring touch to shoulder or hand. Reassure her that what she is feeling is normal; give her information on her progress. Encourage her—tell her how well she is doing, and try the following to help her more: Modify environment—turn down lights, play music (of her choice). Encourage upright positions. Encourage rhythmic movements such as: • Slow-dancing • Walking • Gently bouncing or swaying on a birth ball • Rocking in a chair Encourage her to try a warm bath or shower. Massage (or show her partner how to) shoulders, back, hands, feet, to help her relax. Provide hot packs (shoulders, back) or cold packs (back, cool cloth to forehead, neck). Encourage her to vocalize during contractions (eg, *I can do it, I can do it*). Add aromatherapy (jasmine or lavender scent in bath water, lotion, or essential oil on a cotton ball). If she is experiencing severe back pain: • Encourage her to try an all-fours position, pelvic tilts. • Encourage her to try the lunge. • Do knee press, counterpressure, double hip squeeze. • Provide hot or cold packs for lower back. • Offer intradermal water block.
8–10 She is overwhelmed, unable to cope effectively with her contractions.	Between contractions, try strategies listed above. Reassure her that you will stay with her to help her. Reassure her that what she is feeling is normal; acknowledge her pain. Have partner, other support person provide counterpressure to back as needed. During contractions, use the "Panic Routine": • Position yourself so that you can have eye-to-eye contact with her. • With permission, place your hands on her shoulders or arms. • Breathe with her to help her establish a rhythm.

Form meets JCAHO requirements. Developed by Debby Amis & Jeanne Green for Lamaze International; may be copied with attribution. Available at www.lamaze.org.

- Pain and the mother's response provide clues to progress for the mother and the midwife.
- Working through pain gives the mother a tremendous sense of accomplishment.
- Pain itself facilitates endorphin release (Leap & Anderson, 2004).

Lowe (2001) has studied the differences between the dominant neurophysiologic model of pain that accompanies tissue trauma and the extremely complex pain rooted in sensory and emotional components. Environment, culture, and previous experiences with pain all lead to an individualized interpretation of nociceptive

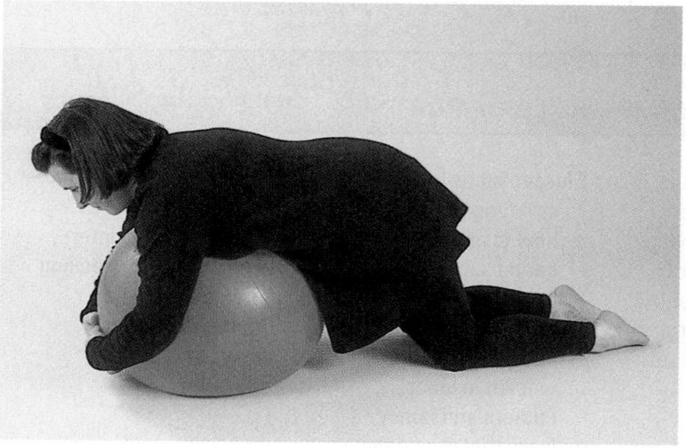

FIGURE 14.2 Some women learn the use of birth balls to help control the pain of labor.

labor stimuli (Lowe, 2001). In a comparative analysis, 61% of Dutch women and 16% of U.S. women in labor received no pain medication; their postpartum ratings of labor pain were similar (Senden et al., 1988). Although the U.S. women in the study expected labor to be more painful, the Dutch participants anticipated birth as a natural process and were less inclined toward interventions (Lowe, 2001).

For nurses attending laboring women, the management of pain is equally important to the way in which women perceive treatment from their health care providers. Simkin (1991, 1992) found that women with positive feelings about their labors and births recalled being well cared for and supported by health care personnel. Up to 20 years later, women with negative feelings associated with childbirth recounted unpleasant and disappointing interactions with hospital staff. Within this context, nurses should never underestimate their ability to increase or diminish a woman's feelings of self-esteem, sense of accomplishment, and overall satisfaction with birth and strive to assist all clients with their transformations to parenthood.

VARIATIONS IN CHILDBIRTH EDUCATION

Childbirth classes today are put forth by various organizations with differing views of the roles of women, partners, and providers. One organization may promote the partner's involvement during labor and birth, whereas another may emphasize deep relaxation on the mother's part alone as the sole method of support. One program may include detailed discussions of birth's physiology, whereas another may emphasize emotional responses to labor. Even when the same organization is involved, information may be quite different in classes taught in home settings rather than in classes taught in hospitals. Educators may complete the same curriculum within a particular organization but differ in approaches because of their own histories with birth, additional education gleaned from workshops or conferences, or cultural or religious backgrounds. Variations may exist related to how much an organization or instructor advocates for parents, attempts to change a facility's policies, or other matters.

Childbirth Education Programs, Providers, and Approaches

Since the 1970s, many organizations have formed to address particular issues in childbirth. Some provide their own classes. For example, Kitzinger's women's network expanded to include fathers, midwives, and doulas. Additionally, programs are evolving to accommodate growing interest in births at home and other alternative settings. The backgrounds of some long-standing methods (eg, Dick-Read, Lamaze) were discussed earlier and are summarized in Table 14.2, which also highlights the characteristics of other common approaches to childbirth education. The following paragraphs explore variations in detail.

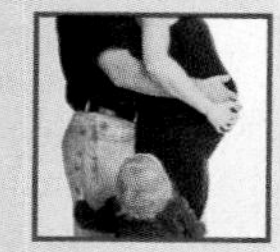

Recall Clarice and her partner Joel from the beginning of the chapter. They reported behavior difficulties with their 3-year-old son that seemed related to Clarice's pregnancy. How might childbirth education benefit this family?

Hypnosis in Labor and Birth

Hypnosis has been found to be a successful pain reduction method of empowering women and their partners during the labor and birth process. Women are educated in the techniques needed to promote a self-trance that alters their perception of reality. Methods may include a series of relaxation techniques consisting of therapeutic suggestions, visualization, and relaxation breathing (Dorothy M. Larkin, October 5, 2006, personal communication). See Box 14.1 on p. 563.

Birthing From Within

Pam England, midwife and artist, founded Birthing From Within to offer a soulful and holistic approach to labor. Expectant couples master a variety of mind-focusing practices that include breath awareness, mindfulness, self-hypnosis, and visualizations; additionally, parents-to-be may explore the wise and compassionate use of drugs and epidurals (Birthing From Within, 2000).

Doulas

In ancient Greek times, the word "doula" meant "slave." Later, it came to describe a woman who goes into the home and assists a new mother by cooking for her, helping with other children, holding the baby, and so forth. She might be a neighbor, a relative, or a friend, and she performs her task voluntarily and on a temporary basis (Raphael, 1976, p. 24). Today, **doula** has come to mean

TABLE 14.2 Common Educational Methods

TYPE	MISSION STATEMENT OR EXPLANATION	ROLE OF WOMAN	ROLE OF PARTNER	ROLE OF PROVIDER
Lamaze	To promote, protect, and support normal birth through education and advocacy (www.lamaze.org)	Women who are fully informed, confident, and supported will want normal birth (Vision Statement, www.lamaze.org).	Classes focus on instructing partners how to provide quiet, gentle support and encouragement and basic comfort measures for most women in labor. Fathers and family learn that their calm, focused presence is the most important thing women need from them (Lamaze International Position Paper: Lamaze for the 21st Century).	Caregivers should respect the physiologic birth process and not intervene without compelling medical indication (Vision statement, www.lamaze.org).
Bradley	Having a baby is an experience that should be rooted in love, supported by a strong husband and sustaining a wife who flowers beautifully in childbirth for the JOY of it. Natural Childbirth works, and families matter (M. Hathaway, personal communication, December 1, 2005).	Women should fully participate in pregnancy, birth, and motherhood as nature intended. Classes help her learn how to nourish her baby and prepare for the birth. Becoming an expert in relaxation, exercise, learning, and trusting the natural process helps her give birth (M. Hathaway, personal communication, December 1, 2005).	The partner should "husband" or protect this woman. He should take classes to learn how to coach her through pregnancy, labor, and birth. He should learn how to participate at birth, bonding as a family and helping to care for the new baby. He needs to be there to help, encourage, and inspire the woman and be man enough to finish what he starts! (M. Hathaway, personal communication, December 1, 2005).	Comparing birthing to swimming, the health care provider is the lifeguard. Both swimming and birthing carry an irreducible minimal risk, and "lifeguards" are necessary but only for complications (Bradley, 1996). Health care providers encourage the family to give birth together. They support and provide backup if medically necessary. Normal birth is not an emergency (M. Hathaway, personal communication, December 1, 2005).
Hypnosis for Labor and Birth	Relaxation techniques (therapeutic suggestions, visualization, relaxation breathing) will result in a self-trance, decreasing the need for medications and minimizing stress during childbirth.	By bringing her body into deep relaxation, the muscles work as naturally meant (Isidro-Cloudas, 2006). Therapeutic suggestions can increase relaxation and promote positive childbirth.	The partner should provide support the woman finds helpful, such as rubbing the back, providing a cool compress, or repeating certain phrases (Dorothy M. Larkin, October 5, 2006, personal communication.	Provide support like that of partner. Recognize and work within the pattern and rhythm of the woman's breathing and movements. For example, before a vaginal examination, allow the woman time to mentally prepare herself.
Birthing From Within	Childbirth is a profound rite of passage, not a medical event (even when medical care is part of the birth). The essence of childbirth preparation is self-discovery, not assimilating obstetric information (Birthing From Within, 2000).	The purpose of childbirth preparation is to help mothers give birth-in-awareness, not to achieve a specific birth outcome (Birthing From Within, 2000).	Fathers help best as birth guardians or loving partners, not as coaches: they also need support (Birthing From Within, 2000).	Parents deserve support for any birth option that might be right for them (eg, drugs, technology, home birth, bottle-feeding). For parents, pregnancy, birth, and postpartum are continuous adjustments during which ongoing holistic support and education should be available (Birthing From Within, 2000).

Continued

TABLE 14.2 Common Educational Methods

TYPE	MISSION STATEMENT OR EXPLANATION	ROLE OF WOMAN	ROLE OF PARTNER	ROLE OF PROVIDER
Boot Camp for New Dads	Give every child the opportunity for a caring and capable father beginning at birth (Boot Camp for New Dads, n.d.).	None found.	Most new fathers are committed at birth and want to do right by their children. Support for them should be offered early in pregnancy. Class activities should include discussion of how partners can support each other; practice in diapering, swaddling, dressing, and feeding infants; information in massages for baby and mom; and relaxation/coaching techniques for labor and birth (Boot Camp for New Dads, n.d.).	Fathers should be made to feel comfortable with their babies. Care providers can invite fathers to cut the umbilical cord (but not pressure them); assist the dads to hold, burp, and change their baby; and encourage dads to come to regular health maintenance visits (Boot Camp for New Dads, n.d.).

a woman who provides continuous physical, emotional, and informational support to the mother before, during, and after childbirth (Klaus et al., 2002, p. vi) (Fig. 14.3).

Doulas of North America (DONA), formed in 1992, was the effort of a small group of birth support experts to promote the importance of continuous emotional and physical support for mothers and their partners during pregnancy, labor, and birth. Peggy and John Kennell, Phyllis and Marshall Klaus, Penny Simkin, and Annie Kennedy based the organization on research that demonstrated statistically significant decreases in cesarean birth,

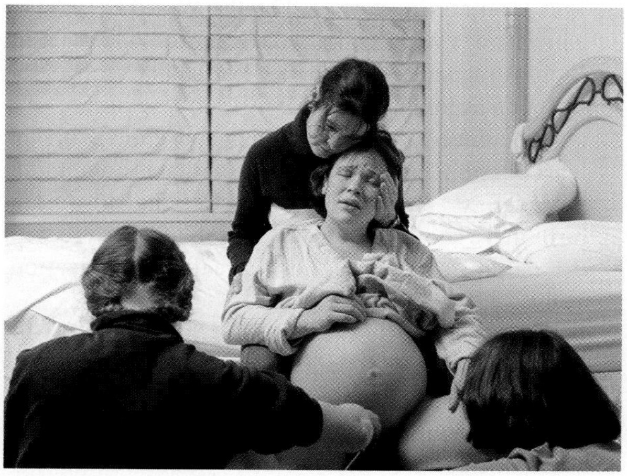

FIGURE 14.3 A woman who is having a home birth is being assisted by a doula.

use of vacuum extractor or forceps, requests for analgesia or anesthesia, and mothers who were dissatisfied with their birth experiences (Simkin & Way, 2005). Increasingly, doulas are combining birth support with childbirth education and are excellent resources for the next generation of birth educators.

Partner-Oriented Approaches

Fathers and other partners have been involved in birth since the formalization of childbirth education in the early 1970s. Many of them attend prenatal classes, learn breathing techniques, and discover how to help mothers during labor (Fig. 14.4). Such partners have adopted the responsibilities of "coaching" the mother.

Dr. Robert Bradley, a Denver obstetrician, moved the role of fathers into prominence in his book *Husband-Coached Childbirth,* first published in 1965. Bradley viewed prepared childbirth as a "humanistic, undrugged approach to parenthood" (1965). He developed the Bradley Method of prenatal training in which mothers and fathers follow nature and give birth without the "terrible indignities of drugs" (Bradley, 1996). The Bradley Method advocates for the father's continuous presence in labor and birth. Fathers prepare so that they understand what their wives are doing, enabling them to coach, guide, and encourage women in their "ennobling work" (Bradley, 1996).

Boot Camp for New Dads emerged in the 1990s as a response to absent, apathetic, or abusive fathers (Boot Camp for New Dads, n.d.). The organization began in

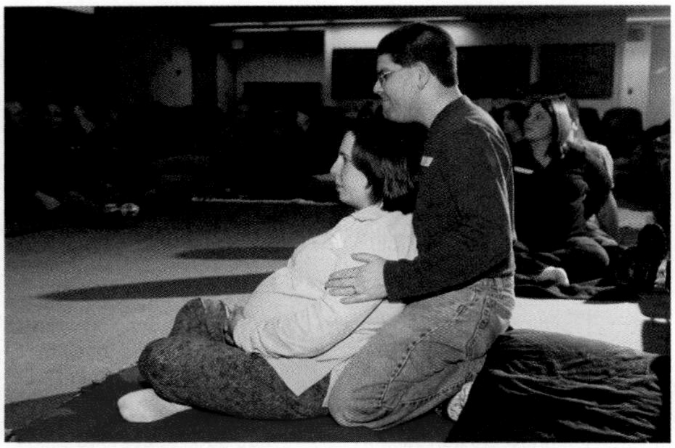

FIGURE 14.4 Many fathers and partners attend prenatal classes and learn the techniques and methods that will help pregnant women have a positive labor and birth experience.

Irvine, California, when a few fathers held an orientation workshop for men who were about to become parents. The nervous rookies learned before birth how to care for their infants, the rewards of being involved, positive communication skills, the labor and birth process, and the appreciation of mothers for paternal involvement. They found that supporting one another is the key to success and that paternal participation in birth and parenting gives mothers strength, encouragement, and calmness (Boot Camp for New Dads, n.d.). The rookies returned, after their babies were born, to orient the next group of men. Mentoring continues today.

QUOTE 14-2

"My husband has benefited so much from the prenatal classes he has attended. I think he knows more about what to expect than I do!"

A first-time mom-to-be

Midwives

A **midwife** is a person who, having been regularly admitted to a midwifery educational program duly recognized in the country of location, has successfully completed the prescribed course of studies in midwifery and has acquired the requisite qualifications to be registered, legally licensed, or both to practice midwifery (International College of Nurse-Midwives, 2005). In the United States, a **certified nurse-midwife (CNM)** is a person educated in the two disciplines of nursing and midwifery who possesses evidence of certification according to the requirements of the American College of Nurse-Midwives (ACNM, 2004).

Midwives are well known for their ability to teach health promotion and illness prevention to expectant women. "Every midwife is a childbirth teacher. Every prenatal appointment is a class" (England & Horowitz, 2001, p. 201). Midwives use their precious prenatal visit time to empower women. Mothers accept responsibility for their prenatal health when they weigh themselves, test their urine, and record the results in their charts. Time with mothers and their partners gives midwives the ability to teach the difference between pain and suffering, the need for breath awareness and relaxation, massage techniques, and the emotional and physical transition toward parenthood. If parents are attending childbirth classes, midwives are available to provide more depth to the information they've received in class.

Cesarean Prevention Approaches

Cesareans/Support, Education and Concern (C/SEC), the International Cesarean Awareness Network (ICAN), and the Cesarean Prevention Movement, Inc. (CPM) are consumer movements promoting specific preparation courses for women desiring vaginal birth after cesarean birth (VBAC) (see Chap. 16). These groups provide information, support, and education for women healing from cesarean birth and those wanting vaginal birth after previous cesarean.

La Leche League

La Leche League was founded in 1956 by women who wanted to make breastfeeding easier and more rewarding for both mother and child. Today, participants gather to share information and experiences about breastfeeding and offer one another support in parenting choices as well.

Birth Networks

Birth networks are the latest wave of parent information resources growing rapidly throughout the United States. Expectant parents, eager to have a healthy pregnancy and newborn, are often at a loss to find health care providers and community resources to assist them toward these ends. In response, these grassroots community organizations have the following goals:

- Promote care practices that support **normal birth.** This terminology was used by the World Health Organization (WHO) at its Task Force Meeting on Monitoring and Evaluation of Perinatal Care, held in Bologna in January 2000, by which "the aim of care is to achieve a healthy mother and child with the least possible level of intervention that is compatible with safety. This approach implies that in normal birth there should be a valid reason to interfere with the natural process" (World Health Organization, 1999).
- Endorse the **Mother-Friendly Childbirth Initiative,** a document that defines mother-friendly services in hospitals, birth centers, and home birth practices
- Provide support, education, and evidenced-based information about normal birth for parents
- Serve as a resource for caregivers that support normal birth (Lamaze Institute for Normal Birth, 2005)

BOX 14.1 Script for Hypnosis in Labor and Birth

> Think about being on the beach. Enjoy the warmth of the sun. Feel your stress and tension melting as you become more relaxed. You may feel your body helping to birth your child. Think about relaxing into the contraction, like riding a wave. Imagine your cervix and vagina opening wide for your child to journey outside into your arms.

Media, Internet, and Other Resources

The mass media serves as a significant source of childbirth education for today's parents, especially as Western cultures emphasize and discuss pregnancy, labor, birth, breastfeeding, and parenting more openly than ever before. For example, television programs that show live births abound on many cable stations. Unfortunately, real-time birth does not fit neatly into a 30-minute time slot, so these programs are edited to focus on drama and trauma that will attract viewers. Some parents-to-be who watch these programs do not find their experiences represented accurately or may become more apprehensive about what lies ahead. Whatever sources of birth information expectant parents may encounter, nurses, midwives, and other health care providers need to give on-site nurturing, caring, and guidance and ensure that they correct any misinformation that might affect the experience of childbirth.

Access to Childbirth Education

Parents attending classes may be old or young, single or married, heterosexual or homosexual, incarcerated, or adoptive. They may have disabilities, have experienced previous pregnancy loss, or have conceived by in vitro fertilization. Their pregnancies may be planned or unplanned, desired or unwanted. They may or may not speak the culture's predominant language. Their religious or cultural backgrounds may dictate their preferences and activities in labor and birth. They may be predominantly left or right brained and will be influenced by the way their families have spoken of birth. They will be limited to the classes available within their geographic location. They also may face limitations related to cost, transportation, employment restrictions, and other family obligations.

Women attending childbirth education classes receive information about labor, pain relief, birth, normal infant care, postpartum adjustment, and breastfeeding. Increasing the proportion of pregnant women who attend formal childbirth classes has been identified as a developmental objective for *Healthy People 2010* (U.S. DHHS, 2000). In the *Listening to Mothers* survey (Declercq et al., 2002), only 36% of women reported taking childbirth education classes. Most new mothers (70%) took classes, whereas only 19% of experienced mothers did so. More women (88%) attended classes in a medical setting than in a home (4%) or community site (7%).

Lu and associates (2003) studied the sociodemographic disparities in attendance at childbirth classes in a telephone survey of 1540 mothers of children aged 4 to 35 months. Overall, 66% of the mothers had ever attended childbirth classes. More than 75% of white, college-educated, and married women had attended at least one childbirth class. Fewer than 50% of Hispanic or African American, poor, unmarried, and minimally educated women had done so.

Shilling (2000) has identified potential barriers to access to childbirth education classes:

- A previous negative experience in an educational setting
- Worries about feeling foolish or ignorant
- Expecting to learn about birth from family or friends
- Anxiety about being in a minority because of race, religion, skin color, or cultural background
- Timing and location of classes interfering with work or requiring unavailable transportation
- Expecting to discuss personal, intimate, or embarrassing matters
- Fear of bad luck resulting from early preparation for the birth
- Discomfort with discussing unexpected outcomes
- Lack of the predominant language skills

Many communities provide alternatives to formal childbirth education classes. For example, outreach workers may conduct teaching in a woman's home on a one-to-one basis. Some clinics offer "bench clinics" in which groups of women learn information as they wait during prenatal appointments. Rising (2005) has developed a model of group education and prenatal care called CenteringPregnancy in which women enter a group after their initial nursing or medical evaluation. At each subsequent session, the woman completes her standard prenatal assessment within the group setting. Women participate actively by taking their own weights and blood pressure readings and recording the findings on their charts. They meet with the same 8 to 12 other women with similar due dates regularly to discuss pertinent physical, emotional, social, and spiritual topics associated with childbirth (Rising, 2005).

Continuity of Health Promotion

Childbirth education is no longer limited to an isolated series of classes during the last trimester. It comes from many sources. For teaching to effectively allay parental fears about trauma or pain, women and their supporters must understand the body's natural abilities for giving birth. They must welcome pain as a sign of the body's activity to bring forth a child. They must understand that medical interventions serve as life-protecting technologic advances.

Mothers and their supporters begin to learn about birth even before they recognize the need for education. The women in their culture describe birth in such a way that builds fear or fosters strength. Women receive education in their school classrooms, from their friends, from health professionals, and from the media (Fig. 14.5). Ideally, each community would collaborate to provide evidence-based information to women and men preconceptually that continues past the birth of their children into parenting. This may not be achievable because of professional differences in opinions about natural versus medicalized birth, as well as the transience of both citizens and professionals. What is achievable is for each and every professional in contact with pregnant or parenting women and men to consider himself or herself an educational resource and to provide the most evidence-based information that the woman needs or desires at that time. Nurses may consider taking a self-assessment of the mother-friendliness of their practice in *Is Your Perinatal Practice Mother-Friendly? A Strategy for Improving Maternity Care* (Hotelling, 2004). An appropriate self-assessment tool for childbirth educators can be found in *A Call to Action and a Challenge to Use a Standard to Measure Mother-Friendly Birth Classes* (Hotelling, 2001).

COLLABORATIVE CARE: EDUCATION FOR PREGNANCY, CHILDBIRTH, AND PARENTING

Many options are available to the woman and her family in preparation for pregnancy, childbirth, and parenting. Information can be provided in formal classes, one-on-one teaching sessions, informal teaching episodes (eg, during health visits), and discussions with family members and friends. Clients and families dealing with this information, however, may find it overwhelming. Nurses play major roles in collaborating with other caregivers to cover many topics, clarify data, and correct any misconceptions so that the woman and her family can make the most appropriate and informed decisions.

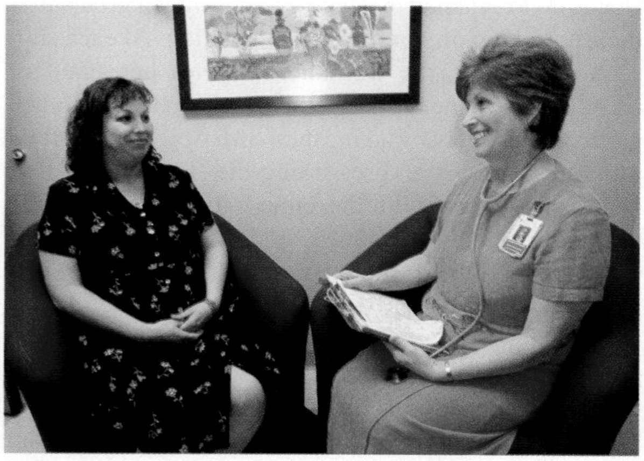

FIGURE 14.5 Health professionals are a primary source of childbirth education for many families.

Assessment

Assessment typically involves determining the client's knowledge about pregnancy, childbirth, and parenting. Ideally, this assessment occurs before the woman becomes pregnant to ensure that she is in the best possible health. Early assessment helps to minimize risks that could complicate pregnancy or jeopardize the fetus, thereby enhancing the success of a positive outcome for all involved.

Once a pregnancy is established, assessment focuses on ascertaining the woman's knowledge level about the physical and psychological changes that accompany gestation, common discomforts that she may experience, and danger signs and symptoms (see Chap. 12). In addition, the client's experiences with any previous pregnancies can help provide clues about areas that need clarification or correction. Another key area of assessment includes the woman's knowledge level about measures to promote a healthy pregnancy.

As the pregnancy continues, assessment focuses on the woman's and family's ability to adapt and preparations for the actual labor and birth. Key areas of focus include the following:

- Understanding of normal labor and birth, including signs and symptoms of true and prodromal labor
- Goals for labor and birth, including involvement of family members (eg, siblings)
- Desire for attending childbirth education classes
- Plans for birth, including birth attendant, support persons, and setting
- Options for pain management
- Plans for feeding the newborn
- Understanding of newborn care, growth, and development
- Plans for the newborn once at home

Assessment continues after the birth to determine the teaching needs of the new parents. Common areas of focus include general newborn care, feeding method, and newborn growth and development. Assessment also addresses the woman's understanding of the events after birth, including the physical and psychological changes that aid in returning her body to its pre-pregnant state. These topics are discussed in detail throughout Unit 5 of this text.

Select Potential Nursing Diagnoses

Nursing diagnoses appropriate for the woman and her family related to education can be numerous, encompassing a wide range of concerns. Some of the more common nursing diagnoses may include the following:

- **Deficient Knowledge** related to the events of pregnancy, labor, and birth; measures for newborn care; newborn feeding methods; or appropriate parenting techniques
- **Deficient Knowledge** related to available methods for managing pain of labor
- **Health-Seeking Behaviors** related to measures to promote optimal pregnancy outcomes
- **Anxiety** related to lack of experience with pregnancy and fear of the unknown
- **Decisional Conflict** related to lack of knowledge, misconceptions, and inaccurate information about labor and birth
- **Readiness for Enhanced Family Processes** related to seeking out information to promote a positive pregnancy and childbirth experience for the entire family

Planning/Intervention

Outcomes are highly individualized based on the client's needs. Some common outcomes may include the following:

- The client and partner will identify measures to promote a healthy outcome.
- The client and partner will choose an appropriate plan for labor and birth, including options for pain management.
- The client and partner will decide on a setting for birth.
- The client and partner will participate in a childbirth education class of their choosing.
- The client and partner will verbalize statements reflecting that they feel prepared for the childbirth experience.
- The client and partner will demonstrate newborn care measures appropriately.
- The family will demonstrate measures to integrate the newborn into the family.

The ultimate goal in preparing for pregnancy, childbirth, and parenting is that the woman and her partner can make informed decisions that meet their needs and promote the most optimal outcome for themselves, their newborn, and their family. See NIC/NOC Box 14.1 for some general interventions and outcomes appropriate to childbirth education.

Client teaching is the primary intervention for preparing the woman and her family for pregnancy, childbirth, and parenting. The nurse should develop an individualized teaching plan based on initial assessment of the client's knowledge level. Together, team members modify or revise this plan as the client's needs change and pregnancy progresses. Important areas of client teaching include information related to healthy behaviors and health promotion, childbirth education programs, and pain management.

NIC/NOC Box 14.1 Education About Pregnancy, Childbirth, and Parenting

Common NIC Labels

- Anticipatory Guidance
- Breastfeeding Assistance
- Childbirth Preparation
- Health Education
- Lactation Counseling
- Pain Management
- Parent Education: Infant
- Preconception Counseling
- Prenatal Care
- Teaching: Infant Nutrition

Common NOC Labels

- Knowledge: Breastfeeding
- Knowledge: Health Behaviors
- Knowledge: Labor and Delivery
- Knowledge: Maternal Child Health
- Knowledge: Preconception
- Knowledge: Pregnancy
- Pain Control
- Parent Infant Attachment
- Prenatal Health Behavior

Healthy Behaviors

Education about healthy behaviors begins early in a person's life, with emphasis on eating properly, getting enough exercise, and reducing factors that may lead to illness. The ultimate goal is to maintain and improve health throughout life. In addition, teaching about healthy behaviors fosters improved awareness for enhanced decision making, which can lead to greater autonomy. Chapter 2 presents a detailed description of major areas of health promotion for women along with numerous suggestions for teaching and recommendations for screening.

Preconception counseling is an optimal time to reinforce previous teaching about healthy behaviors and present new information about pregnancy and ways to promote maternal and fetal well-being. Teaching commonly addresses these areas:

- Nutritional intake, including balanced diet, most nutritious cooking methods
- Exercise and activity
- Medication use, over-the-counter and prescription

- Modifiable risk factors, such as drug and alcohol use, exposure to teratogens
- Stress reduction and coping strategies
- Screening and counseling

See Chapter 11 for more detailed information related to preconceptual health.

Once a woman becomes pregnant, teaching expands to include the woman's partner and the changes that are and will be occurring throughout gestation. Much of this teaching commonly takes place during prenatal visits. In addition, some facilities have group classes that provide antepartal information. In each instance, nurses must be sure to incorporate any religious, sociocultural, or age-related influences into teaching.

Many changes occur in the maternal body during pregnancy. The nurse plays a key role in teaching the woman about these normal changes, both physiologic and psychological, and how to promote self-care. See Chapter 12 for more information. The nurse also teaches the woman how to manage the common discomforts of pregnancy, such as nausea and vomiting, breast tenderness, constipation, fatigue and muscle cramps, urinary frequency, ankle edema, and backache. In addition, he or she instructs the woman and partner about danger signs and symptoms of pregnancy so that they can notify a health care provider immediately, receive early intervention, and possibly reduce the risk for problems.

Throughout pregnancy, the nurse should provide reinforcement and review of instructions. He or she should allow time for the client and partner to ask questions and clarify any concerns or misinformation that they may have (Fig. 14.6).

As the woman progresses through the third trimester, teaching begins to focus on the upcoming events of labor and birth. Although information about settings available for labor and birth, such as hospitals, birthing centers, and home births may be given earlier in the pregnancy, the nurse should be sure to review and reinforce this information with the client and her partner. In this way, the couple can make an informed decision based on their preferences and needs. In addition, this information helps the couple to develop a birth plan that promotes autonomy and fosters feelings of control over the situation.

The nurse needs to explain and review with the client and her partner the process of labor, expected events, procedures, and assessments so that they have a sense of what to expect. Such preparation can alleviate anxiety about the unknown and assist them to make decisions about the events surrounding birth.

Client teaching also addresses preparation for the newborn and his or her care. Typically, the nurse reviews the normal characteristics of the newborn and assists the client in preparing for breastfeeding or bottle feeding. He or she usually gives information about growth and development as well (see Chaps. 20 and 21). In addition, the nurse should teach about what the woman should expect physically and psychologically for herself during the postpartum period (see Chap. 18).

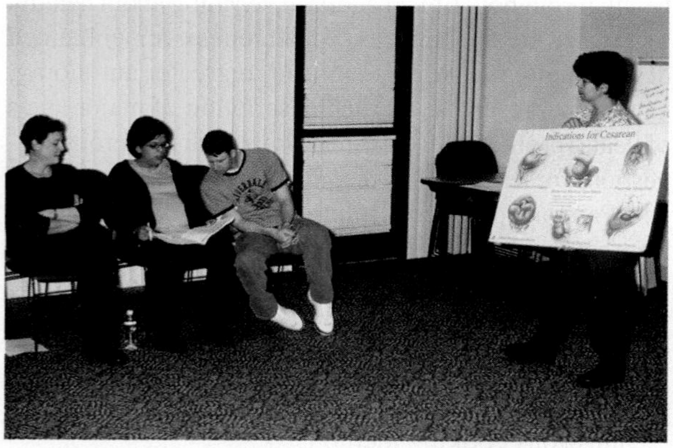

FIGURE 14.6 During individual and group teaching sessions, nurses and other instructors need to provide time to impart information, review understanding, and answer questions.

Pain Management

The degree of discomfort and pain associated with labor and birth can be a major concern for the pregnant woman and her partner. Nurses are instrumental in educating the woman and her partner about the pain of labor and the many nonpharmacologic and pharmacologic options available to manage the pain. Once armed with this knowledge, the client and her partner can choose the methods most appropriate for their situation and beliefs. See Nursing Care Plan 14.1.

Nonpharmacologic Methods

Women can use nonpharmacologic methods for pain relief during labor alone, in combination with other nonpharmacologic methods, or as adjuncts to pharmacologic interventions. Regardless of how such methods are used, the nurse should describe and discuss the various options with the client and her partner so that they can decide on the types that would be most appropriate for them. Examples of nonpharmacologic methods include the following:

- Relaxation
- Imagery
- Music
- Breathing techniques
- Herbal preparations
- Aromatherapy
- Heat and cold applications
- Hydrotherapy
- Therapeutic touch
- Massage
- Hypnosis

NURSING CARE PLAN 14.1

The Couple Preparing for Labor and Birth

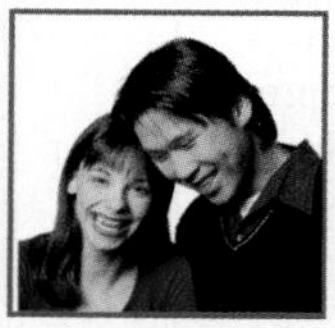

Remember Belinda, the 29-year-old woman at 14 weeks' gestation with her first pregnancy. Upon further assessment, Belinda reveals that her husband's desire for natural childbirth results from his concern about the use of drugs during labor. Belinda says, "My mom was asleep when she had me. And I was fine. I want to do what's best for my baby, but I'm afraid of the pain."

NURSING DIAGNOSES

- **Anxiety** related to inexperience with labor, birth process, and associated pain
- **Deficient Knowledge** related to labor and birth, pain experience, and pain-relief measures
- **Decisional Conflict** related to management of the labor and birth process

EXPECTED OUTCOMES

1. The client will identify areas of concern related to the labor and birth process.
2. The client will state options available for labor management.
3. The client will describe the process of labor and birth accurately.
4. The client and husband will participate in a childbirth education program that addresses their needs.
5. The client and husband will choose the most appropriate method for them to manage labor and birth.

INTERVENTIONS	RATIONALES
Assess the client's level of understanding about the labor and birth process; include her husband in the assessment and discussion/teaching.	Assessment provides a baseline to identify specific client needs and to develop an individualized teaching plan. Participation of the partner provides support to the client, promotes informed decision making, and enhances the chances for a positive experience for both parties.
Explore client's and husband's exposure to labor and birth; assist them to identify potential areas of concern; correct any misconceptions or myths related to labor and birth; allow time for questions.	Information about exposure provides additional foundation for teaching and opportunities to identify concerns, clarify or correct misinformation, and teach new concepts.
Discuss with the couple possible factors, such as culture, religion, and financial status, that may influence their perception of labor and birth and measures to use for pain.	Further knowledge of possible factors influencing perceptions aids in determining appropriate suggestions for the couple.
Teach the couple the various options available for labor and birth, including effectiveness and advantages and disadvantages. Describe different approaches to childbirth, including psychoprophylaxis, Dick-Read method, and Lamaze method.	Such information provides a foundation from which the client and her husband can make an informed decision.

Continued

NURSING CARE PLAN 14.1 ● The Couple Preparing for Labor and Birth *(Continued)*

INTERVENTIONS	RATIONALES
Explain about the phenomenon of pain during labor and birth; review nonpharmacologic and pharmacologic options available. Review the use of close monitoring to prevent complications if pharmacologic agents are used.	An understanding of labor pain provides a foundation for deciding on the most appropriate methods for pain control. Knowledge of measures to prevent complications can alleviate anxiety related to the effects of analgesia on the fetus.
Reinforce with the couple the need for adaptation and adjustment during labor.	Awareness of potential changes helps to prepare them for what to expect and to plan accordingly.
Review with the client and husband childbirth education classes available in the community; encourage them to investigate such classes and enroll in those that meet their needs.	Childbirth education programs vary. Enrollment fosters learning and sharing with others, thereby promoting a positive experience.
Provide written information about labor, birth, childbirth education programs, and approaches to labor and birth. Encourage the couple to investigate the Internet and local community for additional information.	Adequate information is necessary to make an informed decision.
Schedule a return visit for the client and husband to provide follow-up discussion and teaching.	A return visit provides an opportunity to evaluate teaching and success of interventions as well as opportunities for clarification and additional instruction.

EVALUATION

1. The client identifies uncertainty and inexperience with labor as major areas of concern.
2. The couple verbalize labor management options accurately.
3. The couple demonstrate understanding of the events associated with labor.
4. The couple choose a childbirth education program appropriate to their desired goals.
5. The couple decide on an appropriate plan for labor and birth.

- Biofeedback
- Transcutaneous electrical nerve stimulation (TENS)
- Acupressure and acupuncture

The nurse may begin teaching by explaining the physiology of the pain response and the factors that influence pain perception. Next, he or she may describe sources that cause pain during labor and birth (see Chap. 17). Most people are aware that uterine contractions are the major source of pain; however, they also need to understand that stretching of the cervix and perineum may contribute. An additional source of pain can be pressure from the fetus on the surrounding organs and tissues as it moves through the birth canal. The nurse should present such information to the client and partner so that they can understand the nature of the pain. As the nurse reviews the methods for pain relief, the client and partner are better prepared to make selections based on a fully informed understanding of what is happening to the woman's body. During such discussions, the nurse should always keep in mind any sociocultural, religious, or other beliefs and concerns that may influence the reactions and choices of the woman and her partner.

The nurse should explain the methods to the client and her partner and demonstrate specific techniques or steps, such as the different types of breathing that can be used. The client and partner then can return-demonstrate any steps or techniques to ensure that they are performing them properly (Fig. 14.7). Positive feedback for their performance is encouraging, along with suggestions as necessary to enhance their use of techniques. In addition, the nurse should remind the client and her partner that during labor, nurses providing care will be readily available to keep them informed about the progress of labor and provide support and encouragement for the methods chosen.

Pharmacologic Methods

Many different pharmacologic agents may be used during labor and birth to provide pain relief. In addition, they may be administered by different techniques. As with nonpharmacologic methods, pharmacologic methods may be used alone, in combination with other medications, or in combination with nonpharmacologic methods. Nurses need to ensure that clients receive adequate information about the options available related to medications. They must include potential effects on the client and her fetus as part of this teaching. Chapter 17 provides a detailed discussion of pharmacologic methods for pain relief.

Childbirth Education Programs

Childbirth education programs are wide ranging and vary in focus and philosophy, content, and methods of presentation (Table 14.3). Some programs base information on the belief that labor is a physiologic process requiring no medical intervention unless compelling evidence supports it. Other programs present information based on the concepts of relaxation, exercise, learning, and trusting of the natural birth process. One program may cover pregnancy from conception through birth, whereas another may focus solely on labor.

The nurse should be familiar with childbirth education programs offered in the community. He or she should provide the client and partner information about the various classes and encourage them to review their goals for the pregnancy, labor, and birth. The nurse can assist parents to investigate the programs, including talking with instructors and others who have participated in them. Such information helps the couple make an informed decision based on their desires and needs.

Expectant parenting classes are also available and commonly provide information about newborn care, growth and development, and family health. Other types of programs include sibling and grandparent classes and refresher courses for parents who already have a child or children. Nursing Care Plan 14.2 provides an example of a family incorporating sibling education classes into their pregnancy preparations.

Evaluation

Success of the teaching plan is determined by evaluating the client's, partner's, and family's response to the instruction. The nurse should look for observable changes in behavior related to promoting health. For example, a review of the woman's nutritional patterns indicates that she is now ingesting the required amount of fluid daily to promote breast milk production and is consuming the recommended amount of calories to foster appropriate weight gain. Statements also provide clues to the client's understanding of instructions. For example, the client may state that she and her partner are enrolled in a childbirth education course at the local hospital. The couple may report that they have decided on a doula for support or that they are planning to use several nonpharmacologic measures to assist with pain relief during labor. Client satisfaction about the choices made also provides information for evaluation. Demonstration of any techniques such as feeding or newborn care provides additional objective evidence of learning.

(text continues on page 575)

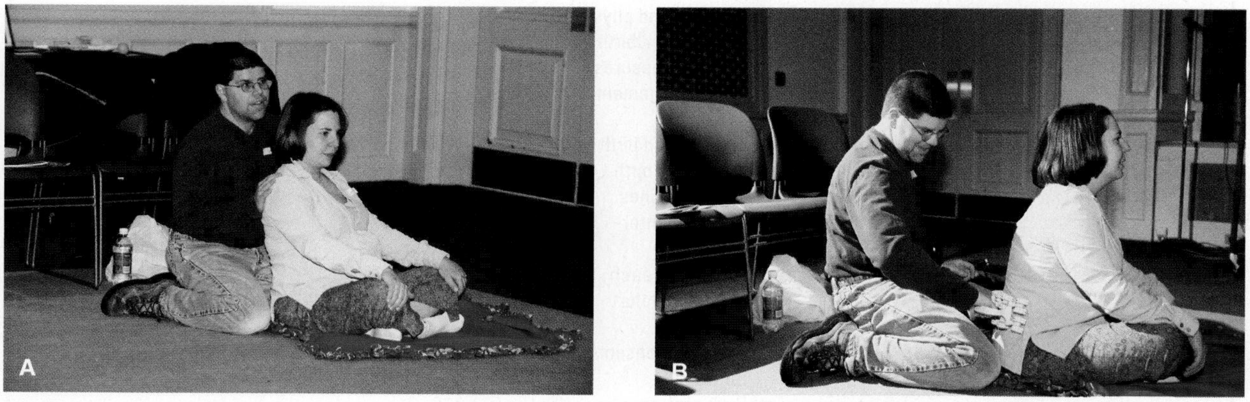

FIGURE 14.7 Ideally, during teaching sessions clients (**A**) learn principles and (**B**) return-demonstrate their understanding of what was conveyed.

● **TABLE 14.3 Common Educational Classes**

TYPE	ATTENDEES	TOPICS COVERED	TIMING	PURPOSE
Preconception	Parents planning a pregnancy	● Emotional and physical changes in early pregnancy ● Physical health for pregnancy ● Emotional health for pregnancy ● Nutrition for healthy pregnancy ● Prevention of birth defects ● Financial planning ● Fertility issues	Anytime an individual or couple is planning pregnancy	To promote healthy lifestyles before becoming pregnant. Specific areas of focus include the following: ● Stress reduction ● Folic acid intake ● Management of health conditions affecting pregnancy and birth ● Smoking cessation ● Avoidance of toxic substances ● Environmental health
Early prenatal	Parents in the first or second trimesters whether planning birth at home, in a birth center, or in a hospital	● Physical and emotional changes of pregnancy ● Sexuality ● Minor discomforts of pregnancy ● Danger signs ● Nutrition ● Rest and sleep ● Exercise ● Use of drugs ● Stress management ● Fetal development ● Finances ● Working within the health care system ● Resources ● Myths ● Choices in caregivers ● Choices in birth sites ● Practice in each class of comfort measures (Nichols & Humenick, 2000)	As early as possible in the first trimester; also valuable in the second trimester	To promote health in pregnancy, as manifested by: ● Term birth ● Adequate birth weight ● Relationship maintenance ● Good maternal health and energy ● Stress relief ● Bonding ● Financial planning ● Support systems
Prenatal	Parents in the third trimester	All of the above, *plus:* ● Common fears and anxieties ● Father involvement in childbirth ● Choice and birth preferences ● Anatomy and physiology of childbirth ● Comfort measures ● Pain management strategies ● Variations in birth ● Hospital or birth center routines ● Obstetric interventions ● Practice in each class of comfort measures ● Informed consent/refusal ● Birth preferences (Nichols & Humenick, 2000)	Third trimester	To promote health in the third trimester, in labor and birth, *plus* ● Develop relaxation awareness ● Plan for support during labor, birth, and postpartum ● Understand hospital or birth center culture and routines ● Promote healthy lifestyles ● Avoid unnecessary interventions ● Prevent complications ● Develop an understanding of the body's natural ability to give birth

Continued

TABLE 14.3 Common Educational Classes

TYPE	ATTENDEES	TOPICS COVERED	TIMING	PURPOSE
Homebirth preparation	Parents planning a homebirth	All of the above, *plus:* ● Supply list ● Nutrition to prevent anemia ● Attendants for siblings ● Birth preferences ● Support systems	Third trimester	Parents choosing homebirth are responsible for healthy lifestyles, supplying the home with needed equipment, and planning for support during and after birth.
Vaginal birth after cesarean (VBAC)	Parents who have had a previous cesarean	● Previous birth experience ● Desire for/confidence about vaginal birth ● Risks for cesarean birth ● Risks for VBAC ● Comparison of primipara and multipara labors ● Support systems ● Variations in labor ● Avoidable factors leading to cesarean ● Vaginal birth planning ● Cesarean birth planning ● Preparation of siblings ● Breastfeeding ● Review of familiar comfort techniques ● Introduction to unfamiliar comfort techniques ● Informed consent/refusal ● Birth preferences	Third trimester	Parents learn of the benefits of trial of labor and vaginal birth after a previous cesarean birth and wish to avoid an unnecessary cesarean birth.
Refresher	Parents who have already had at least one birth	● Review of previous birth experience ● Review of comfort measures used successfully ● Comparison of primipara and multipara labors and birth ● Birth preferences	Third trimester	Parents may enjoy the last-trimester ritual of focusing on the new baby. They also may feel previous classes helped them and wish to refresh their skills. Some parents had a disappointing birth experience and want information to avoid repeating their previous experiences.
Multiple births	Parents expecting multiple births	All prenatal class topics, *plus:* ● Increased nutrition, hydration, and rest needs ● Body mechanics and exercises for posture ● Time management and stress reduction ● Preterm labor symptoms ● Breastfeeding multiples ● Resources for other parents of multiples ● Fetal surveillance ● Birth preferences	Late in the second trimester or early in the third trimester	Parents of multiples want information on how the birth may be different from singleton births and want to prepare for birth and postpartum.

Continued

TABLE 14.3 Common Educational Classes *(Continued)*

TYPE	ATTENDEES	TOPICS COVERED	TIMING	PURPOSE
Breastfeeding preparation	Parents at any time of pregnancy	• Breast milk production • Benefits • Nutrition, hydration, and relaxation for breastfeeding • Proper latch • Fertility • Positions at the breast • Demand versus scheduled feeding • How to tell when the infant is getting enough milk • Hand expression and pumping • Storing breast milk • Complications • The partner's roles • Resources for support	Anytime during pregnancy	Preparation will help decrease the stress of breastfeeding for parents by providing information about the process and resources for questions after they are home.
Fathers' support skills	Fathers in the third trimester	• Mother's emotional changes in labor • Maintaining relaxation, rhythm, and rituals in labor • Options for levels of participation • Positioning for comfort • Maintaining focus, breathing, and rhythmic activity • Helping interpret what is happening • Nutrition and hydration during labor • Active support during transition and birth • Sharing in the joy of the birth	Second or third trimester	Fathers attend childbirth classes that focus primarily on the mother and infant. Hearing information specific to their needs empowers them to participate in the birth in an individualized way and become active in their newborn's care.
Parents with previous pregnancy loss	Parents who have experienced pregnancy loss either by miscarriage, stillbirth, or perinatal death	• Grief • Concerns in this pregnancy • Emotional guarding • Stress and anxiety relief • Openly acknowledging pregnancy loss • Birth planning • Emotions during birth and postpartum	Women can start classes early to deal with emotions of grief and their effects on current pregnancy.	Caregivers don't often recognize the grief that parents are carrying in this pregnancy after a previous loss. This grief can impair attachment and interfere with healthy child development.
Hospital tour	Parents taking prenatal classes	• Facilities • Roles of members of the medical team • Hospital protocols • Comfort amenities (eg, bath, shower, birth balls, healing touch) • Admission procedures • Creating a peaceful environment	Anytime during pregnancy	Familiarity with the hospital environment allows parents to personalize their birth space and improves relaxation.

Continued

TABLE 14.3 Common Educational Classes

TYPE	ATTENDEES	TOPICS COVERED	TIMING	PURPOSE
Grandparents' class	Parents of the expectant mother and father	● Current childbirth practices ● Changing relationships with the new family ● Breastfeeding benefits ● Newborn capabilities	Anytime during pregnancy	Grandparents are an integral part of the newborn's development and can be invaluable support systems for the new family. Bringing them up to date with birth and parenting culture helps them participate in more satisfying ways.
Sibling class	Parents and other children in the family	● Role of sibling as big brother or sister ● Tour of facility ● Characteristics and behavior of newborns	Third trimester (generally)	Involvement of siblings in the birth experience decreases jealousy and acting out.
Parenting	Parents wanting information on newborns	● Adjustment to parenthood ● Infant growth and development ● Basics of infant care ● Soothing the newborn ● Infant massage ● Consumer information ● Sleep–wake states of the newborn ● Mimicry by newborns ● Brain and emotional development in the first 3 years ● Infant cues ● Emotional and physical needs ● Nutrition and hydration needs ● Infant illness ● Styles of parenting ● Anger management ● Support systems	Classes may be structured for expectant parents or for parents with newborns.	Understanding newborn communication can have a positive effect on family development and decrease stress and anxiety in caring for the newborn.
Adoptive parenting	Parents adopting a child	All the above, *plus* integration of the new child into the extended family	Anytime before or after adoption	Adoptive parents usually do not have the benefits of 9 months of exploration and discussion of parenting that frequently accompanies biologic pregnancy. Their needs are different; support comes from group interaction.
Infant massage	Parents, grandparents, and other extended family of infants	● Engagement and disengagement cues ● Physical and psychological benefits for both adults and infants ● Basics of infant massage strokes ● Verbal and nonverbal communication	Anytime during pregnancy or postpartum	Parents want to learn to soothe their infants and to create peaceful children. They also want to participate in the health promotion that comes from nurturing touch such as: ● Enhanced development of the nervous system ● Neurologic stimulation ● Increased alertness/heightened awareness ● Reduced stress hormones ● Improved immune function and digestion

NURSING CARE PLAN 14.2

The Expectant Family With Sibling Adjustment Difficulties

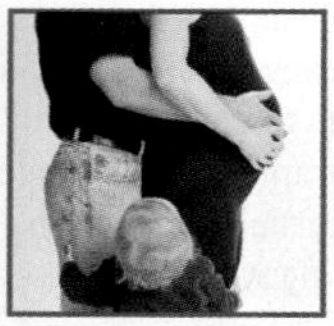

Remember Clarice and her partner Joel from the beginning of the chapter. When questioning the couple further, they mention that their son has regressed somewhat. "He used to be able to dress himself and put on his shoes with no problem. Now he wants me to do it. And I constantly have to tell him to be careful and not jump on me. Then when I tell him to be careful, he throws a tantrum. What can we do?"

NURSING DIAGNOSES

- **Deficient Knowledge** related to growth and development and effect of pregnancy on toddler
- **Readiness for Enhanced Family Processes** related to desire for seeking help with toddler

EXPECTED OUTCOMES

1. The couple will identify the effects of current pregnancy on their son.
2. The couple will implement measures to reduce the threat of the new baby on their son.
3. The couple will state that the son is demonstrating beginning acceptance of pregnancy and birth of the new baby, including fewer regressive and acting-out behaviors.

INTERVENTIONS	RATIONALES
Assess the couple's level of understanding about growth and development of a toddler and effects of pregnancy on children.	Assessment provides a baseline for identifying specific client needs and developing an individualized teaching plan.
Review with the couple the child's struggle for developing autonomy during this period (see Chap. 5).	Knowledge of the child's need to develop independence helps foster an understanding of the child's behavior patterns.
Explain that the child's behavior is a reflection of feelings of jealously or fears of not being loved (eg, not being mommy's or daddy's little boy anymore).	Children may fear the loss of parental love and experience jealousy with the prospect of the birth of a new baby.
Encourage the couple to include their son in age-appropriate activities involving the pregnancy throughout the perinatal period, such as helping to prepare the baby's room, choosing special toys, and reading stories about being a big brother.	Inclusion of the child in activities promotes feelings of security and being loved.
Urge the couple to spend time with their son in activities totally unrelated to the new baby; encourage other family members to spend individualized time with the toddler.	Individualized activities for the toddler promote a sense of security and love.
Suggest that the couple investigate the community for sibling education classes.	Sibling education classes help prepare children in an age-appropriate manner for the birth of the new baby.

Continued

NURSING CARE PLAN 14.2 ● The Expectant Family With Sibling Adjustment Difficulties

INTERVENTIONS	RATIONALES
Have the couple observe the effects of these actions on the child's behavior for improvement.	Improved behavior suggests that the child is adapting to the prospect of a new sibling.
Plan to follow up with the couple by telephone in 2 to 3 weeks.	Follow-up provides a means of evaluating the success of the plan; it also provides opportunities for additional teaching.

EVALUATION

1. The couple verbalize the effects of pregnancy on their son.
2. The couple include their son in age-appropriate preparations for the new baby.
3. The family participates in sibling education classes in preparation for birth of the new baby.
4. The child demonstrates fewer regressive and acting-out behaviors.

Questions to Ponder

1. Based on the statistics presented in Table 14.1, the rate of preterm births has increased from 1993 to 2003. What might be some reasons for this increase?
2. How should a nurse respond to a pregnant woman who states, "I'm not using any medication for pain. I'm doing it natural all the way."
3. A couple pregnant with their second child are concerned about how their 2½-year-old son may respond to the new baby. What suggestions might be appropriate?

SUMMARY

- Childbirth education has changed dramatically over the years from information about pregnancy, birth, parenting, and breastfeeding supplied woman-to-woman, to information supplied by physicians in an authoritative, medicalized fashion, to the current trend combining both models.
- The optimal time to begin childbirth education is when a person or couple makes the conscious decision to become a parent.
- The twilight sleep movement, which began in the early 1900s, involved the combined use of scopolamine and morphine to produce amnesia and anesthesia in the woman.
- Prepared childbirth methods became prominent after World War II. These included psychoprophylaxis emphasizing the use of controlled breathing, abdominal stroking, and pressure application on the hip and back; Dick-Read method addressing the holistic nature of childbirth in which mind and body were connected; and the Lamaze method, which integrated the psychoprophylactic method with medications only as requested.
- Common themes associated with childbirth education include fear of birth, pain management, and desire for control.
- For the nurse attending a laboring woman, pain is a less important issue than how the woman feels she is treated by her care providers. Thus, nurses are in a position to increase or diminish a woman's feelings of self-esteem, sense of accomplishment, and overall satisfaction with birth and to assist her in her transformation to motherhood.
- Childbirth education classes vary widely in their views of the people involved with the birth experience, methods for support and pain control, settings, approaches to birth, teaching methods, experiences of educators, and focus of advocacy.
- A developmental objective for *Healthy People 2010* is to increase the proportion of pregnant women who attend a formal series of prepared childbirth classes.
- Possible barriers to accessing childbirth education classes include previous negative experiences in educational settings; worries about feeling foolish or ignorant; expecting to learn about birth from family or

friends; anxiety about being in a minority; timing and location of classes interfering with work and requiring public transportation; expecting discussion of personal and intimate matters that are embarrassing; fear of bad luck caused by early preparation for the birth; feelings of being uncomfortable with discussing unexpected outcomes; and lack of the predominant language skills.

- Childbirth education is not an isolated series of classes in the last trimester of pregnancy. Health care professionals in contact with pregnant or parenting women and men must view themselves as educational resources for these clients and provide them with the most evidenced-based information desired by the clients at that time.

REVIEW QUESTIONS

1. Which of the following should the nurse identify as a major benchmark for a woman's satisfaction with birth?
   A. The woman's feelings of control during birth
   B. Use of nonpharmacologic pain-relief methods
   C. The extent of childbirth education received
   D. The woman's past experiences with childbirth
2. The nurse is preparing a presentation about the history of childbirth education. Which of the following should the nurse include as characteristic of the colonial period in America?
   A. Most births were attended by colonial physicians.
   B. The mother spent 3 to 4 weeks before the birth lying in.
   C. Attendance at the births of other women provided the education.
   D. Women typically had children spaced closely together.
3. Which of the following medications were used together to produce twilight sleep?
   A. Ether and chloroform
   B. Meperidine and fentanyl
   C. Halothane and lidocaine
   D. Scopolamine and morphine
4. Which of the following should the nurse integrate into the discussion about psychoprophylaxis for prepared childbirth?
   A. Pain is caused by fear that produces tension that leads to pain.
   B. The emphasis is on psychological strategies to prevent pain.
   C. Chemicals are important in removing the pain sensation.
   D. Healthy bodies and attitudes help women cope with strong physical labor sensations.
5. After teaching a group of students about the typical prenatal classes offered in the early 20th century, which type of class, if stated by the group, indicates the need for additional instruction?
   A. Nutrition
   B. Baby care
   C. Maternal hygiene
   D. Partner coaching
6. A pregnant woman plans to remain awake and aware during labor and birth, using deep relaxation to help tune out distractions. The nurse identifies this as the
   A. Dick-Read method.
   B. hypnobirthing approach.
   C. Lamaze method.
   D. Birthing From Within approach.
7. A pregnant woman asks the nurse, "A friend of mine used a doula when she was in labor. What is this?" Which description should the nurse include in the response?
   A. A woman specially trained in the methods of breathing, relaxation techniques, and hypnosis for pain control
   B. A person who provides continuous emotional, physical, and informational support to the mother before, during, and after childbirth
   C. A mentor who teaches the partner about caring for the newborn and supporting the mother during the labor process
   D. A person educated in nursing and childbirth who demonstrates evidence of certification and successful course study completion
8. During discussion with a pregnant woman about childbirth education, the client asks about programs designed to assist with breastfeeding. Which of the following resources should the nurse suggest?
   A. Birth network
   B. Hypnobirthing
   C. La Leche League
   D. Lamaze class
9. When presenting a program to a group of women of childbearing age about the benefits of childbirth education, when should the nurse state that childbirth education should ideally begin?
   A. On the first prenatal visit after pregnancy is confirmed
   B. During the late first trimester or early second trimester
   C. At a preconception visit to the woman's health care provider
   D. When the woman and partner consciously decide to become parents
10. When describing the trend toward natural childbirth, which concept is considered to be most important?
    A. Deconditioning of pain with creation of a new response to pain
    B. Use of antiseptics making hospitals safer for childbirth
    C. Maternal survival as a measure of success in childbirth
    D. Decision related to choosing a male birth attendant over a female birth attendant

REFERENCES

Abushaikha, L., & Oweis, A. (2005). Labour pain experience and intensity: A Jordanian perspective. *International Journal of Nursing Practice, 11,* 33–38.

Amis, D., & Green, J. (2005). Assessment of effective coping during labor. Retrieved January 7, 2006, from http://www.lamaze.org.

Baker, A., Ferguson, S. A., Roach, G., & Dawson, D. (2001). Perceptions of labour pain by mothers and their attending midwives. *Journal of Advanced Nursing, 35*(2), 171–179.

Bass, S. E., Joshi, S. S., Nuttall, D., Sazinsky, S. L., Scharschmidt, T., & Spencer, R. B. (2001). Biotechnology and its social impact. Princeton University. Retrieved April 1, 2006, from http://www.molbio.princeton.edu/courses/mb427/2001/projects/02/antibiotics.htm.

Bing, E., & Colman, L. (2000). *My life in birth.* Washington, DC: Lamaze International.

Birthing From Within. (2000). Philosophical assumptions & guiding principles of Birthing From Within mentors and classes. Retrieved March 12, 2006, from http//:www.birthingfromwithin.com/philosophy.html.

Boot Camp for New Dads. (n.d.) Organizational profile. Retrieved March 19, 2006, from http://bend.org/public?org-newfathers.htm.

Bradley, R. A. (1996). *Husband-coached childbirth: The Bradley method of natural childbirth* (4th ed.). (Revised and edited by Marjie and Jay Hathaway). New York: Bantam Books.

Caton, D., Frolich, M. A., & Euliano, T. Y. (2002). Anesthesia for childbirth: Controversy and change. *American Journal of Obstetrics and Gynecology, 186,* S25–S30.

Charles, D. H., Ness, A. R., Campbell, D., Smith, G. D., Whitley, E., & Hall, M. H. (2005). Folic acid supplements in pregnancy and birth outcome: Re-analysis of a large randomized controlled trial and update of Cochrane review. *Paediatric and Perinatal Epidemiology, 19*(2), 112–124.

Chinn, P. L., & Kramer, M. K. (2004). *Integrated knowledge development in nursing* (6th ed.). St. Louis, MO: Mosby.

Coalition for Improving Maternity Services. (1996). The Mother-Friendly Childbirth™ Initiative. Available at: http://www.motherfriendly.org.

Crosby, R. A., Kegler, M. C., & DiClemente, R. J. (2002). Understanding and applying theory in health promotion practice and research. In R. J. DiClemente, R. A. Crosby, & J. Dahl (Eds.). *New JCAHO pain standards are approved.* American Pain Society. Retrieved April 20, 2006, from http://www.ampainsoc.org/about/annual/1999/annual16.html.

Declercq, E. R., Sakala, C., Corry, M. P., Applebaum, S., & Risher, P. (2002). *Listening to mothers: Report of the first national U.S. survey of women's childbearing experiences.* New York: Maternity Center Association.

England, P., & Horowitz, R. (2001). Midwives as teachers: The 5-minute curriculum. In L. V. Walsh (Ed.), *Midwifery: Community-based care during the childbearing year* (pp. 201–209). Philadelphia: W. B. Saunders.

Hotelling, B. (2001). A call to action and a challenge to use a standard to measure Mother-Friendly birth classes. *Journal of Perinatal Education, 10*(3), 27–33.

Hotelling, B. (2004). Is your perinatal practice Mother-Friendly? A strategy for improving maternity care. *Birth, 31*(2), 143–146.

HypnoBirthing® U.K.: The Mongan method. (n.d.) Retrieved July 23, 2005, from http:www//hypnobirthing.co.uk/history_of_hypnobirthing.shtml.

International College of Nurse-Midwives. (2005). International definition of a midwife. Retrieved January 4, 2006, from http://www.acnm.org/display.cfm?id=437.

International Information Programs. (2005). Glossary. U.S. Department of State's Bureau of International Information. Available at: http://usinfo.state.gov.

Isidro-Cloudas, T. (2006). All about hypnobirthing. Discovery Communications, Inc. Retrieved March 12, 2006, from http://health.discovery.com/centers/pregnancy/americanbaby/hypnobirth.html.

Jiminéz, S. L. M. (2002). Comfort and pain management. In F. H. Nichols & S. S. Humenick (Eds.), *Childbirth education: Practice, research and theory* (2nd ed.). Philadelphia: W. B. Saunders.

Karmel, M. (1981). *Thank you, Dr. Lamaze.* (A new edition of the original work.) New York: Harper & Row Publishers.

Kegler, M. C. *Emerging theories in health promotion practice and research: Strategies for improving public health.* San Francisco: Jossey-Bass.

Klaus, M. H., Kennell, J. H., & Klaus, P. H. (2002). *The doula book: How a trained labor companion can help you have a shorter, easier, and healthier birth* (2nd ed.). Cambridge, MA: Perseus Publishing.

La Leche League International. (2006). *What is La Leche League International?* Retrieved March 31, 2006, from http://www.lalecheleague.org/whatisLLL.html.

Lamaze Institute for Normal Birth. (2005). What is a birth network? Retrieved April 1, 2006, from http://www.lamaze.org/institute/birthnetworks/what.asp?parent=18.

Leap, N., & Anderson, T. (2004). The role of pain in normal birth and the empowerment of women. In S. Downe (Ed.), *Normal childbirth: Evidence and debate.* London: Churchill Livingstone.

Lothian, J., & DeVries, C. (2005). *The official Lamaze guide: Giving birth with confidence.* New York: Meadowbook Press.

Lowe, N. K. (2001). The nature of labor pain. *American Journal of Obstetrics and Gynecology, 186,* S16–24.

Lu, M. C., Prentice, J., Yu, S. M., Inkelas, M., Lange, L. O., & Halfon, N. (2003). Childbirth education classes: Sociodemographic disparities in attendance and the association of attendance with breastfeeding initiation. *Maternal and Child Health Journal, 7*(2), 87–93.

March of Dimes. (2005). Born too soon and too small in the United States. March of Dimes Birth Defects Foundation. Retrieved November 1, 2005, from http://www.marchofdimes.com/peristats.

Maternity Center Association. (2001). Tools for deciding and questions to ask. Retrieved November 1, 2005, from http://www.maternitywise.org/mw/tools.html.

Maternity Center Association. (2004). Informed decision making. Retrieved November 1, 2005, from http://www.maternitywise.org/mw/mid.html.

Merriam-Webster Medical Dictionary. (2005). Trimester. Medline Plus Dictionary. Available at: http://www2.merriam-webster.com.

Midwifery Task Force. (2005). The midwives model of care. Citizens for Midwifery. Retrieved April 5, 2006, from http://www.cfmidwifery.org/mmoc/define.aspx.

National Center for Health Statistics. (2005). U.S. Life Expectancy at all time high but infant mortality increases. *U.S. Department Health and Human Services.* Retrieved February 12, 2006, from http://www.cdc.gov/nchs/pressroom/04news/infantmort.htm.

Nichols, F. H., & Humenick, S. S. (2000). *Childbirth education: Practice, research and theory.* (2nd ed.). Philadelphia, PA: W. B. Saunders.

Nolan, M. L. (1997). Antenatal education—where next? *Journal of Advanced Nursing, 25,* 1198–1204.

Ondeck, M. (2000). Historical development. In F. H. Nichols and S. S. Humenick (Eds.), *Childbirth education: Practice, research and theory* (2nd ed.). Philadelphia: W. B. Saunders.

Pitcock, C. D., & Clark, R. B. (1992). From Fanny to Fernand: The development of consumerism in pain control during the birth process. *American Journal of Obstetrics and Gynecology, 167,* 581–587.

Porth, C. M. (2004). Essentials of pathophysiology: Concepts of altered health states. Philadelphia: Lippincott Williams & Wilkins.

Rising, S. S. (2005). CenteringPregnancy®: A model for group prenatal care. Retrieved March 23, 2006, from http://www.centeringpregnancy.com.

Rothman, B. K. (1991). *In labor: Women and power in the birthplace.* New York: W. W. Norton.

Sagady, M. (1999). The challenge of change: Making mother-friendly care a reality in childbirth education. *International Journal of Childbirth Education.* Retrieved March 19, 2006, from http://www.icea.org/0999samp.htm.

Senden, I. P., Wetering, M. D., Eskes, T. K., Biewrkens, P. B., Laube, D. W., & Pitkin, R. M. (1988). Labor pain: A comparison of parturients in a Dutch and an American teaching hospital. *Obstetrics and Gynecology, 71,* 541–544.

Shilling, T. (2000). Cultural perspectives on childbearing. In F. H. Nichols & S. S. Humenick (Eds.), *Childbirth education: Practice, research and theory* (2nd ed.). Philadelphia: W. B. Saunders.

Simkin, P. (1991). Just another day in a woman's life? Women's long-term perceptions of their first birth experience: Part I. *Birth, 18*(4), 203–211.

Simkin, P. (1992). Just another day in a woman's life? Part II: Nature and consistency of women's long-term memories of their first birth experiences. *Birth, 19*(2), 64–81.

Simkin, P. (1996). The experience of maternity in a woman's life. *Journal of Obstetric, Gynecologic and Neonatal Nursing, 25*(3), 247–252.
Simkin, P. (2000). Commentary: The meaning of labor pain. *Birth, 27*(4), 254–255.
Simkin, P., & Way, K. (2005). Position paper: The birth doula's contribution to modern maternity care. DONA International. Retrieved March 12, 2006, from http://www.dona.org/publications/position_paper_birth.php.
Stamler, L. L. (1998). The participants' views of childbirth education: Is there congruency with an enablement framework for patient education? *Journal of Advanced Nursing, 28*(5), 939–947.
Taylor, S. E., Klein, L. C., Lewis, B. P., et al. (2000). Biobehavioral responses to stress in females: Tend-and-befriend, not fight-or-flight. *Psychological Review, 107*(3), 411–429.
U.S. Department of Health and Human Services. Office of Disease Prevention and Health Promotion. (2000). *Healthy people 2010* (2nd ed.). Washington, DC: U.S. Government Printing Office. Available at: http://www.health.gov.
U.S. Department of Veterans Affairs. (2006). Pain: The 5th vital sign. Section 6: JCAHO. Retrieved April 20, 2006, from http://www.va.gov/oaa/pocketcard/section6_jcaho.asp.
Wertz, R. W., & Wertz, D. C. (1989). *Lying-in: A history of childbirth in America.* New Haven, CT: Yale University Press.
Wikipedia. (2005). HypnoBirthing. Wikipedia, The Free Encyclopedia. Retrieved February 12, 2006, from http://en.wikipedia.org/wiki/Hypnobirthing.
Wirth, F. (2001). *Prenatal parenting.* New York: HarperCollins.
World Health Organization, Department of Reproductive Health and Research. (1999). *Care in normal birth: A practical guide* (p. 3). Geneva: Author.
Zwelling, E. (1996). Childbirth education in the 1990's and beyond. *Journal of Obstetric, Gynecologic and Neonatal Nursing, 25*(5), 425–432.

LABOR AND CHILDBIRTH

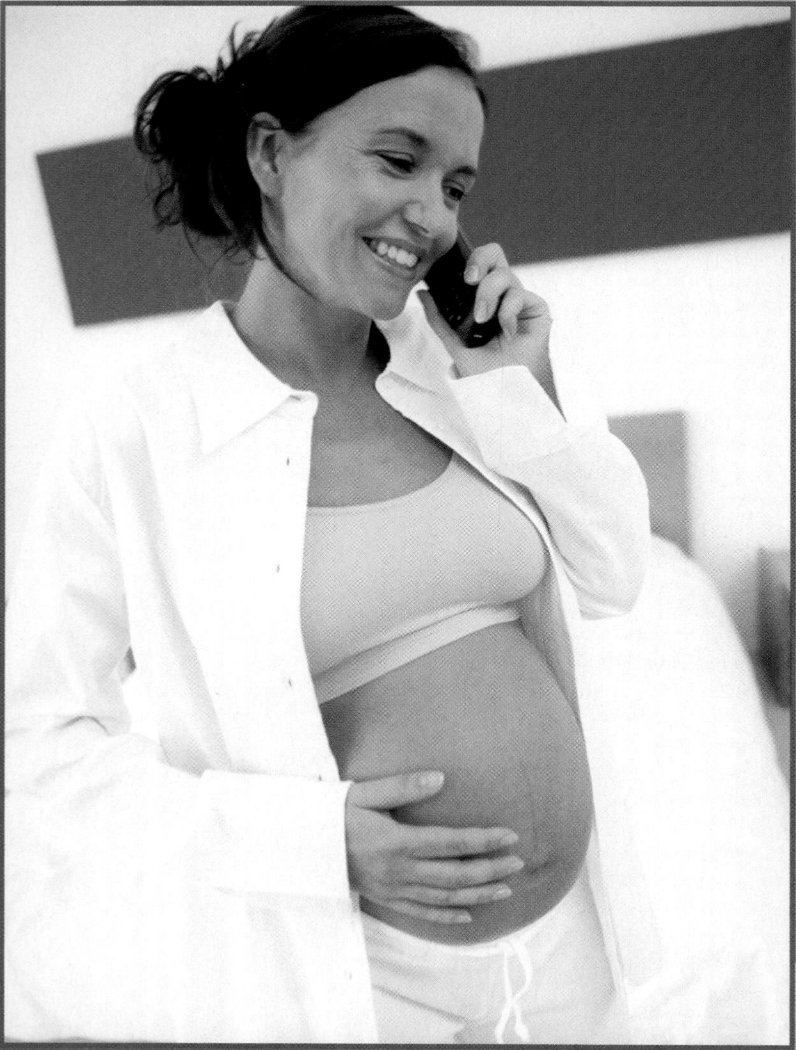

UNIT 4

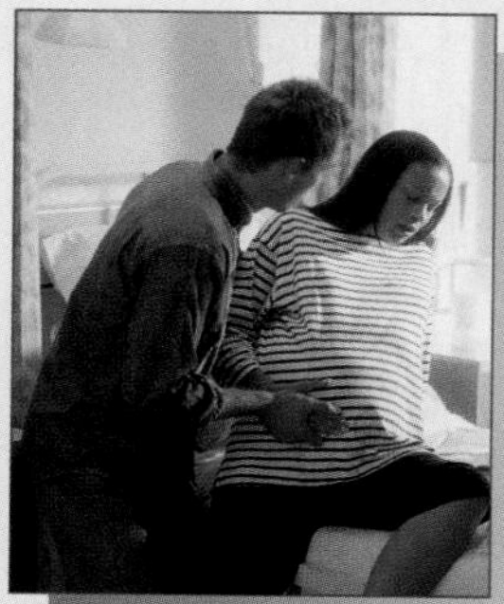
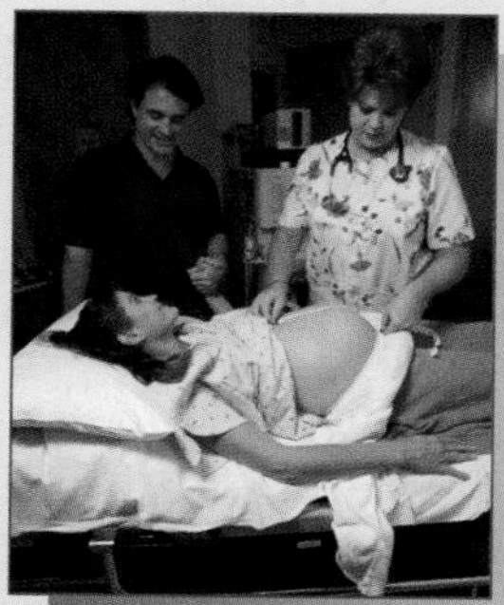
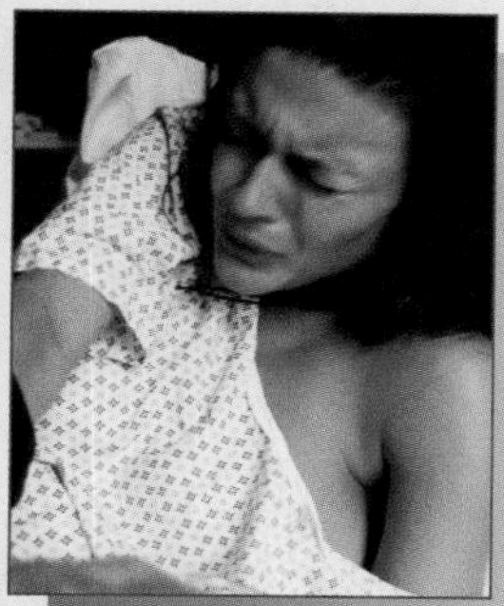
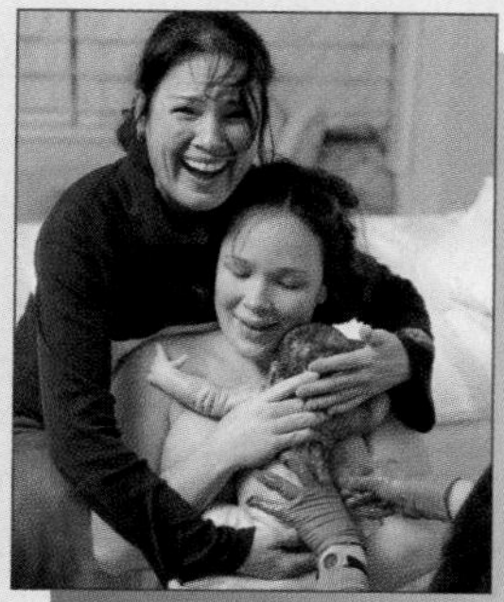

Labor and childbirth represent both an end and a beginning. The experience serves as the culmination of the approximate 9 months that the expectant family has spent preparing to welcome and to incorporate a new member. At the same time, birth represents the first separation between mother and child. It is the initial step in a series of milestones that mark a person's progression toward total independence from his or her parents.

Unit 4 explores the normal processes of labor and the related management to facilitate a healthy vaginal birth. It discusses conditions that pose potential risks during labor, as well as complications that arise only during the process of childbirth itself. The content also presents methods of assisted delivery, including cesarean births. This unit also examines dimensions of pain during labor and various methods that can be implemented to manage it.

CHAPTER 15

Labor and Childbirth

Wendy Budin

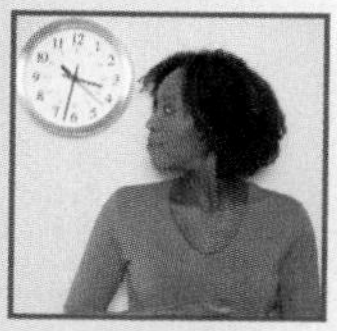

Tyrese, 31 years old and at 38 weeks' gestation with her first pregnancy, comes to the clinic for an appointment. During health history taking, Tyrese states, "The last few days I've been urinating more frequently than I had been. My belly doesn't seem so tight anymore. My back's been aching lately, too."

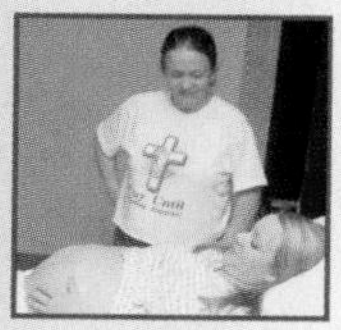

Yolanda, 29 years old and G2P1, arrives at the labor and birth suite at term. Her contractions are moderate, occurring every 7 to 8 minutes and lasting approximately 30 seconds. She is accompanied by her mother. "My husband is on his way home from a business trip," Yolanda says. "I hope he gets here in time."

You will learn more about Tyrese's and Yolanda's stories later. Nurses working with these and similar clients need to understand this chapter's content to manage care and address issues appropriately. Before beginning, consider the following points related to the above scenarios:

- What are nursing care priorities for each client? Explain your response.
- In what stage of labor is each client? What physiologic events happen during these stages?
- How might labor and birth be similar for each woman? How might these processes be different?
- How would you expect each client's circumstances to influence the nurse's approach to assessment, teaching, and follow-up? What other factors would you want to learn?

LEARNING OBJECTIVES

On completion of this chapter, the reader should be able to:

- Describe signs of approaching labor.
- Differentiate prodromal labor from progressive labor.
- Recognize the influence of a client's cultural background on her choices about and responses to labor and birth.
- Discuss current theories explaining the onset of labor.
- Describe the characteristics of the cervix and uterine contractions as labor progresses.
- Identify the landmarks of the fetal skull.
- Define concepts used to describe fetopelvic relationships.
- Describe the mechanisms of labor when the fetus is in a cephalic presentation.
- Explain how maternal position may affect labor and birth.
- Discuss maternal system responses to labor and birth.
- Describe monitoring techniques used to assess fetal well-being.
- Recognize various patterns in fetal heart rate and appropriate nursing implications.
- Identify characteristics of the stages and phases of normal labor.
- Describe emotional and social changes that women experience throughout labor and birth.
- Describe collaborative measures to facilitate the normal course of labor and birth.

KEY TERMS

acceleration
acme
active labor
afterbirth
attitude
baseline bradycardia
baseline tachycardia
baseline variability
Bishop score
bloody show
Braxton-Hicks contractions
bregma
contraction
contraction duration
contraction frequency
contraction intensity
crowning
deceleration
denominator
dilation
doula
early deceleration
early labor
effacement
electronic fetal monitoring (EFM)
engagement
episiotomy
first stage of labor
fontanelles
fourth stage of labor
labor
late deceleration
lie
lightening
mechanisms of labor
molding
occiput
pelvic inlet
pelvic outlet
position
presentation
presenting part
prodromal labor
second stage of labor
spontaneous rupture of membranes (SROM)
station
third stage of labor
transition phase
variable deceleration
vertex

QUOTE 15-1

"It is refreshing to know that for all the billions of times it has occurred, the birth of a child, like the wonder inspired by a sunset, can never be tarnished by repetition."

Anonymous

Childbirth is a transcendent event with meaning far beyond the actual physiologic process (Lee & Lamp, 2005). In addition to the physical sensations and work involved, labor and birth also encompass psychological, spiritual, and social dimensions. The nursing and psychosocial literature consistently describes childbirth as a life-altering experience for women and their families (England & Horowitz, 1998; Kitzinger, 2001; Lundgren, 2004; Vincent, 2002). It forever shapes women's thoughts of themselves and may affect their relationships, both positively and negatively, with children and other family members (Goodman et al., 2004; Simkin, 1996; Waldenstrom, 2004). The care provider and place of birth can enhance or diminish a woman's confidence and ability to give birth (Lamaze International, 2001; Matthews & Callister, 2004). Nurses who provide supportive, competent care during labor can positively influence the quality of a family's childbirth experience, as well as the health and well-being of mothers and babies.

To respond professionally, nurses must understand the basic physiologic and psychological aspects of childbirth. This chapter describes the process of normal labor and birth as well as appropriate collaborative care measures for the various stages and phases of this experience. The nurse's role throughout birthing focuses heavily on assessing maternal and fetal physical status, as well as identifying the learning and psychosocial needs of the client and her significant others. Providing care to families during labor and birth is both a privilege and an opportunity. It allows nurses to participate in a miracle, contributing to the safe arrival of a new human being and guiding the family through a multidimensional, complex, and ongoing journey.

PRELABOR

Most women are unaware of the exact moment that labor begins. Theoretically, labor starts when the cervix begins to dilate; however, this initiating event is difficult to determine (Gross et al., 2005; Ragusa et al., 2005). Therefore, health care providers typically rely on the client's report of signs and symptoms to pinpoint the time of the onset of labor.

During the last few weeks of pregnancy, several premonitory changes may indicate that the mother's body is preparing for childbirth. The cervix begins to soften, thin, and move forward; it also may begin to open. The fetus settles into the pelvis. **Contractions** (intermittent tightening of the uterine muscles) may be noticeable as achy sensations or as pressure in the lower abdomen or lower back. Such contractions are highly variable. They can be irregular—starting and stopping—or regular. Sometimes they are mild; at other times, they may be strong. These early contractions, referred to as **prodromal labor,** can last for hours to a few days.

Signs of Approaching Labor

Signs and symptoms of approaching labor include lightening, increased Braxton-Hicks contractions, backache, bloody show, spontaneous rupture of membranes, diarrhea, spurt of energy, and weight loss (Rouse & St. John, 2003). Most women experience one or more of these events in the weeks and days leading up to labor.

Lightening

Lightening is the lay term used to describe fetal settlement or engagement into the maternal pelvis. Typically, the woman's abdomen changes in shape as the uterus drops forward. Decreased fundal height measurements also indicate that the baby has "dropped" (Fig. 15.1). Lightening may happen suddenly. The woman may arise one morning entirely relieved of the abdominal tightness and diaphragmatic pressure that she experienced previously (see Chap. 12). Relief in one direction, however, often is followed by greater pressure below. She may experience shooting pains down the legs from pressure on the sciatic nerves, increased vaginal discharge, and greater urinary frequency because of uterine pressure on the bladder.

In women nearing childbirth for the first time, lightening may occur approximately 10 to 14 days before labor. In women who have given birth before, lightening is more likely after labor already has started.

Braxton-Hicks Contractions

Women may notice increased **Braxton-Hicks contractions,** which are normal, irregular, usually painless

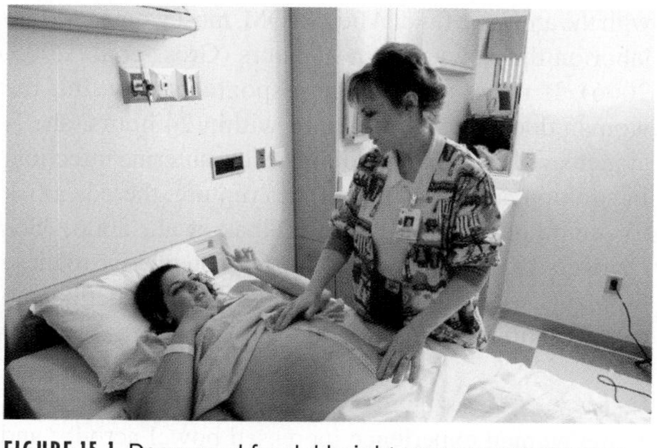

FIGURE 15.1 Decreased fundal height measurements near term indicate that the baby has "dropped" and that the woman is approaching labor.

uterine contractions throughout pregnancy caused by increased estrogen levels and uterine distention (Khan & Razi, 2005). These contractions do not lead to the progressive cervical changes that indicate active labor. More frequent and intense Braxton-Hicks contractions commonly are associated with other subtle signs of approaching labor, such as a low, mild backache.

Backache

By the end of pregnancy, the woman's back may hurt persistently as a result of accumulated postural changes. Such pain also may be from mild and early uterine contractions. Backache also may develop from pressure on the sacroiliac joint, which is related to the influence of relaxin hormone on the pelvic joints. A backache should be considered suggestive of labor if it fluctuates regularly, increases in intensity, or is accompanied by pelvic pressure or cramping.

Bloody Show

Another sign of impending labor is a pink or **bloody show.** This pinkish-tinged vaginal discharge, often mixed with mucus, results from dislodgment of the mucous plug that has sealed the cervical os throughout pregnancy and rupture of the cervical capillaries as effacement and dilation begin (Khan & Razi, 2005). Women may notice this discharge before recognizing any of the other preliminary signs of labor. Some women notice a bloody show following a routine vaginal examination in the last few weeks of pregnancy.

Spontaneous Rupture of Membranes

Spontaneous rupture of membranes (SROM) is the natural breaking of the bag of waters, or amniotic sac, either before or during labor. Occasionally, SROM is the first indication of approaching labor. The woman may experience SROM as a trickle or gush of clear or slightly straw-colored amniotic fluid from the vagina. Sometimes, whitish particles of the vernix are visibly mixed with the amniotic fluid. After SROM, most women go into labor on their own within 24 hours (Gross et al., 2005, 2006). If membranes rupture spontaneously, but the woman does not go into labor within 24 hours, she is at increased risk for developing an intrauterine infection. In addition, any time membranes rupture, there is a risk for umbilical cord prolapse (Dilbaz et al., 2006). See Chapters 13 and 16 for more information relative to these problems, as well as a discussion of labor induction and augmentation.

Diarrhea

Some women experience increased bowel activity and mild diarrhea shortly before labor. Such developments probably are associated with the release of prostaglandin that accompanies labor. They also may be the body's attempt to empty the bowel so that the digestive system is not competing with the woman's other organs for energy during the demanding work of childbirth.

Spurt of Energy

Some women have described anecdotally an unexpected spurt of physical and emotional energy, feeling better than they have in weeks, before the onset of labor. The underlying mechanism may be increased epinephrine resulting from decreased placental progesterone production (Pillitteri, 2007). Other women report a "nesting" instinct, during which they find themselves preparing their home for the newborn (eg, organizing the nursery, cleaning) with a flurry of activity. Some health care providers advise women to ignore this feeling and to conserve energy for the approaching work of labor.

Weight Loss

After months of steady weight gain, the woman nearing labor may lose a few pounds (Fig. 15.2). This weight loss may result from changes in estrogen and progesterone levels, causing electrolyte shifts and decreased body fluid.

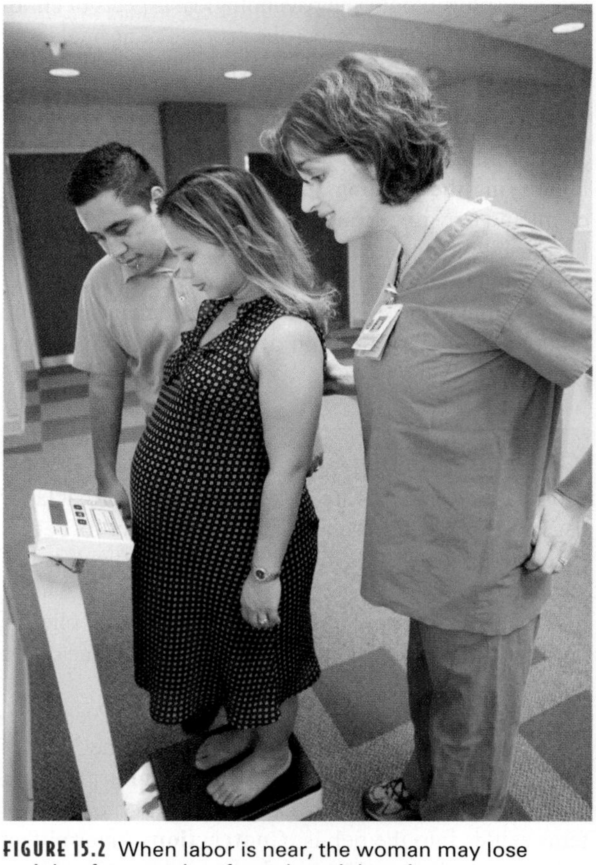

FIGURE 15.2 When labor is near, the woman may lose weight after months of steady weight gain.

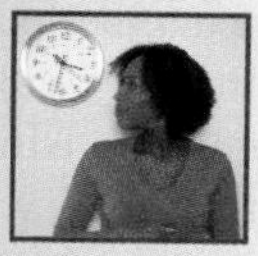

Recall Tyrese, who is at 38 weeks' gestation. Based on the information provided in the opening scenario, which signs would the nurse identify as indicating that Tyrese's labor is approaching? What additional information does the nurse need to assess?

BOX 15.1 Characteristics of True Labor Contractions

- Regular
- Gradually become closer together, eventually occurring every 4 to 6 minutes and lasting 30 to 60 minutes
- Strengthen with time
- Cause vaginal pressure and discomfort starting in the back and radiating to the front
- Continue regardless of position or activity

True Versus "False" Labor

The term "false labor" has been used inaccurately to describe a situation in which women are, in fact, in prodromal or very early labor, which can last from a few hours to a few days. The contractions usually do not progress in frequency, duration, or intensity, and there is usually no progressive cervical dilation. In addition, the contractions of prodromal labor decrease with changes in position or activity.

A client experiencing prodromal labor needs anticipatory guidance and reassurance. The nurse should advise her and her partner to observe and record the characteristics of contractions, especially noting any changes with alterations in position or activity. Also, the nurse should urge the woman to obtain adequate nutrition and fluids (in case contractions become progressive). Fatigue and discouragement are common, especially if prodromal labor is lengthy or recurrent. Care providers should avoid labeling the woman's experience as "false labor" because such terminology tends to invalidate the woman's real experience. Additionally, these early contractions are, in fact, helping to prepare for childbirth.

When the client moves from prodromal to active labor, contractions become rhythmic and regular. Their intervals are constant and decrease in frequency; their duration and intensity increase, and positional or activity changes do not affect them. (Walking may, in fact, enhance their progression.) Progressive contractions often start in the back and then radiate to the lower groin. They usually are associated with pelvic pressure, increased vaginal discharge, loss of the mucous plug (or "bloody show"), and possibly rupture of the membranes. They result in progressive cervical effacement and dilation. See Box 15.1.

Emotional Experience of Impending Labor

Because of the many physical changes women experience late in pregnancy and before labor, restless or sleepless nights are common and may contribute to gradually mounting tension and fatigue. Increased anxiety heightens awareness; therefore, women may become more sensitive to various stimuli. If the fetus is less or more active than usual, the client may worry. The client may question whether the weight loss of 2 to 3 lbs that sometimes precedes the onset of labor is normal. (It is.) She may be concerned about her ability to cope with labor. During this time, the client may be preoccupied with planning last-minute details for the baby. Throughout labor, nurses play a vital role in assisting the client and partner to use effective coping mechanisms to achieve a positive outcome (Simpson, 2005).

QUOTE 15-2

"The days leading up to the birth of my baby were filled with so many mixed emotions. In many ways, they were a good preparation for the time that followed!"

A 27-year-old mother

Sociocultural Aspects Related to Impending Labor and Birth

Although the childbirth experience is universal and so unites women around the world, cultural values and norms exert great influences over it. Culture forms the backdrop for all human behavior and learning. Each person brings her own beliefs, worldview, rituals, attitudes, values, ways of knowing, and learning to every situation (Shade et al., 1997). Clients and families frequently base their coping with childbirth on cultural beliefs, rituals, and traditions (Andrews & Boyle, 2004).

Ethnic and cultural groups vary greatly in their beliefs, values, and behaviors surrounding childbirth. A goal of perinatal nursing is to provide a culturally competent environment in which women and their families feel cared for and that they have been treated with their best interests considered (Callister, 2005). When working with clients from a culture that differs from his or her own, the nurse needs to remain aware of the many possibilities that may exist in that culture and avoid assuming that a particular client will automatically conform to a specific pattern. He or she needs to look for cues, develop skills, acquire knowledge, and maintain objectivity.

Areas that require particular cultural sensitivity from nurses include the meaning of childbirth to the client and the ways she experiences and chooses to deal with pain (Cioffi, 2004). Western medicine tends to convey a message that childbirth is a medical problem fraught with danger and demands assistance from qualified medical professionals (Davis-Floyd & Sargent, 1997). For some women, however, this belief tarnishes the birth experience. Some clients view childbirth as normal, natural, and healthy and face labor confidently, relying on their inner wisdom (Kennedy & Shannon, 2004; Lothian, 2001). Many cultures praise women for their achievement in birthing a baby. Other cultures attribute or give at least partial credit for this accomplishment to the skill of the obstetrician. For example, in the United States, people often use terminology indicating that a woman is "delivered" of her child as opposed to giving birth. Additionally, certain cultures require strict adherence to rituals during labor and birth. These beliefs may influence the position the woman chooses for labor, as well as who is allowed to remain with her during birth (Andrews & Boyle, 2004).

Just as attitudes toward the meaning of birth differ among cultures, so do expressions of pain and feelings about pain management (Callister et al., 2003; McLachlan & Waldenstrom, 2005). For some clients, crying and moaning are culturally appropriate responses to discomfort. For others, remaining stoic and nonverbal about pain is culturally expected. Cultures that view childbirth as a natural experience may prefer nonpharmacologic options for pain relief or complementary and alternative therapies (see Chap. 17). The upbringing, culture, and personal values of the nurse and other health care providers, as well as their own ability to cope with pain, may influence their attitudes toward the clients' responses and choices about the expression and relief of pain.

The nurse also should consider his or her expectations of the role family members are to play in providing labor support (de Montigny & Lacharite, 2004). Gender-determined roles and responsibilities vary among different cultures, as does family decision making. Such influences may contribute to selections of location for and support people during labor and birth (Bashour & Abdulsalam, 2005). For cultural or religious reasons, some fathers cannot touch the woman during labor or birth. Regardless of their degree of participation, male family members need to feel accepted by health care providers during this time. Some women feel that exposing any part of their body is unacceptable. This may influence their choice of health care provider and who can perform procedures during labor and birth. Expectation of the role of health care providers also may vary according to culture. The nurse needs to ascertain what the woman's preferences are about care providers and procedures.

Collaborative Management

During the prelabor phase, collaborative management focuses on providing the client and her significant others with anticipatory guidance and support. The best advice for a client is to be patient and to have confidence that her body is doing exactly what it is supposed to at this time. The nurse should encourage the woman not to worry whether it is really labor. For the vast majority of women, labor eventually becomes quite apparent. As labor approaches, the nurse should encourage the client to eat, drink plenty of fluids, and rest. She and her partner or other support people can do things that they enjoy such as watching television, going for a walk, or visiting with friends. By surrounding herself with people with whom she is comfortable, the woman can stay positively focused and receive reassurance. Nursing Care Plan 15.1 highlights the care of a woman in prelabor.

LABOR AND BIRTH

Labor refers to the series of events by which the products of conception are expelled from the mother's body (Cunningham et al., 2005). This technical definition does not in any way convey the wonder of the process responsible for this beautifully synchronized and salutary achievement. Nature has designed labor and birth simply and elegantly (Lothian, 2001). Although every birth is unique and unfolds in a special way, the process is remarkably and beautifully consistent. Once labor begins, it normally runs its course until its purpose—the birth of the baby—is fulfilled.

The traditional definition of labor is the period when regular uterine contractions are associated with cervical effacement and dilation. This explanation, however, presents many clinical problems. Some facilities arbitrarily define the onset of labor as the time of admission to the birth unit. Other maternity care settings define labor as when a woman's cervix has achieved a dilation of 3 or 4 cm. Yet other facilities use the woman's self-reporting of the onset of symptoms as the time of onset of labor. Unfortunately, none of these interpretations is entirely adequate.

Etiology of Labor

Just what initiates labor is not definitely known (Gross et al., 2005; Ragusa et al., 2005). For many years, researchers have assumed that several factors (either alone or combined) bring about labor. For example, some have attributed labor to the withdrawal of progesterone near the end of pregnancy. Others have supported the idea that marked distention of the uterus and pituitary action lead to the release of oxytocin and thus uterine activity (Simpson & Creehan, 2001).

During the past few decades, new information has challenged several proposed causes of the initiation of labor. Currently, interrelationships between mother and fetus are considered to play important roles, although these relationships are not yet well understood. The following discussion summarizes some of the most common theories of the onset of labor.

Progesterone Withdrawal

The progesterone withdrawal theory suggests that initiation of labor is related to both maternal hormones and fetal status. Progesterone is thought to suppress uterine

NURSING CARE PLAN 15.1

The Client in Prelabor

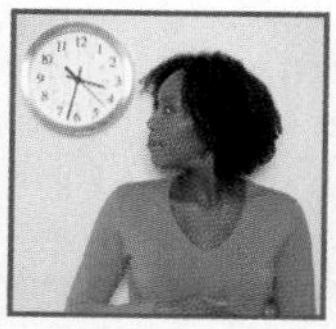

Physical examination of Tyrese reveals cervical dilation of 1 cm and effacement of 30%. Her membranes are intact. The fetus is in a cephalic presentation, vertex position at −2 station. Fetal heart rate is 144 bpm. Tyrese says, "Does this mean I'm in labor? I'm not having contractions."

NURSING DIAGNOSES

- **Deficient Knowledge** related to prelabor signs and symptoms and upcoming labor and events
- **Anxiety** related to first experience with labor and uncertainty of the unknown.

EXPECTED OUTCOMES

1. The client will state the signs and symptoms of true labor.
2. The client will verbalize events related to upcoming labor and birth.
3. The client will identify areas causing her concern.

INTERVENTIONS	RATIONALES
Assess the client's level of understanding about signs and symptoms of approaching labor and the process of childbirth.	Assessment provides a baseline to identify specific client needs and develop an individualized plan.
Discuss her concerns, feelings, and perceptions related to labor and birth.	Talking provides opportunities to emphasize positive aspects of the current situation; verbalization of concerns aids in establishing sources of stress and problem areas to address.
Communicate accurate data and answer questions honestly. Reinforce facts, emphasizing that each pregnancy, labor, and birth is highly individualized.	Open honest communication promotes trust and helps correct any misconceptions. Facts help to dispel unfounded fears, myths, or guilt feelings.
Evaluate the client's past coping strategies to determine which have been most effective.	Use of appropriate coping strategies aids in reducing anxiety.
Correlate the client's current signs and symptoms with those associated with approaching labor; review the signs and symptoms of true labor and actions to take.	Correlation of current status provides insight into changes occurring in preparation for labor. Having knowledge of true labor signs and symptoms and actions to take alleviates stress.
Urge the client to report any spontaneous gush of fluid.	Spontaneous rupture of membranes can lead to cord prolapse. If rupture is prolonged, the risk for infection increases.
Teach the client what to expect relative to contraction strength and frequency and progression of labor.	An understanding of what to expect reduces fear of the unknown.
Review comfort measures, such as music, distraction, hot/cold compresses, massage, and position changes that can be used.	Knowledge of available measures to control pain helps reduce anxiety associated with contractions.
Give the client the phone number of a person to notify when signs of true labor occur.	Availability of a contact person helps reduce anxiety, providing a source for anticipatory guidance once labor begins.

Continued

NURSING CARE PLAN 15.1 ● The Client in Prelabor *(Continued)*

EVALUATION

1. The client states the signs and symptoms of true labor accurately.
2. The client identifies the progression of events associated with labor and birth.
3. The client verbalizes appropriate measures to cope with concerns related to labor and birth.

irritability throughout pregnancy by counterbalancing the increased uterine contractility resulting from increased estrogen levels (Goff, 1993). Changes within the fetal membranes and decidua as the placenta ages and as term approaches may be associated with increased estrogen synthesis and decreased progesterone production. Increased estrogen levels can increase oxytocin in the myometrium (uterine muscles). In addition, a compound called transforming growth factor-β may react in a gene-specific manner that not only decreases progesterone but also increases oxytocin receptors. Research is currently being conducted in this area.

Oxytocin Production

Oxytocin is a hormone released from the posterior pituitary gland in increased amounts during labor. Release of oxytocin alone, however, does not adequately explain what initiates labor. Progesterone during labor tends to inhibit the uterine response to oxytocin. It is only after estrogen has already influenced the uterine muscles that sensitivity to oxytocin increases, as does the number of oxytocin receptors. In fact, oxytocin may be given in large amounts early in pregnancy with little or no effect, and such administration often has little influence on an unripened cervix (Blackburn & Loper, 2003). This finding has major clinical implications for the use of oxytocin as an agent for elective induction of labor. Because oxytocin performs best after oxytocin receptors in the uterus have increased, one of the best ways to determine whether a woman will respond well to labor induction is to perform a pelvic assessment for cervical ripening. A ripe cervix is likely to have many oxytocin receptors and, subsequently, favorable outcomes.

A **Bishop score** is a system for rating cervical ripeness for labor based on assessment of its position, consistency, effacement, and dilation, as well as the fetal station (Table 15.1). A favorable Bishop score indicates that, even without exogenous oxytocin stimulation, labor will most likely begin soon on its own.

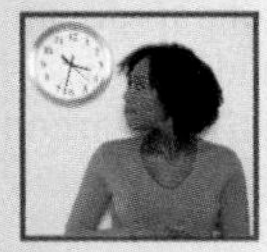

Remember Tyrese, the woman being seen at the prenatal clinic at 38 weeks' gestation. Suppose examination revealed cervical dilation of 1 cm, 30% effacement, –2 station, and a soft cervix at the midposition. What would be Tyrese's Bishop score?

Prostaglandin Production

Prostaglandins are agents formed from fatty acids that act as chemical mediators or local hormones. They stimulate smooth muscle contraction and probably have been the most studied compounds in the past 25 years in relation to labor's onset (Blackburn & Loper, 2003). Unlike oxytocin, administration of prostaglandins appears

TABLE 15.1 Bishop Score System

	FACTOR				
SCORE	**Dilation (cm)**	**Effacement (%)**	**Station**	**Cervical Consistency**	**Cervical Position**
0	Closed	0–30	–3	Firm	Posterior
1	1–2	40–50	–2	Medium	Midposition
2	3–4	60–70	1, 0	Soft	Anterior
3	5 or more	80 or more	+1 or more		

Each factor is given a score, and the subtotals are combined. Scores above 8 indicate cervical ripeness and a high likelihood for labor and successful induction.

From Bishop, E. H. (1964). Pelvic scoring for elective induction. *Obstetrics and Gynecology, 24,* 266.

to initiate labor any time during gestation. The importance of prostaglandins is further enhanced by findings that women who take high doses of antiprostaglandin drugs (eg, aspirin, ibuprofen) may have delayed labor (Blackburn & Loper, 2003; Cunningham et al., 2005).

Estrogen Stimulation

The estrogen stimulation theory is based on increase in estrogen levels that occur at 34 to 35 weeks' gestation. Estrogen appears to promote oxytocin production and the formation of estrogen receptors in the uterine muscles. It also is thought to stimulate prostaglandin production. Researchers have postulated that because estrogen production comes from fetal adrenal precursors, this may be an example of fetal factors contributing to labor initiation (Blackburn & Loper, 2003).

Fetal Influence

The fetus may have roles in both initiation of labor and the process of labor itself, although exact mechanisms are not well understood. For example, the fetal lungs or kidneys may transmit a signal for labor through a mediator secreted into the amniotic fluid (Cunningham et al., 2005). Theorists have suggested that fetal cortisol levels rise to a point that initiates labor. The fact that fetuses with anencephaly tend to be postterm supports this finding. Anencephalic fetuses also have adrenal dysfunction, which in turn decreases available fetal cortisol (Cunningham et al., 2005).

Other Theories

Some other explanations for initiation of labor include overdistention of the uterus and infections. According to the overdistention theory (also termed the "stretch theory"), the uterus reaches a set threshold that leads to synthesis and release of prostaglandins (Rouse & St. John, 2003). Infections may be associated with the initiation of labor, especially preterm labor. In such cases, however, it is likely that labor results not simply from the infectious process but also from the increased level of prostaglandins, which is a natural mediating response to infection.

Processes of Labor and Birth

To understand what labor and birth involve, subdividing the topic into different categories can be helpful. The traditional way of doing so has been to identify the "Ps" of labor (Rouse & St. John, 2003):

- *Powers:* uterine contractions and maternal pushing
- *Passageway:* the maternal pelvis and soft parts
- *Passenger:* fetus

Other influences on labor and birth include maternal psychological status, support from partners and others, and maternal position during labor.

Powers

Uterine Contractions. As mentioned earlier, uterine contractions are intermittent tightenings of the myometrium. Throughout labor, the muscles in the upper uterine segment are more active, contracting more intensely and for longer than those of the lower uterine segment. After the muscles have contracted, they relax, pulling up the cervix and lower uterine segment. The upper segment thickens with time, while the more passive lower segment thins (Rouse & St. John, 2003).

Normal uterine contractions are like waves, composed of an increment (the building up or ascending portion), an **acme** (the peak), and a decrement (the coming down or descending portion). When describing contractions, caregivers refer to their frequency, duration, and intensity (Fig. 15.3). **Contraction frequency** means the time from the beginning of one contraction to the beginning of the next. **Contraction duration** is timed from the beginning to the end of the same contraction. **Contraction intensity** refers to strength.

Contractions, the primary power needed to accomplish labor and birth, are intermittent throughout labor,

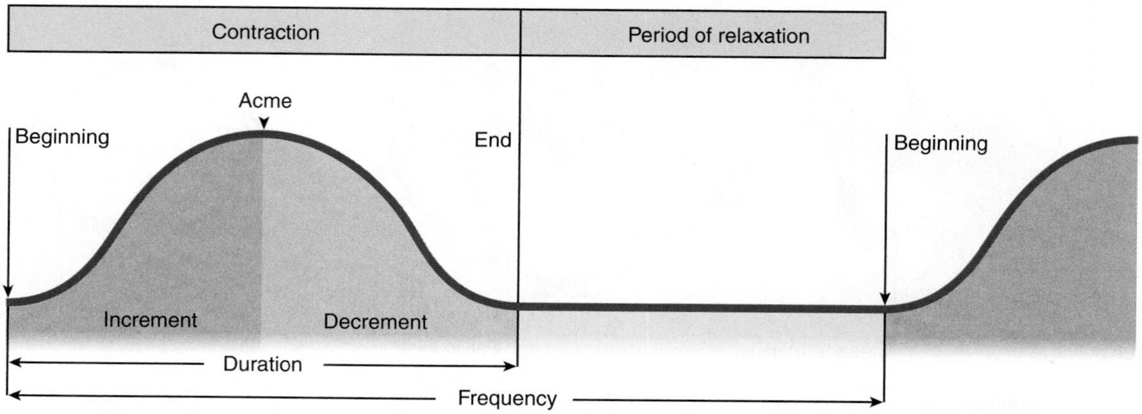

FIGURE 15.3 A uterine contraction has three phases: increment, acme, and decrement.

forming a regular pattern interspersed with rest periods. The intervals of rest between contractions are essential, not only for maternal comfort but also for fetal welfare. Labor contractions are mild at first and then become increasingly more intense as labor progresses.

Pushing. In addition to contractions, the other power is the intra-abdominal force provided by the mother through pushing (Rouse & St. John, 2003). This power is reserved for the second stage of labor, after effacement and dilation are complete. It is commonly referred to as "bearing down." As labor continues, many women begin to experience an involuntary urge to push. With pushing, the woman contracts her abdominal muscles to provide an auxiliary force to the contractions, increasing intra-abdominal pressure to force the fetus through the vagina.

For many years it was suggested that women should push with a closed glottis (also called Valsalva maneuver) and under directed efforts by health care personnel. Research findings, however, questioned both the efficacy and potential harm of these measures. Closed glottis pushing increases intrathoracic pressure and impairs blood return from the lower extremities, leading to an initial increase and then decrease in blood pressure. These changes affect uteroplacental blood flow and perfusion (Simpson & Creehan, 2001). Fetal hypoxia and resultant acidosis have been associated with prolonged and forceful closed glottis pushing (Mayberry et al., 1999). In addition, some studies have shown that coached pushing resulted in only a minimal decrease in the length of the second stage of labor (Bloom et al., 2006; Sampselle et al., 2005). Women have been observed to push effectively by either controlled exhalations or brief breath holding when they are not instructed to do otherwise. Physiologic and spontaneous approaches to pushing avoid risks and allow women to follow their own instincts (Chalk, 2004; Karnng-Edgren, 2001; Mayberry, 2000; Roberts 2002).

Passageway

The passageway consists of both a hard passage (bony pelvis) and a soft passage (maternal soft tissue structures).

Maternal Bony Pelvis. The pelvis is the bony ring known as the hip girdle, which separates the lower extremity from the trunk. It transmits body weight to the lower extremities. In women, the pelvis also serves as the passage for the fetus to be born.

Pelvic Structures. The major pelvic bones include the innominate bones (formed by the fusion of the ilium, ischium, and pubis around the acetabulum), sacrum, and coccyx. For obstetric purposes, the pelvis is arbitrarily divided into halves: the false pelvis and the true pelvis (Fig. 15.4). An imaginary line called the *linea terminalis,* which extends from the symphysis pubis to the sacral prominence, separates them.

The false pelvis is the wide, broad area between the iliac crests. It supports the uterus and directs the fetus into the true pelvis to engage. The true pelvis is below the linea terminalis and actually serves as the bony birth passage. The entrance to the true pelvis is called the **pelvic inlet.** The shape of the true pelvis is curved, not straight, which means that the fetus must first move down and then up over the sacrum as it descends through the **pelvic outlet,** or the lower border of the true pelvis. This has implications for the positioning of women during the expulsion stage.

Pelvic Types. Various methods have been used to predict the adequacy of a pelvis in terms of the ease of passage. Four basic types have been classified according to shape: *gynecoid, android, anthropoid,* and *platypelloid.* The features of these types are discussed in Chapters 12 and 16. In some women, the pelvis is a mixture of two types. Generally, vaginal birth is most easily accomplished with a gynecoid pelvis and is difficult or impossible with an android or platypelloid type (Rouse & St. John, 2003).

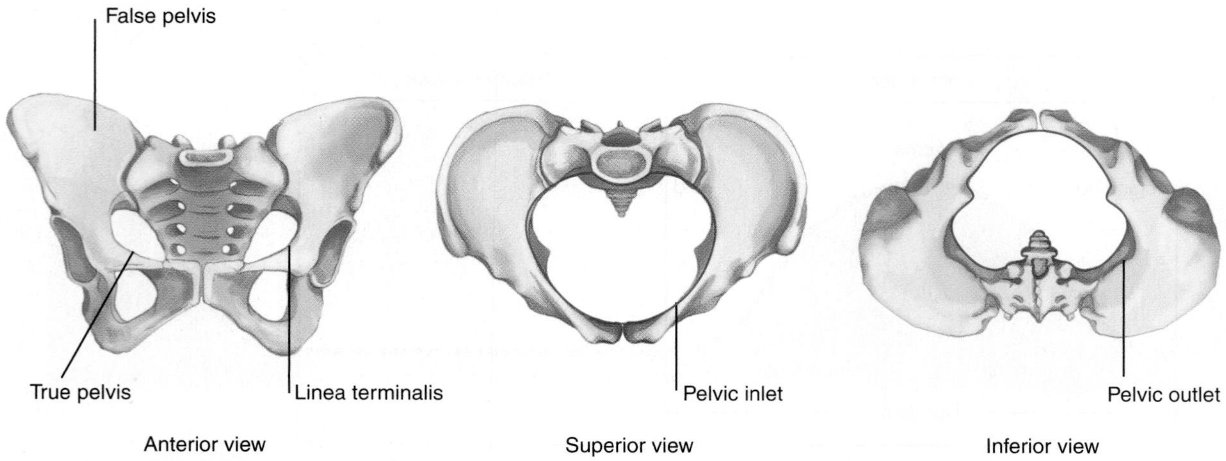

FIGURE 15.4 The maternal bony pelvis: anterior, superior, and inferior view.

Pelvic Diameters. In addition to pelvic shape, fetal ability to pass through depends on the size of the true pelvis. To determine the size, examiners take measurements of diameters of the pelvic inlet, midpelvis, and pelvic outlet early in the antepartal period, often on the first prenatal visit (see Chap. 12).

Maternal Soft Parts. For normal labor and birth, the soft tissues of the cervix, vagina, and perineum must stretch to allow passage of the fetus. Progesterone and relaxin facilitate such softening and increase the elasticity of the muscles and ligaments. During the last few weeks of pregnancy, the cervix softens, effaces, and becomes more elastic. Ripening also results from Braxton-Hicks contractions and engagement of the fetal head, which serves as a wedge against the cervix. Already distensible, the vagina becomes even more stretchable throughout pregnancy. Estrogen promotes growth of the vaginal mucosa and underlying tissues and increases cellular glycogen. Increased vascularity helps to thicken and lengthen the vaginal walls. These changes allow the vagina to accommodate passage of the fetus. The muscles of the perineum also soften and become more stretchable.

Passenger

Fetal Head. Because the fetal head is usually the largest part that must pass through the vaginal opening, its size and relative rigidity are important factors that influence the mechanism of labor. The fetal head is divided into the face and base of the skull and the cranial vault (Fig. 15.5). The bones of the skull are well ossified and firmly united. The bones of the cranial vault, however, are relatively thin, poorly ossified, and loosely connected to one another by membranous attachments. At birth, flexibility of the bones of the cranial vault allows some movement and overriding, so that the fetal head can adapt to the maternal pelvis. This adaptive process is called **molding** and sometimes manifests in the newborn as an elongated head (see Chap. 16). Molding disappears generally within the first few days after birth.

Two frontal bones, two parietal bones, and one occipital bone make up the cranial vault. The associated diameters are important (Fig. 15.6). The biparietal diameter, or the distance between the two parietal bones, is considered the widest transverse diameter of the fetal head. It measures approximately 9.25 cm (Cunningham et al., 2005). Other important fetal diameters include the following:

- Suboccipitobregmatic—approximately 9.5 cm
- Submentobregmatic—approximately 9.5 cm
- Occipitofrontal—approximately 11.75 to 12 cm
- Occipitomental—approximately 13.5 cm (Rouse & St. John, 2003)

The membranous attachments are called *sutures.* The *sagittal suture* joins the two parietal bones. The *lambdoidal suture* joins the parietal and occipital bones. The *coronal suture* joins the parietal and frontal bones. The sutures are considerably enlarged at their point of intersection and are known as **fontanelles.** The two major fontanelles are the diamond-shaped anterior fontanelle (also known as the **bregma**), and the triangular-shaped posterior fontanelle. The anterior fontanelle does not close until a baby is approximately 18 months old. The posterior fontanelle usually closes by 6 to 8 weeks after birth.

The cranial vault is divided into three distinct sections. The **vertex** is the portion that lies between the anterior and posterior fontanelles. The **occiput** constitutes the area of the occipital bone. The *brow* is the portion lying between the large anterior fontanelle and the eye sockets.

Fetopelvic Relationships. To understand the relationship between the fetus and the maternal uterus and pelvis, the nurse needs to be familiar with descriptive terminology (Rouse & St. John, 2003).

- **Lie** is the relationship of the fetal long axis (spine) to the maternal long axis (spine). Lie is *longitudinal* when

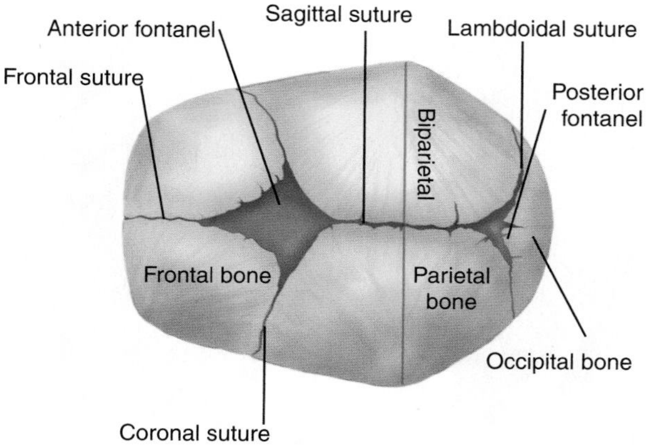

FIGURE 15.5 Landmarks of the fetal skull.

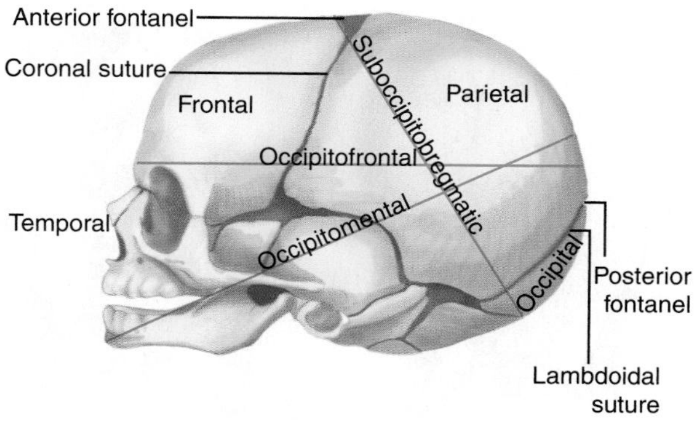

FIGURE 15.6 Diameters of the fetal skull.

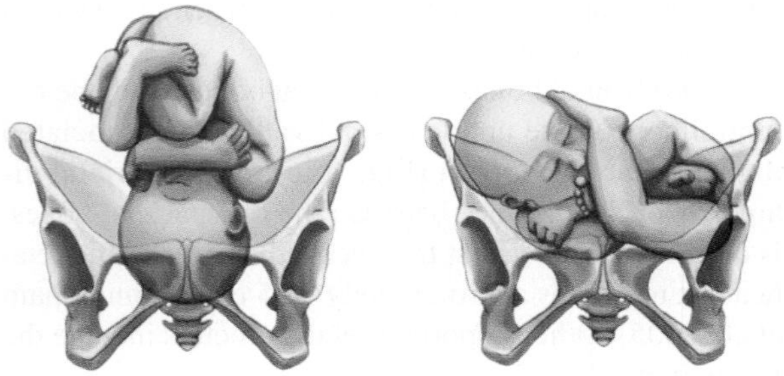

FIGURE 15.7 Fetal Lie. (**A**) Longitudinal lie. (**B**) Transverse lie.

the fetal spine is parallel with the maternal spine. Lie is *transverse* when the fetal spine is perpendicular to the maternal spine (Fig. 15.7).

- **Presentation** refers to the fetal part that lies over the pelvic inlet. The main presentations are *cephalic* (head first), *breech* (pelvis or buttocks first), and *shoulder.* Cephalic presentations are subdivided as vertex, military, brow, and face (Fig. 15.8).
- **Presenting part** refers to the most dependent fetal part lying nearest to the cervix. During a vaginal examination, it is the area with which the examiner's finger first makes contact.
- **Attitude** is the relation of the fetal parts to one another. The basic attitudes are *flexion* and *extension* (Fig. 15.9). The fetal head is in flexion when the chin approaches the chest. It is in extension when the occiput nears the back. The typical fetal attitude is flexion.
- **Denominator,** an arbitrarily chosen landmark on the fetal presenting part, is used when describing position. Each presentation has its own denominator. With a cephalic presentation, the denominator is the occiput.
- **Position** means the relationship of the denominator to the front, back, or sides of the maternal pelvis and is described using the first three letters of these landmarks. To use an example, a fetus in the cephalic presentation has the denominator as the occiput, which in this case is in the right anterior quadrant of the maternal pelvis. The abbreviation assigned is ROA (right occiput anterior) (Box 15.2). Occiput anterior positions facilitate labor because the head acts as a dilating wedge as the contractions help propel the fetus through the smallest pelvic diameters. Occiput posterior positions tend to prolong labor and are associated with other risks (Senecal et al., 2005). The woman usually experiences increased back pain, especially because the fetal head usually is not well flexed (see Chap. 16).

Station. Station refers to the relationship of the fetal presenting part to an imaginary line drawn at the ischial spines within the maternal pelvis. When the largest diameter of the fetal presenting part has passed the pelvic inlet, **engagement** has occurred. Fetal engagement normally accompanies lightening, approximately 2 weeks before labor in a primipara. When the head is the engaged part, not only has the widest diameter passed the pelvic inlet, but also its most forward portion, the vertex, lies approximately at the imaginary line joining the ischial spines. A presenting part at the level of the spines is at 0 station. A part 1 cm below the spines is at +1 station. If it is at 2 cm below, it is at +2 station. A part 1 cm above the spines, it is at −1 station. See Figure 15.10.

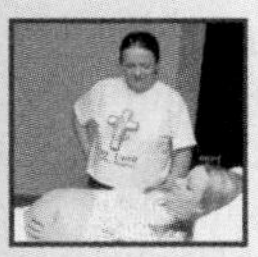

Yolanda arrived at the health care facility complaining of contractions. A vaginal examination reveals that the fetus is in a cephalic presentation in ROP position. What assessments would be priorities?

Mechanisms of Labor

While labor is causing uterine and cervical changes, the fetal presenting part goes through a series of passive movements designed to mold its smallest possible diameter to the irregular shape of the pelvic canal. In this way,

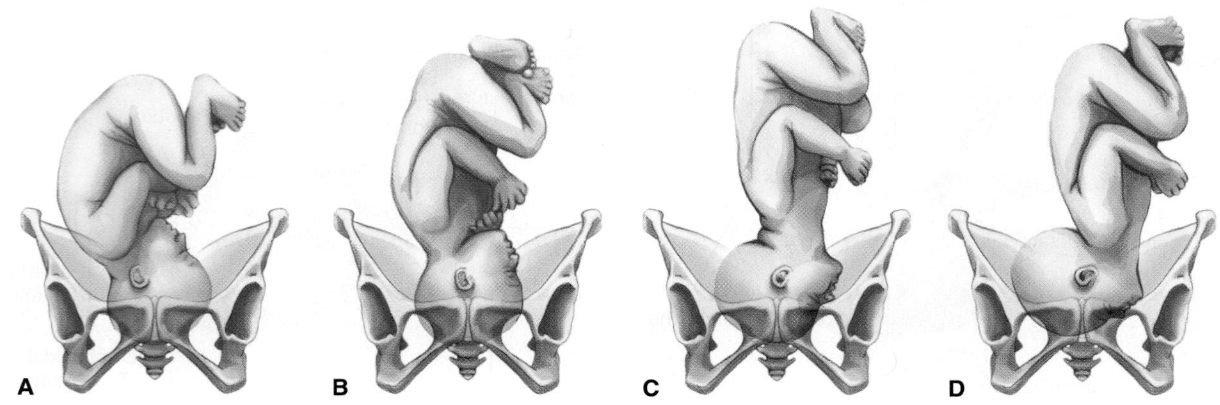

FIGURE 15.8 Cephalic fetal presentations. (**A**) Vertex. (**B**) Military. (**C**) Brow. (**D**) Face.

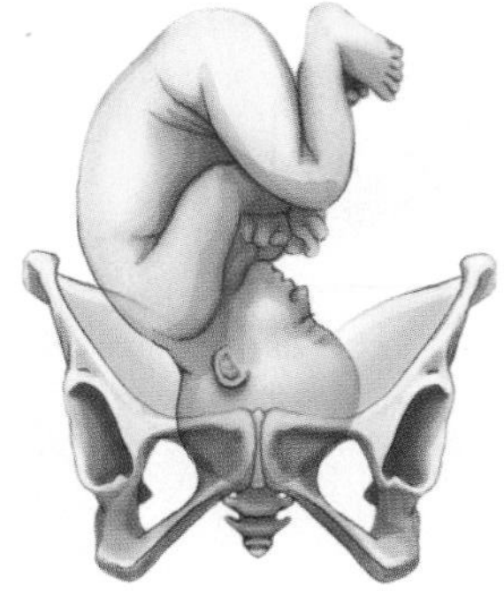

FIGURE 15.9 Full fetal flexion, with the smallest fetal diameter presenting to the maternal pelvis.

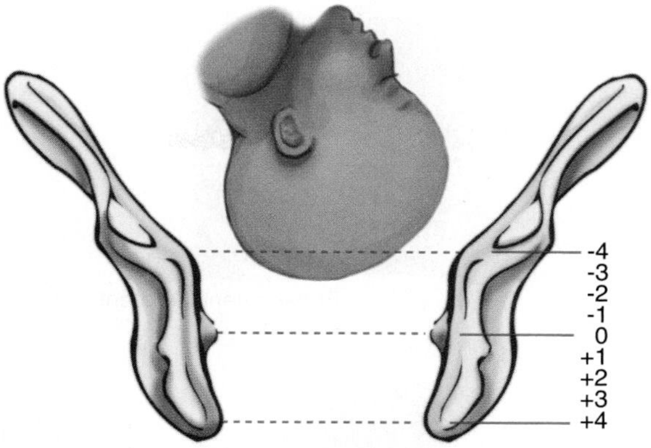

FIGURE 15.10 Fetal stations.

the presenting part will encounter as little resistance as possible. These *cardinal movements,* which usually occur in a smooth sequence, constitute the **mechanisms of labor** (Khan & Razi, 2005). Because a vertex presentation is most common, the next discussion describes the mechanisms of labor for this type (Fig. 15.11).

Descent

When the fetal head presents, it usually enters the pelvis in a transverse position facing the mother's side. This is because the pelvic inlet is widest from side to side, and the oval-shaped fetal head fits best that way.

Descent, the downward movement of the fetus, is attributed to one or more of four forces:

- Pressure of amniotic fluid
- Direct pressure of the uterine fundus on the fetus
- Contraction of the maternal abdominal muscles during pushing
- Extension and straightening of the fetal body

Although descent is said to be continuous, it actually occurs only with contractions. In the intervals of relaxation, the presenting part recedes somewhat, thus relieving pressure on it and maternal soft tissues, as well as restoring circulation diminished temporarily by the contraction.

Flexion

Early in the process of descent, the fetal head encounters sufficient resistance, causing it to flex so that its chin rests on its chest. The head thus presents its narrowest diameter, the suboccipitobregmatic, to the pelvic outlet.

Internal Rotation

When the occiput reaches the pelvic floor, it is rotated 45 degrees anteriorly and comes to lie beneath the symphysis pubis. In this fashion, the shoulders remain in their original position. Internal rotation of the head thus involves a twisting of the fetal neck.

Extension

During extension, the occiput passes out of the pelvis. The nape of the fetal neck moves under the maternal pubic arch, enabling the fetal scalp, brow, eyes, nose, mouth, and chin to push through the vagina.

Restitution

As soon as the head passes through the vaginal opening, the fetal neck untwists, and restitution occurs. The occiput thus returns 45 degrees to its original position.

BOX 15.2 Terminology of Fetal Positions

Vertex Presentation (Occiput)

- Left occipitoanterior (LOA)
- Left occipitotransverse (LOT)
- Left occipitoposterior (LOP)
- Right occipitoanterior (ROA)
- Right occipitotransverse (ROT)
- Right occipitoposterior (ROP)

Face Presentation (Mentum)

- Left mentoanterior (LMA)
- Left mentotransverse (LMT)
- Left mentoposterior (LMP)
- Right mentoanterior (RMA)
- Right mentotransverse (RMT)
- Right mentoposterior (RMP)

Breech Presentation (Sacrum)

- Complete
- Left sacroanterior (LSA)
- Left sacrotransverse (LST)
- Left sacroposterior (LSP)
- Right sacroanterior (RSA)
- Right sacroposterior (RSP)

Shoulder Presentation (Acromion)

- Left acromion dorsal anterior (LADA)
- Left acromion dorsal posterior (LADP)
- Right acromion dorsal anterior (RADA)
- Right acromion dorsal posterior (RADP)

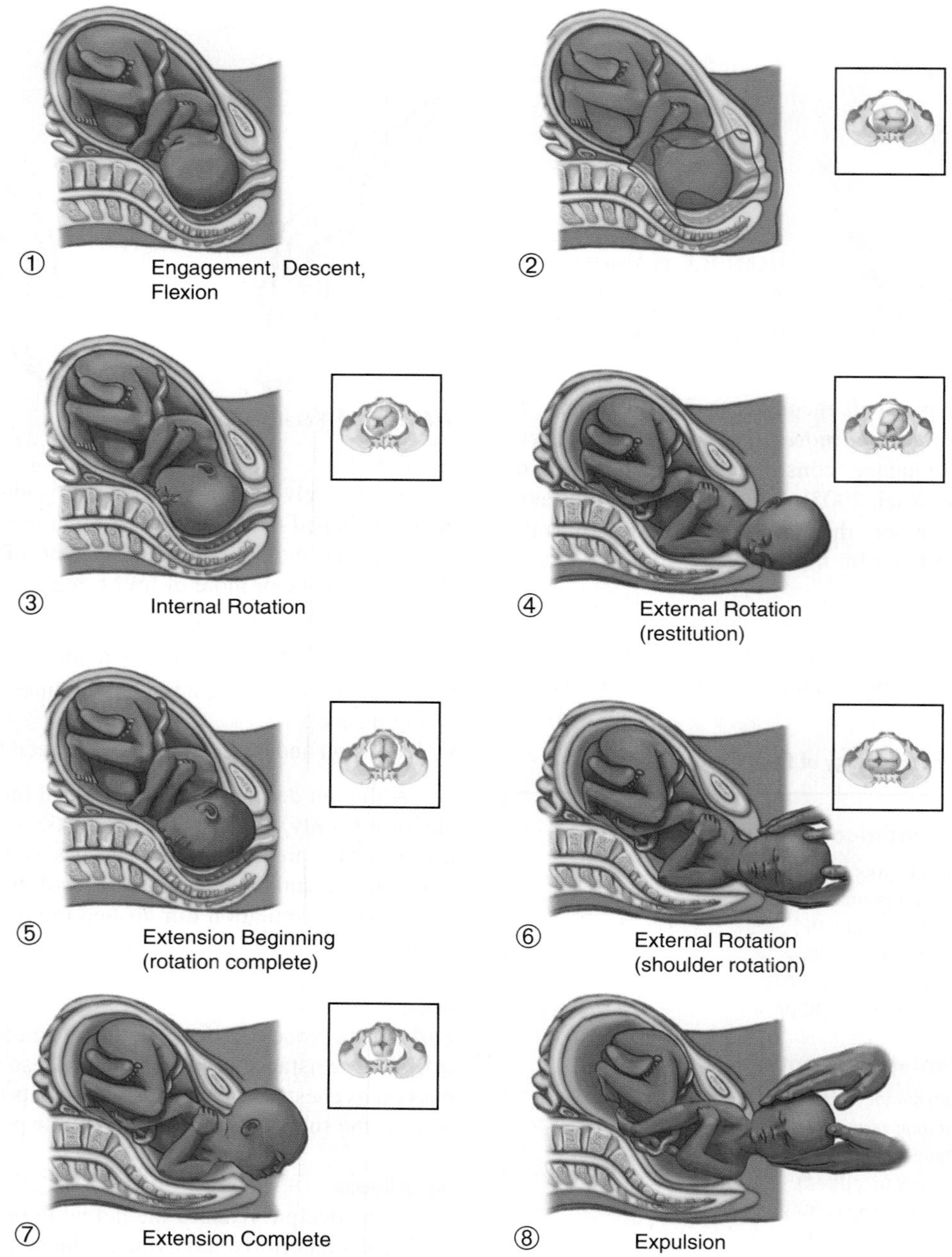

FIGURE 15.11 The cardinal movements of labor, vertex presentation.

External Rotation

When the fetal anterior shoulder meets the resistance of the pelvic floor, it is shunted downward, forward, and inward to the maternal symphysis pubis. This positioning brings the shoulder into the anteroposterior diameter of the outlet and causes the head to rotate externally 45 degrees more.

Birth of the Shoulders and Expulsion

When the anterior shoulder comes into view beneath the pubic arch, it pauses while the posterior shoulder is being born by lateral flexion. Once both shoulders are out of the vagina, the rest of the baby is readily born.

Maternal Responses to Labor

Maintenance of the normal physiologic process of labor is an important goal in the care of a pregnant woman and her fetus. Identifying factors that influence normal labor and how they might be enhanced or altered is important to promoting health and achieving expected outcomes.

Cardiovascular System

Labor has major effects on maternal cardiovascular status. Generally, cardiac output, cardiac workload, heart rate, and blood pressure all increase. Cardiac output elevates as a result of the transfer of maternal blood (300 to

500 mL) from the uterus and placental vascular bed into the maternal systemic vascular system with each contraction. Blood pressure and heart rate may rise with contractions. Fear and anxiety can cause the release of catecholamines, leading to transient tachycardia. Therefore, the nurse should assess blood pressure and pulse between labor contractions.

Hematologic changes include an elevated white blood cell count, which researchers hypothesize may be related to the stress of labor. The physical work of labor may cause blood glucose levels to decrease. Blood coagulation time may decrease, whereas plasma fibrinogen levels increase. Peripheral vascular changes may result in maternal flushed cheeks (malar flush) or hot or cold feet.

Position in labor or at birth may further influence cardiovascular changes. Supine positions can lead to decreased cardiac output and stroke volume with increased heart rate from compression of the inferior vena cava and descending aorta. Extended breath holding (Valsalva maneuver) can increase intrathoracic pressure, decrease venous return, and increase venous pressure. This results in increased cardiac output, increased blood pressure, decreased pulse, and potential fetal hypoxia (Blackburn & Loper, 2003). Anxiety and pain also increase cardiac work and may be a major component of the changes demonstrated with a contraction.

Respiratory System

Uterine muscle activity increases oxygen consumption. Maternal respiratory rates usually rise with anxiety, pain, exertion, or the use of controlled breathing techniques for pain management. The client should try to avoid persistent hyperventilation resulting from fear or pain.

Major changes occur in acid–base relationships during labor, although these appear to quickly reverse themselves after birth. These normal alterations include mild respiratory alkalosis in early first-stage labor and mild metabolic acidosis compensated by respiratory alkalosis at the end of first-stage labor; mild respiratory acidosis during bearing down efforts; and finally metabolic acidosis uncompensated by respiratory alkalosis at birth (Blackburn & Loper, 2003).

Gastrointestinal System

During active labor, gastric motility decreases, whereas the emptying time of the stomach increases. If opioids are administered, the emptying time is likely to be even more prolonged (Cunningham et al, 2005). Traditional practice was to limit food and fluids during labor because of the risk for vomiting and possible aspiration. When the stomach remains relatively empty, however, nausea and vomiting are common intrapartal complaints, particularly during the transition phase. In fact, an empty stomach increases gastric acidity, which may lead to nausea and vomiting. Some women also experience belching during transition. To compensate for restriction of oral fluids, administration of intravenous (IV) fluids has become routine care in many facilities. According to the findings from randomized clinical trials, however, withholding food and fluid from women in labor and giving routine IV infusions are unlikely to be beneficial (Enkin et al., 2000). Clear liquids are absorbed rapidly, so providers can encourage the woman to drink these if no apparent complications exist (Scrutton et al., 1999; Sleutal & Golden, 1999). Caregivers may offer a woman in labor a light or liquid diet according to her preferences (American College of Obstetricians and Gynecologists [ACOG], 2002; Enkin et al., 2000). IV infusions are needed only for high-risk or special cases (eg, use of epidural anesthesia, administration of oxytocin).

Genitourinary and Renal System

Glomerular filtration rate increases during labor with increased cardiac output; therefore, polyuria is common. The nurse should observe the laboring woman closely for bladder distention or inability to void. These findings can result from relaxed bladder tone, analgesia or anesthesia, fetal compression, or trauma. Along with polyuria, diaphoresis, decreased hydration, and increased respirations also can affect electrolyte balance. Proteinuria (trace to 1+) may result from the breakdown of muscle tissue.

Psychosocial Responses

Maternal emotional status before and during labor strongly influences the progression of childbirth. The psyche of a frightened, anxious, or upset client can affect the normal physiology of labor and birth (Fig. 15.12). High levels of catecholamines may interfere with the normal process (Simpson & Creehan, 2001). Norepinephrine and epinephrine may stimulate both α and β receptors of the myometrium and interfere with labor's rhythmic nature, culminating in a pattern of ineffective contractions and, consequently, prolonging childbirth (see Chap. 16).

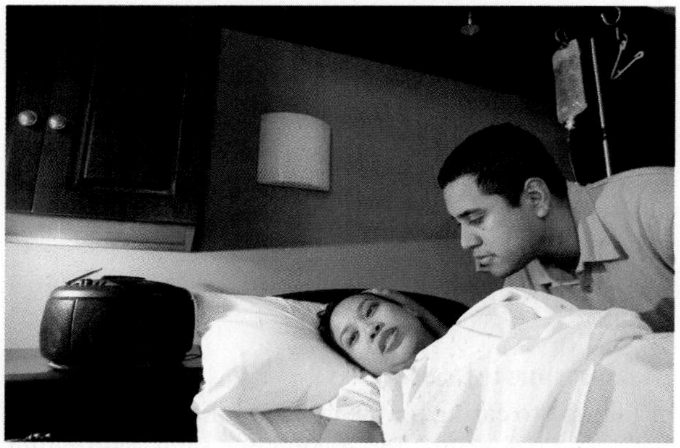

FIGURE 15.12 Fear, anxiety, or distress during childbirth can alter maternal physiology negatively and prolong labor. Support from partners and others during this time can be crucial to assisting women through this emotional time.

Anxiety also can increase pain perception, leading to an increased need for analgesia or anesthesia (see Chap 17).

Many factors contribute to the client's emotional response to birth. Lack of knowledge, fear of pain, personal or family stress, lack of labor support from a significant other, degree of self-confidence, feelings of loss of control, negative attitudes about birth, cultural background, and concerns for personal safety can all serve to block labor's progress (Goodman et al., 2004; Turley, 2004). The birth environment can influence labor as well (Hodnett et al., 2005).

Maternal psychosocial responses vary based on previous coping strategies and associated events. Early in labor, the client may be apprehensive, yet excited. As labor progresses and contractions increase in frequency and intensity, the woman tends to focus on the work at hand. As pain increases, so may discouragement and fatigue, decreasing the client's ability to effectively tolerate contractions (Simpson & Creehan, 2001). For example, during the active phase, the client experiences growing discomfort, including pressure on the bladder and rectum. Strategies she used earlier in labor may be less effective when dealing with the more intense sensations. The client may respond to pain with screaming or crying. Fatigue and exhaustion may further compound these feelings. As a result, the client may fear that she will completely lose control.

Nurses play a key role in ensuring that the client in labor receives adequate support throughout the experience. Research has shown that women with strong self-esteem and support from significant others feel more in control over the sensations and events not previously anticipated (Goodman et al., 2004; Moore, 2001). Encouraging prenatal participation in childbirth education classes helps to prepare women for labor (see Chap. 14). Once in labor, the nurse can urge the client to use techniques and strategies learned in these classes. Providing assistance in the form of emotional support, comfort measures, information, advocacy, and partner support are key (Matthews & Callister, 2004; Simpson & Creehan, 2001).

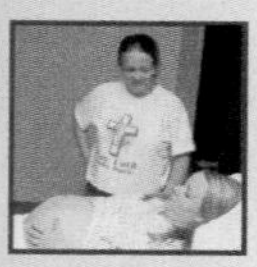

Recall Yolanda, the woman in early labor described at the beginning of the chapter. She voiced concern about whether her husband would arrive in time to attend the birth. What effects might this situation have on her labor?

Fetal Responses to Labor

In addition to caring for the mother during labor, nurses also are responsible for evaluating fetal well-being throughout this time. Although most fetuses respond well to the changing intrauterine environment, contractions, restricted mobility and positioning, and various obstetrical interventions can be potentially stressful. Thus, close monitoring of fetal health is important.

Fetal heart rate (FHR) patterns provide important insights into response to labor; alterations can signal developing problems. The goal of monitoring FHR is to assist care providers to identify fetuses experiencing distress (hypoxia or asphyxia) and to intervene in a timely manner to reduce or relieve that distress. The FHR can be assessed either through intermittent auscultation or continuous electronic fetal monitoring (EFM).

Auscultation of Fetal Heart Rate

For mothers and fetuses with no risk factors, intermittent auscultation provides a safe, noninvasive way to evaluate fetal well-being. Intermittent auscultation of FHR can be done with a fetoscope or more commonly with an ultrasound Doppler device. Current recommendations for auscultation are as follows (Association of Women's Health, Obstetric and Neonatal Nurses [AWHONN], 2000):

- In low-risk pregnancies, auscultate every 30 minutes during the active phase of the first stage of labor.
- In high-risk pregnancies, FHR should be auscultated and documented every 15 minutes during the active phase of the first stage of labor and every 5 minutes during the second stage of labor.
- In addition, the FHR should always be checked and recorded after any invasive procedure or potential changes in the intrauterine environment, such as rupture of membranes, vaginal examinations, or administration of medications.

Before auscultating FHR with a fetoscope or Doppler, the examiner first should determine the location of the back of the fetus, where the strongest heart sounds are transmitted. The examiner can determine the location of the fetal back using Leopold maneuvers to palpate (see Chap. 12). He or she should place the fetoscope or Doppler on the maternal abdomen and listen and count for 60 seconds (Fig. 15.13). Listening to the FHR both during and after a contraction is important to assess for changes in patterns with contractions. If the FHR decreases or does not return to baseline soon after the peak of a contraction, team members should implement measures to enhance uteroplacental perfusion. Examples include a change in maternal position and increased hydration. In cases of suspected fetal distress, continuous EFM (discussed next) may be indicated so that providers can carefully assess the fetal response to contractions (Society of Obstetricians and Gynaecologists of Canada [SOGC], 2002).

Electronic Fetal Monitoring

Electronic fetal monitoring (EFM) involves ongoing evaluation of the FHR and uterine contractions through

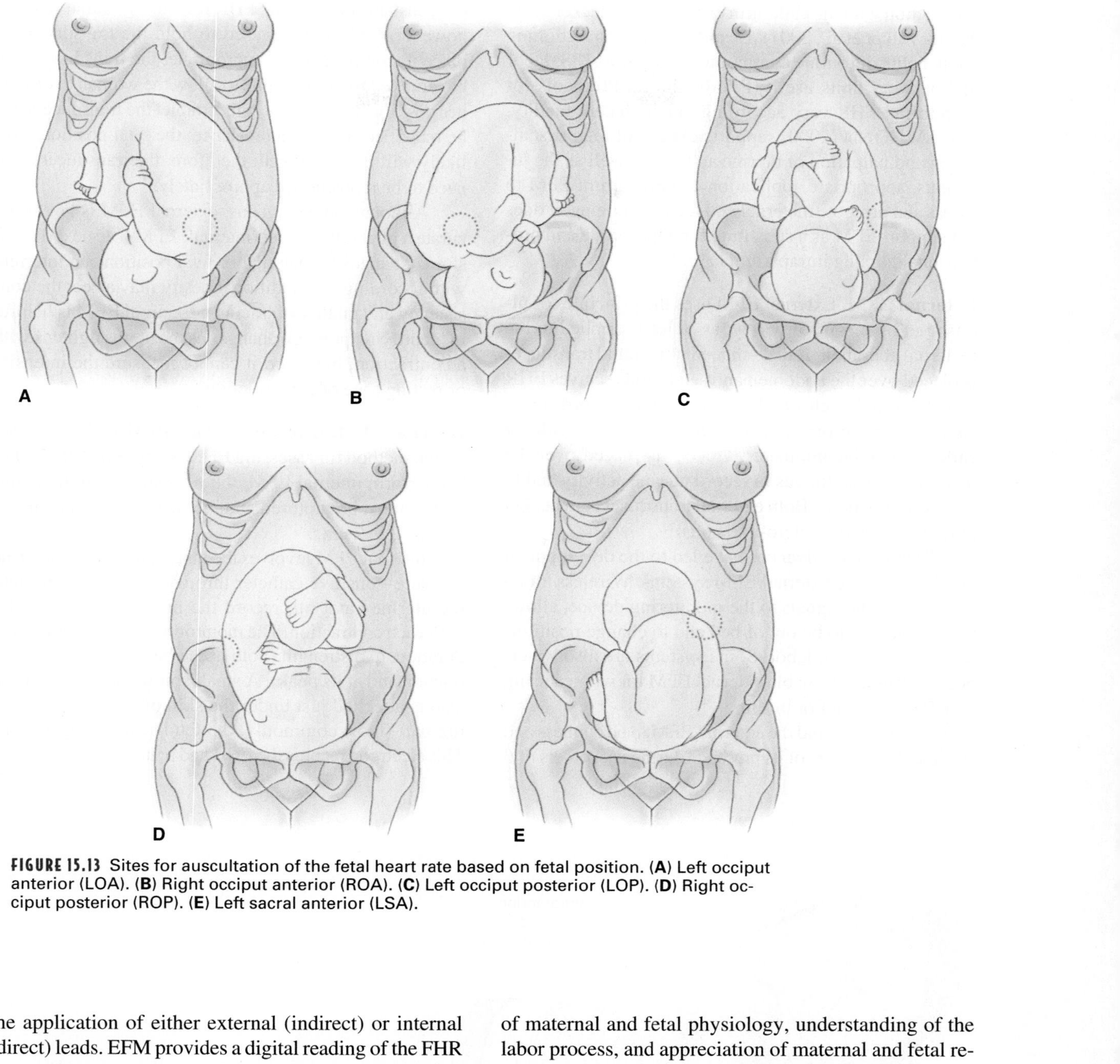

FIGURE 15.13 Sites for auscultation of the fetal heart rate based on fetal position. (**A**) Left occiput anterior (LOA). (**B**) Right occiput anterior (ROA). (**C**) Left occiput posterior (LOP). (**D**) Right occiput posterior (ROP). (**E**) Left sacral anterior (LSA).

the application of either external (indirect) or internal (direct) leads. EFM provides a digital reading of the FHR and uterine contractions in a window display on the unit as well as on printed paper that records tracings over time. The FHR appears as a wavy line at the top of the paper as it prints from the monitor. Contractions appear along the bottom as a series of little hills that gradually become steeper as labor progresses. The fetal monitor printout becomes part of the woman's medical record.

Use of EFM allows care providers to assess fetal well-being by examining the relationship between FHR and maternal uterine activity. The nurse is responsible for ensuring that fetal monitor tracings reflect interpretable FHR and maternal uterine activity. Knowledge of maternal and fetal physiology, understanding of the labor process, and appreciation of maternal and fetal response to labor in normal as well as abnormal circumstances enhance interpretation of fetal monitor tracings and subsequent clinical judgments.

Studies consistently have shown limited benefits in perinatal outcomes using EFM instead of intermittent auscultation (Thacker et al., 2001). Since its introduction into obstetrical care, fetal monitoring has not proved valuable to predicting or preventing fetal neurologic morbidity (Feinstein et al., 2000; Goodwin, 2000; Walker et al., 2001). Although continuous EFM has failed to reduce fetal neurologic morbidity, it has coincided with an increase in cesarean births and has decreased overall maternal satisfaction with the childbirth experience (Thacker et al., 2001; Walker et al., 2001). Despite evidence questioning the benefits of routine continuous EFM, most U.S. labor and delivery units use it (Priddy, 2004). Protocols for monitoring FHR vary according to health care facility. The AWHONN (2000) supports the use of fetal auscultation and palpation of uterine activity as well as the judicious, appropriate application of intrapartum EFM to assess and promote maternal and fetal well-being. It does not support EFM as a substitute for appropriate and professional nursing intrapartum care.

External EFM. External EFM uses the principles of ultrasound by means of two types of leads applied to the maternal abdomen. A disk-shaped ultrasound transducer is placed over the abdomen and sends and receives FHR signals from the fetus to the device, which records these signals as waveforms. A pressure-sensitive transducer called a tocodynamometer ("toco") is placed over the maternal uterine fundus to record uterine activity and to assess contractions. Both external transducers are held in place with elastic Velcro-like belts.

Technologic advances have led to the development of telemetry-like external EFM systems. Wireless transducers send the signals to the monitoring device, allowing the woman to be out of bed and to change positions readily throughout labor. Some systems are also waterproof, designed to enable external EFM for women using tubs for pain relief or birthing.

Some clients find the external EFM to be painless and are actually unaware of its presence during use; others find the constant sound of the FHR reassuring. Some women, however, find the belts used to hold the transducers in place uncomfortable. If appropriate, the transducers can be removed for a short time to allow the woman to change her position. Once she is comfortable, the transducers can be reapplied. In such an instance, the fetal position most likely will have changed; therefore, the transducers will need to be repositioned appropriately.

Although advantageous, external EFM is not as accurate a method as direct (internal) EFM (see next discussion). Changes in maternal or fetal position can interfere with recordings. In addition, obesity may affect the consistency and quality of tracings. External EFM is helpful in identifying pressure changes as the uterus tightens with a contraction; however, it cannot measure the intensity or resting tone of a contraction.

Internal EFM. Direct or internal EFM is the most accurate method for assessing FHR (Feinstein et al., 2003). To perform internal EFM, the woman's amniotic membranes must be ruptured, and her cervix must be dilated at least 2 to 3 cm.

Internal EFM involves the insertion of an intrauterine pressure–sensitive catheter through the vagina and into the uterine cavity to record the pressure of the cavity with each contraction. The monitor records the frequency, duration, and strength (both at the beginning of the contraction and at its peak). A small spiral-shaped electrode also is attached just under the skin of the fetal presenting part (most commonly, the fetal scalp) (Fig. 15.14). This electrode records the FHR and pattern on the monitor.

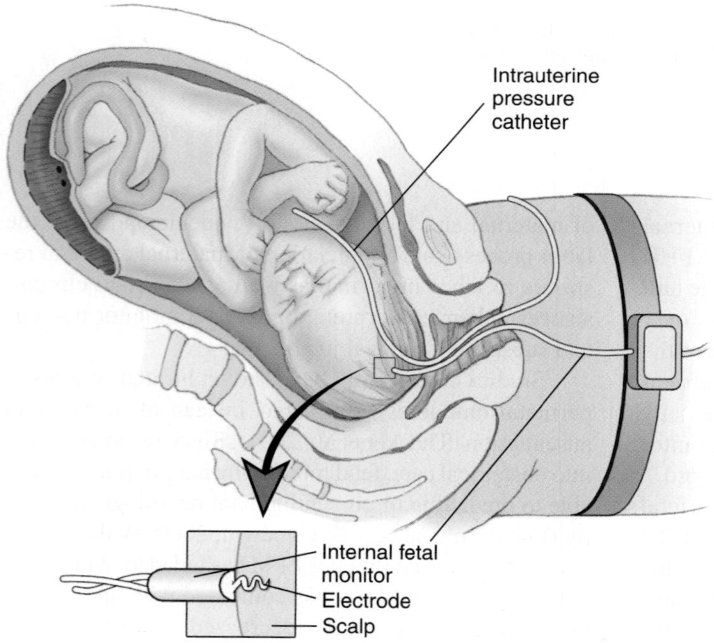

FIGURE 15.14 With internal electronic fetal monitoring, an intrauterine pressure catheter is inserted through the vagina and into the uterine cavity. An electrode is attached just under the skin of the fetal presenting part.

TABLE 15.2 Keys to Interpreting Fetal Heart Rate Patterns

NORMAL/REASSURING INDICATIONS	NONREASSURING INDICATIONS	OMINOUS INDICATIONS
● Baseline 110 to 160 bpm	● Tachycardia	● Tachycardia with lost variability
● Moderate bradycardia with good variability	● Moderate bradycardia with absent or lost variability	● Prolonged marked bradycardia
● Fetal accelerations	● Marked bradycardia	● Severe variable decelerations
	● No beat-to-beat variability	● Persistent late decelerations
	● Moderate variable decelerations	

Internal EFM, although highly accurate, poses some risks. Because the method is invasive, mother and fetus are at risk for infection with use. It also requires the woman to remain in bed throughout labor and childbirth. Internal EFM is contraindicated for use in women who are HIV positive or who have active or chronic hepatitis, herpes simplex virus, or any other known untreated sexually transmitted infection (STI) (Simpson & Creehan, 2001).

Fetal Heart Rate Patterns

Patterns of FHR generally are common and consistent. Table 15.2 compares various FHR interpretations.

Baseline Fetal Heart Rate. Baseline FHR is the typical FHR during a 10-minute period or between uterine contractions in labor. It is the average speed at which the heart is beating and normally ranges from 120 to 160 beats per minute (bpm).

Baseline bradycardia is an FHR less than 120 bpm. Common causes of mild baseline bradycardia include postterm pregnancy and persistent posterior position. Fetal hypoxia and prolonged umbilical cord compression may lead to bradycardia. **Baseline tachycardia,** which is an FHR above 160 bpm, may be associated with acute hypoxia, maternal or fetal fever, and use of certain β-sympathomimetic drugs.

Baseline variability or rhythm is described as the short-term beat-to-beat interval changes in the FHR or the long-term oscillations or undulation of the baseline FHR. Decreased variability is associated with fetal central nervous system depression. Fetal sleep cycles may cause the variability to decrease temporarily (30 to 60 minutes).

Periodic and Episodic Changes. Periodic changes are brief deviations above or below the baseline FHR. Such changes usually occur in relation to uterine contractions or fetal activity. Episodic changes refer to the changes above or below the baseline FHR unrelated to uterine contractions. See Figure 15.15.

An **acceleration** of the FHR is an increase of at least 15 bpm over baseline that lasts at least 15 seconds. An acceleration of FHR often is associated with fetal movement and is considered a sign of fetal well-being.

A **deceleration** of the FHR is a deviation below baseline that persists for at least 10 to 15 seconds but for less than 2 minutes. A *prolonged deceleration* lasts longer than 2 minutes. If the deceleration persists longer than 10 minutes, it becomes a new baseline.

An **early deceleration** is a decrease in the FHR that begins and ends at the same time as the uterine contraction, causing a consistent uniform U-shaped waveform that mirrors the contraction on the EFM tracing. Early decelerations are thought to result from vagal nerve stimulation caused by compression of the fetal head during labor. They are considered a normal physiologic response to labor and need no intervention.

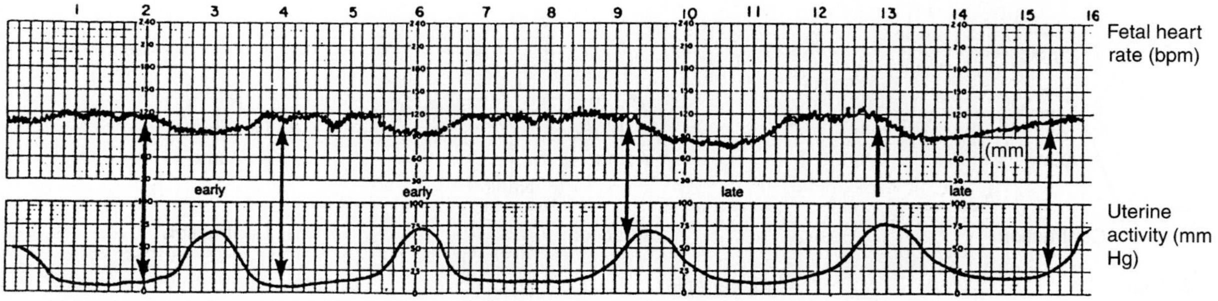

FIGURE 15.15 Electronic fetal monitoring tracing showing early and late decelerations.

A **late deceleration** is a decrease in the FHR that begins after the peak of the contraction and ends after the contraction has ended. Late decelerations are thought to result from uteroplacental insufficiency or compromised uteroplacental perfusion. They often are associated with supine hypotensive syndrome or hyperstimulation of the uterus with oxytocin. Late decelerations are an indication for measures to increase uteroplacental circulation and fetal oxygenation. Maternal position changes can improve maternal venous return. Upright positions also are associated with more efficient uterine activity. Administration of oxygen by a nasal cannula or facemask may raise the mother's PO_2 and oxygen saturation, thereby making more oxygen available for transfer to the fetus. Discontinuing administration of oxytocin should reduce uterine activity and in turn increase uteroplacental perfusion.

A **variable deceleration** is a rapid decrease in the FHR and a rapid return to baseline. It may occur during or between contractions and has a characteristic V shape; prolonged variable decelerations that do not recover quickly may take on a U- or W-shaped appearance, or may not resemble other patterns (Feinstein et al., 2003). Variable decelerations usually are associated with compression of the umbilical cord. Changes in maternal position may correct variable decelerations by relieving cord compression. See Figure 15.16.

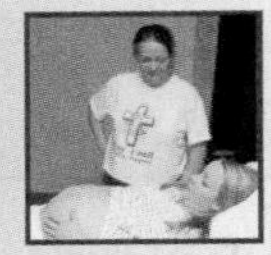

Think back to Yolanda. Suppose that external EFM is being used, and the nurse notes a rapid decrease in the FHR with a rapid return to baseline. This change occurs between contractions; the waveform appears V shaped. What should the nurse do next?

Stages and Phases of Labor

Labor usually is divided into distinct "stages" to portray the typical changes as it progresses. The first stage is subdivided into three "phases." In reality, most women usually move from one "phase" or "stage" to another in a fairly seamless continuum (Table 15.3). A "fourth" stage of labor generally includes the first 4 hours after delivery of the placenta, at which time the mother's body is undergoing dramatic changes (see Chap. 18).

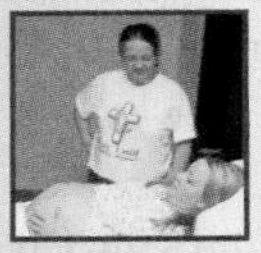

Consider Yolanda, the woman in labor described at the beginning of the chapter. Based on her report of contractions, which stage of labor should the nurse suspect at this time?

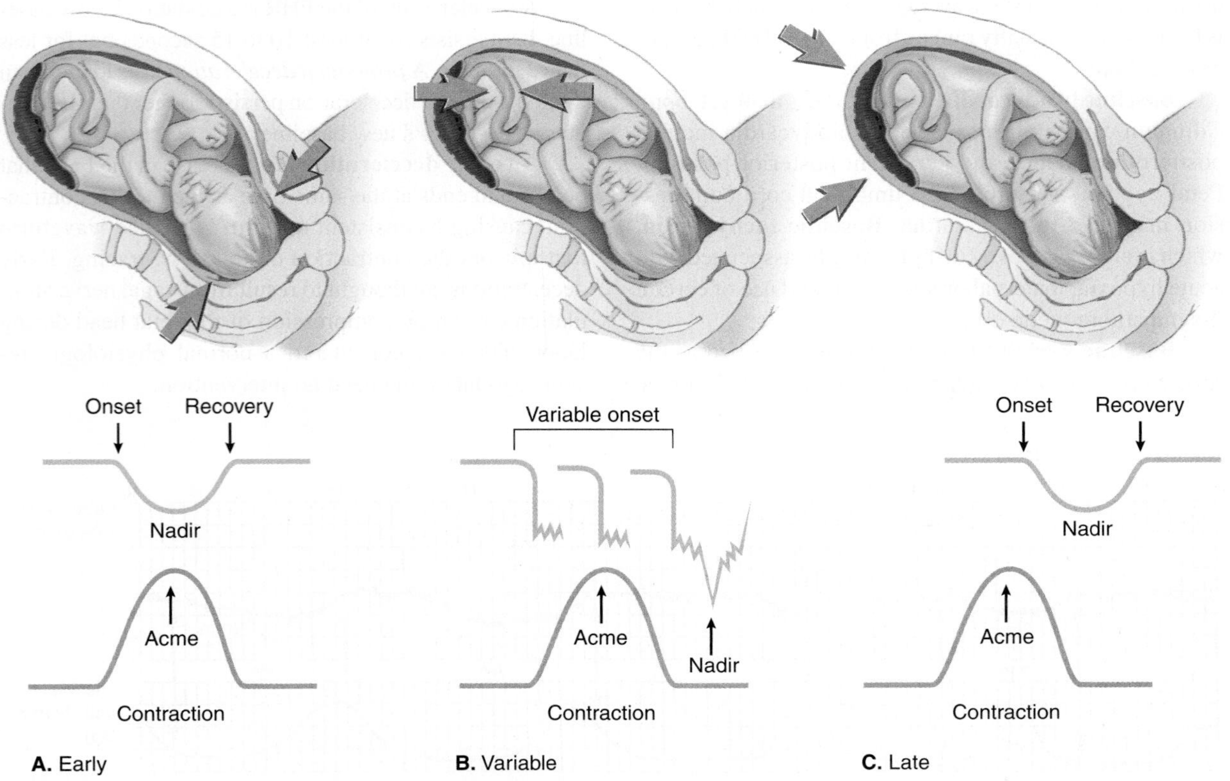

FIGURE 15.16 (**A**) Early deceleration. (**B**) Variable deceleration. (**C**) Late deceleration.

TABLE 15.3 Stages and Phases of Labor

STAGE	CERVICAL DILATION (CM) AND EFFACEMENT (%)	DURATION	CONTRACTIONS
First Stage			
Latent phase	0 to 3 cm; 0% to 40%	Nulliparas: up to 9 hours Multiparas: 5 to 6 hours	Occur every 5 to 10 minutes, lasting 30 to 45 seconds and mild
Active phase	4 to 7 cm; 40% to 80%	Nulliparas: 6 hours Multiparas: 4 hours	Occur every 2 to 5 minutes, lasting 45 to 60 seconds and moderate
Transition phase	8 to 10 cm; 80% to 100%	Nulliparas: 1 hour Multiparas: 30 minutes	Occur every 1 to 2 minutes, lasting 60 to 90 seconds and strong
Second Stage	10 cm; 100%	Nulliparas: 1 hour Multiparas: 30 minutes	Occur every 2 to 3 minutes or less, lasting 60 to 90 seconds and strong
Third Stage	10 cm; 100%	Approximately 30 minutes	Mild to moderate
Fourth Stage	Gradual return to nonpregnant state	1 to 4 hours	Dissipate

First Stage: Effacement and Dilation

The **first stage of labor** is characterized by noticeable cervical changes as a result of uterine contractions. The cervix softens, thins, shortens, and opens to a diameter of 10 cm. These cervical changes are referred to as effacement and dilation.

Effacement is the softening, thinning, and shortening of the cervical canal from a structure 1 or 2 cm long to one in which no canal exists at all. What remains is merely a circular orifice with almost paper-thin edges. During effacement, the edges of the internal os are drawn upward, so that the former cervical mucosa becomes part of the lower uterine segment.

Dilation of the cervix means that the cervical canal or "os" enlarges from an orifice a few millimeters in diameter to an opening large enough (approximately 10 cm) to permit the passage of the fetus. When the cervix no longer can be felt, dilation is said to be complete. Although the forces concerned with dilation are not well understood, several factors appear to be involved. The muscle fibers of the cervix are arranged in such a way that they pull on and tend to draw open the edges. The uterine contractions put pressure on the amniotic sac; through hydrostatic pressure, the sac burrows into the cervix in pouch-like fashion, exerting a dilating action. Without the membranes, the pressure of the presenting part against the cervix and the lower uterine segment has a similar, although less efficient, effect.

In women giving birth for the first time, effacement usually occurs before dilation. In women who have given birth before, effacement and dilation are simultaneous. In other words, the cervix of a woman who has given birth before opens or dilates with rather thick cervical edges (Cunningham et al., 2005).

The first stage of labor is commonly divided into three phases: early (or latent), active (or accelerated), and transition. The first stage often starts slowly with short, infrequent uterine contractions. Over a period of hours or sometimes days, the contractions become stronger and closer together. As contraction intensity increases, the cervix continues to efface and dilate and the fetus descends into the pelvis. The contractions are most intense as the cervix dilates the last few centimeters. At the end of the first stage of labor, the cervix is opened or dilated fully, and the fetus is ready to be born (Fig. 15.17).

Early Labor (Latent Phase). During **early labor,** also called the latent phase of the first stage of labor, the cervix

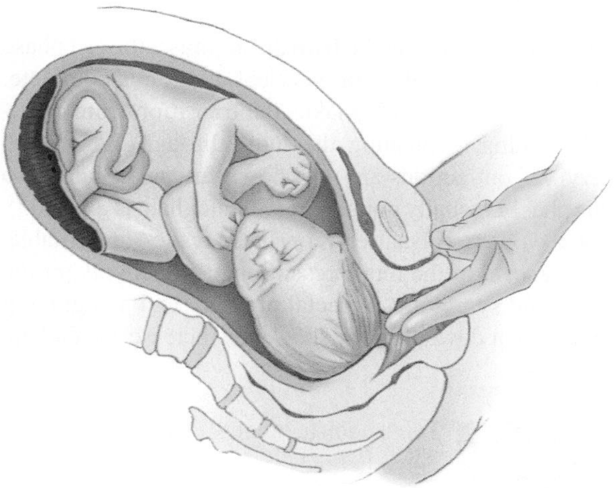

FIGURE 15.17 When performing vaginal examinations, the clinician can check to see the progress of cervical effacement and dilation to ensure that the woman is ready to give birth.

continues to thin and open, dilating to 3 to 4 cm. Contractions in early labor may feel much like the Braxton-Hicks contractions that the woman experienced in late pregnancy, like an intermittent backache, or like menstrual cramps. They begin relatively mildly and do not usually interfere with the woman's activity. This phase is often a time of excitement and anticipation of the events that lie ahead. The woman may be talkative and enthusiastic. Health care providers should encourage the client and her support people to remain at home as long as possible in early labor because relaxation and mobility are easier to accomplish there. Labor is meant to be gradual, so this phase may take some time. Early labor usually accounts for approximately two thirds of the total time spent in labor.

Over several hours, contractions become longer, stronger, more regular, and closer together (approximately 5 minutes apart, each lasting 25 to 45 seconds). Several factors, such as the degree of maternal fatigue, hydration, and nutrition, influence progress during this phase. Maternal emotions and attitudes about labor, as well as the availability and effectiveness of support systems, can affect this phase. Additionally, sedation and regional anesthesia may slow or even halt labor if given at this time.

Active Labor (Accelerated Phase). During **active labor,** contractions become longer and stronger, eventually occurring approximately 3 minutes apart and lasting for up to 1 minute or more. During this phase, which generally takes 2 to 6 hours, the cervix continues to efface and dilate from approximately 4 to 8 cm. These stronger contractions help the fetus rotate into a proper position for birth. The woman may experience additional physical symptoms that add to discomfort. Clients in active labor usually become serious and more focused. Labor is very hard work for women during this phase (Cunningham et al., 2005).

Transition Phase. In the **transition phase,** the last phase of the first stage of labor, cervical dilation is complete, and the maternal body makes the transition from cervical opening to pushing the fetus through the opened cervix. Contractions are now powerful and efficient, so this phase is usually quite short (Cunningham et al., 2005). Some women feel nauseous or shaky, restless, or irritable. The descent of the fetal presenting part accounts for the signs and symptoms of rectal pressure and a beginning urge to bear down. Bloody show may increase and darken.

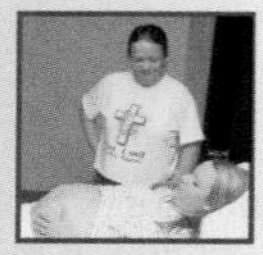

Think back to Yolanda, G2P1, who has come to the labor and birth suite complaining of contractions. How would the nurse expect her contractions to change as she progresses through labor?

COLLABORATIVE CARE: FIRST STAGE OF LABOR

Health care providers, including nurses, have major responsibilities and accountability during labor, birth, and the period immediately following. Clinical management depends on understanding normal physiologic and emotional responses, appreciating and watching for variations and deviations from normal, and individualizing care so that the experience is both safe and satisfying for the childbearing family (Matthews & Callister, 2004). Using the nursing process can help with the formulation of a plan of care that promotes positive labor and birth. See Nursing Care Plan 15.2.

Assessment

Assessment of a laboring woman arriving at the health care facility varies depending on her current phase. Determining how soon birth may occur is a crucial first priority. If birth is imminent, staff members should complete a focused assessment of maternal and fetal well-being and prepare the woman for childbirth. Areas of focus in such cases include the following:

- Pregnancy status (gravida and para status) and expected date of birth, including date of last menstrual period
- Contraction frequency, intensity, and duration, including when contractions first started
- Other signs and symptoms, such as bloody show, rupture of membranes, pressure, or urge to push
- Maternal vital signs and FHR
- Allergies
- Blood type and Rh status
- Oral intake, including the time and what was ingested
- Current pregnancy health care provider
- Past and present obstetric history, including outcomes and any problems encountered
- Birth plans, including personal preferences such as measures for pain relief, people for support, or photographing
- Infant feeding method chosen

Chapter 16 discusses care measures in the event of a precipitous or emergency vaginal birth.

If birth is not imminent, a more detailed assessment is performed that usually includes a maternal history, physical examination, and specimen collection. Assessment Tool 15.1 illustrates a sample assessment form on admission to the labor and birth area. Once initial evaluations are completed, assessment of maternal and fetal well-being continues throughout this stage of labor.

Maternal History

A detailed maternal history includes review of the current gestation, information about estimated date of birth, date of last menstrual period, and progression through-

NURSING CARE PLAN 15.2

The Client in Labor

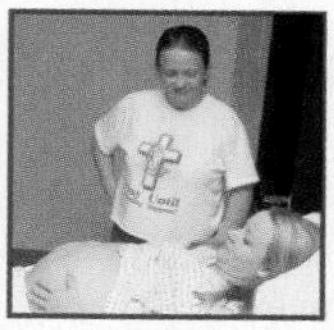

Yolanda's labor has progressed slowly over the past 6 hours. She is experiencing contractions of moderate to strong intensity every 3 to 4 minutes, lasting approximately 50 to 60 seconds each. Cervical effacement is 80%, with dilation at 6 cm. The fetal presenting part is at +1 station; fetal heart rate is averaging 128 to 136 bpm.

Yolanda's husband has just arrived. She states, "I'm so glad you made it. I'm so tired and these contractions are really starting to hurt. My music doesn't seem to be helping the pain anymore."

NURSING DIAGNOSES

- **Pain** related to increased intensity and frequency of contractions and progression of labor
- **Fatigue** related to slow progression of otherwise normal labor events and anxiety about husband's arrival

EXPECTED OUTCOMES

1. The client will report a decrease in pain to a tolerable level.
2. The client will identify appropriate positions to aid in pain relief.
3. The client will demonstrate ability to participate in labor activity with support from her husband.

INTERVENTIONS	RATIONALES
Ask the client to rate her pain on a scale of 1 to 10.	Assessment provides a baseline from which to develop an individualized plan of care and to provide a basis for future comparison.
Question the client about measures she is using currently for pain relief.	Identification of current measures helps determine alternative strategies.
Encourage the client to change positions frequently, such as sitting upright or forward leaning, getting on her hands and knees, or squatting; suggest ambulation.	Sitting promotes perineal relaxation; forward leaning aids in fetal rotation and relief of back pain and pressure; hands-and-knees position enhances placental blood flow and promotes fetal rotation; squatting widens the pelvic outlet and facilitates fetal movement. Ambulation encourages fetal rotation and descent and improves contraction efficiency.
Discourage the supine position; encourage the side-lying position.	Side-lying position prevents supine hypotension syndrome and promotes uteroplacental blood flow.
Suggest use of a birthing ball with a gentle rocking or side-to-side motion.	A birthing ball helps widen the pelvis and enhances fetal descent and rotation.
Encourage the husband to assist with position changes, using stroking and light massage.	Participation promotes sharing of the experience and provides support to the client.
Suggest the use of heat and cold therapy or a warm bath, if appropriate.	Heat aids in muscle relaxation; cold slows pain impulse transmission. Submersion in warm bath water relaxes muscles and promotes buoyancy, allowing the body to float.

Continued

NURSING CARE PLAN 15.2 ● The Client in Labor *(Continued)*

INTERVENTIONS	RATIONALES
Offer analgesics as indicated.	Analgesics alter the sensation of pain.
Give the client time to rest between position changes and contractions; balance activity and rest periods.	A balance of activity and rest reduces the risk for fatigue.
Assess maternal and fetal status before and after each strategy; continue to monitor the client's pain level for changes.	Frequent monitoring is necessary to ensure well-being and to determine the effectiveness of interventions.

EVALUATION

1. The client rates contraction pain at a level of 2 to 3 out of 10.
2. The client uses varying positions to assist with pain relief.
3. The client and her husband participate in labor events.

out pregnancy. The nurse should ask the client about her contractions, including onset, duration, frequency, and intensity. In addition, he or she should inquire about fetal movement and any other signs and symptoms the client has experienced such as bloody show and rupture of membranes (including the time). Questions about weight gain, any problems (eg, elevated blood pressure or blood glucose levels, excessive nausea and vomiting, bleeding, infection), and results of previous testing, such as ultrasounds or biophysical profiles, can provide clues to potential problems during labor and birth. The nurse should note the client's blood type and Rh status.

The nurse also should gather information about maternal psychosocial condition, including the woman's adjustment to this pregnancy, available support people, and possible cultural influences. He or she should review the mother's expectations, plans, and preferences for this labor and birth, such as choice of pain relief measures and presence of support people (including any of her other children), to ensure individualized care.

Past obstetric history also is essential to obtain. This information includes the numbers of previous pregnancies and their progression, problems, and outcomes (eg, preterm birth); abortions; and living children and their birth weights. Questions about previous labor and birth experiences may help to provide clues about any preconceptions or possible factors that may influence how the woman approaches and copes this time.

Other areas to address include the woman's past health history, including any previous illnesses such as tuberculosis, heart disease, kidney disorders, or STIs, as well as a brief family medical history. The nurse also should question the client about the use of cigarettes, alcohol, complementary and alternative therapies, and any prescribed, over-the-counter, or illicit drugs or herbal remedies. Screening for possible abuse also is important.

Physical Examination

Physical examination of the woman in labor begins with measurement of the client's height and weight. The nurse also should obtain the client's vital signs (Fig. 15.18). He or she should complete a review of body systems or head-to-toe examination, as well as checking fetal status.

Maternal Status

Physical examination of maternal status involves assessing contractions and status of the amniotic membranes. The nurse should inspect the abdomen for contour changes and measure fundal height. He or she also should palpate the abdomen for tightening and relaxation with contractions and ask the client to rate current pain level to establish a baseline for future comparison. Leopold's maneuvers can assist team members to determine fetal presentation and position (see Chap. 12). These maneuvers also help to determine the best location for auscultating fetal heart sounds.

The woman's membrane status is evaluated. Typically, a sterile vaginal examination is completed to obtain a sample of fluid for testing. Nursing Procedure 15.1 describes the method for testing for rupture of membranes. During the examination, cervical effacement and dilation also are assessed, and fetal presentation, position, and station are determined. Vaginal examinations

● ASSESSMENT TOOL 15.1 Sample Documentation Form Used for Admission to the Perinatal Unit

ADMISSION ASSESSMENT OBSTETRICS

▲ PATIENT IDENTIFICATION ▲

ADMISSION DATA

Date	Time	Via ☐ Ambulatory ☐ Wheelchair ☐ Stretcher					
Grav.	Term	Pre-term	Ab.	Living	EDC	LMP	GA

Prev. adm. date ______ Reason ______
Obstetrician ______ Pediatrician ______
Ht.______ Wt. ______ Wt. gain ______
Allergies (meds/food) ☐ None ______ ☐ Hx latex sensitivity
BP______ T______ P______ R______
FHR ______ Vag exam ______

Reason for Admission

☐ Labor / SROM ☐ Induction ______
☐ Primary C/S ______ ☐ Repeat C/S
☐ Observation ______
☐ OB / Medical complication ______

Onset of labor: ☐ Not in labor
Date ______ Time ______
Membranes: ☐ Intact
☐ Ruptured / Date ______ Time ______
☐ Clear ☐ Meconium ☐ Bloody ☐ Foul
Vaginal bleeding: ☐ None
☐ Normal show ☐ ______

Current Pregnancy Labs ☐ NPC

☐ POL ☐ PPROM ☐ Cerclage
☐ PIH ☐ Chr. HTN ☐ Other ______
☐ Diabetes ______ Diet ______
☐ Insulin ______
☐ Amniocentesis ______ Results ______
Bld type / RH ____ Date Rhogam ____
Antibody screen ☐ Neg ☐ Pos
Rubella ☐ Non-immune ☐ Immune
Diabetic screen ☐ Normal ☐ Abnormal
Recent exposure to chick pox ☐
Current meds: ______

	Pos	Neg	Tested
Hepatitis B	☐	☐	☐ No
HIV	☐	☐	☐ No
Group B strep	☐	☐	☐ No
GC	☐	☐	☐ No
Chlamydia	☐	☐	☐ No
RPR	☐	☐	☐ No

Previous OB History

☐ POL ☐ Multiple gestation
☐ Prev C/S type ______ Reason ______
☐ PIH ☐ Chronic HTN ☐ Diabetes ______
☐ Stillbirth/demise ☐ Neodeath ☐ Anomalies
☐ Precipitous labor (<3 H) ☐ Macrosomia
☐ PP Hemorrhage
☐ Hx Transfusion reaction ☐ Yes ☐ No
☐ Other ______

Latest risk assessment ☐ None
1. ______ 3. ______
2. ______ 4. ______

Date ______
Signature ______ Time ______

NEUROLOGICAL

☐ WNL
Variance: ☐ HA
☐ Scotoma / visual changes
Reflexes ☐ < 2 + ☐ > 2 +
☐ Clonus___ bts
☐ Numbness ☐ Tingling
☐ Hx Seizures
☐ ______

RESPIRATORY

☐ WNL
Variance: ☐ Hx Asthma ☐ URI
Respirations: ☐ < 12 ☐ > 24
Effort: ☐ SOB
☐ Shallow ☐ Labored
Auscultation:
☐ Diminished ☐ Crackles
☐ Wheezes ☐ Rhonchi

	No	Yes
Cough for greater than 2 weeks?	☐	☐
Is the cough productive?	☐	☐
Blood in the sputum?	☐	☐
Experiencing any fever or night sweats?	☐	☐
Ever had TB in the past?	☐	☐
Recent exposure to TB?	☐	☐
Weight loss in last 3 weeks?	☐	☐

If the patient answers yes to any three of the above questions implement policy and procedure # 5725-0704.

GASTROINTESTINAL

☐ WNL
Variance: ☐ Heartburn
☐ Epigastric pain Nausea
☐ Vomiting ☐ Diarrhea
☐ Constipation ☐ Pain
☐ Wt. Gain < 2lbs / month**
☐ Recent change in appetite of < 50% of usual intake for > 5 days
☐ ______

INTEGUMENTARY

☐ WNL
Variance: ☐ Rash ☐ Lacerations
☐ Abrasion ☐ Swelling
☐ Urticaria ☐ Bruising
☐ Diaphoretic/hot
☐ Clammy/cold
☐ Scars
☐ ______

FETAL ASSESSMENT

☐ WNL
Variance:
☐ NRFS
FHR ☐ < 110 ☐ > 160
LTV ☐ Absent ☐ Minimal
☐ Increased
STV Absent
Decelerations: ______
☐ Decreased fetal movement
☐ IUGR
☐ ______

CARDIOVASCULAR

☐ WNL
Variance:
☐ MVP
Heart rate: ☐ < 60 ☐ > 100
B/P: Systolic: ☐ < 90 ☐ > 140
Diastolic: ☐ < 50 ☐ > 90
☐ Edema ______
☐ Chest pain / palpitations
☐ ______

MUSCULOSKELETAL

☐ WNL
Variance:
☐ Numbness ☐ Tingling
☐ Paralysis ☐ Deformity
☐ Scoliosis
☐ ______

GENITOURINARY

☐ WNL
Variance: ☐ Albumin ______
Output: ☐ < 30 cc/Hr.
☐ UTI ☐ Rx ☐ Frequency
☐ Dysuria ☐ Hematuria
☐ CVA Tenderness
☐ Hx STD
☐ Vag. discharge ______
☐ Rash ☐ Blisters
☐ Warts ☐ Lesions
☐ ______

EARS, NOSE, THROAT, AND EYES

☐ WNL
Variance:
☐ Sore throat ☐ Eyeglasses
☐ Runny nose ☐ Contact lenses
☐ Nasal congestion
☐ ______

PSYCHOSOCIAL

☐ WNL
Variance: ☐ Hx depression
☐ Yes ☐ No
☐ Emotional behavioral care
Affect: ☐ Flat ☐ Anxious
☐ Uncooperative ☐ Combative
Living will ☐ Yes ☐ No
☐ On chart
Healthcare surrogate ☐ Yes ☐ No
☐ On chart
Are you being hurt, hit, frightened by anyone at home or in your life? ☐ Yes ☐ No
Religious preference ______

Tobacco use	☐ Denies	☐ Yes	Amt ______
Alcohol use	☐ Denies	☐ Yes	Amt ______
Drug use	☐ Denies	☐ Yes	Amt type ______
Primary language	☐ English	☐ Spanish	☐ ______

PAIN ASSESSMENT

1. Do you have any ongoing pain problems? ☐ No ☐ Yes
2. Do you have any pain now? ☐ No ☐ Yes
3. If any of the above questions are answered yes, the patient has a positive pain screening.
4. *Patient to be given pain management education material. Complete pain / symptom assessment on flowsheet.*
5. *Please proceed to complete pain assessment.*

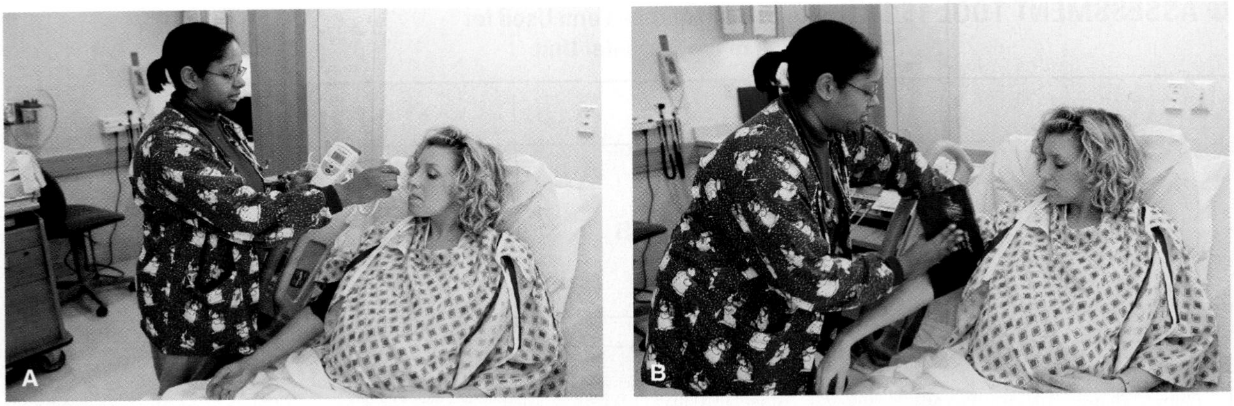

FIGURE 15.18 The nurse assesses maternal vital signs upon admission to the health care facility for childbirth.

NURSING PROCEDURE 15.1

Testing for Rupture of Membranes

PURPOSE

To determine the status of the amniotic membranes during labor and to differentiate amniotic fluid from urine and bloody show

ASSESSMENT AND PLANNING

- Assess the client's knowledge of and previous exposure to the procedure.
- Questions the client about any report of a sudden gush of fluid or slow trickle of fluid.
- Inspect fluid for color if possible.
- Gather the necessary equipment:
  - Nitrazine test paper
  - Sterile speculum
  - Glass slide
  - Sterile cotton-tipped applicator
  - Microscope
  - Sterile gloves

IMPLEMENTATION

1. Explain the procedure to the client and answer any questions *to help allay her anxiety.*
2. Position the client for a vaginal examination.
3. Wash hands.
4. Expose the perineal area, making sure to keep the client covered as much as possible *to ensure privacy and promote adequate access to the perineum.*
5. Put on sterile gloves; obtain a small strip of Nitrazine paper, approximately 2 inches in length, making sure that bare hands do not come in contact with the paper *to prevent contaminating the test strip.*
6. Spread the labia with the nondominant hand and apply a small section of the Nitrazine paper to the vaginal opening near the cervical os until it is wet to obtain a sample of fluid. *An adequate sample is needed to ensure the accuracy of the results.*
7. Compare the color of the test strip with the color guide on the paper container *to determine the pH of the secretions.*

Continued

NURSING PROCEDURE 15.1

Testing for Rupture of Membranes

8. Interpret the findings; if the test strip turns blue (blue-green, blue-gray, or deep blue), then the pH is alkaline and suggests rupture of membranes; if the test strip is yellow or olive-yellow or olive-green, then the pH is acidic and membranes are probably intact.
9. *Alternatively,* perform or assist with a sterile vaginal examination to obtain a specimen of fluid with a sterile cotton-tipped applicator to ensure collection of an accurate specimen without contamination; apply the fluid to a glass slide and allow to dry.
10. Observe the slide under the microscope for a ferning appearance, *which indicates a high estrogen content suggestive of amniotic fluid and ruptured membranes.*
11. Provide perineal care *to promote client comfort.*
12. Remove gloves and wash hands.
13. Report and document the findings.

EVALUATION

- The client tolerated the procedure without difficulty.
- Rupture of membranes confirmed

AREAS FOR CONSIDERATION AND ADAPTATION

Perinatal Considerations

- *If necessary, use a sterile cotton-tipped applicator to obtain a specimen of fluid from the posterior vagina during a sterile vaginal examination. Then apply the applicator to the test strip.*
- *Be aware that false test results may occur if inadequate fluid is obtained.*

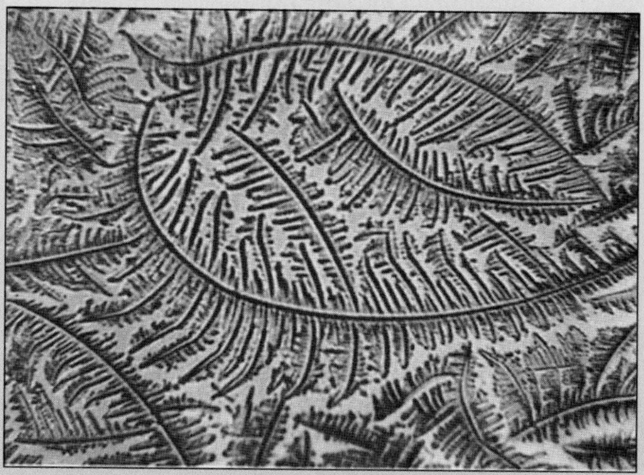

typically are more painful when performed during a contraction. In addition, there is an increased risk for rupturing the membranes also at this time (Pillitteri, 2007).

Fetal Status

Physical examination of the fetus focuses on assessing the rate and pattern of the fetal heart either intermittently by auscultation or continuously by electronic monitoring. Using electronic monitoring also provides objective information about the client's contraction pattern and intensity. Nursing Procedure 15.2 describes the steps in applying an external EFM.

Specimen Collection

Collection of urine and blood specimens commonly is part of initial intrapartal assessment. Protocols for specific testing vary among health care facilities. Generally, a clean-catch urine specimen for urinalysis is collected. Other laboratory tests may include blood specimens for hemoglobin and hematocrit, complete blood count, blood type and Rh factor, and serologic testing (Rouse & St. John, 2003).

Select Potential Nursing Diagnoses

Nursing diagnoses commonly included in the care of a woman experiencing the first stage of labor are as follows:

- **Pain** related to increasing intensity of uterine contractions and progression of labor
- **Risk for Injury** (maternal or fetal) related to potential complications associated with labor

NURSING PROCEDURE 15.2

Applying an External Electronic Fetal Monitor

PURPOSE

To assess fetal heart rate and uterine contractions continuously during labor

ASSESSMENT AND PLANNING

- Assess the client's knowledge of and previous exposure to the procedure.
- Auscultate FHR and maternal vital signs; assess contractions by palpation.
- Perform Leopold's maneuvers to determine the location of the fetal back and best area to assess FHR.
- Gather the necessary equipment:
    - Electronic fetal monitor with paper installed
    - Tocodynamometer
    - Ultrasound transducer
    - Belts or Velcro to secure transducers
    - Conductive gel
- Plug in the monitor and insert the transducer lines into the appropriate outlets on the front of the monitor.
- Turn on the monitor and run a test strip.

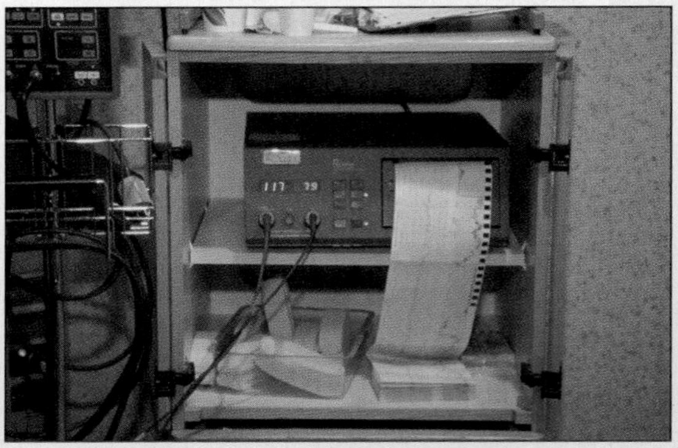

IMPLEMENTATION

1. Wash hands.
2. Place the client in a comfortable position, elevating the head of the bed approximately 30 degrees; if appropriate, place the client in a side lying position *to maximize utero-placental blood flow.*
3. Place one belt under the woman at the upper part of her abdomen and the other at her lower abdomen and bring the edges of the belt out to the side *to facilitate securing the transducers once in they are in place.*
4. Apply conductive gel to the ultrasound transducer *to ensure sound transmission* and place in on the client's abdomen in the area of the fetal back *to hear the FHR.*
5. Increase the volume on the monitor and reposition the transducer to the area where the FHR sounds are loudest.
6. Secure the transducer with the lower belt.
7. Palpate the uterine fundus to determine where it is the firmest and apply the tocodynamometer at that location.
8. Secure the tocodynamometer with the upper belt.
9. Observe the recording from the monitor *to ensure that the monitor is recording the events.* Record the date and time of initiating EFM along with the client's vital signs and identifying information.

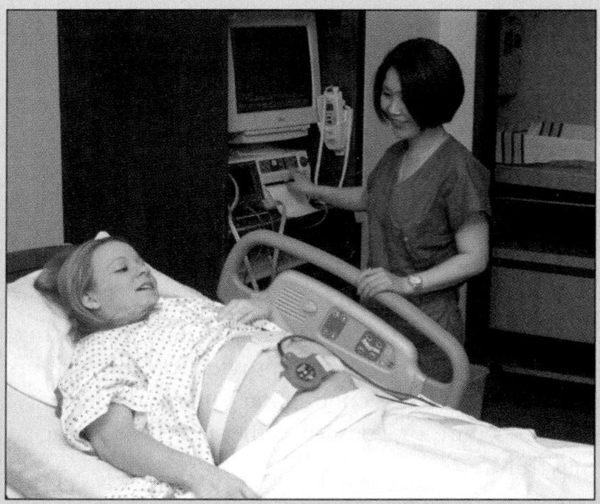

Continued

NURSING PROCEDURE 15.2

Applying an External Electronic Fetal Monitor

10. If necessary, reposition the woman comfortably, making sure that the EFM is working correctly.
11. Place the client's call light within easy reach.
12. Wash your hands.
13. Document the procedure.

EVALUATION

- Client tolerated procedure without difficulty
- External EFM applied
- FHR and uterine contractions within acceptable parameters

AREAS FOR CONSIDERATION AND ADAPTATION

Perinatal Considerations

- Be aware that telemetry-like units are available for external EFM so that the woman can ambulate and get out of bed without disrupting the monitoring.
- Warn the woman that the conductive gel may feel cold to her skin.
- Assess FHR patterns frequently for periodic and episodic changes that might indicate fetal distress.

- **Anxiety** related to uncertainty of the progression of labor and anticipated birth
- **Anxiety** related to first experience with labor and birth
- **Powerlessness** related to inability to cope with demands and work of labor
- **Deficient Knowledge** related to labor process and events
- **Risk for Deficient Fluid Volume** related to limited fluid intake, increased insensible fluid loss, or fluid replacement
- **Ineffective Breathing Pattern** related to inappropriate use of breathing techniques
- **Fatigue** related to duration of the labor process and energy expenditure

Planning/Intervention

NIC/NOC Box 15.1 highlights some common interventions and outcomes for the woman in labor. As with all care, goal setting and implementation need to be individualized to the client's specific circumstances. Assessment Tool 15.2 provides a sample of a chart used to document labor's progress over time.

Early Labor

During early labor, the woman may have difficulty believing that she is really in labor. The best thing for her to do is to take good care of herself. Alternating between rest and activity may be helpful (eg, a long walk followed by a warm shower). The nurse should encourage her to eat easily digested foods (eg, tea and toast) and to drink plenty of fluids. The American Society of Anesthesiologists (ASA, 1998) recommends "that oral intake of modest amounts of clear liquids be allowed for uncomplicated laboring patients. Examples of clear liquids include, but are not limited to, water, juice, fruit juices without pulp, carbonated beverages, clear tea, and black coffee." Withholding food and drink may lead to dehydration and ketosis, poor progress in labor, a diagnosis of dystocia, and a cascade of interventions leading to cesarean birth (American College of Nurse–Midwives [ACNM], 1999; Scrutton et al., 1999). A recent study found no difference in rates of medical interventions, adverse birth outcomes, or vomiting between eating and noneating groups of laboring women; however, the same study showed that eating during early labor may increase labor's total duration (Parsons et al., 2006).

Many women find that home is the best place to be during this phase because they can move about easily and do things for themselves. When contractions become so strong that she cannot talk through them, the client should begin using relaxation and breathing techniques. She may find it comforting to have support people nearby, helping her to stay calm and confident. Ongoing assessment of maternal and fetal well-being is essential.

NIC/NOC Box 15.1 Labor

Common NIC Labels

- Admission Care
- Analgesic Administration: Intraspinal
- Anxiety Reduction
- Anticipatory Guidance
- Decision-Making Support
- Intrapartal Care
- Surveillance: Late Pregnancy
- Vital Signs Monitoring

Common NOC Labels

- Coping
- Decision Making
- Endurance
- Fetal Status: Intrapartum
- Health Beliefs: Perceived Control
- Knowledge: Labor and Delivery
- Maternal Status: Intrapartum
- Pain Control
- Vital Signs Status

Active Labor

During contractions in active labor, many women find it helpful to develop a rhythmic response, using breathing, movement, and sound, followed by rest between contractions. Birthing balls can be valuable tools (Fig. 15.19). While leaning or sitting on the ball, the woman can rock, move, or circle her hips to decrease discomfort. Movement also encourages the release of endorphins, the body's natural painkiller (Simkin & Ancheta, 2000).

Ambulation during labor has many benefits. It facilitates progress by stimulating more effective contractions, increases pressure of the presenting part against the cervix to facilitate effacement and dilation, and promotes fetal rotation and descent. It may promote comfort and offer diversion and stimulation. Many women find walking beneficial during early and even active labor (Fig. 15.20).

Although ambulation during labor has many benefits, clients in U.S. health facilities may not walk frequently during labor. The Listening to Mothers survey consisted of phone or electronic mail interviews about women's labor and birth experiences. Of the 1583 women who responded, 71% reported that they did not walk around even once after regular contractions began. The primary reason given for not walking was that they were "connected to things." Other reasons reported for staying in bed were pain drugs "that made them unable to support themselves," being told by care providers not to walk around, and grogginess from pain medication. Twenty percent chose to stay in one place (Declercq et al., 2002).

As long as there are no maternal or fetal contraindications, the nurse is responsible for suggesting walking and providing assistance as needed because the client in labor may not consider this option. If the woman has an IV line inserted, she can take the IV pole with her as she ambulates. If EFM is being used, the nurse can disconnect the leads for short intervals if FHR and variability are normal. An alternative is the use of wireless transducers for external EFM as described earlier. Ambulation should not be used for clients receiving medication or when concern exists about maternal or fetal status.

Laboring women may find a warm bath relaxing. The buoyancy of water helps relieve discomfort; warmth may relieve tension (Cluett et al., 2004). Relaxation and warmth also may help labor progress (Primeau et al., 2003). Using a handheld showerhead to direct water onto the abdomen also may be soothing. The tingling water stimulates the skin, resulting in less awareness of pain. Sometimes alternating applications of warm and cold compresses is more effective than using just one or the other. Cold packs are particularly useful for musculoskeletal and joint pain; thus, back pain usually responds particularly well to cold therapy.

As contraction strength increases, so does the woman's need for continuous support. Thus, companionship from a birth partner or family members becomes more important as labor progresses (Gilliland, 2002) (Fig. 15.21). One successful measure for reducing labor pain is the continuous presence of a professionally trained, supportive companion who focuses on the woman throughout each contraction. This person can softly speak words of reassurance and encouragement, stroke the client, hold her hand, walk with her, suggest position changes, instruct her, and reassure her partner. Controlled trials have shown that such a person, often called a **doula** from the Greek word meaning "woman's servant," improves obstetric outcomes and client satisfaction compared with usual hospital care (Berg & Terstad, 2006; Declercq et al., 2002; Pascali-Bonaro & Kroeger, 2004). Clear evidence demonstrates the effectiveness of physical, emotional, and psychological support for women during childbirth (Gilliland, 2002). Research also has demonstrated consistently that birth satisfaction is linked to the amount of support a woman receives from caregivers, the quality of her relationship with them, her involvement with decision making, and her personal expectations (Goodman et al., 2004; Hodnett, 2002) (Research Highlight 15.1). The AWHONN (2000) maintains that continuous available labor support by professional registered nurses is a critical component to achieving positive birth outcomes.

Changing positions frequently not only helps the woman stay more comfortable but also encourages labor

(text continues on page 616)

● ASSESSMENT TOOL 15.2 Sample Labor Flow Sheet

Labor Progress Chart

Maternal/Newborn Record System

Admit date	Admit time	Blood type and Rh	Age	G	T	Pt	A	L	EDD___/___/___ LMP___/___/___	Membranes	☐ Intact ☐ Bulging	☐ Ruptured Date___/___/___	SROM	AROM Time___
/ /														

Current date / /	Time →																		
Vital signs	Temperature																		
	Pulse																		
	Respiration /O_2 saturation																		
	Blood pressure																		
Maternal	Deep tendon reflexes (L/R)	/	/	/	/	/	/	/	/	/	/	/	/	/	/	/	/	/	/
	Urine (protein/sugar)	/	/	/	/	/	/	/	/	/	/	/	/	/	/	/	/	/	/
	Vaginal bleeding																		
	Pain																		
	Edema (site, extent)																		
Uterine activity	Monitor mode																		
	Frequency																		
	Duration																		
	Peak IUP																		
	Resting tone																		
	Intensity																		
	MVUs																		
Fetal assessment	Monitor mode (Strip #____)																		
	Baseline (FHR)																		
	STV																		
	LTV																		
	Accelerations																		
	Decelerations																		
	Membranes/fluid																		
	Scalp pH																		
Intake/output (mL's/Hr)	IV																		
	PO																		
	Urine																		
	Emesis																		
Cont meds	Pitocin mU/min																		
	Magnesium sulfate gms/hr																		
Intervention	Treatments																		
	Teaching/support																		
	Touch																		
	Position/activity																		
	Physical care																		
Initials																			

Abbreviations/ key	Deep tendon reflexes	Vaginal bleeding	Pain	Uterine activity monitor mode	MVUs Montevideo units	Fetal monitor mode	STV short-term variability
	0 = No response +1 = Sluggish +2 = Normal +3 = Hyperactive +4 = Brisk + hyperactive C = Clonus	NS = Normal show ABN = Frank vaginal bleeding	0 = No pain ⋮ 5 = Distressing pain ⋮ 10 = Highest intensity	P = Palpation E = External I = Internal	The sum of the peak of each uterine contraction minus its resting tone, in a 10-minute period.	A = Auscultation (fetoscope) D = Doppler E = External I = Internal	+ = Present (roughness of tracing line present) ∅ = Absent (tracing line is smooth) **LTV long-term variability** ∅ = 0– 2 BPM = Absent ↓ = 3– 5 BPM = Minimal + = 6–25 BPM = Absent ↑ = greater than 25 BPM = Marked

Continued

● ASSESSMENT TOOL 15.2 Sample Labor Flow Sheet *(Continued)*

Labor Progress Chart
Maternal/Newborn Record System

Current date / /

Allergy/sensitivity ☐ None ☐ Latex ☐ Other______

Chart______of______

Accelerations
++ = 15 BPM ↑X 15 sec
+ = less than 15 BPM ↑+/or less than 15 sec
0 = None

Decelerations
N = None
L = Late
E = Early
P = Prolonged
V = Variable

Membranes
I = Intact
B = Bulging
R = Ruptured

Fluid
C = Clear
M = Meconium stained
B = Bloody
F = Foul odor
NF = No foul odor

Treatments
O_2 = O_2 L/min
IVB = IV bolus
SC = Straight catheterization
FC = Foley catheterization
ABD = Abdominal hair removal

Teaching/support
O = Orient to unit
SR = Safety review
LR = Labor review
F = Focusing
BRT = Breathing/relaxation techniques
PrO = PreOp.

Touch
E = Effleurage
B = Backrub
CP = Counterpressure
M = Massage

Position/activity
w = Walking
C = Chair
SQ = Squatting
JR = Jet hydrotherapy
SH = Shower
K = Kneeling
LS = Left side
RS = Right side
KC = Knee chest
T = Trendelenburg

Physical care
MC = Mouth care
SC = Superficial cold
SH = Superficial heat
PC = Peri care
BP = Bedpan

Continued

● ASSESSMENT TOOL 15.2 Sample Labor Flow Sheet

Labor Progress Chart

Maternal/Newborn Record System

TIME →

Mark X ●

STATION	DILATATION
	10
−4	9
−3	8
−2	7
−1	6
0	5
+1	4
+2	3
+3	2

Effacement % and/or position

Examined by:

COMPOSITE NORMAL DILATATION CURVES

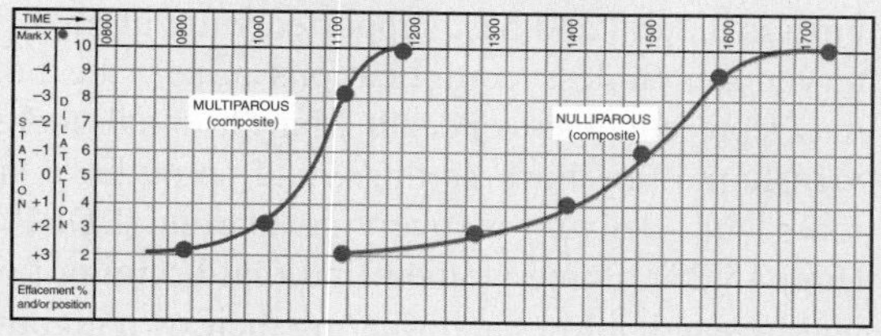

COMPOSITE CURVES OF ABNORMAL LABOR PROGRESS—MULTIPAROUS

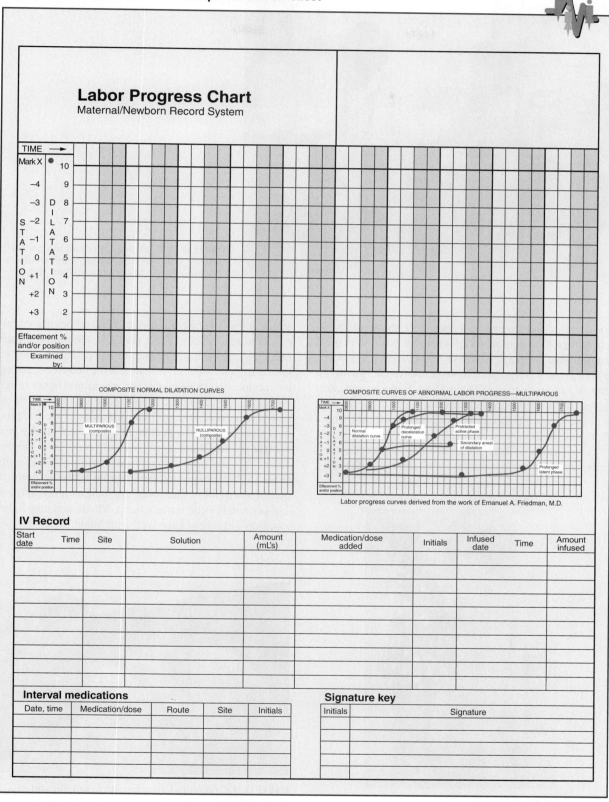

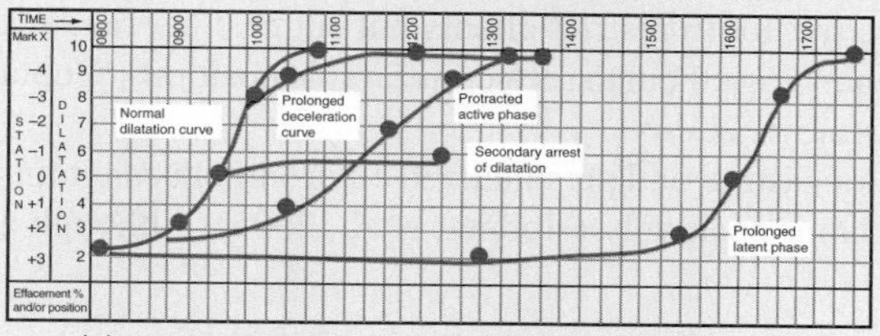

Labor progress curves derived from the work of Emanuel A. Friedman, M.D.

IV Record

Start date	Time	Site	Solution	Amount (mL's)	Medication/dose added	Initials	Infused date	Time	Amount infused

Interval medications

Date, time	Medication/dose	Route	Site	Initials

Signature key

Initials	Signature

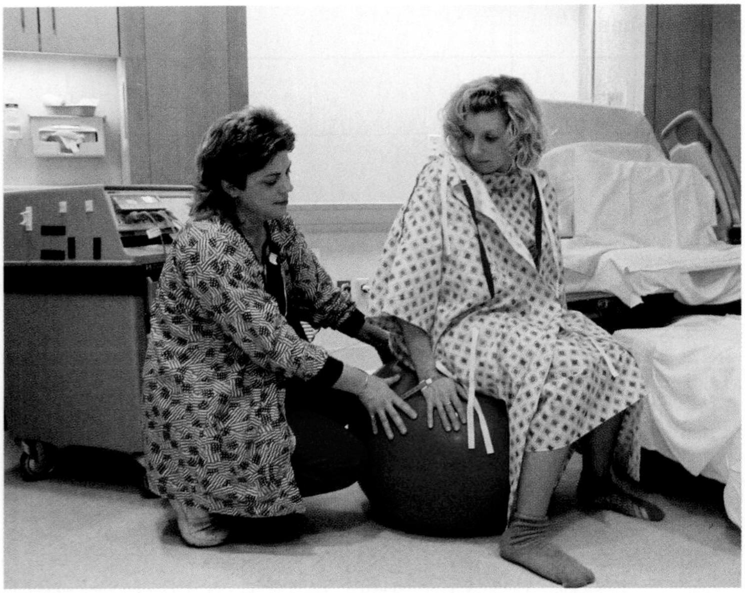

FIGURE 15.19 While leaning or sitting on the birthing ball, the laboring woman can move in various ways to decrease discomfort.

to progress. Under normal circumstances, the nurse should encourage the client to adopt whatever position is most comfortable (Gupta & Hofmeyr, 2004). If progress slows, a change of position and movement often help without causing excessive pain (Table 15.4). Experienced caregivers try not to restrict clients but suggest alternatives and encourage them to seek comfortable positions (Gupta & Hofmeyr, 2004).

A peaceful and personalized environment can influence labor positively (Hodnett et al., 2005). Although a small but increasing number of U.S. labors are occurring in nonhospital settings, the most common birth site remains the hospital. The hospital environment may be very different from the woman's home or a free-standing birth center. To some clients whose cultural belief is that birth is natural and best supported without medical intervention (unless complications arise), the hospital may represent illness or death. Many hospitals today provide home-like birth settings, and some have single-room labor-delivery-recovery-postpartum (LDRP) units (Fig. 15.22). Some women find that bringing favorite pictures and pillows and wearing their own nightgowns can personalize the environment. Music and dim lights also may help them cope well with labor.

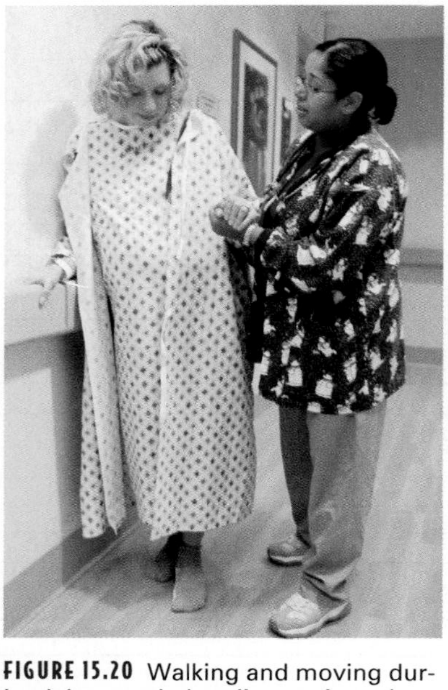

FIGURE 15.20 Walking and moving during labor can help relieve pain and may assist with moving labor forward.

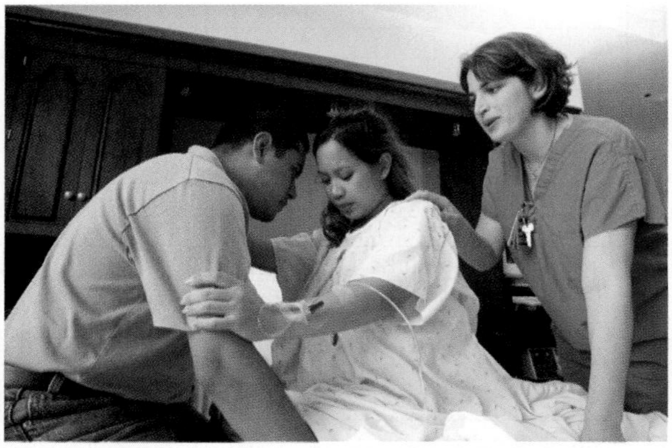

FIGURE 15.21 Ongoing assistance with breathing and pain management techniques from partners, support people, nurses, and doulas can be of great benefit to women in labor.

● RESEARCH HIGHLIGHT 15.1 Why Do Some Women Change Their Opinion About Childbirth Over Time?

PURPOSE: To study women's memories of childbirth, compare their immediate feelings with recollections at various stages, and determine influential variables in changed perceptions.

DESIGN: The investigator analyzed questionnaires completed by women 2 months postpartum and 1 year postpartum and grouped findings into two subsamples: those who said childbirth was positive and those who said it was negative at 2 months postpartum. Within each sample, the researcher then compared psychosocial background, labor outcomes, infant health outcomes, and experiences of intrapartum care for those whose 1-year assessment was consistent with their 2-month report, as well as those whose views had changed.

RESULTS: Evaluations of childbirth that became more negative with time were associated with labor complications, dissatisfaction with intrapartum care, psychosocial problems, and depression. Improved assessments with time were associated with positive interactions with and support from birth attendants.

NURSING IMPLICATIONS: Supportive care from those who work with women giving birth can have long-term effects whose influence grows with time. Such assistance also may protect against negative memories and general dissatisfaction.

Waldenstrom, U. (2004). *Birth, 31*(2), 102–107.

Transition

During transition, the client may find it helpful to focus on one contraction at a time. She should continue breathing during contractions. Even though rest between contractions becomes shorter, the nurse should encourage the client to relax and to use the time to restore her energy. Those providing labor support should offer close, undivided attention; gentle, unwavering encouragement; and praise. As with earlier phases of this first stage, ongoing assessment of maternal and fetal well-being is crucial.

Evaluation

Interventions during the first stage of labor are effective if the client progresses without developing any complications. The fetus should demonstrate reassuring FHR patterns between 120 and 160 bpm. Additionally, the client uses various techniques to achieve a tolerable level of pain and participates in decision making. If problems develop, appropriate interventions are instituted to ensure maternal and fetal well-being.

Second Stage: Pushing or Expulsion

Once the cervix is dilated fully, the woman is said to move into the **second stage of labor** and begins pushing. At this time, the fetus maneuvers through the maternal pelvis, rotating and slowly descending through the birth canal. This stage can last from 15 minutes to several hours (Cunningham et al., 2005). For some women, initial contractions during this stage are strong and powerful, causing an overwhelmingly strong urge to push. As they experience this feeling, many clients become very focused on the task at hand. For some women, however, second-stage contractions increase gradually, similarly to those of first-stage labor. Pressure grows as the fetus descends. Women may grunt or groan with contractions. It is not unusual for clients to hold their breath instinctively as they bear down (Roberts, 2002).

When the fetus reaches the maternal perineum, contractions are intense and often accompanied by burning or stretching. The perineum begins to bulge outward, the labia separate, and the presenting fetal part (usually the head) gradually becomes visible. After each contraction, the fetal head recedes somewhat until the next contraction, when it bulges a little more. Eventually the fetal head reaches a point at which it no longer recedes. This is called **crowning.** As the head descends, the pelvic floor becomes thin and shiny, and the anus protrudes. When the head emerges, the woman usually experiences tremendous relief and some pressure with delivery of the shoulders. Then the rest of the fetus moves out easily (Fig. 15.23).

The time for all this to happen varies widely, depending partly on fetal size and position, as well as on the woman's freedom to move into different positions. Breathing that the woman uses for pushing (ie, prolonged breath holding versus controlled exhalation) also can influence the effectiveness of her efforts. Fear may influence expulsion. A woman who is scared of birth or anticipated pain may be reluctant to push.

See Figure 15.24 for an illustrated sequence of a normal vaginal birth.

COLLABORATIVE CARE: SECOND STAGE OF LABOR

Assessment

Assessment during the second stage involves monitoring of maternal vital signs, as frequently as every 15 to

● **TABLE 15.4 Positions for Labor**

POSITION	DESCRIPTION
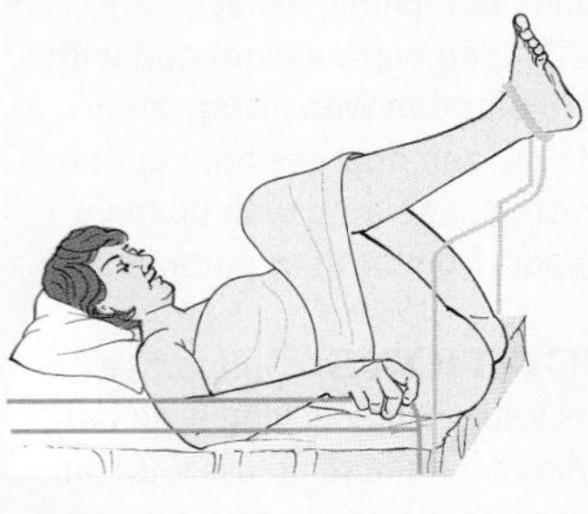 Lithotomy	The woman is flat with her legs in stirrups. This position provides the birth attendant with good access to the perineum and allows him or her to control the birth. Risks for supine hypotensive syndrome and injury are increased.
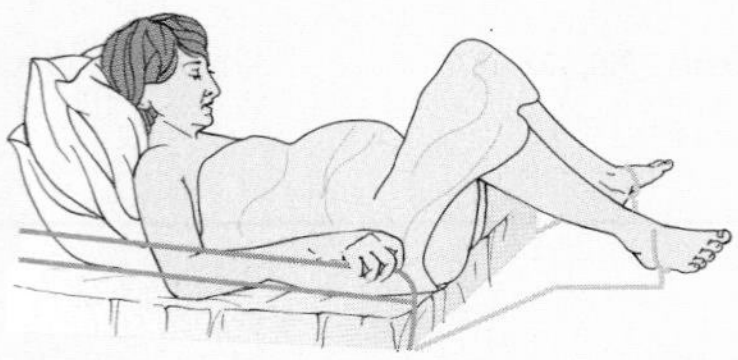 Modified dorsal recumbent	The woman is sitting up in bed with her feet placed on pedals. This position provides the birth attendant with good access to the perineum and allows him or her to control the birth. It is not comfortable for the woman and does not assist with fetal expulsion.
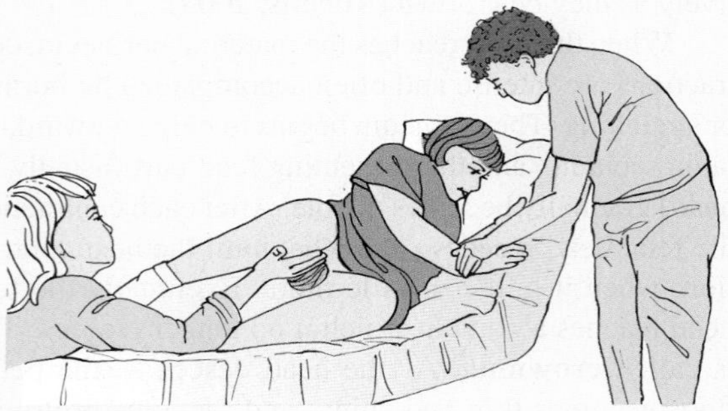 Side-lying	The woman lies on her side. This position may increase maternal comfort; however, it may be awkward for the birth attendant and require assistance from a third party to hold the woman's upper leg during birth.
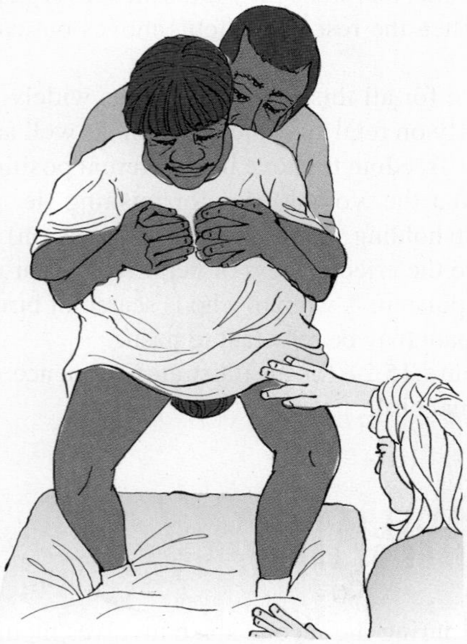 Squatting	The woman squats. This position can enhance maternal comfort and relies on gravity to facilitate fetal expulsion. The woman is at risk for losing her balance and thus needs support from another person behind her or the use of a birthing bar or stool.

Continued

● **TABLE 15.4** **Positions for Labor**

POSITION	DESCRIPTION
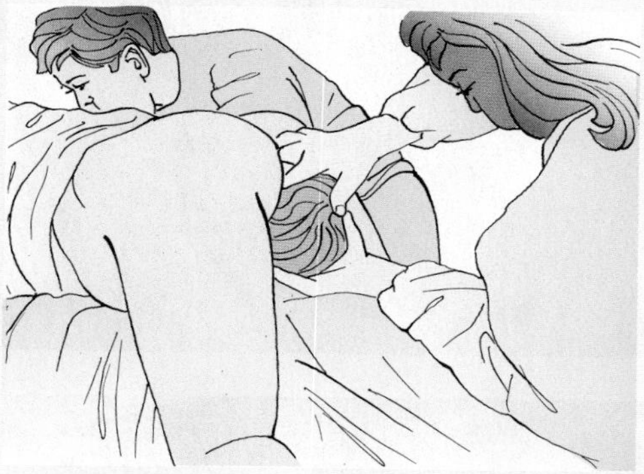 **Hands and knees**	The woman gets on her hands and knees with assistance from others. This position encourages rotation of the fetal head and perineal stretching and provides the best access to the perineum for the birth attendant. The woman may become tired. This position usually prohibits the use of instruments for assistance.

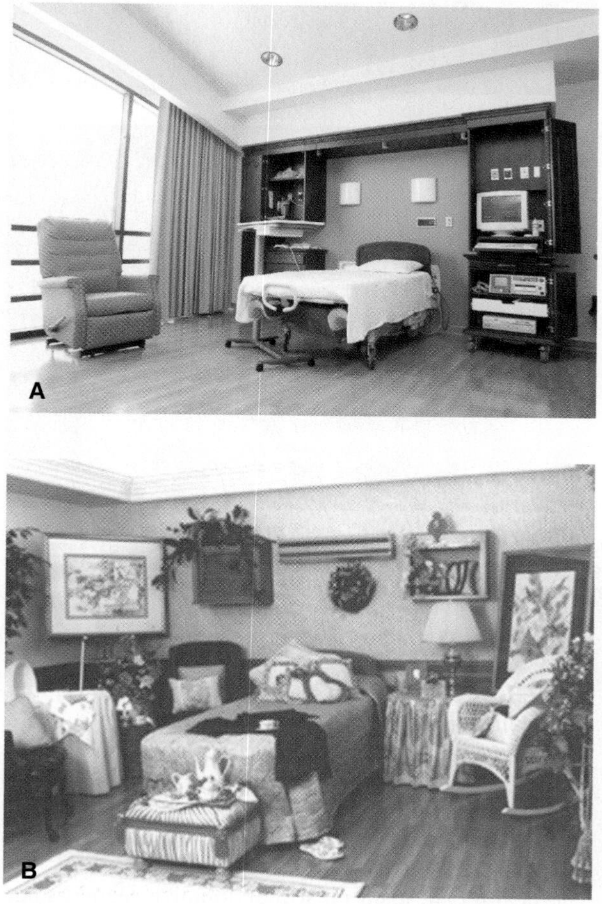

FIGURE 15.22 (**A**) An LDRP (labor, delivery, recovery, postpartum) unit in a hospital. (**B**) A home-like unit in a birthing center. (Photos courtesy of Joe Mitchell.)

30 minutes. In addition, the nurse continues to regularly evaluate cervical dilation and effacement and fetal station. The nurse also should check uterine contractions every 15 minutes. At this time, the woman may voice a strong urge to push because of pressure from the fetal head.

For pregnancies considered to be low risk, FHR patterns are monitored every 15 minutes; for those considered high risk, monitoring occurs every 5 minutes (AWHONN, 2000). The nurse should observe the FHR pattern for early or variable decelerations, which may result from compression of the umbilical cord with contractions. These patterns are not problematic as long as the pattern returns to baseline after the contraction.

The nurse should consider the woman's psychosocial status and ability to handle the increased physical and emotional stress of this time. Because of the increased intensity and frequency of contractions, she may find coping difficult. On the other hand, she may have less

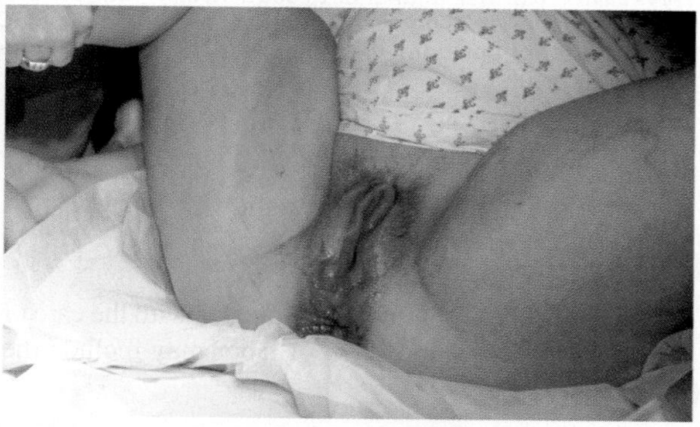

FIGURE 15.23 As the fetal head pushes down, the perineum bulges. This sign indicates that birth is imminent. (Copyright © Barbara Proud.)

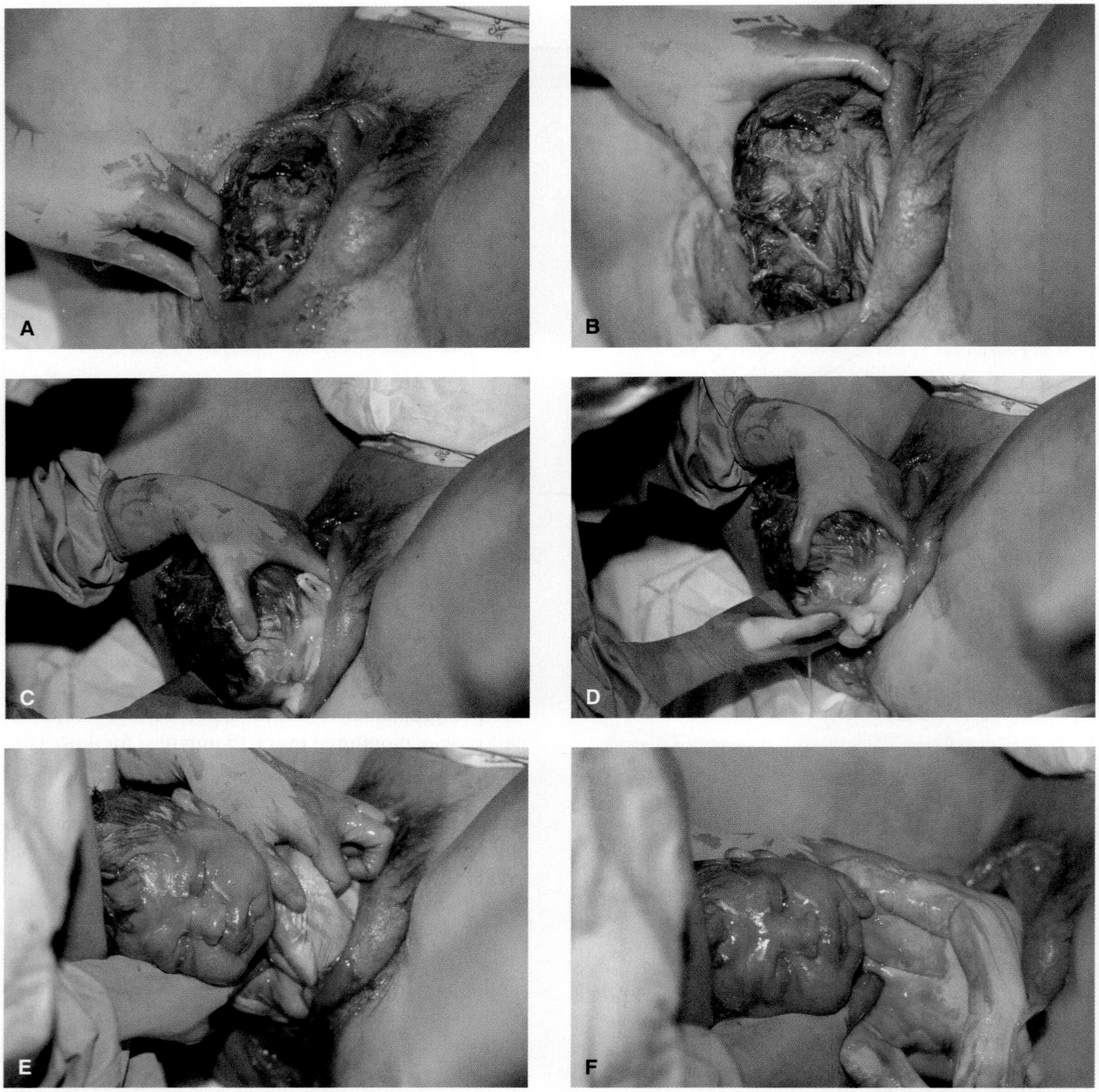

FIGURE 15.24 Normal vaginal birth sequence. (**A**) Early crowning. (**B**) Late crowning. The fetal head is face down, in normal occiput anterior position. (**C, D**) Extension of the fetal head (right occiput anterior position). (**E**) Birth of the shoulders. (**F**) Emergence of the rest of the fetal body, including the umbilical cord.

apprehension or feel relieved now that she can sense the urge to push and sees an end in sight.

Select Potential Nursing Diagnoses

Nursing diagnoses commonly associated with the care of a woman in the second stage of labor may include the following:

- **Pain** related to the increased intensity and frequency of contractions
- **Ineffective Coping** related to unfamiliar sensations and increased intensity of contractions
- **Fatigue** related to prolonged efforts of pushing
- **Risk for Injury** (maternal or fetal) related to inappropriate pushing techniques, umbilical cord compression

Planning/Intervention

The health care team must individualize second-stage management. Nevertheless, certain universal interventions are recommended (AWHONN, 2000):

- Teach women prenatally about the benefits of upright positions.
- During labor, encourage women to change positions frequently. Suggested positions include squatting, semirecumbent, standing, and upright kneeling.
- Allow women to rest until they feel an urge to push.
- Encourage spontaneous bearing down.
- Support, rather than direct, the client's involuntary pushing efforts.
- Discourage prolonged maternal breath holding (more than 6 to 8 seconds).
- Validate the normalcy of sensations and sounds the woman is voicing.

During the second stage, the urge to push usually feels strongest at the peak of the contraction and then fades toward the end. Women should follow along and do what feels right. For most clients, this means taking normal breaths as the contraction builds and then pushing when the urge becomes irresistible (Hansen et al., 2002). Some women find it helps to make sounds in response to what they are feeling. Low-pitched groaning, sighing, and moaning may help release tension, which may assist in coping with pain (Roberts, 2002). Labor supporters should validate the normalcy of sensations and sounds she makes and provide quiet, reassuring encouragement. Some women may find cheering and coaching helpful, but this behavior may annoy others. Individualized support for the client and her partner is most important (Bloom et al., 2006). If progress is slow, the nurse can encourage the client to change positions. For example, benefits of upright or lateral positions as compared with supine or lithotomy positions include reduced duration of second-stage labor, reduced assisted deliveries, reduced episiotomies, and smaller increases in second-degree perineal tears (Carroli & Belizan, 2000; Easton et al., 2000). The nurse should urge the client to release tension in the perineum. Warm compresses may help with relaxing this area. It is most important for the woman to rest between contractions. Pushing is hard work.

Episiotomy is a surgical incision into the perineum to enlarge the outlet (Fig. 15.25). It was introduced as an obstetric intervention in the late 1800s based on a belief that it would protect the perineum from severe lacerations. Historically, obstetricians also proposed that the use of episiotomy improves future sexual function and reduces urine and fecal incontinence. Research findings, however, suggest otherwise. Episiotomy is associated with increased third- and fourth-degree lacerations and increased postpartum pain when compared with spontaneous lacerations (Easton & Feldman, 2000; Hartmann et al., 2005). Research shows no reliable evidence that routine use of episiotomy has any beneficial maternal effect (Carroli & Belizan, 2000). On the contrary, clear evidence shows that it may cause harm, such as greater need for surgical repair and poorer future sexual capacity (Nager & Helliwell, 2001). Although hospitals vary widely in their use of episiotomies, in recent years it appears that the number of routine episiotomies has decreased (Goldberg et al., 2002; Webb & Culhane, 2002).

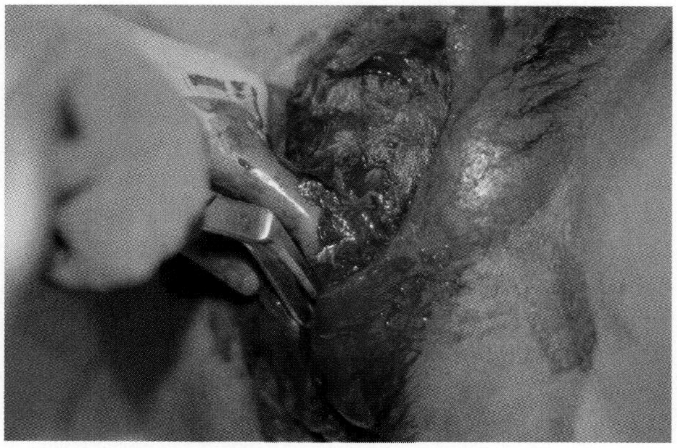

FIGURE 15.25 Episiotomy.

Although there is no maternal indication for routine episiotomy, there are sometimes fetal indications for the procedure. Because episiotomy does shorten the second stage of labor, it may be indicated in cases of fetal distress.

Evaluation

Interventions during the second stage of labor are effective when the woman pushes successfully without experiencing fatigue and maternal and fetal well-being are maintained in preparation for birth.

QUOTE 15-3

"It was hard work. Really, really tough. But look at my little one! Yes, it was worth it."

From a woman who just gave birth after 13 hours of labor

Third Stage: Afterbirth

The **third stage of labor** refers to the separation and expulsion of the **afterbirth,** or placenta and membranes. This stage usually occurs spontaneously within 5 to 30 minutes of the fetus emerging from the birth canal (Smith & Brennan, 2004). After this time, the uterus relaxes for a few minutes. Then contractions begin again. This causes the placenta to fold and separate from the uterus. Bleeding on the maternal side of the placenta occurs, further helping the placenta to separate. Separation leads to movement of the placenta to the lower uterus or upper vagina.

Indications that placental expulsion is imminent include the following:

- Lengthening of the umbilical cord
- A sudden gush of blood

- Change in uterine shape to globular and ascent into the abdomen

These signs usually occur within 5 to 10 minutes of birth. Maternal bearing-down efforts may lead to actual expulsion of the placenta. When examined, the placenta may present with the shiny, glistening fetal side (indicating separation first at the center and then at the edges; called Schultze's mechanism) or the red, raw, rough-shaped maternal side (indicating that the placenta separated at the edges first; called Duncan's mechanism). See Figure 15.26.

Contractions during third-stage labor are mild to moderate. They usually feel like strong menstrual cramps. Many women overlook them because they are focused on seeing their babies. Some women experience generalized shivering during this stage, which may result from a low environmental temperature, the sudden release of pressure on the pelvic nerves, or excess epinephrine production during labor (Smith & Brennan, 2004). The woman also may experience a range of other physical symptoms, such as hunger, thirst, exhaustion, or bladder distention.

After expulsion of the placenta, the birth attendant examines the woman's cervix, vaginal tract, and perineum for lacerations. Lacerations are common in women who experience a difficult or precipitate birth, a birth with a newborn weighing more than 9 lbs, or a birth that involves the use of the lithotomy position and instrumentation, such as forceps (see Chap. 16). Lacerations may occur anywhere along the birth canal, commonly affecting the perineum. Perineal lacerations are classified as first, second, third, or fourth degree, depending on the extent and depth of tissue involvement. See Table 15.5.

One of the most important issues during this time is protecting the woman against the dangers of postpartum hemorrhage. This problem is discussed in detail in Chapters 18 and 19.

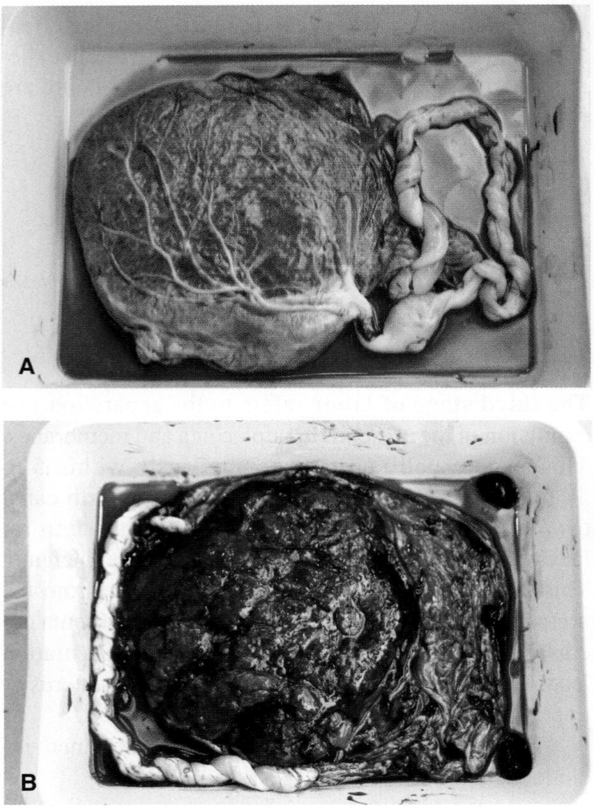

FIGURE 15.26 Placenta. (**A**) Schultze's mechanism—fetal side. (**B**) Duncan's mechanism—maternal side.

COLLABORATIVE CARE: THIRD STAGE OF LABOR

Assessment

Assessment continues throughout the third stage of labor and becomes especially important because immediately after birth nurses frequently are responsible for both the woman and her newborn (see Chap. 20). When the placenta has been delivered in the third stage of labor, the birth attendant assesses the status of uterine contractility, inspects the placenta, membranes, and cord, and inspects and repairs the episiotomy or any lacerations of the cervix, vagina, or perineum. The umbilical cord should contain two arteries and one vein. Blood samples from the umbilical cord arteries or vein may be drawn promptly after delivery of the placenta and sent for cord blood analysis. Analysis of cord blood may be done for blood typing should the newborn require emergency blood replacement therapy. In newborns who demonstrated abnormal FHR patterns during labor, exhibited respiratory depression or low Apgar scores at birth, or had meconium-stained amniotic fluid, cord blood may be used to evaluate for acidemia secondary to possible cord compression or placental hypoperfusion. An umbilical cord blood sample also may be obtained for a direct Coombs' test to detect the presence of maternal Rh-positive antibodies (see Chap. 22).

TABLE 15.5 Lacerations

DEGREE	CHARACTERISTICS
First-degree	Involve the fourchette, perineal skin, and vaginal mucous membrane, but no muscle
Second-degree	Involve all of the above and the muscles of the perineum, but not the rectal sphincter
Third-degree	Involve all of the above, and the rectal sphincter
Fourth-degree	Involve all of the above and extend through the rectum

Select Potential Nursing Diagnoses

Nursing diagnoses that may be applicable during the third stage of labor are similar to those for the second stage of labor, with the following additions:

- **Risk for Injury** (maternal and newborn) related to birth process, possible hemorrhage
- **Risk for Deficient Fluid Volume** related to blood loss during birth
- **Deficient Knowledge** related to birth and body system changes after birth
- **Risk for Infection** related to perineal lacerations, creation of episiotomy
- **Readiness for Enhanced Parenting** related to birth of newborn and immediate bonding

Planning/Intervention

After birth of the baby, the woman needs continued support for delivery of the placenta, examination of the genital tract, and repair of the episiotomy or lacerations. Ongoing assessment of the uterine fundus is essential. Relaxation techniques and breathing strategies she used throughout first-stage labor will be helpful at this time as well to deal with any discomforts.

Evaluation

The desired outcomes associated with the third stage of labor include birth of a healthy newborn, expulsion of an intact placenta, and evidence of beginning uterine involution. In addition, the woman experiences blood loss less than 500 mL and reports a significant decrease in pain (Cunningham et al., 2005). Moreover, the mother and her partner demonstrate beginning bonding behaviors with their newborn.

Fourth Stage: Immediate Postpartum

The **fourth stage of labor** refers to the period immediately after delivery of the placenta. It typically lasts 1 to 4 hours and may be referred to as the recovery phase (Cunningham et al., 2005). During this period, the woman's body begins to undergo several major physiologic changes as it starts returning to a nonpregnant state. Intra-abdominal pressure decreases markedly from birth of the baby and delivery of the placenta. The uterus should be well contracted, in the midline of the abdomen, and between the symphysis and umbilicus. Uterine contraction is a major means of achieving hemostasis. If inadequate, postpartum hemorrhage can occur. Therefore, frequent continued assessment of the uterine fundus is essential.

Major hemodynamic changes result from normal blood loss at delivery and decreased intra-abdominal pressure. With placental expulsion, blood flow to the placenta is no longer needed. As a result, blood is shunted to the maternal systemic venous circulation. In addition, blood volume decreases because of the blood loss and diuresis. Cardiac output initially increases, most likely from increased stroke volume related to the increased venous return. It then gradually returns to prelabor levels within 1 hour after birth.

In addition to mild uterine cramping, some women experience generalized shivering. They may experience urinary retention, especially if they received regional anesthesia. Women also may feel fatigue, muscle aches, and hunger and thirst. Emotional reactions vary from overwhelming joy and relief to temporary disbelief and withdrawal.

Chapter 18 discusses care of the family during the fourth stage of labor in detail. See Chapter 19 for discussion of maternal complications during the postpartum period.

Questions to Ponder

1. A client, G1P0, comes to the labor and birth suite stating, "I think I'm in labor." After several hours, her contractions continue to be mild and irregular with no increase in frequency, duration, or intensity. Her cervical dilation remains at 1 cm and membranes are intact. She is discharged home to wait. What information would the nurse include in the discharge teaching?
2. A couple in the fourth stage of labor is inspecting their newborn. The father says, "His head looks so funny. It's so oblong." How would the nurse explain this condition?
3. A nurse is teaching a childbirth education class to a group of expectant parents. As part of this class, the nurse is planning to describe how the fetus moves through the pelvic canal for birth. Develop a teaching plan that explains these movements.

SUMMARY

- Prelabor refers to the period before the actual onset of labor associated with signs such as lightening, Braxton-Hicks contractions, backache, bloody show, spontaneous rupture of membranes, a spurt of energy, and weight loss.
- Labor is typically defined as the series of processes that result in the expulsion of the products of conception from the mother's body. The exact cause of labor is not known, but several theories have attempted to explain the cause. Some of the more common theories include progesterone withdrawal, oxytocin production, prostaglandin production, estrogen stimulation, and fetal influence.
- The process of labor and birth involves powers (uterine contractions and maternal pushing), passageway (maternal pelvis and soft parts), passenger (fetus),

and position (maternal). Additionally, psychosocial factors play a role.

- Normal uterine contractions are composed of an increment, acme, and decrement. Frequency refers to the time from the beginning of one contraction to the beginning of the next. Duration is measured from the beginning to the end of the contraction. Intensity refers to the strength of the contraction.
- The four basic shapes of the female pelvis are gynecoid, android, anthropoid, and platypelloid. Vaginal birth is most easily accomplished with a gynecoid pelvis.
- Fetal lie, presentation, attitude, and position are key factors involved in the relationship between the fetus and the maternal pelvis.
- A fetus is engaged when the presenting part is at station 0, at the level of the ischial spines. Measurements of the presenting part above the ischial spines are identified as a negative station (eg, −1, −2); measurements below are identified as a positive station (eg, +1, +2).
- For birth, the fetus goes through a series of passive movements so that the smallest diameter of the presenting part presents to the irregular shape of the pelvis. These movements are called the cardinal movements or mechanisms of labor: descent, flexion, internal rotation, extension, restitution, external rotation, and birth of the shoulders and expulsion.
- During labor, the woman's body undergoes physiologic and psychological changes to meet the demands of labor. The fetus also must respond to the changing intrauterine environment.
- Fetal heart rate can be monitored by auscultation or electronic monitoring. Electronic monitoring may be external (indirect) or internal (direct).
- Baseline fetal heart rate is the typical FHR during a 10-minute period or between uterine contractions in labor. It normally ranges from 120 to 160 bpm. Baseline variability refers to the short-term beat-to-beat interval changes in FHR or the long-term oscillations or undulation of the baseline. Decreased variability is associated with fetal central nervous system depression.
- Periodic changes involve brief deviations in FHR above or below the baseline, usually in response to uterine contractions or fetal activity. Episodic changes are deviations above or below baseline unrelated to uterine contractions.
- Accelerations of FHR are associated with fetal activity and are usually considered signs of fetal well-being. Early decelerations are thought to result from vagal nerve stimulation from fetal head compression during labor and are considered a normal physiologic response. Late decelerations are thought to result from uteroplacental insufficiency or compromised uteroplacental perfusion and require intervention to increase uteroplacental circulation and fetal oxygenation. Variable decelerations usually are associated with compression of the umbilical cord and typically require a change in maternal positioning.
- Labor is divided into four stages based on the degree of cervical dilation, cervical effacement, and contraction pattern.
- The first stage of labor is further divided into three phases: early (latent) phase, active phase, and transition phase. During the first stage of labor, the cervix softens, thins, shortens, and dilates to a diameter of 10 cm. Contractions become regular, frequent, and intense.
- Care of the woman during the first stage of labor focuses on assessing maternal and fetal well-being, assisting the woman to cope with the increased contraction frequency and intensity, providing support to the woman and her partner, and ensuring adequate pain relief.
- The second stage of labor involves the woman's pushing efforts and movement of the fetus through the birth canal, resulting in the birth of a newborn.
- During the second stage of labor, care focuses on more frequent assessment of maternal and fetal well-being, position changes, and support of pushing efforts.
- The third stage of labor involves separation and expulsion of the placenta. Care focuses on continued support of the woman as the placenta is delivered.
- The fourth stage of labor refers to the period immediately after delivery of the placenta, typically lasting from 1 to 4 hours. At this time, care focuses on monitoring the woman and her newborn, promoting maternal comfort, providing adequate education and support, and facilitating attachment behaviors.

REVIEW QUESTIONS

1. During a sterile vaginal examination of a woman in labor, the nurse identifies the buttocks as lying over the pelvic inlet. The nurse should document this presentation as
   A. cephalic.
   B. breech.
   C. shoulder.
   D. transverse.
2. Examination reveals that the presenting part of the fetus in the cephalic presentation has passed the pelvic inlet and is at the level of the ischial spines. The nurse interprets this to mean that the presenting part is
   A. engaged.
   B. floating.
   C. at −1 station.
   D. crowning.
3. Which method would be most effective for the nurse to use when assessing the intensity of a client's uterine contractions?

A. Auscultating with a Doppler ultrasound
B. Observing the woman's facial expression
C. Asking the woman to rate the intensity
D. Palpating the uterine fundus

4. When assessing contractions by the recording from an EFM, the nurse measures from the beginning of the contraction to the end of that contraction to determine
A. frequency.
B. duration.
C. acme.
D. intensity.

5. A woman in labor states, "I think my water just broke." On inspection, the nurse notes a large amount of clear straw-colored fluid on the bed. Which action should the nurse do first?
A. Test the fluid with Nitrazine paper
B. Call the primary care provider
C. Provide perineal care
D. Assess FHR

6. The nurse is preparing to auscultate the fetal heart rate with a Doppler device. Assessment reveals that the fetal back is toward the mother's left side, fetal arms are toward the mother's right side, and the fetus is in a vertex presentation. Where should the nurse position the device initially?
A. Left upper quadrant
B. Left lower quadrant
C. Right upper quadrant
D. Right lower quadrant

7. EFM reveals a baseline FHR of 144 bpm, which slows to 128 bpm as the client's contraction peaks. The FHR then returns to baseline by the end of the contraction. The nurse interprets this finding as indicating
A. compression of the fetal head.
B. uteroplacental insufficiency.
C. umbilical cord compression.
D. uterine hyperstimulation.

8. A woman admitted to the labor and birth suite is accompanied by her partner and a doula. The nurse includes the doula in the client's plan of care based on the understanding that the doula's primary role is to
A. assist the primary care provider in the birth.
B. provide for client comfort and continuous support.
C. act as major decision maker during labor.
D. care for the client's partner during labor.

9. A woman arrives at the labor and birth area. Assessment reveals moderate contractions every 5 minutes and lasting approximately 45 seconds. Cervical dilation is 3 cm; cervical effacement is approximately 50%. The nurse determines that the client is in which stage of labor?
A. First stage, latent phase
B. First stage, transition phase
C. Second stage
D. Third stage

10. The labor and birth record of a client who gave birth to a healthy newborn approximately 45 minutes ago reveals the need for an episiotomy. The nurse explains this to the client, describing it as which of the following?
A. Artificial rupture of the membranes
B. Use of medication to enhance contractions
C. A perineal incision to enlarge the outlet
D. Thinning of the cervical tissue

REFERENCES

American College of Nurse–Midwives (ACNM). (1999). Clinical bulletin No. 3: Intrapartum nutrition. *Journal of Nurse-Midwifery, 44*(2), 124–128.

American College of Obstetricians and Gynecologists (ACOG). (2002). *ACOG Practice bulletin #36 (July 2002): Obstetric analgesia and anesthesia.* Washington, DC: Author.

American College of Obstetricians and Gynecologists (ACOG). (2000). *Evaluation of cesarean delivery.* Washington, DC: Author.

American Society of Anesthesiologists (ASA). (1998). *Practice guidelines for obstetrical anesthesia.* Available at the American Society of Anesthesiologists website: http://www.asahq.org.

Andrews, M., & Boyle, J. (2004). *Transcultural concepts in nursing care* (3rd ed.). Philadelphia: Lippincott.

Association of Women's Health, Obstetric and Neonatal Nurses (AWHONN). (2000). *AWHONN position statement, issue: Professional nursing support of laboring women.* Washington, DC: Author.

Bashour, H., & Abdulsalam, A. (2005). Syrian women's preferences for birth attendant and birth place. *Birth, 32*(1), 20–26.

Berg, M., & Terstad, A. (2006). Swedish women's experiences of doula support during childbirth. *Midwifery,* in press.

Blackburn, S., & Loper, D. (2003). *Maternal, fetal, and neonatal physiology: A clinical perspective* (2nd ed.). Philadelphia: W. B. Saunders.

Bloom, S. L., et al. (2006). A randomized trial of coached versus uncoached maternal pushing during the second stage of labor. *American Journal of Obstetrics and Gynecology, 194*(1), 10–13.

Caldeyro-Barcia, R. (1979). The influence of maternal bearing-down efforts during second-stage on fetal well-being. *Birth and the Family Journal, 6*(1), 17–21.

Callister, L. C. (2005). What has the literature taught us about culturally competent care of women and children? *MCN—American Journal of Maternal and Child Nursing, 30*(6), 380–388.

Callister, L. C., Khalaf, I., Semenic, S., Kartchner, R., & Vehvilainen-Julkunen, K. (2003). The pain of childbirth: Perceptions of culturally diverse women. *Pain Management Nursing, 4*(4), 145–154.

Carroli, G., & Belizan, J. (2000). Episiotomy for vaginal birth. Cochrane Review. In *The Cochrane Library, Issue 3.* Oxford, UK: Update Software.

Chalk, A. (2004). Spontaneous versus directed pushing. *British Journal of Midwifery, 12,* 626–630.

Cioffi, J. (2004). Caring for women from culturally diverse backgrounds: Midwives' experiences. *Journal of Midwifery and Women's Health, 49*(5), 437–442.

Cluett, E. R., Nikodem, V. C., McCandlish, R. E., & Burns, E. E. (2004). Immersion in water in pregnancy, labour, and birth. *Cochrane Database of Systematic Reviews, 2,* CD000111.

Cunningham, F. G., Gant, N. F., Leveno, K. J., Bloom, S. L., Hauth, J. C., Gillstrap, L. C., III, & Wenstrom, K. D. (2005). *Williams obstetrics* (22nd ed.). New York: McGraw-Hill.

Davis-Floyd, R., & Sargent, C. (Eds.) (1997). *Childbirth and authoritative knowledge.* Berkeley, CA: University of California Press.

Declercq, E., Sakala, C., Corry, M., Applebaum, S., & Risher, P. (2002). *Listening to mothers: Report of the first national U.S. survey of women's childbirth experiences.* New York: Maternity Center Association.

de Montigny, F., & Lacharite, C. (2004). Fathers' perceptions of the immediate postpartal period. *Journal of Obstetric, Gynecological, and Neonatal Nursing, 33*(3), 328–339.

Dilbaz, B., Ozturkoglu, E., Dilbaz, S., Ozturk, N., Sivaslioglu, A. A., & Haberal, A. (2006). Risk factors and perinatal outcomes associated with umbilical cord prolapse. *Archives of Gynecology and Obstetrics, 274*(2), 104–107.

Easton, E., et al. (2000). Preventing perineal trauma during childbirth: A systematic review. *Obstetrics & Gynecology, 95*(93), 464–471.

Easton, E., & Feldman, P. (2000). Clinical commentary. Much ado about a little cut: Is episiotomy worthwhile? *Obstetrics & Gynecology, 95*(4), 616–618.

England, P., & Horowitz, R. (1998). *Birthing from within.* Albuquerque, NM: Pantera Press.

Enkin, M., et al. (2000). *A guide to effective care in pregnancy and childbirth* (3rd ed.). New York: Oxford University Press.

Feinstein, N., Torgersen, K. L., & Atterbury, J. (2003). *AWHONN's fetal heart monitoring principles and practices* (3rd ed.). Dubuque, IA: Kendall-Hunt Publishing Company.

Feinstein, N., Sprague, A., & Trepanier, M. (2000). Fetal heart rate auscultation. *AWHONN Life-lines, 4*(3), 35–44.

Gilliland, A. (2002). Beyond holding hands: The modern role of the professional doula. *Journal of Obstetric, Gynecologic, and Neonatal Nursing, 31*(6), 762–769.

Goer, H. (1999). *The thinking woman's guide to a better birth.* New York: Perigree.

Goer, H. (1995). *Obstetric myths versus research realities: A guide to the medical literature.* Westport, CT: Bergin & Garvey.

Goff, K. (1993). Initiation of parturition. *American Journal of Maternal Child Nursing, 18,* Suppl: 7(13).

Goldberg, J., Holtz, D., Hyslop, T., & Tolosa, J. (2002). Has the use of routine episiotomy decreased: Examination of episiotomy rates from 1983 to 2000. *Obstetrics & Gynecology, 99*(3), 395–400.

Goodman, P., Mackey, M. C., & Tavakoli, A. S. (2004). Factors related to childbirth satisfaction. *Journal of Advanced Nursing, 46*(2), 212–219.

Goodwin, L. (2000). Intermittent auscultation of the fetal heart rate: A review of general principles. *Journal of Perinatal and Neonatal Nursing, 14*(3), 53–61.

Gross, M. M., Drobnic, S., & Keirse, M. J. (2005). Influence of fixed and time-dependent factors on duration of normal first stage labor. *Birth, 32*(1), 27–33.

Gross, M. M., Hecker, H., Matterne, A., Guenter, H. H., & Keirse, M. J. (2006). Does the way that women experience the onset of labour influence the duration of labour? *British Journal of Obstetrics and Gynecology, 113*(3), 289–294.

Gupta, J. K., & Hofmeyr, G. J. (2004). Positions for women during second stage of labour. *Cochrane Database of Systematic Reviews, 1,* CD002006.

Hansen, S., Clark, S., & Foster, J. (2002). Active pushing versus passive fetal descent in the second-stage of labor: A randomized controlled trial. *Obstetrics & Gynecology, 99*(1), 29–34.

Hartmann, K., Viswanathan, M., Palmieri, R., Gatlehner, G., Thorp, J. Jr., & Lohr, K. N. (2005). Outcomes of routine episiotomy: A systematic review. *JAMA, 293*(17), 2141–2148.

Hodnett, E. (2002). Caregiver support for women during childbirth. In *The Cochrane Library, Issue 4.* Oxford, UK: Update Software.

Hodnett, E., et al. (2002). Effectiveness of nurses as providers of birth labor support in North American hospitals. *Journal of the American Medical Association, 288*(11), 1373–1381.

Hodnett, E. D., Downe, S., Edwards, N., & Walsh, D. (2005). Home-like versus conventional institutional settings for birth. *Cochrane Database of Systematic Reviews, 1,* CD000012.

Karnng-Edgren, S. (2001). Using evidence-based practice to improve intrapartum care. *Journal of Obstetric, Gynecologic, and Neonatal Nursing, 30*(4), 371–375.

Kennedy, H. P., & Shannon, M. T. (2004). Keeping birth normal: Research findings on midwifery care during childbirth. *Journal of Obstetrical, Gynecological, and Neonatal Nursing, 33*(5), 554–560.

Khan, F. O., & Razi, M. S. (2005). Normal labor and delivery. *E-medicine.* Retrieved June 1, 2006, from http://www.emedicine.com/med/topic3239.htm.

Kitzinger, S. (2001). *Rediscovering birth.* New York: Pocket Books.

Lamaze International. (2001). *Lamaze International position paper: Lamaze in the 21st century.* Washington, DC: Author.

Lee, C. J., & Lamp, J. K. (2005). The birth story interview: Enhancing student appreciation of the personal meaning of pregnancy and birth. *Nurse Educator, 30*(4), 155–158.

Lothian, J. (2001). Back to the future: Trusting normal birth. *Journal of Perinatal Education, 15*(3), 13–22.

Lundgren, I. (2004). Releasing and relieving encounters: Experiences of pregnancy and childbirth. *Scandinavian Journal of Caring Sciences, 18*(4), 368–375.

Matthews, R., & Callister, L. C. (2004). Childbearing women's perceptions of nursing care that promotes dignity. *Journal of Obstetric, Gynecologic, and Neonatal Nursing, 33*(4), 498–507.

Mayberry, L., et al. (1999). Maternal fatigue: Implications of second stage labor nursing care. *Journal of Obstetric, Gynecologic, and Neonatal Nursing, 28*(2), 175–181.

Mayberry, L. (2000). *Second-stage labor management: Promotion of evidence-based practice and a collaborative approach to patient care.* Washington, DC: AWHONN.

Mayberry, L., Clemmens, D., & De, A. (2002). Epidural analgesia side effects, co-interventions, and care of women during childbirth: A systematic review. *American Journal of Obstetrics & Gynecology, 186*(Suppl. 95), S81–S93.

McLachlan, H., & Waldenstrom, U. (2005). Childbirth experiences in Australia of women born in Turkey, Vietnam, and Australia. *Birth, 32*(4), 272–282.

Moore, M. (2001). Adopting birth philosophies to guide successful birth practices and outcomes. *Journal of Perinatal Education, 10*(2), 43–45.

Nager, C., & Helliwell, J. (2001). Episiotomy increases perineal laceration length in primiparous women. *American Journal of Obstetricians and Gynecologists, 185*(2), 444–450.

Parsons, M., Bidewell, J., & Nagy, S. (2006). Natural eating behavior in latent labor and its effect on outcomes in active labor. *Journal of Midwifery and Women's Health, 51*(1), e1–6.

Pascali-Bonaro, D., & Kroeger, M. (2004). Continuous female companionship during childbirth: A crucial resource in times of stress or calm. *Journal of Midwifery and Women's Health, 49*(4 Suppl. 1), 19–27.

Pillitteri, A. (2007). *Maternal and child health nursing* (5th ed.). Philadelphia: Lippincott Williams & Wilkins.

Priddy, K. D. (2004). Is there logic behind fetal monitoring? *Journal of Obstetric, Gynecologic, and Neonatal Nursing, 33*(5), 550–553.

Primeau, M. R., Lucey, K. A., & Crotty, P. M. (2003). Managing the pain of labor. *Advance for Nurses, 4*(12), 15–19.

Ragusa, A., Mansur, M., Zanini, A., Musicco, M., Maccario, L., & Borsellino, G. (2005). Diagnosis of labor: A prospective study. *Medscape General Medicine, 7*(3), 61.

Roberts, J. (2002). The push for evidence: Management of the second-stage. *Journal of Midwifery & Women's Health, 47*(1), 2–15.

Rooks, J., Sakala, C., & Corry, M. (Eds.) (2002). The nature and management of labor pain: Peer reviewed papers from an evidence-based symposium. *American Journal of Obstetrics and Gynecology, 186*(Suppl. 5).

Rouse, D. J., & St. John, E. (2003). Normal labor, delivery, newborn care, and puerperium. In J. R. Scott, R. S. Gibbs, B. Y. Karlan, & A. F. Haney (Eds.), *Danforth's obstetrics and gynecology* (9th ed., pp. 35–56).

Sampselle, C. M., Miller, J. M., Luecha, Y., Fischer, K., & Rosten, L. (2005). Provider support of spontaneous pushing during the second stage of labor. *Journal of Obstetric, Gynecologic, and Neonatal Nursing, 34*(6), 695–702.

Scrutton, M., Metcalfe, G., Lowy, C., Seed, P., & O'Sullivan, G. (1999). Eating in labor: A randomized controlled trial assessing the risks and benefits. *Anaesthesia, 54*(4), 329–344.

Senecal, J., Xiong, X., Fraser, W. D., et al. (2005). Effect of fetal position on second-stage duration and labor outcome. *Obstetrics and Gynecology, 105*(4), 763–772.

Shade, B., Kelly, C., & Oberg, M. (1997). *Creating culturally responsive classrooms.* Washington, DC: American Psychological Association.

Simkin, P. (1996). The experience of maternity in a woman's life. *Journal of Obstetric, Gynecologic, and Neonatal Nursing, 25*(3), 247–252.

Simkin, P., & Ancheta, R. (2000). *The labor progress handbook: Early interventions to prevent and treat dystocia.* Malden, MA: Blackwell Science.

Simkin, P., & O'Hara, M. (2002). Nonpharmacologic relief of pain during labor: Systematic reviews of five methods. *American Journal of Obstetrics & Gynecology, 186*(5), S131–S151.

Simpson, K. R. (2005). The context and clinical evidence for common nursing practices during labor. *MCN—American Journal of Maternal Child Nursing, 30*(6), 356–363.

Simpson, K. R., & Creehan, P. A. (2001). *AWHONN perinatal nursing* (2nd ed.). Philadelphia: Lippincott Williams & Wilkins.

Sleutal, M., & Golden, S. (1999). In review. Fasting in labor: relic or requirement. *Journal of Obstetric, Gynecologic, and Neonatal Nursing, 28*(5), 507–512.

Smith, J. R., & Brennan, B. G. (2004). Management of the third stage of labor. *E-Medicine.* Retrieved June 6, 2006, from: http://www.emedicine.com/med/topic3569.htm.

Society of Obstetricians and Gynaecologists of Canada (SOGC). (2002). Fetal health surveillance in labor (SOGC Clinical Practice Guidelines No. 112). *Journal of Obstetrics and Gynecology in Canada, 112*(March), 1–13.

Thacker, S. B., Stroup, D., & Chang, M. (2001). Continuous electronic heart rate monitoring for fetal assessment during labor. *Cochrane Database of Systematic Reviews, 2,* CD000063.

Turley, G. M. (2004). Essential forces and factors in labor. In S. Mattson & J. E. Smith (Eds.), *AWHONN: Maternal–newborn nursing* (3rd ed., pp. 227–270). Philadelphia: Elsevier.

Vincent, P. (2002). *Baby catcher: Chronicles of a modern midwife.* New York: Scribner.

Waldenstrom, U. (2004). Why do some women change their opinion about childbirth over time? *Birth, 31*(2), 102–107.

Walker, D., Shunkwiler, S., Supanich, J., Williamsen, J., & Yensch, A. (2001). Labor and delivery nurses' attitudes toward intermittent fetal monitoring. *Journal of Midwifery & Women's Health, 46*(6), 374–380.

Webb, D., & Culhane, J. (2002). Hospital variation in episiotomy use and the risk of perineal trauma during childbirth. *Birth, 29*(2), 132–136.

Zhang, J., Troendle, J., & Yancey, M. (2002). Reassessing the labor curve in nulliparous women. *American Journal of Obstetrics & Gynecology, 187*(4), 824–828.

CHAPTER 16

High-Risk Labor and Childbirth

Nancy Watts

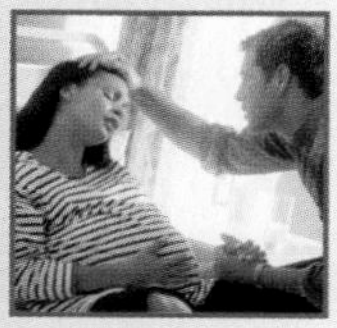

Beverly, a 35-year-old client (G3P2), arrives at the labor and birth suite with her husband. She is at term and experiencing contractions approximately every 5 minutes. Her cervix is 3 cm dilated and 50% effaced. Beverly states, "I have a lot of pain in my back. It feels like the baby is pressing on my spine. This happened with my last pregnancy, too."

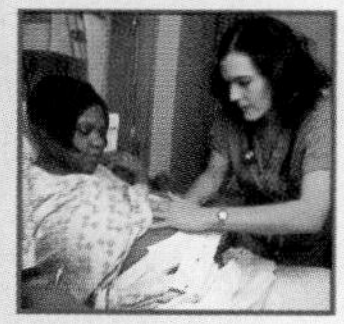

Carlotta (G1P0) is at 42 weeks' gestation. She and her boyfriend have come to the labor and delivery area for a scheduled induction of labor. Carlotta appears tired, saying, "I really haven't slept much because I've been a bit worried about what's next." She adds that she is really hoping to use the Jacuzzi during labor and that she won't need an epidural.

You will learn more about these stories later in this chapter. Nurses working with these and similar clients need to understand the material in this chapter to manage care and address issues appropriately. Before beginning, consider the following points:

- Does anything about either case qualify as an emergency? Explain your answer.
- Would you consider each client to be at high risk during labor and birth? Why or why not?
- How might each client's specific situation influence the nurse's approach to care?
- What details will the nurse need to investigate with Beverly about her complaints? What about Carlotta?
- What areas of teaching would the nurse need to address with both women and their families?

LEARNING OBJECTIVES

On completion of this chapter, the reader should be able to:

- Explain what is meant by dystocia.
- Identify the general causes of problems with the powers of labor and ways that health care providers intervene to resolve them.
- Discuss common fetal positions, presentations, and circumstances that may halt labor's progress and appropriate related nursing measures.
- Identify problems with the maternal pelvis or vaginal outlet that may pose risks during childbirth.
- Describe the risks associated with preterm labor, contributing factors, and associated management parameters.
- Explain complications that can accompany postterm pregnancy and alternatives for resolving this circumstance.
- Identify conditions that can result in hemorrhage during labor and childbirth.
- Discuss why quick interventions for cord prolapse and amniotic fluid embolism are so important.
- Describe necessary adaptations during labor in cases of multiple gestation, maternal obesity, and women who have undergone circumcision.
- Outline the process of labor induction and related nursing care.
- Identify indications for amnioinfusion.
- Explain when forceps or a vacuum extractor might be used, related processes, and appropriate nursing care.
- Discuss general reasons for increasing rates of cesarean birth.
- Outline the process of cesarean birth and appropriate nursing interventions during the preoperative, intraoperative, and postoperative stages.

KEY TERMS

amnioinfusion
amniotic fluid embolism
arrest disorder
breech presentation
cephalopelvic disproportion (CPD)
constriction rings
cord prolapse
dystocia
external cephalic version
failure to progress
forceps
hydrocephalus
hyperstimulation
hypertonic uterine contractions
hypotonic uterine contractions
macrosomia
molding
occipitoposterior (OP) positioning
pathologic retraction ring
Piper forceps
postterm pregnancy
precipitous labor
preterm labor
protraction disorder
shoulder dystocia
uterine rupture
vacuum extractor
vaginal birth after cesarean (VBAC)

This chapter focuses on those conditions that pose risks during the process of labor and birth. It explores difficulties related to labor that fails to progress and problems with labor's timing—either too early or too late in gestation. The chapter covers hemorrhagic problems in labor, as well as difficulties with the umbilical cord and amniotic fluid. It focuses on some special conditions that require adaptations in labor, such as maternal obesity, female circumcision, and multiple gestation. The last section focuses on common interventions employed when labor and birth are at risk, including cervical ripening and labor induction, amnioinfusion, assisted birth, and cesarean birth.

RISK ASSESSMENT AND IDENTIFICATION

A fundamental component of quality perinatal care is the identification of pregnancies at increased risk for complications, whether maternal, fetal, or both (Herzig et al., 2006). Various systems have been used to determine such risks. As discussed in Chapter 13, previous obstetric history, medical health, current pregnancy, anxiety, social support, age, and socioeconomic background are critical components of assessment for each pregnant woman.

Risk factors related specifically to labor and birth may be identified early in pregnancy when the mother has an established health problem such as preexisting cardiac disease or diabetes (see Chap. 13). Other concerning circumstances are known about before labor's onset but do not pose significant problems until that time. Examples may include breech presentation and placenta previa. Still other problems manifest only during labor and birth, such as shoulder dystocia and hypotonic uterine contractions. Regardless of when the situation is determined to be at high risk, the nurse's role involves multidisciplinary collaboration to facilitate health and healing for the client and her family. The overarching goal is to minimize fetal, maternal, and neonatal complications (Gilbert & Harmon, 2003).

Although pregnancy is always a situational stressor, high-risk gestation, labor, and childbirth pose increased concerns for all family members. Expectant parents normally complete several developmental tasks and psychological adjustments to facilitate their future attachment with the newborn. When parents are anxious about maternal and fetal safety, health, well-being, and outcomes, bonding processes may be delayed or impeded (Sittner et al., 2005). Common emotions include ambivalence, anxiety, frustration, low self-esteem, decreased preparation for the newborn, increased unmet expectations, and increased risk for postpartum depression (Gilbert & Harmon, 2003). The client and her partner or support person may feel guilty about an inability to protect the fetus, which also may compromise bonding. See Research Highlight 16.1.

The nurse needs to consider the client's and family's response to a high-risk diagnosis and develop a plan of care to support them. Assessment of stress level and support systems is important (Coffman & Ray, 2002; Sittner et al., 2005). Formulating diagnoses based on individual needs facilitates family-centered care. Encouraging family members to express concerns regarding the high-risk status, providing explanations regarding the normal process of labor, teaching how the high-risk problem might alter the course of labor and birth, and clarifying misconceptions can be supportive interventions. Keeping the client informed of her progress and the results of monitoring that she and the fetus are receiving is encouraging and helpful. Advocating on the family's behalf for appropriate goals may alleviate any feelings of ambivalence members may have. Referrals as appropriate to social work, public health nurses, clinical nurse specialists, or physicians may be critical for appropriate follow-up.

RESEARCH HIGHLIGHT 16.1 Effects of High-Risk Pregnancies on Families

PURPOSE: To describe the psychosocial effects that high-risk gestation can have on the entire family and to examine what strengths can assist families to cope with the special challenges inherent in such situations

SAMPLE AND DESIGN: Researchers employed a descriptive study with naturalistic inquiry to interview pregnant women who had various high-risk concerns. They collected data using semistructured, one-on-one audiotaped interviews, observations, and autobiographical profiles directly from the participants. The researchers then transcribed, examined, and clustered data to arrive at specific themes.

RESULTS: The participants consistently identified having mixed emotions throughout their pregnancies. Family strengths that assisted them through the experience included an ability to manage stress and crisis, commitment, appreciation, affection, spiritual well-being, and enjoyable time together. The least common strength identified was positive communication.

CONCLUSIONS: Nurses can help families coping with high-risk pregnancies to identify strengths and to use them during difficult stages, including the labor and birth itself.

Sittner, B. J., DeFrain, J., & Hudson, D. B. *MCN—American Journal of Maternal Child Nursing, 30*(2), 121–126.

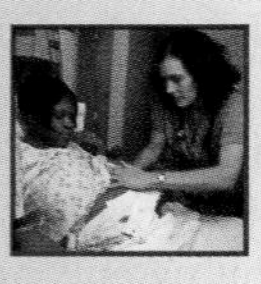

Think back to Carlotta, the client with a postterm pregnancy scheduled for induction of labor. What types of stress might she and her family be experiencing?

DYSFUNCTIONAL LABOR (DYSTOCIA)

Dystocia (abnormal or dysfunctional labor) can happen for many reasons. It occurs in approximately 10% of all labors and is the leading cause of cesarean births (Ressel, 2004). Dystocia can develop during any of labor's phases (see Chap. 15). Normally, the latent phase lasts 5 to 9 hours; a latent phase beyond 14 to 20 hours is considered prolonged (Dudley, 2003). The active phase of labor begins once the cervix is dilated 3 to 4 cm and normally lasts 2 to 5 hours. Active labor beyond 5 hours would be considered prolonged (Dudley, 2003).

One classification of dysfunctional labor is a **protraction disorder,** which is characterized by delayed cervical dilation and slowed descent of the fetal head. Protraction disorders may develop in labor's latent phase, active phase, or second stage. In some women who experience a protracted latent phase, cervical dilation can progress normally once they receive supportive fluids, reassurance, and minimum sedation, although some providers opt to manage labor in such cases more aggressively with augmentation or induction (Dudley, 2003).

Arrest disorders generally happen during active labor and are characterized by the following:

- *Prolonged deceleration phase* (at least 3 hours in a nullipara and 1 hour in a multipara)
- *Secondary arrest of cervical dilation* (no progress for more than 2 hours)
- *Arrest of the descent of the fetal head* (more than 60 minutes in a nullipara and 30 minutes in a multipara)
- *Failure of the descent of the fetal head* (none during the first stage, deceleration phase, or second stage of labor) (Dudley, 2003)

Arrest disorders frequently are associated with **cephalopelvic disproportion (CPD),** or inability of the fetal head to pass through the maternal pelvis because of shape, size, or position (Cunningham et al., 2005).

When the cervix does not dilate normally despite normal uterine contractions and no CPD, the condition is called **failure to progress.** When early labor fails to progress despite uterine contractions, the health care team should evaluate carefully whether the client is experiencing true or false labor.

As discussed in Chapter 15, several elements must interact successfully for labor and birth to progress normally. The *powers* (contractions and pushing) must be sufficient for the cervix to thin and open and to propel the fetus through the birth canal. The *passageway* (maternal vagina) and *passenger* (fetus) must be sized, shaped, and positioned in such a way to allow the fetus to pass through unharmed. Causes leading to dystocia can involve any of the three "P's":

- *Powers.* During the first stage of labor, uterine contractions are too weak or uncoordinated to facilitate adequate cervical effacement and dilation. During the second stage, contractions and pushing are insufficient to promote adequate fetal descent. Another problem involves uterine contractions that are so rapid and strong that labor progresses more quickly than normal.
- *Passenger.* These problems include such issues as fetal malpresentation, malposition, or macrosomia.
- *Passageway.* Difficulties related to the passageway involve abnormalities of maternal pelvic shape or size.

PROBLEMS WITH THE POWERS

When problems with uterine contractions or maternal bearing-down efforts lead to prolonged labor, maternal and fetal complications can ensue. For example, risks for intrauterine infection are increased if labor continues for an extended time after the membranes have ruptured (Cunningham et al., 2005). Other potential difficulties include exhaustion and dehydration. Examples of problems with the powers include hypertonic and hypotonic contractions, inadequate expulsion forces, pathologic retraction and constriction rings, and precipitous birth.

Hypertonic Uterine Contractions

Normally, contractions start at the superior aspect of the uterus and proceed downward to the cervix. In contrast, **hypertonic uterine contractions** are distorted. The uterine midsegment may contract with more force than the fundus, or the impulses in each upper corner of the uterus may not be synchronized (Fig. 16.1). This problem is associated most commonly with a prolonged latent phase (Dudley, 2003).

Hypertonic uterine contractions fail to promote normal cervical dilation. They can be extremely painful, lead-

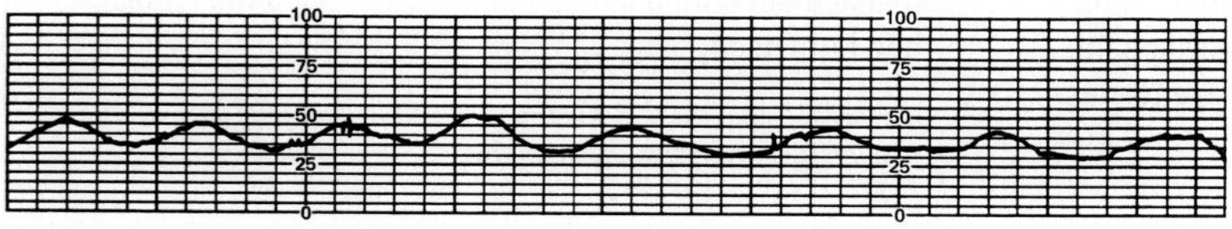

Uterine activity

FIGURE 16.1 With hypertonic uterine contractions, tracings will show a high resting pressure (35 to 40 mm Hg).

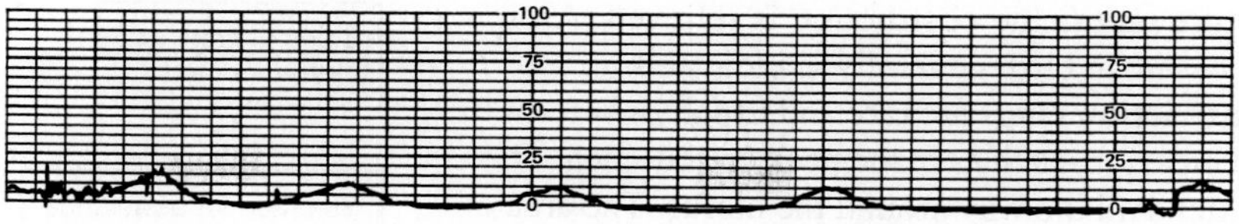

FIGURE 16.2 With hypotonic uterine contractions, tracings reflect a low resting pressure (less than 10 mm Hg).

ing to uterine tenderness even between contractions. A common contributing factor is placental abruption, which must be considered and ruled out or managed aggressively, depending on the findings.

Treatment usually involves fluid administration to maintain hydration and electrolyte balance, as well as rest. Intramuscular morphine may be administered to inhibit the uncoordinated contraction pattern. A short-acting barbiturate may be given to promote rest. Oxytocin usually is contraindicated because it could compound uterine resting tension, which might interfere with fetal oxygenation. When this pattern of contractions persists despite the above interventions, cesarean birth usually is indicated, especially if the fetus shows signs of distress (Cunningham et al., 2005).

QUOTE 16-1

"I remember feeling so frustrated when my labor started but failed to progress adequately. I felt like I had been running a marathon only to find at the last mile that they were extending the race just for fun!"

A woman who experienced a total labor that lasted 22 hours

Hypotonic Uterine Contractions

Hypotonic uterine contractions have no basal tone, are infrequent, and fail to dilate the cervix satisfactorily (Fig. 16.2). They usually appear during the active phase of labor; however, this pattern also may develop during the second stage. Common causes include uterine overdistention (eg, multiple gestation, macrosomic fetus), fetal malposition, incorrect timing of analgesic administration, and use of regional anesthesia (see Chap. 17).

Treatment generally involves pinpointing and managing the underlying cause. For example, if the problem is uterine overdistention related to macrosomia, a cesarean birth might be elected. If no cause can be found, the next step is clinical rupture of the membranes to facilitate labor progression. Oxytocin may be administered as well. Labor that fails to progress despite these measures generally indicates the need for cesarean birth.

Pathologic Retraction and Constriction Rings

When the membranes have ruptured and labor is prolonged, a **pathologic retraction ring** (Bandl's ring) may develop in the uterus. This finding manifests as an exaggeration of the normal physiologic retraction ring found at the junction of the upper and lower uterine segments (Fig. 16.3). The area above the ring thickens, whereas the lower segment thins. A pathologic retraction ring is a medical emergency because the lower segment

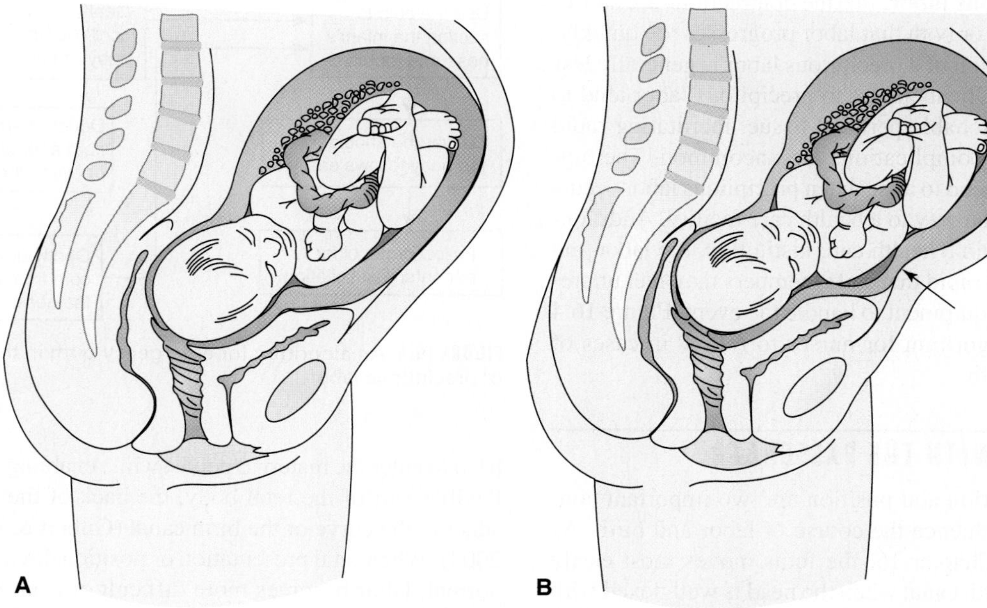

FIGURE 16.3 (**A**) In normal labor, the upper uterine segment thickens, whereas the lower segment thins. (**B**) With a pathologic retraction (Bandl's) ring, the abdomen shows an indentation where the wall below the ring is thin. Unrectified, this problem can lead to uterine rupture.

will rupture unless the obstruction is relieved. An immediate cesarean birth generally is indicated.

Constriction rings are rare and usually conform to a fetal depression, such as in the neck or abdomen. They do not extend all the way around the uterus. The area of spasm is thick, but the lower uterine segment does not become stretched or thinned. Cesarean birth is usually the treatment of choice with constriction rings.

Inadequate Voluntary Expulsive Forces

During uterine contractions, most women with a fully dilated cervix cannot resist the urge to push. Under normal circumstances, the force of the maternal abdominal muscles helps propel the fetus through the birth canal. Certain factors, however, can interfere with sensing or responding to the urge to push. Examples include fatigue, pain, fear, and anxiety. Pharmacologic agents used to manage labor pain also may pose problems if administered at the wrong time or in an incorrect dose (see Chap. 17). Rarely, spinal cord injury or other physical problems render maternal expulsive efforts inadequate.

Treatment measures vary and depend on the underlying cause. For example, the client whose pushing efforts are inhibited because of pain may require analgesia. Conversely, if a client has received too strong a dose of epidural anesthesia, time simply may need to pass for the effects of the medication to wear off sufficiently for her to push adequately. Careful selection and timing of pharmacologic pain management can help prevent this problem.

Precipitous Labor

With **precipitous labor,** uterine contractions are so frequent, intense, or both that labor progresses too quickly. The total duration of a precipitous labor is generally less than 3 hours. Clients prone to precipitous labor tend to have soft, stretchable perineal tissue, facilitating rapid fetal descent. Complications are uncommon. The biggest problems tend to arise when precipitous labor occurs outside or on the way to a health care facility. Additionally, even within a health care institution, the labor and birth can be so rapid that staff members may feel unprepared or lack equipment to handle the event. Figure 16.4 presents an algorithm for nurses to follow in cases of emergency birth.

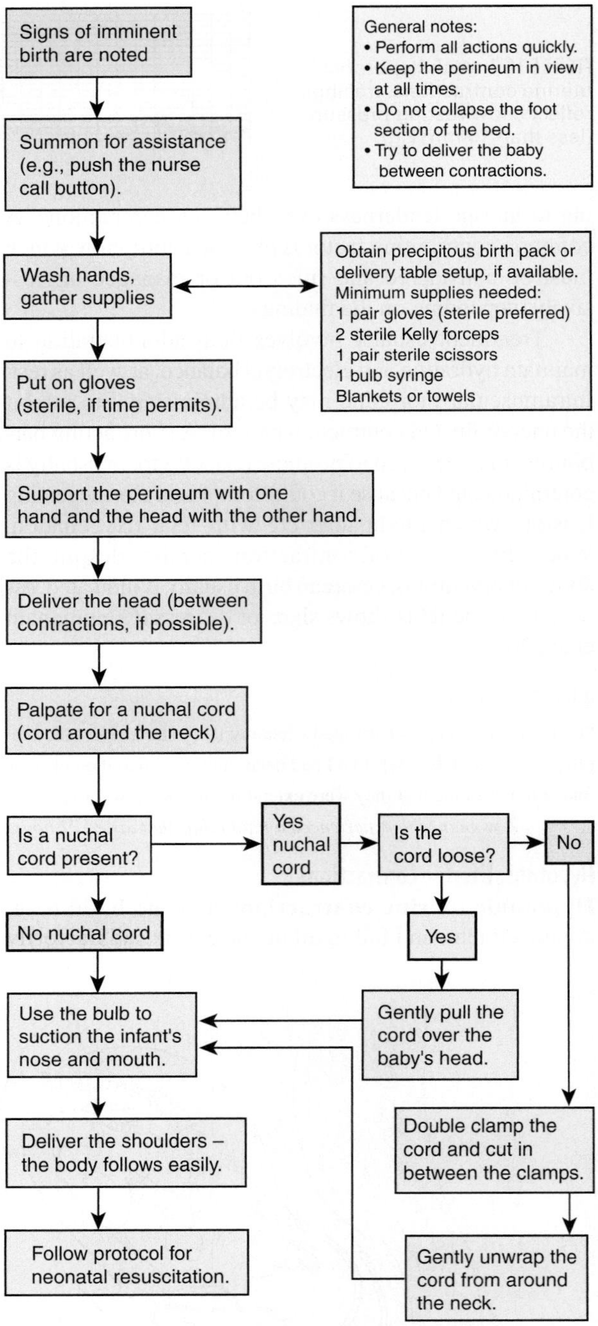

FIGURE 16.4 An algorithm for emergency birth in the case of precipitous labor.

PROBLEMS WITH THE PASSENGER

Fetal presentation and position are two important conditions that influence the course of labor and birth. As discussed in Chapter 15, the fetus moves most easily through the birth canal when the head is well flexed with the chin resting on the thorax and when the occipital area of the skull presents anterior to the maternal pelvis. These conditions allow the smallest diameter of the fetal head to enter the maternal pelvis, while enabling the most flexible part of the fetal body, the back of the neck, to adapt to the curve of the birth canal (Gilbert & Harmon, 2003). When fetal presentation or position deviates from normal, labor becomes more difficult or even impossible. Other problems in labor may result when the fetus is large or has abnormalities that significantly alter body size or shape.

Breech Presentation

In **breech presentation,** the fetal buttocks are the presenting part, a circumstance that develops in approximately 3% to 4% of all births (Fischer, 2005). The following different attitudes can be included with breech presentation:

- *Frank breech:* the thighs are flexed and the legs lie alongside the fetal body.
- *Complete breech:* the legs are flexed at the thighs and the feet present with the buttocks.
- *Footling (incomplete) breech:* one foot (single) or both feet (double) present before the buttocks (Fig. 16.5).

Factors that increase the risk for breech presentation include prematurity, intrauterine growth restriction (IUGR), congenital anomalies (eg, hydrocephaly), multiple pregnancy, and oligohydramnios (Cruikshank, 2003; Fischer, 2005).

The Term Breech Trial has changed the guidelines for labor and birth in cases of breech presentation. Results have indicated that vaginal birth of a fetus presenting as breech increases risks for overall morbidity and mortality; thus, cesarean birth is recommended as part of the care in such circumstances (Ghosh, 2005). This opinion remains controversial, however, and some obstetricians attempt vaginal breech births depending on the specific attitude involved and other maternal and fetal risk factors (Doyle et al., 2005; Hellsten et al., 2003).

Close to the end of pregnancy but before labor, the health care team should discuss with the client carrying a fetus with breech presentation the possibility of **external cephalic version** (ECV), the need to schedule a cesarean birth, and the risks and benefits of these procedures to both mother and fetus. The ECV procedure is a method of manipulating the fetus to turn from breech to vertex presentation (Hutton & Hofmeyr, 2006). The ideal time to carry out ECV is after 36 completed weeks' gestation because the fetus may still turn spontaneously before term. Additionally, by 37 weeks' gestation, the fetus is sufficiently mature to survive if complications develop that require emergency cesarean birth. The client and her family should receive information about ECV, its possibility of success (30% to 50%), its risks (eg, rupture of membranes, fetal bradycardia), and discomfort associated with the procedure (Hutton & Hofmeyr, 2006). ECV should be performed in a hospital triage setting with staff and resources to accommodate emergency cesarean birth as necessary. During the procedure, the fetus should be turned so that he or she "follows its nose" (Fig. 16.6). A nonstress test for fetal well-being should be completed at the beginning of and immediately after ECV. Ultrasound imaging may be used concurrently to determine the presence of nuchal cord and the volume of amniotic fluid (Skupski et al., 2003).

Occasionally, a client presents in labor and the examiner discovers during abdominal palpation that the fetus is in breech presentation. In such an event, the woman's primary care provider should be contacted as soon as possible so that appropriate interventions and adjustments can be enacted. For a client with a multiple pregnancy, one or both fetuses may be breech. Ultrasound imaging may assist in this determination before birth; again, development of an individualized plan of care is essential.

COLLABORATIVE CARE: BREECH PRESENTATION

Assessment

If a breech presentation has not been identified previously by ultrasound or other methods, indications in a laboring client include a palpable head in the uterine fundus during Leopold's maneuvers, fetal heart tones audible

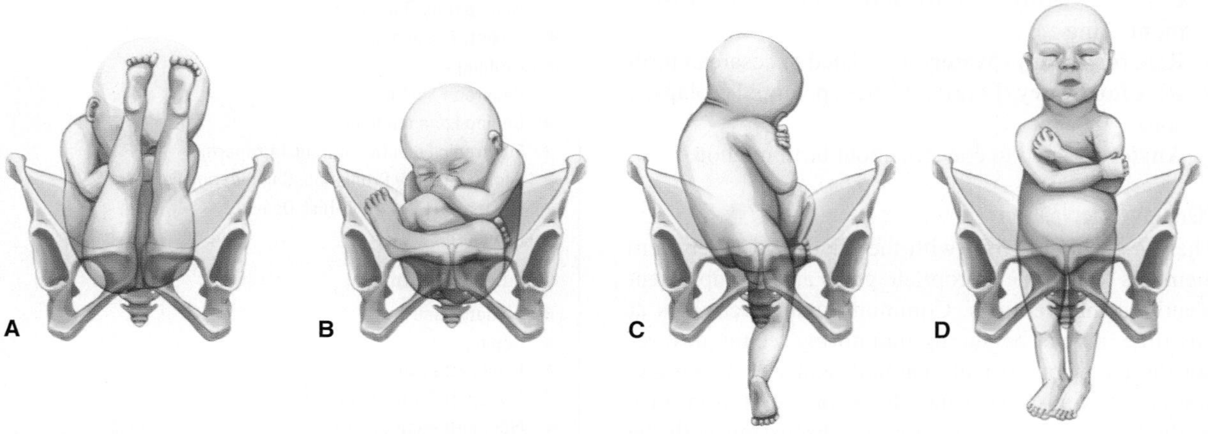

FIGURE 16.5 (**A**) Frank breech presentation. (**B**) Complete breech presentation. (**C**) Single footling breech presentation. (**D**) Double footling breech presentation.

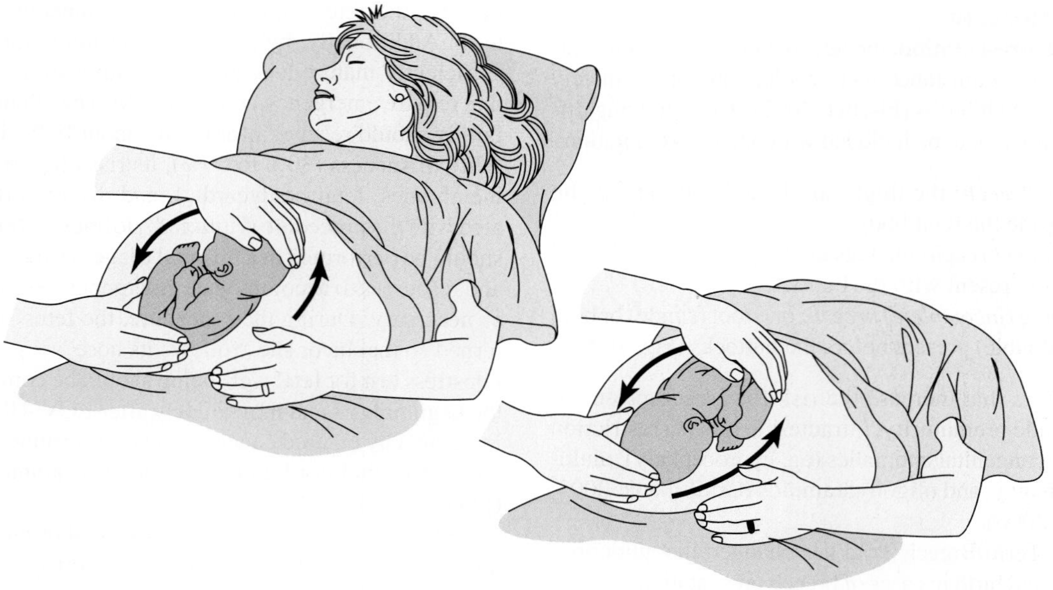

FIGURE 16.6 To perform external cephalic version, the provider uses external pressure to rotate the fetus to a cephalic lie.

slightly above the umbilicus, palpable buttocks during a vaginal examination, and passage of meconium after rupture of the membranes. Once ultrasound confirms breech presentation, the nurse should continue to monitor maternal and fetal status while the team makes decisions about the method of birth. The nurse usually plays an important role in communicating information among team members and with the client and family during this time. Continuous fetal assessment is especially important because breech presentation increases the possibility of cord prolapse (see later discussion). Electronic fetal monitoring generally is used in cases of breech presentation.

Select Potential Nursing Diagnoses

The following nursing diagnoses are likely:

- **Risk for Injury (Maternal)** related to invasive monitoring
- **Risk for Injury (Maternal)** related to cesarean birth
- **Risk for Injury (Fetal)** related to potential prolapsed cord
- **Anxiety** related to concern about birth method

Planning/Intervention

The nurse should work with the client and other team members to outline appropriate goals and to implement identified interventions. Common nursing activities at this time include beginning monitoring techniques; reporting the status of maternal and fetal well-being and any changes; preparing the client for the chosen birth method (vaginal or cesarean); and discussing with the client and her support people what is happening. Explanations and reassurance may be particularly helpful because anxiety and fear related to concern over a breech presentation may compromise the client's ability to participate effectively during labor. NIC/NOC Box 16.1 outlines common interventions and outcomes in cases of breech presentation.

Pudendal or epidural anesthesia generally are used during vaginal breech births because they do not interfere with labor and facilitate the client's active participation.

NIC/NOC Box 16.1 Breech Presentation

Common NIC Labels

- Anticipatory Guidance
- Anxiety Reduction
- Birthing
- Cesarean Section Care
- Coping Enhancement
- Electronic Fetal Monitoring: Intrapartum
- Family Integrity Promotion: Childbearing Family
- Intrapartal Care: High-Risk Delivery
- Newborn Care

Common NOC Labels

- Anxiety Control
- Coping
- Fetal Status: Intrapartum
- Maternal Status: Intrapartum
- Newborn Adaptation
- Risk Control

With a vaginal breech birth, the mechanism of labor is similar to that for vertex presentations (see Chap. 15 and Fig. 16.7). Although some vaginal breech births are spontaneous, they usually require assisted methods, generally to extract the fetal head. An example is the application of Piper forceps, which is discussed later in this chapter.

The procedure for cesarean birth is described and illustrated in detail toward the end of this chapter.

Evaluation

Desired outcomes with a breech presentation include the following:

- The client and fetus show no indications of distress.
- The client verbalizes minimal anxiety and fear.
- The client demonstrates positive coping strategies.
- The client verbalizes understanding of the chosen method of birth.
- The client gives birth to a healthy newborn.

Other Malpresentations

Other abnormal fetal presentations that affect labor's progress include shoulder, face, brow, and compound presentations.

- *Shoulder presentation* (transverse lie) occurs when the fetus lies crosswise rather than longitudinally in the uterus. The shoulder usually is in the brim of the inlet. Depending on positioning, the back, abdomen, ribs, or flank also can be the presenting part. Common risk factors include multiparity, prematurity, placenta previa, and contracted pelvis (Cunningham et al., 2005). This serious complication increases risks for uterine rupture and perinatal mortality for both mother and child. ECV in late pregnancy or early labor occasionally is successful in alleviating this problem (Cruikshank, 2003). Generally, however, this presentation in a client in active labor is an indication for cesarean birth.
- With *face presentation,* the chin usually enters the pelvic inlet first. A contracted pelvis is the most common

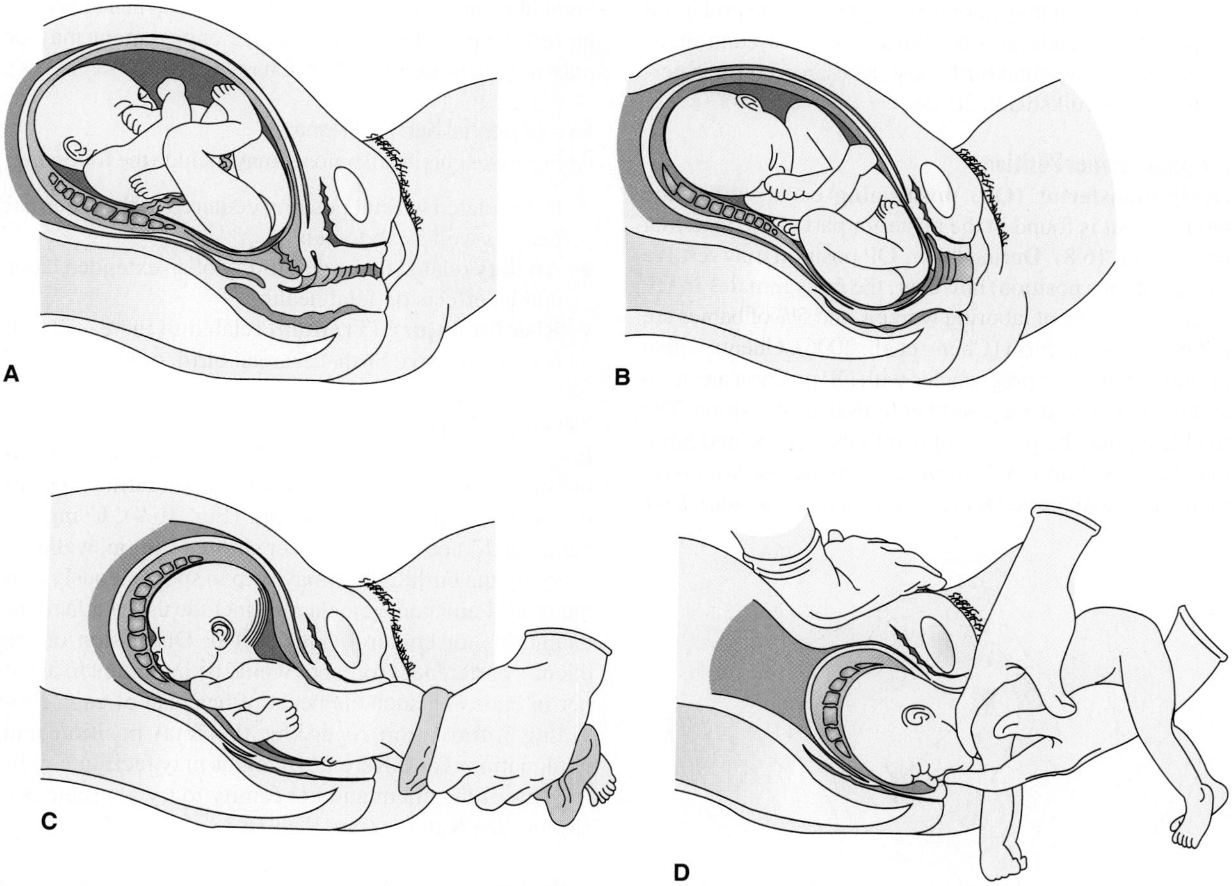

FIGURE 16.7 Steps in a vaginal breech birth. (**A**) The fetus is in the left sacroposterior position. (**B**) The fetus begins to descend and rotate internally. (**C**) The birth attendant uses a cloth to hold the fetal legs, helping to turn the shoulders. (**D**) Using gentle pressure, the attendant flexes the fetal head fully and applies traction to move the shoulders upward and outward. The nurse may apply pressure to the maternal abdomen to help facilitate flexion of the fetal head.

cause. If labor is effective and the maternal pelvis is adequate, spontaneous vaginal birth is possible. A cesarean birth is indicated when the fetus shows signs of distress or the maternal pelvis is contracted.

- In *brow presentation,* the largest diameter of the fetal head presents at the pelvic inlet. Again, the underlying factor usually is a contracted pelvis. Unless the fetus is small and the pelvis is large, vaginal birth is impossible. Frequently, however, this unstable presentation spontaneously converts to an occiput or face presentation. Principles of management are the same as for face presentations. Labor progressing normally without fetal distress requires no intervention. Erratic or hyperactive labor and failure of the presentation to change are indications for cesarean birth.
- *Compound presentations* occur when an extremity prolapses and enters the pelvis with the presenting part. The most common development is for a fetal arm to prolapse with the head. The major complication is increased incidence of prolapsed umbilical cord. Many compound presentations correct themselves spontaneously. If the progress of labor is arrested, the birth attendant may attempt to reposition the prolapsed part. If such attempts are unsuccessful or contraindications to a vaginal birth exist, a cesarean birth is performed (Cruikshank, 2003).

Occipitoposterior Position

Occipitoposterior (OP) positioning occurs when the fetal occiput is found in the posterior part of the maternal pelvis (Fig. 16.8). During labor, OP position may resolve to the anterior position; however, the fetus remains in OP position for 10% of laboring women, and 5% of babies are in OP position at birth (Cheng et al., 2006). Clients with a previous history of pregnancies with OP position are at increased risk for carrying another fetus in this position. The fetal head may be poorly applied to the cervix, and labor may be slow. Labor induction or augmentation with oxytocin may have limited success (see later discussion). Risk factors associated with persistent OP position include a 5-minute Apgar score less than 7, meconium-stained amniotic fluid, birth trauma, and longer neonatal stay in the hospital (Cheng et al., 2006).

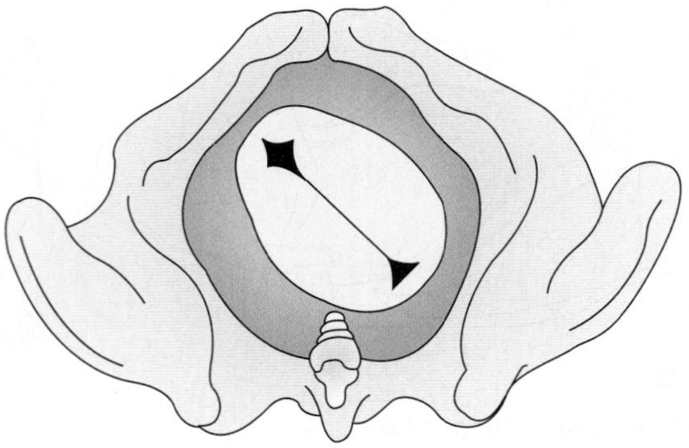

FIGURE 16.8 View from the vaginal outlet of a fetus in the left occipitoposterior position with a cephalic presentation.

COLLABORATIVE CARE: OP POSITION

When labor occurs with a fetus in OP position, the major finding generally is maternal back pain with contractions. The underlying cause is internal pressure from the fetal skull against the maternal spine. Monitoring of this woman's progress in labor and the ongoing position of the fetus is critical to care.

Assessment

When a client arrives at the obstetrical unit describing her labor primarily as "back pain," health care providers should suspect that the fetal position is OP. They can use abdominal palpation for verification. A space or dip at the maternal umbilicus might indicate the space between the fetal arms and legs. Palpating the fetal back may be difficult; the fetal heart rate may be auscultated at the level of the umbilicus or laterally. The fetal head may not be felt deep in the pelvis because engagement may or may not occur before labor (Chadwick, 2002).

Select Potential Nursing Diagnoses

Appropriate nursing diagnoses may include the following:

- **Pain** related to fetal position centered in the maternal back as well as abdomen
- **Anxiety** related to the possibility of an extended labor and its effects on fetal health
- **Risk for Injury (Trauma)** related to increased risk for an operative birth, cesarean birth, or both

Planning/Intervention

For the woman, encouraging different positions and ambulation that may allow the pelvis to open further and encourage a fetal shift is essential (Fig. 16.9). Using the hands-and-knees, side-lying, or sitting position, walking, or trying the birthing ball may help to spontaneously turn the fetus. Pain management may include use of a Jacuzzi, analgesics, or epidural (Fig. 16.10). Discussion of the client's preferences for labor would be important to assist her in choosing such elements of her plan of care. Providing information regarding the fetal position and explanations for different strategies may facilitate willingness of the client and her family to try alternate positions. See Nursing Care Plan 16.1.

Evaluation

Desired outcomes include normal progress in labor, fulfillment of the client's wishes as per her birth plan, and achievement of a spontaneous vaginal birth.

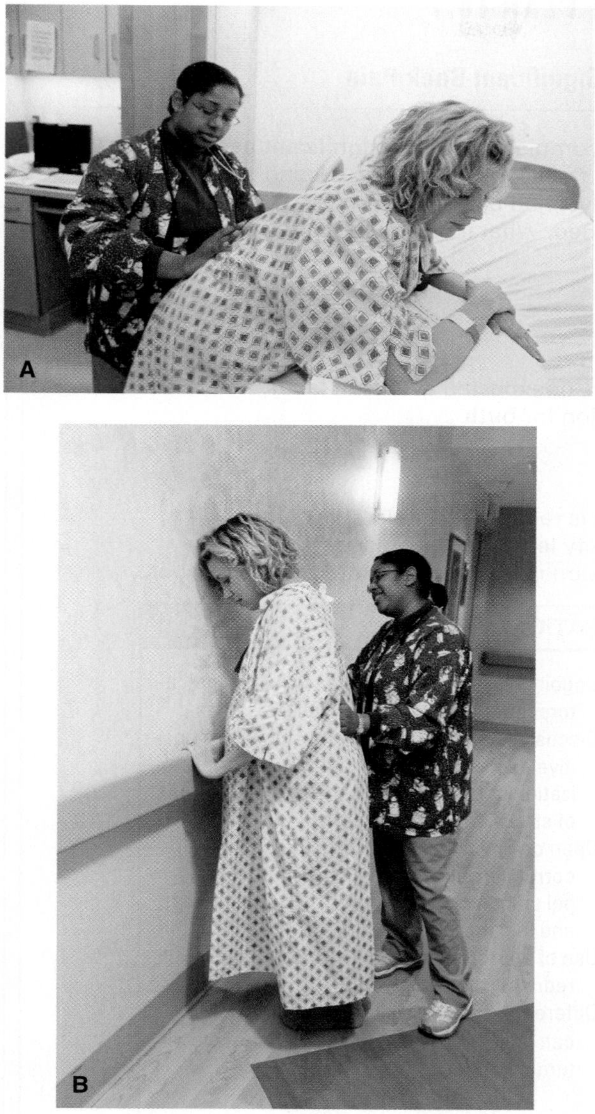

FIGURE 16.9 To help ease the pain of back labor and facilitate a fetal shift in position, the nurse may encourage the woman to (**A**) try different positions and (**B**) ambulate.

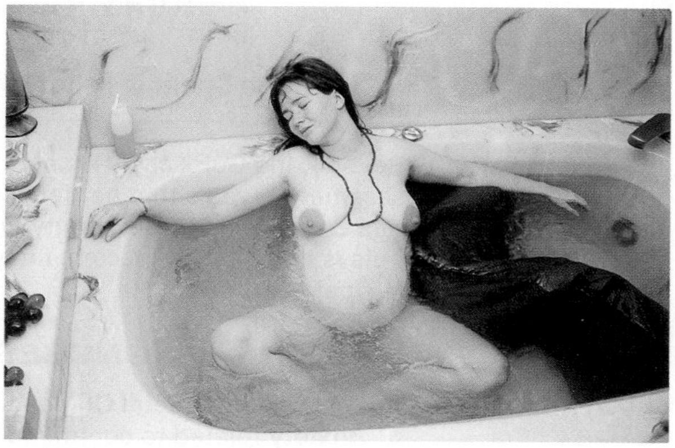

FIGURE 16.10 One method of easing pain during back labor may include the use of a Jacuzzi or bath. (Photo courtesy of Kaye Bullock, CPM.)

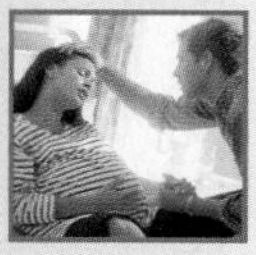

Remember Beverly, the G3P2 client from the beginning of the chapter who is complaining of back pain. Assessment reveals that the fetus is in the OP position. What measures might the care team use to help turn the fetus?

Shoulder Dystocia

Shoulder dystocia, or inability of the fetal shoulders to move through the maternal pelvis following the birth of the head, occurs in approximately 1% of all births (Jevitt, 2005). Risk factors include maternal diabetes, maternal obesity, postterm pregnancy, fetal macrosomia, previous history of shoulder dystocia, and multiparity (Sheiner et al., 2006). Often shoulder dystocia is unexpected and presents only as slow extension of the fetal head with the chin remaining tight against the maternal perineum. The fetal head may appear to be trying to return into the vagina ("*turtle sign*").

Care of all laboring women during the second stage includes prevention of shoulder dystocia. Careful monitoring of labor's progress, particularly of ongoing descent during the second stage, is a crucial preventive measure. Clear ongoing communication among team members enhances assessment of the client's progress and the need for interventions as appropriate.

COLLABORATIVE CARE: SHOULDER DYSTOCIA

Once shoulder dystocia is diagnosed, the health care team usually attempts several steps to assist with birth. It is crucial for members to remain calm, attempt different strategies in a timely fashion, and move on at the right point. Potential maternal complications include vaginal, cervical, or perineal lacerations requiring extensive repair; bladder injury; hematoma; uterine rupture; and postpartum hemorrhage (see Chap. 19). Potential fetal complications include brachial plexus injury; fractures; and asphyxia (Gurewitsch et al., 2006).

Assessment

Nursing assessment of the second stage of labor should include awareness of the descent of the fetal head and time. If the client has received epidural anesthesia (see Chap. 17), she may not push until after her cervix has become fully dilated. Rather, she may wait for the "urge to push" to ensure that her efforts work with her body sensations. The nurse should assess fetal health as well as

NURSING CARE PLAN 16.1

The Client in Labor With Significant Back Pain

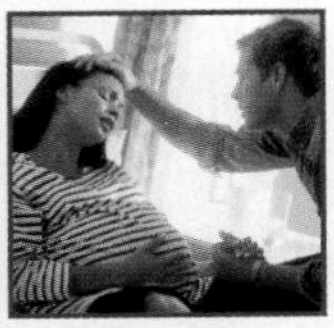

Beverly, the G3P2 client in labor, is complaining about significant back pain. Assessment reveals that her fetus is in the OP position. "My second baby also was this way, but he turned pretty quickly. I had back pain for a bit, but not like now. This is not what I expected. I'm worried. What if he doesn't turn?" The client rates her pain as 9 out of 10.

NURSING DIAGNOSES

- **Pain** related to fetal OP position
- **Anxiety** related to continued pain, unexpected events of labor, and failure of the fetus to turn to the anterior position for birth

EXPECTED OUTCOMES

1. The client will verbalize that pain is reduced to a tolerable level.
2. The client will state that her anxiety level has decreased.
3. The client will participate in decision making about preferences for labor.

INTERVENTIONS	RATIONALES
Frequently assess the client's level of pain, asking her to rate it on a scale of 1 to 10.	Ongoing assessment provides valuable indicators for effectiveness of relief strategies.
Discuss with the client her concerns, feelings, and perceptions related to changes in expectations about labor and birth and current pain level.	Discussion allows the nurse to emphasize positive aspects of the current situation; verbalization of concerns helps to identify sources of stress and problem areas.
Communicate accurate data and answer questions honestly. Reinforce facts, emphasizing that each pregnancy, labor, and birth is highly individualized.	Open communication promotes trust and helps correct any misconceptions. Facts can dispel unfounded fears, myths, misconceptions, and feelings of guilt.
Evaluate the client's past coping strategies to determine which have been effective.	Use of appropriate coping strategies aids in reducing anxiety.
Explain to the client and her partner measures that facilitate spontaneous turning of the fetus. Encourage frequent position changes and ambulation. Suggest the use of a birthing ball, hands-and-knees position, or sitting.	Different maternal positions and ambulation can help open the pelvis and facilitate fetal turning.
Teach the client's partner how to provide pressure or massage to the lower back. Suggest applying ice or heat to the area.	Fetal head rotation may compress the sacral nerve. Pressure, massage, or heat or cold may help alleviate this painful sensation.
Offer pharmacologic measures for pain relief.	Medications can reduce or decrease pain.
Frequently assess the abdomen for fetal position; perform Leopold's maneuvers; monitor fetal and maternal status as indicated.	Leopold's maneuvers aid in determining fetal presentation and position. Frequent monitoring provides information about maternal and fetal well-being.
Update the couple regularly about the progress of labor and the fetus. Offer continuing support and guidance to them.	Frequent communication promotes the couple's participation and reinforces the effectiveness of their activities, thus enhancing a sense of accomplishment.

EVALUATION

1. The client verbally rates pain as a 2 or 3.
2. The client states that she is more comfortable.
3. The client identifies preferences and choices for labor and birth.
4. The client progresses through labor without additional problems.

maternal vital signs to ensure stability. Once pushing efforts begin, it is important to monitor duration and to communicate with the client's care provider if progress, fetal descent, or both are not occurring.

Select Potential Nursing Diagnoses

Common nursing diagnoses in the care of shoulder dystocia include the following:

- **Anxiety** related to unexpected emergency measures required to facilitate birth
- **Deficient Knowledge** related to measures being done to assist with this birth
- **Risk for Injury (Trauma)** related to fetal and maternal measures required to facilitate birth

Planning/Intervention

The sense of urgency present in any obstetrical emergency accompanies shoulder dystocia. The nurse should begin by calling for additional help and then working with the obstetrician and other team members to facilitate birth.

1. The first step is usually to assist the client into McRobert's maneuver (Fig. 16.11). This procedure involves hyperflexing the woman's legs into a knee-chest position, allowing elevation of the anterior fetal shoulder while flexing the fetal spine. Assistance with holding the woman's legs if she has had an epidural may be required.

2a. After McRobert's maneuver, the next step is suprapubic pressure (Fig. 16.12). This gentle pressure with the palm or heel of the hand against the fetal back directs the pressure toward the fetal midline. The nurse and all care providers must know the difference between fundal and suprapubic pressure to apply them appropriately. Generally, McRobert's maneuver and suprapubic pressure resolve 50% of cases of shoulder dystocia when the episiotomy has been adequate (Kwek & Yeo, 2006).

2b. Another alternative is to assist the woman into a hands-and-knees position with the objective of dislodging the shoulder. (This measure is not possible with an epidural in place.)

3. The next attempt is the Woods screw rotational maneuver, which is to move the posterior fetal shoulder through a 180-degree turn, allowing the anterior fetal shoulder to present for birth.

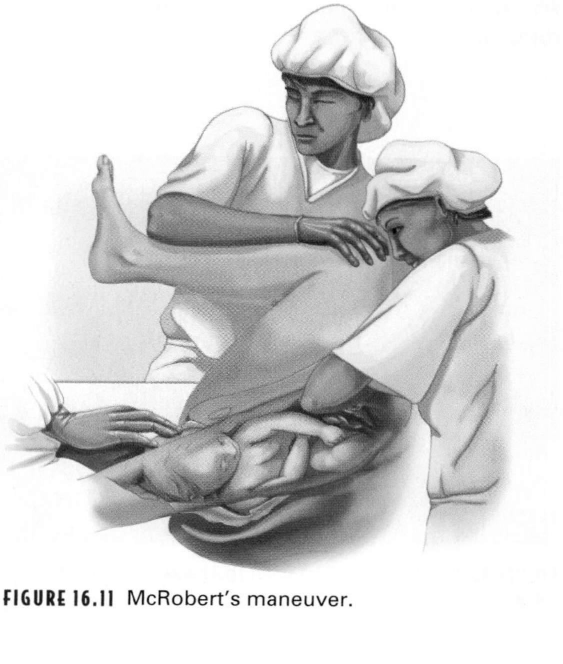

FIGURE 16.11 McRobert's maneuver.

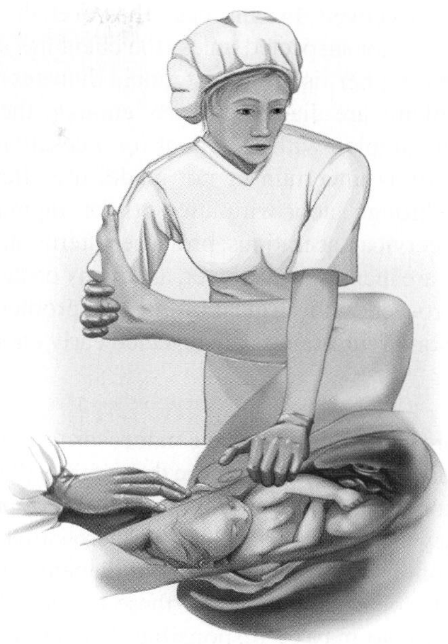

FIGURE 16.12 Application of suprapubic pressure.

After birth is complete, examinations for maternal injury and hemorrhage and appropriate neonatal resuscitation efforts are crucial. Documentation of all appropriate medical and nursing interventions is vital, as is communication with the family to describe what was done and why.

Evaluation

Birth without extensive injury to either mother or infant is the desired outcome of care. Team members who work together in a calm and organized fashion can assist in decreasing stress perceived by the client and her family under these circumstances.

Excessive Fetal Size or Fetal Abnormalities

Other passenger-related problems include excessive fetal size and fetal abnormalities. Usually, these problems are determined in utero based on ultrasound findings and

Leopold's maneuvers. In many cases, however, these complications are not suspected unless the client has a condition increasing her risk (eg, gestational diabetes). When such problems are diagnosed early enough, the health care team can plan with the client for a cesarean birth. If diagnosis is uncertain or not made, the client may progress through labor with attempts for vaginal birth. Risks for cervical lacerations, prolapsed uterus, and other problems are increased, however, and many obstetricians elect to proceed with surgical birth when problems with fetal size or circumstances are detected early enough.

Macrosomia

A newborn is considered to have **macrosomia** (excessive size) when he or she weighs more than 4500 g (9.9 lbs) at birth, a complication in approximately 10% of pregnancies (Jazayeri & Contreras, 2005). Macrosomia usually results from uncontrolled gestational diabetes, genetics, multiparity, or a combination of these factors. Postterm pregnancy also may be responsible. Fetuses weighing more than 11 lbs are rare.

Macrosomia can cause cephalopelvic disproportion. It also can cause uterine overdistention, reducing the strength of contractions, prolonging labor, and increasing the risk for overall maternal and fetal complications. When the fetal biparietal diameter (usually 9.5 to 9.8 cm at term) of a macrosomic fetus attempts to fit through the maternal pelvis, **molding** (overlapping of the skull bones at major suture lines) occurs, decreasing the biparietal diameter up to 0.5 cm without fetal injury (Fig. 16.13). Severe molding may lead to tearing, intracranial hemorrhage, or scalp edema. Molding generally disappears within the newborn's first few days, but severe pressure between fetus and pelvis may cause skull fracture.

Birth trauma frequently associated with macrosomia increases risks for fetal or newborn mortality. Macrosomic newborns may have a difficult extrauterine transition because of problems during labor and birth, such as bruising, cephalohematoma, and brachial plexus injury.

QUOTE 16-2

"I wound up having an unexpected cesarean birth because my son weighed 10 lbs and my labor was going on too long. Fortunately, the cause wasn't diabetes—he just was a big boy! I think about that sometimes now when he's at his high chair refusing to eat dinner. . . ."

The mother of a healthy toddler who is at the 70th percentile for height and weight

Fetal Abnormalities

Fetal abnormalities that can contribute to dystocia include such problems as hydrocephalus, neck masses, a large and swollen fetal abdomen from excessive bladder distention, enlarged liver or kidneys, and, rarely, conjoined twins. Any of these problems can interfere with fetal descent or passage through the birth canal.

The most common fetal anomaly causing dystocia is **hydrocephalus,** or excess accumulation of cerebrospinal fluid in the brain ventricles and subsequent cranial enlargement (Fig. 16.14). Hydrocephalus accounts for approximately 12% of all birth-related malformations (Cunningham et al., 2005) and is associated frequently with other congenital defects (eg, spina bifida) (see Chap. 22). Breech presentations are common with cases of hydrocephalus because the distended cranium cannot fit into the pelvic inlet.

Obstructed labor associated with hydrocephalus may lead to uterine rupture, particularly if the problem is not detected before labor begins. The nurse should suspect hydrocephalus when palpation for the fetal head reveals an enlarged symmetric mass in the uterine fundus. Such detection can be challenging, however, because excessive amniotic fluid commonly makes such palpation more difficult.

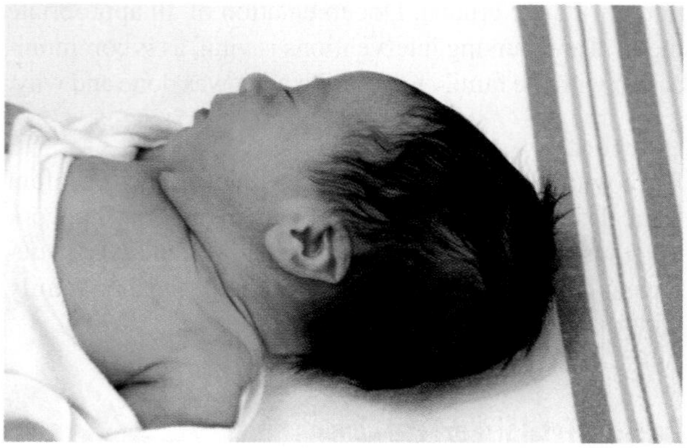

FIGURE 16.13 A macrosomic newborn may have cranial molding if the presenting part was too big for the maternal outlet.

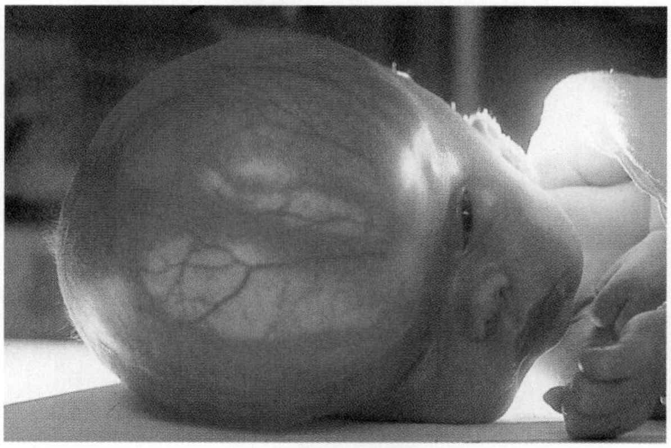

FIGURE 16.14 One problem with the passenger that may cause dystocia is hydrocephalus.

When ultrasound reveals hydrocephalus in advance of labor and birth, a cranial shunt may be inserted in utero to minimize brain damage and to delay birth until gestation advances closer to term. Fetal surgery to treat hydrocephalus is becoming more common. The labor will be difficult, and risks for newborn morbidity and mortality are high. Nursing interventions should focus on providing significant maternal support. See Chapter 22 for additional information.

PROBLEMS WITH THE PASSAGEWAY

Generally, problems related to the passageway involve the maternal pelvis. Many of these concerns can be predicted and prepared for when a woman has received adequate prenatal care; however, if a woman arrives at the health care facility for the first time in labor, passageway problems may need to be addressed as an obstetric emergency.

Pelvic Shape Problems

As discussed in Chapter 12, the maternal pelvis is one of four types: gynecoid, anthropoid, android, and platypelloid. Vaginal birth usually is successful when the maternal pelvis is gynecoid or anthropoid. The chances for vaginal birth usually are poor for women with the other two pelvic types, generally indicating a need for cesarean birth.

Contracted Pelvis

With a contracted pelvis, one or more of the pelvic diameters are reduced to the point of interference with labor's progress. Pelvic contraction can occur at the inlet, midpelvis, or outlet.

- *Inlet contraction.* The pelvic anteroposterior diameter is less than 10 cm, the pelvic transverse diameter is less than 12 cm, or both. This problem may result from small maternal body size, rickets, or delayed maternal development. It is difficult for the fetal presenting part to fit well at the cervix, leading to the complications inherent with prolonged labor.
- *Midpelvic contraction.* The distance between the ischial spines is less than 9 cm or the sum of the interspinous and posterior sagittal distance is less than 13.5 cm. The presenting part can engage in the pelvis, making this problem harder to recognize and manage than inlet contraction.
- *Outlet contraction.* The distance between the ischial tuberosities is less than 8 cm. Although this problem increases the risks for perineal tears and forceps-assisted birth, vaginal birth usually can be accomplished.

Interventions depend on the specific problems involved and other maternal and fetal risk factors.

PRETERM LABOR

Preterm labor is considered true labor that begins before 37 completed weeks of gestation. The rate of preterm birth is approximately 7% (Newton, 2004). Avoidance, early detection, and management of this problem are major foci of prenatal and antepartal care because preterm labor accounts for 75% of neonatal deaths not caused by congenital malformations (Newton, 2004).

U.S. hospital costs associated with prematurity exceed $2 billion annually (Gilbert & Danielsen, 2003) (see Chap. 22). IUGR is increased in women who present with preterm labor and progress to premature childbirth (Gilbert & Danielsen, 2003). Other complications include cerebral palsy, neurodevelopmental delay, respiratory complications (eg, bronchopulmonary dysplasia), and blindness (Society of Obstetricians and Gynecologists in Canada [SOGC], 2000).

Etiology and Risk Factors

The causes of preterm labor are not well identified or clear. Common contributing factors include preterm prelabor rupture of membranes (pPROM) (see Chap. 13), multiple pregnancy, incompetent cervix, and maternal disease. Frequently, the cause remains unknown. Research has shown several conditions to increase risks for preterm labor. See Box 16.1.

BOX 16.1 Risk Factors for Preterm Labor

- Adolescent pregnancy
- African American race
- Alcohol or drug use, especially cocaine
- Anemia
- Bacterial vaginosis
- Cervical insufficiency
- Chorioamnionitis
- Cigarette smoking
- Closely timed pregnancies
- Diabetes mellitus
- Domestic violence
- History of previous preterm birth
- Hydramnios
- Hypertension
- Low socioeconomic status
- Malnutrition
- Multiple gestation
- Periodontal disease
- Placental problems
- Sexually transmitted infections
- Stress
- Urinary tract infections
- Uterine abnormalities

In all pregnancies, health care providers exert significant effort to detect and treat any risk factors aggressively. Although actual cervical changes are necessary for preterm labor to be diagnosed, any premature uterine activity requires immediate evaluation to ensure that nothing more serious is developing. The anticipated success rate of delaying labor in such instances depends on the stage of labor at which interventions are implemented. Ideally, however, labor is postponed for as long as possible to advance the gestation closer to 37 weeks. See the section, Preterm Premature Rupture of the Membranes, in Chapter 13 for more discussion of measures commonly used to halt labor. Also see Teaching Tips 16.1.

Bacterial infection of the lower genital tract may contribute to preterm labor (Guinn & Gibbs, 2003). Thus, experts have recommended prenatal screening of urine and cervical cultures for group B streptococcus, with appropriate antibiotics and follow-up cultures for those women who test positive (see Chap. 13). Abstinence from sexual intercourse is another preventive measure in clients susceptible to preterm labor. Tocolytic agents are used for management of early preterm labor because the effectiveness of these drugs decreases as labor advances.

Assessment Findings

Early diagnosis is often difficult. Possible signs and symptoms include menstrual-like cramps or abdominal pain; diarrhea; pressure in the pelvis or lower back; and increased vaginal discharge. Because these symptoms are nonspecific, however, they may not concern the woman until a real problem has developed. Diagnosis of preterm labor occurs with regular uterine contractions and rupture of the membranes.

COLLABORATIVE CARE: PRETERM LABOR

Health care providers must work together to assess a client who presents to the labor and birth area before term to identify her risk factors for preterm labor, establish her gestation, and evaluate her contractions. If she is found to be in true labor, traditional treatments of bedrest, intravenous (IV) fluid administration, and tocolytic medications (eg, magnesium sulfate) may be employed; however, little evidence shows that these measures effectively arrest labor. Nevertheless, even moderate prolongation of pregnancy can be beneficial and provide sufficient time to administer antenatal steroids that can assist with fetal lung maturity. A typical regimen is 12 mg intramuscular (IM) betamethasone every 12 hours or 6 mg IV/IM dexamethasone every 6 hours (SOGC, 2000). Tocolytics with research support include ritodrine and indomethacin (Table 16.1).

Health care providers need to determine the best location for this client depending on gestation and other risk factors. If labor continues to progress, admission of the client to a center with advanced neonatal facilities may be necessary.

Assessment

The nurse who first sees this client and her family in the obstetrical assessment area should approach them calmly to decrease anxiety. Depending on institutional policy, labor assessment may include vaginal examination; eval-

● TEACHING TIPS 16.1 Preventing Premature Birth

Babies born before 37 weeks' completed gestation can suffer lifelong health consequences such as chronic lung disease, cerebral palsy, and blindness. Being born too soon is the leading cause of death in newborns. Because ways to prevent preterm labor are not clearly established, the best approach is for pregnant women to try to preserve and maintain their overall health and to know the signs of preterm labor. Early treatment may reduce problems.

Measures to preserve and to optimize maternal health include the following:

- Schedule and attend regular prenatal appointments.
- Take a prenatal vitamin daily throughout pregnancy.
- Give the health care provider a comprehensive medical history including any other instances of preterm labor and birth.
- Stop smoking or cut back as much as possible.
- Stop drinking alcohol.
- Avoid illegal drugs; inform the health care provider of any over-the-counter medications or herbal remedies used.
- Avoid stress as much as possible; talk to family and friends about ways that they can help.
- Call the health care provider if any burning or pain accompanies urination or if vaginal discharge is increased and whitish.
- Be aware of the signs of preterm labor; call the health care provider if they develop.

  Signs for women to be aware of and to report to providers are as follows:
  - Contractions every 10 minutes or more often
  - Clear, pink, or brownish fluid (water) leaking from the vagina
  - The feeling that the baby is pushing down
  - A low, dull backache
  - Menstrual-like cramps
  - Cramps with or without diarrhea

TABLE 16.1 Common Medications Used in Preterm Labor

DRUG	ACTION	NURSING CONSIDERATIONS
Betamethasone (Celestone)	Stimulates production of surfactant, which promotes fetal lung maturity and protects against respiratory distress (in fetuses younger than 34 weeks' gestation)	Teach the client and family about the medication's potential benefits to the fetus. Monitor the client for any signs of edema or infection. Regularly assess maternal lung sounds.
Indomethacin (Indocin)	Inhibits uterine activity	Continually assess vital signs, fetal heart rate, and uterine activity. Administer the oral form with food to reduce gastric irritation. Be alert for adverse maternal effects, including rash, nausea and vomiting, heartburn, oligohydramnios, and hypertension; and adverse fetal effects, including heart problems, pulmonary hypertension, and necrotizing enterocolitis.
Magnesium sulfate	Relaxes uterine muscles and arrests contractions	The initial loading dose of 4 g is given intravenously over 15 to 30 minutes. Infusion then is maintained at 1 to 2 g/hr. Report any signs of hypotension or absent deep tendon reflexes. Monitor the client's level of consciousness and report any deviations from normal. Regularly evaluate vital signs and fetal heart rate. Ensure that calcium gluconate is readily available as an antidote in cases of magnesium toxicity.

uation of contraction frequency, intensity, and duration; and monitoring of fetal well-being. The nurse should record presence of amniotic fluid, vaginal bleeding, or bloody show, along with information about the onset of contractions, maternal well-being, and past medical history.

Select Potential Nursing Diagnoses

Nursing diagnoses commonly included in the care of the woman experiencing preterm labor are as follows:

- **Deficient Knowledge** related to treatment plan for preterm labor
- **Anxiety** related to maternal and fetal health
- **Risk for Injury (Trauma)** related to preterm labor and birth (particularly fetal)

Planning/Interventions

Once the nurse has collected assessment information, he or she should notify the client's primary obstetric provider as soon as possible. Depending on the stage of labor and progress, staff members may need to arrange transport to another location to facilitate the safest care for the newborn.

Indications for labor inhibition involve considerations related to gestational age. Because fetal lungs usually are mature by 36 completed weeks, the baby born between 36 and 38 weeks and weighing more than 2500 g usually does not need pulmonary support. Tocolytic therapy for a fetus older than 35 weeks is unlikely to be instituted. Tocolytic therapy generally is employed in the following situations:

- Preterm labor has been diagnosed definitively.
- Gestational age is more than 20 but less than 36 weeks.
- Fetal weight is estimated as less than 2500 g.
- Fetal lung profile shows signs of immaturity (inadequate alveolar surfactant) (SOGC, 2000).

If tocolytic management stops labor, drug administration needs to continue until contractions have decreased or ceased, according to the health care provider's preferences and the client's ability to tolerate the medications. Antenatal steroids should be administered during this time per normal dosages. If labor stops spontaneously, the client needs ongoing monitoring in the assessment area (based on facility protocol), with plans made about when to return:

- If contractions begin again
- If she experiences low backache
- With any presence of show, rupture of the membranes, vaginal bleeding, or a combination of these problems

In early labor (cervical dilation of 2 to 3 cm), bedrest, hydration, and sedation frequently stop uterine activity by increasing intravascular volume and uterine blood flow, as well as by reducing pressure of the fetal head on the cervix. Tocolytic therapy further enhances success.

If the client gives birth spontaneously, staff must be available to care for the newborn. Ideally, personnel from the neonatal intensive care unit attend the birth. Explaining to the family the procedures employed and the care provided helps alleviate anxiety. If transport of the newborn is required following birth, taking pictures with the baby, holding the baby, or even briefly touching the baby can assist parents with bonding. Establishing communication with the transport team and the institution where the baby will be transferred for care is essential; if possible, the mother should be transported to the same site as the baby. See NIC/NOC Box 16.2 for common interventions and outcomes in cases of preterm labor.

Evaluation

Ideal outcomes include early diagnosis of labor and identification and treatment of the cause. If preterm labor cannot be controlled or delayed, desired outcomes are having appropriate resources and personnel present during the birth and a healthy newborn and mother.

POSTTERM PREGNANCY AND LABOR

Establishment of an accurate due date is a critical element in effective prenatal care. A woman's last menstrual period, together with her obstetric history, including the length of her menstrual cycle, and an initial ultrasound (usually between 16 and 20 weeks of pregnancy), helps primary care providers determine an accurate due date (see Chap. 12). The fetal biparietal diameter obtained at the initial ultrasound normally is accurate to within 5 days (Schmidt, 1999).

Approximately 90% of women give birth within 14 days after their due date (Wilkes & Galan, 2002). Significant concern arises with **postterm pregnancy** (a pregnancy that extends beyond 42 weeks' gestation) (Moore & Martin, 2003):

- After 40 weeks, the overall fetal mortality rate of 1% to 2% begins to increase.
- By 42 weeks, the mortality rate doubles.
- Morbidity increases exponentially as gestation exceeds 40 weeks, particularly when other risk factors (eg, gestational diabetes) exist.
- Placental function peaks at 36 weeks and begins to deteriorate by 38 weeks. This deterioration may lead to inadequate fetal nutrition and IUGR, oligohydramnios, and inadequate fetal oxygenation. Efficient placental function beyond 38 weeks may contribute to macrosomia and subsequent birth trauma.
- Meconium staining occurs in 25% to 30% of all prolonged pregnancies (twice the rate of term pregnancies). Causes include hypoxic events or maturity of the fetus with vagal reflex. Fresh meconium occurs most often with umbilical cord compression and impaired maternal–fetal blood flow. With oligohydramnios, meconium thickens and increases the risk for aspiration.

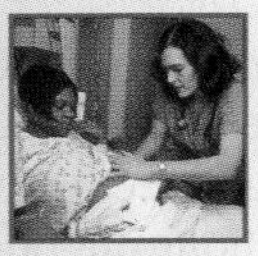

Consider Carlotta, who is at 42 weeks' gestation and scheduled for induction of labor. What would be the rationale for inducing her labor?

Women with postterm pregnancy generally experience various emotions. Impatience, frustration, fatigue, depression, and pressure from family and friends may cause them to become anxious about labor and birth and concerned for fetal safety and health. These emotions may accumulate with ongoing prenatal visits and questions from interested others. Setting a date for induction of labor and then having to change that date (eg, because of an unexpected increase in activity at the birthing center) may lead to anger and sadness. Allowing the client to express her feelings, come to the health care facility for a fetal health evaluation (nonstress test), and reschedule at the soonest available time may help mitigate negative feelings in such circumstances.

Factors when deciding whether to induce labor include the following:

- Cervical ripeness
- Fetal pulmonary maturity
- Fetal ability to tolerate labor
- Uterine sensitivity to the proposed induced method
- Maternal condition
- Gestational age
- Fetal size and gestation

Contraindications to labor induction include the following:

NIC/NOC Box 16.2 Preterm Labor

Common NIC Labels

- Anticipatory Guidance
- Anxiety Reduction
- Decision-Making Support
- Family Support
- High-Risk Pregnancy Care
- Intrapartal Care: High-Risk Delivery
- Labor Suppression
- Medication Administration
- Medication Management
- Teaching: Procedure/Treatment
- Ultrasonography: Limited Obstetric

Common NOC Labels

- Coping
- Decision Making
- Fetal Status: Intrapartum
- Knowledge: Treatment Regimen
- Maternal Status: Intrapartum

- Complete placenta previa or vasa previa (see Chap. 13)
- Classical uterine incision from a previous cesarean birth
- Pelvic structural deformities
- Active genital herpes infection
- Abnormal fetal presentation (eg, transverse lie)

Labor is most likely to occur when the cervix displays readiness to progressively efface and dilate. The Bishop's score is used to assess cervical readiness (see Chap. 15). Low numbers indicate an unfavorable cervix and an increased likelihood of prolonged labor and cesarean birth. A score of 8 or more indicates an increased likelihood of a successful vaginal birth. Another method of cervical assessment is transvaginal ultrasound. Tests for fetal fibronectin also may be used—this substance is found in the endocervix when cervical ripening has begun. Presence of fetal fibronectin is associated with a shorter time from induction to birth and a decreased need for prostaglandin administration.

Detailed discussion of the methods of labor induction is found later in this chapter.

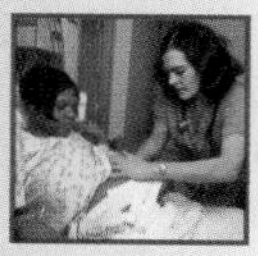

The health care provider obtained the following scores when evaluating Carlotta's cervical readiness: dilation = 2; effacement = 2; station = 2; cervical consistency = 1; position = 2. What would these findings indicate?

HEMORRHAGIC PROBLEMS

Vaginal bleeding at any time during pregnancy is physically and emotionally stressful for clients and their health care providers. Pregnant women are repeatedly told during childbirth education classes, prenatal appointments, and preadmission visits to be vigilant for this problem. The nurse in the labor and birth area must be aware of the different causes of vaginal bleeding at this time so that he or she can assess and communicate other appropriate signs and symptoms to the obstetrician or midwife. Initial assessment focuses on the severity of bleeding and stability of the woman and fetus.

PLACENTAL PROBLEMS

Bleeding associated with labor may involve the placenta and its membranes. Problems of placental attachment are presented in detail in Chapter 13; they are described briefly here in terms of their role in labor and birth.

Placenta Previa

Painless, bright red vaginal bleeding is the defining characteristic of *placenta previa* (see Chap. 13). If such bleeding has not been identified or does not develop until after labor starts, bloody show and uterine contractions may further confuse the situation (Oyelese & Smulian, 2006). Accurate identification depends on thorough assessment of the extent of vaginal bleeding. In cases of hemorrhage, blood loss is not difficult to diagnose. When the amount of bleeding is ambiguous, review of the prenatal history for placental location, vaginal bleeding, or maternal–fetal tachycardia can assist with a diagnosis. The nurse should immediately report any excessive vaginal bleeding during labor. Vaginal examination in clients with potential or actual placenta previa should be avoided.

Evaluations during labor would include the following:

- Bleeding: amount, presence of clots, color, and ability to stop spontaneously
- Pain and contractions
- Vital signs: pulse, temperature, respiratory rate, and blood pressure
- Fetal heart rate
- Leopold's maneuvers to determine fetal position and presentation

The nurse should report any findings outside of the normal range to the client's health care provider. Other communication issues include progress in labor and need for pain management.

A cesarean birth should be anticipated. General anesthesia is likely if the client is hypovolemic, bleeding, or both; spinal anesthesia would be considered if bleeding stops and volume status is within normal limits. The mother will need close monitoring during the postpartum period for signs of hemorrhage.

Placental Abruption

As discussed in Chapter 13, *placental abruption* (premature separation of a normally implanted placenta) can be a minor or life-threatening problem. Women with a previous placental abruption have a 10-fold increased risk for recurrence (Carter, 1999). Because of the pregnant state, maternal vital signs may not be valid indicators of the degree of blood loss or shock.

Care of the client and family depends on the gestation and maternal and fetal status. The goal is to stabilize both mother and fetus; if the fetus is alive and near or at term, the team focuses on a cesarean birth as quickly as possible. Blood loss may be substantial during birth; medications such as oxytocin, ergometrine, and Hemabate should be readily available at this time (Palmer, 2002). Ongoing assessment of vital signs, pain, bleeding, and fetal monitoring for reassuring signs would be essential components of the plan of care. In some cases of severe abruption, the fetus dies in utero. In such cases, the decision for vaginal or cesarean delivery is based on the risks for hemorrhage or other complications related to optimizing maternal health.

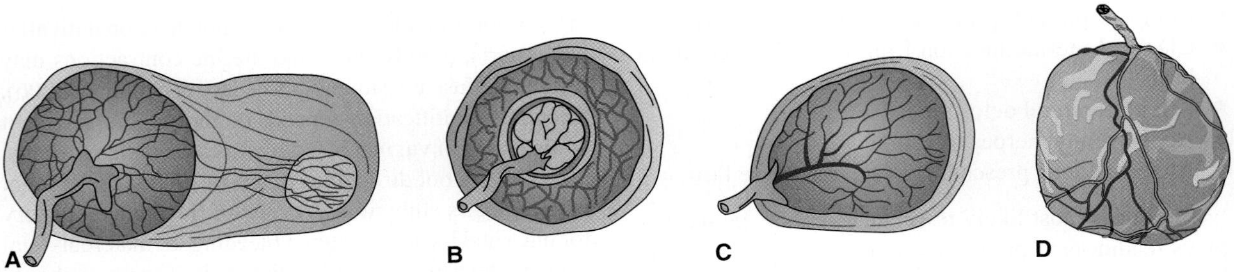

FIGURE 16.15 (A) Succenturiate placenta. (B) Circumvallate placenta. (C) Battledore placenta. (D) Velamentous placenta.

Other Placental Anomalies

Some placental problems are not identified until labor begins or after birth (Fig. 16.15):

- With *succenturiate placenta,* one or more small accessory lobes develop in the membranes at a distance from the main placenta. Connecting vessels may tear during birth or when the membranes rupture. After placental expulsion, one or more lobes may be retained in the uterus, resulting in maternal postpartum hemorrhage (see Chap. 19).
- In *circumvallate placenta,* the membranes are folded back on the fetal surface of the placenta, exposing part of the umbilical cord. Such exposure increases risks for small prenatal hemorrhages leading to preterm birth, as well as of retained placenta leading to postpartum hemorrhage.
- In a *battledore placenta,* the umbilical cord inserts at the placental margin rather than in the center. This variation is not considered clinically significant.
- With a *velamentous placenta,* umbilical blood vessels course unprotected for long distances through the membranes to insert into the placental margin. If they pass over the internal cervical os, they are at risk for compression by the presenting fetal part. Another risk is tearing when the membranes rupture. Both problems can cause fetal death.

UTERINE RUPTURE

Uterine rupture means separation of the uterine wall with or without fetal expulsion. Spontaneous uterine rupture is rare and associated with scar dehiscence or incomplete rupture usually secondary to a previous cesarean birth. Risk is increased if the time between the previous surgery and the current labor is less than 18 months (Cunningham et al., 2005). Risk is higher in clients who have had a classical uterine incision (vertical scar), which involves the contractile portion of the uterus. Other contributing factors include the following:

- Poor management of induction or augmentation of labor
- Instrument-assisted birth
- Manipulation during pregnancy (eg, ECV)
- Shoulder dystocia
- Use of fundal pressure in the second stage of labor
- Multiparity
- Placental implantation over a previous uterine scar

Common signs and symptoms include severe abdominal pain that continues between contractions, fresh vaginal bleeding, fetal heart rate abnormalities (eg, variable or late decelerations, tachycardia), cessation of labor, and hematuria. Team members must be aware of the need to palpate the contractions of a woman in labor receiving epidural anesthesia whose resting tone is not present between contractions. Assessment for resting tone ensures that the uterus is contracting, with relaxation between uterine activity.

As soon as a diagnosis of uterine rupture is established, preparations for emergency abdominal surgery must begin to control the bleeding. A cesarean birth usually occurs, and neonatal well-being largely depends on the age of gestation when the rupture happened. In most cases, the client must undergo a hysterectomy. Depending on the woman's condition, age, and desire for additional children, débridement of the rupture site and primary closure may be attempted. Team members give blood transfusions and IV fluids to replace lost blood and to alleviate shock. The client receives antibiotics to prevent or to combat infection.

PROLAPSED UMBILICAL CORD

When a portion of the umbilical cord falls in front of, lies beside, or hangs below the fetal presenting part, it is defined as **cord prolapse** (Fig. 16.16). This development occurs in 1 in 300 to 600 births (Boyle & Katz, 2005). Cord prolapse can be as follows:

- *Occult or hidden:* The cord cannot be seen or felt during a vaginal examination; diagnosis is based on ultrasound.
- *Complete and palpable:* The cord cannot be seen but can be felt during vaginal examination as a pulsating mass.
- *Presenting and visible:* The umbilical cord precedes the fetal head or feet and can be seen protruding from the maternal vagina.

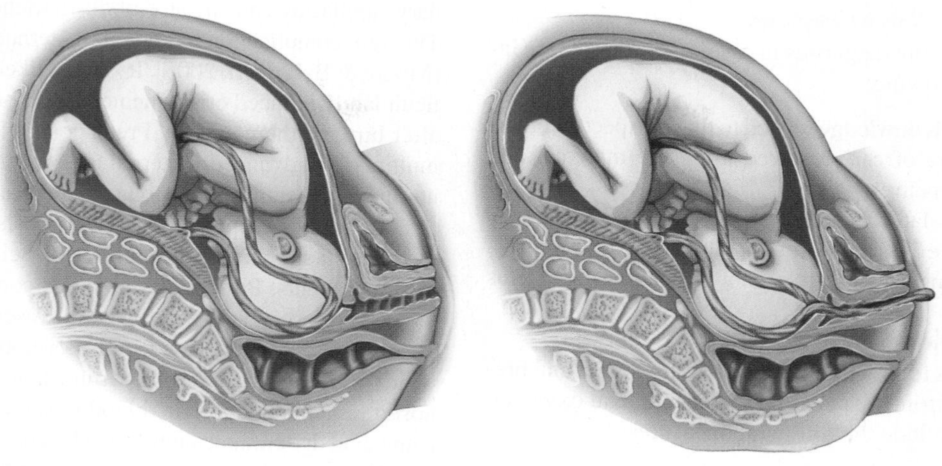

A B

FIGURE 16.16 Cord prolapse may be (**A**) contained within the uterus or (**B**) visible at the vulva.

Cord prolapse is related directly to an abnormally long umbilical cord, as well as to those conditions that result in the fetus not filling the maternal pelvis (eg, malpresentation). Common contributing factors include transverse lie and breech presentation. Other risk factors include preterm labor, fetal abnormalities, polyhydramnios, amniotomy (particularly if the presenting part is high), premature rupture of the membranes, placenta previa, pelvic tumors, and obstetric procedures such as ECV (Dilbaz et al., 2006).

COLLABORATIVE CARE: CORD PROLAPSE

Perinatal mortality associated with cord prolapse is at least 10% to 20% and is related to the interval between detection and birth (Baskett, 1999). Rapid action is most likely to have a favorable outcome. Compression of the umbilical cord between the presenting part and maternal pelvis decreases or cuts off fetal circulation. Fetal hypoxia can occur quickly; if uncorrected, umbilical cord compression leads to damage to the fetal central nervous system, fetal death, or both.

Prevention of cord prolapse is the best form of management and includes bedrest for a woman with ruptured membranes if the presenting part is high (unengaged). Amniotomy should not be done until the presenting part is engaged. If prolapse occurs while providing care, preparations for prompt cesarean birth should begin immediately (unless the maternal cervix is fully dilated, in which case vaginal birth may be attempted). Oxygen is administered, and continuous fetal monitoring is begun. Saline-soaked gauze at room temperature can be applied to any portion of the umbilical cord outside the vagina (a vagal response can be stimulated with chilling of the cord). The priority should be to keep pressure off of the cord until birth. To do so, the Trendelenburg position is employed to manually elevate the presenting part from the pelvis, or the maternal bladder may be filled to tolerance (approximately 500 mL), which raises the presenting part off the compressed cord.

If the cord prolapses before initiation of care, the first question to consider is whether the fetus is viable. Viability depends on gestation, presence of any lethal anomaly, and fetal heart rate on auscultation or ultrasound. This assessment should occur as quickly as possible, and information should be provided to the woman and family members.

Assessment

Assessment findings may include the following:

- Sudden appearance of a loop of umbilical cord at the introitus after rupture of amniotic membranes
- Variable or prolonged fetal heart decelerations following rupture of amniotic membranes that does not resolve with position change (spontaneous or with an amniotomy)
- Fetal bradycardia in conjunction with rupture of amniotic membranes
- Presence of the umbilical cord in the vagina on vaginal examination
- Any combination of these factors

A perinatal nurse working in a triage or admission area of a birthing unit should be alert to any risk factors for cord prolapse when assessing each laboring woman. Determining fetal station and status of the amniotic membranes is important and should be documented for each client. Regular observations of the perineum should be part of every woman's assessment, particularly after rupture of the membranes.

Select Potential Nursing Diagnoses

Common nursing diagnoses in cases of cord prolapse include the following:

- **Deficient Knowledge** related to the unexpected, emergent nature of care required to ensure maternal and fetal well-being
- **Anxiety** related to maternal and fetal well-being
- **Ineffective Tissue Perfusion** related to cord compression causing decreased placental circulation to the fetus

Planning/Implementation

Interventions focus on relieving pressure of the fetal presenting part from the cord and increasing fetal oxygenation. They include the following measures:

- Assist the woman into a knee-chest, Trendelenburg, or Sims lateral position, using pillows to elevate the buttocks.
- Place a hand into the vagina to elevate the presenting part and separate the cord from the presenting part and pelvis.
- Continuously assess fetal heart rate for ominous changes.
- Keep the exposed portion of the umbilical cord moist with prewarmed normal saline (do not reinsert) while assessing for pulsation and color.
- Administer oxygen at 8 to 12 L/min.
- Administer IV fluids.
- Notify the health care provider.
- Initiate ultrasound or real-time scanning as needed.
- Provide information to the woman and her family regarding the plan for care and rationales.
- Provide constant emotional and physical support (nursing presence).
- Document all care provided.
- Prepare for an emergency cesarean birth (as required) (Nichols & Zwelling, 1997).

Evaluation

Ongoing evaluation of care is based on fetal vital signs and maternal pain and anxiety and continues until birth, usually cesarean, is completed. Desired outcomes are as follows:

- Fetal gas exchange is normal, as evidenced by normal fetal heart rate patterns (average variability, no decelerations, and baseline within normal limits).
- The client and family verbalize understanding of the condition and the plan of care.
- The client expresses a decrease in pain and anxiety.
- A healthy infant is born.

AMNIOTIC FLUID EMBOLISM

With **amniotic fluid embolism,** a tear in the amnion and chorion provides a mechanism by which amniotic fluid can enter the maternal circulation and reach the pulmonary capillaries, causing an embolism (Schoening, 2006). This rare complication has a high maternal mortality rate (Moore & Baldisseri, 2005). It is most likely during a difficult labor, induced or augmented labor, or during or just after birth of the newborn. Predisposing factors include multiparity, advanced maternal age, macrosomia, intrauterine fetal death, and meconium in the amniotic fluid.

Signs and symptoms include cyanosis, hypotension, dyspnea, tachypnea, and chest pain. Seizures develop in some clients. Pulmonary edema is common in those women who survive the initial cardiovascular insult, and many of these clients subsequently develop coagulopathy, which may manifest as postpartum hemorrhage. Diagnostic tests include arterial blood gases, complete blood count, and disseminated intravascular coagulation profile.

The general goals of management are to maintain oxygenation, blood pressure, and cardiac output and to manage any coagulopathy (Moore & Baldisseri, 2005). Treatment may include intubation and mechanical ventilation with 100% oxygen if the client is unconscious. Monitoring of central venous pressure and blood transfusions may be implemented as necessary. IV fluids in normotensive clients should be restricted to avoid pulmonary edema (Perozzi & Englert, 2004).

The nurse should monitor the client's responses, anticipate possible therapies, and provide supportive care for her and her family. The nurse should place the client in Fowler's position and administer oxygen, medication, and blood products as ordered. The nurse should regularly monitor intake and output and not leave the client alone. If the client has not yet given birth, the nurse is responsible for monitoring the fetal heart rate and preparing for emergency birth. Because risk for maternal mortality is high with this condition, the nurse also may need to prepare to help the family through the grieving process (Perozzi & Englert, 2004).

MULTIPLE PREGNANCY

As discussed in Chapter 13, the number of multiple pregnancies is increasing for various reasons, including increased maternal age, increased use of reproductive-assisted technologies, and hereditary factors (Healy & Gaddipati, 2005; Watson-Blasioli, 2001). During labor and birth, the care of clients carrying more than one fetus can be particularly challenging. Potential perinatal complications include preterm labor, hypertension, anemia, placental dysfunction, cord abnormalities, congenital anomalies, IUGR, and low birth weight (Ellings et al., 1998).

During pregnancy, ultrasounds are used to determine fetal chorionicity, which is one of the most important determinants of pregnancy outcome (Taylor, 2006). Ultrasound also is used to determine gestation, fetal growth, and amniotic fluid volume. Planning for the birth of multiple fetuses usually occurs during pregnancy and should include education regarding the many possibilities and options that may become part of the client and her family's care. A birth plan discussed with health care providers should be flexible enough to include interventions such as cesarean birth as necessary but also to allow as much choice and decision making as possible over such things as feeding method, support people, and early labor comfort measures. The team providing care should give realistic information that dispels any myths regarding labor and birth, such as amount of pain and time between births of the newborns. The nurse should openly discuss with the client fears and concerns and should document findings for team members to review upon admission (Ellings et al., 1998; Ramsey & Repke, 2003).

Labor requires ongoing assessment and may progress differently than with a single gestation (Ellings et al., 1998). The early first stage may be shorter and the active stage longer because of uterine overdistention, malpresentation, or both. The second stage of labor also may be longer than with a singleton pregnancy because of a slower descent of the first presenting fetus (Ellings et al., 1998; Silver et al., 2000).

Method of childbirth depends on the position of the first fetus. If the presenting fetus is in the cephalic position, vaginal birth would most likely be the plan. If the first fetus is in a breech position, a cesarean birth would be encouraged. The presenting fetus may be in a transverse position or malposition; in this case, cesarean birth usually is the plan of care. If the second fetus is in a breech position, the health care team may discuss with the client the best plan for the birth. Concerns may include size of the fetuses and the ability to complete ECV at some point in labor.

Assessing the client's preference for pain medication or nonpharmacologic relief options would be important at the beginning of labor. An epidural has been suggested as beneficial if conditions exist that require an operative or cesarean birth (SOGC, 2000).

Throughout labor, the nurse should monitor presence of show; evaluate contraction frequency, intensity, and duration; and assist with vaginal examinations. Ensuring that the client is comfortable is important, as is encouraging her to voice her fears and concerns. Enabling her support person to stay with her and assist with comfort measures and encouragement is beneficial.

Care between births of the fetuses is also important because risks for cord entanglement, fetal compromise, and placental abruption are increased. Continuing to monitor subsequent fetuses after the birth of the first, as well as maternal bleeding and vital signs, is important to ensure maternal and fetal health.

Each infant must be identified clearly, as must each cord blood sample. Times of birth must be recorded for each infant and documented. Average time between vaginal births of multiple gestations is 30 minutes, whereas it is only approximately 1 minute if the birth is cesarean (Ellings et al., 1998).

The SOGC (2000) recommends that future health care providers' workshops and educational sessions focus on the special needs of families with twins and higher-order multiples (Research Highlight 16.2). Achievement of healthy infants and ongoing maternal health are the desired care outcomes.

MATERNAL OBESITY

The woman in labor who is obese faces some special challenges. Her care includes all normal admission blood work, assessments, and information. Depending on her weight, the team may need to review the weight restrictions of certain pieces of equipment such as labor beds,

● RESEARCH HIGHLIGHT 16.2 Mothering Multiples: A Metasynthesis of Qualitative Research

PURPOSE: To assist nurses to develop "a richer understanding" and to successfully apply clinical knowledge when working with women who give birth to multiple newborns

SAMPLE AND DESIGN: The researchers synthesized findings from six separate qualitative studies focused on mothering multiples in the first year of life. They performed a seven-stage process to pull out and compare themes from these studies in a documented format.

RESULTS: Many of the participants reported that providing child care 24 hours a day, 7 days a week was simply overwhelming. Emotions fluctuated from wonder and gratitude to depression and despair. Many of these mothers identified a need for a support network. They also expressed concern that they would not always be able to treat their children equally and reported challenges in learning how to adapt to the differences of their children.

CONCLUSIONS: While clients are pregnant and during postpartum teaching in cases of multiple gestation, nurses should be aware of the unique needs of this experience and assist families to develop supportive networks. Community resources may be helpful. Further research is needed with women of different cultural and demographic groups.

Beck, C. (2002). *Journal of Maternal Child Nursing, 27,* 214–221.

chairs in the birthing room, and stretchers. Correct assessments regarding whether such equipment can support the woman are vital for safety; however, it is critical that team members make such judgments factually and with sensitivity to avoid communicating judgment or negative reactions about this woman's weight to her and her family.

Accurate weight assessment also is important to ensure that doses of analgesics and anesthesia are sufficient and to determine the size of monitoring equipment to use. An appropriately sized blood pressure cuff is essential to obtain correct readings.

Because obese women are at increased risk for prolonged labor, macrosomia, blood loss, cesarean birth, and other problems, regular assessments of the progress of labor and early communication about any abnormalities are essential (Robinson et al., 2005). Any significant blood loss during labor should be reviewed for color, amount, and cause.

Accurate assessments of uterine activity, auscultation, and position changes may be challenging. The client may require internal monitoring. Ideally, the client is placed in an upright or semi-Fowler's position to increase her lung capacity and decrease her cardiac workload (Cesario, 2003). Macrosomia should be anticipated by assisting the client into a hyperflexed position for birth and ensuring that newborn resuscitative equipment and pediatric staff are available and ready if needed (Ehrenberg et al., 2004).

If the client requires a cesarean birth, the anesthetic of choice is epidural or spinal. Insertion of the needle may be difficult, however, because of additional adipose tissue. Helping the client curl her back as tightly as possible for insertion is important. Attempting to intubate her for general anesthesia is difficult because of her weight; however, it may be necessary if emergency complications develop. Placing a folded blanket under her head may facilitate access to the anterior airway and more rapid intubation (James, 2001). Goals for care include sensitive treatment, accurate weights, regular assessment of vital signs and progress of labor, and a healthy mother and newborn.

FEMALE CIRCUMCISION

As discussed in Chapter 6, female circumcision has a history estimated to be more than 5000 years (Box 16.2). It continues to be practiced in many countries. Long-term and short-term health problems associated with female circumcision include hemorrhage, infection, increased risk for HIV, urinary retention, and frequent urinary tract infections. Circumcised women may experience dysmenorrhea, pelvic inflammatory disease, incontinence, depression, and sexual dysfunction.

With increasing cultural diversity being found in the United States and Canada, encounters with clients who have undergone female circumcision are becoming more frequent (Whitehorn et al., 2002). In caring for circumcised women, the nurse should try to view these clients within the context of their culture, values, and beliefs to provide empathetic and nonjudgmental care. The first time that a nurse sees the external genitalia of such a client, she may be shocked, upset, or angry. Sometimes the term "female genital mutilation" is used to describe female circumcision, which suggests the Western view of this practice as abusive. Nurses must remember, however, that the client may not have been part of the decision making about the procedure. Or, the client may value the procedure and see it as positive.

BOX 16.2 Types of Female Circumcision

- Circumcision/Sunna, the least severe form, consists of pricking, slitting, or removing part of the clitoris.
- Excision (intermediate) is removal of the entire clitoris, occasionally with part of the labia majora.
- Infibulation is removal of the clitoris, labia minora, and adjacent aspect of the labia majora. The edges of the labia majora are then sewn together with sutures, thorns, or herbal paste, leaving only a small opening for passage of urine and menstrual flow by the insertion of a matchstick-size reed left in place until healing has occurred (Auscherman, et al., 1999).

Many cultures that practice female circumcision tend to encourage women to receive information about pregnancy, labor, and birth from other women in their community. Such clients who receive antepartal care in a health facility may arrive in labor with normal anxiety inherent to the unknown, as well as additional fear because of a lack of familiarity with the hospital environment or Western health care practices.

Clients who have not been defibulated before labor require immediate assessment. The scar may be opened early in labor or during the second stage to facilitate progress toward birth. Evaluation of the client's anxiety and knowledge regarding labor and birth is important. Discussing her wishes regarding labor support people, pain medications, comfort measures, and health care providers can decrease anxiety and increase culturally sensitive care provision.

If preferred or necessary, interpretative services should be arranged to enhance communication, which is key to culturally sensitive care. Normal vaginal examinations are extremely difficult to perform in infibulated women, so an experienced practitioner should modify the procedure to use a single finger with extensive lubrication. The nurse should pay close attention to labor's progression because female circumcision may increase the risk for dysfunctional labor. The nurse should rely on behavioral cues instead of vaginal examinations to assess progress, such as expressions of an "urge to push," increased number or length of contractions, increased maternal focus, and presence of "show." He or she should explain all procedures and how they will be completed while the woman is in labor. Labor support as per the woman's wishes should be provided.

An episiotomy may be necessary depending on the degree of circumcision. The nurse should teach about this process. Suturing afterward will be completed to repair the tissue but cannot replace what was removed (Omar-Hashi, 1994). Postpartum explanations regarding anatomy and repair will help the client understand and be comfortable with her recovery. The client needs preparation for postpartum pain that results from reversal of the infibulation. Pain management interventions may include analgesics, sitz baths, and application of witch hazel to the area (Omar-Hashi, 1994).

BIRTH-RELATED PROCEDURES COMMON IN HIGH-RISK LABOR AND BIRTH

Cervical Ripening and Labor Induction

During pregnancy and labor, the uterine cervix goes through changes in physical appearance and biochemical composition often preceding uterine contractions (Hadi, 2000). Cervical ripening is a series of events similar to those seen with tissue inflammation (Arias, 2000). A ripe cervix is shortened, softened, partly dilated, and centered. This type of cervix is necessary for the full dilation needed to accommodate passage of the fetus. See Chapter 15 for a review of Bishop scoring.

Methods of Cervical Ripening

Various methods can be used to ripen the cervix (Table 16.2) (Tenore, 2003). For example, the client may be advised to try sexual intercourse, breast stimulation, or both to promote the release of endogenous oxytocin. Current research, however, has not validated the safety or effectiveness of these methods (Kavanagh & Kelly, 2005; Kavanagh et al., 2005). Some clients use herbal treatments, such as black and blue cohosh or evening primrose oil. Such agents have not been studied, and nurses need to carefully document the client's use of these or any other complementary/alternative modalities for safety.

Mechanical Methods. One mechanical method of cervical ripening involves the insertion of an indwelling (Foley) catheter into the endocervical canal, with direct pressure from the balloon applied to the lower uterine segment (Rai & Schreiber, 2005). Another method is the use of hygroscopic dilators such as laminaria and synthetic products containing magnesium sulfate. These dilators can be inserted on an outpatient basis because they provide slow progressive cervical ripening over 12 to 24 hours.

Cervical ripening also can be done by "stripping" the membranes or performing an amniotomy. With stripping of the membranes, the care provider inserts a finger through the cervical os and moves it in a circular direction to detach the membranes. With an amniotomy, the care provider inserts a device called an amniohook through the os to rupture the membranes.

Pharmacologic Methods. Prostaglandins are frequently used to help ripen the cervix (Baxley, 2003). Currently, three types of prostaglandins are administered: dinoprostone inserts (Cervidil), dinoprostone gel (Prepidil), and misoprostol (Cytotec) (Pharmacology Box 16.1). Misoprostol is a drug used commonly to treat peptic ulcers; its use in cervical ripening is not currently approved by the U.S. Food and Drug Administration (FDA).

TABLE 16.2 Common Approaches to Labor Induction

INDUCTION AGENT	DOSAGE	ACTION
Prostaglandin E_2 (Cervidil, Prepidil)	Inserted vaginally (Cervidil) providing 0.3 mg/hr for 12 hours (total of 10 mg) or intracervically (Prepidil gel) providing 0.5 mg total	Facilitates cervical maturation and ripening Decreases time to active labor and possible amniotomy
Mechanical agents such as a Foley catheter	Inserted into cervix and then the balloon is inflated with 30–40 mL sterile water	Physical stretching of the cervix
Membrane sweeping or digitally stripping the membranes from the lower uterine segment	May be performed with a vaginal examination by a health care provider	Releases prostaglandin from the membranes and decidua
Prostaglandin E_1 (Misoprostol)	25–50 μg p.v. q4h	Significantly improves Bishop's score, decreases time to active labor and birth (Magtibay et al., 1998)
Amniotomy (ARM)	May be performed together with oxytocin infusion	May achieve uterine contractions alone in a woman with a high Bishop's score

● PHARMACOLOGY 16.1 Misoprostol (Cytotec)

INDICATION: Misoprostol is a synthetic prostaglandin.

ACTION: It produces dilation of the cervix.

PREGNANCY RISK CATEGORY: X

DOSAGE: 25 to 50 μg orally or placed intravaginally in the posterior fornix

POSSIBLE ADVERSE EFFECTS: Nonreassuring fetal heart rate patterns, uterine hyperstimulation, nausea, headache, diarrhea

NURSING IMPLICATIONS

- Ensure that the client does not have any problems or risk factors that would contraindicate use of this drug.
- Continuously monitor uterine activity and fetal heart rate.
- Check that a tocolytic agent and an IV fluid line are readily available in the event of uterine hyperstimulation.

From Karch, A. (2005). *2005 Lippincott's nursing drug guide.* Philadelphia: Lippincott Williams & Wilkins.

Oxytocin Pharmacology

Oxytocin increases uterine contractility by increasing the circulation of free intracellular calcium. There are two types of oxytocin: endogenous (naturally secreted by the fetus and woman in labor) and exogenous (synthetic hormone used to induce or augment labor) (Clayworth, 2000). Oxytocin receptors in the uterine myometrium and decidua increase during pregnancy, particularly in the third trimester and during the latent phase of labor as a result of the hormonal influences of estrogen, progesterone, and prostaglandin. With the increased number of receptors, the amount of oxytocin required to produce uterine contractions decreases. Uterine activity is rhythmic and coordinated but not constant.

In normal spontaneous labor, the highest concentrations of oxytocin are found in the umbilical cord blood. Maternal blood levels reach what would approximately be achieved with an exogenous oxytocin infusion of 2 to 4 mU/min while the fetus secretes another 2 mU/min. These levels increase in the second stage of labor to accomplish birth. Therefore, the total oxytocin concentration is in the range of 4 to 6 mU/min.

Exogenous oxytocin is the drug most commonly used when the cervix is ripe and labor is being induced or augmented. A continuous IV infusion of oxytocin is administered at an ordered starting dose (Pharmacology Box 16.2). Then, the dose is increased until an adequate contraction pattern is achieved (Clayworth, 2000). A continuous oxytocin infusion raises the circulating blood level slowly: 20 to 30 minutes are required. The client usually feels a uterine response within 3 to 5 minutes (increase in uterine contractions) (Fig. 16.17). The half-life of oxytocin is 7 to 15 minutes, so its effect is diminished quickly if it is discontinued or decreased.

Goal of Oxytocin Administration. The goal of oxytocin administration is to produce uterine contractions with a

● PHARMACOLOGY 16.2 Oxytocin

INDICATION: Oxytocin is a synthetic form of the naturally occurring hormone.

ACTION: It is used to facilitate uterine contractions.

PREGNANCY RISK CATEGORY: C

DOSAGE: Initially 1 to 2 mU/min by IV infusion, increased at a rate of no more than 1 to 2 U/min every 15 to 30 minutes until a regular contraction pattern is established

POSSIBLE ADVERSE EFFECTS: Cardiac dysrhythmia, uterine hypertonicity, nausea and vomiting, fetal bradycardia, water intoxication

NURSING IMPLICATIONS

- Use an infusion pump to ensure control of accurate administration.
- Monitor the frequency, duration, and strength of each contraction.
- Assess maternal vital signs, especially blood pressure for signs of hypotension. If hypotension develops, the oxytocin needs to be discontinued, and the primary care provider needs to be alerted.
- Check the fetal heart rate regularly for any nonreassuring characteristics.

From Karch, A. (2005). *2005 Lippincott's nursing drug guide.* Philadelphia: Lippincott Williams & Wilkins.

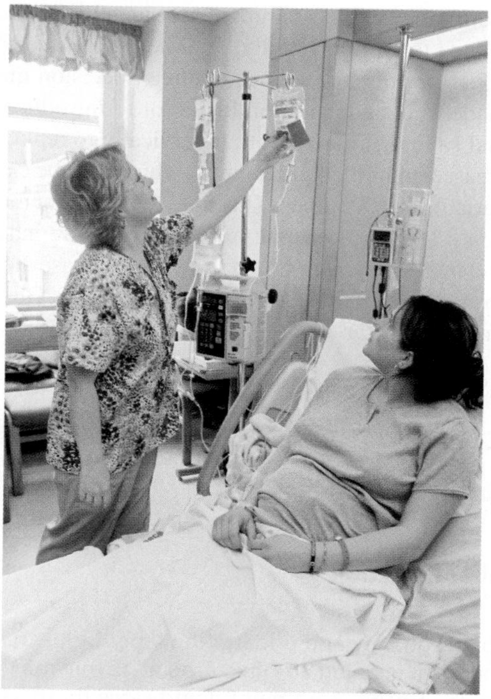

FIGURE 16.17 During IV infusion of oxytocin, the nurse uses an infusion pump to regulate flow, which has been piggybacked into the main IV line.

frequency of every 2 to 3 minutes, lasting 40 to 60 seconds. The desired intrauterine pressure (IUP) is 50 to 60 mm Hg above baseline, with a palpated resting tone between contractions (less than 20 mm Hg).

Formula for Calculation of an Oxytocin Dosage. The following formulas can be used to calculate dosages of oxytocin:

1. Determine mU oxytocin/mL by:
   Units of oxytocin
   mL of IV fluid × 1000 = milliunits per (mU/mL)
2. Determine mU of oxytocin/min by
   (mU/mL)/1 × (mL/hr)/60 min = milliunits per min (mU/min)
3. Confirm administration rate in mL/hr by
   (mU/min × 60 min/hr)/mU/mL = ___ mL/hr

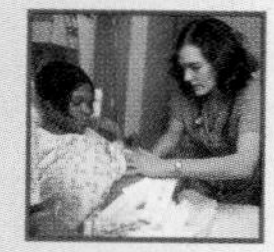

Suppose the health care provider initially orders an IV infusion of oxytocin at 2 mU/min. The pharmacy supplies an infusion that contains 10 mU/mL. How much solution would Carlotta receive in 1 hour?

Associated Complications. Several complications are associated with the use of oxytocin to induce or augment labor:

- Uterine **hyperstimulation** refers to increased number of contractions or increased myometrial tone causing uteroplacental hypoperfusion and fetal hypoxia. Excessive uterine contractions also can lead to uterine rupture or abruptio placentae. Problems may stem from an overdosage of oxytocin, increased sensitivity to oxytocin by increased number of oxytocin receptors, or increased exogenous oxytocin production by maternal or fetal components. Management of oxytocin in cases of hyperstimulation is a common question among health care providers. During labor, the exchange of oxygen and carbon dioxide for the fetus occurs primarily between contractions. Placental function decreases when intrauterine pressures are greater than 35 mm Hg and severely reduced when intrauterine pressures are at 50 to 60 mm Hg. This means that there is some reduction of maternal fetal blood flow in almost all contractions. Fetal compromise from hypoxia, uterine rupture, or both may occur with uterine hyperstimulation, particularly with a uterine resting tone above 20 mm Hg (Clayworth, 2000).
- Oxytocin administered over long periods, at high dosages, or both can result in hyponatremia (water intoxication), confusion, convulsion, and congestive heart failure. Detailed records of intake and output are essential to prevent these problems or manage them if they develop.
- Oxytocin administered for a prolonged period has a hypotensive effect; blood pressure monitoring is required in the nursing care management.

Collaborative Management. Nursing care of the client before oxytocin infusion begins should include the following:

- Assess baseline vital signs and fetal heart rate.
- Explain the physiology of uterine contractions and pharmacology of oxytocin.
- Describe the process of induction to the woman and family (complementary to the health care provider's initial description in arranging an induction).
- Assess for uterine contractions and rupture of membranes.
- Ensure the presence of written orders for the oxytocin.
- Complete an obstetrical nursing history of the woman before starting the induction.

During oxytocin infusion, the nurse should perform the following interventions:

- Continuously monitor fetal heart rate and uterine activity.
- Palpate the abdomen for uterine activity (the goal is contractions every 2 to 3 minutes lasting 45 to 60 seconds with adequate resting tone). If an IUP catheter is in place, resting tone should not be above 20 mm Hg; contraction intensity should not exceed 60 mm Hg.

- Assess blood pressure and pulse hourly and more often if these values are increasing.
- Maintain records of intake and output.
- Communicate with the woman and her support people and other care providers about labor progress.
- Provide encouragement and support as the woman progresses through labor.
- Provide comfort measures and pain management as per the woman's wishes.
- Continue oxytocin infusion with increases as per the contraction pattern and the birth attendant's orders.
- Document oxytocin dosages, uterine activity, fetal heart rate, vital signs, and the woman's response.
- Notify the health care provider of identified concerns related to uterine activity, fetal heart rate, labor progress, or presence of meconium. A decision may be made to include amnioinfusion or to introduce normal saline during labor transcervically to replace decreased amniotic fluid volume, which may be causing variable decelerations. This fluid replacement must be done slowly as per unit protocols to ensure maternal and fetal safety; it has been shown to decrease the need for cesarean birth (ACOG Committee on Obstetric Practice, 2002).

See Nursing Care Plan 16.2 for more information.

NURSING CARE PLAN 16.2

The Client Undergoing Labor Induction

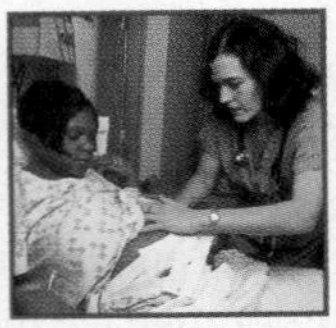

Recall Carlotta, who is in her 42nd week of pregnancy and undergoing labor induction. Four hours after induction begins, oxytocin is being administered at 12 mU/min. Carlotta reports that the contractions are becoming more painful and rates them as 7 on a scale of 1 to 10. They are approximately 3 minutes apart and lasting 90 seconds each. Her cervix is 4 cm dilated. An amniotomy was performed with the last vaginal examination; clear fluid was obtained. Fetal heart rate ranges from 134 to 146 beats/min with a reassuring pattern.

NURSING DIAGNOSES

- **Deficient Knowledge** related to process of induction, labor and birth experience, and pain relief measures
- **Anxiety** related to fear of the unknown and lack of familiarity with labor progression

EXPECTED OUTCOMES

1. The client will demonstrate understanding of the events associated with induction, labor, and birth.
2. The client will identify appropriate options other than the use of a Jacuzzi for comfort during labor and birth.
3. The client will verbalize specific areas of concern.
4. The client will identify positive strategies to cope with her concerns.

INTERVENTIONS	RATIONALES
Assess the client's level of understanding about induction, labor, and birth.	Such data provide a baseline for identifying specific client needs and developing an individualized plan.
Discuss with the client her concerns, feelings, and perceptions related to labor and birth and expectations about pain.	Discussion allows the nurse to emphasize positive aspects of the current situation; verbalization of concerns can establish sources of stress and problem areas.

Continued

NURSING CARE PLAN 16.2 ● The Client Undergoing Labor Induction

INTERVENTIONS	RATIONALES
Communicate accurate facts; answer questions honestly. Reinforce true information, emphasizing that each pregnancy, labor, and birth is highly individualized.	Open, honest communication promotes trust and helps correct misinformation. Facts help dispel unfounded fears, myths, misconceptions, or guilt feelings.
Evaluate the client's past coping strategies to determine which have been effective.	Use of appropriate coping strategies aids in reducing anxiety.
Review measures used during labor and birth to monitor maternal and fetal well-being.	Knowledge of ongoing fetal surveillance aids in alleviating stress related to the unknown.
Encourage the client to include her partner in this experience.	His participation promotes sharing, provides support, and enhances the chances for success.
Teach the client and partner about oxytocin, preparing them for what to expect relative to contraction strength and frequency.	Understanding the need for monitoring related to use of oxytocin will facilitate appropriate choices of pain management.
Explain the need for continuous monitoring of maternal and fetal well-being.	Continuous monitoring allows for early detection and prompt intervention should problems arise.
Review comfort measures, such as music, distraction, hot/cold compresses, massage, and position changes that the client can employ other than use of the Jacuzzi.	Pharmacologic and nonpharmacologic measures can help control pain.
Provide opportunities for the client and partner to practice various comfort measures; allow the client to select the methods best for her.	Practice reinforces learning. Allowing the client to choose the best methods for her promotes decision making and feelings of control.
Assist the client and partner to adapt measures or try alternatives for pain relief should previous choices prove ineffective.	Events and pain level vary throughout labor. Adapting methods or selecting alternatives helps to ensure effectiveness.
Continually update the client and partner about the client's progress. Provide positive reinforcement related to methods used and labor progression.	Ongoing information helps prevent unnecessary fear and anxiety about the unknown and promotes progress toward the goal of a healthy newborn. Positive reinforcement promotes the couple's involvement and feelings of control, thereby enhancing self-esteem.

EVALUATION

1. The client verbalizes accurate information related to events of induction and labor.
2. The client identifies nonpharmacologic and pharmacologic options for pain relief.
3. The client states that her concerns and fears have decreased.
4. The client demonstrates use of appropriate coping strategies to deal with anxiety and fear.

NURSING DIAGNOSES

- **Risk for Injury** related to the use of oxytocin and effects on mother and fetus
- **Pain** related to increased uterine contractions

Continued

NURSING CARE PLAN 16.2 ● The Client Undergoing Labor Induction *(Continued)*

EXPECTED OUTCOMES

1. The client will remain free of adverse effects of oxytocin administration.
2. The client will progress through labor without complications.
3. The client will report a decrease in pain to a tolerable level.
4. The client will demonstrate use of appropriate pain-relief measures.

INTERVENTIONS	RATIONALES
Assess vital signs, especially blood pressure, fetal heart rate and pattern, and contractions, continuously.	Continuous assessment provides a baseline for comparisons and allows for early detection of problems.
Reinforce explanations about oxytocin infusion, equipment, and monitoring.	Anxiety can contribute to pain perception. Continued explanations help to reduce anxiety.
Assess the oxytocin infusion rate by infusion pump; gradually increase rate as ordered. Ensure that oxytocin is administered as a secondary infusion piggybacked into the main IV line.	The goal of oxytocin administration is to produce uterine contractions lasting 45 to 60 seconds approximately every 2 to 3 minutes. Administering oxytocin as a secondary infusion allows for prompt discontinuation if complications develop.
Palpate the abdomen between contractions; note resting tone.	Increased resting tone can cause problems with placental perfusion. Oxytocin can lead to hypertonic uterine contractions.
Encourage the client to lie on her side.	A side-lying position promotes placental perfusion.
Assess pain level; ask the client to rate it.	Such rating objectively quantifies the level of pain.
Review options for pain relief; assist the client with measures per her request; administer pharmacologic agents as indicated and ordered.	Increased pain may compound anxiety and tension, leading to enhanced pain perception. Immediate assistance to control pain is important at this time.
Continue to assess pain level and vital signs, as well as fetal heart rate and patterns.	Ongoing assessment provides indicators about the effectiveness of chosen pain relief methods and oxytocin administration.
Monitor intake and output closely; obtain laboratory tests as ordered; assess for changes in mental status (such as confusion); be alert for signs and symptoms of heart failure.	Oxytocin can lead to hyponatremia, confusion, convulsion, and congestive heart failure. Close monitoring is essential to prevent these problems.

EVALUATION

- The client exhibits vital signs and other assessment findings (including fetal heart rate and pattern and uterine contractions) within acceptable parameters.
- The client progresses through the stages of labor without incident.
- The client states that pain is tolerable, rating it as a 2 to 3 with appropriate pain relief measures.

Amnioinfusion

With **amnioinfusion,** a volume of warmed, sterile, Ringer's lactate solution or normal saline is infused through an intrauterine pressure (IUP) catheter to increase fluid volume. The infusion improves fetal and placental oxygenation, helps cushion the umbilical cord, and dilutes any meconium that may be found. Indications for amnioinfusion include severe variable decelerations resulting from cord compression, oligohydramnios (decreased amniotic fluid), postmaturity, preterm labor with rupture of the membranes, and thick meconium fluid (Gramellini et al., 2003). Contraindications to this procedure include cord prolapse, vaginal bleeding of unknown cause, hypertonic uterine contractions, amnionitis, and severe fetal distress.

The client must be given an explanation of the procedure and how it will solve the problem. Informed consent must be obtained. The client will need to remain on bedrest during the procedure. The birth attendant should perform a vaginal examination to establish dilation, confirm presentation, and ensure that the umbilical cord has not prolapsed. An infusion pump is used to instill 250 to 500 mL of the chosen solution over 20 to 30 minutes. Close monitoring of fluid volume and uterine contractions is required to prevent uterine overdistention or increased uterine tone. Team members should regularly assess maternal vital signs, pain, and intake and output, as well as the fetal heart rate pattern. The team and the client should be prepared to begin the procedure for cesarean birth if fetal heart rate does not improve after the amnioinfusion.

Forceps-Assisted Birth

When a woman's expulsive forces are not sufficient to push the fetus through the birth canal, forceps may be used to rotate, provide traction, or both to the fetal head (Patel & Murphy, 2004). **Forceps** are stainless-steel instruments that look like tongs; they can fit around the head of the fetus to help pull the baby through the vaginal outlet (Fig. 16.18). Forceps consist of two parts that cross each other like a pair of scissors. Each part has a handle, lock, shank, and blade (Belfort, 2003). The lock may be of a sliding type or a screw type. The blade usually consists of two curves. The cephalic curve conforms to the shape of the fetal head, whereas the pelvic curve conforms to the shape of the birth canal. The two blades are designated as left and right. The left blade is placed into the vagina on the mother's left side; the right blade is inserted on the right side.

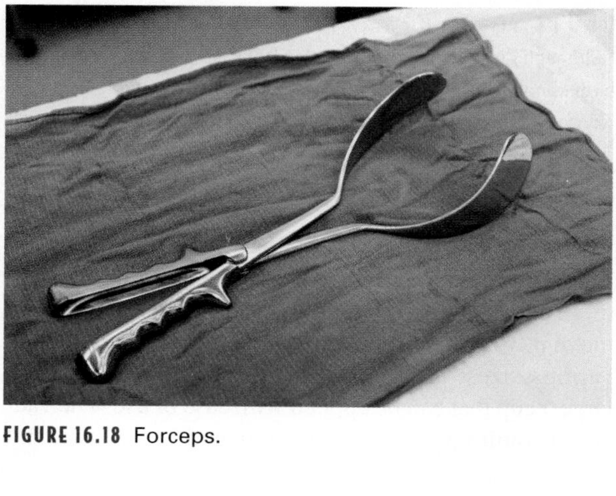

FIGURE 16.18 Forceps.

Indications for use include a prolonged second stage; failure of the fetal presenting part to rotate fully, descend in the pelvis, or both; non-reassuring fetal heart rate patterns; compromised maternal pushing sensations from anesthesia; intrapartum infection; and maternal heart disease, acute pulmonary edema, or fatigue.

Criteria for Use

Certain criteria are necessary to justify the safe use of forceps (Ross et al., 2006):

- The woman is having uterine contractions. Her membranes have ruptured, and the cervix is dilated fully.
- The maternal bladder is empty. (Urinary catheterization may be used to drain the bladder as necessary before forceps are implemented.)
- The woman is receiving adequate anesthesia. Type of anesthesia depends on the forceps used, which is related to fetal position and presentation.
- The team providing care have determined that birth is mechanically feasible based on an adequate maternal pelvis, engaged fetal head, and sufficient level of the presenting part.
- The presenting part is vertex, face with anterior chin, or after-coming head in vaginal breech.
- The fetal head position is known.

Under no circumstances should forceps be applied to an unengaged presenting part.

Types of Applications

The ACOG (1989) revised their classification system for station and type to better define those applications that posed a significant level of fetal risk (Ross et al., 2006). The following types of applications are according to the station and position of the fetal presenting part at the time of application (ACOG & AAP, 2002):

- *Outlet forceps:* The fetal skull has reached the pelvic floor, with the fetal head at the perineum and the fetal scalp visible at the introitus without spreading the labia. Rotation of 45 degrees or less is required. The sagittal suture is in the anteroposterior diameter or the right or left anterior or posterior position.
- *Low forceps:* The leading point of the fetal skull is at or above station +2 and not on the pelvic floor. This category is subdivided into rotation requiring less or more than 45 degrees.

- *Mid forceps:* These are applied when the fetal head is engaged but the leading point of the skull is less than +2.

Collaborative Management

Several pairs of different approved types of forceps are autoclaved, encased in suitable wrappings, and kept in the delivery room for immediate use as needed. The other instruments needed for forceps-assisted birth are the same as for any vaginal birth.

When use of forceps is indicated and the type has been selected, the client is placed in the lithotomy position and draped. The nurse should explain the procedure and its rationale to the client and family. He or she should tell the woman that she will feel pressure and pulling but should not feel any pain with adequate regional or spinal anesthesia. The nurse should encourage the client to use any breathing techniques and other labor-coping mechanisms she has learned to prevent muscle tensing during application of the forceps. Usually, an episiotomy is performed to provide adequate room for maneuvering the forceps without tearing the maternal tissues (see Chap. 15).

The birth attendant performs a vaginal examination to check the exact position of the fetal head. He or she then introduces two or more fingers of one hand into the left side of the vagina to guide the left blade of the forceps into place while protecting the maternal vagina and cervix from injury. The attendant uses the other hand to gently place the left blade of the forceps into the left side of the vagina between his or her fingers and the fetal head. The attendant then carries out the same procedure on the right side. He or she attaches the blades together at the shank, applying traction intermittently, not continuously (Fig. 16.19). Between traction, the attendant partly disarticulates the blades of the forceps to ease pressure on the fetal head. During application, the nurse should monitor uterine contractions and report findings, so that the birth attendant can coordinate the timing of the contractions with forceps traction. Team members should encourage the mother to continue with pushing efforts as traction is applied.

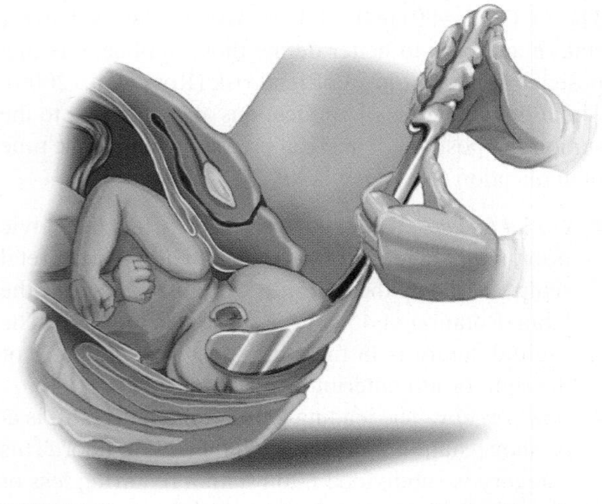

FIGURE 16.19 Application of the forceps to the fetal head.

Fetal bradycardia is common with forceps-assisted birth, generally related to the increased pressure of the fetal head, umbilical cord compression, or both. Continuous fetal monitoring is thus required, and appropriate newborn resuscitation equipment should be available. A pediatrician also should attend the birth in case fetal distress has prompted the need for forceps.

Piper forceps (a special type of forceps used in breech presentations with an after-coming head) are applied after the shoulders have been delivered and after gentle traction combined with suprapubic pressure has brought the fetal head into the maternal pelvis (Locksmith et al., 2001). The body and arms are suspended with a towel to facilitate application of the blades (Fig. 16.20). The birth attendant introduces the left blade upward along the fetal head on the left side and then applies the right blade in the same fashion. After locking the forceps in place, the attendant uses palpation to confirm their position on the head. Following an episiotomy, traction is applied, and the chin, mouth, and nose emerge over the perineum.

Complications

Forceps-assisted birth can pose risks for both mother and newborn. Forcible rotation can injure the maternal uterus, vagina, or cervix, causing potential lacerations and bleeding. Injury to the anal sphincter also is common (Christianson et al., 2003). If forceps are applied incorrectly and one blade overlies the fetal face, the newborn may exhibit unsightly bruising, which usually disappears after a few days. Excessive force may cause more serious injury to the newborn's head, including skull fracture, scalp lacerations, or subdural hematoma (Patel & Murphy, 2004).

QUOTE 16-3

"Although I understood the rationale for the use of forceps in giving birth to my baby, I was so terrified while it was happening. I kept worrying they would scrape the baby's face or hurt us in some way."

A client who required a forceps-assisted birth

Vacuum-Assisted Birth

The **vacuum extractor** is a cup-shaped device attached to a suction pump and applied to the fetal head to remove it from the birth outlet (Fig. 16.21). Cups come in various sizes; usually, the birth attendant selects the largest cup that can be applied with ease of use. The vacuum is built up slowly to create negative pressure, and

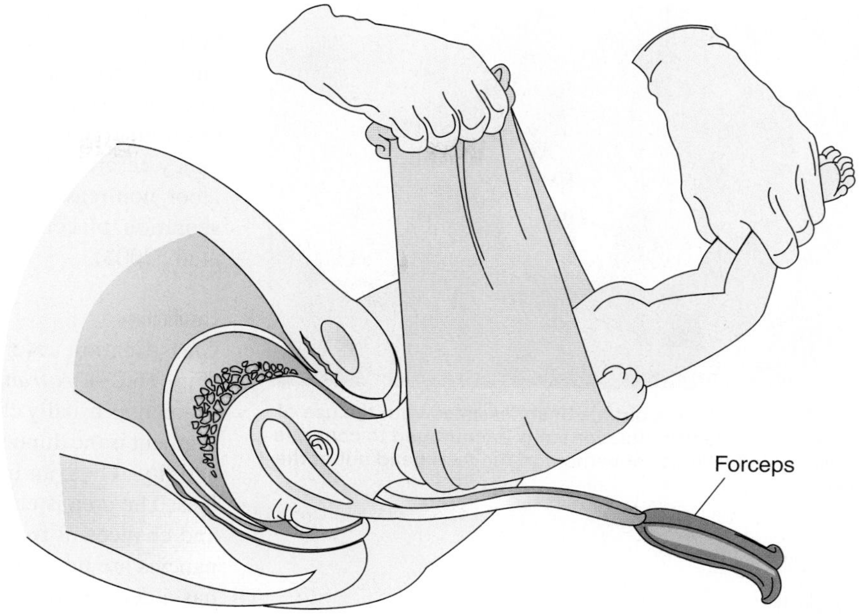

FIGURE 16.20 The Piper forceps are occasionally used to assist with vaginal breech births.

the suction creates an artificial caput within the cup, providing firm attachment to the fetal scalp. The birth attendant applies traction until the head emerges from the vagina.

Indications for use are the same as with forceps. The rate of vacuum-assisted births is approximately 6% of all U.S. births (Pope et al., 2004). Although vacuum extractors are growing in popularity, they currently are used less frequently than forceps (Pope et al., 2004). Some believe that vacuum extractors are safer because they pose less risk for maternal injury, although findings also show the use of forceps to pose fewer risks to the fetus (Caughey et al., 2005; Johanson & Menon, 2000).

Criteria for Use

Criteria for using the vacuum extractor are the same as those for using forceps, with the following exceptions:

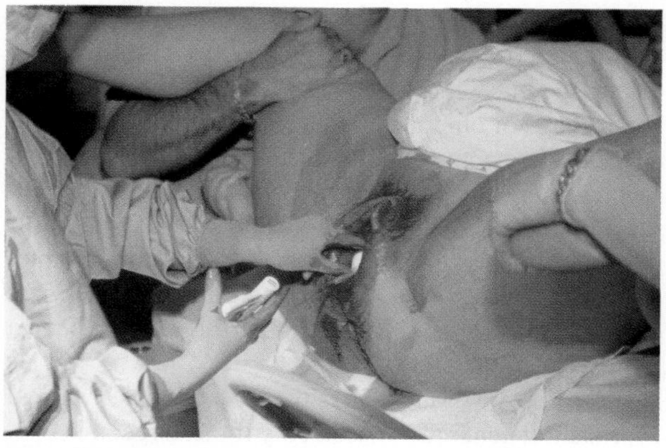

FIGURE 16.21 Application of the vacuum extractor.

- The vacuum extractor can be used in multiparous women who have only a small rim of cervix that is stretched easily over the remaining fetal head.
- The vacuum extractor should never be used in cases of preterm birth because the suction cup can injure the fetal head and scalp.
- It should never be used in cases of breech or face presentation.

Collaborative Management

When a vacuum extractor is being used, the nurse should briefly explain the procedure and its necessity to the client and family. He or she should advise the woman that she will feel pressure and pulling; however, with adequate regional or spinal anesthesia, the client should not feel pain. The client should employ breathing techniques and other labor management techniques she has learned to cope with labor.

After the birth attendant assembles the appropriate-size cup and sterile tubing, the nurse should attach the distal end to suction. Once the cup has been applied to the fetal head, the suction should be activated. To prevent damage to the maternal tissues, suction must be released if the cup slips off the fetal head. The team should encourage the client to push during contractions, while the birth attendant applies the device (Fig. 16.22).

Fetal heart rate during the procedure requires ongoing monitoring. Newborn resuscitation equipment should be available, and the pediatrician should be called if neonatal complications are expected. Team members should advise the parents that the newborn's head will have edema or bruising where the cup was applied, but that this will disappear within a few days (McQuivey, 2004).

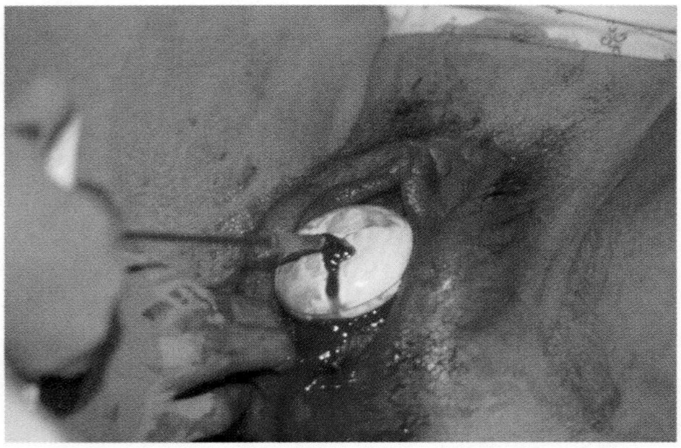

FIGURE 16.22 When a birth is being assisted with the use of a vacuum extractor, the woman is encouraged to continue pushing to facilitate movement of the fetal head out of the vaginal outlet.

Complications

As with forceps, use of the vacuum extractor can result in maternal and fetal injuries (Johnson et al., 2004). One measure to prevent vaginal lacerations is to perform a digital examination of the entire circumference of the suction cup after application but before initiation of the vacuum. Use of the device should be kept as brief as possible to prevent fetal scalp injuries. Generally, if traction on the suction cup during three contractions does not produce encouraging descent of the fetal head, the team should abandon the use of vacuum extraction and move to plans for a cesarean birth.

Cesarean Birth

Cesarean birth is moving from being considered surgery with significant risks for maternal morbidity and mortality to surgery that many women are actively requesting. Contributing factors to this shift in views include advances in surgical techniques, antibiotic therapy, anesthesia, and thromboprophylaxis (Jibodu, 2000; Wax et al., 2004). The number of cesarean births is rising both in the United States and Canada; approximately 20% of all U.S. births occur this way (Mackenzie et al., 2003). The increase can be partially accounted for by increases in multiple gestations and maternal requests. Reasons a woman may want to undergo cesarean birth without trying vaginal birth include fear of labor pain, fetal morbidity, or maternal pelvic floor damage, as well as finding it more convenient to have a planned date of birth. Other factors that may be contributing to the rising incidence of cesarean birth include the use of electronic fetal monitoring, which provides earlier indications of fetal distress than in the past; increased malpractice suits, leading birth attendants to elect for surgery rather than attempting difficult or assisted vaginal births; and more frequent use of labor induction and augmentation (Youngkin & Davis, 2004).

When working with clients undergoing cesarean birth, perinatal nurses must be skilled in providing care during surgery, either in the scrubbing or circulating role. The client being cared for may be having an anticipated or an emergency cesarean birth. Reasons for an emergency cesarean birth may include failure to progress in labor, non-reassuring fetal heart rate tracings, breech presentation, placenta previa, and fetal malposition (Kolas et al., 2003).

Classification

Classification refers to the type of uterine incision (Fig. 16.23). A *transverse incision* in the lower uterine segment is usually chosen for several reasons. The lower segment is the thinnest portion of the uterus with the least activity. Thus, an incision at this site minimizes blood loss. The area is easier to repair than the upper portion, and chances of rupture of the scar in subsequent pregnancies are minimized. Use of this type of incision also has a decreased risk for paralytic ileus, peritonitis, and bowel adhesions. After opening the abdominal cavity, the surgeon makes the initial incision transversely across the uterine peritoneum, where it is attached loosely just above the bladder. He or she then dissects the lower peritoneal flap and bladder from the uterus and incises the uterine muscle. The membranes are ruptured, the fetus is removed, the placenta is extracted, and intravenous oxytocin is administered to facilitate uterine contractions. Suturing of the uterine wall occurs in two layers, which seals off the incision and helps prevent lochia from entering the peritoneal cavity. A layer of absorbable suture is used to reapproximate the visceral peritoneum. Packs are removed from the abdominal cavity, with the abdomen closed in layers.

With a classic cesarean, the surgeon makes a vertical incision directly into the wall of the uterine body. After extraction of the uterine contents, three layers of absorbable sutures are used to close the incision. This approach requires cutting into the full thickness of the uterine corpus. Indications for this type of incision are extensive adhesions involving the bladder and lower uterine segment from previous cesarean births, transverse lie, and anterior placenta previa. Because it provides rapid access to the fetus, it also may be chosen in cases of acute hemorrhage or other emergencies that threaten maternal or fetal safety. Other conditions that may warrant a classic incision include a fetus of less than 34 weeks who presents by breech, maternal fibroids that restrict the lower uterine segment, need for maternal hysterectomy immediately following the birth, invasive maternal cervical cancer, and cesarean birth being performed to rescue a living fetus from a dead woman.

A rare type of incision is the low (cervical) vertical approach. It generally is used only if the surgeon is having difficulty extracting the fetus through other methods.

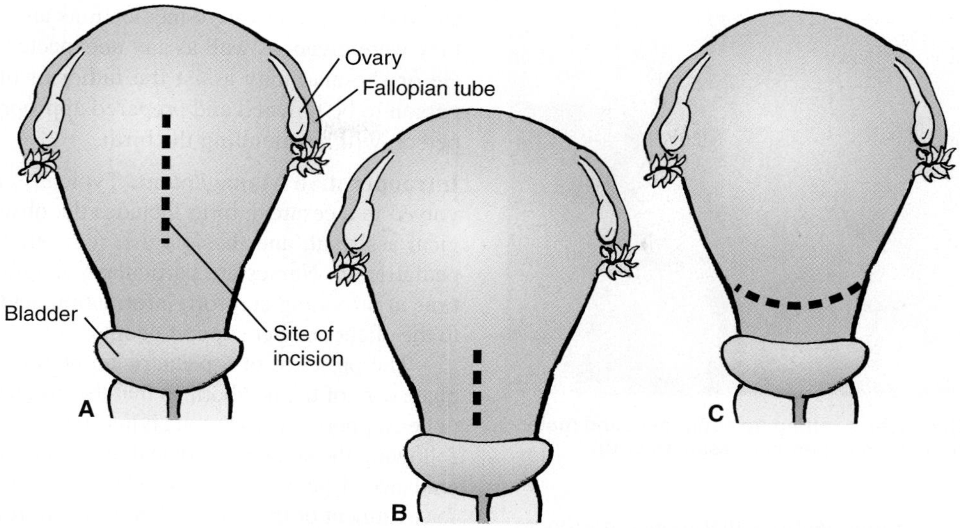

FIGURE 16.23 (A) The classical cesarean incision is vertical and used in emergencies when quick removal of the fetus is critical or when the fetus is so large that this method is the only way to enable delivery. (B) The low cervical vertical approach is used rarely. (C) The most common method is the low transverse approach because the scar has a decreased risk for rupture during subsequent pregnancies.

Collaborative Management

Standards of care for clients undergoing cesarean birth should be included within each institution's perioperative and obstetric program. A family-centered approach is vital and should accommodate involvement of the client's support person to facilitate the woman's participation. Preadmission should include discussion of postoperative pain management, realistic understanding of pain and surgical recovery, and warning signs of infection. NIC/NOC Box 16.3 reviews appropriate interventions and outcomes for cesarean births.

Preoperative Management. Even if the cesarean birth is an elective procedure, the experience of surgery can be anxiety producing for the client and her family. Such anxiety can be heightened when the cesarean birth is unanticipated or an emergency. Team members need to concentrate on alleviating fears, correcting misperceptions, teaching normal procedures and likely outcomes, and communicating findings. If the surgery is elective, providers should verify the pregnancy's gestation and review the maternal and pregnancy history.

Preparation for the surgery itself is extensive. Common diagnostic studies performed to ensure maternal and fetal well-being include complete blood count; urinalysis; blood type and cross-match (in case blood for transfusion is needed); and ultrasound to evaluate fetal position and placental location. If the gestation is preterm, an amniocentesis may be needed to check fetal lung maturity. The health care provider usually discusses the need for the surgery, the risks, and the type of anesthesia that will be used (spinal, epidural, or general) (see Chap. 17). Epidural anesthesia is used most frequently so that the mother can remain awake and aware of the birth experience.

The nurse should document the mother's last oral intake and what was eaten. He or she assists with preparing the necessary equipment, including newborn resuscitation equipment and a warm crib (Fig. 16.24). The nurse

NIC/NOC Box 16.3 Cesarean Birth

Common NIC Labels

- Bleeding Reduction
- Cesarean Section Care
- Fluid/Electrolyte Management
- Incision Site Care
- Infection Protection
- Intravenous Therapy
- Skin Surveillance
- Wound Care

Common NOC Labels

- Fluid Balance
- Hydration
- Hydration Status: Food and Fluid Intake
- Knowledge: Labor and Delivery
- Knowledge: Treatment Procedure
- Tissue Integrity: Skin and Mucous Membranes
- Wound Healing: Primary Intention

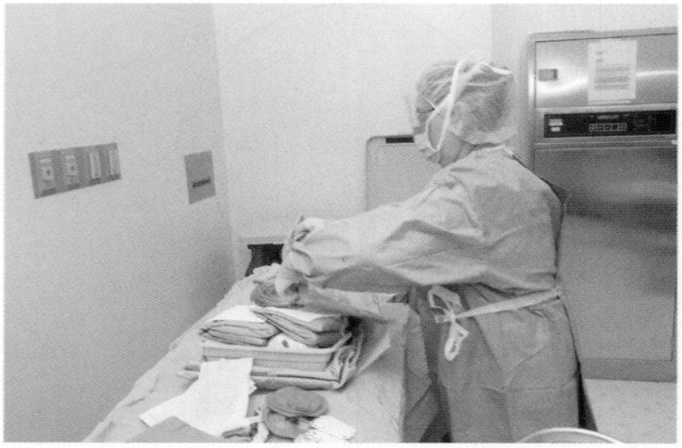

FIGURE 16.24 The nurse is setting up equipment and material in preparation for an impending cesarean birth.

can begin teaching interventions that reduce postoperative complications, including use of deep-breathing exercises and the incentive spirometer. Team members will prepare the surgical site and begin an IV infusion for fluid replacement therapy as ordered. The client will need an indwelling (Foley) catheter, which will remain in place for approximately 24 hours. The nurse should administer any ordered preoperative medications and record when they were given, as well as any unexpected side effects. He or she also may assist the father or other support person to be gowned and prepared appropriately if this person will be attending the birth.

Intraoperative Management. Typically, the team involved in a cesarean birth includes the obstetrician, surgical assistant, anesthesiologist, registered nurses, and pediatrician. Nurses are particularly helpful during this time at providing comfort, information, and reassurance to the client and her support people.

The presence of a pediatrician helps to ensure adequate care of the newborn so that the obstetrician and his or her supports can focus on giving attention to the woman following the surgery. Neonatal nurses also may be in attendance, depending on the newborn's condition and need for treatment or transport. After removal from the uterus, the newborn who is experiencing no complications may be shown to the mother or given to the support person to hold before general newborn care procedures are initiated (see Chap. 20). Figure 16.25 depicts a cesarean birth sequence.

Postoperative Management. Maternal postpartum care is similar to that for women who have undergone vaginal

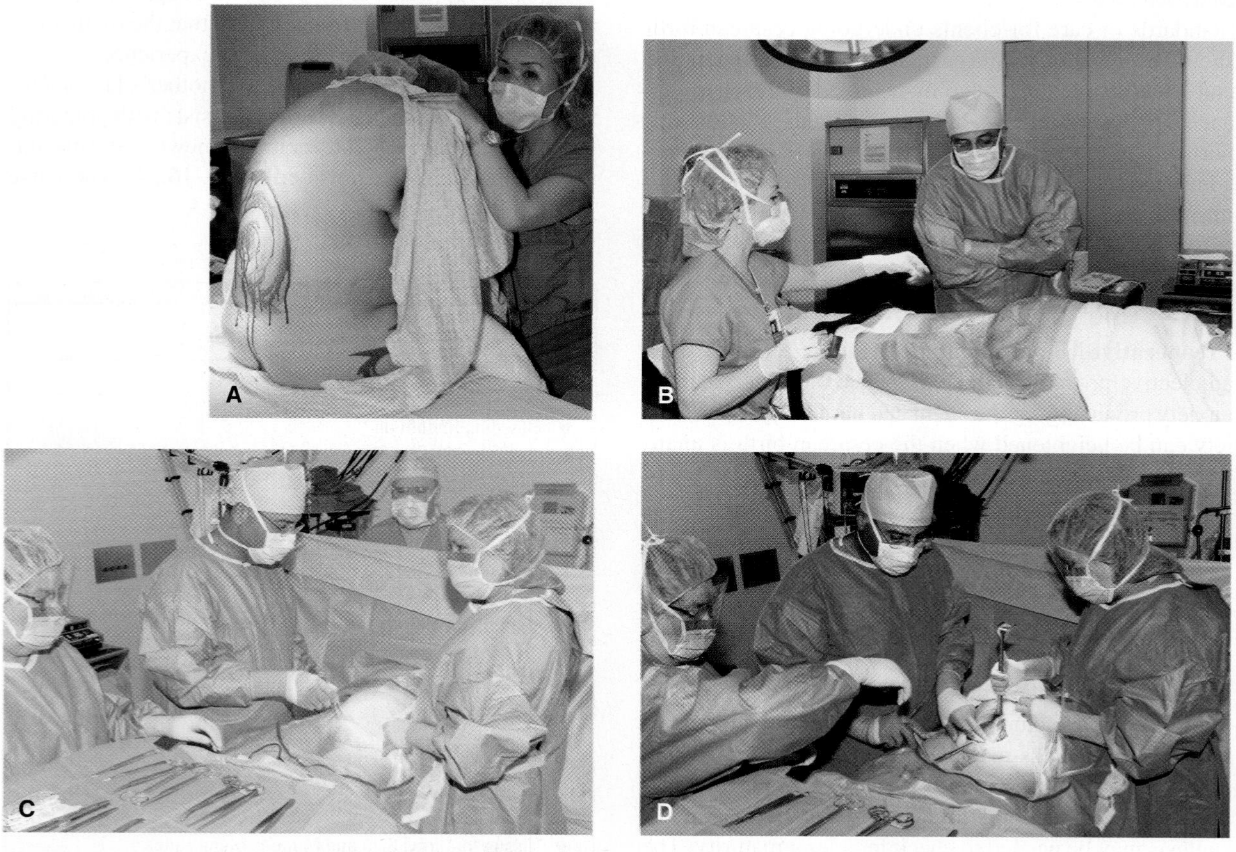

FIGURE 16.25 A cesarean birth sequence. (**A**) The client is receiving anesthesia. (**B**) The surgical area is being cleaned and prepared. (**C**) The obstetrician begins cutting. (**D**) The uterus has been opened.

(Continued)

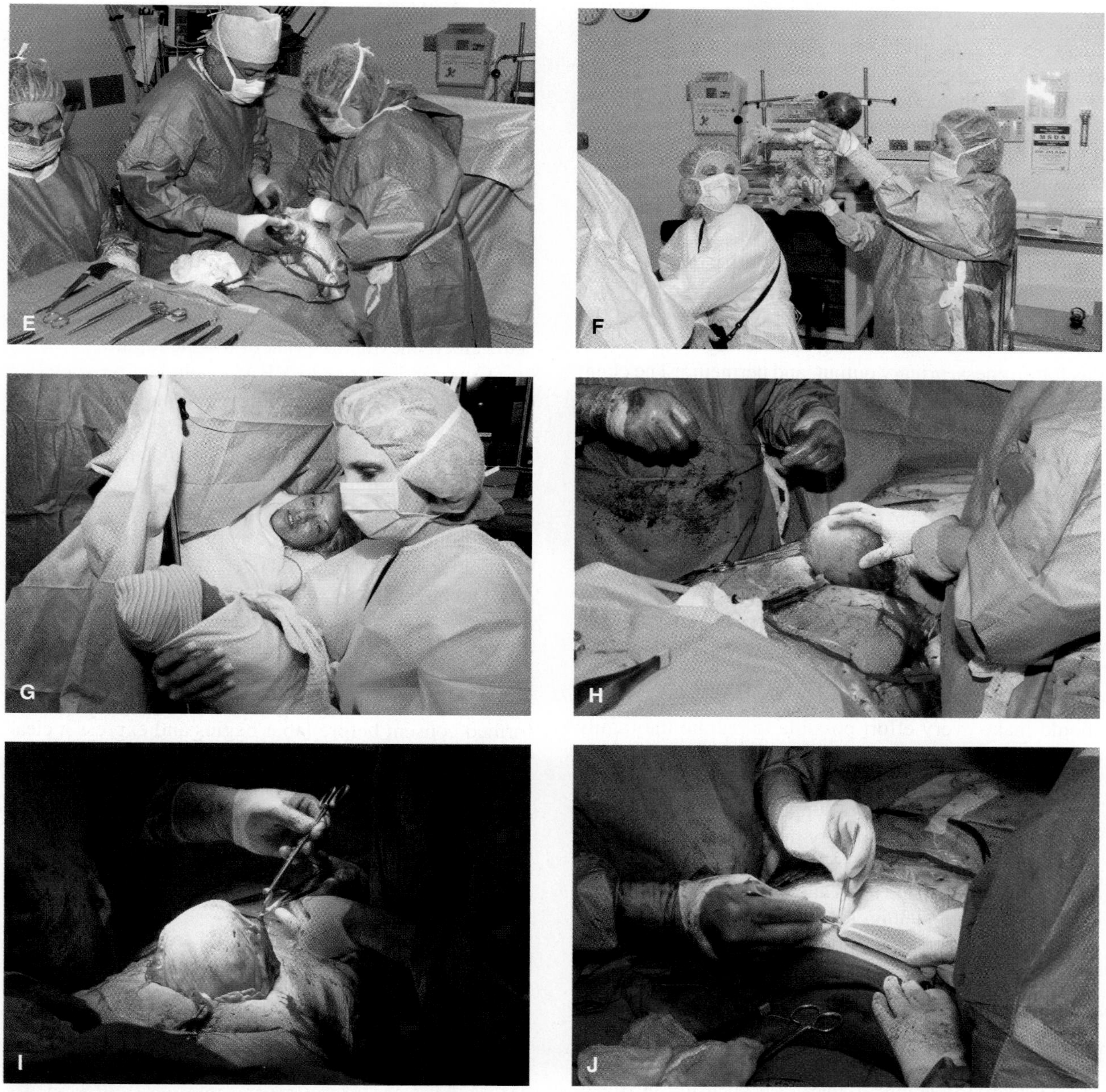

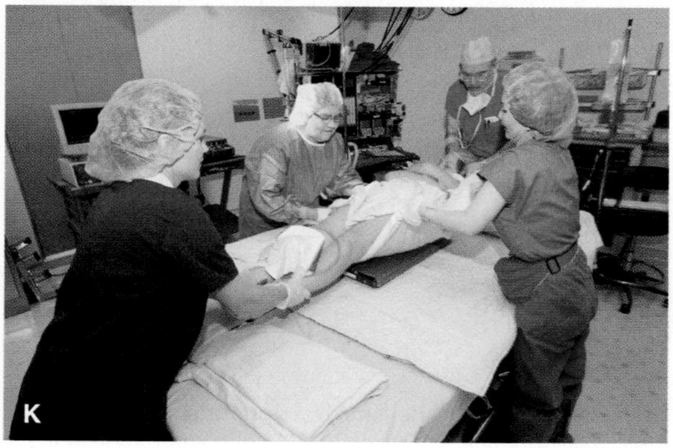

FIGURE 16.25 *(Continued)* A cesarean birth sequence. (**E**) Team members begin extracting the fetus from the uterus. (**F**) The newborn emerges successfully. (**G**) The nurse holds the newborn and shows her to the mother. (**H**) The uterus is being pushed back into the woman's body. (**I**) The surgeon is repairing the uterus. (**J**) The incision site is sutured. (**K**) The client is being prepared for transfer from the operating area to a recovery area.

birth. The experience of major surgery, however, necessitates some added measures. The nurse should check this client's vital signs and lochia flow every 15 minutes for the first hour, every 30 minutes for the next hour, and every 4 hours thereafter if stable. If the client received sedation, her level of consciousness needs to be monitored; if she received regional anesthesia, the nurse needs to document when sensation to the legs returns. The client should cough, perform deep-breathing exercises, and use the incentive spirometer every 2 hours.

The client likely will be in the health care facility for 2 to 3 days longer than the client who undergoes a vaginal birth. During this time, regular assessments will be done of her abdominal dressing and drainage, uterine fundus for firmness, urinary output, and perineum. The client likely will receive a regimen of pain medication tailored to be tapered with time as the incision heals. Pain from the incision may require the client to need assistance with moving in bed and turning from side to side. The nurse will need to check any IV infusions and monitor intake and output per orders. Although standards of introducing solid foods vary, some clients are able to eat regular food within 12 to 18 hours postpartum.

One major difference between vaginal and cesarean birth is that the surgery imposes a forced separation between mother and newborn in the first few hours. Depending on the condition of both parties, team members should make every effort possible to reunite the family quickly and to facilitate early touching and holding of the newborn to promote bonding. Clients who intend to breastfeed may require extra support because postpartum pain and recovery from surgery may make the initial experience more challenging. Special involvement from a lactation consultant and extra attention to this area may be helpful. Early ambulation is important to prevent cardiovascular and respiratory problems. If the surgery was unanticipated, follow-up regarding the disparity between the family's expectations (ie, vaginal birth) and actuality and how they are adjusting to that is an important emotional consideration.

Discharge teaching focuses on ensuring adequate rest, knowing signs of infection to report, and adhering to restrictions about lifting and performing household tasks like vacuuming. The client should avoid sexual intercourse until lochia has ceased and she no longer has any abdominal or perineal discomfort. As with all postpartum clients, contraception education should be provided. Protocols for follow-up appointments vary, but many clients who undergo cesarean birth are seen 6 weeks after discharge from the hospital, which is similar to women who undergo vaginal birth.

Vaginal Birth After Cesarean

Vaginal birth after cesarean (VBAC) is the term used for a vaginal birth after the client has undergone at least one previous cesarean birth. Factors associated with a positive VBAC experience include spontaneous labor, an initial favorable pelvic examination, and no use of oxytocin (Durnwald & Mercer, 2004). Although many health care providers emphasize the possibility of VBAC to clients who have had transverse incisions (Fig. 16.26), the reality is that the expression "Once a cesarean, always a cesarean" still largely holds true today (Coleman et al., 2005; Dauphinee, 2004). Arguments against VBAC focus on the increased risks of uterine rupture and hemorrhage. In most cases of attempted VBAC, women go through a trial of labor to see how they progress; such trial must occur in an environment capable of switching to manage acute emergency in the event of uterine rupture.

Contraindications to VBAC include a prior classic cesarean birth, prior myomectomy, uterine scar other than low transverse cesarean scar, contracted pelvis, and inadequate staff or facility available should emergency cesarean birth be required (SOGC, 2005). Cervical ripening increases the risk for uterine rupture; thus, this procedure is contraindicated in clients attempting VBAC (ACOG Committee on Obstetric Practice, 2002). Labor induction in a woman who has experienced previous cesarean birth also poses risk for uterine rupture and needs to be discussed with the client before the induction takes place (Dauphinee, 2004; Kayani & Alfirevic, 2005).

The client attempting VBAC must give fully informed consent before labor begins and express a clear understanding of the risks and benefits. The nurse must keep detailed and accurate records of the client's plan of care, the timing of interventions, the client's response, and fetal status. Such records provide the details necessary to ensure prompt attention is given to any emergency development. Nonreassuring fetal monitoring tracing is

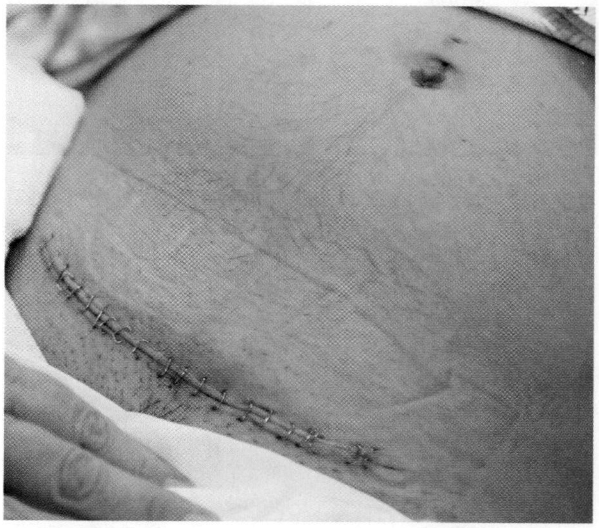

FIGURE 16.26 A low transverse incision for a cesarean birth provides options for future attempts at a vaginal birth in subsequent pregnancies.

an indication of potential uterine rupture and should lead the team to begin the process of emergency cesarean birth. According to ACOG criteria for a safe trial of labor for VBAC, the obstetrician, anesthesia provider, and operating room team must be immediately available (ACOG, 1999; Dauphinee, 2004).

Questions to Ponder

1. A client is attending a regular prenatal visit. She is at 24 weeks' gestation. During a discussion with the nurse, the client reports that a few weeks ago, she had some light pink vaginal spotting that lasted for 1 day only. She says, "It went away, and I can still feel the baby moving, so I didn't think it was anything to worry about."
   - What is your reaction to this scenario? How would you respond to the client?
   - What teaching needs do you identify? What would be your next steps?
2. One of your close family members is in the 14th week of a normally progressing second pregnancy. Her first pregnancy ended with a low transverse cesarean birth of a healthy baby. The surgery was unplanned and occurred because of failure to progress after several hours of labor. Your relative says to you, "My obstetrician has been telling me that I can attempt a vaginal birth with this pregnancy, but I'm really not sure if that would be for the best. It seems in some ways that it would be easier and more convenient for me to just schedule another surgery—at least I'll know what to expect! What do you think?"
   - How do you feel about the growing rates of cesarean births? When do you think they should be indicated for clients?
   - What risks and benefits of both vaginal and cesarean birth in these circumstances can you outline for your relative? What things would you consider in responding to her statements?

SUMMARY

- Dystocia is abnormal or dysfunctional labor. It can develop at any point in labor and may involve a problem with the powers of labor, passenger (fetus), or passageway (maternal birth canal).
- Problems with the powers of labor usually involve uterine contractions or maternal bearing-down efforts. Examples include hypertonic and hypotonic contractions, inadequate expulsion forces, pathologic retraction and constriction rings, and precipitous birth. Many of these conditions necessitate surgical birth.
- Breech presentation means that the fetal buttocks are the presenting part. In most cases, a breech presentation is an indication for cesarean birth. If the fetus is at term, providers may initiate external cephalic version (ECV) to rotate the fetus and facilitate vaginal birth. Vaginal breech birth is becoming less common but sometimes happens and often requires the use of forceps.
- In addition to the buttocks in breech presentation, other abnormal fetal presentations include shoulder, face, brow, and compound presentations.
- With occipitoposterior (OP) positioning, the fetal occiput lies in the posterior part of the maternal pelvis. As a result, the fetal head does not apply well to the cervix, which may delay the progress of labor. This problem also can result in significant back pain for the mother. To resolve the problem, the client might try changes in position or ambulation to encourage the fetus to move.
- When shoulder dystocia develops, the fetal shoulders cannot move through the maternal pelvis after the fetal head has emerged. A calm cooperative team approach to intervention is necessary and requires a stepwise approach. Techniques to alleviate shoulder dystocia include McRobert's maneuver, suprapubic pressure, assisting the woman into a hands-and-knees position to dislodge the shoulder, and finally the Woods screw rotational maneuver.
- Other problems with the fetus that may pose risks for labor and childbirth include macrosomia and fetal abnormalities.
- Many problems with the maternal pelvis can be anticipated when a woman has received adequate prenatal care.
- True labor that starts before 37 completed weeks of gestation is considered preterm. This problem is responsible for most neonatal deaths unrelated to congenital anomalies. Health care providers focus heavily on teaching clients the signs of preterm labor and, when it occurs, working to halt or delay progress for as long as possible to get the gestation closer to 37 weeks.
- Postterm pregnancy is pregnancy that extends beyond 42 completed weeks' gestation. This situation poses significant risks for fetal morbidity and mortality and usually necessitates labor induction.
- Hemorrhage during labor can result from problems with the placenta or because of a ruptured uterus. Excessive bleeding is always a medical emergency requiring prompt and focused interventions.
- Cord prolapse occurs when part of the umbilical cord falls in front of, lies beside, or hangs below the fetal presenting part. It is a common cause of fetal death and thus mandates quick attention and management.
- Amniotic fluid embolism can occur during labor or postpartally and poses significant risks for maternal mortality. General treatment goals include maintaining oxygenation, blood pressure, and cardiac output and managing any coagulopathy. Regular monitoring of the client is essential.

- The birth process in cases of multiple gestation may require some adjustments based on the number of fetuses and their individual presentations, weights, and other factors.
- The obese woman in labor requires special considerations, such as intensively monitoring her vital signs, ensuring equipment can accommodate her safely, and regularly checking the progress of her labor.
- Growing diversity in North America is exposing more health care providers to women in labor who have previously undergone various forms of female circumcision. Nurses and other caregivers need to treat circumcised women with sensitivity and respect and assist them through their labor process with enhanced attention to managing their pain and risks for hemorrhage and infection.
- Various factors may require assisted labor through cervical ripening and induction. Methods to ripen the cervix include mechanical, surgical, and pharmacologic interventions.
- Exogenous administration of oxytocin is used to increase uterine contractility. Administration of a continuous IV infusion of oxytocin begins with a starting dose that is increased until an adequate contraction pattern is achieved. Nursing care during oxytocin administration focuses on monitoring maternal vital signs and fetal heart rate; explaining how oxytocin facilitates uterine contractions to the client and family; monitoring the progress of uterine contractions; checking for any complications; providing comfort and assistance with pain management; and documenting findings.
- Amnioinfusion may be used in cases of cord compression, oligohydramnios, postmaturity, preterm labor with rupture of the membranes, and thick meconium fluid to improve fetal and placental oxygenation, help cushion the umbilical cord, and dilute any meconium that may be found.
- Rates of cesarean births are increasing for several reasons. Regardless of whether the surgery is planned or unexpected, this type of birth requires expert nursing care during all phases of the operation to protect maternal and fetal health and to optimize long-term outcomes for the family.
- Women who receive low transverse incisions during cesarean birth may be candidates for vaginal birth in future pregnancies.

REVIEW QUESTIONS

1. A woman in labor is experiencing hypertonic uterine contractions. The nurse would be least likely to prepare the client for which intervention?
   A. Intravenous fluid therapy
   B. Intramuscular morphine
   C. Administration of short-acting barbiturate
   D. Intravenous oxytocin (Pitocin)
2. A client has undergone ECV successfully. Which of the following would the nurse do next?
   A. Prepare the client for an ultrasound
   B. Plan for an immediate cesarean birth
   C. Have the client undergo a nonstress test
   D. Perform McRobert's maneuver
3. Which finding would lead the nurse to suspect that the fetus of a client in labor is in OP position?
   A. Complaints of significant back pain with contractions
   B. Auscultation of fetal heart sounds in the lower abdomen
   C. Fetal back easily palpated with Leopold's maneuvers
   D. Fetal buttocks identified as the presenting part
4. Which of the following assessment findings would indicate the need for tocolytic therapy in a client with preterm labor?
   A. Fetus at 37 weeks' gestation
   B. Immature fetal lung profile
   C. Fetal weight of 2700 grams
   D. Intact membranes
5. A woman who is at 41 weeks' gestation is being evaluated for possible labor induction. The nurse assesses the client's cervical readiness using the Bishop scoring method. Which score would indicate that the cervix is favorable for labor induction?
   A. 3
   B. 5
   C. 7
   D. 9
6. After teaching a group of students about placental anomalies, the instructor determines that the teaching was successful when the students identify which anomaly as least problematic?
   A. Battledore placenta
   B. Velamentous placenta
   C. Circumvallate placenta
   D. Succenturiate placenta
7. Which position would be least effective for a pregnant woman in labor who is experiencing umbilical cord prolapse?
   A. Knee-chest
   B. Trendelenburg
   C. Semi-Fowler's
   D. Sims lateral
8. A client is to receive a continuous intravenous infusion of oxytocin. The nurse determines that the client is receiving the intended effect as evidenced by:
   A. uterine resting tone of 35 mm Hg.
   B. contractions occurring every 2 to 3 minutes.
   C. contractions lasting approximately 2 minutes.
   D. contraction intensity of 70 mm Hg.
9. The nurse is describing the types of uterine incisions that may be used with a client who is to have an elective cesarean birth. Which of the following

should the nurse include as characteristics of a transverse incision?

A. Reduces the amount of blood lost during the procedure
B. Promotes rapid access to the fetus if problems develop
C. Allows for birth of a fetus younger than 34 weeks in breech presentation
D. Uses three layers of absorbable sutures to close the incision

REFERENCES

American College of Obstetricians and Gynecologists (ACOG). (1989). *Obstetric forceps. Committee opinion No. 71.* Washington, DC: Author.

American College of Obstetricians and Gynecologists (ACOG). (1999). ACOG practice bulletin. Vaginal birth after previous cesarean delivery. Number 5, July 1999 (replaces practice bulletin number 2, October 1998). Clinical management guidelines for obstetrician-gynecologists. *International Journal of Gynaecologists and Obstetricians, 66*(2), 197–204.

American College of Obstetricians and Gynecologists (ACOG) Committee on Obstetric Practice. (2002). Committee opinion. Induction of labor for vaginal birth after cesarean delivery. *Obstetrics and Gynecology, 99*(4), 679–680.

Arias, R. (2000). Pharmacology of oxytocin and prostaglandins. *Clinical Obstetrics and Gynecology, 43,* 455–468.

Auscherman, J., Welshimer, K., & Black, J. (1999). Female genital mutilation: What health educators should know. *Journal of Health Education, 30*(4), 222–228.

Baskett, T. (1999). *Essential management of obstetric emergencies* (3rd ed.). Bristol: Clinical Press Ltd.

Baxley, E. G. (2003). Labor induction: A decade of change. *American Family Physician, 67*(10), 2076–2080.

Belfort, M. A. (2003). Operative vaginal delivery. In J. R. Scott, R. S. Gibbs, B. Y. Karlan, & A. F. Haney (Eds.), *Danforth's obstetrics and gynecology* (9th ed., pp. 419–447). Philadelphia: Lippincott Williams & Wilkins.

Boyle, J. J., & Katz, V. L. (2005). Umbilical cord prolapse in current obstetric practice. *Journal of Reproductive Medicine, 50*(5), 303–306.

Carter, S. (1999). Overview of common obstetric bleeding disorders. *Nurse Practitioner, 24*(3), 50–73.

Caughey, A. B., Sandberg, P. L., Zlatnik, M. G., Thiet, M. P., Parer, J. T., & Laros, R. K., Jr. (2005). Forceps compared with vacuum: Rates of neonatal and maternal morbidity. *Obstetrics and Gynecology, 106*(5 Pt. 1), 908–912.

Cesario, S. (2003). Obesity in pregnancy: What every nurse needs to know. *AWHONN Lifelines, 7*(2), 118–125.

Chadwick, J. (2002). Malpresentations and malpositions. In M. Boyle (Ed.), *Emergencies around childbirth: A handbook for midwives.* Oxon, UK: Radcliffe Medical Press.

Cheng, Y. W., Shaffer, B. L., & Caughey, A. B. (2006). The association between persistent occiput posterior position and neonatal outcomes. *Obstetrics and Gynecology, 107*(4), 837–844.

Christianson, L. M., Bovbjerg, V. E., McDavitt, E. C., & Hullfish, K. L. (2003). Risk factors for perineal injury during delivery. *American Journal of Obstetrics and Gynecology, 189*(1), 255–260.

Clayworth, S. (2000). The nurse's role during oxytocin administration. *Journal of Maternal–Child Nursing, 25,* 80–85.

Coffman, S., & Ray, M. A. (2002). African American women describe support processes during high-risk pregnancy and postpartum. *Journal of Obstetrical, Gynecological, and Neonatal Nursing, 31*(5), 536–544.

Coleman, V. H., Erickson, K., Schulkin, J., Zinberg, S., & Sachs, B. P. (2005). Vaginal birth after cesarean delivery: Practice patterns of obstetrician-gynecologists. *Journal of Reproductive Medicine, 50*(4), 261–266.

Cruikshank, D. P. (2003). Breech, other malpresentations, and umbilical cord complications. In J. R. Scott, R. S. Gibbs, B. Y. Karlan, & A. F. Haney (Eds.), *Danforth's obstetrics and gynecology* (9th ed., pp. 381–395). Philadelphia: Lippincott Williams & Wilkins.

Cunningham, F. G., Gant, N. F., Leveno, K. J., Bloom, S. L., Hauth, J. C., Gilstrap, L. C., III, & Wenstrom, K. D. (2005). *Williams obstetrics* (22nd ed). New York: McGraw-Hill.

Dauphinee, J. D. (2004). VBAC: Safety for the patient and the nurse. *Journal of Obstetrical, Gynecological, and Neonatal Nursing, 33*(1), 105–115.

Dilbaz, B., Ozturkoglu, E., Dilbaz, S., Ozturk, N., Sivaslioglu, A. A., & Haberal, A. (2006). Risk factors and perinatal outcomes associated with umbilical cord prolapse. *Archives of Gynecology and Obstetrics, 274*(2), 104–107.

Doyle, N. M., Riggs, J. W., Ramin, S. M., Sosa, M. A., & Gilstrap, L. C. 3rd. (2005). Outcomes of term vaginal breech delivery. *American Journal of Perinatology, 22*(6), 325–328.

Dudley, D. J. (2003). Complications of labor. In J. R. Scott, R. S. Gibbs, B. Y. Karlan, & A. F. Haney (Eds.), *Danforth's obstetrics and gynecology* (9th ed., pp. 397–417). Philadelphia: Lippincott Williams & Wilkins.

Durnwald, C., & Mercer, B. (2004). Vaginal birth after cesarean delivery: Predicting success, risk of failure. *Journal of Maternal, Fetal, and Neonatal Medicine, 15*(6), 388–393.

Ehrenberg, H. M., Mercer, B. M., & Catalano, P. M. (2004). The influence of obesity and diabetes on the prevalence of macrosomia. *American Journal of Obstetrics and Gynecology, 191*(3), 964–968.

Ellings, J., Newman, R., & Bowers, N. (1998). Intrapartum care for women with multiple pregnancy. *Journal of Obstetrical and Neonatal Nursing, 27*(4), 466–472.

Fischer, R. (2005). Breech presentation. [E-Medicine]. Retrieved May 19, 2006, from http://www.emedicine.com/med/topic3272.htm.

Ghosh, M. K. (2005). Breech presentation: Evolution of management. *Journal of Reproductive Medicine, 50*(2), 108–116.

Gilbert, E., & Harmon, J. (2003). *Manual of high risk pregnancy and delivery* (3rd ed.). St. Louis: Mosby.

Gilbert, W., & Danielsen, B. (2003). Pregnancy outcomes associated with intrauterine growth restriction. *American Journal of Obstetrics and Gynecology, 188*(6), 1596–1601.

Gramellini, D., Fieni, S., Kaihura, C., Faiola, S., & Vadora, E. (2003). Transabdominal antepartum amnioinfusion. *International Journal of Gynaecology and Obstetrics, 83*(2), 171–178.

Guinn, D. A., & Gibbs, R. S. (2003). Preterm labor and delivery. In J. R. Scott, R. S. Gibbs, B. Y. Karlan, & A. F. Haney (Eds.), *Danforth's obstetrics and gynecology* (9th ed., pp. 173–190). Philadelphia: Lippincott Williams & Wilkins.

Gurewitsch, E. D., Johnson, E., Hamzehzadeh, S., & Allen, R. H. (2006). Risk factors for brachial plexus injury with and without shoulder dystocia. *American Journal of Obstetrics and Gynecology, 194*(2), 486–492.

Hadi, H. (2000). Cervical ripening and labor induction: Clinical guidelines. *Clinical Obstetrics and Gynecology, 43,* 524–536.

Healy, A. J., & Gaddipati, S. (2005). Intrapartum management of twins: Truths and controversies. *Clinics in Perinatology, 32*(2), 455–473.

Hellsten, C., Lindqvist, P. G., & Olofsson, P. (2003). Vaginal breech delivery: Is it still an option? *European Journal of Obstetrical, Gynecological, and Reproductive Biology, 111*(2), 122–128.

Herzig, K., Danley, D., Jackson, R., Petersen, R., Chamberlain, L., & Gerbert, B. (2006). Seizing the 9-month moment: Addressing behavioral risks in prenatal patients. *Patient Education and Counseling, 61*(2), 228–235.

Hutton, E. K., & Hofmeyr, G. J. (2006). External cephalic version for breech presentation before term. *Cochrane Database of Systematic Reviews, Jan 25*(1), CD000084.

James, C. (2001). Obesity and pregnancy: Obstetric and anesthetic implications. *Current Reviews for Perianaesthesia Nurses, 23*(19), 221–232.

Jazayeri, A., & Contreras, D. (2005). Macrosomia. *E-Medicine.* [Online] Available at: http://emedicine.com/med/topic3279.htm.

Jevitt, C. M. (2005). Shoulder dystocia: Etiology, common risk factors, and management. *Journal of Midwifery and Women's Health, 50*(6), 485–497.

Jibodu, O. (2000). Caesarean section on request. *Journal of the Society of Obstetricians and Gynaecologists of Canada, 22*(9), 684–689.

Johanson, R. B., & Menon, B. K. (2000). Vacuum extraction versus forceps for assisted vaginal delivery. *Cochrane Database of Systematic Reviews, 2,* CD000224.

Johnson, J. H., Figueroa, R., Garry, D., Elimian, A., & Maulik, D. (2004). Immediate maternal and neonatal effects of forceps and vacuum-assisted deliveries. *Obstetrics and Gynecology, 103*(3), 513–518.

Kavanagh, J., & Kelly, A. J. (2005). Sexual intercourse for cervical ripening and induction of labor. *Cochrane Database of Systematic Reviews,* CD003093. DOI: 10.1002/24651858. CD003393.

Kavanagh, J., Kelly, A. J., & Thomas, J. (2005). Breast stimulation for cervical ripening and induction of labor. *Cochrane Database of Systematic Reviews,* CD003092. DOI: 10.1002/24651858. CD003392.

Kayani, S. I., & Alfirevic, Z., (2005). Uterine rupture after induction of labour in women with previous caesarean section. *British Journal of Obstetrics and Gynecology, 112*(4), 451–455.

Kolas, T., Hofoss, D., Daltveit, A. K., Nilsen, S. T., Henriksen, T., Hager, R., et al. (2003). Indications for cesarean deliveries in Norway. *American Journal of Obstetrics and Gynecology, 188*(4), 864–870.

Kwek, K., & Yeo, G. S. (2006). Shoulder dystocia and injuries: Prevention and management. *Current Opinion in Obstetrics and Gynecology, 18*(2), 123–128.

Locksmith, G. J., Gei, A. F., Rowe, T. F., Yeomans, E. R., & Hankins, G. D. (2001). Teaching the Laufe-Piper forceps technique at cesarean delivery. *Journal of Reproductive Medicine, 46*(5), 457–461.

Mackenzie, I. Z., Cooke, I., & Annan, B. (2003). Indications for cesarean section in a consultant obstetric unit over three decades. *Journal of Obstetrics and Gynecology, 23*(3), 233–238.

Magtibay, P., Ramin, K., Harris, D., Ransey, P., & Ogburn, P. (1998). Misoprostol as a labor induction agent. *Journal of Maternal–Fetal Medicine, 7,* 15–18.

McQuivey, R. W. (2004). Vacuum-assisted delivery: A review. *Journal of Maternal, Fetal, and Neonatal Medicine, 16*(3), 171–180.

Moore, J., & Baldisseri, M. R. (2005). Amniotic fluid embolism. *Critical Care Medicine, 33*(10 Suppl), S279–285.

Moore, L., & Martin, J. N. Jr. (2003). Prolonged pregnancy. In J. R. Scott, R. S. Gibbs, B. Y. Karlan, & A. F. Haney (Eds.), *Danforth's obstetrics and gynecology* (9th ed., pp. 219–223). Philadelphia: Lippincott Williams & Wilkins.

Newton, E. R. (2004). Preterm labor. [E-Medicine]. Retrieved May 19, 2006, from http://www.emedicine.com/med/topic3245.htm.

Nichols, J., & Zwelling, E. (1997). *Maternal–newborn nursing: Theory and practice.* Philadelphia: W. B. Saunders.

Omar-Hashi, K. (1994). Female genital mutilation: Perspectives from a Somalian midwife [commentary]. *Birth, 21*(4), 224–226.

Oyelese, Y., & Smulian, J. C. (2006). Placenta previa, placenta accreta, and vasa previa. *Obstetrics and Gynecology, 107*(4), 927–941.

Palmer, C. (2002). Obstetric emergencies and anesthetic management. *Current Reviews for Perianesthesia Nurses, 24*(11), 121–132.

Patel, R. R., & Murphy, D. J. (2004). Forceps delivery in modern obstetric practice. *British Medical Journal, 328*(7451), 1302–1305.

Perozzi, K. J., & Englert, N. C. (2004). Amniotic fluid embolism: An obstetric emergency. *Critical Care Nurse, 24*(4), 54–61.

Pope, C. S., O'Grady, J. P., & Hoffman, D. (2004). Vacuum extraction. [E-Medicine]. Retrieved April 28, 2006, from http://www.emedicine.com/med/topic3389.htm.

Rai, J., & Schreiber, J. R. (2005). Cervical ripening. [E-Medicine]. Available at: http://www.emedicine.com/med/topic3282.htm.

Ramsey, P. S., & Repke, J. T. (2003). Intrapartum management of multifetal pregnancies. *Seminars in Perinatology, 27*(1), 54–72.

Ressel, G. W. (2004). ACOG releases report on dystocia and augmentation of labor. *American Family Physician, 69*(5), 1290–1291.

Robinson, H. E., O'Connell, C. M., Joseph, K. S., & McLeod, N. L. (2005). Maternal outcomes in pregnancies complicated by obesity. *Obstetrics and Gynecology, 106*(6), 1357–1364.

Ross, M. G., Beall, M. H., & Bonni, A. (2006). Forceps delivery. [E-Medicine]. Retrieved April 28, 2006, from http://www.emedicine.com/med/topic3284.htm.

Schmidt, J. (1999). Prolonged pregnancy. In L. Mandeville & N. Troiano (Eds.), *High-risk and critical care intrapartum nursing* (2nd ed.). Philadelphia: Lippincott Williams & Wilkins.

Schoening, A. M. (2006). Amniotic fluid embolism: Historical perspectives and new possibilities. *MCN—American Journal of Maternal Child Nursing, 31*(2), 78–83.

Sheiner, E., Levy, A., Hershkovitz, R., Hallak, M., Hammel, R. D., Katz, M., & Mazor, M. (2006). Determining factors associated with shoulder dystocia: A population-based study. *European Journal of Obstetrics, Gynecology, and Reproductive Biology, 126*(1), 11–15.

Silver, R. K., Haney, E. I., Grobman, W. A., MacGregor, S. N., Casele, H. L., & Neerhof, M. G. (2000). Comparison of active phase labor between triplet, twin, and singleton gestations. *Journal of the Society for Gynecologic Investigation, 7*(5), 297–300.

Simpson, K. (2002). *Cervical ripening and induction and augmentation of labor* (2nd ed.). Washington, DC: AWHONN.

Sittner, B. J., DeFrain, J., & Hudson, D. B. (2005). Effects of high-risk pregnancies on families. *MCN—American Journal of Maternal Child Nursing, 30*(2), 121–126.

Skupski, D., Harrison-Restelli, C. & Dupont, R. (2003). External cephalic version. *Gynecologic and Obstetric Investigation, 56,* 83–88.

Society of Obstetricians and Gynaecologists in Canada. (2005). SOGC clinical practice guidelines. Guidelines for vaginal birth after previous caesarean birth. Number 155 (replaces guideline Number 147), February 2005. *International Journal of Gynaecology and Obstetrics, 89*(3), 319–331.

Society of Obstetricians and Gynaecologists in Canada, (2000). *Advances in labor and risk management* (7th ed.). Ottawa: Author.

Taylor, M. J. (2006). The management of multiple pregnancy. *Early Human Development 82*(6), 365–370.

Tenore, J. L. (2003). Methods for cervical ripening and induction of labor. *American Family Physician, 67*(10), 2123–2128.

Watson-Blasoli, J. (2001). Double-take: Defining the need for specialized prenatal care for women expecting twins: A Canadian perspective. *AWHONN Lifelines, 5*(2), 34–42.

Wax, J. R., Cartin, A., Pinette, M. G., & Blackstone, J. (2004). Patient choice cesarean: An evidence-based review. *Obstetrics and Gynecology Survey, 59*(8), 601–616.

Whitehorn, J., Ayonrinde, O., & Maingay, S. (2002). Female genital mutilation: Cultural and psychological implications. *Sexual and Relationship Therapy, 17*(2), 161–170.

Wilkes, P. T., & Galan, H. (2002). Postdate pregnancy. [E-Medicine]. Retrieved May 19, 2006, from http://www.emedicine.com/med/topic3248.htm.

Youngkin, E. Q., & Davis, M. S. (2004). Women's health: A primary care clinical guide. Upper Saddle River, NJ: Prentice Hall.

CHAPTER 17

Pharmacologic Pain Management of Labor

Judy Kaye Smith, MSN, RN, BC

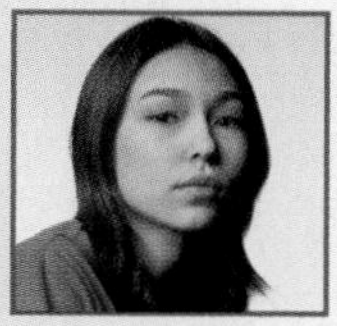

Marnie is a 20-year-old gravida 1, para 0 client admitted to the labor and delivery unit. She is experiencing contractions that last approximately 30 seconds every 5 to 6 minutes. She denies taking any drugs or medications during the pregnancy except for prenatal vitamins. Marnie is using relaxation breathing that she learned during her expectant childbirth classes but states, "When my contractions get stronger, I definitely want something for the pain."

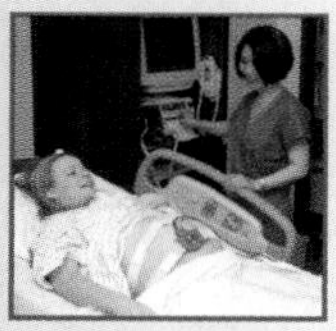

Felicia, 36 years old, is admitted to the health care facility in active labor. Her husband, Chuck, is with her. This is Felicia's third pregnancy. Her cervix is 80% effaced and 5 cm dilated. She is experiencing moderately strong contractions that last for 60 seconds every 4 minutes. Health history reveals the use of pudendal blocks during her two previous vaginal births.

You will learn more about these stories later in this chapter. Nurses working with these clients and others like them need to understand this chapter to manage care and address issues appropriately. Before beginning, consider the following points related to the above scenarios:

- What care is appropriate for clients experiencing pain related to uterine contractions during labor?
- What aspects of the two clients' histories and pregnancies are similar? What components are different?
- What factors might be contributing to each client's pain?
- What behavioral manifestations might each client exhibit in response to pain?
- What medications would be most appropriate for Marnie? For Felicia?

LEARNING OBJECTIVES

On completion of this chapter, the reader should be able to:

- Define the relevant terms that describe pain management strategies within a multicultural perspective.
- Describe the two major theories related to pain.
- Identify methods of pharmacologic pain management.
- Compare and contrast the different methods used to achieve analgesia and anesthesia.
- Discuss complications of regional anesthesia.
- Describe the processes involved in the administration of general anesthesia.
- Describe collaborative care related to specific forms of pain management.

KEY TERMS

ambulatory epidural pump
analgesia
anesthesia
client-controlled analgesia
epidural anesthesia block
epidural blood patch
general anesthesia
local anesthesia
narcotic agonist-antagonists
narcotic antagonist
pain threshold
pain tolerance
referred pain
sedative hypnotics
somatic pain
spinal anesthesia
transition
visceral pain

Pain is a unique experience that varies for each person. What one woman may describe as mild, cramping, achy discomfort, another might describe as the most excruciating feeling she has ever known. The Joint Commission on Accreditation of Healthcare Organizations (JCAHO) Standard RT.1.2.7 (2001) states that clients have the right to appropriate assessment and management of their pain. For this reason, most health care facilities now require nurses to initially assess each client for level of pain on admission and to perform further pain evaluations with each subsequent physical assessment.

Because pain is so subjective, nurses need to develop an understanding of not only the physiology and psychology of pain, but also the pharmacology behind pain relief methods and how cultural beliefs about pain can affect client perceptions. Nurses and clients need to discuss plans regarding pain management. Ideally, such discussion can occur at or before the client's admission to the health care facility. Through assessment of the client's understanding of the different methods of relief, nurses can identify areas for which additional education and collaborative care may be necessary. Nurses should provide information and act as client advocates to gather needed information regarding the various methods of pain relief. If clients express interest in having epidural anesthesia during labor, informed consent is essential, with thorough explanations and the client's signature on the facility's form to confirm understanding.

Nursing interventions generally begin with nonpharmacologic measures such as client teaching and emotional and physical support (see Chap. 14). When pain exceeds the client's threshold for coping, she may require pharmacologic measures to facilitate pain relief. This chapter explores the various facets of collaborative care related to the phenomenon of pain during labor and childbirth.

PHYSIOLOGY OF LABOR PAIN

Pain is considered an unpleasant, subjective sensory and emotional experience associated with actual or potential tissue damage (Falk, 2006). This universally recognized phenomenon is caused by some type of noxious stimuli and is a frequent and compelling reason for seeking health care. From a behavioral perspective, pain is a pattern of response that functions to protect a person from harm.

Pain Terminology

Pain threshold is the point at which a person physically perceives a sensation as painful. **Pain tolerance** is the maximum amount of pain that a person is willing to endure (Munoz & Luckmann, 2005).

Pain can be described as visceral, somatic, or referred. **Visceral pain** refers to a superficial type of pain. An example is the pain most clients usually experience with contractions during the first stage of labor (see Chap. 15), starting over the lower portion of the abdomen and radiating to the lumbar region and down the thighs. **Somatic pain** is usually deeper than visceral pain and is similar to the pain during the late phases of the first stage of labor and the second stage of labor. Somatic pain in labor results from stretching of the perineal tissues to allow passage of fetus. **Referred pain** is felt at a site different from the injured or diseased organ or part of the body responsible for the pain. An example is pain during labor that a woman may feel in the back, flank, or thighs.

Variations in Labor Pain

Pain during labor generally results from normal physiologic processes and obstetrical factors, including progressive cervical dilation, perineal distention, intensity and duration of contractions, and fetal position and size. Labor pain is an example of acute pain, which varies greatly among people and changes at various points.

Sympathetic and parasympathetic nerve fibers link the uterus to the autonomic nervous system, which has both inhibitory and excitatory cell bodies in the nerve ganglia. The uterine nerve receptors are sensitive to pressure or stretching, thus creating contraction of the smooth muscle in the uterus. As pressure and stretching of the uterine tissues increase, actual or potential damage occurs, which releases the substances that cause pain.

First Stage of Labor

During the first stage, the cervix dilates, and the lower uterine segment stretches (Fig. 17.1). Hypoxia develops, and lactic acid accumulates in the uterine muscle. Cervical dilation and lower uterine stretching create traction on the ovaries, fallopian tubes, and uterine ligaments. Pressure on the maternal pelvis causes afferent pain impulses to travel along the sympathetic nerves that enter the neuroaxis between the 10th and 12th thoracic and first lumbar spinal segment (Simpson & Creehan, 2001). Stimulation of these nerves causes chemical mediators to release substances into the extracellular fluid surrounding the pain fibers. The substances include histamine, bradykinin, cholecystokinin, serotonin, potassium ions, norepinephrine, prostaglandins, leukotrienes, and substance P (Falk, 2006). The first six substances stimulate pain sensation at nociceptors in the skin, bone periosteum, joint surfaces, and arterial walls. The latter three substances (prostaglandins, leukotrienes, and substance P) actually sensitize the large myelinated a-delta and small unmyelinated C fibers along which the pain impulse is transmitted to the spinal cord. The C fibers conduct impulses slowly and tend to carry duller, low-level discomfort, whereas the a-delta fibers carry sharper, more localized pain.

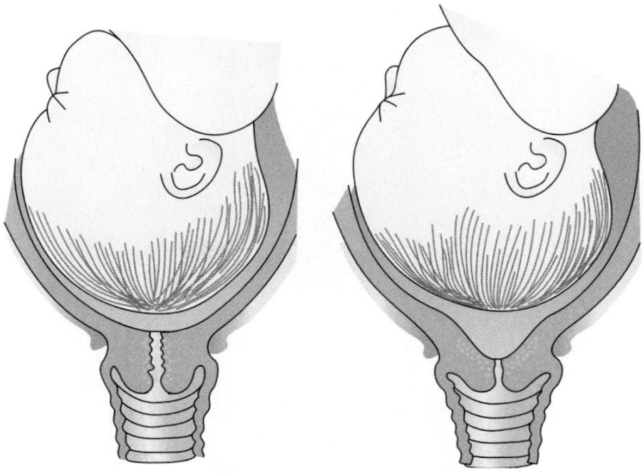

FIGURE 17.1 During the first stage of labor, progressive cervical dilatation and lower uterine stretching create traction on the maternal reproductive structures, which can lead to pain.

In the dorsal horn of the spinal column, somatostatin, cholecystokinin, and substance P serve as neurotransmitters for the pain impulse across the synapse between the peripheral and spinal nerves. The sensation then ascends the spinal column to the brain cortex, which interprets the sensation as pain (Fig. 17.2).

The degree of pain in labor changes as dilation progresses, but the client's ability to tolerate the changes varies with the duration of labor. Exhaustion from lack of sleep or prolonged labor can contribute to increased pain perception. If the fetal presenting part is descending in the occipital-posterior position, the force of the contractions may push the presenting part into the client's sacrum and coccyx, producing lower back pain.

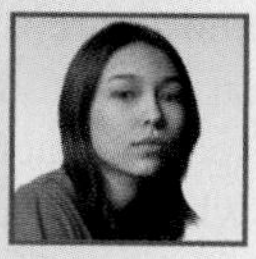

Think back to Marnie, the client in labor from the beginning of the chapter, who is using breathing techniques to help manage her discomfort. How might Marnie's pain level change as she progresses through the first stage of labor?

Second Stage of Labor

During the second stage of labor, descent of the fetal presenting part exerts pressure on the pelvic floor muscles,

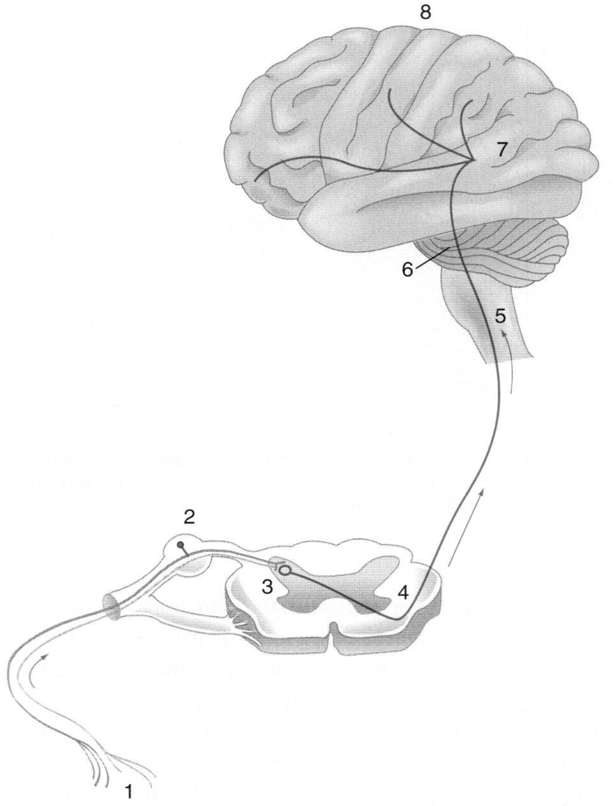

FIGURE 17.2 (1) Pain receptors transmit the sensation of pain through sensory nerves into the dorsal root ganglia. (2) The pain impulse enters the spinal cord. (3, 4) Signals cross the cord and ascend to (5) the reticular formation, (6) midbrain, (7) thalamus, and (8) cerebral cortex.

vagina, perineum, and vulva. This pressure, in turn, places stress on the urethra, bladder, and rectum. As a result, all these areas are likely to be painful and in discomfort (Fig. 17.3).

In response to the physical discomfort produced by labor contractions, physiologic responses to the pain occur over which the woman has little control. Labor pain often causes anxiety (Lang et al., 2006). When anxiety is unrelieved, cortisol, glucagons, and catecholamines naturally multiply, leading to increased metabolism and oxygen consumption. The increased levels of catecholamines also cause hypoperfusion of the uterus and decreased blood flow to the placenta, which can in turn lead to increased uterine contractility. Such increased contractility can place the fetus at risk for asphyxia, which appears as nonreassuring fetal heart rate changes on fetal monitoring (Britt & Pasero, 1999).

As labor continues, the period between uterine contractions becomes gradually shorter. As the client prepares to push, intervals between contractions may be only a few seconds. The point at which the cervix is at 7 to 10 cm and uterine contractions are occurring every minute is known as **transition** and is likely to be the peak intensity of labor pain.

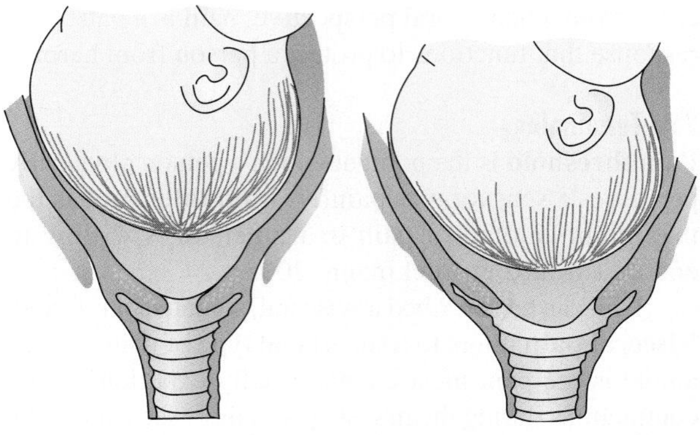

FIGURE 17.3 In the second stage of labor, much pain comes from pressure of the fetal presenting part on the maternal pelvis, genitalia, and perineum.

Third and Fourth Stages of Labor

At birth, afferent pain impulses travel along the sympathetic nerve fibers that enter the neuroaxis between the second and fourth sacral spinal segments and follow much the same pathway as outlined during the first stage of labor. Although pushing can be exhausting and taxing, many clients find the experience of pushing out the newborn and placenta a relief from pain. Obviously, the amount of pain will be related to how quickly the client moves from crowning to expulsion, whether the birth needs to be assisted through use of forceps or other devices, whether lacerations develop or an episiotomy is necessary, and other variables. Additionally, these and other aspects are likely to influence the client's experience of pain during the fourth stage of labor (the first hour after childbirth). At this time, however, the client's recovery also may be facilitated by distraction and stronger emotions as she interacts with her newborn for the first moments of life (Fig. 17.4).

QUOTE 17-1

"My mother always told me that you forget the pain of childbirth once your baby is born. I wouldn't say I've forgotten it, but holding my little one in my arms and interacting with her every day definitely makes up for the pain!"

A client recounting her experiences with labor, childbirth, and postpartum

PSYCHOLOGY OF PAIN

All pain involves both physical and psychological components. A person's thoughts, feelings, and beliefs are interconnected with her perceptions of pain (Fig. 17.5). People may experience more pain when they focus on it, if they have been told to expect one thing but experience

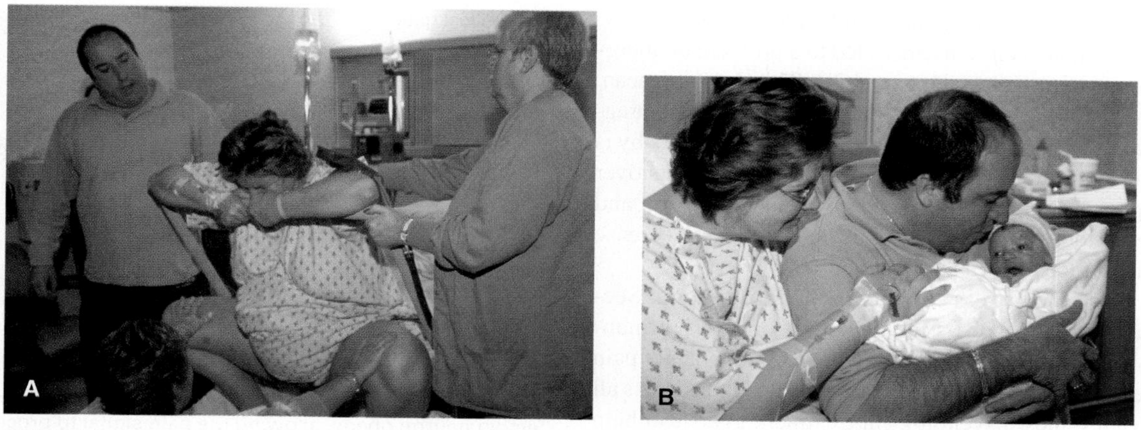

FIGURE 17.4 (**A**) Many women find pushing to be a relief of pain, although it is challenging and exhausting. (**B**) During the postpartum recovery period, initial bonding with the newborn and the positive emotions it engenders can help mitigate residual pain and discomfort from childbirth.

something different, or if they expect a high level of pain and are tense as well as being under stress (Alehagen et al., 2005). Researchers believe that stimuli are filtered through the limbic-hypothalamic system and that the frontal cortex in the brain influences rational interpretation and response to pain (Falk, 2006).

Acute pain, such as labor pain, is primarily physical in nature. It usually has a finite duration and can be relieved by various nonpharmacologic methods (see Chap. 14) and pharmacologic agents. Chronic pain has a distinctly significant psychological component that needs both physical and psychological interventions. Chronic pain generally results from ongoing physical damage or the body's inability to heal (eg, arthritis, cancer, trauma). Clients usually develop emotional symptoms when medical treatment does not eliminate pain.

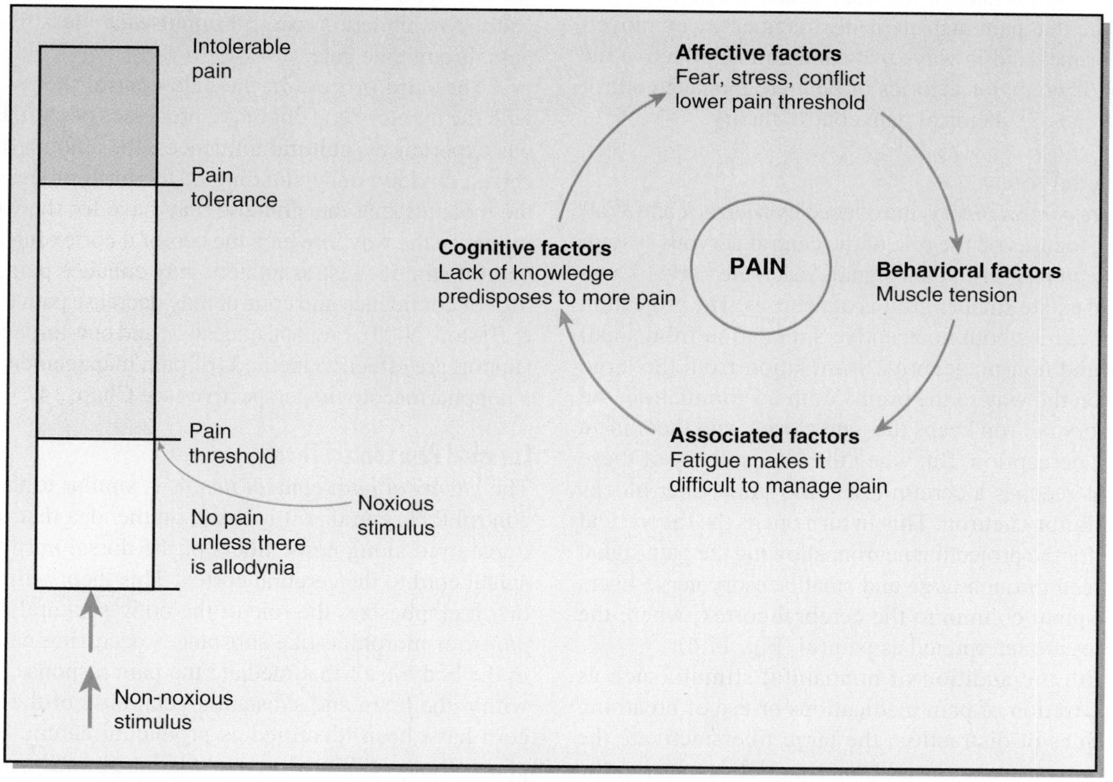

FIGURE 17.5 Many factors at various levels can interact to produce an individual pain response.

Chronic pain following labor and childbirth is unlikely, unless a client's circumstances led to a problem or abnormality requiring special intervention. This does not mean, however, that all pain or discomfort associated with pregnancy and childbirth will disappear as soon as the baby is born. The maternal body makes many adjustments over the postpartum weeks and months, and exhaustion and other emotions during that time actually may decrease her tolerance of pain at this time.

Emotional stress can increase pain intensity. Secondary factors such as the degree of disability, financial stress, or loss of work are also part of a client's pain experience, and treatment must be designed to address all relevant issues. Psychological treatment goals can help clients to learn how to predict and manage the pain cycle, use coping skills to minimize pain, and maximize active involvement in positive life experiences, despite pain.

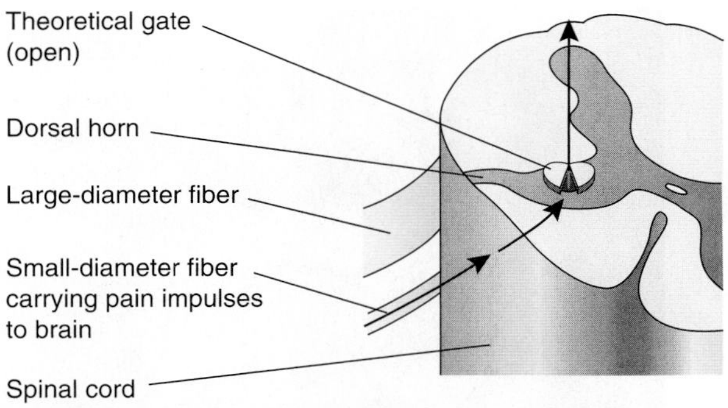

FIGURE 17.6 In the gate control theory, the small fiber blocks the inhibitory neuron that normally preserves a pain-free state. In turn, the theoretical "gate" for the projection neuron opens, allowing the pain signal to proceed through large and small sensory nerve fibers in the spinal column to the cerebral cortex, where the impulses are interpreted as painful.

THEORIES OF PAIN

Each client's experience with pain is different; furthermore, each pain experience for that particular client also may be unique. For example, a woman may experience significant pain during labor in her first pregnancy, but less pain in a subsequent pregnancy. A host of factors influence pain experiences, including physiologic, psychosocial, cultural, and environmental aspects.

Understanding theories about what causes pain perception is important for nurses, because it can help them to ensure that pain management strategies are employed during times and in ways that can be most effective for clients. Two major theories of pain are the gate control theory and the chemical pain control theory.

Gate Control Theory

The *gate control theory,* introduced by Melzack and Wall (1965), focuses on the role of the central nervous system in the pain response. Pain signals reach the nervous system and excite smaller groups of neurons. The projection neuron carries both nociceptive stimulation from small fibers and non-nociceptive stimulation from the large fibers on the way to the brain. With no stimulation, the inhibitory neuron keeps the gate closed, and there is no painful perception. But when the total activity of these neurons reaches a certain level, the small fiber blocks the inhibitory neuron. This in turn opens the theoretical "gate" for the projection neuron, allowing the pain signal to proceed through large and small sensory nerve fibers in the spinal column to the cerebral cortex, where the impulses are interpreted as painful (Fig. 17.6).

With the addition of nonpainful stimuli, such as administration of pain medications or use of breathing techniques or distraction, the large fibers activate the inhibitory neuron, partially or completely closing the gate, depending on the strength of the stimulation competing with the painful stimuli for access to the projection neuron (Falk, 2006). Physical, emotional, and behavioral injury or anxiety may potentiate pain, whereas relaxation techniques and distraction may alleviate pain (Simkin & Bolding, 2004). The areas in which the gates operate are usually in the dorsal horn of the spinal cord and the brainstem.

A second process in the gate control theory is the stimulation of the reticular activating system (RAS) in the brainstem. The RAS interprets visual, auditory, and painful stimuli. When the cerebral cortex is focused on visual or auditory stimulation, painful impulses are less likely to pass through the gate.

The third process in the gate control theory deals with the memory and cognitive processes of pain. Previous experiences, cultural influences, the amount of perceived anxiety, understanding of the birth process, and the meaning that the situation may have for the woman influence the way in which the cerebral cortex interprets painful stimuli. Just as anxiety may enhance pain, feelings of confidence and control may decrease pain (Green & Baston, 2003). Prenatal education and one-to-one labor support are effective methods of pain management from a nonpharmacologic perspective (see Chap. 14).

Chemical Pain Control Theory

The *chemical pain control theory* is similar to the gate control theory in that it is based on the idea that pain is transferred along nerve fibers of the dorsal horn of the spinal cord to the cerebral cortex. This theory differs in that it emphasizes the role of the body's natural *endorphins,* or morphine-like substances occurring naturally in the body itself that mediate the pain response. Areas within the brain and substantia gelatinosa of the spinal cord have been identified as producing natural endorphins (Yerby, 2000). These endorphins generally increase during pregnancy and the postpartum period and may help clients who choose to use nonpharmacologic pain relief methods only to move through the labor and childbirth experience without needing medications. The body's ability to produce and maintain endorphins also influences a client's perception of pain at any given time as well as her overall ability to tolerate pain.

INFLUENCES ON PAIN AND PAIN MANAGEMENT

For centuries, discomfort during labor and birth was considered inevitable and something that women simply had to endure. Nevertheless, people searched for many remedies to provide labor pain relief. Early Chinese writings mention the use of opiates and herbs such as hemp and mandrake; Persian writings discuss the drinking of wine by women in labor, and wine, beer, and brandy were commonly self-administered in Europe during the Middle Ages (Yerby, 2000). The greatest strides in labor pain management, however, occurred during the past 200 years.

In the mid-19th century, the use of anesthesia was introduced in Great Britain and the United States. The early use of ether and chloroform in obstetrical practice has been credited to Dr. James Simpson, professor of midwifery at Edinburgh University (Cohen, 1996). During this period, the American Medical Association Committee on Obstetrics justified the use of anesthesia during labor and birth (Morrison et al., 1996); however, great debate existed over its validity. Some physicians felt that anesthesia masked the mother's response to labor, which was considered to be a valuable guide in determining labor progress. Religious objections also were prominent, based on interpretations of God's decree to Eve in the Garden of Eden (Genesis Chapter 3, Verse 16) that pain for women shall be greatly multiplied during childbirth (Cohen, 1996). The controversy was minimized, however, when a doctor in 1853 administered chloroform to Queen Victoria during the birth of her ninth child, Prince Leopold (Morrison et al., 1996). By 1862, chloroform and ether had become widely used anesthetics in obstetrical practice.

During this same period, other methods of pain relief, including parenteral opioids (eg, morphine and meperidine [Demerol]), as well as parenteral and inhalation anesthesia, were being developed. In the early 1900s, twilight sleep produced by the addition of scopolamine to morphine became an accepted method for pain relief during childbirth. A high incidence of neonatal respiratory distress following its administration, however, led to its discontinuation (Morrison et al., 1996).

In the 1930s, a focus on natural childbirth techniques began with the work of Dr. Grantley Dick Read, who believed that women could use *psychoprophylaxis* (mind over physical matter) to control the pain of childbirth (Yerby, 2000). Dick Read felt that relief of fear and tension could diminish pain to a level at which women would be able to cope or that the pain would possibly even cease. In the 1960s, the Lamaze method of patterned breathing techniques to promote relaxation during labor became popular. These and other nonpharmacologic methods of pain control are discussed in more detail in Chapter 14.

More recently, agonist-antagonist drugs such as nalbuphine (Nubain) and butorphanol (Stadol) have been used to produce sedation, dizziness, and relaxation during the latent phase of the first stage of labor. More refined techniques of epidural anesthesia administration, however, have led to the widespread contemporary use of drugs for pain during active labor.

Cultural Considerations

When clients are asked if any cultural or religious beliefs affect their health care, their response is frequently "No." Nevertheless, nurses should recognize that every client has cultural beliefs and values that influence his or her perceptions, regardless of whether he or she openly recognizes these factors. For example, culture often dictates what a person considers appropriate verbal behavior or body language in response to pain (Munoz & Luckmann, 2005). Therefore, nurses should identify the most frequently seen ethnic and religious groups within their geographic location and develop profiles of their culturally specific responses to pain. Understanding these various cultural responses to pain can assist nurses greatly to recognize and support individual client responses.

Client responses to pain generally can be classified into two broad categories: stoic and emotive. Stoic responses generally are characterized by fewer verbal and nonverbal expressions, with clients seldom complaining or showing emotion. Conversely, emotive responses are frequent, often verbal, and expressive.

First- and second-generation immigrants to the United States and Canada tend to respond to pain in ways that are conventional within their culture of family origin. Later generations who may have assimilated the values of the culture into which they have moved, however, are less likely to retain traditional views about pain (Munoz & Luckmann, 2005). Some clients consider pain a natural part of labor, whereas others view it as excruciating and inhumane (Table 17.1). Additional information on cultural health assessment is provided in the reference list at the end of this chapter.

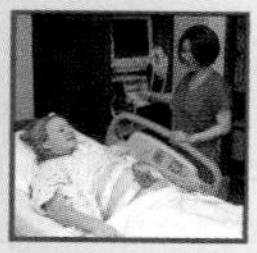

Remember Felicia, the woman in labor with her third child described at the start of the chapter. How might the pain she experienced in previous labors currently influence her perception of her pain?

● **TABLE 17.1 Cultural Views of Pain**

CULTURE	VIEWS
Asian/Pacific Islanders (Japanese, Chinese, Thai, Filipino, Vietnamese, Hawaiian)	Pain is considered a serious symptom of illness for which medical care is sought. Pain is excruciating, but women in labor believe it is disgraceful to verbally express or act out because of pain. Some will moan to express pain. Some believe that pain and illness are a punishment from God and that it is not appropriate to interfere with God's plan. They may refuse pain medications because of their religious beliefs. Some will dislike IM injections and prefer oral or IV routes of administration.
European-American European-Canadian	Pain is a physical experience with personal, social, cultural, and spiritual dimensions. They generally regard pain as a symptom of illness or injury, express pain readily, and are likely to seek pain relief.
Native Americans	Pain generally is undertreated in this population. Clients often tend to be stoic, tolerate a high level of pain, and use meditation, self-control, and traditional herbs for pain management. They make complaints of pain usually in general terms (eg, uncomfortable, doesn't feel good). They may complain more to trusted family than health care workers.
African Americans	Some clients deny or avoid dealing with pain until it is unbearable and only then seek medical attention. Others are more vocally expressive about pain with tears and lamentations.
Scandinavian (Finland, Sweden, Switzerland)	They demonstrate hardiness and resilience and are often stoic about pain. Health care workers must pay close attention to nonverbal cues, changes in conduct, and somatic complaints such as nausea and dizziness when evaluating pain. These clients tend to view pain as a natural part of labor.
Hispanic	They view pain as necessary and an indicator of serious illness. They may see enduring sickness as a sign of strength. They tend to seek health care later than some other cultures. Clients tend not to verbalize complaints of pain, but expression of pain in women is more socially acceptable.
Middle Eastern	They are more expressive about pain, particularly around family members with whom they feel comfortable. Some may have low pain threshold. They can better cope with pain if they understand its source and prognosis. They believe that injections are more effective than pills.

Legal and Ethical Perspectives

Because methods of pain relief available during labor are constantly evolving, clients need to make informed decisions about their preferences. The real challenge for health care providers is to provide optimal care, enabling clients to feel satisfaction with the birth experience, while ensuring that they attain the maximum relief possible. Satisfaction with pain management is difficult to measure, however, because each woman is unique.

Nurses should understand that a client's personal ethical or moral views, shaped through past events, life experiences, thoughts, and actions, need to be considered as influences on her decision making relative to pain management modalities. Clients have the right to make informed decisions based on their ability to take personal responsibility for their decisions, to understand the consequences of their actions, and to make choices apart from coercive or obstructive controlling influences (Lowe, 2004). Informed choice and consent are key factors in the partnership between clients and health care providers.

Choice of pain management methods is personal. Informed consent, however, is a universal legal element for all clients, especially in relation to invasive procedures such as epidural or spinal anesthesia. Three main elements must be present for consent to be considered truly informed:

- The client must receive unbiased information before giving consent.
- Consent must be a voluntary decision.
- The client must be mentally competent and capable of accepting responsibility for the selected decision.

The timing for providing information about pain relief can be difficult. Obviously, giving information during active labor would be least optimal. When at all possible, health care providers must ensure that they give adequate information to the client before she reaches the active phase of labor. Ideally, such discussion occurs well in advance of labor, and at least as soon as labor is suspected. For example, ideal times to discuss and plan for pain management options would be during prenatal appointments. Effective collaborative communication is the key to providing satisfactory pain management for pregnant and childbearing women (Yerby, 2000).

QUOTE 17-2

"During appointments with clients, I really try to discuss with them the different options and techniques available for managing pain in labor. It's much easier with women who have already been through the experience, but many first-time parents can be overwhelmed by the options, risks, and benefits. Still, I find those clients who have been educated about labor pain management tend to have better experiences during the actual event, regardless of what specific methods they choose to employ."

A nurse practitioner/midwife

Drug Pharmacokinetics

Pharmacokinetics refers to drug absorption, metabolism, distribution, and excretion in the body. Physiologic changes during pregnancy and childbirth, such as increased cardiac output, alter a woman's normal pharmacokinetics. Weight gained during pregnancy, although partly the result of fetal growth, also occurs because of changes in fluid balance within the body compartments, which alters the distribution and plasma concentrations of drugs. As progesterone and pregnanediol increase in late pregnancy, the ability of the maternal liver to conjugate drugs may be diminished.

The optimum goal of pharmacologic pain management during labor is to provide maximum pain relief to the mother while ensuring minimum risks to both mother and fetus. Three factors must be considered when determining whether analgesic medications are appropriate for use during labor:

- *Possible effects on the woman.* The effect of pharmacologic agents in labor on the woman poses the greatest concern because fetal well-being depends on adequate functioning of the maternal homeostatic mechanism that maintains adequate oxygenation and circulation to the fetus.
- *Possible effects on the fetus.* All drugs given for pain relief during labor cross the placental barrier by simple diffusion. Some drugs cross more readily than others. The action of drugs depends on the rate at which the medication is metabolized by liver enzymes and excreted by the kidneys. Because the fetal liver and kidneys are too immature to metabolize analgesics, high doses of medications may remain active in the fetal circulation for prolonged periods.
- *Possible effects on the strength and frequency of labor contractions.* Incorrect dosages or medications given at the wrong time can negatively affect the course of labor and childbirth.

TYPES OF PHARMACOLOGIC PAIN MANAGEMENT

Knowledge of the changes that occur during pregnancy, labor, and birth enables health care providers to determine which pharmacologic methods to use as well as the proper dosage to relieve pain without causing severe maternal or fetal side effects. Pain control methods work best when administered as soon as possible after the pain is recognized as uncomfortable.

Sedative Hypnotics

Sedative hypnotics relieve anxiety and induce sleep. They are not a specific drug classification but a description of the effects produced by this group of drugs. In low doses, they cause sedation and rest; higher doses produce a hypnotic effect. Two classifications of sedative hypnotics are barbiturates and histamine-1 (H_1) receptor antagonist (antihistamine) ataractics.

Barbiturates

Barbiturates include secobarbital sodium (Seconal) and pentobarbital (Nembutal). Such medications do not relieve pain but usually are given during early labor to induce sleep, decrease anxiety, and depress the central nervous system.

Clients in prolonged early labor sometimes benefit from a brief period of therapeutic rest or sleep. If clients admitted to the triage area in an obstetrical unit are not dilated to 3 cm but a reactive fetal heart rate strip is present, the health care provider may elect to give an oral dose of secobarbital or pentobarbital and send the client home to await more active labor. Usually after having some rest, true labor with a more coordinated, effective contraction pattern is established.

Ninety percent of secobarbital or pentobarbital is absorbed through the gastrointestinal tract. These drugs have an onset of action within 10 to 15 minutes for oral doses and duration of effect of 3 to 4 hours. The medications are metabolized in the liver and have a half-life of 30 hours with excretion through the urinary tract. They do cross the placenta, possibly affecting the newborn's central nervous system (Karch, 2005). Thus, the newborn may experience decreased responsiveness and ability to suck. Respiratory and vasomotor depression of both mother and fetus also may occur. When these drugs are given without an analgesic, they potentially can create a paradoxical increase in apprehension, causing hyperactivity and disorientation.

Histamine-1 Receptor Antagonist Ataractics

Promethazine hydrochloride (Phenergan) and hydroxyzine hydrochloride (Vistaril) are H_1 receptor antagonist ataractics frequently administered with narcotics during labor to relieve anxiety, increase sedation, and decrease the narcotic side effects of nausea and vomiting. Promethazine is absorbed readily from the gastrointestinal tract and has an onset of action within 20 minutes when administered by the intramuscular (IM) route and within 5 minutes when administered by the intravenous (IV) route. The duration of effect lasts up to 12 hours after administration, and most clients describe feeling sedated or groggy after administration (Karch, 2005). Promethazine is metabolized in the liver and excreted by urine and feces. It crosses the placental barrier and can cause cardiorespiratory depression in the newborn if birth occurs soon after administration.

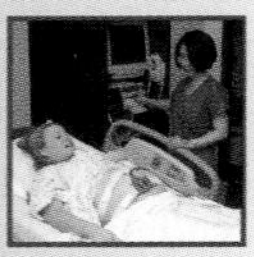

Think back to Felicia, the woman in labor with her third child, discussed at the chapter opening. What if Felicia received promethazine 3 hours ago and now requests to ambulate to the bathroom to urinate. Should the nurse support this request?

Analgesic Compounds

Analgesia means the use of agents to reduce or decrease awareness of pain. Opioid analgesics possess properties derived from or similar to morphine. The other commonly used form of analgesia is narcotic agonist-antagonist compounds.

To provide pain relief, the individual health care provider selects the medication, usually based on his or her preference. Table 17.2 summarizes the most common analgesics used during labor and childbirth.

Opioid Analgesics

Morphine provides excellent analgesia, but its long duration of action (up to 7 hours) after administration and its depressive effects on the newborn limit its use to the latent phase of labor when birth is not anticipated for several hours. Side effects frequently include nausea, vomiting, possible histamine release that causes orthostatic hypotension, and occasional bradycardia (Karch, 2005).

A synthetic morphine-like compound, *meperidine* (Demerol), is one of the most commonly used opioid analgesics in labor (Pharmacology Box 17.1). Meperidine has been found effective in relieving severe, persistent, or recurrent pain. In labor, it helps to relax the cervix and stimulates a feeling of maternal euphoria and well-being. Meperidine is metabolized by the liver to an active form, normeperidine, and excreted through the urine. Peak effect usually occurs 40 to 50 minutes after IM administration. With IV administration, onset of action is rapid (within 30 seconds), reaching peak effects in 5 to 10 minutes. Effects can last up to 3 hours (Karch, 2005).

Meperidine also may be administered in low doses by **client-controlled analgesia,** which is a system of drug dispensing in which a preset IV dose of narcotic agent is delivered when the client presses a button. Use of client-controlled analgesia facilitates more frequent dosing (Fig. 17.7).

The most frequent side effects of meperidine are nausea and vomiting. To minimize them, promethazine (Phenergan) often is given prophylactically with meperidine. In an attempt to minimize effects on the newborn, maternal IV injections should be given during a contraction because blood flow to the fetus is minimal at this point. If birth occurs soon after administration or during peak effect periods, the newborn may experience respiratory depression. Therefore, 0.1 mg/kg of a **narcotic antagonist** (a drug primarily used to treat narcotic-induced respiratory depression) must be readily available for administration to the newborn after birth (Karch, 2005). A commonly used narcotic antagonist is naloxone (Narcan) (Pharmacology Box 17.2). Naloxone can be given intramuscularly, intravenously, or subcutaneously. Its duration of effect is considerably shorter than the analgesic medication for which it is being given. Therefore, nurses should remain alert for the return of respiratory depression and the need for repeated doses of naloxone.

When meperidine is used during labor, implications for breastfeeding mothers during the postpartum period are significant because it may take 2 to 3 days for the body to excrete 95% of the medication. The meperidine that remains within the mother's system is transferred to the baby through the breast milk (Karch, 2005). Because the newborn liver is immature and cannot readily metabolize the residual medication, the baby tends to exhibit neurobehavioral depression for at least 3 days (see Chaps. 20 and 22). Manifestations include general sleepiness and increased problems with latching on for breastfeeding (Beech, 1999). Infants who have been exposed to high doses of meperidine are more likely to cry when handled. Additionally, ability to self-console is reduced for as long as 3 to 6 weeks after administration (Beech, 1999). Thus, before administration, the nurse should find out whether the client intends to breastfeed and advocate for the use of drugs with fewer residual effects.

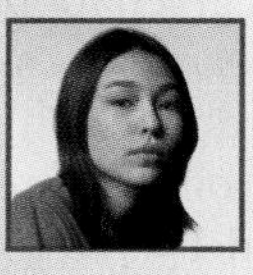

Suppose Marnie, described at the beginning of the chapter, received meperidine for pain during labor. She is breastfeeding her newborn and asks why the newborn is sleepy. How should the nurse respond?

Narcotic Agonist-Antagonist Compounds

Narcotic agonist-antagonists are analgesic agents that stimulate opiate receptors, resulting in pain relief, and block specific opiate receptors, alleviating maternal and neonatal respiratory depression. The latter antagonist property, however, could lead to withdrawal symptoms in opioid-dependent clients and their newborns. Two narcotic agonist-antagonists becoming increasingly popular are butorphanol tartrate (Stadol) and nalbuphine hydrochloride (Nubain). Their major advantage is that they exhibit a *ceiling effect,* which means that once dosages

TABLE 17.2 Analgesic Medications During Labor

ANALGESIA MEDICATION AND DRUG CLASSIFICATION	USUAL DOSAGE/ROUTES	OPTIMAL TIME FOR ADMINISTRATION AND WHEN TO STOP MEDICATION	INDICATION FOR USE/ DESIRED EFFECTS/ NURSING IMPLICATIONS	MATERNAL–FETAL SIDE EFFECTS
Seconal (secobarbital sodium) or Nembutal (pentobarbital) Barbiturate Sedative hypnotic	100–200 mg PO	Early prodromal labor	Sedation; to induce sleep, decrease anxiety, CNS depression	Maternal paradoxical apprehension, hyperactivity, and disorientation Neonatal CNS depression Decreases neonatal ability to suck
Phenergan (promethazine hydrochloride) or Vistaril (Hydroxyzine) Hydrochloride Histamine-1 receptor antagonist (antihistamines) ataractics	12.5–25 mg IM/IV 25–50 mg IM	Early phases of labor	Adjunct therapy to decrease nausea and vomiting associated with opioid narcotic analgesics	Maternal sedation Neonatal cardiopulmonary sedation if birth occurs too soon after administration
Demerol (meperidine) Opioid agonist analgesic/ narcotic analgesic	25–50 mg IV, 50–100 mg IM Usually given with Phenergan IV or Vistaril IM, which potentiate the narcotic effects and decrease nausea and vomiting	Early labor during the first phase of the first stage Pain relief after cesarean birth	Decreases pain impulse transmission by opioid receptors Effective analgesic that produces a sense of well-being Promotes relaxation, which possibly aids cervical relaxation Have Narcan readily available to reverse adverse effects	Can slow labor contractions if given too soon in labor Nausea, vomiting, sedation, neonatal respiratory depression Decreased beat-to-beat variability of the fetal heart rate
Morphine (morphine sulfate) Opioid narcotic analgesic	Intrathecally 0.2–1 mg; 5 mg epidurally	After client is in active labor or in preparation for a cesarean birth	Effective analgesia, relaxation, and pain relief Have Narcan available	Itching Can possibly slow labor progress
Nubain (nalbuphine) or Stadol (butorphanol tartrate) Mixed agonist-antagonist analgesics	10–20 mg IM; 5–10 mg slow IV push 1–2 mg IV/IM	Usually given during the early stages of labor when birth is not imminent	Effective for relief of mild to moderate pain Have Narcan readily available	Mild maternal sedation and some neonatal respiratory depression Dizziness, weakness, nausea and vomiting

Source: Karch, A. M. (2005). *Lippincott's nursing drug guide.* Philadelphia: Lippincott Williams & Wilkins.

PHARMACOLOGY 17.1 Meperidine (Demerol)

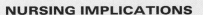

ACTION: Meperidine acts as an agonist at specific opioid receptors in the central nervous system to produce analgesia, sedation, and euphoria.

PREGNANCY CATEGORY: C

DOSAGE: When contractions are regular, 50 to 100 mg IM or SC every 1 to 3 hours.

POSSIBLE ADVERSE EFFECTS: Lightheadedness, dizziness, facial flushing, irregular heart beat, palpitations, pruritus, nausea, vomiting, sweating

NURSING IMPLICATIONS

- Have opioid antagonist and facilities for assisted or controlled respirations available with parenteral administration.
- Use with extreme caution in patients with renal problems.

From: Karch, A. (2005). 2005 *Lippincott's nursing drug guide.* Philadelphia: Lippincott Williams & Wilkins.

pass a certain level, there is no increase in the severity of respiratory distress as a newborn side effect. Therefore, these drugs are considered safer alternatives for clients. There is, however, a negative ceiling effect on the analgesic level, which means that once dosages are given beyond a certain level, there is no further increase in the amount of pain relief obtained from them. Major side effects include drowsiness, dizziness, weakness, nausea, and vomiting. In some clients, these drugs can cause a psychomimetic reaction of dysphoria and unease.

Butorphanol (Stadol). Butorphanol (Stadol) has an analgesic potency 30 to 40 times that of meperidine and 7 times that of morphine (Karch, 2005). It can be given through IM or IV administration, usually in dosages of 1 to 2 mg. Butorphanol takes effect in approximately 5 minutes, peaks in 30 to 60 minutes, and has duration of action of approximately 3 to 4 hours. This drug may cause both maternal and neonatal respiratory depression, but effects may be reversed by administration of naloxone. Butorphanol also has been shown to produce a sinusoidal fetal heart rate pattern before birth (Karch, 2005). Less risk for nausea and vomiting is associated with administration of butorphanol than with meperidine. Butorphanol is considered safer for women who intend to breastfeed because it is metabolized more readily than meperidine. Butorphanol should not be used with clients who have a known dependence on opiates; it should be used with caution in cases of suspected drug dependence because it may precipitate withdrawal symptoms. Urinary retention, although not common, may occur. Therefore, the nurse should be vigilant in assessing for bladder distention. Butorphanol should be stored at room temperature and away from light (Karch, 2005).

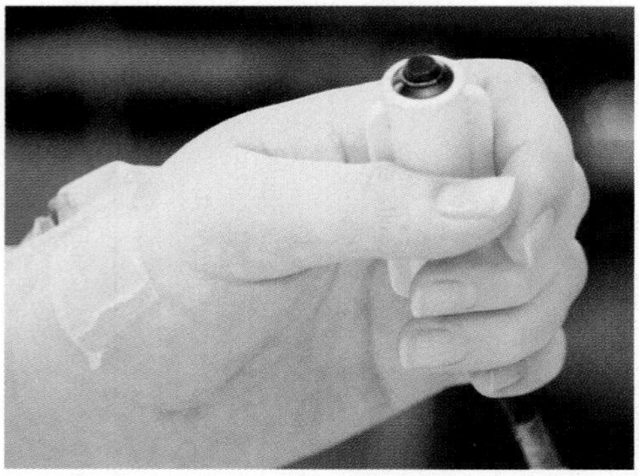

FIGURE 17.7 Client-controlled analgesia.

Nalbuphine. Nalbuphine can be given by IM, subcutaneous, or IV push routes in doses of 5 to 10 mg. With IV administration, the drug produces effects in approximately 2 to 3 minutes, peaks within 15 to 20 minutes, and lasts approximately 3 to 6 hours. IV administration should occur over 3 to 5 minutes; therefore, it should be given over two contractions (Karch, 2005). Adverse effects include respiratory depression, drowsiness, dizziness, crying, blurred vision, diaphoresis, and urinary urgency. Nausea and vomiting also may occur but to a lesser degree than noted with meperidine and other narcotic agents. Nurses need to review the client's history to identify the possibility of contraindications. Examples include a history of past or current drug dependence, sensitivity to sulfites, and asthma (Karch, 2005). If there are no contraindications, the IV route is used most commonly. As with other narcotics and synthetic narcotic derivatives, health care providers should evaluate the client's respiratory status and the fetal heart rate characteristics carefully after administration. Common side effects include dizziness, sedation, confusion, and respiratory depression. Naloxone may be used to reverse the effects of both maternal and neonatal respiratory depression. Nalbuphine is metabolized more readily than meperidine and therefore is safe for clients who intend to breastfeed.

Anesthesia

When analgesics no longer are effectively managing labor pain or when labor progresses to the second stage, alternative methods of relief may need to be considered.

PHARMACOLOGY 17.2 Naloxone Hydrochloride (Narcan)

ACTION: Naloxone hydrochloride is a narcotic antagonist that counteracts the effect of narcotic analgesics.

PREGNANCY CATEGORY: B

DOSAGE: 0.01 mg/kg, administered either IV by umbilical vein, SC, or IM; repeated at 2- to 3-minute intervals until response is obtained.

POSSIBLE ADVERSE EFFECTS:
Hypotension, hypertension, tachycardia, diaphoresis, tremulousness

NURSING IMPLICATIONS

- Anticipate the need for resuscitative measures; have resuscitative equipment and emergency drugs readily available.
- If no IV access is available, prepare for possible administration by endotracheal tube.
- If no response is seen after two or three doses, question whether respiratory depression is caused by narcotics.
- Continuously monitor all vital signs for changes.
- Remember that the pain-relieving effect of narcotics will be reversed; assess for pain in the neonate.

Source: Karch, A. M. (2005). *Lippincott's nursing drug guide.* Philadelphia: Lippincott Williams & Wilkins.

These methods involve anesthesia. **Anesthesia** means the use of agents that cause partial or complete loss of sensation with or without loss of consciousness.

Table 17.3 summarizes the most common anesthetic agents used during labor and childbirth. The various categories of anesthesia have different applications, actions, effects, and requirements. The obstetrician or certified nurse midwife initiates local and pudendal anesthesia, whereas an anesthesiologist or certified nurse anesthetist is responsible for administration of regional (epidural) and general anesthesia. Regardless of the type of anesthesia used, the single most important aspect of care is to ensure client safety. The most optimum way to avert complications involves adequately and thoroughly assessing the client in advance of administering any anesthetic medications.

Local Anesthesia

Local anesthesia is used during vaginal birth to induce loss of sensation in the perineum and vagina during cutting, repair, or both of the episiotomy. Local anesthetic agents injected into the perineum and posterior vagina block the conduction of nerve impulses between the perineum and the central nervous system. The types of nerve fibers react differently to various anesthetic agents. The smaller nerve fibers (small C and a-delta fibers) are more sensitive to local anesthetics, whereas the larger A-alpha, A-beta, and A-gamma fibers continue to retain pressure sensation, muscle tone, sense of position, and motor function.

Absorption of anesthetic agents primarily depends on the vascularity of the area being injected. Such anesthetic agents also increase blood flow to the injected area by causing vasodilation. If the client is healthy or has a high metabolic rate, absorption is expedited. If the client is malnourished, dehydrated, has an electrolyte imbalance, or has a history of cardiovascular or pulmonary problems, toxic side effects are possible. If the anesthetic agent contains a vasoconstrictor such as epinephrine, absorption is delayed, and the anesthetic effect is prolonged. Agents containing vasoconstrictors decrease uteroplacental blood flow, however, which makes it an undesirable additive in most situations. The liver and plasma esterase break down local anesthetics, and the byproduct is excreted by the kidneys. The drug is administered in the weakest possible concentration and the smallest amount necessary to produce the desired numbness. Most agents used for local anesthesia are rapidly metabolized and have little or no effect on the mother or breastfeeding newborn after birth.

Three local anesthetics are currently available for use:

- **Esters.** These include procaine hydrochloride (Novocain), chloroprocaine hydrochloride (Nesacaine), and tetracaine hydrochloride (Pontocaine). They are rapidly metabolized, thereby reducing the potential for maternal toxicity and preventing placental transfer to the fetus.
- **Amides.** Examples include lidocaine hydrochloride (Xylocaine), mepivacaine hydrochloride (Carbocaine), and bupivacaine hydrochloride (Marcaine). These agents are more powerful and longer acting than the esters. They readily cross the placenta and can actually be measured in the fetal circulation.
- **Opiates.** Generally, opiates are reserved for epidural anesthesia but may be used as local anesthetics in select cases. They include morphine (Duramorph) and fentanyl (Sublimaze). When opiates are used in isolation, the amount of pain relief is less effective than when they are combined with a low-dose local anesthetic. The mechanism of action is specific to opiate receptors in the spinal column (Russell & Reynolds, 1997).

Reactions to local anesthetics range from mild, transient symptoms to total cardiovascular collapse. Mild side

TABLE 17.3 Obstetric Anesthesia

ANALGESIA MEDICATION AND DRUG CLASSIFICATION	USUAL DOSAGE/ROUTES	OPTIMAL TIME FOR ADMINISTRATION AND WHEN TO STOP MEDICATION	INDICATION FOR USE/ DESIRED EFFECTS/ NURSING IMPLICATIONS	MATERNAL–FETAL SIDE EFFECTS
Fentanyl (Sublimaze) Opioid Analgesic/ narcotic analgesic	50–100 mcg or 25–50mcg IV; can also be continuously administered epidurally with bupivacaine at 8–12 mL/hr	Generally given epidurally after the client has reached 4–5 cm dilation and is in active labor	For epidural of intrathecal analgesia, usually given in combination with a local anesthetic or given IV to induce relaxation for general anesthesia Monitor client vital signs closely. Preload client with IV fluids.	Maternal hypotension; maternal, fetal respiratory depression; slowing of labor if given too early
Bupivacaine (marcaine) Local anesthetic	Administered with Fentanyl or morphine as a continuous epidural agent in titrated doses based on client's weight	Generally given epidurally after the client has reached 4–5 cm dilation and is in active labor	Rapid onset; loss of pain perception	Maternal hypotension; slowing of labor if given too early; may obliterate pushing sensation; possibly prolongs the second stage of labor
Xylocaine (Lidocaine)	Local anesthetic	Administered just before birth	Produces perineal anesthesia of the perineum, vagina, and vulva in pudendal anesthesia or for local infiltration of perineum just before episiotomy incision	None apparent
Pentothal (thiopental) Short-acting barbiturate	Administered IV by an anesthesiologist or nurse anesthetist	Just before a cesarean birth to obtain a rapid anesthetic effect to enable placement of an endotracheal tube and inhalation anesthetic administration	Emergency cesarean birth when it is imperative to delivery the neonate quickly. Position client in left lateral tilt to prevent vena caval compression. Oxygenate client at 100%.	Maternal pulmonary aspiration, pneumonitis, pulmonary edema, uterine atony postpartum
Anectine (succinylcholine) Depolarizing muscle relaxant	Administered IV by an anesthesiologist or nurse anesthetist	Same as above	Same as above	Same as above; triggering mechanism in clients with hereditary tendency for developing malignant hyperthermia

Source: Karch, A. M. (2005). *Lippincott's nursing drug guide.* Philadelphia: Lippincott Williams & Wilkins.

effects generally include heart palpitations, ringing in the ears, itching, apprehension, and confusion. The client also may complain of a metallic taste in the mouth. High concentrations can cause a local reaction, with tissue edema forming on the perineum. Moderate reactions are characterized by more intense degrees of the mild symptoms. In addition, nausea, vomiting, hypotension, and muscle twitching that can possibly progress to convulsions with a loss of consciousness can occur. The severest reaction involves laryngeal edema, joint pain, swelling of the tongue, bronchospasm, sudden loss of consciousness, coma, severe hypotension, and potentially cardiac arrest.

Systemic lethal reactions are most common when an excessive dose (either too great a concentration or too large a volume) has been administered. Accidental injection into the venous system potentially can cause vasomotor and respiratory depression as well as depression of the medullary centers in the brain. With a massive intravascular dose, sudden circulatory collapse can occur within 1 minute of administration. Therefore, close monitoring of the client following administration of any local anesthetic is essential. To ensure that resuscitative medications can be administered readily in the event of a systemic reaction, anesthetic agents should never be given without having an IV access in place.

With mild symptoms of toxicity, oxygen is administered by facemask. An IV injection of short-acting barbiturates is given to decrease anxiety. If the client develops convulsions, maintenance of a patent airway and administration of 100% oxygen are essential. Thiopental (Pentothal) or diazepam (Valium) may be used to stop convulsions.

Pudendal Anesthesia

Pudendal anesthesia typically is administered during the second stage of labor to anesthetize the lower vagina, vulva, and perineum. The obstetrician or certified nurse midwife injects the anesthetic agent, such as Xylocaine, Procaine, Marcaine, Nesacaine, or Carbocaine, through the lateral vaginal walls into the area near both the right and left pudendal nerve behind the sacrospinous ligament at the level of the ischial spines (Fig. 17.8). The injection is made through the vagina with the woman in lithotomy or dorsal recumbent position. Pudendal anesthesia can provide pain relief within 2 to 10 minutes after administration that lasts for approximately 1 hour. The procedure provides adequate anesthesia for vaginal births, application of outlet forceps or vacuum extraction, and perineal repair. Frequently, local infiltration of the perineum is combined with pudendal anesthesia because it is possible for pudendal anesthesia to be ineffective if that is the only area of injection. Although the injection is localized to the involved area, the fetal heart rate and the mother's blood pressure are checked immediately after the injection to identify possible hypotension.

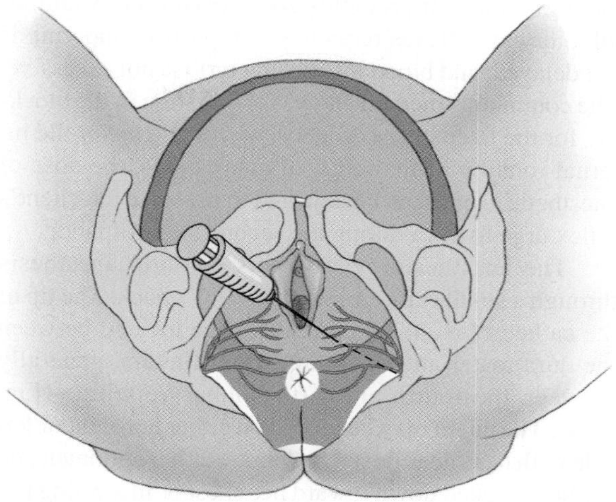

FIGURE 17.8 Administration site for pudendal analgesia.

Epidural Anesthesia Block

Epidural anesthesia block is one of the most common methods of intrapartum pain management currently used in the United States. It is controversial. Some observers believe that epidurals undermine natural childbirth; others believe that their use affirms a woman's inalienable right to pain relief during labor (Nystedt et al., 2004). Whichever viewpoint one ascribes to, most experts agree that the rate of epidurals is increasing (Gaiser, 2005). As a result, many clients now go into labor and childbirth expecting to receive an epidural block.

Although it is possible for an epidural to be unsuccessful or partly successful in providing relief, generally it is considered the most effective and flexible method of pain management during labor (Simpson & Creehan, 2001). Epidurals usually cause less depression of the central nervous system for mother and fetus than do sedative hypnotics, opioids, and narcotic agonist-antagonist compounds.

Clients receiving epidurals generally should be in the active phase of the first stage of labor with cervical dilation of 4 to 5 cm. The fetal head should be engaged at zero station, with fetal monitoring showing a stable and reassuring fetal heart rate pattern. Nevertheless, the American College of Obstetrics and Gynecology (2002) emphasizes that, provided no medical contraindications exist, a maternal request for pain relief during labor is sufficient reason to initiate the procedure.

Epidurals usually are administered continuously throughout the active and transitional phases of labor, vaginal birth, and repair of the episiotomy. The primary goal is to provide sufficient anesthesia with as little blockage to the sensory and motor nerves as possible. Doing so enables the client to retain the ability to sense pressure in the vagina and to push during the second stage of labor.

The epidural block alters the client's physiologic responses to pain but enables her to be fully awake during labor and birth. It promotes good relaxation. Additionally, airway reflexes remain intact, gastric emptying is not delayed, and blood loss during birth is not excessive. The continuous method allows for variation in the blocking for the later stages of labor, which allows for the internal rotation of the fetus. In many cases, the dose of anesthetic agents can be adjusted to preserve the client's reflex urge to push during the second stage of labor.

The anesthesiologist injects epidural anesthesia through a small catheter into the client's back. The tip of the catheter lies in the epidural space located between the dura mater and the ligamentum flavum, generally between the fourth and fifth lumbar vertebrae (Fig. 17.9). The client may be placed on either her right or left side with her knees flexed upward near her abdomen and her head tucked down toward her chest or in a sitting position on the side of the bed with her head tucked down toward the chest. A small pillow may be placed in front of her chest and abdomen for support to help the client maintain positioning. Such positioning facilitates the opening of the epidural space between the vertebrae and minimizes the risk for inadvertent puncture of the spinal column.

Initially, an epidural needle makes the puncture for insertion. Then a small catheter is threaded through the needle into the space, and the needle is removed, leaving the catheter in place for administration of medications. Once the needle has been inserted into the client's back, she must be encouraged and supported to remain in as stable a position as possible until the Silastic catheter has been threaded and the needle has been removed.

Epidurals are used most frequently to provide continuous analgesia and anesthesia from the T10 to the S5 levels, which is necessary for relieving pain during the remainder of labor and vaginal birth. For a cesarean birth, the block must extend from at least T8 and to S1 to be effective. The diffusion of epidural anesthesia depends on the location of the catheter tip, the dose and volume of the anesthetic agent used, and the woman's position.

Epidurals may be administered in various ways. Blocks can be administered as a one-time single dose through an epidural needle that is inserted and then removed; as a single dose through an epidural catheter, with additional doses given periodically if the client begins to experience discomfort; or as a continuous infusion. One form of continuous infusion is an **ambulatory epidural pump,** in which the pump is connected to the catheter and titrated doses of pain medication are delivered to the client based on her height and weight until she has given birth. Some types of administration require that the client remain in bed, whereas ambulatory epidurals allow the client with sufficient motor control to be out of bed.

QUOTE 17-3

"When my labor wasn't progressing and the obstetrician decided to do a c-section, I felt so sad, because I thought I would not be able to experience the actual birth. I was so pleased to know that my birth could be done with epidural anesthesia and that I would be able to see him when they pulled him out. I crashed for a few hours as soon as he was born, and I don't remember much about the initial recovery, but I remember the important part!"

A woman who had epidural anesthesia during cesarean birth

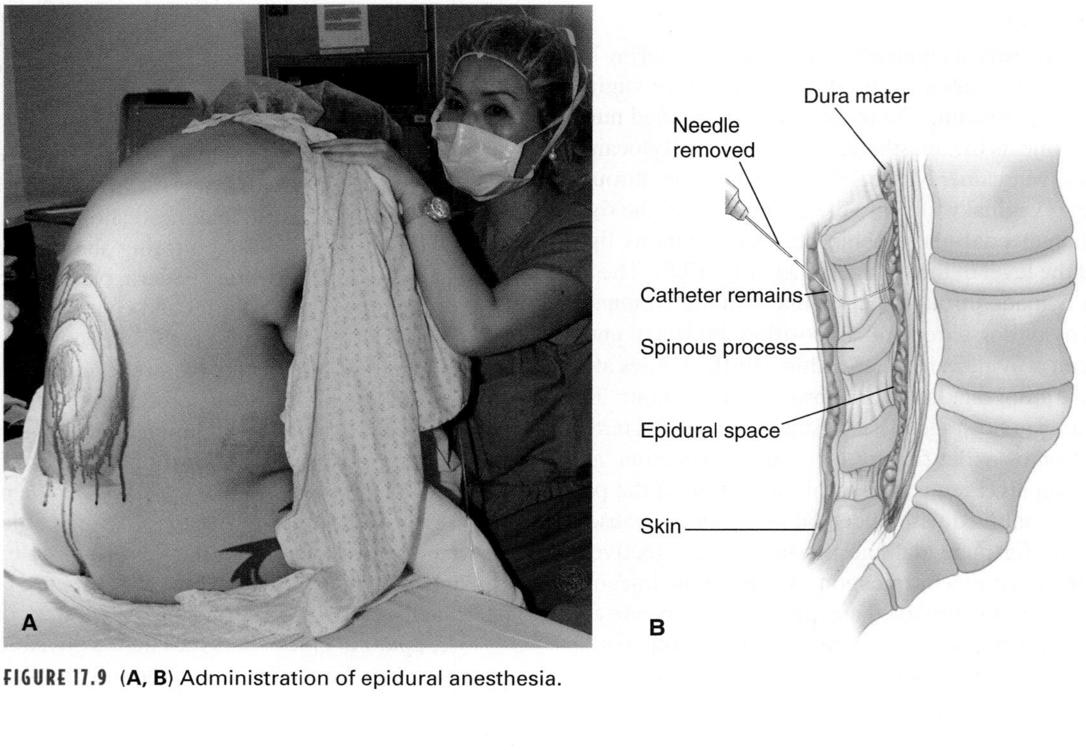

FIGURE 17.9 (**A, B**) Administration of epidural anesthesia.

Combined Spinal Epidural Anesthesia

Combined spinal epidural anesthesia may be accomplished through much the same procedure as for epidural anesthesia except that the needle is inserted into the subarachnoid space and an injection of fentanyl (Sublimaze) and bupivacaine (Marcaine) is given. The spinal needle is removed, and the Silastic epidural catheter is threaded through the epidural needle.

Combined spinal epidural anesthesia has a faster onset of pain relief than epidural anesthesia. The synergistic effect of opioids and local anesthesia, in addition to a lower total dose of required medication, reduces the motor blockade response. This enables the woman to feel pressure and have the sensation to push during the second stage of labor. Occasionally, especially when combined spinal epidural anesthesia is used during cesarean births, a one-time injection of an opioid such as morphine (Duramorph) into the epidural space immediately after birth provides analgesia for approximately 24 hours. Morphine takes effect within 30 to 60 minutes after the injection and peaks at approximately 14 to 16 hours. Side effects are possible, however, including respiratory depression, itching, rash, nausea, vomiting, and urinary retention.

If the client has received epidural morphine immediately after birth, vital signs are monitored hourly for 24 hours. No narcotic medications can be given to the client because they will potentiate the narcotic effect of the morphine. If the client develops itching and a rash, comfort measures, such as back rubs, the use of lotion, cool or warm compresses, and diversional activities are implemented. If the itching cannot be tolerated, diphenhydramine hydrochloride (Benadryl) can be given.

Spinal Anesthesia

In **spinal anesthesia,** a local anesthetic agent is injected directly into the subarachnoid space between the dura and the spinal cord (Fig. 17.10). Here the agent mixes with the cerebrospinal fluid to provide anesthesia from the region of T10 (hip) to the feet for a vaginal birth and from the region of T6 (nipples) to the feet for a cesarean birth.

The advantages of spinal anesthesia include the immediate onset of effect, relative ease of administration, need for a smaller dose volume to produce anesthesia, excellent muscle relaxation, and retention of the drug in the mother's body (ie, no passage through the placenta). The onset of action is usually within 1 to 2 minutes after administration, lasting approximately 1 to 3 hours depending on the type of agent used.

Spinal anesthesia has some disadvantages. The client cannot sense the urge to push, which results in the need for an episiotomy, low forceps, or vacuum extraction. The incidence of bladder and uterine atony as well as post-spinal headache is also higher than that associated with epidural anesthesia (see later discussion).

General Anesthesia

Occasionally, life-threatening complications such as severe pre-eclampsia, abruptio placentae, non-reassuring

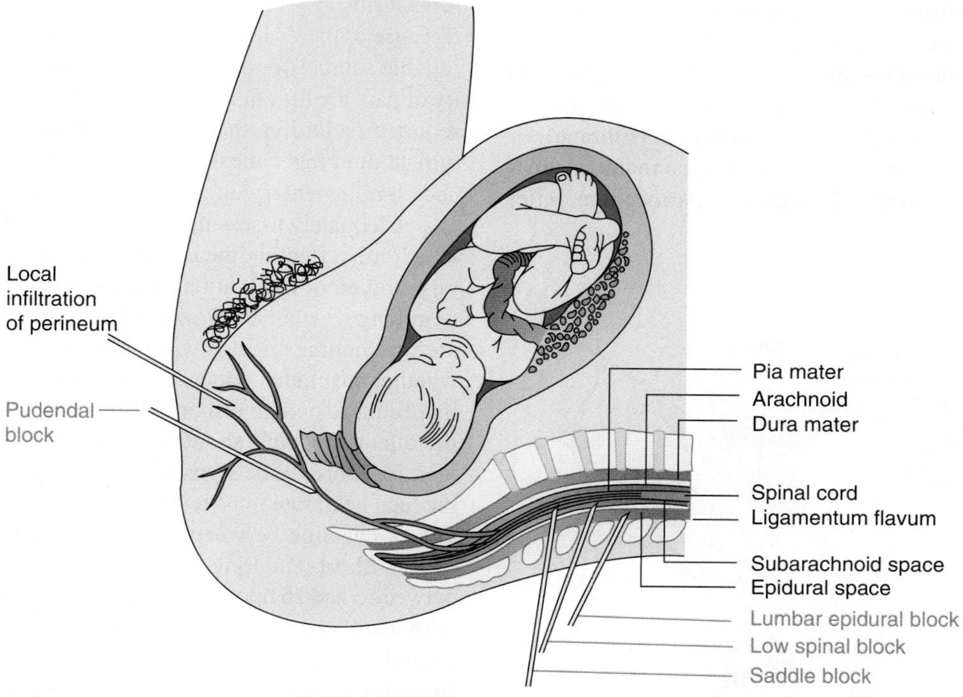

FIGURE 17.10 Injection of spinal anesthesia directly into the subarachnoid space between the dura and the spinal cord.

fetal heart rate patterns, or hemorrhagic conditions in obstetrics, arise that necessitate an expeditious emergency cesarean birth to facilitate the best possible outcome. The procedure for spinal and epidural anesthesia generally takes several minutes to perform properly. Then it takes several more minutes to achieve maximum pain control. As a result, precious minutes can be lost during which the fetus could suffer irreparable damage or even die in utero. Therefore, general anesthesia is often the method of choice for emergency births. **General anesthesia** actually involves rendering the client totally unconscious.

Induction is accomplished through IV injection. The drugs of choice for induction are as follows:

- Thiopental sodium (Pentothal), an ultrashort-acting barbiturate
- Succinylcholine chloride (Anectine), a neuromuscular blocking agent that usually exerts its effect rapidly but has a brief duration of action

After induction, the anesthesiologist inserts a cuffed endotracheal tube into the trachea. During the insertion of the endotracheal tube, the nurse should apply and maintain cricoid pressure just below the "Adam's apple." The nurse should use the thumb and forefinger to firmly compress the cricoid ring (the first and only tracheal cartilage ring that is a complete circle) 2 to 3 cm posteriorly. This pressure occludes the esophagus to prevent passive regurgitation and possible aspiration during the procedure (Fig. 17.11). The pressure is maintained until the anesthesiologist has inserted the endotracheal tube, inflated the cuff, and confirmed proper placement or has indicated that the pressure can be released.

After securing the airway, the obstetrician proceeds with the cesarean birth. The use of inhalation anesthetics such as halothane (Fluothane), enflurane (Ethrane), or methoxyflurane (Penthrane), and oxygen maintains maternal unconsciousness throughout the procedure. After childbirth, nitrous oxide often is added to enhance the anesthetic effect. Additional doses of muscle relaxants may be given as needed to maintain appropriate surgical conditions.

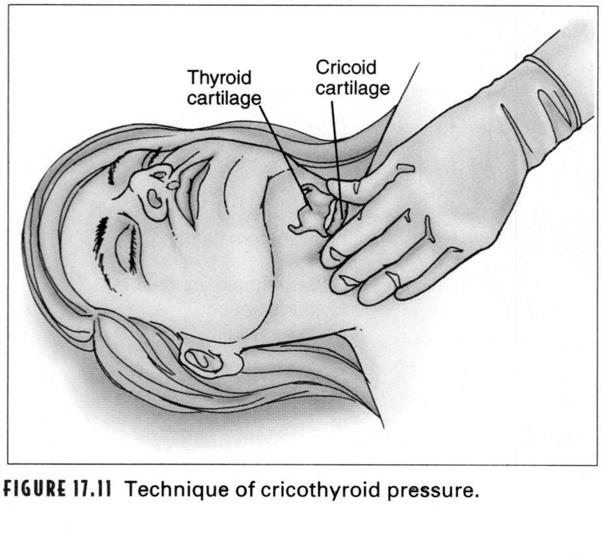

FIGURE 17.11 Technique of cricothyroid pressure.

COLLABORATIVE CARE: PHARMACOLOGIC PAIN MANAGEMENT

Clients in labor have many choices available for pain management. Some clients prefer to totally use nonpharmacologic methods (see Chap. 14). Others choose to use pharmacologic methods, and the discussions that follow focus on collaborative care oriented toward the various types available. Some women use a combination of nonpharmacologic and pharmacologic techniques. Nurses must be continuously aware of and sensitive to individual variations that clients choose for dealing with pain.

If a client asks for a pharmacologic pain intervention, the nurse should inform her of what to expect about the onset, duration, and side effects that she may experience after administration. Determining the optimum time for administration depends on a thorough assessment of numerous factors. If given too early in labor, contractions may become less frequent, thus prolonging labor, or result in depression of the fetal central nervous system. If given too late, the woman has no or minimal pain relief, and the newborn may experience respiratory depression.

Assessment

Because of pain's highly subjective nature, the two most reliable sources for determining the existence and severity of pain are the client's vital signs and the client's self-report. In addition, the nurse should assess the client's typical pain relief measures, including the use of drugs and complementary/alternative therapies.

Adequately assessing level of pain and the extent to which it is affecting the client are key to the proper administration of medications. Factors to include when determining whether analgesics are necessary for pain relief are whether the client is willing to take medications and whether the client's vital signs are stable and within normal limits. The nurse should listen very closely to what the client is saying about her level of pain and remain alert for more subtle signs of discomfort. Assessment of the fetal heart rate must reveal a stable, reassuring pattern with a baseline between 120 to 160 beats per minute (bpm). Short- and long-term variability should average between 5 and 25 bpm. The client should be in active labor with a well-established contraction pattern and demonstrated progression in cervical dilation and fetal descent. In addition, before any medication is given, the nurse should ascertain whether the woman has any history of drug reactions or allergies. The nurse also should ensure that activities such as changing position or assisting the client to the bathroom to urinate are completed before the administration of any analgesic.

Vital Signs

Usually, when pain is present, the client demonstrates changes in her vital signs. Pulse rate, respiratory rate, and blood pressure may significantly increase above the client's baseline. Once pain is relieved, the vital signs generally return to baseline (Fig. 17.12).

Client Self-Report

Various scales that rely on a client's self-reports have been developed to assist nurses and other health care providers to uniformly measure levels of pain. These pain-rating scales provide a measure for quantifying the severity of pain. Commonly used rating scales include the 0 to 10 simple rating scale and the visual analog descriptive pain intensity scale. Both scales ask the client to rate her level of pain between 0 (no pain) and 10 (excruciating, the worst pain that can be imagined). Assessment Tool 17.1 illustrates the numerical pain-rating scale.

The Wong-Baker FACES pain-rating scale is a pictorial representation used to assess pain (Assessment Tool 17.2). This tool contains a series of six faces that depict six levels of pain. The first face is a happy face. Subsequent faces increase in intensity to the last face, depicting tears. Each face is numbered from 0 to 5 with a corresponding description ranging from "no hurt" to "hurts worst." The tool is easy to use, especially with non–English-speaking clients. The health care provider shows the scale to the client and asks her to choose which face best represents her level of pain.

Another assessment scale for determining pain, especially with clients who cannot verbalize their level of pain is the Face, Legs, Activity, Cry, and Consolability (FLACC) 10-point scale. See Assessment Tool 17.3 for an example. Another detailed assessment scale for determining pain is the McGill-Melzac Pain Questionnaire (Assessment Tool 17.4).

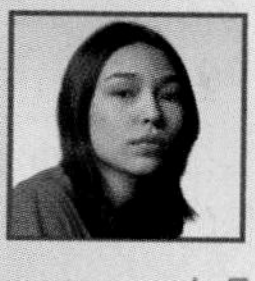

Consider Marnie, the young woman from the beginning of the chapter experiencing contractions every 5 to 6 minutes. Imagine that Marnie does not speak English and an interpreter is not readily available. How could the nurse assess Marnie's pain?

Medication Use

Assessment to determine appropriate selection of pharmacologic agents also includes obtaining a thorough history of medication use at home, including legal prescription drugs, illicit drugs, and complementary/alternative therapies. When clients have used certain drugs, interactions with analgesics and anesthetics that may be administered during labor can have serious implications. Although not recommended for pregnant women because of mutagenic effects to developing cells in early pregnancy, clients at times elect to take illicit and herbal drugs without discussing the ramifications of such use with their physician or nurse midwife. For example, St. John's wort (*Hypericum perforatum*) to treat mild to moderate depression can decrease the sedative effects of barbiturates, increase the sedative effects of narcotics, and prolong the bleeding time of clients receiving general anesthesia, increasing the risk for hemorrhage during a surgical procedure such as cesarean birth (Gallen, 2001). Most anesthesiologists generally prefer that the woman discontinue medications and herbs that pose problems in labor and birth for at least 30 days before having an invasive procedure performed.

Drugs such as butorphanol (Stadol) and nalbuphine (Nubain) should be used with extreme caution in clients with a recent history of drug abuse because they can precipitate a withdrawal type of reaction. To collaborate with the client's primary care provider regarding methods of pain management and to provide a safe, therapeutic environment, nurses should refer to appropriate resources such as drug handbooks and the *Nursing Herbal Medicine Handbook* (Gallen, 2001) when the client's history reveals drugs or herbs not commonly used in pregnancy.

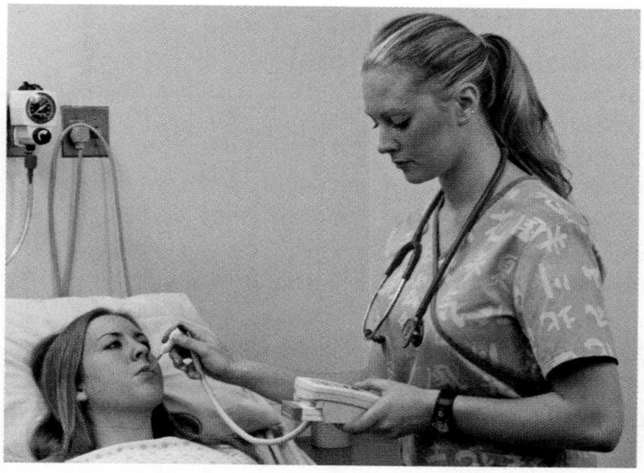

FIGURE 17.12 The nurse should regularly assess the client's vital signs to evaluate the effectiveness of pain-relieving measures.

Select Potential Nursing Diagnoses

The most obvious nursing diagnosis for the woman in labor is **Pain** related to increasing intensity and frequency of uterine contractions and perineal tissue pressure and

● ASSESSMENT TOOL 17.1 Pain Distress Scales

SIMPLE DESCRIPTIVE PAIN DISTRESS SCALE[1]

None	Annoying	Uncomfortable	Dreadful	Horrible	Agonizing

0–10 NUMERIC PAIN DISTRESS SCALE[1]

No pain — Distressing pain — Unbearable pain

0	1	2	3	4	5	6	7	8	9	10

VISUAL ANALOG SCALE (VAS)[2]

No distress — Unbearable distress

[1]If used as a graphic rating scale, a 10-cm baseline is recommended.
[2]A 10-cm baseline is recommended for VAS scales.
(From AHCPR, Acute Pain Management Guide Panel, 1992.)

● ASSESSMENT TOOL 17.2 Wong-Baker Faces Rating Scale

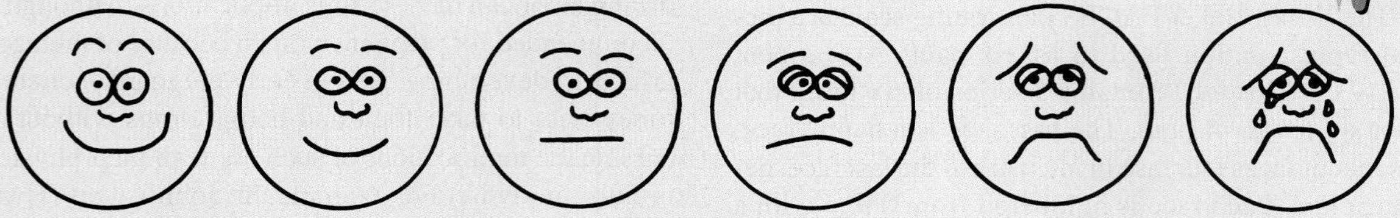

1. Explain to the child that each face is for a person who feels happy because he or she has no pain (hurt, or whatever word the child uses) or feels sad because he or she has some or a lot of pain.
2. Point to the appropriate face and state, "This face . . .":
   0—"is very happy because he [or she] doesn't hurt at all."
   1—"hurts just a little bit."
   2—"hurts a little more."
   3—"hurts even more."
   4—"hurts a whole lot."
   5—"hurts as much as you can imagine although you don't have to be crying to feel this bad."
3. Ask the child to choose the face that best describes how he or she feels. Be specific about which pain (eg, "shot" or incision) and what time (eg, Now? Earlier before lunch?)

(From Wong, D. L., et al. [2001]. *Wong's essentials of pediatric nursing* [6th ed.]. St. Louis: Mosby.)

● ASSESSMENT TOOL 17.3 Face, Legs, Activity, Cry, and Consolability (FLACC) Scale

Category	0	1	2
Face	No particular expression or smile	Occasional grimace or frown	Frequent to constant quivering chin, clenched jaw
Legs	Normal position or relaxed	Uneasy, restless, tense	Kicking or drawing legs up
Activity	Lying quietly, normal position, moves easily	Squirming, shifting back and forth, tense	Arched, rigid, or jerking
Cry	No cry awake or asleep	Moans or whimpers, occasional complaint	Crying steadily, screams, sobs, frequent complaints
Consolability	Content, relaxed	Reassured by occasional touching, hugging, or being talked to; distractible	Difficult to console or comfort

● ASSESSMENT TOOL 17.4 McGill-Melzack Pain Questionnaire

McGill - Melzack Pain Questionnaire

Patient's Name ______ Date ______ Time ______ am/pm

Analgesic(s) ______ Dosage ______ Time Given ______ am/pm

______ Dosage ______ Time Given ______ am/pm

Analgesic Time Difference (hours): +4 +1 +2 +3

PRI: S ______ (1-10) A ______ (11-15) E ______ (16) M(S) ______ (17-19) M(AE) ______ (20) M(T) ______ (17-20) PRT(T) ______ (1-20)

1 FLICKERING, QUIVERING, PULSING, THROBBING, BEATING, POUNDING

2 JUMPING, FLASHING, SHOOTING

3 PRICKING, BORING, DRILLING, STABBING, LANCINATING

4 SHARP, CUTTING, LACERATING

5 PINCHING, PRESSING, GNAWING, CRAMPING, CRUSHING

6 TUGGING, PULLING, WRENCHING

7 HOT, BURNING, SCALDING, SEARING

8 TINGLING, ITCHY, SMARTING, STINGING

9 DULL, SORE, HURTING, ACHING, HEAVY

10 TENDER, TAUT, RASPING, SPLITTING

11 TIRING, EXHAUSTING

12 SICKENING, SUFFOCATING

13 FEARFUL, FRIGHTFUL, TERRIFYING

14 PUNISHING, GRUELING, CRUEL, VICIOUS, KILLING

15 WRETCHED, BLINDING

16 ANNOYING, TROUBLESOME, MISERABLE, INTENSE, UNBEARABLE

17 SPREADING, RADIATING, PENETRATING, PIERCING

18 TIGHT, NUMB, DRAWING, SQUEEZING, TEARING

19 COOL, COLD, FREEZING

20 NAGGING, NAUSEATING, AGONIZING, DREADFUL, TORTURING

PPI

0 No pain

1 MILD

2 DISCOMFORTING

3 DISTRESSING

4 HORRIBLE

5 EXCRUCIATING

PPI ______ COMMENTS:

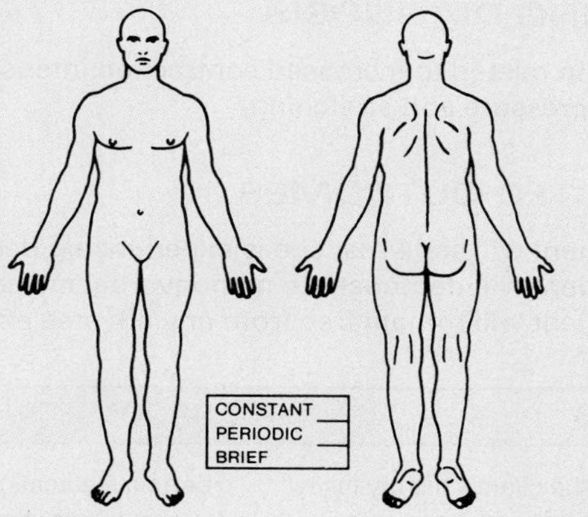

CONSTANT ___
PERIODIC ___
BRIEF ___

ACCOMPANYING SYMPTOMS: NAUSEA, HEADACHE, DIZZINESS, DROWSINESS, CONSTIPATION, DIARRHEA

COMMENTS:

SLEEP: GOOD, FITFUL, CAN'T SLEEP

COMMENTS:

ACTIVITY: GOOD, SOME, LITTLE, NONE

FOOD INTAKE: GOOD, SOME, LITTLE, NONE

COMMENTS:

COMMENTS:

Key:
PPI = present pain intensity
PRI = pain rating index
S = sensory components of pain
A = affective, or emotional, components of pain
E = evaluative terms
M = miscellaneous terms

Combinations of words can be identified: M(S) and M(AE) and the entire number totaled: PRI(T). (Copyright 1970. Ronald Melzack)

stretching. Other appropriate nursing diagnoses may include the following:

- **Deficient Knowledge** related to lack of familiarity with pain relief methods
- **Anxiety** related to stress of labor progression and concern about fetal well-being
- **Ineffective Coping** related to stress of labor and pain
- **Situational Low Self-Esteem** related to feelings of inadequacy and lack of control over pain

Planning/Intervention

Outcomes are highly individualized based on the woman's situation. Ideally the outcome for the woman in pain is relief of that pain. Nursing Care Plan 17.1 provides information about a general approach to managing pain in labor, and NIC/NOC Box 17.1 provides an overview of common interventions and outcome labels for the client experiencing pain during labor and birth. The following sections focus on specific collaborative interventions and considerations for each type of pharmacologic pain relief available.

Administering Sedative Hypnotics and Analgesic Compounds

When medications are administered, the nurse should document drug dose, route, and site according to the agency's policy. In addition, he or she should document the client's vital signs and fetal heart rate (Fig. 17.13).

NURSING CARE PLAN 17.1

The Client Experiencing Pain During Labor

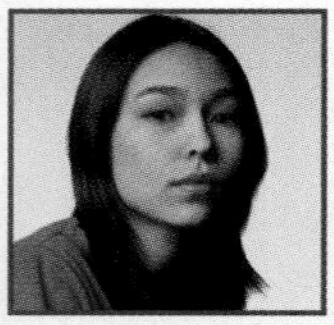

Recall Marnie, the gravida 1, para 0 client described at the beginning of the chapter. Marnie has progressed in labor and is now experiencing moderately strong contractions every 3 minutes, lasting 60 seconds. She is now 6 cm dilated and 90% effaced. She is holding on tightly to the side rail of the bed, crying softly and grimacing. She states, "I'm really uncomfortable." Her vital signs are stable; the fetal heart rate is 140 bpm.

NURSING DIAGNOSIS

Acute Pain related to increased contraction intensity and frequency and increased perineal pressure and stretching

EXPECTED OUTCOMES

1. The client will state that she is experiencing decreased pain.
2. The client will demonstrate no nonverbal indicators of pain.
3. The client will remain free from any adverse effects of analgesia administration.

INTERVENTIONS	RATIONALES
Thoroughly review the client's history for use of prescription, illegal, herbal, or homeopathic medications.	Certain medications interact with analgesics and anesthetics, with serious implications for client care.
Ask the client to rate her pain using a rating scale of 0 to 10 (with 0 being no pain and 10 being the worst pain imaginable). Assess for evidence of behavioral responses to pain such as grimacing, crying, or wringing of hands. Assess pain location and characteristics.	These data provide information about the etiology and characteristics of pain. Rating allows for objective reassessment of the client's pain.
Accept the client's interpretation of pain; assess for possible factors influencing the pain level.	Pain is a unique experience for each person. Physical, social, psychological, cultural, and spiritual norms influence the expression of pain.
Promote a comfortable environment with one-to-one support for the client. Reinforce and encourage her use of breathing and nonpharmacologic methods of pain relief during early labor.	A comfortable environment reduces stressors from influencing pain. One-to-one support assists the client to use techniques learned in any childbirth education classes to cope with discomfort during labor.
Explain the physiology of the client's discomfort (eg, back labor). Explain pharmacologic methods of pain management, including advantages and disadvantages of each option.	Explanations decrease fear and anxiety as well as assist the client to cope with discomfort. Information empowers the client to make some decisions when she may feel that she has little control over anything.
Administer analgesia as ordered.	Administration of analgesia promotes pain relief.

Continued

NURSING CARE PLAN 17.1 ● The Client Experiencing Pain During Labor

INTERVENTIONS	RATIONALES
Monitor maternal and fetal responses to medications. Observe for adverse reactions.	All drugs given to the mother potentially carry risks for the client and also cross the placental barrier and can affect the fetus adversely. Prompt recognition and treatment to minimize maternal–fetal responses to medications is critical to producing an optimum outcome.
Re-evaluate the client's perception of pain after drugs have been administered.	Re-evaluation helps determines the effectiveness of the method of pain relief employed.
Monitor the mother's vital signs and the fetal heart rate as ordered.	Medications can pass through the placenta and affect the fetus.
Change the client's position frequently as tolerated. Assist with ambulation if allowed.	Position changes promote comfort. Ambulation helps to reduce pain. Because of possible central nervous system depression with pharmacologic agents such as sedatives and narcotics, the client needs assistance with balance and ambulation to promote safety.
If the client wants an epidural or spinal anesthesia, ensure that she is fully informed of all potential complications and that she signs a consent form. Notify appropriate personnel if the client desires such pain relief.	Informed consent is necessary for any invasive procedure. All consents should be signed in advance of receiving sedatives, hypnotics, opioids, and agonists-antagonist medications, which can cause sedation and drowsiness. Early notification facilitates organization of the anesthesia provider's time to promote the quickest administration of the epidural possible when the client is ready for one.
Continually reassess the client's level of pain, vital signs, and fetal status. Administer additional doses of analgesia as ordered.	Continued reassessment is necessary to determine the effectiveness of interventions and to identify possible adverse effects on mother and fetus. Additional medication may be necessary to achieve desired results.

EVALUATION

1. The client states that pain is tolerable and that she is comfortable.
2. The client rates her pain as 2 to 3 on a pain rating scale of 0 to 10.
3. The client demonstrates no crying, grimacing, or other nonverbal indicators of pain.
4. The client's vital signs and fetal heart rate are within acceptable parameters.

When medications begin to take effect, the client may sleep between contractions. This short period of rest can facilitate relaxation and restore the client's energy level. In some cases, the client's pain may be so intense that she may not want to do anything except get the medication. Subsequently, drug administration should be facilitated as expeditiously as possible to be helpful. The nurse also should caution any family members or other support people that the client might become disoriented and confused after administration of analgesic medications.

NIC/NOC Box 17.1 Pharmacologic Pain Management in Labor

Common NIC Labels

- Analgesic Administration
- Analgesic Administration: Intraspinal
- Anesthesia Administration
- Anxiety Reduction
- Distraction
- Pain Management
- Patient-Controlled Analgesia (PCA) Assistance
- Postanesthesia Care
- Sedation Management
- Vital Signs Monitoring

Common NOC Labels

- Anxiety Level
- Client Satisfaction: Symptom Control
- Comfort Level
- Pain Control
- Pain Level
- Rest
- Sleep
- Vital Signs

Managing Care During Epidural Anesthesia

Before the administration of epidural analgesia, health care providers must obtain the client's informed consent, with all potential side effects fully explained. IV access is established to provide a route for administration of resuscitative drugs should the epidural create an adverse reaction. Most anesthesiologists prefer that the client receive a preparatory loading dose of solution, usually a minimum of 500 to 1000 mL of IV lactated Ringer's or normal saline solution over 15 to 30 minutes before epidural administration. If at all possible, this loading dose should be given early, when beginning to provide care for the client, rather than waiting until just before the epidural is going to be administered. See Nursing Care Plan 17.2 for care of the client receiving epidural anesthesia.

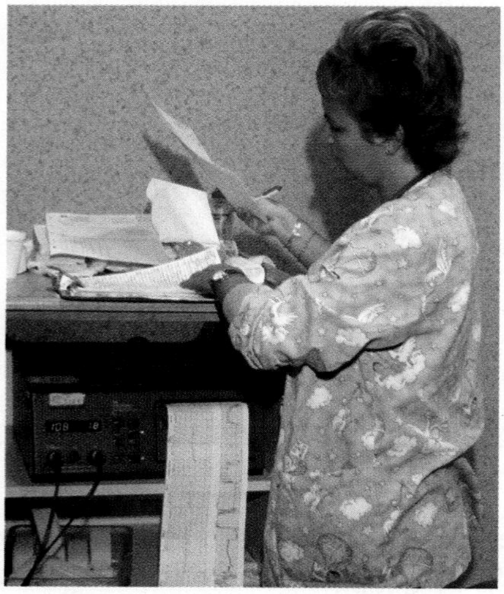

FIGURE 17.13 Following the administration of analgesic medications for labor pain, the nurse should document maternal vital signs and fetal heart rate.

Some clients have difficulty maintaining the stable position required during epidural anesthesia because of the severity and duration of their contractions. The nurse, along with the client's significant other (if possible), should be diligent in providing stable support for the client during the procedure as well as in encouraging the client to remain calm. Catheter insertion is performed between contractions as often as possible to prevent movement during this time, which can increase the risk for inadvertent perforation of the subarachnoid space containing the cerebrospinal fluid.

Ongoing Monitoring. Regardless of how the epidural is administered, close observation of both the maternal and fetal heart patterns and rates are essential components of care. The nurse should assess vital signs every 2 minutes initially for the first 20 to 30 minutes, and then every 5 to 15 minutes depending on the client's status and agency policy. Oxygen saturation levels are monitored by pulse oximetry. In addition to frequent blood pressure readings, the pulse oximeter reading may reveal one of the first signs of a complication related to the epidural anesthesia. The client preferably is placed in a semi-reclining position tilted laterally to keep the gravid uterus from compressing the ascending vena cava and descending aorta, which can impair venous return and decrease placental perfusion. The nurse should change the woman's position every 15 to 30 minutes to facilitate even dispersion of the anesthetic agent and to prevent a one-sided dose effect. The nurse should keep in mind that onset of anesthesia can take 20 to 30 minutes to be effective. Therefore, ongoing provision of comfort measures and encouragement in relaxation techniques are essential.

Addressing Adverse Reactions and Complications. Although their incidence is relatively low, the client receiving epidural anesthesia is at risk for possible adverse reactions and complications.

(text continues on page 697)

NURSING CARE PLAN 17.2

The Client Who Receives Epidural Anesthesia

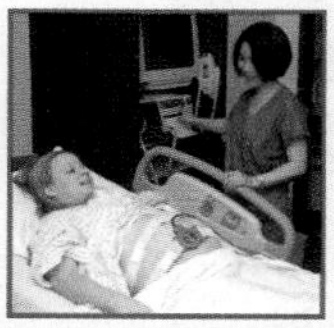

Recall Felicia, the client from the beginning of the chapter admitted to the health care facility in active labor. During the interview, she states, "I tried natural childbirth with my other two children, but eventually I needed something for pain. The contractions were just too strong. Chuck and I talked this over with our physician, and we all agreed that I would get an epidural for the pain."

NURSING DIAGNOSIS

Risk for Injury related to the effects of epidural anesthesia, including hypotension, prolongation of labor, neurologic injuries, and systemic toxicity

EXPECTED OUTCOMES

1. The client will experience complete relief of discomfort with minimal to no adverse effects.
2. The client will demonstrate progression through the second stage of labor within 2 hours of the initiation of epidural anesthesia.
3. The client will exhibit a return of sensation and ability to void in the postpartum period after epidural anesthesia is discontinued.

INTERVENTIONS	RATIONALES
Obtain baseline maternal vital signs and fetal heart rate before the procedure.	Baseline assessment ensures that the client's values are within normal limits and allows for comparison with future assessments to detect changes.
Check to make sure that the client has signed an informed consent.	Informed consent is necessary because the procedure is invasive and the client is at risk for potential adverse effects. A signed informed consent indicates that the client understands the procedure and associated risks.
Provide adequate hydration, including a 500-mL to 1000-mL bolus of fluid before the procedure.	Adequate hydration ensures adequate intravascular fluid volume, which minimizes the risk for hypotension after administration.
Assist the client to assume either a sitting or side-lying position with the back arched to open the spaces between the spinal vertebrae.	Such positioning facilitates opening of the epidural space and minimizes the risk for inadvertent puncture of the spinal column.
Provide ongoing encouragement and support, assisting the client to remain stable during the procedure.	Proper positioning minimizes the potential for spinal cord injury from inadvertent client movement during the critical point when the spinal needle has been inserted into the client's back.
Monitor blood pressure, pulse, and respirations every 2 minutes after initial injection of an anesthetic agent for a minimum of 20 minutes and then every 5 to 15 minutes until stable. Repeat monitoring of vital signs every 2 minutes after additional doses for 20 minutes. Evaluate results against the baseline readings.	Changes in vital signs, especially blood pressure, indicate a possible adverse reaction. Blocking of the sympathetic nerve fibers in the epidural space causes decreased peripheral resistance, resulting in hypotension. Systolic blood pressure less than 100 mm Hg can lead to fetal hypoxia.

Continued

NURSING CARE PLAN 17.2 ● The Client Who Receives Epidural Anesthesia (*Continued*)

INTERVENTIONS	RATIONALES
Monitor maternal temperature every 2 hours until birth.	Epidural anesthesia can temporarily elevate the mother's temperature.
Observe for signs of local anesthetic/analgesic toxicity: tinnitus, tingling, or unexplained confusion. If toxicity occurs, medications should be discontinued, and emergency interventions should be implemented.	Such observation aids in early detection and prompt intervention should any problems occur, minimizing risks to mother and fetus.
Monitor maternal oxygen saturation levels by pulse oximetry.	Adequate maternal oxygenation promotes adequate fetal oxygenation. Changes in oxygen saturation levels aids in detecting hypoxia related to suppression of respirations secondary to high anesthesia.
Assist the client to a semi-reclining position in a lateral tilt.	Proper positioning promotes a more even distribution of the medication bilaterally and prevents the anesthetic effect from rising too high; lateral tilt aids in keeping the gravid uterus from compressing the ascending vena cava and the descending aorta, which can impair venous return and decrease placental perfusion.
Assess the level of anesthesia.	The higher the level of anesthesia, the greater the risk for respiratory depression from paralysis of the diaphragm.
Monitor uterine contractions closely. Carefully check the fetal heart rate and progress of labor; notify the health care provider if the second stage becomes prolonged (more than 3 hours in a primipara or more than 2 hours in a multipara).	No contractions may indicate that the anesthesia is rising too high. The client may not be able to feel the pressure of the fetal head descending in the pelvis. Fetal distress is rare after an epidural but can occur if the medication is absorbed rapidly or with severe maternal hypotension. Epidural anesthesia is associated with an increased risk for prolonged second stage of labor.
Check to ensure that the pump is functioning properly and that tubing is not kinked or compressed by maternal weight or positioning. Assess for hot spots and breakthrough pain. Notify anesthesiology personnel of any of these problems.	A patent infusion is necessary to provide adequate pain relief. Hot spots may require removal of the catheter and reinsertion. Breakthrough pain typically indicates the infusion is below the therapeutic dose or interrupted integrity of the epidural line.
Anticipate insertion of an indwelling (Foley) catheter.	Use of a catheter prevents bladder distention, which may interfere with fetal descent.
Provide comfort measures for nausea, vomiting, and shivering.	Comfort measures are important to provide relief from troublesome effects.
If hypotension is noted, administer oxygen by facemask at the prescribed rate and increase IV fluids. Reposition the client as necessary to maintain adequate oxygenation to the fetus.	Oxygen administration ensures that maternal blood is well oxygenated, leading to adequate fetal oxygenation. Increasing IV fluids helps to restore intravascular fluid volume, thereby increasing blood pressure.

Continued

NURSING CARE PLAN 17.2 ● The Client Who Receives Epidural Anesthesia

INTERVENTIONS	RATIONALES
Elevate the client's legs on a pillow for 2 to 3 minutes but avoid a Trendelenburg position.	Placing the client in the left lateral tilt position improves placental blood flow. Elevating the legs can increase venous blood return from the extremities to the heart and circulation to the brain. The Trendelenburg position should be avoided following an epidural because it can cause the anesthesia level to rise too high, leading to possible respiratory paralysis.
Notify the health care provider and anesthesia personnel if measures are ineffective.	If the above measures are ineffective, the anesthesiologist may need to administer ephedrine to increase the client's blood pressure.
After birth, remove the epidural catheter, verifying that the tip of the catheter is intact.	Confirmation of the catheter tip ensures that all the catheter has been removed and hasn't broken off.
Maintain the client on bedrest with an indwelling urinary (Foley) catheter in place until effects of epidural anesthesia have worn off. Assess for return of sensation, range of motion, and ability to control lower extremities.	Bedrest helps to ensure client safety with ambulation after birth; the catheter aids in reducing the risk for bladder distention that can interfere with uterine involution, which can lead to postpartum hemorrhage.

EVALUATION

1. The client remains free of any adverse effects of epidural anesthesia.
2. The client gives birth to a healthy newborn within 2 hours of initiating epidural anesthesia.
3. The client demonstrates a return of bodily functions upon discontinuation of epidural anesthesia after birth.

Therefore, nurses should be thoroughly prepared to handle any and all potential complications.

Maternal hypotension is one of the most frequent effects of epidural anesthesia. If the client's blood pressure drops significantly, fetal distress can occur. Rapid administration of the loading dose of the IV solution, however, generally can minimize this effect. Continuous IV access is maintained throughout labor to allow for repeated bolus doses of fluids as needed to maintain maternal homeostasis. The IV access also provides a means for drug administration should an emergency arise. If hypotension occurs, oxygen is administered by facemask, and a bolus of IV fluid is given. If these measures fail to stabilize the client's blood pressure, ephedrine, a vasopressor, should be readily available for administration.

Epidurals are at risk for failure because the catheter has to be placed properly within the epidural space to produce adequate anesthesia. Potentially distressing complications include an inadequate block, a one-sided block, and a hot spot. In an *inadequate block,* the epidural fails to minimize the client's pain sufficiently. If the block is inadequate, the anesthesiologist can inject a bolus dose of medication through the catheter, possibly increase the continuous ordered dose, or both. With a *one-sided block,* pain is only managed on one side. In such cases, the nurse can turn the woman to the unaffected side. In rare cases, the anesthesiologist may have to re-administer the drug through the catheter with the client lying on her unaffected side. With a *hot spot* (window of pain), the epidural provides effective relief except for one small area of the abdomen, in which pain is intense. If this occurs, the anesthesiologist should be notified. The catheter may need to be removed and reinserted.

Breakthrough pain can occur any time the epidural infusion is below the therapeutic dose required or the integrity of the epidural line is interrupted. The nurse should first ascertain whether the infusion pump is functioning properly and check that maternal body weight or positioning is not kinking or compressing the tubing. If nursing care measures fail to rectify the problem, the anesthesiologist may need to provide a bolus injection of the anesthetic agent.

Itching and rash can occur during the epidural infusion. Typically, these begin on the client's face, neck, or torso and usually result from the anesthetic agent used. If an allergic reaction occurs, comfort measures such as back rubs, application of lotion, cool or warm compresses, and diversion are implemented. If the itching becomes too uncomfortable for the client, an order for diphenhydramine hydrochloride (Benadryl) may be obtained from the anesthesiologist. The usual dose is 25 to 50 mg every 4 to 6 hours as needed to control the symptoms.

Epidural anesthesia may slow the progress of labor and extend the duration of the second stage. The health care team working with the client needs to monitor the client's motor and sensory function carefully as she prepares to start pushing. If the client lacks motor and sensory function, pushing should be delayed until some of the sensation returns, thus facilitating her ability to push effectively.

A less frequent problem with epidural anesthesia is elevation of the maternal temperature to 100.7°F (37.8°C) or greater. It is believed that the temperature elevation may result from a decrease in heat loss because of reduced sweating secondary to sympathetic nerve blockade. Also, women in labor are generally NPO except for ice chips. Subsequently, they may experience fluid imbalance and dehydration. Increasing IV fluids and providing comfort measures can help reduce the temperature. Nevertheless, the nurse needs to differentiate the cause of the temperature elevation, determining whether it is a rebound effect of the anesthesia or an indication of infection.

Short-term localized tenderness at the puncture site and backache are common during the first postpartum week. The discomfort is thought to result from muscle tension during stressful times in labor as well as the required positioning during the administration of the epidural.

Other possible complications include urinary retention, shivering, nausea, and vomiting. After total relief of the client's discomfort has been achieved through the administration of the epidural, an indwelling urinary (Foley) catheter frequently is inserted to prevent bladder distention from inadvertently impeding fetal descent. The nurse should monitor urinary output hourly. Shivering generally results from irritation of the nerve endings by the injection of the epidural agent. Covering the client with a warm blanket may help reduce the shivering. If the client becomes nauseous and experiences vomiting, application of a cool cloth to the forehead or throat may help.

Neurologic injuries also may result from epidural anesthesia. Because of the resulting relaxation and decreased pain sensation, the client's legs may be excessively flexed when positioned during pushing. Overstretching of the pelvic nerves may result. Clients may report numbness, tingling, and paresthesia in one foot or leg that can be severe or last long enough to require the use of a cane or a walker for weeks to months. Any report of such symptoms that last longer than the expected duration for an epidural should be referred to the anesthesiologist for further evaluation.

A serious complication of epidural anesthesia is a systemic toxic reaction. This usually results from inadvertent injection of anesthetic agents into the spinal column, excessive doses of medications injected into the epidural space, or accidental intravascular injection of medications. The client who experiences a toxic reaction generally complains of numbness and tingling that rises progressively higher to the arms and chest. If the reaction is severe, the nerves supplying the respiratory muscles may be blocked, thus causing severe respiratory depression or arrest, oxygen desaturation, and loss of consciousness. Such clients may require endotracheal intubation and emergency resuscitation measures until their condition stabilizes. If respiratory stability is achieved, a vaginal birth may still be possible.

The effect of epidural anesthesia on postpartum breastfeeding is controversial. Some observers suggest that epidurals are safer than other forms of analgesia and anesthesia with minimal long-term side effects (Chang & Heaman, 2005; Halpern et al., 1999; Nystedt et al., 2004). Breastfeeding also may be hampered, however, by drugs used during epidural anesthesia (Baumgarder et al., 2003; Volmanen et al., 2004). The "caine" anesthetic agents enter the maternal circulation by diffusion and cross the placenta to the fetus. The newborn's liver is too immature to break down the medication, so the effects can linger for prolonged periods, often causing the newborn to be sleepy, have difficulty latching on, and have an inefficient, disorganized sucking and swallowing ability. When such problems occur, mothers may become discouraged, which may lead to early unintentional weaning. The nurse should work to provide additional assistance and support to the mother and the baby to promote and acquire successful, efficient breastfeeding skills. See Research Highlight 17.1.

Discontinuing Use. After childbirth, the epidural infusion and pump are discontinued, and the catheter is removed

RESEARCH HIGHLIGHT 17.1 Epidural Analgesia During Labor and Delivery: Effects on the Initiation and Continuation of Effective Breastfeeding

OBJECTIVES: Epidural anesthesia used frequently during labor commonly is regarded as a safe procedure. The purpose of this study was to determine whether epidural anesthesia is associated with problems initiating or continuing breastfeeding in newborns.

DESIGN: The research design was a prospective cohort study examining a sample of normal women who gave vaginal birth to healthy infants. One group received epidural analgesia. The other group did not. Each mother in both groups was assessed 8 to 12 hours postpartum and in a telephone follow-up interview 4 weeks after childbirth.

RESULTS: No significant differences were found in either group relative to immediate success at beginning breastfeeding or in the number of women who continued breastfeeding at 4 weeks postpartum.

NURSING IMPLICATIONS: The findings of this study indicate that epidural anesthesia should not negatively influence outcomes of breastfeeding. In evaluating the causes of problems with breastfeeding after administration of epidural anesthesia, health care providers should carefully assess all the specific dynamics of the client's situation to help address problems and facilitate an effective experience.

Chang, Z. M., & Heaman, M. I. (2005). *Journal of Human Lactation, 21*(3), 305–314.

from the client's back. The intactness of the black tip of the catheter must be confirmed with a physician or another nurse. The epidural amount administered through the pump is calculated and charted on the appropriate agency flow sheet such as a narcotic control record. Client ambulation usually is delayed until the effects of the anesthesia have worn off and the client has full sensation and the ability to control leg movements. The obstetrician may elect to leave the urinary catheter in place until full sensation has returned. Doing so helps to prevent urinary retention because the client may be unable to determine when her bladder is full as a result of residual anesthetic effects. Adequate bladder emptying also promotes effective uterine contraction.

Managing Care During Spinal Anesthesia

When spinal anesthesia is used, the client is positioned in much the same way as for epidural anesthesia to ensure that the intravertebral space is widened. After insertion, the client may be positioned upright to provide anesthesia to the desired level for a vaginal birth or more supine if the level desired is for a cesarean birth. Because spinal anesthesia generally is used during cesarean births, positioning the client flat in bed with a small, flat pillow under her head for at least 8 hours after administration is highly recommended.

Addressing Adverse Reactions and Complications. Marked hypotension, decreased cardiac output, decreased placental perfusion, and respiratory distress may occur during spinal anesthesia. Systemic allergic drug reactions and respiratory paralysis resulting in the need for cardiopulmonary resuscitation are more severe potential complications. If signs of serious maternal distress, fetal compromise, or both occur, emergency care must be implemented. The client is turned to the left side or placed in a left lateral tilt position. Oxygen is administered through facemask according to the agency's protocol. The nurse should monitor maternal vital signs and fetal heart rate every 2 to 5 minutes until stable. In addition, the nurse should notify the anesthesiologist and primary care provider. The anesthesiologist may administer or order ephedrine per protocol.

Hematoma in the spinal column is a rare complication that can result in spinal cord compression or ischemia. Neurologic damage may range from sensory or motor weakness to quadriplegia and death. Presenting symptoms generally include lower-body motor weakness, back pain, and sensory deficits. Delays in symptom identification, diagnosis, and treatment can result in more severe damage. Concern about hematoma in the spinal column is one of the primary reasons that epidural and spinal anesthesia methods are contraindicated in cases of severe coagulopathy.

Addressing Postdural Spinal Headache. Headaches after childbirth are not unusual and can be from several causes, including dehydration, prolonged labor, pushing, or regional anesthesia. The distinguishing characteristic of a postdural spinal headache is the association between the client's position and headache severity. A true postdural spinal headache causes severe pain when the client is upright (ie, sitting or standing), but the pain is minimal or disappears completely when the client is recumbent. A postdural spinal headache usually begins within 5 days after the procedure. The headache can last for several days and is usually unresponsive to minor analgesics.

Leakage of cerebrospinal fluid from the inadvertent puncture or actual puncture into the spinal column is thought to be the major cause of a postdural spinal headache. With postural changes during the postpartum period, the diminished volume of cerebrospinal fluid allows the brain to shift more than usual. This shifting exerts traction on the pain-sensitive structures of the brain, resulting in a severe headache with visual and auditory disturbances when the client is upright. Left untreated, the problem may persist for days to several weeks.

The likelihood of a postdural spinal headache can be minimized if the anesthesiologist uses a small-gauge spinal needle and avoids puncturing the meninges. If a postdural headache does occur, treatment generally includes hydration measures. The nurse should encourage the client to increase her intake of water and caffeinated beverages. In addition, an IV infusion of lactated Ringer's solution may be administered at 150 mL/hour to assist the body in replacing the cerebrospinal fluid loss. Caffeine is encouraged because it causes cerebral vasoconstriction. The client is placed on bed rest. Analgesics for the headache may be beneficial in some instances. Such therapy, however, is not always effective in relieving a postdural spinal headache. Sometimes, the leakage of the cerebrospinal fluid is excessive to the point that an **epidural blood patch** may be required. However, this invasive procedure carries additional risks. The spinal column may be punctured again, which will result in worsening of the headache and arachnoiditis if the blood is inadvertently injected into the subarachnoid space.

The technique for an epidural blood patch involves insertion of an epidural needle, preferably in the same vertebral interspace as the original puncture. A venipuncture is performed, and 20 mL of the client's blood is obtained. The autologous blood without an anticoagulant present is then injected through the epidural needle into the epidural space by an anesthesiologist.

The epidural blood patch seems to work in two ways: first, the blood clots and plugs the hole in the spinal column to stop the leakage of cerebrospinal fluid. Second, the volume of the blood in the epidural space exerts pressure within the spinal column, which increases the cerebrospinal fluid level surrounding the brain.

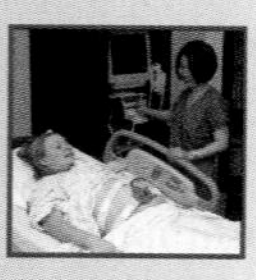

Think back to Felicia from the beginning of the chapter and Nursing Care Plan 17.2. Suppose Felicia develops a postdural headache following epidural anesthesia during labor. What measures would the nurse implement?

Managing Care During General Anesthesia

Before induction of general anesthesia, the nurse should place a wedge under the client's right hip to displace the uterus to the left, which prevents compression of the vena cava. The client is then preoxygenated for 3 to 5 minutes with 100% oxygen. This is followed by induction.

Addressing Adverse Reactions and Complications. Although general anesthesia is an expeditious method of providing pain control, it is never the preferred method during childbirth because it carries added risks for both mother and fetus. Increased pressure on the stomach from the weight of the gravid uterus, in conjunction with more production of gastric acid and pepsin, places pregnant clients at risk for gastric reflux. In addition, physiologic changes in the gastrointestinal system during labor increase the likelihood of regurgitation and aspiration. These changes include decreased bowel motility, delayed stomach emptying, and decreased barrier pressure at the gastroesophageal junction. As a result, the client receiving general anesthesia has an increased risk for possible aspiration of vomitus and hypoxia during administration. Pulmonary aspiration of gastric contents can cause lower airway obstruction, pneumonitis, pulmonary edema, and death. Therefore, before receiving general anesthesia, the client should receive a nonparticulate antacid such as sodium citrate (Bicitra). Additional medications such as histamine-2 blockers, for example, cimetidine (Tagamet), or ranitidine (Reglan) also may be given to help decrease the gastric pH level and volume of stomach acid.

Thiopental (Pentothal) and inhalation anesthetics rapidly cross the placenta. Therefore, the obstetrician has only an 8-minute window from induction of anesthesia to birth to get the fetus out without causing severe respiratory depression. Infants born to women under general anesthesia may be slow to respond at birth and may require resuscitative measures. Therefore, adequate equipment and personnel, including a pediatrician, must be present during birth.

Two other complications of general anesthesia include awareness during the procedure and uterine atony. It is possible for some clients to have some degree of awareness during the procedure, which may be attributed to an attempt to minimize drug-induced respiratory depression of the newborn. The addition of nitrous oxide after birth of the infant can decrease maternal awareness. If the client describes instances of awareness, the nurse should seriously explore the implications and notify the anesthesiologist so that the client can receive further assessment and explanation of the incident.

Uterine atony is a potential complication in all births regardless of whether analgesia or anesthesia is used. With general anesthesia, the use of inhalation anesthetic agents can produce decreased uterine contractility and tone after birth. Therefore, IV oxytocin (Pitocin) is administered to facilitate uterine contraction. Checking fundal firmness and lochia each time vital signs are taken is imperative during the postoperative period.

Controlling Malignant Hyperthermia. Malignant hyperthermia is an uncommon but concerning complication of general anesthesia. This autosomal-dominant inherited disorder of the skeletal muscles is characterized by a hypermetabolic response to all commonly used inhalation anesthetics such as halothane and depolarizing muscle relaxants such as succinylcholine chloride (Wappler, 2001). The exact mechanism by which different substances initiate malignant hyperthermia is essentially unknown; however, research has shown that a defect in intracellular calcium-2 ion homeostasis plays an important role in the process (Wappler, 2001). Family history generally reveals unexplained or sudden deaths during surgery as well as history of cardiac disease. When anesthesiologists interview clients before administering anesthesia, this is a key point that they assess before determining which method of pain control will be the most beneficial during the surgical procedure.

The clinical syndrome of malignant hyperthermia includes muscle rigidity, jaw rigidity, hypercapnia, tachycardia, hyperpyrexia, and myoglobinuria. Hypoxia results from increased carbon dioxide production, oxygen consumption, and muscle membrane breakdown. The disruption of the cell membranes leads to electrolyte imbalances (hyperkalemia). Malignant hyperthermia is suspected when the client displays the following:

- Temperature greater than 101.7°F (38.7°C)
- Difficulty with intubation from muscle rigidity, jaw rigidity, and laryngospasm
- Oxygen desaturation
- Blood loss that changes in color from bright red to dark maroon
- Cyanosis
- Tachycardia
- Dysrhythmias
- Cardiac arrest
- Respiratory and metabolic acidosis

Once malignant hyperthermia is recognized, volatile inhaled anesthetics and depolarizing muscle relaxants must be discontinued. In addition, all the breathing circuits and IV lines need to be changed immediately. Primary care measures include reversing the muscle rigidity with dantrolene sodium (Dantrium). Dosages are generally 2 to 3 mg/kg initially to a total of 10 mg/kg until rigidity is absent. Other measures include the symptomatic relief of the elevated temperature by placing the client on a cooling blanket, placing ice packs at the axillary and groin areas, continuously monitoring core body temperature, correcting acidosis with administration of sodium bicarbonate, 1 to 2 mEq/kg, and restoring electrolyte balance. In addition, intake and output are closely assessed. Isotonic IV solutions are used instead of lactated Ringer's, which may worsen the acidosis rather than correcting it. IV furosemide (Lasix) and continuous infusion of glucose and insulin are used to force diuresis, which is geared to 1 to 2 mL/kg of body weight. Arterial and central venous catheters are inserted to monitor hemodynamic status. Specimens obtained periodically for laboratory testing include arterial blood gases, electrolyte levels, complete blood count, coagulation studies, and renal function tests. Low-dose heparin therapy should also be initiated as soon as possible (Wappler, 2001). After stabilization is accomplished, the client is transferred to the intensive care unit for follow-up.

Discontinuing Use. After general anesthesia is completed, the client is awakened. Once she is responsive and spontaneously breathing with sufficient rate and tidal volume, and has the protective airway reflexes of swallowing, the mouth is suctioned, the endotracheal cuff is deflated, and the client is extubated. Once the tube has been removed, the client is transferred to the recovery room.

Clients who have received general anesthesia require close observation and monitoring after giving birth. Nurses should thoroughly assess all major body systems and prepare to provide immediate responses to any problems encountered.

Respirations should be observed closely for rate and depth. Oxygen can be administered by nasal cannula or facemask (when higher concentrations are needed). Pulse oximetry is used to determine oxygen saturation. Frequent intermittent blood pressure monitoring and electrocardiograms (ECGs) are performed until the client is stable. Suction equipment also must be readily available for use should the client vomit. The client must not be left alone during the critical point of recovery, which is the first hour after birth. The client should be stimulated and oriented to time and place frequently to prevent her from being too sleepy and hypoventilating. Vigilance by the nursing staff is the most important aspect in promoting a safe recovery period after administration of general anesthesia.

Evaluation

The nurse should monitor to ensure that the client's pain is managed effectively during labor and birth and that complications or problems postpartally are minimized. Each client's outcomes are further individualized based on the particulars of her situation.

Questions to Ponder

1. An Asian American woman is admitted to labor and birth in active labor. She is quiet and reserved but looks apprehensive.
   - From a cultural perspective, what might be some behaviors expected of Asian American women in pain?
   - What would be the most therapeutic way to assist the client in managing her pain during labor?
   - What types of pain relief methods and drugs would be appropriate for a client of this culture?
2. A client received epidural anesthesia 15 minutes ago, and her systolic blood pressure drops from a baseline of 120 mm Hg to 88 mm Hg.
   - What complication is the client most likely experiencing?
   - How would you expect to intervene?
   - What follow-up nursing care measures would be appropriate?

SUMMARY

- Pain, a truly unique experience, varies for each woman.
- JCAHO mandates that clients have the right to appropriate assessment and management of pain.
- Because pain is so subjective, nurses need to understand not only the physiology and psychology of pain, but also the pharmacology of pain relief methods and how cultural beliefs affect client perceptions of pain.
- Factors that produce pain during labor include the progression of cervical dilation, perineal distention, intensity and duration of contractions, and fetal position and size.
- During the first stage of labor, the uterine muscle experiences hypoxia and lactic acid accumulation from cervical dilation and stretching of the lower uterine segment. These in turn create traction on the ovaries, fallopian tubes, and uterine ligaments. Pressure on the maternal pelvis causes afferent pain impulses to travel along the sympathetic nerves that enter the spinal column.
- In the dorsal horn of the spinal column, somatostatin, cholecystokinin, and substance P serve as neurotransmitters for the pain impulse across the synapse between peripheral nerves and the spinal nerves. The pain then ascends the spinal column to the brain cortex, where it is interpreted as pain.
- During the second stage of labor, descent of the fetal presenting part exerts pressure on the pelvic floor muscles, vagina, perineum, and vulva, which in turn exerts pressure on the urethra, bladder, and rectum. The pain impulses ascend the spinal column in the same manner as during the first stage of labor.
- The gate control theory suggests that pain signals reach the nervous system and excite small groups of neurons. When the total activities of these neurons reach a certain level, a theoretical gate opens up and allows the pain signal to proceed through large and small sensory nerve fibers in the spinal column to the cerebral cortex, where the impulses are interpreted. Depending on the influence of physical, emotional, and behavioral factors, the gate also can close, which blocks the pain impulse from reaching the brain.
- β Endorphins are naturally occurring pain-moderating substances in the spinal column, which generally increase during pregnancy and the postpartum period. This may explain why various forms of massage, water therapy, or transcutaneous electrical nerve stimulation (TENS) may reduce the discomfort of pain.
- It is important for nurses to identify the most frequently seen ethnic groups within one's geographic location and to develop a profile of culturally specific responses to pain. Having an understanding of various cultural responses to pain can greatly assist nurses to be more attuned to client-specific needs during labor and birth.
- The real challenge for health care providers is to give optimum care, which enables clients to feel satisfaction with the birth experience while attaining the maximum pain relief possible.
- Choice of pain management methods is based on personal beliefs. Implementation of a client's desired methods is an ethical responsibility for health care providers, whereas informed consent is the prevailing legal consideration, especially related to invasive procedures such as epidural or spinal anesthesia.
- Three main elements must be present to be considered a truly informed consent: unbiased information should be given before giving consent; consent must be a voluntary decision; and the client must be competent and capable of accepting responsibility for the selected decision.
- Pharmacokinetics is the study of drug absorption, metabolism, distribution, and excretion in the body. The increased cardiac output of pregnancy and childbirth and its concomitant physiologic changes alter these processes.
- For centuries, discomfort during labor and birth has been considered inevitable and something to be endured. The desire for pain relief during childbirth has led to the trial of many remedies; however, the greatest strides in pain management have occurred during the past 200 years.
- Determining the optimum time for giving analgesics depends on the performance of a complete assessment of various factors. If given too early in labor, contractions may become less frequent, thus prolonging labor, or it may cause fetal central nervous system depression. If given too late, the woman will experience minimal or no pain relief, and the newborn may experience respiratory depression.

- Analgesia reduces or decreases awareness of pain, whereas anesthesia can cause partial or complete loss of sensation with or without loss of consciousness.
- Sedative hypnotics relieve anxiety and induce sleep. Common sedative hypnotics include secobarbital (Seconal), pentobarbital (Nembutal), promethazine (Phenergan), and hydroxyzine (Vistaril).
- Common opioid drugs include morphine and meperidine (Demerol). Common narcotic agonist-antagonists include butorphanol (Stadol) and nalbuphine (Nubain). Naloxone (Narcan) is a narcotic antagonist used to reverse the effects of opioid and narcotic agonist-antagonist agents.
- Local anesthesia is used in obstetrics to induce a loss of sensation in the perineum and vagina during a vaginal delivery to facilitate the cutting, repair, or both of the episiotomy.
- An epidural block is the injection of local anesthetic agents into the epidural space between the dura mater and the ligamentum flavum between the fourth and fifth lumbar vertebrae through a small catheter inserted into the client's back by an anesthesiologist. The catheter may be connected to a pump, which delivers titrated doses of pain medication until birth is accomplished. Common drugs used with epidurals are bupivacaine (Marcaine) and fentanyl (Sublimaze).
- With spinal anesthesia, a local anesthetic agent is injected directly into the subarachnoid space between the dura and the spinal cord, where it mixes with the cerebrospinal fluid to provide anesthesia from the T10 region (hip) to the feet for a vaginal delivery and from the T6 region (nipples) to the feet for a cesarean birth.
- General anesthesia renders the client unconscious with short-acting IV sedation followed by endotracheal intubation and the use of inhalation anesthetics such as nitrous oxide, halothane (Fluothane), enflurane (Ethrane), or methoxyflurane (Penthrane) and oxygen.
- The two most reliable sources for determining the existence of pain and its severity are the client's vital signs and the client's self-report.
- Client self-report of pain can be determined through the use of various measurement scales, including the Wong-Baker FACES scale and the Face, Legs, Activity, Cry, and Consolability (FLACC) scale.
- Assessment to determine appropriate selection of analgesic and anesthetic agents also entails obtaining a thorough history of medication use at home, including legal prescription drugs, illegal drugs, homeopathic remedies, and herbal derivatives. When homeopathic, herbal, or illicit drugs have been used, interactions with analgesics and anesthetics can occur that may have serious implications for client care.
- The most common complication of epidural anesthesia is maternal hypotension. Failure to correct hypotension in the mother can result in fetal hypoxia.
- Postdural spinal headache is a frequent complication of spinal anesthesia. It also can be a result of an inadvertent spinal administration occurring during epidural insertion. The postdural spinal headache causes severe pain when the client is in an upright position such as sitting or standing but is minimal or disappears completely when the client assumes a recumbent position.
- Common complications of general anesthesia include nausea, vomiting, and aspiration. A less common complication is malignant hyperthermia.

REVIEW QUESTIONS

1. The nurse should be alert for the development of malignant hyperthermia in a client who has received
   A. epidural anesthesia.
   B. general anesthesia.
   C. pudendal anesthesia.
   D. local anesthesia.
2. Three hours after giving vaginal birth to a healthy newborn with the aid of epidural anesthesia, a client complains of a headache unrelieved by medication. The nurse suspects that the client is possibly suffering from
   A. exhaustion and needs more rest in a quiet environment.
   B. dehydration and needs to drink more decaffeinated fluids.
   C. migraine with a low tolerance for pain and needs stronger medication.
   D. effects of an inadvertent spinal anesthetic requiring additional intervention.
3. A client in the first phase of labor whose cervix is dilated to 3 cm is complaining of pain. The nurse would anticipate an order for pain management at this point in time that involves
   A. continuing nonpharmacologic pain relief techniques.
   B. giving secobarbital by mouth.
   C. giving nalbuphine and promethazine by IV push.
   D. assisting with epidural anesthetic administration.
4. The nurse identifies the pain occurring during the late phase of the first stage and second stage of labor that results from stretching of the perineal tissues to allow passage of the fetus as which of the following?
   A. Somatic pain
   B. Visceral pain
   C. Referred pain
   D. Psychosomatic pain
5. When assessing a client, the nurse determines that the client's particular culture views injections as more effective for pain relief than pills. This is a description of the cultural beliefs of
   A. Middle Eastern culture.
   B. Hispanic culture.
   C. Far Eastern Asian/Pacific culture.
   D. American Indian culture.

6. The two most reliable sources for determining the existence of pain and severity are the client's vital signs and
   A. self-report of the client using the FLACC scale.
   B. subjective client observation using the Wong-Baker FACES pain scale.
   C. self report of the client using a 0- to 10-point scale rating for the level of pain.
   D. evaluating the client's verbal complaints using the FLACC scale.
7. The health care provider administers an injection of local anesthetic into a space between the dura mater and the ligamentum flavum. The nurse documents this
   A. pudendal block.
   B. spinal block.
   C. local block.
   D. epidural block.
8. If used for analgesia in labor, which drug has a significant impact on breastfeeding during the postpartum period?
   A. Secobarbital (Seconal)
   B. Meperidine (Demerol)
   C. Promethazine (Phenergan)
   D. Nalbuphine (Nubain)
9. Following an epidural, the client's systolic blood pressure drops from a baseline of 118 mm Hg to 75 mm Hg. The nurse's most immediate response should be to
   A. administer ephedrine IV.
   B. inform the anesthesiologist.
   C. increase the IV fluid rate.
   D. administer oxygen by nasal cannula.

REFERENCES

Alehagen, S., Wijma, B., Lundberg, U., Wijma, K. (2005). Fear, pain and stress hormones during childbirth. *Journal of Psychosomatic Obstetrics and Gynecology, 26*(3), 153–165.

American College of Obstetrics and Gynecology (ACOG) Committee on Obstetric Practice. (2002). ACOG Committee Opinion No. 269, February 2002. Analgesia and cesarean delivery rates. *Obstetrics and Gynecology, 99*(2), 369–370.

Baumgarder, D. J., Muehl, P., Fischer, M., & Pribbenow, B. (2003). Effect of labor epidural anesthesia on breast-feeding of healthy full-term newborns delivered vaginally. *Journal of the American Board of Family Practice, 16*(1), 7–13.

Beech, B. (1999). Drugs in labour: What effect do they have twenty years hence? *Midwifery Today, 50,* 31–33, 65.

Britt, R., & Pasero, C. (1999). Pregnancy, childbirth, postpartum, and breastfeeding. In M. McCaffery & C. Pasero (Eds.), *Pain: Clinical manual* (2nd ed., pp. 608–625). St. Louis: Mosby.

Chang, Z. M., & Heamon, M. I. (2005). Epidural analgesia during labor and delivery: Effects on the initiation and continuation of effective breastfeeding. *Journal of Human Lactation, 21*(3), 305–314.

Cohen, J. (1996). Doctor James Young Simpson, Rabbi Abraham De Sola, and Genesis Chapter 3, verse 16. *Obstetrics and Gynecology, 88,* 895–898.

Falk, K. M. (2006). Pain management. National Center of Continuing Education. Retrieved April 3, 2006, from http://www.nursece.com/onlinecourses/9004.html.

Gallen, E. *Nursing herbal medicine handbook.* (2001). Springhouse, PA: Springhouse Publishers.

Gaiser, R. R. (2005). Labor epidurals and outcome. *Best Practice and Research: Clinical Anaesthesiology, 19*(1), 1–16.

Green, J. M., & Baston, H. A. (2003). Feeling in control during labor: Concepts, correlates, and consequences. *Birth, 30*(4), 235–247.

Halpern, S. H., Levine, T., Wilson, D. B., MacDonell, J., Katsiris, S. E., & Leighton, B. L. (1999). Effect of labor analgesia on breastfeeding success. *Birth, 26*(2), 83–88.

Joint Commission on Accreditation of Healthcare Organizations. (2001). Pain assessment and management standards: Ambulatory care. Retrieved April 4, 2006, from http://www.jcrinc.com/subscribers/perspectives.asp?durki=3240&site=10&return=2897.

Karch, A. M. (2005). *2005 Lippincott's nursing drug guide.* Philadelphia: Lippincott Williams & Wilkins.

Lang, A. J., Sorrell, J. T., Rodgers, C. S., & Lebeck, M. M. (2006). Anxiety sensitivity as a predictor of labor pain. *European Journal of Pain, 10*(3), 263–270.

Lowe, N. K. (2004). Context and process of informed consent for pharmacologic strategies in labor pain care. *Journal of Midwifery and Women's Health, 49*(3), 250–259.

Melzack, R., & Wall, P. D. (1965). Pain mechanisms: A new theory. *Science, 150,* 971–979.

Morrison, L. M., Wildsmith, J. A., & Ostheimer, G. W. (1996). History of pain in childbirth. In A. Van Zundert & G. W. Ostheimer (Eds.), *Pain relief and anesthesia in obstetrics.* New York: Churchill Livingstone.

Munoz, C., & Luckmann, J. (2005). *Transcultural communication in nursing* (2nd ed.). Albany, NY: Thompson Delmar Learning.

Nystedt, A., Edvardsson, D., & Willman, A. (2004). Epidural analgesia for pain relief in labour and childbirth: A review with a systematic approach. *Journal of Clinical Nursing, 13*(4), 455–466.

Physician's desk reference: Nurse's drug handbook. (2003). Boston: Blackwell.

Russell, R., & Reynolds, F. (1997). Pain relief and anesthesia during labor. In R. K. Creasy (Ed.), *Management of labor and delivery.* Malden, MD: Blackwell.

Simkin, P., & Bolding, A. (2004). Update on nonpharmacologic approaches to relieve labor pain and prevent suffering. *Journal of Midwifery and Women's Health, 49*(6), 489–504.

Simpson, K. R., & Creehan, P. A. (2001). *Perinatal nursing.* Philadelphia: Lippincott Williams & Wilkins.

Volmanen, P., Valanne, J., & Alahuhta, S. (2004). Breast-feeding problems after epidural analgesia for labour: A retrospective cohort study of pain, obstetrical procedures and breast-feeding practices. *International Journal of Obstetric Anesthesia, 13*(1), 25–29.

Wappler, F. (2001). Malignant hyperthermia. *European Journal of Anaesthesiology, 18,* 632–652.

Yerby, M. (2000). *Pain in childbearing: Key issues in management.* New York: Bailliere Tindall.

POSTPARTUM PERIOD AND NEWBORN CARE

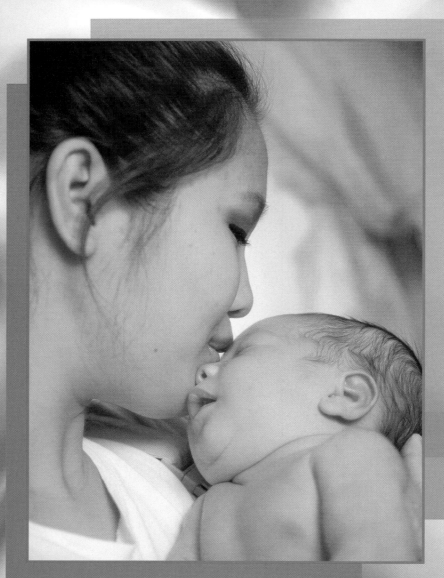

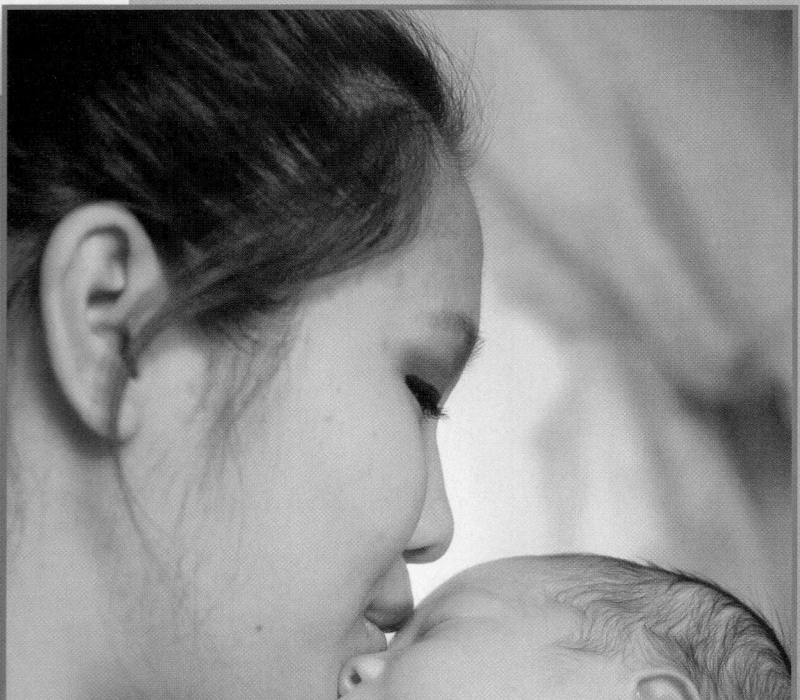

UNIT 5

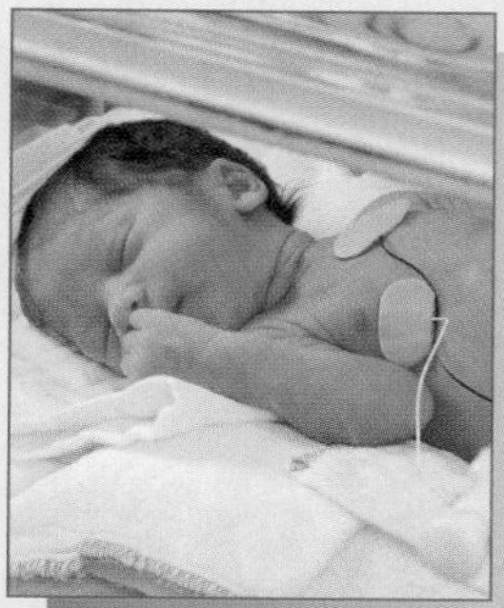
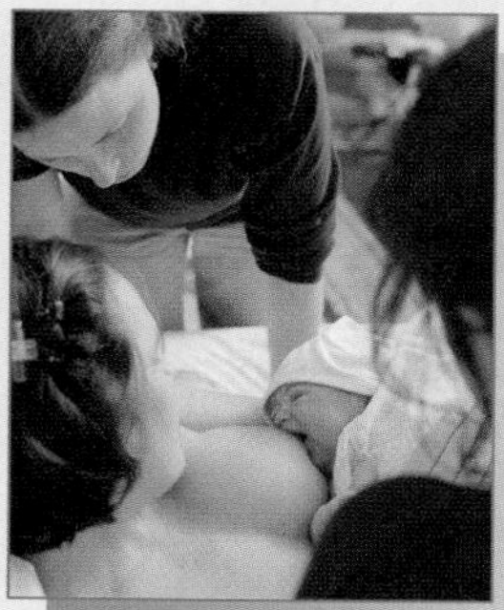
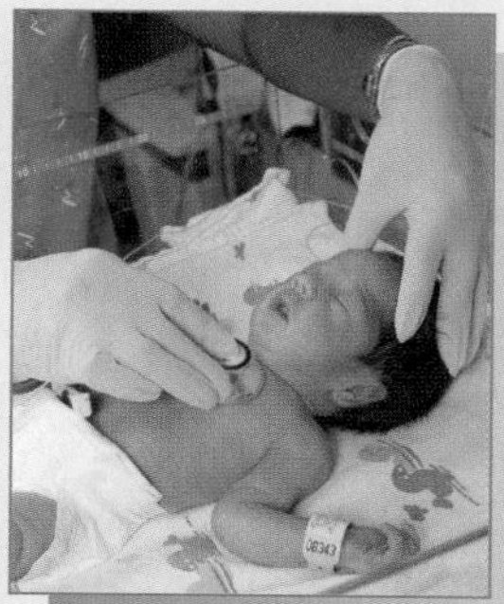
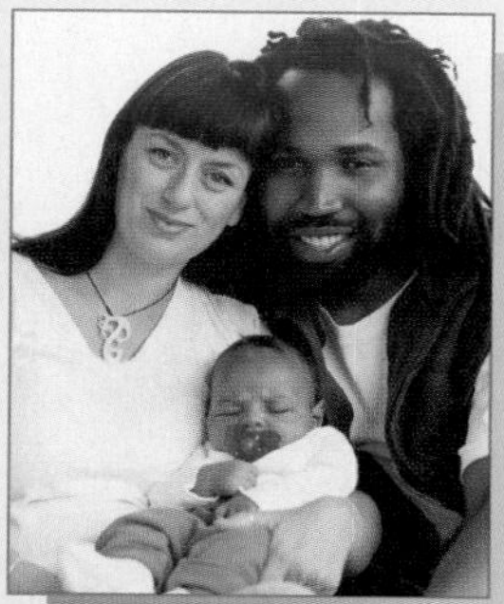

Rapid changes mark the first days and weeks after a baby enters the world, both for mother and newborn, as well as for their family and support people. The maternal body begins its gradual return to the nonpregnant state, with variations in duration influenced by the choice of newborn feeding method, the woman's own unique physiology, the conditions under which she is making the transition to motherhood, and other factors. Under normal circumstances, the newborn is embarking on a series of rapid and remarkable changes that allow him or her not only to survive but also to thrive in the extrauterine environment.

This unit describes normal and unexpected maternal physiologic and psychological changes throughout the first 6 weeks after childbirth, as well as collaborative care provisions for the new family. It explores the healthy baby's immediate post-birth transitions, as well as topics of importance to new parents for their child's initial weeks of life. The unit reviews important details about newborn feeding for both nursing and non-nursing families. It also covers common problems that newborns can face as a result of size, gestational age, congenital or acquired conditions, or other factors and collaborative strategies for managing them.

CHAPTER 18

Fourth Stage of Labor and Postpartum Period

Robin Evans

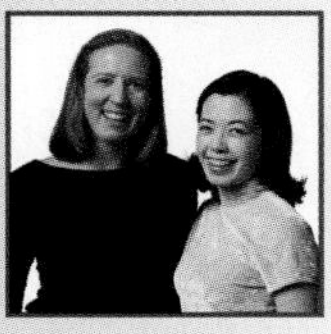

Nadia, 27 years old, has just given vaginal birth to a viable, healthy boy after 18 hours of labor. Nadia required a midline episiotomy. The placenta was delivered intact. Nadia's life partner, Chelsea, is in the labor suite attending the birth. Chelsea asks, "What happens now?"

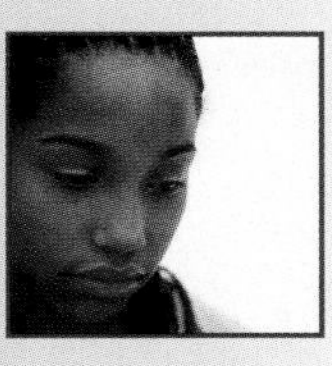

Jody, 32 years old, is a single primipara who gave birth 3 days ago in the local hospital. Jody and her daughter were discharged home on the second postpartum day. The nurse from the health care facility's early discharge program arrives at Jody's house for a routine follow-up visit 4 days later. A tearful Jody states, "The baby's been really fussy and has hardly slept since we got home. I don't know how to make her stop crying." Jody also reports that her "bottom" is sore and that her breasts "hurt a fair amount."

Nurses working with these and similar clients need to understand this chapter to care adequately for clients immediately after they have given birth and in the weeks that follow. Before beginning, consider the following points related to the above scenarios:

- What care is appropriate for the maternal client immediately after giving birth? How can health care providers appropriately involve spouses, partners, and other support people?
- What physical, psychological, emotional, and other effects might early discharge from health care facilities have on new mothers and their families? How can nurses help prepare clients for the challenges ahead?
- What behaviors and responses by clients and their families during the postpartum period would you consider "normal" reactions? What behaviors and responses would require nursing intervention?

LEARNING OBJECTIVES

On completion of this chapter, you should be able to:

- Discuss expected physiologic and psychological variations during the fourth stage of labor and postpartum.
- Identify the etiologies of physical and psychological changes during the fourth stage of labor and postpartum.
- Summarize the areas of focus in assessment during the fourth stage of labor.
- Explain comprehensive collaborative care of the woman during the postpartum period.
- Discuss teaching strategies to enhance the health, comfort, and psychological well-being of the postpartum woman.

KEY TERMS

afterpains
boggy uterus
colostrum
couplet care
engorgement
episiotomy
fourth stage of labor
hemorrhoids
Homans' sign
involution
Kegel's exercises
lochia
lochia alba
lochia rubra
lochia serosa
postpartum blues
puerperium
subinvolution
uterine atony

The birth of an infant signals the beginning of a new chapter in the life of the mother and her significant others. It also initiates several changes within the client's body, with both physiologic and psychological effects.

This chapter focuses on maternal physiologic and psychological changes during the fourth stage of labor and puerperium (postpartal period). The fourth stage of labor begins after delivery of the placenta and lasts until 1 hour postpartum (see Chap. 15). The **puerperium** consists of the first 42 days following childbirth. The content in this chapter provides information important in assisting nurses to conduct appropriate assessments and interventions for both prevention of maternal complications and promotion of a healthy mother and baby. Chapter 19 describes care in high-risk postpartum situations in detail.

PHYSIOLOGIC CHANGES

During pregnancy, all maternal body systems experience many progressive changes over 9 months. Starting with the fourth stage of labor and for several weeks to months after, these changes revert as the client's body returns to a nonpregnant state.

Weight

Immediately following birth, clients lose approximately 11 to 13 lb (5 to 6 kg), which is largely a combination of uterine contents and blood (Cunningham et al., 2005). They lose an additional 4.5 to 6.5 lb (2 to 3 kg) from diuresis in the first postpartum week. One study found that total weight loss during the first 6 weeks postpartum is similar for most women, regardless of body mass index (BMI) or weight gained during pregnancy (Gunderson et al., 2001). This same study showed that women with a BMI of greater than 29 have the least weight loss postpartum, even though they also usually have the least net weight gain during pregnancy (Gunderson et al., 2001; Walker et al., 2005).

By 6 to 18 months postpartum, women weigh an average of 8 lb (3.6 kg) more than they did before pregnancy (Gore et al., 2003; Olson et al., 2003). Factors associated with increased postpartum weight include excess weight prior to pregnancy, smoking cessation during pregnancy, reduced postpartum physical activity, lifestyle changes that may contribute to obesity, and weight gain during pregnancy (Lederman, 2001; Olson, 2003). Although a popular notion is that lactation accelerates postpartum weight loss, studies have not shown this method to have statistically significant effects (Dewey, 2004; Goldberg, 2005; Haiek et al., 2001).

QUOTE 18-1

"I was so disappointed when I went home from the hospital after giving birth. I thought I'd look the same as before I was pregnant. Was I in for a shock! I was still wearing maternity clothes a month later. Even though I lost most of the weight I had gained during pregnancy pretty quickly, it took months to be able to get into my old jeans. No one warned me how dramatic the changes would be on my body for a long time to come."

A first-time mother

Cardiovascular System

Once the fetus and placenta are delivered, the maternal body begins to return to its pre-pregnant state. The blood flow to the uteroplacental unit that increased during pregnancy is diverted to the systemic maternal circulation immediately after delivery of the placenta (James, 2001). The woman loses approximately 500 mL of blood with a vaginal birth, and 1000 mL or more with a cesarean birth (MacMullen et al., 2005; Magann et al., 2005). Plasma volume decreases initially by as much as 1000 mL from this blood loss but increases again by the third postpartum day as fluid shifts from the extracellular space into the vascular space (Bowes & Katz, 2002). Overall blood volume in the postpartum client is decreased, resulting from blood loss during birth and diuresis in the first postpartum week (James, 2001). Blood volume returns to pre-pregnant values by approximately 1 week postpartum (Cunningham et al., 2005).

Cardiac output, which increased as much as 40% during pregnancy, remains elevated for approximately 48 hours postpartum. The cause is thought to be primarily increased stroke volume from venous return (Cunningham et al., 2005). Cardiac output returns to pre-pregnancy values by 1 to 3 weeks postpartum (Cunningham et al., 2005).

Pulse rate remains stable or decreases following birth (James, 2001). A pulse rate higher than 100 beats/minute may indicate postpartum hemorrhage or infection (see Chap. 19). A rise in blood pressure of approximately 6 mm Hg systolic and 4 mm Hg diastolic is common in the first 4 days postpartum (Tan & de Swiet, 2002). Blood pressure may remain elevated, however, in women who had gestational hypertension or pre-eclampsia, hypertension before pregnancy, or late onset pre-eclampsia (see Chap. 13).

Within the first 48 hours postpartum, clients have increased blood coagulability, although research has shown that the number of platelets in relation to antepartum values varies (Bowes & Katz, 2002). This increased coagulability corresponds with an increased risk for thromboembolism in the puerperium.

Hematologic System

Following birth, the client's hemoglobin value remains close to that during pregnancy. By 6 weeks postpartum, hemoglobin will have risen to nonpregnant values (12 to 16 g/dL) (Cunningham et al., 2005; Fischbach, 2004). Any significant blood loss during labor and birth results in a decreased hemoglobin value that will take longer to return to normal. The amount of hemoglobin added during pregnancy also affects the degree and rate of fluctuation (Cunningham et al., 2005).

Most women experience no postpartum decrease in hematocrit (Cunningham et al., 2005). Because of increased blood volume during pregnancy, clients can withstand the normal blood loss that accompanies birth with little or no change in hematocrit; plasma volume decreases to a greater extent than do red blood cells (James, 2001). In some instances, hematocrit may be increased several days postpartum, as a result of the diuresis that follows birth (Rouse & St. John, 2003). By 6 weeks postpartum, the hematocrit value should have returned to normal pre-pregnancy values (36% to 48%) (Samuels, 2002).

Most women regain normal serum iron levels (50 to 170 μg/dL) by the second week of the puerperium (Fischbach, 2004). The return of hemoglobin and hematocrit values to their level before pregnancy depends on whether the woman had adequate iron stores (Samuels, 2002). The most common causes of postpartum anemia are iron deficiency and hemorrhage (Cunningham et al., 2005; Samuels, 2002). These causes may be linked, in that significant hemorrhage in one pregnancy with subsequent depletion of iron stores may contribute to iron-deficiency anemia in a later pregnancy (Cunningham et al., 2005). Iron-deficiency anemia is common in clients who took an iron supplement during pregnancy (James, 2001); therefore, they should continue the supplement for some time postpartum as well.

Abruptio placentae, placenta previa, and **uterine atony** (failure of the uterus to contract) are all significant causes of postpartum hemorrhage (see Chap. 19). Because of the risk for decreased perfusion to vital organs, hemorrhage requires aggressive collaborative management. Once hypovolemia is under control, the primary health care provider usually orders the administration of iron supplements for the resulting anemia.

Leukocytosis is common in the postpartum period, with white blood cell (WBC) counts elevated to 25,000 to 30,000/μL (James, 2001). This leukocytosis is nonpathologic, with granulocytes predominant. The relative lymphopenia (decreased lymphocytes) and absolute eosinopenia (decreased eosinophils) that may be seen, along with an elevated erythrocyte sedimentation rate (ESR), may complicate assessment of infections. A 30% increase in WBC count over a 6-hour period requires further investigation for possible infection.

Respiratory System

Following childbirth, maternal progesterone levels, intra-abdominal pressure, and diaphragmatic pressure all decrease. These changes result in the respiratory system returning quickly to a pre-pregnant state. Breathing becomes easier as the client expels the uterine contents. With more cesarean births being done with spinal or epidural anesthesia, effects on the respiratory system that previously resulted from the use of general anesthesia are decreasing.

Gastrointestinal System

After birth, maternal abdominal muscles that were stretched during pregnancy remain relaxed. This relaxation, combined with decreased gastrointestinal motility that may result from labor and birth, may lead to gaseous distention (James, 2001). This finding may be especially prevalent in women who have had a cesarean birth, following manipulation of the abdominal contents. Decreased motility may predispose the woman to paralytic ileus. Thus, clients who undergo cesarean birth usually receive only clear fluids until bowel sounds are present, followed by solids (James, 2001). Heartburn during pregnancy usually resolves by approximately 6 weeks postpartum as pressure on the esophageal sphincter and stomach decrease following birth.

Women may continue to experience constipation in the postpartum period, although the underlying reasons for it differ from those during the antepartum period. Postpartally, fear of pain or tearing of sutures may lead to reluctance to defecate, increasing the incidence of constipation. Other contributing factors may include dehydration, immobility, and use of medications such as iron preparations and codeine. **Hemorrhoids** (rectal varicose veins that protrude from the anus or are hidden internally) during pregnancy may be more prominent following labor and birth. They may cause discomfort and also contribute to constipation. Women usually have a bowel movement within the first several days after childbirth. Normal bowel function returns in approximately 2 weeks.

Integumentary System

Following childbirth, skin hyperpigmentation that resulted in chloasma (mask of pregnancy) disappears. Chloasma may reappear, however, if the woman experiences excessive sun exposure or takes oral contraceptives (Goodheart, 2003). Striae gravidarum, or "stretch marks," begin to fade to a silvery white.

Abdominal muscle distention during pregnancy that results in separation of the rectus muscles may persist after birth. With proper exercise and limited stress placed on these muscles, they usually reapproximate and heal by the late postpartum period.

Endocrine System

During pregnancy, the placenta produces large amounts of estrogen and progesterone, causing significant elevations of these hormone levels from the nonpregnant state. With delivery of the placenta, estrogen and progesterone levels sharply decrease (Cunningham et al., 2005). Prolactin, a hormone secreted by the anterior pituitary gland, promotes milk secretion (Guyton & Hall, 2006). The concentration of prolactin begins to rise in the fifth week of pregnancy and continues until birth, when it reaches a level 10 to 20 times that of the nonpregnant level (Guyton & Hall, 2006). The high levels of estrogen and progesterone during pregnancy inhibit secretion of milk; their decrease at birth initiates the client's ability to lactate (Guyton & Hall, 2006). Plasma prolactin levels fall to the pre-pregnant state over the first few weeks following birth; however, the levels surge and rise with each act of suckling by the infant (Cunningham et al., 2005; Guyton & Hall, 2006).

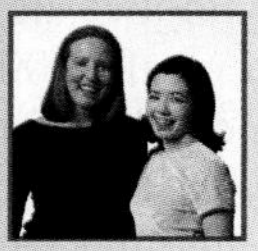

Remember Nadia, who has just given birth to a son. What hormonal changes would the nurse expect Nadia to be experiencing at present?

During pregnancy, the thyroid gland increases up to 50% from its pre-pregnancy state, with a corresponding rise in production of thyroxine, primarily from placental secretion of human chorionic gonadotropin (hCG) (Guyton & Hall, 2006). Thyroid hormone levels normally return to pre-pregnancy values approximately 4 to 6 weeks postpartum (Bowes & Katz, 2002). Immunosuppression, a normal physiologic consequence of pregnancy, may result in the development of transient thyroiditis and hypothyroidism, which can become permanent (Sarvghadi et al., 2005). Accompanying symptoms include memory loss, lack of concentration, and depression (Lazarus, 2005). The basal metabolic rate (BMR), which was elevated during pregnancy partly because of increased adrenocortical hormones and increased thyroxin levels, returns to normal within 7 to 14 days postpartum.

Postpartum glucose levels often fall as a result of delivery of the placenta and the resulting loss of its hormones, such as human placental lactogen (hPL). As the client loses the insulin resistance produced by hPL, her blood glucose levels also decrease. The client with type 1 diabetes mellitus experiences reduced insulin requirements postpartum and will need adjustments to her insulin dosages. Breastfeeding may contribute to hypoglycemia.

Reproductive System

The reproductive system probably experiences the greatest postpartum changes of all. As during pregnancy, the most noticeable changes occur in the uterus (see Chap. 12).

Uterus

The uterine body consists primarily of myometrium covered by serosa and lined by basal decidua (Cunningham et al., 2005; Marchant, 2003). Once its contents are expelled with birth of the newborn and delivery of the placenta, the uterine cavity collapses. The uterus contracts, and the myometrial cells begin to decrease (Cunningham et al., 2005; James, 2001). This process of contraction and decreased size is referred to as **involution.**

The uterus weighs approximately 1000 g after birth. With involution, it decreases to 500 g by 1 week postpartum, 300 g at 2 weeks postpartum, and finally to 100 g or less by 6 weeks postpartum (Bowes & Katz, 2002; Cunningham et al., 2005; James, 2001). Immediately after birth, the uterine fundus is palpable slightly below the level of the umbilicus. After the first 2 days, the fundus descends into the pelvis at a rate of approximately 1 cm/day until it returns to its previous pre-pregnant size by approximately 4 to 6 weeks postpartum (Bowes & Katz, 2002; Cunningham et al., 2005). This rate is highly individualized, however, and thus may not follow a specific schedule (Marchant, 2003) (Fig. 18.1).

During the first few days postpartum, the uterus continues to contract. In primiparas, contractions usually are tonic, meaning that they are continuous. In multiparas, the uterus periodically contracts vigorously, causing cramps referred to as **afterpains.** Although primarily seen in multiparas, some primiparas also experience afterpains (Marchant, 2003). Women tend to feel afterpains more severely during breastfeeding, probably because the process of nursing stimulates the release of oxytocin from the posterior pituitary gland (Cunningham et al., 2005).

The decidua basalis separates into two layers: basal and superficial (James, 2001). As the superficial layer is sloughed off, vaginal discharge, termed **lochia,** results (Cunningham et al., 2005). Erythrocytes, shreds of decidua, epithelial cells, and bacteria are visible microscopically in lochia (Cunningham et al., 2005). For the first 3 to 4 days, enough blood is in the lochia to make it appear dark red (**lochia rubra**). By 4 to 5 days, less blood is present, and the lochia becomes progressively paler (**lochia serosa**). By approximately the 10th day, increased leukocytes and decreased fluid content combine to give the lochia a white or yellowish white appearance (**lochia alba**). Lochia may continue for up to 4 weeks postpartum; it may reappear up to 56 days postpartum (Cunningham et al., 2005). The total volume of lochia is approximately 150 to 400 mL (James, 2001). Its flow may increase concurrently with breastfeeding and afterpains, probably from the secretion of oxytocin, which stimulates uterine contraction.

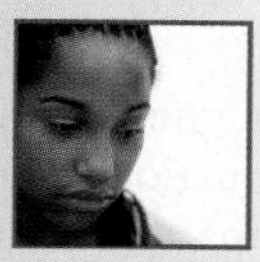

Think back to Jody, the single mother who was discharged home on her second postpartum day and is receiving routine follow up 4 days later. Where would the nurse expect to assess Jody's uterine fundus? What type of lochia would be expected?

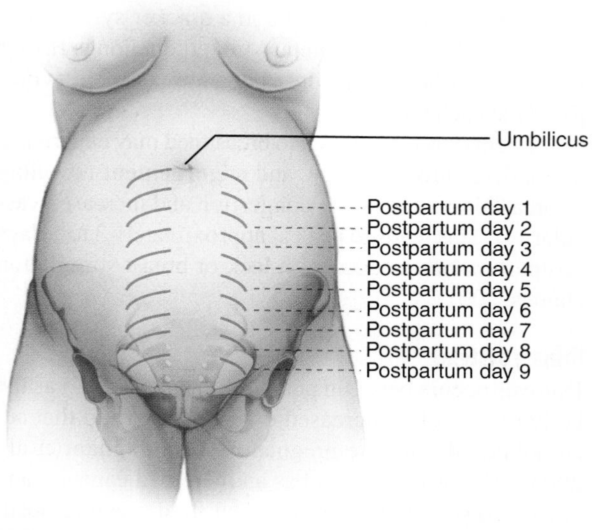

FIGURE 18.1 Progression of uterine involution during the postpartal period.

The endometrium regenerates by the third week postpartum, and the placental site takes approximately 6 weeks to heal (Cunningham et al., 2005). Immediately after birth, the site measures approximately 8 to 10 cm, decreasing rapidly until the end of the second week, when it is approximately 3 to 4 cm in diameter (James, 2001). The placental site heals from the margins, preventing formation of scar tissue. During this process, necrotic tissue is exfoliated and sloughed off, sometimes resulting in a limited increased vaginal flow that lasts only 1 to 2 hours (Cunningham et al., 2005). If the site does not heal properly, postpartal hemorrhage may occur (see Chap. 19).

Subinvolution, an arrest or slowing of involution, is characterized by prolonged lochia, irregular or excessive uterine bleeding, and sometimes profuse hemorrhage (MacMullen et al., 2005). The primary cause of subinvolution is failure of the uterus to contract effectively, resulting in a **boggy uterus.** The main contributors to a boggy uterus are retention of placental tissue and exposure of large blood vessels after placental separation (Cunningham et al., 2005; MacMullen et al., 2005).

Cervix

The cervix and lower uterine segment are thin following birth. Cervical lacerations may be present, especially along the lateral outer margin, which corresponds with the external os (Cunningham et al., 2005). Women who have had a precipitous labor or an instrument-assisted birth (eg, forceps or vacuum extractor) are at greatest risk for cervical lacerations (Poole et al., 2001).

The cervical os contracts slowly, continuing to admit two fingers until the end of the first postpartum week, when it narrows to 1 cm. By this time, the cervix has begun to thicken and elongate. Cervical edema may be present for several months following childbirth (Bowes & Katz, 2002).

The cervix never returns to its pregravid state (Fig. 18.2). The os continues to be slightly wider than previously, with depressions where lacerations occurred (Cunningham et al., 2005). The lower uterine segment contracts much less forcefully than does the remainder of the uterus. It does, however, eventually return to a smaller isthmus between the uterine body and the internal cervical os (Cunningham et al., 2005).

Ovaries

For the first several weeks following birth, gonadotropin activity is minimal (James, 2001). Menstruation usually returns approximately 6 to 10 weeks postpartum for the nonlactating client and 8 weeks to 18 months postpartum for the breastfeeding client (Cunningham et al., 2005). Researchers hypothesize that elevated prolactin levels in lactating women partly account for the delayed return of menstruation (James, 2001). Approximately 25% of women ovulate before the first menses (James, 2001); the remainder do not ovulate until after menses returns. The chance for ovulation within the first 6 months postpartum in a woman who is breastfeeding exclusively is 1% to 5% (Bowes & Katz, 2002).

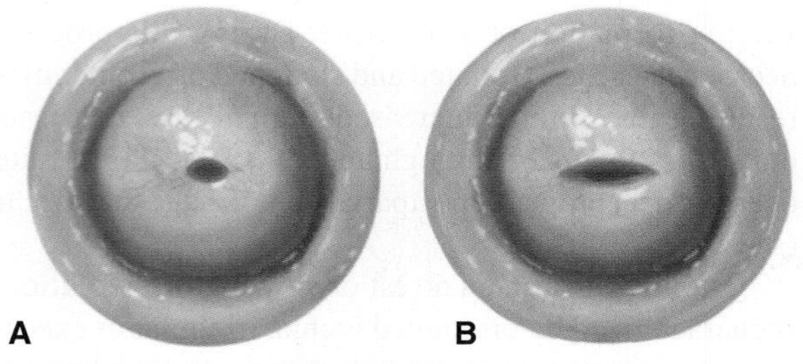

FIGURE 18.2 The cervical os in a client who has never been pregnant (**A**) and after giving birth (**B**).

Vagina

The vagina and vaginal wall may appear smooth and bruised in the early postpartum period. The bruising tends to disappear quickly, partly from decreased pelvic congestion. Rugae reappear in the vagina approximately 3 weeks postpartum (James, 2001). The voluntary muscles of the pelvic floor, often lax in the early puerperium, regain their tone after approximately 6 weeks. Because the lactating woman often has a high circulating estrogen level as a result of ovarian suppression, the return of rugae may be delayed.

Breasts

Postpartum changes in the breasts primarily are related to the client's newborn feeding decision. Delivery of the placenta and the subsequent sudden decrease in circulating progesterone and estrogen stimulate the anterior pituitary to secrete prolactin (see Chap. 21). Repeated sucking by the infant stimulates the release of prolactin and affects the intensity and duration of lactation (Cunningham et al., 2005). Prolactin levels are high for approximately the first 10 days postpartum before declining slowly over the next 6 months (Walker & Creehan, 2001).

The neurohypophysis secretes oxytocin, which stimulates contractions of the uterus, myoepithelial cells in the alveoli, and small milk ducts (Cunningham et al., 2005) (Fig. 18.3). Women sometimes feel the "let-down reflex," the sensation that accompanies the release of oxytocin and contractions of the alveoli and small milk ducts in the breast, as a tingling or heaviness in the breast (Walker & Creehan, 2001). It is primarily stimulated by the infant sucking on the breast, but it also may be stimulated by the sound of the infant's cry. See Chapter 21 for further discussion of breastfeeding.

Production of milk is related closely to the infant's demands. Efficient nursing, in which the breasts are emptied with each feeding, results in a quicker synthesis of milk with a higher fat content. Milk production is slower in the client whose infant does not empty the breast completely at each feeding.

Clients who choose not to breastfeed may experience breast discomfort, leakage, and **engorgement** (swelling of breast tissue caused by congestion and increased vascularity). This tends to peak at approximately 3 to 5 days postpartum but recedes with lack of breast stimulation (James, 2001).

Urinary System

Diuresis occurs between postpartum days 2 and 5 as the body reverses the increased extracellular fluid that accumulated during the pregnancy (Cunningham et al., 2005). The bladder often has an increased capacity and decreased sensation to intravesical fluid pressure, leading to problems of urinary retention and overdistention. Other contributing factors include any anesthesia used

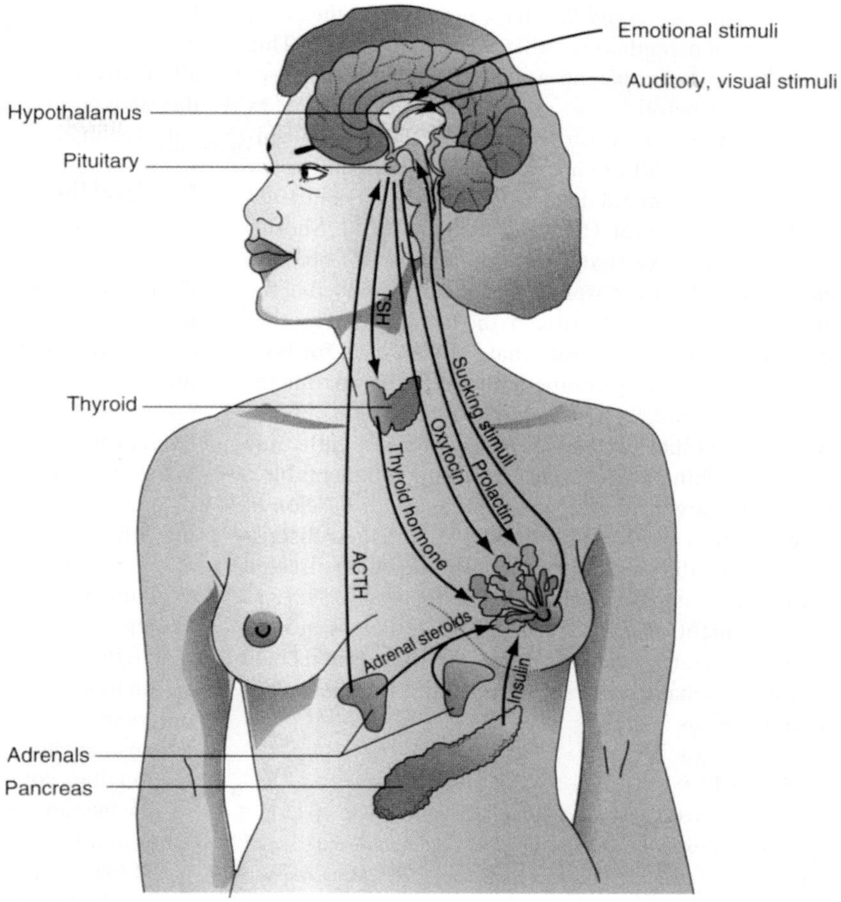

FIGURE 18.3 Stimulation of the hormones responsible for lactation by the newborn's suckling. ACTH, adrenocorticotropic hormone; TSH, thyroid-stimulating hormone.

during labor and birth, as well as alterations in bladder neural function. Bladder distention is evident when the fundus is found higher in the abdomen and off to the right as the full bladder displaces the uterus. Spontaneous voiding should resume within 8 hours after birth. Bladder tone should return by postpartum day 5 to 7. Carpal tunnel syndrome that the woman may have experienced during pregnancy resolves as diuresis reverses the edema that caused pressure on the median nerve (Pazzaglia et al., 2005).

The dilated ureters and renal pelves associated with pregnancy return to their pre-pregnant state by approximately 2 to 8 weeks postpartum (Cunningham et al., 2005). Glomerular filtration rate (GFR) and renal blood flow return to normal pre-pregnant values within 6 weeks (James, 2001).

Postpartum clients may develop or continue to have stress incontinence. This finding occurs primarily in clients who had a prolonged second stage of labor, gave vaginal birth to an infant with a large head circumference, gave vaginal birth to a large-for-gestational-age (LGA) baby, or required an **episiotomy** (see Chap. 15) resulting in impaired muscle function around the urethra (Glazener et al., 2006; Schytt et al., 2004).

Glycosuria disappears; creatinine clearance usually is normal by 1 week postpartum. Mild proteinuria, however, may persist for the first day or two. Blood urea nitrogen (BUN) may be increased because of the sloughing of necrotic tissue during involution (James, 2001).

PSYCHOLOGICAL CHANGES AND MATERNAL ADJUSTMENT

Many primipara clients anticipate that life following birth will be a modified version of their usual circumstances. Adequately preparing for the physical, psychological, social, and emotional changes they will undergo, particularly during the early postpartal period, is challenging (George, 2005; Nelson, 2003). Even a client with previous children who is somewhat prepared for what to expect after a new baby arrives may sense expectations from others to quickly "pick up the pieces" and carry on with her life, experiencing only joy and delight in her baby (O'Reilly, 2004). While many clients relish their new roles and responsibilities, several challenges, both physiologic and psychological, influence reactions. Various factors can cause the postpartum period to unfold differently than initially expected. Regardless of how much the client and her family may have prepared for the baby, the reality of parenthood is still a significant change. This is true for first-time parents as well as for those who have been parents before.

The time that a postpartum client spends in hospital following childbirth has decreased significantly over recent years: from 3.8 days in 1980 to 2.4 days in 1997 (National Center for Health Statistics, 2002). Shorter hospital stays have significant implications for both the care provided in the hospital and the care provided in the community. During the time in the hospital, the mother is expected to demonstrate that she can care for both herself and her baby competently, at the same time recovering physically (Bowman, 2005; Martin, 2002). Because this shortened hospital stay provides little time for new teaching, prenatal classes and appointments have assumed a larger role as opportunities for discussion of care for both mother and infant. Established discussions during the prenatal period allow teaching directed toward the postpartum client in the hospital to serve as reinforcement of prior learning. Nevertheless, not all pregnant clients participate in prenatal classes or receive adequate prenatal care, so the potential for substantial learning needs is high.

QUOTE 18-2

"The first few weeks after I had the baby were a rollercoaster. I was happy, scared, excited, sad, exhausted, and energized all at the same time. I loved my baby so much, but sometimes I felt jealous, because all the attention that had been on me for several months immediately moved to her."

A first-time mother

Immediate Reactions

Directly following birth, the mother often views her newborn in wonderment, closely inspecting and counting fingers and toes (Fig. 18.4). If she intends to breastfeed, initiation at this point is beneficial to both her and the baby. The newborn is in a quiet wakeful state, usually ready to feed. Success in initiating breastfeeding at this time provides positive feedback to the client and instills feelings of confidence.

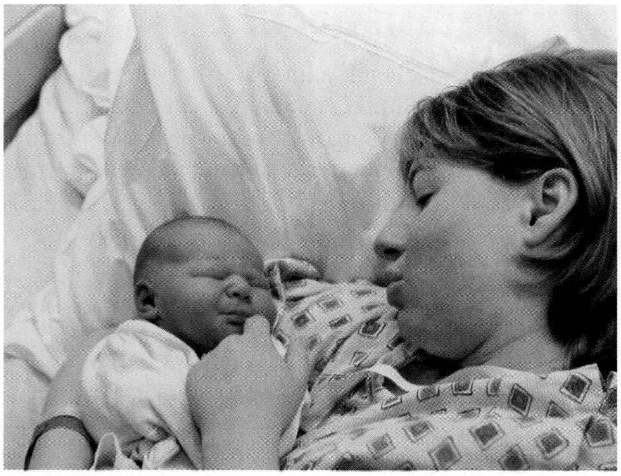

FIGURE 18.4 The new mother bonds with her baby immediately after giving birth.

Theories of Change

Development of the maternal role begins during pregnancy and continues in the early postpartum period. Dominant theories of postpartum change suggest that the process is composed of distinct phases that the client progresses through in a linear fashion, completing each before moving into the next. Although some researchers have suggested that these theories are outdated, others believe the tasks involved remain valid. What they consider invalid is viewing each phase as discrete and the process as linear. Studies indicate that the processes clients experience are much more fluid and continuous (Fenwick et al., 2005; Martell, 2001; Waldenstrom, 2004) (Research Highlight 18.1). For example, Rubin's theory, developed in 1961, indicated that in the first 3 postpartum days, the new mother often wants to share her experiences of labor and birth with others in an effort to understand and resolve inconsistencies between expectations and reality. This generalization does not apply to all women. Some clients need to discuss and resolve any developments during the labor and birth that did not happen as they had anticipated (eg, the client who anticipated a vaginal birth but instead had a cesarean birth).

Clients also tend to focus on food and sleep during this time. They spend the next few days focusing on regaining control of their lives and adjusting to the responsibilities of caring for their infants. Because clients may spend only a small part of this time in a hospital where supports are directly available to assist with caring for self and baby, the availability of supports in the home and community for the initial period after discharge assumes new importance (Jack et al., 2005).

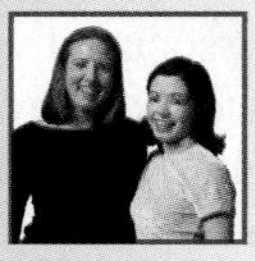

Think back to Nadia and her partner Chelsea who have just become parents of a new baby boy. Chelsea asks, "What happens now?" How would you respond?

Sleep Deprivation and Exhaustion

While the mother is working to accept her new reality, she also is concerned with her newborn. Depending on the length and timing of labor and birth, the new mother may be coping with sleep deprivation, which may be aggravated as she contends with multiple interruptions and expectations while tending to the needs of herself and

RESEARCH HIGHLIGHT 18.1 Heading Toward the New Normal: A Contemporary Postpartum Experience

OBJECTIVE: To develop a theoretical description about contemporary first-time mothers' experiences during the first 2 to 3 weeks following a vaginal birth.

DESIGN: This qualitative descriptive study used grounded theory methodology and constant comparison to develop a theoretical description from the data.

PARTICIPANTS AND SETTING: Thirty-two primiparous women who had a vaginal birth completed an initial questionnaire and were interviewed within the week following discharge from the hospital and again 1 to 2 weeks later. The first interview focused on the early postpartum experience. The second interview provided an opportunity for the mothers to discuss what had happened since the previous interview and to verify and clarify initial findings. The researcher also used the second interview to saturate the emerging themes. All interviews took place in the women's homes.

RESULTS: The core theme was reorganization of the women's lives as mothers, what the researcher referred to as "heading toward the new normal." Within this core theme, three processes were identified, each with three subcategories:

1. Appreciating the body
   a. Restoring the body
   b. Connecting to the newborn
   c. Thinking differently
2. Settling in
   a. Becoming competent
   b. Developing confidence
   c. Accommodating/integrating the newborn into their lives
3. Becoming a new family
   a. Realigning relationships
   b. Developing new routines
   c. Delineating boundaries

Identified nursing implications included helping the client feel that she and her newborn are safe and cared for; assuring the client that nursing assistance is available around the clock for any help needed; keeping explanations simple and based on a few essential topics; adapting teaching to suit the client's usual problem-solving strategies; maintaining a positive focus during discharge teaching on how to determine whether the baby is healthy; providing information about support services that the mother may access if she needs help or feels that she can't handle the situation; and supporting decisions appropriate for the mother's lifestyle and within developmental and safety parameters for the newborn.

CONCLUSION: Previous theories of puerperal change suggested that women experienced discrete and linear stages, completing one phase before moving to the next. Findings from this study suggest, however, that contemporary women experience a fluid and continuous process.

Martell, L. K. (2001). *Journal of Obstetric, Gynecologic, and Neonatal Nursing, 30,* 496–506.

baby. Sleep deprivation may lead to such problems as seeming disinterest in the baby, mood swings, and difficulty coping (Dennis & Ross, 2005; George, 2005; Ross et al., 2005). Health care providers need to critically assess for signs of sleep deprivation to differentiate behaviors resulting from exhaustion from those caused by true attachment problems. The health care provider may seek information about the amount of sleep that the client is getting, both during the night and with any naps taken during the day. If behaviors such as disinterest or excessive crying are evident despite sufficient sleep, the health care provider may consider alternate reasons for challenges to attachment with the baby.

Emotional State

Society in general often has unrealistic expectations of motherhood that are difficult, if not impossible, to attain (Beck, 2002). The client may expect to be a perfect mother, happy with her child and able to cope with the baby and all the changes with little or no help; in short, the fairy tale mother. She or others close to her may assume that the client will have no difficulty in adapting to her multiple roles, bonding with her baby, or coping with the amount of time and the unpredictability required to care for the tiny, helpless newborn. Such expectations tend to be inconsistent with reality (George, 2005). Clients who believe that they should meet these expectations are at risk for compromising their mental health (Mazzeo et al., 2006).

Estimates are that 30% to 75% of women experience **postpartum blues** (feelings that cause them to cry frequently, often for what they consider no reason), usually within 2 to 3 weeks after giving birth (Seyfried & Marcus, 2003; Vieira, 2003). Symptoms are mild and may include increased emotional lability, crying, and emotional sensitivity (Chaudron, 2003). Lack of sleep can compound the woman's inability to cope with these symptoms; conversely, the associated emotional

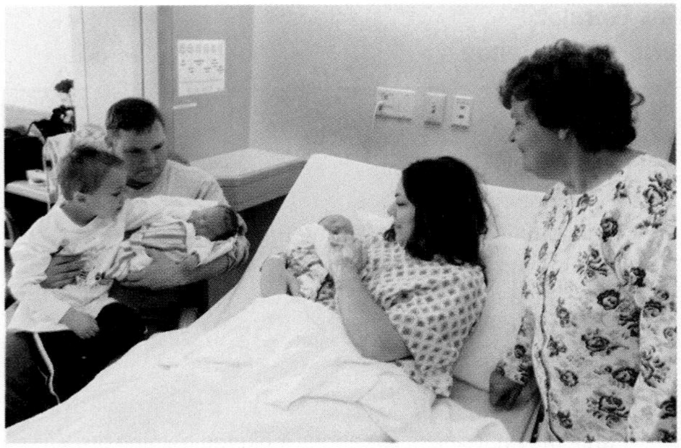

FIGURE 18.5 Couplet care allows the family to bond with the newborn during the period of recovery in the health care facility.

lability and crying may affect the woman's ability to achieve a satisfactory amount and quality of sleep to meet her needs. Thus, health care providers should urge women to nap and rest as much as possible whenever the baby is quiet.

Postpartum depression is a more serious condition (Beck, 2002). Women with postpartum depression experience many different emotions including anger, guilt, anxiety, irritability, loneliness, sleep disorders, feelings of being overwhelmed, a sense of failure, and feelings of harming themselves or their babies (Beck, 2002; Chaudron, 2003; Edhborg et al., 2005). There seems to be no absolute set of symptoms that any woman experiences; each woman's combination of feelings and emotions is unique. Other psychological problems during the postpartum period include postpartum psychosis and postpartum anxiety disorders. See Chapters 5 and 19 for more detailed discussion.

COLLABORATIVE CARE: THE FOURTH STAGE OF LABOR AND POSTPARTUM PERIOD

Many facilities today primarily base nursing care for mothers and newborns on the concept of **couplet care.** In couplet care, nurses care for mother and baby as a unit. This is in contrast to previous models of care that separated mothers and newborns for extended periods. The couplet model provides the mother and significant others with time to interact with the infant, becoming attuned to his or her schedules and habits (Fig. 18.5).

Most facilities also employ one of two models of care for the overall process of labor through postpartum. The first model is referred to as *labor, delivery, recovery, and postpartum (LDRP).* In LDRP, the client remains in the same room throughout all four phases. In the second model, the client is in one room to experience labor, childbirth, and recovery. She then moves to another room, often on another unit, for her postpartum stay.

Immediate Assessment

Health care providers conduct a focused maternal assessment during the **fourth stage of labor,** the period from delivery of the placenta until 1 hour after birth (Table 18.1). Vital signs, including pulse and blood pressure, require assessment every 15 minutes for the first hour following delivery of the placenta (James, 2001; Weathersby, 2002). More frequent monitoring may be required if the woman's condition is unstable. Nursing Care Plan 18.1 highlights the assessment and care of a client in the fourth stage of labor.

The nurse should assess the client's temperature at least once in this first hour. Many clients develop gener-

(text continues on page 721)

TABLE 18.1 Expected Findings and Alterations During the Fourth Stage of Labor

ASSESSMENT	EXPECTED FINDINGS	ALTERATIONS	POSSIBLE CAUSES
Pulse	May be slightly decreased from labor	Rate > 100 beats/min	Postpartum hemorrhage
Blood pressure	Mild rise of approximately 6 mm Hg systolic, 4 mm Hg diastolic	Increases above levels mentioned	Gestational hypertension Pre-eclampsia Hypertension before pregnancy Late-onset pre-eclampsia
Temperature	May be slightly increased	>100.4°F, 38°C	Early postpartum infection
Uterus	Fundus usually approximately one to two fingerbreadths below umbilicus, firm and midline	Fundus above umbilicus, deviated from midline Fundus boggy	Distended bladder, clots retained in uterus Uterine atony, retained placental fragments
Lochia	Moderate rubra	More than two pads saturated in 1 hour	Bleeding from lacerations, uterine atony, postpartum hemorrhage
Bladder	Should not be palpable	Distention	Urinary retention
Perineum	Pink, no signs of bruising or edema	Bruising, edema, hematoma	Tissue trauma during delivery

NURSING CARE PLAN 18.1

The Postpartum Mother during the Fourth Stage of Labor

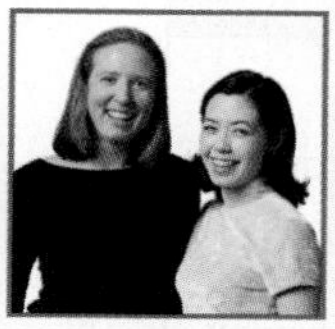

Recall Nadia and her partner, Chelsea, the new parents of a healthy baby boy. Nadia is in the fourth stage of labor, and Chelsea is at her bedside. They have decided that Natalie will breastfeed the newborn. Maternal assessment reveals that Nadia's fundus is firm and midline at the level of her umbilicus. She states, "I feel cold and tired. I'm a bit sore." Chelsea asks, "Is this normal?"

NURSING DIAGNOSIS

Risk for Injury related to possible complications associated with the fourth stage of labor

EXPECTED OUTCOMES

1. The client will remain free of injury during the fourth stage of labor.

INTERVENTIONS	RATIONALES
Assess vital signs every 15 minutes, including temperature at least once during the first hour.	Fluctuating vital signs provide clues to changes in the client's physiologic status.
Palpate fundus for height, location, and firmness every 15 minutes.	After childbirth, the uterus should be firm and located at the midline.
Massage the uterus if it feels boggy, soft, or difficult to locate; administer medications such as oxytocin as ordered.	A uterus that is not well contracted can predispose the client to hemorrhage. Oxytocin aids in contracting the uterus.
Inspect the lochia for amount, color, and clots every 15 minutes.	Saturation of more than two perineal pads during this time suggests hemorrhage; clots may suggest uterine atony or retention of placental fragments, predisposing the client to hemorrhage.
Inspect the perineum every 15 minutes for edema, appearance of episiotomy, and possible evidence of lacerations; inspect the episiotomy for intactness and approximation.	Perineal inspection provides clues to possible areas of infection or hematoma formation or unsuspected areas of bleeding. The episiotomy should be intact with well-approximated edges to prevent possible complications.
Apply ice to the perineum.	Ice provides comfort and promotes vasoconstriction.
Palpate the client's bladder for distention; encourage her to void if possible.	A distended bladder interferes with uterine involution, increasing risk for hemorrhage.
Offer the client a warm blanket; change bed clothes and linens frequently.	A warm blanket promotes comfort; chilling and shaking are common after childbirth. Frequent linen changes prevent further chilling from diaphoresis, also common postpartally.
Provide the client with fluids (intravenously or orally as indicated); provide diet as tolerated and ordered.	The postpartum client is often hungry after childbirth because of energy expended during labor and limited oral intake. Fluids aid in maintaining fluid balance.

Continued

NURSING CARE PLAN 18.1 ● The Postpartum Mother during the Fourth Stage of Labor *(Continued)*

INTERVENTIONS	RATIONALES
Assess the lower extremities for redness, swelling, and warmth. Check Homans' sign.	Postpartum clients are at risk for thrombophlebitis and thrombus formation from an increased hypercoagulable state.
Encourage the client to put the newborn to her breast to feed.	Breastfeeding in this early period helps stimulate milk production and promote attachment.

EVALUATION

1. The client exhibits vital signs and assessment findings within acceptable parameters.
2. The client remains free of any signs and symptoms of complications.

NURSING DIAGNOSIS

Deficient Knowledge related to client's and partner's inexperience with labor, birth, and parenthood

EXPECTED OUTCOMES

1. The client and partner will verbalize understanding of events associated with labor and birth.
2. The client and partner will demonstrate beginning attachment behaviors with the newborn.

INTERVENTIONS	RATIONALES
Assess understanding of postpartum events and care; recognize the client, partner, and newborn as a family unit.	Assessment provides a baseline from which to develop appropriate interventions.
Explore the family's exposure to postpartum and newborn care; ascertain their participation in childbirth education classes; correct any misconceptions or myths related to these methods; allow time for questions.	Information about exposure provides additional foundation for teaching and provides opportunities to clarify or correct misinformation and teach new information.
Explain the various assessments and monitoring that will be done and the information that each can reveal.	This information will help alleviate anxiety about unknown aspects of the process.
Review the measures to facilitate physiologic adjustment during the postpartum period, including self-care measures and the need for adequate rest and nutrition.	Numerous physiologic changes occur during the postpartum period as the client's body returns to her pre-pregnancy state.
Assist the family with initial efforts at putting the newborn to the breast; encourage en face positioning, touching, stroking, and talking.	Breastfeeding immediately after birth and interaction with the newborn promote bonding and attachment.

Continued

NURSING CARE PLAN 18.1 ● The Postpartum Mother during the Fourth Stage of Labor

INTERVENTIONS	RATIONALES
Encourage the partner to assist the client with measures and provide necessary support; discuss ways the partner can participate in breastfeeding, such as the client pumping her breasts and the partner feeding the newborn.	Partner participation promotes sharing of the experience and feelings of control over the situation.
Begin teaching the family newborn care measures as appropriate; when possible, have them demonstrate care.	Initial teaching helps foster independence and self-esteem; return demonstration aids in determining the effectiveness of the teaching.
If necessary, initiate referral for community services to assist with transition.	Additional support from community services may be necessary to promote a positive experience for the family.

EVALUATION

1. The client and partner verbalize understanding of events associated with labor and birth.
2. The client and partner use appropriate behaviors to interact with newborn.
3. The client and partner verbalize positive statements about their newborn and about themselves as parents.
4. The client and partner demonstrate beginning ability to care for their newborn.

alized shaking and teeth chattering, as though they were cold, even though temperature remains stable during this time. This response is normal following the stress of labor and birth, and a warmed blanket can provide comfort. If the client underwent a cesarean birth under general anesthesia, assessment of her vital signs also should include evaluation of her respiratory rate.

The nurse should assess the client's uterus every 15 minutes during the fourth stage of labor for fundal height and tone (Nursing Procedure 18.1). The examiner should place one gloved hand just above the symphysis pubis, either with the medial side of the hand or the area between the thumb and other fingers in a "V" shape against the client's skin. This positioning guards the uterus and prevents any downward displacement that may result in prolapse or inversion. With the other gloved hand, using the flat side of the fingers and hand and beginning above the umbilicus, the nurse should firmly palpate the abdomen and feel for the uterine fundus. The fundus will feel like a hard round object within the abdominal cavity. In the period immediately following birth, the fundus is easily palpable within the abdomen. The examiner should assess position of the fundus in relation to the umbilicus and measure it in fingerbreadths (eg, one fingerbreadth above the umbilicus). Immediately following birth, the uterus should be one to two fingerbreadths under the umbilicus, although it is normal to find it up to the height of the umbilicus. The fundus should be in the midline of the abdomen.

During palpation for tone, the fundus should feel hard as a result of uterine contraction. If the uterus is not well contracted, the fundus will feel boggy, soft, or difficult to find. The nurse should gently massage a boggy fundus with his or her hand, maintaining the position of the second hand that is guarding the uterus until the uterus returns to firm. Once the fundus regains firmness, the nurse should discontinue massage. The postpartum woman is at greatest risk for hemorrhage within the first hour following birth because of the exposure of large venous sinuses after placental separation (James, 2001; Weathersby, 2002).

The nurse should assess the woman's lochia every 15 minutes during the fourth stage of labor for color, amount, and any clots. During this first hour, the expected finding is moderate lochia rubra with no clots. Saturation of more than two pads within this first hour

(text continues on page 724)

NURSING PROCEDURE 18.1

Assessing the Uterus, Lochia, and Perineum after Vaginal Childbirth

PURPOSE

To evaluate uterine involution after vaginal birth and reduce the risk for postpartum hemorrhage

ASSESSMENT AND PLANNING

- Review the client's intrapartal record for time of childbirth and any possible complications during labor and birth, including the presence of episiotomy.
- Assess the amount of blood loss during birth.
- Determine the time of the last uterine assessment.
- Ask the client about any pain.
- Gather equipment
    - Clean gloves
    - Perineal pads (if not at the client's bedside)
    - Light source (overhead light, penlight, or flashlight)
    - Waterproof linen saver pad
    - Perineal care supplies, such as squeeze bottle with warm water and bedpan

IMPLEMENTATION

1. Explain the procedure and rationale to the client, informing her that she may feel some discomfort, *to aid in alleviating anxiety.*
2. Ask the client when she last voided; have her empty her bladder *to prevent bladder from interfering with uterine involution;* help the client ambulate to the bathroom or offer a bedpan as indicated.
3. Provide for client privacy by drawing the curtain, closing the door, and covering the client with a bath blanket or sheet.
4. Have the client lie supine with her head flat or on a pillow *to assist in accurate assessment of fundal height.* Allow the client to flex her knees if appropriate *to help relax the abdominal muscles.*
5. Put on gloves and expose the abdominal and perineal areas.
6. Place the nondominant hand in a slightly cupped position at the lower fundus just above the symphysis pubis *to help stabilize and support the uterus.*
7. Working from the umbilicus down, gently move the dominant hand down the abdomen until the top of the fundus is located. It should be at the midline and feel hard and round.
8. If the fundus does not feel firm, gently massage the uterus using the dominant hand while maintaining the position of the nondominant hand on the lower uterus *to stimulate uterine contraction and prevent uterine inversion.* Continue to massage the uterus until it becomes firm; avoid too vigorous massaging or overmassaging *to prevent uterine muscle exhaustion.*

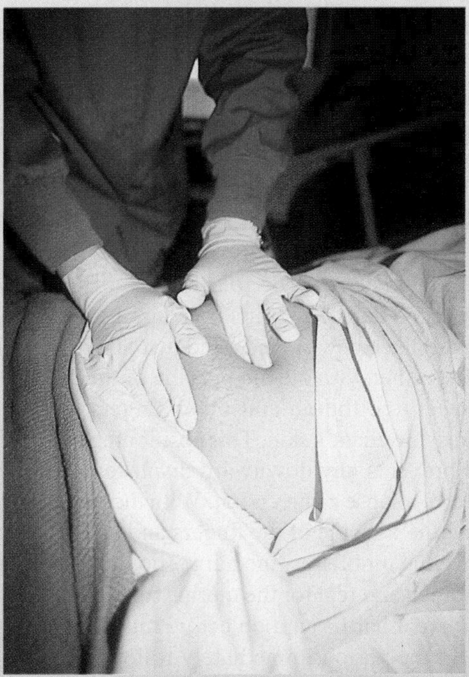
Step 7. Locating the position of the fundus.

Continued

NURSING PROCEDURE 18.1 CONTINUED

Assessing the Uterus, Lochia, and Perineum after Vaginal Childbirth

9. Using the fingers as a guide, measure the distance from the umbilicus to the top of the fundus in fingerbreadths *to determine the progression of involution.*
10. Remove and inspect the client's perineal pad; note the amount, color, and character of the drainage.
11. Check under the client's buttocks *to evaluate for any blood that may be pooling there.*
12. Inspect the perineal area *to assess for possible complications.* Include the episiotomy line as appropriate. Note the approximation of the episiotomy edges and the appearance of any drainage from the stitches. Report any redness, edema greater than minimal, ecchymosis, or hematomas.
13. Assist the woman to turn on her left side; lift the upper buttock to reveal the perineal area. Inspect the area for changes.
14. Assist the client back to the supine position and provide or assist with perineal care. Replace the waterproof linen saver pad. Provide the woman with a clean perineal pad.
15. Remove gloves and discard all used equipment and supplies appropriately.
16. Document findings.

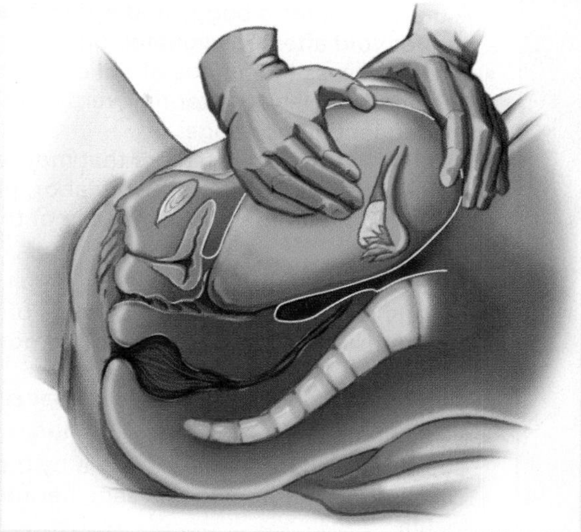

Step 8. Massaging the fundus.

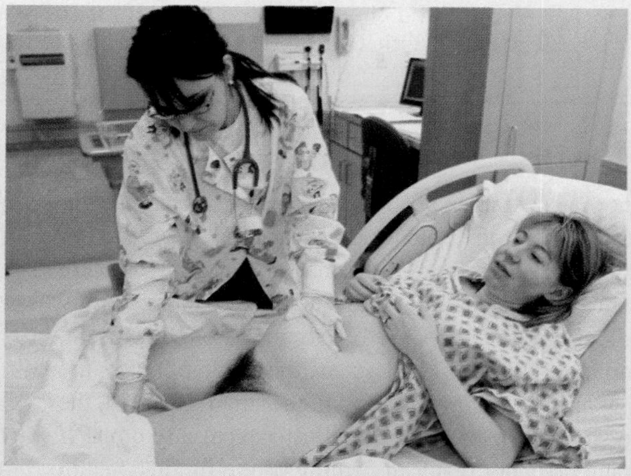

Step 10. Assessing the perineal pad for lochia.

EVALUATION

1. Fundus was firm and midline at the appropriate height for the client's postpartum day.
2. The client exhibited moderate lochia rubra, with minimal to no clots.
3. The episiotomy site was clean, dry, and intact with well-approximated edges.

AREAS FOR CONSIDERATION AND ADAPTATION

Perinatal Considerations

- Encourage the client to void before palpation of the fundus. A full bladder can interfere with uterine involution.

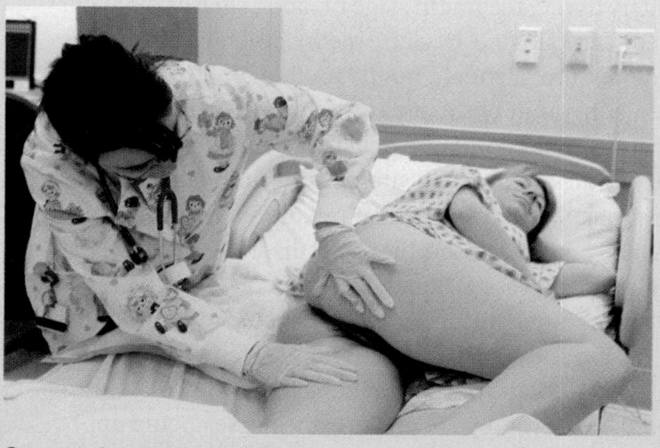

Step 13. Inspecting the perineum.

Continued

NURSING PROCEDURE 18.1 CONTINUED

Assessing the Uterus, Lochia, and Perineum after Vaginal Childbirth

A uterus that feels boggy and is displaced from midline suggests a full bladder. If the client cannot void after a designated time (eg, 6 to 8 hours), anticipate the need for catheterization.

- Closely assess the fundus of a client who has given birth to more than one newborn. Multiple gestation can lead to uterine overdistention, placing the client at risk for uterine atony and subsequent hemorrhage.
- Be alert for other risk factors that may lead to uterine atony and postpartum hemorrhage, including prolonged or difficult labor, placenta previa or abruption, labor augmentation or stimulation with oxytocin, and use of tocolytics.

Lifespan Considerations

- Closely assess the fundus and lochia of a multiparous client because multiparity is a predisposing risk factor for postpartum hemorrhage.

Community-Based Considerations

- Expect to continue to assess a client's fundus, lochia, and perineum at home visits. The fundus should no longer be palpable by the 10th day postpartum.
- Teach the client how to massage her uterus, inspect her episiotomy site, and monitor her lochia.
- Review signs and symptoms associated with uterine subinvolution, which may lead to late postpartum hemorrhage.
- Instruct the client to notify her primary care provider about any changes in lochia amount, characteristics, and odor or if she experiences any fever.

is abnormal (Weathersby, 2002). Excessive lochia may indicate uterine atony, retention of placental fragments, or lacerations of the perineum, vagina, or cervix. Assessment of the uterine fundus should reveal whether uterine atony is the cause of the excessive bleeding; if atony is present, the nurse should begin to massage the fundus. If clots are present and the fundus is found higher than expected, the nurse should massage it carefully to expel any clots. If massage does not result in firming of the fundus, health care personnel may administer medications often ordered routinely during the fourth stage of labor, such as oxytocin or methylergonovine. Because methylergonovine elevates blood pressure, it should not be used in any woman with pre-existing high blood pressure. If bleeding continues, the nurse should notify the physician. Bleeding that continues with a contracted uterus may indicate cervical lacerations that have not been repaired adequately or a previously undiagnosed bleeding disorder such as von Willebrand's disease (James, 2006).

The nurse should assess the perineum every 15 minutes during the fourth stage of labor. He or she should identify any edema or signs of hematoma (a swollen, discolored area). If they are present, the nurse should apply ice to the affected area. Additionally, the nurse should evaluate the site of episiotomy or laceration for edema and approximation.

Ongoing Assessment

Ongoing assessments involve those measures performed during the first hour postpartum as well as several additional components (Table 18.2). Following a systematic regimen that the nurse can repeat multiple times for many clients is most efficient. One of the most common methods is to use the acronym BUBBLES to organize a head-to-toe assessment (Assessment Tool 18.1). When working with postpartum clients, it is important for the nurse to recognize not only any alterations and their significance, but also the interrelationship between changes in body systems and their different manifestations in different assessments.

Vital Signs

Protocols for assessment of pulse and blood pressure vary among institutions; however, most include a schedule of more frequent assessments for the first 24 hours postpartum, which is when the client is at greatest risk for hemorrhage (James, 2001; Weathersby, 2002) (Fig. 18.6). An example may include assessment of vital signs every 30 minutes for 1 hour after the first hour of assessments, then every 4 to 6 hours for the remainder of the 24 hours postpartum. Indications for more frequent monitoring will dictate any necessary variations.

Nurses usually take the client's temperature every 4 to 6 hours postpartum. Temperature may increase

TABLE 18.2 Expected Findings and Alterations in the Postpartum Period

ASSESSMENT	EXPECTED FINDINGS	ALTERATIONS	POSSIBLE CAUSES
Pulse, blood pressure, and temperature	Within normal limits	Increased pulse Increased or decreased blood pressure Increased temperature	Postpartum hemorrhage Puerperal infection Late onset pre-eclampsia
Breasts	Soft for first 48 to 72 hr If breastfeeding, fuller, firmer breasts, intact nipples If not breastfeeding, breasts may be engorged and leaking by the third day	Engorgement if breastfeeding Painful, reddened, bruised nipples	Incorrect latch Tongue tie
Uterus	Fundus firm, midline, height decreasing approximately one fingerbreadth below umbilicus each day	Fundus higher in abdomen than expected Fundus boggy	Full bladder Retention of placental fragments Subinvolution Uterine atony
Bladder	Voiding, not palpable, diureses	Decreased sensation to void	Prolonged effects of anesthesia Altered bladder neural function
Bowels	Bowel sounds Bowel movements	Absent or decreased bowel sounds Constipation	Decreased motility Paralytic ileus Fear of pain, tearing of any sutures Hemorrhoids Dehydration Immobility Medications
Lochia	Gradually decreasing amount, which may increase after breastfeeding or rising from recumbent position Rubra for 3 to 4 days, serosa until day 10, then alba	Increased amount from expected or previously assessed	Uterine atony Retention of placental fragments Postpartum hemorrhage
Episiotomy/perineum	No ecchymosis or edema, sutures (if present) intact and well approximated	Ecchymosis, edema, sutures missing, episiotomy reddened, with discharge, dehiscence, or both	Trauma to tissues during delivery Infection of episiotomy/laceration
Homans' sign	Negative	Positive (pain felt in calves on dorsiflexion of foot) Redness, swelling, and heat on back of calf	Thrombophlebitis or thrombus formation
Psychosocial	Shares experiences of labor and birth Looks directly at infant (en face position) Touches and talks to baby Interprets baby's behavior appropriately May have increased emotional lability and sensitivity and cry more between day 3 and week 2	Interacts very little with infant Rarely talks or touches infant Feels angry, guilty, anxious, irritable, lonely, overwhelmed Has difficulty sleeping Feels sense of failure Has thoughts of harming self or baby Palpitations	Fatigue Thyroid dysfunction Postpartum depression Anxiety disorder Postpartum psychosis

ASSESSMENT TOOL 18.1
Postpartum Assessment Guide

B—breasts
U—uterus
B—bladder
B—bowel
L—lochia
E—episiotomy/perineum
S—homans' sign

minimally in the initial 24 hours postpartum as a result of the dehydration that accompanies prolonged labor. The nurse should instruct the client to report any elevation in temperature above 100.4°F (38°C) once she is discharged. This finding may indicate a postpartum infection, especially if it occurs in the first 10 days.

Breasts

Assessment of the breasts primarily is related to the client's newborn feeding decision. For example, slight engorgement in a client who has chosen to breastfeed has

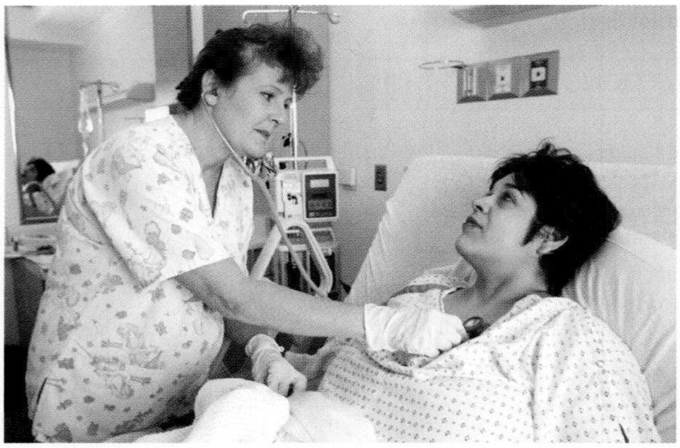

FIGURE 18.6 The nurse checks the client's vital signs as part of postpartum assessment.

different significance than in a client who has chosen to formula feed. The subsequent plan for nursing actions also differs for each.

The nurse should assess any postpartum client's breasts for symmetry, consistency, and lumps. If the client is breastfeeding, the breasts initially are soft, usually for approximately the first 48 to 72 hours (Walker & Creehan, 2001). After this time, milk begins to form, and the breasts fill. As milk production increases, the breasts become fuller and firmer. Veins become more prominent. Some clients experience engorgement, in which the breasts, nipples, or both become hard and distended. Engorged breasts usually are extremely uncomfortable and may create breastfeeding difficulties because the infant may have trouble latching onto the distended nipple.

If the client is breastfeeding, the nurse should assess the nipples for intactness. He or she should note any signs of redness, bruising, or cracking. Bruising appears as black or blue patches, often toward the periphery of the nipple. Cracking usually develops following redness as the nipple is subjected to continued suction pressure from an incorrectly positioned infant's mouth. Assessment of the latch during feeding may reveal reasons for these conditions and provide cues to the nurse for additional teaching that may assist the woman to correct latching issues. See Chapter 21 for further discussion.

If the client is formula feeding, the nurse should check the nipples for any discharge and the breasts for any lumps or hardness. The client may experience some fullness of her breasts and leaking 1 to 4 days following the birth of her baby (Walker & Creehan, 2001). The swelling is usually less pronounced than in the mother who is breastfeeding; however, it can be equally painful and disturbing.

Uterus

As discussed earlier, the nurse should assess the client's uterus for fundal height and tone (Weathersby, 2002). He or she should check the position of the fundus in relation to the umbilicus and measure it in fingerbreadths (eg, one fingerbreadth above the umbilicus). By approximately 12 hours after childbirth, the fundus is found at the level of the umbilicus (Weathersby, 2002). It usually decreases by approximately one fingerbreadth per day beginning on day 2 until it can no longer be palpated by approximately day 8 to 10. By that time, it is too low in the abdomen to be felt. The nurse should feel the fundus in the midline of the abdomen. A fundus palpable above the level of the umbilicus and to the right is most frequently the result of a full bladder. For this reason, it often is advantageous for the nurse to encourage the client to void before assessment.

Other factors that the nurse should consider when assessing and interpreting uterine findings include vital signs, particularly the pulse and blood pressure, lochia, and the bladder.

Bladder

The nurse should assess the client's bladder for amount, frequency, and any difficulties initiating voiding or emptying the bladder. Some women experience problems with retention, either an inability to void at all or retaining residual urine. Such difficulties often relate to pressure on the bladder during labor and birth, perineal trauma and resulting edema, or the continuing effects of anesthesia (Groutz et al., 2004). If the course of childbirth suggests a risk for these problems, the nurse should measure the client's initial voidings until output is adequate (Zaki et al., 2004).

Urinary frequency typically accompanies diuresis. It also may be present, however, as overflow if the woman does not empty the bladder completely. The nurse should palpate the bladder to assess for adequate emptying. A full bladder usually pushes the uterus up in the abdomen, resulting in a fundus higher than expected and shifted to the client's right side. A full bladder is implicated in uterine atony and increased vaginal discharge. Critical thinking in performing any postpartum assessment includes ensuring that the woman has voided prior.

Bowels

The bowels are the next area for assessment. The nurse should auscultate the client's abdomen for bowel sounds; especially in cases of cesarean birth, manipulation of abdominal contents may increase the potential for an ileus. Sounds should be audible in all four abdominal quadrants. The nurse should ask the client whether she has had a bowel movement and if any problems or complications accompanied it. Clients may have some apprehension about having a bowel movement. Expressed concerns often relate to fear of associated discomfort or pain and, for women with episiotomy or lacerations, "ripping my stitches." Teaching about potential effects of postponing elimination, such as that retaining feces in the large intestine promotes further absorption of water leading to more difficult passage, may provide the information necessary to make an informed decision. Information also may have the added benefit of providing reassurance.

Lochia

The nurse should assess the lochia for color, amount, and any clots (see Nursing Procedure 18.1). If the woman has voided just before the assessment, she usually will have changed her perineal pad, necessitating adaptation in evaluation of the lochia. The nurse can manage this process in several ways. He or she may request that the client refrain from discarding the pad in the garbage, instead leaving it in the bathroom for assessment. Alternatively, the nurse may ask the client to describe her flow. The nurse should base this decision primarily on an individual basis, considering the client's ability to perform this assessment and his or her experience. For example, the nurse will be less likely to consult the client who has given birth a short time before assessment, but more likely to consult with the client who is several days postpartum and familiar with the characteristics of her flow. Documentation of lochia includes the color (rubra, serosa, or alba), any odor, and amount (Fig. 18.7).

The nurse should look for and document any clots, including size and consistency. He or she should further examine findings to differentiate between true clots and tissue. The nurse may attempt to separate the material, using either gloves or tongue depressors. Material that can be separated easily confirms a clot. If separation is difficult or impossible, the nurse should suspect the presence of tissue. In this case, he or she should collect the specimen and send it to the laboratory for histologic examination.

Assessment of lochia is tied closely to assessment of the fundus, bladder, and vital signs, particularly pulse and blood pressure. The nurse should assess the lochia for amount, color, any clots, and odor. He or she should base the significance of expected findings contextually according to the course of the postpartum period.

During the fourth stage of labor, lochia is usually rubra, moderate, and without clots. The client should not saturate more than two pads in the first hour. If the client's flow is heavier or contains clots, the fundus may be atonic. Assessment and appropriate intervention are required.

Although the greatest risk for postpartum hemorrhage is within the first hour after birth, clients also may develop late postpartum hemorrhage (between 24 hours and 6 weeks postpartum). Typically, flow decreases over time. The color of lochia should change from rubra (red) to serosa (pink) by approximately postpartum day 4 or 5. The serosa lochia should change to alba (yellowish white) by approximately day 10.

Perineum

Before assessing the perineum, the nurse should collect information about whether the client had an episiotomy, a laceration, or an intact perineum to individualize and guide findings. If the client received an episiotomy, the nurse should check whether it was midline or mediolateral. If midline, the nurse may ask the client to lie on either side for the assessment. If the episiotomy is either right medi-

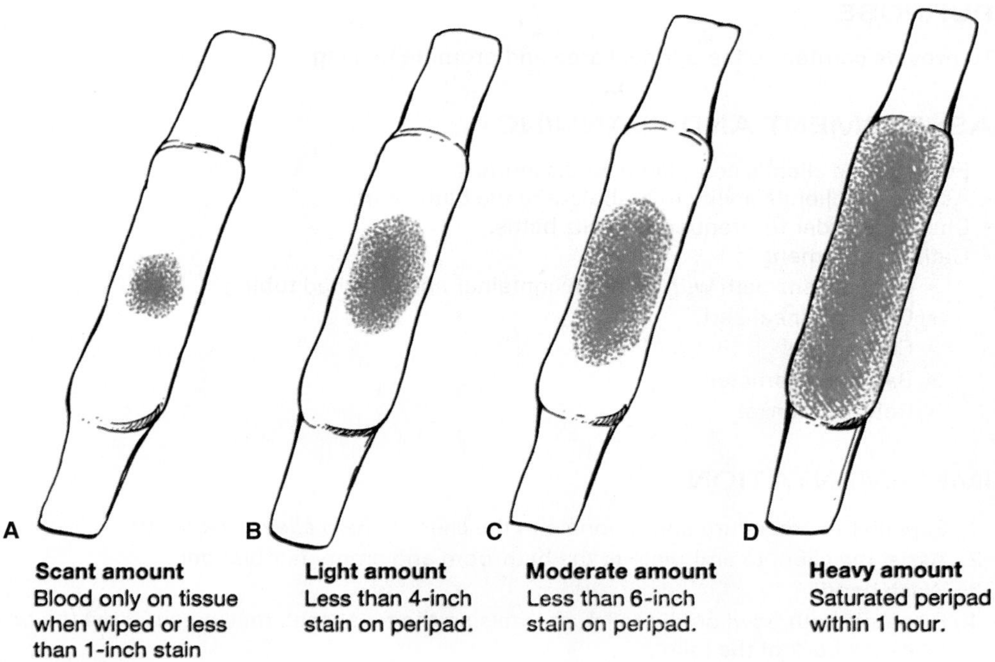
A
Scant amount
Blood only on tissue when wiped or less than 1-inch stain on peripad.
B
Light amount
Less than 4-inch stain on peripad.
C
Moderate amount
Less than 6-inch stain on peripad.
D
Heavy amount
Saturated peripad within 1 hour.

FIGURE 18.7 (**A**) With scant lochia, just a little bit of coloring or darkening appears to be on the top. (**B**) With light lochia, approximately one third of the pad is covered centrally. (**C**) With moderate lochia, approximately two thirds of the pad is covered centrally. (**D**) With heavy lochia, the whole pad is covered.

olateral (RML) or left mediolateral (LML), the client should lie on the side that puts the episiotomy next to the bed. For example, if a client had an LML episiotomy, she should lie on her left side for the assessment; if the client had an RML, she should lie on her right side. Such positioning prevents the application of tension to the episiotomy and sutures, as the nurse lifts the upper cheek of the buttocks to facilitate inspection.

Collection of information about any perineal laceration, including the degree assigned, prepares the nurse for what will be seen. Cervical, first-degree, and second-degree lacerations are rarely visible because the sutures are usually hidden within the vagina, making direct assessment impossible. Visible lacerations, most frequently third and fourth degree, involve structures that the nurse can assess more easily.

To check the episiotomy or lacerations, the nurse should don clean gloves. He or she should ask the client to assume a side-lying position on the bed. The nurse should lift the client's upper buttock cheek to allow for adequate light and visualization. Assessment of episiotomy and lacerations follows the same guidelines as for any incision. These include evaluations for redness, edema, ecchymosis, discharge, and approximation (REEDA). The nurse also should check to ensure that sutures are intact. See Nursing Procedure 18.1.

If the client has no episiotomy or laceration, the nurse should assess the perineum for edema and bruising. Even though the perineum is intact, the client may still experience edema, resulting from prolonged pushing during the second stage or a large baby. Cool compresses or ice packs are most effective in reducing edema and promoting comfort if applied during the first 24 hours postpartum (Weathersby, 2002). The nurse should take care to ensure that the cold is not applied directly to the skin, but that a barrier is used for application. After 24 hours, warmth is more appropriate. The nurse should encourage the client to use a sitz bath to provide warm, moist heat. Alternatively, the client may prefer a tub bath for the same outcome. See Nursing Procedure 18.2.

Calves

Because the postpartum woman is at increased risk for thrombophlebitis and subsequent development of a

NURSING PROCEDURE 18.2

Assisting the Postpartum Client with a Sitz Bath

PURPOSE

To provide comfort to the perineal area and promote healing

ASSESSMENT AND PLANNING

- Evaluate the client's complaints of discomfort.
- Assess the client's ability to ambulate to the bathroom.
- Check the order for frequency of sitz baths.
- Gather equipment:
  - Portable sitz bath with solution container and attached tubing
  - Clean perineal pad
  - Clean towel
  - Bath thermometer
  - Robe or blanket

IMPLEMENTATION

1. Explain the procedure and rationale to the client *to help alleviate anxiety.*
2. Assist the client to ambulate to the bathroom and empty her bladder.
3. Wash hands.
4. Place sitz bath bowl on the toilet after raising the toilet seat, making sure that the opening faces the back of the toilet.
5. Attach the tubing to the slot on the bowl with the end of the tubing in the bowl with the openings facing up. Clamp the tubing.

Continued

NURSING PROCEDURE 18.2

Assisting the Postpartum Client with a Sitz Bath

6. Fill the solution container with warm water at a temperature from 102°F to 105°F; check temperature with a bath thermometer as necessary *to prevent thermal injury to the client.*
7. Secure the container closed; hang it a few feet above the level of the sitz bath *to ensure a constant flow by gravity when the tubing is unclamped.*
8. Unclamp the tubing and allow the warm water to fill the bowl, then reclamp the tubing.
9. Have the client remove her perineal pad; assist her to sit on the sitz bath so that her perineum is in the warm water.
10. Unclamp the tubing and allow the warm water to flow. Advise the client to adjust the flow of water using the clamp on the tubing. The water will flow from front to back, exiting at the opening in the back of the bowl.
11. Provide the client with a blanket or robe *to prevent chilling.*
12. Provide for privacy; place the emergency call bell within the client's reach *to ensure safety.*
13. Advise the client to remain seated on the sitz bath for approximately 20 minutes.
14. Instruct the client to press the call bell if she feels lightheaded or dizzy or experiences any problems.
15. After 20 minutes, assist the client to pat herself dry with a clean towel using a front to back motion *to prevent contamination of the area.*
16. Assist the client to put on a new perineal pad and then to ambulate back to her bed.
17. Clean equipment for reuse following standard precautions.
18. Document the interventions, including any teaching completed and the client's ability to tolerate and assist with the procedure.

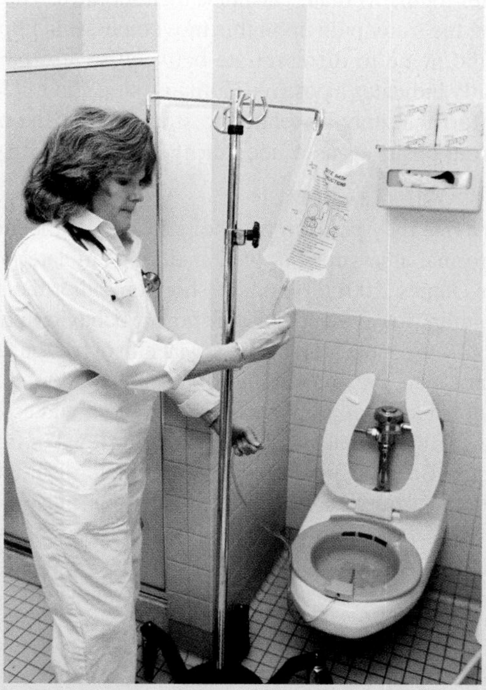

Step 8. Clamping the tubing for the sitz bath.

EVALUATION

- The client tolerated the procedure without any complaints of fatigue, dizziness, or lightheadedness.
- The client participated in setting up and performing the procedure.
- The client verbalized relief of perineal discomfort after the sitz bath.
- The client experienced no evidence of thermal injury.

AREAS FOR CONSIDERATION AND ADAPTATION

Perinatal Considerations

- Pregnant clients may use sitz baths to deal with hemorrhoids that can develop during pregnancy from increased venous pressure from the expanding uterus.
- Be aware that some health care providers are prescribing cool water sitz baths to provide comfort. Check with the health care provider about which type of bath is ordered.

Community-Based Considerations

- Be sure to teach the woman how to perform the sitz bath so that she can continue the treatment at home.
- Instruct the woman to perform the sitz bath at home approximately 3 to 4 times per day.
- Urge the woman to check the temperature of the water carefully to ensure her safety.

thrombus, the nurse should direct assessment toward early detection of these problems (James, 2001). He or she initially should check the client's lower legs for any redness, swelling, or warmth that may indicate early thrombophlebitis. If findings are normal, he or she should proceed with checking for **Homans' sign** (Fig. 18.8). The client should assume the supine position and dorsiflex each ankle. Alternatively, the nurse may dorsiflex the ankles for the woman. The nurse then should ask the client if she feels any pain upon this movement. It is important for the nurse to differentiate between severe pain that usually indicates a positive Homans' sign and milder discomfort that may be related to stretching of the muscle or from positions assumed during labor and birth.

Psychological and Emotional State

The nurse may perform psychological assessment during the formal assessment as well as during any later interactions (James, 2001). He or she should monitor the mother and infant for evidence of attachment behaviors: holding the baby to enable looking directly at him or her (en face position); touching and talking to the baby; and interpreting infant behavior appropriately. The nurse should assess the mother's emotional lability as well as the level of maternal fatigue (Beck & Indman, 2005). Her state of fatigue can have direct implications for behaviors that may be incorrectly assessed as emotional lability. The nurse should evaluate the client's teaching needs on an ongoing basis, taking opportunities to educate whenever needs are apparent.

Rectus Muscle

The nurse should assess the client's rectus muscle at least once in the early postpartum period for any diastasis or separation. This diastasis may result from the growing uterus and fetus during pregnancy that forces the muscles apart. To do so, the client should lay supine on the bed without a pillow under her head. The nurse should place the index and middle fingers across the muscle and ask the woman to raise her head. This movement results in the rectus abdominis muscles becoming more prominent (Bickley, 2007), making any separation in the muscles easily palpable. If the nurse feels a separation of more than two fingers' width, or if "peaking" of the abdominals is visible, he or she should caution the woman to avoid any exercises that put stress on the abdominal muscles (Brayshaw, 2003) and to avoid any heavy lifting or vacuuming for at least 6 weeks until the muscle can heal. Failure to follow this guideline could result in a hernia.

Rh Status

The RH antigen is inherited as a dominant factor. Rh incompatibility exists when the mother is Rh negative (lacks Rh antigen) and the biological father is Rh positive. If the couple's first fetus is Rh positive, the mother may be sensitized by exposure to the antigen through mixing of fetal and maternal blood. The woman's body recognizes the antigens as foreign and thus begins to make antibodies against them (isoimmunization). Because this process takes time, this fetus is usually not at any risk for complications. Problems may develop, however, with subsequent pregnancies. If the fetus is Rh positive, the antibodies can cross the placenta, attach to fetal RBCs, and begin to hemolyze them (Harrod et al, 2003). This can lead to a fetal anemia called **hemolytic disease of the newborn.** Hemolytic disease of the newborn may be possible in a first fetus if the mother was exposed to the antigen because of a fetal maternal hemorrhage during a miscarriage or abortion (Cunningham, 2005).

To prevent hemolytic disease of the newborn, anti-D gamma globulin (RhoGAM) is given routinely to all Rh-negative women at 28 weeks' gestation or after any invasive procedures that could result in mixing of maternal and fetal blood (eg, amniocentesis) (Cunningham, 2005). Nevertheless, isoimmunization can still happen in clients who receive late or no prenatal care. For this reason, the nurse should review the client's Rh status and proceed to administer RhoGAM if necessary, as described in Nursing Procedure 18.3.

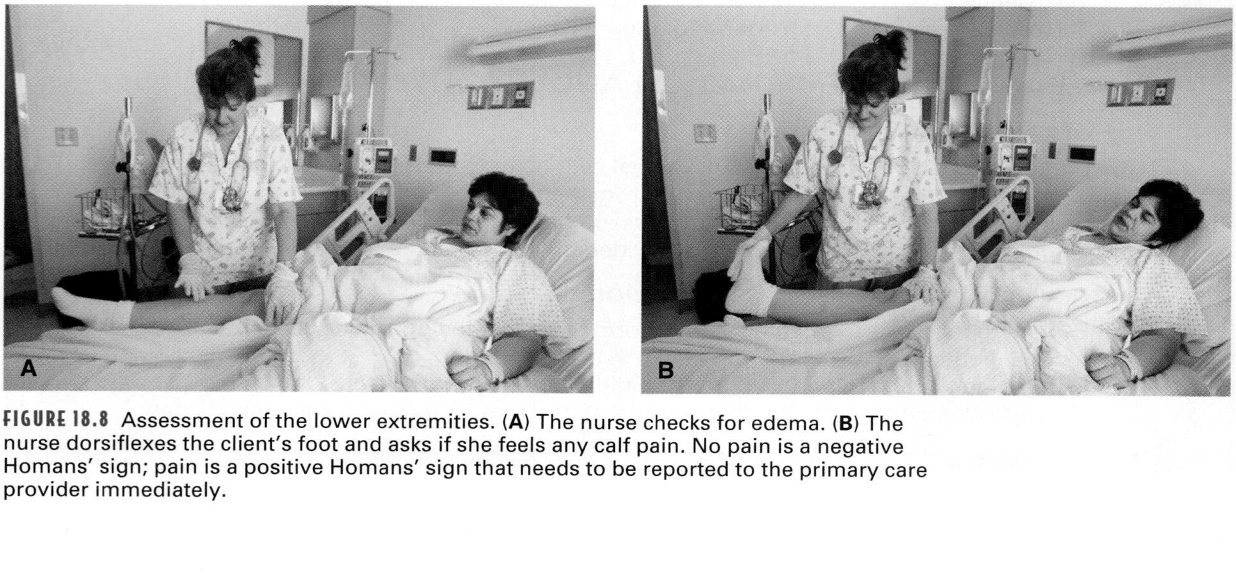

FIGURE 18.8 Assessment of the lower extremities. (**A**) The nurse checks for edema. (**B**) The nurse dorsiflexes the client's foot and asks if she feels any calf pain. No pain is a negative Homans' sign; pain is a positive Homans' sign that needs to be reported to the primary care provider immediately.

NURSING PROCEDURE 18.3

Administering Rh Immune Globulin (RhoGAM)

PURPOSE

To prevent Rh isoimmunization in future pregnancies for a woman who is Rh negative with an Rh-positive newborn

ASSESSMENT AND PLANNING

- Assess the maternal blood type to determine whether the client is a candidate for therapy. A candidate for therapy is Rh-D negative and has never been sensitized to RhD-positive blood (evidenced by a negative result on the indirect Coombs' test), and has given birth within the past 72 hours to an Rh-positive newborn who is not sensitized (evidenced by positive direct Coombs' test).
- Verify the time of newborn birth.
- Check for any possible allergies to immunoglobulins, blood, or blood products.
- Ascertain that the client has signed an informed consent, if required by the health care facility.
- Gather the necessary equipment:
  - Rh immune globulin (standard dose [300 μg])
  - Appropriate-sized syringe and needle for intramuscular injection
  - Alcohol wipes
- Cross-check the vial with another nurse for identification number and correct dosage; sign the triplicate form that accompanies the vial.
- Assess the deltoid site for appropriateness of injection; if the client is extremely thin or a dose larger than standard is ordered, the ventrogluteal or gluteal site may be used.

IMPLEMENTATION

1. Explain the purpose of RhoGAM administration. Inform the client that RhoGAM is a blood product; answer any questions.
2. Inform the client that the drug is given by intramuscular injection.
3. Prepare the standard dose as ordered in syringe.
4. Confirm the client's identity *to ensure that the right drug is being administered to the right client.*
5. Identify the proper site for injection *to promote optimal absorption.*
6. Prepare the site for injection by wiping with an alcohol wipe using a circular direction *to ensure cleanliness.*

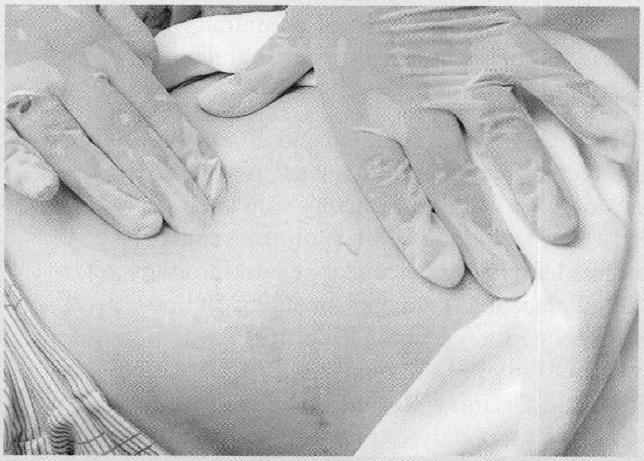

Step 5. Locating the correct site for intramuscular injection of RhoGAM.

7. Administer the dose intramuscularly into the appropriate site.
8. Discard syringe and needle into sharps container.
9. Document administration of injection, including vial identification number, route, dose, and the client's response.
10. Attach the top copy of the triplicate form to the client's chart; send the remaining two copies back to the laboratory or blood bank with the empty vial.
11. Give the client an identification card identifying her Rh status and use of RhoGAM; encourage her to keep it with her or in a convenient location.

Continued

NURSING PROCEDURE 18.3 CONTINUED

Administering Rh Immune Globulin (RhoGAM)

EVALUATION

1. The client demonstrated understanding of the need for RhoGAM administration.
2. The client tolerated the injection without incident.

AREAS FOR CONSIDERATION AND ADAPTATION

Perinatal Considerations

- Administer a standard dose of RhoGAM routinely at 28 weeks' gestation as prophylaxis to prevent isoimmunization.
- Expect to administer larger than standard doses as ordered in situations involving large amounts of bleeding, such as severe abruptio placentae.
- Administer microdoses of RhoGAM after spontaneous abortion, elective abortion, ectopic pregnancy, and gestational trophoblastic disease occurring during the first trimester.
- Give RhoGAM after any maternal trauma, chorionic villi sampling, amniocentesis, and percutaneous umbilical blood sampling.

Community-Based Considerations

- If the client has been discharged early from the health care facility, check to ensure that she has received RhoGAM before discharge. If not, expect to administer RhoGAM on the first home visit, which must occur within 72 hours of childbirth.

Select Potential Nursing Diagnoses

The following are examples of commonly applicable NANDA diagnoses during the fourth stage of labor and postpartal period:

- **Pain** related to engorgement and nipple discomfort
- **Ineffective Breastfeeding** related to maternal anxiety, lack of knowledge, or difficulty with latch
- **Risk for Deficient Fluid Volume** related to postpartum hemorrhage secondary to uterine atony, retention of placental fragments, or subinvolution
- **Pain** related to continued uterine contractions secondary to involution after delivery
- **Risk for Urinary Retention** related to decreased sensation secondary to pressure on the bladder during labor and childbirth or lingering anesthesia
- **Risk for Infection** related to urinary retention
- **Risk for Stress Incontinence** related to weak pelvic muscles
- **Risk for Injury** related to possible hemorrhage secondary to uterine atony and resulting increased lochia
- **Risk for Infection** related to organism invasion of placental site
- **Pain** related to edema, bruising, hematoma, episiotomy or laceration
- **Risk for Infection** related to organism invasion of episiotomy or laceration
- **Fatigue** related to sleep deprivation during labor and postpartum
- **Risk for Impaired Parent–Infant Attachment** related to fatigue, unrealistic expectations, and depression

Planning/Intervention

Expected outcomes for the postpartum woman are highly individualized based on her particular circumstances. Certain outcomes are appropriate for any postpartum woman, however, during the fourth stage of labor and then throughout the postpartum period:

- The client will remain free of any signs and symptoms of infection or injury after delivery.
- The client will exhibit vital signs, uterine involution, and lochia within acceptable parameters.
- The client will rate her pain as tolerable.
- The client will void within 8 hours of childbirth without any signs and symptoms of urinary retention or fluid imbalance.
- The client will demonstrate ability to provide care for herself and her newborn.
- The client will exhibit ability to provide adequate nutrition to the newborn.
- The client will demonstrate appropriate bonding and attachment behaviors with the newborn.

NIC/NOC Box 18.1 highlights common interventions and outcomes for the postpartum period. Initially, the client most likely needs close, frequent assessments and additional instruction and support to achieve these outcomes during the fourth stage of labor. As the postpartum period progresses, the nurse should expect that the client will develop increasing independence in caring for herself and her newborn and will demonstrate continued behaviors to foster attachment and bonding with the newborn, thereby promoting the development of trust. In addition, the client should demonstrate a return to her pre-pregnancy level of function, incorporating healthy lifestyle practices to address any pre-pregnancy areas of concern and measures to balance the need for activity and rest. See Nursing Care Plan 18.2, which addresses the care of a new mother in the postpartum period.

Caring for the Breasts in the Breastfeeding Client

For the breastfeeding client, engorgement often results from vascular congestion and milk stasis, primarily caused by the infant not fully emptying the mother's breasts at each feeding. Encouraging the infant to feed every 2 or 3 hours may help prevent or decrease engorgement. Application of warm compresses to the breasts also may alleviate engorgement. The client can avoid lumps that result from milk stasis in the ducts by ensuring that the infant empties the breast at feedings. Expressing a small amount of breast milk may help to soften the breasts enough to allow the infant to latch on successfully.

The client who is nursing may experience some nipple tenderness that may progress to redness, bruising, or cracking. Some nipple pain in the first week postpartum is common, but pain beyond this time usually indicates a problem requiring significant intervention (Morland-Schultz & Hill, 2005). The most common cause of nipple pain is improper positioning and latch (Morland-Schultz & Hill, 2005). The client who is breastfeeding for the first time often needs support and teaching when starting. Although most babies latch on and nurse well from the beginning, many take time to be able to nurse efficiently. Breastfeeding is a learned activity for mother and infant, a fact that clients don't always recognize or internalize. Clients whose newborns are not feeding well need additional support because their difficulties are inconsistent with their image of what the breastfeeding experience should be like. See Chapter 21 for a discussion of positioning for breastfeeding.

Pain or bruising on the upper portion of the nipple may result from the infant pinching the nipple with his or her gums. The mother can correct this problem by lifting the infant's head up so that he or she faces the nipple directly. If the infant has received a pacifier or bottle nipple, he or she may repeat the different action required to suck on these when returning to feed at the breast. The different sucking action used may lead to nipple pain as the infant uses the same actions to breastfeed. Failure to revert back to the necessary sucking motions may require suck training. A short frenulum also prevents the infant from using the proper sucking motions, again leading to sore nipples. In this instance, the nurse notifies the physician, who may "clip" the baby's "tongue tie" to allow the movement necessary to feed (Wallace & Clarke, 2006).

Infectious organisms also may cause nipple pain, the most common being *Candida albicans.* Nipples infected with candida appear bright red and shiny and are extremely sore during breastfeeding. Women often describe the pain as shooting or burning. The nurse notifies the physician of this development: treatment consists of application of an antifungal cream to the nipples following feedings and the infant receiving oral nystatin (Wiener, 2006).

Several remedies for nipple pain have been suggested, including the application of a small amount of expressed **colostrum** or breast milk, tea bags, warm-water compresses, lanolin cream, and air drying the nipples after feedings (Morland-Schultz & Hill, 2005). The use of hydrogel dressings both prophylactically and as a treatment option for nipple pain has been effective (Dodd & Chalmers, 2003).

(text continues on page 736)

NIC/NOC Box 18.1 Postpartum Care

Common NIC Labels

- Anticipatory Guidance
- Attachment Promotion
- Bleeding Reduction
- Breastfeeding Assistance
- Infection Control
- Infection Protection
- Pain Management
- Parent Education: Infant
- Parenting Promotion
- Postpartal Care
- Teaching: Infant Nutrition

Common NOC Labels

- Comfort Level
- Hydration
- Knowledge: Infection Control
- Knowledge: Postpartum
- Maternal Status: Postpartum
- Pain Control
- Pain: Disruptive Effects
- Parent–Infant Attachment
- Parenting
- Tissue Integrity: Skin and Mucous Membranes
- Urinary Continence
- Urinary Elimination

NURSING CARE PLAN 18.2

The Postpartum Mother and Newborn at Home

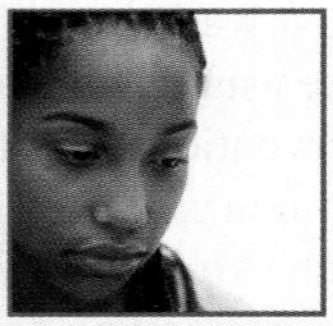

Recall Jody and her newborn, who were presented at the beginning of this chapter. On inspection, the nurse notices that Jody's episiotomy area is reddened and edematous. Her uterus is firm and approximately 6 cm below the umbilicus. Lochia is moderate and reddish pink. The client's breasts are firm and tender on palpation. Other findings of the physical examination are normal.

Jody is bottle-feeding her newborn. Jody's mother, Olivia, has just arrived to stay at the home for the next 2 weeks. Olivia tells the nurse that she is concerned about Jody and wants to know what she can do to best help her.

NURSING DIAGNOSES

- **Pain** related to breast engorgement and episiotomy
- **Deficient Knowledge** related to measures to promote comfort

EXPECTED OUTCOMES

1. The client will state that breast and episiotomy discomfort has decreased.
2. The client will identify two strategies to decrease discomfort.

INTERVENTIONS	RATIONALES
Ask the client to rate her breast pain on a scale of 1 to 10, with 1 being no pain and 10 being the worst pain; have the client rate her perineal pain in the same manner.	Use of a pain rating scale helps quantify subjective information about the client's pain and provides a baseline from which to plan interventions.
Explain the current physiologic changes and how the body is attempting to heal.	Information about the underlying events associated with pain helps the client understand the normal processes and helps alleviate fears that something is wrong.
Inform the client that breast engorgement typically subsides within 2 to 3 days from the lack of breast stimulation; instruct the client in measures to decrease discomfort, such as applying cool compresses and using a supportive, well-fitting bra.	Knowledge that breast engorgement is a short-term problem along with strategies to promote comfort can assist the client to cope with the situation.
Suggest strategies to alleviate episiotomy discomfort, such as perineal care with warm-water sitz baths or tub baths; encourage the client to perform perineal care after each voiding or bowel movement; assist her to plan time for the use of sitz or tub baths during the day.	The warmth and moisture provided by the baths increase circulation to the area, which facilitates healing and decreases edema. These measures also will help keep the area clean and prevent infection, which could prolong healing and increase discomfort.
Assist the client to identify ways to decrease discomfort, such as tightening the buttocks before sitting. Urge the client to avoid using inflated rings or similar devices.	Tightening the buttocks before sitting will prevent placing direct pressure on the episiotomy. Avoiding the use of an inflated ring will prevent circulatory compromise to the perineum.

Continued

NURSING CARE PLAN 18.2 ● The Postpartum Mother and Newborn at Home

INTERVENTIONS	RATIONALES
Instruct the client in signs and symptoms to report to her health care provider: elevated temperature, foul-smelling vaginal drainage, or change in color or amount of lochia.	Knowledge of potential signs and symptoms of complications promotes early detection and prompt intervention.
Contact the client within 2 days (either by phone or in person) to assess if pain is decreased.	Follow-up client contact aids in determining the success of strategies and if further planning and intervention are necessary. If pain is unchanged or worsened, further assessment is warranted to rule out infection or other complications.

EVALUATION

1. The client verbalizes understanding of the body's healing process.
2. The client demonstrates strategies to decrease discomfort.
3. The client reports that pain is controlled at a tolerable level.

NURSING DIAGNOSES

- **Fatigue** related to demands of caring for newborn, early discharge, and postpartal status
- **Health-Seeking Behaviors** related to fatigue, discomfort, and anxiety
- **Risk for Impaired Parent–Infant Attachment** related to fatigue and unrealistic expectations

EXPECTED OUTCOMES

1. The client will identify measures to relieve fatigue and obtain adequate rest.
2. The client will verbalize activities to promote positive interactions with her newborn.
3. The client will identify areas for additional support.

INTERVENTIONS	RATIONALES
Question the client about her usual day, including the newborn's typical routine; assess the client's emotional state and interaction with the newborn.	Assessment provides a baseline from which to develop appropriate individualized interventions. Evaluation of the client's emotional state is important to identify evidence of postpartum blues and to differentiate this from postpartum depression or psychosis.
Teach the client about behaviors to watch for in the newborn that can assist in anticipating routines.	Knowledge of the newborn's developing routines aids in improved anticipation of and planning for time for herself and the baby's needs.
Use both oral and written materials to assist the client to identify common behaviors in newborns.	Helping the client understand newborn behaviors and their causes fosters realistic expectations of both baby and herself.

Continued

NURSING CARE PLAN 18.2 ● The Postpartum Mother and Newborn at Home *(Continued)*

INTERVENTIONS	RATIONALES
Assist the client to identify newborn patterns of sleeping and waking; help her identify times when she can plan for rest or naps; involve the client's mother in the discussion.	Understanding the newborn's patterns helps the client plan times to obtain additional rest; short naps throughout the day will assist the client to supplement sleep she may be missing at night. Including the mother in the discussion allows her to provide support.
Question the client about any measures she uses to promote sleep; encourage her to use these measures.	Drinking warm milk, listening to soothing music, and maintaining a dark room can help promote sleep.
Assist the client to identify things that her mother can do that will help her.	Doing so will allow the client to maintain control but receive support that will promote coping and adequate rest.
Monitor the client and newborn for evidence of attachment behaviors; reinforce using the en face position, touching, and talking to the newborn during interactions.	Fatigue can directly affect the client's ability to interact with her newborn. Positive interactions with the newborn foster attachment and promote a sense of well-being in the mother.
Provide the client and her mother with available community resources and encourage their use.	Additional support can be effective in helping the client adapt to her new role.
Plan a follow-up telephone call to the client in the next few days and a return home visit within 3 days to evaluate status.	Follow-up is essential to determine the effectiveness of interventions and to determine the need for additional instruction and possible referrals.

EVALUATION

1. The client verbalizes understanding of infant sleep–wake cycles.
2. The client identifies times during the day when she can nap while her mother assumes care of the newborn.
3. The client participates in a community support group for new single parents.
4. The client demonstrates positive attachment behaviors with her newborn.

Caring for the Breasts in the Formula-Feeding Client

The client who is not breastfeeding may begin to experience some engorgement at approximately 1 to 4 days postpartum, with the problem peaking at 3 to 5 days postpartum (James, 2001; Weathersby, 2002). Application of cool compresses will assist with vasoconstriction, which can help eliminate discomfort. Another helpful measure is to wear a well-fitting bra. This engorgement usually disappears approximately 48 to 72 hours later as the lack of stimulation prevents the production of milk (Walker & Creehan, 2001). Avoiding nipple or breast stimulation may assist in comfort.

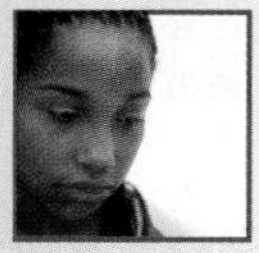

Recall Jody, the single mother discharged home with her newborn on the second postpartum day. She is experiencing breast discomfort. Jody states, "I thought since I wasn't breastfeeding, I wouldn't have this problem." How should the nurse respond?

Monitoring the Fundus

If the examiner finds the uterine fundus boggy or cannot feel it, he or she initially should gently massage the fundus, which should become firm within a short time. If this does not happen, the nurse should notify the primary care provider. Intravenous administration of 10 to 20 units of oxytocin added to 1000 mL crystalloid often is ordered routinely in the immediate postpartum period, when the client is at highest risk for hemorrhage. Methylergonovine or 15-methylprostaglandin F_{2a}, a prostaglandin, also may be ordered.

If the fundus continues to remain uncontracted, other factors may be contributing to atony. Retained placental fragments could be the cause. In addition to uterine atony, the client may pass pieces of tissue vaginally. The examiner can differentiate tissue from blood clots by attempting to tear them apart with gloved hands or tongue depressors. Blood clots are easily pulled apart; tissue does not readily tear. If the woman passes tissue, the examiner puts it into a container with a preservative and sends the material to the laboratory for analysis. If the client continues to present with uterine atony, the nurse should notify the primary care provider. In some instances, clients require surgical removal of placental fragments.

There may be several causes for a fundus found above expected height in relation to the length of time postpartum. The underlying cause would dictate the appropriate intervention. The most common cause is a distended bladder or blood clots within the uterus (Weathersby, 2002). The nurse encourages the woman to empty her bladder. Some women have difficulty voiding postpartum as a result of anesthesia used intrapartally or alterations in neural function of the bladder. Catheterization may be indicated in these instances. Fundal massage may be used to dispel uterine clots.

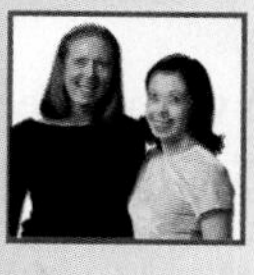

Remember Nadia, the new mother from the beginning of the chapter. Initially the nurse assessed her fundus midline, immediately below the umbilicus. Her lochia was moderate and dark red, without any clots. Now, 30 minutes later, assessment reveals a fundus that is 2 cm above the umbilicus, boggy, and displaced to the right. What would the nurse suspect? How should the nurse intervene?

Assisting With Elimination

The nurse should assist the client to the bathroom (unless contraindicated by her condition), which often helps initiate voiding. The nurse should measure the client's first voiding postpartum to ensure that it is sufficient (Zaki et al., 2004). The first voiding should occur within 8 hours of childbirth (Cunningham et al., 2005). A client who cannot void with a distended bladder requires catheterization. Health care practitioners should not allow the bladder to become distended; this can lead to loss of muscle tone and continued difficulty voiding. At the same time, catheterization should not be used indiscriminately because it increases the risk for urinary tract infection.

The client may continue to experience stress incontinence postpartum, primarily because of loss of pelvic muscle tone. Routinely doing **Kegel's exercises,** in which the woman alternately contracts and relaxes the perineal muscles as though stopping urination, may assist with preventing incontinence (see Chap. 24).

Monitoring Lochia

If the nurse assesses that a woman's lochia is excessive, he or she also must evaluate the uterus and bladder. The nurse should check the uterus for tone and position to rule out atony as the cause of the increased lochia. If the nurse finds that the client's uterus is atonic, he or she should institute actions to reverse this problem, which will most likely result in decreased lochia to expected amounts. The nurse also should check the bladder for distention.

The nurse should inform the client about expected changes in lochia color and amount throughout the postpartum period. Education includes the importance of contacting the health care provider immediately if flow significantly increases or returns to rubra after changing to serosa.

The nurse should assess the odor of the lochia. Normal lochia is not foul smelling. Foul-smelling lochia usually indicates endometritis and is frequently accompanied by an elevation in the woman's temperature, most commonly after the third postpartum day (James, 2001).

Caring for the Episiotomy

The nurse should plan interventions for the perineal area based on the client's point in the postpartum period. Shortly after childbirth, perineal care with warm water provides a feeling of comfort and facilitates visualization of the area. If the postpartum client develops perineal edema during the first 24 hours, she can apply ice to the perineum to decrease swelling. Ice is also soothing when applied after repair of episiotomy or laceration.

For edema that appears or continues after the first 24 hours, warmth, especially moist heat, is appropriate. Methods of heat application include the use of a sitz bath or a tub bath (see Nursing Procedure 18.2). Both cause vasodilation, increasing circulation to the area that aids in comfort, healing, and cleanliness. A client whose perineum is quite tender, or who has either a laceration or episiotomy repair, should use such baths two or three times a day.

Educating the Client and Family

Women and their significant others often have many learning needs as they seek information to care for themselves and the new baby. The short time that many new families spend in the hospital, however, often prevents many questions and issues from being addressed adequately. Prenatal education has begun to incorporate many aspects of postpartum and newborn care in an effort to ensure that families are informed before childbirth. Information is also readily available in books, on the Internet, and in classes (see Chap. 14). Nevertheless, it remains important for nurses to assess learning needs of mothers themselves. Research has shown that new mothers may identify different learning needs than do nurses during the early postpartum period (Bowman, 2005; Ruchala, 2000). Prenatal and postpartum support groups are available to provide instruction and discussion. Nurses must keep in mind that hormonal changes that may affect the woman's attention span and thinking, as well as the large volume of new material that she is exposed to and expected to learn and remember (Martell, 2001), can compound her ability to understand and retain new material. Fatigue and discomfort also may compromise her learning abilities.

The new mother needs support to get enough rest to meet her needs. Education focuses on needs identified by the client and her significant others; the nurse should implement teaching at the time of identification (Fig. 18.9). Rather than attempting to cover everything that the new mother might need to know, the nurse may find it more appropriate to concentrate on a few essential topics, keeping explanations simple and reinforcing learning through repetition (Martell, 2001). The nurse should try to individualize teaching to the client's preferred learning style and usual problem-solving strategies. He or she should inform the client of available community resources and provide supplementary data in a written format. These may include supports such as a visiting program offered from the public health offices for mothers who are discharged early from the hospital, La Leche League support for breastfeeding, parenting groups and hotlines, and other similar resources that may be available in the community. It also may be helpful for the nurse to assist the woman to recognize the need to sort through all the available information and advice that she may obtain and assist her to develop strategies to match selections to her lifestyle and problem-solving approaches (Martell, 2001).

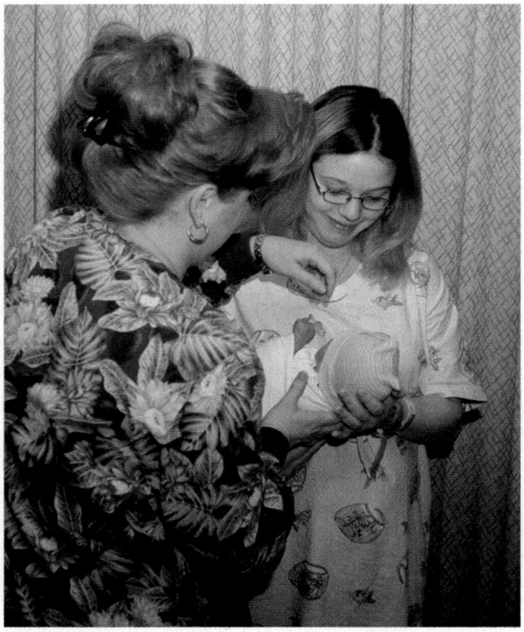

FIGURE 18.9 The nurse provides teaching according to the new mother's learning readiness and needs.

As mothers are in the hospital for short periods following birth, the time available to complete teaching is decreased. The shorter time has implications for both the amount of information that the nurse can provide and the amount that the client can take in and remember. The role of the nurse as educator within the acute care setting is evolving to focus on facilitating information that focuses on essential material. The role of the community nurse in educating is continuing to evolve. Provision of information about support services, as well as support in developing skills in evaluating information and advice that is provided in and by a multitude of sources, assists the new mother to cope. See Research Highlight 18.2.

Assisting Lesbian Parents

Expectations attached to the concepts of family and motherhood in U.S. and Canadian society are linked to traditional Euro-American values: families include children with two parents of the opposite sex. Many health care providers share this expectation. Because the idea of lesbian parenthood is antithetical to this belief, health care providers can easily avoid acknowledging the existence of these clients and hence any recognition of their needs (McManus et al., 2006).

One of the first decisions that a lesbian woman needs to make, once she is pregnant, is whether to "come out" to her health care provider. This dilemma continues not only throughout pregnancy but also following birth. Wilton and Kaufmann (2001) found that lesbian women wanted understanding of their needs from their health care providers as well as inclusion of their partners, just as do heterosexual women. Lesbian women, unlike heterosexual women, have to decide whether disclosure would facilitate or impede this. Additional concerns surrounded whether this knowledge would affect the quality of care provided and whether the information would produce a prejudiced reaction. Regardless of their decision, most women wanted to be able to share this information.

Another stressor that lesbian women have identified during the postpartum period is the lack of support provided to their partners. In some cases, clinicians have not recognized partners as part of the family unit and have

RESEARCH HIGHLIGHT 18.2 First-Time Mothers: Social Support and Confidence in Infant Care

OBJECTIVE: To examine the relationship between social support for first-time mothers and their confidence in caring for their infants, as well as to identify their sources of postpartum support

DESIGN: The study used a descriptive, correlational design, with a 28-item questionnaire.

PARTICIPANTS AND SETTING: The researcher recruited 135 first-time mothers, 74% of whom completed questionnaires 6 weeks after childbirth.

RESULTS: Appraisal support had moderate relationship with confidence in infant care practices ($r = 0.4$, $p < 0.01$). Informational support had a weaker but statistically significant relationship ($r = 0.2$, $p < 0.05$). The participants identified husbands/partners and their own mothers as primary sources of appraisal support. They identified nurses and other mothers as primary sources of informational support.

CONCLUSION: Because women rely so heavily on them for support, it is vital for mothers' husbands/partners to actively participate in antenatal and postnatal care and teaching. The development of interdisciplinary education programs that allow public health nurses and midwives to work collaboratively in facilitating social support for first-time mothers is critical.

Leahy Warren, P. (2005). *Journal of Advanced Nursing, 50*(5), 479–488.

mistreated them accordingly (Wilton & Kaufmann, 2001). This lack of respect creates anxiety for the postpartum woman as well as depriving her of her source of support. Most lesbian mothers want to be treated the same as all mothers, regardless of sexual orientation (Lauderdale, 2003). For example, it is always appropriate to ask a pregnant woman about support available to her and whether she has a partner who will be co-parenting with her. Research has shown, however, that these questions have been significantly absent when the mother is lesbian (Wilton & Kaufmann, 2001).

Acknowledging the partner as a support for the mother and recognizing the family unit are essential nursing activities, whether in the hospital or community setting. Nurses must be careful with the language that they use. The mother and nurse may assign different meanings to "partner" and "parent." Health care providers should be sensitive to all women's right to have their choice of partner and family unit respected. They should facilitate inclusion of partners and encourage their participation.

Evaluation

Evaluation of changes in assessment and the effectiveness of interventions is important to ensuring appropriate maternal progress in the postpartum period. Nursing mothers should attend to any nipple pain quickly; such pain can progress rapidly to tissue breakdown and cracking of the nipples. This causes increased discomfort, potential for infection, and prolonged healing. All these potential outcomes can have a discouraging effect on the mother and may result in the discontinuation of breastfeeding. The nurse should provide assistance to all clients experiencing difficulties with breastfeeding or problems with the breasts postpartum. Lactation consultants are available in the hospital and community; nurses and clients should consult them when problems persist or are exacerbated.

The uterus should continue to remain well contracted and be found further down in the abdomen over time. The client should understand how her flow will change over time and to notify her health care practitioner immediately if the flow changes inappropriately.

An empty bladder should not be palpable above the symphysis pubis. The client should be able to sense a full bladder and have no difficulty emptying her bladder. Any burning or frequency, which may indicate a urinary tract infection, should not accompany urination. The client may, however, experience some frequency as diuresis takes place in the early postpartum.

In some instances, a transient increase in lochia is normal, such as following breastfeeding as a reaction to uterine contraction caused by the release of oxytocin stimulated by the infant sucking. Women's lochia also may increase when they initially rise after having been recumbent for some time. Such positioning can result in lochia pooling in the uterus; when the client sits or stands, the lochia then flows. In other instances, increased lochia or a return to lochia rubra from lochia serosa requires investigation to rule out late postpartum hemorrhage.

Sutures, if present, should remain intact. The nurse should tell the client that the sutures are dissolvable and will not need removal. Signs that an episiotomy or laceration is not healing properly include redness, edema, ecchymosis, and discharge. With normal healing, the edges are well approximated.

Questions to Ponder

1. A client who gave birth to her first baby 14 hours ago asks to be discharged home. She indicates that her mother and mother-in-law are both at home to help.
   - What are your personal feelings about a first-time mother going home early in the puerperium?

- What additional information might be helpful for the nurse to have before responding?
- What specific supports might the nurse want to ensure are in place before discharge?

SUMMARY

- Women lose approximately 5 to 6 kg of weight following childbirth. By 6 to 18 months postpartum, clients tend to weigh 1 to 2 kg more than they did before pregnancy.
- Approximately 500 mL of blood is lost with a vaginal birth, and approximately 1000 mL of blood is lost with a cesarean birth. Plasma volume decreases by as much as 1000 mL. Blood volume returns to pre-pregnant values by approximately 1 week postpartum.
- Cardiac output remains elevated for 48 hours. The pulse rate remains stable or decreases slightly. A mild rise in blood pressure has been seen as a common phenomenon in the first 4 days postpartum.
- Hemoglobin usually fluctuates near pregnancy values for several days and then rises to nonpregnancy values. Most clients do not experience any change in hematocrit postpartum. Normal serum iron levels are regained by the second week postpartum. Nonpathologic leukocytosis is seen in the postpartum period.
- After childbirth, intra-abdominal pressure decreases, as does diaphragmatic pressure. Abdominal muscles remain in a relaxed state. Gaseous distention and decreased motility may result. Constipation may be a problem related to fear, dehydration, immobility, or medications. Hemorrhoids may be more prevalent.
- Chloasma disappears after delivery. Striae gravidarum fade to a silvery white.
- Estrogen and progesterone levels decrease. Plasma prolactin level falls lower than during pregnancy but increases with each act of sucking by the infant. Thyroid hormone levels return to pre-pregnant levels by 6 weeks postpartum. Basal metabolic rate returns to normal approximately 7 to 14 days postpartum. Glucose levels fall as a result of removal of placenta.
- The uterus weighs approximately 1000 g after birth and decreases to 100 g or less by 6 weeks postpartum. The fundus is felt one fingerbreadth below the umbilicus immediately after childbirth, decreasing approximately one fingerbreadth each day following. The uterus remains contracted.
- Lochia is sloughed off up to 4 weeks postpartum. Lochia rubra is dark red and lasts for the first 3 to 4 days. Lochia serosa is paler and lasts from day 4 or 5 until day 9. Lochia alba is yellowish white and lasts from the 10th day until the flow stops.
- The endometrium regenerates by the 3rd week postpartum. The placental site takes approximately 6 weeks to heal.
- Subinvolution may occur because of failure of the uterus to contract, most commonly caused by retention of placental tissue or exposed blood vessels after placental separation.
- The cervical os contracts slowly. Cervical edema may be present for several months. The cervix never returns to the pregravid state.
- Menstruation returns for the woman who is not breastfeeding by approximately 6 to 10 weeks postpartum, and from the 8th week to 18 months postpartum for the woman who is breastfeeding. Approximately 25% of women ovulate before the first menses.
- Rugae reappear in the vagina approximately 3 weeks postpartum. The voluntary muscles of the pelvic floor regain their tone approximately 6 weeks postpartum.
- Changes in the breasts primarily are related to the breastfeeding decision.
- Diuresis occurs between the 2nd and 5th day postpartum. Spontaneous voiding should resume within 8 hours after birth. Bladder tone should return by 5 to 7 days.
- Many clients experience postpartum blues, usually between 3 and 14 days postpartum. Symptoms may include increased emotional lability, crying, and sensitivity. Postpartum depression and psychosis are more serious but have significantly lower incidences.
- A focused assessment is done during the fourth stage of labor, including vital signs, uterus, lochia, and perineum.
- A more complete assessment is done less frequently for the remainder of the postpartum. This assessment includes breasts, uterus, bladder, bowels, lochia, episiotomy and perineum, Homans' sign, and psychological state.

REVIEW QUESTIONS

1. A client who is 2 days postpartum tells the nurse that she is voiding frequently. Further assessment reveals that the client's temperature is 37.8°C, her fundus is at the umbilicus and firm, and she is voiding 500 mL at a time. Which of the following would the nurse recognize as a potential cause for urinary frequency?
   A. Urinary overflow
   B. Postpartum diuresis
   C. Urinary tract infection
   D. Trauma to pelvic muscles
2. A client just gave birth to her second child 30 minutes ago. The newborn boy weighs 3800 g. The client is currently breastfeeding. Which of the following

findings would the nurse recognize as most significant in her next assessment?
   A. Lochia is moderate rubra.
   B. Pulse rate has decreased by 10 beats/minute.
   C. The client reports abdominal pains.
   D. The fundus is two fingerbreadths above the umbilicus.

3. The nurse is examining the results of laboratory blood testing for a client who is 2 days postpartum. Which of the following findings would the nurse recognize as most significant?
   A. WBC count = 27,000/μL
   B. Hematocrit = 0.40
   C. Hemoglobin = 10 g/dL
   D. Serum iron = 85 μg/dL

4. The nurse is assessing a client who is 2 days postpartum. During attempted examination of the fundus, the nurse cannot find it. Which of the following nursing actions would be most appropriate next?
   A. Assess the lochia.
   B. Massage the fundus.
   C. Administer ordered oxytocin.
   D. Nothing, it is probably already too low to be felt.

5. A postpartum client who is breastfeeding asks when she can expect menses to return. Which response from the nurse would be most appropriate?
   A. "Your menses will return at 8 weeks postpartum whether you breastfeed or formula feed."
   B. "Women who breastfeed can expect menstruation to return at 6 weeks postpartum."
   C. "Women who breastfeed can expect menstruation to return at 8 weeks postpartum."
   D. "Women who breastfeed may not experience menstruation until 18 months postpartum."

6. A client who is 3 days postpartum is breastfeeding her baby girl. The client reports that her breasts are very swollen and sore. Which of the following interventions would be the most appropriate for the nurse to recommend?
   A. Lanolin ointment
   B. Warm compresses
   C. Cool compresses
   D. Expression of the excess milk

7. During a home visit to a postpartum client, the nurse suspects early signs of postpartum depression based on initial conversation. Which intervention would be most important to consider when completing a full assessment?
   A. Assess for signs of bipolar disorder.
   B. Assess for shortness of breath and sensations of smothering.
   C. Consider that the client may show unique signs.
   D. Refrain from questions to which the client might be sensitive.

8. A nurse is admitting a client from the labor and delivery unit who gave birth to a baby girl 3 hours ago. During initial assessment, the client reports that she is a lesbian with a supportive female partner. Which of the following would be most important for the nurse to include as part of her care?
   A. Ask the client how she got pregnant.
   B. Include the client's partner in all care.
   C. Act as though there is nothing different about her.
   D. Tell the other nurses to promote sensitivity.

9. The nurse is teaching a new mother who is 1 day postpartum. The client indicates that she is planning to go home the next day. Which of the following principles would be most important?
   A. Implement teaching whenever the nurse is with the client.
   B. Sit with the client to review everything she will need to go home.
   C. Identify what the client thinks she needs to know.
   D. Reinforce information every time the nurse has an opportunity.

10. During a routine assessment, the nurse finds that the fundus of a client who is 14 hours postpartum is two fingerbreadths above the umbilicus and slightly boggy. The flow is large rubra. Which of the following actions would the nurse consider taking next?
   A. Notify the physician.
   B. Palpate the bladder for distention.
   C. Massage the uterus to expel clots.
   D. Administer oxytocin to stimulate uterine contractions.

REFERENCES

Beck, C. T. (2002). Postpartum depression: A metasynthesis. *Qualitative Health Research, 12*(4), 453–472.

Beck, C. T., & Indman, P. (2005). The many faces of postpartum depression. *Journal of Obstetrical, Gynecological, and Neonatal Nursing, 34*(5), 569–576.

Bickley, L. S. (2007). *Bates' guide to physical examination and history taking* (9th ed.). Philadelphia: Lippincott Williams & Wilkins.

Bowes, W. A., & Katz, V. L. (2002). Postpartum care. In S. G. Gabbe, J. R. Niebyl, & J. L. Simpson (Eds.), *Obstetrics: Normal and problem pregnancies* (4th ed., pp. 701–728). Philadelphia: Churchill Livingstone.

Bowman, K. G. (2005). Postpartum learning needs. *Journal of Obstetrical, Gynecological, and Neonatal Nursing, 34*(4), 438–443.

Brayshaw, E. (2003). Special exercises for pregnancy, labour and the puerperium. In D. M. Fraser & M. A. Cooper (Eds.), *Myles textbook for midwives* (14th ed., pp. 231–250). Philadelphia: Churchill Livingstone.

Chaudron, L. (2003). Is postpartum psychosis a bipolar variant? A phenomenological question. *Psychiatric Times, 20*(7), 54–61.

Cunningham, F. G., Gant, N. F., Leveno, K. J., Bloom, S. L., Hauth, J. C., Gillstrap, LC. III, & Wenstrom, K. D. (2005). *Williams obstetrics* (22nd ed). New York: McGraw-Hill.

Dennis, C. L., & Ross, L. (2005). Relationships among infant sleep patterns, maternal fatigue, and development of depressive symptomatology. *Birth, 32*(3), 187–193.

Dewey, K. G. (2004). Impact of breastfeeding on maternal nutritional status. *Advances in Experimental Medical Biology, 554,* 91–100.

Dodd, V., & Chalmers, C. (2003). Comparing the use of Hydrogel dressing to lanolin ointment with lactating mothers. *Journal of Obstetric Gynecology and Neonatal Nursing, 32*(4), 486–494.

Edhborg, M., Friberg, M., Lundh, W., & Widstrom, A. M. (2005). "Struggling with life": Narratives from women with signs of postpartum depression. *Scandinavian Journal of Public Health, 33*(4), 261–267.

Fenwick, J., Hauck, Y., Downie, J., & Butt, J. (2005). The childbirth expectations of a self-selected cohort of Western Australian women. *Midwifery, 21*(1), 23–35.

Fischbach, F. (2004). *A manual of laboratory and diagnostic tests* (7th ed.). Philadelphia: Lippincott Williams & Wilkins.

George, L. (2005). Lack of preparedness: Experiences of first-time mothers. *MCN—The American Journal of Maternal and Child Nursing, 30*(4), 251–255.

Glazener, C. M., Herbison, G. P., MacArthur, C., Lancashire, R., McGee, M. A., Grant, A. M., & Wilson, P. D. (2006). New postnatal urinary incontinence and other risk factors in primiparae. *British Journal of Obstetrics & Gynecology, 113*(2), 208–217.

Goldberg, G. (2005). Maternal nutrition in pregnancy and the first postnatal year—2. After the birth. *Journal of Family Health Care, 15*(5), 137–138, 140.

Goodheart, H. P. (2003). *Goodheart's photoguide of common skin disorders: Diagnosis and management* (2nd ed.). Philadelphia: Lippincott Williams & Wilkins.

Gore, S. A., Brown, D. M., & West, D. S. (2003). The role of postpartum weight retention in obesity among women: A review of the evidence. *Annals of Behavioral Medicine, 26*(2), 149–159.

Groutz, A., Hadi, E., Wolf, Y., Maslovitz, S., Gold, R., Lessing, J. B., & Gordon, D. (2004). Early postpartum voiding dysfunction: Incidence and correlation with obstetric parameters. *Journal of Reproductive Medicine, 49*(12), 960–964.

Gunderson, E. P., Abrams, B., & Selvin, S. (2001). Does the pattern of postpartum weight change differ according to pregravid body size? *International Journal of Obesity, 25,* 853–862.

Guyton, A. C., & Hall, J. E. (2006). *Textbook of medical physiology* (11th ed.). Philadelphia: W. B. Saunders.

Haiek, L. N., Kramer, M. S., Ciampi, A., & Tirado, R. (2001). Postpartum weight loss and infant feeding. *Journal of the American Board of Family Practice, 14*(2), 85–94.

Harrod, K. S., Hanson, L., Vanderosse, L., & Heywood, P. (2003). Rh-negative status and isoimmunization update. *Journal of Perinatal and Neonatal Nursing, 17*(3), 166–178.

Jack, S. M., DiCenso, A., & Lohfeld, L. (2005). A theory of maternal engagement with public health nurses and family visitors. *Journal of Advanced Nursing, 49*(2), 182–190.

James, A. H. (2006). Von Willebrand disease. *Obstetrics and Gynecology Survey, 61*(2), 136–145.

James, D. C. (2001). Postpartum care. In K. R. Simpson & P. A. Creehan (Eds.), *AWHONN's perinatal nursing* (2nd ed., pp. 446–472). Philadelphia: Lippincott Williams & Wilkins.

Lauderdale, J. (2003). Transcultural perspectives in childbearing. In M. M. Andrews & J. S. Boyle (Eds.), *Transcultural concepts in nursing care* (4th ed., pp. 95–131). Philadelphia: Lippincott Williams & Wilkins.

Lazarus, J. H. (2005). Thyroid disorders associated with pregnancy: Etiology, diagnosis, and management. *Treatments in Endocrinology, 4*(1), 31–41.

Lederman, S. A. (2001). Pregnancy weight gain and postpartum loss: Avoiding obesity while optimizing the growth and development of the fetus. *Journal of the American Medical Women's Association, 56*(2), 53–58.

Luppi, C. J. (2001). Physiologic changes of pregnancy. In K. R. Simpson & P. A. Creehan (Eds.), *AWHONN's perinatal nursing* (2nd ed., pp. 96–114). Philadelphia: Lippincott Williams & Wilkins.

MacMullen, N. J., Dulski, L. A., & Meagher, B. (2005). Red alert: Perinatal hemorrhage. *MCN—The American Journal of Maternal and Child Nursing, 30*(1), 46–51.

Magann, E. F., Evans, S., Hutchinson, M., Collins, R., Howard, B. C., & Morrison, J. C. (2005). Postpartum hemorrhage after vaginal birth: An analysis of risk factors. *Southern Medical Journal, 98*(4), 419–422.

Marchant, S. (2003). Physiology and care in the puerperium. In D. M. Fraser & M. A. Cooper (Eds.), *Myles textbook for midwives* (14th ed., pp. 625–638). Philadelphia: Churchill Livingstone.

Martell, L. K. (2001). Heading toward the new normal: A contemporary postpartum experience. *Journal of Obstetric Gynecology and Neonatal Nursing, 30*(5), 496–506.

Martin, E. J. (2002). *Intrapartum management modules: A perinatal education program* (3rd ed.). Philadelphia: Lippincott Williams & Wilkins.

Mazzeo, S. E., Slof-Op't Landt, M. C., Jones, I., Mitchell, K., Kendler, K. S., Neale, M. C., et al. (2006). Associations among postpartum depression, eating disorders, and perfectionism in a population-based sample of adult women. *International Journal of Eating Disorders, 39*(3), 202–211.

McManus, A. J., Hunter, L. P., & Renn, H. (2006). Lesbian experiences and needs during childbirth: Guidance for health care providers. *Journal of Obstetric, Gynecologic, and Neonatal Nursing, 35*(1), 13–23.

Morland-Schultz, K., & Hill, P. D. (2005). Prevention of and therapies for nipple pain: A systematic review. *Journal of Obstetrical, Gynecological, and Neonatal Nursing, 34*(4), 428–437.

National Center for Health Statistics. (2002). *Longer hospital stays for childbirth.* Retrieved October 30, 2003, from http://www.cdc.gov/nchs/products/pubs/pubd/hestats/hospbirth.htm.

Nelson, A. M. (2003). Transition to motherhood. *Journal of Obstetrical, Gynecological, and Neonatal Nursing, 32*(4), 465–477.

Olson, C. M., Strawderman, M. S., Hinton, P. S., & Pearson, T. A. (2003). Gestational weight gain and postpartum behaviors associated with weight change from early pregnancy to 1 y postpartum. *International Journal of Obesity and Related Metabolic Disorders, 27*(1), 117–127.

O'Reilly, M. M. (2004). Achieving a new balance: Women's transition to second-time parenthood. *Journal of Obstetrical, Gynecological, and Neonatal Nursing, 33*(4), 455–462.

Pazzaglia, C., Caliandro, P., Aprile, I., Modelli, M., Foschini, M., Tonali, P. A., et al. (2005). Multicenter study on carpal tunnel syndrome and pregnancy incidence and natural course. *Acta Neurochirurgica Supplement, 92,* 35–39.

Pedersen, C. A. (1999). Postpartum mood and anxiety disorders: A guide for the nonpsychiatric clinician with an aside on thyroid associations with postpartum mood. *Thyroid, 9*(7), 691–697.

Poole, J. H., Burke Sosa, M. E., Freda, M. C., Kendrick, J. M., Luppi, C. J., Krening, C. F., & Dauphinee, J. D. (2001). High risk pregnancy. In K. R. Simpson & P. A. Creehan (Eds.), *AWHONN's perinatal nursing* (2nd ed., pp. 173–194). Philadelphia: Lippincott Williams & Wilkins.

Ross, L. E., Murray, B. J., & Steiner, M. (2005). Sleep and perinatal mood disorders: A critical review. *Journal of Psychiatry and Neuroscience, 30*(4), 247–256.

Rouse, D. J., & St. John, E. (2003). Normal labor, delivery, newborn care and puerperium. In J. R. Scott, R. S. Gibbs, B. Y. Karlan, & A. F. Haney (Eds.), *Danforth's obstetrics and gynecology* (9th ed., pp. 35–56). Philadelphia: Lippincott Williams & Wilkins.

Ruchala, P. (2000). Teaching new mothers: Priorities of nurses and postpartum women. *Journal of Obstetric Gynecology and Neonatal Nursing, 29,* 265–273.

Samuels, P. (2002). Hematologic complications of pregnancy. In S. G. Gabbe, J. R. Niebyl, J. L. Simpson (Eds.), *Obstetrics: Normal and problem pregnancies* (4th ed., pp. 1169–1194). Philadelphia: Churchill Livingstone.

Sarvghadi, F., Hedayati, M., Mehrabi, Y., & Azizi, F. (2005). Follow up of patients with postpartum thyroiditis: A population-based study. *Endocrine, 27*(3), 279–282.

Schytt, E., Lindmark, G., & Waldenstrom, U. (2004). Symptoms of stress incontinence 1 year after childbirth: Prevalence and predictors in a national Swedish sample. *Acta Obstetrica and Gynecologica Scandinavia, 83*(10), 928–936.

Seyfried, L. S., & Marcus, S. M. (2003). Postpartum mood disorders. *International Review of Psychiatry, 15*(3), 231–242.

Sharma, V., & Mazmanian, D. (2003). Sleep loss and postpartum psychosis. *Bipolar Disorders, 5*(2), 98–105.

Tan, L. K., & de Swiet, M. (2002). The management of postpartum hypertension. *British Journal of Obstetrics and Gynecology, 109*(7), 733–736.

Vieira, T. (2003). When joy becomes grief: Screening tools for postpartum depression. *AWHONN Lifelines, 6*(6), 506–513.

Waldenstrom, U. (2004). Why do some women change their opinion about childbirth over time? *Birth, 31*(2), 102–107.

Walker, L. O., Sterling, B. S., & Timmerman, G. M. (2005). Retention of pregnancy-related weight in the early postpartum period: Implications for women's health services. *Journal of Obstetrical, Gynecological, and Neonatal Nursing, 34*(4), 418–427.

Walker, M., & Creehan, P. A. (2001). Newborn nutrition. In K. R. Simpson & P. A. Creehan (Eds.), *AWHONN's perinatal nursing* (2nd ed., pp. 550–574). Philadelphia: Lippincott Williams & Wilkins.

Wallace, H., & Clarke, S. (2006). Tongue tie division in infants with breast feeding difficulties. *International Journal of Pediatric Otorhinolaryngology, 70*(7), 1257–1261.

Weathersby, A. M. (2002). Assessment of the newborn and newly delivered mother. In E. J. Martin (Ed.), *Intrapartum management modules: A perinatal education program* (3rd ed., pp. 571–600). Philadelphia: Lippincott Williams & Wilkins.

Wiener, S. (2006). Diagnosis and management of Candida of the nipple and breast. *Journal of Midwifery and Women's Health, 51*(2), 125–128.

Wilton, T., & Kaufmann, T. (2001). Lesbian mothers' experiences of maternity care in the UK. *Midwifery, 17,* 203–211.

Zaki, M. M., Pandit, M., & Jackson, S. (2004). National survey for intrapartum and postpartum bladder care: Assessing the need for guidelines. *British Journal of Obstetrics and Gynecology, 111*(8), 874–876.

CHAPTER 19

The High-Risk Postpartum Woman

Debbie Raines and Della Campbell

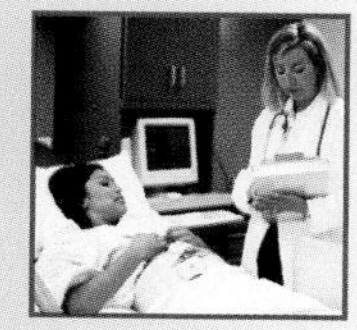

Rosanna, 36 years old, gave birth vaginally to her fourth child, a healthy boy, 6 hours ago. She received oxytocin to augment her labor, which was prolonged. She states, "I think something might be wrong. I haven't urinated yet, but I feel like I have to. And I've been changing my pad quite frequently. I don't remember this happening after giving birth to my other children."

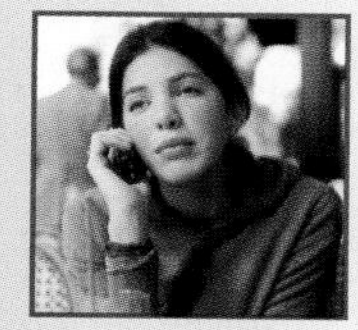

Ten days ago, Leslie, 26 years old, underwent a planned cesarean birth. Her recovery in the health care facility was unremarkable, and she was discharged home with her healthy daughter on postpartum day 5. Today, she calls the health care provider to report that she has had a fever ranging from 100.8°F to 101.5°F (38.2°C to 38.6°C) for the past 2 days. She also states that her incision is reddened and very sore. "I just don't feel well," she reports.

You will learn more about Rosanna's and Leslie's stories throughout this chapter. Nurses working with such clients need to understand the content in this chapter to adequately care for postpartum clients who may be experiencing complications. Before beginning, consider the following points related to the above scenarios:

- What issues are similar for each client? What issues are different?
- What additional information would the nurse need to obtain from each client?
- What factors might be contributing to each client's risk for developing a postpartum complication?
- How can nurses help to prevent maternal postpartum complications? What circumstances might cause the appearance of postpartum complications to be delayed?
- How would the nurse respond to each woman? What steps would the nurse take next?

LEARNING OBJECTIVES

On completion of this chapter, the reader should be able to:

- Discuss potential maternal complications following childbirth.
- Identify factors, both congenital and acquired, that place a client at risk in the postpartum period.
- Summarize the components of the nursing process (assessment, diagnosis, planning, intervention, and evaluation) for specific maternal postpartum conditions.
- Describe the perinatal nurse's role in assisting clients and their families in both the acute and long-term resolution of maternal postpartum complications.

KEY TERMS

cystocele
deep venous thrombosis
early postpartum hemorrhage
hematoma
hypofibrinogenemia
late postpartum hemorrhage
multiparity
pelvic relaxation
peripartum cardiomyopathy (PPCM)
peritonitis
postpartum blues
postpartum depression (PPD)
postpartum hemorrhage
puerperal infection
pulmonary embolism
rectocele
subinvolution
superficial venous thrombosis
thromboembolic disorder
uterine displacement
uterine inversion
uterine prolapse

Maternal postpartum complications are a possibility following any pregnancy and may be related to problems that started before or during pregnancy, during labor, or during or after birth. For example, they may be related to preexisting or coexisting medical problems such as diabetes, cardiac disease, HIV infection, or sickle cell disease (see Chaps. 4 and 13). They may have resulted specifically from the birth itself, such as with cases of hemorrhage or infection. Psychological complications, which may not manifest until weeks or months after the birth, may be influenced by situations such as teenage or mature motherhood, homelessness, and domestic or community violence (Apgar et al., 2005; Birkeland et al., 2005; Dearing et al., 2004). All maternal physiologic and psychological complications during the postpartum period can affect not only the health status of the mother, but also that of the newborn by potentially interfering with the maternal–newborn attachment process. Furthermore, they can disrupt the dynamics of the entire family, with health-related, fiscal, and emotional effects and costs (Box 19.1).

With the current practice of short stays in health facilities, many infections and other postpartum complications do not become apparent until after the mother and newborn have been discharged home (Bowes & Katz, 2002). Not only does this circumstance potentially interfere with recognition and treatment, but it also may require rehospitalization of the new mother, imposing separation between her and the newborn. Thus, client teaching about the signs and symptoms of potential postpartum problems and the importance of contacting the health care provider in case they develop is a vital component of discharge planning for all postpartum families.

Nurses need skill and expert judgment in differentiating variations of normal from true postpartum complications. They also should actively educate clients and families about those alterations that may appear after discharge and necessitate follow-up with a health care provider. Many conditions described in this chapter occur in clients who had no complications during pregnancy or childbirth. Therefore, comprehensive history taking, physical examination, and ongoing assess-

BOX 19.1 Postbirth Hemorrhage and Maternal Death

- About 515,000 women die during pregnancy and childbirth each year.
- About 130,000 women bleed to death each year while giving birth.
- Two thirds of women with postpartum hemorrhage have no identifiable risk factors.
- Ninety percent of cases of postpartum hemorrhage result from uterine atony.

From Maternal Neonatal Health. (2004). Preventing postpartum hemorrhage: Active management of the third stage of labor. Available at: http://www.mnh.jhpiego.org.

ment of all postpartum clients are essential to quality nursing care.

FOCUSED ASSESSMENTS FOR CLIENTS WITH POSTPARTUM COMPLICATIONS

General nursing assessment of postpartum clients who develop a complication involves comprehensive health history taking and physical examination (see Chap. 18). When the postpartum client manifests a problem, the nurse should review carefully her pregnancy, intrapartum, and birth histories and events to identify potential risk factors and to implement strategies that promote the safety and well-being of the client, newborn, and family.

Attributes of particular focus include the following:

- Pregnancy factors
  - Infections, especially urinary tract infections (UTIs)
  - History of preterm labor or preterm rupture of membranes
  - Abnormal placental implantation (ie, placenta previa, placenta accreta, placenta increta)
  - Intrapartal and birth factors
  - Length of labor
  - Mode of birth
  - Use of invasive technologies: internal uterine and fetal monitoring, fetal pulse oximetry, urinary catheterization, frequent vaginal examinations
  - Type of analgesia and anesthesia
- General health status factors
  - Chronic conditions or preexisting disease states such as hypertension or sickle cell disease (see Chap. 4)
  - Nutritional status
  - Use of drugs, alcohol, and other substances
  - Access to health care systems

BLEEDING COMPLICATIONS

Bleeding complications are a leading cause of postpartum morbidity and mortality; more than 50% of all maternal deaths occur within 24 hours of childbirth, most frequently from excessive bleeding (Baskett & O'Connell, 2005; Wainscott, 2004). Consequently, knowledge of the risk factors for postbirth bleeding complications, early identification of assessment parameters indicating such alterations, and prompt intervention are important components of promoting client safety and well-being.

Many clients can tolerate a certain amount of blood loss following birth because the body uses compensatory mechanisms related to the normal expansion of blood volume during pregnancy (see Chaps. 12 and 18). **Postpartum hemorrhage** is defined as blood loss greater than 500 mL during or after the third stage of labor (Wainscott, 2004). This excessive bleeding may cause or result in hemodynamic instability if left untreated. Health care personnel need to identify the etiology of the hemorrhage so that they can initiate prompt and effective interventions to eliminate it and halt the blood loss.

The anatomic origin of postpartum hemorrhage can be the contractile tissue of the upper uterine segment at the site of placental implantation, or the noncontractile or poorly contractile tissue of the lower uterine segment, cervix, vagina, or broad ligament. Most cases of postpartum hemorrhage are avoidable (Wainscott, 2004). Risk factors include the following:

- Uterine fibroids or anomalies
- Placental anomalies including placenta previa, placenta abruptio, or abnormal implantation
- Previous uterine surgery: cesarean birth or myomectomy scar
- Difficult births or manual removal of the placenta
- Retained placental fragments
- Altered uterine contractility
- **Multiparity** (a woman who has had two or more births at greater than 20 weeks' gestation)
- Uterine overdistention: polyhydramnios, a macrosomic fetus or newborn (greater than 4000 g), or a multifetal gestation in current pregnancy
- Prolonged or precipitous labor
- Labor induced with oxytocin, or oxytocin augmentation during labor
- Intrauterine infection: chorioamnionitis
- Abnormal coagulopathy
- History of hemorrhage

Postpartum hemorrhage can be further classified as early (within the first 24 hours of birth) or late (24 hours or more after birth) (Box 19.2). Figure 19.1 depicts the various problems leading to early and late postpartum hemorrhage.

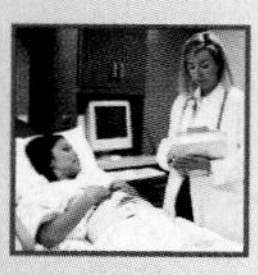

Consider Rosanna, the 36-year-old woman who has given birth to her fourth child. What factors might be contributing to her increased risk for postpartum hemorrhage?

● **BOX 19.2 Etiology of Early and Late Postpartum Hemorrhage**

Abnormal coagulopathy
Altered maternal anatomy
Altered uterine contractility
Hematoma
Infection
Lacerations of the genitourinary tract
Retained products of conception

Early Postpartum Hemorrhage

Early postpartum hemorrhage occurs within 24 hours of birth and usually results from uterine atony and continued bleeding from the placental implantation site. Other causes include lacerations of the genital tract, hematomas, and uterine inversion.

Uterine Atony

Uterine atony (lack of normal uterine muscle tone) can result from hypotonia and lead to early postpartum hemorrhage. Normally, uterine contraction results in vascular compression and homeostasis at the placental insertion site, an effect similar to a tourniquet. Without uterine contraction, blood continues to seep from the placental implantation site.

Specific causes of uterine atony include the following:

- Uterine overdistention
- Preexisting uterine anomaly

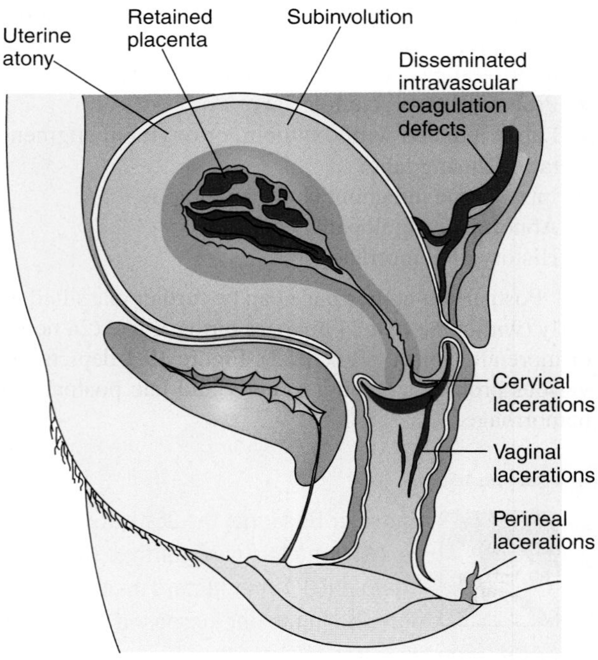

FIGURE 19.1 Postpartum hemorrhage can develop from various causes.

- Poor uterine contractility secondary to high multiparity, rapid or prolonged labor, Pitocin-induced or augmented labor, or use of muscle-relaxing medications (eg, magnesium sulfate, general anesthetics)

COLLABORATIVE CARE: HEMORRHAGE AND UTERINE ATONY

Assessment

The earliest sign of early postpartum hemorrhage from uterine atony is excessive vaginal bleeding. Further assessment is necessary to identify the cause, estimate the blood loss, and control the bleeding. Estimating the blood loss is critical to ongoing assessment of the client's hemodynamic status. A pad count and, more specifically, weighing pads and other blood-soaked articles to calculate the quantity of blood loss is appropriate. To quantify the amount of blood loss, the nurse should weigh the dry pad before placing it on the woman. Immediately upon removing the blood-soaked pad, the nurse should weigh it again. The difference in weight in grams between the blood-soaked pad and the dry weight of the pad is the number of milliliters of blood absorbed by that pad (500 mL approximates 454 g).

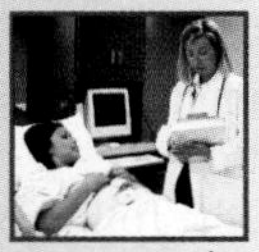

Remember Rosanna, the postpartum client described at the beginning of the chapter, who complains of bleeding and being unable to urinate. The nurse assesses her perineal pad and notices that it is saturated with dark red blood. While helping Rosanna to change her position, the nurse also notices that the protective pad under the client's buttocks is wet with blood. How would the nurse estimate Rosanna's blood loss?

Because the source of bleeding is the former placental site, blood may pool in the lower uterine segment and become evident only with positional change or manual pressure to the uterus, resulting in expression of the pooled blood. Bleeding from an atonic uterus is generally dark red and flows in a steady stream, possibly with clots. Bleeding related to laceration of the genital tract is bright red and appears "spurting." If clots are present, the nurse should differentiate whether they are simple clots or remnants from retained placental tissue. Retained placental tissue impedes uterine contraction and causes excessive bleeding.

Palpation of the uterine fundus reveals a soft "boggy" uterus secondary to the lack of muscular contraction. In addition, the uterine fundus may be displaced from midline. In such an event, the nurse should assess the bladder for distention. A distended bladder will displace an otherwise contractile uterus and can cause uterine atony.

If bleeding is excessive with a firm uterine fundus, the nurse should investigate causes for the bleeding other than uterine atony. Examples include a genital tract laceration or **hypofibrinogenemia.** Hypofibrinogenemia is a congenital or acquired condition of a low level of fibrinogen, a necessary protein in the clotting cascade.

Changes in vital signs are a late sign of blood loss related to postpartum hemorrhage. Because of the increased blood volume in pregnancy, which remains during the first 24 to 48 hours postpartum, the maternal heart rate and blood pressure may demonstrate minimal changes until the woman has lost a significant volume of blood. Frequent monitoring of maternal vital signs during the first 2 hours after birth, however, may reveal subtle trends related to blood loss (Bowes & Katz, 2002). In addition, the nurse should assess the client's skin for color, warmth, and promptness of capillary refill.

The first symptoms that many clients experiencing postpartum hemorrhage report include nausea, lightheadedness, dizziness, and headache. Laboratory studies include evaluation of hemoglobin and hematocrit as a baseline for comparison of the client's hemodynamic status as it equilibrates during subsequent recovery. If blood loss is excessive or hypofibrinogenemia is suspected, a complete clotting profile may be done.

Ongoing assessment includes observation for signs of hypovolemic shock:

- Hypotension: lower blood volume leading to decreased stroke volume and cardiac output
- Tachycardia and thready pulse: systemic vasoconstriction and decreased cardiac output (early)
- Decreased pulse pressure: decreased stroke volume (late)
- Cold, pale, clammy skin: decreased peripheral perfusion resulting from vasoconstriction
- Cyanosis: vasoconstriction and red blood cell loss, leading to decreased hemoglobin available for oxygen transport
- Oliguria: decreased renal perfusion
- Extreme thirst: excessive loss of extracellular fluids
- Apathy, lethargy, and confusion: decreased oxygen perfusion to brain and altered cerebral blood flow

Select Potential Nursing Diagnoses

The following nursing diagnoses may be appropriate in cases of early postpartum hemorrhage related to uterine atony:

- **Ineffective Tissue Perfusion** related to decreased oxygen-carrying capacity and oxygen transport to vital organs and tissues
- **Deficient Fluid Volume** related to excessive blood loss
- **Risk for Injury** related to decreased circulation volume
- **Fear** related to excessive blood loss
- **Fear** related to lack of understanding of what is happening

Planning/Intervention

The goal of interventions is to decrease blood loss. NIC/NOC Box 19.1 provides common interventions and outcomes related to postpartum hemorrhage. Prompt identification of the cause of the blood loss is critical. Following birth, the nurse should massage the uterus until it becomes firm. Fundal massage needs to be vigorous but gentle to prevent injury to the uterine anatomy (see Chap. 18). Once firm, excessive massage can lead to overstimulation of the uterine muscle, resulting in relaxation manifested as excessive bleeding. Thus, the nurse should avoid excessive uterine massage. If he or she finds a previously firm fundus to be relaxed, displaced, and boggy, the nurse should assess for bladder distention and encourage the woman to void or initiate catheterization as indicated. Simple emptying of a full bladder may facilitate uterine contraction and decreased bleeding. In severe cases, the nurse may insert a Foley catheter to keep the bladder empty and to facilitate bimanual compression. A nurse midwife or an obstetrician would perform bimanual compression of the uterine structure to decrease bleeding.

NIC/NOC Box 19.1 Postpartum Hemorrhage

Common NIC Labels

- Anxiety Reduction
- Blood Products Administration
- Cerebral Perfusion Management
- Coping Enhancement
- Decision Making Support
- Fluid/Electrolyte Management
- Fluid Monitoring
- Fluid Resuscitation
- Hemodynamic Regulation
- Hemorrhage Control
- Hypovolemia Management
- Shock Management
- Shock Management: Cardiac
- Vital Signs Monitoring

Common NOC Labels

- Anxiety Control
- Circulation Status
- Coagulation Status
- Fear Control
- Fluid Balance
- Hydration
- Tissue Perfusion: Cardiac
- Tissue Perfusion: Cerebral
- Vital Sign Status

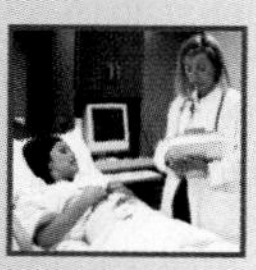

Think back to Rosanna, the client who gave birth to her fourth child 6 hours ago. Fundal assessment reveals a boggy uterus displaced to the right. How would the nurse intervene?

To perform bimanual compression, the examiner should insert a gloved hand into the vagina and press a closed fist against the uterus. He or she should place the other hand on the client's abdomen to grasp the uterine fundus and push it down toward the symphysis pubis. The examiner may maintain compression for as long as 20 to 30 minutes.

Pharmacologic agents are used to control early postpartum hemorrhage from uterine atony (Table 19.1). Oxytocin (Pitocin) frequently is added to the intravenous (IV) fluids immediately after the third stage of labor or delivery of the placenta to stimulate uterine contraction. If bleeding becomes excessive, the primary care provider may order additional oxytocin and continuation of the IV infusion. Concentrations of oxytocin above 30 to 40 U/L of IV fluid, however, do not promote more effective uterine contraction and increase the risk for fluid overload secondary to the antidiuretic effects of the medication (Strong, 1997).

Methylergonovine maleate (Methergine) is administered intramuscularly. Nurses must administer it with caution in women who have elevated blood pressure or cardiovascular disease because it causes a sudden increase in blood pressure and could initiate a cerebral vascular accident in clients at risk with preexisting conditions. In cases of severe hemorrhage, nurses may administer an intramuscular injection of 15-methyl derivative of prostaglandin F2-α carboprost tromethamine (Hemabate). Use of this prostaglandin-based agent is reserved for the most severe cases of hemorrhage because of the associated side effects, including diarrhea, hypertension, vomiting, fever, and tachycardia.

Clients experiencing postpartum hemorrhage need an IV line with a large-bore needle to accommodate large-volume fluid replacement and possible blood transfusion. Initiating IV access early is important because waiting until blood loss has been excessive may lead to vascular collapse. Nursing Care Plan 19.1 highlights some key strategies when caring for a client experiencing early postpartum hemorrhage from uterine atony.

(text continues on page 753)

● **TABLE 19.1 Drugs Used to Control Postpartum Hemorrhage**

DRUG	ACTION/INDICATION	NURSING IMPLICATIONS
Oxytocin (Pitocin)	Stimulates the uterus to contract/ to contract the uterus to control bleeding from the placental site	Assess fundus for evidence of contraction and compare amount of bleeding every 15 minutes or according to orders. Monitor vital signs every 15 minutes. Monitor uterine tone to prevent hyperstimulation. Reassure client about the need for uterine contraction and administer analgesics for comfort. Offer explanation to client and family about what is happening and the purpose of the medication. Provide nonpharmacologic comfort measures to assist with pain management. Set up the IV infusion to be piggybacked into a primary IV line. This ensures that the medication can be discontinued readily if hyperstimulation or adverse effects occur while maintaining the IV site and primary infusion.
Methylergonovine maleate (Methergine)	Stimulates the uterus/to prevent and treat postpartum hemorrhage due to atony or subinvolution	Assess baseline bleeding, uterine tone, and vital signs every 15 minutes or according to protocol. Offer explanation to client and family about what is happening and the purpose of the medication. Monitor for possible adverse effects, such as hypertension, seizures, uterine cramping, nausea, vomiting, and palpitations. Report any complaints of chest pain promptly.
Ergonovine maleate (Ergotrate)	Stimulates uterine contractions/ to control postpartum or postabortion hemorrhage	Assess baseline bleeding, uterine tone, and vital signs every 15 minutes or according to protocol. Offer explanation to client and family about what is happening and the purpose of the medication. Monitor for possible adverse effects, such as nausea, vomiting, weakness, muscular pain, headache, or dizziness.
Prostaglandin (PGF-2a, Prostin/15m, Hemabate)	Stimulates uterine contractions/ to treat postpartum hemorrhage due to uterine atony when not controlled by other methods	Assess vital signs, uterine contractions, client's comfort level, and bleeding status as per protocol. Offer explanation to client and family about what is happening and the purpose of the medication. Monitor for possible adverse effects, such as fever, chills, headache, nausea, vomiting, diarrhea, flushing, and bronchospasm.

NURSING CARE PLAN 19.1

The Client With Postpartum Hemorrhage

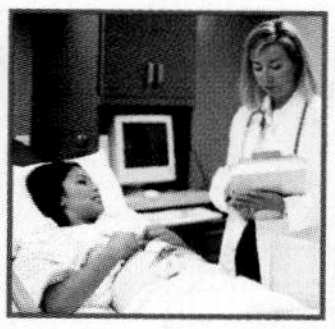

Recall Rosanna, who gave birth to her fourth child 6 hours ago. She is complaining of an inability to void and vaginal bleeding greater than expected. Further assessment reveals a boggy uterus displaced to the right. Her bladder is distended. She has saturated two perineal pads in the last hour. When inspecting her lochia, the nurse notices moderate blood on the protective underpad, pooling under her buttocks. The area is approximately 10 inches in diameter and saturating the protective pad. The client's skin is pale and cool. Pulse rate and blood pressure are slightly decreased from baseline but within acceptable parameters.

NURSING DIAGNOSIS

Impaired Urinary Elimination related to effects of vaginal birth

EXPECTED OUTCOMES

1. The client will identify measures to promote voiding.
2. The client will state that she has voided on her own.

INTERVENTIONS	RATIONALES
Assess the abdomen for bladder distention.	Bladder distention indicates urinary retention and interferes with uterine involution.
Assist the client to the bathroom to sit on the toilet to void; provide privacy.	Sitting on the toilet helps the client maintain the normal anatomic position for urination.
Run water in the sink, run warm water over the perineum, or place client's hand in a basin or sink filled with warm water; if necessary, fill a sitz bath with warm water and have the client sit on it.	The sound of running water or the sensation of warm water stimulates urination and also helps promote client relaxation.
Allow the client sufficient time to void.	Rushing increases anxiety and contributes to urinary retention.
If the client cannot void, prepare to catheterize her.	Bladder distention must be relieved to prevent further interference with uterine involution.
Measure the amount of urine voided.	Voiding less than 100 mL suggests incomplete bladder emptying.

EVALUATION

1. The client uses measures to stimulate voiding.
2. The client voids at least 100 mL clear yellow urine.

NURSING DIAGNOSES

- **Risk for Injury** related to postpartum hemorrhage secondary to uterine atony
- **Ineffective Tissue Perfusion: Cardiopulmonary** related to effects of blood loss from postpartum hemorrhage

Continued

NURSING CARE PLAN 19.1 ● The Client With Postpartum Hemorrhage *(Continued)*

EXPECTED OUTCOMES

1. The client will remain free of injury from postpartum hemorrhage.
2. The client will exhibit a firm uterus with moderate lochia rubra.
3. The client will demonstrate vital signs and cardiopulmonary status within acceptable parameters.

INTERVENTIONS	RATIONALES
Assess the fundus for location and firmness.	Fundal assessment provides information about the contraction of the uterus after birth.
Inspect the perineal area; assess lochia amount and color; check for evidence of clots.	Lochia from uterine atony is dark red and steady, possibly with some clots.
Reposition the client to inspect for pooling of blood.	Blood may pool in the lower uterine segment and become evident only with positional changes.
Perform pad count and weigh perineal pads and any other blood-soaked articles.	Pad count and weight provide an estimate of the amount of blood loss.
Assess the client's ability to void and encourage voiding; monitor amounts voided. If necessary, insert a urinary catheter.	Urinary retention leads to bladder distention, which interferes with uterine involution. Urinary catheterization, although a last resort, can help keep the bladder empty.
Massage the uterus gently but vigorously until firm.	Uterine massage aids in uterine contraction. Too vigorous massage can overstimulate the uterine muscle, leading to uterine relaxation and further bleeding.
Anticipate bimanual compression by the nurse midwife or obstetrician.	Bimanual compression promotes uterine contraction.
Insert a large-bore IV line if one is not already in place; administer fluid replacement as ordered.	Fluid replacement helps to maintain vascular volume.
Administer oxytocin IV or methylergonovine maleate IM as ordered.	Oxytocin and methylergonovine stimulate uterine contraction.
Monitor vital signs frequently for changes; administer oxygen as ordered.	Continued blood loss can lead to hypovolemic shock. Oxygen administration ensures adequate tissue perfusion.
Continue to assess uterine fundus and lochia for changes.	Ongoing assessment is necessary to determine effectiveness of interventions and identify signs and symptoms of possible hypovolemic shock.
Provide emotional support and teaching to the client and family about what is happening, including measures to prevent further problems.	Emotional support and information help to reduce anxiety and fear.

EVALUATION

1. The client demonstrates reduced bleeding to within acceptable parameters.
2. The client exhibits moderate lochia rubra with a uterus that remains firm and contracting.
3. The client demonstrates vital signs and cardiopulmonary status within acceptable limits.
4. The client and family verbalize understanding of events.

If the previously described interventions are ineffective in controlling uterine bleeding, an invasive intervention may be indicated. Surgical options include utero-ovarian, uterine, and hypogastric vessel ligation to interrupt blood flow to the uterus while sparing removal of the uterus. An interventional radiology procedure is angiographic embolization of selected pelvic arteries, which has been proved a safe and effective treatment for intractable postpartum uterine hemorrhage that also preserves future fertility (Ornan et al., 2003). As a last resort to stop massive blood loss and resulting hypovolemic shock, a hysterectomy can be performed.

Evaluation

Successful immediate outcomes include a firm fundus and decreased uterine bleeding. Ongoing evaluation requires monitoring for developing signs of hypovolemic shock as noted previously.

Even after resolution of the acute bleeding episode, clients who experience postpartum hemorrhage are at risk for anemia. Long-term evaluation includes a plan to decrease the possibility of anemia. In cases of mild hemorrhage, dietary counseling and iron supplements are used to rebuild the client's blood volume and hemoglobin stores. Fatigue associated with anemia combined with exhaustion resulting from the newborn's round-the-clock demands places women who have experienced hemorrhage at particular risk for coping and adjustment problems. Therefore, support in the home environment and assistance with infant care activities are essential components of the follow-up plan. If anemia is severe or results in symptoms of hypovolemia, a blood transfusion may be ordered.

Lacerations

Laceration of the genital tract is suspected when postpartum bleeding continues despite a firm, well-contracted uterine fundus. Bleeding associated with genital laceration usually is bright red. Lacerations may occur despite attentive and skilled care during labor and birth. Risk factors for lacerations include forceps or vacuum delivery, precipitous second stage and rapid expulsion, and birth of large infants (Bowes & Katz, 2002). In addition, scarring from prior gynecologic or birth events and vulvar, perineal, or vaginal varicosities increase the incidence of lacerations (Bowes & Katz, 2002). Nevertheless, lacerations can occur during any vaginal birth from the excessive stretching and pulling on the tissue that the birth process imposes, which leads to tissue thinning and friability. Tissue changes combined with increased vascularity of the labia and vaginal areas during pregnancy can lead to profuse postpartum bleeding.

COLLABORATIVE CARE: LACERATIONS

Lacerations may be present on perineal, vaginal, or cervical tissue (Fig. 19.2). Those that are extensions of an episiotomy are classified as first, second, third, or fourth degree (see Chap. 15). Genital bleeding from lacerations usually is present during the first hours following birth.

Assessment

The nurse should initially assess the uterine fundus to note its position and consistency and determine whether the bleeding is being caused by uterine atony. If the fundus is firm and midline, the nurse should begin seeking other clues to the cause, such as laceration. Some lacerations, such as of the cervix, do not cause massive external bleeding; rather, they cause a slow and steady bleeding leading to significant hemorrhage.

Vaginal examination is often necessary to visualize the upper vagina and cervix to inspect for laceration. The client may report localized discomfort in the area of the tear. In addition, her vital signs, fluid status, elimination function, skin pallor, and temperature are important assessment parameters. Blood work, including a complete blood count (CBC) and platelet count, is necessary to evaluate hemodynamic status, provide a baseline for comparison, and rule out a platelet disorder as the cause of the bleeding.

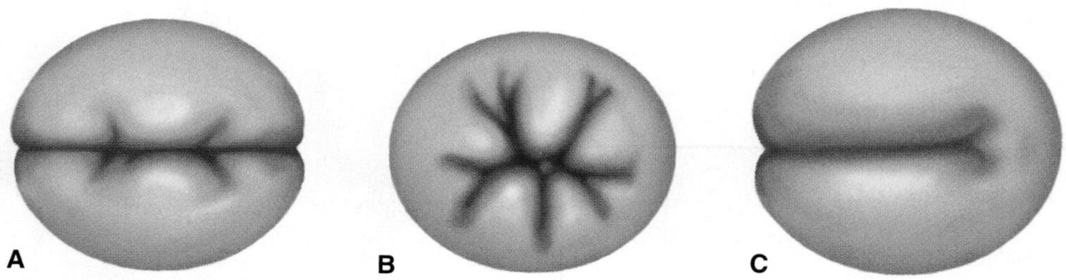

FIGURE 19.2 Cervical lacerations can lead to bleeding during the first hours following birth. They may be visible as healed areas and considered a normal assessment finding over time. Examples include unilateral transverse lacerations (**A**), bilateral transverse lacerations (**B**), and stellate lacerations (**C**).

Select Potential Nursing Diagnoses

The following nursing diagnoses may be appropriate in cases of postpartum lacerations:

- **Ineffective Tissue Perfusion** related to blood loss
- **Risk for Injury**
- **Impaired Tissue Integrity** related to laceration

Planning/Intervention

Resolution of active bleeding and pain are priority goals. After identification of a genital tract laceration, treatment depends on location and severity. Many lacerations need suturing. After surgical repair, nursing care is similar to episiotomy care: application of an ice pack for 12 to 24 hours to minimize swelling, followed by sitz baths to enhance circulation and healing. Maintaining perineal hygiene decreases the risk for a secondary infection at the site of the tissue damage. See Box 19.3.

The nurse should offer analgesics as prescribed by the primary care provider to minimize perineal discomfort. Depending on the location of the laceration and amount of tissue trauma, the client may have fears about or difficulty involving elimination. Nursing measures to monitor adequate urinary and fecal output are a component of the plan of care. Once the client has passed the acute recovery period, the nurse should teach her Kegel's exercises (see Chap. 23) to assist with healing as well as to restore tone to the injured tissue (Mason et al., 2001).

Evaluation

Evaluation parameters vary based on the location of the laceration and the client's clinical condition. Ongoing expected outcomes include maintenance of hemodynamic stability and urinary function and prevention of secondary infections. As previously mentioned, the client needs evaluation for the onset of hypovolemic shock as well as anemia because she has lost the expanded blood volume that accompanies pregnancy.

Hematoma

A **hematoma** is a localized collection of blood that results from bleeding into the connective tissue beneath the vaginal mucosa or vulvar skin as a consequence of tissue injury or trauma. It can develop rapidly with no visual evidence of external bleeding.

Types. The most common hematoma following birth is a *vulvar hematoma* and results when ruptured arteries and veins in the superficial fascia seep into the nearby tissue. Because the bleeding is into an enclosed area, localized pressure, discoloration, and pain result. Trauma to the soft tissue during birth may result in a *vaginal hematoma.* A vaginal hematoma can obstruct the urethra, making urination difficult. *Retroperitoneal hematomas* are rare but extremely dangerous. Because of their location, they may not be evident until a large amount of blood loss results in hypotension and hypovolemic shock.

Assessment Findings. The characteristic sign of hematoma is severe, localized pain inconsistent with that expected following birth. The pain does not go away despite administration of analgesics and other supportive measures. Other indicators include difficulty voiding or inability to void and complaints of rectal pressure similar to the sensation during second-stage labor. On inspection, the vulvar area appears ecchymotic, and an outline of the hematoma is visible (Fig. 19.3).

Hematomas present as tense fluctuant masses. Those located in the vaginal area may require vaginal examination for visualization. Changes in vital signs and blood work may not immediately identify acute bleeding because of the physiologic adaptations and expansion of total blood volume that accompany pregnancy.

Collaborative Management. The priority goal is prevention of hematoma. The best method of prevention is application of ice to the perineum following difficult or traumatic birth. When a hematoma has already developed, the goals become cessation of the bleeding, reabsorption or drainage of the blood mass, and attention to the client's need for pain management and elimination care.

BOX 19.3 Good Perineal Hygiene

Frequent perineal care
Sitz baths
Frequent pad changes
Warm compress to area
Good handwashing technique
Wipe or pat perineal area front to back

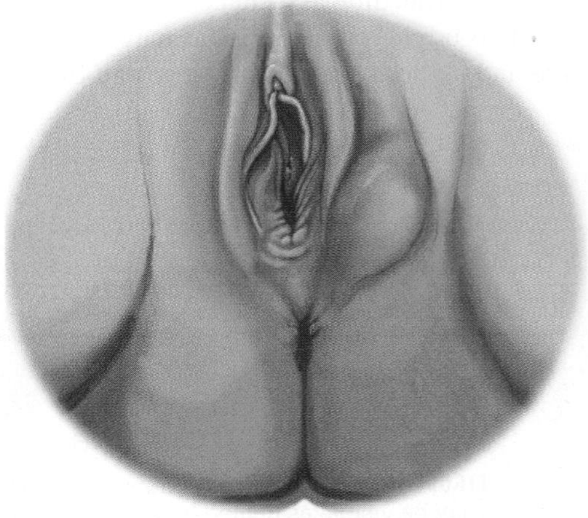

FIGURE 19.3 With a hematoma, the area is ecchymotic, and an outline of the swollen area is visible.

Small vulvar hematomas often absorb spontaneously. Comfort measures of localized ice and heat application may help reduce swelling and discomfort and facilitate reabsorption of the hematoma. Hematomas that are large or increasing in size need incision, evacuation, and drainage of the blood and clots. Any bleeding vessels are sutured to prevent reformation of the hematoma. After incision, the area usually is packed to promote hemostasis and drainage. The packing usually remains in place for 12 to 18 hours and is then removed before it becomes a reservoir for bacterial proliferation. A Foley catheter often is inserted to promote urinary elimination.

The amount of blood lost from hematoma may be considerable and is difficult to estimate because of its enclosed nature. Therefore, fluid and blood replacement may be indicated to prevent hypovolemic shock. In addition, broad-spectrum antibiotics often are prescribed to prevent secondary infection.

Comprehensive and ongoing inspection of the perineal tissue facilitates early identification and intervention. Indicators of effective interventions are resolution of the bleeding as evidenced by decreasing size of the mass, decreasing pain, returning perfusion to area, and no secondary infection.

Uterine Inversion

Uterine inversion, a relatively rare complication of childbirth (Hostetler & Bosworth, 2000), is when the uterine fundus drops into the endometrial cavity. The fundus may or may not extend beyond the external cervical os. The etiology is clear and usually involves rapid expulsion of the uterine contents (fetus and amniotic fluid) coupled with excessive traction on the umbilical cord (Rocconi et al., 2002). Other contributing factors include excessive fundal pressure during the second stage of labor or during postpartum fundal palpation, a short umbilical cord, uterine anomalies, use of oxytocin, primiparity, rapid uterine decompression, and placental anomalies (eg, placental accreta).

Classification. Uterine inversion is classified by degree:

- *Incomplete inversion:* The uterine fundus drops into the endometrial cavity but does not extend beyond the cervical os.
- *Complete inversion:* The uterine fundus extends beyond the external cervical os.
- *Prolapsed inversion:* The inverted fundus extends beyond the vaginal introitus.
- *Total inversion:* The uterus and vaginal wall are inverted, not usually as related to the puerperal period.

Assessment Findings. Identification is based on clinical signs and symptoms. Characteristic findings include a nonpalpable fundus, profuse bleeding, and obvious alterations in the abdominal examination. With incomplete inversion, the poorly contracted fundus may be palpable in the lower uterine segment; with complete inversion, the inverted fundus is palpable at the cervical os. Evidence of hypovolemic shock with severe hypotension may provide additional diagnostic clues. Sonographic imaging reveals characteristic findings to support the diagnosis of uterine inversion.

Collaborative Management. The ultimate goals are repositioning the uterine fundus, promoting uterine contraction, and controlling uterine bleeding. This emergency requires attendance by the primary care provider in addition to nursing care. Once inversion is suspected, health care personnel should stop the administration of all oxytocin agents until anatomic alignment of the uterus is corrected. Manual manipulation is used to reposition the uterus. To assist with repositioning, the nurse may administer prescribed medications such as magnesium sulfate or terbutaline to facilitate myometrial relaxation. Some studies have examined the use of low-dose nitroglycerin because of its faster onset, quicker dissipation, and decreased effects on hemodynamics compared with magnesium sulfate or terbutaline (Dayan & Schwalbe, 1996). The mechanism of action for all these drugs is to relax the uterus by vascular smooth muscle relaxation. After replacement of the uterine fundus, the nurse administers prescribed oxytocin agents to cause uterine contraction, which will prevent reinversion and decrease blood loss.

When attempts at manual reduction of inversion are unsuccessful, surgical correction is needed. Whether assisting with manual manipulation or preparing the woman for surgery, nursing interventions focus on supporting circulating volume, enhancing tissue oxygenation, monitoring vital signs and urinary output as indicators of the onset of hypovolemic shock, and implementing pain management strategies.

As with other bleeding complications, monitoring for the effects of hypovolemia (eg, acute renal failure, Sheehan's failure), as well as for anemia, is an appropriate evaluation parameter.

Late Postpartum Hemorrhage

Late postpartum hemorrhage is excessive vaginal bleeding 24 hours or more after birth. Often, it develops 7 to 14 days following birth but can occur as late as 1 month after birth. It often is associated with infection or retained placental fragments, both of which lead to **subinvolution** of the uterus (see Chap. 18). Placental fragments, which remain attached to the uterine wall after the third stage of labor, begin to undergo necrosis as the uterine blood supply decreases postpartally. As retained placenta necroses, a fibrin deposit and placental polyp form. Eventually the polyp detaches from the uterine wall, resulting in hemorrhage. A typical scenario in late postpartum hemorrhage is a new mother at home beginning to regain energy and resume daily activities, who suddenly experiences a gush of foul-smelling uterine bleeding, which may or may not be accompanied by uterine tenderness and low-grade fever. Signs that may follow actual hemorrhage include increased uterine cramping, lochia rubra, and malodorous vaginal discharge.

COLLABORATIVE CARE: LATE POSTPARTUM HEMORRHAGE

Because late postpartum hemorrhage usually occurs after the woman returns home, initial recognition is by the woman herself. Therefore, all postpartum women need education about normal patterns and changes in uterine involution and lochial flow.

Assessment

Abnormalities such as bright red bleeding; excessive clot passage; persistent lochia rubra; foul-smelling lochia; pain or tenderness in the lower abdomen, back, or perineum; or a low-grade, persistent fever need referral to a health care provider.

The uterine fundus may be palpable beyond the first 7 to 10 days after birth as a result of subinvolution. When palpable, the fundus is usually tender. Bimanual examination confirms a uterus larger than expected for the specific stage of the postpartum recovery period. A uterine ultrasound is useful to identify additional remnants of tissue in the uterine cavity.

An order for a complete blood count is important, because the white blood cell (WBC) count and differential are used to assess for infection, and the hemoglobin and hematocrit are examined for quantity of blood lost.

Select Potential Nursing Diagnoses

Appropriate nursing diagnoses in cases of late postpartum hemorrhage may include the following:

- **Deficient Fluid Volume** related to excessive blood loss
- **Ineffective Maternal Role Performance** related to rehospitalization and sick role
- **Infection** related to retention of necrotic tissue and bacterial proliferation
- **Risk for Injury** related to blood loss, infection, and altered hemodynamics
- **Impaired Parenting** related to rehospitalization of mother and separation from infant

"It was terrifying to be at home and to start bleeding so profusely. But the hardest part of all was having to go back to the hospital and be away from my child."

A client recalling her experience with late postpartum hemorrhage

Planning/Intervention

The client experiencing late postpartum hemorrhage needs treatment at a health care facility. Physiologic needs related to blood loss resulting in potential hemodynamic changes are the highest priority; however, these clients also have significant psychological needs related to the unexpected emergency. Nursing care focuses on measures to provide a sense of maternal safety and well-being, as well as methods to help her deal with separation from the newborn.

On admission, the client should receive a large-bore IV tube to infuse crystalloid solutions (eg, normal saline, lactated Ringer's) to expand circulating volume. Pharmacologic agents such as oxytocin or methylergonovine maleate may be administered to stimulate uterine contraction, which is necessary to decrease bleeding as well as to push out any remaining necrotic tissue. If bleeding continues despite pharmacologic interventions and uterine massage, the primary care provider may perform bimanual compression.

Curettage of the uterine lining is used only when nonsurgical interventions are ineffective. Surgical curettage further traumatizes the uterine lining and may result in increased bleeding. When surgical intervention is used, the client and her family need to be aware that a hysterectomy may be necessary if the bleeding cannot be controlled with less invasive measures.

Intrauterine infection and late postpartum hemorrhage are highly correlated; therefore, the nurse should administer prescribed broad-spectrum antibiotics (Bowes & Katz, 2002). Ongoing monitoring of vital signs and laboratory values provide data related to the client's hemodynamic and febrile status.

Evaluation

Resolution of the bleeding, elimination of the causative factors, and resolution of any infection are indicators of effective treatment. Monitoring the client's laboratory test results (ie, WBC and differential) and temperature provides useful evaluation parameters related to coexistence of an infection. In addition, decreases in uterine size and lochia indicate involution. Follow-up includes evaluation of hematocrit and hemoglobin for signs of anemia and treatment with dietary counseling and iron supplementation as needed.

POSTPARTUM INFECTIONS

The classic definition of **puerperal infection** is a temperature of 100.4°F (38.0°C) or higher on any two of the first 10 days following birth exclusive of the first 24 hours. The Joint Commission on Maternal Welfare originally developed this definition in 1919; with minor revisions, it is still the standard in practice today. In addition, a temperature of 101°F or higher during the first 24 hours is considered a parameter for identification of early infection.

The timing of the increased temperature may provide cues to the source and cause of the infectious process. Elevated temperatures during the first 24 hours indicate infections that are preexisting or began before the birth. For example, the client who had premature rupture of membranes 7 days before birth was susceptible to ascending infection and may manifest signs of endometrial infection in the first 24 hours after birth. Infections directly related to the birth generally appear 24 to 72 hours later. The most common sites for these infections are the uterus and vagina. Finally, infections related to an incision (episiotomy or cesarean section), blood clots, or the breasts usually do not develop until 4 days or more after birth. Infections can be classified according to site as shown in Box 19.4.

Although fever is the primary finding suggesting a postpartum complication, in some situations, increased temperature indicates another problem, such as dehydration during the first 24 hours or breast engorgement at postpartum days 3 to 5. Therefore, comprehensive assessment and critical analysis of collected data are essential nursing roles.

Infection of the Uterus and Surrounding Tissues

Endometritis is the primary cause of postpartum infections (Cunningham et al., 2005). During pregnancy, the uterine cavity and endometrial lining are sterile, and the intact amniotic membrane protects them from bacterial organisms. After rupture of the membranes, anaerobic and aerobic bacteria that normally reside in the female cervix, vagina, perineum, and bowel can ascend into the uterus and contaminate its lining. The introduction of these bacteria, combined with an open wound in the decidua at the site of placental attachment, results in a favorable environment for bacterial growth and infection. When endometritis presents 1 to 2 days after birth, the causative organism is usually group A streptococcus. Anaerobic organisms such as *Escherichia coli* usually cause later-appearing infections (3 to 4 days after birth) (Duff, 2002). According to a study in the Cochrane Database, the incidence of endometritis following cesarean births was reduced by two thirds in women who received prophylactic antibiotics (French & Small, 2002).

Endometritis is an ascending infection, meaning that the normally sterile uterine lining becomes contaminated with organisms from the lower reproductive tract. Situational factors such as PROM, long labor, and cesarean birth, and frequent invasive interventions, such as multiple vaginal examinations, placement of intrauterine catheters or fetal scalp electrodes or fetal pulse oximetry, and manual removal of the placenta, are known risk factors. These risk factors enhance the opportunity to introduce bacterial organisms into the uterine cavity. Endometritis complicates 1% to 3% of vaginal births, 5% to 15% of scheduled cesarean births, and 30% to 35% of cesarean births after a period of labor (Franzblau & Witt, 2003).

BOX 19.4 Classification of Postpartum Maternal Infections According to Site

- Uterus and surrounding tissues
  - Endometritis: infection of the uterine lining
  - Parametritis: infection extending to the broad ligament of the uterus
  - Peritonitis: infection of the abdominal cavity
- Pelvic thrombophlebitis: infection spreading along the pelvic venous structures
- Bladder and kidneys
  - Cystitis: infection of the bladder and urethra
  - Pyelonephritis: infection of the kidneys (renal pelves)
- Skin infections
- Episiotomy/laceration: infection of the perineal incision or damaged tissue
- Abdominal: infection of the surgical incision
- Blood clots
  - Thrombophlebitis: infection within the peripheral vascular system leading to clot formation
- Breasts
  - Mastitis: infection in the milk glands

COLLABORATIVE CARE: UTERINE INFECTIONS

Assessment

Classic signs of endometritis are temperature of 100.4°F (38°C) or greater, tachycardia, and fundal tenderness. The pattern of temperature elevation in cases of severe infection usually is characterized by jagged, irregular spikes, with peaks usually in the evening (Fig. 19.4). The initial characteristic client presentation includes generalized symptoms of fever, chills, anorexia, malaise, tachycardia, and "just not feeling well." Specific subsequent assessment findings consistent with postpartum endometritis include lower abdominal pain, subinvolution of the uterus, tenderness on fundal palpation, malodorous lochia, and prolonged or painful afterpains.

Significant laboratory data include a CBC with differential; lochial, cervical, and endometrial cultures; and blood culture. To provide accurate data, all cultures need to be collected before antimicrobial therapy begins. Blood work that shows an elevated leukocyte count with a shift to the left is consistent with endometritis. The most common time frame for presentation of endometritis is 24 to 48 hours after birth.

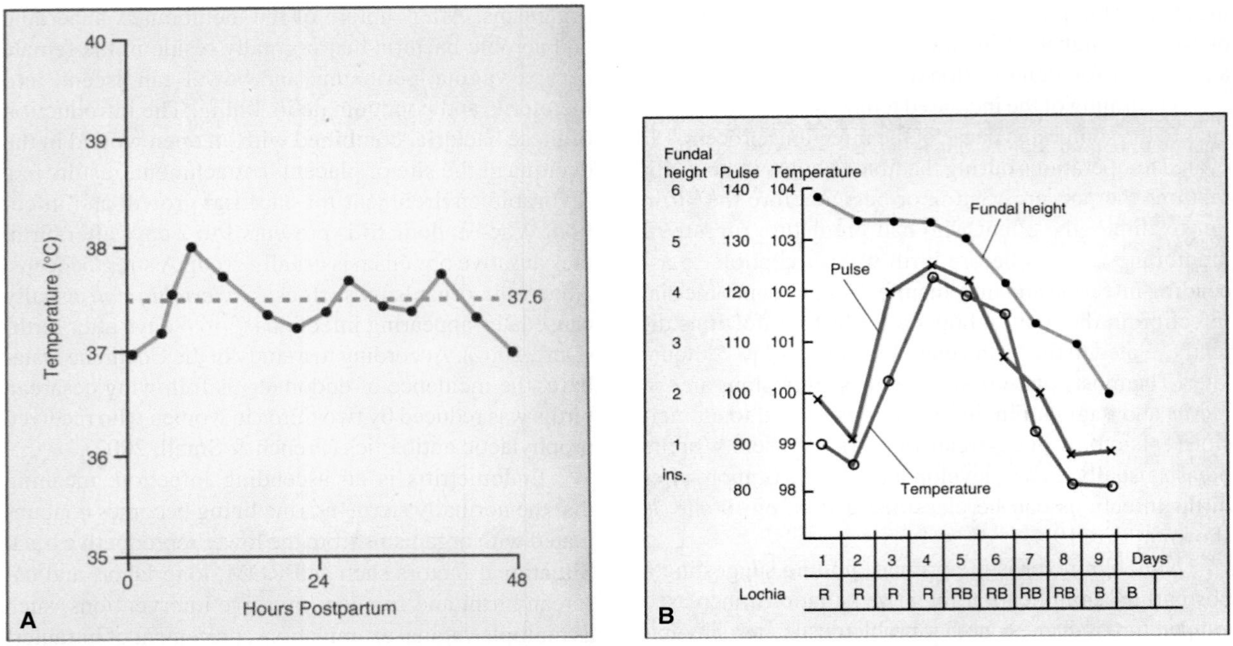

FIGURE 19.4 (**A**) In normal postpartum recoveries, the client's temperature shows characteristic resolution within 48 hours of childbirth. (**B**) With endometritis, temperature remains elevated for several days. Other signs of endometritis include increased pulse, uterine subinvolution, and malodorous lochia, which remains red. (R, red; B, brown)

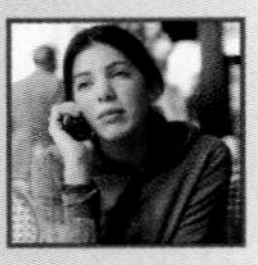

Think back to Leslie, the client described at the beginning of the chapter who had a cesarean birth 1 week ago. What assessment information would be important to obtain to aid in ruling out the possibility of endometritis?

Select Potential Nursing Diagnoses

The following nursing diagnoses may be appropriate for the client with infection of the uterus and surrounding tissues:

- **Impaired Tissue Integrity** related to bacterial invasion of endometrial tissue
- **Imbalanced Body Temperature** related to intrauterine infection
- **Impaired Parenting** related to lack of energy to engage in child care activities
- **Impaired Parenting** related to maternal–newborn separation
- **Risk for Impaired Urinary Elimination** related to decreased bladder sensation secondary to pain and inflammation
- **Risk of Impaired Bowel Elimination** related to decreased activity and dietary intake

Planning/Intervention

After the collection of blood, tissue, and lochia for cultures, the nurse should initiate IV antibiotic treatment as prescribed. Pending identification of the specific causative organism, the client receives a combination of antibiotics proven effective against a broad range of aerobic and anaerobic organisms known to cause endometritis. The current standard is a combination of gentamicin and clindamycin, which demonstrates a cure rate of approximately 90% (Kennedy, 2001). Most endometrial infections respond to IV antibiotics within 48 to 72 hours (Looney et al., 1999). If a client's fever and other symptoms persist despite 48 hours of antimicrobial treatment, other causes of the symptoms need investigation. IV antimicrobial therapy usually continues until the client has been afebrile and without symptoms for 48 hours. NIC/NOC Box 19.2 provides common interventions and outcomes related to infection of the uterus and surrounding tissues.

Nursing responses specific to the care of the client with postpartum endometritis include use of semi-Fowler's position to encourage uterine drainage, good perinatal hygiene to prevent reintroduction of bacterial organisms, and general care and support of the client with a fever and generalized infection such as hydration, nutrition, and comfort management. Inflammation and pain from the infected uterus may lead to incomplete

NIC/NOC Box 19.2 Infections of the Uterus and Surrounding Tissues

Common NIC Labels

- Fever Treatment
- Fluid Management
- Infection Protection
- Medication Administration
- Perineal Care
- Postpartal Care
- Temperature Regulation
- Vital Signs Monitoring

Common NOC Labels

- Thermoregulation
- Tissue Integrity: Skin and Mucous Membranes
- Vital Sign Status
- Wound Healing

bladder emptying, urinary retention or infection, and sluggish peristalsis. Thus, the nurse should monitor fluid status and urine and bowel elimination to prevent secondary complications.

Evaluation

Expected outcomes reflecting effective collaborative treatment include afebrile status, progressive uterine involution and lochial changes, and enhanced client well-being. Most clients respond to antimicrobial treatment within 48 to 72 hours as evidenced by resolution of symptoms.

Sequelae of unresolved endometritis include peritonitis, gastrointestinal tract compromise or paralytic ileus, and septic shock. Ongoing nursing assessment and client education are critical to identifying any recurrence of endometritis, which mandates reestablishing aggressive management of the complication to prevent long-term morbidity and mortality.

Other Genital Tract Infections

Parametritis or parametrial cellulitis is extension of a uterine infection into the broad ligament (Fig. 19.5). Lymphatic transmission of bacteria or direct exposure of the tissue to the invading organism disseminates the infection. The following manifestations develop on approximately the 10th postpartum day:

- Prolonged fever with fluctuations
- Lateral extension of abdominal pain
- Subinvolution, hypotension, chills, decreased bowel sounds, nausea, and vomiting
- Positive rebound tenderness on abdominal palpation

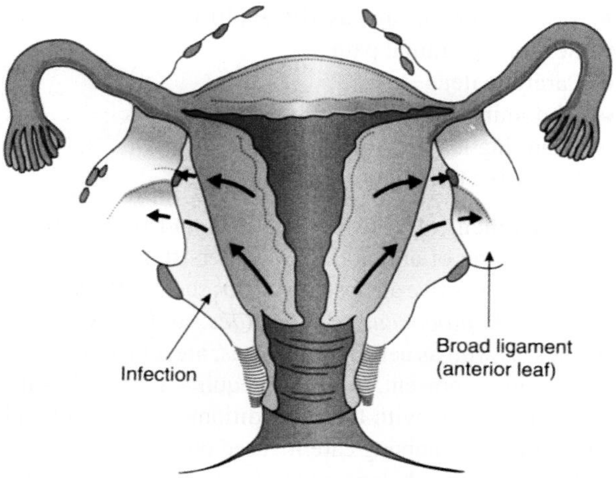

FIGURE 19.5 With parametritis (parametrial cellulitis), uterine infection spreads into the broad ligament, with symptoms developing usually after the first postpartum week.

- Pain and tenderness in both iliac fossae
- Firm, tender mass felt in one adnexa, or both adnexa pushing the uterus to the opposite side or restricting its mobility

Peritonitis, infection of the peritoneum or abdominal cavity, is a life-threatening postpartum complication (Fig. 19.6). The client with peritonitis exhibits assessment findings such as the following:

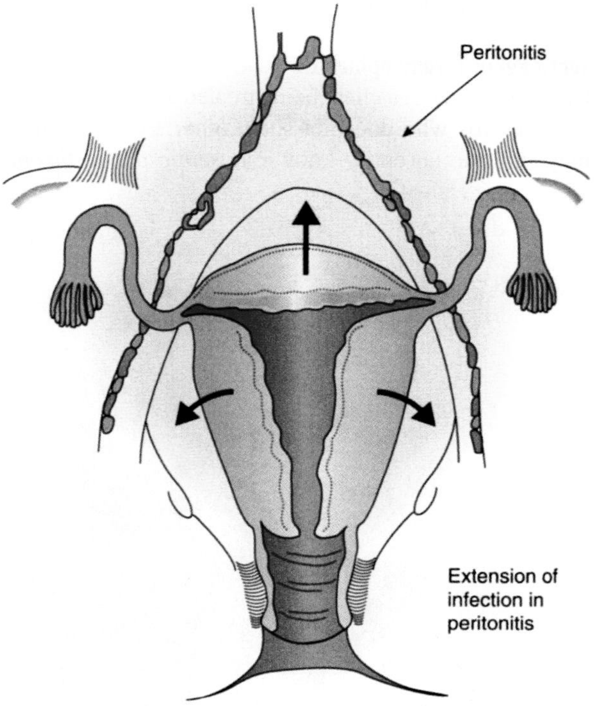

FIGURE 19.6 Life-threatening peritonitis can develop from spread of a postpartum uterine infection into the abdominal cavity.

- Temperature as high as 105°F (40°C)
- Severe abdominal pain
- Paralytic ileus
- Abdominal rigidity
- Vomiting leading to dehydration
- Excessive thirst and anxiety

Treatment of both parametritis and peritonitis is administration of antibiotics. With persistent fever, antimicrobials effective against organisms such as *Peptostreptococcus, Peptococcus, Bacteroides,* and *Clostridium* species, as well as aerobic coliforms, are added. If a paralytic ileus is present, the client requires gastric decompression. Clients with these conditions are quite ill and require vigilant nursing care focused on the regulation of body temperature, balancing fluids and electrolytes, management of nutrition, and administration of antibiotics.

Ongoing nursing assessment focuses on the possible development of septic shock caused by bacteremia; such assessment is critical to early intervention and to decreasing the risk for morbidity and mortality. *Bacteremia* is invasion of the blood by bacteria from the uterus entering the circulatory system through the lymphatics or vascular system. Assessment parameters indicative of bacteremia include the following:

- Rapid temperature elevation
- Profuse foul-smelling lochia
- Symptoms of shock
- Oliguria (decreasing urinary output is an early sign of impending shock)

Septic Pelvic Thrombophlebitis

Persistent fever in a client being treated appropriately for endometritis who does not show other signs of illness may indicate an entity known as *septic pelvic thrombophlebitis* (SPT). This problem results when an infection spreads along the pelvic venous structures. The usual portal of entry into the vascular system is the placental site. Bacteria lead to infection of the myometrial veins, thrombosis formation, and further growth of anaerobic bacteria (Brown et al., 1999). Blood clots may form in these veins and embolize to the lungs.

Clients diagnosed with a puerperal infection are at increased risk for SPT. The common manifestation is a prolonged, spiking fever that continues despite antibiotic therapy. Complaints of pain in the flank or lower abdomen also may be present. In many cases, however, the persistent, spiking fever is the only sign of this complication.

Traditional treatment is a course of IV heparin. Some sources recommend additional diagnostic imaging to confirm venous clots, whereas others emphasize the initiation of anticoagulation treatment based on the client's clinical presentation (Danilenko-Dixon et al., 2001; Spritzer et al., 1995). If the client is started on heparin therapy, monitoring clotting profiles, assessing for bleeding, and teaching about self-care during anticoagulation therapy are all components of the nurse's role.

Resolution of the previously resistant fever is the initial sign of effective treatment. Signs of effective anticoagulation therapy include a partial thromboplastin time (PTT) two times normal (according to the reference laboratory used by the facility) and no evidence of abnormal bleeding. The progression of uterine involution is evident as the pelvic thrombosis resolves.

Wound Infections

Postpartum wound infections include those of the perineum (lacerations or episiotomy site) following vaginal birth and of the abdomen following cesarean birth (Fig. 19.7). Perineal infection is relatively rare (0.35% to

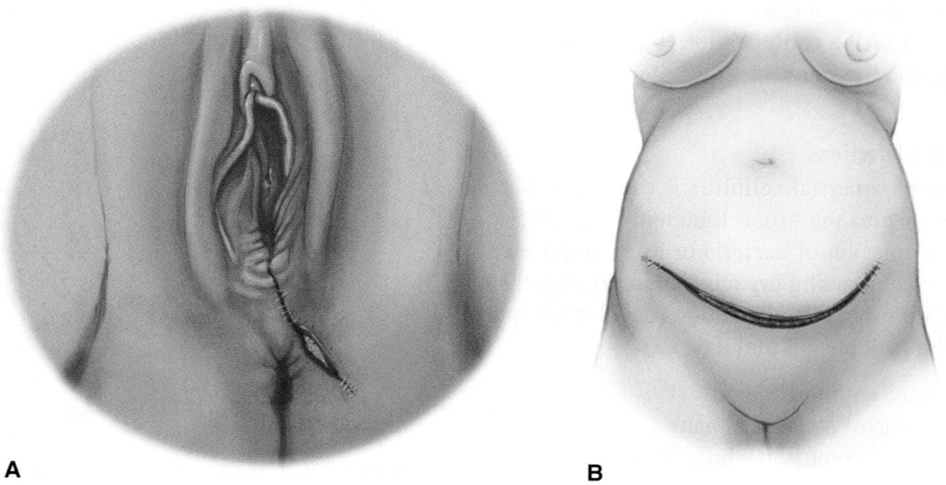

FIGURE 19.7 Wound infections can develop following vaginal or cesarean births. (**A**) Postpartum vaginal wound infection may stem from the episiotomy site. (**B**) Postpartum cesarean wound infection may arise at the site of the surgical incision.

3%) (Franzblau & Witt, 2003) and is related to infected lochia, fecal contamination, and poor hygiene. Extensive perineal trauma, such as a fourth-degree laceration, and instrument-assisted births, such as forceps and vacuum extractions, place the woman at increased risk for perineal infection. Abdominal incision infection (3% to 15%) usually results from contamination of the wound with organisms from the vaginal flora; however, *Staphylococcus aureus* from the skin or other sources is identified in 25% of cases (Franzblau & Witt, 2003). The most common complication of a wound infection is prolonged hospitalization.

Wound dehiscence ranges from 0.1% to 2.3% (Baggish & Lee, 1975; Chukudebelu & Okafor, 1978; Hendrix et al., 2000). Approximately 45% of all abdominal wound dehiscence is attributed to infected abdominal incisions that then lead to additional surgical intervention, complex wound care therapies, and prolonged healing time (Hendrix et al., 2000). Primary prevention of wound infections includes keeping incisions clean and dry to eliminate the opportunity for bacterial growth and proliferation. See Teaching Tips 19.1.

COLLABORATIVE CARE: WOUND INFECTIONS

Assessment

Erythema, induration, warmth, tenderness, and purulent drainage at the site with or without fever are indicative of a wound infection. A draining wound often presents without fever. Early clues of a developing wound infection include edema, skin discoloration, or poor approximation of the skin edges.

Clients with a perineal infection frequently complain of excruciating pain, malodorous discharge, and vulvar edema. On inspection, the perineal area is edematous and red. Thorough inspection of the surrounding area is necessary to evaluate for the coexistence of a hematoma or perineal abscess as the reservoir of the infection.

Abdominal wound infections do not present until 4 to 5 days postoperatively and are often preceded by endometritis. On examination, the incision line may be erythematous, warm and tender to touch, and indurated. Drainage may not be immediately evident. Fluid collection pockets, however, may be found near the wound. When probed, the pockets may release serosanguineous or purulent fluid.

Laboratory data include serial CBC with differentials and cultures of the wound drainage.

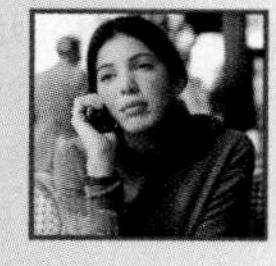

Consider Leslie, the client from the beginning of the chapter who called to report a fever and incisional complaints 10 days after giving birth. The nurse instructs Leslie to come to the health care facility for an evaluation because the client might have an incisional infection. During assessment of Leslie, what would the nurse look for?

Select Potential Nursing Diagnoses

The following nursing diagnoses may be appropriate for the client with a wound infection:

- **Impaired Skin Integrity** related to fluid accumulation
- **Disturbed Body Image** related to draining wound or wound healing by secondary intention
- **Pain** related to wound care procedures
- **Ineffective Protection** related to open abdominal incision

Planning/Intervention

Treatment is based on facilitating drainage of the infected area. An infected incision may open spontaneously and begin to drain; in other cases, the skin incision is intentionally opened to allow drainage. Once the infected area is drained and cleaned, antibiotic treatment is initiated to

● TEACHING TIPS 19.1 Postpartum Infections

The nurse teaches the client recovering from postpartum infections the following:

- Follow the antibiotic regimen exactly as described. Be sure to self-administer the medication precisely as described. Even if you begin to feel better, be sure to finish the entire set of drugs.
- Monitor your temperature at least once daily; report to your health care provider any reading above 100.4°4 (38°C).
- Alert your health care provider if you develop abdominal pain, chills, changes in the odor or color of lochia, or abnormalities at a specific site, such as warmth, redness, or swelling.
- Wash your hands thoroughly before and after eating, newborn care, using the bathroom, or wiping/touching the genitals and anal area.
- Use a front-to-back motion when changing your perineal pad.
- Drink adequate fluids; follow a diet that is high in protein and vitamins.
- Strive to get as much rest as possible.

eradicate the bacterial organism. In addition to antibiotic administration, ongoing nursing care of an infected abdominal incision involves keeping the area clean and packed with saline-moistened gauze pads. Most infected wounds are left open and heal by secondary intention. As a result, client and family teaching about ongoing wound care and potential referral for home care and support are also necessary components of the nursing plan of care. Nursing Care Plan 19.2 highlights the care of a woman with an infection of an incision.

Pharmacologic treatment of perineal and wound infections includes antibiotics to eradicate the bacterial organism and symptomatic relief including nonsteroidal anti-inflammatory drugs and local anesthetic sprays. Antimicrobials are selected based on the culture of the organism demonstrating sensitivity to the tested class of antibiotic. A broad-spectrum antibiotic generally is initiated until this laboratory report has been completed (24 to 48 hours). For perineal infections, in addition to facilitating drainage, sitz baths every 4 to 6 hours are used to maintain cleanliness, enhance circulation, and provide comfort (see Nursing Procedure 18.2 in Chap. 18). Ongoing care includes teaching about perineal hygiene and teaching Kegel's exercises to enhance circulation and tissue strength (see Chap. 23).

Evaluation

After wound drainage, most clients respond rapidly to antibiotics. Interventions are considered effective when the woman has been afebrile for 24 to 48 hours. Other signs of effective nursing interventions are decreasing pain and site inflammation. If the wound is left open, the base and surrounding tissue should appear pink and healthy throughout healing. Ongoing evaluation after discharge to monitor ongoing wound healing and to identify early indicators of a secondary infection is important to overall client well-being.

Urinary Tract Infection

UTIs are the most common medical complication during pregnancy and the postpartum period (McDermott et al., 2000). Up to one third of postpartum women have bacteriuria; however, only 2% of these women develop symptomatic infections (Clark, 1995). Postpartum clients are at increased risk for UTI for several reasons:

- Trauma to the bladder from passage of the fetus from uterus to perineum
- Hypotonicity of the lower urinary tract leading to urinary stasis
- Frequency of urinary catheterization and vaginal examinations during labor (associated with a higher incidence of UTIs)
- Instrument-assisted births, including cesarean, forceps, and vacuum births, and induction of labor

A UTI is diagnosed when significant bacteruria, defined as 100,000 bacteria of the same species milliliter, is present on a clean-catch or catheterized specimen. Bacteria counts between 10,000 and 100,000 are considered equivocal and indicate that the test needs to be repeated. Common guidelines state that for a single isolate, a density greater than 10^5 colony-forming units (CFU)/mL indicates infection, less than 10^4 CFU/mL indicates urethral or vaginal contamination, and between 10^4 and 10^5 CFU/mL requires further evaluation based on clinical information.

Obtaining a clean-catch urine culture during the postpartum period is difficult because of lochial discharge, which contaminates the urine specimen. The risk for introducing bacteria into the urinary tract and promoting an ascending infection is associated with obtaining a catheterized specimen. Therefore, the benefits and limitations of each specimen collection procedure need to be evaluated based on the individual client situation and client-specific data.

Inflammation of the lower urinary tract (bladder and urethra) is known as *cystitis,* whereas inflammation of the upper urinary tract (kidneys and ureters) is known as *pyelonephritis.*

COLLABORATIVE CARE: POSTPARTUM URINARY TRACT INFECTIONS

Assessment

The primary early sign of postpartum cystitis is elevated temperature. Consequently, when the client has a temperature of 100.4°F (38.0°C) or higher, a UTI needs to be considered. UTIs often are characterized by a lingering low-grade fever. Clients also may report symptoms of urinary frequency, urgency, dysuria, hematuria, and suprapubic or lower abdominal pain. Many of these symptoms, however, are difficult to distinguish from some expected renal system adaptations during the early postpartum period.

On inspection, the urine frequently is dark with particulate matter and a foul odor. Relevant laboratory assessments include urinalysis, CBC, and urine culture. Voided urine specimens during the postpartum period are not useful because of contamination with lochial discharge and other vaginal secretions.

Cystitis can appear anytime during the postbirth period. Inflammation of the renal pelves or pyelonephritis usually does not appear until the end of the first postpartum week. The client with pyelonephritis exhibits an extremely high temperature (104°F or 40°C) accompanied by chills, anorexia, and flank pain, and feels extremely ill. In addition to urinary signs of frequency and dysuria, the kidney finding of costovertebral angle tenderness is also present. Pyelonephritis is more common

NURSING CARE PLAN 19.2

The Postpartum Client Who Develops a Wound Infection

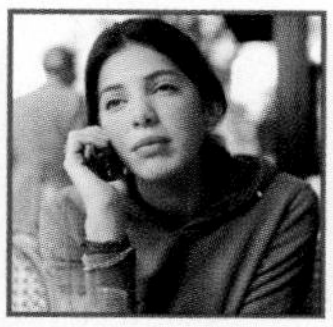

Remember Leslie, who had a cesarean birth approximately 1 week ago. She reports to the emergency department at the nurse's instructions. Assessment reveals that the client's temperature is 101.1°F (38.4°C). Other vital signs are within acceptable parameters. Her low transverse incision is reddened, edematous, and warm to the touch. A 1½-inch area at the right end of her incision is bulging and tense. On palpation, the area opens and drains approximately 45 mL of serosanguineous and purulent drainage.

NURSING DIAGNOSES

- **Impaired Skin Integrity** related to postpartum wound infection
- **Deficient Knowledge** related to wound care

EXPECTED OUTCOMES

1. The client will exhibit indications of wound healing such as decreased redness, warmth, and inflammation.
2. The client will identify measures to care for the wound to promote healing.

INTERVENTIONS	RATIONALES
Assess the incisional wound closely; note drainage amount, color, and character.	This information provides a baseline from which to determine appropriate interventions.
Obtain a culture of the wound; send it to the laboratory.	Wound culture identifies the causative organism for initiating appropriate antibiotic therapy.
Clean the wound using aseptic technique; pack the open area with saline-moistened gauze pads.	Wound cleansing and packing promote healing and prevent abscess formation.
Administer prescribed antibiotics.	Antibiotic therapy is necessary to treat the underlying cause of the wound infection.
Institute wound care, such as irrigation, as ordered.	Specific wound care measures help to promote healing.
Encourage the client to consume a diet high in protein.	She needs additional protein for wound healing.
Instruct the client in the wound care procedure; have her participate in wound care.	Client participation enhances learning and feelings of control over the situation.
Continue to assess the wound and drainage for changes.	Ongoing assessment is necessary to determine the effectiveness of treatment and identify possible progression of infection.
Have the client return demonstrate the procedure for wound care.	Return demonstration of the procedure indicates client learning.
Anticipate referral for home care services after discharge.	Home care provides opportunities for additional teaching, follow-up, and care.

EVALUATION

1. The client exhibits a clean dry wound with pink base and surrounding tissue.
2. The client demonstrates the procedure for wound care appropriately.

Continued

NURSING CARE PLAN 19.2 ● The Postpartum Client Who Develops a Wound Infection *(Continued)*

NURSING DIAGNOSIS

Hyperthermia related to inflammatory process and wound infection

EXPECTED OUTCOME

The client will exhibit temperature within acceptable parameters.

INTERVENTIONS	RATIONALES
Assess the client's temperature at least every 4 hours for changes.	Temperature assessment provides information about the client's current infection.
Administer antipyretics as ordered.	Antipyretics aid in reducing fever.
Encourage fluid intake.	Fluid intake helps to replace fluids lost from fever.
Administer IV fluids and antibiotics as ordered.	IV fluids help maintain fluid balance and provide an access route for antibiotic therapy, which treats the underlying cause of the infection.
Institute measures to promote rest and relaxation.	Fever and infection can stress the body's reserves.

EVALUATION

The client remains afebrile.

in the right renal pelves and results from bacteria ascending from the lower urinary tract. Anaerobic organisms such as *Escherichia coli* are the most frequent causative agents for ascending infection (Duff, 2002).

Select Potential Nursing Diagnoses

The following nursing diagnoses may apply to the client with postpartum UTIs:

- **Impaired Urinary Elimination** related to infection and pain
- **Ineffective Thermoregulation** related to bacterial infection
- **Pain** related to dysuria or CVA tenderness
- **Risk for Deficient Fluid Volume** related to elevated body temperature and decreased oral intake to avoid painful urination

Planning/Implementation

The best treatment is prevention, beginning with teaching self-care practices and encouraging healthy behaviors immediately postpartum. Examples of such practices and behaviors include good perineal hygiene, wiping from meatus to rectum to prevent bacterial contamination, and frequent bladder emptying. NIC/NOC Box 19.3 provides common interventions and outcomes related to a postpartum urinary tract infection.

Once a UTI is diagnosed, medical treatment consists of antimicrobial therapy and analgesia. Choice of

NIC/NOC Box 19.3 Postpartum Urinary Tract Infections

Common NIC Labels

- Fever Treatment
- Fluid Management
- Medication Management
- Infection Prevention
- Pain Management
- Temperature Regulation
- Urinary Elimination Management
- Vital Signs Monitoring

Common NOC Labels

- Comfort Level
- Pain Control
- Thermoregulation
- Urinary Elimination

antibiotic is usually made before urine culture and sensitivity results are available but needs to be adjusted once the culture results identify the causative organism. Initially most antibiotics are administered intravenously but then are switched to an oral form for completion of a 10-day course. Urinary tract analgesics are prescribed to relieve symptoms of dysuria. In addition the woman needs to maintain high fluid intake to provide a "bladder flush."

Clients with pyelonephritis are acutely ill and require bedrest, IV fluids for hydration, parenteral antimicrobial therapy, and a cooling blanket for a high fever. Follow-up diagnostic procedures such as renal ultrasounds or IV pyelograms may be indicated for those with continuing urinary tract problems.

Evaluation

At the completion of treatment, the client should have a follow-up urine culture to evaluate effectiveness. Bacteria counts will be decreased if the treatment was effective. Continuing high counts may indicate a persistent infection. Following treatment of UTI, the nurse should teach self-care practices to prevent future infections:

- Good perineal and bladder hygiene
- Adequate fluid intake, including cranberry juice
- Kegel's exercises

Mastitis

Mastitis is inflammation of the mammary glands caused by milk stasis and bacterial invasion of breast tissue. Common pathogens include normal skin flora and resident flora of the infant's oronasal pharynx such as *S. aureus.* Other common pathogens include group A and B hemolytic streptococci, *Escherichia coli,* and *Bacteroides* species (Barbosa-Cesnik et al., 2003). Cracked nipples provide a portal of entry for the organism; once the bacteria enter the breast tissue milk, stasis provides a medium for proliferation.

Proper self-care and breastfeeding technique prevent mastitis (see Chap. 21). Primary prevention strategies include the following:

- Performing handwashing before breastfeeding
- Breastfeeding frequently to prevent engorgement and milk stasis
- Avoiding constant pressure on the breast tissue, such as tight clothing, poorly fitting bras, or pressure on the nipple or areola to stop milk flow
- Latching the infant to areola and nipple and changing positions to prevent sore and cracked nipples
- If the breast is distended before feeding, applying warm, moist heat to the breast, gently massaging the area, and changing the infant's nursing position to ensure emptying of the breast after each feeding

COLLABORATIVE CARE: MASTITIS

Assessment

Identification of mastitis is based completely on clinical presentation. Onset is usually sudden and may mimic that of influenza. A short history of fever, chills, and complaints of localized warmth, swelling, and tenderness of the breast are common symptoms.

Mastitis usually does not develop until the second to fourth week after birth. On inspection, a painful, hardened, red area is seen on the breast (Fig. 19.8). The axillary glands may be enlarged on the affected side, and the breast may be engorged. Mastitis usually is unilateral; however, if left untreated, it can progress to abscess formation and systemic infection. Blood work reveals leukocytosis, consistent with an infection, but does not provide specific indicators of the source of infection. Cultures of breast milk may be obtained to identify the causative organism but are not of much use in establishing the diagnosis or in guiding treatment decisions.

Select Potential Nursing Diagnoses

The following nursing diagnoses may be appropriate for the client with mastitis:

- **Infective Breastfeeding** related to pain or discomfort, malaise, and fear of transmitting infection to the infant
- **Imbalanced Infant Nutrition** related to interrupted breastfeeding because of maternal illness and discomfort

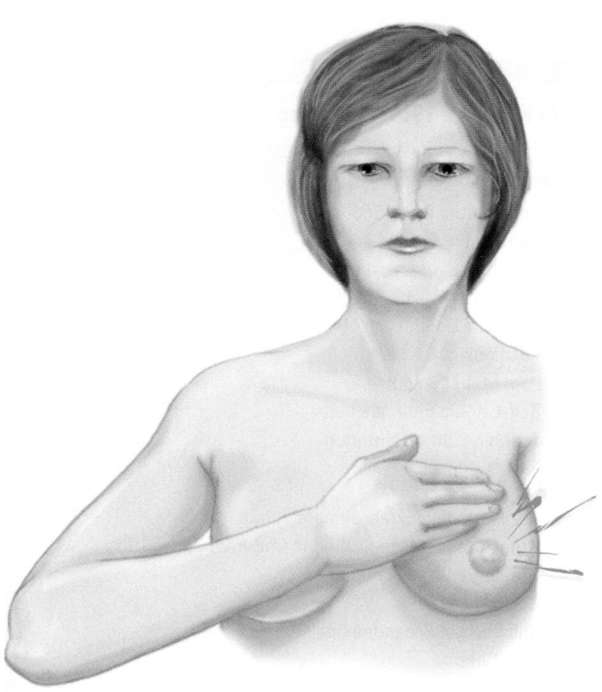

FIGURE 19.8 Mastitis is characterized by a hard, reddened, and painful area on an engorged breast.

- **Disturbed Self-Image** related to self-perceived inability to meet basic infant care needs

Planning/Intervention

Treating the infection, preventing milk stasis (incomplete emptying of the breast), and maintaining nipple integrity are the primary goals. Little evidence-based research has been done on the type or duration of antibiotic treatment because cultures of breast milk are rarely performed. The primary care provider generally prescribes a penicillinase-resistant penicillin or cephalosporin, both of which will cover staphylococci and streptococci (Barbosa-Cesnik et al., 2003). Most antimicrobials used to treat mastitis are safe during breastfeeding. Resolution of the infection is usually evident following 48 hours of treatment with an appropriate antibiotic. NIC/NOC Box 19.4 provides common interventions and outcomes related to mastitis.

To prevent milk stasis, the nurse should encourage continued breastfeeding. Infant suckling at the breast is a more effective means of breast emptying than is use of a breast pump or manual expression. Analgesics, application of intermittent ice packs to the affected breast followed by a warm pack immediately before feeding, and a supportive bra are useful adjuncts in decreasing maternal discomfort.

The nurse should also assess and evaluate the infant for signs and symptoms of bacterial colonization. If the infant is colonized, treatment of the infant is indicated.

The nurse also should educate the woman to avoid practices that place pressure on the breast tissue and may impede milk flow, such as wearing tight clothing or underwire bras, gripping the breast tightly when nursing, using pressure on the breast tissue to move it away from the infant's nose while nursing, sleeping on her stomach, and stopping milk flow by applying pressure to the areola. Finally, clients need to know the importance of good hygiene, complete emptying of the breast, and care of nipples to prevent cracking as measures that can prevent mastitis.

Evaluation

Resolution of the maternal febrile state and elimination of breast pain and inflammation are indicators of effective treatment. In addition, the nurse should evaluate breastfeeding technique, specifically infant positioning, latch-on technique, and sucking behavior (see Chap. 21).

NIC/NOC Box 19.4 Mastitis

Common NIC Labels

- Anticipatory Guidance
- Attachment Promotion
- Breastfeeding Assistance
- Heat/Cold Application
- Lactation Counseling
- Positioning
- Pain Management
- Self-Esteem Enhancement
- Teaching: Infant Nutrition

Common NOC Labels

- Breastfeeding Establishment: Infant
- Breastfeeding Establishment: Maternal
- Breastfeeding Maintenance
- Comfort Level
- Knowledge: Breastfeeding
- Pain Control
- Self-Esteem

THROMBOEMBOLIC COMPLICATIONS

The hypercoagulability associated with pregnancy places the postpartum client at increased risk for thromboembolic disorders. A **thromboembolic disorder** is the formation of a clot or clots inside a blood vessel caused by inflammation or partial obstruction of the vessel (Fig. 19.9). Thromboembolic disorders of concern during the postpartum period include the following:

- **Superficial venous thrombosis:** Inflammation, clot formation, and resulting flow obstruction are confined to the superficial saphenous venous system. This condition also is referred to as *phlebitis* because it is associated with inflammation of the vascular structures.
- **Deep venous thrombosis:** This involves the deep veins of the legs and can extend from the foot to the iliofemoral region. This condition is not associated with inflammation but with obstruction and clot formation.
- **Pulmonary embolism:** A rare complication of deep venous thrombosis, this occurs when a portion of the clot (emboli) breaks free and is carried through the circulatory system until it lodges in the pulmonary artery, where it occludes the vessel and obstructs pulmonary blood flow.

The pathophysiology of thromboembolic disease is based on the presence of Virchow's triad: (1) venous stasis resulting in decreased blood flow; (2) vascular mechanical, chemical, or traumatic injury; and (3) hypercoagulability.

Specific risk factors that increase the incidence of clot formation during the postpartum period include the following:

- Delayed ambulation
- History of venous thrombosis or varicosities
- Obesity
- Maternal age older than 35 years

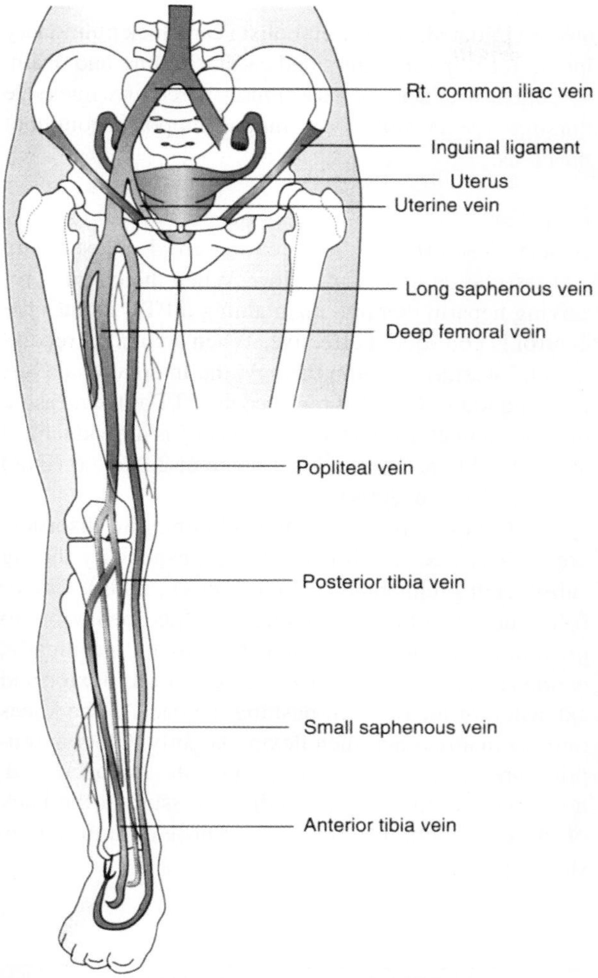

FIGURE 19.9 Common sites of postpartum thrombophlebitis.

- Preexisting cardiopulmonary disease or diabetes
- Route of birth (increased risk with cesarean births)

COLLABORATIVE CARE: THROMBOEMBOLIC COMPLICATIONS

The incidence of thromboembolic complications has decreased with the acceptance of maternal ambulation early in the postpartum period (Floortje et al., 2004). Deep venous thrombosis and pulmonary embolism, however, remain leading sources of maternal mortality and morbidity (Falter, 1997).

Assessment

Phlebitis or superficial venous thrombosis is characterized by unilateral pain and tenderness in the lower extremity. It usually is below the knee and rarely leads to serious complications such as pulmonary embolism. On inspection, the affected area appears reddened and enlarged. Palpation reveals warmth and an enlarged vein over the site of the thrombus. Superficial venous thromboses above the knee need further diagnostic testing to rule out deep venous thrombosis. The hypercoagulable state of pregnancy, combined with traumatic childbirth and extended periods of inactivity, bedrest, and obesity, are risk factors.

Deep venous thrombosis is also characterized by unilateral leg pain, swelling, and warmth. Calf tenderness on ambulation is associated with deep venous thrombosis. Palpation of the extremity reveals unequal leg warmth and unequal size related to vascular congestion in the affected leg. Clinically observable signs may be absent in several clients with deep venous thrombosis.

Assessment of Homans' sign is a procedure used to identify potential thrombophlebitis (see Chap. 18). The feeling of calf pain on flexion of the foot is a positive Homans sign. Although a positive Homans sign requires further evaluation, a negative Homans sign does not rule out deep venous thrombosis. Because of the highly variable presentation of thromboembolic disorders and the inaccuracy of clinical symptoms alone, additional diagnostic testing is needed.

Doppler studies and impedance plethysmography (IPG) are common noninvasive diagnostic tests to confirm deep venous thrombosis. Doppler studies use a combination of ultrasound and Doppler technology to visualize the veins and to detect their compressibility. If the vein is not compressible, thrombosis is likely. Impedance plethysmography measures the rate of emptying of the deep veins in the calf after occlusion of the deep veins in the thigh. A venogram is an invasive technique, involving injections of radiopaque dye into the vein and using x-ray to follow the dye as it travels through the vein.

Signs of pulmonary embolism include dyspnea, tachypnea, sudden chest pain, tachycardia, cardiac dysrhythmia, apprehension, and hemoptysis. Without prompt intervention, death may result from cardiac failure and hypoxia. Laboratory tests include indirect measures such as serial blood gases, blood coagulation studies, electrocardiogram, and chest x-ray, but the definitive diagnostic procedure is a ventilation-perfusion scan of the lung using radioisotopes.

Select Potential Nursing Diagnoses

The following nursing diagnoses may be appropriate for the client with thromboembolic disorders:

- **Pain** related to venous obstruction and altered tissue oxygenation
- **Impaired Tissue Integrity** related to obstructed blood flow and tissue oxygenation
- **Impaired Mobility** related to bedrest

- **Impaired Gas Exchange** related to clot in pulmonary artery
- **Risk for Disuse Syndrome** related to bedrest and activity restriction
- **Risk for Injury** related to the clot dislodging and becoming a pulmonary emboli and bleeding sequela secondary to anticoagulation administration
- **Impaired Parenting** related to activity restriction, pain, and treatment plan

Planning/Intervention

Superficial venous thrombosis is treated conservatively with nonsteroidal anti-inflammatory drugs (eg, ibuprofen) for pain, combined with rest and elevation of the affected extremity to promote venous return. Elastic compression stockings are used to support the venous structures and prevent further stasis. Local application of heat may enhance circulation and comfort and relieve inflammation. A bed cradle prevents pressure from the bed covers on the legs.

When a deep venous thrombosis is diagnosed, anticoagulation therapy is added. Initially, IV heparin therapy is started, usually with a bolus dose followed by a continuous infusion. Heparin administration is adjusted to coagulation studies; specifically, a PTT 2 times the control. The nurse should also monitor the client's platelet count to assess for the development of heparin-induced thrombocytopenia.

After stabilization of her condition and evidence of adequate anticoagulation, the client will be switched to oral warfarin sodium (Coumadin) therapy. She continues on oral therapy for 3 to 6 months. Although warfarin sodium is contraindicated during pregnancy because it crosses the placenta and has potential teratogenic effects, it is safe during the postpartum period. Nevertheless, the drug is secreted in breast milk, and parents must be educated to the potential warning signs requiring pediatric attention (ie, infant bleeding, bruising, or petechiae) (Colman-Brochu, 2004). For these reasons, subcutaneous heparin may be a replacement consideration for use in mothers who wish to continue breastfeeding.

All clients using any type of anticoagulant therapy need monitoring. The nurse should make them aware of signs and symptoms of hemorrhage including epistaxis, blood in urine or stool, ecchymosis, or petechiae. In the immediate postpartum period, the nurse should evaluate the effect of anticoagulant therapy on uterine bleeding. He or she also should caution clients receiving anticoagulation therapy to avoid products containing aspirin, which inhibits the synthesis of clotting factors and can further prolong clotting time and precipitate bleeding.

When a pulmonary embolism is suspected, prompt intervention is needed. Heparin therapy and oxygen therapy are initiated. A large embolism can block pulmonary blood, resulting in right-sided cardiac failure and death. The client with a pulmonary embolism requires intensive nursing care as well as continuous support throughout the crisis.

Evaluation

Indicators of effective intervention are decreased pain and restoration of vascular flow. When the client is receiving heparin therapy, maintaining a PTT 2 times the control is considered effective. When a client is receiving oral warfarin sodium therapy, the International Normalizing Ratio (INR) has replaced the PTT as the measure of anticoagulation effectiveness. Dosing is individualized and titrated to achieve a target range of 2.0 to 3.0 (INR) (Colman-Brochu, 2004).

All clients treated for thromboembolic disorders are at increased risk for recurrence, especially during subsequent pregnancies (Floortje et al., 2004). Therefore, client teaching about exercises and behaviors to prevent future clot formation is important. Specifically, women need to perform leg exercises such as flexion and extension of the feet and pushing the back of the knees into the mattress and then flexing slightly. Other appropriate preventive measures are keeping the legs uncrossed, not flexing at the groin, avoiding pressure at the back of the knees, and wearing support hose or antiembolic stockings.

PERIPARTUM CARDIOMYOPATHY

Peripartum cardiomyopathy (PPCM) is a rare but serious complication (Lampert & Lang, 1995). It may present during the last month of pregnancy until 6 months after birth, but most cases appear in the early postpartum period. Clients with PPCM have a 25% to 50% risk for dying within the first 3 months (Dorbala et al., 2005). The exact etiology is unknown, but its frequent emergence in the immediate postpartum period supports a theory of autoimmune pathogenesis triggered by pregnancy, viral infection, or, in susceptible clients, prolonged use of tocolysis (Goli et al., 2004).

Adaptive changes in the maternal immune system during pregnancy include the reduction of suppressor cells. In the immediate postpartum period, restoration of the nonpregnant maternal immune system results in increased activity of the autoimmune system. Additionally, the hemodynamic stress of pregnancy (increases in cardiac output, intravascular volume, and stroke volume) may contribute to PPCM. Clients with hypertension and specifically pregnancy-induced hypertension have a higher frequency of PPCM (Goli et al., 2004).

COLLABORATIVE CARE: PERIPARTUM CARDIOMYOPATHY

Assessment

Assessment findings are consistent with acute heart failure and hemodynamic compromise. Common presenting symptoms are shortness of breath, orthopnea, and paroxysmal nocturnal dyspnea. Fatigue is also a common but frequently overlooked finding that may be confused with normal discomfort during the postpartum adjustment.

Chest x-rays reveal interstitial and alveolar edema and some cardiomegaly. Electrocardiogram findings are generally nonspecific and include poor R-wave progression, intraventricular conduction delay, and nonspecific ST- and T-wave changes. Laboratory studies reveal little or no elevation of cardiac proteins. Evaluation of liver function tests and renal function tests provides an indication of organ perfusion. The absence of fever and leukocytosis eliminates the diagnosis of myocarditis secondary to sepsis. An echocardiogram is used to evaluate left ventricular function.

Select Potential Nursing Diagnoses

The following nursing diagnoses may be appropriate for the client with PPCM:

- **Decreased Cardiac Output** related to heart failure
- **Ineffective Tissue Perfusion** related to hemodynamic changes

Planning/Intervention

Medical management is similar to that for other forms of heart failure. When PPCM presents in late pregnancy, health care personnel also need to consider the risk that the management protocol poses to the fetus.

Angiotensin-converting enzyme (ACE) inhibitors are the main medical therapy for postpartum clients. ACE inhibitors are contraindicated during pregnancy because of an increased association with fetal loss, especially in late pregnancy, secondary to fetal hypotension resulting from maternal hypotension and decreased uteroplacental perfusion. Oligohydramnios, anuria, and renal tubular dysplasia also have been reported (Qasqas et al., 2004).

Like other forms of heart failure, PPCM can lead to thrombotic and embolic complications. Thus, clients often are started concurrently on anticoagulant therapy; appropriate nursing care and teaching are indicated.

The client's functional status determines her activity level. She should not perform aerobic activities and heavy lifting, however, until her provider evaluates the degree of left ventricular failure recovery. Because of the increased metabolic demands of lactation and the passage into breast milk of many of the pharmacologic agents used to manage PPCM, breastfeeding is discouraged.

Evaluation

There is no "cure" for PPCM. The outcomes and needs for further treatment vary. Some clients remain stable for long periods, some deteriorate gradually, and some deteriorate rapidly and may be candidates for heart transplantation.

If the client's heart returns to normal size within 6 months postpartum, her prognosis is good. In contrast, if the heart remains enlarged, future pregnancy may result in progression of the heart failure (Felker et al., 2000). The risk for mortality is increased when clients with chronic cardiomyopathy become pregnant. It is not known how to predict who will recover and who will develop severe heart failure and need extreme treatment measures.

REPRODUCTIVE ANATOMIC COMPLICATIONS

Anatomic complications usually begin soon after childbirth and have long-term consequences. They include problems such as loss of urine when laughing or sneezing or "dropping" of the bladder, uterus, or rectum. Childbirth or hard manual labor also can lead to prolapse of the uterus, bladder, or rectum.

Pelvic Problems

Pelvic relaxation is a broad term encompassing the stretching, pushing, and straining of the structures supporting the organs of reproduction and elimination. Pelvic relaxation is actually a complex problem because weaknesses can occur in various support structures. The defects are understood based on the area of weakness relative to the vaginal walls. Pregnancy and birth, as well as the anatomic changes that accompany the loss of ovarian hormone function during menopause, make these key times for discovery of pelvic relaxation anomalies (Fig. 19.10).

During pregnancy, elevated progesterone levels facilitate relaxation of the pelvic support structures to prepare the lower reproductive tract for expulsion of the fetus. Although attributes of pregnancy and birth often are associated with these alterations, nulliparous women also can be affected. In fact, preexisting factors (eg, altered hormone levels, obesity, family history) and structural complications (eg, anatomic alterations of the uterus, vagina, bladder, and rectum) are associated with pelvic relaxation (Markinkovic & Stanton, 2004).

During pregnancy, labor, and birth, the female reproductive organs undergo various anatomic and physiologic adaptations, stresses, and traumas. The increased volume and weight of the uterus during pregnancy displaces and stretches the supporting structures and adjacent organs. In the actual processes of labor and birth, these structures are exposed to stretching, pressure, and

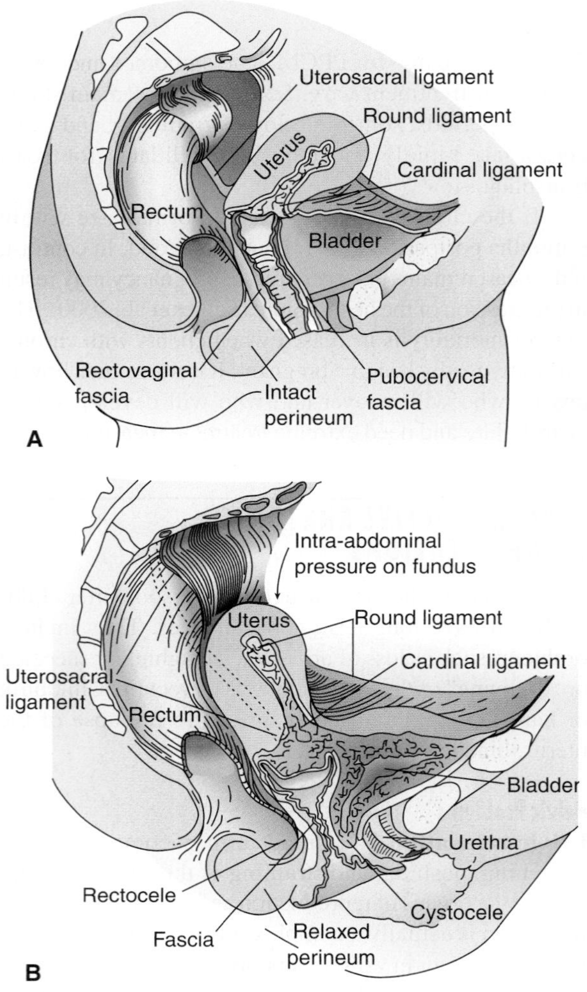

FIGURE 19.10 (**A**) Normal support of the vagina and uterus. (**B**) Problems of relaxation and support in the female reproductive system.

trauma as the fetus descends and clears a pathway to the outside world. Large infants, prolonged labors, and precipitous births can result in excessive stretching of and injury to the vaginal wall. In addition, the descending fetal head can exert downward pressure on the bladder neck and urethra, resulting in soft tissue damage. These alterations, although expected, may lead to anatomic complications during both the immediate postpartum period and later in the client's life. Structural changes related to pregnancy and birth may be present after birth but are often asymptomatic until later, often the perimenopausal years. These conditions alter the position and function of the uterus, bladder, and rectum.

Nursing care of pregnant and postpartum clients needs to include teaching exercises and other strategies that maintain and support the tone and strength of the pelvic support structures during this time of increased abdominal weight and stress.

Uterine Alterations

Pregnancy alters the uterine position to accommodate the growing fetus. The round ligaments attached to the uterine sidewall and the uterosacral ligaments extending from the cervix support the uterus and determine its positions. In the nonpregnant state, the position of the uterus is anteverted, with the cervix pulled posterior and upward. During pregnancy, the uterus becomes retroverted to facilitate its enlarging size, and the cervix moves anteriorly to create a physical barrier between the flora of the posterior vaginal fornix of the female genital tract and to facilitate birth. The enlarging uterine contents cause stretching and tension on the round and uterosacral ligaments. Usually by 2 months postpartum, these ligaments have regained their tone, and the uterus returns to its nonpregnant position.

In a small percentage of women, the uterus remains retroverted following birth; this condition is known as **uterine displacement.** The most common types of uterine displacement are retroversion and anterior displacement (Markinkovic & Stanton, 2004) (Fig. 19.11). The common feature of uterine displacement is anterior positioning of the cervix (Dougherty et al., 2000). Uterine displacement has implications for the woman's future reproductive capacity because the cervix is near the anterior vaginal wall and not the posterior fornix, where seminal fluids pool after coitus (Markinkovic & Stanton, 2004).

Uterine prolapse is a more serious type of uterine displacement and results in the cervix and body of the uterus protruding through the vagina. The degree of prolapse is described as mild, moderate, or severe or as first-degree, second-degree, or third-degree, depending on the amount of the uterine body protruding into the vagina

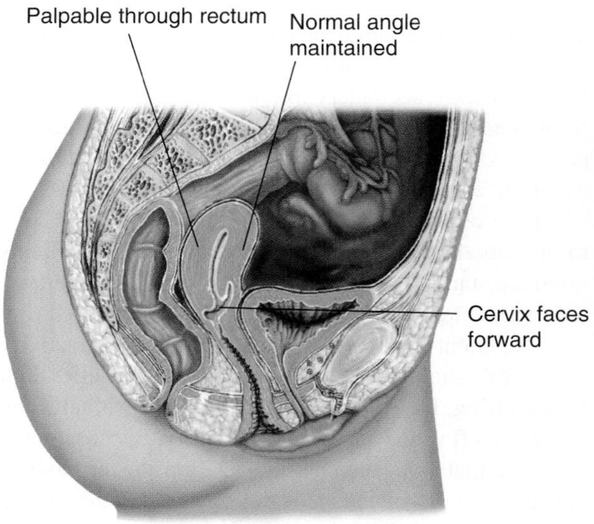

FIGURE 19.11 Uterine retroversion can be a normal anatomic variant or can develop as a complication after childbirth.

(Fig. 19.12). As more of the uterus is descending, the vagina becomes inverted.

COLLABORATIVE CARE: UTERINE DISPLACEMENT OR PROLAPSE

Assessment

Uterine displacement can block the flow of blood, lymph, and nerve impulses through the pelvic structures. This altered circulation manifests in various symptoms, including dysmenorrhea (painful periods), irregular periods, low back pain, infertility, recurrent vaginal infections, urinary incontinence, dyspareunia (painful intercourse), varicose veins, and aching legs.

One of the first signs of uterine displacement is secondary infertility. When the uterus does not return to the nonpregnant position (ie, cervix posterior), conception becomes difficult because the cervix is near the anterior vaginal wall and not in the posterior fornix, where seminal fluids accumulate.

Uterine prolapse is seen more often during perimenopause as the effects of ovarian hormones on the tissue decrease, resulting in decreased tone of pelvic supports and atrophic tissue changes. The most common complaints are a sensation of fullness or protrusion into the vagina, as well as low back pain and fatigue. Prolonged periods of standing and deep penetration during intercourse aggravate symptoms.

On physical examination, the protruding mass is palpable and visible in the vaginal vault (Fig. 19.13). Vaginal discharge is often present, and the upper vagina appears beefy red during visualization on speculum examination.

Select Potential Nursing Diagnoses

The following nursing diagnoses may apply to the client with postpartum uterine alterations:

- **Disturbed Self-Esteem** related to change in reproductive organs and sexual function
- **Activity Intolerance** related to leg pain and discomfort
- **Sexual Dysfunction** related to anatomic changes in vaginal area and sensations during coitus

Planning/Intervention

Although extensive damage to the supporting structures may be identified and repaired immediately after birth, most symptoms of uterine relaxation do not appear until perimenopause. At this time, loss of ovarian hormone function leads to additional relaxation and atrophy of pelvic tissue, leading to symptoms of pelvic relaxation. Preventative nursing care includes teaching the client to perform pelvic-strengthening exercises, such as Kegel's exercises, throughout the childbearing years (see Chap. 23).

Evaluation

Evaluation of effectiveness is based on the client's presenting symptoms and situation. Measures of effectiveness include elimination of symptoms through successful repositioning of the prolapsed organ. In premenopausal clients attempting additional childbearing, fertility interventions such as artificial insemination may be useful therapies to assist in conception (see Chap. 10).

Cystocele and Rectocele

A coexisting finding with uterine prolapse may be a cystocele or rectocele (see Chap. 4) (Fig. 19.14). A **cystocele** occurs when the wall between the bladder and vagina weakens and the bladder drops into the vagina. A **rectocele** is a weakening between the front wall of the rectum and vagina, resulting in the rectum ballooning into the vagina during defecation. The underlying cause

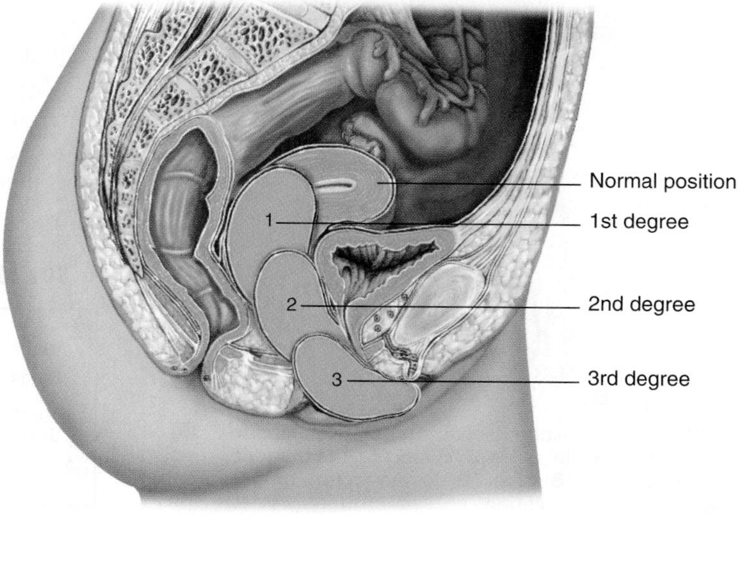

FIGURE 19.12 Uterine prolapse. In first-degree or mild prolapse, the cervix remains in the vagina. In second-degree or moderate prolapse, the cervix is at the vaginal introitus. In third-degree or severe prolapse, the cervix and vagina bulge out of the uterus entirely.

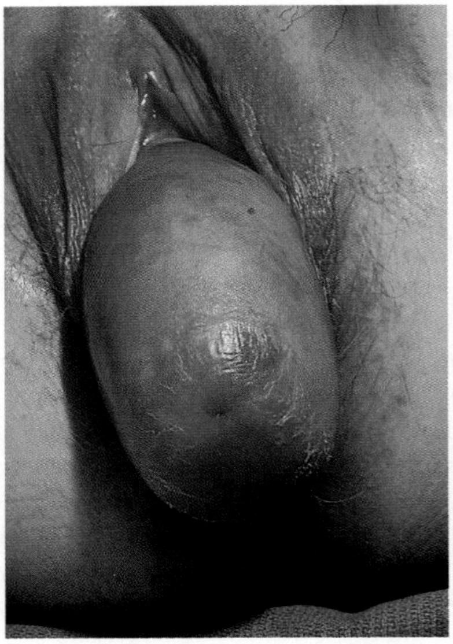

FIGURE 19.13 Physical appearance of a uterine prolapse.

of both cystocele and rectocele is weakening of the pelvic supports. Contributing factors include birth trauma, prolonged second stage, instrument-assisted births (forceps or vacuum extractions), and lacerations or episiotomies that extend into the rectum or anal sphincter. Related factors not specific to pregnancy include heavy lifting, obesity, repeated straining during bowel movements, low estrogen levels, and congenital vaginal wall weakness.

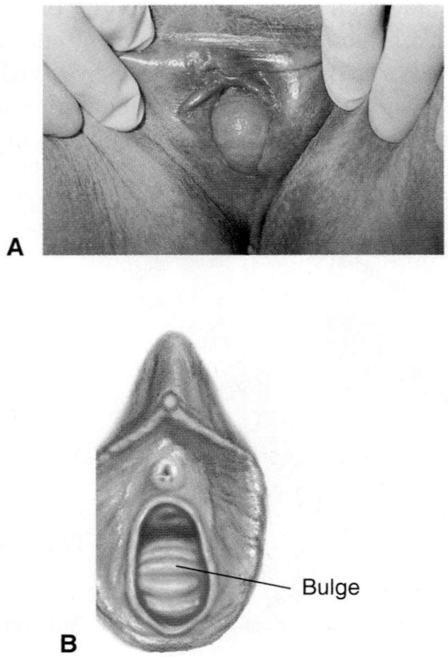

FIGURE 19.14 Weakened pelvic supports can lead to cystocele and rectocele. (**A**) With cystocele, the bladder drops into the vagina. (**B**) In rectocele, the rectum bulges into the vagina during defecation.

COLLABORATIVE CARE: CYSTOCELE AND RECTOCELE

Assessment

The client with a cystocele frequently complains of discomfort and problems emptying the bladder. Bulging of the bladder into the vagina results in a feeling of fullness or a bearing-down sensation. Urinary symptoms include frequency and retention, resulting in numerous and recurrent UTIs. If there is damage to the bladder neck, the client may experience incontinence. The loss of support of the bladder neck (where the bladder and urethra meet) is the most common cause of female urinary incontinence. With increased abdominal pressure, such as during lifting, coughing, sneezing, or even just laughing, the natural mechanism for holding urine is lost, so the urine leaks. On pelvic examination, palpation of the anterior vaginal wall reveals a bulge when the client is asked to bear down. A cystocele is graded on a scale of 1 to 3 based on severity of the protrusion into the vagina (Box 19.5). If a cystocele is suspected, a voiding cystourethrogram may be ordered to show the shape of the bladder and any obstructions to urinary flow.

Rectoceles are often asymptomatic. If present, vaginal symptoms are similar to those of uterine or bladder prolapse: fullness and pain on intercourse. Rectal symptoms include bleeding, constipation, and difficult evacuation with straining. Usually symptoms are associated with a large rectocele, which is uncommon in the immediate postpartum period. The exception is clients who experience a fourth-degree laceration or extension of the episiotomy; they have high potential for a weakened area at the suture line.

Select Potential Nursing Diagnoses

The following nursing diagnoses may apply to the woman with a cystocele or rectocele:

- **Impaired Urinary or Bowel Elimination** related to anatomic position of bladder or rectum
- **Risk for Infection** related to incomplete emptying of body's waste products providing a reservoir of bacterial proliferation.
- **Social Isolation** related to changes in anatomy and elimination functions

BOX 19.5 Subjective Grading of Cystoceles

Grade 1: Mild—bladder creates bulging into the vagina
Grade 2: Severe—bladder has reached the opening of the vagina
Grade 3: Advanced—bladder bulges out through the opening of the vagina

- **Disturbed Self-Esteem** related to loss of control of basic elimination functions
- **Anxiety** related to fear of loss of control bodily fluids in public (ie, stress or urge incontinence)

Planning/Intervention

For a cystocele, treatment ranges from none to surgery. In the immediate postpartum period, clients may experience mild vaginal wall relaxation. The nurse should instruct these clients in the use of levator muscle exercises (Kegel's exercises) to restore pelvic floor muscle tone. He or she should also instruct clients to avoid heavy lifting or straining, which could aggravate the loss of support.

Asymptomatic rectoceles are treated supportively. Activities to avoid constipation, such as a high-fiber diet and plenty of fluids, are the basics of any treatment plan. Fiber keeps the stool moist as it moves along the colon, resulting in stools that are larger, softer, and easier to pass. The nurse should instruct clients with rectocele to avoid prolonged straining during defecation to minimize additional strain and protrusion. Clients at high risk for development of a rectocele, based on contributing factors during birth or a fourth-degree episiotomy or laceration, also benefit from teaching about diet and avoiding straining during the postpartum period when the body is healing and restoring tone.

Evaluation

Evaluation focuses on the degree of anatomic alteration and the prescribed treatment. Priority nursing concerns focus on control of elimination functions, comfort, and strategies to enhance the client's sense of well-being and participation in activities of daily living.

PSYCHOLOGICAL COMPLICATIONS

Because the postpartum client is at increased risk for various psychological disorders, nurses in health care settings need to be familiar with their prevalence and onset, especially in the time surrounding childbirth. Women in their childbearing years constitute the highest population at risk for depressive disorders (Altshuler et al., 2001) (see Chap. 5).

The birth of a child is not always a happy event for every new mother. The postpartum client with depressive feelings may be filled with loneliness. She lacks emotions and cannot take interest in things she previously enjoyed (Beck, 1992; Beck & Indman, 2005). This experience is in contrast to the societal images of the happy mother and infant and growing family unit.

All clients need to understand that following childbirth, they are likely to experience physiologic and psychological changes that will affect daily life (George, 2005) (see Chap. 18). Normal but at times bothersome experiences during the postpartum period include the following:

- Fatigue as a result of getting up repeatedly in the middle of the night to tend to the infant
- Breast discomfort or leakage as a result of lactation and breastfeeding
- Pain and discomfort related to episiotomy, hemorrhoids, or other birth-related entities
- Uncertain time of the return of menses
- Pressure to be a good mother and wife or partner and to meet everyone's expectations

New mothers have been known to say, "Nobody told me it would be like this" and "I didn't realize it was going to be every minute of the day and night." In addition to the above physical alterations, many clients report experiencing tension, anxiety, mood variations, and negative thinking (Clemmens et al., 2004).

Because of the numerous and dramatic individual and family changes during this period, nurses must be aware of the common postpartum psychological conditions that signify a problem beyond the normal adjustment period. Several screening tools are available for psychological alterations during the postbirth period. Nurses need to use these tools in the practice setting to identify clients with indicators of evolving conditions (Assessment Tool 19.1). The Edinburgh Postnatal Depression Scale (EPDS) is an example of a tool widely available to practitioners as well as the public (Assessment Tool 19.2). This simple 10-item questionnaire can assist in identifying mothers suffering from postpartum depression. The authors are clear in stating that clinical evaluation must be carried out to confirm a diagnosis and initiate intervention.

Tragic events portrayed in the international media have drawn much needed attention to postpartum psychological conditions that have been inadequately addressed in the past (Spinelli, 2004). Events of mothers committing suicide, homicide, or both related to postpartum psychological problems have heightened the awareness of the public and the health care industry. Many insurers offer postpartum telephone screening for their members, member health newsletters address the warning signs for new parents, and continuing medical and nursing educational offerings attempt to provide current assessment and therapeutic intervention strategies for professionals.

As these clients recover and regain energy, they often begin to recognize that their relationship with the newborn, other children, or both may have suffered as a result of the illness. Studies have noted that children of women diagnosed with postpartum psychiatric conditions have a higher incidence of interaction difficulties with their mothers (Clemmens et al., 2004). Postpartum psychiatric conditions are total family illnesses; the condition and the

● ASSESSMENT TOOL 19.1 Postpartum Depression Screening Tools

Tool	Purpose	Format	Scoring	Interpretation	Critique
Beck Depression Inventory (BDI)	To measure behavioral manifestations of postpartum depression	21 multiple-choice items, each with four options	Item scoring: 0 = neutral score 3 = maximum score Tool Score: range, 0–63	Score of 10 or higher indicate postpartum depression	Acceptable reliability and validity Widely used in the depression literature Poor sensitivity A generalized depression scale that doesn't address all the specifics of postpartum depression
Edinburgh Postnatal Depression Scale (EPDS)	To detect postpartum depression through self-report. The scale will not detect mothers with anxiety neuroses, phobias, or personality disorder.	10 short statements regarding common depressive symptoms with four replies matched to the statement	Each statement is scored on a scale of 0 to 3. Total possible score ranges from 0 to 30.	Scores above a threshold of 12/13 indicate the woman is suffering a depressive illness of varying severity.	Simple to complete Acceptable to women who do not consider themselves unwell Does not provide mothers with an opportunity to fully describe their symptoms Obstacles to use include limited literacy and writing skills
Postpartum Depression Checklist (PDC)	A checklist of symptoms arranged in order of severity and used to make a diagnosis of postpartum depression.	11 symptoms of postpartum depression arranged in a checklist format	No score is calculated. Positive responses indicate the need for further assessment and possible referral.	Women contemplating harming herself or others need immediate referral to a psychiatric facility.	Mothers may give "socially acceptable answers" to conform with societal expectations.

resulting changes in family dynamics affect everyone in the family. Therefore, the entire family also needs support.

The most common psychiatric conditions specific to the postbirth period are postpartum blues, postpartum depression, postpartum panic disorders, and postpartum psychosis.

Postpartum Blues

Postpartum blues is the term used for a self-limited, transitory mood disorder that usually resolves by the end of the second or third postpartum week. Postpartum blues can occur anytime between the 3rd and 10th day after birth. Approximately 30% to 75% of new mothers experience postpartum blues, but the degree and severity are highly variable (Seyfried & Marcus, 2003). Several causes of postpartum blues, including biochemical, psychological, social, and cultural factors, have been investigated, but none has been identified as the etiology. Some new mothers experience a loss of support from family and friends as the focus of attention and concern

● ASSESSMENT TOOL 19.2 Edinburgh Postnatal Depression Scale (EPDS)

INSTRUCTIONS FOR USERS

1. The mother is asked to underline the response that comes closest to how she has been feeling in the previous 7 days.
2. All 10 items must be completed.
3. Care should be taken to avoid the possibility of the mother discussing her answers with others.
4. The mother should complete the scale herself, unless she has limited English or has difficulty with reading.
5. The EPDS may be used at 6–8 weeks to screen postnatal women. The child health clinic, postnatal checkup, or a home visit may provide suitable opportunities for its completion.

Name: ____________________

Address: ____________________

Baby's Age: ____________________

As you have recently had a baby, we would like to know how you are feeling. Please UNDERLINE the answer that comes closest to how you have felt IN THE PAST 7 DAYS, not just how you feel today.

1. I have been able to laugh and see the funny side of things.
As much as I always could
Not quite so much now
Definitely not so much now
Not at all

2. I have looked forward with enjoyment to things.
As much as I ever did
Rather less than I used to
Definitely less than I used to
Hardly at all

3. *I have blamed myself unnecessarily when things went wrong.
Yes, most of the time
Yes, some of the time
Not very often
No, never

4. I have been anxious or worried for no good reason.
No, not at all
Hardly ever
Yes, sometimes
Yes, very often

5. *I have felt scared or panicky for no very good reason.
Yes, quite a lot
Yes, sometimes
No, not much
No, not at all

6. *Things have been getting on top of me.
Yes, most of the time I haven't been able to cope at all
Yes, sometimes I haven't been coping as well as usual
No, most of the time I have coped quite well
No, I have been coping as well as ever

7. *I have been so unhappy that I have had difficulty sleeping.
Yes, most of the time
Yes, sometimes
Not very often
No, not at all

8. *I have felt sad or miserable.
Yes, most of the time
Yes, quite often
Not very often
No, not at all

9. *I have been so unhappy that I have been crying.
Yes, most of the time
Yes, quite often
Only occasionally
No, never

10. *The thought of harming myself has occurred to me.
Yes, quite often
Sometimes
Hardly ever
Never

Response categories are scored 0, 1, 2, and 3 according to increased severity of the symptoms. Items marked with an asterisk are reverse scored (ie, 3, 2, 1, and 0). The total score is calculated by adding together the scores for each of the ten items.

Source: Cox, J. L., Holden, J. M., & Sagovsky, R. (1987). *British Journal of Psychiatry, 150.*

Users may reproduce the scale without further permission providing they respect copyright by quoting the names of the authors, the title, and the source of the paper in all reproduced copies.

shift from the previously pregnant woman to the newborn. Others mourn the special relationship lost between the pregnant woman and her unborn child, whereas still others experience a feeling of being let down when the excitement of labor and birth are over. Although the exact etiology is unknown, research has shown a decreased incidence of postpartum blues in cultures that encourage open expression of emotions and that surround the postpartum woman with supportive and loving care (Dennis & Creedy, 2004).

Nevertheless, some cultures have a societal norm that *all* new mothers are happy and welcome and celebrate the birth of a child. When a woman does not experience overwhelming feelings of joy, she feels depressed and guilty, assuming "something is wrong with her." Husbands, partners, family, and friends expect her to be happy; combined with their own joy about the new baby, they may not recognize the mother's sadness and progressively unusual behaviors. The client's thoughts of not being a "good mother" undermine her confidence because she feels unable to meet the generally accepted expectations of her family. Being sad and asking for help caring for herself are inconsistent with the norms and expectations for a new family. Nurses can help eliminate these barriers by asking new mothers, "How are you feeling?" and providing a safe and trusting environment for women to seek help and counseling.

"I just can't help it . . . he is so beautiful and I should be so happy but I just start to cry over the littlest things . . ."

A woman 5 days postpartum holding her newborn son and sobbing uncontrollably

COLLABORATIVE CARE: POSTPARTUM BLUES

Assessment

Emotional swings, crying easily and often for no reason, and feelings of restlessness, fatigue, difficulty sleeping, headache, anxiety, loss of appetite, decreased ability to concentrate, irritability, sadness, and anger are common findings. These clients are physically healthy, and the onset of the blues is believed to be unrelated to their own or their babies' health or well-being (Clemmens et al., 2004).

Perinatal nurses can initiate conversations that encourage the new mother to openly discuss her feelings. A therapeutic communication approach from the nurse might be, "Many women have shared with me that they have a difficult time with emotions during the postpartum period. Are you having any difficulties, problems, or feelings that you would like to talk about?" (Clemmens et al., 2004). With this simple question, the nurse not only attempts to assess the woman's emotional state but also provides her with information that not all new mothers are happy all the time. It validates her emotions as real and starts to build a relationship that allows her the freedom to share these emotions without fear or shame.

Select Potential Nursing Diagnoses

The following nursing diagnoses may apply to the woman with postpartum blues:

- **Anxiety** related to new role expectations and responsibilities
- **Ineffective Coping** related to fatigue, physical discomforts, and demands of caring for infant
- **Disturbed Sleep Pattern** related to physiologic changes of the immediate post-birth period and demands of caring for a newborn

Planning/Intervention

Primary interventions related to postpartum blues are teaching anticipatory guidance, providing opportunities for the client to share and express her emotions about her birth experience, and identifying and activating support systems. One of the most important postbirth educational strategies is to provide the client and family with information about the signs and symptoms of postpartum blues. The nurse should emphasize that postpartum blues are common and help the family to recognize the importance of encouragement and support for the new mother. Having family members, friends, support people, or doula do the laundry, fix meals, and perform other household tasks so the new mother can rest and care for the infant may help decrease the client's fatigue and the severity of the blues.

Evaluation

Most cases of postpartum blues resolve spontaneously. Having support and assistance with household responsibilities will assist the client to make a successful transition. Indicators of resolution of the "blues" are increased energy and feeling more in control of the situation and her role as mother.

Postpartum Depression

Postpartum depression (PPD) is more serious and persistent than postpartum blues. Unlike the limited nature of postpartum blues, PPD may last for weeks or months. It usually begins in the fourth week postpartum and evolves slowly over several weeks (Apgar et al., 2005). The complete presentation of PPD can develop any time in the first year after childbirth. Although PPD is considered underreported, 10% to 15% of women suffer from it worldwide (Hanna et al., 2004); a meta-analysis of published research reports a prevalence of 13% (Dennis & Creedy, 2004). The exact etiology remains unclear, but it appears to be a multifactorial disorder with a higher incidence observed in clients with a past history of psychiatric disorders, interpersonal difficulties, lingering postpartum blues, or life-event problems (Bloch et al., 2006; Dennis & Creedy, 2004). Other factors linked to PPD include the following:

- Prenatal anxiety or depression
- Child care stress
- Stressful life events
- Unstable relationships with husband or partner, parents, or both (marital conflicts)
- Lack of social support. This factor is of importance because women lacking sufficient social support have been twice as likely to suffer from PPD (Dennis & Creedy, 2004).

Clients who have suffered from PPD have described the state as a downward spiral and an emotionally painful experience for themselves and their families (Edhborg et al., 2005). For them, feeling depressed at a time when family and friends anticipate happiness further intensifies anxiety and a sense of lost support. Societal norms that the birth of a new family member is a joyous event may lead to the client's reluctance to discuss her symptoms or feelings toward the infant. Sometimes, the infant is the source of the client's depressive feelings. She may feel jealous that the infant has displaced her in her partner's affections or that all the attention is now focused on the child. She also may feel resentful that the baby has "taken away" her former life. Clients rarely share these feelings because of embarrassment or fear of negative reactions from family, friends, and health care professionals.

COLLABORATIVE CARE: POSTPARTUM DEPRESSION

Assessment

Clients who continue to show signs and symptoms of postpartum blues beyond 7 to 10 days after giving birth have a higher incidence of developing PPD (Clemmens et al., 2004). Those experiencing PPD feel their lives are rapidly tumbling out of control: feelings of guilt and inadequacy intensify their sense of being an incompetent parent (Edhborg et al., 2005). The nurse should assess clients for the following signs of PPD:

- Inability to sleep or rest
- Crying that is uncontrollable and unprovoked
- Change in appetite, especially a craving for sweets
- Decreased energy and fatigue
- Feelings of worthlessness and a negative outlook on the future
- Sense of isolation
- Lack of concern for personal appearance
- Feelings of uncontrollable anxiety, irritability, and loss of control; obsessive thoughts of being a failure
- Hostility or anger directed toward others
- Problems with maternal–infant interaction, perception of the infant as difficult, and feeling guilty about not being able to care for the baby
- Feeling of being an inadequate mother and of being trapped

There is no perfect time to assess the woman for signs of PPD (Apgar et al., 2005). Assessment needs to be continuous, beginning during pregnancy and continuing throughout the infant's first year of life (Garg et al., 2005; Ryan et al., 2005). During pregnancy, the nurse should perform a comprehensive health history focused on family and personal history of psychiatric or depressive disorders. If the client has given birth previously, exploring her psychological adaptation after pregnancy can reveal important clues. The nurse should document risk factors or altered perceptions related to the pregnancy and communicate findings to care providers during the postbirth period.

During the birth and immediate postpartum period, assessment and evaluation of mother–baby attachment behaviors (including how she holds, talks to, and interacts with the baby and how she describes the infant to others), the interactions between the parents or mother and other family members, availability of support systems, and identification of community resources are all important. The nurse should reevaluate these assessment parameters throughout follow-up visits during the traditional 6-week postpartum period (Apgar et al., 2005; Garg et al., 2005).

Initial symptoms of PPD may be subtle. Health care providers, especially in pediatric health care settings where clients bring their infants for ongoing care, must be attuned to assessing women for signs of PPD and identify subtle pleas for help (Fig. 19.15). Maternal nursing assessment through the first year after childbirth needs to include asking clients, "How are you feeling?" and providing a safe and trusting environment for them to seek help and counseling.

Select Potential Nursing Diagnoses

The following nursing diagnoses may apply to the woman with PPD:

- **Impaired Parenting** related to negative feelings about the infant and mothering role

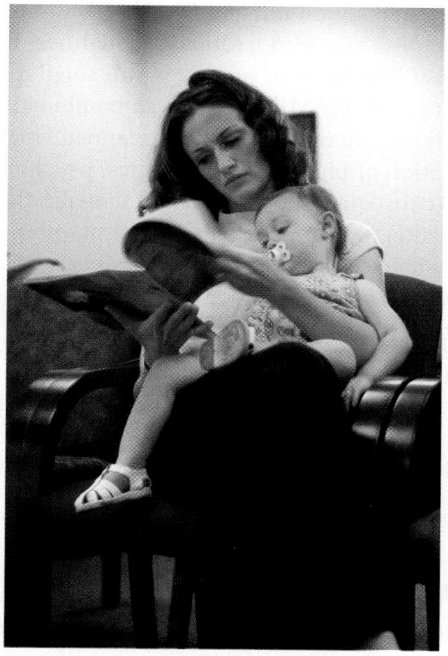

FIGURE 19.15 All health care providers, including nurses working in general practice, family health, and pediatric settings, should remember to ask about signs and symptoms of postpartum depression in mothers throughout the child's first year of life.

- **Anxiety** related to overwhelming demands of motherhood and meeting newborn's needs
- **Self-Care Deficit** related to changes in nutrition, sleep, hygiene, and other activities of daily living secondary to depression
- **Risk for Injury:** Harm to self, infant, or both

Planning/Intervention

Early referrals for clients with a history or evidence of depression are essential. Nevertheless, the client with PPD may lack the energy to follow through on information that the nurse provides. Therefore, simply giving the client the name or phone number of a support group or provider is not enough. A critical component of nursing intervention is actually getting her to the support group or involved with the appropriate mental health professional. Assisting the client to make contact and conscious follow-up to be certain she keeps appointments and attends support sessions is within the scope of the nurse's responsibility.

Complementary/Alternative Medicine Modalities

Complementary/alternative medicine (CAM) has been growing in popularity in the United States during the past several decades. Clients may pursue various CAM treatments for PPD (Complementary/Alternative Medicine 19.1). The client needs to discuss the use of all CAM modalities, particularly if she is breastfeeding her newborn.

For clients with mild PPD, CAM is simply complementary to standard treatment modalities, not a replacement. The body of science is still small regarding the efficacy of CAM when used in combination with conventional therapy. Standard treatment includes a combination of pharmacotherapeutics, psychotherapy, and psychosocial (support groups) modalities. Before the initiation of pharmacologic treatment, other physiologic parameters such as thyroid dysfunction must be ruled out (McCoy et al., 2003).

Pharmacotherapeutics

Tricyclics and selective serotonin reuptake inhibitors are effective for treatment of PPD. For the breastfeeding mother, these drugs are considered safe (based on limited scientific studies) because little of the medication passes into the breast milk (Weier & Beal, 2004). Providers need to balance the risk for drug ingestion through breast milk with the benefits of the maternal–infant attachment gained through the closeness of continued breastfeeding. Perhaps for this reason, lactating mothers may turn to CAM as part of their treatment routine. If medication is the treatment of choice, the client must continue it for at least 6 months, even if depressive symptoms improve.

Psychotherapy

Individual counseling and group therapy are successful interventions. Recognizing that the client's feelings are real and identifying coping strategies are the focus of these sessions. The client must identify and verbalize her fears and concerns regarding her mothering role and responsibilities. She also needs to be asked about suicidal or homicidal thoughts during each session. In addition, if the couple is having marital difficulties, marriage counseling also may be indicated.

Support Groups

Support groups provide the client with an outlet for learning that she is not the only one having difficulty during the postbirth period. They help her find ways to cope within her family and situation. Additionally, they provide many clients with an opportunity to interact with other women as a means to decrease social isolation.

Evaluation

Some clients require hospitalization to protect them from harm, whereas others are treated in the community setting. Evaluation is a long-term and ongoing process. The client with PPD needs continuous support and care. Signs of effective interventions include decreased depressive symptoms and increased coping abilities concurrent with resumptions of mothering role and activities of daily living.

Postpartum Panic Disorder

Sudden terror and a sense of impending doom are characteristic of postpartum panic disorders. These disorders involve full-blown panic attacks during the postpartum period. The onset of panic disorder may be related to the changing PCO_2 level during the period after childbirth. During pregnancy, elevated progesterone levels lead to

● COMPLEMENTARY/ALTERNATIVE MEDICINE 19.1

Common CAM Modalities for Postpartum Depression

- Traditional Chinese medicine
- Omega-3 dietary supplements
- Massage
- Aromatherapy
- Acupuncture

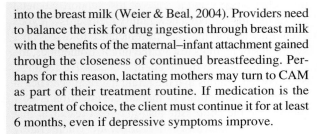

greater minute ventilation volume and lower maternal PCO_2 levels to facilitate diffusion across the placenta and elimination of fetal waste products. In the postbirth period, progesterone levels decline and PCO_2 levels increase, possibly predisposing women to panic attacks (Altshuler et al., 2001). Physical symptoms accompanying the sense of terror include shortness of breath, dizziness, nausea, palpitations, and chest pain. Panic disorder is defined as panic attacks followed by at least 1 month of worry about another or its implications (American Psychiatric Association [APA], 2000).

Anxiety is a common symptom in postpartum disorders and often is a foreboding sign of the advent of postpartum panic disorders (Matthey et al., 2003). Typical signs and symptoms that women with panic disorders exhibit include the following:

- Extreme anxiety
- Heart palpitations
- Chest pain and sensation of choking or suffocation
- Hot or cold flashes, trembling
- Restlessness, agitation, irritability
- Fear of losing control or going crazy
- Sudden awakening from sleep
- Excessive or obsessive worry or fears

Panic attacks often have no identifiable trigger; the onset is sudden and unanticipated.

Treatment of panic disorders includes a combination of cognitive and behavioral therapies. Medications are also appropriate in some cases. The most important aspect is supporting the client in seeking and following through with treatment. Initially treatment is helping her to understand what a panic disorder is and that having one does not mean she is going crazy. Cognitive therapy can assist the client to identify possible triggers for attacks and to understand that the attack is separate from the trigger event. Cognitive restructuring or changing ways of thinking assists the client to replace panic-inducing thoughts with more realistic and positive ones (APA, 2003). Relaxation techniques can help some clients manage an attack. Useful relaxation techniques include patterned or paced breathing and positive visualization.

Medications such as antidepressants and antianxiety agents are prescribed in some cases. If medication is the treatment of choice, the nurse should learn the implications of the chosen medication on lactation if the client is breastfeeding. Finally, these clients need referral to a support group as an adjunct to the previously described therapies.

Commitment and follow-through are essential to success. The client will not experience a change in attacks after only one or two sessions. After extended treatment programs of usually 6 to 9 months, however, many clients experience significant improvement in the frequency and intensity of the attacks (American Academy of Family Physicians, 2000).

Postpartum Psychosis

Postpartum psychosis is a severe condition occurring in less than 2% of postpartum clients (Dennis & Creedy, 2004; Seyfried & Marcus, 2003). The clinical picture resembles PPD with the additional symptoms of delusional thought processes and thoughts of harming self, infant, or both. Postpartum psychosis is of great concern because the mother's behavior presents a real and significant threat to the safety of her infant, herself, and others.

Symptoms of postpartum psychosis often begin to manifest during the third trimester of pregnancy. Women with a history of postpartum psychosis have a 35% to 60% recurrence rate in subsequent pregnancies (APA, 2000).

Psychosis arising for the first time in pregnancy is uncommon (Winans, 2001). Psychosis is a condition occurring in the context of an underlying psychiatric disorder like bipolar affective disorder, schizophrenia, or major depression. For some clients, postpartum psychosis is the only psychotic episode they will experience. For others, postpartum psychosis may be the first episode of a psychiatric disorder or an acute exacerbation of an underlying disorder.

During a psychotic episode, the client losses touch with reality. She may experience the following:

- Hallucinations (eg, hear voices when nobody is around)
- Delusions, or ideas she believes despite all proof that they are false (eg, that someone is trying to harm her, or that her baby is the devil)
- Disordered thoughts or illogical or chaotic thought processes

Psychosis is a very frightening condition and needs immediate treatment. Postpartum psychosis occurs usually within 2 to 4 weeks after childbirth.

COLLABORATIVE CARE: POSTPARTUM PSYCHOSIS

Assessment

Signs and symptoms of postpartum psychosis may develop at any time from immediately after birth to 3 months later, but the average onset is 2 to 4 weeks postpartum (Winans, 2001). They include the following:

- Disturbed sleep
- Emotional lability
- Confusion and disorientation
- Disorganized thoughts and behavior
- Hallucinations (hearing voices when there is no one there)
- Delusions (thinking that people are trying to harm her or that she has special powers)
- Withdrawal

The client often complains of being unable to stand, move, or work. As the condition progresses, she exhibits suspicious and incoherent behavior, confusion, irrational statements, and obsessive concerns about the baby's health and welfare. Delusions, often specific to the infant, are present in approximately 50% of cases (Winans, 2001). Clients suffering from postpartum psychosis often relate having auditory hallucinations in which they hear that the infant is possessed by evil or doomed to a terrible fate.

Select Potential Nursing Diagnoses

The following nursing diagnoses may apply to the client with postpartum psychosis:

- **Disturbed Thought Processes** related to perception of hallucinations and delusional thoughts
- **Risk for Violence** related to delusional thinking

Planning/Intervention

Postpartum psychosis is a medical emergency and requires immediate hospitalization and treatment. These clients need to be hospitalized for their own safety and to prevent potential harm to the infant. Because of confusion, the client may not have the insight to recognize how ill she is and the need for treatment. Treatment options for women with postpartum psychosis include the following:

- Biologic approach: rule out medical conditions that may present as psychosis (eg, infection, seizure disorder, electrolyte disturbance); include the use of antipsychotic and mood-stabilizing medications
- Psychological approach: interpersonal therapy, supportive psychotherapy (individual or group), couple counseling
- Social approach: psychoeducation and support involving the significant other, friends, and family; teaching the client how to build social networks and supports; creating a supportive living environment

Evaluation

Following treatment, most clients can return to their daily activities but may fluctuate between remissions and exacerbations. Like any other person, the client will have good days and not-so-good days. The problem is an inability to cope with not-so-good days. The presence of an ongoing support network is invaluable.

Questions to Ponder

1. A client comes to the health care facility for her 6-week postpartum checkup. She looks sad, tired, and pale. The nurse asks the client how her mood is and how well she has been coping with the changes having a newborn brings. The client shrugs and says she's doing "as well as could be expected." When the nurse tries to gather more information, the client's responses are similarly unrevealing.
   - What other methods could the nurse employ to gather more information?
   - If the nurse can determine evidence of a postpartum mood disorder, what methods might prove effective in working with this client?
   - What things might be happening other than PPD?

SUMMARY

- Postpartum maternal complications can develop in any pregnancy from conditions that existed before or during pregnancy, during labor, or during or after birth.
- Risk factors for postpartum complications include infections, history of preterm labor or preterm rupture of membranes, abnormal placental implantation, prolonged labor, assisted labor, chronic conditions or preexisting disease states, poor nutritional status, substance abuse, and inadequate prenatal care.
- Postpartum hemorrhage means loss greater than 500 mL during or after the third stage of labor. It can develop early (within the first 24 hours of birth) or late (24 hours or more after birth).
- Causes of early hemorrhage include uterine atony, lacerations of the genital tract, hematomas, and uterine inversion. The goals of care in all cases are to identify the underlying cause of and to stop the bleeding.
- Late postpartum hemorrhage usually is associated with infection or retained placental fragments, both of which lead to uterine subinvolution. The client will need care for this problem in a health care facility to manage the bleeding, eliminate the cause, and cure any infection.
- Puerperal infections involve a temperature of 100.4°F (38.0°C) or higher on any 2 of the first 10 days following birth exclusive of the first 24 hours. They can occur in the uterus and surrounding tissues (endometritis), the broad ligament of the uterus (parametritis), peritoneum or abdominal cavity (peritonitis), wounds of the perineum or abdomen, urinary tract, or breasts (mastitis).
- Pregnancy-related hypercoagulability increases the client's risk for thromboembolic disorders.
- A rare but serious postpartum complication is peripartum cardiomyopathy (PPCM), which has no cure.
- Reproductive anatomic complications can have long-term consequences. Pelvic relaxation, uterine displacement, uterine prolapse, cystocele, and rectocele can interfere with a woman's urinary elimination, enjoyment of intercourse, future fertility, and other areas. In some cases, surgical repair is necessary.

- Psychological complications can range from the mild and self-limited postpartum blues to the more concerning postpartum depression, postpartum panic disorder, and postpartum psychosis. Ongoing assessment and evaluation of the client's mood starting in pregnancy and continuing throughout the infant's first year of life is necessary to prevent unfortunate consequences related to emotional instability.

REVIEW QUESTIONS

1. Which of the following factors would be least likely to contribute to the development of endometritis?
   A. Use of fetal scalp electrodes
   B. Prolonged rupture of membranes
   C. Urinary catheterization
   D. Manual removal of the placenta
2. The nurse should suspect a laceration of the genital tract in a postpartum client who exhibits
   A. dark red, steady bleeding.
   B. spurting of bright red blood.
   C. purulent lochia.
   D. boggy uterus.
3. The nurse is performing a pad count on a postpartum client and weighs the pads to estimate the amount of blood loss. Which of the following totals for weight would indicate that the client is experiencing hemorrhage?
   A. 250 grams
   B. 325 grams
   C. 450 grams
   D. 675 grams
4. Inspection of the perineum of a postpartum client reveals ecchymosis and a tense fluctuant mass of the vulva. The nurse interprets this finding as consistent with
   A. uterine prolapse.
   B. parametritis.
   C. vulvar hematoma.
   D. uterine inversion.
5. Which of the following interventions would be a priority for a client who is readmitted to the health care facility with a diagnosis of late postpartum hemorrhage?
   A. Administration of broad spectrum antibiotics to prevent infection
   B. Intravenous fluid therapy to expand circulating volume
   C. Preparation for surgical curettage to remove the source of bleeding
   D. Application of ice to the perineum to promote vasoconstriction
6. After teaching a postpartum client about measures to prevent urinary tract infections, which statement would lead the nurse to suspect that the client needs additional teaching?
   A. "I will drink plenty of fluids throughout the day to flush out my bladder."
   B. "I will try to limit the number of times that I go to the bathroom to urinate."
   C. "I will change my perineal pad often, keeping the area as clean as possible."
   D. "I will use a front to back wiping motion when cleaning my perineal area."
7. A client diagnosed with mastitis asks the nurse, "Should I continue to breastfeed my baby?" Which response if made by the nurse, would be most appropriate?
   A. "We had better ask your health care provider if you should continue to breastfeed."
   B. "Well, that's really a decision for you to make. But, you can stop if you like for now."
   C. "Continuing to breastfeed will keep your breasts empty so that organisms can't grow."
   D. "You are receiving an antibiotic that could be transmitted to the baby so you shouldn't breastfeed right now."
8. Which of the following should the nurse expect to find when assessing a postpartum woman with deep vein thrombosis?
   A. Dyspnea
   B. Sudden chest pain
   C. Hemoptysis
   D. Calf tenderness on ambulation
9. Which agent would the nurse expect to administer as the drug of choice to a postpartum woman diagnosed with peripartum cardiomyopathy?
   A. Angiotensin-converting enzyme (ACE) inhibitors
   B. Nonsteroidal anti-inflammatory drugs (NSAIDs)
   C. Anticoagulant therapy
   D. Cephalosporin antibiotics
10. Assessment of a client with postpartum depression would reveal which of the following?
    A. Hallucinations
    B. Delusions
    C. Uncontrolled crying
    D. Confusion

REFERENCES

Altshuler, L. L., Cohen, L. S., Moline, M. L., Kahn, D. A., Carpenter, D., & Docherty, J. P. (2001). The Expert Consensus Guideline Series. Treatment of depression in women. *Post-graduate Medicine, Mar*(Spec No), 1–107.

American Academy of Family Physicians. (2000). *Panic disorder: Panic attacks and agoraphobia.* Retrieved March 7, 2003, from http://familydoctor.org/handouts/137.html.

American Psychiatric Association. (2003). Answers to your questions about panic disorder. Retrieved March 7, 2003, from http://www.apa.org/pubinfo/panic.html.

Apgar, B. S., Serlin, D., & Kaufman, A. (2005). The postpartum visit: Is six weeks too late? *American Family Physician, 72*(12), 2443–2444.

Baggish, M. S., & Lee, W. K. (1975). Abdominal wound disruption. *Obstetrics & Gynecology, 46,* 530–534.

Barbosa-Cesnik, C., Schwartz, K., & Foxman, B. (2003). Lactation mastitis. *Journal of the American Medical Association, 289*(13), 1609–1612.

Baskett, T. F., & O'Connell, C. M. (2005). Severe obstetric maternal morbidity: A 15-year population-based study. *Journal of Obstetrics and Gynaecology, 25*(1), 7–9.

Beck, C. T. (1992). The lived experience of post-partum depression: A phenomenological study. *Nursing Research, 41*(3), 166–170.

Beck, C. T., & Indman, P. (2005). The many faces of postpartum depression. *Journal of Obstetrical, Gynecological, and Neonatal Nursing, 34*(5), 569–576.

Birkeland, R., Thompson, J. K., & Phares, V. (2005). Adolescent motherhood and postpartum depression. *Journal of Clinical Child and Adolescent Psychology, 34*(2), 292–300.

Bloch, M., Rotenberg, N., Koren, D., & Klein, E. (2006). Risk factors for early postpartum depressive symptoms. *General Hospital Psychiatry, 28*(1), 3–8.

Bowes, W. A., & Katz, V. L. (2002). Postpartum care. In S. G. Gabbe, J. R. Niebyl, & J. L. Simpson (Eds.), *Obstetrics: Normal and problem pregnancies* (4th ed., pp. 701–726). New York: Churchill Livingstone.

Brown, C. E., Stettler, R. W., Twickler, D., et al. (1999). Puerperal septic pelvic thrombophlebitis: Incidence and response to heparin therapy. *American Journal of Obstetrics and Gynecology, 181*(1), 143–148.

Chukudebelu, W. O., & Okafor, E. I. (1978). Burst abdomen following cesarean section. *International Journal of Gynaecology & Obstetrics, 15,* 532–534.

Clark, R. A. (1995). Infections during the post-partum period. *Journal of Obstetrical, Gynecological, and Neonatal Nursing, 24*(6), 542–548.

Clarridge, J. E., Pezzlo, M. T., & Vosti, K. L. (1987). *Laboratory diagnosis of urinary tract infections. Cumulative techniques and procedures in clinical microbiology.* Washington, DC: American Society of Microbiology.

Clemmens, D., Driscoll, J. W., & Beck, C. T. (2004). Postpartum depression as profiled through the depression screening scale. *MCN—The American Journal of Maternal/Child Nursing, 29*(3), 180–185.

Colman-Brochu, S. (2004). Deep vein thrombosis in pregnancy. *MCN—The American Journal of Maternal Child Nursing, 29*(3), 186–192.

Cox, J. L., Holden, J. M., & Sagovsky, R. (1987). Edinburgh Postnatal Depression Scale (EPDS). *British Journal of Psychiatry, 150.*

Cunningham, F. G., Gant, N. F., Leveno, K. J., Gilstrap, L. C. III, Hauth, J. C., & Wenstrom, K. D. (2001). *Williams obstetrics* (21st ed.). New York: Lippincott Williams & Wilkins.

Danilenko-Dixon, D. R., Heit, J. A., Silverstein, M., Yawn, B. P., Petterson, T. M., Lohse, C. H., & Melton, L. J. (2001). Risk factors for deep vein thrombosis and pulmonary embolism during pregnancy or post partum: A population-based, case-control study. *American Journal of Obstetrics and Gynecology, 184*(2), 104–110.

Dayan, S. S., & Schwalbe, S. S. (1996). The use of small-dose intravenous nitroglycerin in a case of uterine inversion. *Anesthesia and Analgesia, 82,* 1091–1093.

Dearing, E., Taylor, B. A., McCartney, K. (2004). Implications of family income dynamics for women's depressive symptoms during the first 3 years after childbirth. *American Journal of Public Health, 94*(8), 1372–1377.

Dennis, C-L., & Creedy, D. (2004). Psychosocial and psychological interventions for preventing postpartum depression. *The Cochrane Database of Systematic Reviews, 4.*

Dorbala, S., Brozena, S., Zeb, S., Galatro, K., Homel, P., Ren, J. F., & Chaudhry, F. A. (2005). Risk stratification of women with peripartum cardiomyopathy at initial presentation: A dobutamine stress echocardiography study. *Journal of the American Society of Echocardiography, 18*(1), 45–48.

Dougherty, M., Burns, P., Campbell, D. A., Johnson, C., & Wyman, J. (2000). Continence for women, evidence-based clinical practice guideline, *AWHONN.*

Duff, P. (2002). Maternal and perinatal infections. In S. G. Gabbe, J. R. Niebyl, & J. L. Simpson (Eds.), *Obstetrics: Normal and problem pregnancies* (4th ed., pp. 1293–1345). New York: Churchill Livingstone.

Edhborg, M., Friberg, M., Lundh, W., & Widstrom, A. M. (2005). "Struggling with life": Narratives from women with signs of postpartum depression. *Scandinavian Journal of Public Health, 33*(4), 261–267.

Falter, H. J. (1997). Deep vein thrombosis in pregnancy and the puerperium: A comprehensive review. *Journal of Vascular Nursing, 15*(2), 58–62.

Felker, G. M., et al. (2000). Underlying causes and long-term survival in patients with initially unexplained cardiomyopathy. *New England Journal of Medicine, 342,* 1077–1084.

Floortje, M., Vandenbrouke, J. P., Buller, H. R., Colly, L. P., & Bloemenkamp, K. W. (2004). Estimates of risk of venous thrombosis during pregnancy and puerperium are not influenced by diagnostic suspicion and referral basis. *American Journal of Obstetrics and Gynecology, 191*(3), 825–829.

Franzblau, N., & Witt, K. (2003). Normal and abnormal puerperium. *E-Medicine.* Retrieved March 7, 2003, from http://www.emedicine.com/med/topic3240.htm.

French, L. M., & Small, F. M. (2002) *Antibiotic regimens for endometritis after delivery* (Cochrane Review). In The Cochrane Library, Issue 2 2002. Oxford: Update Software.

Garg, A., Morton, S., & Heneghan, A. (2005). A hospital survey of postpartum depression education at the time of delivery. *Journal of Obstetrical, Gynecological, and Neonatal Nursing, 34*(5), 587–594.

George, L. (2005). Lack of preparedness: Experiences of first-time mothers. *MCN—The American Journal of Maternal and Child Nursing, 30*(4), 251–255.

Goli, A. K., Koduri, M., Smith, S., & Fahrig, S. A. (2004). Peripartum cardiomyopathy underreported in primiparas. *Southern Medical Journal, 97*(10), S18–S19.

Hale, T. W. (2002). *Medications and mothers' milk: A manual of lactational pharmacology* (10th ed.). Amarillo, TX: Pharmasoft Publishing.

Hanna, B., Jarman, H., & Savage, S. (2004). The clinical application of three screening tools for recognizing post-partum depression. *International Journal of Nursing Practice, 10*(2), 72–79.

Hendrix, S. L., Schimp, D. O., Martin, J., Singh, A., Kruger, M., & McNeeley, S. G. (2000). The legendary superior strength of the Pfannenstiel incision: A myth? *American Journal of Obstetrics and Gynecology, 182*(6), 1446–1451.

Hostetler, D. R., & Bosworth, M. F. (2000). Uterine inversion: A life threatening emergency. *Journal of the American Board of Family Practice, 13*(2), 120–123.

Kennedy, E. (2001). Pregnancy, postpartum infections. *E-Medicine.* Retrieved March 7, 2003, from http://www.emedicine.com/emerg/topic482.htm.

Lampert, M. B., & Lang, R. M. (1995). Peripartum cardiomyopathy. *American Heart Journal, 130,* 860–870.

Looney, J. R., Lewis, R., Prevost, R., Hoppe, J., & Sibai, B. (1999). Clindamycin therapy in postpartum endometritis: The efficacy of daily versus every 8-hour dosing. *Obstetrics & Gynecology, 93*(4, Suppl. 1), S48.

Markinkovic, S. P., & Stanton, S. L. (2004). Incontinence and voiding difficulties associated with prolapse. *Journal of Urology, 171*(3), 1021–1028.

Mason, L., Glenn, S., & Watson, I. (2001). The instruction in pelvic floor exercises provided to women during pregnancy or following delivery. *Midwifery, 17*(1), 55–64.

Matthey, S., Barnett, B., Howie, P., & Kavanagh, D. J. (2003). Diagnosing postpartum depression in mothers and fathers: Whatever happened to anxiety. *Journal of Affective Disorders, 74*(2), 139–147.

McCoy, S. J., Beal, J. M., & Watson, G. H. (2003). Endocrine factors and postpartum depression. A selected review. *Journal of Reproductive Medicine, 48*(6), 402–408.

McDermott, S., Callaghan, W., Szwejbka, L., Mann, H., & Daguise, V. (2000). *Obstetrics & Gynecology,* 96(1), 530–534.

Maternal Neonatal Health. (2003). Preventing postpartum hemorrhage: Active management of the third stage of labor. Retrieved March 7, 2003, from http://www.mnh.jhpiego.org/best/pphactmng.asp.

Ornan, D., White, R., Pollak, J., et al. (2003). Pelvic embolization for intractable postpartum hemorrhage: Long-term follow-up and implications for fertility. *Obstetrics & Gynecology, 102*(3), 904–910.

Qasqas, S. A., McPherson, C., Frishman, W. H., & Elkayam, U. (2004). Cardiovascular pharmacotherapeutic considerations during pregnancy and lactation. *Cardiology in Review, 12*(5), 240–261.

Rocconi, R., Huh, W. K., & Chiang, S. (2002). Postmenopausal uterine inversion associated with endometrial polyps. *Obstetrics & Gynecology, 102*(3), 521–523.

Ryan, D., Milis, L., & Misri, N. (2005). Depression during pregnancy. *Canadian Family Physician, 51,* 1087–1093.

Seyfried, L. S., & Marcus, S. M. (2003). Postpartum mood disorders. *International Review of Psychiatry, 15*(3), 231–242.

Spinelli, M. G. (2004). Maternal infanticide associated with mental illness: Prevention and the promise of saved lives. *American Journal of Psychiatry, 161*(9), 1548–1557.

Spritzer, C. E., Evans, A. C., & Kay, H. H. (1995). Magnetic resonance imaging of deep venous thrombosis in pregnant women with lower extremity edema. *Obstetrics & Gynecology, 85*(4), 603–607.

Strong, T. H. (1997). Obstetric hemorrhage. In M. Foley & T. Strong (Eds.), *Obstetric intensive care* (pp. 30–46). Philadelphia: W. B. Saunders.

Vieira, T. (2003). When joy becomes grief. *AWHONN's Lifelines, 6*(6), 506–513.

Wainscott, M. P. (2004). Pregnancy, postpartum hemorrhage. Retrieved March 15, 2006, from http://www.emedicine.com.

Weier, K. M., & Beal, M. W. (2004). Complementary therapies as adjuncts in the treatment of postpartum depression. *Journal of Nurse Midwifery & Women's Health, 49*(2), 96–104.

Winans, E. (2001). The galactopharmacopedia. Antipsychotics and breastfeeding. *Journal of Human Lactation, 17*(4), 344–347.

CHAPTER 20

The Healthy Newborn

Jeanette Zaichkin

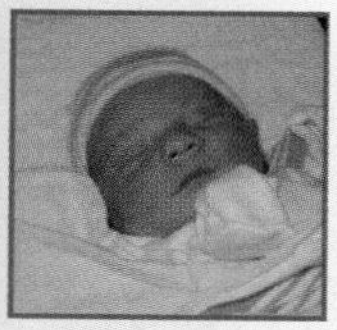

Thomas was born 8 hours ago at 40 weeks' gestation to a 34-year-old married primipara. His mother had ongoing prenatal care and experienced no complications during pregnancy, labor, or birth. Upon entering the room during a routine assessment, the nurse finds Thomas lying on the bed, clothed in a shirt and diaper. His mother sits in the bed next to him. As the nurse begins to take vital signs, Thomas has a small emesis of breast milk. He gags and coughs; mucus comes through his nose. His mother is visibly upset. "What is happening?" she asks worriedly. "Is he choking?"

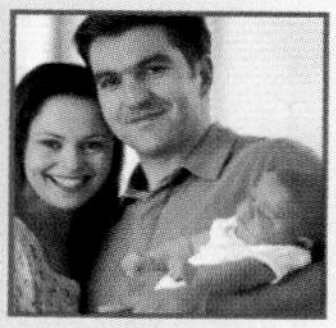

William is a full-term newborn whose parents have chosen to circumcise him. The nurse is providing the parents with instructions about the procedure. William's father seems concerned about how the circumcision will be done and the pain that the baby will experience. He tells the nurse that he thinks it is important that he and his son are physically similar, but he feels bad about causing his child to experience any trauma. The same nurse is providing care before, during, and after the procedure.

You will learn more about these clients as the chapter progresses. Nurses working with these and similar families need to understand the material in this chapter to manage care effectively and address issues appropriately. Before beginning, consider the following points related to the above scenarios:

- How should the nurse individualize care to ensure that each family's needs are met—not only in terms of physical care, but also in terms of emotional and psychological care?
- What factors may be contributing to parental behavior and reactions in these scenarios?
- Are any additional assessment data or questions in order?
- What teaching might be appropriate for each family?
- What other health care personnel might assist in these scenarios?

LEARNING OBJECTIVES

On completion of this chapter, the reader should be able to:

- Identify the major differences between fetal circulation and newborn circulation.
- List three cardiopulmonary changes that must occur at birth for successful extrauterine transition.
- Discuss immediate nursing interventions at birth for active and healthy full-term newborns who are breathing and have pink mucous membranes.
- Describe appropriate calculation and use of Apgar scores.
- Identify signs of abnormal newborn transition.
- Describe collaborative strategies to promote normal newborn transition.
- Discuss the relationship between birth weight and gestational age.
- Describe normal and abnormal physical examination findings in newborns.
- Discuss four types of heat loss in newborns and preventive interventions for each.
- Identify two classifications of newborns at risk for hypoglycemia and six signs of neonatal hypoglycemia.
- Explain why most healthy full-term newborns experience jaundice in the first week of life.
- Describe why newborns are susceptible to infection.
- Identify infant behavioral states and cues.
- Identify risk factors for Sudden Infant Death Syndrome (SIDS).
- Describe an approach for assessing cultural differences in newborn care with clients not from the United States or Canada.
- List newborn care topics for parent education.

KEY TERMS

acid mantle
acrocyanosis
Apgar score
apnea
approach cues
avoidance cues
Ballard Gestational Age Assessment Tool
bilirubin
bradycardia
brick dust spots
brown adipose tissue (BAT)
circumcision
circumoral cyanosis
cyanotic
ductus arteriosus
foramen ovale
free-flow oxygen
functional residual capacity (FRC)
grunting
hypoglycemia
hypoxemia
hypoxia
indirect bilirubin
jaundice
lanugo
large for gestational age (LGA)
low birth weight (LBW)
meconium
meconium-stained amniotic fluid
nasal flaring
neutral thermal environment (NTE)
nonshivering thermogenesis (NST)
occipital–frontal circumference (OFC)
periodic breathing
petechiae
phototherapy
physiologic jaundice
pink
plethoric
postterm
premature/preterm
pseudomenses/pseudomenstruation
radiant warmer
retractions
small for gestational age (SGA)
Sudden Infant Death Syndrome (SIDS)
surfactant
tachycardia
tachypnea
term
total bilirubin
unconjugated bilirubin
vagal reflex
vernix caseosa
very low birth weight (VLBW)
witch's milk

The birth of a baby is a significant life event influenced by cultural norms and expectations. Nurses responsible for newborn care need to balance the expectations of the new mother and her family with astute assessment and timely interventions.

Nursing care for newborns should begin with critical examination of the maternal prenatal and intrapartal history. At birth, the nurse should assess the newborn's well-being and ensure that critical extrauterine adaptations are happening. During the complete physical examination, the nurse should distinguish normal findings and variations from abnormalities. He or she should evaluate the newborn continuously thereafter, taking every opportunity to monitor the infant's condition, as well as to teach parents how to care for their baby and appreciate his or her amazing innate abilities.

QUOTE 20-1

"It's an incredible honor to be present at the birth of a new baby. The family always thanks me for being there, but I feel like I am the one who should be thanking them."

From a neonatal nurse

FROM FETUS TO NEWBORN

The newborn's cry signifies the beginning of life outside the womb. New mothers, their families, and health care providers of all cultures eagerly anticipate this cry as an initial signal of wellness. The more complex mechanics underlying a successful transition from intrauterine to extrauterine life are discussed below. Knowledge of them provides a foundation for understanding the principles of neonatal resuscitation and anticipating abnormalities.

Review of Fetal Circulation

To better understand newborn pulmonary physiology, the nurse needs to appreciate the differences between fetal circulation and extrauterine circulation. Chapter 11 discusses and illustrates fetal anatomy and physiology in detail. The next paragraphs provide a quick review.

In utero, the placenta acts as a low-resistance circulatory pathway for gas exchange. Blood flows from areas of higher to areas of lower pressure. The fetal lungs do not oxygenate tissues or excrete carbon dioxide; they are filled with fluid consisting of secretions from the alveolar epithelium, not air. The blood vessels that perfuse the fetal lungs are tightly constricted.

Two shunts (detours) within the fetal heart are essential to fetal circulation (see Fig. 11-12 in Chap. 11). The **foramen ovale** and **ductus arteriosus** divert oxygenated blood away from the fetal lungs to the brain and other vital organs. The foramen ovale allows blood to pump directly from the right to the left ventricle. The ductus arteriosus connects the pulmonary artery and descending aorta, causing most of the blood to detour the fetal lungs (Blackburn, 2003).

The fetal lungs maintain a state of pulmonary arterial vasoconstriction. The small amount of relatively hypoxic blood that reaches the fetal lungs helps maintain this constricted state. In addition, fetal pulmonary arteries have smaller lumens and more muscle mass than adult pulmonary arteries, limiting blood flow through them. As the fetus matures, these blood vessels prepare for extrauterine life by become increasingly reactive to changes in oxygenation and acid–base levels (Blackburn, 2003).

Finally, resistance to blood flow is different in the fetal pulmonary blood vessels. Blood flows most easily from areas of high pressure to low pressure. Fetal circulation functions so that the high pulmonary vascular resistance (PVR) in the lungs encourages blood to bypass them and shunt from the right side of the heart to the left. The blood passes through the foramen ovale and ductus arteriosus to the fetal aorta and returns to the low-pressure placenta for gas exchange. In contrast, adult PVR is low to permit easy blood circulation from the pulmonary arteries into the lungs. In the adult, systemic vascular resistance (SVR) is fairly high, allowing the aorta to distribute oxygenated blood throughout the body (Blackburn, 2003).

Respiratory and Circulatory Transitions at Birth

The fetal system of high PVR and low aortic SVR allows the placenta to be a low-resistance medium for gas exchange, which works well for the fetus. Critical transitions must occur within moments of birth, however, if transition to extrauterine life is to be successful (Fig. 20.1). If all goes correctly, three critical changes happen:

- Respiration begins and continues effectively.
- Fluid is cleared from the airways.
- SVR increases, shunts close, and blood circulates through the lungs (Blackburn, 2003; Kattwinkel, 2006; Lockridge, 1999).

Respiration

Several factors induce respiration. During vaginal birth, the maternal birth canal compresses the fetal chest. As the chest emerges, the thorax recoils, and air is sucked into the lung fields. Additionally, clamping of the umbilical cord affects chemoreceptors sensitive to changes in arterial oxygen and carbon dioxide content, contributing to the onset of respirations.

Temperature also is influential. The sudden cooling of the wet newborn as he or she emerges from the warm intrauterine environment causes sensory receptors on the skin to transmit impulses to the respiratory center (Blackburn, 2003). Finally, normal handling and drying of the newborn stimulates respirations; however, tactile stimulation does not always induce respirations in a newborn compromised at birth (Kattwinkel, 2006).

Clear Airways

First breaths must be strong enough to move the thick fluids that filled the fetal airway from the trachea to the

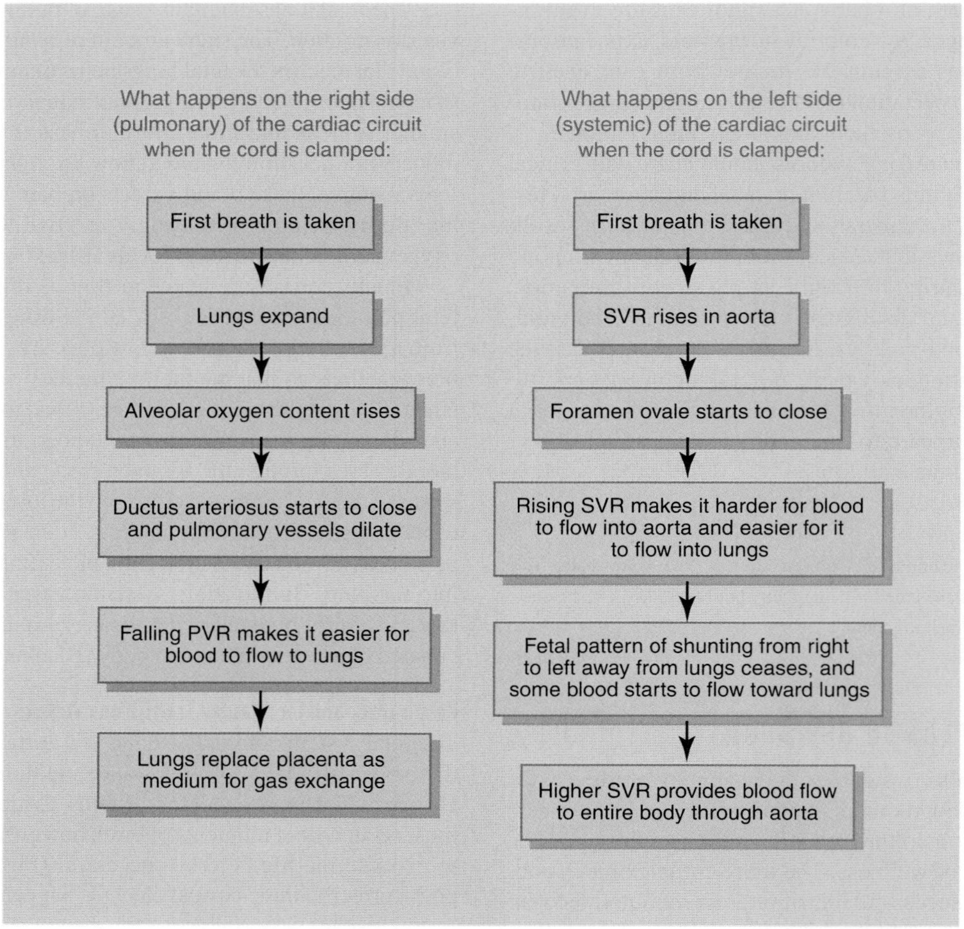
What happens on the right side (pulmonary) of the cardiac circuit when the cord is clamped:
First breath is taken
Lungs expand
Alveolar oxygen content rises
Ductus arteriosus starts to close and pulmonary vessels dilate
Falling PVR makes it easier for blood to flow to lungs
Lungs replace placenta as medium for gas exchange
What happens on the left side (systemic) of the cardiac circuit when the cord is clamped:
First breath is taken
SVR rises in aorta
Foramen ovale starts to close
Rising SVR makes it harder for blood to flow into aorta and easier for it to flow into lungs
Fetal pattern of shunting from right to left away from lungs ceases, and some blood starts to flow toward lungs
Higher SVR provides blood flow to entire body through aorta

FIGURE 20.1 Transition from fetal to neonatal circulation. PVR, pulmonary vascular resistance; SVR, system vascular resistance. (From Lockridge, T. [1999]. Persistent pulmonary hypertension of the newborn. *Mother Baby Journal, 4*[2], 22.)

terminal air sacs. Fetal lungs hold approximately 10 to 30 mL/kg of fluid. Thus, the lungs of a newborn weighing 3 kg (6 lbs, 11 oz) hold approximately 30 to 90 mL (1 to 3 oz) of fluid (Blackburn, 2003).

Fortunately, production of fetal lung fluid begins to decrease before labor begins (Blackburn, 2003). Release of catecholamines is associated with labor and may stimulate the lungs to stop secreting fluid (Askin, 2002), so that the baby must clear only a fraction of the original lung fluid volume at birth (Blackburn, 2003). In those cases in which the mother does not experience labor and concomitant exposure to catecholamines, the newborn is at risk for retaining lung fluid and developing transient tachypnea (Askin, 2002; Cooper & Goldenberg, 1990; Polin & Fox, 2004) (see Chap. 22).

For breathing to begin, liquid in the lungs must be replaced with an equal volume of air, and **functional residual capacity (FRC)** must be established (Blackburn, 2003). This means that the newborn's first breaths must be deep enough to displace the liquid in the airways and to retain some air in the alveoli so that subsequent breaths are less difficult. A fatty substance called **surfactant** causes retention of air in the lungs, decreasing surface tension at the air–liquid interface (Perinatal Continuing Education Program [PCEP], 1999c). Surfactant consists of phospholipids and proteins produced by type II cells in the lining of the alveoli and secreted onto the alveolar surface. Surfactant is essential to normal lung function because it allows the alveoli to remain open instead of collapsing completely during exhalation. By 28 to 32 weeks' gestation, the number of type II cells increases. Surfactant production peaks at about 35 weeks' gestation. By 32 weeks, 60% of fetuses have adequate surfactant to support extrauterine respiration. Surfactant deficiency results in respiratory distress syndrome (Blackburn, 2003) (see Chap. 22).

With the first few breaths, alveolar fluid is absorbed into the lung tissue, and the alveoli fill with air. The lymphatic system reabsorbs 10% to 20% of the lung fluid (Polin & Fox, 2004). Aeration and increased oxygen tension increase alveolar blood flow and the capillaries' ability to remove fluid. When these systems work efficiently, they disperse lung fluid in the first few hours after birth (Blackburn, 2003). This explains why newborns have audible crackles for a short time after birth. Residual air is retained in the lungs from the early breaths; within 1 hour after birth, 80% to 90% of FRC is created (Blackburn, 2003).

Blood Circulation

Clamping of the umbilical cord shuts off the placental circuit and causes rapid changes in PVR and SVR. With the low-resistance pathway removed, SVR increases. Other contributors to increased SVR include increased arterial blood volume because the blood that previously had a placenta to return to remains in the vascular system (Blackburn, 2003).

This increased SVR reduces right-to-left shunting and sends blood through the lungs rather than allowing it to detour through the foramen ovale and ductus arteriosus. The foramen ovale closes and seals as changes in circulatory pressures reduce pressure on the right side of the heart and increase pressure on the left side. Rising oxygen levels cause the other fetal shunt, the ductus arteriosus, to begin to constrict almost immediately after birth of a healthy newborn. In most cases, the ductus arteriosus functionally is closed by 96 hours of life; full anatomic closure with formation of a fibrous strand known as the *ligamentum arteriosus* is complete within 2 to 3 months (Blackburn, 2003). The ductus can reopen, however, in response to **hypoxia** (abnormally low oxygen concentration in tissues) or increased PVR. This return to fetal circulation, called pulmonary hypertension, results in a dangerous cycle of hypoxia and pulmonary vasoconstriction (Fig. 20.2). Thus, attaining and maintaining adequate ventilation and oxygenation in newborns and avoiding procedures that cause hypoxia, such as deep suctioning, are important concerns (see Chap. 22).

With gaseous distention and increased oxygen in the alveoli, the pulmonary blood vessels begin to dilate and relax. Vasodilation of these arterial vessels decreases PVR in the newborn by nearly 80%, which increases blood flow through the lungs and minimizes blood flow through the fetal shunts (Blackburn, 2003). Adequate oxygen is now available from the lungs and enters the bloodstream. As the baby continues to take deep breaths, adequate oxygen moves from the lungs into the bloodstream. The baby changes from a gray-blue color to pink. Note that this

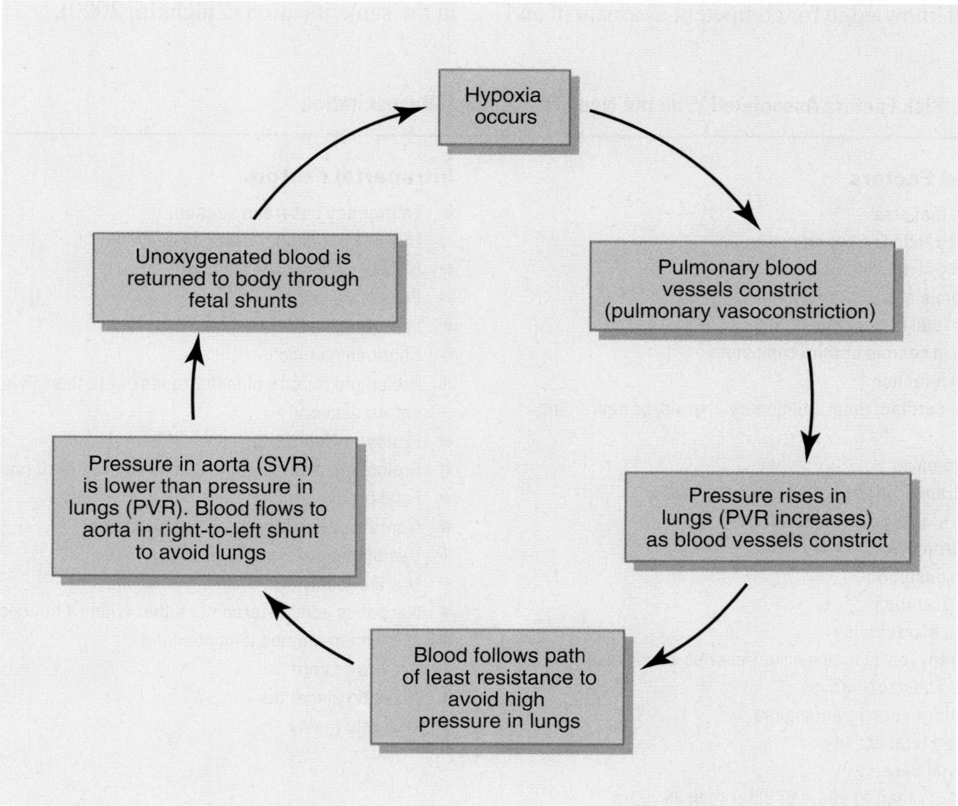

FIGURE 20.2 Cycle of inadequate ventilation/oxygenation at or shortly after birth. PVR, pulmonary vascular resistance; SVR, system vascular resistance. (From Lockridge, T. [1999]. Persistent pulmonary hypertension of the newborn. *Mother Baby Journal, 4*[2], 23.)

chapter uses the term **pink** to denote adequate oxygenation and perfusion for newborns of all racial and ethnic backgrounds. In newborns with dark complexions, pink mucous membranes (lips, tongues, and gums) denote adequate oxygenation and perfusion. In light-skinned newborns, providers assess the color of the face, trunk, and mucous membranes.

IMMEDIATE NURSING MANAGEMENT OF THE NEWBORN

QUOTE 20-2

"I never realized how much in love I would be with my baby."

(From a new mother)

Most pregnancies result in the birth of a healthy full-term newborn who requires little assistance from health care personnel. Nevertheless, nurses must be prepared for any deviation from normal. Nursing actions in a compromised newborn's first moments can have lifetime consequences (Kattwinkel, 2006). Therefore, nurses who attend births and are responsible for newborn resuscitation and admission need to assess prenatal and intrapartal history to determine risk factors for receiving a compromised newborn, ensure that all equipment for resuscitation and admission is present and working, possess skills and knowledge for competent assessment and intervention, and communicate with colleagues and the newborn's family to ensure that the plan of care incorporates any special circumstances.

Prenatal and Intrapartal History

The nurse responsible for newborn admission should assess the prenatal and intrapartal history for any risk factors. Many maternal conditions can influence the course of labor and birth, the initial transition period, and beyond (Box 20.1). After the nurse checks the history, he or she should know whether to prepare for admission of a healthy newborn or to anticipate complications that will require interventions to stabilize an at-risk or sick newborn.

Preparedness for Resuscitation

At least 90% of newborns make a smooth extrauterine transition; approximately 10% need some assistance to begin breathing; the rare 1% require complex resuscitation procedures to survive (AHA, 2006). Although the need for resuscitation is usually evident before birth, a newborn may require resuscitation for an unknown or unanticipated reason. Therefore, all equipment necessary for complete resuscitation must be readily available and operational at all births. Supplies should be visible and arranged identically in every room to ensure that any member of the resuscitation team can always find them in the same location (Zaichkin, 2000).

BOX 20.1 Risk Factors Associated With the Need for Neonatal Resuscitation

Antepartal Factors

- Maternal diabetes
- Pregnancy-induced hypertension
- Chronic hypertension
- Fetal anemia or isoimmunization
- Previous fetal or neonatal death
- Bleeding in second or third trimester
- Maternal infection
- Maternal cardiac, renal, pulmonary, thyroid, or neurologic disease
- Polyhydramnios
- Oligohydramnios
- Premature rupture of membranes
- Fetal hydrops
- Postterm gestation
- Multiple gestation
- Size–date discrepancy
- Drug therapy (eg, magnesium, adrenergic-blocking drugs)
- Maternal substance abuse
- Fetal malformation or anomalies
- Diminished fetal activity
- No prenatal care
- Age younger than 16 years or older than 35 years

Intrapartal Factors

- Emergency cesarean section
- Forceps or vacuum-assisted delivery
- Breech or other abnormal presentation
- Premature labor
- Precipitous labor
- Chorioamnionitis
- Prolonged rupture of membranes (more than 18 hours before delivery)
- Prolonged labor (more than 24 hours)
- Prolonged second stage of labor (more than 2 hours)
- Fetal bradycardia
- Nonreassuring fetal heart rate patterns
- Use of general anesthesia
- Uterine tetany
- Narcotics administered to mother within 4 hours of delivery
- Meconium-stained amniotic fluid
- Prolapsed cord
- Abruptio placentae
- Placenta previa

From American Heart Association. (2006). *Textbook of neonatal resuscitation* (5th ed.). Elk Grove Village, IL: AAP/American Heart Association. Permission comes from Wendy Simon, Manager, Life Support Programs, AAP, Elk Grove Village, IL.

Ideally, every birth is attended by at least one person whose primary responsibility is the baby and who is capable of initiating resuscitation. Either that person or someone else who is immediately available should have the skills required to perform a complete resuscitation (Assessment Tool 20.1). This means that the person designated to attend the newborn has no other responsibilities at this time, is capable of assessing the need for resuscitation, and can perform competently initial steps of resuscitation, bag-and-mask ventilation, and chest compressions. This person may be able to perform advanced resuscitation procedures, or another person, such as a physician or nurse practitioner, should be available immediately who can perform procedures such as endotracheal

● ASSESSMENT TOOL 20.1 Algorithm for Neonatal Resuscitation

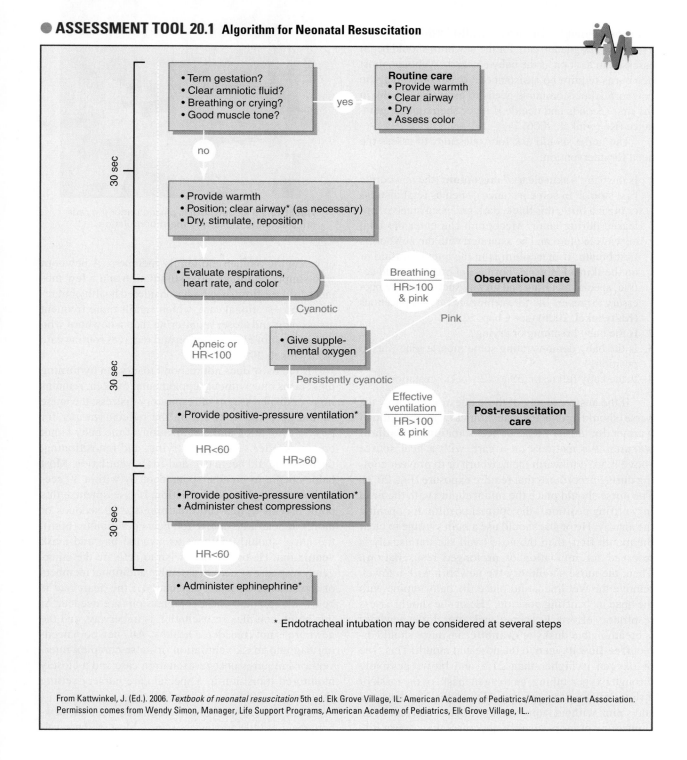

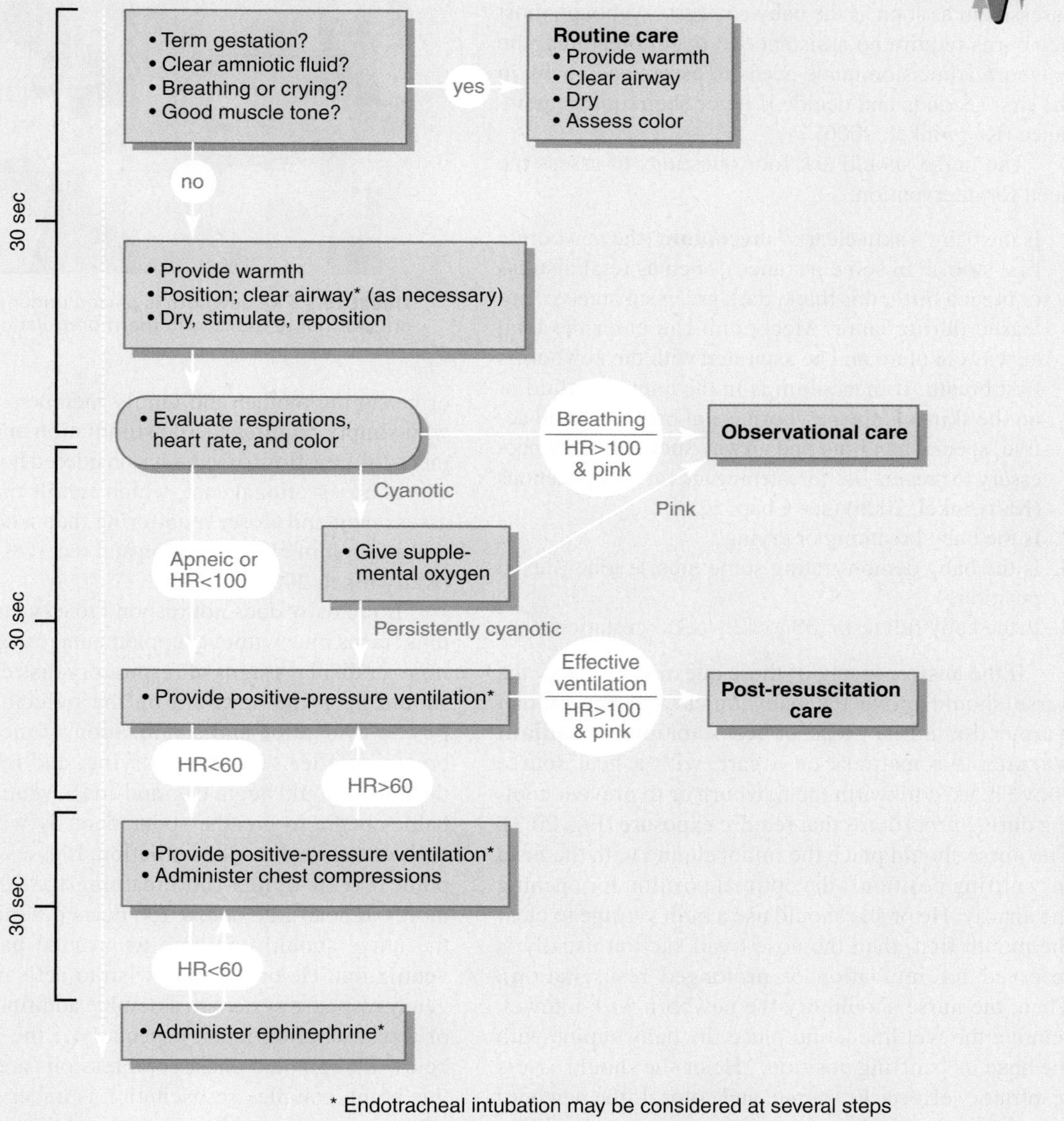

From Kattwinkel, J. (Ed.). 2006. *Textbook of neonatal resuscitation* 5th ed. Elk Grove Village, IL: American Academy of Pediatrics/American Heart Association. Permission comes from Wendy Simon, Manager, Life Support Programs, American Academy of Pediatrics, Elk Grove Village, IL..

intubation or medication administration when complex resuscitation is necessary (Kattwinkel, 2006).

If a high-risk birth is anticipated, the nurse should follow the health care facility's protocol for assembling a team of skilled resuscitation providers to attend the birth. Team composition varies, but may include a pediatrician, neonatologist, neonatal nurse practitioner, respiratory therapist, and neonatal nurses.

Assessment During the First Moments After Birth

The nurse assigned to care for the newborn should begin assessment as soon as the baby emerges. Although most newborns require no assistance to begin breathing, the newborn admission nurse needs to assess each baby in the first seconds and decide if he or she requires assistance (Kattwinkel, 2006).

The nurse should ask four questions to assess the need for intervention:

1. Is the baby's skin clear of **meconium** (the newborn's first stool)? In some instances, such as fetal distress or breech birth, this thick, dark green substance is released during labor. Meconium can enter the fetal airways in utero and be aspirated with the newborn's first breath. If meconium is in the amniotic fluid or on the skin and the newborn is not breathing and active, special handling and airway suctioning are necessary to prevent life-threatening airway complications (Kattwinkel, 2006) (see Chap. 22).
2. Is the baby breathing or crying?
3. Is the baby demonstrating some muscle tone (flexed position)?
4. Is the baby full term (38 to 42 weeks' gestation)?

If the answer to any of these questions is "no," the nurse should move the baby quickly to the radiant warmer for initial steps of resuscitation. A **radiant warmer** is a mattress on a cart, with a heat source above it, used to warm the newborn or to prevent cooling during procedures that require exposure (Fig. 20.3). The nurse should place the infant supine with the head in "sniffing position," the optimal position for opening the airway. He or she should use a bulb syringe to clear the mouth first, then the nose (wall suction usually is reserved for intubation or prolonged resuscitation). Then, the nurse should dry the newborn with a towel, remove the wet linen, and place the baby supine with the head in "sniffing position." He or she should assess respiratory efforts, heart rate, and color. If the newborn is breathing but dusky or **cyanotic,** the nurse should direct **free-flow oxygen** to the nose and mouth. This type of oxygen is higher than 21% and blows passively through oxygen tubing, an oxygen mask, or the mask of a flow-inflating oxygen bag. If the baby becomes and stays pink without supplemental oxygen and shows no signs of respiratory distress, the nurse may return him

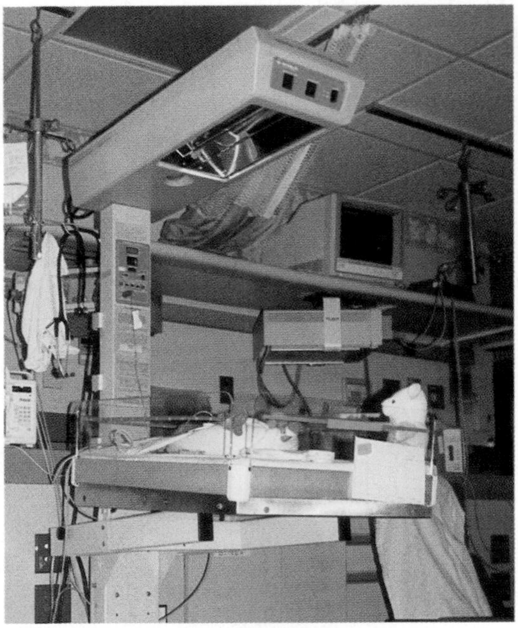

FIGURE 20.3 The newborn is placed under the radiant warmer to assist with thermoregulation.

or her to the mother and family members. A newborn who simply requires tactile stimulation and a few moments of free-flow oxygen is considered healthy but receives observational care, which entails more frequent assessment and closer monitoring than a newborn who requires minimal intervention and receives routine care (Kattwinkel, 2006).

If the baby does not respond to oxygen by turning pink, turns blue without supplemental oxygen, remains limp, or displays signs of respiratory distress, the nurse should keep the newborn on the radiant warmer for further evaluation and stabilization. If the baby is not breathing after suctioning, drying, and repositioning, the nurse should begin bag-and-mask ventilation. Most babies begin to breathe spontaneously within 30 seconds of bag-and-mask ventilation. If assessment at this point reveals **apnea** (no breathing for 20 seconds or more) or heart rate below 100 beats per minute (bpm), the nurse should continue to provide bag-and-mask ventilation. He or she may wish to activate the emergency response system to assemble additional members of a resuscitation team, especially if the heart rate is below 60 bpm and chest compressions are needed. At this point, complex resuscitation is underway, and the newborn is not considered healthy. Any newborn needing bag-and-mask ventilation or more complex interventions requires post-resuscitation care and a closely monitored transition in a special care nursery setting (Kattwinkel, 2006) (see Chap. 22).

If the answers to all four questions are "yes," the newborn requires little nursing assistance. Most mothers welcome their babies onto their chest or abdomen, where a health care provider positions the newborn prone to help drain any remaining fluids from the mouth and nose. If the baby is not making gurgling sounds or draining fluid from the nose or mouth, repeated suctioning is unnecessary. Deep suction, by placing the tip of the bulb syringe deep in the throat or using a suction catheter, may elicit a gag and vagal reflex. This leads to apnea, **bradycardia,** and resulting hypoxia, which unnecessarily complicates the baby's transition. All that is required is to ensure that the newborn's airway is clear, which is accomplished by suctioning with a bulb syringe the mouth first and then the nose, or wiping both clear with a towel (Kattwinkel, 2006) (Fig. 20.4).

The nurse dries the baby as thoroughly as possible to prevent further heat loss and remove birth fluids. A towel is usually more efficient for drying than a baby blanket (Zaichkin, 2006). Hospital towels and blankets for newborn care need not be sterile (American Academy of Pediatrics [AAP], 2002).

Vaginal Birth

A newborn doing well following vaginal birth requires only routine care (Kattwinkel, 2006). The nurse should provide warmth, clear the airway, and dry the baby quickly and thoroughly. Unless the mother has emergent medical needs or requests otherwise, there is no reason to separate her from a healthy newborn. A policy of taking a healthy newborn immediately to a radiant warmer or other location for observation and admission is outmoded and hinders attachment. The nurse can place the baby directly on the mother's abdomen or chest, covering both with a dry, warm blanket. Skin-to-skin contact can maintain warmth (Kattwinkel, 2006).

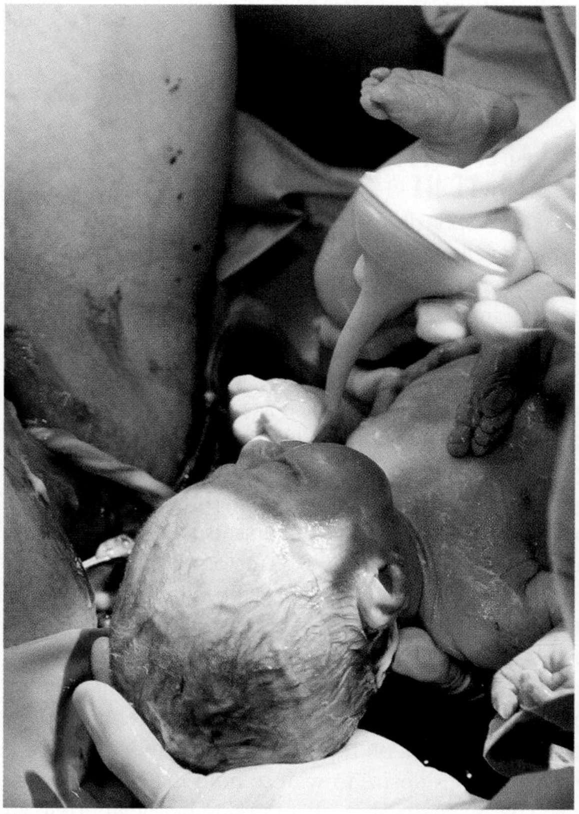

FIGURE 20.4 Use of the bulb syringe immediately after birth to suction the newborn.

Cesarean Birth

The nurse should follow the same resuscitation and admission procedures in cases of cesarean birth. He or she should immediately receive this newborn at the radiant warmer and suction, dry, and position the baby for further assessment. If the newborn requires no special care, the father or birth partner may use warm blankets to hold and show the newborn to the mother (Fig. 20.5).

Apgar Scoring

While the nurse handles the newborn and assesses progress in the first minute of life, he or she also assesses the 1-minute **Apgar score** (Assessment Tool 20.2). Created by anesthesiologist Virginia Apgar in 1952, the Apgar score became the standard of practice for assessing and documenting the infant's response to birth (Apgar, 1953). In 1962, the acronym APGAR was proposed to recall the components of the scoring system (Butterfield, 1962):

- **A:** Appearance (color)
- **P:** Pulse (heart rate)
- **G:** Grimace (reflex irritability)
- **A:** Activity (muscle tone)
- **R:** Respiration (respiratory effort)

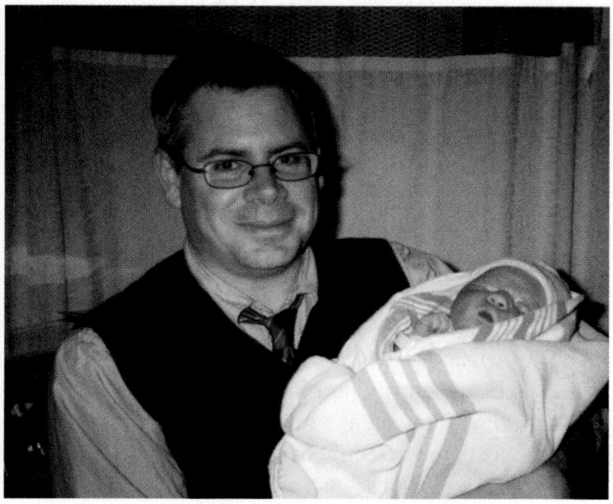

FIGURE 20.5 This father is preparing to present his newborn to the baby's mother following a cesarean birth.

● ASSESSMENT TOOL 20.2 Apgar Scoring System

	Score		
Sign	**0**	**1**	**2**
Color	Blue or pale	Acrocyanotic	Completely pink
Heart rate	Absent	Slow (<100 bpm)	≥ 100 bpm
Reflex irritability	No response	Grimace	Cry or active withdrawal
Muscle tone	Limp	Some flexion	Active motion
Respirations	Absent	Weak cry: hypoventilation	Cry or active withdrawal

Source: AAP & ACOG (2006). The Apgar Score. *Pediatrics, 117*(4), 1446.

Each component is assigned a value of 0, 1, or 2; the five numbers then are added for a total. Scoring is done 1 minute and 5 minutes after birth. To help ensure accuracy, scoring should occur at the 1-minute and 5-minute marks, not retrospectively (Apgar, 1966). The Apgar score does not determine resuscitation efforts; therefore, resuscitative efforts are not delayed until the 1-minute Apgar is determined. If the newborn does not attain a 5-minute score of at least 7, additional scores are assigned every 5 minutes up to 20 minutes (Kattwinkel, 2006).

Because Apgar scoring is somewhat objective, Dr. Apgar suggested that an impartial observer, not the delivering practitioner, assign the scores (Apgar, 1966). In most cases, the person responsible for newborn resuscitation and admission assigns the Apgar scores of a healthy newborn, and the delivering practitioner does not contest them. If the newborn requires resuscitation, a collaborative effort from all resuscitation team members, in conjunction with narrative documentation of interventions and their timing, ensures an accurate record of events.

Most healthy full-term newborns receive 1-minute scores of 7 to 9 and 5-minute scores of 8 or 9. Because pink hands and feet are rare in the first few minutes of life, a perfect score of 10 is unusual.

New criteria appear on the revised and expanded Apgar chart introduced by the American Academy of Pediatrics (AAP) and American College of Obstetricians and Gynecologists (ACOG) in 2006. The criteria allow for the different responses expected at birth from a preterm newborn or a baby requiring resuscitation, and more accurately describe the newborn's responses resulting from a resuscitation intervention (AAP & ACOG, 2006).

The Apgar score alone is not sufficient evidence on which to base neurologic outcomes in term newborns. The difference between 1-minute and 5-minute Apgar scores reflects the effectiveness of resuscitation efforts. An Apgar score of 0 to 3 at 5 minutes may correlate with neonatal mortality but alone does not predict later neurologic dysfunction (AAP & ACOG, 2006).

Apgar scoring is a U.S. standard and a useful tool for documenting the newborn's responses to the extrauterine environment and resuscitation efforts. In addition to Apgar scores, complete documentation, including a narrative description of the newborn's behavior and responses to interventions, is essential to a complete medical record.

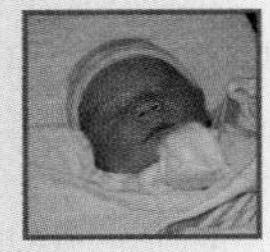

Recall Thomas, the 8-hour-old newborn described at the beginning of the chapter. Suppose he had an Apgar score of 5 at 1 minute and 6 at 5 minutes. How would the nurse proceed?

COLLABORATIVE CARE: IMMEDIATE NEWBORN CARE

The team responsible for the newborn needs to ensure that the plan of care is clear and agreed on before birth and well in advance of the final moments of labor. The nurse who has been involved in maternal intrapartum care and shifts her responsibilities to the newborn should already have assessed family preferences for involvement in the first few minutes after birth. The nurse assigned to perform newborn admission may need to clarify the plan with the family and the labor and delivery team; he or she should check the prenatal and intrapartal history and clarify any risk factors. The newborn admission nurse usually asks the labor nurse if there are any new risk factors with implications for the newborn, such as abnormalities in fetal heart rate, meconium staining, maternal fever, prolonged rupture of membranes, or recent maternal narcotic administration.

Family preferences may include the partner's wish to cut the umbilical cord, the mother's preference to receive the newborn on her chest immediately after birth, or the family's desire to wait to hold the baby until he or she has been dried. A client giving her newborn to an adoptive family may have specific wishes about seeing and holding the baby. The nurse should ask the family about cultural or spiritual beliefs that influence admission procedures and adapt routine policies to accommodate reasonable requests. The nurse's responsibility to facilitate integration of the newborn into the family begins immediately at birth; however, if the newborn requires resuscitation or intervention, nursing and medical care take precedence. Following such an emergency, the nurse should make sure to include the mother and support partners in the newborn's plan of care.

Assessment

At birth, the nurse should assess many parameters simultaneously (Kattwinkel, 2006):

- Any meconium on the newborn's skin
- Breathing
- Muscle tone
- Heart rate (by palpating the umbilical pulse)
- Reflex irritability (grimacing response to bulb suction or gagging on mucus)
- Approximate gestational age
- Color

The experienced neonatal nurse also should assess approximate weight and, by doing so, compare it to expected gestational age. If the newborn appears smaller or larger than average, the nurse should be prepared to address risk factors requiring immediate intervention, before a complete physical examination. He or she also should quickly inspect the baby, scanning for unusual variances or congenital anomalies that might interfere with normal transition.

Select Potential Nursing Diagnosis

The following nursing diagnosis may be appropriate during the first few moments after birth:

- **Ineffective Breathing Pattern** related to obstructed airway, neuromuscular immaturity, perinatal compromise, or physiologic inability to transition to extrauterine circulation

Planning/Intervention

The nurse should ensure that the baby's airway is clear and dry fluids from the skin. The following findings and interventions may be appropriate:

- Breathing but not pink—provide free-flow oxygen.
- Limp or having acute respiratory distress—take infant to radiant warmer for more thorough assessment, remembering that ventilation is the most important intervention.
- Apneic—stimulate the baby briefly by drying or flicking the soles of the feet. If there is no response, immediately begin bag-and-mask ventilation (Kattwinkel, 2006).

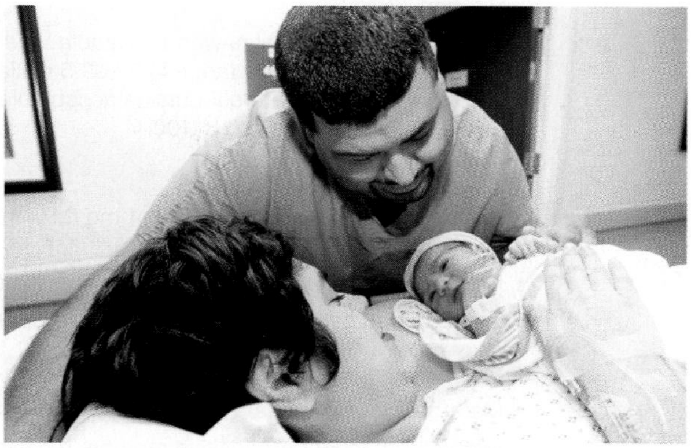

FIGURE 20.6 A family is bonding following labor and birth. (Photo courtesy of Joe Mitchell.)

Newborns requiring no resuscitation or brief free-flow oxygen usually can stay with their mothers under close nursing supervision. If all appears well after assignment of the 5-minute Apgar score, the nurse can leave the newborn on the mother's chest, covered with a warm dry blanket, and maintain vigilance from a short distance. The nurse should remain alert to the newborn's needs while the family enjoys a few minutes of privacy with their new relative (Fig. 20.6). NIC/NOC Box 20.1 highlights some common nursing interventions and outcomes for the healthy newborn.

Evaluation

The healthy newborn is term, pink, and active and has minimal signs of respiratory distress soon after birth.

EARLY NEWBORN CARE PROCEDURES

The first hours after a baby's birth are busy for perinatal and neonatal staff. The timing of the following procedures varies with institutional protocols and family preferences (Fig. 20.7).

NIC/NOC Box 20.1 Care of the Newborn

Common NIC Labels

- Kangaroo Care
- Newborn Care
- Newborn Monitoring
- Nonnutritive Sucking

Common NOC Labels

- Newborn Adaptation
- Thermoregulation: Neonate

1. **Vital signs**
   - TPR q 30 minutes until newborn is stable WNL for 2 hours after birth; TPR q 4-6 hours thereafter. Acceptable temperature range is 97-99.5 axillary.
   - Check rectal temperature if outside acceptable range. Notify physician if rectal temperature is <97 and resistant to warming or 100.4.

2. **Routine medications**
   - **Phytonadione** (Aqua Mephyton) 1 mg IM within 1 hour of birth for infants > 2500 gms. If < 2500 gms, give 0.5 mg IM. (Parent can refuse.)
   - **Erythromycin Ophthalmic** 0.5% ointment to each eye within 1 hour of birth.
   - **Triple dye** to cord x 1. Alcohol to cord q 8 hours. (Parent can refuse.)

3. **Hepatitis B vaccine/HBIG:** Administer according to criteria below, after obtaining parental consent
   - Maternal HbsAg status: ______________________________
   - Infants born to HbsAg-positive mothers receive, within 12 hours of birth and at 2 IM sites: Hepatitis B Immune Globulin (HBIG) 0.5 ml IM x 1 **AND** Recombivax HB preservative free 5.0 mcg/0.5 ml IM x 1
   - Infants born to HbsAg-negative mothers receive before discharge: Recombivax -HB preservative free 5.0 mcg/0.5 ml IM x 1 **OR** Engerix-B 10 mcg/0.5 ml x 1
   - If maternal status unknown, call physician for orders.

4. **Blood glucose monitoring**
   - Implement Neonatal Hypoglycemia policy for infant at risk, including infants > 4200 gms and infants < 2500 gms.
   - Order STAT blood glucose, notify physician and initiate IV therapy if glucose screen is
     ≤ 20,
     < 40 and baby is unable to feed due to immaturity, respiratory distress, other
     OR < 40, thirty minutes after feeding for a preceding glucose screen < 40

5. **Cord blood studies** Maternal blood type: ☐
   - Collect cord blood at delivery and send to lab; hold cord blood for seven days.
   - Order blood type: Rh and Coombs test if mother is Rh negative or little *'c'* negative.
   - Order Total Bilirubin, Reticulocyte count, Hgb and Hct if Coombs text is positive.

6. **Jaundice monitoring**
   - Implement Hyperbilirubinemia Protocol for infants at risk.
   - Order total bilirubin if any jaundice is noted in the first 24 hours of life.
   - Screen for hyperbilirubinemia risk prior to discharge.

7. **Toxicology screening**
   - Order urine toxicology screen if indicated per perinatal screening criteria. Notify newborn's mother, physician, and social worker.

8. **Feeding:** If infant weighs < 2500 gms, feed q 3 hours
   - Breastfeeding: May initiate breastfeeding immediately if stable. Subsequent feedings on demand or at least every 3-4 hours. Do not supplement with glucose or formula without medical indication and physician's orders.
   - Formula feeding: use formula brand of parent's choice; feed 20-calorie formula with iron q 3-4 hours.

9. **Discharge**
   - Metabolic screen after 12 hours of age or prior to discharge, or by 5 days if still hospitalized.
   - Universal newborn hearing screen prior to discharge.

10. **Infant with complicated transition: NOTIFY PHYSICIAN**
    - Follow American Academy of Pediatrics NRP Textbook Guidelines for resuscitation.
    - Admit to Special Care Nursery for post-resuscitation care or for evaluation of abnormal transition.

Physician signature:______________________________ Date/time: ____________________

Nurse signature:______________________________ Date/time: ____________________

FIGURE 20.7 Sample routine hospital orders for the newborn.

Identification

Identical identification bands should be written for mother and newborn with information including the mother's hospital number, the baby's sex, and the date and time of birth. For multiple births, each baby's band should denote birth order; for example, "Twin A" signifies the firstborn of twins. Another team member present in the delivery room verifies the accuracy of information printed on the bands. The nurse should place one band on the mother's wrist and usually one on the newborn's wrist and ankle. Banding the mother and newborn must occur before separating them for any reason. Each time the newborn is reunited with the mother, the nurse should compare their identification bands to ensure a match (Fig. 20.8). This is important to avoid inadvertently giving a mother an infant who does not belong to her (AAP & ACOG, 2002).

Weight

Parents and family members are usually eager to learn the newborn's weight. The nurse should take care to obtain an accurate weight while protecting the newborn from cold and undue stress (Nursing Procedure 20.1). He or she should record the weight shortly after birth (the infant may breastfeed first, if desired) and daily thereafter (AAP & ACOG, 2002).

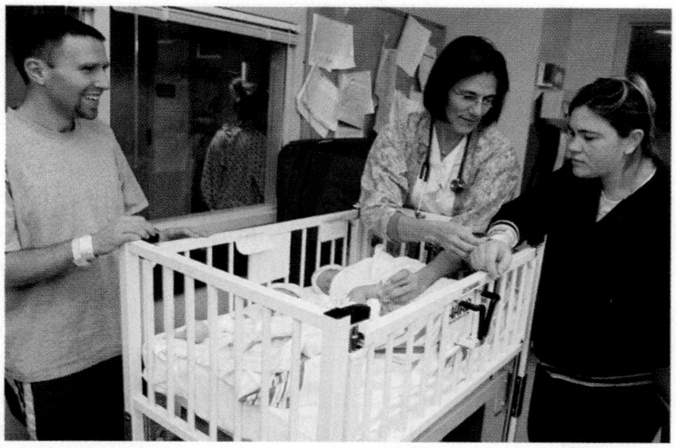

FIGURE 20.8 The nurse is checking the newborn's and mother's identification bands to ensure a match.

Measurements

Measurement of length and occipital–frontal circumference (OFC) is necessary to assess appropriateness of size for gestational age and future growth. The nurse should use a nonstretchable measuring tape. He or she can measure length by either of the following methods (Tappero, 2003):

- Place the infant supine, with the legs extended and the infant looking straight up. Mark on the bed to indicate

NURSING PROCEDURE 20.1
Weighing the Newborn

PURPOSE

To measure the newborn to help determine gestational age and to establish a baseline for use in evaluating growth and development

ASSESSMENT AND PLANNING

- Assess the newborn's Apgar scores at 1 and 5 minutes *to determine newborn's transition to extrauterine life.*
- Assess the newborn's temperature and determine whether he or she is experiencing cold stress; if so, delay the procedure until temperature stabilizes.
- Calibrate the scale if necessary.
- Explain the procedure to the parents.
- Gather the necessary equipment:
    - Calibrated scale
    - Prewarmed blanket or disposable scale covering
    - Clean gloves

IMPLEMENTATION

1. Wash hands and put on gloves.
2. Place prewarmed blanket or covering on scale *to minimize risk for heat loss from conduction.*
3. Reset the scale to zero *to ensure accuracy of measurement.*

Continued

NURSING PROCEDURE 20.1 CONTINUED

Weighing the Newborn

4. Place naked newborn on the covering. Position the newborn on the scale *to minimize stress;* keep one hand over the newborn body without touching the newborn *to ensure safety.*
5. Quickly note the weight in pounds, ounces, and grams as appropriate.
6. Remove the newborn from the scale, and continue with care, removing gloves and washing hands when care is completed.
7. Document the weight in the newborn's medical record.

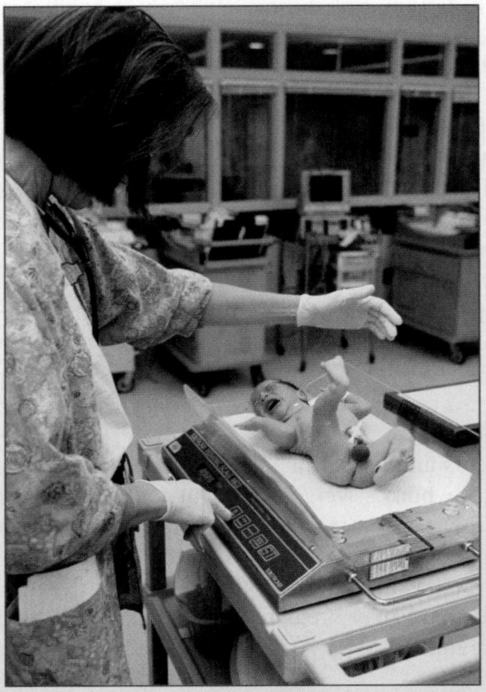

Step 4. Weighing the newborn while carefully guarding with the other hand.

EVALUATION

- Newborn is weighed without difficulty.
- Newborn experiences no evidence of cold stress.

AREAS FOR CONSIDERATION AND ADAPTATION

Lifespan Considerations

- Keep in mind that while the newborn remains at the facility, weights are obtained daily.
- Avoid placing the naked newborn directly on the scale's cold surface in the supine position. The newborn is more likely to be startled, to cry and move about, interfering with obtaining an accurate weight. Additionally, placing the naked newborn on a cold surface facilitates heat loss.

Community-Based Considerations

Obtain newborn weights at each visit. Typically, parents do not have a baby scale in their home. The home care nurse needs to bring a scale to the visit.

the crown of the head and the infant's heel. Measure the distance between the two marks (Fig. 20.9).

- Position the infant as described above. Place the zero point of the tape measure at the heel and run it alongside the infant to the head. Mark the end spot on the tape with a finger and read the measurement.

The nurse should measure OFC by wrapping the tape around the infant's head, over the occipital, parietal, and frontal prominences, avoiding the ears. He or she should measure three times and record the largest finding (Fig. 20.10). Cranial molding or scalp edema may affect OFC. The nurse should note such findings in the medical record (Tappero & Honeyfield, 2003).

Chest circumference measurement is now optional, but many institutions perform it (Fig. 20.11). The nurse should measure the chest circumference around the nipples during newborn expiration (Tappero & Honeyfield, 2003). If using a paper tape measure, he or she should make sure that it does not stick and tear when the infant is lying against it, which could result in an incorrect measurement. Also, the nurse should lift the infant's torso off the mattress to remove the tape measure from the back; pulling the tape measure out from under the supine infant can result in paper cuts on the infant's torso.

Gestational Age Assessment

Gestational age assessment is performed to estimate a newborn's postconceptual age (Tappero & Honeyfield, 2003). The nurse needs to know the gestational age and

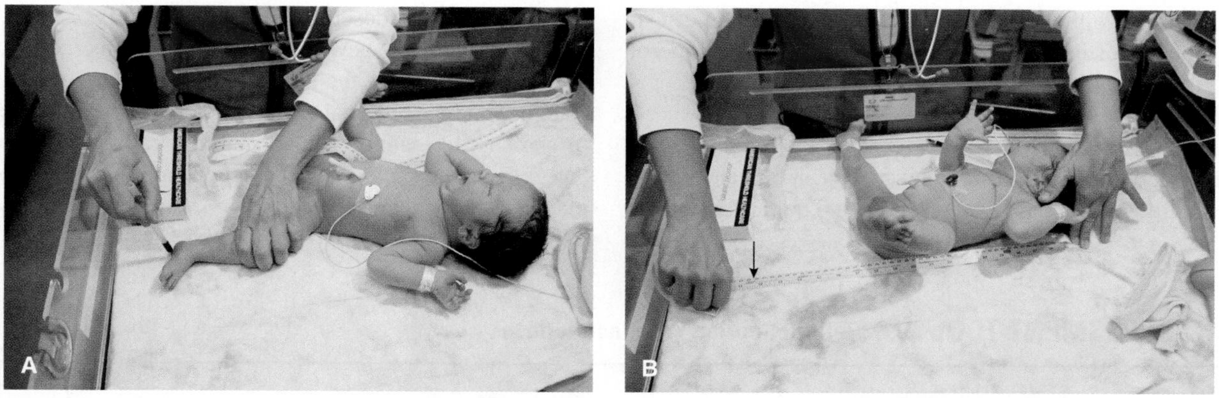

FIGURE 20.9 To measure the newborn's length, the nurse extends the baby's leg and marks the pad at the heel (**A**) and measures from the newborn's head to the heel mark (**B**).

the growth parameters appropriate to it because neonatal risks for each classification are different. A newborn's gestational age is not evident by assessing weight alone. An infant who weighs 4 lbs at 39 weeks' gestation has a vastly different set of risk factors and management interventions than an infant who weighs 4 lbs at 35 weeks' gestation.

Gestational age can be assessed in four ways:

1. **Maternal menstrual history:** An average term pregnancy is 266 days (38 weeks after ovulation) or 280 days (40 weeks from the first day of the last menstrual period) (Blackburn, 2003). Assessing gestational age by using the date of the last ovulation or menstrual period depends on the regularity of maternal menstrual cycles. Irregular cycles, failed contraception, and inaccurate recall by the woman can affect this method.
2. **Ultrasound examination:** Gestational age by ultrasound before 12 weeks is accurate to ±5 days. Ultrasound between 12 and 18 weeks is accurate to ±7 days. Between 18 and 28 weeks' gestation, ultrasound is accurate to ±12 days (Dodd, 1996).
3. **Ballard assessment:** The **Ballard Gestational Age Assessment Tool** originated from the Dubowitz Assessment of Gestational Age (Dubowitz et al., 1970). The Dubowitz scale consists of 11 external physical characteristics and 10 neurologic signs. Ballard and colleagues (1979) simplified the Dubowitz tool using six physical and six neuromuscular criteria. Studies have shown that the Dubowitz and Ballard scales may overestimate gestational age by 2 weeks (Alexander et al., 1992). The new Ballard gestational tool, expanded to include the very preterm infant, is purported to overestimate gestational ages less than 37 weeks by only 2 to 4 days (Ballard et al., 1991).
4. **Lens vascularity:** This method used to a limited extent can help determine gestational age when differences among other methods are significant. The developing lens of the eye has a vascular system that invades and nourishes the eye during fetal growth. The vascular system appears at approximately 27 weeks' gestation and disappears after 34 weeks' gestation. The stages of atrophy are divided into four grades according to the pattern and presence of blood vessels visualized on the eye lens

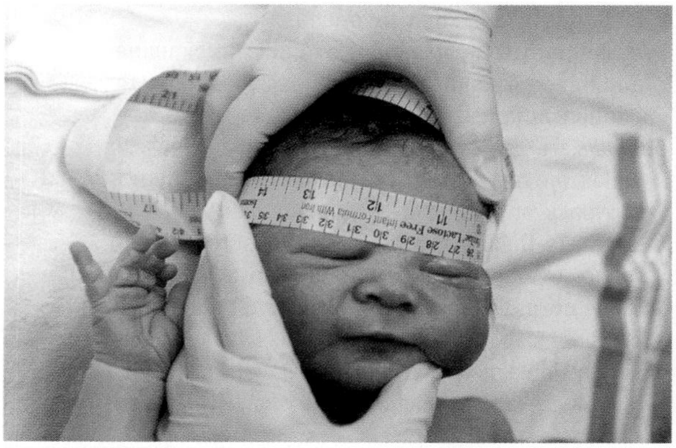

FIGURE 20.10 Measuring head circumference.

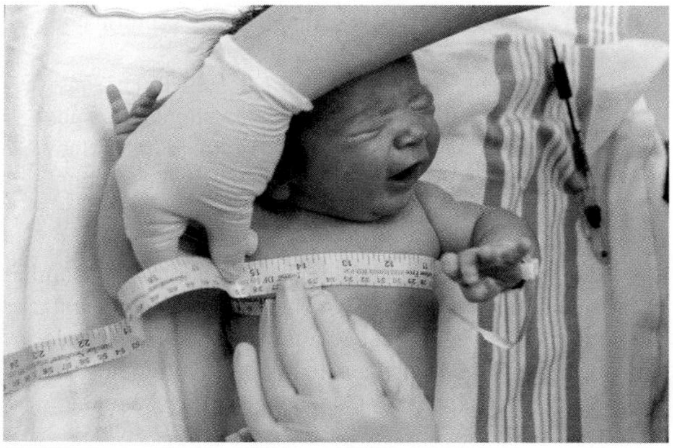

FIGURE 20.11 Measuring chest circumference.

with an ophthalmoscope. The grading system must be performed within 24 to 48 hours of age (Tappero & Honeyfield, 2003).

Infant Classification

To determine infant gestational age, the nurse can use the Ballard Gestational Age Assessment Tool according to the directions and descriptors (Assessment Tool 20.3). After examining the newborn and scoring each criterion, the nurse should add the two scores for neuromuscular category and the physical category to obtain the total. He or she should match the final maturity rating with the "weeks" on the same line. Instructions are unclear as to which gestational age score to assign when the total falls

● ASSESSMENT TOOL 20.3 Ballard Scoring With Instructions

Instructions for Use of the Ballard Gestational Age Assessment Tool

Neuromuscular Maturity

Posture is the position the baby naturally assumes when lying quietly on his back. A very premature infant will lie with arms and legs extended in whatever posture he is placed. As intrauterine development progresses, the fetus is capable of more and more flexion. When born at term, an infant lies with his arms flexed to his chest, his hands fisted, and his legs flexed towards his abdomen.

Square window (wrist) is the angle achieved when the infant's palm is flexed toward his forearm. A premature infant's wrist exhibits poor flexion and makes a 90-degree angle with the arm. An extremely immature infant has no flexor tone and cannot achieve even 90-degree flexion. A term infant's wrist will flex completely against the forearm. This can also be done with the ankle, but ankle flexion was excluded from the Ballard tool because it duplicates the wrist flexion and may not be possible or accurate in babies with intrauterine positional effects.

Arm recoil is elicited by first flexing the arms at the elbows to the chest, then fully extending them and releasing. Term infants will resist extension and briskly return their arms to the flexed position. Very preterm infants will not resist extension and respond with weak and delayed flexion in a small arc. The flexion angle of the elbow is estimated.

Popliteal angle is assessed with the infant lying supine. Keeping his pelvis flat, flex his thigh to his abdomen and hold it there while extending his leg at the knee. The angle at the knee is estimated. The preterm infant will achieve greater extension.

Scarf sign is elicited by moving the baby's arm across his chest as far toward the opposite shoulder as possible while he is lying supine. The term infant's elbow will not cross midline, but it will be possible to bring the preterm infant's elbow much farther toward the opposite shoulder.

Heel to ear is similar to popliteal angle, but the knee and thigh are not held in place. The baby's foot is drawn as near to the head or ear as possible. Scoring is based on the distance from heel to head. The premature baby will be able to get his foot close to his head.

Physical Maturity

Skin is assessed for thickness, transparency and texture. Premature skin is thin, with visible vessels, and smooth. Extremely preterm infants have sticky, transparent skin. A term infant's skin is thick, veins are difficult to see and the texture may be flaky.

Lanugo is the fine hair seen over the back of premature babies by 24 weeks. It begins to thin over the lower back first and disappears last over the shoulders.

Plantar creases are the deep folds and creases seen over the bottom of the foot. One or two appear over the pad of the foot at approximately 32 weeks. At 36 weeks, the creases cover the anterior two-thirds of the foot. At term, they cover the whole foot. At very early gestation, the length of the sole is measured. For extremely immature infants, this item was expanded to include foot length measured from the tip of the great toe to the back of the heel.

Breast tissue is examined for visibility of nipple and areola and size of bud when grasped between thumb and forefinger. The very premature infant will not have visible nipples or areola. These become more defined and then raised by 34 weeks, with a small bud appearing at 36 weeks and growing to 5–10 mm by term.

Ear formation includes the development of cartilage and the curving of the pinnae. Lack of cartilage in earlier gestation results in the ear folding easily and retaining this fold. As gestation progresses, soft cartilage can be felt with increasing resistance to folding and increasing recoil. The pinnae are flat in very preterm infants. Incurving proceeds from the top down toward the lobes as gestation advances.

Eyes in the extremely immature infant are examined, and the degree of eyelid fusion is assessed with gentle traction.

Genitalia are virtually indistinguishable at 20 weeks. In males, the testes are in the inguinal canal around 28 weeks, and rugae are beginning to be visible. By 36 weeks, the testes are in the upper scrotum, and rugae cover the anterior portion of the scrotum. At term, rugae cover the scrotum, and at postterm the testes are pendulous. In females, the clitoris is initially prominent and the labia minora are flat. By 36 weeks, the labia majora are larger and the clitoris is nearly covered.

Continued

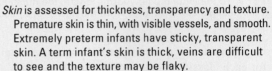

● ASSESSMENT TOOL 20.3 Ballard Scoring With Instructions

NEUROMUSCULAR MATURITY

NEUROMUSCULAR MATURITY SIGN	SCORE −1	0	1	2	3	4	5	RECORD SCORE HERE
POSTURE								
SQUARE WINDOW (Wrist)	>90°	90°	60°	45°	30°	0°		
ARM RECOIL		180°	140°–180°	110°–140°	90°–110°	<90°		
POPLITEAL ANGLE	180°	160°	140°	120°	100°	90°	<90°	
SCARF SIGN								
HEEL TO EAR								
						TOTAL NEUROMUSCULAR MATURITY SCORE		

SCORE

Neuromuscular ____

Physical ____

Total ____

MATURITY RATING

Score	Weeks
−10	20
−5	22
0	24
5	26
10	28
15	30
20	32
25	34
30	36
35	38
40	40
45	42
50	44

PHYSICAL MATURITY

PHYSICAL MATURITY SIGN	SCORE −1	0	1	2	3	4	5	RECORD SCORE HERE
SKIN	sticky, friable, transparent	gelatinous, red, translucent	smooth, pink, visible veins	superficial peeling and/or rash, few veins	cracking pale areas, rare veins	parchment, deep cracking, no vessels	leathery, cracked, wrinkled	
LANUGO	none	sparse	abundant	thinning	bald areas	mostly bald		
PLANTAR SURFACE	heel-toe 40–50 mm: −1 <40 mm: −2	>50 mm no crease	faint red marks	anterior transverse crease only	creases ant. 2/3	creases over entire sole		
BREAST	impercep-tible	barely perceptible	flat areola no bud	stippled areola 1–2 mm bud	raised areola 3–4 mm bud	full areola 5–10 mm bud		
EYE-EAR	lids fused loosely: −1 tightly: −2	lids open pinna flat stays folded	sl. curved pinna; soft; slow recoil	well-curved pinna; soft but ready recoil	formed and firm instant recoil	thick cartilage, ear stiff		
GENITALS (Male)	scrotum flat, smooth	scrotum empty, faint rugae	testes in upper canal, rare rugae	testes descending, few rugae	testes down, good rugae	testes pendulous, deep rugae		
GENITALS (Female)	clitoris prominent and labia flat	prominent clitoris and small labia minora	prominent clitoris and enlarging minora	majora and minora equally prominent	majora large, minora small	majora cover clitoris and minora		
						TOTAL PHYSICAL MATURITY SCORE		

between those listed. It has been suggested that the "gestational age that most closely approximates the maturity rating is chosen. For example, if the maturity rating score is 23, a gestational age of 33 weeks is assigned" (Tappero & Honeyfield, 2003).

- A preterm infant is less than 37 completed weeks' gestation (less than 38 weeks' gestation).
- A term infant is 38 to 41 weeks' gestation.
- A postterm infant is more than 42 weeks' gestation.
- A low-birth-weight infant weighs less than 2500 g (5 lbs, 8 oz) and can be preterm, term, or postterm.

Chapter 22 provides an illustrated comparison of the differences in Ballard screening characteristics for preterm and term infants.

Next, the nurse should plot the infant's weight on the growth curve chart (Fig. 20.12). Weight is on the vertical axis; gestational age is on the horizontal axis. He or she notes whether the plot point falls into the shaded area denoting less than the 10th percentile (small for gestational age [SGA]), between the 10th and 89th percentile (average for gestational age [AGA]), or above the 90th percentile (large for gestational age [LGA]). For example, if the infant is 37 weeks' gestation and weighs 1800 g, the infant is preterm and SGA. Any newborn whose plot point falls into the SGA shading is below the 10th percentile for growth, which means that the newborn is smaller than 90% of all other babies of the same gestational age.

Weight and gestational age combine to describe an infant who is:

- Preterm and SGA, AGA, or LGA
- Term and SGA, AGA, or LGA
- Postterm and SGA, AGA, or LGA

After plotting the weight, the nurse should mark the length and head circumference on the corresponding charts. He or she should note if an SGA infant has not grown at the expected rate for one, two, or all three growth parameters. The SGA newborn who experienced growth restriction late in gestation is usually SGA for weight only. This is termed *asymmetric growth restriction.* The infant less than the 10th percentile for weight and length suffered from limited growth earlier in gestation than the newborn lacking in weight only. If all three parameters are in the 10th percentile, the infant

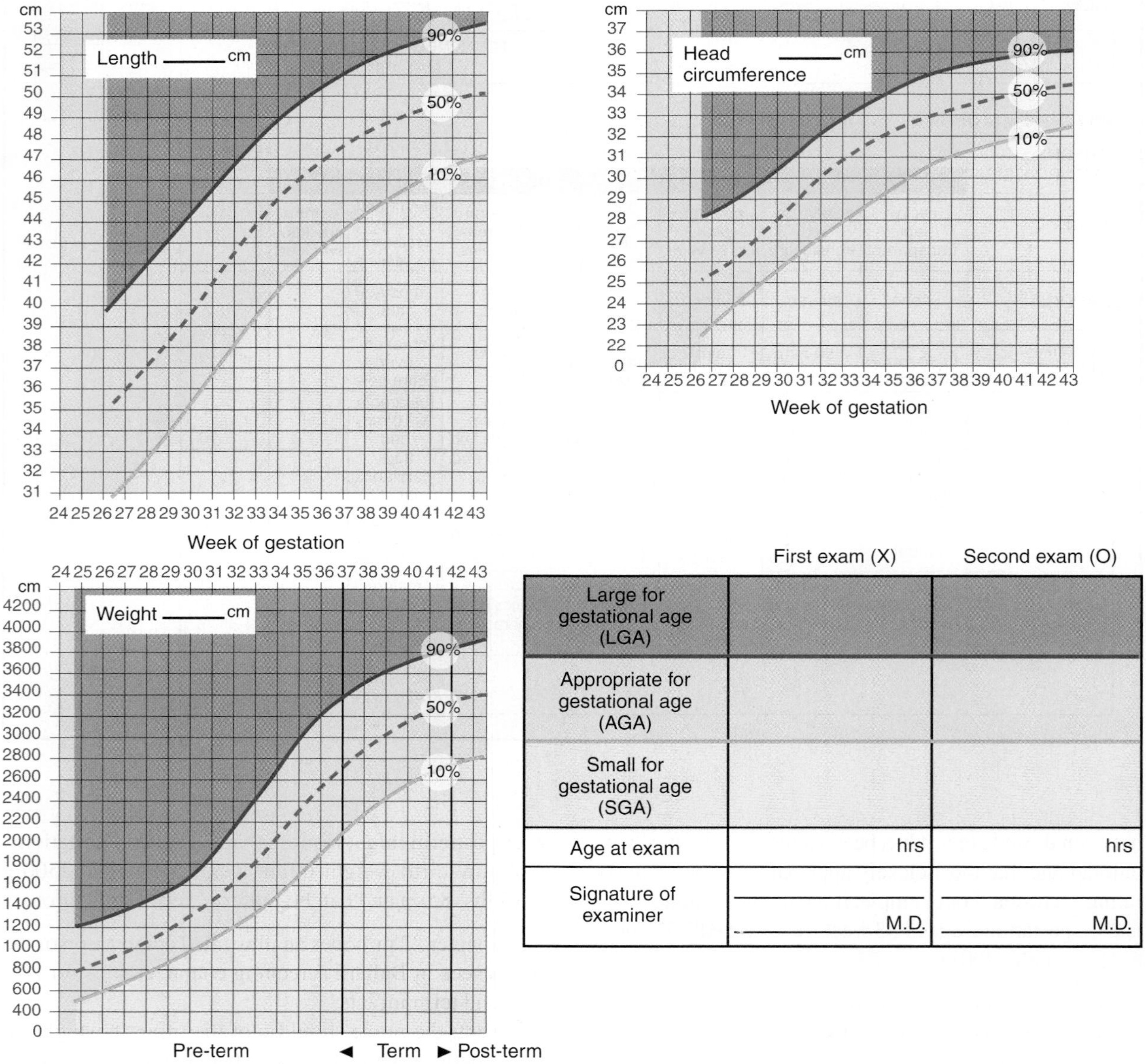

FIGURE 20.12 Sample growth curve charts for newborns.

is referred to as having *symmetric* or *proportionate growth restriction.* This usually reflects factors that caused diminished growth beginning early in gestation, such as viral infections, single-gene defects, and chromosome disorders (Tappero & Honeyfield, 2003). Although the asymmetric group is likely to catch up in growth, babies with symmetric growth restriction are at risk for continued small size and behavioral and intelligence problems (Dodd, 1996).

An infant at 36 weeks' gestation who weighs 3200 g is LGA and preterm, likely to be the infant of a mother with diabetes, and at risk for hypoglycemia, respiratory distress syndrome (RDS), and slow feeding. An infant of 40 weeks' gestation weighing 1200 g is term and SGA and at risk for fetal distress, hypoglycemia, congenital anomalies, congenital infection, and polycythemia.

The experienced neonatal nurse should quickly and accurately assess gestational age during initial newborn assessment. If the estimated date of delivery (EDD) is based on the last menstrual period, ultrasound examination, or both, the nurse should use his or her own initial assessment results to confirm the obstetrical estimation. If estimated gestational age is unclear, the nurse can quickly assess four physical parameters: ear, nipples, genitalia, and plantar creases. These findings should give enough information to develop an initial assessment and management plan. From these four criteria, the nurse can determine whether the newborn appears preterm, term, or postterm. Using an experienced eye for estimating weight, the nurse then can link the gestational age assessment to estimated weight to decide if the newborn is AGA, SGA, or LGA. This information is critical for assessing medical risks, preventing complications, assessing developmental capabilities, and implementing nursing care (Dodd, 1996). Therefore, by the time the nurse has ensured that the newborn's airway is clear, wiped the baby dry, assigned the first Apgar score, and done a quick visual assessment to rule out major anomalies, he or she also has estimated gestational age and size for age and begun to formulate a plan of care based on this initial assessment.

The First Bath

The first bath is an additional opportunity to closely examine newborn skin and behavioral responses to stimuli. Parents often assist with the first bath and gain important information about their newborn and caregiving skills. In addition, a bath can improve the newborn's appearance and is important for infection control (AAP & ACOG, 2002). See Research Highlight 20.1.

Timing and procedure vary among institutions. The initial bath is now given sooner than in the past to decrease the possibility of transmitting blood-borne pathogens through contact with maternal body fluids on the newborn's skin. Early bathing (1 to 2 hours after birth) of the stable term newborn also decreases the use of latex gloves, which are required for health care personnel handling newborns before and during the first bath. Decreased latex exposure may minimize latex allergies (Varda, 2000).

Until the first bath has been given, health care team members need to use standard precautions when handling

● RESEARCH HIGHLIGHT 20.1 Tub Bathing vs. Sponge Bathing

OBJECTIVE: To compare the effects of tub bathing and sponge bathing on newborn temperature, state control, and condition of the umbilical cord.

PARTICIPANTS AND SETTING: Twenty infants 1 to 4 days old participated in this hospital-based study. The same nurse sponge-bathed 10 babies and tub-bathed the 10 remaining babies. The nurse took the axillary temperature of all babies before and after the bath and measured and maintained the temperature of the bath water between 100° to 103°F (37.8° to 39.4°C). The nurse recorded behavioral states. Cord care followed hospital protocol.

RESULTS: The axillary temperatures of 90% of the sponge-bathed infants dropped 0.2° to 1°F, but still remained within the normal range of 97° to 98°F (36.1° to 36.7°C). All the tub-bathed infants maintained their temperature, whereas 80% of them increased their temperatures 0.2° to 1.2°F. All the temperatures of the tub-bathed infants remained within normal range. Ninety percent of the sponge-bathed babies cried during the procedure. Seventy percent of the tub-bathed babies were drowsy or quiet alert. Cord care did not differ between the two groups.

CONCLUSION: In this small group, tub bathing was more beneficial than sponge bathing in comparisons of temperature and behavioral state. Assessing the effect of tub bathing on umbilical cord condition and time of separation is difficult because this study did not follow the babies after discharge. Parents may prefer giving a tub bath to a sponge bath if the baby seems less stressed by a tub bath. More research is required using larger populations.

Cole, J. G., Brissette, N. J., & Lunardi, B. (1999). *Mother Baby Journal, 4*(3), 39–43.

the newborn (AAP & ACOG, 2002). They delay the first bath until the newborn's temperature is within normal limits. Because bathing can be stressful, providers delay the first bath for any baby exhibiting distress during transition, such as respiratory distress, temperature instability, or hypoglycemia.

Research regarding the timing of the first bath has demonstrated no negative effects on temperature stability. For a healthy term newborn protected from thermal stress before, during, and after washing, the first bath may occur as early as 60 minutes of age (Behring et al., 2003; Nako et al., 2000; Penny-MacGillivray, 1996; Varda & Behnke, 2000).

Warm tap water is adequate. Water temperature should be only slightly cooler than an adult would find acceptable for bathing and not lower than infant body temperature (36.7°C or 98.6°F). One research study found that the water temperature nurses used for newborn bathing ranged from 36.1°C (97°F) to 38.9°C (102°F) (Behring et al., 2003).

Most health care facilities use either a mild, nonmedicated soap or a mild antiseptic solution for the first bath, because of the risk for percutaneous absorption of the chemicals in these products (Blackburn, 2003). Alkaline soap destroys the skin's acid mantle by neutralizing the pH, which disturbs the balance of protective skin flora. The term infant recovers the acid mantle approximately 1 hour after bathing. Most hospitals use some type of soap for the initial bath because of concerns about pathogens in maternal fluids, such as hepatitis B and HIV. Some hospitals even use a mild antiseptic solution for the first bath, which they should rinse thoroughly from the infant's body (Blackburn, 2003).

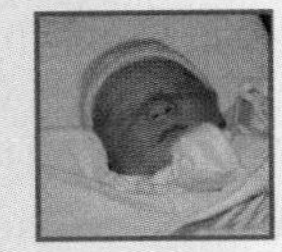

Remember Thomas, the newborn from the beginning of the chapter. Imagine that he is 2 hours old and is to receive his first bath. The nurse is demonstrating the bath to his mother, who says, "I found a really nice fragrant soap at the bath shop that I'm going to use when I bathe him at home." How should the nurse respond?

The bathing procedure exposes the newborn to cooling and stress. Nurses take every precaution to limit adverse reactions. An efficient and organized procedure ensures that the bath, including hair washing, is complete in less than 10 minutes.

Illustrated guidelines for the initial bath appear in Nursing Procedure 20.2. The newborn may be bathed under the protection of a radiant warmer. In this procedure, the infant's temperature has been taken to ensure stability within normal limits, and no transitional distress is present (Teaching Tips 20.1).

NURSING PROCEDURE 20.2

Bathing the Newborn

PURPOSE

To clean the newborn

ASSESSMENT AND PLANNING

- Organize supplies for bathing:
  - Basin of warm water
  - Several washcloths
  - Several towels at one end of the radiant warmer
  - Soap
  - Comb
  - Small cup for pouring water at or very near to the sink

IMPLEMENTATION

1. Wash hands and put on gloves. Keep gloves on until you have dried the baby.
2. Lay the infant under the prewarmed radiant warmer; unwrap and unclothe him or her. Change the wet or soiled diaper, if necessary. Rediaper and swaddle the newborn in a warm blanket, leaving only the head exposed.

Continued

NURSING PROCEDURE 20.2

Bathing the Newborn

3. Take the infant to the sink and regulate the running water temperature.
4. Use a clean washcloth to gently wash the face without soap. Include behind and inside the ears. Gently pat the face dry.
5. Wash the head and hair. Because of the possibility of fluctuating water temperature and pressure, do not hold the head directly under the running water. It is safer to collect the water in a cup or small pitcher and slowly pour it onto the infant's head over the sink. If the parent is uneasy about pouring, thoroughly soak a washcloth in running water and use it to wet the hair.
6. Use a small amount of soap and massage it gently into the scalp. Do not rub vigorously to remove tenacious **vernix.** (Some vernix may remain firmly attached to the baby's skin.) Comb soap through the hair to loosen and remove blood, if necessary.
7. Rinse the hair thoroughly and gently dry the head with a towel. Cover the baby's head with the towel and return the infant to the radiant warmer.
8. Wash the body:
   a. Lay the infant under the radiant warmer. Positioning the infant with the head and feet across the width of the warmer provides room for a basin of clean water and supplies at the head of the warmer. Remove the baby's blanket and diaper. Expose the head to the radiant heat to help ensure drying by the end of the bath.
   b. Quickly moisten the infant's body with a wet washcloth. Do not worry about wetting the blanket underneath the baby. Work quickly and finish washing the baby's body within 1 or 2 minutes.
   c. Rub the soap into a lather with your gloved hands. Quickly massage the soap over the infant's body with your gloved hands (hands reach into infant folds faster and more efficiently than a bulky washcloth), starting at the neck creases and working down. Wash the arms, armpits, and fingers. Wash the chest. Roll the infant onto the side to wash the back. Then wash the legs and feet. Do not wash the buttocks or genitals yet.
   d. Thoroughly wet a clean washcloth and rinse the infant, ensuring that you rinse soap from neck and armpit creases. If the infant is lying on top of soaked towels at this time, remove those towels and place the baby on a dry towel.
   e. Now use this clean wet washcloth to wash the genital area. Wipe vernix and secretions out of thigh creases. For girls, separate the labia and wipe front to back to remove secretions. Always use a clean portion of the washcloth for a front-to-back maneuver. For uncircumcised boys, do not attempt to retract the foreskin.

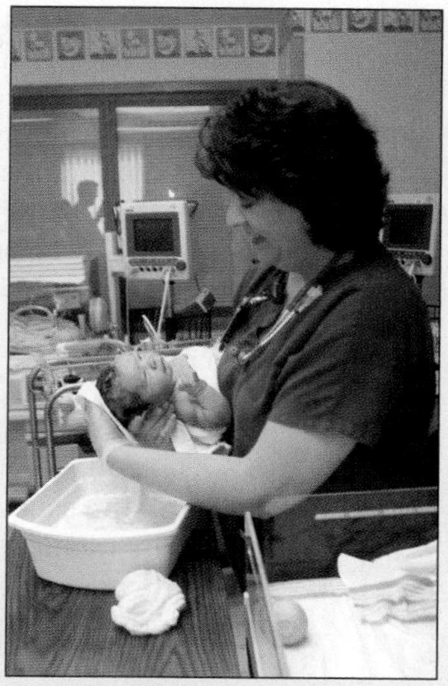

Step 5. Using a washcloth to wet the baby's hair.

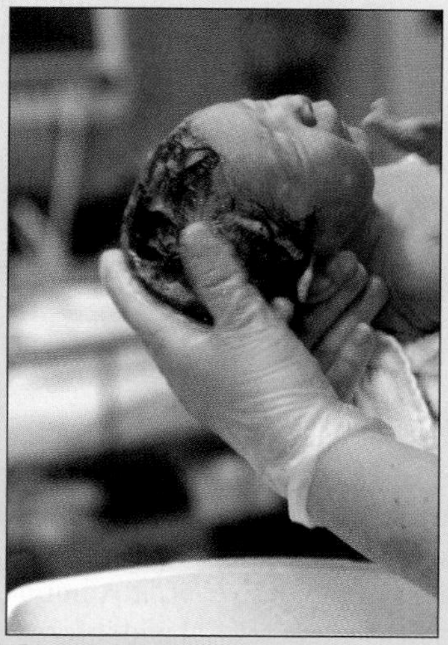

Step 6. Massaging the soap into the baby's scalp.

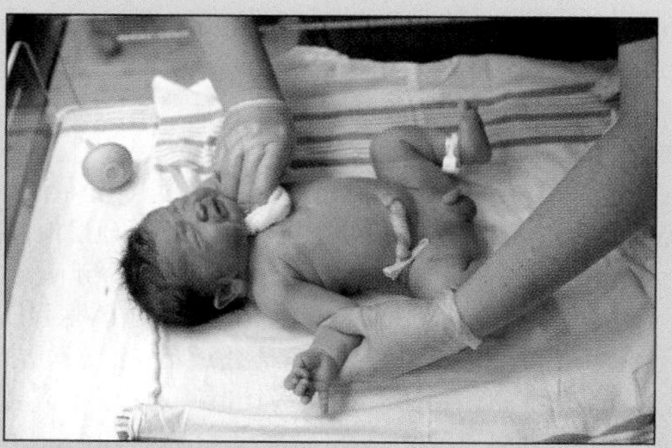

Step 8b. Bathing under the newborn's neck.

Continued

NURSING PROCEDURE 20.2 CONTINUED

Bathing the Newborn

Gently and quickly move around the genital area, remembering to lift the scrotal sac and clean the skin underneath.

f. Clean the bottom last. Rinse any soap remaining in this area.

9. Lift the newborn off the radiant warmer to remove the waterproof pad (and with it, the wet linen on top); lay it aside or place it inside a nearby linen receptacle. Do not throw linen on the floor.
10. Lay the baby down on the dry towel underneath the radiant warmer. Finish drying the baby gently and thoroughly. Do not vigorously rub the skin. Discard the towel.
11. Diaper the infant.
12. Complete any necessary admission procedures, such as the vitamin K injection and cord care, if prescribed.
13. Place the newborn skin to skin with the mother or her partner if desired, with a head covering and a warm blanket over the baby. Or attach a thermistor probe to the newborn for rewarming on the radiant warmer for 10 to 15 minutes.
14. Check the baby's temperature 15 to 30 minutes after the bathing procedure is complete to monitor thermal recovery.

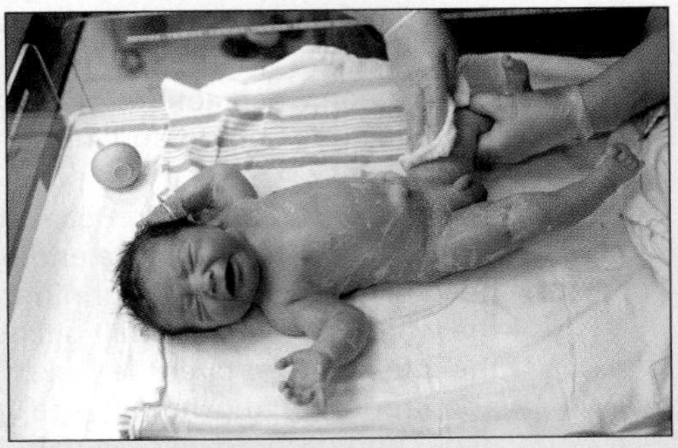
Step 8e. Cleaning the thighs and leg creases.

EVALUATION

- Newborn is bathed without difficulty.
- Newborn experiences no evidence of cold stress.

Medication Administration

U.S. and Canadian newborns routinely receive two medications at birth: intramuscular (IM) vitamin K and an antibiotic agent for eye prophylaxis. Parents may refuse either or both; however, it is important to document the reasons for any refusal and information given to parents about the risks of foregoing recommended treatment. Some facilities have specific forms for parents to sign should they refuse standard procedures recommended for newborn care.

Vitamin K

The nurse should administer vitamin K (phytonadione) within 1 hour of birth (AAP & ACOG, 2002) (Nursing Procedure 20.3). A single parenteral dose of vitamin K prevents vitamin K–deficiency bleeding (VKDB), formerly known as *classic hemorrhagic disease of the newborn* (HDN) (Miller, 2003). Vitamin K is not actually required to make clotting factors. It is required to convert precursor proteins made in the liver into activated proteins with coagulant properties. Fetal vitamin K levels are low because of poor placental transport and because the fetus lacks intestinal flora that synthesize vitamin K. Without administration of vitamin K at birth, bleeding can occur from the gastrointestinal (GI) tract, umbilicus, circumcision site, and any puncture sites in some newborns (Blackburn, 2003).

Vitamin K deficiency may cause unexpected bleeding during the first week of life in apparently healthy newborns. Early VKDB occurs in 0.25% to 1.7% of newborns. Late VKDB occurs primarily in exclusively breastfed infants 2 to 12 weeks old who received no or inadequate neonatal vitamin K prophylaxis. Infants with intestinal malabsorption defects are also at risk. Late VKDB often manifests as sudden central nervous system hemorrhage and occurs in 4.4 to 7.2 per 100,000 births (Motohara et al., 1987; von Kreis & Hanawa, 1993). Oral vitamin K administration at birth decreases this rate to 1.4 to 6.4 per 100,000 births, but parenteral vitamin K administration prevents the development of late VKDB in infants, except for those with severe malabsorption defects (von Kreis & Hanawa, 1993).

TEACHING TIPS 20.1 Newborn Nursing Care

- Practice newborn resuscitation skills before you need them! Palpate the umbilical pulse at the base of the umbilicus at every birth, even if the baby is pink, active, and crying. Estimate the heart rate by palpating the pulse for 3 or 4 seconds. Then double-check your estimation by counting the pulse rate for 6 seconds and multiplying by ten. Competence at palpating the umbilical pulse and quickly estimating a heart rate is important during assessment of a depressed newborn in need of resuscitative measures.
- When using the bulb syringe, suction the **M**outh first, then the **N**ose to prevent aspiration. Remember to suction the mouth first because **M** comes alphabetically before **N.**
- Parents often wish to take a photo of the baby being weighed at admission, with the digital readout of pounds and ounces showing on the scale. The baby will be warm and comfortable for this photo if he is in a warm blanket and placed prone on the scale for this procedure.
- "Dress" the radiant warmer in layers that facilitate the admission and bathing process. Layering your linen on the radiant warmer prevents multiple errands to obtain linen during this busy time.
- Radiant warmer "dressing"
  - Layer 1: A baby blanket covers the mattress
  - Layer 2: Two baby blankets are spread out and ready to wrap the newborn.
  - Layer 3: Two towels are spread out and ready to dry the newborn after bathing.
  - Layer 4: waterproof pad
  - Layer 5: Two baby blankets ready to wrap the newborn after birth
  - Top layer: Two towels ready to dry the newborn at birth.
  - A clean T-shirt and two blankets are folded and set to the side on the warmer, ready to dress the infant after bathing.
  - Admission and bathing supplies are within easy reach or kept in the supply drawer of the warmer.
- Perform the physical assessment in front of parents and talk through what you are seeing, hearing, and touching. Although parents may not understand everything you are doing, they will learn about things they would not have asked about, and many of their other questions will be answered as they listen. Sharing your knowledge increases parental confidence in your ability to care for their baby.
- If the physical assessment reveals a defect or variance in the midline of the body, look carefully for additional midline defects. For example, if a cleft palate is present, look closely for accompanying defects such as a two-vessel umbilical cord, hypospadias, or an imperforate anus.
- Assess degree of jaundice in natural light, near a window if possible. Gently pressing and releasing the tip of the newborn's nose will reveal jaundice on the nose (therefore, on the face), if it is present.

Oral vitamin K has been shown to be as effective as parenteral vitamin K in the prevention of early VKDB (McNinch et al., 1985; O'Connor & Addiego, 1986). Surveillance data from four countries, however, reveal oral prophylaxis failures of 1.2 to 1.8 per 100,000 live births, compared with no reported cases after parenteral administration of vitamin K (Cornelissen et al., 1997). In addition, newborns who receive incomplete oral prophylaxis are at a higher risk for developing late VKDB, with rates of 2 to 4 per 100,000 (Miller, 2003).

Parenteral vitamin K has been investigated as a link to an increased incidence of childhood leukemia. The AAP (1993) has found no association between IM administration of vitamin K and childhood leukemia or other cancers.

Because parenteral vitamin K prevents VKDB in newborns and young infants, the AAP currently recommends parenteral instead of oral vitamin K to newborns (Miller, 2003). Although the Canadian Paediatric Society (CPS) concurs, an option is available for those parents who refuse the IM injection (CPS & College of Family Physicians of Canada, 1997). In cases in which parents refuse parenteral vitamin K, the CPS recommends an oral dose of 2 mg vitamin K with the first feeding. The parenteral form is used for oral administration because that is all that is available. This is repeated at 2 to 4 weeks and 6 to 8 weeks of age. Parents who choose this option are warned that their infants remain at an increased risk for late VKDB.

Even though it is possible that not all newborns require vitamin K, it is difficult to identify which infants require prophylaxis and which do not. Therefore, IM administration of vitamin K remains the standard of practice (AAP & ACOG, 2002; CPS & College of Family Physicians of Canada, 1997).

Eye Prophylaxis

Three topical medications are acceptable for prevention of gonococcal ophthalmia in all infants (AAP & ACOG, 2002).

- Tetracycline (1%)
- Erythromycin (0.5%)
- Ophthalmic solution of povidone-iodine (2.5%)

Within 1 hour of birth, the nurse should deposit a 1- to 2-cm ribbon of sterile ophthalmic ointment into the

NURSING PROCEDURE 20.3

Administering Vitamin K to a Newborn

PURPOSE

To prevent Vitamin K deficiency bleeding in the newborn

ASSESSMENT AND PLANNING

- Assess the newborn for time of birth to ensure that medication is given within 1 hour of birth.
- Check the medical record for the medication and dose ordered.
- Prepare the prescribed dose of medication in the syringe using the appropriate size needle.
- Ensure the environment is well lit.
- Explain the reason for the procedure to the parents.
- Assess the newborn's thigh to determine an appropriate injection site.
- Gather the necessary equipment:
  - Syringe with appropriate size needle attached containing prescribed dose of vitamin K (25-gauge needle recommended)
  - Alcohol wipes
  - Clean gloves
  - Clean cotton balls, gauze pads, or washcloth

IMPLEMENTATION

1. Wash hands and put on clean gloves.
2. Confirm the newborn's identity.
3. Clean the skin of the newborn's thigh with warm water *to reduce maternal body fluids on the skin.*
4. Swaddle the newborn's upper body *to minimize movement and possible injury during injection.*
5. Locate the vastus lateralis muscle and select the injection site.
6. Clean the area with an alcohol wipe working from the center outward in a circular pattern and allow to air dry.
7. Using the nondominant hand, grasp the newborn's thigh *to stabilize it.*
8. Remove the cap from the syringe and quickly insert the needle using a dart-like motion into the selected site at a 90-degree angle.

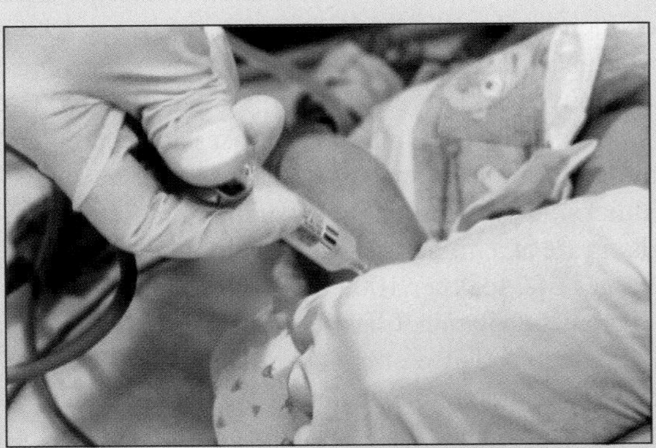

Step 8. Injecting vitamin K IM.

9. Stabilize the syringe with the nondominant hand and pull back on the plunger *to aspirate for blood.*
10. If no blood appears in the syringe, slowly inject the medication; if blood appears, quickly remove the syringe and discard; prepare a new syringe and restart the procedure.
11. When all of the medication has been injected, remove the syringe and cover the site with an alcohol wipe. Apply pressure and massage the site to promote distribution of the drug into the muscle.
12. Inspect the injection site *to check for any signs of bleeding or bruising.*
13. Discard syringe and used equipment appropriately.
14. Document administration on the newborn's medical record.

Continued

NURSING PROCEDURE 20.3
Administering Vitamin K to a Newborn

EVALUATION

- The newborn receives the prescribed vitamin K injection without difficulty.
- Injection site is free of any redness, bruising, or hematoma.
- Newborn tolerates procedure well.

AREAS FOR CONSIDERATION AND ADAPTATION

Lifespan Considerations

- If appropriate, enlist the aid of an additional person, such as support person, parent, or other health care team member *to help contain the newborn and prevent movement that could result in injury during the injection.*
- Keep in mind that a 1-inch needle may be necessary to reach the muscle tissue, depending on the newborn's size.
- Always double-check the dosage to be administered.
- Assess the newborn for signs and symptoms of bleeding, such as tarry stools, hematuria, blood oozing from sites such as the umbilical cord base, and decreased hemoglobin and hematocrit levels. This may indicate the need for additional vitamin K.

Community-Based Considerations

- At the follow-up home visit, question the parents about any possible signs and symptoms of bleeding and notify the health care provider if any occur.
- If the newborn was delivered at home, expect to administer vitamin K as soon as possible after the home birth.

conjunctival sac (Nursing Procedure 20.4). He or she should not irrigate the eyes with sterile water or saline. The nurse should wipe away excess ointment with sterile cotton after 1 minute, if necessary (AAP & ACOG, 2002).

Administration of eye prophylaxis is often challenging. It is nearly impossible to force open the eyelids of a newborn who is crying or lying under bright lights; therefore, the infant should be in a quiet alert state. This behavioral state is most likely in a somewhat upright position under dimmed lights.

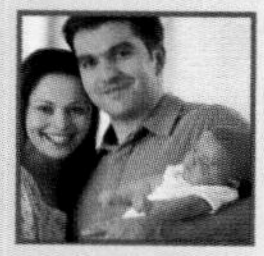

Think back to William, the newborn about to be circumcised. The nurse should check William's medical record to determine whether he has received which medication?

Full Physical Examination

Physical examination begins at birth and continues throughout the hospital stay. Table 20.1 summarizes the complete newborn physical examination, which should occur by 2 hours of age (AAP & ACOG, 2002). Table 20.2 reviews newborn reflexes, and Box 20.2 summarizes an approach to newborn assessment. The astute nurse recognizes signs of abnormalities quickly and intervenes before further compromise develops.

When preparing to participate in the physical examination, the nurse should proceed as follows (Tappero & Honeyfield, 2003):

- Wash your hands before beginning. If parents are present, teach the importance of good handwashing to prevent illness. If the examination takes place before the initial bath, standard precautions mandate that the nurse wear gloves (AAP & ACOG, 2002).
- Gather necessary equipment before beginning.
- Keep the newborn warm. A radiant warmer provides a thermally safe environment and easy access to the exposed newborn. Warm hands and a warm stethoscope help decrease newborn stress.
- Look and listen before touching or handling the infant. Observe posture, muscle tone, color, respiratory efforts, and behavioral state. Listen for expiratory grunting, stridor, or other audible signs of respiratory distress before disturbing the infant.
- Keep the newborn as calm as possible. Start with the least invasive and obtrusive maneuvers (observation,

NURSING PROCEDURE 20.4
Performing Eye Prophylaxis

PURPOSE

To prevent the development of severe eye infections (ophthalmia neonatorum) from gonorrhea or chlamydia

ASSESSMENT AND PLANNING

- Check the newborn's medical record for maternal history of sexually transmitted infections.
- Review the order for prescribed agent and check to ensure that the agent is for ophthalmic use only.
- Assess the newborn's state of reactivity, ensuring that the newborn is in a quiet alert state.
- Explain the rationale for the procedure to the parents.
- Gather equipment.
  - Prescribed sterile ophthalmic ointment
  - Sterile cotton balls or dry sterile gauze pads
  - Clean gloves

IMPLEMENTATION

1. Wash hands and put on gloves.
2. Gently wipe the newborns' face with a soft gauze pad or cotton ball *to dry the face and prevent the hand from slipping.*
3. Open the prescribed ointment, making sure to keep the tip of the tube sterile.
4. Open one eye by gently separating the upper and lower lids, exposing the conjunctiva of the lower lid *to allow placement of the ointment.*
5. Lay a thin ribbon of ointment, approximately 1 to 2 cm in length, along the conjunctival sac, from the inner to outer canthus.
6. Release the eyelids and allow the newborn to close his or her eyes *to permit the ointment to be dispersed within the eye.*
7. After 1 minute, wipe away an excess ointment with a sterile cotton ball or gauze.
8. Repeat the steps with the other eye *to ensure complete prevention.*
9. Document the procedure in the newborn's medical record according to agency policy.

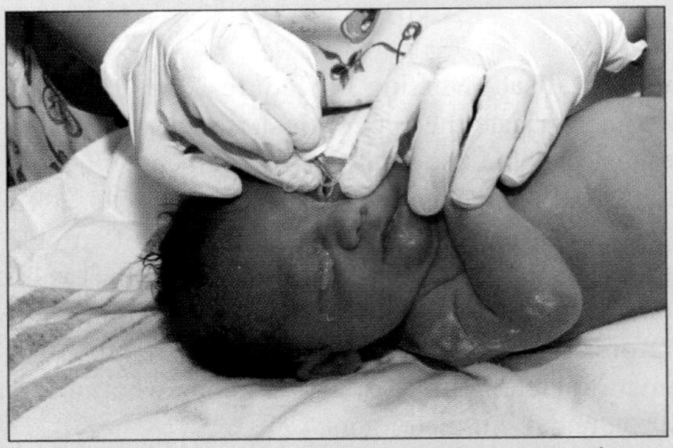

Step 5. Administering antibiotic ointment to the newborn's eye.

EVALUATION

- Ophthalmic ointment was applied to both eyes without difficulty.
- Newborn tolerated procedure without any problems.

AREAS FOR CONSIDERATION AND ADAPTATION

Lifespan Considerations

- Check the specific agency policy for the timing of eye prophylaxis. In some agencies, eye prophylaxis is performed immediately after birth. In other agencies, it may be postponed for

Continued

NURSING PROCEDURE 20.4
Performing Eye Prophylaxis

about 1 hour to allow the parents to bond with their newborn immediately after birth without interference from the ointment, which could blur the newborn's vision.

- If necessary, dim the lights to prevent the newborn from experiencing undue discomfort and upset due to the glare of the lights.
- After instilling the ointment, do not irrigate with eyes with sterile water or saline.

Community-Based Considerations

- When making the first home visit, check with the parents to ensure that the newborn received eye prophylaxis before he or she was discharged.

auscultation); finish with those assessments that may be more upsetting (assessment of Moro reflex). Handle the newborn gently. If parents are present, use teachable moments to point out newborn developmental capabilities.

- Choose a quiet environment for auscultation.
- Establish a routine. Performing the physical assessment approximately the same way each time decreases the risk for forgetting any aspect of the examination.

THE NEWBORN TRANSITIONAL PERIOD

Full-term healthy newborns demonstrate a predictable pattern of behavioral changes, behavioral states and cues, sensory abilities, and physiologic adaptations during the first 6 to 8 hours of life. This time frame is referred to as the *transitional period* (Desmond et al., 1963).

Behavioral Changes

The transitional period is divided into an initial period of reactivity and inactivity and a second period of reactivity. Time periods vary depending on labor management, maternal medications, and initial feeding (Bakewell-Sachs et al., 1997).

Initial Period of Reactivity

The initial period of reactivity occurs in the first 30 to 60 minutes of life and is characterized by an alert, intensely exploratory newborn. At this time, the healthy term newborn is fully alert and active and has a strong desire to suck. This period is optimal to give the newborn the opportunity to breastfeed for the first time. It also is good for interaction (Fig. 20.13). The nurse can facilitate parent–child eye contact by minimizing unnecessary bright lights and delaying installation of prophylactic eye medication.

Adaptation to extrauterine life allows for wide swings in normal parameters. The newborn may be tachypneic (up to 80 breaths per minute) and tachycardic (up to 180 bpm). The nurse may observe mild to moderate chest wall retractions, nasal flaring, and expiratory grunting; he or she may hear crackles. The nurse may note **periodic breathing** (pauses in breathing of less than 15 seconds). **Acrocyanosis** (bluish hands and feet) is also normal (see Table 20.4, given later). Bowel sounds are active.

Abnormal transition may be manifested by any signs of increasing distress instead of steady resolution. Signs that require immediate intervention include central cyanosis; apnea greater than 15 seconds, especially if accompanied by pallor, cyanosis, or bradycardia (heart rate less than 100 bpm); asymmetric chest wall movement; unequal breath sounds; excessive salivation or mucus; and hypotonia or lethargy.

Period of Relative Inactivity

This period occurs 2 to 3 hours after birth. The newborn becomes less interested in external stimuli and falls asleep for a few minutes to several hours. The baby becomes less responsive. During deep sleep, the baby is difficult to arouse. Feeding is difficult if not impossible. Heart rate should stabilize at 120 to 140 bpm; respiratory rate decreases to 40 to 60 breaths per minute. The newborn should be centrally pink with clear breath sounds and show no signs of respiratory distress. The temperature may fall.

Second Period of Reactivity

The second period of reactivity lasts approximately 4 to 6 hours and begins when the newborn fully awakens from the first sleep. He or she is alert and responsive once again. Heart and respiratory rates may increase but should remain within normal limits. The newborn may pass urine and his or her first meconium.

Behavioral States

Assessment of infant state enables caregivers to measure the newborn's response to external stimuli and to interpret

(text continues on page 817)

TABLE 20.1 Physical Examination of the Newborn

ASSESSMENT AREA AND TECHNIQUE	NORMAL FINDINGS	NORMAL VARIATIONS	SIGNIFICANT DEVIATIONS*
General Appearance			
Color	Consistent with genetic background; pink mucous membranes Mottled with cooling Bruises over presenting part	Pigmentation: pink, ruddy especially over face; olive; yellowish-pink; black **Acrocyanosis** (blue palms and soles) **Circumoral cyanosis** (blue around mouth): normal for first 24 hours, then evaluate **Jaundice** (yellow skin color): mild jaundice normal after day 1 of life **Harlequin color change** (in side-lying position, red color demarcated on dependent side, pale color on upper half; persists 1–30 minutes; color reverses if infant is rotated to other side)	**Pallor** (gray color could indicate hypotension) **Plethora** (deep red color could denote polycythemia) **Central cyanosis** (blue trunk, lips, mucous membranes denote hypoxia) **Jaundice,** especially in first 24 hours of life
Respiratory effort	Diaphragmatic and abdominal breathing Rate: 40–60 breaths/min; may decrease in deep sleep and increase after crying Periodic breathing: pauses in breathing up to 20 seconds without bradycardia or color change	Expiratory **grunting, nasal flaring,** and mild **retracting** in initial part of transition (with rapid resolution)	**Grunting, flaring, retracting** that worsens or does not resolve quickly in transition **Apnea** (cessation of breathing > 20 seconds with decreased heart rate and color change to pale or dusky) **Gasping** (intermittent rapid inhalation) **Stridor** (high-pitched sound during breathing indicates obstruction)
Tone/neuromuscular	Term infant flexed, fists clenched Term infant with healthy tone can be pulled up to sitting position using elicited palmar grasp reflex Head moves side to side Moves all extremities Moves smoothly between behavioral states (term infant)	Mild tremors with startling Frank breech: extended legs for brief time	Marked jitteriness (could indicate low blood glucose level) Tremors that continue when care provider touches or holds area (suspect seizure activity); marked hypertonia or extension Marked hypotonia
Gestational Age (see gestational assessment information on pages 798–803)			
VITAL SIGNS: **Temperature** (broad range of normal; standard varies regionally)			Fever is rare sign of infection; unstable temperature in stable environment is more worrisome. **Hyperthermia** or **hypothermia** is stressful and dangerous; requires evaluation of etiology such as environmental threat, sepsis, or neurologic abnormality
● Axillary (preferred)	36.5°–37.3°C or 97.5°–99.1°F		
● Skin (usually used for special care infant)	36°–36.5°C or 96.8°–97.5°F (term) 36.2°–37.2°C or 97.2°–98.7°F (preterm)		
● Rectal (not preferred, risky)	36.5°–37.5°C or 97.5°–99.5°F		
● Tympanic (not recommended)			
Heart rate (apical)	120–160 bpm; increases with and after crying	Term infant's heart rate may increase to 180 bpm during crying and decrease to 80–100 bpm during deep sleep.	**Bradycardia** (persistent resting rate < 100 bpm, unless term in deep sleep without distress) **Tachycardia** (resting rate 180–200 bpm) Persistent irregular rhythm

Continued

TABLE 20.1 Physical Examination of the Newborn

ASSESSMENT AREA AND TECHNIQUE	NORMAL FINDINGS	NORMAL VARIATIONS	SIGNIFICANT DEVIATIONS*
Respiratory rate	Shallow, irregular 40–60 breaths/min; may decrease when in deep sleep and increase after crying **Periodic breathing** (a series of respirations followed by a pause of up to 20 seconds)	Transient **tachypnea** (fast rate) after stress or crying Rate may slow when sleeping.	**Tachypnea** (resting respiratory rate > 60 breaths/min) **Bradypnea** (respiratory rate < 25–30 breaths/min) **Apnea** (cessation of breathing > 15 seconds with decreased heart rate and color change to pale or dusky) **Gasping** (intermittent rapid inhalation)
Blood pressure not routinely required; oscillometric measurement preferred	Varies with weight, gestational age, and infant state; approximately 78/42 mm Hg		**Capillary refill time** > 3 seconds: press on skin of trunk until it blanches and count seconds until color returns Weak pulses Pallor, gray color Mottling Cool skin
Measurements: **Weight**	Varies with genetic composition 2500–3800 g (5 lbs, 8 oz to 8 lbs, 6 oz)	Weight, length, and OFC must be assessed with gestational age to determine whether the newborn is SGA, AGA, or LGA. An infant is classified as SGA, AGA, or LGA *and* preterm, term, or postterm.	
Length	45–52 cm (17–22 inches)		
OFC (occipital-frontal circumference)	32–37 cm (12.5–14.5 inches)		
Chest circumference (not routinely required)	30–35 cm (12–14 inches)	Usually 2 cm smaller than the OFC; however, cranial molding can influence OFC and chest measurements.	
Skin	Soft, smooth, elastic Hydrated skin springs back into shape if pinched Initially edematous Flaky and dry by day 2–3 **Vernix caseosa** (greasy yellow-white substance) **Lanugo** (fine hair on cheeks, shoulders, forehead, pinna of ears) **Milia** (tiny white papules on brow, cheeks, nose) **Erythema toxicum** or "**newborn rash**" (small white or yellow papules on a red base; lasts several hours to several days) **Sucking blisters** (vesicles on lips, hands from in utero or postnatal sucking) **Stork bite or nevus simplex** (pink macule on nape of neck, upper eyelids, bridge of nose or upper lip that usually fades)	**Meconium staining** (cord, nails, skin may be stained greenish-brown from meconium-stained amniotic fluid) **Forceps marks** on cheek(s) Petechiae over presenting part **Port wine nevus** (flat pink or purple lesion on white skin and solid black on black skin, usually on face; does not blanch, grow, or fade) **Mongolian spots or hyperpigmented macule** (bluish or gray-blue areas of pigmentation on dorsum and buttocks) commonly found on Asian, African, or dark-skinned races. **Café-au-lait patches** (less than six) Pigmented nevus (dark brown or black macule) **Strawberry hemangioma** (bright red, raised, soft, grows then regresses over years; most appear by 6 mo of age)	Loose, wrinkled skin may indicate growth aberration or dehydration. Widespread **petechiae** not associated with presenting part Rash, especially if vesicular **Skin tags** (depending on positioning and associated physical findings) **Webbing** of hands, feet **Laceration** infrequently occurs during cesarean birth. More than 6 **café-au-lait** patches may indicate **neurofibromatosis.**

Continued

TABLE 20.1 Physical Examination of the Newborn *(Continued)*

ASSESSMENT AREA AND TECHNIQUE	NORMAL FINDINGS	NORMAL VARIATIONS	SIGNIFICANT DEVIATIONS*
Head	Fontanels: Anterior palpated as 5-cm diamond Posterior palpated as smaller triangle Palpate sutures; should be unjoined Generally symmetric shape Full range of motion	Cranial **molding and asymmetry,** difficulty palpating fontanels and suture lines because of molding **Scalp lesion or abrasion** (from scalp electrode, vacuum extractor) **Cephalhematoma** (hematoma between periosteum and skull bone; raised lump does not cross suture lines and resolves in months) **Caput succedaneum** (tissue swelling may cross suture lines and resolves quickly) **Petechiae** (if breech birth or cord around neck) **Torticollis** (head held immobile at angle) Hispanic babies may have low hairline over forehead and down neck	Severe molding, especially if accompanied by abnormal transition Indentation on cranium (fracture) Full, bulging fontanels Remarkable pulsation of fontanels Unusually large or small head in relation to body size Unusual hair pattern or texture
Eyes	Eyes placed at same level Eyelids above pupils but within iris Edema in first days of life Lashes and eyebrows present Eyes open and eyeballs present Eyes move freely, fix, and follow Eyes close in response to bright light Blinking present Occasional **strabismus** (crossed eyes) Slight **nystagmus** (involuntary eye movements) Blue color in light-skinned baby and brown color in dark-skinned baby (eye color established at approximately 3 months)	**Subconjunctival hemorrhage** (red spot on sclera; resolves) Slightly blue sclera No tears when crying	Unusually wide set eyes Eyes never seen open, even in dim light Constant strabismus, nystagmus, or both Purulent drainage Ulceration Unusual lashes (absent, bushy, unusually long) Upward slant in non-Asian (may indicate Down syndrome) Jaundiced sclera (hyperbilirubinemia)
Ears	Well-formed cartilage Visibly open auditory canal Placement: line drawn through inner and outer canthi of eye lines up with top notch of ear Responds to voices, loud noises when awake	**Darwin's tubercle** (nodule on posterior helix)	**Preauricular skin tag,** especially if accompanied by other variances **Sinus tract** near ear Low-set ears (may require assessment after cranial molding has resolved) Abnormal ear attachment to head
Nose	Midline placement Normal breathing when mouth is closed Frequent sneezing	Asymmetric appearance because of birth trauma	Cyanosis or respiratory distress when mouth is closed (**choanal atresia**) **Nasal flaring** (respiratory distress) Persistent or marked nasal drainage Unusual nose, such as pointed or upturned

Continued

TABLE 20.1 Physical Examination of the Newborn

ASSESSMENT AREA AND TECHNIQUE	NORMAL FINDINGS	NORMAL VARIATIONS	SIGNIFICANT DEVIATIONS*
Mouth and Throat	Symmetric movement of mouth Coordinated breathing, sucking, and swallowing during feeding Pink gums Free-moving tongue Sucking pads inside cheeks Dome-shaped hard palate Midline, single uvula Lusty cry of moderate pitch and tone	Sucking blisters on lips **Epstein's pearls** (small white epithelial cysts) on hard palate	Mouth pulls to one side (asymmetric strength or movement) **Cleft palate** (hard or soft palate) Large or deeply ridged tongue Excessive drooling; frequent choking (evaluate for esophageal atresia or tracheoesophageal fistula) Shrill, weak, or absent cry Cheesy coating on tongue that does not wipe off or bleeds when wiped (indicative of oral thrush—*Candida albicans*) Teeth (may be predeciduous or deciduous): aspiration risk if loose Small jaw and recessive chin, especially if accompanied by respiratory distress (Robin syndrome)
Neck	Short, straight Creased anterior Clavicles intact Head held in midline with free range of motion	Fractured clavicle(s) from difficult birth: popping or crackling felt or heard when palpated	Abnormally short neck Hyperextended or arched neck Webbing (Turner's syndrome) Excessive skin folds Hypotonia (no head control)
Chest	Circular, barrel shape Symmetric respiratory movement Well-formed, symmetric nipples Clear, bilateral breath sounds	Xiphoid cartilage (lower end of sternum) may protrude Supernumerary (extra) nipples Breast enlargement (from maternal hormones) **"Witch's milk"** (milky substance from breast) Rales normal first few hours of life	**Intercostal and/or sternal retractions** (ribs and/or sternum suck inward with inhalation due to use of accessory muscles during respiratory distress) Decreased or asymmetric breath sounds, especially with respiratory distress
Heart **(see also Vital Signs section)**	**PMI** (point of maximal impulse) heard lateral to midclavicular line at 3rd or 4th intercostal space **Regular rate and rhythm**	Heart murmur without accompanying symptoms	PMI shifted to right or left, especially if accompanied by respiratory distress (**pneumothorax**) Distant heart sounds Extra heart sound(s) PMI on right side of chest (**pneumothorax** or **dextrocardia**) Dysrhythmia (irregular rate), tachycardia, bradycardia Heart murmur with accompanying symptoms such as edema, irregular rate/rhythm, pallor or duskiness, respiratory distress, other anomalies **Audible bowel sounds in chest, especially if accompanied by respiratory distress** (diaphragmatic hernia)
Abdomen	Cylindrical and protruding Abdominal skin color congruent with genetic background Soft bowel sounds present 1 to 2 hours after birth No protrusion of umbilicus (*Note: palpation of liver and kidneys is not considered a nursing assessment activity in some settings.*)		**Scaphoid** (sunken) abdomen (diaphragmatic hernia) Bowel sounds in chest (diaphragmatic hernia) Palpable masses or bulges front or back Marked distention, shiny appearance, or visible bowel loops Inaudible bowel sounds Projectile vomiting

Continued

TABLE 20.1 Physical Examination of the Newborn *(Continued)*

ASSESSMENT AREA AND TECHNIQUE	NORMAL FINDINGS	NORMAL VARIATIONS	SIGNIFICANT DEVIATIONS*
	Liver palpable 1–2 cm below right costal margin at mid-clavicular line (use caution) A healthy spleen is not normally palpable. Kidneys are difficult to palpate; left more evident than right. Femoral pulses palpable, equal, bilateral Two arteries and one vein visible at birth		Bilious (greenish) vomit Failure to pass meconium in 48 hours Hyperperistalsis or visible peristalsis (bowel obstruction) Absent or diminished femoral pulses (coarctation of aorta). Suspect coarctation if four-limb blood pressure demonstrates upper extremities systolic pressure is > 20 points higher than systolic of lower extremities.
Umbilicus	No intestinal structures visible inside cord Drying without bleeding, odor	Protruding umbilicus common in black babies Yellow-green staining of cord (from meconium-stained amniotic fluid)	Two vessel umbilical cord (single artery) Bleeding around cord Red or swollen umbilical area Purulent drainage from umbilical area **Omphalocele** (abdominal contents herniated into area of cord) **Gastroschisis** (abdominal contents herniated through abdominal wall)
Extremities	Term baby assumes in utero flexed positioning Symmetric full range of motion Extension limited Muscle tone congruent with gestational age Ten fingers, ten toes appropriately spaced Dry flaky hands and feet Flat sole of foot Fingernails and toenails present Fists clenched	Positional deformities (usually resolve) Polydactyly (extra digits) may be familial. **Simian crease** (single horizontal crease across palm) sometimes found in normal infants; also related to Down syndrome	Absent movement Asymmetric movement, strength, or range of motion Hypotonia Hyperflexion Limited range of motion Hypermobility of joints Polydactyly (extra digits) or syndactyly (webbed digits), especially if accompanied by additional anomalies Short fingers, incurved little finger, low-set thumb, and a simian crease (suggests Down syndrome) Persistent cyanotic nail beds Suspect dislocated or **subluxated** hip: Limited hip abduction, Unequal gluteal or leg folds, Unequal knee height, Positive Ortolani's sign (audible clunk on hip abduction)
Genitalia	First void within 24 hours (most babies) to 48 hours (all babies) of birth Urine has mild odor	Rust-stained urine (uric acid crystals)	**Ambiguous genitalia** (sex not clearly discernible from visible anatomy) Failure to void within 48 hours of birth Foul-smelling or bloody urine
MALE	Slender penis, 2.5 cm long Urethral meatus at tip of penis Voids within 24 hours with adequate stream and volume Foreskin adheres to glans and tight 2–3 months Erection possible because of erectile tissue Scrotal skin can be loose or tight	Scrotal bruising and edema if breech birth **Epithelial pearls** (small, firm, white lesion at tip of penis)	Undescended testes (may be in inguinal, femoral, perineal, or abdominal areas) **Hydrocele** (enlarged scrotum due to fluid Discolored testes **Hypospadias** (urinary meatus on ventral surface of penis) **Epispadias** (urinary meatus on dorsal surface of penis) Fecal discharge from penis

Continued

● **TABLE 20.1 Physical Examination of the Newborn**

ASSESSMENT AREA AND TECHNIQUE	NORMAL FINDINGS	NORMAL VARIATIONS	SIGNIFICANT DEVIATIONS*
	Rugae consistent with gestation Two palpable testes Testes descended but not consistently in scrotum Smegma		
FEMALE	Edema common Development of labia consistent with gestational age Clitoris usually large Area pigment consistent with genetic background Smegma, vernix present Open vaginal orifice Urinary meatus difficult to see Mucoid discharge Bloody discharge (**pseudomenses** from maternal hormones)	Area bruised if breech birth Vaginal tag (usually disappears in first month of life)	Absent vaginal orifice Fecal discharge from vagina
Back	Spine straight, no openings, masses Term infant can raise and support head for a moment when prone Symmetric buttocks Patent single anus Meconium stool followed by transitional, then soft, yellow stool		Limited movement or flexion Nevus with tuft of hair along spine (associated with **spina bifida**) Sinus anywhere along spine **Meningocele** (lesion associated with spina bifida where meninges protrude through vertebral defect, covered by thin atrophic skin). **Myelomeningocele** (lesion associated with spina bifida, most often in the lumbar spine, characterized by protrusion of meninges, spinal roots, and nerves, remnants of spinal cord fusion and exposed neural tube). No meconium passage in first 48 hr No anus **Imperforate** anus Anal fissures or fistulas

*Conditions noted in this column require further assessment and evaluation. Some conditions, such as central cyanosis or gastroschisis, require immediate life-saving interventions, including support of ventilation and oxygenation, thermoregulation, perfusion, and metabolic needs. Other conditions listed in this column are less urgent, but still require evaluation and special care. See Chapter 22 for a more complete discussion of selected high-risk neonatal topics.

physiologic and behavioral changes. The caregiver assesses infant state to evaluate the newborn's ability to control it, move smoothly from one state to another, and maintain alertness (Tappero & Honeyfield, 2003).

Brazelton's Neonatal Behavioral Assessment Scale (NBAS) describes two sleep and four awake states (Brazelton, 1978): deep sleep, light sleep, drowsy, quiet alert, active alert, and crying. Table 20.3 describes characteristics of each state and the implications for caregiving and interaction. Full-term, healthy newborns should move easily from one state to another and eventually demonstrate a unique and organized pattern of control. The nurse should assess state as an indicator of overall well-being and central nervous system integrity (Tappero & Honeyfield, 2003).

The nurse should teach parents infant states to help them identify their newborn's unique characteristics and to facilitate optimal interactions. For example, the parent should be able to recognize the light sleep state as one in which the newborn is asleep but may make brief fussy sounds. The parent who recognizes this state knows to wait until the infant is more fully awake before interpreting these sounds as meaning that the baby is ready to interact or feed. The parent who does not recognize light

● **TABLE 20.2 Developmental Reflexes in the Newborn**

NAME OF REFLEX	FIGURE	TO ELICIT REFLEX	EXPECTED NEONATAL RESPONSE	DISAPPEARANCE
Moro	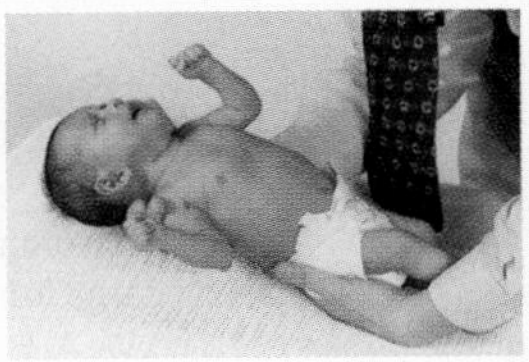	Hold the infant supine with the head a few inches above the mattress. Remove the hand supporting the infant's head and allow the head to fall back onto mattress.	Infant first extends and abducts the arms and opens the hands. Then the arms adduct with some flexion and closing of the fists. The infant may cry.	12 mo
Palmar grasp	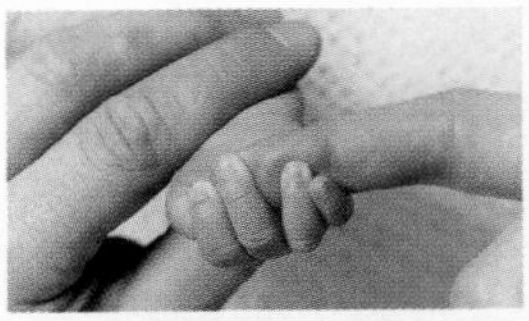	Press the palmar surface of the infant's hand with a finger.	Infant grasps the finger and holds tighter with attempts to withdraw. Full-term neonate can support full body weight if lifted slightly.	2 mo
Rooting	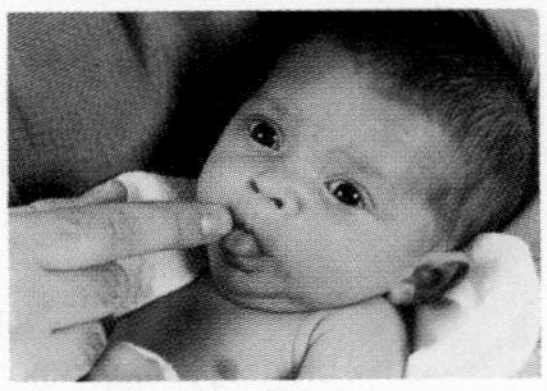	Stroke the infant's cheek and corner of the mouth.	The infant's head turns toward the stimulus and the mouth opens.	3–4 mo
Stepping	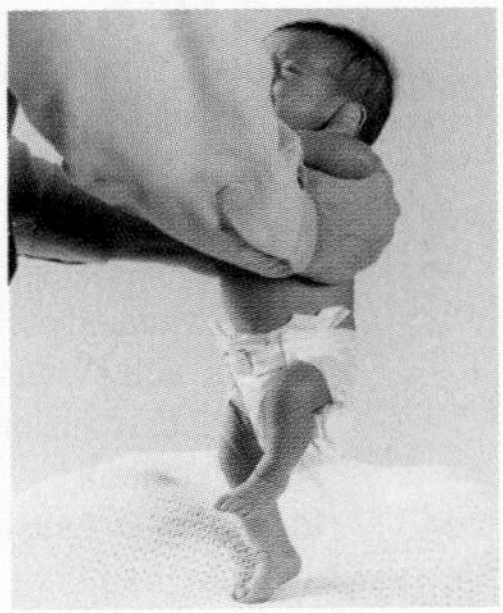	Hold the infant upright and touch the soles of the feet to a flat surface.	Infant makes alternating stepping movements.	3–4 mo
Sucking	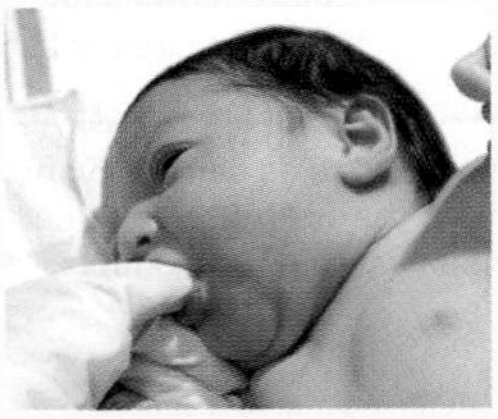	Touch or stroke the baby's lips.	Mouth opens and sucking movements begin.	12 mo
Tonic neck	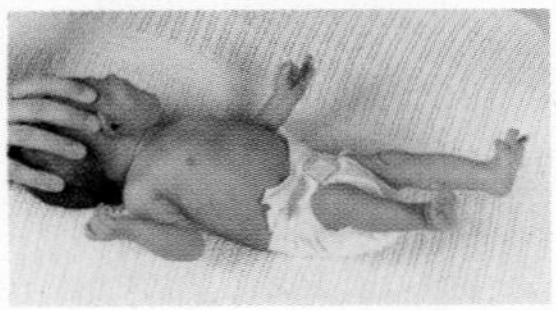	Place infant supine and turn his or her head to one side.	Infant extends the arm on the side in which the head is turned and flexes the upper extremity on the opposite side (fencing position).	7 mo
Truncal incurvation (Galant)	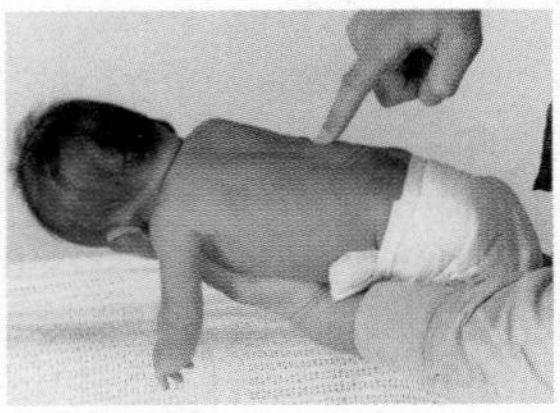	Hold infant prone, in suspended position, with palm of hand against infant's chest. Apply firm pressure with the thumb or cotton swab parallel to the spine in the thoracic region.	The infant flexes the pelvis toward the side of the stimulus.	3–4 mo

BOX 20.2 A Sample Approach to Newborn Physical Examination

This box describes one method of organizing the newborn physical examination reviewed in Table 20.1 as a guide for inexperienced examiners. With practice, each examiner develops a personal style. It is assumed that the infant is unclothed and supine under a radiant warmer.

Observation

It can be very difficult for a practitioner to just stand at the crib and observe an infant. The immediate inclination is to touch and talk to the infant. The practitioner must delay this natural response until later in the examination, however, because observation alone produces important information about every organ system. These initial observations allow the practitioner to develop a visual differential diagnosis before employing other assessment techniques.

If these multiple observations prove normal, the examiner is less likely to find a significant abnormality upon auscultation and palpation. Each observation of normality serves to reassure the examiner—just as an observation of abnormality should heighten the examiner's suspicion that further inspection is necessary.

Observation is not an isolated technique for use only at the outset of the examination. Although spending a moment or two observing the infant at the bedside before touching him or her is important, observation of the infant's responses takes place throughout the assessment. The examiner must learn to take advantage of every opportunity the infant's behavior offers for observation. If, for example, the infant awakens spontaneously during the examination, the practitioner should use that opportunity to examine the baby's eyes.

Hands-on inspection includes measurements and tactile inspection of the skin. It also includes maneuvers to assess symmetry and reflexes.

Auscultation

After observing the infant closely, many examiners next auscultate the chest, heart, and abdomen. To separate the sounds of the heart from those of the lungs, concentration is important. Listen first to one type of sound, then to the other. For example, listen first to the heart—its rate, rhythm, regularity, and any added sounds. Then listen to breath sounds, ignoring the cardiac sounds.

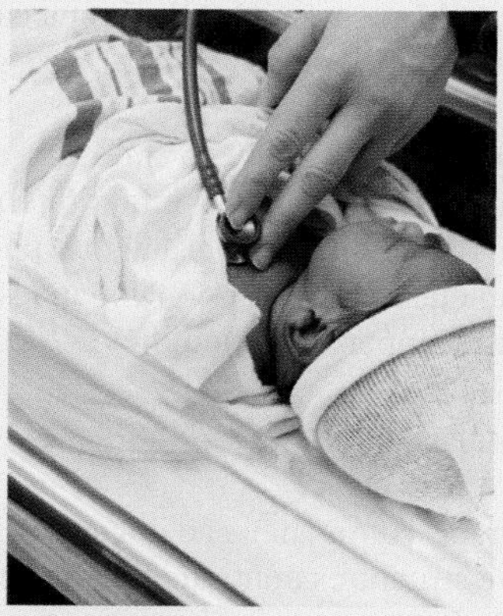

Auscultating the newborn's lungs.

Palpation

Continue with palpation. Palpating certain parts of the body disturbs the infant more than others. An ordered approach keeps the infant calm through much of the process.

Because femoral pulses are difficult to assess in a crying infant, palpate them first. Then palpate the brachial pulses. Next palpate the abdomen, beginning with the more superficial liver and spleen. (Learning to palpate the liver and spleen with the tips of the fingers as well as the lateral edges of the index fingers facilitates examination from either side of the bassinet.) Palpate for abdominal masses; then use deeper palpation for the kidneys. At this point, the infant may be disturbed and crying, but this will not impede the remainder of the examination.

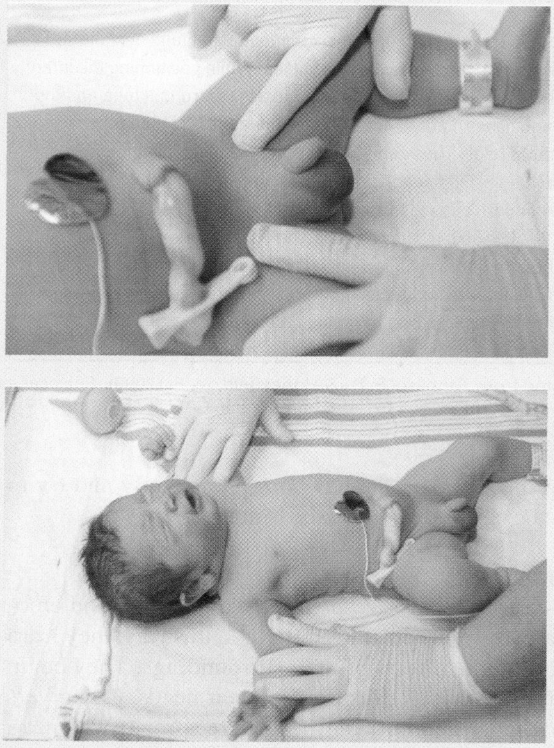

Top: Palpating the femoral pulse. **Bottom:** Palpating the brachial pulse.

The Integrated Examination

The skilled examiner integrates examination tasks. For example, after palpating the head, neck, clavicles, arms, and hands, he or she can perform the pull-to-sit maneuver to assess palmar grasp, arm strength, and tone. At that point, the clinician is holding the infant in an appropriate position to elicit the Moro

Continued

BOX 20.2 A Sample Approach to Newborn Physical Examination (*Continued*)

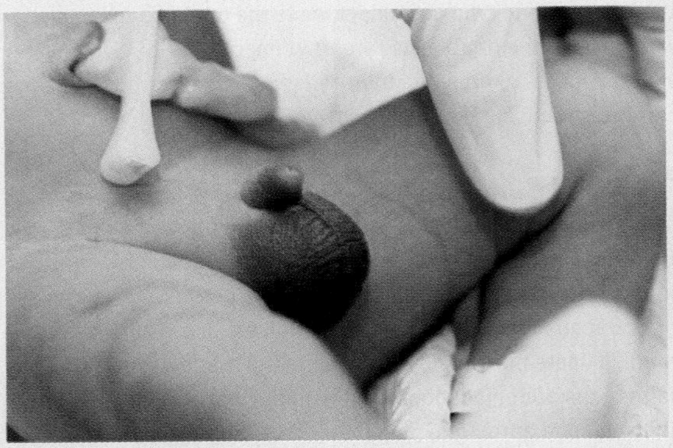

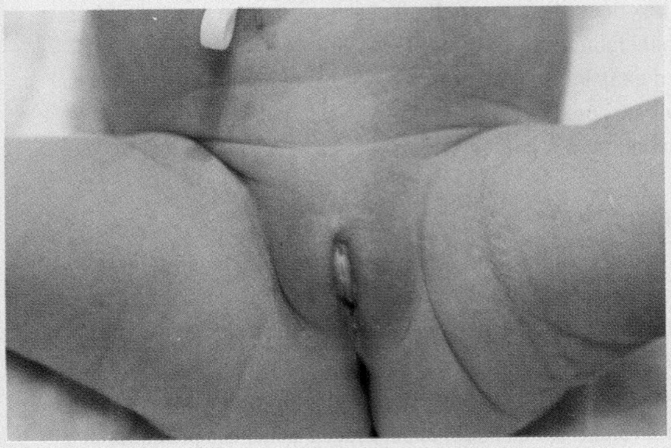

Left: Male newborn genitalia. **Right:** Female newborn genitalia.

reflex. The practitioner can examine the genitalia next, before progressing to the lower extremities. While positioning the infant prone on the practitioner's hand to assess truncal tone and the truncal incurvation reflex, the examiner also can check the baby's back. These shortcuts facilitate multiple inspections and save time. Examination of the hips should be last because this procedure causes the most stress to the infant.

It is usually not necessary to assess reflexes separately. The examiner will most likely have observed root and suck by this point. He or she can incorporate Moro and palmar grasp into the upper extremity examination, as just explained.

Although an extremely cooperative infant may sleep through the entire process, the assessment is not complete until the infant has been observed through the various behavioral states. Facial asymmetry, for example, cannot be seen until the infant cries.

Ideally, the parents should observe the first complete examination. They appreciate demonstration of their infant's normality and uniqueness as well as early identification of unusual or abnormal findings.

Adapted from Tappero, E. P., & Honeyfield, M. E. (2003). *Physical assessment of the newborn: A comprehensive approach to the art of physical examination* (3rd ed.). Santa Rosa, CA: NICU INK Book Publishers.

sleep may awaken the newborn prematurely and try to feed the child when he or she is not ready.

Behavioral Cues

Full-term newborns respond physiologically and emotionally to environmental stimuli. In this way, they learn to control the effects of their surroundings. They begin to display various cues to meet their needs. Caregivers who respond appropriately develop reciprocity with newborns and reinforce behavioral organization (Tappero & Honeyfield, 2003).

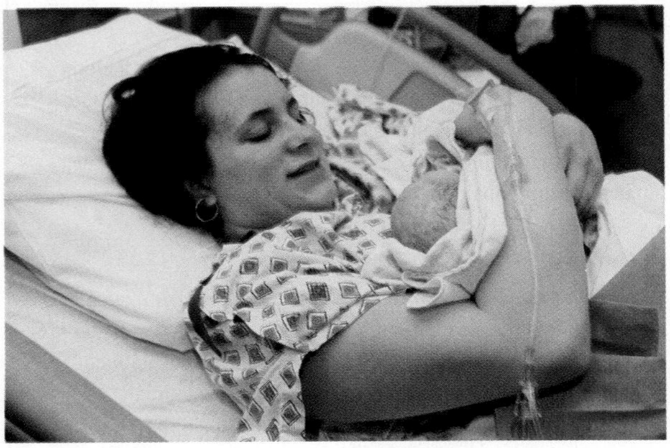

FIGURE 20.13 Maternal–infant bonding during a period of reactivity.

Behavioral cues consist of approach and avoidance cues (Box 20.3). **Approach cues** indicate a readiness to interact with the environment. **Avoidance cues** (time-out signals) indicate that the newborn is tired or overstimulated and needs a break from interaction. The caregiver who proceeds with interaction may exceed the infant's sensory threshold, meaning that the infant cannot respond appropriately and displays signs of stress and fatigue (Tappero & Honeyfield, 2003).

Parents who learn how to interpret their infant's behavior have stronger parent–infant interaction during the first year of life. The newborn whose parents respond to behavioral cues can better control and respond to the environment (Tappero & Honeyfield, 2003).

Neonatal Sensory Abilities

Vision

Healthy term newborns have adequate visual abilities at birth, but eye structures continue to mature over the first 6 months. At birth, newborns can fix on an object and track its movement. They can see objects up to 2½ feet away but prefer high-contrast or highly contoured objects 8 to 12 inches away (Blackburn, 2003). It is interesting to

TABLE 20.3 Infant States and Implications for Caregiving

STATE	BODY ACTIVITY	EYE MOVEMENTS	FACIAL MOVEMENTS	BREATHING PATTERN	LEVEL OF RESPONSE	IMPLICATIONS FOR CAREGIVING
Sleep States						
Quiet (deep) sleep	Nearly still, except for occasional startle or twitch	None	Without facial movements, except for occasional sucking movement at regular intervals	Smooth and regular	Threshold to stimuli very high so that only very intense and disturbing stimuli will arouse	Caregivers trying to feed infants in quiet sleep will probably find the experience frustrating. Infants will be unresponsive, even if caregivers use disturbing stimuli to arouse infants. Infants may arouse only briefly and then become unresponsive as they return to quiet sleep. If caregivers wait until infants move to a higher, more responsive state, feeding or caregiving will be much more pleasant.
Active (light) sleep	Some body movements	Rapid eye movement (REM); fluttering of eyes beneath closed eyelids	May smile and make brief fussy or crying sounds	Irregular	More responsive to internal and external stimuli; when these stimuli occur, infants may remain in active sleep, return to quiet sleep, or arouse to drowsy	Active sleep makes up the highest proportion of newborn sleep and usually precedes awakening. Because of brief fussy or crying sounds made during this state, caregivers who are not aware that these sounds occur normally may think it is time for feeding and may try to feed infants before they are ready to eat.
Awake States						
Drowsy	Activity level variable, with mild startles interspersed from time to time; movements usually smooth	Eyes open and close occasionally; are heavy lidded with dull, glazed appearance	May have some facial movements but often there are none and the face appears still	Irregular	Infants react to sensory stimuli, although responses are delayed; state change after stimulation frequently noted	From the drowsy state, infants may return to sleep or awaken further. To awaken, caregivers can provide something for infants to see, hear, or suck, as this may arouse them to a quiet alert state, a more responsive state. Infants who are left alone without stimuli may return to a sleep state.
Quiet alert	Minimal	Brightening and widening of eyes	Faces have bright, shining, sparkling looks	Regular	Infants attend most to the environment, focusing attention on any stimuli that are present	Infants in this state provide much pleasure and positive feedback for caregivers. Providing something for infants to see, hear, or suck will often maintain a quiet alert state. In the first few hours after birth, most newborns commonly experience a period of intense alertness before going into a long sleep period.
Active alert	Much body activity; may have periods of fussiness	Eyes open with less brightening	Much facial movement; faces not as bright as in quiet alert state.	Irregular	Increasingly sensitive to disturbing stimuli (hunger, fatigue, noise, excessive handling)	Crying is the infant's communication signal. It is a response to unpleasant stimuli from the environment or within infants (eg, fatigue, hunger, discomfort). Crying says that infants' limits have been reached. Sometimes infants can console themselves and return to lower states. At other times, they need help from caregivers.
Crying	Increased motor activity with color changes	Eyes may be tightly closed or open	Grimaces		Extremely responsive to unpleasant external or internal stimuli	Caregivers may need to intervene at this state to console and bring the infant to a lower state.

Source: Blackburn, S. T. (2003). *Maternal, fetal, and neonatal physiology: A clinical perspective* (2nd ed.). St. Louis: Elsevier.

BOX 20.3 Approach and Avoidance Cues

Signs of Attention (Approach)

- Dilated pupils
- Focused gaze
- Hand-to-mouth movements
- Quiet alert state
- Reaching or grasping
- Regular heart rate
- Regular respirations
- Rhythmic sucking

Signs of Overstimulation (Time-Out)

- Apnea
- Arching
- Finger splaying
- Frowning
- Fussing, crying
- Gaze aversion
- Heart rate changes
- Hiccuping
- Increased oxygen requirement
- Irregular respirations
- Mottled skin
- Sneezing
- Stiffening
- Vomiting
- Yawning

From Tappero, E. P., & Honeyfield, M. E. (2003). *Physical assessment of the newborn: A comprehensive approach to the art of physical examination* (3rd ed., p. 165). Santa Rosa, CA: NICU INK Book Publishers.

note that the traditional cradle hold positions a newborn perfectly for focusing on the adult's face.

Hearing

Healthy term newborns hear best in the low and mid-range frequencies but prefer high intonation and rhythmic vocalizations. They can recognize and will turn the head in response to their mother's voice. They react negatively to loud or offensive noises (Blackburn, 2003).

Newborn hearing loss is the most common diagnosable defect at birth (AAP, 1999a; Hyde, 2005). Auditory screening before hospital discharge is discussed later.

Smell

Sense of smell is fairly well developed in healthy term newborns, enabling them to detect and identify various odors. Breastfed newborns can differentiate the odor of their mother's breast pad from pads soaked in water or from another woman (Blackburn, 2003; Tappero & Honeyfield, 2003). Newborns grimace, sniff, or startle in response to strong odors (eg, anise, mint) (Tappero & Honeyfield, 2003).

Touch

The fetus responds to touch as early as 2 months' gestational age; by birth, the sense of touch is well developed (Vanhatalo, 2000). Tactile stimulation such as rubbing the baby's back, trunk, or extremities with a towel or flicking the soles of the feet helps initiate respirations at birth (Kattwinkel, 2006).

Taste

The fetus has taste receptors by 16 weeks' gestation and a full complement of taste receptors by term. Newborns can discriminate different tastes; for example, they prefer glucose water over sterile water (Lecanuet & Schaal, 1996).

Physiologic Adaptations

During the stabilization–transition period (AAP & ACOG, 2002), the newborn makes dramatic adaptations to extrauterine life. Thorough assessment is required to monitor his or her progress and to identify abnormalities. This section presents the adaptations made in several body systems and is followed by an explanation of collaborative care for the areas discussed.

Thermoregulation

The uterine environment maintains fetal body temperature approximately 0.5°C (0.9°F) higher than maternal body temperature. At birth, the newborn may lose heat through evaporation at a rate of 0.5°F per minute (skin temperature) (Blackburn, 2003). Maintenance of normal body temperature is critical to survival. A large ratio of surface area to body mass and decreased insulating subcutaneous fat make newborns more vulnerable to temperature variations than adults. This vulnerability increases with decreasing gestational age (Blackburn, 2003).

The nurse strives to maintain a **neutral thermal environment (NTE)** for every newborn. An NTE minimizes heat production and oxygen consumption. In other words, body temperature stays within normal range without requiring physiologic mechanisms that increase metabolic rate and oxygen consumption (National Association of Neonatal Nurses [NANN], 1997).

Range of Normal Temperature. Neonatal body temperature has a fairly broad range of normal (MacDonald et al., 2006; NANN, 1997; Rutter, 1999):

- Axillary: 36.5°–37.3°C (97.5°–99.1°F)
- Skin:
  - Full-term infant: 36°–36.5°C (96.8°–97.5°F)
  - Preterm infant: 36.2°–37.2°C (97.2°–98.7°F)
- Rectal: 36.5°–37.5°C (97.5°–99.5°F)

The AAP cites normal axillary temperature for a full-term infant as 36.1° to 37.0°C (97° to 98.6°F) in an open crib with appropriate clothing (AAP & ACOG, 2002).

Methods of Taking Newborn Temperatures. The nurse can assess newborn temperature as follows (Blackburn, 2003; NANN, 1997):

- **Axillary:** This method is safe and approximates core temperature.
- **Skin:** This method is used frequently to assess continuously the skin temperature of preterm infants or those at risk for temperature instability. Healthy newborn skin temperature is displayed when the radiant warmer is used anytime the infant must be unclothed and exposed for more than a short period. A thermistor probe is placed on the surface of the skin and displays temperature electronically. The optimal location for the thermistor probe is not known (Blackburn, 2003). It is usually recommended to place the probe over the liver or abdomen, or on the back of a prone infant. The nurse should make sure that the probe is in full contact with the skin and covered with a foil reflector to avoid radiant or convective cooling of the thermistor probe (see Chap. 22).
- **Tympanic:** Infrared tympanic thermometry is safe and noninvasive. Because of unproven accuracy in newborns, however, it is not yet recommended for use (Bakewell-Sachs et al., 1997).
- **Rectal:** This method is no longer recommended to assess core temperature and rectal patency. Skin temperature drops before core temperature, so a rectal temperature does not reflect stability of the newborn's temperature. In addition, rectal perforation is a risk (Blackburn, 2003; NANN, 1997).

How Newborns Lose and Gain Heat. Newborns transfer heat to and from the body surface in four ways (Blackburn, 2003) (Fig. 20.14).

- **Evaporation**
  - **Heat is lost** when moisture from the skin and respiratory tract converts to vapor. *Example: A warm, wet newborn is exposed to cool air in the delivery room.*
- **Conduction**
  - **Heat is lost** from the body surface to a cooler solid surface touching the newborn. *Example: Newborn is placed on the surface of a cold scale for weighing.*
  - **Heat is gained** from a surface warmer than the infant. *Example: Newborn is placed on a warm blanket or chemical thermal mattress.*
- **Convection**
  - **Heat is lost** from the body surface to the surrounding air. *Example: An exposed newborn is placed in a bassinet near a door that is opened and closed frequently.*
  - **Heat is gained** if the surrounding air temperature is higher than the infant's skin temperature. *Example: An infant is placed in an incubator with circulating air at a higher temperature than the infant's skin temperature.*
- **Radiation**
  - **Heat is lost** from the body surface to a cooler solid surface not touching the newborn. *Example: A newborn is placed near a cold window on an exterior wall.*
  - **Heat is gained** when the solid surface is warmer than the infant's skin temperature. *Example: A cool infant is placed under an infant warmer (radiant heat source).*

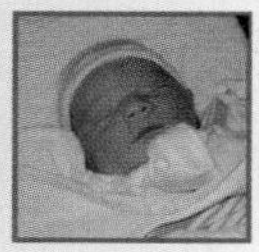

Thomas is lying on the mother's bed, clothed in a shirt and diaper. How might he be losing heat?

Newborns make heat in four ways (Blackburn, 2003; NANN, 1997):

- *Metabolic processes:* The amount of heat this method produces varies with activity, state, health status, and environmental temperature. The brain, heart, and liver produce the most metabolic energy by oxidative metabolism of glucose, fat, and protein (Blackburn, 2003).
- *Voluntary muscle activity:* Increased muscle activity during restlessness and crying generates some heat. In addition, the newborn may attempt to conserve heat by assuming a flexed position to decrease surface area. Shivering, the most important method to generate heat in adults, is less important in newborns. Most likely, this is because the shivering threshold is lower in newborns than in adults and occurs as a very late response associated with decreased spinal cord temperature after prolonged exposure (Blackburn, 2003).
- *Peripheral vasoconstriction:* In response to cooling, peripheral vasoconstriction reduces blood flow to the skin and therefore decreases loss of heat from the skin's surface (NANN, 1997).
- ***Nonshivering thermogenesis (NST):*** This mechanism is the main source of heat production in the newborn triggered at a mean skin temperature of 35°–36°C (95–96.8°F) (Blackburn, 2003). Thermal receptors transmit impulses to the hypothalamus, which stimulates the sympathetic nervous system and causes norepinephrine release in **brown adipose tissue (BAT).** Found around the scapulae, kidneys, adrenal glands, head, neck, heart, great vessels, and axillary regions, BAT, or brown fat, is highly vascular and accounts for 2% to 7% of the newborn's weight (Bruck, 1978). BAT generates more energy than any other body tissue (Fisher & Polk, 1994). Norepinephrine in BAT activates lipase, which results in lipolysis and fatty acid oxidation. This chemical process generates heat, which is transferred to the perfusing blood and tissues near the BAT. This increases local temperature

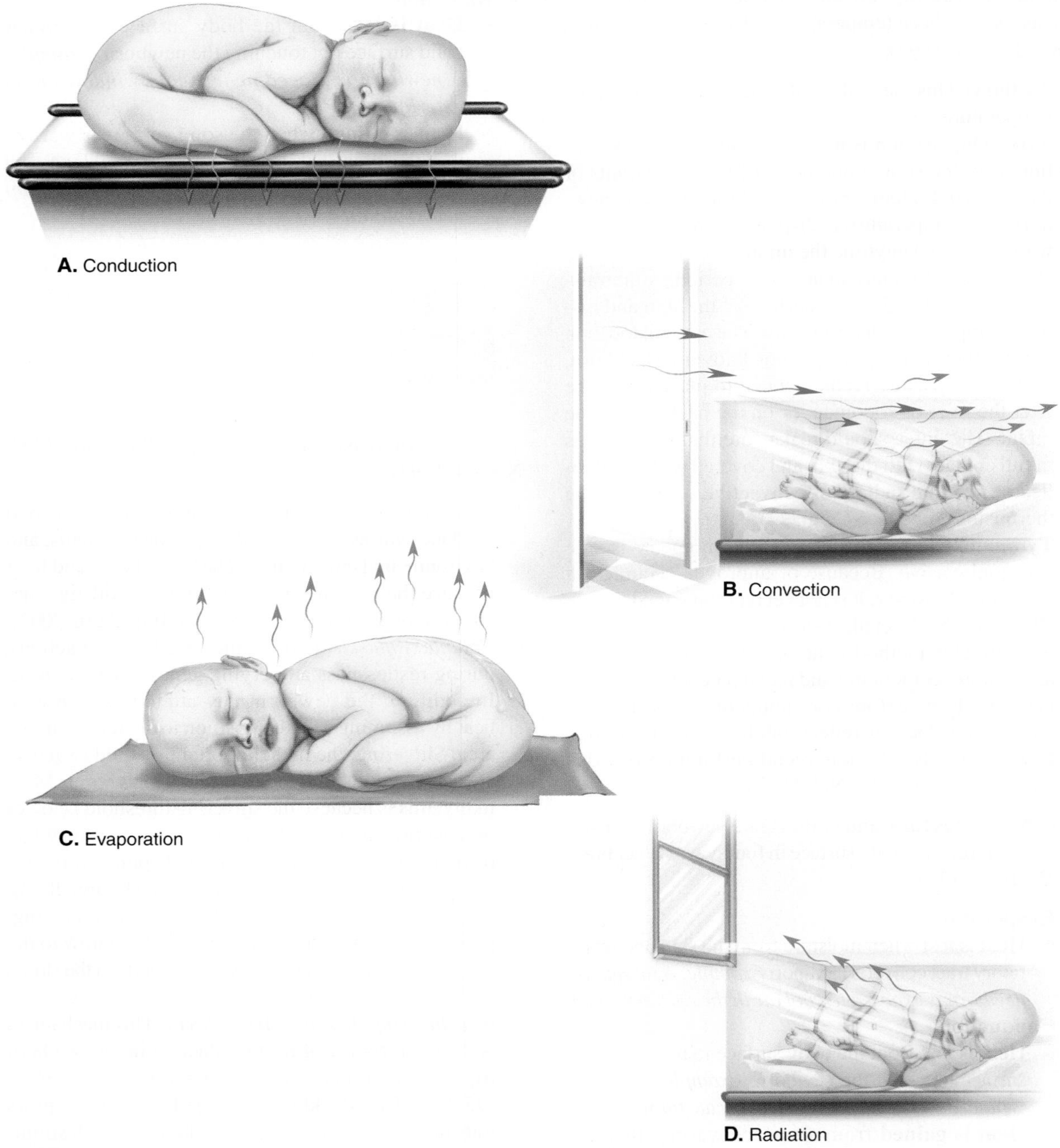

FIGURE 20.14 Heat loss in newborns occurs in four ways: (**A**) conduction, (**B**) convection, (**C**) evaporation, (**D**) radiation.

and eventually results in increased axillary temperature (Blackburn, 2003).

Cold Stress. When heat loss overwhelms the newborn's ability to compensate, cold stress occurs (Fig. 20.15). Clinical signs include peripheral vasoconstriction, resulting in **acrocyanosis** and cool, mottled, or pale skin. The term newborn may become restless, agitated, or hypoglycemic. Signs of increased oxygen consumption include clinical signs of respiratory distress such as **tachypnea, grunting,** or lethargy (Bakewell-Sachs et al., 1997). The compensatory mechanisms of the newborn with cold stress initiate a chain of metabolic events that can result in **hypoxemia,** metabolic acidosis, glycogen depletion, hypoglycemia, and altered surfactant production.

Heat Stress. The newborn is equally vulnerable to overheating. Hyperthermia (temperature above 37.5°C

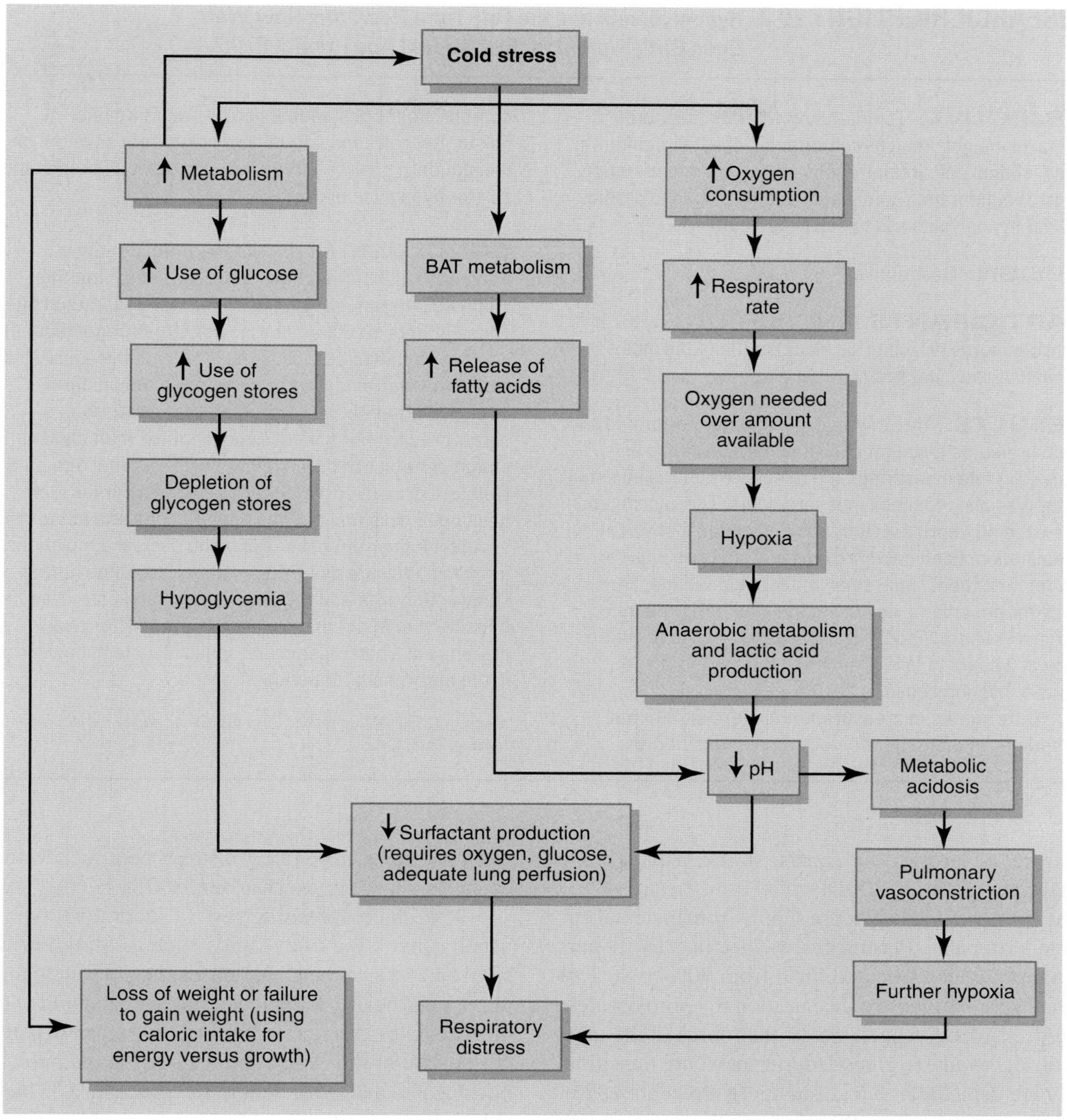

FIGURE 20.15 Physiologic consequences of cold stress. BAT, brown adipose tissue. (From Blackburn, S. T. [2003]. Maternal, fetal, and neonatal physiology: A clinical perspective [2nd ed.]. St. Louis: W. B. Saunders.)

[99.5°F]) usually results from overheating (Blackburn, 2003). Consequences include increased heart, respiratory, and metabolic rates (increased oxygen consumption); dehydration from insensible water loss; and peripheral vasodilation that may cause hypotension (NANN, 1997). Clinical signs may include tachypnea, apnea, tachycardia, hypotension, flushing, irritability, sweating (in term and older preterm newborns), poor feeding, lethargy, hypotonia, extended posture, and weak cry (NANN, 1997).

Glucose Metabolism

Maintenance of normal blood glucose concentration can be a major problem for sick or low-birth-weight infants; however, the nurse caring for healthy full-term newborns should be aware that hypoglycemia is always possible. Because untreated hypoglycemia may result in long-term neurologic complications, immediate identification of and intervention for it are essential. See Research Highlight 20.2.

Definitions of neonatal **hypoglycemia** have been controversial over the years; no uniform standard exists. At present, a plasma glucose concentration of less than 45 mg/dL appears to be abnormal for term and preterm infants and requires intervention (Cowett & Loughead, 2002). Newborns at risk for hypoglycemia include those who are SGA, LGA, born to mothers with diabetes (IDM),

● RESEARCH HIGHLIGHT 20.2 Hypoglycemia and the Full-Term Newborn: How Well Does Birth Weight for Gestational Age Predict Risk?

OBJECTIVE: To determine whether measurements of weight, head circumference, chest circumference, abdominal circumference, mid-arm circumference, thigh circumference, and length could be used to predict risk for hypoglycemia in full-term newborns.

DESIGN: Descriptive

PARTICIPANTS AND SETTING: 157 full-term newborns (94 white, 63 black) participated in this community hospital setting.

RESULTS: The principal investigator performed all measurements twice on each newborn, using an unmarked, white measuring tape to ensure that the investigator was blind to these measurements. The investigator knew the newborn's weight and completed a physical examination. Each newborn was classified as appropriate for gestational age, small for gestational age, or large for gestational age using the standard growth curve. Newborn blood glucose was measured by heel stick at 2 hours of age or sooner if the newborn had signs of hypoglycemia.

Differences in measurements were significant based on race and gender. A subset classified as appropriate for gestational age had an increased risk for hypoglycemia. Plotting the newborn's weight on the standard growth curve did not accurately predict the risk for hypoglycemia.

CONCLUSION: Providers often identify a newborn's risk for hypoglycemia by classifying the infant as appropriate, small, or large for gestational age. Those infants identified as small or large for gestational age are identified as most at risk for hypoglycemia. This study provides evidence, however, that the midarm circumference–to–head circumference ratio was a better predictor of risk for hypoglycemia than classification of newborn birth weight by gestational age on a standard growth curve. Standard growth curves were developed from homogenous populations and not tested to validate their effectiveness in the clinical populations for which they are used. This author advocates further study in this area and the development of a user-friendly bedside tool to accurately assess the risk for hypoglycemia in a heterogeneous population of term newborns in the early postbirth period.

Johnson, T. S. (2003). *Journal of Obstetric, Gynecologic, and Neonatal Nursing, 32*(1), 48–57.

premature, or stressed by sepsis, shock, asphyxia, or hypothermia (Karlsen, 2001).

At birth, the steady glucose supply from maternal circulation terminates. Plasma glucose declines by 2 hours after a term, uncomplicated birth from 60% to 80% of maternal serum glucose concentration to approximately 50 mg/dL. Liver glycogen stores, the source of the most immediately available glucose during newborn transition, usually are depleted in 3 to 12 hours (Karp et al., 1995). The nadir occurs at 60 to 90 minutes of age (Cornblath et al., 2000).

Diminished hepatic glucose production causes most neonatal hypoglycemia. In these infants, hypoglycemia is associated with decreased availability of glycogen, lactate, glycerol, and amino acids—the substrates necessary to make glucose available to cells. In addition, the hypoglycemic newborn may have altered responses to neural or hormonal factors and immature or altered enzymatic pathways (Cowett & Loughead, 2002).

Symptoms of hypoglycemia are not unique to that condition. For example, hypothermia, lethargy, and respiratory distress are also symptoms of neonatal sepsis. In addition, some infants with hypoglycemia are totally asymptomatic. Thus, identifying risk factors and screening those newborns most likely to develop hypoglycemia are important. Signs of hypoglycemia include jitteriness, hypothermia, lethargy, hypotonia, high-pitched or weak cry, apnea, respiratory distress, poor suck, vomiting, cyanosis, and seizures (Karlsen, 2001).

A bedside screening test (a laboratory-type test, usually involving body fluids such as blood, urine, or stool and done at the client's bedside, not sent to the laboratory) is the usual method of initial evaluation of blood glucose level. Accuracy of the initial screen depends on correct use of the evaluation method, so the nurse must be educated and proficient in the procedure. If the bedside screen reveals a low blood glucose value, the nurse usually draws a blood sample by heelstick or venipuncture for laboratory confirmation. Providers do not delay treatment of suspected hypoglycemia while waiting for test results. Interventions can include oral feeding for relatively healthy babies or intravenous (IV) therapy for more compromised or severely hypoglycemic newborns (Assessment Tool 20.4).

Prevention of hypoglycemia in term newborns is essential. Minimizing stress, maintaining normal body temperature, and initiating feeding as soon as the newborn is stable facilitate successful transition, including normal blood glucose homeostasis.

Hematopoietic System

Timing of Cord Clamping. The timing of clamping of the umbilical cord influences neonatal blood volume; however, no standard exists for when to clamp. Early

● ASSESSMENT TOOL 20.4 Sample Glucose Screening Protocol

Date: ______________________

Time: ______________________

Note: Please line through any items not desired or check appropriate box. All items will be implemented unless otherwise ordered

1 Routine newborn admission per protocol

2 If positive risk factors (SGA, LGA, IDM, premature or septic), check blood glucose with monitor (BGM) within 30 minutes of birth or STAT if symptomatic.

3 If blood glucose 40 - 120 mg/dl:
- Feeding per parent's choice
- Recheck at 90 minutes and 4 hours of life

4 If blood glucose <40 mg/dl and asymptomatic:
- Breast feed or give 30 ml formula of parent's choice
- Recheck BGM 30 minutes after feeding is completed, then every hour x 3

5 If blood glucose <40 mg/dl and symptomatic:
- Give 30 ml formula
- Recheck BGM 30 minutes after feeding is completed, then every hour x 2, then before feedings
- Feed every 3 hours

6 If followup BGM is < 40 mg/dl
- Draw STAT glucose via laboratory method *(LAB/GLU)*
- Give 30 ml formula
- Recheck BGM 30 minutes after feeding is completed
- Notify physician if STAT glucose is abnormal
- IV glucose management for IDM and hypoglycemia:
  - Acute: 2 ml/kg D10W IV push (4mg/kg D10W IV if seizures are present)
  - Maintenance: 3-4 ml/kg/hr over 24 hours to prevent rebound hypoglycemia
  - Follow blood glucose every 4 hours while IV infusion is present

7 If infant is symptomatic after the initial blood glucose monitoring period:
- Check BGM STAT
- If < 40 mg/dl, follow protocol above
- Notify physician if symptoms continue

8 For infants of insulin-dependent diabetic mothers:
- Check BGM every half hour x 4
- Check BGM before breast or formula feeding once every 8 hours
- Feed every 3 hours x 24 hours

9 Discontinue protocol when 3 consecutive BGM checks are 40 -120 mg/dl

Physician signature: ______________________ Date: ______________

Noted by: ______________________ Date: ______________ Time: ______________

Physician's orders

Addressograph

Glucose Screening: Full Term Neonates with Hypoglycemia and Newborns of Diabetic Mothers

MS 211 Approved: 8/02

Permission from Norma Cooper, RN, Manager, Obstetrics Department, Olympic Medical Center, 939 Caroline Street, Port Angeles, WA 98362 clamping (30 to 40 seconds) versus late clamping (after 3 minutes) can make a 30% difference in blood volume (Wardrop & Holland, 1995). Research cites advantages and disadvantages to both techniques (Ceriani Cernadas et al., 2006; Ibraham et al., 2000; Mercer et al., 2000). By 3 days after birth, differences in blood volume between early and late clamped umbilical cords are almost negligible in healthy term newborns as a result of a normal decrease in plasma volume (Blackburn, 2003).

Blood Components. Blood components begin to form as early as 2 to 3 weeks' gestation. By term, blood volume averages 80 to 100 mL/kg (Blackburn, 2003). The transition from fetal to neonatal hematologic system involves numerous changes in the structure and function of blood components, particularly those of the red blood cells (RBCs).

Red Blood Cells. Hemoglobin molecules have binding sites for oxygen molecules. When oxygen fills all the binding sites, the hemoglobin is said to be 100% saturated.

Fetal hemoglobin (HbF) differs from adult hemoglobin (HbA). HbF is saturated more readily with oxygen molecules than HbA, which is essential to fetal survival because of the low-oxygen intrauterine environment. This high affinity for oxygen molecules exists because HbF does not have binding sites for a substance called 2,3-DPG, which enables HbF to attract and hold oxygen molecules more readily than HbA. The increased affinity for oxygen molecules facilitates oxygen transfer across the placenta but reduces oxygen release to the tissues. Thus, at any given oxygen content, the oxygen saturation of the hemoglobin molecule is greater with HbF than with HbA (Blackburn, 2003).

At term, newborn cord blood contains 50% to 80% HbF and 15% to 40% HbA (Blackburn, 2003). The more preterm the newborn, the more HbF remains. This works against preterm infants, whose HbF results in a diminished ability to respond to hypoxia by releasing oxygen molecules into the tissues. The higher proportion of HbA in term newborns compared with preterm newborns makes an efficient response to oxygen needs a less significant problem. Conversion from HbF to HbA continues over the first 6 months of life, as HbA production takes over and reaches 90% (Blackburn, 2003).

Because intrauterine oxygen exchange is less efficient than extrauterine oxygen exchange through the lungs, fetuses and newborns have a higher RBC count and hemoglobin level than children and adults. Hemoglobin levels average approximately 17 g/dL; the RBC count is 4.6 (Blackburn, 2003). Hemoglobin can increase up to 6 g/dL in the first hours of life, resulting from the decrease in plasma volume and the net increase in RBCs. Hematocrit ranges from 51.3% to 56%, with the aforementioned increase in the first few hours of life. Hemoglobin and hematocrit fall again to levels near the cord blood values by the end of the first week (Blackburn, 2003).

White Blood Cells. The white blood cell (WBC) count is approximately 10,000 to 26,000/mm^3 in term infants and less in preterm infants (Oski & Naiman, 1982). It increases on the first day of life, perhaps as a result of the stress of birth, and decreases to approximately 12,000/mm^3 by 4 or 5 days in both term and preterm newborns (Hathaway & Bonnar, 1987; Oski, 1982). Immature forms of WBCs (eg, neutrophils, eosinophils) can be elevated in the first 3 or 4 days of life (Blackburn, 2003). Intense crying may increase the WBC count 146% and result in a left shift in the differential (more immature cells present, which indicates mobilization of WBCs to fight infection) (Christensen, 2000). A complete blood count (CBC) with differential is not routine for a healthy newborn, so additional diagnostic procedures, such as chest radiography, and initiation of IV therapy may occur in the same period. The infant's behavioral state just before and during a CBC with differential is helpful to note on the medical record, especially if the blood draw is difficult, stressful, or prolonged. Personnel performing neonatal laboratory tests should be proficient and comfort newborns as much as possible during procedures by holding or swaddling them or providing a pacifier for sucking.

Platelets. Platelet counts range from 150,000 to 450,000/mm^3, which is similar to adult counts. Platelet counts below 150,000/mm^3 are abnormal in newborns (Del Vecchio & Sola, 2000). Platelet function may be hypoactive in the first few days of life, which is protective because of increased risk for thrombosis; however, this increases the risk for bleeding and bleeding disorders for preterm and compromised newborns (Blackburn, 2003). Platelet count also may be used to look for infection.

Blood Sampling. Venous sampling (blood drawn from a vein) will yield lower hemoglobin, hematocrit, and RBC values than a capillary (heelstick) sample (Blackburn, 2003). The nurse can minimize differences between capillary and venous results by prewarming the heel before drawing a capillary sample, obtaining a brisk blood flow, and discarding the first few drops of blood (Blackburn, 2003). The nurse also should document the site of the sample in the medical record.

Hepatic System

The liver accounts for 5% of the newborn's weight (Blackburn, 2003). The maternal liver handles fetal metabolic functions, but after birth, liver function becomes essential to neonatal survival (Blackburn, 2003). The liver is responsible for metabolism of hormones, drugs, proteins, and carbohydrates (Blackburn, 2003). It also stores vitamins and iron and synthesizes proteins and blood clotting factors (Slater, 1998). Although all liver functions are important, this discussion focuses on energy storage, digestive function, and filtration and waste management.

Functions of the Liver. In late gestation, the fetal liver increases glycogen storage in preparation for the newborn transition. Glycogen maintains glucose homeostasis immediately after birth. With the loss of the maternal glucose supply at birth, neonatal blood glucose level falls. The baby uses approximately 90% of liver glycogen stores in the first 24 hours as a result of rapid *glycogenolysis* (the release of glucose from glycogen). Neonatal blood glucose usually reaches its lowest level 60 to 90 minutes after birth. Steady hepatic release of glucose occurs by 3 to 4 hours of life. As glycogen levels fall, the healthy term infant mobilizes free fatty acids and ketones to stabilize blood glucose. In the first several days, blood glucose homeostasis is glucose dominant; thereafter, it becomes insulin dominant, as in adults (Blackburn, 2003).

Production and excretion of bile, which is essential for digestion and nutrition, is another important liver function. Bile helps emulsify fats and transports fatty acids and fat-soluble vitamins to the surface of the intestinal mucosa for absorption (Slater, 1998).

The liver has 50,000 to 100,000 microscopic functional units called lobules. Between the cords of lobules are spaces called sinusoids. Sinusoids are lined with Kupffer cells, which phagocytosize old blood cells, bacteria, and other materials (Slater, 1998).

Bilirubin Metabolism. In newborns, the liver plays a major role in the metabolism of **bilirubin,** a yellow pigment formed from hemoglobin as a byproduct of RBC breakdown. In high concentrations, bilirubin is toxic to the brain and body tissues (AAP & ACOG, 2002). Bilirubin production is almost twice as much in newborns as in adults because of the low-oxygen intrauterine environment and because the lifespan of RBCs is shorter (Blackburn, 1995). These factors place newborns at risk for hyperbilirubinemia.

Cord blood bilirubin levels are approximately 2 mg/dL (Maisels, 1999). Clamping of the umbilical cord decreases circulation to the liver. Preterm or sick newborns also may experience intermittent patency of the ductus venosus, resulting in shunting of the blood past the liver sinusoids, which interferes with bilirubin removal from the plasma (Blackburn, 2003).

Unconjugated bilirubin, also called **indirect bilirubin,** is bound to circulating albumin in the bloodstream and has not yet been metabolized by the liver. Each gram of albumin binds approximately 8.5 to 10 mg of bilirubin. As bilirubin production increases, all the albumin sites may be taken up, and the free (unbound) bilirubin can move into fatty tissue, such as the skin, where it causes jaundice, or the brain, where it can cause neurologic damage (Blackburn, 1995).

The liver removes unconjugated (indirect) bilirubin from the albumin and "conjugates" it. The conversion of indirect bilirubin to direct bilirubin depends on glucose and oxygen. This process involves an important enzyme called glucuronyl transferase, in which unconjugated (indirect) bilirubin interacts with glucose and glucuronic acid to produce direct bilirubin, which is water soluble. Next, direct bilirubin is excreted into the small intestine, which processes bilirubin into urobilinogen. When oxidized, urobilinogen forms orange urobilin, giving the stool its characteristic color. Most urobilinogen is excreted in stool, whereas some is reabsorbed in the colon and excreted in urine (Blackburn, 2003).

It is possible for urobilinogen to be converted back into indirect bilirubin, a process known as *enterohepatic shunting*. In this process, unconjugated (indirect) bilirubin is absorbed across the intestinal mucosa, reenters the circulation, and ends up back in the liver. Any delay in intestinal movement or decrease in intestinal flora increases the risk for direct bilirubin to convert to indirect bilirubin, thus necessitating the need to reenter the liver and begin the excretion process again (Blackburn, 2003).

Serum bilirubin levels are expressed as three values: total, indirect, and direct. Total bilirubin is simply the sum of the indirect and direct values. Most elevated bilirubin in newborns results from elevated unconjugated, or indirect, bilirubin. Therefore, indirect and total bilirubin values are usually nearly the same (PCEP, 1999a). On the other hand, direct bilirubin values do not usually exceed 1.5 mg/dL. Marked elevation of direct bilirubin usually indicates cholestatic liver disease, which may develop from other liver disease, anatomic obstruction, genetics, or metabolic disorders (Slater, 1998).

Newborn jaundice progresses from head to toe. Jaundice may be more evident in dark-skinned babies by pressing a finger on their skin. Jaundice in a baby is noticeable before capillary refill (PCEP, 1999a). A newborn becomes visibly jaundiced as bilirubin levels reach a total serum value of 5 to 7 mg/dL in the first few days after birth. This normal event is called **physiologic jaundice** and occurs in 45% to 60% of term newborns (Blackburn, 2003). See Chapters 21 and 22 for detailed discussions of other types of jaundice and their treatment.

Gastrointestinal System

Oral Feeding. The beginning of oral feeding is critical to the development of immature gastrointestinal function (Blackburn, 2003). Enteral feeding causes surges in plasma concentrations of gastric hormones and enteric neuropeptides. Human milk is rich in these factors, as well as being the preferred source of energy and fluid (Blackburn, 2003). Healthy term babies may be breastfed as soon as possible after birth and 8 to 12 times per day thereafter (AAP & ACOG, 2002). Formula-fed babies should eat within 6 to 8 hours of birth or sooner if indicated by hunger cues or risk for hypoglycemia (see Chap. 21). The term newborn's gastric capacity is approximately 6 mL/kg, which means that a newborn weighing 3400 g

(7 lbs, 8 oz) has a gastric capacity of approximately 20 mL, or a little more than ½ oz of fluid (Blackburn, 2003). See Chapter 21.

Meconium

QUOTE 20-3

"On the second day, meconium came from my baby like a lava flow. I found it unnerving, but my nurse reassured me, saying that the more the baby stooled, the less problem he would have with jaundice."

(From a mom)

Meconium, the newborn's first stool, begins to form at approximately 16 weeks' gestation (Blackburn, 2003). This black, sticky substance consists of vernix caseosa, lanugo, squamous epithelial cells, occult blood, bile, and other intestinal secretions. Bacteria appear in meconium by 24 hours of life. Almost all newborns pass meconium by 24 to 48 hours. Failure to pass meconium is a sign of intestinal obstruction and places the newborn at high risk for hyperbilirubinemia (Blackburn, 2003).

Immunologic System

Susceptibility to Infection. Immature immunologic responses make the newborn susceptible to infection. In addition, lack of exposure to common organisms results in a delayed or decreased immune response. Preterm infants, especially those born before 32 to 33 weeks' gestation, are especially susceptible to infection because of a markedly immature immune response (Blackburn, 2003).

Newborns can become infected while in utero (through transplacental passage of an organism from mother to fetus), during labor (through contact or aspiration of organisms in the birth canal), or after birth (from organisms in the environment or, less commonly, breast milk) (Remington & Klein, 2006). The nurse should be aware of prenatal, intrapartal, and neonatal risk factors for infection, use standard precautions and excellent handwashing technique, and teach parents basic preventive hygiene procedures.

Departure from the sterile uterine environment exposes the newborn to a host of potential pathogens. The birth process, hospital environment, and ingested and inhaled substances expose the skin, respiratory system, and gastrointestinal tract. Skin flora increases immediately after birth; in term healthy newborns, the skin achieves a balance of colonized bacteria that protects them from invading pathogens. Gastric acidity initially protects the gut from gram-positive and gram-negative bacteria; breastfeeding infants receive the added benefit of antimicrobial substances in human milk (Blackburn, 2003).

Term newborns have temporary passive immunity from transplacental transfer of maternal immunoglobulins, especially immunoglobulin G (IgG). IgA levels are decreased, however, and place them at risk for viral and gram-negative bacteria (Blackburn, 2003). The inexperienced immune system fails to produce detectable type-specific antibodies. Newborns cannot localize infection because of their inability to produce adequate neutrophils and other phagocytes and transport them to infection sites. For this reason, signs of sepsis can be diffuse and nonspecific instead of localized; for example, temperature instability is a more common sign of neonatal sepsis than is fever (Blackburn, 2003) (see Chap. 22).

Infection Prevention Strategies. The best strategy for preventing nosocomial infections is thorough handwashing. The nurse's work shift begins with a 3-minute scrub of the hands and arms above the elbow with an antiseptic soap and brush. Thereafter, the nurse should wash her hands for at least 10 seconds with bacteriocidal soap before and after contact with the infant and after touching objects. This rule applies regardless of whether the nurse wears gloves. The nurse should remove rings, watches, and bracelets and trim fingernails short. No false fingernails or opaque nail polishes should be permitted because they increase the likelihood of inadequate cleansing. Alcohol-based foams or gels, although not appropriate when hands are soiled, kill bacteria when applied to clean hands and given sufficient contact time (follow manufacturer's guidelines) (AAP & ACOG, 2002).

Nursery personnel managing healthy term newborns do not need to wear cover gowns as long as the facility strictly enforces handwashing. People with respiratory, gastrointestinal, or skin infections should *not* have contact with newborns. In addition, any staff member with a skin condition or appliance that prevents or impairs handwashing should not have contact with newborns (AAP & ACOG, 2002).

Hospitals vary in their approach to staff members with herpes simplex virus. Transmission from infected personnel to infants is rare. If an infected staff member is allowed to work with newborns, he or she should cover lesions and perform meticulous handwashing. Nevertheless, any staff member with herpetic hand infections (herpes whitlow) may not have contact with any client until the infection has resolved (AAP & ACOG, 2002).

Ideally, each newborn has individual supplies, such as a digital thermometer and stethoscope, in his or her bassinet. If these supplies travel from baby to baby, staff members must follow strict procedures for cleaning after each use to prevent infection (AAP & ACOG, 2002).

Parents also share responsibility for protecting infants. They also must wash their hands thoroughly before providing newborn care, before preparing formula, and, of course, after using the bathroom. Siblings with fever, symptoms of acute illness, or recent exposure to a known communicable disease (eg, chickenpox) should not be allowed to visit the newborn at the hospital (AAP & ACOG, 2002).

Integumentary System

Skin Functions. Newborn skin has three functions: to limit transepidermal water loss, to prevent absorption of chemicals, and to protect against pathogens (Polin & Fox, 2004). The epidermal thickness of the term newborn is as well developed as in an adult; however, the more preterm the infant, the more immature the barrier (Blackburn, 2003).

Transepidermal water loss is not a significant risk factor for healthy term infants. Term infants lose 6 to 8 g/mL^2/hr, similar to that of nonsweating adults (Polin & Fox, 2004). Transepidermal water loss in term infants requires consideration when their care requires a radiant warmer, an incubator, or phototherapy (Blackburn, 2003).

Skin Characteristics. A newborn's skin is more permeable than an adult's to substances such as drugs and chemicals. Skin permeability increases with decreasing gestational age. Obviously, skin disease and injury increase the risk for permeability. Permeability is illustrated by the historical practice of bathing newborns with hexachlorophene to prevent colonization with staphylococci. This practice was later found to increase the risk for neurologic damage (Kopelman, 1973). In addition, neonatal skin can absorb both povidone-iodine and isopropyl alcohol. Elevated blood plasma levels of iodine have been found in newborns when the agent was not completely cleansed from the skin following use (Pyati, 1977). Isopropyl alcohol, depending on its concentration, duration of exposure, condition of the skin, pressure to the skin, and quality of skin perfusion, can cause drying, irritation, and burns (Blackburn, 2003). Table 20.4 depicts various skin findings in newborns.

The skin's **acid mantle** has a surface pH lower than 5 and acts as a bacteriostatic barrier. After birth, colonization of the skin begins immediately, and "friendly" bacteria grow in balance to protect against infectious pathogens. Disturbance of the acid mantle (eg, through frequent bathing with alkaline soaps or application of emollients) disrupts the balance and changes the species of colonizing bacteria (Lund, 1997).

Renal System

Fetal Development. At birth, the kidneys must take over from the placenta fluid and electrolyte balance, metabolic excretion, and other functions. Although the newborn has the same number of nephrons by 34 to 35 weeks' gestation as an adult, the kidneys are less functional and do not approach full maturation until the second year of life (Blackburn, 2003).

Newborn Kidney Function. Glomerular filtration rate (GFR) is low in comparison to an adult's. This means that the newborn's kidneys favor resorption of sodium and cannot dispose of water rapidly when necessary. The newborn is therefore at risk for water retention and edema (Blackburn, 2003).

Tubular function is altered so that the kidneys have less ability to concentrate urine, putting newborns at risk for dehydration. Limited ability to concentrate urine also puts the newborn at risk for acid–base abnormalities, hyperkalemia, hypocalcemia, and hypoglycemia (Blackburn, 2003).

With advancing gestational age, extracellular water and total body water decrease, and intracellular water increases. Diuresis occurs shortly after birth and accounts for the loss of 5% to 10% of birth weight in the term infant's first week of life (Blackburn, 2003).

Urine. Healthy term infants urinate 15 to 60 mL/kg/day (Blackburn, 2003). The initial void occurs in the delivery room for 13% to 21% of newborns; 95% of all newborns void in the first 24 hours, and all newborns should have voided by 48 hours (Clark, 1977). A newborn who has not voided by 24 hours requires further evaluation (AAP & ACOG, 2002).

The urine is usually straw colored but may be cloudy with mucus. Specific gravity is low (1.008 to 1.012) (Martin et al., 2006). Female infants sometimes have small amounts of bloody mucus from **pseudomenses/pseudomenstruation,** resulting from the withdrawal of maternal hormones (Tappero & Honeyfield, 2003). Pink stains (**brick dust spots**) may appear in the urine of both males and females; they result from uric acid crystals and are not a cause for concern (Blackburn, 2003).

Promoting Normal Transition

No one knows exactly what the experience of birth is like for the fetus-newborn. He or she likely feels the mother's muscular uterine contractions. Each contraction may lead to mild hypoxia and a transient drop in blood pressure (Blackburn, 2003). During vaginal birth, contractions and maternal pushing efforts propel the baby through the narrow birth canal and out the vaginal opening. Cesarean birth abruptly exposes the newborn to handling and light as the baby is pulled from the uterus into the extrauterine environment. For the first time, the newborn experiences cool room temperature, tactile stimulation, bright light, loud noises, and new feelings of gravity and proprioception. He or she discovers what may be a surprising ability to extend the head, arms, and legs, and reacts to this startling lack of containment around the body.

The incredible forces of the birth process may be evident during physical examination. The newborn's eyes may be puffy and bruised and the skull molded into an elongated shape. Boggy areas of fluid may be palpable under the scalp. In some instances, the nose is flattened or pushed to one side. A large baby may even suffer a fractured clavicle as the shoulders make the tight fit through the vaginal opening.

TABLE 20.4 Common Skin Manifestations of the Normal Newborn

SKIN MANIFESTATION	FAMILY TEACHING TIPS
Acrocyanosis	A bluish color to the hands and feet of the newborn is normal in the first 6 to 12 hours after birth. Acrocyanosis results from slow circulation in the extremities.
Milia 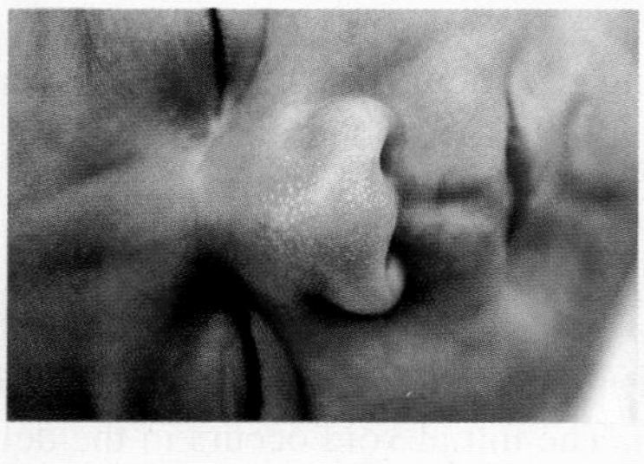	Small white spots on the newborn's face, nose, and chin that resemble pimples are an expected observation. Do not attempt to pick or squeeze them. They will subside spontaneously in a few days.
Erythema toxicum 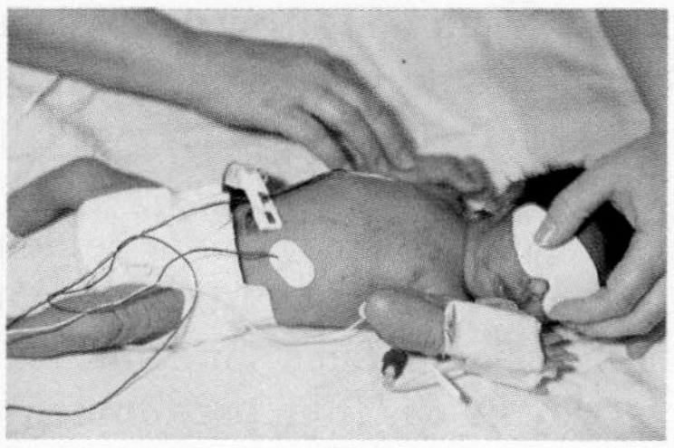	The so-called newborn rash commonly appears on the chest, abdomen, back, and buttocks of the newborn. It is harmless and will disappear.
Mongolian spot 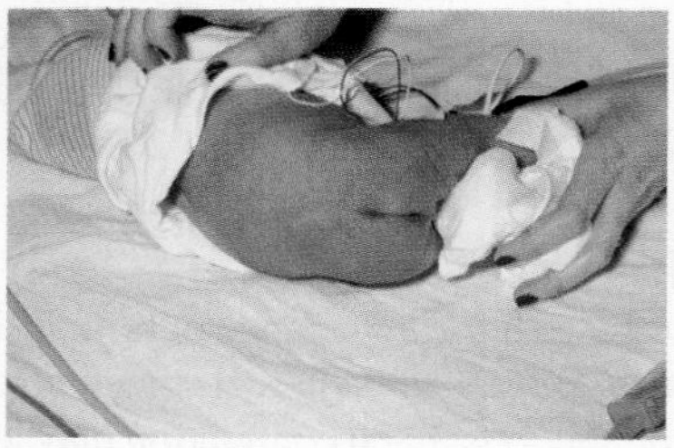	These bluish black areas of discoloration are commonly seen on the back, buttocks, or extremities of African American, Hispanic, Mediterranean, or other dark-skinned newborns. These spots should not be mistaken for bruises or mistreatment and gradually fade during the first year or two of life.
Telangiectatic nevi 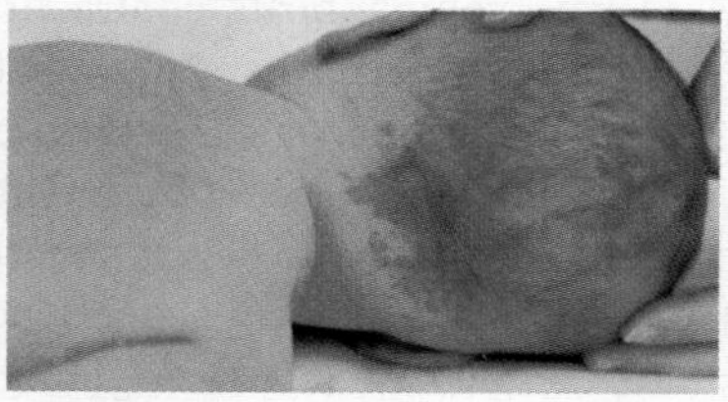	These pale pink or red marks ("stork bites") are sometimes found on the nape of the neck, eyelids, or nose of fair-skinned newborns. Stork bites blanch when pressed and generally fade as the child grows.
Nevus flammeus or port-wine stain 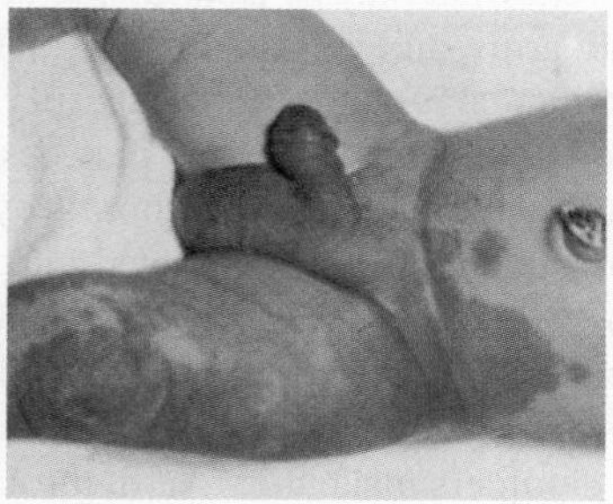	A port-wine stain is a dark reddish purple birthmark that most commonly appears on the face. It is caused by a group of dilated blood vessels. It does not blanch with pressure or fade with time. There are cosmetics available that help cover the stain if it is disfiguring. Laser therapy has been successfully used to fade port-wine stains.

Experienced and thoughtful neonatal nurses recognize that transition is more likely to be successful if unnecessary stressors are eliminated. Nurses who handle the newborn gently, protect the baby from unnecessary and invasive procedures, and treat him or her in accordance with developmental abilities promote successful extrauterine transitions, model excellent caregiving skills to parents, and promote parent–infant attachment. Strategies for a "gentle" newborn transition include the following:

- ***Gentle handling:*** Move newborns calmly and gently. Do not twist the extremities or change resting position abruptly. Speak to babies before touching them and while providing care.
- ***Use of containment:*** Newborns are accustomed to containment within the uterus and comforted by boundaries on the extremities, top of the head, and feet and legs. Swaddling is an example of containment; however, newborns are comforted by containment during caregiving that precludes swaddling. Examples include "nesting" the newborn if radiant warmer use is required, asking the mother's partner or support person to gently hold the newborn's arms across its chest during the vitamin K injection, and quieting a newborn who is escalating from an active alert state to a crying state.
- ***Avoidance of gastric suction:*** Vigorous or deep suctioning, especially with a suction catheter, may elicit a vagal response, slowing heart rate and causing apnea, bradycardia, and resultant hypoxia. Nurses can remove secretions at birth with a towel, bulb syringe, or suction catheter. Thereafter, in a healthy newborn, the bulb syringe is usually the only suction device needed to clear the mouth or nares and then only to remove visible vomitus or mucus. Sick newborns may require gastric suctioning to remove gastric contents to facilitate assisted ventilation and prevent aspiration; however, routine gastric suctioning for healthy newborns is unnecessary and invasive (Zaichkin, 2000).
- ***Use of ambient or dim light:*** Newborns are accustomed to a dark intrauterine environment. Physical examination is best performed when newborns are in a quiet alert state. A bright overhead light causes infants to close the eyes, grimace, and become uncomfortable. Transient bright light may be required to check a blink reflex or to better visualize an aspect of anatomy. The nurse should prevent continuous bright light from shining in the baby's face.
- ***Use of axillary temperature:*** Routine rectal temperature measurement is now rare. Axillary temperature measurement is noninvasive and approximates core temperature (Blackburn, 2003). Placement of a thermometer in the newborn's rectum does not prove rectal patency because anal stenosis or atresia may occur at any point along the anorectal canal (Tappero & Honeyfield, 2003). Rectal temperature can be uncomfortable and requires removal of blankets and the diaper, exposing the newborn to chilling. Most importantly, rectal temperatures place newborns at risk for trauma, perforation, and cross-contamination (Blackburn, 2003).

If the baby is term, stable, and in good condition, and in accordance with the mother's birth plan, health care providers should separate mother and baby as little as possible. The nurse may take the baby's axillary temperature while the mother or partner is holding the child. The nurse also can assess heart rate and breath sounds easily while parents hold the baby. Some nurses instill prophylactic eye medication and give the IM injection of vitamin K with the baby in a parent's arms.

COLLABORATIVE CARE: THE TRANSITIONAL PERIOD

Transition goes well for 85% to 90% of newborns, and these infants emerge from the first 4 to 6 hours of life healthy and ready to interact with the environment. The remaining 10% to 15% develop potentially life-threatening complications that require immediate identification and intervention (Askin, 2002). The nurse caring for the infant in transition must be alert for signs of abnormal transition, and the experienced nurse can assess the differences between an infant experiencing a "rocky" transition and an infant who is truly ill.

The newborn can be classified as well, at risk, or sick (PCEP, 1999b):

- The *well newborn* is term and AGA with no history of prenatal or intrapartal risk factors. The nurse would anticipate a smooth transition for this infant.
- The *at-risk newborn* is near term or term and has one or more risk factors relating to size for gestation, prenatal and intrapartum risk factors, or both. The nurse is alert for problems that may develop in transition. With appropriate nursing support and minimal interventions, the at-risk newborn may overcome initial challenges and become a well newborn. Conversely, the at-risk newborn may develop problems that require special care for a sick newborn.
- The *sick newborn* has clear risk factors relating to gestational age, size for gestation, and prenatal or intrapartal history. The nurse anticipates care of a sick newborn who will require evaluation and support in a special care nursery environment.

Because of the incredible complexity of adaptation necessary for the transition to extrauterine life, the term healthy newborn is allowed a short period to resolve initial challenges during transition. The nurse must know the prenatal and intrapartum risk factors that could place the newborn at risk. If such factors are present, the nurse anticipates potential neonatal implications and prepares to intervene during transition as necessary. For the at-risk newborn, the nurse defers stressful procedures such as bathing until the newborn is stable. For a sick newborn, the nurse defers both bathing and feeding (see Chap. 22).

Duration and severity of symptoms differentiate normal from abnormal transition. Respiratory distress is the most common manifestation of abnormal transition (Askin, 2002). If present, signs of respiratory distress (expiratory grunting, nasal flaring, and retracting) should be mild and intermittent, unaccompanied by additional problems (eg, pallor, heart murmur, lethargy), and steadily resolve in the first 30 to 60 minutes of life (Thureen et al., 2005). It is not uncommon for near-term newborns or those born by cesarean to exhibit mild to moderate respiratory distress for several hours after birth. With appropriate nursing care to ensure adequate oxygenation, thermoregulation, and blood glucose levels, most of these infants improve over the course of a few hours (Askin, 2002). Any newborn with moderate or severe respiratory distress requires immediate evaluation in a setting prepared to support his or her thermal, pulmonary, cardiovascular, and metabolic requirements (see Chap. 22). See Box 20.4.

Assessment

The nurse should assess axillary temperature every 30 minutes after birth until the newborn's condition has remained stable for 2 hours (AAP & ACOG, 2002). Thereafter, he or she should take the temperature during routine assessments every 3 to 4 hours, preferably when the newborn is awake for care and feeding. The nurse should assess temperature more often if the newborn is at increased risk for heat loss from prematurity or a central nervous system anomaly, if temperature is unstable, or if the newborn shows other signs of distress related to temperature instability, such as cool or mottled skin, respiratory distress, jitteriness, or sweating (in term and postterm babies).

The nurse caring for the infant should check the prenatal and intrapartal history to identify risk factors for hypoglycemia and follow the hospital's screening protocol. Blood glucose screening is part of assessment for any infant showing signs of hypoglycemia or respiratory or central nervous system distress. Bedside glucose monitoring is not a routine part of admission for healthy newborns with no known risk factors or symptoms (AAP & ACOG, 2002).

Inspection of color is part of routine newborn assessment and lends information about blood volume and perfusion. Color variations should be congruent with the newborn's genetic makeup; however, a newborn with persistently pale mucous membranes or one who is plethoric requires further evaluation. Heel-stick or venous blood sampling of the hemoglobin and hematocrit is indicated for these newborns to rule out anemia and polycythemia.

The nurse should assess for jaundice by pressing the newborn's skin firmly with a finger and evaluating how much jaundice appears where the skin blanches. Many settings use a transcutaneous bilirubin meter as a bedside screen. Bilirubin advances from head to foot, so a baby with jaundice to the knees has a higher bilirubin level than a baby with jaundice to the nipples. The newborn who appears slightly jaundiced by day 2 or 3 may require a laboratory evaluation of bilirubin, especially if he or she is being discharged. Follow-up examination, laboratory testing, or both are indicated; the nurse may make necessary arrangements before discharge. The newborn with jaundice in the first 24 hours requires immediate evaluation by a pediatric provider. The newborn at risk for pathologic jaundice requires more intensive blood work, such as blood typing and Coombs' testing (see Chap. 22). A baby whose bilirubin level rises faster than his or her capacity to metabolize it may require phototherapy (see Chap. 22).

The newborn has audible bowel sounds in the first few hours of life. The nurse should observe and assess ability to suck, swallow, and breathe, which ensure effective feeding every 2 to 4 hours and adequate fluid intake. The newborn should pass stool by 48 hours (AAP & ACOG, 2002).

The nurse should routinely and periodically assesses vital signs, appearance, feeding, and activity. Signs of infection may be nonspecific and subtle. If the nurse suspects developing signs of infection, he or she should perform more frequent assessments.

The healthy newborn voids by 24 hours (AAP & ACOG, 2002). The nurse should document in the medical

BOX 20.4 Signs of Abnormal Transition

- Abdominal distention
- Central cyanosis or duskiness requiring continuous or intermittent supplemental oxygen
- Frequent choking or drooling, especially if accompanied by apnea or cyanosis
- Hypotonia or lethargy
- Marked jitteriness or tremors
- Pale, gray, or mottled appearance, which indicates poor perfusion
- Respiratory distress that does not steadily resolve in the first 30 to 60 minutes of life or increases over time, with expiratory grunting, nasal flaring, retracting, tachypnea, gasping, or apnea
- Unstable temperature in a stable thermal environment
- Unusual neurologic activity
- Vomiting of bilious material
- Weak or high-pitched cry

record assessment of urine output and any variances. He or she should instruct parents to report the number of wet diapers that they change or how to document them. The nurse should notify the pediatric provider of delayed or abnormal urination (AAP & ACOG, 2002).

Select Potential Nursing Diagnoses

The following nursing diagnoses may be appropriate:

- **Risk for Imbalanced Body Temperature** related to larger body surface in relationship to mass and decreased subcutaneous fat
- **Risk for Injury** related to hypoglycemia
- **Risk for Injury** related to blood volume excess or deficit
- **Risk for Injury** related to excess byproducts of RBC breakdown and concurrent hepatic immaturity
- **Risk for Injury** related to delayed or abnormal GI function secondary to immaturity or pathology
- **Risk for Infection** related to immature immunologic defenses and environmental exposure
- **Risk for Impaired Skin Integrity** related to immature skin structure and environmental exposure
- **Risk for Deficient/Excess Fluid Volume** related to immature renal physiology

Planning/Intervention

No health care team member should ever leave a newborn exposed after unwrapping or undressing the baby for a physical examination or procedure such as a blood draw. Parents, who naturally unwrap the newborn to count fingers and toes, to look for familial characteristics, or to make sure that "everything is there," should be allowed this important examination, but encouraged to make it brief. To avoid hyperthermia, staff must be educated in correct use of warming interventions, such as radiant warmers, chemical warmers, heat lamps, and incubators. Strategies to promote thermoregulation include drying the newborn immediately after birth; dressing the newborn in clothing, blankets, and a hat to conserve body temperature; ensuring that linen, blankets, and clothing are dry; positioning the newborn in a draft-free area; and using necessary warming interventions, such as the radiant warmer, appropriately and safely.

Clear and complete communication among team members is essential to identify newborns at risk for hypoglycemia. The nurse caring for the mother should notify nursery personnel, the pediatric care provider, or both when she admits a laboring woman at risk for giving birth to a baby predisposed to blood glucose instability. Risk factors include prematurity, maternal diabetes, SGA newborn, or intrapartal fetal stress. Laboratory confirmation of aberrant bedside glucose screening test results should occur quickly. Interventions vary depending on the etiology and degree of hypoglycemia. Feeding by breast, nipple, or gavage is effective in most cases. Newborns in distress, those with acute hypoglycemia, and infants born before 35 to 36 weeks' gestation are managed with IV therapy. Thermal and oxygen support are important adjuncts because thermal stress and respiratory distress increase glucose metabolism (Karp et al., 1995).

The nurse caring for the newborn should be aware of any risk factors for anemia or polycythemia and communicate them to the pediatric provider. Communication with labor and delivery staff is important to obtain late intrapartum information, such as suspected partial placenta previa or placental abruption, which places the newborn at risk for decreased blood volume and anemia. Evidence of discordant placental circulation may explain anemia or polycythemia in twins. Laboratory blood work to ascertain the newborn's hemoglobin, hematocrit, or CBC and differential is not required routinely; however, any infant at risk for or showing evidence of anemia, polycythemia, or infection requires evaluation. The pale or plethoric newborn also requires support to ensure thermal stability and adequate perfusion and oxygenation.

Because healthy newborns and mothers usually are discharged by day 2 or 3, collaborative efforts are necessary to identify those babies who require treatment for hyperbilirubinemia. The nurse should teach parents when to call the health care provider (when the baby is jaundiced head to toe, or when lethargy, poor feeding, or both accompany jaundice). He or she should recommend a system of follow-up examination, either in the home or clinic, within 48 hours of discharge, especially for those infants discharged before 48 hours old (AAP & ACOG, 2002). Early and effective feeding promotes excretion of bilirubin; therefore, the baby should stay with the mother as much as possible so that feeding can occur at the first opportunity.

The nurse should document bowel sounds, feeding activity, feeding tolerance, and bowel activities. He or she should instruct parents about how to discuss infant feeding and stooling or how to document them. The nurse should notify the pediatric provider of delayed or abnormal stooling, abdominal distention, or bilious vomiting (AAP & ACOG, 2002). Early and effective feeding helps promote intestinal motility and stooling. The nurse should alert the pediatric provider of abnormalities, and, when appropriate, stop feeding until medical evaluation is complete.

The infant's medical records should be complete and identify all factors that would place him or her at risk for infection. Examples include foul-smelling amniotic fluid or maternal fever late in labor. The nurse should communicate such information both verbally and in the record to the infant's care provider. All team members, including the baby's parents, should practice meticulous handwashing and protect the newborn from exposure to pathogens.

A newborn with developing sepsis can become critically ill within hours. A CBC with differential is necessary for those at high risk or with abnormal transition or clinical signs of infection (see Chap. 22). In addition, the plan of care usually includes IV antibiotics and support of thermoregulation, oxygenation, perfusion, and glucose metabolism. Parents of a sick newborn require information and support during this stressful time (see Chap. 22).

Every team member should work to protect the newborn's skin from damage and chemical exposure. The nurse should report any skin abnormalities or breaks to the pediatric care provider in a timely manner. He or she should thoroughly wash off any soap used for bathing to prevent absorption of chemicals through the skin. He or she should point out skin characteristics to parents. The nurse should discourage use of perfumed baby products.

Early and effective feeding helps promote adequate voiding. Accurate documentation ensures adequate assessment of renal activity and prevents unnecessary interventions and diagnostic tests. The nurse should notify the pediatric provider of delayed or abnormal voiding.

Evaluation

Standards for normal newborn temperature vary regionally; however, axillary temperature should be stable and between 97.5° and 99.1°F (36.5° and 37.3° C). The newborn should be wrapped in dry clothing and blankets in a warm, draft-free environment. The nurse should document temperature and any interventions to adjust it and re-evaluate periodically to ensure stability or to identify instability that requires additional assessment and intervention.

Blood glucose level should be at least 45 mg/dL while weaning IV fluids or advancing oral feedings (Cowett & Loughead, 2002). The nurse should document results of bedside screening and laboratory tests and symptoms of hypoglycemia, such as jitteriness or lethargy.

The healthy term newborn has no apparent risk factors for alterations in quantity or function of blood components. In addition, he or she is pink and well perfused and shows no signs of sepsis. RBC (including hemoglobin and hematocrit), WBC, and platelet counts vary considerably among newborns, depending on gestational age and environmental factors; however, laboratory values should be within normal limits.

Physiologic jaundice should resolve in the first week of life. Evidence of resolution includes disappearance of visible jaundice and decreasing serum bilirubin levels to normal limits.

The healthy term infant can coordinate sucking, swallowing, and breathing to feed effectively 8 to 12 times per day. He or she has audible bowel sounds, a soft protruding abdomen, and no bilious vomiting; the baby passes meconium by 12 to 24 hours of birth.

The nurse should evaluate blood work for diagnostic confirmation of infection. An infant responding positively to interventions has stable vital signs within normal limits, adequate oxygenation and perfusion, normal laboratory blood test results, and normal voiding and stooling. He or she also tolerates feedings when appropriate.

The skin overall should be dry and flaking in a term newborn by the second or third day of life. The newborn should have voided straw-colored urine. Female infants may have small amounts of bloody mucus from pseudomenses. The nurse should document each wet diaper and weigh the newborn daily. A loss of 5% to 10% of birth weight is expected in the first week of life from normal diuresis.

ONGOING ASSESSMENTS

The nurse's vigilance does not end when the newborn transition period is over. Although this chapter focuses on performance of the most thorough newborn physical assessment, it is important to know that the nurse observes and assesses the newborn to some degree *every* time he or she sees the baby. Even when the nurse simply passes by the bassinet, the nurse should glance at and assess the newborn's resting position, respiratory status, color, and state to ensure ongoing safety and well-being.

The nurse should record periodic assessment of vital signs and indicators of well-being such as color, activity, feeding, and elimination on the infant's hospital record. (See Fig. 20.16 for a sample of a basic well-baby daily flowsheet.) He or she should note any deviations from normal, which may necessitate a narrative note for further explanation. The nurse should describe interventions and their associated outcomes.

Infant safety parameters are also part of periodic assessment. The sample in Figure 20.16 has a prompt to check that newborn identification bands are secure and that mother and baby bands match. Variations on infant hospital flowsheets include such items as a space to record the infant's position (eg, supine) and that the bulb syringe is present in the bassinet.

BASIC CARE OF THE HEALTHY NEWBORN

Basic nursing care of the healthy newborn usually differs little from care that parents render after discharge. In most cases, the healthy mother and newborn are separated as little as possible during the hospital stay; therefore, basic newborn care that the nurse performs usually is an opportunity to teach parents these skills (Nursing Care Plan 20.1). Hospital lengths of stay often

(text continues on page 841)

Well baby daily flow sheet

* Indicates additional information in nursing progress notes = normal	Date: Time:							
Crib (C), Radiant Warmer (RW)								
Temperature: Axillary (A), Skin (S), Rectal (R)								
Pulse								
Respirations								
Assessment								
General Appearance: Tone, activity, cry, reflexes								
Skin: color/lesion								
Head/neck								
Eyes/ears/nose/throat								
Lungs/breath sounds/thorax/heart								
Abdomen/bowel tones								
Genitalia/anus								
Trunk/spine								
Extremeties/joints								
Nutrition								
Breast — Quality of feeding: Well (W), Fair (F), Poor (P)								
Breast — Length of time per side: left/right								
Formula — Type amount:								
Formula — Method: Nipple (N), Finger (F), Dropper (D), Cup (C), Tube at breast (T)								
Regurgitation								
Output								
Void								
Stool: Yellow (Y), Seedy (S), Green (G), Mustard-like (M), Transitional (T)								
Treatments								
Circumcision: physician/checked								
Lab work drawn: HCT, CBC, Lytes, Bili, PKU, Glucose strip (G), other (O)								
Clamp removed (CR), Bath (B)								
Physician visit/exam								
Parental contact/visit: Mother (M), Father (F)								
Matching ID bands on: Admission (A), Transfer (T), Q shift (Q)								
Hearing Screen: Pass/Referred								
Caregiver's initials								
Signatures and initials								

Newborn Care Record

FIGURE 20.16 Sample well-baby daily flowsheet.

NURSING CARE PLAN 20.1

The Healthy Newborn and Family

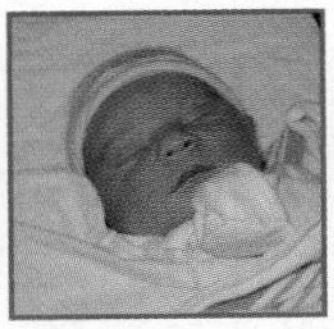

Recall Thomas, the 8-hour-old newborn from the beginning of this chapter. Further assessment reveals the following: weight, 8 lbs, 4 oz; pink color; alert and active; axillary temperature, 97.2°F; heart rate, 148 bpm and steady with appropriate PMI and no audible murmur; respirations 52 breaths/min, with no grunting, nasal flaring, or retractions; clear and equal bilateral breath sounds. Bowel sounds are present. Thomas voided at birth and has passed his first meconium stool. The nurse notes a small red puncture mark on the occipital part of the scalp from a fetal monitor electrode. He was lying on the bed when the nurse arrived.

NURSING DIAGNOSES

- **Ineffective Airway Clearance** related to excess mucus, gagging, and choking
- **Deficient Knowledge (Maternal)** related to newborn care and airway maintenance

EXPECTED OUTCOMES

1. The newborn will maintain a patent airway.
2. The newborn will exhibit no signs of continuing respiratory distress.
3. The mother will demonstrate beginning skill with use of the bulb syringe.

INTERVENTIONS	RATIONALES
Turn the newborn on his side.	This position promotes fluid drainage from the nose and mouth to prevent aspiration.
Suction the mouth first, then the nares with the bulb syringe.	Gentle suctioning promotes a patent airway. The baby may gasp upon placement of the bulb syringe in the nares; therefore, suctioning the mouth first prevents aspiration.
Assess for signs and symptoms of respiratory distress, such as nasal flaring or grunting respirations. Auscultate the lungs after any choking episode.	Assessment provides information to determine the effect of and recovery from choking episodes.
Replace the bulb syringe in the bassinet where it is visible.	The syringe should be available for immediate use as necessary.
Continue to assess the newborn's respiratory status frequently.	Continued assessment is necessary to allow for early identification of and prompt intervention for any additional problems.
Instruct the mother in how to use the bulb syringe; have her identify situations in which she may need the bulb syringe; have her return-demonstrate the procedure; offer praise and positive reinforcement.	Teaching assists the mother to gain necessary skills to care for her son. Return demonstration indicates the effectiveness of teaching. Positive reinforcement and praise promote feelings of confidence.

Continued

NURSING CARE PLAN 20.1 ● The Healthy Newborn and Family

EVALUATION

1. The newborn experiences full recovery.
2. The newborn maintains a patent airway with minimal to no mucus present.
3. The mother demonstrates the ability to use the bulb syringe appropriately and correctly.

NURSING DIAGNOSIS

Risk for Imbalanced Body Temperature related to immature temperature control, change in environmental temperature, and large body surface in relation to mass

EXPECTED OUTCOME

The newborn will maintain an axillary temperature of 97.5° to 99.1°F clothed in a shirt, diaper, and two blankets.

INTERVENTIONS	RATIONALES
Assess the newborn's temperature as per agency policy.	Assessment provides a baseline from which to make future comparisons. Thomas's current axillary temperature is at the low end of the normal range.
Institute measures to conserve the newborn's heat; use warmed blankets and the overhead radiant warmer. Double-wrap the infant in a blanket and place a thermally insulated hat on his head.	Newborns need additional measures to conserve heat because of their immature ability to regulate body temperature.
Avoid situations that may promote heat loss; dry skin thoroughly, avoid placing bassinet near doorways or drafts, and avoid placing newborn on cold surfaces.	Heat is lost through conduction, convection, radiation, and evaporation.
Continue to monitor temperature as indicated; recheck temperature 30 minutes after instituting warming measures.	Temperature should respond to warming measures and stabilize.

EVALUATION

The newborn maintains an axillary temperature within expected parameters.

NURSING DIAGNOSIS

Deficient Knowledge (Maternal) related to care of healthy newborn

EXPECTED OUTCOMES

1. The mother will demonstrate safe caregiving practices for her newborn.
2. The mother will demonstrate how to use the bulb syringe during choking episodes.
3. The mother will identify strategies to protect the infant from infection and injury.
4. The mother will demonstrate beginning confidence in caring for her newborn.

Continued

NURSING CARE PLAN 20.1 ● The Healthy Newborn and Family *(Continued)*

INTERVENTIONS	RATIONALES
Assess maternal knowledge of newborn care. Provide facts; clarify misconceptions.	Assessment provides a baseline from which to develop an individualized teaching plan.
Use written, verbal, and audiovisual information to teach the mother about safe caregiving practices, such as keeping the infant in the bassinet or in her arms instead of on the bed.	Providing nonjudgmental supportive information about infant safety helps ensure that the mother will listen and learn about strategies to prevent injury to her infant.
Reassure the mother that infants are competent at clearing their airways. Explain that the bulb syringe is necessary when fluids coming from the baby's mouth or nose accompany choking.	Helping the mother to perceive her infant as competent will minimize undue fear and anxiety. Additional teaching about the bulb syringe helps to promote confidence when using it.
Demonstrate the use of the bulb syringe to her. Ask for a return demonstration by placing the syringe gently inside the infant's cheek and near the nares, using correct technique to aspirate fluids.	Asking for a return demonstration during a calm moment will increase the mother's feelings of competence.
Explain that infants are vulnerable to infection. Demonstrate handwashing technique to mother after infant caregiving, and remind the mother to wash her hands regularly before giving newborn care. Show the small scalp abrasion to the mother and explain signs to report that would indicate infection (redness, drainage, swelling, signs of illness in the newborn).	Teaching the mother about the infant's vulnerability to infection facilitates her involvement in protecting the infant from infection.
Reinforce additional measures for newborn care including bathing, diapering, clothing, using car seats, comforting, and sleeping position.	Adequate knowledge related to care measures helps to promote their use.
Review the signs and symptoms of newborn illness; encourage the mother to notify the health care provider should any occur.	Signs and symptoms of newborn illness can be vague; knowledge of when to notify the health care provider promotes early detection and prompt intervention.
Arrange for possible referral to social services and home care if indicated.	Support from additional sources helps to ease the transition and provides opportunities for additional follow-up and teaching.

EVALUATION

1. The mother demonstrates measures to provide safe newborn care.
2. The mother demonstrates calm and efficient use of the bulb syringe, identifying situations when use is necessary.
3. The mother implements appropriate measures to protect the newborn from infection and injury.
4. The mother states that she feels more confident when providing care to her newborn.

are fewer than 48 hours, so it is important for the mother and her partner or support person to provide much newborn care, calling on the nurse to answer questions and assist as necessary. (For newborn feeding and nutrition information, see Chap. 21.)

Cultural Aspects

The nurse should consider cultural aspects of newborn care while teaching parents relevant skills. Knowing how ethnic practices may differ from standard hospital practices is helpful. It is not safe to assume that the hospital protocol or pediatric provider's orders will be congruent with the family's cultural practices. Neither is it safe to stereotype the behavior of ethnic groups by assuming that literature about cultural practices applies to everyone within each culture. The nurse should observe parental responses to teaching and ask if they have a different preference. For example, the nurse who teaches umbilical cord care to a Russian immigrant may approach the situation by saying, "The way I just showed you is how many mothers in the United States do this. Is this what you expected? Would you like to talk about other methods?"

No health care professional can assume that information related to culture or ethnicity applies to each specific client just because he or she comes from that background. For more information about caring for clients of different cultures and ethnicities, see the following:

- Ottani, P. A. (2002). Embracing global similarities: A framework for cross-cultural obstetric care. *Journal of Obstetrical, Gynecological, and Neonatal Nursing, 31*(1), 33–38.
- Enang, J. E., Wojnar, D., & Harper, F. D. (2002). Childbearing among diverse populations: How one hospital is providing multicultural care. *AWHONN Lifelines, 6*(2), 153–158.

Table 20.5 provides some broad parameters for aspects related to newborn care across various cultures. These guidelines do not apply to every client from a culture, which nurses must keep paramount in mind when delivering care.

Care of the Newborn Following Home Birth

Newborn care for an infant born at home follows the same principles applied to care rendered in the hospital. A multidisciplinary team provides care, with the nurse coordinating the plan. The scope of nursing practice "is limited to practices deemed safe and appropriate to be carried out in an environment that is physically separated from a health care institution and its resources" (Association of Women's Health, Obstetric and Neonatal Nurses [AWHONN], 1998, p. 36). Concepts important to home care of the newborn include the following:

- Women and newborns receive the same level of nursing care and expertise in the home as would be expected in a licensed birth setting.
- The nurse, health care provider, and family members develop the plan of care collaboratively with the client, with consideration of various aspects of the home life.
- Nursing practice in a home care setting is consistent with federal, state, and provincial regulations that direct practice. Standards of newborn care are the same in the home setting as in the hospital setting. For example, vitamin K administration, eye prophylaxis, administration of hepatitis B immunoglobulin (HBIG) and hepatitis B vaccine if appropriate, and newborn metabolic screening should be offered to (but may be refused by) parents in the home birth setting. The nurse should document timely assessments, the plan of care, interventions, evaluation, and outcomes.

The primary focus of home care is safety. Appropriate client selection, sound clinical judgment, and prompt transfer to a receptive environment when necessary help ensure good perinatal outcomes (American College of Nurse-Midwives [ACNM], 2003).

Infant Security

Infant abduction from hospital settings is uncommon but not outside the realm of possibility. Hospital personnel need education regarding abductor profiles (Box 20.5), abductor behavior, means of abduction, and their facility's emergency plan in the event of abduction. Every obstetrical unit must have policies and procedures in place to reduce the risk for abduction (American Health Consultants, 1998). Components may ensure that:

- Only those family members or support people who bear an identification bracelet matching the newborn's may transport the newborn.
- The newborn is described accurately in the newborn record, foot-printed properly, and photographed for the medical record.
- All hospital personnel wear photo identification above the waist.
- Client names are visible only to hospital personnel, not to visitors.
- All newborns are transported in their cribs. Anyone walking with a newborn in their arms is stopped and questioned.
- A staff member accompanies the newborn and parents to their car at discharge. Any person with a newborn outside the obstetrical unit and unaccompanied by staff is questioned.
- Newspaper and Internet birth announcements use only the parents' first names. (Publication of last names enables an abductor to find the parent's address.)
- Unit access is controlled, unit and stairway exits have alarms, and video cameras record the faces of people leaving the unit (Shogan, 2002).

TABLE 20.5 Tips for Newborn Care of Selected Cultures

CULTURE	GREETING	CONSENTS FOR TREATMENT	FATHER'S ROLE IN BIRTH PROCESS AND NEWBORN CARE	INFANT FEEDING	CIRCUMCISION	OTHER
American Indian	Handshake	May involve family consensus	Varies	Breast and bottle	No	May save remnant of umbilical cord
Arab American	Handshake may be related to gender; use title and first name; smile, eye contact acceptable	Verbal consent preferred; explain need for written consent	Not expected to participate Female family member provides support.	Believe colostrum is harmful Need support to breastfeed	Males: yes, but may delay until school age Females: unusual, although female family members may have been circumcised in home country	Children are sacred, obedient.
Black/African American	Handshake with Mr./Mrs. and last name	Varies with level of education	Varies with health education	Varies with education; most are willing to breastfeed	Varies	Respect elders, considering them a source of wisdom
Cambodian (Khmer)	Handshake for acculturated	May be uncomfortable with written consents; ensure translation	Varies; father may be involved, but women may prefer their mothers	Delay breastfeeding to avoid colostrum; bottle feeding denotes higher status	No	Cuddling uncommon; sniffing instead of kissing
Central American	Friendly handshake	Consent procedure may be unfamiliar	May be present; passive role	Varies by social class; may combine methods; higher income prefer bottle feeding	Male circumcision not traditional; however, parents may wish to acculturate through circumcision.	Mother and baby may use herbal teas and baths.
Chinese American	Friendly greeting, use Mr./Mrs. and last name	Involve oldest male of family; assess understanding	Female family members present; fathers usually not active	Breastfeeding preferred. Mother prefers hot foods while breastfeeding.	Male circumcision common.	New baby is highly valued.
Cuban	Formal at first introduction, then familiar tone and address.	Client may consult with most respected or eldest member before consenting.	Traditionally, fathers not involved; however varies with acculturation	Breastfeeding rates increasing among Cubans.	Male circumcision common.	Family members may wish to be present at all times.
Gypsy (Roma)	Varies. Greet each other with palm up.	Generally understood and acceptable.	Mother or aunt preferred at birth.	Cultural norm is breastfeeding; however, young mothers may prefer bottle feeding.	Male circumcision not traditional, but may be requested.	Extended family valued. Anxious when separated from family.

Jewish American	Varies	Varies	Varies depending on belief. Orthodox men may not be in physical contact with mother but may be physically present during newborn period (Rosner & Tendler, 1980).	Varies	Male circumcision (bris) is a religious rite on the newborn's 8th day; it usually is performed by a mohel, who may or may not be a physician.	Adoption is acceptable.
Mexican American	Formal greeting, include children	Varies; consider literacy level	Varies; father or female relatives provide support	Breastfeeding is most common.	Male circumcision not traditional, but may be requested.	Wide diversity in beliefs and practices.
Russian	Serious, formal. Use Mr./Mrs. and last name	Often require family consensus	Traditionally passive role.	Breastfeeding expected and highly valued.	Male circumcision varies with religious affiliation.	Cover baby's head; keep baby warm.
Vietnamese	Varies with degree of familiarity. Client offers her hand first for handshake.	May nod yes but not understand; try to verify understanding.	Varies; female family member may be birth coach and support but father is accessible.	Breastfeeding is traditional but bottle feeding may be used.	Male circumcision varies with economic status and beliefs.	Mother rarely separated from new baby.

From Lipson, J. G., Dibble, S. L., & Minarik, P. A. (Eds.) (1996). *Culture & nursing care: A pocket guide.* San Francisco: UCSF Nursing Press; and Bank, R. D. (2002). *The everything Judaism book.* Avon, MA: Adams Media Corporation.

BOX 20.5 Abductor Profile

Characteristics

- Female between the ages of 12 and 50 years
- Large build or overweight for height
- Married or involved in a failing relationship
- May have experienced a pregnancy loss (miscarriage, stillbirth, adoption)
- Lives in the community where the abduction takes place
- Often emotionally immature, compulsive, with low self-esteem
- May be feigning a pregnancy and have told acquaintances that she is pregnant

Typical Abduction Strategies

- Visits birthing centers asking detailed questions about procedures and unit layout
- Plans the abduction and then acts quickly when opportunity arises
- Impersonates medical, nursing, laboratory, volunteer, social work, or photography personnel
- With an accomplice or alone, may create a disturbance, such as pulling fire alarm or starting a fire, to distract staff
- Calls mother by her first name, learned from crib card or unsecured medical record
- Befriends the mother and stays for several hours to establish her trust
- Removes the newborn from the baby mother's room by saying the baby needs lab tests, vital signs, photographs, weight, etc.
- Removes the baby from the unit in a sport bag or under a coat
- Once the abduction has occurred, considers the baby to be her own

From Rabun, J. (ed). (2000). *For healthcare professionals: Guidelines on prevention of and response to infant abductions* (6th ed.). Alexandria, VA: National Center for Missing and Exploited Children.

Parents play a major role in ensuring their infant's security. They must learn the basics of hospital security for their infant to help prevent abduction. See Teaching Tips 20.2 for a sample instruction sheet.

Temperature Assessment

Once the term newborn has been discharged, parents have no reason to take his or her temperature at home unless they suspect illness. Because the nurse models the axillary method of temperature assessment, the parent usually learns this procedure. If a caregiver voices a preference for rectal temperature assessment, the nurse can teach that method in addition to the axillary method. Because of the potential for trauma and injury to the newborn during rectal assessment, however, nurses may advise parents to use the axillary method as their initial screen. If parents determine that the axillary temperature is abnormal and their pediatric provider wants a rectal temperature, parents can proceed cautiously with a rectal temperature.

The nurse should take the axillary temperature by placing the thermometer deep into the baby's axilla and holding the arm down gently against the baby's chest (Fig. 20.17). The reading will be inaccurate if the thermometer tip extends past the axilla (exposed to air) or if the thermometer touches clothing instead of skin.

Use of the Bulb Syringe

The bulb syringe clears the upper airways of mucus and gastric secretions. Personnel first use it at birth to clear the mouth and nose to facilitate initial respirations. The bulb syringe then stays in the bassinet for use in the event of emesis. Healthy newborns have an active gag reflex and are adept at clearing their upper airways, however, and the bulb syringe often is not needed after the transitional period.

The nurse should teach parents to use the bulb syringe when secretions are visible in the baby's nose or

TEACHING TIPS 20.2 Instructions for Keeping Your Baby Safe in the Hospital

- Give the baby only to hospital personnel wearing a hospital photo name tag.
- Go with any staff person who takes the baby from your room, if you wish.
- Never let the baby out of sight or leave him or her alone. Call the staff to take the baby when you shower, need to close the bathroom door, or plan to nap.
- Keep the baby on the far side of the room away from the door. This will help prevent people from moving the baby without your notice.
- Question any stranger who enters the room if the reason for the visit is unclear or strange.
- Call the nurse's station immediately to report a stranger or to check the identity of anyone who claims to work at the hospital.

Adapted from Shogan, M. G. (2002). Emergency management plan for newborn abduction. *Journal of Obstetric, Gynecologic, and Neonatal Nursing, 31*(3), 340–346.

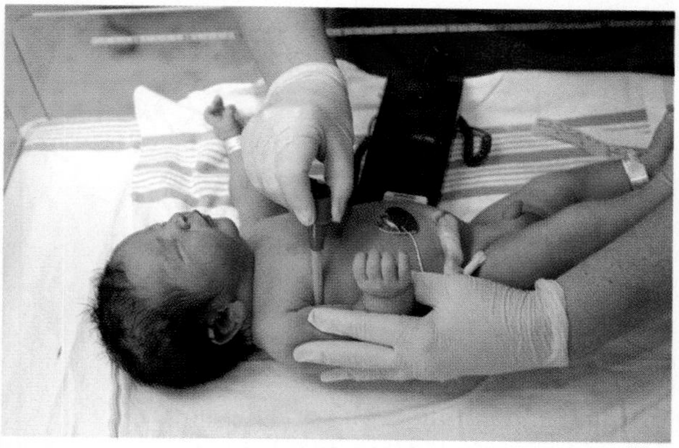

FIGURE 20.17 Taking axillary temperature in a newborn.

mouth or if the newborn is gagging or gurgling through oral fluids. Because the baby is likely to gasp when the syringe is placed into the nares, parents should suction the mouth before the nose to prevent aspiration (Kattwinkel, 2006). See Nursing Procedure 20.5.

During a gagging or choking episode, a calm but swift response is required. Parents gain confidence in their ability to handle this situation if the nurse can talk them through the skill, or, if necessary for a more timely intervention, demonstrate efficient use of the syringe. After the baby has recovered, the entire family may require comforting and reassurance!

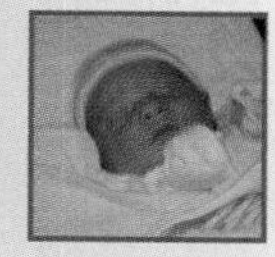

Thomas, the 8-hour-old term newborn, started gagging and choking after vomiting some breast milk. His mother was visibly upset. How would the nurse calm her?

Voiding and Stooling

Urine output may be low for the first 2 days of life. The baby should void by 24 hours of age. By the third or fourth day, parents should note a wet diaper with every feeding—about 6 to 8 wet diapers per day.

The appearance of the first stool, called **meconium,** may surprise parents. This sticky black substance usually passes in the first 24 hours, although some infants do not pass meconium stool until 48 hours. Meconium stools persist for up to 3 days, then gradually change to the seedy yellowish color of normal newborn stool (Fig. 20.18). Breastfed babies have softer, more liquid stools than formula-fed infants. Breastfed babies' stools are also less malodorous than stools from formula-fed babies.

Stooling patterns vary depending on whether the infant is breastfed or formula fed. Some breastfed infants stool at every feeding. Parents need to be concerned only if their baby's stool is malodorous and liquid (diarrhea stool) or if it contains mucus or blood. Newborns are rarely constipated, but parents should consult their care provider if the newborn seems to strain or cry during bowel movements or produces hard, pellet-like stools.

Diapering

Cloth or disposable diapers may be used for newborn care. Parents should check the diaper when the infant awakens for a feeding. Stooling may occur during feeding, especially for the breastfeeding baby, which may necessitate a diaper change after feeding as well. Parents can prevent diaper rash by keeping the diaper area clean and dry. They should wash the buttocks and perianal region with plain or soapy water as necessary. Stool and skin secretions can hide in vaginal folds and under the scrotum, so nurses teach parents to wipe the vaginal area from front to back with a clean cloth, or to clean under and around the scrotal sac. Commercial diaper wipes are an unnecessary added expense; if parents use them, however, they should choose a brand without alcohol or added fragrance. They should fold the diaper down to keep the umbilicus exposed to air until after the cord falls off and the umbilical site heals (Fig. 20.19). With practice, parents soon will be able to secure a diaper that is not so tight as to press into the baby's abdomen, and not so loose as to allow the diaper to leak or fall off during handling.

Cord Care

Cord care practices vary by institution and region and include no care, isopropyl alcohol, triple dye, and antimicrobial ointments. No one method has been proved superior in preventing colonization and disease (AAP & ACOG, 2002). The nurse should teach parents the method at his or her institution, with consideration for cultural differences. He or she should tell parents that the cord may become gooey before separation. Most importantly, the nurse should ensure that parents know how to call the health care provider if the umbilical site becomes red or swollen, or has purulent or malodorous discharge.

Clothing

While in the hospital, the newborn usually is clothed in a cotton T-shirt, diaper, and two blankets. The newborn's head is poorly insulated and accounts for significant heat loss; therefore, a hat protects vulnerable newborns from heat loss (Blackburn, 2003). The stockinette hats commonly used in hospitals are poor insulators. Preferred fabrics include insulated fabrics, wool, or polyolefin, or hats lined with Gamgee or a plastic liner (Blackburn, 2003).

Parents often worry that the newborn will become chilled at home and therefore tend to overheat the house and overdress their newborn. The healthy newborn requires about one layer more of clothing than the parent, in a house heated or cooled for the parent's comfort.

NURSING PROCEDURE 20.5

Suctioning with a Bulb Syringe

PURPOSE

To remove visible mucus, secretions, and vomitus from the newborn's mouth or nares

ASSESSMENT AND PLANNING

- Review the newborn's medical record for a history of antepartal or intrapartal problems.
- Assess the newborn's gag reflex; assess for gagging and gurgling with oral feedings.
- Auscultate the newborn's lungs *to evaluate for evidence of crackles and wheezes.*
- Inspect the newborn's mouth and nose for visible secretions or vomitus.
- Explain the procedure and its rationale to the parents.
- Gather the necessary equipment:
    - Bulb syringe (in newborn's bassinet)
    - Receptacle or tissue for discarding secretions
    - Clean gloves

IMPLEMENTATION

1. Wash hands and put on gloves.
2. Position the newborn on the side with the head slightly lower than the rest of the body *to facilitate drainage by gravity.*
3. Compress the bulb before insertion *to prevent injury to the newborn's oral mucosa.*
4. Gently insert the tip of the bulb syringe into the dependent side of the newborn's mouth *to collect drainage.*
5. Release the compression on the bulb *to allow for re-expansion and the collection of secretions.*
6. Remove the bulb syringe from the newborn's mouth and gently squeeze the bulb *to release the collected drainage into the appropriate receptacle or onto a tissue.*
7. Turn the newborn to the other side and repeat the steps to suction the other side of the newborn's mouth; if necessary, repeat the steps to suction each nares.
8. Discard the collected secretions and clean the receptacle as necessary.
9. Wash the bulb syringe in warm soapy water and rinse. Place the bulb syringe back in the newborn's bassinet for future use. Remove gloves and wash hands.
10. Reassess the newborn's lungs; provide reassurance and comforting to the parents and the newborn.

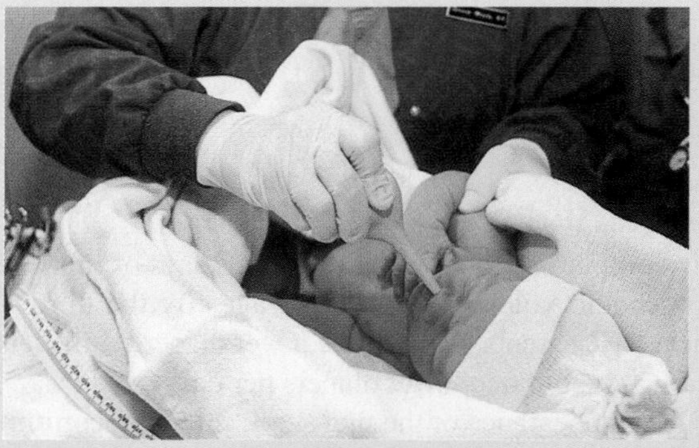

Step 7. Suctioning the newborn with a bulb syringe.

EVALUATION

- Newborn tolerated the procedure without difficulty.
- Excess secretions are removed and no longer evident.
- Lungs remained clear on auscultation.

Continued

NURSING PROCEDURE 20.5
Suctioning with a Bulb Syringe

AREAS FOR CONSIDERATION AND ADAPTATION

Lifespan Considerations

- As an alternative to positioning the newborn on the side during suctioning, use the football hold with the newborn positioned on the side.
- Always suction the newborn's mouth before the nose to prevent possible aspiration of secretions as the newborn gasps when the nostril is touched.
- Never insert the bulb syringe into the middle of the newborn's mouth, toward the back of the mouth, or toward the roof of the mouth to prevent stimulating the gag reflex.
- Teach the parents how to perform suctioning with bulb syringe and signs and symptoms observed that indicate the need for suctioning; have the parents return demonstrate the procedure.
- If suctioning with bulb syringe is ineffective, anticipate the need for additional suction measures.
- Keep in mind that use of the bulb syringe is typically not necessary after the newborn's transitional period.

Community-Based Considerations

- Have the parents return-demonstrate the procedure for using the bulb syringe.
- If the infant has copious or tenacious nasal secretions, teach the parents how to instill normal saline to help loosen the secretions and aid in their removal.
- If the parents are using a humidifier in the home, review the procedure for cleaning the device to prevent growth of microorganisms.

Wrapping

Swaddling provides containment, security, and warmth. Parents need not worry that their swaddling technique is less neat or efficient than that of the hospital staff. The nurse teaches parents how to swaddle, allowing the newborn's hands to be in close proximity to the mouth (Fig. 20.20). Hand-to-mouth behavior is calming and an important developmental achievement.

Parents can swaddle by following these steps:

- Place a blanket on a flat surface with one corner of the blanket pointing away. Fold that corner down a few inches.
- Place the baby face up on the blanket, with the neck on the top folded edge of the blanket.
- Fold the left corner over the baby's body and tuck it under the back.
- Fold the bottom corner up over the feet and chest. Fold down any excess over the chest.
- Fold the right corner around the infant's body.

The nurse should remind parents that the baby's legs need to be free of swaddling when placed in a car seat. The infant must wear an outfit that allows the crotch strap to separate the legs (not a sleeping-bag style outfit). Some outfits have a slit that allows parents to push the buckle through. If needed, parents can place blankets over the baby once he or she is secured in the car seat.

Holding

There are two basic ways to hold a baby:

- *Cradle hold:* The baby is held supine across the adult's chest, with one arm supporting the head and neck, and the other supporting the back and lower body.
- *Football hold:* The baby is held supine along the inner aspect of the adult's forearm. The adult's hand and wrist support the baby's head and neck, and the rest of the forearm supports the baby's back and lower body. The baby is tucked securely against the adult's body, but not squeezed tightly. The football hold leaves the adult's other hand free.

Variations on these holds include the following:

- *The one-handed cradle hold:* The baby is held prone on the adult's arm, cradled against the adult's body.
- *Against the shoulder:* The baby is held upright, prone against the adult's chest, while the adult supports the baby's head and bottom.

The nurse can reassure parents that any holding position that supports the infant's head, neck, and back, and prevents dangling or dropping the infant, is acceptable.

Comforting

QUOTE 20-4

"My baby was crying hard in his bassinet, and I felt like crying, too. The nurse came in, picked the baby up and positioned him up against

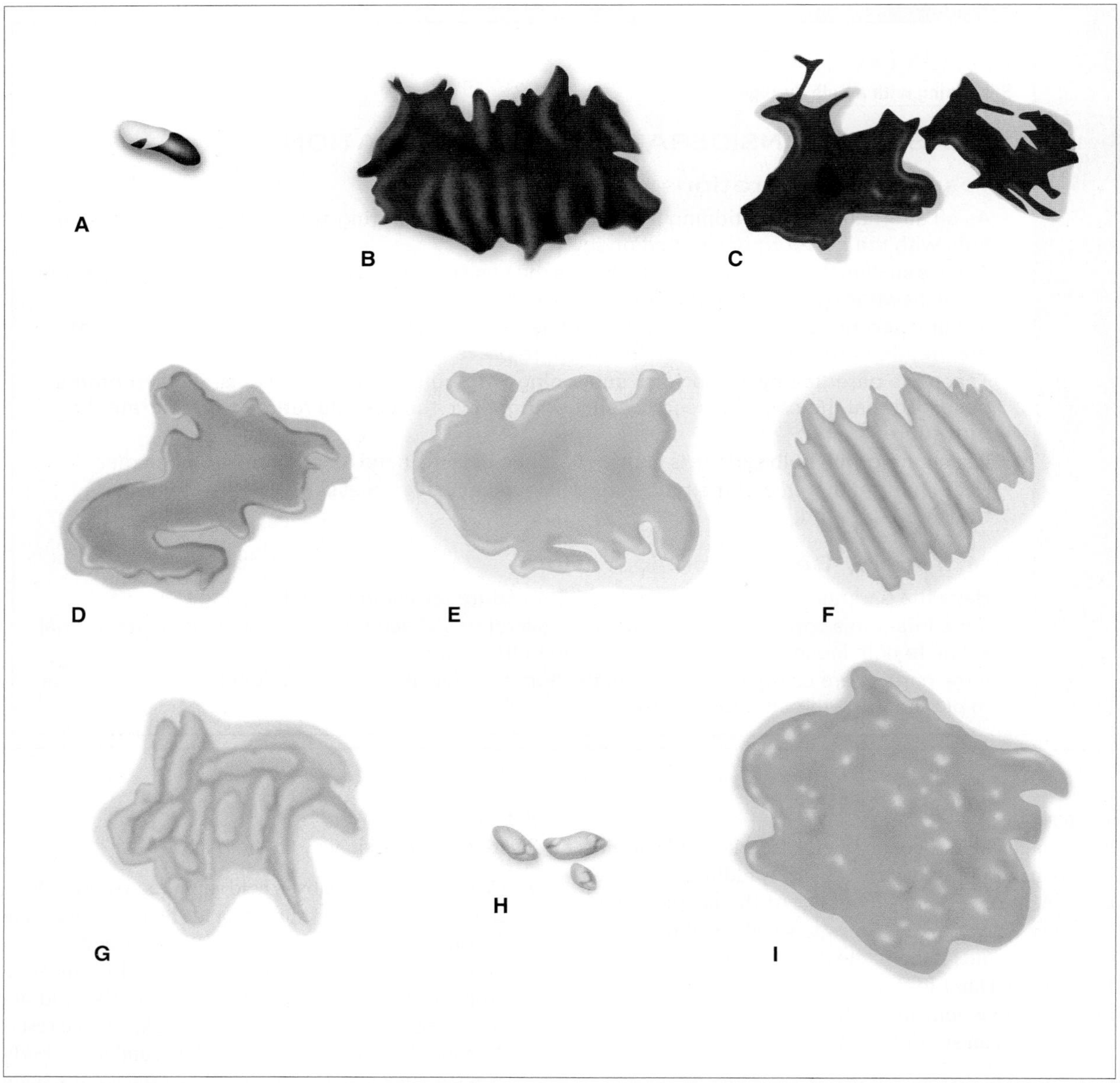

FIGURE 20.18 Characteristics of newborn stool: (**A**) meconium plug, (**B**) first meconium stool, (**C**) meconium after breastfeeding, (**D**) first transitional breastfed stool, (**E**) second transitional breastfed stool, (**F**) normal breastfed stool, (**G**) cow-milk stool, (**H**) constipated stool, (**I**) diarrheal stool.

my shoulder. I said, "What now?" and the nurse said, "Hold him close and talk softly in his ear." I didn't quite know what to say, but I murmured something and the baby immediately quieted and turned to look at me. It was amazing. I felt like his mother."

From a mom

A baby's cry is a loud distress signal designed to elicit caregiving. Acoustical spectrometry reveals distinct signature cries for boredom (in term infants), hunger, pain, stress, fatigue, and maternal separation (Christensson et al., 1995). Most parents can distinguish these different cries within 2 weeks of birth (Ludington-Hoe et al., 2002).

Prolonged crying has detrimental physiologic effects. It decreases arterial oxygen tension (Rooth et al., 1987), increases blood pressure (Dinwiddie et al., 1979), fills the stomach with air (Shaker et al., 1979), depletes energy reserves (Ludington, 1990), and increases WBC count (Christensen & Rothstein, 1979). The nurse should encourage parents to answer their baby's cry immediately, every time. A complete response includes touching, talking, and positioning oneself in the newborn's field of vision when answering the cry (Ludington-Hoe et al., 2002). A newborn is not spoiled by receiving immediate attention in response to crying. In fact, one study

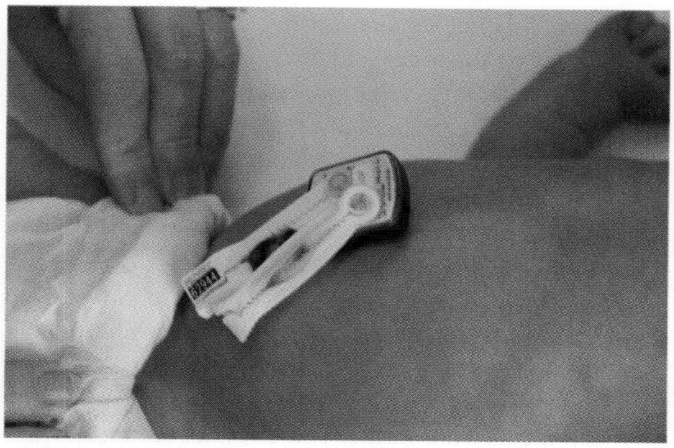

FIGURE 20.19 Diapering to avoid irritation to the umbilical area.

showed that babies whose cries were met consistently and completely in the first 6 months were found to cry less later (Barr et al., 2001). In one study, infant crying was reduced by 60% when parents learned to respond immediately and completely every time (Dihigo, 1998). Infants whose cries are answered in this way learn that their needs will be met.

Skin-to-skin holding (kangaroo care) is one way to prevent crying (Ludington, 1990; McCain et al., 2005; Michelsson et al., 1996). Traditional holding is the next best method to reduce crying (Taylor et al., 2000). Heartbeat sounds, lullabies, music, mother's voice, and rhythmic rocking movements should be in the parental repertoire of comfort strategies.

The newborn who is especially sensitive to environmental stimuli may escalate crying in response to too many simultaneous quieting attempts. He or she may be overwhelmed when confronted all at once by the visual stimulation of the mother's face, as well as her voice, touch, and rocking and patting. For these newborns, the parent must experiment with a softer approach, such as briefly looking at and speaking to the newborn, then swaddling the infant or holding him or her skin to skin against her shoulder in a quiet environment. Avoiding simultaneous talking, rocking, and patting may help the newborn regain control.

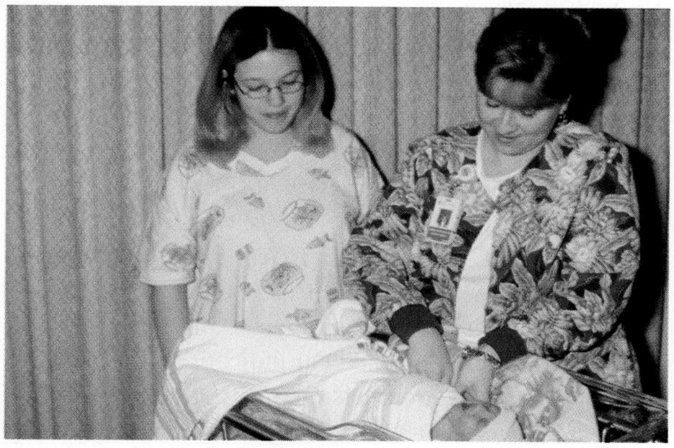

FIGURE 20.20 This nurse is teaching swaddling of a newborn to a mother.

Parental Stress

Parents should know that a baby's constant demands are stressful for them. Sometimes parents may feel angry and at risk for losing their temper. The nurse should acknowledge that these feelings are normal on a tough day and a signal that the parent requires some time away. He or she should help parents plan for these times by encouraging them to arrange for a trusted friend or family member to take over baby care for a few hours as needed. A walk around the block, warm bath, or nap can be restorative.

If no such respite care is available when the parent is losing control, the nurse should teach the parent to put the infant safely in the crib and move to another room. It is better to allow the infant to cry in the crib than to strike or shake the baby, which can cause fatalities. A parent with a fussy baby and few support systems is at risk for neglecting or abusing the newborn. The nurse is responsible for educating the parent about community resources to assist after discharge, such as parent support groups, parenting classes, and mother-to-mother mentoring programs.

Sleep Positioning and Sudden Infant Death Syndrome

Sudden infant death syndrome (SIDS) is defined as "the sudden death of an infant under 1 year of age, which remains unexplained after a thorough case investigation, including performance of a complete autopsy, examination of the death scene, and review of the clinical history" (AAP, 2005, p. 1). SIDS is a leading cause of mortality after 1 month and before 1 year (AAP, 2005). The cause is unknown. Risk factors for SIDS include prone sleep position, sleeping on a soft surface, maternal smoking during pregnancy, overheating, late or no prenatal care, young maternal age, prematurity or low birth weight, and male sex. Blacks and Native Americans and Alaskan Natives have two to three times the national average of SIDS deaths (AAP, 2005).

In 1992, the AAP recommended that infants be placed supine for sleeping to reduce the risk for SIDS (Fig. 20.21). Because prone sleep positioning was a modifiable risk factor, the Back to Sleep campaign was initiated in the United States in 1994. The campaign disseminates information to hospital nurseries and physicians, to child care education programs, and through public media campaigns. Since 1992, use of the prone sleeping position for infants has decreased from more than 70% to approximately 13% in 2004, and the SIDS rate has decreased by more than 50% (AAP, 2005).

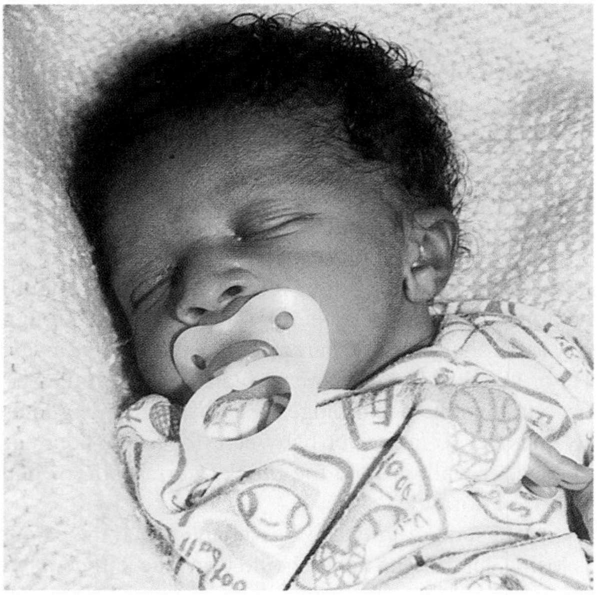

FIGURE 20.21 Newborns should be placed in the supine position when sleeping to help reduce risk of SIDS.

Recommendations to reduce risk of SIDS include the following (AAP, 2005):

- Place infants in a supine position (wholly on the back) for every sleep. Side sleeping is less safe than supine sleeping and is not advised.
- Use a firm sleep surface without soft materials or objects (eg, pillows, quilts, comforters, sheepskins) under a sleeping infant. A firm crib mattress covered by a sheet is recommended.
- Do not allow soft objects and loose bedding in the crib. Bumper pads should be thin, firm, and secure. Tuck any blankets in around the crib mattress.
- Avoid smoking during pregnancy, which has emerged as a major risk factor in almost every epidemiologic study of SIDS. Avoid exposing the infant to secondhand smoke.
- Sleep in a separate but proximate sleeping environment with the baby. Risk for SIDS is lower when the baby sleeps in the same room as the mother. A sleeping apparatus (crib) that conforms to Consumer Product Safety Commission standards is recommended. Standards for "co-sleepers" (infant beds that attach to the mother's bed) have not yet been established.
- Offer a pacifier at naps and bedtime. Reduced risk for SIDS associated with pacifier use during sleep is compelling.
- Avoid overheating the infant, who should be lightly clothed for sleep.

Bathing the Newborn

Only a few rules are important for infant bathing:

- Current practice dictates sponge bathing until the umbilical cord separates and heals.
- The baby requires a bath only once or twice a week. Parents can keep the baby's face, neck creases, and perianal area clean between baths by washing them with a cloth and plain water.
- Organize supplies before starting baths. Everything should be within arm's reach. Wash cloths and towels. An extra towel is helpful to keep nearby if the parent needs to take the baby out of the water to deal with an intervention.
- The bath should be in a warm location, free of drafts.
- If bathing on a flat surface without sides or rails, always keep one hand on the baby.
- Never leave the infant alone. If it is necessary to get the phone or retrieve a towel from the linen closet, take the infant with you.
- After the initial bath, soap rarely is needed for a newborn bath. Options should be discussed with the pediatric care provider.
- Avoid use of lotions, oils, and talcum powders. All contain chemicals that the infant's skin can absorb. The baby can inhale powder, resulting in respiratory problems. Dry flaking skin is normal. Cracks and fissures require pediatric evaluation.
- Fingernails grow quickly. Parents can file them with a soft emery board or cut them straight across with baby nail clippers or blunt edged scissors. *Never* bite off the baby's nails—doing so can cause injury and infection. Nail care is easiest when the baby is asleep.

ADDITIONAL PARENT EDUCATION

Circumcision

Circumcision is the surgical removal of the foreskin from the end of the penis. Since ancient Egypt, a major rationale for circumcision has been maintenance of penile hygiene; however, data fail to support this association (AAP, 1999b). Jewish circumcision traditionally takes place on the eighth day of the male child's life and is practiced as a religious ritual, not for health (Bank, 2002). Religious circumcision also is performed for Islamic boys.

Although circumcision remains common in the United States, it is uncommon in Asia, South America, Central America, and northern Europe (AAP, 1999b). Estimates are that approximately 30% of U.S. male newborns were circumcised in the 1930s, with the number rising to nearly 80% by the early 1970s (American Medical Association [AMA], 1999). In 1971 and 1975, the AAP recommended against circumcision. In 1975, the CPS agreed, citing no valid medical indications for neonatal circumcision. U.S. circumcision rates appeared to decline in the 1970s and early 1980s, but incidence varies by location, religious affiliation, and socioeconomic classification (AMA, 1999). The AAP (1999) estimates that

1.2 million U.S. males are circumcised annually. In addition, circumcision rates vary among U.S. racial and ethnic groups, with estimates at 81% for whites, 65% for blacks, and 54% for Hispanics (Laumann et al., 1997). Approximately 48% of Canadian males are circumcised (Leitch, 1970).

Routine circumcision remains controversial. Although some studies show reduced rates of sexually transmitted and urinary tract infections in circumcised men (Moses et al., 1990; Wiswell & Roscelli, 1986), others do not (Poland, 1990; Wallerstein, 1985). "Existing scientific evidence demonstrates potential medical benefits of newborn male circumcision; however, these data are not sufficient to recommend routine neonatal circumcision" (AAP & ACOG, 2002, p. 205).

Nonreligious circumcision may be done in the hospital or clinic setting. Cultural beliefs, the circumcision status of the infant's father and male siblings, and the opinions of the care provider all influence the decision of parents. Health care professionals should give parents unbiased information, a chance to ask questions, and a discussion of the decision. Surgical consent is required. Risks include bleeding and infection, with the complication rate estimated at approximately 0.2% to 0.6% (Gee & Ansell, 1976; Harkavy, 1987). The true incidence of complications is unknown, but most complications are minor (AAP & ACOG, 2002). See Box 20.6.

Until recently, many physicians performed circumcision without considering pain management (Geyer et al., 2002). Several interventions may be used for pain; however, acetaminophen, the sucrose pacifier, and swaddling are not recommended as sole agents for managing operative pain (AAP & ACOG, 2002). The AAP recommends the provision of anesthesia (a dorsal penile block or ring block) to the infant undergoing circumcision (AAP & ACOG, 2002). Additional analgesic interventions are listed below (Geyer et al., 2002):

- Acetaminophen: Administer 10 to 15 mg/kg 1 hour before circumcision and every 4 to 6 hours for 24 hours following circumcision.
- EMLA cream (eutectic mixture of local anesthetic): Apply topical cream made of a 1:1 oil emulsion of lidocaine and prilocaine 1 hour before surgery.
- Sucrose pacifier: Dip a pacifier in 25% oral sucrose and give to the neonate during the circumcision procedure. Sweet tasting substances provide opioid-mediated analgesia.
- Swaddling and padding: Swaddle the newborn's upper body for warmth and containment. Place him on a padded circumcision board to help decrease discomfort during circumcision.

Postoperative care includes observing the site for bleeding and greenish exudate and documenting the first postoperative void. The nurse should teach parents the postoperative care practices that their pediatric care provider recommends. Nursing Care Plan 20.2 provides more information. See also Figure 20.22.

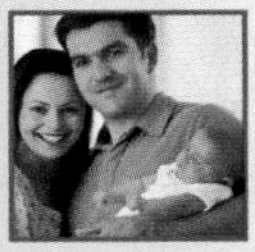

William's father is concerned about having his son experience trauma during the upcoming circumcision. What interventions would be essential in this situation?

Immunizations

Immunizations saved millions of lives in the 20th century and are an important health practice today (Table 20.6). Without immunizations, now rare diseases will return and infect infants and children (Atkinson & Wolfe, 2002). Immunizations are safe, but not risk-free. Most side effects are mild, such as pain or soreness at the injection site. Anaphylaxis is rare, occurring approximately once in every 500,000 doses (Atkinson & Wolfe, 2002).

Parents may voice two concerns regarding childhood vaccinations. The first is the proposed link between vaccinations and *autism,* a chronic developmental disorder usually identified between 18 and 30 months. This concern tends to result from information in the media in the late 1990s regarding a possible link between the measles, mumps, rubella (MMR) vaccine and autism. Because vaccines, including MMR, are administered just before the peak age of onset for autism, a temporal relationship between diagnosis of autism and vaccination is expected. At this point, health care professionals can assure parents that no convincing evidence has been

(text continues on page 856)

BOX 20.6 Risks and Benefits of Circumcision

Risks

- Pain
- Bleeding
- Injury to penis
- Meatitis

Benefits

- Lower incidence of urinary tract infections
- Decreased incidence of swelling and fluid around the foreskin
- Decreased incidence of phimosis (inability to retract foreskin)
- Decreased incidence of penile cancer

From Geyer, J., Ellsbury, D., Kleiber, C., Litwiller, D., Hinton, A., & Yankowitz, J. (2002). An evidence-based multidisciplinary protocol for neonatal circumcision pain management. *Journal of Obstetric, Gynecologic, and Neonatal Nursing, 31*(4), 403–410.

NURSING CARE PLAN 20.2

The Newborn Undergoing Circumcision

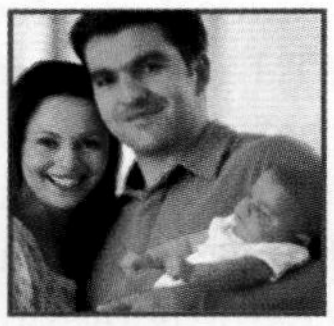

Remember baby William from the beginning of the chapter. After more discussions with the nurse, the family continues with its plan to circumcise him.

NURSING DIAGNOSES

- **Pain** related to the surgical procedure
- **Risk for Injury** related to the invasive surgical procedure and potential for hemorrhage
- **Deficient Knowledge (Parental)** related to care of the circumcision site

EXPECTED OUTCOMES

1. The newborn will undergo a circumcision without any complications.
2. The newborn will experience minimal to no pain during and after the circumcision.
3. The parents will identify appropriate measures to care for the circumcision site.

INTERVENTIONS	RATIONALES
Check the circumcision clamps for mismatch and expired sterility.	Mismatched equipment can cause injury and disfigurement to the penis. Sterilized equipment is required to maintain surgical asepsis of the surgical field and to prevent infection of the surgical wound.
Support and facilitate the chosen method of anesthesia. ● Dorsal penile nerve block (DPNB) and local anesthesia and a subcutaneous ring block. ● A subcutaneous ring block alone. ● Apply local anesthesia according to agency policy. (EMLA is recommended as a local anesthetic cream applied 60–90 minutes before the surgery.)	DPNB is the injection of two local anesthetics into the base of the penis, which effectively blocks pain impulses. The infant is pain free during the circumcision. Subcutaneous ring block is the injection of 1% lidocaine into the midshaft of the penis. This procedure blocks pain impulses and is more effective than EMLA (AAP Circumcision Policy). EMLA is used to inhibit conduction of nerve impulses; however, it is ineffective for pain during circumcision and has been implicated in causing methemoglobinemia in several cases (AAP Circumcision Policy).
Check the newborn's chart for administration of vitamin K.	Administration of vitamin K is given to all newborns to reduce the risk for bleeding. This is especially important because hemorrhage is an associated risk with circumcision.
Check the newborn's identity with orders for circumcision, medical record number on the chart, and the signed consent.	Checking identity is essential to ensure that the procedure is performed on the correct newborn.
Position the infant on a padded surface in preparation for circumcision.	A padded surface promotes comfort and that no bony prominences are exposed to a hard surface, preventing loss of blood flow and oxygenation to the tissues over them.
Provide a sucrose pacifier.	The sucrose pacifier serves as a distraction, which is an alternative pain-relieving strategy.

Continued

NURSING CARE PLAN 20.2 ● The Newborn Undergoing Circumcision

INTERVENTIONS	RATIONALES
Provide emotional support to the parents during the procedure; keep them informed about how their newborn is doing.	Support helps to allay parents' anxiety.
If ordered, apply light pressure on the penis for 3–5 minutes after circumcision.	This measure provides hemostasis and permits efficient clotting with minimal bleeding.
Administer acetaminophen before and after the procedure as ordered.	Acetaminophen produces peripherally acting analgesia by raising the pain threshold. It is intended for simple pain of short duration and is especially recommended for infants and children.
Apply a topical anesthetic cream to the penis postoperatively, according to agency policy.	Topical anesthesia agents relieve pain by stabilizing neurons and inhibiting the conduction of impulses.
Assess vital signs and for signs and symptoms of hemorrhage every 15 minutes for the first hour after the procedure.	Frequent postprocedure assessment is essential for early detection of possible hemorrhage or infection.
Allow the parents to hold and comfort the newborn after the procedure.	Bonding and attachment help allay the parents' anxieties and fears and promote the newborn's feelings of comfort and security.
Follow agency policy for daily care of the site. Note that most agency policies do not permit wrapping of the penis with Vaseline gauze.	Site care is recommended to reduce harmful bacterial flora. A circumferential wrap with Vaseline gauze could become a tourniquet if the penis becomes edematous.
Monitor the newborn's vital signs after the procedure as ordered; assess time and amount of first voiding after the circumcision.	Monitoring provides information about the possible development of complications. The local anesthetic and surgical trauma to the penis and perineal area may interfere with voiding. It is extremely important to ensure patency of the urethra. Significant urinary output also provides an indication of adequate hydration.
Check the penis and perineal area frequently postoperatively for swelling and color.	Excessive redness and edema in the perineal area or penis may indicate beginning infection. Bluish color and swelling may indicate a hematoma formation from the DPNB.
Ensure that the newborn has sufficient fluids.	Hydration is necessary to maintain fluid balance and to produce a dilute urine, minimizing irritation to penis.
Teach the parents how to care for the circumcision at home: ● Cleanse the penis with warm saline or follow the agency's policy for site care. ● Apply anesthetic creams as directed. ● Give acetaminophen as directed. ● Monitor voiding and report any fever, bleeding, swelling, urinary retention, or bruising to the health care provider. ● Provide adequate fluids according to the feeding hydration schedule developed for the infant preoperatively.	Teaching empowers parents and increases confidence in caring for their newborn. Providing appropriate care reduces the risk for infection, dehydration, pain, and other complications.

Continued

NURSING CARE PLAN 20.2 ● The Newborn Undergoing Circumcision *(Continued)*

EVALUATION

1. The newborn undergoes a circumcision without any difficulty.
2. The newborn demonstrates vital signs within age-acceptable parameters, feeds well, and sleeps undisturbed.
3. The newborn shows no evidence of bleeding or infection from the circumcision site; the penile area is red but without any odor or discharge.
4. The newborn voids adequate urine within 5 hours of the procedure.
5. The parents demonstrate measures to properly care for the circumcision site.

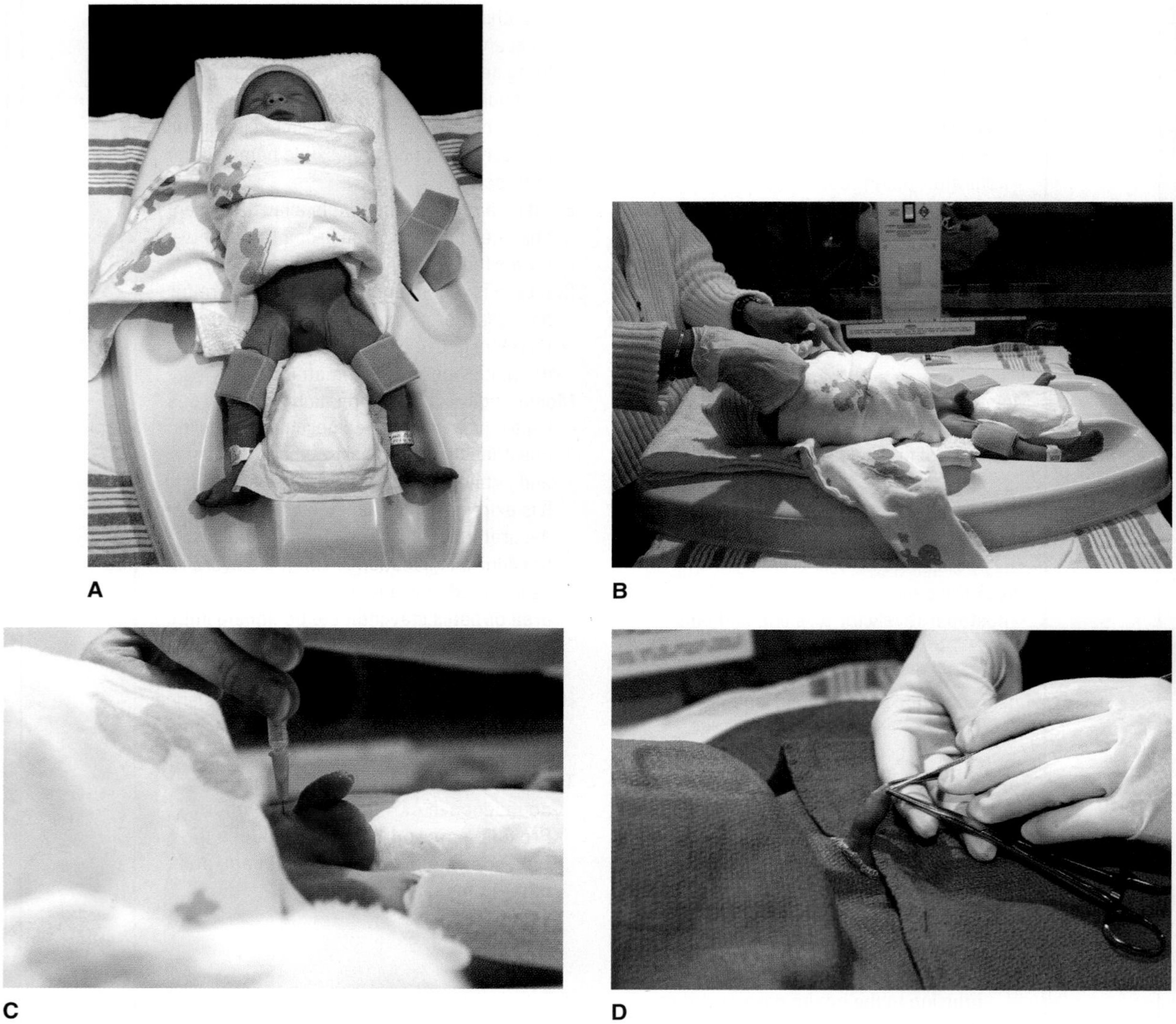

FIGURE 20.22 Circumcision using the Gomco (Yellen) clamp. (**A**) The baby's upper body is swaddled, while his legs are strapped to the circumcision board. (**B**) The nurse gives the baby a sucrose pacifier to provide pain relief during the procedure. (**C**) The physician injects local anesthesia into the area where the procedure will be performed. (**D**) Forceps are applied to pull the foreskin forward as the incision is made into the prepuce.

Continued

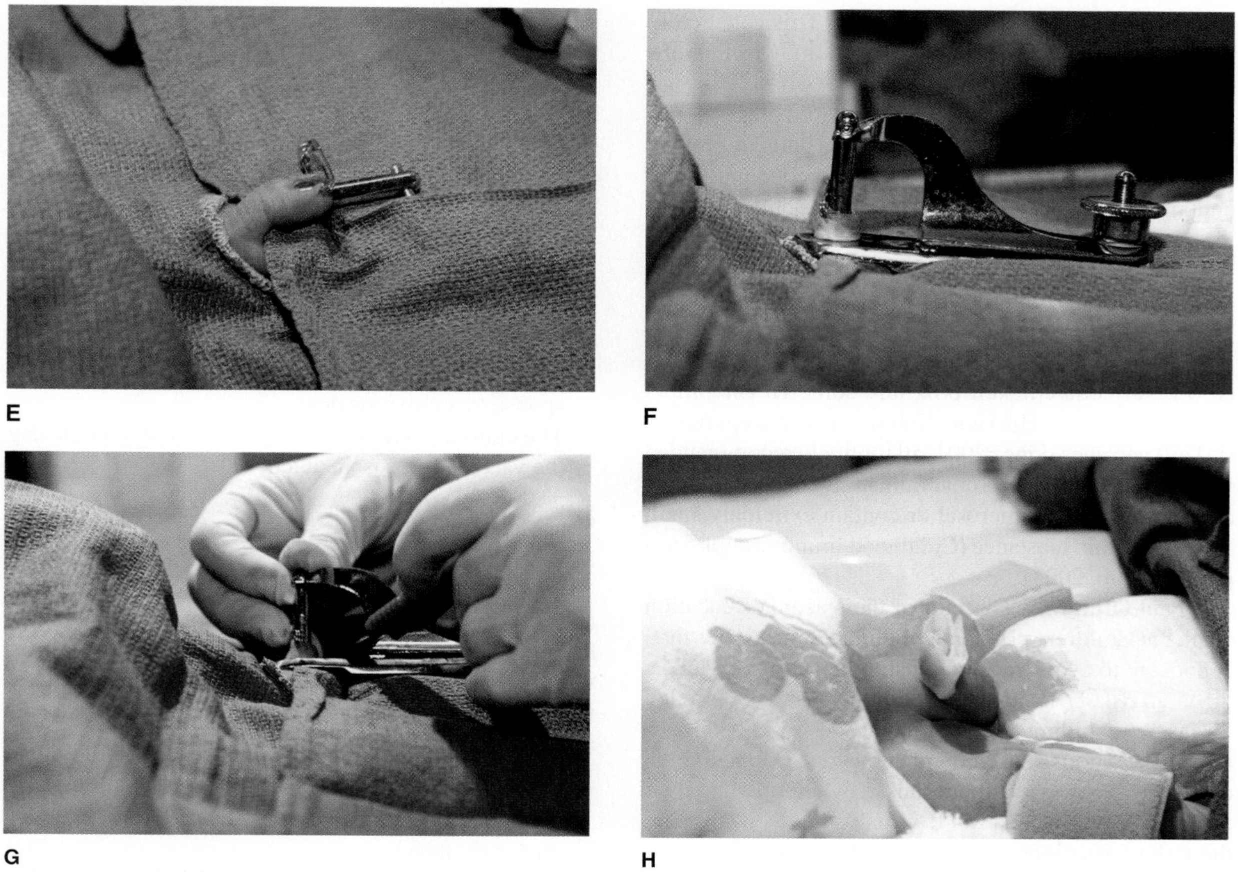

FIGURE 20.22 (*Continued*) Circumcision using the Gomco (Yellen) clamp. (**E**) The prepuce is drawn over the cone. (**F**) The clamp is applied. (**G**) After application of pressure for 3 to 4 minutes, the physician uses a scalpel to remove any excess foreskin. (**H**) The clamp has been removed, and a petroleum gauze dressing is loosely applied to promote healing, according to institutional protocol.

TABLE 20.6 Impact of Vaccines in the 20th Century

DISEASE	20TH-CENTURY ANNUAL MORBIDITY	2001 PROVISIONAL TOTAL	DECREASE (%)
Smallpox	48,164	0	100
Diphtheria	175,885	2	100.0
Pertussis	147,271	5,396	96.3
Tetanus	1,314	27	97.9
Polio (paralytic)	16,316	0	100
Measles	503,282	108	100
Mumps	152,209	231	99.8
Rubella	47,745	19	100
Congenital rubella	823	2	99.8
Haemophilus influenzae (< 5 yr)	20,000 (est)	183	99.1

From Centers for Disease Control and Prevention (CDC). (1999).

Impact of vaccines universally recommended for children—United States, 1900–1998. *Morbidity and Mortality Weekly Report, 48*(12), 243–248; and CDC. (2002). Provisional cases of selected notifiable diseases preventable by vaccination, United States, weeks ending December 29, 2001, and December 30, 2000 (52nd week). *Morbidity and Mortality Weekly Report, 50*(52), 1174–1175.

found that any vaccine causes autism. This genetically based disorder has not been linked to vaccinations (Demicheli et al., 2005).

Thimerosal, an organic mercury-based preservative, had been added to vaccines since the 1930s to prevent bacterial and fungal contamination in opened multidose containers. With recent efforts to reduce children's environmental mercury exposure, the Public Health Service and the AAP recommended removal of thimerosal from vaccines. Thimerosal was never found to be dangerous and was not linked to autism; in fact, vaccines that never contained thimerosal include MMR, polio (IPV), varicella/chicken pox, and some *Haemophilus influenzae* type b (Hib) and diphtheria/tetanus/pertussis (DTaP) vaccines. Since 2001, all routinely recommended vaccines manufactured for administration to U.S. infants either are free of thimerosal or contain extremely small amounts of this substance (Childhood Immunization Support Program, 2003).

Paul Offit, MD, Director of the Vaccine Education Center at Children's Hospital of Philadelphia, states that, "choosing to avoid vaccines is simply a choice to take a different risk. Unvaccinated children are at risk for many diseases, including meningitis caused by Hib, bloodstream infections caused by pneumococcus, pneumonia caused by measles, deafness caused by mumps, and liver cancer caused by hepatitis B virus. When you compare the risk of vaccines and the risk of diseases, vaccines are the safer choice" (Washington State Department of Health, 2002, p. 7).

Most vaccines are administered before children are 2 years old. Many vaccinations require boosters throughout life (Fig. 20.23).

Prenatal blood testing for hepatitis B status is the obstetrical standard of care. Women who are hepatitis B surface antigen (HBsAg) negative may be immunized safely during pregnancy. Women not tested during pregnancy, those at high risk for infection, and those with clinical hepatitis should be tested on hospital admission (AAP & ACOG, 2002). Transmission of hepatitis B virus (HBV) from an HBsAg-positive mother to her newborn occurs primarily during childbirth. Approximately 70% to 90% of babies who become infected become chronic carriers of HBV. Preventing transmission from mother to infant, however, is possible. Perinatal HBV infection can be prevented in approximately 95% of exposed newborns who receive hepatitis B immune globulin (HBIG) within 12 hours of birth. HBIG is made of antibodies that protect against the HBV, therefore providing passive immunity and immediate, although not long-term, protection. For lasting protection against HBV, the newborn must complete the three-dose immunization series (AAP & ACOG, 2002). The baby may receive HBIG and HBV vaccine at the same time but at different sites (eg, in anterolateral thigh muscle of the right and left leg). Maternal blood should be removed from the infant's skin before injection to prevent inoculation of the virus on the skin.

Parental informed consent is required before administration of HBIG or hepatitis B vaccine. Like any vaccine or medication, an adverse or allergic reaction may result. Nevertheless, HBIG and hepatitis B vaccine are very safe. The only reasons a care provider might delay or decide not to give a child a hepatitis B vaccination include the following (Childhood Immunization Support Program, 2003):

- The child or family has a severe allergy to baker's yeast.
- The child has had a life-threatening reaction in response to a previous dose.
- The child has a moderate or severe illness on the day the vaccination is scheduled.

Signs of Newborn Illness

Many pediatric providers give parents a list of circumstances that merit a phone call or office visit. Parents need to recognize and evaluate signs of illness in a newborn immediately because newborns can develop life-threatening complications quickly. The nurse should instruct parents to call their pediatric provider immediately if their baby exhibits:

- Respiratory distress, including fast breathing (more than 60 breaths/min), grunting, nasal flaring, retracting, or cyanosis
- Abdominal distention, especially if the belly is hard or if distention is accompanied by vomiting or no bowel movement for more than 1 day
- Forceful vomiting that shoots out several inches
- Diarrhea (watery stools up to eight times per day)
- Fever (more than 100°F or 37.8°C)
- Lethargy and poor feeding
- Muscle weakness
- Jitters of the whole body
- Blue color of face, tongue, and lips
- Persistent coughing or choking during feedings
- Excessive crying
- Watery white or mucous discharge from the eyes; sticky eyelashes from eye discharge
- Head-to-foot jaundice
- Umbilical cord that is red or exuding pus at the base, or that elicits a cry from the baby when touched
- Umbilicus that swells and does not dry after the umbilical cord has fallen off (Trubo et al., 2004)

Car Seats

All 50 states require use of a car seat or infant safety seat (AAP, 2002) during any motor vehicle trips with a baby. The nurse is in the tenuous position of offering advice and providing teaching that may affect newborn safety in the car while risking potential legal liability for such information if the newborn is injured in a subsequent

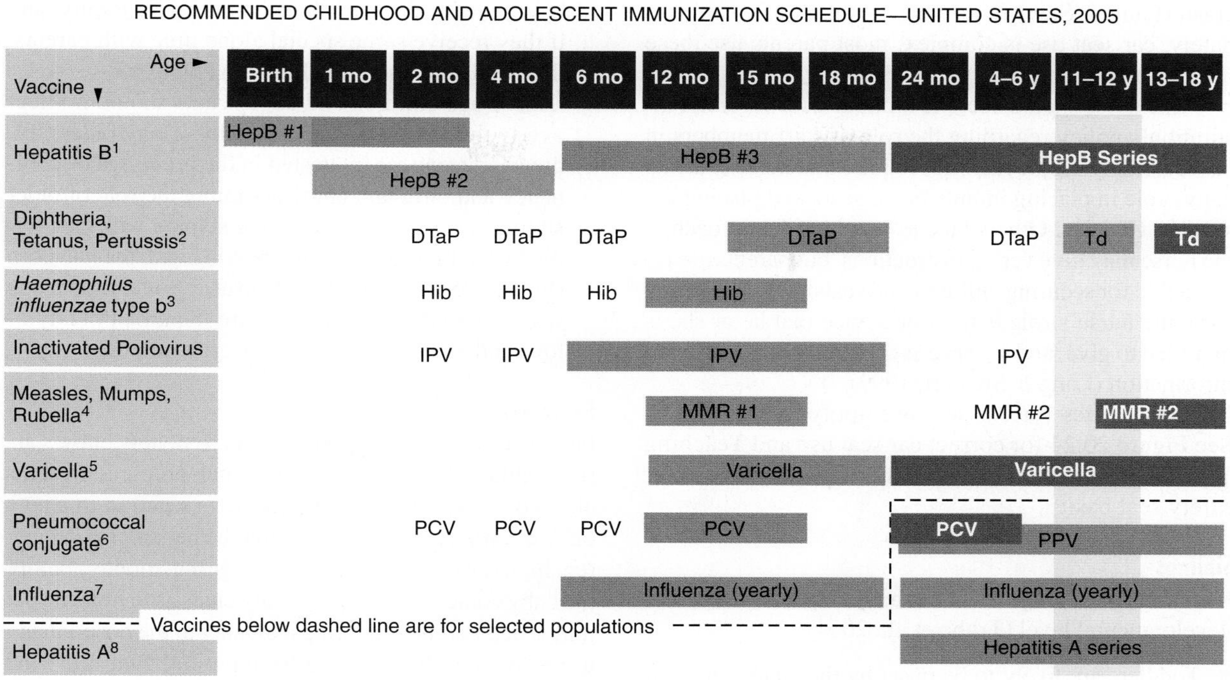

This schedule indicates the recommended ages for routine administration of currently licensed childhood vaccines, as of December 1, 2004, for children through age 18 years. Any dose not administered at the recommended age should be administered at any subsequent visit when indicated and feasible.

Indicates age groups that warrant special effort to administer those vaccines not previously administered. Additional vaccines may be used whenever any components of the combination are indicated and other components of the vaccine are not contraindicated.

Providers should consult the manufacturers' package inserts for detailed recommendations. Clinically significant adverse events that follow immunization should be reported to the Vaccine Adverse Event Reporting System (VAERS). Guidance about how to obtain and complete a VAERS form is available at www.vaers.org or by telephone, 800-822-7967.

- **Range of recommended ages**
- **Preadolescent assessment**
- **Only if mother HBsAg(–)**
- **Catch-up immunization**

FOOTNOTES

1. Hepatitis B (HepB) vaccine. All infants should receive the first dose of HepB vaccine soon after birth and before hospital discharge; the first dose may also be administered by age 2 months if the mother is hepatitis B surface antigen (HBsAg)-negative. Only monovalent HepB may be used for the birth dose. Monovalent or combination vaccine containing HepB may be used to complete the series. Four doses of vaccine may be administered when a birth dose is given. The second dose should be given at least 4 weeks after the first dose, except for combination vaccines which cannot be administered before age 6 weeks. The third dose should be given at least 16 weeks after the first dose and at least 8 weeks after the second dose. The last dose in the vaccination series (third or fourth dose) should not be administered before age 24 weeks.

Infants born to HBsAg-positive mothers should receive HepB and 0.5 mL of hepatitis B immune globulin (HBIG) at separate sites within 12 hours of birth. The second dose is recommended at age 1–2 months. The final dose in the immunization series should not be administered before age 24 weeks. These infants should be tested for HBsAg and antibody to HBsAg (anti-HBs) at age 9–15 months.

Infants born to mothers whose HBsAg status is unknown should receive the first dose of the HepB series within 12 hours of birth. Maternal blood should be drawn as soon as possible to determine the mother's HBsAg status; if the HBsAg test is positive, the infant should receive HBIG as soon as possible (no later than age 1 week). The second dose is recommended at age 1–2 months. The last dose in the immunization series should not be adminstered before age 24 weeks.

2. Diphtheria and tetanus toxoids and acellular pertussis (DTaP) vaccine. The fourth dose of DTaP may be administered as early as age 12 months, provided 6 months have elapsed since the third dose and the child is unlikely to return at age 15–18 months. The final dose in the series should be given at age ≥4 years. **Tetanus and diphtheria toxoids (Td)** is recommended at age 11–12 years if at least 5 years have elapsed since the last dose of tetanus and diphtheria toxoid-containing vaccine. Subsequent routine Td boosters are recommended every 10 years.

3. *Haemophilus influenzae* type b (Hib) conjugate vaccine. Three Hib conjugate vaccines are licensed for infant use. If PRP-OMP (PedvaxHIB® or ComVax® [Merck]) is administered at ages 2 and 4 months, a dose at age 6 months is not required. DTaP/Hib combination products should not be used for primary immunization in infants at ages 2, 4, or 6 months but can be used as boosters after any Hib vaccine. The final dose in the

4. Measles, mumps, and rubella vaccine (MMR). The second dose of MMR is recommended routinely at age 4–6 years but may be administered during any visit, provided at least 4 weeks have elapsed since the first dose and both doses are administered beginning at or after age 12 months. Those who have not previously received the second dose should complete the schedule by age 11–12 years.

5. Varicella vaccine. Varicella vaccine is recommended at any visit at or after age 12 months for susceptible children (i.e., those who lack a reliable history of chickenpox). Susceptible persons aged ≥13 years should receive 2 doses administered at least 4 weeks apart.

6. Pneumococcal vaccine. The heptavalent **pneumococcal conjugate vaccine (PCV)** is recommended for all children aged 2–23 months and for certain children aged 24–59 months. The final dose in the series should be given at age ≥12 months. **Pneumococcal polysaccharide vaccine (PPV)** is recommended in addition to PCV for certain high-risk groups. See *MMWR* 2000;49(RR-9):1-35.

7. Influenza vaccine. Influenza vaccine is recommended annually for children aged ≥6 months with certain risk factors (including, but not limited to, asthma, cardiac disease, sickle cell disease, human immunodeficiency virus [HIV], and diabetes), healthcare workers, and other persons (including household members) in close contact with persons in groups at high risk (see *MMWR* 2004;53[RR-6]:1-40). In addition, healthy children aged 6–23 months and close contacts of healthy children aged 0–23 months are recommended to receive influenza vaccine because children in this age group are at substantially increased risk for influenza-related hospitalization. For healthy persons aged 5–49 years, the intranasally administered, live, attenuated influenza vaccine (LAIV) is an acceptable alternative to the intramuscular trivalent inactivated influenza vaccine (TIV). See *MMWR* 2004;53(RR-6):1-40. Children receiving TIV should be adminstered a dosage appropriate for their age (0.25 mL if aged 6–35 months or 0.5 mL if aged ≥3 years). Children aged ≤8 years who are receiving influenza vaccine for the first time should receive 2 doses (separated by at least 4 weeks for TIV and at least 6 weeks for LAIV).

8. Hepatitis A vaccine. Hepatitis A vaccine is recommended for children and adolescents in selected states and regions and for certain high-risk groups; consult your local public health authority. Children and adolescents in these states, regions, and high-risk groups who have not been immunized against hepatitis A can begin the hepatitis A immunization series during any visit. The 2 doses in the series should be

FIGURE 20.23 Childhood immunization schedule.

crash (Lang & Stewart, 1999; Lincoln, 2005). Unfortunately, car seat use is complex; most parents use these devices incorrectly (Taft et al., 1999).

The nurse should become familiar with his or her institution's policy regarding the role of staff members in car seat safety. Some facilities require that nurses play an active role in placing infants in car seats and placing car seats in vehicles. Others take a "hands-off" approach—the nurse may give verbal instructions, but parents are responsible for securing children and seats into cars. In any case, the nurse's role is to offer advice that he or she is qualified to give, and to serve as a resource for additional information (Lang & Stewart, 1999).

Basic rules for car seat use apply in every case. See Figure 20.24 for correct car seat use and Teaching Tips 20.3 for written information for parents about car safety seat basics.

Siblings

Reactions of siblings to a new baby depend on age and developmental level (Trubo et al., 2004):

- Toddlers are likely to be upset by the change in their routine when their mother is hospitalized. They may be frightened by the unfamiliarity of the hospital environment and confused at seeing their mother in a hospital bed. Toddlers probably will be jealous of and feel displaced by the new baby. They may seek attention by misbehaving or displaying regressive behaviors, such as soiling themselves after having been successfully toilet-trained or sucking the baby's pacifier. Toddlers need extra loving attention and reassurance that they maintain their special place in the family.
- Preschoolers may feel jealousy and resentment, but discussion before the baby is born may help temper these feelings. Parents should include preschoolers in preparations for the newborn, such as readying the crib and helping choose an outfit for the baby to wear home. If preschoolers are reassured that their status as "big sister or brother" benefits the entire family, and if they receive some special alone time with parents, they will cope more readily with changes.
- School-age children and adolescents should not feel overly threatened by the new baby. Many older children and teens are interested in the processes of pregnancy and birth and enjoy assuming the role of older sibling. They probably will like helping with caregiving by feeding, holding, and playing with the newborn (Fig. 20.25). Parents should ensure special time alone with older siblings, and reassure them that plenty of love and attention for everyone are available.

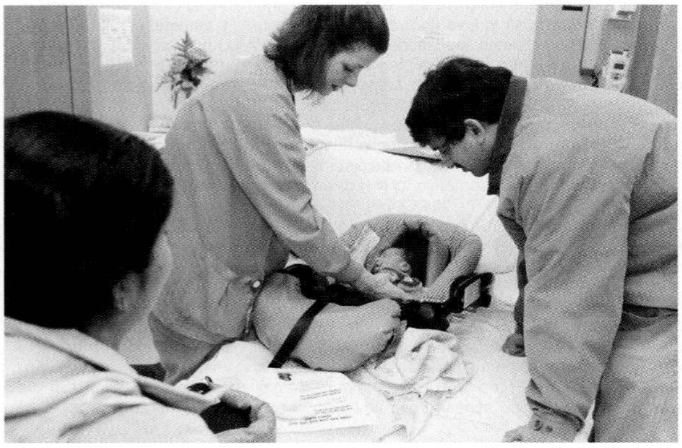

FIGURE 20.24 This nurse is checking to make sure the newborn is secured in the car seat correctly.

Pet Safety

Parents can attempt to prepare pets for a new baby's arrival, although knowing whether such preparation actually works is impossible. Every pet's reaction to a new baby is unique, although knowing the pet's temperament (eg, high-strung, demanding, easy-going, moody) before the baby comes home yields many clues as to how the pet may react. Parents can bring a blanket to the hospital and use it to wrap the newborn for a period, then bring the blanket home to the pet and "introduce" the baby's scent to the animal. In any event, if the pet is used to being the center of attention in the household, the pet may feel jealous and misbehave or act aggressively toward other pets, family members, or the newborn.

Parents are usually eager to introduce the new baby to the family pet. This process should be gradual, and adults must closely supervise the behavior of a pet that could potentially bite or injure the baby. They should never leave the animal alone with the baby. The animal usually grows accustomed to the newborn in 2 to 3 weeks; however, parents must be observant and cautious whenever the animal is around the baby (AAP, 1998).

Dangers of Secondhand Smoke

Passive smoking is harmful to children's respiratory health. Children exposed to environmental tobacco smoke have increased rates of lower respiratory illness, middle ear effusion, asthma, SIDS, and development of cancer in adulthood (AAP, 1997).

If the baby is in an environment with smokers, certain precautions can help protect the baby's health:

- No one should smoke in any area where the baby is living. The smoker must smoke outside the baby's living environment.
- If the smoker takes care of the baby, the smoker should cover his or her clothing while smoking. The smoker may use a designated overblouse or jacket, which he or she wears only while outside smoking.
- No one should smoke in a car that the baby rides in, even when the baby is not in the car.

TEACHING TIPS 20.3 Car Safety Seat Basics

- Always use a car safety seat, starting with your baby's first ride home from the hospital. Help your child form a lifelong habit of buckling up.
- Read the car safety seat manufacturer's instructions and always keep them with the car safety seat.
- Read your vehicle owner's manual for important information on how to install the car safety seat correctly in your vehicle.
- The safest place for all children to ride is in the back seat.
- Never place a child in a rear-facing safety seat in the front seat of a vehicle that has a passenger airbag.
- The harness system holds your child in the car safety seat and the seat belt or anchor system holds the seat in the car. Attach both snugly to protect your child.
- Do not use a car safety seat that
  - Is too old. Look on the label for the date it was made. If it is more than 10 years old, it should not be used. Some manufacturers recommend that seats only be used for 5–6 years. Check with the manufacturer to find out when the company recommends getting a new seat.
  - Was in a crash. It may have been weakened and should not be used, even if it looks fine. Do not use a seat if you do not know its full history.
  - Does not have a label with the date of manufacture and seat name of model number. Without these, you cannot check on recalls.
  - Does not come with instructions. You need them to know how to use the car safety seat. Do not rely on the former owner's directions. Get a copy of the instruction manual from the manufacturer before you use the seat.
  - Has any cracks in the frame of the seat.
  - Is missing parts. Used seats often come without important parts. Check with the manufacturer to make sure you can get the right parts

Has the car safety seat been recalled? You can find out by calling the manufacturer or the Auto Safety Hot Line at 888/DASH-2-DOT (888-327-4236) from 8 AM to 10 PM ET, Monday through Friday. This information is also available on the NHTSA Web site at: http://www.nhtsa.dot.gov/cars/problems/recalls/index.cfm.

If the seat has been recalled, be sure to follow instructions to fix it or get the necessary parts. You also may get a registration card for future recall notices from the hot line.

Be sure to register the car seat upon purchase.

Adapted from the American Academy of Pediatrics. (2002). *Car safety Seats: A guide for families.* Available at http://www.aap.org/family/carseatguide.htm.

The nurse caring for infants or new mothers plays a vital role in identifying families at risk from tobacco exposure. His or her role is to motivate, advise, and assist parents in starting a smoking cessation program.

Household Safety

The parent of a newborn may not be thinking yet of "child-proofing" the home. Nevertheless, it is never too early to begin to identify potential safety hazards. Even a young infant can grasp a dangerous object or roll off a bed or changing table (Table 20.7).

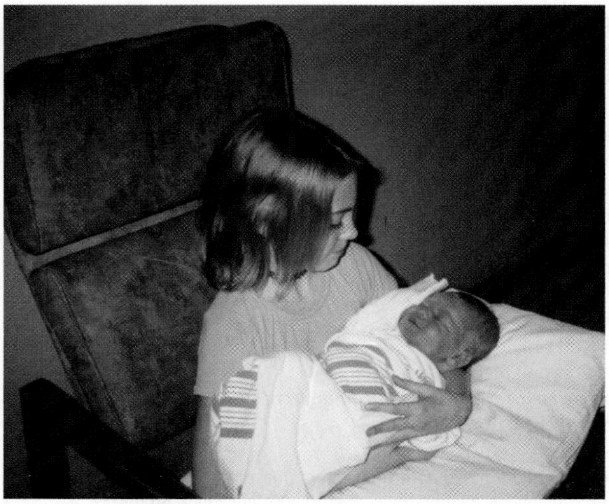

FIGURE 20.25 This older school-age child is enjoying holding her new baby sibling.

READINESS FOR HOSPITAL DISCHARGE

The healthy term AGA newborn is ready for discharge when (AAP & ACOG, 2002):

- The postpartum courses for both mother and baby are uncomplicated.
- Vital signs are normal and stable.
- The neonate has urinated and defecated at least once.
- The neonate has completed at least two successful feedings with coordinated sucking, swallowing, and breathing.
- Results of the physical examination are within normal limits.
- Any circumcision site shows no evidence of bleeding for at least 2 hours.
- There is no evidence of significant jaundice in the first 24 hours of life.
- The mother or both parents demonstrate adequate caregiving skills, including breastfeeding (if appropriate), and have received information about signs of illness, proper use of a car seat, proper sleep positioning, and whom to call in case of complications or emergencies.

TABLE 20.7 Newborn Injury Prevention

TYPE OF INJURY	PREVENTION MEASURES
Airway obstruction	*Never* prop the baby's bottle.
Choking	Use only one-piece pacifiers; *do not* "make" a pacifier from a baby bottle nipple.
	Keep small objects out of the baby's reach (this includes such items as button eyes glued or sewn onto stuffed animals that may be pulled off).
	Learn first aid for a choking baby.
Strangulation	*Do not* place the crib close to window drapery cords; gather cords up and out of reach on hooks.
	Never tie pacifiers or other items (eg, jewelry) around the baby's neck.
	Remove drawstrings from the baby's clothing.
	Do not place electrical cords or extension cords where infants or children can become entangled in them.
Suffocation	Place the baby on her back to sleep if not contraindicated.
	Learn infant CPR (or pediatric basic life support).
	Do not place pillows or other soft objects in the baby's crib (especially large stuffed animals).
	Do not place the baby on a water bed or a beanbag chair.
	Store and dispose of plastic bags safely.
Car crash related	Follow instructions on proper use of car seats.
	"The back is where it's at!" All infants and children under the age of 12 should be placed in the back seat whenever possible as long as the backseat permits them to be secured with a restraint that is appropriate for their age and size.
Crib related	*Never* leave the baby in a crib with the side rail lowered.
	Cornerposts should *not* extend above the crib end panels because older infants can use them to climb up and over the railing.
	The headboard and footboard should *not* have cutouts.
	Spacing between crib slats should not exceed 2 ⅜ inches.
	Crib hardware should be secure.
	The mattress should be firm and snug fitting (*no* gaps between the frame and mattress to entrap the infant).
	Remove mobiles, crib gyms, and bumper pads from crib rails as soon as the infant can crawl or kneel.
	Check for peeling paint and rough edges or splinters.
Drowning	*Never* leave the baby alone in the bath or any body of water.
	Empty buckets or containers of fluid immediately after use; *never* leave them unattended.
	Keep the bathroom door closed; use doorknob covers.
	Use lid-locks for toilets.
	Install a barrier between the swimming pool and house.
Falls	*Do not* use a baby walker unless it has a label stating that it meets the new safety standard.
	When your baby is on a high surface (eg, changing table, couch, bed), always place one hand on the baby, and *never* leave her unattended.
	Use gates at the top and bottom of stairways.
	Use window guards.
	Never put a crib or playpen near a window.
	Use nonslip area rugs.
	Use a rubber mat or another nonslip device in the bathtub.
	Remove coffee tables with sharp edges from the center of the room as soon as the child pulls to stand.
	Stabilize or remove from tables or shelves heavy items that a child could pull down on herself—such as lamps, TV sets, VCRs.
Fire, scald burns, and electrical injuries	*Do not* carry the baby and hot items at the same time.
	Keep hot beverages out of the baby's reach.
	Do not use placemats or tablecloths—infants and children can tug on them.
	Keep the baby in a safe place while you are cooking.
	Turn pot handles to the stove's back or side so the child can't pull down pots.
	Keep small appliances out of reach and unplugged.
	Have a fire extinguisher handy.
	Have working smoke detectors in your home.
	Maintain the hot-water heater temperature at 120°F.
	When preparing a bath, turn cold water on first, and then add hot water.
	Block fireplaces, space heaters, and kerosene lamps with gates or another barrier.
	Keep lighters and matches out of children's reach.
	Use safety plugs on all outlets.
	Install ground fault circuit interrupters in electrical outlets in bathrooms, kitchens, and laundry rooms.
	Do not place electrical cords or extension cords where infants or children can bite or chew on them.

Continued

TABLE 20.7 Newborn Injury Prevention

TYPE OF INJURY	PREVENTION MEASURES
Poisoning	Store household cleaners, medicines, cosmetics, toiletries, and chemicals in high, locked cabinets. *Do not* store these items near food. Keep all of these items in their original containers (*do not* transfer to soda or other food bottles). Use child-protective caps whenever possible. Flush old medicines down the toilet. Keep syrup of ipecac out of reach in your medicine cabinet (used to induce vomiting when appropriate—check with your local poison control center first). Place household plants out of reach—some are poisonous (check with your local poison control center or American Heart Association, Pediatric Basic Life Support Program). Keep the local poison control center phone number by your phones. Install carbon monoxide detectors in your home.
Other injuries	Keep handguns locked up and out of reach of children of all ages (preferably out of the house). Install safety latches on cabinets, particularly those containing sharp utensils and poisons. Make basements, utility rooms, and garages off limits.

Courtesy of Kathleen Southerton, RNC, PhD, University Hospital, Stony Brook, New York. Adapted by permission.

- Family members or health care professionals knowledgeable in newborn care, lactation, and recognition of jaundice and dehydration are available to the mother for the first few days following discharge.
- Laboratory data such as maternal syphilis, HBsAg, and HIV status have been reviewed, and newborn blood type and direct Coombs' test result are known, if clinically indicated.
- Screening tests, such as metabolism and hearing, have been performed in accordance with state laws.
- The first in the series of hepatitis B vaccines has been administered, or a follow-up appointment has been scheduled to administer the vaccine.
- A pediatric care provider has been identified for continuing medical care, and a follow-up appointment has been made.
- Family, environment, and social risk factors have been assessed, such as untreated parental substance abuse; history of child abuse or neglect; mental illness in a parent who is in the home; lack of social support, particularly for single, first-time mothers; no fixed home; history of untreated domestic violence; or adolescent mother, particularly if other risk factors are present.

Newborn Metabolic Screening

Each state's Department of Health regulates newborn genetic screening tests. The purpose of every metabolic screening program is to prevent complications of genetic diseases through early identification and treatment. Some states test for as many as 15 genetic disorders; others screen for as few as four. With evolving technology, the number of genetic metabolic illnesses for which screening can be done is growing constantly, and new variants of disease conditions continue to be found. The March of Dimes recommends that all babies receive screening for at least nine metabolic disorders for which proven treatments are available (Table 20.8). As of this writing, only nine states are following this recommendation (March of Dimes, 2003).

Nurses should understand that metabolic screening tests are not diagnostic. That is, these blood tests simply identify infants whose results indicate a need for further testing and diagnostic evaluation (Kenner & Moran, 2005).

Each hospital has established procedures to ensure that newborn metabolic screening tests occur before hospital discharge in accordance with state law. Each state's Department of Health can provide information regarding the timing of initial screening before discharge and the necessity for repeat screening (AAP & ACOG, 2002).

Parents can refuse testing based on religious or personal beliefs. In such cases, they must sign a waiver to document their understanding of the risks involved in refusing testing. Health care personnel place the waiver in the newborn's medical record. Some states also require additional documents.

Umbilical cord blood is not adequate for testing disorders that exhibit metabolite accumulation after birth or after feeding (AAP & ACOG, 2002). Ideally, the blood sample is collected between 48 and 72 hours of age; however, some healthy term newborns are discharged from the hospital before this time. Babies tested earlier than 24 hours of age (and, in some states, all babies) usually are retested by a pediatric care provider by 2 weeks of age to ensure detection of phenylketonuria (PKU) and congenital hypothyroidism. A heel-stick sample most often is obtained; however, some states allow a venous sample. See Nursing Procedure 20.6 for an example of the heel-stick collection technique.

Auditory Screening

Permanent childhood hearing loss (PCHL) occurs in 2 to 4 of every 100 NICU graduates and in 1 to 3 of every 1000

TABLE 20.8 Core Group of Newborn Screening Tests Recommended by the March of Dimes

TEST/DISORDER SCREENED	INCIDENCE	CHARACTERISTICS	TREATMENT
Medium-chain acyl-CoA dehydrogenase (MCAD) deficiency	1 in 15,000	An inherited disorder of fatty acid metabolism caused by lack of an enzyme required to convert fat to energy. Seemingly well infants or children can suddenly develop seizures, respiratory failure, cardiac arrest, coma, and death. Identifying affected children before they become ill is vital to preventing a crisis and averting these consequences.	Steady food or glucose intake and avoidance of fasting
Phenylketonuria (PKU)	1 in 12,000	An inability to properly process the essential amino acid phenylalanine, which then accumulates and damages the brain. PKU can cause severe mental retardation unless detected soon after birth and treated with a special formula.	A low phenylalanine diet at least throughout childhood and adolescence and, for females, during pregnancy
Congenital hypothyroidism	1 in 4000	Thyroid hormone deficiency that severely retards both growth and brain development	Oral doses of thyroid hormone
Congenital adrenal hyperplasia	1 in 5000	A set of inherited disorders resulting from defects in the synthesis of hormones produced by the adrenal gland. Certain severe forms can cause life-threatening salt loss from the body.	Salt and hormone replacement
Biotinidase deficiency	1 in 70,000	Deficiency of biotinidase, an enzyme that recycles the B vitamin biotin. Complications include frequent infections, uncoordinated movement, hearing loss, seizures, mental retardation, coma, and death.	Extra biotin
Maple syrup urine disease	1 in 250,000	Rare inborn error of metabolism that ranges from mild to severe. Severely affected babies rarely survive for more than 1 month; those who do survive usually have irreversible mental retardation. Early detection and treatment are vital for normal outcomes.	A special diet that requires frequent monitoring and must be continued indefinitely
Galactosemia	1 in 50,000	Lack of the liver enzyme needed to convert galactose into glucose. Galactose accumulates in and damages vital organs, leading to blindness, mental retardation, infection, and death.	Elimination of milk and other dairy products from diet
Homocystinuria	1 in 275,000	Deficiency of the enzyme that converts homocysteine into cystathionine, needed by the brain for normal development. Can lead to mental retardation, eye problems, skeletal abnormalities, and stroke.	Special diet with high doses of vitamin B_6 or B_{12}
Sickle cell anemia	1 in 400 African Americans	Blood disease that can cause severe pain, damage to vital organs, stroke, and early death.	Vigilant medical care, treatment with penicillin

NURSING PROCEDURE 20.6

Performing a Heel Stick on a Newborn

PURPOSE

To obtain a blood specimen for analysis

ASSESSMENT AND PLANNING

- Check the medical record to ensure that the newborn has received vitamin K.
- Assess the lower extremities for color and warmth; if necessary, apply a warm moist pack or compress to the heel area for several minutes *to promote vasodilation.*
- Review the order for type of testing to be performed; ensure that an appropriate laboratory request form has been completed.
- Explain the reason for the procedure to the parents if appropriate.
- Gather the necessary equipment.
    - Alcohol wipes
    - Clean gloves
    - Specimen container
    - Lancet or skin puncturing device
    - Sterile 2- × 2-inch gauze pads
    - Tape

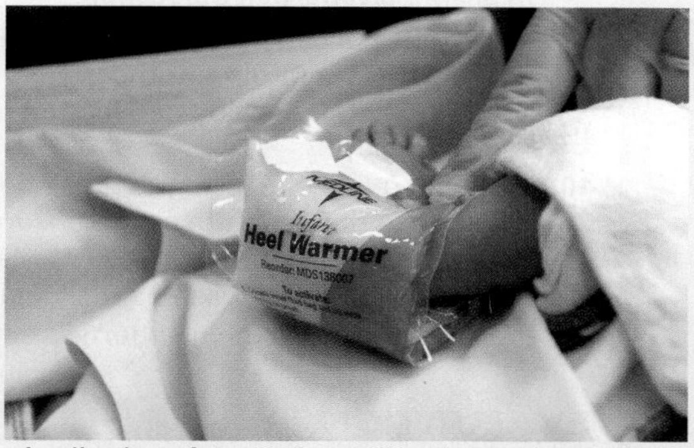

Application of a warming pad to the newborn's heel.

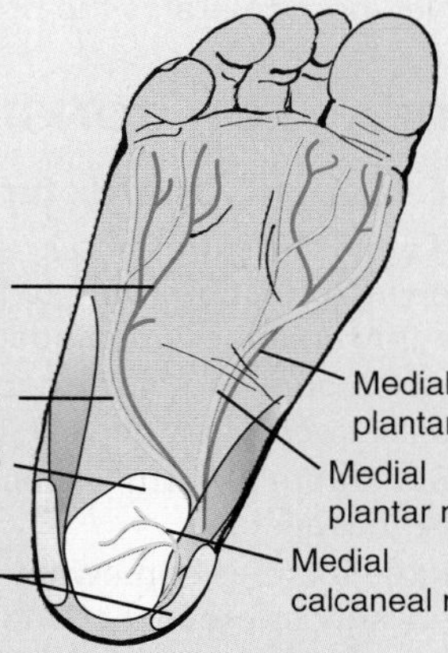

Step 3. Areas of the heel and foot with nerves and arteries.

IMPLEMENTATION

1. Wash hands and put on clean gloves.
2. Remove the warm moist pack if applied.
3. Inspect the lateral aspects of the newborn's foot *to select a site that is free of nerves and major arteries.*
4. Support the foot with one hand covering the palmar aspect *to prevent inadvertent puncture to an area rich in nerves and major blood vessels.*
5. Palpate the selected site *to ensure that adequate padding is over the bone.*
6. Clean the site with an alcohol wipe or according to agency policy; allow to air dry.
7. Holding the lancet device, quickly insert the device into the intended site to a depth no greater than 2 mm *to prevent puncturing the bone.* Discard the lancet device in the sharps container.

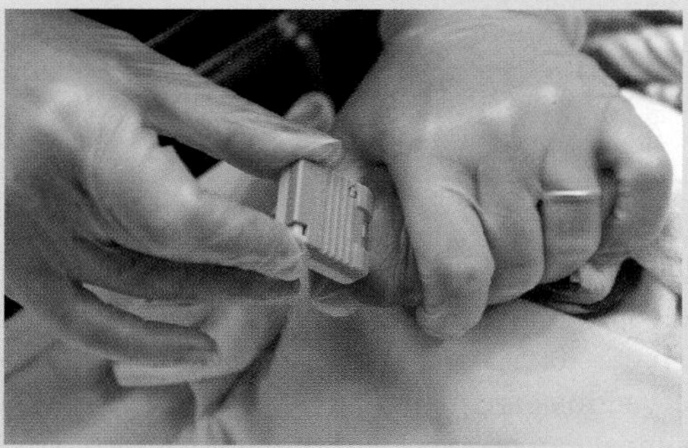
Step 7. Inserting the lancet device.

Continued

NURSING PROCEDURE 20.6 CONTINUED

Performing a Heel Stick on a Newborn

8. Obtain the first drop of blood and wipe away with a dry gauze pad *to prevent contaminating or diluting the specimen.* Obtain a second drop of blood and, if necessary, gently milk the foot instead of squeezing to obtain this drop of blood *to ensure accuracy of the results.*

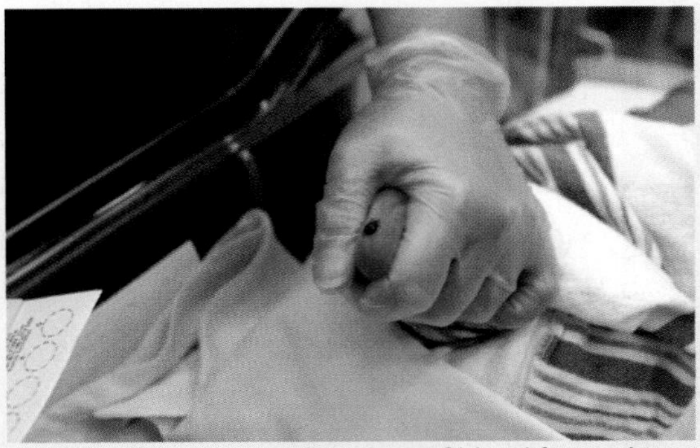

Step 8. Obtaining the first drop of blood for testing.

9. Collect the specimen as indicated and send to the laboratory or process the specimen at the bedside depending on agency policy.
10. Apply a pressure dressing of gauze and tape to the puncture site *to ensure hemostasis.*
11. Remove gloves and wash hands; document procedure and disposition of the specimen.
12. Provide comfort to the newborn after the procedure.

EVALUATION

- Specimen is obtained without undue pain or discomfort to the newborn and sent to the laboratory.
- Newborn tolerates the procedure well.

AREAS FOR CONSIDERATION AND ADAPTATION

Lifespan Considerations

- If a pressure dressing is unavailable, use an alternate means of ensuring hemostasis by applying direct pressure to the site for several minutes until the bleeding has ceased; then apply an adhesive bandage to the site.
- When applying a warm moist pack to the newborn's heel area, check the temperature of the pack to prevent thermal injury.
- Substitute a warm washcloth, towel, or diaper for the warm moist pack if a commercial pack is unavailable.
- If the infant is somewhat older, anticipate the need to gently immobilize the lower leg temporarily to prevent sudden movements during the procedure, which may cause injury.

Community-Based Considerations

- Heel sticks may be used in the home setting to obtain blood specimens in newborns and infants. Always check with the laboratory for any specific requirements or modifications that may be necessary.
- Instruct the parents to apply topical anesthetic if ordered at the specified time before the procedure to minimize pain.

healthy newborns, making it the most common diagnosable defect at birth (AAP, 1999a; Finitzo & Crumley, 1999; Hyde, 2005). If PCHL is detected and appropriate interventions are made by 6 months of age, normal development can be expected. If diagnosis or treatment is delayed for longer than 6 months, however, permanent developmental delays can occur in otherwise normal babies (Joint Commission on Infant Hearing, 2000).

Newborn hearing screening is becoming the hospital standard of care. The AAP recommends that every hospital with an obstetrical service develop and implement universal newborn hearing screening. Doing so involves testing all newborns during their hospital stay, retesting before discharge those newborns who fail their initial test, and ensuring tracking and follow-up for newborns who require additional evaluation (AAP & ACOG, 2002).

Hearing loss detected in the neonatal period results from various causes:

- Heredity
- Perinatal factors such as congenital malformations of the head and neck
- Very low birth weight (below 1500 g)
- Congenital infections (eg, cytomegalovirus, rubella, herpes, syphilis, toxoplasmosis)
- Hyperbilirubinemia requiring exchange transfusion
- Apgar score of 0 to 4 at 1 minute or 0 to 6 at 5 minutes
- Mechanical ventilation lasting 5 days or longer
- Any syndrome known to include hearing loss
- Bacterial meningitis
- Ototoxic drugs (eg, gentamicin, furosemide)

Two types of technology are available for newborn hearing testing. Both screen each ear separately and require the environment to be relatively quiet. *Auditory brain stem response* (ABR), also called brainstem auditory evoked response (BAER), measures variations in electric brain activity in response to tones or clicks. ABR involves placing electrodes on the baby's scalp. A click or a tone is delivered through earphones, and the neural response from the cochlea to the brainstem is measured. The other technology available is the *oto-acoustic emissions* (OAE) test, also called the evoked otoacoustic emissions (EOAE) test. A small probe that contains a microphone is placed in the ear canal, and click sounds are introduced. The test measures outer hair cell function in response to a stimulus. Echo responses are measured in healthy ears (UNHS Project Team, 2001).

Hearing loss ranges in degree from minimal to profound. Two types are possible. If a problem lies in the outer or middle ear, the hearing loss is termed *conductive,* which can be corrected medically or surgically. If the problem is detected in the cochlea, the hearing loss is called *sensorineural.* To date, no cure exists for sensorineural hearing loss. Sometimes, hearing loss is a mix of the two types (Knott, 2001).

Re-evaluation of hearing is necessary throughout childhood to detect progressive or late-onset hearing loss. Routine checkups include assessment of the child's ear, as well as asking the child's caregiver about any concerns related to the child's speech development or response to sounds (Purdy, 2000).

Hospital-based screening is not diagnostic. Hospital auditory screening of all newborns should result in a referral rate below 4%. This evaluation occurs as soon as possible but by 3 months of age. Babies diagnosed with hearing loss require intervention no later than 6 months (AAP & ACOG, 2002).

Postdischarge Follow-Up

Any newborn discharged before 48 hours of age should be examined again within 48 hours of discharge. For healthy term newborns, the frequency of subsequent visits varies by region but should follow the AAP recommendations for preventive health care. Early visits include important assessments of growth (weight gain, OFC, and length), general health, and attainment of developmental milestones. Immunizations should be administered according to the Childhood Immunization schedule (see Fig. 20.22). Pediatric visits also give providers an opportunity to assess parent–infant attachment; parenting skills, including breastfeeding; any remarkable stressors such as postpartum depression, intimate partner violence, or substance abuse; and any evidence of child neglect or abuse. Every state mandates health care professionals to report cases of suspected child abuse (AAP & ACOG, 2002).

Questions to Ponder

1. Laurie was born by scheduled repeat cesarean section to a 32-year-old G3 P2. The mother had a healthy uneventful pregnancy of 38 weeks' gestation by ultrasound. Apgar scores were 7 at 1 minute and 8 at 5 minutes. Laurie required less than 1 minute of free-flow oxygen for central cyanosis after delivery. Free-flow oxygen gradually was withdrawn, and her lips and mucous membranes remained pink in room air. Laurie appeared to be in good condition and was wrapped in a warm blanket, given to her father to hold in the operating room, and viewed and touched by her mother.

   Laurie is now 15 minutes old. She is lying supine on the radiant warmer with the thermistor probe in place. Her temperature is 97.5°F (36.5°C) axillary, heart rate is 152 bpm without murmur, respiratory rate is 80 breaths per minute with mild intermittent expiratory grunting, nasal flaring, and intercostal retracting. She has bilateral breath sounds and crackles. She has active bowel sounds. She is active and alert with symmetric movement and good muscle tone.
   - Would you expect Laurie to be a well, at-risk, or sick baby?
   - Are any assessment findings of concern at this time?
   - Would any further assessment information be helpful in determining Laurie's status?
2. Ms. Chung comes to the nurses' station with her baby in her arms. You are not familiar with the Chung family. Ms. Chung asks for a warm blanket for her baby because he is shivering. You accompany Ms. Chung back to her room and assess the infant. The baby is mottled, cool to the touch, and jittery. His cry is high-pitched. His T-shirt is wet in a large area on the front. He appears to weigh about 2500 g (5 lbs, 8 oz).
   - How do you explain Baby Chung's "shivering" to his mother?
   - What are Baby Chung's possible problems?

- What further information do you want to know about Baby Chung?
- What are immediate nursing interventions for Baby Chung?

3. Ms. Taylor is 19 years old, a G1 P0-1, single woman with an uncomplicated pregnancy and delivery. Her mother is with her. Sierra is a 2-day-old, 38-week, AGA healthy girl. You walk into Ms. Taylor's room just as Sierra begins to stir and cry. Ms. Taylor picks her up immediately and holds her under the armpits. Sierra dangles, without a blanket around her, about 12 inches away from her mother's face. "Why are you crying now?" she asks loudly, peering at Sierra intensely. The baby turns her head and cries louder and harder. Ms. Taylor rearranges her, holding her head in one hand, and supporting her bottom in the other. She bounces Sierra up and down rapidly and repeatedly speaks her name into her face. The baby arches away from her and cries louder. Grandmother Taylor then takes the baby from her daughter and begins her own bouncing, up and down and sideways in a face-to-face position, just as her daughter had done. Then she begins to walk quickly back and forth across the room as she bounces and speaks directly into her face.

   Sierra is screaming frantically now, waving her arms and legs. Ms. Taylor and her mother glare at each other, then turn and look at you.
   - What is your assessment of Sierra's behavioral state and cues?
   - What are your observations about how Sierra, her mother, and her grandmother are interacting?
   - What is your approach to supportive teaching in this situation? What interventions might help Sierra regain state control?

SUMMARY

- Fetal lungs are filled with fluid, not with air.
- Fetal circulation involves two important cardiac shunts, the ductus arteriosus and the foramen ovale. These shunts divert oxygenated blood to the brain and other vital organs, away from fetal lungs.
- Blood vessels in the fetal lungs are tightly constricted, and blood pressure is high (high pulmonary vascular resistance). The systemic blood pressure in the fetus is low (low systemic vascular resistance). With the newborn's first strong breaths, oxygen entering the lungs causes the vessels in the lungs to relax and allows blood to perfuse the newborn's lungs, and blood pressure in the baby's body increases. This rise in systemic vascular resistance closes the cardiac shunts and establishes newborn circulation.
- Surfactant is a fatty substance produced by cells in the lungs. Surfactant is essential to lung function because it allows the alveoli to remain open instead of collapsing during exhalation. Surfactant production peaks at about 35 weeks' gestation, which is why babies born before this time are likely to have surfactant deficiency, resulting in respiratory distress syndrome.
- A baby at birth whose skin is clear of meconium, breathes or cries, demonstrates good muscle tone, becomes pink, and appears to be term gestation requires little resuscitative assistance. The nurse need only provide warmth, clear the airway with a bulb syringe if necessary, and dry the baby to prevent cold stress.
- The Apgar score is a system used to evaluate the newborn at 1 and 5 minutes of age by assigning 0 to 2 points to each of five components: color, heart rate, reflex irritability, muscle tone, and respiratory effort. Most healthy term newborns receive a score between 7 and 9.
- The Apgar score reflects the newborn's response to extrauterine transition and resuscitative efforts but is not used to determine the need for resuscitation. The Apgar score is not predictive of neurologic outcome.
- A newborn is term, preterm, or postterm, depending on gestational age. In addition, the newborn is small for gestational age (SGA), appropriate for gestational age (AGA), or large for gestational age (LGA), depending on weight, head circumference, and length in relation to the gestational age.
- A physical assessment should proceed with observation, auscultation, and palpation, in that order.
- The nurse can quickly approximate gestational age by assessing maturational characteristics of the infant's ear pinna, nipples, genitalia, and sole creases.
- The newborn has two sleep and four awake states: deep sleep, light sleep, drowsy, quiet alert, active alert, and crying. Each state has implications for caregiving.
- The newborn learns to control his or her environment by displaying approach cues, indicating a readiness to interact, and avoidance cues, indicating the need to disengage from interaction.
- Some newborns exhibit signs of respiratory distress immediately after birth, but a healthy newborn steadily improves and stabilizes over a short period of time.
- A newborn with abnormal transition shows signs of distress and does not improve or deteriorates. Signs of abnormal transition include respiratory distress, poor perfusion, hypotonia, marked jitteriness, temperature instability, abdominal distention, vomiting of bilious material, and frequent choking accompanied by apnea or cyanosis.
- The newborn transfers heat to and from the body surface in four ways: evaporation, conduction, convection, and radiation.
- The ill or the low-birth-weight newborn is at risk for hypoglycemia.

- Signs of neonatal hypoglycemia include jitteriness, hypothermia, lethargy, hypotonia, high-pitched or weak cry, apnea, respiratory distress, poor suck, vomiting, cyanosis, and seizures. A hypoglycemic newborn may be asymptomatic.
- Forty-five to 60% of term newborns become jaundiced in the first week of life owing to RBC hemolysis and immature liver function. Jaundice in the first 24 hours of life is never normal.
- The newborn is susceptible to infection due to immature immunologic responses to infection and because of delayed or decreased immune response due to the newborn's lack of exposure to common organisms.
- The best infection prevention strategy is thorough handwashing.
- The nurse promotes normal transition by avoiding mother–infant separation, by handling the newborn gently, using containment, avoiding frequent and deep suction, avoiding bright light in the infant's face, and avoiding rectal temperature assessment.
- Acyanosis is normal in the few days of life, especially if the baby is exposed to cool temperatures; central cyanosis indicates hypoxia and an emergent need for supplemental oxygen.
- A healthy newborn has pink lips and mucous membranes, an axillary temperature congruent with the community standard in the range of 97.5° to 99.1°F (36.5° to 37.3°C), a heart rate of 120 to 160 bpm, and a respiratory rate of 40 to 60 breaths per minute. The healthy newborn urinates by 24 hours of age and stools by 48 hours of age.
- The cause of SIDS is unknown. Risk factors for SIDS include prone sleep position, sleeping on a soft surface, maternal smoking during pregnancy, overheating, late or no prenatal care, young maternal age, prematurity or low birth weight, and male sex.
- The health care provider must assess the cultural and spiritual beliefs of the client. It is not safe to stereotype the behavior or beliefs of a person from a designated ethnic group by assuming that literature about cultural practices applies to everyone within the specified ethnic group.
- Parent education before discharge includes temperature taking, use of the bulb syringe, normal amounts voiding and stooling, diapering, dressing, and bathing, cord care, sleep position, car seat use, dangers of secondhand smoke, circumcision care, and signs of newborn illness.

REVIEW QUESTIONS

1. The nurse educator is teaching a group of student nurses the differences between fetal and newborn circulation. Which statement about fetal circulation would indicate that the educator's teaching plan has been successful?
   A. "Fetal circulation is characterized by high pulmonary vascular resistance and high systemic vascular resistance."
   B. "Fetal circulation is characterized by low pulmonary vascular resistance and low systemic vascular resistance."
   C. "Fetal circulation is characterized by high pulmonary vascular resistance and low systemic vascular resistance."
   D. "Fetal circulation is characterized by low pulmonary vascular resistance and high systemic vascular resistance."
2. When performing an initial newborn assessment, which parameters would be most important to assess in the first minute of life?
   A. Color, respirations, heart rate
   B. Gestational age, sex, muscle tone
   C. Weight, length, head circumference
   D. Color, respirations, temperature
3. Oxygen administration would most likely be required at the birth of a newborn with:
   A. Acrocyanosis
   B. Jaundice
   C. Central cyanosis
   D. Circumoral cyanosis
4. The nurse is reporting a newborn's Apgar scores to the baby's parents. The father asks what the information means. Which response, if made by the nurse, would be most appropriate?
   A. "Apgar scores help determine which steps of resuscitation are required."
   B. "Apgar scores reflect the newborn's response to extrauterine transition and resuscitation efforts."
   C. "Apgar scores are assessed at 1, 3, and 5 minutes of age."
   D. "Apgar scores are the best predictor of neurologic outcome."
5. A nurse is collecting data for a baby with suspected neonatal hypoglycemia. Which set of findings would support this diagnosis?
   A. Jitteriness, high-pitched cry, lethargy
   B. Plethora, excess mucus production, dysrhythmia
   C. Blood glucose level of 50 mg/dL, no crying, fever
   D. Apnea, bradycardia, fever
6. Which of the following scenarios most clearly depicts abnormal newborn transition?
   A. Term baby; vaginal birth; Apgar scores 5 (1 minute), 8 (5 minutes); required brief free-flow oxygen for central cyanosis after birth; now 20 minutes old and pink in room air; respiratory rate 68 breaths per minute; bilateral crackles heard with auscultation.
   B. Term baby; vaginal birth; Apgar scores 8 (1 minute), 9 (5 minutes); now 10 minutes old; pink when active and crying; dusky when quiet.

C. Term baby; scheduled repeat cesarean birth; now 15 minutes old; pink with marked acrocyanosis; respiratory rate 72 breaths per minute; intermittent expiratory grunting and nasal flaring.
D. Term baby; emergency cesarean birth for fetal distress; Apgar scores 6 (1 minute), 8 (5 minutes); required free flow oxygen until 3 minutes of age, now 25 minutes old; pale pink and quiet alert; respiratory rate 68 breaths per minute with periodic breathing noted.

7. When educating parents of a newborn regarding when to contact the newborn's care provider, the best statement by the nurse would be:
A. Contact the provider if the newborn has not voided within 24 hours and stooled within 48 hours of birth.
B. Contact the provider if the newborn has not voided within 12 hours and stooled within 24 hours of birth.
C. Contact the provider if the newborn has not voided and stooled within 4 hours after the first feeding.
D. Contact the provider if the newborn has not voided and stooled at least once every 8 hours times three.

8. Which statement by the father of a newborn diagnosed with physiologic jaundice indicates that teaching has been effective?
A. "Physiologic jaundice is a normal result of immature liver function."
B. "Physiologic jaundice is uncommon in term infants like my baby."
C. "I should have noticed the jaundice in the baby's first 24 hours."
D. "The baby will have ongoing problems with his skin coloring."

9. When providing anticipatory guidance to a group of expectant parents, the nurse correctly identifies the preferred sleeping position for a term healthy newborn as:
A. Prone
B. Supine
C. Dorsal recumbent
D. Side-lying with a blanket roll for support

10. The nurse is teaching a new mother about common signs of newborn illness. Which of the following sets of findings would the nurse alert the mother to look for and to report?
A. Respiratory distress and temperature instability
B. Fever and soft frequent stools
C. Sweating and shivering
D. Periodic breathing and nevus simplex

REFERENCES

Alexander, G. R., et al. (1992). Validity of postnatal assessments of gestational age: A comparison of the method of Ballard JL, et al. and early ultrasonography. *American Journal of Obstetrics and Gynecology, 166*(3), 891–895.

American Academy of Pediatrics, Vitamin K Ad Hoc Task Force (1993). Controversies concerning vitamin K and the newborn. *Pediatrics, 91,* 1001–1003.

American Academy of Pediatrics. (1997). Environmental tobacco smoke: A hazard to children (RE9716). *Pediatrics, 99*(4), 639–642.

American Academy of Pediatrics. (1998). Safety outside the home. In S. P. Shelov (Ed.), *Caring for your baby and young child: Birth to age 5.* Elk Grove Village, IL: Author.

American Academy of Pediatrics. (1999a). Newborn and infant hearing loss: Detection and intervention. *Pediatrics, 103*(2), 527–530.

American Academy of Pediatrics (1999b). Circumcision policy statement (RE9850). *Pediatrics, 103*(3), 686–693.

American Academy of Pediatrics (2002). Car safety seats: A guide for families 2002. Available at: http://www.aap.org/family/carseatguide.htm.

American Academy of Pediatrics, Task Force on Sudden Infant Death Syndrome. (2005). The changing concept of sudden infant death syndrome: Diagnostic coding shifts, controversies regarding the sleeping environment, and new variables to consider in reducing risk. *Pediatrics, 116*(5), 1245–1255.

American Academy of Pediatrics & American College of Obstetricians and Gynecologists. (2006). The Apgar score. *Pediatrics, 117*(4), 1444–1447

American Academy of Pediatrics & American College of Obstetricians and Gynecologists. (2002). *Guidelines for perinatal care* (5th ed.). Elk Grove Village, IL: American Academy of Pediatrics.

American College of Nurse-Midwives. (2003). Criteria for provision of home birth services. ACNM Clinical Bulletin Number 7. *Journal of Midwifery & Women's Health, 48*(4), 299–301.

American Health Consultants. (1998). Prepare for the worst: Fortify newborn security. *Hospital Peer Review, 23*(10), 180.

American Medical Association. (1999). Neonatal circumcision: Report 10 of the Council on Scientific Affairs (1–99). Available at: http://www.ama-assn.org.

Apgar, V. (1953). A proposal for a new method of evaluation of the newborn infant. *Anesthesia and Analgesia, 32,* 260.

Apgar, V. (1966). The newborn (Apgar) scoring system: Reflections and advice. *Pediatric Clinics of North America, 113,* 645–650.

Askin, D. F. (2002). Complications in the transition from fetal to neonatal life. *Journal of Obstetric, Gynecologic, and Neonatal Nursing, 31*(3), 318–327.

Association of Women's Health, Obstetric and Neonatal Nurses (AWHONN). (1998). *Standards and guidelines for professional nursing practice in the care of women and newborns* (5th ed.). Washington, DC: Author.

Atkinson, W., & Wolfe, C. (2002). *Epidemiology and prevention of vaccine-preventable diseases* (7th ed.). Atlanta: Centers for Disease Control.

Bakewell-Sachs, S., Shaw, V. D., & Tashman, A. L. (1997). *Assessment of risk in the term newborn.* White Plains, NY: March of Dimes Birth Defects Foundation.

Ballard, J. L., Novak, K. K., & Driver, M. (1979). A simplified score for assessment of fetal maturation of newly born infants. *Journal of Pediatrics, 95*(5), 769–774.

Ballard, J. L., et al. (1991). New Ballard score, expanded to include extremely premature infants. *Journal of Pediatrics, 119*(3), 417–423.

Bank, R. D. (2002). *The everything Judaism book.* Avon, MA: Adams Media Corporation.

Barr, R. G., St. James-Roberts, I., & Keefe, M. (2001). Johnson & Johnson Pediatric Round Table Scientific Conference. New evidence on unexplained early infant crying: Its origin, nature, and management. Skillman, NJ: Johnson & Johnson Pediatric Institute.

Behring, A., Vezeau, T. M., & Fink, R. (2003). Timing of the newborn first bath: A replication. *Journal of Obstetric, Gynecologic, and Neonatal Nursing, 22*(1), 39–46.

Blackburn, S. (1995). Hyperbilirubinemia and neonatal jaundice. *Neonatal Network, 14*(7), 15–25.

Blackburn, S. T. (2003). *Maternal, fetal, & neonatal physiology: A clinical perspective* (2nd ed.). St. Louis: W. B. Saunders.

Brazelton, T. B. (1978). The Brazelton Neonatal Behavior Assessment Scale. Introduction. *Monographs of the Society for Research in Child Development, 43*(5–6), 1–13.

Bruck, K. (1978). Non-shivering thermogenesis and brown adipose tissue in relation to age, and their integration in the thermoregulatory system. In O. Lindberg (Ed.), *Brown adipose tissue* (pp. 117–154). New York: Elsevier.

Butterfield, L. J. (1962). Practical epigram of the Apgar score. *Journal of the American Medical Association, 208,* 353.
Canadian Paediatric Society. (1975). Circumcision in the newborn period. *CPS News Bulletin,* 8(2), 1–4.
Canadian Paediatric Society and College of Family Physicians of Canada. (1997). Routine administration of vitamin K to newborns. *Paediatrics & Child Health, 2*(6), 429–431.
Carter, B., Haverkamp, A., & Merenstein, G. (1993). The definition of acute perinatal asphyxia. *Clinics in Perinatology, 20,* 287–304.
Ceriani Cernadas, J. M., Carroli, G., Pellegrini, L., Otano, L., Ferreira, M., Ricci, C., et al. (2006). The effect of timing of cord clamping on neonatal venous hematocrit values and clinical outcome at term: A randomized controlled trial. *Pediatrics, 117*(4), 779–786.
Childhood Immunization Support Program. (2003). What parents should know about thimerosal: From the American Academy of Pediatrics. Available at: http://www.cispimmunize.org.
Christensen, R. D. (2000). Expected hematologic values for term and preterm neonates. In R. Christensen (Ed.), *Hematologic problems of the neonate.* Philadelphia: W. B. Saunders.
Christensen, R. D., & Rothstein, G. (1979). Pitfalls in the interpretation of leukocyte counts of newborn infants. *American Journal of Clinical Pathology, 72*(40), 608–611.
Christensson, K., et al. (1995). Separation distress call in the human neonate in the absence of maternal body contact. *Acta Paediatrica, 84*(5), 468–473.
Circumcision Information Resource Page. (1997). What were the original motivations behind routine infant circumcision in the West? Available at: http://www.cirp.org.
Clark, D. A. (1977). Time of first void and first stool in 500 newborns. *Pediatrics, 60,* 457.
Cooper, R., & Goldenberg, R. (1990). Catecholamine secretion in fetal adaptation to stress. *Journal of Obstetric, Gynecologic, and Neonatal Nursing, 19,* 223–226.
Cornblath, M., et al. (2000). Controversies regarding definition of neonatal hypoglycemia: Suggested operational thresholds. *Pediatrics, 105,* 1141.
Cornelissen, M., von Kries, R., Loughnan, P., Schubiger, G. (1997). Prevention of vitamin K deficiency bleeding: Efficacy of different multiple oral dose schedules of vitamin K. *European Journal of Pediatrics, 156,* 126–130.
Cowett, R. M., & Loughead, J. L. (2002). Neonatal glucose metabolism: Differential diagnosis, evaluation, and treatment of hypoglycemia. *Neonatal Network, 21*(4), 9–19.
Del Vecchio, A., & Sola, M. C. (2000). Performing and interpreting the bleeding time in the neonatal intensive care unit. *Clinics in Perinatology, 27,* 643.
Demicheli, V., Jefferson, T., Rivetti, A., & Price, D. (2005). Vaccines for measles, mumps and rubella in children. *Cochrane Database of Systematic Reviews, 19*(4), CD004407.
Desmond, M. M., Franklin, R. R., Valbona, C., Hill, R. M., Plumb, R., Arnold, H., & Watts, J. (1963). The clinical behavior of the newly born: 1. The term baby. *Journal of Pediatrics, 62,* 307–325.
Dihigo, S. K. (1998). New strategies for treatment of colic: Modifying the parent/infant interaction. *Journal of Pediatric Health Care, 12*(5), 256–262.
Dinwiddie, R., et al. (1979). Cardiopulmonary changes in the crying neonate. *Pediatric Research, 13*(8), 900–903.
Dodd, V. (1996). Gestational age assessment. *Neonatal Network, 15*(1), 27–36.
Dubowitz, L. M. S., Dubowitz, V., & Goldberg, C. (1970). Clinical assessment of gestational age in the newborn infant. *Journal of Pediatrics, 77*(1), 1–10.
Finitzo, T., & Crumley, W. S. (1999). The role of the pediatrician in hearing loss: From detection to connection. *Pediatric Clinics of North America, 46*(1), 15–34.
Fisher, D. A., & Polk, D. H. (1994). The ontogenesis of thyroid function and activity. In D. Tulchinsky & A. B. Little (Eds.), *Maternal–fetal endocrinology* (2nd ed.). Philadelphia: W. B. Saunders.
Gee, W. F., & Ansell, J. S. (1976). Neonatal circumcision: A ten-year overview with comparison of Gomco clamp and Plastibell device. *Pediatrics,* 58, 824–827.
Geyer, J., Ellsbury, D., Kleiber, C., Litwiller, D., Hinton, A., & Yankowitz, J. (2002). An evidence-based multidisciplinary protocol for neonatal circumcision pain management. *Journal of Obstetric, Gynecologic, and Neonatal Nursing, 31*(4), 403–410.
Greer, F. R. (1995). Vitamin K deficiency and hemorrhage in infancy. *Clinics in Perinatology, 22,* 759.
Harkavy, K. L. (1987). The circumcision debate. *Pediatrics, 79,* 649–650.
Hathaway, W. E., & Bonnar, J. (1987). *Hemostatic disorders of the pregnant woman and newborn infant.* New York: Elsevier.
Hyde, M. L. (2005). Newborn hearing screening programs: Overview. *Journal of Otolaryngology, 34*(Suppl 2), S70–78.
Ibraham H., et al. (2000). Placental transfusion: Umbilical cord clamping and preterm infants. *Journal of Perinatology, 20,* 351.
Joint Commission on Infant Hearing. (2000). Joint Commission on Infant Hearing 2000 Position Statement: Principles and guidelines for early hearing detection and intervention programs. *American Journal of Audiology, 9*(1), 9–29.
Juretschke, L. J. (2000). Apgar scoring: Its use and meaning for today's newborn. *Neonatal Network, 19*(1), 17–19.
Karlsen, K. A. (2005). *The S.T.A.B.L.E. program* (5th ed.). Park City, UT.
Karp, T. B., Scardino, C., & Butler, L. A. (1995). Glucose metabolism in the neonate: The short and sweet of it. *Neonatal Network, 14*(8), 17–23.
Kattwinkel, J. (Ed.) (2006). *Textbook of neonatal resuscitation* (5th ed.). Elk Grove Village, IL: American Academy of Pediatrics/American Heart Association.
Kenner, C., & Moran, M. (2005). Newborn screening and genetic testing. *Journal of Midwifery and Women's Health, 50*(3), 219–226.
Knott, C. (2001). Universal newborn hearing screening coming soon: "Hear's" why. *Neonatal Network, 20*(8), 25–33.
Kopelman, A. E. (1973). Cutaneous absorption of hexachlorophene in low-birth-weight infants. *Journal of Pediatrics, 82,* 972.
Lang, N. J., & Stewart, D. D. (1999). Child passenger safety: Clear reflections on gray areas. *Mother Baby Journal, 4*(4), 9–11.
Laumann, E. O., Masi, C. M., & Zuckerman, E. W. (1997). Circumcision in the United States. *JAMA,* 277, 1052–1057.
Lecanuet, J. P., & Schaal, B. (1996). Fetal sensory competencies. *European Journal of Obstetrics and Gynecology, 68,* 1.
Leitch, I. O. (1970). Circumcision: A continuing enigma. *Australian Paediatrics Journal, 6,* 59–65.
Lincoln, M. (2005). Car seat safety: Literature review. *Neonatal Network, 24*(2), 29–31.
Lockridge, T. (1999). Persistent pulmonary hypertension of the newborn. *Mother Baby Journal, 4*(2), 19–32.
Ludington, S. M. (1990). Energy conservation during skin-to-skin contact between premature infants and their mothers. *Heart & Lung, 19*(5), 445–451.
Ludington-Hoe, S., Cong, X., & Hashemi, F. (2002). Infant crying: Nature, physiologic consequences, and select interventions. *Neonatal Network, 21*(2), 29–36.
Lund, C. H., et al. (1997). Prevention and management of infant skin breakdown. *Nursing Clinics of North America, 34,* 907.
MacDonald, M. G., Seshia, M. M., & Mullet, M. D. (2006). *Avery's neonatology: Pathophysiology and management of the newborn* (6th ed.). Philadelphia: Lippincott Williams & Wilkins.
Maisels, M. J., (1999). Jaundice. In G. B. Avery, M. A. Fletcher, & M. G. MacDonald (Eds.), *Neonatology* (5th ed.). Philadelphia: Lippincott Williams & Wilkins.
March of Dimes. (2003). Few states offer adequate newborn screening: Most fall short of March of Dimes recommendations. *March of Dimes (About Us) News,* July 29, 2003. Available at: http://www.modimes.org.
Martin, R., Fanaroff, A., & Walsh, M. (2006). *Fanaroff and Martin's neonatal-perinatal medicine: Diseases of the fetus and infant.* Philadelphia: Lippincott Williams & Wilkins.
McCain, G. C., Ludington-Hoe, S. M., Swinth, J. Y., Hadeed, A. J. (2005). Heart rate variability responses of a preterm infant to kangaroo care. *Journal of Obstetric, Gynecologic, and Neonatal Nursing, 34*(6), 689–694.
McNinch, A. W., Upton, C., Samuels, M., et al. (1985). Plasma concentrations after oral or intramuscular vitamin K1 in neonates. *Archives of Disease in Childhood, 60,* 814–818.
Mercer, J. S., Nelson, C. C., & Skovgaard, R. L. (2000). Umbilical cord clamping: Beliefs and practices of American nurse-midwives. *Journal of Midwifery and Women's Health, 45,* 58.

Michelsson, K., et al. (1996). Crying in separated and non-separated newborns: Sound spectrographic analysis. *Acta Paediatrica, 85*(4), 471–475.

Miller, C. A. (2003). Controversies concerning vitamin K and the newborn. *Pediatrics, 112*(1), 191–192.

Moses, S., Bradley, J., Nagelkerke, N., Ronald, A., Ndinya-Achola, J., & Plummer, F. (1990). Geographical patterns of male circumcision practices in Africa: Association with HIV seroprevalence. *International Journal of Epidemiology, 19*(3), 693–697.

Motohara, K., Endo, F., & Matsuda, I. (1987). Screening for late neonatal vitamin K deficiency by acarboxyprothrombin in dried blood spots. *Archives of Disease in Childhood, 62,* 370–375.

Nako, Y., et al. (2000). Effects of bathing immediately after birth on early neonatal adaptation and morbidity: A prospective randomized comparative study. *Pediatrics International, 42*(5), 517–522.

National Association of Neonatal Nurses. (1997). *Neonatal thermoregulation: Guidelines for practice.* Petaluma, CA: Author.

Niermeyer, S., et al. (2000). International guidelines for neonatal resuscitation: An excerpt from the guidelines 2000 for cardiopulmonary resuscitation and emergency cardiovascular care: International consensus on science. *Pediatrics, 106*(3), e29.

O'Connor, M. E., & Addiego, J. E. Jr. (1986). Use of oral vitamin K_1 to prevent hemorrhagic disease of the newborn infant. *Journal of Pediatrics, 108,* 616–619.

Oski, F. A., & Naiman, J. L. (1982). *Hematologic problems in the newborn* (3rd ed.). Philadelphia: W. B. Saunders.

Perinatal Continuing Education Program (PCEP). (1999a). *Book II: Neonatal care.* Charlottesville, VA: University of Virginia.

Perinatal Continuing Education Program (PCEP). (1999b). *Book III: Complex perinatal care.* Charlottesville, VA: University of Virginia.

Perinatal Continuing Education Program (PCEP). (1999c). *Book IV: Specialized newborn care.* Charlottesville, VA: University of Virginia.

Penny-MacGillivray, T. (1996). The newborn's first bath: When? *Journal of Obstetric, Gynecologic, and Neonatal Nursing, 25*(6), 481–487.

Poland, R. (1990). The question of routine neonatal circumcision. *New England Journal of Medicine, 322*(18), 1312–1315.

Polin, R. A., & Fox, W. W. (2004). *Fetal and neonatal physiology* (3rd ed.). Philadelphia: W. B. Saunders.

Purdy, I. B. (2000). Newborn auditory follow-up. *Neonatal Network, 19*(2), 25–33.

Pyati, S. P., et al. (1977). Absorption of iodine in the neonate following topical use of povidone iodine. *Journal of Pediatrics, 91,* 825.

Remington, J. S., & Klein, J. O. (2006). *Infectious diseases of the fetus and newborn infant* (6th ed.). Philadelphia: W. B. Saunders.

Rooth, G., Huch, A., & Huch, R. (1987). Transcutaneous oxygen monitors are reliable indicators of arterial oxygen tension (if used correctly). *Pediatrics, 79*(2), 283–286.

Rutter, N. (1999). Thermal adaptation to extrauterine life. In C. H. Rodeck & M. J. Whittle (Eds.), *Fetal medicine: Basic science and clinical practice.* London: Churchill Livingstone.

Shaker, I. J., et al. (1979). Aerophagia, a mechanism for spontaneous rupture of the stomach in the newborn. *Annals of Surgery, 39*(11), 619–623.

Shogan, M. G. (2002). Emergency management plan for newborn abduction. *Journal of Obstetric, Gynecologic, and Neonatal Nursing, 31*(3), 340–346.

Slater, R. (1998). Liver function tests in the newborn. *Neonatal Network, 17*(6), 75–78.

Taft, C. H., Mickalide, A. D., & Taft, A. R. (1999). *Child passengers at risk in America: A national study of car seat misuse.* Washington, DC: National SAFE KIDS Campaign.

Tappero, E. P., & Honeyfield, M. E. (2003). *Physical assessment of the newborn: A comprehensive approach to the art of physical examination* (3rd ed.). Santa Rosa, CA: NICU Ink Book Publishers.

Taylor, A., Fisk, N. M., & Glover, V. (2000). Mode of delivery and subsequent stress response. *Lancet, 355*(9198), 120.

Thureen, P. J., Deacon, J., Hernandez, J. A., & Hall, D. (2005). *Assessment and care of the well newborn* (2nd ed.). Philadelphia: Elsevier.

Trubo, R., Shelov, S. P., Hannemann, R. E., Agran, P. F., Remer, T., Baker, S. S., et al. (2004). *Caring for your baby and young child: Birth to age 5* (4th ed., revised). New York: Bantam.

UNHS Project Team. (2001). *Universal newborn hearing screening: Frequently asked questions.* Seattle: Children's Hospital & Regional Medical Center.

U.S. Consumer Product Safety Commission (2003). Crib safety tips. Available at: http://www.cpsc.gov.

Vanhatalo, S., & van Nieuwenhuizen, O. (2000). Fetal pain? *Brain Development, 22,* 145.

Varda, K. E., & Behnke, R. S. (2000). The effect of timing of initial bath on newborn temperature. *Journal of Obstetric, Gynecologic, and Neonatal Nursing, 29*(1), 27–32.

von Kreis, R., & Hanawa, Y. (1993). Neonatal vitamin K prophylaxis: Report of scientific and standardization subcommittee on perinatal haemostasis. *Thrombosis and Haemostasis, 69,* 293–295.

Wallerstein, E. (1985). Circumcision: The uniquely American medical enigma. *Urologic Clinics of North America, 12*(1), 123–132.

Wardrop, C. A., & Holland, B. M. (1995). The roles and vital importance of placental blood to the newborn infant. *Journal of Perinatal Medicine, 23,* 139.

Washington State Department of Health. (2002). *Plain talk about childhood immunizations* (5th ed.). DOH publication #348-080. Seattle: Public Health-Seattle & King County.

Wiswell, T., & Roscelli, J. (1986). Corroborative evidence for the decreased incidence of urinary tract infections in circumcised male infants. *Pediatrics, 78*(1), 96–99.

Zaichkin, J. (Ed.). (2006). *Instructor's manual for neonatal resuscitation* (4th ed.). Elk Grove Village, IL: AAP/American Heart Association.

Resources

American Academy of Neonatal Nursing
1410 Neotomas Avenue, Suite 107
Santa Rosa, CA 95405-7533
707-569-1415

American Academy of Pediatrics
141 Northwest Point Blvd.
P.O. Box 927
Elk Grove Village, IL 60009-0927
www.aap.org

American Academy of Pediatrics/American Heart Association Neonatal Resuscitation Program (NRP)
141 Northwest Point Blvd.
P.O. Box 927
Elk Grove Village, IL 60009-0927
www.aap.org/nrp

Association of Women's Health, Obstetric and Neonatal Nurses (AWHONN)
2000 L Street, N.W., Suite 740
Washington, DC 20036
800-673-8499

Back to Sleep (information about SIDS)
800-505-CRIB

National Association of Neonatal Nurses
4700 West Lake Avenue
Glenview, IL 60025-1485
800-451-3795

National Center for Missing and Exploited Children
699 Prince Street
Alexandria, VA 22314-3175
800-THE-LOST
www.missingkids.com

National Highway Traffic Safety Administration
AAP Care Safety Seats: A Guide for Families
www.aap.org/family/carseatguide.htm

National Information Center on Deafness
Gallaudet University
800 Florida Avenue, N.E.
Washington, DC 20002-3695
202-651-5051

CHAPTER 21

Newborn Nutrition

Michelle Johnson

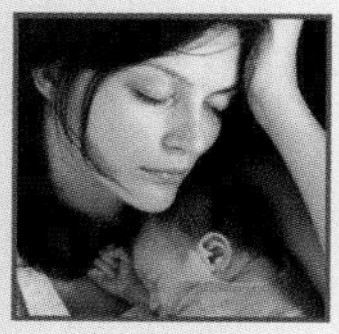

Lindsay, a 35-year-old G1P1001, is 6 weeks postpartum after cesarean birth of a son. She is at the clinic for her scheduled follow-up appointment. The infant is thriving, but Lindsay's recovery has been rough. During discussions with the nurse, Lindsay states that she understands the benefits of breastfeeding, but that the physical demands are overwhelming her. She reports that she would prefer to switch to formula feeding, but that she feels like if she does so, she's being selfish and inadequate.

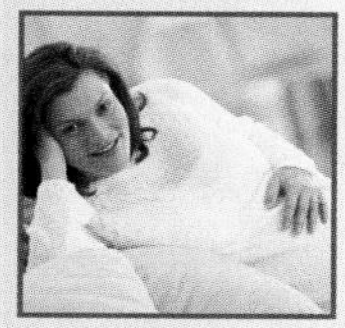

Joelle, a 24-year-old multigravida (G2P1001), is at 25 weeks' gestation. Although she had positive results with bottle-feeding formula to her first infant, Joelle has been reading about the benefits of breastfeeding and wants to pursue this method for the baby she is expecting. She asks the nurse for more information about the positive aspects of breastfeeding and ways to ensure a successful experience.

Nursing interactions with these clients are discussed in more detail later in this chapter. Before beginning this chapter, consider the following points related to the above scenarios:

- How will the nurse working with both clients tailor care to best suit the needs of the women and their families?
- What aspects of teaching do these women require? What issues are similar? What issues are different?
- Which points or considerations might these clients have overlooked or not know about? What other types of information will the nurse require?
- How might the nurse involve the clients' families in care?

LEARNING OBJECTIVES

On completion of this chapter, the reader should be able to:

- Discuss with parents and other caregivers pertinent information needed to make informed decisions about infant feeding.
- Discuss the benefits of and contraindications for breastfeeding newborns.
- Outline collaborative care strategies for women who choose breastfeeding.
- Discuss the benefits of and contraindications for using formula as a primary source of newborn nutrition.
- Identify various types of formula and their indications for use.
- Outline collaborative care strategies for women who choose bottle feeding.
- Evaluate the adequacy of infant nutritional intake.
- Identify common problems associated with infant feeding and provide supportive measures for their resolution.

KEY TERMS

colic
colostrum
foremilk
gastroesophageal reflux
hindmilk
infant formula
jaundice
mastitis
mature human milk
meconium
milk bank
nursing supplementer
plugged milk duct
protein hydrolysate
rooting reflex
thrush
transitional milk

Nurses are well positioned in the health care field to ensure that parents and other caregivers receive accurate information about and use appropriate techniques for newborn and infant feeding. Nurses need to be aware of the many related problems that can develop. They often are the first or only people of whom clients ask feeding-related questions. For this reason, nurses need thorough understanding of the various feeding techniques and strategies to overcome feeding challenges so that they can help clients appropriately (Spatz, 2005).

THE FEEDING DECISION

Method of feeding is one of the most important choices parents or other caregivers must make for their newborn. Many factors influence the decision about infant nutrition, including the attitudes of the primary caregivers and significant others, health care professionals, the media, and personal values and choices (Kong & Lee, 2004; Labarere et al., 2005). See Research Highlight 21.1.

Maternal breast milk has unique nutritional, immunologic, developmental, and economic advantages; additionally, women who breastfeed their children experience unique health benefits (Leung & Sauve, 2005). Such women frequently cite its advantages over commercially prepared formulas as a factor in their decision. Other factors that influence the decision to breastfeed include higher socioeconomic levels, higher education attainment, occupation, and white race (Chezem et al., 2003; Kong & Lee, 2004; Li et al., 2005). Donor human milk is a viable alternative when the use of maternal milk is contraindicated or the volume of maternal milk is insufficient to meet the newborn's needs (Tully et al., 2004).

Commercially prepared formulas are another feeding option that provides sole-source nutrition to meet the newborn's demands. These formulas have adequate

RESEARCH HIGHLIGHT 21.1 Why Do Women Stop Breastfeeding? Findings From the Pregnancy Risk Assessment and Monitoring System

OBJECTIVE: To evaluate contributing factors to breastfeeding cessation and associations between prenatal feeding intentions and actual breastfeeding results.

DESIGN: The researchers assessed 2 years of data from the Pregnancy Risk Assessment and Monitoring System for the percentage of women who began breastfeeding, continued for less than 1 week, continued for 1 to 4 weeks, and continued for more than 4 weeks. They also examined the reports of the women for not beginning or stopping, as well as the clients' breastfeeding intentions before birth and subsequent outcomes.

RESULTS: Findings showed that 32% of women never started breastfeeding, 4% started but stopped within 1 week, 13% stopped within 1 month, and 51% continued for more than 1 month. Younger clients and those with limited socioeconomic resources were most likely to stop or never start breastfeeding. Participants cited sore nipples, newborn difficulties, inadequate milk supply, and hungry infant as reasons for stopping. Those clients who planned to breastfeed were more likely to initiate and continue with nursing.

CONCLUSIONS: For breastfeeding to be successful, clients need awareness and understanding of breastfeeding prenatally, as well as extensive support after birth, particularly for those at risk.

Ahluwalia, I. B., Morrow, B., & Hsia, J. (2005). *Pediatrics, 116*(6), 1408–1412.

nutrient composition and are appropriate for children up to 12 months old. Some women choose to make their own, noncommercial formulas. In such instances, it is important for health care providers to discuss the materials being used and amounts being given, to ensure adequate nutrition for these infants.

Women who choose formula for their babies do so for various reasons, some of which are as follows:

- Breastfeeding contraindications
- Desire to maintain a sense of "freedom"
- Illness in newborns
- Problems trying to maintain nursing
- Time constraints
- Viewing the breasts sexually
- Desire to avoid physical changes (eg, weight gain from needing extra calories)
- Strong sense of modesty
- Fear of milk leaking at inopportune times (Colin & Scott, 2002; Wagner & Wagner, 1999)

It is important for clients to consider all factors influencing them when making a decision about a newborn feeding method. The next sections explore such factors in more detail and provide the information needed for nurses to address concerns, correct misperceptions, and support clients in making informed choices. See Figure 21.1 for an algorithm of assisting clients in decision making for newborn and infant feeding.

Practical Considerations

Feeding Demands

Breast milk, formula, or a combination can meet newborn nutritional needs. Breast milk is convenient, requires no special preparation, and is the type of nutritional substance most suited for human newborns (Leung & Sauve, 2005; Oddy, 2002). In addition, it comes in a relatively easy-to-use "package," although it may take a few weeks for clients to become comfortable and skilled with the process of breastfeeding. A mother who desires to breastfeed exclusively needs to be prepared to do so every 2 to 3 hours, including through the night, for several weeks to months. The American Academy of Pediatrics (AAP, 2005) emphasizes that during the early weeks of breastfeeding, 8 to 12 feedings at the breast every 24 hours are recommended, with the mother offering her breast whenever the infant shows early signs of hunger (eg, increased alertness or activity, mouthing, rooting). For women who desire breastfeeding but worry that they will not be able to meet its physical or time demands, or who want to involve other family members in newborn feeding, the nurse might suggest supplementing breastfeeding with expressed breast milk provided through an alternative method, such as a bottle or special cup.

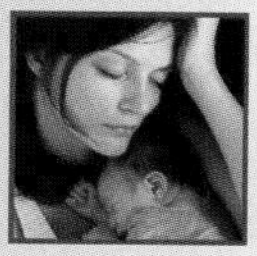

Recall Lindsay, the woman at the beginning of the chapter who is having difficulty breastfeeding her newborn. What issues and alternatives might the nurse want to investigate?

Family Involvement

The attitudes of family and friends in newborn feeding can play a major part in feeding choices. Just as some people feel pressure not to bottle-feed, others may experience similar pressures related to breastfeeding. One study revealed positive correlations between partner support, family knowledge about breastfeeding, and positive family attitudes about breastfeeding with a successful

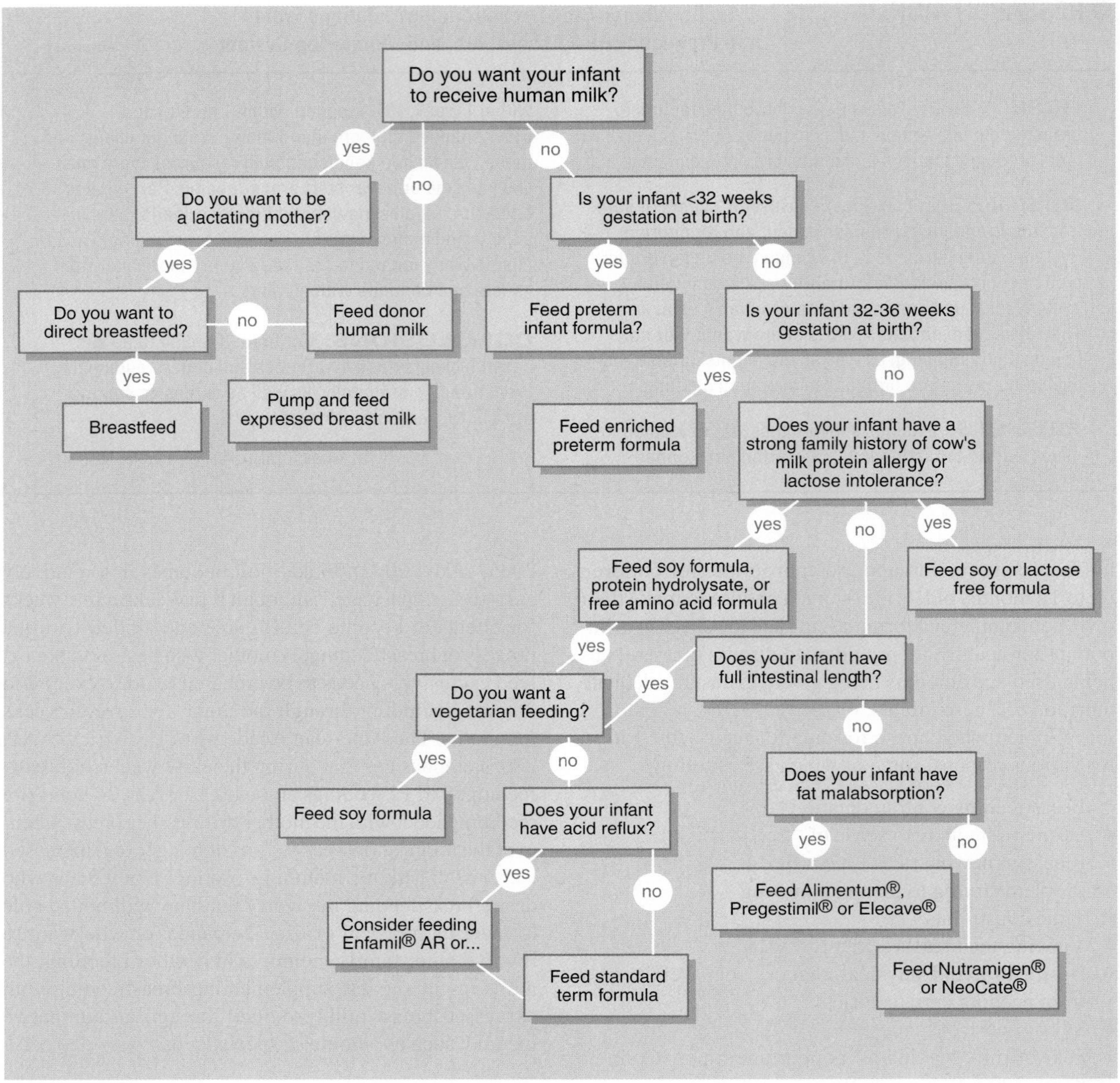

FIGURE 21.1 An algorithm for assisting clients with the newborn feeding decision.

breastfeeding experience (Rose et al., 2004). Both breastfeeding and formula feeding can involve multiple people in the feeding experience. All interested parties can easily accomplish formula feeding, which is simple to learn and easy to maintain. Some fathers who wish to participate in feeding their babies may be concerned that they will be unable to do so if the woman chooses to nurse. Despite this fear, people other than the biologic mother can be involved in giving breast milk to newborns. This requires some additional work because the mother will need to express the milk and store it in either the refrigerator or freezer. The breasts of the breastfeeding woman should be stimulated every 2 to 3 hours as per her child's demand for the first 4 to 6 weeks after birth (AAP, 2005). This may include direct breastfeeding or expressing the breast milk. This constant stimulation of the breast helps to ensure adequate breast milk production. In addition, nipple confusion may occur if bottle feeding is introduced too soon in the breastfeeding process (Dewey et al., 2003; Neifert et al., 1995). Regardless of the type of feeding chosen, family members can also participate in nonnutritional activities, such as preparing the newborn for feeding, changing the diaper or clothes as needed, and, most importantly, cuddling (Fig. 21.2).

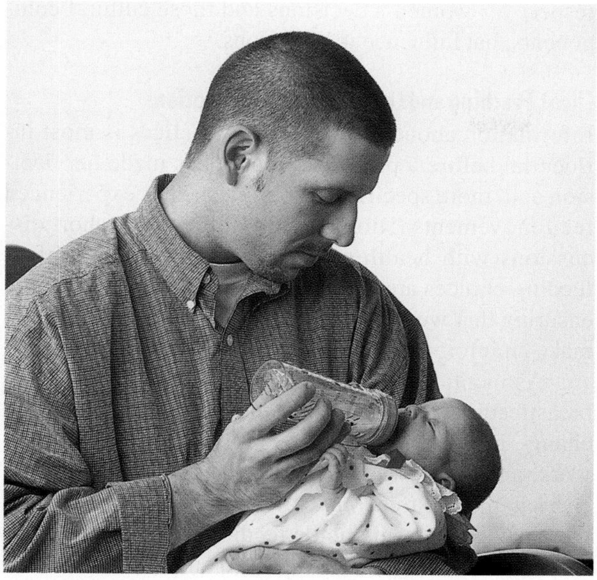

FIGURE 21.2 This father is feeding his newborn formula. Fathers and other caregivers can participate in nutritional activities for both breastfed and bottle-fed babies.

QUOTE 21-1

"When our son needs to eat, both my wife and I lie down together on the bed, with our son between us. It really makes me feel part of the special bond that develops during breastfeeding."

A father discussing his family's experience of feeding their newborn

Concerns About Body Exposure and Personal Comfort Level

Inherent in breastfeeding is the challenge of potentially exposing a part of the body usually covered under clothing. Although societal mores—and laws—are changing, a number of societal issues continue to be related to breastfeeding in public (Li et al., 2004). Additionally, some women are uncomfortable breastfeeding in front of other people. They may fear perceived indecency, or they simply might feel embarrassed (Biancuzzo, 2003; Heath et al., 2002). Nurses may suggest that the client try a variety of tops that she owns to see if there is a particular style that would facilitate her comfort during a feeding session. Additionally, the nurse should be sure that the client is aware of the availability of clothing specifically made for lactating women. Another alternative is to cover the breastfeeding infant with a light blanket that also drapes over the mother's shoulder.

In 1999, the U.S. Congress protected the woman's right to breastfeed on federal property (Humenick & Gwayi-Chore, 2001); state legislators also have fought to protect the right to breastfeed in public places. Nurses should be aware of the specific laws of the state in which they practice regarding breastfeeding. They are key players in promoting societal and legislative changes that support breastfeeding practices. State and local task forces exist for the promotion of breastfeeding. Nurses can appeal to their legislators to sponsor bills that protect breastfeeding practices and volunteer to testify during pertinent hearings.

QUOTE 21-2

"I went out to lunch with a close relative who suggested that instead of breastfeeding my son at the table, I should use a bathroom stall. I asked her if that was where she would like to eat her lunch. We did not go out again until after my son weaned himself."

A first-time breastfeeding mother

Returning to Work Outside the Home

Some countries have legislation mandating prolonged maternity leave. In other countries, such as the United States, maternity policies vary from organization to organization (Waldfogel, 2001). Breastfeeding following the return to work can be successful, but it does require flexibility and additional effort on the part of the mother and her significant others (Rojjanasrirat, 2004). If feasible, the client should try to feed the newborn directly at some time during the work day. For example, some places of employment have on-site day care facilities where parents are encouraged to come and feed or play with their children during work breaks. Another option is for the child to be brought to the woman at work so that she can breastfeed during breaks.

Using a breast pump at work is a viable option for many women because it fosters continuation of breast milk production, provides breast milk to use in bottles for future feedings, and is practical for women who do not have the flexibility or caregiving arrangements to facilitate direct breastfeeding of their newborns while working. Of course, the availability of a private place and time to pump is sometimes at a premium in work environments. Support from employers is essential, or the pumping, and subsequently breastfeeding, process may deteriorate (Slusser et al., 2004). High stress over job-related or other issues also may affect the woman's milk supply.

Nurses who encounter women with questions about the best ways to pump milk at work and other places outside the home can encourage clients to lobby their employers for written policies regarding breastfeeding and pumping in the workplace. They also can assist clients to devise ways to approach employers for support in establishing a place and time to do this, with adequate privacy and minimal disruptions (Slusser et al., 2004; Wyatt, 2002).

Sexual and Emotional Considerations

Some women choose one type of feeding method over another because of sexual and emotional concerns. Women who breastfeed their babies have different, individualized reactions during the process. Some feel an increased emotional attachment (either immediately or eventually) with the infant as a result of breastfeeding. Other women find the sensations unexpected and uncomfortable. Although many women closely associate their breasts with their sexuality, some have difficulty incorporating a view of their breasts as also having a biologic role in infant nutrition (Wagner & Wagner, 1999). They may feel awkward sharing their breasts with their baby or become uncomfortable and conflicted when their breasts are given attention during sexual stimulation. Some women become sexually aroused during the physical act of infant suckling and have varying responses to this experience. These highly personal reactions affect a woman's attitude about feeding and may influence her decision. Nurses should listen when women bring up such concerns and provide reassurance and support to help clients deal with their feelings and reach decisions appropriate for their situation.

Racial, Ethnic, and Cultural Influences

Cultural values and attitudes contribute to a woman's choice of feeding type and methodology. A woman's culture influences the initiation, frequency, and duration of breastfeeding (Kannen et al., 2004; Lawrence & Lawrence, 2005; Sharps et al., 2003). Women may feel ostracized if they choose to break social or cultural normative behaviors regarding infant feeding practices. Populations differ by ethnicity in their feeding practices. According to the 2002 National Immunization Survey (NIS), 71.4% of U.S. children were breastfed for some period; at 3 months, 42.5% were exclusively breastfed, with 51.5% receiving some breast milk; at 6 months, 13.3% of infants were exclusively breastfed, with 35.1% of infants receiving some breast milk; and at 1 year, 16.1% of infants were receiving some breast milk (Li et al., 2005). This study revealed significant racial and ethnic differences, with mothers of non-Hispanic black children less likely to begin and continue breastfeeding than mothers of non-Hispanic white children (51.5% versus 72.1% for ever breastfeeding, 19.7% versus 36.6% for continuing at 6 months) (Li et al., 2005). In New Zealand, 88% of women were found to have initiated breastfeeding, with 42% continuing exclusive breastfeeding by 3 months (Heath et al., 2002). Breastfeeding rates in Sweden have been reported to be 60% at 6 months and 20% at 12 months (Koçtürk & Zetterström, 1999). Native American mothers who participated in the Women, Infants, and Children (WIC) program in eastern Washington were found to have breastfeeding initiation rates of 62%, with a mean duration of breastfeeding of 21 weeks (Dellwo Houghton & Graybeal, 2001).

Nurses must consider cultural influences on feeding choices. They should ask questions about the reasons for beliefs and explore sources of information and knowledge. Although nurses should strive to correct misperceptions and give alternatives, they ultimately should show respect for women's decisions and those cultural components that influence their options.

Client Teaching and Collaborative Interventions

Information about infant feeding practices is most influential before a pregnant woman has made her decision and, more specifically, before she has experienced fetal movements (Riordan, 2004). Frequent, short discussions with health care providers regarding infant feeding choices are preferable to lengthy discussions in ensuring that women have the necessary information to make an informed decision (Taveras et al., 2004).

As mentioned, many women have concerns about breastfeeding, including convenience, modesty, fear of a change in lifestyle, paternal involvement, returning to work, and their own as well as others' negative experiences with breastfeeding. Others may be concerned that they may be choosing bottle feeding for selfish reasons, rather than making a decision based on the child's needs. Health care professionals including nurses are well positioned to listen to women and to address their concerns during each office visit or telephone call. An important health promotion activity for nurses is to educate the mother and family about the nutritional, immunologic, psychological, and developmental benefits of the different feeding strategies (Fig. 21.3). Nurses should put aside personal beliefs and provide unbiased information regarding both types of feeding methods.

Support for women is necessary to ensure adequate nutritional intake for the newborn. Resources provid-

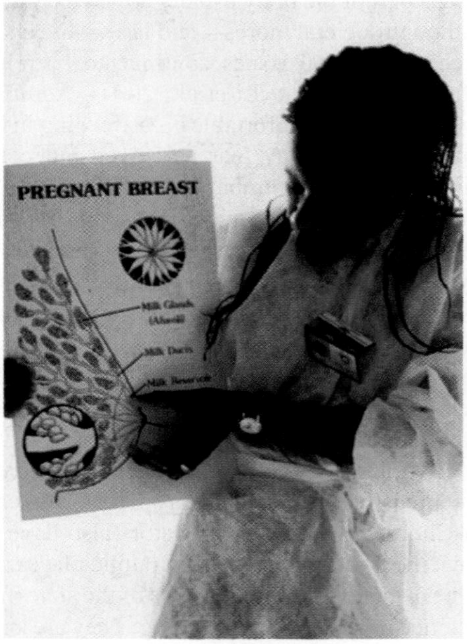

FIGURE 21.3 This nurse is teaching a group of clients about the physiology of lactation and the unique benefits of breastfeeding.

ing support for different feeding methods are available in different venues. They may include formal classes, written information, and health care providers. Women who choose to breastfeed may be referred to certified lactation consultants. These consultants frequently are registered nurses who have successfully completed additional education and achieved certification in the specialty (Bonuck et al., 2005). Wright (2001) has published *Part 2: The Management of Breastfeeding, Appendix B, Resources for Physicians,* which includes resources for professionals and parents, including a list of breast milk banks with their contact information in the United States, Canada, and Mexico. The AAP has published *Ten Steps to Support Parents' Choice to Breastfeed Their Baby* (Box 21.1). Other examples of groups with resources to help medical professionals in their pursuit of breastfeeding education and increased community awareness include the Bright Future Lactation Resource Center (www.bflrc.com), the U.S. Department of Health and Human Services National Women's Health Information Center (www.4woman.gov), the National Alliance for Breastfeeding Advocacy (www.hometown.aol.com/marshalact/), the Coalition to Improve Maternity Services (www.motherfriendly.org), and the National Perinatal Association (www.nationalperinatal.org).

Clients may take nutrition classes during or after pregnancy. Classes may focus on all feeding options or one specific method. Most classes center on strategies for successful breastfeeding. Techniques such as positioning, objective measures to evaluate breastfeeding effectiveness, management of sore nipples, returning to work or school, and feeding in public may be discussed (see later sections). Classes that include bottle feeding may explore the differences among formulas, the use of breast milk in bottles, preparing and caring for bottles, and holding techniques for feeding.

BOX 21.1 Ten Steps to Support Parents' Choice to Breastfeed Their Baby

1. Make a commitment to the importance of breastfeeding.
2. Educate all health care providers in skills necessary to support breastfeeding.
3. Inform women and families about the benefits and management of breastfeeding.
4. Schedule early follow-up visits for all newborns.
5. Show mothers how to breastfeed and how to maintain lactation during periods of separation from their infants.
6. Encourage breastfeeding on demand.
7. Use appropriate anticipatory guidance that supports exclusive breastfeeding until the infants are approximately 6 months old and encourage the continuation of breastfeeding as long as mutually desired by the mother and baby.
8. Support breastfeeding by providing accurate information about maternal issues.
9. Communicate support for breastfeeding in the health care environment.
10. Expand the network of support for breastfeeding.

From AAP Work Group on Breast-feeding (2001). Part 2: The management of breast-feeding. Appendix A: Ten steps to support parents' choice to breast-feed their baby. *Pediatric Clinics of North America, 48*(2).

BREASTFEEDING

The unique and evolving composition of breast milk is well suited to meet the nutrient and growth demands of almost all newborns. To this standard, all commercially prepared formulas are held.

Benefits of Breastfeeding

Human milk contains a host of dynamic and unique feeding properties not found in formula (Lawrence & Lawrence, 2005). Studies have demonstrated that the health benefits of breast milk are associated with how long an infant receives it and whether breast milk is given exclusively or supplemented with other feedings (Oddy, 2002). The AAP (2005), the American Academy of Family Physicians (AAFP, 2001), the National Association of Pediatric Nurse Practitioners (NAPNAP, 2001), and the American Dietetic Association (ADA, 2001) advocate at least 12 months of breastfeeding, with complementary foods introduced at approximately 6 months of age.

Physical and Immunologic Benefits to Newborns

Secretory immunoglobulin A, lactoferrin, and α-lactalbumin account for 60% to 80% of the protein found in breast milk (Biancuzzo, 2003). Secretory immunoglobulin A protects the infant's respiratory system from viral and bacterial infection and the gastrointestinal tract from foreign proteins and viral and bacterial compromise (Biancuzzo, 2003). This property is particularly beneficial to infants with a family history of allergies, especially when breast milk provision is prolonged. Lactoferrin binds iron. Additional enzymes and bifidus factor found only in human milk help colonize protective gut flora in the newborn intestine. Unique binding proteins in human milk bind vitamin B_{12}, which further protects the gastrointestinal tract from pathogens. Lymphocytes and neutrophils in colostrum aid the infant's immature immune system to fight infection, whereas macrophages found in mature human milk enhance immunity as well.

Several studies have shown the long-range enhancements that the above elements of breast milk give to children. With up to 6 months of exclusive consumption of breast milk, infants show decreased upper and lower respiratory tract infections and cases of otitis media (Lawrence & Lawrence, 2005). Those who breastfeed after 6 months of age enjoy ongoing continued protection from otitis media, diarrhea, colds, and wheezing (Chantry et al., 2006; Morrow & Rangel, 2004). A meta-analysis of 12 studies found that consuming breast milk during the first months of life is associated with lower rates of asthma during childhood (Gdalevich, 2001). The protective effect of breast milk for infants at risk for asthma and protein allergy is compounded when the mother avoids dietary allergens such as cow milk, peanuts, tree nuts, eggs, and fish (AAP, 2000; Gdalevich, 2001). The AAP recognizes additional immune-enhancing benefits of breast milk to include reduced incidence and severity of bacteremia, bacterial meningitis, botulism, urinary tract infection, and necrotizing enterocolitis (2005). Other potential benefits include enhanced cognitive development and reduced cases of sudden infant death syndrome (SIDS), type 1 diabetes mellitus, Crohn's disease, ulcerative colitis, lymphoma, and other chronic digestive diseases (AAP, 2005; Schack-Nielsen et al., 2005).

Developmental Benefits

Benefits to cognitive development and visual acuity are attributable to the fatty acids inherent in breast milk. Premature infants fed breast milk have faster brainstem maturation than preterm infants fed preterm infant formula (Amin et al., 2000). Children who were breastfed as infants showed significantly increased cognitive development test scores (Horwood & Fergusson, 1998; Horwood et al., 2001). In addition, low-birth-weight infants fed breast milk showed greater differences in cognitive development scores than normal-birth-weight infants fed breast milk when both were compared with formula-fed infants (Anderson et al., 1999; Slykerman et al., 2005).

The ingestion of human milk enhances physical development. Epidermal growth factor has been shown to contribute to the growth of intestinal cells in vitro. It is thought that epidermal growth factor also promotes intestinal cell growth in living infants.

Nutritional Benefits

One nutritional advantage of human milk is its superior absorption as a result of its high bioavailability. Protein, sodium, potassium, chloride, and phosphorus are nutrients that contribute to potential renal solute load (Fomon & Ziegler, 1999). Compared with infant formulas, the lower values of these nutrients (with greater bioavailability) in breast milk give breast milk the distinction of having the lowest potential renal solute load. This is particularly important for infants with renal impairment or immature kidneys (eg, preterm babies).

Breast milk also is superior because it is a species-specific formulation: its nutrients are uniquely suited to support growth and development for healthy human infants. The protein in human milk is whey dominant, which forms soft, easily digested curds. Enzymes in breast milk aid digestion, enhance development of beneficial intestinal flora, and destroy harmful bacteria. Growth factors and hormones (primarily prolactin) found in human milk are presumed to affect organ development beneficially; however, their specific functions have not yet been elucidated (Biancuzzo, 2003).

Health Benefits to Mothers

The health advantages of breastfeeding to mothers include enhanced uterine involution. Oxytocin, a maternal hormone, triggers the milk ejection reflex in response to the baby suckling at the breast. Oxytocin also increases the rate of uterine contractions; thus, breastfeeding decreases the risk for maternal postpartum hemorrhage (Labbok, 1999).

In general, lactating women lose approximately 0.8 kg per month throughout the first 6 months of lactation. Weight stability is typical for breastfeeding women beyond 6 months of lactation (National Academy of Sciences, 2002), although outcomes depend on many circumstances related to each individual woman.

In a review of 20 studies related to breastfeeding, 11 showed significantly decreased rates of premenopausal breast cancer (Labbok, 2001a). The protective effect of breastfeeding against premenopausal breast cancer generally improves with the total number of months of lifetime spent breastfeeding (Labbok, 2001a, Lawrence & Lawrence, 2005; Schack-Nielsen et al., 2005). A separate analysis using data from 47 studies in 30 countries found that for each year of breastfeeding, the woman's risk for breast cancer decreases by 4.3%; additionally, risk for breast cancer decreased 7% for each birth (Collaborative Group on Hormonal Factors in Breast Cancer, 2002). A review of the literature regarding breastfeeding and ovarian cancer showed that breastfeeding for 2 to 7 months postpartum exerted an average 20% decrease in risk for ovarian cancer (Labbok, 2001a). Although current research has yielded conflicting results, women who breastfeed their infants may be at decreased risk for osteoporosis. Other health benefits include reduced severity of anemia and potential protection against bladder and other infections (Labbok, 2001a).

Economic Benefits

Breast milk undoubtedly is the most economical choice for families of all cultures. It can cost up to $1200 to feed a name-brand formula in the first year of life (Educational Symposium, 2000b). In addition to the costs incurred by purchasing commercially prepared formulas, studies have shown that formula-fed infants require more office visits, hospitalizations, and prescriptions to treat their increased incidence of lower respiratory tract infections, otitis media, and gastrointestinal illness (Howard et al., 1999). Families of breastfed infants spend less money on health care and lose less work time to care for their sick infants (Gartner et al., 1997). Prolonged breast milk feedings also can potentially decrease environmental waste caused by disposal of formula containers, bottles, bags, and nipples.

Bonding Benefits

Breastfeeding offers the mother–infant dyad a unique opportunity for skin-to-skin contact 8 to 12 times each day, which contributes to emotional bonding and trust building. A review of the Cochrane Pregnancy and Childbirth Group trials register found that early breastfeeding (within 30 minutes of birth) enhanced communication between mothers and newborns compared with later initiation (between 4 to 8 hours after birth) (Renfrew et al., 2000). Additionally, breastfeeding duration may increase by as much as 50% with mother–baby contact in the immediate postnatal period (ADA, 2001).

Contraindications to Breastfeeding and Conditions Requiring Adjustments

Earlier discussions explored the many factors that influence the newborn feeding decision. Although nurses should encourage and support breastfeeding, they must treat families that choose formula feeding for reasons other than contraindications with understanding and respect.

Despite the advantages of feeding human milk to infants, situations exist in which either a mother's or infant's medical condition warrants review of the risks versus benefits of feeding mother's own milk.

Medical Contraindications

- The largest challenge to universal breastfeeding practices is the increase in HIV. A meta-analysis determined that the rate of maternal–infant transmission of HIV through breast milk was 26% (Michie & Gilmour, 2001). Breastfeeding by HIV-positive mothers poses a dilemma because even though the rate of transmission is a risk, breastfeeding is important to child survival, the ideal way to feed an infant, and a unique bonding opportunity for child development (Coutsoudis, 2005). Additionally, in developing countries with populations at risk for other infections and nutritional problems contributing to increased infant mortality, the risks of relying on formula feeding may outweigh the risk of transmitting HIV (AAP, 2005). Strategies could be developed and implemented (eg, administration of antiretroviral therapy to mothers, infants, or both) to reduce the risk for HIV transmission in breast milk from mothers to infants. Until further research is conducted, HIV-positive women should avoid breastfeeding (Coutsoudis, 2005). The AAP (2005) advises U.S. women with HIV not to breastfeed their infants, and states a need for additional studies before any changes would be made to their recommendations.
- Human T-cell lymphotrophic virus (HTCV) is transmitted through breast milk. Health care providers should advise HTCV-seropositive mothers not to breastfeed (AAP, 2005; Centers for Disease Control and Prevention [CDC] and the USPHS Working Group, 1993).
- Although cytomegalovirus (CMV) is in the breast milk of CMV-positive mothers, infants who acquire CMV after birth exhibit few, if any, complications (CDC, 2002). Breast milk transmission of CMV has the most serious consequences for CMV-seronegative or preterm infants (AAP, 2005; Lawrence & Lawrence, 2001). Breast milk from CMV-positive mothers should not be fed to infants without maternal antibodies to CMV (Hale, 2002).
- Mothers with herpes simplex virus (HSV) on the breast should temporarily pump and discard their breast milk until the lesion has healed (AAP, 2005; Lawrence & Lawrence, 2001).
- Maternal varicella-zoster virus infection requires temporary isolation of mother and baby until the mother is no longer infectious, there are no new lesions in 72 hours, and existing lesions have crusted over. During this time, the infant having received varicella-zoster immunoglobulin may consume expressed breast milk (Lawrence & Lawrence, 2001).
- The use of the rubella virus vaccine for mothers of preterm or ill infants may warrant a risk-versus-benefits analysis. Vaccinating lactating women with the live rubella virus who are breastfeeding healthy, full-term infants is not a contraindication to breastfeeding (Hale, 2002).
- Breastfeeding mothers with measles should be isolated from their infants for 72 hours after appearance of the rash. As a precaution, they may feed expressed breast milk to infants who have received immunoglobulin (Lawrence & Lawrence, 2001). Although the measles vaccine virus itself passes into breast milk, it has not been reported to cause problems for the breastfed infant (Micromedex, 2003).
- Women with Lyme disease should discontinue breastfeeding temporarily and resume after they begin treatment (Lawrence & Lawrence, 2001).
- For a woman with active tuberculosis (TB), breast lesions may result. Isolation from her infant is indicated until she is considered noncontagious. During isolation, the infant may receive expressed breast milk if there is no active TB breast lesion. After the woman is noncontagious, the breastfeeding dyad may be reunited for direct breastfeeding (AAP, 2005; Lawrence & Lawrence, 2001).
- Women should report unusual maternal exposure to heavy metals or environmental hazards to their physician and to their children's pediatrician so that breast milk can be analyzed for contaminant concentration and milk safety (AAP, 2005).

Nutrition- and Drug-Related Contraindications

Nutritional causes that warrant discontinued use of breast milk include infantile disorders of metabolic origin. Provision of some breast milk is possible with infantile phenylketonuria, maple syrup urine disease, and mild galactosemia. Infants who present with the classic variant of galactosemia are lactose intolerant and must receive a lactose-free formula (AAP, 2005). Infants with tyrosinemia do not tolerate this amino acid and must receive a feeding devoid of this protein (Hall & Carroll, 2000). Maternal Wilson's disease is a contraindication to breastfeeding because treatment therapy is with penicillamine, which adversely alters the infant's mineral status (Lawrence & Lawrence, 2001).

Because of the high rate of transfer of substances in breast milk from mother to infant, women who use illegal drugs and some prescription drugs should not breastfeed (AAP, 2005; Lawrence & Lawrence, 2005). Women who require chemotherapy for cancer should not breastfeed. Antineoplastic agents are toxic to the infant, suppress bone marrow, and may cause epithelial cell damage (AAP, 2005). Tamoxifen therapy is presently a contraindication to breastfeeding because of the lack of information about its transfer into human milk and effects on infants (Hale, 2002; AAP Committee on Drugs, 2001).

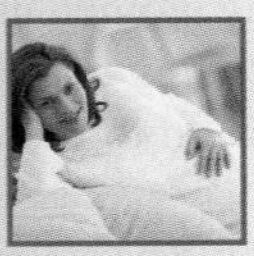

Think back to Joelle, the pregnant woman who is deciding whether to breastfeed. Suppose that the nurse, when reviewing Joelle's medical record, determines that Joelle has a history of herpes simplex virus infection. Would breastfeeding be contraindicated for Joelle?

Physiology of Milk Production

In the first trimester of pregnancy, estrogen and progesterone cause the duct system in breast tissue to multiply. The Montgomery glands (on the areola and around the nipple) enlarge and begin oily secretion that helps protect the nipple and areola (Lauwers & Shinskie, 2005). By 6 to 7 months' gestation, the pregnant woman's breasts increase in secretory activity, and the acini and alveoli within the mammary tissue swell with colostrum (Cahill & Wagner, 2002a). The increased number of alveoli and body fluids that support lactation may increase the weight of the breast by as much as 1 to $1\frac{1}{2}$ lbs (Lauwers & Shinskie, 2005). See Figure 21.4. Following childbirth, a mother's breasts continue the process that allows her to provide her newborn with human milk. The expulsion of the placenta enables the reversal of the inhibitory effect of estrogen and progesterone on lactation, and prolactin levels increase (Cahill & Wagner, 2002a).

Suckling by the infant sends nerve impulses that ascend the spinal cord and stimulate the hypothalamus. In response, the anterior pituitary gland releases prolactin, which is the primary hormone for milk production (Fig. 21.5). Additionally, the posterior pituitary gland releases oxytocin, which causes the cells around breast tissue alveoli to contract, causing the milk ejection reflex (Groh-Wargo et al., 2000). Upon milk removal, the alveoli in the breasts continue the process of refilling the ductal system with human milk in preparation for the next breastfeeding or breast milk pumping session. When emptying of accumulated milk is inadequate, levels of prolactin and oxytocin decrease, causing milk production to decrease as well (Cahill & Wagner, 2002a).

Composition

Box 21.2 provides an overview of the components of human milk. This section describes the different types of

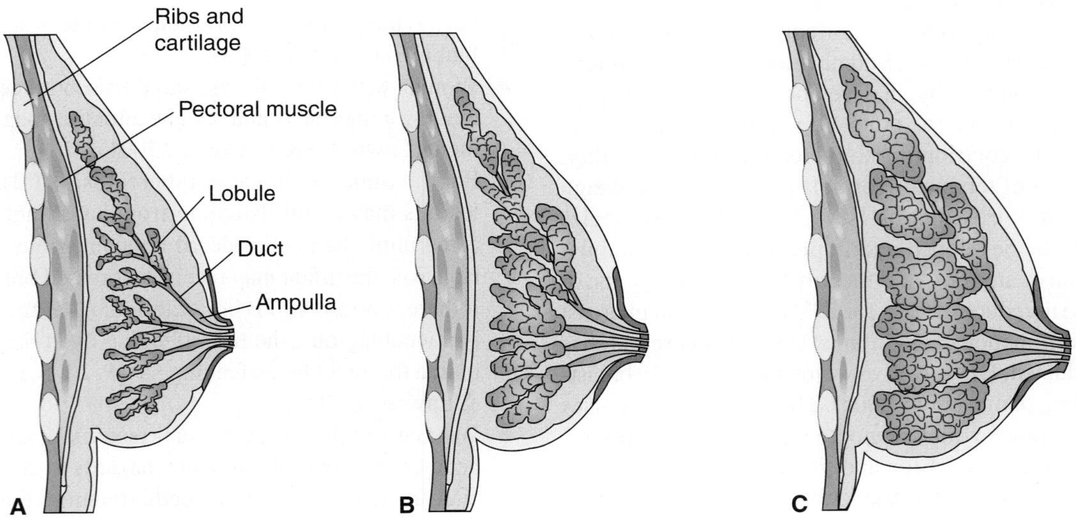

FIGURE 21.4 Comparison of the nonpregnant, nonlactating, adult breast (**A**); pregnant breast (**B**); and lactating breast (**C**). In part C, note the increased size of the overall breast, as well as its ducts and lobules.

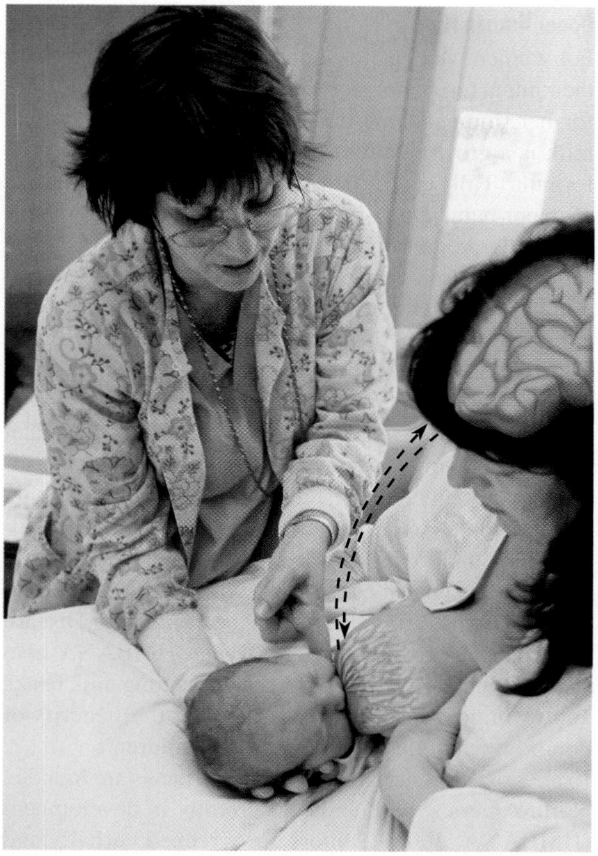

FIGURE 21.5 During breastfeeding, the infant's suckling stimulates the anterior pituitary gland to secrete prolactin, which in turn stimulates the breasts to secrete milk. Suckling also causes the posterior pituitary gland to secrete oxytocin, which in turn stimulates the breasts to eject milk into the ducts for removal by the newborn.

milk found by stage, as well as the different milk found according to feeding session.

Stages of Milk

In the first few postpartum weeks, the type of milk the woman produces changes. **Colostrum,** the milk produced in the first 1 to 4 days of lactation (Labbok, 2001b), is often slightly yellow and high in protein, sodium, potassium, iron, and fat-soluble vitamins (vitamins A, E, and K). It contains large amounts of antibodies and immunoglobulins, which help boost the newborn's immature immune system.

Transitional milk, produced at approximately 7 to 10 days of lactation (Labbok, 2001b), serves as a bridge between colostrum and mature breast milk. It has increased lactose, fat, and calories, but fewer immunoglobulins and total proteins, than colostrum.

Mature human milk contains more energy from lactose and fat than does colostrum. It begins approximately 2 weeks postpartum and lasts until 7 to 8 months of lactation. Milk produced after this time has reduced amounts of some vitamins and minerals.

● BOX 21.2 Constituents of Human Milk

Carbohydrates
- Bifidus factors
- Glycopeptides
- Lactose
- Oligosaccharides

Cells
- Epithelial cells
- Leukocytes
- Lymphocytes
- Macrophages
- Neutrophils

Lipids
- Carotenoids
- Fat-soluble vitamins (A, D, E, and K)
- Fatty acids
- Phospholipids
- Sterols and hydrocarbons
- Triglycerides

Mineral and Ionic Constituents
- Bicarbonate
- Calcium
- Chloride
- Citrate
- Magnesium
- Phosphate
- Potassium
- Sodium
- Sulfate

Nonprotein Nitrogen
- α-Amino nitrogen
- Creatine
- Creatinine
- Glucosamine
- Nucleic acids
- Nucleotides
- Polyamines
- Urea
- Uric acids

Proteins
- α-Lactalbumin
- β-Lactoglobulin
- Caseins
- Enzymes
- Growth factors
- Hormones
- Immunoglobulins
- Lactoferrin
- Lysozyme

Trace Minerals
- Chromium
- Cobalt
- Copper
- Fluoride
- Iodine
- Iron
- Manganese
- Molybdenum
- Nickel
- Selenium
- Zinc

Water-Soluble Vitamins
- B_{12}
- B_6
- Biotin
- C
- Choline
- Folate
- Inositol
- Niacin
- Pantothenic acid
- Riboflavin
- Thiamin

Other Milk Variations

Not only does breast milk vary in nutrient content by stage of lactation, but it also varies for each woman, according to time of day, and as a result of the stage of the feeding session. For example, breast milk fat content is higher in the evening than in the morning (Biancuzzo, 2003). Mothers of premature infants produce breast milk that is higher in iron, sodium, and energy as a result of increased levels of protein and fat.

Foremilk, breast milk delivered during the first 5 to 10 minutes of a feeding, is lower in calories than is later breast milk. **Hindmilk,** breast milk at the end of a feeding session, is higher in fat and energy. Because of the different properties of the milk found throughout a feeding session, it is important to allow the infant to empty entirely at least one breast during a feeding (Kent et al., 2006).

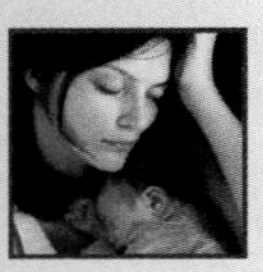

Recall Lindsay, the young woman returning for her 6-week clinic appointment. What type of breast milk is her newborn receiving?

Medicinal Supplementation for Breastfed Infants

Select supplementary vitamins and minerals may be advisable for breastfed infants. Deficiencies in vitamin D and iron are possible if the baby does not obtain an exogenous source in addition to breast milk. Deficiencies of other vitamins and minerals are rare; in such cases, supplementation may be deemed necessary (Greer, 2001).

Vitamin D

The vitamin D stores of full-term infants born to women with adequate vitamin D status are depleted within 2 months of birth (Hoogenboezen et al., 1989). Infants whose face and hands only are exposed to sunlight for 30 to 120 minutes per week receive adequate exposure to make the available form of vitamin D (Hoogenboezen et al., 1989). Dark-skinned infants, because of decreased absorption of ultraviolet B as a result of their pigmentation (Specker et al., 1985), and infants who continually wear protective clothing that shields sunlight are at particular risk for vitamin D deficiency, which can lead to nutritional rickets. The AAP (2005) recommends daily supplementation of 200 IU of vitamin D starting within the first 2 months of life until the daily consumption of vitamin D–fortified formula or milk is 500 mL. An oral dose of a multivitamin containing vitamins A, C, and D plus iron at 0.5 mL/day would provide approximately 250 mg of vitamin D and 5 mg of elemental iron. This dose, plus what the infant gets from breast milk, would be appropriate supplementation (Fomon, 2001).

Iron

According to the AAP (2005), caregivers should introduce breastfed infants to iron-rich complementary foods gradually beginning around 6 months of age. Preterm infants, low-birth-weight infants, infants with hematologic disorders, and infants with inadequate iron stores at birth generally require iron supplementation before 6 months. Iron may be administered while continuing exclusive breastfeeding.

Donor Human Milk

For women who cannot supply their own breast milk to their infant (eg, a mother who cannot pump adequate milk for her immunocompromised newborn), donor human milk is a growing alternative to the use of commercial formula (Tully et al., 2004). Other indications for the use of donor human milk include prematurity, feeding intolerance, burns, gastrointestinal surgery, immunodeficiency diseases, and prevention or treatment of allergies. Immunologic benefits, enhanced nutrient absorption, low allergenicity, growth factors, and maturation of organ systems contribute to the development of the infants who receive donor human milk (Tully et al., 2004).

A **milk bank** is an agency that operates to collect donor human milk, verify its safety for use, and distribute it to those who request it. The Human Milk Banking Association of North America (HMBANA) was established in 1985 to develop standards for the operation of donor milk banks in cooperation with the U.S. Food and Drug Administration (FDA) and the Centers for Disease Control and Prevention (CDC). The HMBANA also serves to increase information sharing among milk banks and to improve societal awareness of the benefits of donor human milk for ill infants and children.

As of this writing, 10 human milk banks are found in North America, with another currently in development (HMBANA, 2005). Donors are screened verbally and serologically for infectious diseases. Donors must follow specific procedures during pumping, storing, and transit to ensure the quality of the donated milk. Once the frozen milk is at the milk bank, aliquots are pooled to promote a more homogeneous mixture, as each woman's breast milk differs slightly in composition. The milk is heat treated at 56° to 62.5°C for 30 minutes by the Holder method. It is then repackaged and refrozen until distribution. Pasteurization and freezing affect several vitamins, minerals, immunoglobulins, enzymes, and lipids (Lawrence & Lawrence, 2005); however, the risk for viral or bacterial contamination outweighs the benefit of preservation of more human milk components. The milk is shipped in an insulated box and may contain dry ice when moved over long distances. The U.S. cost of donor human milk averages $2.50 per fluid ounce (Riordan, 2004). Third-party payers, WIC, and Medicaid are potential sources of financial support. Efforts are made to match the donor's stage of lactation to the recipient infant's physiologic age.

Dilemmas concerning wet-nursing practices still have implications in today's society. Women who wish to directly donate milk to the infant of a friend or family member must consider the legal ramifications if such milk contains harmful bacteria or viruses. They also should consider whether the nutritive quality of breast milk, which varies with stage of lactation, matches the needs of the infant (Arnold, 1994).

COLLABORATIVE CARE: BREASTFEEDING

Breastfeeding classes taken before a baby's birth introduce parents to techniques that help ensure breastfeeding success. Involvement of the woman's partner in breastfeeding education helps to build a supportive environment for the mother contemplating lactation (Pisacane et al., 2005). Peer counseling from mothers, sisters, aunts, or close friends with lactating experience can help the woman as she encounters situations that are new and different to her related to breastfeeding. The lactation consultant is an invaluable professional resource to the breastfeeding dyad (Bonuck et al., 2005).

Professional organizations exist in support of breastfeeding such as La Leche League International (www.lalecheleague.org) and LactNews (www.jump.net/~bwc/lactnews.html). For example, La Leche League International's Web site has an interactive message board, directory of resources, and information about meeting dates and times in a variety of languages. Local branches and support groups also may be available.

Assessment

Breastfeeding requires nutritional and lifestyle considerations to facilitate optimal results for both mother and baby. Exploring areas such as rest, nutrition, and hydration can identify potential problems or concerns and be a good opportunity for nurses to involve the baby's father or other family members in facilitating an optimal environment. Encouraging the infant's siblings to participate in feeding sessions by sitting close to the nursing couple, asking questions, and even holding the infant's hand may help them become more comfortable with a new feeding process in the home. Assessment Tool 21.1 provides a foundation for obtaining information about the woman's knowledge and understanding of breastfeeding that the nurse can use to shape education and interventions.

Rest and Environment

Nurses should evaluate the woman's patterns of rest to ensure that she is getting sufficient sleep to facilitate milk production. This can be difficult because the woman is adjusting to the erratic sleep–wake cycles of the newborn. Nurses should remind breastfeeding mothers to get appropriate rest, which often means sleeping when the infant is sleeping.

Nutrition

Some of a pregnant woman's nutrient reserves may be tapped during pregnancy to support nutrient provision to the fetus. A lactating mother who is in generally good health and consumes a variety of nutritious foods to satisfy hunger can replete the nutrient stores that she used to support her pregnancy.

The nurse should perform a detailed nutritional history and review of the client's dietary behaviors to ensure adequate intake and to correct any problems. During the first 6 months of lactation, women 14 to 50 years require approximately 330 calories/day more than nonlactating women of the same age (see Chap. 3). Estimated energy requirements for a lactating woman in her 7th to 12th months of breastfeeding are approximately 400 calories/day more than nonlactating women (National Academy of Sciences, 2002). A lactating woman's Recommended Dietary Allowance for protein is that of a nonpregnant, nonlactating woman plus 25 g/day of protein (National Academy of Sciences, 2002). This equates to approximately 71 g/day of protein (Trumbo et al., 2002).

● ASSESSMENT TOOL 21.1 Breastfeeding

ASSESSMENT BEFORE BREASTFEEDING

- Has the client ever breastfed before?
  - If yes, what was her experience like?
  - If no, has she had close contact with anyone who has breastfed?
- Has the client taken prenatal classes?
- Has she attended any specific breastfeeding classes?
- What books, Web sites, or other materials has she read about breastfeeding?
- How long ago did the client give birth?
- What kind of birth did the client have?
- What is the client's mood, physical condition, and overall state of health?
- What are the client's breasts like?
- What are the client's nipples like?
- What is the infant's physical condition and overall state of health?
- Does the mother seem confident in handling the newborn?

ASSESSMENT DURING BREASTFEEDING

- Has the mother assumed a comfortable position for herself?
- Is the mother holding the newborn correctly?
- Is the infant opening the mouth wide?
- Does the mother bring her breast to the infant?
- Does the mother feed the newborn every 2 to 3 hours?
- Are the mother's breasts engorged?
- Do the breasts show any signs of bruises, cracks, or abrasions?
- Does the mother report any signs of pain or discomfort?

A lactating woman should consume nutritious foods she enjoys. A host of micronutrients are higher for lactating women than for nonpregnant, nonlactating women and pregnant women (Table 21.1). Conversely, two key nutrients are of interest because nutrient needs are not higher for lactating women. Calcium needs are the same as for the nonpregnant, nonlactating woman: 1300 mg/day for those 18 years or younger and 1000 mg/day for those 19 to 50 years. Iron needs are actually less during lactation than for nonpregnant, nonlactating women and pregnant women: 10 mg/day for women 18 years or younger, and 9 mg/day for women 19 to 50 years (Trumbo et al., 2002). The lactating woman's dietary intake influences the amounts of some nutrients in her breast milk (Box 21.3).

Fluid Intake. The nurse should review the client's fluid intake. Breastfeeding mothers should drink 64 to 80 fl oz/day (the same as any other healthy adult) (Spicer, 2001). One

TABLE 21.1 Dietary Reference Intakes for Nutrients That are Higher for Lactating Women Than for Pregnant or Nonpregnant, Nonlactating Women

NUTRIENT	AMOUNT	FOODS HIGH IN SPECIFIED NUTRIENT
Carbohydrate (g/day)	**210**	Breads, cereal, pasta, rice
Fiber (g/day)	29	Whole grain breads and cereals
Protein (g/day)	**71**	Meats, poultry, fish, eggs, legumes
Vitamin A (μg/day)	**1200**–2800* for ≤ 18 years of age **1300**–3000* for 19–50 years of age	Butter, milk, cheese, liver
Vitamin C (mg/day)	**115**–1800* for ≤ 18 years of age **120**–2000* for 19–50 years of age	Citrus fruit, berries, melon, tomatoes, green vegetables, potatoes
Vitamin E	**19**–800* for ≤ 18 years of age **19**–1000* for 19–50 years of age	Vegetable oils, leafy vegetables, eggs, meat, cereal, milk
Vitamin B_1 (mg/day), also known as thiamin	1.4	Whole or enriched grains, legumes, pork, beef, liver
Vitamin B_2 (mg/day), also known as riboflavin	**1.6**	Milk, milk products, liver, meat, fish, eggs, whole or enriched grains
Vitamin B_3 (mg/day), also known as niacin	**17**–30* for ≤ 18 years of age **17**–35* for 19–50 years of age	Meat, poultry, fish, whole and enriched grains and cereals
Vitamin B_6 (mg/day), also known as pyridoxine	**2**–80* for ≤ 18 years of age **2**–100* for 19–50 years of age	Whole grains and cereals, seeds, legumes, nuts, bran, corn, green leafy vegetables, fish, poultry
Folate (μg/day)	**500**–800* for ≤ 18 years of age **500**–1000* for 19–50 years of age	Liver, green leafy vegetables, yeast
Vitamin B_{12} (μg/day)	**2.8**	Fortified soy milk, cereals, milk, cheese, eggs, meat, liver, fish, meat substitutes
Pantothenic acid (mg/day)	7	Organ meats, whole grain cereals, most foods
Biotin (μg/day)	35	Egg yolk, milk, organ meats, legumes
Choline (mg/day)	550	
Chromium (μg/day)	44 for ≤ 18 years of age 45 for 19–50 years of age	Whole grains, legumes, brewer's yeast, animal protein
Copper (μg/day)	**1300**–8000* for ≤ 18 years of age **1300**–10,000* for 19–50 years of age	Whole grains, legumes, shellfish, meats
Iodine (μg/day)	**290**–900* for ≤ 18 years of age **290**–1100* for 19–50 years of age	Seafood, iodized salt
Manganese (mg/day)	2.6–9* for ≤ 18 years of age 2.6–11* for 19–50 years of age	Legumes, whole grains, nuts, fruits, vegetables, tea, cocoa powder, instant coffee
Molybdenum (μg/day)	**50**–1700* for ≤ 18 years of age **50**–2000* for 19–50 years of age	Milk, whole grains, liver, legumes, leafy vegetables
Selenium (μg/day)	**70**–400*	Seafood, whole grains, legumes, meat, dairy products
Zinc (mg/day)	**13**–34* for ≤ 18 years of age **12**–40* for 19–50 years of age	Meat, liver, eggs, oysters

Recommended Dietary Allowances in bold type; Tolerable Upper Intake Levels followed by an asterisk; all others are Adequate Intake values.
Data from Biancuzzo, 2003; Lauwers & Shinskie, 2005; Mitchell, 2003; Trumbo, Schlicker, Yates, & Poos, 2002.

● **BOX 21.3 Vitamins and Minerals in Breast Milk Influenced by Maternal Diet**

Vitamins

- Vitamin A
- Vitamin D
- Vitamin C
- Thiamin
- Riboflavin
- Niacin
- Vitamin E
- Pyridoxine
- Biotin
- Pantothenic acid
- Cyanocobalamin

Minerals

- Manganese
- Iodine
- Fluoride
- Selenium

of the body's chemical responses to breastfeeding is thirst. A woman who is nursing will likely find it essential to have something to drink available while breastfeeding to quench the sometimes overwhelming need to drink. Carrying a container of water at all times can be helpful.

Allergens, Potentially Offending Foods, and Substances to Avoid. A lactating woman may notice changes in her infant's behavior after consumption of a particular food and subsequent provision of breast milk to her infant. Foods such as peanuts, milk or milk products, chocolate, and cruciferous vegetables (broccoli, cabbage, cauliflower, onion) are associated with infantile fussy behavior (Biancuzzo, 2003) because they tend to produce allergic reactions, gas, or both when transferred to infants in breast milk. For infants with a family history of atopic dermatitis or eczema, evidence exists that as the lactating mother avoids potentially allergenic foods, her children's risk for developing atopic dermatitis decreases (McNamara & Mazurek Melnyk, 2000). The lactating woman should not eliminate all these foods from her diet simply because of the potential for changes in the behavior of her infant. The nurse should advise her to eliminate one food at a time from her diet to determine which, if any, food seems to be causing irritability in the newborn. Once identified, the woman can eliminate or replace that food with another that is less offending and offers the same nutrients.

Caffeine. Breastfeeding mothers do not need to drink milk to make milk; however, they should drink to thirst regularly from noncaffeinated beverages. Women secrete peak levels of caffeine into breast milk 60 to 120 minutes after consumption; the infant receiving caffeine excretes it slowly (Hale, 2002). Maternal caffeine intake greater than 3 cups/day can result in an irritable infant and an altered sleeping pattern (AAP Committee on Drugs, 2001). Caffeinated coffee, soft drinks, tea, and chocolate contribute to daily caffeine intake.

Alcohol. Alcohol secreted into breast milk can be harmful to the breastfed infant, causing symptoms in the baby such as drowsiness, weakness, diaphoresis, and decreased weight and length gain. Maternal consumption of 1 g/kg body weight per day of alcohol decreases milk production (AAP Committee on Drugs, 2001). This equates to four 12-oz beers, 16 oz of table wine, or 4 to 5 oz of liquor per day for a woman who weighs 60 kg (Biancuzzo, 2003). The AAP (2005) recommends that breastfeeding mothers avoid alcoholic beverages because alcohol is concentrated in breast milk and can inhibit milk production. Although the client can have an occasional single, small alcoholic drink, she should avoid breastfeeding for 2 hours after consumption (AAP, 2005). Peak alcohol concentrations in breast milk occur approximately 30 to 60 minutes after ingestion. Lactating women who want to consume an alcohol-containing beverage may drink it shortly after nursing to allow peak concentrations to rise and fall before the next breastfeeding.

Nicotine. Nicotine and its primary metabolite, cotinine, are present in human milk of lactating women who smoke. It has not been determined whether nicotine, other compounds in tobacco, or environmental exposure to tobacco smoke is responsible for increased infant respiratory illness, decreased infant weight gain, or decreased maternal milk production (AAP, 2001). Although there is not enough evidence that nicotine itself causes health risks for breastfeeding infants, health care providers should consider lactation an opportunity to encourage cessation of smoking (AAP, 2005). Eliminating infantile smoke exposure from tobacco products decreases the likelihood of apnea, SIDS, asthma, and pneumonia (Orenstein, 1999).

Contraceptives. Maternal oral contraceptives that contain a combination of estrogen and progesterone may decrease milk production (AAP Committee on Drugs, 2001). Oral contraceptives that contain only progestin do not have the same inhibitory effect on milk production. Injectable depot medroxyprogesterone acetate (DMPA), Depo-Provera, and norethindrone enanthate (NET-ED, NORISTERAT) cause an increase in human milk protein production, whereas fat is decreased and steroids are present. Levonorgestrel (Norplant System) causes a small amount of steroid secretion in human milk. The long-term effects of vaginal rings that contain some progesterone are currently unknown (Biancuzzo, 2003) (see Chap. 8).

Herbs and Galactalogues. Certain substances have been identified as increasing milk production by increasing prolactin levels. These substances are known as *galactogogues* and include herbs, typically in the form of pills or teas. Little research exists to support their efficacy, safety, mechanism of action, or potential side effects. As well, currently no regulations enforce herbal labeling or dosing. See Complementary/Alternative Medicine 21.1 for further discussion.

Select Potential Nursing Diagnoses

The following nursing diagnoses may apply to the care of the breastfeeding woman and newborn:

- **Pain** related to engorged breasts, sore nipples, or both
- **Deficient Knowledge** related to lack of knowledge about breastfeeding techniques and the process of lactation
- **Anxiety** related to concern about infant feeding patterns
- **Effective Breastfeeding** as evidenced by correct technique, content infant, and mother's reports of satisfaction
- **Ineffective Breastfeeding** related to poor infant sucking reflex
- **Ineffective Breastfeeding** related to sore nipples

Planning and Intervention

Nursing Care Plan 21.2 highlights the care of a pregnant woman who is deciding to breastfeed. NIC/NOC Box 21.1 highlights some of the more common nursing interventions and outcomes related to breastfeeding. Although the nurse should tailor care to be appropriate for the specific client's circumstances, the following sections explain appropriate general interventions for various stages and issues related to breastfeeding.

Support of Initial Breastfeeding

When a woman puts her newborn to breast immediately after birth, the posterior pituitary gland releases oxytocin, which causes myoepithelial cells to contract, including the uterus and ductule system of the breast. Uterine contraction in response to infant suckling following birth promotes the expulsion of the placenta (Biancuzzo, 2003), as well as decreasing the risk for maternal hemorrhage. The delivery of the placenta promotes a hormonal milieu low in estrogen and high in prolactin levels. The infant suckling at the breast also stimulates the release of prolactin, which is essential for milk production.

Newborns may lick or explore the nipple without nutritive sucking during the first attempt at the breast. The nurse should help mothers to interpret this experience as positive and as a way for mother and baby to begin bonding.

The nurse should assist with breastfeeding by helping secure privacy for the family by pulling the privacy curtain or closing the door to the room. He or she should assist the woman to find a comfortable breastfeeding position. Pillows are helpful in offering adequate physical support for the mother and baby. The nurse may place a pillow where the mother's body does not support the baby's body. Common bed pillows can be manipulated to accommodate positioning. Some companies manufacture pillows that are curved much like a C shape: the mother places the pillow around her abdomen and uses it to support her arms, which are supporting the infant. Two examples are the Boppy and My Breast Friend. Pillows are also useful to support the arms, feet, or legs of the mother who is upright in bed.

Support of Ongoing Breastfeeding

Holds. Several holds are used for successful breastfeeding (Fig. 21.6). In most holds, the mother supports her breast with one hand while supporting the newborn's head with the other hand.

- The *cradle hold* may be most intuitive for new mothers; however, it offers less control of the baby's head (see Fig. 21.6A). The *cross-cradle hold* works better, because it allows the mother to support the baby's head with one hand and support the breast with the other hand.

(text continues on page 889)

● COMPLEMENTARY/ALTERNATIVE MEDICINE 21.1

Galactogogues

Lactating mothers discuss the intake of herbal teas with their health care providers because some herbs may be transferred to their infants or affect milk production (Hale, 2002). Herbs purported to enhance milk production include alfalfa, blessed thistle, fenugreek, hops, and anise (Ayers, 2000; Cahill & Wagner, 2002a). Although blessed thistle has medicinal properties, as of the 2002 printing of *Medications in Mothers' Milk,* no studies could be found supporting its use as a galactogogue (Hale, 2002). A medicinal galactogogue prescribed in the United States is metoclopramide (Reglan) to improve milk production (Cahill & Wagner, 2002a). Oxytocin nasal spray enhances the milk ejection reflex; however, it is no longer available in the United States (Hale, 2002). As well, whereas domperidone (Motilium) as a galactogogue is not approved for use in the United States, it may be obtained in Canada, Mexico, and some sites within the United States (Cahill & Wagner, 2002a). Consultation with a lactation consultant can help identify causes of insufficient milk production or impaired milk ejection reflex. The solution to a particular woman's problem may be rectified by a change of position, environment, or other behaviors unrelated to the need for a galactogogue.

NURSING CARE PLAN 21.1

The Client Overwhelmed by Feeding Decisions

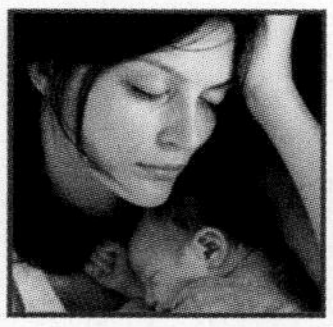

Recall Lindsay, 35 years old, whose dilemma related to feeding was presented at the beginning of the chapter. While inspecting Lindsay's cesarean incision, which is healing well, the client states, "First, I had to have surgery instead of a vaginal birth. I wasn't ready for that. And now, I'm having problems breastfeeding. I feel like such a failure."

NURSING DIAGNOSIS

Situational Low Self-Esteem related to the need for cesarean birth and difficulties breastfeeding

EXPECTED OUTCOMES

1. The client will verbalize positive feelings about herself by end of the visit.
2. The client will identify the effects of cesarean birth on her current feelings.

INTERVENTIONS	RATIONALES
Attempt to identify the meaning of the cesarean birth to the client.	This measure assists in determining the effect on the client's feelings.
Encourage the client to verbalize her feelings and thoughts about herself, her abilities, and her current situation.	Sharing feelings provides a safe outlet for emotions and helps the client gain awareness of how her situation is affecting her self-esteem.
Convey an accepting, positive, nonjudgmental attitude with the client.	This approach is essential for fostering trust.
Review and reinforce the client's positive attributes about herself and her abilities; reinforce with her that the cesarean birth was not "her fault."	Identification of positive attributes provides a foundation for enhancing self-esteem.
Provide suggestions for ways to cope with the physical demands of her situation.	These suggestions aid in relieving the stress associated with outside variables and events and promote feelings of control.
Question the client about available support systems in the family and community; provide her with information about community resources available.	Additional support is helpful in alleviating the stress of the client's current situation.
Review the advantages and disadvantages of breastfeeding and formula feeding including optional methods for holding the newborn during feeding (eg, football hold, side-lying position).	Review of information is necessary to establish a firm foundation from which the client can make an informed decision. After a cesarean birth, certain feeding positions may promote comfort.
Support the client's choice of feeding method nonjudgmentally.	Nonjudgmental support is necessary to foster self-esteem.
Arrange for continued follow-up of client in the home.	Continued follow-up provides further opportunities for assessment, teaching, and support.

EVALUATION

1. The client will actively and openly discuss feelings and concerns.
2. The client will make an informed decision about the best method for feeding her newborn.
3. The client will demonstrate comfort with her decision.
4. The client will demonstrate self-confidence in her abilities to care for herself, her newborn, and her family.

NURSING CARE PLAN 21.2

The Client Who Is Deciding to Breastfeed

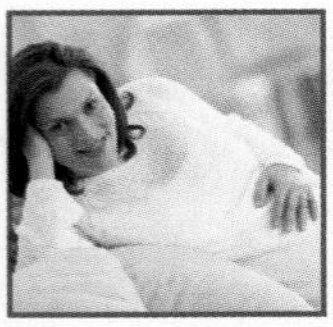

Recall Joelle from the start of this chapter. Further conversation reveals that she will be taking a leave of absence from work for approximately 6 months. She states, "I really would like to try breastfeeding, and my husband is supportive and thinks we should try it, too. But I'm a bit nervous. This is all so new to me."

NURSING DIAGNOSIS

Deficient Knowledge related to lack of experience with breastfeeding

EXPECTED OUTCOMES

1. The client will identify advantages and disadvantages of breastfeeding.
2. The client will state appropriate information related to measures to promote effective breastfeeding.

INTERVENTIONS	RATIONALES
Assess the client's level of understanding about breastfeeding.	Assessment provides a baseline to identify specific client needs and develop an individualized teaching plan.
Explore the client's exposure to breastfeeding in previous pregnancy, including her rationale for choosing formula feeding; correct any misconceptions or myths; allow time for questions.	Information about previous exposure helps to identify possible reasons for her choice and provides opportunities to clarify or correct misinformation and teach new information.
Describe the advantages and disadvantages of breastfeeding.	This information provides additional knowledge from which the client can make an informed effective choice.
Teach the client about the need for proper nutrition and measures needed to prepare for breastfeeding; demonstrate breast care techniques.	Proper nutrition is essential to ensure an adequate milk supply. Preparation for breastfeeding helps the client to become comfortable with handling her breasts; teaching about breast care techniques reduces the risk for future problems.
Demonstrate positions for breastfeeding and review measures for stimulating the neonate to suck and latch on, and for alternating breasts for feedings; allow the client time to practice.	Practice promotes understanding and opportunities to trouble-shoot any problems that may arise; practice also helps to increase self-confidence.
Include the client's partner in teaching sessions.	Participation of the client's partner provides support and enhances the chances for a successful experience.
Arrange for the client to meet with a lactation consultant.	This referral provides additional opportunities for teaching and learning and allows for feedback and positive reinforcement, thus promoting a positive experience.

EVALUATION

1. The client states rationale for choosing breastfeeding.
2. The client demonstrates measures to prepare for breastfeeding.
3. The client demonstrates measures to promote effective breastfeeding.

Continued

NURSING CARE PLAN 21.2 ● The Client Who Is Deciding to Breastfeed

NURSING DIAGNOSIS

Anxiety related to inexperience with breastfeeding

EXPECTED OUTCOMES

1. The client will express concerns related to breastfeeding.
2. The client will identify strategies to cope with the new experience of breastfeeding.

INTERVENTIONS	RATIONALES
Assess the client's current understanding about breastfeeding; communicate accurate facts and answer questions honestly.	Assessment of current understanding provides direction for individualized care targeted to the client's needs; honest communication promotes trust.
Discuss with client her concerns related to breastfeeding; encourage client to verbalize her feelings, concerns, and perceptions.	Discussion provides opportunities to emphasize positive aspects and correct any misconceptions or misinformation; verbalization of fears and concerns aids in establishing sources of stress and problem areas that need to be addressed.
Include client and her partner in discussion about breastfeeding.	Client participation increases feelings of control over the situation and promotes support and sharing.
Evaluate client's past coping strategies to determine which strategies have been most effective.	Use of appropriate coping strategies aids in reducing anxiety.
Question the client about available support systems, such as family, friends, community.	Additional sources of support are helpful in alleviating anxiety.
Provide client with information about support groups, Web sites, and other sources of information related to breastfeeding.	Shared experiences and knowledge of similar situations can aid in preparing the client and her partner for what to expect with breastfeeding.

EVALUATION

1. The client states she is comfortable with her decision to breastfeed.
2. The client verbalizes decreased anxiety when discussing breastfeeding.
3. The client uses appropriate resources for support.

- The mother who has had a cesarean birth may find the football (see Fig. 21.6B) or side-lying (see Fig. 21.6C) hold comfortable. Side-lying also may be a convenient position for feeding during patterns of sleep for the mother and infant. An over-the-shoulder position of the baby while the mother lies down is another option.
- The C-hold refers to supporting the breast by the mother's thumb resting above the areola with the other fingers under the breast. In this way she can lift the breast and help the baby take as much of the areola into the mouth as possible (Lauwers & Shinkskie, 2005).
- The scissor grasp allows for some compression of the areola, although it is less effective if the mother's breast is small or hand is large. The woman places her thumb on top of the breast, close to the thorax, with her index finger above the areola, and places the other fingers beneath the breast for support.

The nurse should instruct the woman that, once the baby is sucking, the mother should continue to support the breast so that its weight does not break the seal that the baby's mouth has made around the breast.

NIC/NOC Box 21.1 Breastfeeding

Common NIC Labels

- Anticipatory Guidance
- Breastfeeding Assistance
- Family Involvement Promotion
- Lactation Counseling
- Nutrition Management
- Parent Education: Infant
- Positioning
- Teaching: Infant Nutrition

Common NOC Labels

- Breastfeeding Establishment: Infant
- Breastfeeding Establishment: Maternal
- Breastfeeding Maintenance
- Knowledge: Breastfeeding

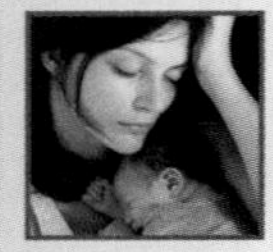

Lindsay reports difficulties with breastfeeding. Which positions might the nurse suggest to enhance Lindsay's comfort during feeding sessions?

Infant Hunger Cues. With the **rooting reflex,** infants open their mouths and turn their heads in search of a nipple, or suck on their fingers or hands to indicate they are preparing for a feeding (see Table 20.5 in Chap. 20). Inducing the rooting reflex may include stroking the baby's cheek in the direction of the mouth with the nipple or a finger to get the baby to turn toward the breast. Getting the baby to open the mouth to accept the breast may include stroking the baby's lower lip with the nipple until the mouth opens wide. Another technique is for the nurse to advise the woman to express a little colostrum from the nipple and to place it on the baby's lips to elicit interest in the stimulus.

A hungry baby may present with clenched fists, flexed arms, and moving legs as though riding a bicycle. Crying is a late sign of hunger (AAP, 2005; Biancuzzo, 2003). Arousing a sleeping baby to eat can be a challenge. The nurse should suggest unwrapping the baby from blankets or even removing some of his or her clothing to help keep the child awake long enough to complete a feeding. Stroking the baby's feet, changing his or her diaper, or applying a warm, moist washcloth may help stimulate the baby as well. The father or other family members eager for involvement in feeding may be good candidates for helping to ready a baby for feeding.

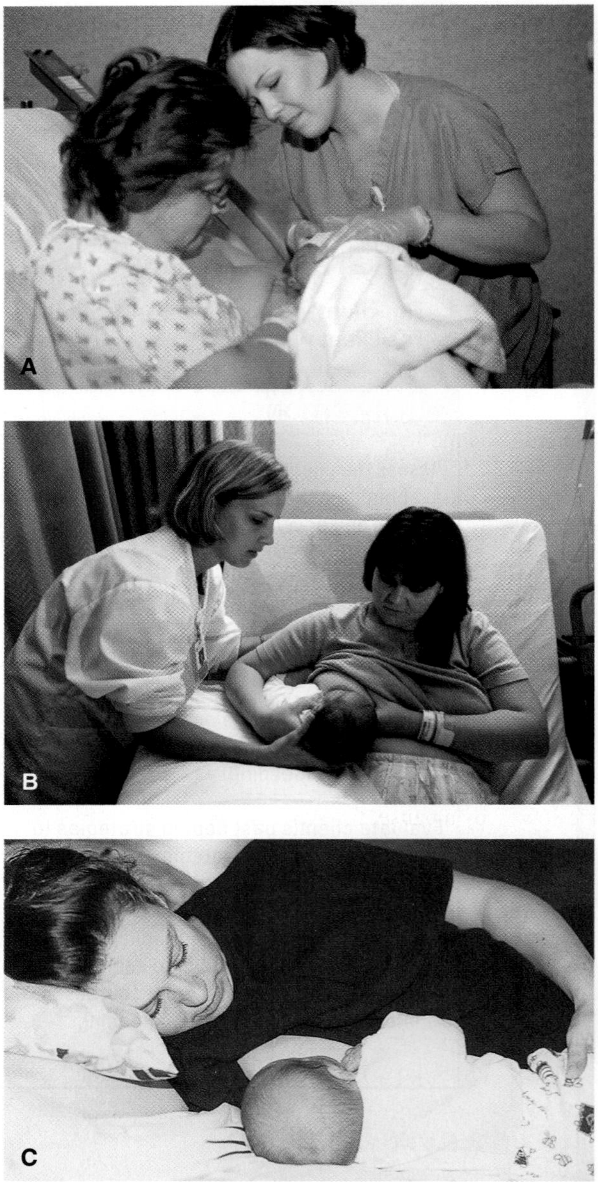

FIGURE 21.6 (**A**) Cradle hold. (**B**) Football hold. (**C**) Side-lying hold.

Latching. When an infant is latched correctly, his or her lips are flanged out over the areola, with nose and chin touching the breast (Fig. 21.7). The mother should hold her newborn close to her, with the infant's head extended slightly and tilted back. When the baby opens his or her mouth wide, the nurse advises the mother to quickly pull the baby onto the areola (with the nipple in the center), without pushing the baby's head, which will cause the baby to arch away from the breast. Approximately 3.8 cm of areolar tissue should be centered in the infant's mouth (Biancuzzo, 2003). Most infants suck rapidly for 30 to 90 seconds (Cahill & Wagner, 2002b) until the mother

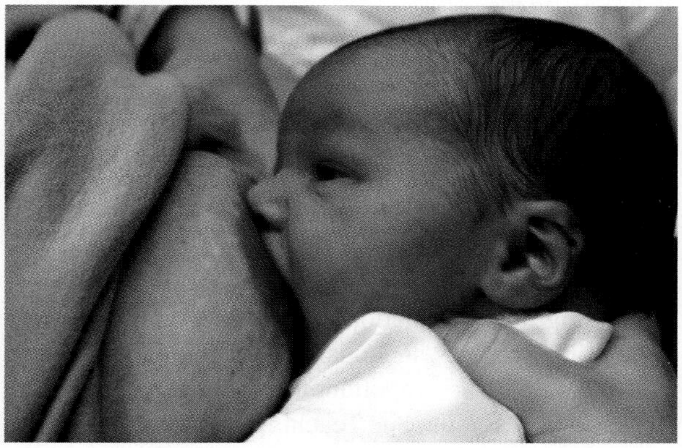

FIGURE 21.7 With correct latching, the newborn's lips flange out over the mother's areola, and the baby's nose and chin touch the mother's breast.

experiences the milk ejection reflex, also known as the let-down reflex. The nurse should advise the mother that she will feel as though the baby is tugging on her breast tissue, but that a good latch is not painful. Audible assessment of swallowing in the first 24 to 48 hours is likely after three to four high-powered sucks and may sound like small puffs of air (Lauwers & Shinskie, 2005). After the mother's milk supply is established, the baby will develop a series of deeper and more rhythmic sucks followed by a pause, for swallowing and breathing (Lau & Hurst, 1999). This series often is referred to as the *suck–swallow–breathe sequence.*

Infant Satiety Cues. Once the baby is latched onto the breast correctly, the mother should allow the infant to suckle until he or she falls off the breast, pushes the nipple from the mouth, or stops sucking entirely. These behaviors are *satiety cues.* The nurse should instruct the mother to watch for the infant's satiety cues to determine when to stop the nursing session rather than concentrating on how long the baby has been breastfeeding. Other signs of satiety include having seen the infant's lower jaw moving deeply and rhythmically, hearing the swallow, and soft maternal breast tissue. A satisfied postprandial baby has relaxed arms and legs, appears drowsy, or falls asleep (Biancuzzo, 2003). A breastfed infant should eat 8 to 12 times in a 24-hour period (AAP, 2005; Hall & Carroll, 2000).

When a mother requests a general timeframe to gauge the length of a breastfeeding session, the nurse can suggest 20 to 30 minutes on the first breast (or until the infant provides satiety cues) and then offering the other breast (Riordan, 2004). Lawrence and Lawrence (2005) suggest offering a guideline of 10 to 15 minutes per feeding during the first days because this plan allows small frequent feeds without stressing the mother. The nurse should encourage the mother to offer both breasts during each early feeding session to stimulate milk production. Breasts produce a chemical inhibitor, which responds to incomplete milk removal by decreasing further milk production (Wilde et al., 1998).

The nurse should remind the client to allow the baby to completely empty at least one breast during a feeding session, and then to offer the other breast if the baby desires. He or she should instruct the client to alternate the breast offered first so that each breast continues to make as much milk as the baby needs. Another technique is to offer just one breast during a feeding, and to alternate the breast with each feeding. If the client must break the suction during a feeding, the nurse should instruct her to insert her finger into the corner of the baby's mouth between the gums.

Burping. The primary reason to burp an infant is to help the baby expel air ingested during feeding or crying. Breastfed infants create a suction on the breast that, when accomplished properly, does not allow for ingestion of air during suckling. Some breastfed infants, however, may benefit from burping during feeding if they swallowed air during crying before breastfeeding.

Use of Artificial Nipples. When establishing breastfeeding, nurses should advise families to delay the introduction of artificial nipples from pacifiers and bottles until the infant has breastfed exclusively for 3 to 6 weeks (AAP, 2005). Newborns begin to recognize their mothers through touch, taste, and smell. They are forming both a nipple preference and comfort with sucking during this time; introduction of more than one nipple may impede breastfeeding. Howard and associates (1999) found that introducing a pacifier before 6 weeks of life was associated with a significantly decreased duration of breastfeeding. Furthermore, the sucking mechanism for breastfeeding differs from that of bottle feeding. The breastfed infant's mouth must open wide to take in breast tissue, while the tongue protrudes over the lower lip, which curls outward. Bottle-fed infants have a partially closed mouth, and the tongue does not protrude quite so far.

Pumping. Most lactating women can anticipate occasions when they will need to express breast milk to be fed during their absence to their babies. Breastfeeding mothers do not need to be present for every infant feeding. *Breast pumping* allows lactating women to express breast milk through a mechanical device; they can store and subsequently feed the milk to their infants. Breast pumping is useful for women who return to work or school. Expressing breast milk affords other caregivers the opportunity to nurture their babies through nourishment. Furthermore, mothers of breastfeeding infants can increase their milk supply by pumping in addition to directly breastfeeding, and some infants benefit from additional feeding volume beyond direct breastfeeding. Examples include slow weight gain, hyperbilirubinemia, and preterm infants who fatigue during breastfeeding.

The nurse also can encourage breast pumping when a woman would like to provide breast milk for her newborn but the baby cannot suckle at the breast. Breast pumping for a new mother should commence 6 to 24 hours after birth (Spicer, 2001). Milk removal must commence by the third postpartum day to promote the likelihood of successful lactation (Labbok, 2001b). A hospital-grade, electric pump is most efficient at extracting milk from the breasts (Fig. 21.8). Features of breast pumps that increase maternal comfort and the effectiveness of milk expression include hospital-grade electric capability, double breast shields that enable pumping both breasts at the same time, adjustment for suction, and adjustment for number of cycles per minute. Other pumps available include piston-style manual pumps, battery-powered pumps, and low-grade electric pumps without enough power for adequate suction or adjustment of suction or cycles.

Some insurers reimburse the cost of a breast pump when infants are born prematurely. The nurse should encourage the client to inquire about insurance coverage for a breast pump, where to obtain the breast pump, and the documentation required for reimbursement. Additionally, local WIC programs may provide a breast pump to babies born preterm. Breast pumps are often available where other baby supplies are sold, with a large variety of pumps found at stores dedicated to baby supplies. The Internet is another resource for mothers who wish to purchase a breast pump.

The client should pump both breasts simultaneously to yield the most volume and to decrease time spent pumping each breast consecutively (Auerbach, 1993) (Fig. 21.9). She should set the level of suction on low and increase suction throughout the session as comfort allows. The breast pump should provide cycles of suction and release as many times as the infant would suckle. This equates to 40 to 90 cycles/min (Spicer, 2001).

Milk supply is stimulated by demand. The stress of the necessity to pump and having a baby someplace other than the well-baby nursery can impair milk production, release, or both. Teaching Tips 21.1 provide suggestions to improve the volume of milk expression.

The nurse should encourage the client to pump every 2 to 3 hours during the day, and minimally once or twice during the night (much the same timing as if the baby were nursing). Pumping sessions should last 10 to 15 minutes. The frequency of pumping sessions is more important to stimulating milk production than is extending the length of pumping sessions. Personal hygiene and pump equipment cleanliness are important to avoid contamination of expressed breast milk. See Teaching Tips 21.2 for details.

Milk Storage. The duration at which breast milk can be stored for use depends on storage conditions. Mothers should feed freshly expressed breast milk to the infant or chill it as soon as possible to retain maximum immunologic and nutritional benefits and to decrease the possibility of bacterial contamination. Expressed breast milk may be refrigerated before use for a maximum of 2 to 3 days. Breast milk stored in the freezer of a refrigerator–freezer combination unit must be used within 3 months. Breast milk stored in a deep freezer may be used within 6 to 12 months (Lauwers & Shinskie, 2005). Refrigerated and frozen human milk should be placed toward the back of the cooling unit to avoid partial warming with repeated opening of the unit's door.

Optimal storage containers for breast milk include specialized disposable breast milk storage bags or plastic or glass containers. Some of breast milk's nutrients and cellular components adhere to the sides of the container into which it was stored. Glass containers help retain human milk's nutrients and antibodies by allowing more cells to become released into solution after thawing and vigorous shaking (Biancuzzo, 2003). Glass has a durable, smooth surface for cleaning and is reusable, making it economical. The interior of soft plastic (polypropylene) bottles is prone to scratches during the cleaning process,

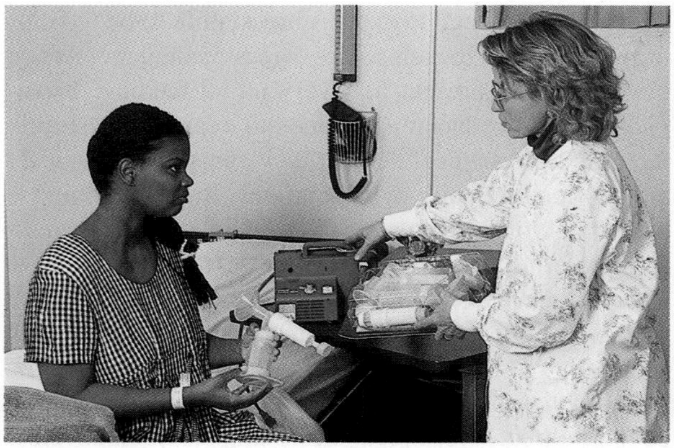

FIGURE 21.8 This nurse is teaching a client about the differences between a hand-held breast pump and an electric breast pump (shown on the table).

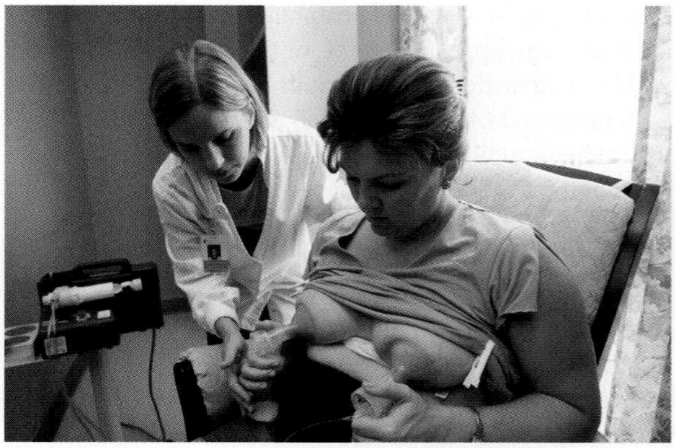

FIGURE 21.9 Pumping both breasts simultaneously will provide the most milk volume and minimize the time the client must spend performing the activity.

TEACHING TIPS 21.1 Improving Milk Volume and Expression

- Use an electric, double pump.
- Pump 8 times in a 24-hour period, allowing for 4 to 5 hours of continuous sleep through the night.
- Provide a comfortable and private environment.
- Play soft music.
- Use imagery to imagine your baby successfully breastfeeding.
- Use imagery to imagine milk flowing from your breasts.
- Apply clean, warm, and moist compresses to breasts before pumping.
- Maintain adequate fluid and nutrient intake.
- Maintain adequate rest.
- Massage shoulders.
- Promote skin-to-skin contact with the baby before pumping ("kangaroo care").
- Place a picture of the baby or an article that belongs to him or her within sight.

making adequate cleaning difficult. Bacteria thrive in scratches. Hard plastic (polycarbonate) bottles are less prone to acquiring scratches during cleaning and allow for the maintenance of the nutrients and cellular components of breast milk (Tully, 2000). Soft, plastic bottle liners (polyethylene bags), the kind used inside hard plastic bottles, are prone to leaking breast milk during freezing and thawing. Use of bottle liner bags also reduces antibody retention. In addition, these bags may alter the smell and taste of human milk, causing the infant to refuse it (Lauwers & Shinskie, 2005).

Management of Problems Related to Breastfeeding

Nipple Protractility. Women who desire to breastfeed should check the protractility of their nipples. A nipple that everts on stimulation helps the infant to find and to center on the nipple, as well as to grasp and stretch the tissue upward against the hard palate for effective milk extraction. The nurse can teach a simple pinch test, which consists of grasping at the base of the nipple with the forefinger and thumb several times. A protracting nipple moves outward; an inverted nipple moves inward. Women with nipples that remain inverted into the third trimester can do several things to evert their nipples. They should consult with their practitioner about the safety of such techniques because nipple stimulation can cause preterm labor in some women by liberating oxytocin from the posterior pituitary gland.

One method of nipple eversion is use of an inverted syringe slightly larger than the nipple. The syringe is cut at the tapered end, and the plunger direction is reversed to provide a soft surface against the nipple. The woman places the smooth (not cut) end of the syringe over her nipple and gently pulls on the plunger. She holds the pressure for 30 seconds, and then releases. She may perform the technique two or three times per day, two or three times per session. After the baby is born, she may perform the technique before each feed. The woman should clean the syringe in hot soapy water and rinse and air-dry it after each use (Kesaree, 1993).

Gentle suction from a breast pump may have the same effect as the syringe. Frequency of the technique is similar (Lauwers & Shinskie, 2005). Another technique is to cut a small hole in the bra at the place of the nipple and allow the pressure around the nipple to push it forward (Lauwers & Shinskie, 2005). A mother may manually

TEACHING TIPS 21.2 Maintaining Breast and Equipment Hygiene

- Cleanse the breast area every day with warm water only; avoid soap on the breast because it can dry the skin.
- Wear a clean bra daily.
- Change breast pads as they become damp.
- Wash hands with warm water and soap just before pumping.
- Express milk into a sterile bottle or container.
- Maintain a "clean" area for equipment. Do not place equipment into sink for cleaning.
- Wash flange and one-way valve with hot water and dish soap (not antibacterial); rinse well with hot water.
- Allow equipment to air-dry.
- Once daily, sterilize equipment that comes in contact with milk by boiling for 3 to 5 minutes in a covered pan or washing in the top rack of a dishwasher.
- Take care not to allow backflow of milk into tubing.
- Label container with baby's name, date, and time of expression.
- Store expressed milk in the refrigerator toward the back for use within 72 hours.
- Store expressed milk in the freezer for use after 72 hours of pumping. Cool milk in refrigerator first.
- Thaw frozen expressed milk in a warm water bath, taking care not to allow water to spill into the container.
- Use previously frozen expressed milk within 24 hours.

form the nipple or apply ice to the nipple before each feed to promote protractility (Lauwers & Shinskie, 2005). Breast shells have not been proved an effective means of everting nipples prenatally (Lauwers & Shinskie, 2005).

Plugged Ducts. A **plugged milk duct** results from accumulation of milk or dead cells that have not been expelled from the breast. The affected breast may present with a tender lump that feels hot to the touch. The lactating woman is afebrile and does not have signs of infection (Biancuzzo, 2003).

The nurse should instruct the client that offering the breast with the plugged duct first may help remove the plug, as a result of the infant's vigorous sucking at the beginning of a feed. Changing the infant's feeding position to point his or her nose in the direction of the plugged duct may be beneficial (Riordan, 2004). Other helpful measures include massaging the affected area while the baby is latched on or during a hot shower. The nurse should advise the woman to avoid wearing constrictive clothing (eg, underwire bras) and baby carriers. If the baby cannot directly breastfeed, the nurse can suggest hand expression while leaning over a container of warm water. The heat from the water causes vasodilation, whereas gravity caused by leaning forward aids in drainage (Biancuzzo, 2003). Alternatively, the woman may apply warm, moist compresses followed by hand expression to release the plug (Lauwers & Shinskie, 2005).

Mastitis. Mastitis means inflammation of a mammary gland (usually unilateral); it may involve bacterial infection. Detection of infection may be through breast milk culturing; causative organisms vary and include common nasal and skin flora such as *Staphylococcus aureus*. Mastitis may be associated with a plugged milk duct, inadequate milk removal, maternal fatigue and stress, or maternal flu-like symptoms (eg, fever. The breast tissue appears red and inflamed and is tender (Barbosa-Cesnik et al., 2003).

Mastitis is most likely after the breastfeeding dyad has been discharged from the hospital. Nurses should advise mothers to continue to breastfeed. Women can position their infants so that the chin points toward the site of infection (Lauwers & Shinskie, 2005). Treatment may include the application of warm, moist compresses before and during feeds, plenty of maternal rest and fluids, and maternal analgesics. Antibiotics may be prescribed, although not necessarily. Penicillinase-resistant penicillins or cephalosporins often are prescribed to cover staphylococci and streptococci (Barbosa-Cesnik et al., 2003). Mothers who require antibiotic therapy should complete the entire course of medication and continue to breastfeed. Mastitis may develop into an abscess, in which needle aspiration or drain placement is necessary to remove the pus.

Evaluation

Expected outcomes are a satisfying, comfortable, feeding relationship for mother and child, providing sufficient newborn nutrition.

FORMULA FEEDING

Infant formula is patterned after the composition of breast milk or the outcomes of the postprandial breastfed infant (Carver, 2003). The Federal Department of Agriculture Infant Formula Act of 1980, revised in 1985, established minimum levels of 29 nutrients and maximum levels of 9 nutrients in commercially prepared infant formulas (Public Law 96-359, 1980). In addition, the Life Sciences Research Office (1998) prepared expert analysis of the scientific literature since 1985 to make updated recommendations on nutrient content for infant formulas. Many nutrient levels in infant formulas are higher than in breast milk because of the lower bioavailability of the formulas. Infant formulas fall into several main classes: standard term, soy, protein hydrolysate, free amino acid based, metabolic, and preterm. Table 21.2 contains indications for the different formulas.

Composition

Standard-term infant formulas are 20 calories/oz standard dilution made from cow milk protein and contain lactose and a blend of fats. Infant soy formulas are made using a soy protein isolate and are lactose free. **Protein hydrolysate** formulas contain short peptide chains and free amino acids from the casein or whey component of cow milk for the protein source. Some hydrolysates contain medium-chain triglycerides (MCTs) in addition to long-chain triglycerides as the fat source. Free amino acid formulas are designed for term infants, composed of synthetic amino acids and containing all long-chain triglycerides as their fat source.

Preterm infant formulas are made with intact cow milk protein and dual sources of carbohydrates and fats to increase absorption. Commercially prepared preterm infant formulas are made in 20, 22, and 24 calories/oz. The main features of preterm formulas are higher levels of protein, vitamins, minerals, and electrolytes than formulas designed for term infants. In addition, there are breast milk fortifiers that enhance the composition of expressed breast milk and better meet the high nutrient needs of premature newborns. They are in liquid or powdered form, and are added to breast milk or the liquid form may be fed alternately with breast milk.

See Table 21.3 for a comparison of constituents and nutrient levels of breast milk and formulas.

Considerations Related to Formula Type

Most healthy full-term infants benefit from a standard cow milk–based, iron-containing infant formula (eg, Similac

TABLE 21.2 Indications for Various Feeding Types

FEEDING TYPE	BRAND NAME	INDICATIONS FOR USE
Human milk		Healthy, full-term infants; most sick term infants; most healthy and sick preterm infants, with supplementation
Standard cow milk–based formula	Similac With Iron Enfamil With Iron	Healthy, full-term infants
	Carnation Good Start	Same as above, with family history of atopy
	Similac Lactose Free	Healthy, full-term infants with lactose intolerance
	Lacto-Free	Same as above
Soy	Isomil	Family history of allergy to cow milk protein, lactose intolerance, galactosemia, vegetarianism
	ProSobee	Same as above, and with sucrose intolerance
	Isomil DF	Decreases duration of loose stools
Protein hydrolysate	Nutramigen	Family history of allergy to cow milk protein, multiple food allergies, idiopathic defects of protein digestion or absorption
	Alimentum, Pregestimil	Same as above, and fat malabsorption
Free amino acid	Neocate	Infants sensitive to intact proteins, multiple food allergies, severe gastroesophageal reflux, Kosher feeding
Metabolic	RCF 3232A 80056 Pro-Phree ProViMin	Used under the precise direction of a physician and dietitian for malabsorptive syndromes requiring protein, carbohydrate, or fat manipulations
Preterm	Similac Special Care With Iron Enfamil Premature With Iron	Preterm infants, until a weight of ~2500–3600 g
	Similac NeoSure Enfamil EnfaCare	Preterm infants ready for hospital discharge who weigh ~1800 g; to be fed until 9 to 12 months corrected gestational age
Human milk fortifier as a supplement to human milk	Similac Human Milk Fortifier (powder), Enfamil Human Milk Fortifier (powder), Similac Natural Care (liquid)	Preterm infants fed human milk in the hospital

With Iron, Enfamil With Iron, Carnation Good Start). Store-brand formulas adhere to the FDA regulations regarding nutrition and manufacturing of infant formulas. Wyeth Nutritionals produces store-brand infant formula in the United States that the retailer then labels as its own. They promote appropriate growth for full-term babies and cost approximately 40% less than brand-name formulas (Educational Symposium, 2000b).

Infants born with iron overload syndrome accumulate dangerously high levels of iron. Iron overload syndrome is not an indication for a low-iron formula (AAP Committee on Nutrition, 1999); the primary therapy for infants with this syndrome is chelation therapy. The chelator dose can be titrated to be effective with the use of iron-containing formula.

Soy formulas (eg, Isomil, ProSobee) are appropriate for infants with galactosemia or primary lactase deficiency, caregivers desiring a vegetarian formula, babies with postacute gastroenteritis with documented lactose intolerance (AAP Committee on Nutrition, 1998), and infants older than 6 months with cow milk allergy (Klemola et al., 2002; Seppo et al., 2005). The AAP Committee on Nutrition (1998) does not support the use of soy formulas for infants with birth weights less than 1800 g. Preterm infants fed soy formula have delayed growth in weight and length; their bones do not mineralize well; and their biochemical indices of protein are less than preterm infants fed cow milk–based infant formulas (AAP Committee on Nutrition, 1998).

Cow milk protein formulas that contain no lactose (eg, Similac Lactose Free, Enfamil LactoFree) are appropriate for infants with primary lactase deficiency. Formula with added rice starch (eg, Enfamil A.R.) may be helpful to infants who require thickened feedings, such as those with gastroesophageal reflux. The formula is only slightly thicker than regular formula during feeding. Upon entering the acidic environment of the stomach, the formula becomes more viscous, which decreases the amount of emesis expelled from the mouth (Mead Johnson Nutritionals, 2000).

TABLE 21.3 Composition of Infant Feedings

NUTRIENTS PER 100 ML FEEDING CHOICE	ENERGY (CAL)	PROTEIN (G/SOURCE/ % OF TOTAL CALORIES)	FAT (G/SOURCE/ % OF TOTAL CALORIES)	CARBOHYDRATE (G/SOURCE/ % OF TOTAL CALORIES)
Mature term Human milk	69.9	0.9/ Mature term human milk/ 5%	4.2/ Mature term human milk/ 54%	7.3/ Lactose/ 42%
Mature preterm Human milk	67.1	1.4/ Preterm human milk/ 8%	3.9/ Mature preterm human milk/ 52%	6.6/ Lactose/ 40%
Similac With Iron	67.6	1.4/ Nonfat milk & whey protein concentrate/ 8%	3.6/ High-oleic saf-flower, coconut, & soy oils/ 49%	7.3/ Lactose/ 43%
Enfamil With Iron	68	1.5/ Whey and nonfat milk/ 9%	3.6/ Palm olein, soy, coconut, & high oleic sunflower oils/ 48%	7.3/ Lactose/ 43%
Carnation Good Start	67	1.8/ Nonfat milk/ 10%	2.8/ Palm olein, soy, coconut, & high-oleic safflower oils/ 37%	8.9/ Corn syrup solids & maltodextrin/ 53%
Similac Lactose Free	67.6	1.4/ Milk protein isolate/ 9%	3.6/ Soy & coconut oils/ 49%	7.2/ Corn syrup solids & sucrose/ 43%
LactoFree	68	1.4/ Milk protein isolate/ 9%	3.1/ Palm olein, soy, coconut, & high oleic sunflower oils/ 48%	7.4/ Corn syrup solids/ 43%
Isomil	67.6	1.7/ Soy protein isolate & L-methionine/ 10%	3.7/ High oleic safflower, coconut, & soy oils/ 49%	7/ Corn syrup & sucrose/ 41%
ProSobee	68	2/ Soy protein isolate & L-methionine/ 12%	3.6/ Palm olein, soy, coconut & high oleic sunflower oils/ 48%	6.8/ Corn syrup solids/ 40%
Isomil DF	67.6	1.8/ Soy protein isolate & L-methionine/ 11%	3.7/ Soy & coconut oils/ 49%	6.8/ Corn syrup & sucrose/ 40%
Nutramigen	68	1.9/ Casein hydro-lysate & added amino acids/ 11%	3.4/ Palm olein, soy, coconut, & high oleic sunflower oils/ 45%	7.4/ Corn syrup solids & modified corn starch/ 44%
Alimentum	67.6	1.9/ Casein hydro-lysate, L-cystine, L-tyrosine, & L-tryptophan/ 11%	3.7/ Safflower, MCT[a], & soy oils/ 48%	6.9/ Sucrose & modified tapioca starch/ 41%
Pregestimil	67.6	1.9/ Casein hydro-lysate & added amino acids/ 11%	3.8/ MCT[a], corn, soy, & high oleic sunflower oils/ 48%	6.9/ Corn syrup solids, modified corn starch, & dextrose/ 41%
Neocate	67.7	2.1/ Synthetic-free amino acids/ 12%	3/ Hybrid safflower, coconut, & soy oils/ 47%	7.8/ Corn syrup solids/ 41%
Similac Special Care With Iron*	80.6	2.2/ Nonfat milk & whey protein concentrate/ 11%	4.4/ MCT[a], soy, & coconut oils/ 49%	8.6/ Corn syrup solids & lactose/ 42%
Enfamil Premature With Iron*	81	2.4/ Whey and nonfat milk/ 12%	4.1/ MCT[a], soy, & coconut oils/ 44%	9/ Corn syrup solids & lactose/ 44%

Continued

TABLE 21.3 Composition of Infant Feedings

NUTRIENTS PER 100 ML FEEDING CHOICE	ENERGY (CAL)	PROTEIN (G/SOURCE/ % OF TOTAL CALORIES)	FAT (G/SOURCE/ % OF TOTAL CALORIES)	CARBOHYDRATE (G/SOURCE/ % OF TOTAL CALORIES)
Preterm human milk & Similac HMF[b,c] (25 mL:1 pkt)	78.9	2.3/ Preterm human milk, nonfat milk, & whey protein concentrate/ 12%	4.1/ Preterm human milk & MCT[a] oil/ 47%	8.2/ Lactose & corn syrup solids/ 42%
Preterm human milk & Enfamil HMF[b,c] (25 mL:1 pkt)	81	2.5/ Preterm human milk, whey protein concentrate, & sodium caseinate/ 12%	4.9/ Preterm human milk, soy, & MCT[a] oils/ 54%	7/ Preterm human milk, corn syrup solids, & lactose/ 35%
Similac NeoSure	74.6	1.9/ Nonfat milk & whey protein concentrate/ 10%	4.1/ Soy, coconut, & MCT[a] oils/ 41%	7.7/ Maltodextrin & lactose/ 41%
EnfaCare With Iron	74	2.1/ Whey & nonfat milk/ 11%	3.9/ High oleic sunflower, MCT[a], & coconut oils/ 46%	7.9/ Maltodextrins, lactose, & citrates/ 43%

[a]Data from Ross Products Division, Abbott Laboratories. (March 2001). *Pediatric nutritionals product guide* (No. A8138). Columbus, OH; Ross Products Division, Abbott Laboratories. (June 1999). *Composition of feedings for infants and young children.* (No. A7368). Columbus, OH; Mead Johnson Nutritionals. (October, 2000). *Enfamil® family of products handbook* (No. LB6 revised 10/00). Evansville, IN; NEONOVA Nutrition Optimizer Version 4.5. Ross Products Division, Abbott Laboratories, Columbus, OH; J. W. Hansen (personal communication, April 15, 2002). Carnation® Good Start per Hendricks, K., Duggan, C., Walker, W. (2000). *Manual of pediatric nutrition;* (3rd ed.). Hamilton, Ontario: B.C. Decker Inc. Scientific Hospital Supplies North America. Retrieved October 20, 2002, from http://www.shsna.com/html/neocate.

[b]Human milk fortifier.

[c]Available in 0.68 cal/mL (20 calories/oz) and 0.8 cal/mL (24 calories/oz).

Protein hydrolysate formulas (eg, Alimentum, Pregestimil, Nutramigen) have proteins that have been cleaved into short peptide chains and free amino acids. They are appropriate for infants with multiple food allergies, a family history of allergy to cow milk protein, or impaired protein metabolism (Hays & Wood, 2005). The AAP (2000) recommends extensively hydrolyzed protein formula or a free amino acid–based formula for allergic infants as an alternative to breast milk. Soy formulas may be a suitable feeding for allergic infants in select cases, depending on the type of allergy manifested (Seppo et al., 2005). Some allergic infants may become sensitized to the soy protein as well (AAP, 2000). In the case of fat malabsorption, a protein hydrolysate that contains both long-chain fatty acids and medium-chain triglycerides as its fat source (eg, Alimentum, Pregestimil) would provide alternate pathways for metabolism of fat and increase absorption. The most elemental formulas (eg, Neocate, EleCare) contain free amino acids and are appropriate for infants sensitive to intact or hydrolyzed proteins, or those who have multiple food allergies or severe gastroesophageal reflux.

Preterm formulas (eg, Similac Special Care With Iron, Enfamil Premature With Iron) were designed to meet high nutrient needs of the preterm infant weighing less than 2500 g. Enriched formulas (eg, Similac NeoSure, Enfamil EnfaCare) are appropriate for preterm infants ready for discharge from the hospital and should be fed until 9 months corrected gestational age (AAP, 2003). Also see Figure 21.1 for guidance on choosing a feeding type.

The AAP does not support infant feedings made from evaporated or sweetened condensed milk because of nutrient inadequacy. These feedings are not sufficient in iron and vitamins C, A, and D to promote normal growth and development. Some evaporated milks are fortified with vitamins A and D. In a prospective study of infants fed breast milk, formula, or evaporated milk formula, researchers found abnormal ferritin and thiamin blood values and decreased copper and selenium in the group who received evaporated milk (Friel et al., 1997; Friel et al., 1999). Although medicinal supplements may be provided, the fat content of evaporated milk is digested poorly, and the sodium and phosphorus contents are excessive. In addition, infants should not receive cow milk because of the possibility of excessive protein load, allergic response, microintestinal blood loss, inferior protein absorption with increased renal solute load, low iron bioavailability, and dehydration.

Additives

The FDA has approved two fatty acids found in breast milk, docosahexanoic acid (DHA) and arachidonic acid (ARA), for inclusion in infant formulas. Literature supporting their use in infant formula shows that their symbiotic relationship can help stimulate infant mental development and visual acuity (Birch et al., 2000; Birch et al., 1998; Clandinin et al., 2005; Innes, 2004). Controversy remains as to what amounts of DHA and ARA may be beneficial in infant formula (Auestad et al., 2001). Presently, store brands do not add DHA or ARA to infant formula. Brand name formulas with added DHA and ARA are available; examples include canned Advance (Ross Pediatrics) and Lipil.

Most U.S. infant formulas contain iron, which is important for cognitive development. Infants who have experienced iron deficiency have shown behavior, motor, and developmental impairment (Akman et al., 2004; Eden, 2005; Lozoff, 1988). Reversal of cognitive deficits does not occur with appropriate iron intake (Lozoff et al., 1991; Walter et al., 1989). Iron deficiency is associated with enhanced lead absorption, which can lead to neurologic and developmental deficits (AAP Committee on Nutrition, 1999). Thus, informing caregivers of the importance of feeding iron-fortified infant formula and addressing their concerns about feeding iron-containing formulas are vital interventions. Iron-fortified infant formulas do not change the consistency or frequency of stools; they simply darken them (Nelson et al., 1988). Medicinal iron and iron from fortified infant cereals may contribute to constipation. Nearly all preterm and full-term formula-fed infants should be fed iron-fortified formulas (AAP Committee on Nutrition, 1998). Preterm infants require supplemental iron at an earlier age and in larger doses than do full-term babies. Medicinal iron doses for preterm infants are based on birth weight, with infants of smallest birth weight requiring higher doses (AAP Committee on Nutrition, 1999). The absorption of iron from breast milk has been estimated to be greater than 50%, compared with iron absorption from cow milk–based formulas at 5% to 12%. Iron absorbed from soy protein-based formulas is 1% to 7% (AAP Committee on Nutrition, 1999).

Client Teaching and Collaborative Interventions

Women who choose to bottle-feed require nursing-led instruction regarding physical delivery of the feeding (Fig. 21.10). Caregivers need to develop new feeding skills and begin to understand the feeding relationship they are developing with the infant. All caregivers will benefit from nursing advice that feeding should be a time to enjoy the newest family member. Nurses can give assistance and reassurance regarding reading hunger cues and feeding cues that signal the infant's need to be burped, fatigue, or the end of a feeding session.

Artificial Nipples

Most infants of term gestation suck well from standard yellow rubber nipples stocked in most well-baby nurseries and stores. Preterm infants benefit from softer nipples with smaller holes. Orthodontic nipples have a flattened appearance, and some infants show a preference for them. Other nipples are marketed as being most like a breast, based on a similar shape to the human breast. Silicone nipples are available in different artificial nipple shapes. Infants with congenital anomalies that involve the tongue, palates, lips, or chin may feed successfully using feeding devices specifically designed for that population. A speech pathologist or an occupational therapist is best trained to make recommendations for safe and effective oral feeding programs.

If an infant does not do well with the choice of artificial nipple, a different shape or material may result in more effective bottle feeding. Once the oral cavity of the infant has grown, he or she may benefit from a nipple with a bigger overall size as well as a larger hole from which the feeding flows.

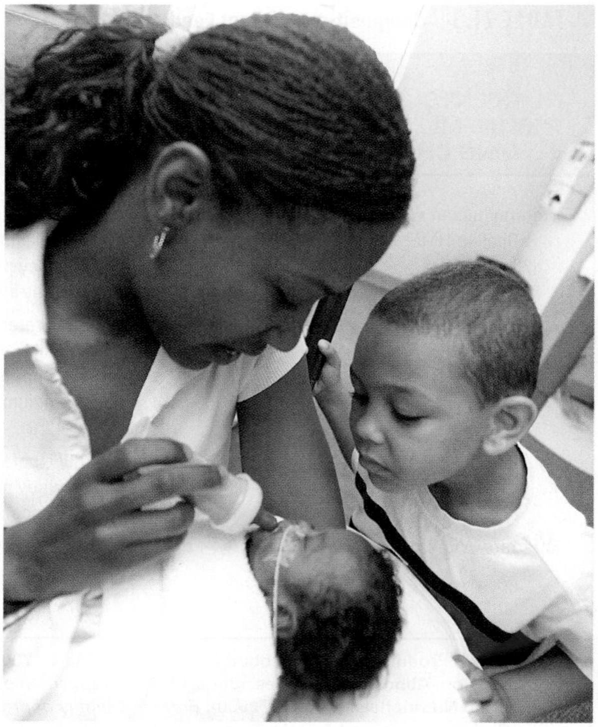

FIGURE 21.10 Nurses should teach clients who bottle-feed their newborns about the importance of correct feeding position, eye contact, and appropriate hygiene measures.

Formula Preparation

Preparation of infant formula depends on the type used. Ready-to-feed bottles and cans (8 or 32 fl oz) are the most convenient and most expensive. Concentrated liquid formulas come in 13 fl oz cans; this form is recommended most often for WIC participants because of its ease of preparation. Powdered formula is available in 12 to 30 oz cans and is the most economical choice. *Preparation of Formula for Infants: Guidelines for Health-Care Facilities* suggests that liquid infant formula should be made in a separate area using aseptic technique for neonatal intensive care settings unless no comparable product is available other than in powdered form (ADA, 2003).

Before preparing formula, caregivers should wash their hands with warm, soapy water to decrease the risk for contamination of formula with bacteria or viruses. They should use a clean, damp cloth to wipe the top of the can and a clean punch-type can opener for puncture. They must shake ready-to-feed and concentrated liquid formulas before opening them to suspend any particles that have settled out of solution. Caregivers reconstitute concentrated liquid formulas by adding an equal amount of water, ounce for ounce, to the formula and shaking or stirring. The empty can that contained the concentrated liquid can serve as the measuring device to ensure that the appropriate amount of water is added (Educational Symposium, 2000a). A glass liquid measuring cup may be the best device to use because plastic bottles and measuring devices tend to shrink over time with repeated exposure to high temperatures from dishwashers or sterilization.

When making powdered formula, caregivers should use the scoop included in the can to measure the powder. Household measures may seem like a good way to make a large volume of formula at once without losing count of the number of scoops; however, they are less accurate than scoops and, if made of plastic, household measurement devices shrink over time. Stirring the formula powder slightly will make it free flowing. Caregivers should dip the scoop into the powder, draw the scoop up the side of the can, and tap or re-dip the scoop to release any air pockets. The powder should be level with the side of the scoop. Caregivers should pack or unpack scoops according to label directions.

Formula may be prepared in a clean pitcher or individual bottles. Prepared formula may be kept in the refrigerator and covered for use within 48 hours. Caregivers should discard an unused can of powdered formula within 30 days of opening, according to label directions.

Sterilization

Water may be sterilized before reconstituting infant formula. Some pediatricians advise sterilization of the water and equipment used to make formula during the first 3 months of life, when the infant's immature immune system is not fully equipped to fight infection. After 3 months, it is assumed that the baby's increased activity and exploration will expose him or her to the pathogens that could cause illness from bottle feeding. Preterm infants or babies with an impaired immune system stand to benefit the most from a sterile water source. Baby or nursery waters are unnecessary and expensive. If caregivers choose nursery water, they should remember that it is not a sterile water source. If well water or pond water is used to prepare formula, it should be sterilized before use (Hall & Carroll, 2000). Well water also should be tested to make sure it does not contain toxic levels of lead (Educational Symposium, 2000a).

To sterilize water or equipment, caregivers should boil it for 1 to 5 minutes, allowing the water to cool before making formula. Extremely hot temperatures may alter the nutrient composition of formula, rendering some of it non-nutritive. An alternative to boiling equipment for sterilization includes countertop electric steam sterilizers. Caregivers should clean the equipment used to make formula, sterilize it if they desire, and allow it to air-dry. The nurse should discuss the importance of adequately cleaning away debris that may support the growth of harmful pathogens from equipment. Pathogens can survive the sterilization process if the equipment is cleaned improperly.

Warming

When warming a feeding for an infant, caregivers should allow it to come to temperature slowly under a running warm water bath (ADA, 2003). The level of the water should not be so close to the opening to allow water to seep into the container. Electric bottle warmers use steam to warm the feeding. Care must be taken to ensure even heating to avoid burning the baby with the formula that's been heated the most on the outside of the bottle. The nurse should instruct caregivers to not warm feedings in microwave ovens because the uneven heating of microwaves can cause hot spots, which can burn a baby's mouth. In addition, the buildup of steam can cause hot liquid to seep or spray out of the bottle.

Positioning and Burping

When discussing with caregivers positioning for bottle-fed babies, the nurse should instruct as follows:

- Wash hands before feeding to limit the transmission of infectious microorganisms to the baby.
- Hold the infant semi-upright and close to promote eye contact. Eye contact increases both the caregiver's and the infant's sense of attachment and promotes bonding. Infants who are bottle-fed also benefit from skin-to-skin contact to promote physical closeness and bonding. Wearing short-sleeved shirts or placing the diapered baby on a parent's bare chest ("kangaroo care") can accomplish this (Educational Symposium, 2000a). See Figure 21.11.
- Take care to interact with the baby during feedings because feeding can evoke feelings of nurturing and attachment. As much as possible, feedings should be in a quiet environment without distractions for caregiver or baby. Without removing the bottle from the infant's mouth, or during times of rest, the caregiver can talk to the infant in soft, sing-song tones, which infants respond to favorably. Some infants are calmed by their mother's voice and may show interest in her singing.

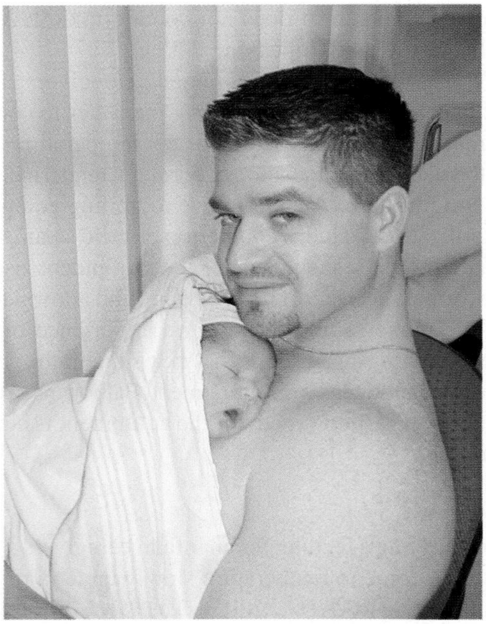

FIGURE 21.11 One measure to promote parent—infant bonding is kangaroo care, in which the newborn is held against a parent's bare chest.

- Tilt the bottle so that the nipple fills with formula or breast milk.
- Never prop a bottle. It is possible for prolonged exposure to carbohydrate from infant formula or juice to damage the unexposed teeth. For this same reason, a child should never be put to sleep with a bottle. Additionally, a baby with a propped bottle or the baby left to self-feed does not benefit from the bonding that a caregiver and infant develop during the feeding relationship.

Caregivers must allow infants to pace themselves with bursts of sucking and periods of rest. During a feeding, the infant may push the nipple out of the mouth, pull away from the bottle, or turn the head to indicate that he or she has swallowed some air before or during the feed and that a burp is appropriate.

Burping

Placing the infant over the shoulder creates abdominal pressure that helps to expel air. The nurse should teach those feeding the baby receiving a bottle to use one hand to support the baby's head or neck and the other hand to pat the baby's back. Other positions that create the same effect are to place the prone infant over the lap, or in a sitting position on the lap, while patting the infant's back with one hand and supporting the chin and head with the other hand (Fig. 21.12).

Feeding Cues

Caregivers never should force infants to finish a bottle, unless indicated for a specific purpose, such as poor weight gain or dehydration. Most infants will finish bottles if encouraged to do so, which could lead to extra spitting and excessive weight gain (Educational Symposium, 2000a). Caregivers should watch for satiety cues (eg, pushing the nipple from the mouth, pulling away

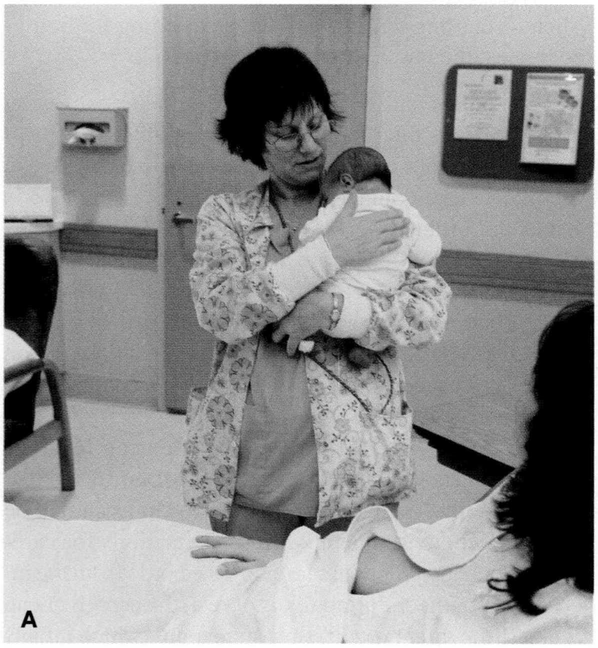

A

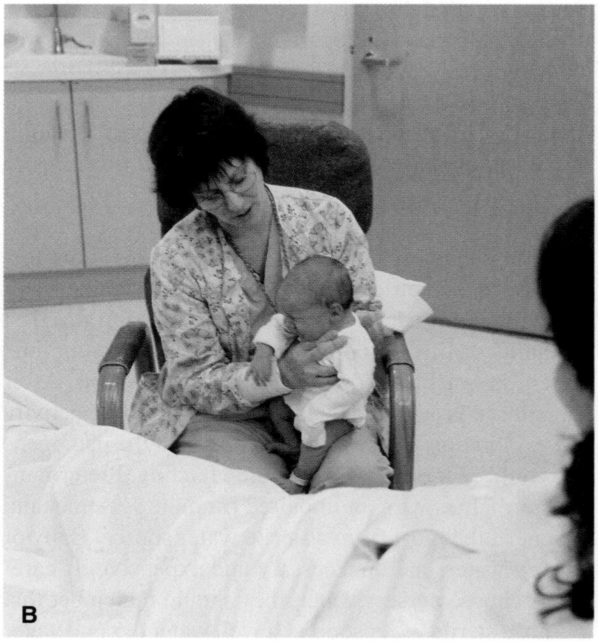

B

FIGURE 21.12 (A) Burping over the shoulder. (B) Burping with the newborn on the lap, while the nurse supports the head and neck.

from the bottle) that the feeding is complete. Additionally, if an infant does not finish a feeding and it appears that the baby wants more later, it is acceptable to give the same bottle to the baby as long as it is no longer than 90 minutes from the start of the original feeding.

OTHER FEEDING DELIVERY STRATEGIES

Parenteral and Enteral Nutrition

Several conditions warrant parenteral nutrition (Box 21.4). Examples include babies born sick or premature. Preterm infants may begin to suck on their tongues, feeding tubes, or hands and fingers as early as 30 to 32 weeks' postconceptual age (Lemons & Loughead, 2001) and have the ability to suck nutritively at approximately 34 to 37 weeks' gestational age (Herbst, 1989; Medoff-Cooper et al., 2001). Such behavior may not be coordinated, however, in terms of the suck–swallow–breathe pattern required for oral eating. Other indications for tube feedings include anatomic anomalies of the gastrointestinal tract (eg, tracheoesophageal fistula); cleft lip, cleft palate, or both; neurologic impairment; and short bowel syndrome.

Initially, the goals of parenteral nutrition are to minimize catabolism and to provide glucose in amounts that will prevent *glycogenolysis* (the breakdown of the body's stores of glucose) and *gluconeogenesis* (the formation of glycogen from fat and protein). Dosing with 4 to 6 mg dextrose/kg/min is adequate to prevent both glycogenolysis and gluconeogenesis.

Parenteral nutrition consists of carbohydrates combined with a crystalline amino acid solution. Lipid infusions either are hung separately or are part of the crystalline solution. The newborn loses 1 g/kg/day of protein to the nitrogen requirements of postnatal life (Auld et al., 1966). Initial dosing of amino acids should meet or slightly exceed this demand (Thureen & Hay, 2000). Initial lipid provision usually is dosed at 1 g/kg/day. Incremental advancement of dextrose, crystalline amino acid, and lipid may be increased according to the infant's tolerance as evidenced by laboratory values of serum glucose, bedside heel sticks, or urine glucose; serum blood urea nitrogen or ammonia; and serum triglyceride levels. Maximum levels are typically 3 to 3.5 g/kg/day of crystalline amino acids and 3 g/kg/day of lipids. The AAP (2003) recommends maximum levels of dextrose up to 15 mg/kg/min, with the specific amount determined by line access and the infant's tolerance.

For newborns receiving parenteral nutrition, small-volume (enteral) feedings (less than 20 to 30 mL/kg/day) should start as soon as they are medically stable. These small-volume feeds are not nutritive; rather, they prime the gut for future success with enteral feeding. Generally, small-volume feeds are initiated as an adjunct to intravenous (IV) fluids or parenteral nutrition, and feeds are advanced while the contribution from IV fluids is decreased.

Whenever possible, enteral nutrition is preferable to parenteral nutrition. After several days without enteric stimulation, mucosal cell damage results. The villi of the intestinal wall become blunted, and feeding progression becomes more difficult. Secretion of sucrase and lactase decreases, absorption of amino acids declines, and bacterial translocation from increased gut permeability is possible, which may lead to necrotizing enterocolitis.

In addition to the physical benefits of enteral feeds for nourishment, monetary savings are significant. Per day, it costs approximately $4.49 to feed a baby formula made from concentrated liquid (KidSource Online, 2002), compared with hundreds of dollars for total parenteral nutrition. Enteral nutrient needs are available as Adequate Intakes set to meet the needs of most infants up to 6 months of age. Adequate Intakes for infant macronutrients and micronutrients are provided in Table 21.4. See Box 21.5.

BOX 21.4 Indications for Parenteral Nutrition

- Gastrointestinal tract anomalies
- Inadequate enteral nutrition for 3 days or more, sooner if possible
- Intractable diarrhea of infancy
- Meconium ileus
- Necrotizing enterocolitis
- No enteral tolerance or availability
- Postoperative correction for gastrointestinal tract anomalies

Cup Feeding

Cup feeding evolved as a methodology from the needs of infants who could not breastfeed directly or suck from a bottle. It is used most often to feed preterm and low-birth-weight infants until they can breastfeed (Collins et al., 2004). It is not an ideal method for full-term infants, who tend to dribble the feeds from the cup and may show a strong preference for the cup when presented with the opportunity to breastfeed directly again.

When doing a cup feeding, the infant is held semi-upright. A cup specifically developed for infant feedings may be used, as may a small cup without a spout, such as a pliable medicine cup, shot glass, or plastic condiment cup used at fast-food restaurants. The cup is placed on the infant's lower lip so that it touches the corners of the mouth. This tactile stimulation, as well as olfactory sense, tells the infant that feeding is about to commence. The caregiver allows the infant to lap milk with the tongue into the mouth (Lauwers & Shinskie, 2005). First attempts should be with a quiet, alert infant who is not overly hungry or crying. Infants may require practice and patience from their caregivers in establishing cup feeding. As infants become more proficient at cup feeding, they may use a sipping technique. Feedings are never poured into the mouth. The infant may hold the breast milk or

TABLE 21.4 Adequate Intakes for Infants 0 to 6 Months of Age

NUTRIENT	AMOUNT PER DAY
Carbohydrate	60 g
Protein	9.1 g
Fat	31 g
Vitamin A	400 μg
Vitamin C	40 mg
Vitamin D	200 IU
Vitamin E	4 mg
Vitamin K	2 μg
Vitamin B_1 (thiamin)	0.2 mg
Vitamin B_2 (riboflavin)	0.3 mg
Vitamin B_3 (niacin)	2 mg
Vitamin B_6	0.1 mg
Folate	65 μg
Vitamin B_{12}	0.4 μg
Pantothenic acid	1.7 mg
Biotin	5 μg
Choline	125 mg
Calcium	210 mg
Chromium	0.2 μg
Copper	200 μg
Fluoride	0.01 mg
Iodine	110 μg
Iron	0.27 mg
Magnesium	30 mg
Manganese	0.003 mg
Molybdenum	2 mg
Phosphorus	100 mg
Selenium	15 μg
Zinc	2 mg

From Trumbo, P., Schlicker, S., Yates, A., & Poos, M. (2002). Dietary Reference Intakes for energy, carbohydrate, fiber, fat, fatty acids, cholesterol, protein and amino acids. *Journal of the American Dietetic Association, 102*(11), 1621–1630.

formula in the mouth until ready to swallow. The infant controls the total amount fed.

At approximately 30 weeks' gestation, preterm infants can effectively move their tongue, swallow, and breathe during cup feeding as evidenced by heart rates, respiratory rates, and oxygen saturations. When comparing cup feeding and bottle feeding, Marinelli and associates (2001) found that bottle feeders had a 10-fold increase in desaturations less than 90%, higher heart rates, and lower mean oxygen saturations. Of note is that the duration of feeding was longer and the volume consumed was smaller for cup feeding than for bottle feeding. Howard and colleagues (1999) found that full-term infants who were cup-fed maintained respiratory stability and consumed comparable volumes in comparable time when compared with bottle feeding. Lang and colleagues (1994) stated that the time required to cup-feed varies as widely as the time it takes to bottle-feed or tube-feed an infant.

BOX 21.5 Calculation of Fluid and Calorie Intake

Calculation of fluid intake

$$\frac{\text{Volume received over 24 hours}}{\text{Weight in kg}} = \text{mL/kg/day}$$

Calculation of calorie intake

Fluid Intake (mL/kg/day) × Caloric density of formula (cal/ml) = cal/kg/day

Finger Feeding

Another feeding methodology is *finger feeding*. One end of a small-bore tube extending ¼ inch beyond the tip of the finger is secured to the caregiver's finger. The other end is placed in a syringe containing the feeding, with the plunger removed (Lauwers & Shinskie, 2005). The caregiver places the finger pad side up and allows the infant to suck the finger, while the nutrient delivery is through the tube. Another variation is to use the plunger of the syringe to deliver approximately 0.5 mL of feeding with every third suck (Biancuzzo, 2003). Caregivers should maintain caution not to allow infants to become accustomed to this mode of feeding so that they begin to prefer it to the exclusion of all other feeding methodologies. They also must be sure to assess the integrity of the roof of the infant's mouth where the tubing is placed.

Nursing Supplementer

When a breastfed infant requires more feeding volume than direct breastfeeding is providing, or for adopted babies, a nursing supplementer may be a good option. A **nursing supplementer** is a device that contains breast milk or formula and delivers the feeding by a tube placed near the mother's nipple and into the infant's mouth (Fig. 21.13). While the infant is breastfeeding, one end of a tube is taped to the mother's breast so that it goes into the baby's mouth. The other end of the tube is connected to a feeding container filled with additional breast milk or infant formula. The container may be pinned to the mother's shirt or hung around her neck. In this way, the infant can continue to breastfeed and stimulate milk production while receiving the additional nutrients required for growth. Consultation with a lactation consultant can provide answers on how to physically manage the baby and the supplementary nursing system. A neonatal nutritionist can provide guidance on how much additional feeding to infuse.

Syringe Feeding

Another possibility is to syringe-feed an infant. This may be dangerous for the baby, however, especially when an untrained caregiver administers the feed. Syringe tips easily can injure the oral cavity. The infant needs to be

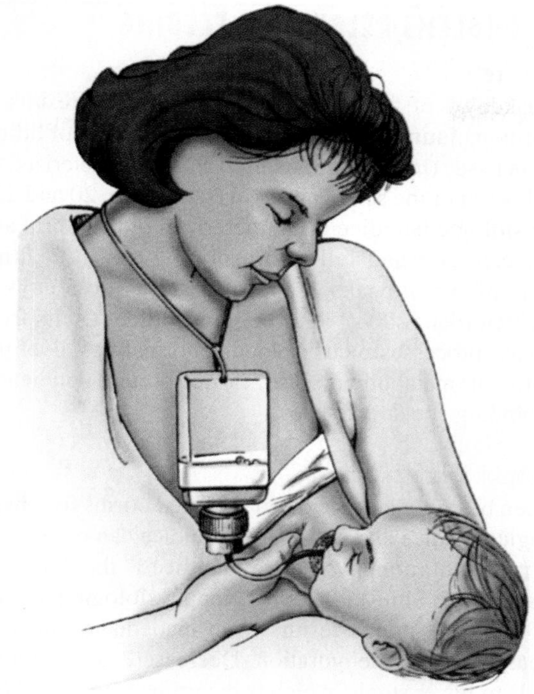

FIGURE 21.13. By using a nursing supplementer, the client can simulate the breastfeeding experience with a formula-fed infant, or with an infant who cannot take breast milk directly from the mother's nipple.

able to coordinate swallowing and breathing because this means of nourishment is caregiver led, and the baby cannot anticipate the milk until it is already in the mouth. The infant cannot control the amount or rate of feeding being delivered into the oral cavity, which could lead to aspiration. Placing the tip of the syringe into the cheek area or under the tongue decreases this risk, as does feeding in a semi-upright position (Lang, 2002).

MEASURES OF SUCCESSFUL FEEDING

Signs of a good breastfeeding session include seeing the baby's lower jaw moving deeply, hearing the baby swallow, having a soft breast after feeding, and viewing behaviors of a satisfied baby. Other ways to measure the success of feeding are discussed in the following sections.

Fluid Intake

Fluid needs in the first 24 hours of life for a full-term newborn are as low as 60 ml/kg/day. A preterm newborn requires approximately 80 mL/kg/day in the first 24 hours of life. Fluid needs increase to 120 to 160 mL/kg/day as babies mature (Groh-Wargo et al., 2000). Dr. William Sears suggests an intake of 2 oz per infant weight (in pounds) per day as a rough guide for how much a baby should ingest in the first 6 months of life (Educational Symposium, 2000b).

Wet Diapers

By the end of the first day of life, the newborn should have voided. If within the first 24 hours of life the infant has not voided, health care providers must consider and investigate causes. By days 2 and 3 of life, the newborn should urinate two to three times per day. The urine should not have a strong odor. By days 4 to 7 of life, the newborn should have six to eight voids in a 24-hour period (Biancuzzo, 2003) (see Box 21.6). In a hospital setting, nurses may be required to quantify urine output by weighing the diaper. Typical urine output for a 24-hour period is 1 to 3 mL/kg/hour (Groh-Wargo et al., 2000).

Stools

Infants develop uniquely recognizable, characteristic, and individual stool patterns. Daily bowel movements do not characterize a stool pattern as normal. When counseling parents on the type of stool they may expect from their infants, nurses should be aware of the various typical colors and consistencies. Additionally, nurses should know that when an infant changes from one feeding type to another, stool habitus also may change.

Meconium is the first stool that the newborn produces; it is black, tar-like, and sticky. Meconium consists largely of bilirubin and biliverdin, substances that accumulate during gestation. The baby eliminates meconium during the first 48 to 72 hours of life (Lauwers & Shinskie, 2005).

By day 3 of life, the breastfed newborn usually has at least three stools per day (Biancuzzo, 2003). Once milk supply is established (days 4 to 7 postpartum), the breastfed newborn usually stools at least three to four times in a 24-hour period (Biancuzzo, 2003). Fewer than four stools per day might indicate inadequate caloric intake and should alert the nurse to evaluate the effectiveness of breastfeeding more closely (Lauwers & Shinkskie, 2005). As breastfeeding progresses, many babies fed breast milk stool with each feeding as a result of a strong gastrocolic reflex.

The bottle-fed baby should have approximately four stools per day during the first week of life (Samour et al.,

BOX 21.6 Evaluation of Output for Breastfed Newborns

- By day of life 1: one stool and one void
- By day of life 3: three stools and three voids per day
- By day of life 4: three to four stools and six to eight voids per day

From Biancuzzo, M. (2003). *Breastfeeding the newborn: Clinical strategies for nurses* (2nd ed.). St. Louis: Mosby.

2003). As bottle-feeding proceeds beyond the first week, the number of stools likely will decline to approximately two per day (Samour et al., 2003).

The stools of breastfed infants are yellow, seedy, very soft, or liquid. Hyams and associates (1995) found that infants fed breast milk or Nutramigen had twice as many stools as infants fed other formulas. Stools of infants fed iron-fortified formulas may be green in color. Additionally, infants fed ProSobee may have harder stools more often than other feeding groups (Hyams and associates, 1995).

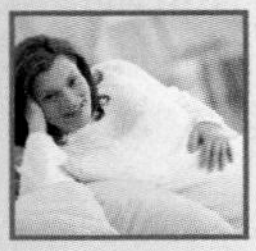

Joelle says, "When I bottle-fed my first baby, I knew exactly how much milk she took. But how will I know if the baby is getting enough when I'm breastfeeding?" How would the nurse respond?

Weight Gain and Growth

Appropriate gains in weight, length, and head circumference give everyone caring for an infant the opportunity to take pride in a thriving baby with good nutritional status. Conversely, too small or too large gains can alert the health care team to genetic, metabolic, physiologic, or iatrogenic complications. Nurses often are expected to weigh infants and measure length and head circumference. Serial measurements are invaluable tools in evaluating infant growth and subsequent development. Newborns lose approximately 5% to 10% of their birth weight as interstitial fluid in the first 5 to 7 days (Biancuzzo, 2003), whereas head circumference may decrease as much as 0.5 cm during this same period (Groh-Wargo et al., 2000). By day 10 of life, the newborn should begin to regain weight (Biancuzzo, 2003). Full-term infants should gain approximately 20 to 30 g/day during the first 3 months of life. Infantile length gains should average 0.69 to 0.75 cm/week. Head circumference should increase by approximately 0.5 cm/week through 3 months of age (Groh-Wargo et al., 2000).

The growth curves from the CDC in collaboration with the National Center for Chronic Disease Prevention and Health Promotion (2000) represent a more ethnically diverse population than did previous charts. These percentile charts include the 3rd and 97th percentiles for better assessment of growth at the extremes of normal distribution. For these reasons, the nurse should use age- and sex-appropriate NCHS 2000 growth curves when evaluating the growth of infants and children. When an infant's growth parameters channel upward or downward sharply by crossing percentiles for weight, length, or head circumference, the nurse should suggest a consultation with a pediatric dietitian to determine a suitable course of action.

PROBLEMS RELATED TO FEEDING

Jaundice

Breakdown of fetal red blood cells (RBCs) results in bilirubin. **Jaundice** results from accumulation of bilirubin in tissue (hyperbilirubinemia) and is characterized by yellowing of the sclera and skin (see Chaps. 20 and 22). Physiologic jaundice is characterized by a natural and expected rise and fall in bilirubin levels in healthy, term infants; it peaks at approximately 3 to 5 days of life (Riordan, 2004). Pathologic jaundice results from disease processes such as blood abnormalities, liver impairment, metabolic disease, carrier protein deficiency, or binding site deficiencies.

Nonphysiologic Jaundice

When bilirubin levels exceed accepted norms for physiologic jaundice and pathologic jaundice can reasonably be ruled out, nonphysiologic jaundice is the diagnosis (Lauwers & Shinskie, 2005). Nonphysiologic jaundice in breastfed infants results from inadequate intake of breast milk, not dehydration. Decreased caloric intake leads to fewer stools, which is the primary means of biliary excretion. The infant may appear lethargic and weak. The danger of high levels of circulating bilirubin is that it is not attached to carrier proteins, which would prevent its passage through the blood–brain barrier, skin, muscle tissue, and mucous membranes. Neurologic damage, known as kernicterus, can result.

Primary treatment includes unlimited access to breastfeeding; evaluation of appropriate positioning, latch, and intake; and possibly supplementary tube feeds of expressed breast milk or infant formula while infant energy levels and successful breastfeeding are reestablished. Phototherapy (artificial light) may be directed to the infant's exposed skin to convert bilirubin to a form that can be excreted without assistance from the liver (see Chaps. 20 and 22).

Late-Onset Jaundice

Late-onset jaundice, also known as breast milk jaundice, is thought to result from a rare factor in some breast milk. Identification of this factor has been met with controversy and conflicting outcomes. Late-onset jaundice develops slowly; peak bilirubin levels do not appear until the second or third week of life. Treatment includes increased breastfeeding and possibly increased light exposure (Riordan, 2004).

Thrush

Thrush is an oral yeast infection, commonly colonized as *Candida albicans* or *Candida parapsilosis* (Mattos-Graner et al., 2001). Also known as candidiasis, thrush results from an overgrowth of or infection with the yeast-like fungus candida. Modes of person-to-person transmission include saliva, mucosa, breast milk, and stool. The characteristic manifestation is white patches on the mucous membranes of the mouth and vagina. Yeast infections on the diaper area or breasts or under the arms may be red or bright pink. The rash is macular and raised. Patches of yeast appear darker on dark skin. The breastfeeding mother may experience extreme pain, described as burning or acidic, which could lead to premature weaning (Morrill et al., 2005).

Both mother and infant require concomitant treatment. Nurses should advise women to apply a prescription topical antifungal cream to water-cleansed breasts after each breastfeeding (Wiener, 2006). Mothers should rinse off any residue left on the breast before the next feeding. In severe cases of recurrent yeast, providers should consider a systemic antifungal medication for the mother (Wiener, 2006). Palliative treatment for the mother may include ibuprofen. Breast shells may protect sore nipple areas from friction caused by clothing. Women should wear clean bras daily and change breast pads at least with every feeding to deprive yeast of a moist environment, which promotes growth. When directly breastfeeding, the infant should not be so hungry that he or she nurses ravenously. The mother should offer the less sore breast first to promote let-down. Breast pumping may be more comfortable than direct breastfeeding. Women should feed expressed breast milk the same day to avoid possible infant recolonization. Maternal dietary addition of acidophilus from yogurt or cottage cheese may help replace appropriate bacteria in the intestines. Temporary maternal dietary restriction of refined sugars and dairy products may help resolve persistent infections. Some women consume additional garlic, zinc, water, and the vitamin B complex to discourage growth of yeast.

Caregivers should thoroughly swab the infant's oral cavity (including the cheek and pouches) with oral nystatin suspension every 3 hours. They should keep the diaper area clean with clear water, allowing the area to air-dry several times a day. They also should apply a prescription topical antifungal cream before rediapering.

Other family members with yeast infections should receive treatment as well. All family members should perform handwashing before and after handling feeding and breast pump equipment, feeding the baby, changing diapers, using the restroom, or handling toys mouthed by the infant. They should wash the hands of infants frequently as well. They should use paper towels to dry hands and bath towels only once before laundering. Laundry must be washed in hot water (122°F or more) and dried in the sun or high heat of an electric clothes dryer. Each day, the infant's toys and pacifier, artificial nipples, breast pump equipment in contact with breast milk, and breast shells require washing in hot soapy water, rinsing, and boiling for 5 minutes. Any medicine droppers that come in contact with the infant's mouth require washing in hot soapy water and thorough rinsing before storing them in the bottle. After 1 week, families should use new artificial nipples, pacifiers, toothbrushes, and teething toys.

Gastroesophageal Reflux

Gastroesophageal reflux (GER) may be characterized by occasional burps, emesis, or nonregurgitant reflux. It is associated with failure to thrive, irritability with feeding, anemia, hematemesis, pneumonia, and apnea. Regurgitation, more than once a day, occurs in up to 50% of healthy infants and does not necessitate intervention, depending on the caregiver's anxiety (Craig et al., 2004).

Changes in caregiver practices can eliminate or reduce symptoms of GER. Small frequent feeds (every 2 to 3 hours) decrease the volume presented to the stomach at one time. In infants who require tube feedings, transpyloric continuous feeds may help reduce GER symptoms (AAP, 2003). Thickened feeds will increase viscosity to decrease episodes of reflux (Craig et al., 2004; Wenzl et al., 2003). Thickened formula feeds may be appropriate for infants with failure to thrive as a result of GER from increased caloric density, decreased emesis, decreased crying time, and increased postprandial sleep (Orenstein et al., 1999). Breast milk contains the enzyme amylase, which breaks down the starch in most thickening agents. Nutritionally, extra calories from thickened feeds with absorbable carbohydrate increases the percentage of calories from carbohydrate, which decreases the percentage of calories from protein and could serve to make an infant overweight from overfeeding. This also could make it difficult for them to achieve age-appropriate physical milestones. Additionally, the viscosity of thickened feeds may not flow freely from the artificial nipple on a bottle, making it necessary to slit the nipple for a larger opening. Conversely, making the slit too big could cause the feeds to flow too quickly, and the infant would not be able to control the volume extracted.

One of the most traditional therapies for GER has been to change positioning of the infant. Studies have shown that prone or left-lateral positioning is preferable to elevated head of the bead or seated positioning for reducing GER symptoms (Ewer et al., 1999; Orenstein, 1990, 1996). Infants with GER possibly caused by a nasogastric tube benefit from small-bore tubing (8-French) versus large bore tubing (12-French) to assist with clearance of the refluxed acid from the esophagus (Noviski et al., 1999). Pharmacologic therapy or Nissen fundoplication is indicated for the infant with GER and resultant failure to thrive, apnea, or recurrent pneumonia (AAP, 2003).

Colic

Wessel (1954) described **colic** as "unconsolable crying for which no physical cause can be found, which lasts more than 3 hours a day, occurs at least 3 days a week, and continues for at least 3 weeks; spasmodic contractions of smooth muscle, causing pain and discomfort."

The etiology of colic has not been determined (Roberts et al., 2004). Gastrointestinal symptoms include sensitivity to dietary intake, excessive flatulence, and gastric and colonic hypermotility. The infant's legs may be drawn up into the abdomen, fists may be clenched, and facial grimaces may be noted, with body stiffening. Colic appears in breastfed and bottle-fed infants, with peak crying in breastfed infants occurring at 6 weeks, and peak crying in bottle-fed infants occurring at 2 weeks (Lucas & St. James-Roberts, 1998). Crying periods may last 3 to 4 hours and are high pitched.

Treatments to reduce colicky behavior include elimination of dairy products from the breastfeeding mother's diet with gradual, weekly reintroduction of specific products (Riordan, 2004); cessation of smoking for the breastfeeding mother; and complete emptying of one breast during a feeding to allow the infant to receive high-fat hindmilk. Weaning a colicky breastfed infant does not improve symptoms of colic (Roberts et al., 2004). Soy protein–based formulas have not been proved to provide relief from symptoms (AAP Committee on Nutrition, 1998). Relief from symptoms appears to be achieved by holding the infant over the shoulder and thereby applying some pressure on the infant's abdomen. Rocking the infant and rubbing his or her back may have a soothing effect. The infant's father or other close family member best accomplishes these palliative measures. Palliative measures attempted by the breastfeeding mother are often met with an infant who is being cued to eat, whether hungry or not, and do not result in relief of colicky behaviors. White noise may soothe some infants. Bottle-fed infants may benefit from a change in the size of the nipple opening. Encouraging the bottle-fed infant to burp during a feeding may decrease the amount of air that the infant swallows.

Water Intoxication

Water intoxication, which can lead to brain injury, seizures, hypothermia, and edema, can result from feeding too much water, either enterally or parenterally. Inappropriately diluting infant formula, feeding water in place of formula, or giving extra water in hot weather can have negative outcomes, especially during the first month of life, when the newborn's glomerular filtration rate and ability to excrete excess water are decreased. Nurses should mention the inappropriateness of feeding excess water to a baby, especially in warm climates where the practice may be more commonplace.

Questions to Ponder

1. During an appointment with her obstetrician, a 22-year-old pregnant woman confides that she would like to breastfeed her newborn. She shares that one of her biggest obstacles is her fear of breastfeeding in public places. Specifically, her father-in-law has voiced his opinion that he does not feel it is an appropriate thing to do in public.
   - What are your personal feelings about mothers breastfeeding in public? What is the state law about public breastfeeding?
   - What type of dialogue might the nurse suggest for the woman to have with her father-in-law?
   - What might the nurse suggest to the woman that might make breastfeeding in a public place more comfortable?
2. During a well-baby visit, a mother shares with her nurse that her newborn has been constipated for the past 2 weeks. The mother reports that her baby strains with bowel movements, turns red in the face, and has clenched fists, and that her infant's stool is formed, soft, and brown. After talking with the baby's grandmother, the mother changed to a low iron-containing formula and started giving the infant 2 fl oz of apple juice in a bottle every day. The mother reports that the baby appears happier.
   - What additional information would the nurse need to gather?
   - What guidance could the nurse give the mother regarding this problem?
   - Ideally, who would be involved in the counseling session?

SUMMARY

- Feeding a baby is an opportunity for the caregiver and infant to begin developing a personal relationship of trust and affection.
- The nurse is positioned well to assist families with making their choice of how to nourish their baby a successful reality. The sharing of feeding techniques for the chosen feeding methodology is an important part of successful feeding and subsequent growth and development.
- The nutritional benefits of breast milk include high bioavailability and ease of digestion, low potential renal solute load, and epidermal growth factor.
- The immunologic benefits of human milk include factors that help fight infection and prevent allergic diseases.
- Developmental advantages of breastfeeding are psychological and neurologic. Breastfeeding offers the mother and infant dyad a unique opportunity to nurture a trust relationship. Neurologic benefits from feeding breast milk include cognitive development and visual acuity.
- Health advantages to the breastfeeding mother include earlier return to pregravida weight, less risk for osteoporosis and premenopausal ovarian and breast cancers, and protection against anemia and some infections.
- Economically, breast milk offers families substantial savings over the cost of purchasing infant formulas. Additionally, there is no environmental waste, and caregivers lose less work time because of fewer infant illnesses.

- Some maternal infectious diseases, metabolic disorders, and drugs are contraindications to feeding human milk. Sometimes a short separation and breast milk substitute are indicated during maternal illness. HIV and human T-cell lymphotrophic virus are known absolute contraindications to feeding mother's own milk in the United States.
- Alternatives to feeding mother's own milk include donor human milk, commercially prepared infant formulas, and parenteral nutrition. Indications for each feeding type have been established; care should be taken to choose the appropriate means of nutrition.
- Feeding methodologies include direct breastfeeding, bottle feeding, cup feeding, tube feeding, finger feeding, syringe feeding, and parenteral nutrition.
- Nurses can assess the adequacy of infant feeding through infant feeding cues, assessment of intake and output, and growth and weight trends.
- Common problems in the newborn period include jaundice, gastroesophageal disease, colic, thrush, and water intoxication. The nurse can be instrumental in making recommendations to the physicians and parents that are consistent with current literature and in providing supportive measures for infants with these complications.

REVIEW QUESTIONS

1. During a 2-week well-baby visit to the baby's primary physician, the infant's mother explains that she's not sure how often to feed her baby based on the baby's cues. The mother shares the following cues with the nurse. Which cue would the nurse correctly identify as a late sign of hunger?
   A. Crying
   B. Sucking on fingers
   C. Sleeping
   D. Licking or smacking lips
2. A woman at 29 weeks' gestation with her first pregnancy is not sure she should breastfeed her newborn. Which statement, if made by the nurse, would be most accurate in describing a benefit of breastfeeding?
   A. "You'll lose more weight than with bottle feeding."
   B. "The baby will gain more weight more quickly with breast feeding."
   C. "Breast milk will provide the baby with maternal antibodies."
   D. "Maternal–child bonding occurs only with breastfeeding."
3. A bottle-feeding primipara calls the nurse help line at the primary pediatrician's office stating that her 2 week old is "throwing up" after every feeding. The mother states that she feeds him soy formula, 5 fl oz every 3 hours, and that she has to work to get him to finish each bottle. Based on the information, the nurse should suggest that the mother
   A. Make an appointment with the pediatrician to explore antireflux medications.
   B. Feed the baby until he appears satisfied instead of making him finish the bottle.
   C. Consider switching to a low-iron formula.
   D. Come to the emergency department to rule out anatomic abnormalities.
4. The mother of a 6-week-old calls the pediatrician's office stating that her baby is constipated. She describes the stool as hard and pellet-like. Which of the following actions should the nurse suggest that the mother take next?
   A. Give the baby 2 oz of water daily.
   B. Weigh urine output at home for 24 hours and call back with the results.
   C. Change to a low-iron-containing formula.
   D. Keep a list of what the baby consumes in 24 hours.
5. When teaching a new mother about warming formula for a feeding, the nurse should include that the new mother should:
   A. Run warm water over the base of the closed feeding container.
   B. Place the bottle in the microwave for 20 seconds.
   C. Pour the feeding into a saucepan and place on the stove on low heat.
   D. Allow the formula to come to room temperature on the counter.
6. The mother of a 2-day-old in the newborn intensive care unit tells the nurse that she's not getting any milk when she pumps her breasts. She shares that she is pumping four times a day for 5 to 10 minutes each pumping session. Which of the following recommendations should the nurse share with the client?
   A. Increase pumping time to 30 minutes per session.
   B. Stop pumping because her milk is not coming in quickly enough.
   C. Take 1 day off from pumping and try again the next day.
   D. Pump every 3 hours and once through the night for 10 to 20 minutes each session.
7. The mother of a newborn, 24 hours old, states that her baby is falling asleep after just 3 to 5 minutes of breastfeeding. The baby has awakened himself to eat only once since birth. Based on this information, the nurse should advise the woman to
   A. wake the baby up to eat every 3 hours.
   B. allow the baby to sleep as much as possible to regain strength.
   C. start formula feeds and monitor for improved hunger cues.
   D. express human milk and try bottle feeding.
8. A lactating mother calls the maternity nurse with complaints of right-sided breast pain with breastfeeding. The woman describes her breast as warm to the touch with a palpable lump; she is afebrile. Based on this information, the nurse should advise the client to

A. stop breastfeeding immediately and take 299 mg ibuprofen every 4 hours as needed for pain.
B. continue to breastfeed 8 to 12 times per day to pass a likely plugged milk duct.
C. schedule a mammogram immediately.
D. see her primary care provider for an antibiotic prescription.

9. The nurse is caring for a newborn in the transitional nursery who drank 358 mL of a 20 kcal/oz (0.67 kcal/mL) formula. The infant's current weight is 2.98 kg. How many milliliters and calories per kilogram did the infant consume?
A. 120 mL/kg/d, and 2403 kcal/d
B. 120 mL/kg/d, and 80 kcal/kg/d
C. 358 mL/d, and 240 kcal/kg/d
D. 120 mL/kg/d, and 240 kcal/kg/d

REFERENCES

Akman, M., Cebeci, D., Okur, V., Angin, H., Abali, O., & Akman, A. C. (2004). The effects of iron deficiency on infants' developmental test performance. *Acta Paediatrica, 93*(10), 1391–1396.

American Academy of Family Physicians. (2001). *Breastfeeding (position paper).* Retrieved March 1, 2006, from http://www.aafp.org.

American Academy of Pediatrics (AAP). (2000). Hypoallergenic infant formulas. *Pediatrics, 106*(2), 346–349.

American Academy of Pediatrics (AAP). (2003). *Pediatric nutrition handbook* (5th ed.). Elk Grove Village, IL: Author.

American Academy of Pediatrics (AAP). (2005). Policy statement: Breastfeeding and the use of human milk. *Pediatrics, 115*(2), 496–506.

American Academy of Pediatrics (AAP) Committee on Drugs. (2001). Transfer of drugs and other chemicals into human milk. *Pediatrics, 108*(3), 776–789.

American Academy of Pediatrics (AAP) Committee on Nutrition. (1999). Iron fortification of infant formulas. *Pediatrics, 104*(1), 119–123.

American Academy of Pediatrics (AAP) Committee on Nutrition. (1998). Soy protein-based formulas: Recommendations for use in infant feeding. *Pediatrics, 101,* 148–153.

American Academy of Pediatrics (AAP) Work Group on Breastfeeding. (2001). Part 2: The management of breast-feeding. Appendix A: Ten steps to support parents' choice to breast-feed their baby. *Pediatric Clinics of North America, 48*(2).

American Dietetic Association (ADA). (2001). Position of the ADA: Breaking the barriers to breast-feeding. *Journal of the American Dietetic Association, 101*(10), 1213–1219.

American Dietetic Association (ADA). (2003). Guidelines for preparation of formula and breastmilk in health care facilities. Retrieved March 2, 2006, from http://www.eatright.org/cps/rde/xchg/ada/hs.xsl/nutrition_5441_ENU_HTML.htm.

Amin, S., Merle, K., Orlando, M., Dalzell, L., & Guillet, R. (2000). Brainstem maturation in premature infants as a function of enteral feeding type. *Pediatrics, 106*(2), 318–322.

Anderson, J., Johnstone, B., & Remley, D. (1999). Breast-feeding and cognitive development: A meta-analysis. *American Journal of Clinical Nutrition, 70*(4), 525–535.

Arnold, L. (1994). Informal sharing of human milk: Not-so-hypothetical questions, concrete answers. *Journal of Human Lactation, 10,* 43–44.

Auestad, N., Halter, R., Montalto, M., Jacobs, J., Burks, W., Erickson, J., et al. (2001). Growth and development in term infants fed long-chain polyunsaturated fatty acids: A double-masked, randomized, parallel, prospective, multivariate study. *Pediatrics, 108*(2), 372–381.

Auerbach, K. (1993). Sequential and simultaneous breast pumping: A comparison. *International Journal of Nursing Studies, 27,* 257.

Auld, P., Bhangananda, P., & Mehta, S. (1966). The influence of an early caloric intake with IV glucose on catabolism of premature infants. *Pediatrics, 37,* 592–596.

Ayers, J. (2000). The use of alternative therapies in the support of breastfeeding. *Journal of Human Lactation, 16*(1), 52–55.

Barbosa-Cesnik, C., Schwartz, K., & Foxman, B. (2003). Lactation mastitis. *Journal of the American Medical Association, 289*(13), 1609–1612.

Biancuzzo, M. (2003). *Breastfeeding the newborn: Clinical strategies for nurses* (2nd ed.). St. Louis: Mosby.

Birch, E., Garfield, S., Hoffman, D., Uauy, R., & Birch, D. (2000). A randomized controlled trial of early dietary supply of long-chain polyunsaturated fatty acids and mental development in term infants. *Developmental Medicine and Child Neurology, 42,* 174–181.

Birch, E., Hoffman, D., Uauy, R., Birch, D., & Prestidge, C. (1998). Visual acuity and the essentiality of docosahexaenoic acid and arachidonic acid in the diet of term infants. *Pediatric Research, 44,* 201–209.

Bonuck, K. A., Trombley, M., Freeman, K., & McKee, D. (2005). Randomized, controlled trial of a prenatal and postnatal lactation consultant intervention on duration and intensity of breastfeeding up to 12 months. *Pediatrics, 116*(6), 1413–1426.

Cahill, J., & Wagner, C. (2002a). Challenges in breastfeeding: Maternal considerations. *Contemporary Pediatrics, 5,* 94.

Cahill, J., & Wagner, C. (2002b). Challenges in breastfeeding: Neonatal concerns. *Contemporary Pediatrics, 5,* 113.

Carver, J. D. (2003). Advances in nutritional modifications of infant formulas. *American Journal of Clinical Nutrition, 77*(6), 1550S–1554S.

Centers for Disease Control and Prevention (CDC). (2002). National Center for Infectious Diseases: Guidelines for counseling persons infected with human T-lymphotrophic virus type I (HTLV-1) and type II (HTLV-II). *Annals of Internal Medicine, 118,* 448–454.

Centers for Disease Control and Prevention (CDC) and the U.S. Public Health Service (USPHS) Working Group. (1993). Cytomegalovirus (CMV) Infection. Retrieved May 4, 2003, from http://www.cdc.gov/ncidod/diseases/cmv.htm.

Chantry, C. J., Howard, C. R., & Auinger, P. (2006). Full breastfeeding duration and associated decrease in respiratory tract infection in U.S. children. *Pediatrics, 117*(2), 425–432.

Chezem, J., Friesen, C., & Boettcher, J. (2003). Breastfeeding knowledge, breastfeeding confidence, and infant feeding plans: Effects on actual feeding practices. *Journal of Obstetric, Gynecological, and Neonatal Nursing, 32*(1), 40–47.

Clandinin, M. T., Van Aerde, J. E., Merkel, K. L., Harris, C. L., Springer, M. A., Hansen, J. W., & Diersen-Schade, D. A. (2005). Growth and development of preterm infants fed infant formulas containing docosahexaenoic acid and arachidonic acid. *Journal of Pediatrics, 146*(4), 461–468.

Colin, W. B., & Scott, J. A. (2002). Breastfeeding: Reasons for starting, reasons for stopping and problems along the way. *Breastfeeding Review, 10*(2), 13–19.

Collaborative Group on Hormonal Factors in Breast Cancer. (2002). Breast cancer and breastfeeding: Collaborative reanalysis of individual data from 47 epidemiological studies in 30 countries, including 50 302 women with breast cancer and 96 973 women without the disease. *Lancet, 360,* 187–195.

Collins, C. T., Ryan, P., Crowther, C. A., McPhee, A. J., Paterson, S., & Hiller, J. E. (2004). Effect of bottles, cups, and dummies on breast feeding in preterm infants: A randomized controlled trial. *British Medical Journal, 329*(7459), 193–198.

Coutsoudis, A. (2005). Breastfeeding and the HIV positive mother: The debate continues. *Early Human Development, 81*(1), 87–93.

Craig, W. R., Hanlon-Dearman, A., Sinclair, C., Taback, S., & Moffatt, M. (2004). Metoclopramide, thickened feedings, and positioning for gastro-oesophageal reflux in children under two years. *Cochrane Database of Systematic Reviews, 4,* CD003502.

Dellwo Houghton, M., & Graybeal, T. (2001). Breast-feeding practices of Native American mothers participating in WIC. *Journal of the American Dietetic Association, 101*(2), 245–247.

Dewey, K. G., Nommsen-Rivers, L. A., Heinig, M. J., & Cohen, R. J. (2003). Risk factors for suboptimal breastfeeding behavior, delayed onset of lactation, and excess neonatal weight loss. *Pediatrics, 112*(3 Pt. 1), 607–619.

Eden, A. N. (2005). Iron deficiency and impaired cognition in toddlers: An underestimated and undertreated problem. *Paediatric Drugs, 7*(6), 347–352.

Educational Symposium. (2000a). Key issues to address with bottle-feeding. *Pediatric Nursing, 27*(1), 50–51.

Educational Symposium. (2000b). Store brand formulas: A new alternative for bottle-feeding moms. *Pediatric Nursing, 27*(1), 56–57, 60.
Ewer, A., James, M., & Tobin, J. (1999). Prone and left lateral positioning reduce gastro-esophageal reflux in preterm infants. *Archives of Disease in Childhood, Fetal and Neonatal Edition, 81,* F201–F205.
Fomon, S. (2001). Feeding normal infants: Rationale for recommendations. *Journal of the American Dietetic Association, 101*(9), 1002–1005.
Fomon, S., & Ziegler, E. (1999). Renal solute load and *potential* renal solute load. *Journal of Pediatrics, 134,* 11.
Friel, J. K., Andrews, W. L., Edgecombe, C., McCloy, U. R., Belkhode, S. L., L'Abbe, M. R., et al. (1999). Eighteen-month follow-up of infants fed evaporated milk formula. *Canadian Journal of Public Health, 90*(4), 240–243.
Friel, J., Andrews, W., Simmons, B., L'Abbe, M., Mercer, C., & MacDonald, A. (1997). Evaluation of full-term infants fed an evaporated milk formula. *Acta Paediatrica, 86,* 448–453.
Gartner, L., Black, S., Eaton, A., Lawrence, R., Naylor, A., Neifert, M., et al. (1997). American Academy of Pediatrics Work Group on Breast-feeding: Breast-feeding and the use of human milk. *Pediatrics, 100*(6), 1035–1038.
Gdalevich, M. (2001). Breast-feeding and the risk of bronchial asthma in childhood: A systematic review with meta-analysis of prospective studies. *Journal of Pediatrics, 139*(2), 261–262.
Groh-Wargo, S., Thompson, M., & Hovasi Cox, J. (2000). *Nutritional care for high-risk newborns* (3rd ed., revised). Chicago: Precept Press.
Hale, T. (2002). *Medications and mothers' milk* (10th ed.). Amarillo, TX: Pharmasoft Publishing.
Hall, R., & Carroll, R. (2000). Infant feeding. *Pediatrics in Review, 21*(6), 191–199.
Hays, T., & Wood, R. A. (2005). A systematic review of the role of hydrolyzed infant formulas in allergy prevention. *Archives of Pediatric and Adolescent Medicine, 159*(9), 810–816.
Heath, A., Reeves Tuttle, C., Simons, M., Cleghorn, C., & Parnell, W. (2002). A longitudinal study of breast-feeding and weaning practices during the first year of life in Dunedin, New Zealand. *Journal of the American Dietetic Association, 102,* 937–943.
Herbst, J. J. (1989). Development of suck and swallow. In: Lebenthal, E., ed. *Human gastrointestinal development* (pp. 229–239). New York: Raven Press.
Hoogenboezen, T., Degenhart, H., & De Muninch Keizer-Schrama, S. (1989). Vitamin D metabolism in breast-feeding infants and their mothers. *Pediatric Research, 25,* 623–628.
Horwood, L., Darlow, B., & Mogridge, N. (2001). Breast milk feeding and cognitive ability at 7–8 years. *Archives of Disease in Childhood, Fetal and Neonatal Edition, 84,* F23–F27.
Horwood, L., & Fergusson, D. (1998). Breast-feeding and later cognitive and academic outcomes. *Pediatrics, 101*(1), e9.
Howard, C., de Blieck, A, ten Hoopen, C., Howard, F., Lanphear, B., & Lawrence, R. (1999). Physiologic stability of newborns during cup- and bottlefeeding. *Pediatrics, 104,* 1204–1207.
Human Milk Banking Association of North America (HMBANA). (2005). Milk bank locations. Retrieved March 2, 2006, from http://www.hmbana.org/index.php?mode=locations.
Humenick, S., & Gwayi-Chore, M. (2001). Leader or left behind: National and international policies related to breastfeeding. *Journal of Obstetric, Gynecologic, and Neonatal Nursing, 30,* 529–540.
Hyams, J., Treem, W., Etienne, N., Weinerman, H., MacGilpin, D., & Hine, P. et al. (1995). Effect of infant formula on stool characteristics of young infants. *Pediatrics, 95,* 50–54.
Innis, S. M. (2004). Polyunsaturated fatty acids in human milk: An essential role in infant development. *Advances in Experimental Medical Biology, 554,* 27–43.
Kent, J. C., Mitoulas, L. R., Cregan, M. D., Ramsay, D. T., Doherty, D. A., & Hartmann, P. E. (2006). Volume and frequency of breastfeedings and fat content of breast milk throughout the day. *Pediatrics, 117*(3), e387–e395.
Kesaree, N. (1993). Treatment of inverted nipples using a disposable syringe. *Journal of Human Lactation, 9,* 27–29.
KidSource Online. (2002). Retrieved October 20, 2002, from http://www.kidsource/maternal.conn/cost.feeding.html.
Klemola, T., Vanto, T., Juntunen-Backman, K., Kalimo, K., Korpela, R., & Varjonen, E. (2002). Allergy to soy formula and to extensively hydrolyzed whey formula in infants with cow's milk allergy: A prospective, randomized study with a follow-up to the age of 2 years. *Journal of Pediatrics, 140*(2), 219–224.
Koçtürk, T., & Zetterström, R. (1999). Editorial commentary: Thoughts about rates of breast-feeding. *Acta Paediatrica, 88,* 356–358.
Kong, S. K., & Lee, D. T. (2004). Factors influencing decision to breastfeed. *Journal of Advanced Nursing, 46*(4), 369–379.
Labarere, J., Gelbert-Baudino, N., Ayral, A. S., Duc, C., Berchotteau, M., Bouchon, N., et al. (2005). Efficacy of breastfeeding support provided by trained clinicians during an early, routine preventive visit: A prospective, randomized, open trial of 226 mother–infant pairs. *Pediatrics, 115*(2), e139–e146.
Labbok, M. (2001a). The evidence for breastfeeding: Effects of breastfeeding on the mother. *Pediatric Clinics of North America, 48*(1).
Labbok, M. (2001b). The evidence for breastfeeding: Lactogenesis, the transition from pregnancy to lactation. *Pediatric Clinics of North America, 48* (1).
Lang, S., Lawrence, C., & Orme, R. (1994). Cup feeding: An alternative method of infant feeding. *Archives of Disease in Childhood, 71,* 365–369.
Lang, S. (2002). *Breastfeeding special care babies* (2nd ed., pp. 194, 197). China: Harcourt Publishers Limited.
Lau, C. & Hurst, N. (1999). Oral feeding in infants. *Current Problems in Pediatrics, April,* 105–125.
Lauwers, J., & Shinskie, D. (2005). *Counseling the nursing mother: A lactation consultant's guide* (4th ed.). Sudbury, MA: Jones and Bartlett.
Lawrence, G., Greer, F., et al. (2003). American Academy of Pediatrics: Clinical report, guidance for the clinician in rendering pediatric care. *Pediatrics, 111*(4), 908–910.
Lawrence, R. A., & Lawrence, R. M. (2005). *Breast-feeding: A guide for the medical profession* (6th ed.). St. Louis, MO: Mosby.
Lawrence, R. M., & Lawrence, R. A. (2001). The evidence for breastfeeding; given the benefits of breast-feeding, what contraindications exist? *Pediatric Clinics of North America, 48*(1).
Lemons, P., & Loughead, J. (2001). From gavage to oral feedings: Just a matter of time. *Neonatal Network, 20*(3), 7–14.
Leung, A. K., & Sauve, R. S. (2005). Breast is best for babies. *Journal of the National Medical Association, 97*(7), 1010–1019.
Li, R., Darling, N., Maurice, E., Barker, L., & Grummer-Strawn, L. M. (2005). Breastfeeding rates in the United States by characteristics of the child, mother, or family: The 2002 National Immunization Survey. *Pediatrics, 115*(1), e31–e37.
Li, R., Hsia, J., Fridinger, F., Hussain, A., Benton-Davis, S., & Grummer-Strawn, L. (2004). Public beliefs about breastfeeding policies in various settings. *Journal of the American Dietetic Association, 104*(7), 1162–1168.
Life Sciences Research Office. (1998). LSRO Report: Assessment of nutrient requirements for infant formulas. *Journal of Nutrition, 128,* 2059S–2078S.
Lozoff, B. (1988). Behavioral alterations iron deficiency. *Advances in Pediatrics, 35,* 331–359.
Lozoff, B., Jimenez, E., & Wolf, A. (1991). Long-term developmental outcome of infants with iron deficiency. *New England Journal of Medicine, 325,* 687–694.
Lucas, A., & St. James-Roberts, I. (1998). Crying, fussing and colic behaviour in breast- and bottle-fed infants. *Early Human Development, 53*(1), 9–18.
Mattos-Graner, R., Bento de Moraes, A., Rontani, R. & Birman, E. (2001). Relation of oral yeast infection in Brazilian infants and use of a pacifier. *Journal of Dentistry for Children, January–February,* 33–36.
McNamara, T., & Mazurek Melnyk, B. (2001). The effect of food intake on atopic disease in high-risk infants and young children. *Pediatric Nursing, 26*(6), 602–604.
Mead Johnson Nutritionals. (2000, Oct.). *Enfamil® family of products handbook (*No. LB6 revised 10/00). Evansville, IN: Author.
Medoff-Cooper, B., Bilker, W., & Kaplan, J. (2001). Suckling behavior as a function of gestational age: A cross-sectional study. *Infant Behavior & Development, 24,* 83–94.
Michie, C., & Gilmore, J. (2001). Breast feeding and the risks of viral transmission. *Arch Dis Child, 84,* 381–382.
Micromedex. (2003). Measles virus vaccine live (systemic). Retrieved May 4, 2003, from http://www.nlm.nih.gov.

Mitchell, M. (2003). *Nutrition across the life span* (2nd ed.). Philadelphia: W. B. Saunders.

Morrill, J. F., Heinig, M. J., Pappagianis, D., & Dewey, K. G. (2005). Risk factors for mammary candidosis among lactating women. *Journal of Obstetric, Gynecologic, and Neonatal Nursing, 34*(1), 37–45.

Morrow, A. L., & Rangel, J. M. (2004). Human milk protection against infectious diarrhea: Implications for prevention and clinical care. *Seminars in Pediatric Infectious Diseases, 15*(4), 221–228.

National Academy of Sciences. (2002). Dietary Reference Intakes for energy, carbohydrate, fiber, fat, fatty acids, cholesterol, protein, and amino acids. Retrieved April 27, 2003, from http://www.nap.edu.

National Association of Pediatric Nurse Associates and Practitioners (NAPNAP). (2001). NAPNAP position statement on breastfeeding. Retrieved March 1, 2006, from http://www.napnap.org/index.cfm?page=54&sec=57.

Neifert, M., Lawrence, R., & Seacat, J. (1995). Nipple confusion: Toward a formal definition. *Journal of Pediatrics, 126*(6), S125–129.

Nelson, S., Ziegler, E., Copeland, A., Edwards, B., & Fomon, S. (1988). Lack of adverse reactions to iron-fortified formula. *Pediatrics, 81*(3), 360–364.

Noviski, N., Yehuda, Y., Serour, F., & Gorenstein, A. (1999). Does the size of nasogastric tubes affect gastroesophageal reflux in children? *Journal of Pediatric Gastroenterology and Nutrition, 29*, 448–451.

Oddy, W. H. (2002). The impact of breast milk on infant and child health. *Breastfeeding Review, 10*(3), 5–13.

Orenstein, S. (1990). Effects of behavior state of prone versus seated positioning for infants with gastroesophageal reflux. *Pediatrics, 85*(5), 765–767.

Orenstein, S. (1996). Prone positioning in infant gastroesophageal reflux: Is elevation of the head worth the trouble? *Journal of Pediatrics, 117*, 184–187.

Orenstein, S. (1999). Consultation with the specialist, gastroesophageal reflux. *Pediatrics in Review, 20*(1), 24–28.

Pisacane, A., Continisio, G. I., Aldinucci, M., D'Amora, S., & Continisio, P. (2005). A controlled trial of the father's role in breastfeeding promotion. *Pediatrics, 116*(4), 494–498.

Renfrew, M., Lang, S., & Woolridge, M. (2000). Early versus delayed initiation of breastfeeding. *Cochrane Database Systematic Reviews [Computer File]*. Retrieved March 28, 2003, from MD Consult.

Riordan, J. (Ed.) (2004). *Breast-feeding and human lactation* (3rd ed.). Sudbury, MA: Jones and Bartlett.

Roberts, D. M., Ostapchuk, M., & O'Brien, J. G. (2004). Infantile colic. *American Family Physician, 70*(4), 735–740.

Rojjanasrirat, W. (2004). Working women's breastfeeding experiences. *MCN—The American Journal of Maternal and Child Nursing, 29*(4), 222–227.

Rose, V. A., Warrington, V. O., Linder, R., & Williams, C. S. (2004). Factors influencing infant feeding method in an urban community. *Journal of the National Medical Association, 96*(3), 325–331.

Ross Products Division, Abbott Laboratories. (2001, March). *Pediatric Nutritionals Product Guide* (A8138). Columbus, OH: Author.

Samour, P. Q., Helm, K. K., & Lang, C. E. (2003). *Handbook of pediatric nutrition* (2nd ed.). Sudbury, MA: Jones & Bartlett.

Schack-Nielsen, L., Larnkjaer, A., & Michaelsen, K. F. (2005). Long term effects of breast feeding on the infant and mother. *Advances in Experimental Medicine and Biology, 569*, 16–23.

Seppo, L., Korpela, R., Lonnerdal, B., Metsaniitty, L., Juntunen-Backman, K., Klemola, T., et al. (2005). A follow-up study of nutrient intake, nutritional status, and growth in infants with cow milk allergy fed either a soy formula or an extensively hydrolyzed whey formula. *American Journal of Clinical Nutrition, 82*(1), 140–145.

Sharps, P. W., El-Mohandes, A. A., Nabil El-Khorazaty, M., Kiely, M., & Walker, T. (2003). Health beliefs and parenting attitudes influence breastfeeding patterns among low-income African-American women. *Journal of Perinatology, 23*(5), 414–419.

Slusser, W. M., Lange, L., Dickson, V., Hawkes, C., & Cohen, R. (2004). Breast milk expression in the workplace: A look at frequency and time. *Journal of Human Lactation, 20*(2), 164–169.

Slykerman, R. F., Thompson, J. M., Becroft, D. M., Robinson, E., Pryor, J. E., Clark, P. M., et al. (2005). Breastfeeding and intelligence of preschool children. *Acta Paediatrica, 94*(7), 827–829.

Spatz, D. L. (2005). The breastfeeding case study: A model for educating nursing students. *Journal of Nursing Education, 44*(9), 432–434.

Specker, B., Tsang, R., & Hollis, B. (1985). Effect of race and diet on human milk vitamin D and 25-hydroxyvitamin D. *American Journal of Diseases in Children, 139*, 1134–1137.

Spicer, K. (2001). What every nurse needs to know about breast pumping: Instructing and supporting mothers of premature infants in the NICU. *Neonatal Network, 20*(4), 35–41.

Taveras, E. M., Li, R., Grummer-Strawn, L., Richardson, M., Marshall, R., Rego, V. H., et al. (2004). Mothers' and clinicians' perspectives on breastfeeding counseling during routine preventive visits. *Pediatrics, 113*(5), e405–e411.

Thureen, P., & Hay, W. Jr. (2000). Intravenous nutrition and postnatal growth of the micropremie. *Clinics in Perinatology, 27*(1), 197–219.

Trumbo, P., Schlicker, S., Yates, A., & Poos, M. (2002). Dietary Reference Intakes for energy, carbohydrate, fiber, fat, fatty acids, cholesterol, protein and amino acids. *Journal of the American Dietetic Association, 102*(11), 1621–1630.

Tully, M. R., Lockhart-Borman, L., & Updegrove, K. (2004). Stories of success: The use of donor milk is increasing in North America. *Journal of Human Lactation, 20*(1), 75–77.

Tully, M. (2000). Recommendations for handling of mother's own milk. *Journal of Human Lactation, 16*(2), 149–151.

Wagner, C., & Wagner, M. (1999). The breast or the bottle? Determinants of infant feeding behaviors. *Clinics in Perinatology, 26*(2), 505–525.

Waldfogel, J. (2001). International policies toward parental leave and child care. *Future Child, 11*(1), 98–111.

Walter, T., De Andraca, I., Chadud, P., & Perales, C. (1989). Iron deficiency anemia: Adverse effects on infant psychomotor development. *Pediatrics, 84*(1), 7–17.

Wenzl, T. G., Schneider, S., Scheele, F., Silny, J., Heimann, G., & Skopnik, H. (2003). Effects of thickened feeding on gastroesophageal reflux in infants: A placebo-controlled crossover study using intraluminal impedance. *Pediatrics, 111*(4 Pt. 1), e355–e359.

Wessel, M., et al. (1954). Paroxysmal fussing in infancy, sometimes called "colic." *Pediatrics, 114*, 421–434.

Wiener, S. (2006). Diagnosis and management of Candida of the nipple and breast. *Journal of Midwifery and Women's Health, 51*(2), 125–128.

Wilde, C., Addey, C., Bryson, J., et al. (1998). Autocrine regulation of milk secretion. *Biochemistry Society Symposium, 63*, 81–90.

Wright, N. (2001). Part 2: The management of breast-feeding. Appendix B, Resources for physicians, Web sites, books, and organizations. *Pediatric Clinics of North America, 48*(2).

Wyatt, S. N. (2002). Challenges of the working breastfeeding mother. Workplace solutions. *Journal of the American Association of Occupational Health Nurses, 50*(2), 61–66.

CHAPTER 22

The High-Risk Newborn

Mary F. King

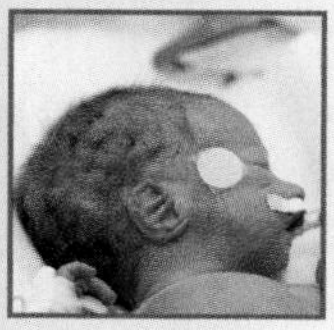

Baby Mitchell was born at 30 weeks' gestation 48 hours after his mother experienced premature rupture of membranes (PROM). His birth weight was 3 lbs, 8 oz (1590 g), considered average for gestational age (AGA). Mitchell was placed on a ventilator because of difficulty establishing respirations.

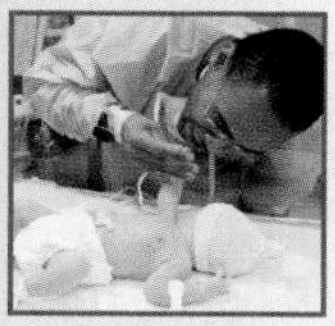

Baby Madeline was born at 39 weeks' gestation following an uneventful labor and vaginal birth. Her weight was 9 lbs, 1 oz, considered large for gestational age (LGA); her length was 21.5 inches. Madeline's parents, Louie and Danita, learned during a routine antepartal ultrasound that Madeline had congenital cleft lip and palate. The early diagnosis provided an opportunity for the parents to research the defect and to receive counseling and teaching about it. Nevertheless, actually seeing Madeline at birth came as "a shock" to Danita. While holding Madeline, she said "Oh, my poor baby." Louie tried to comfort them both.

You will learn more about these stories later in this chapter. Nurses working with such families need to understand the content presented here to manage care and address issues appropriately. Before beginning, consider the following points related to the above scenarios:

- What aspects present issues of immediate concern? What interventions are needed? Explain your answers.
- What are the priorities of care for Baby Mitchell? For Baby Madeline?
- How might the nurse promote parental attachment in each situation?
- What long-term effects related to each newborn's condition does the nurse need to address when teaching the parents? How might these factors affect family functioning?

LEARNING OBJECTIVES

On completion of this chapter, the reader should be able to:

- Correlate small for gestational age (SGA) and large for gestational age (LGA) status with precipitating factors and common complications.
- Prioritize the needs of newborns experiencing complications related to size, gestational age, or both.
- Discuss collaborative care for newborns with complications related to size, gestational age, or both.
- Identify major congenital anomalies experienced by newborns and their underlying factors and conditions.
- Analyze physiologic stressors related to congenital anomalies that may affect newborn extrauterine adaptation negatively.
- Establish immediate priorities for care and provisions for transfer home when congenital anomalies lead to alterations in oxygenation, nutrition, growth, and development.
- Discuss the effects that newborn complications may have on family role attachment and coping.
- Describe collaborative management strategies for newborns with common congenital anomalies.

KEY TERMS

bronchopulmonary dysplasia (BPD)
congenital diaphragmatic hernia
developmental dysplasia of the hip (DDH)
esophageal atresia (EA)
gastroschisis
hydrocephaly
hyperbilirubinemia
hypoglycemia
imperforate anus
intrauterine growth restriction (IUGR)
kernicterus
large for gestational age (LGA)
meningocele
myelomeningocele
omphalocele
oral–facial cleft
phototherapy
postterm newborn
preterm newborn
respiratory distress syndrome
retinopathy of prematurity (ROP)
small for gestational age (SGA)
spina bifida
talipes equinovarus
tracheoesophageal fistula
trophic feedings

With the first cry at birth, newborns begin the transition from fetal to extrauterine life, which involves marked cardiovascular and respiratory changes (see Chap. 20). In addition, newborns must have energy to consume and metabolize nutrients as well as to maintain and produce heat. Preparations for these changes begin in utero, with the maternal body normally providing an optimal environment for fetal growth. For example, during gestation, the fetus develops fat for insulation against heat loss and stores liver glycogen for energy. The fetal lungs produce surfactant to facilitate breathing (see Chap. 11). Primitive neurologic reflexes support future adaptation.

Unfortunately, not all newborns have the necessary physiologic reserves for an uneventful extrauterine transition. Certain complications can affect the newborn's ability to successfully adapt, grow, and not only survive, but also *thrive.* For example, birth asphyxia immediately threatens oxygenation and usually requires immediate resuscitation (see Chap. 20). Congenital anomalies may interfere with the ability to make necessary adjustments. For example, cleft lip, palate, or both compromise the baby's ability to feed optimally and also may impose problems with parental–newborn attachment.

Antepartal and intrapartal health history taking and physical examination can help nurses identify risk factors that may contribute to neonatal complications, thus forewarning the health care team attending a birth to be prepared to accommodate special needs (see Chaps. 13 and 16). In some cases, however, risk factors or problems are not readily apparent at birth, and by poor adaptation, complications, or congenital defects catch the healthcare team by surprise. Thus, vigilant ongoing newborn assessment is essential to detect any gradually evolving problems. Nurses should be alert to subtle changes in newborn behavior, crying, and feeding and be prepared to intervene promptly and aggressively, as a family advocate.

All parents hope for and expect their newborn to be perfect in every way. When a newborn has an obvious or visible congenital anomaly, injury from birth trauma, or other complication requiring aggressive management, nurses need to intervene therapeutically with the entire family to facilitate grieving over the loss of what was expected and healthy coping with the real situation. Nurses also should assist families to accept the outcome and to adjust psychosocially, making the necessary role adaptations to accommodate their new relative.

Occasionally, problems or deviations from normal cause no symptoms or manifest slowly. In such cases, family members may deny or ignore these emerging problems. Nurses need to be aware of individual and collective needs to interact effectively in such cases and to develop with families a culturally sensitive and acceptable plan of care. Knowledge of available resources and community and agency contacts is crucial for collaborative long-term planning.

NEWBORN RISK IDENTIFICATION

Many different factors can present fetal risks and lead to newborn complications. Attempts to identify such risks begin as early as possible, with genetic screening, risk assessments, and early prenatal care and testing (see Chap. 11). Ongoing nursing assessments and evaluations during the first hours of life also help identify newborns at risk (see Chap. 20). A careful and complete nursing history reviews pre-pregnancy and antepartal maternal health, labor and birth history, and the family's cultural and lifestyle practices.

With all clients, the nurse should strive to establish rapport during the initial antepartal visit, regardless of timing. Rather than admonishing a client who is late seeking prenatal care, the nurse should praise her current initiative and use verbal and nonverbal communication to make the client feel that her own needs and those of the fetus are priorities. The nurse should first establish credibility; through active listening, positive attention, eye contact, and touch (when appropriate), the nurse can establish trust. During subsequent antepartal visits, a trusting relationship between nurse and client facilitates acceptance of such things as community support systems for nutrition and transportation when personal resources are limited or absent.

Nurses interact with pregnant clients in various settings and collaborate with other members of the health team to provide education and interventions for expectant parents, the fetus, the newborn, and other important parties (eg, siblings). Chapters 13 and 16 cover in detail problems in pregnancy, labor, and birth that can have ramifications. See Table 22.1 for a summary of common risk factors and their possible neonatal consequences.

PROBLEMS RELATED TO SIZE AND GESTATIONAL AGE

Newborns vary in size and how long they spend in utero. Differences in size can result from genetics or be related to alterations in the quantity and quality of nutrients and growth hormone transferred to the fetus through the placenta during gestation. Differences in duration of gestation vary based on several factors, including whether this is a woman's first pregnancy, any complications that occurred during gestation, problems with estimating correct due date, genetics, and reasons yet unidentified. As discussed in Chapter 20, a baby born between 38 and 42 weeks' gestation is considered *term.* When gestation is less than 38 completed weeks, the newborn is considered a **preterm newborn;** when gestation is more than 42 weeks, the newborn is considered a **postterm newborn.** Both preterm and postterm newborns are at risk for complications (see later discussion).

Birth weights vary normally and can be correlated with gestational week. Soon after birth, the nurse weighs the newborn and estimates gestational age (see Chap. 20). Typical weight for a term newborn ranges from 6.6 to 8.8 lbs (3000 to 4000 g). Weights below this range indicate a problem related to size and may be categorized as follows:

- Low birth weight (LBW): The newborn weighs less than 5.5 lbs (2500 g).
- Very low birth weight (VLBW): The newborn weighs less than 1500 g.
- Extremely low birth weight (ELBW): The newborn weighs 1000 g or less (Tyson & Saigal, 2005).

Major problems associated with an ELBW include intracranial hemorrhage and pulmonary dysfunction. Neurosensory impairments in ELBW newborns include

TABLE 22.1 Pregnancy Risk Factors and Potential Newborn Complications

PROBLEM	POSSIBLE NEONATAL CONSEQUENCES
Maternal Infections	
Toxoplasmosis	Cranial deformity Microcephaly Hydrocephaly
Rubella	Cataracts Deafness Cardiac anomalies Cognitive and motor deficits Cleft lip and palate Intrauterine growth restriction (IUGR)
Syphilis	Cognitive deficits and orthopedic deformities Congenital syphilis
Cytomegalovirus	Severe disability Cranial nerve damage Blindness Deafness Hepatic dysfunction
Herpes	Congenital herpes simplex virus infection Encephalitis Convulsions Shock Neurologic damage Death
Gonorrhea	Severe eye infection (ophthalmia neonatorum) Blindness (if untreated) from corneal damage
Hepatitis B virus (HBV)	Hepatitis B infection with potential for becoming a chronic carrier
Chlamydia	Eye infection
Candidiasis	Thrush (oral *Monilia*)
Human immunodeficiency virus (HIV)	Possible HIV infection resulting from placental transmission, perinatal exposure, or breast milk
Group B streptococcus	Early onset (day of birth): Rapidly progressing pneumonia Respiratory distress Late onset (2–4 wks): Meningitis Intracranial pressure Bulging fontanels Neurologic deficits
Maternal Substance Abuse	
Alcoholism	Fetal alcohol syndrome Spontaneous abortion Low birth weight Low Apgar scores
Cocaine abuse	Congenital anomalies of the brain, kidneys, and urogenital tract SGA IUGR Prematurity Necrotizing enterocolitis Birth asphyxia secondary to placental abruption Brain infarcts Neurobehavioral abnormalities
Smoking or exposure to secondhand tobacco smoke	Spontaneous abortion SGA Low birth weight Increased risk for sudden infant death syndrome (SIDS) Birth defects including congenital urinary tract anomalies

Continued

TABLE 22.1 Pregnancy Risk Factors and Potential Newborn Complications

PROBLEM	POSSIBLE NEONATAL CONSEQUENCES
Heroin	IUGR SGA Increased risk for SIDS Newborn withdrawal Poor feeding Dehydration and electrolyte imbalance related to vomiting and diarrhea
Marijuana	Preterm birth Decreased birth weight and length Possible delays in growth and development
Common Maternal Conditions	
Adolescent pregnancy	Low birth weight Preterm birth IUGR secondary to gestational hypertension, pre-eclampsia Higher death rate in first year of life, in particular if mother's age is younger than 15 years at birth
Maternal–newborn blood group/Rh incompatibility	Kernicterus Hyperbilirubinemia Erythroblastosis fetalis
Hypertensive disorders	IUGR SGA Preterm birth Hypoglycemia Intrauterine hypoxia Birth asphyxia
Diabetes mellitus	Hypoglycemia Congenital anomalies Macrosomia with increased risk for birth injury (shoulder and neck) IUGR or SGA from poor placental perfusion

cerebral palsy, deafness, and blindness, which create long-term health and educational needs.

Size, gestational maturity, and condition are variables that help predict how well a newborn will adapt to the extrauterine environment. The newborn whose growth and development are average for gestational age (AGA) meets the normal expected size for weeks' gestation. The newborn whose growth pattern is at either extreme, either **small for gestational age (SGA)** or **large for gestational age (LGA),** may be at risk for predictable complications. Mortality and morbidity rates are linked directly with birth weight and completed weeks' gestation (Newburn-Cook et al., 2002; Porth, 2005). See Figure 22.1 for a comparison of the appearances of SGA, AGA, and LGA newborns.

Classifications of SGA, AGA, and LGA are independent from classifications of preterm, term, and postterm newborns. For example, a baby born at 40 weeks' gestation would be considered term. If he or she also weighed less than 5.5 lbs (2500 g), the newborn would be considered SGA. Similarly, a baby born at 34 weeks' gestation who weighed 5.5 lbs would be LGA, despite his or her preterm status.

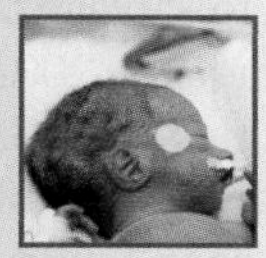

Consider baby Mitchell, described at the beginning of the chapter. How would the nurse classify Mitchell based on gestational age? Suppose Mitchell was born at 40 weeks' gestation. How would the nurse then classify him based on his birth weight?

SGA Newborn

The weight of the SGA newborn typically is below the 10th percentile on the intrauterine growth chart for gestational age (see Chap. 20). SGA newborns near or at term typically weigh less than 5.5 lbs (2500 g).

Etiology

Some newborns have genetically small stature and thus are SGA. Many SGA newborns, however, experienced growth problems in utero. **Intrauterine growth restriction (IUGR)** is the name given when fetal growth is below normal because the fetus is not receiving necessary nutrients and oxygen required for development. IUGR

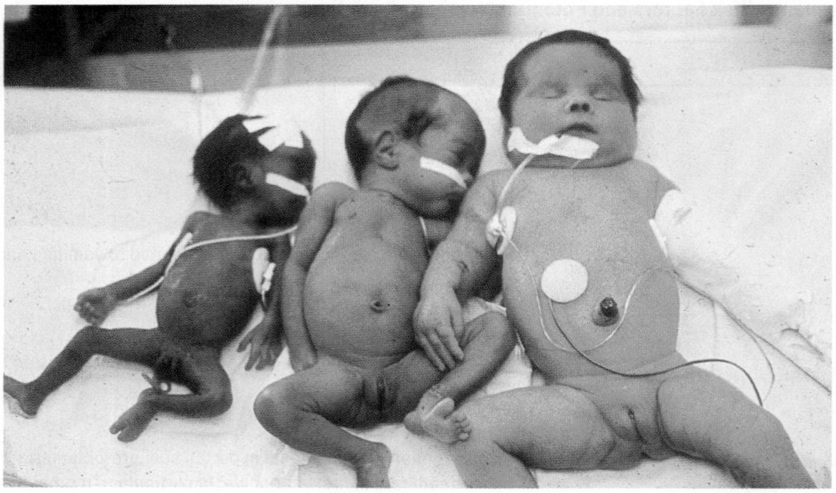

FIGURE 22.1 Comparison of SGA, AGA, and LGA newborns. Reprinted with permission from Korones, S. B. (1986). *High-risk newborn infants: The basis for intensive nursing care* (4th ed.). St. Louis: C. V. Mosby.

can develop any time in pregnancy, but its point of onset can have different effects. With *symmetric (early-onset) IUGR,* the fetus tends to lag behind in growth for most of the pregnancy, resulting in a newborn proportionally small all over. This condition usually results from a long-term or chronic prenatal problem, such as placental dysfunction, maternal substance abuse, phenylketonuria, or chromosomal abnormalities. With *asymmetric (late-onset) IUGR,* the fetus typically grows normally until the third trimester. Subsequent growth problems cause the head to continue normal development, but body size falls behind normal parameters as a result of "brain sparing" (nutrients and oxygen are diverted away from the body to salvage the brain at the expense of other organs) (Akera & Ro, 2003).

Box 22.1 lists risk factors contributing to SGA, IUGR, or both. Some of these conditions are modifiable. For example, smoking in pregnancy has been found to double the incidence of IUGR, with infants displaying birth weights considerably less than newborns of nonsmoking women (Newburn-Cook et al., 2002).

Newborn Characteristics

SGA newborns are similar in physical appearance to and share some needs with preterm newborns (see later discussion). Both types of infants appear scrawny and underdeveloped with little subcutaneous fat for insulation and scant brown fat for heat production, making hypothermia a common problem. The head may appear large in proportion to the body; poorly developed suck pads give the head an oval appearance. The face is angular and pinched. Decreased muscle mass is most evident in the buttocks, thighs, and cheeks.

The stomachs of SGA newborns have a small capacity. Unlike preterm newborns, however, term SGA newborns with no additional complications are gestationally and physically mature and therefore have coordinated suck and swallow (Jones et al., 2002). This enables them to tolerate early oral feedings safely. Because they tend to be weak, however, they may benefit from nasogastric tube feedings to conserve energy and promote weight gain.

BOX 22.1 Risk Factors Associated With IUGR, SGA, or Both

Maternal Factors

- Adolescent pregnancy
- Anemia
- Cardiac disease
- Chronic renal disease
- Cigarette smoking
- Diabetes
- Hypertension
- Infection
- Malnutrition
- Residence at high altitude
- Respiratory disease
- Sickle cell disease
- Substance use (alcohol, drugs)

Uterine/Placental Factors

- Abruptio placentae
- Decreased blood flow in uterus and placenta
- Infection in the tissues around the fetus
- Placenta previa

Fetal Factors

- Birth defects
- Chromosomal abnormalities
- Infection
- Multiple gestation

Typically, SGA newborns do not demonstrate "catch up" growth. Stunted growth and problems related to poor development of vital organs may persist beyond the preschool years.

LGA Newborns

Excessive body weight is the defining criterion for LGA (also called *macrosomia*) (see Chap. 16). Depending on the assessment tool used, adjustments may be considered for gestational age and sex. Typically, newborns above the 90th percentile on growth charts, which equals approximately two standard deviations above the mean for weight, are considered LGA (Akera & Ro, 2003). In some cases, birth weight above 4000 g alone has been used to classify a newborn as LGA. Regardless of preterm, term, or postterm status, any birth weight exceeding 4500 g is considered excessive (Lapunzina et al., 2002). See Box 22.2 for risk factors.

Newborn Characteristics

LGA newborns typically have rounded flushed faces and prominent chin pads. Shoulders are large and broad; abdomens are round and protuberant with increased body mass. Because of their physical size, they may be mistaken at first glance for "older" infants.

LGA newborns may be healthy and normal pending physical appraisal for gestational age and neurologic maturity. Nevertheless, they are at risk for such complications as birth trauma, hypoglycemia, and congenital anomalies.

Associated Complications

Birth Trauma. Trauma can result during vaginal or cesarean birth of the LGA newborn (see Chap. 16). Ecchymosis and erythema may develop from birth injuries related to poor fit of passenger with passageway or from use of forceps. Subcutaneous bleeding or extensive bruising can lead to jaundice. Observation and inspection of the newborn's symmetry of movement may reveal neurologic trauma or paralysis.

Head trauma may result in increased intracranial pressure (ICP). Close monitoring of the newborn's behavior may provide clues for detecting subtle and insidious signs of increased ICP, which include altered sleep–wake cycles, crying, and pain. Later signs of increased ICP are more ominous and include bulging fontanels, high-pitched crying, and seizure activity.

Vaginal birth of the LGA newborn with very wide shoulders commonly results in clavicular fracture (Akera & Ro, 2003). Supraclavicular edema and ecchymosis may be apparent on inspection; crepitus can be palpated over the fractured clavicle. Swaddling, careful handling, and gentle cuddling promote comfort for the newborn with birth trauma.

Hypoglycemia. LGA newborns are at risk for **hypoglycemia** (serum blood glucose level below normal values; in term newborns, it ranges from 40 to 60 mg/dL). This common and dangerous complication usually develops within 2 to 6 hours of birth.

Newborn hypoglycemia is related closely to size and condition as well as to complications of labor and birth that interfere with placental perfusion (Johnson, 2003). A close relationship between maternal and fetal glucose concentrations during both early and late gestation has been well documented (Yariv et al., 2004), so a drop in maternal glucose level affects the fetus as well.

When the laboring woman is on prolonged NPO status, her body uses its glucose stores for energy. Once these stores are depleted, the maternal body metabolizes fat. In addition, emergency cesarean birth at any time may be necessary, and reliable venous access must be maintained throughout labor. The nurse administers intravenous (IV) fluids with dextrose to the laboring woman; and also may offer concentrated glucose by mouth in the form of clear hard lollipops, which do not jeopardize NPO status. The concentrated sugar source is absorbed rapidly into the sublingual vessels and can help prevent glucose depletion, yet will not contribute to risk for aspiration should emergency surgery be required. Lollipops are preferred over hard candies because a woman in labor could become startled by a sudden and unusually strong contraction, possibly resulting in foreign body aspiration. A lollipop on a paper stick does not pose the choking hazard associated with hard candies. These nursing interventions provide a quick glucose source for the laboring woman and may prevent undiagnosed, asymptomatic fetal hypoglycemia (Yariv et al., 2004).

Many times, low blood glucose levels in newborns have no accompanying clinical signs or symptoms. Indications of hypoglycemia include a change in level of consciousness (eg, fretfulness, lethargy, stupor) and poor feeding despite previous successful efforts. The nurse should be alert for a whimpering or weak cry, tremors or jitteriness, respiratory difficulties, and central cyanosis. Untreated hypoglycemia may result in cardiac failure (Cornblath et al., 2000).

Congenital Anomalies. LGA newborns are at increased risk for skeletal deformities such as hip subluxation and talipes calcaneovalgus (Lapunzina et al., 2002). These

BOX 22.2 Risk Factors for LGA Newborn

- Excessive pregnancy weight gain
- Fetal exposure to high estrogen levels
- High maternal birth weight
- LGA in previous infants
- Maternal diabetes
- Maternal pregravid obesity
- Multiparity

problems are thought to be related to mechanical factors secondary to a cramped intrauterine environment with little amniotic fluid to facilitate movement and positioning. Incidence of hydrocephaly increases with birth weight; however, this probably is related to the heaviness of fluid volume rather than true LGA (Lapunzina et al., 2002). Minor skin conditions, such as pigmented nevi, angiomas, and vascular birthmarks, also are associated with LGA status (Lapunzina et al., 2002).

Preterm Newborn

A classification of preterm (premature) is used when a baby is born any time before the 38th week of gestation, independent of birth weight. Birth before 30 weeks' gestation is considered "very preterm" (Pressler et al., 2001). LBW typically accompanies preterm status because the untimely birth interrupts normal growth and development.

Ongoing technologic advances have enabled babies born as young as 23 to 25 weeks' gestation to survive (Jones et al., 2002). Nevertheless, such newborns may have impaired vision and hearing, chronic lung disorders, and lifelong cognitive impairment (Newburn-Cook et al., 2002). See Box 22.3 for factors associated with preterm birth.

Newborn Characteristics

Characteristics of preterm newborns are related to gestational age. The Ballard Gestational Age assessment tool correlates findings with gestational age, including VLBW newborns (see Chap. 20).

The appearance of preterm newborns often differs significantly from that of term babies. Generally, the preterm newborn's skin is ruddy, thin, and permeable, with visible blood vessels. Fine, downy lanugo covers the skin; vernix is scant unless the newborn is close to term. Heels and palms are shiny and gelatinous with few creases. The head appears large in proportion to the body; the eyelids may still be fused in very preterm newborns. Eyelids may be edematous, and eye rolling may be noted with wakefulness and spontaneous eye opening. Fontanelles are large; cranial suture lines are prominent and moveable. The chest is small with little to no breast tissue. The abdomen has a "pot belly" appearance. In females, the external genitalia appear large with widely separated labia and a large clitoris. In males, the scrotal sac is loose and possibly empty (undescended testes) with few rugae.

The cry of preterm newborns may be weak and whimpering. Respirations are typically rapid, irregular, possibly shallow, and diaphragmatic with periods of apnea. Respiratory distress is evidenced by sternal retractions, inspiratory lag, flared nostrils with inspiration, and grunting on expiration.

Posture is reflective of limp, weak muscles. Preterm newborns tend to stay in place when positioned. Seizure activity may be evidenced by stiffness.

Preterm newborns also demonstrate specific behavioral responses to stress. Examples include averting gaze, tremors, and splaying of fingers of one or both hands. In some cases, they may simply sigh and become flaccid. Such behaviors, in conjunction with physiologic indicators of poor tolerance to stress (eg, tachycardia), brief periods of apnea, and color changes, are cues that the newborn is becoming overstressed and needs rest.

Figure 22.2 compares in detail typical physical examination and reflex characteristics in preterm versus term infants.

BOX 22.3 Factors Associated With Preterm Birth

- Previous preterm birth
- Uterine anomalies: bicornate uterus, incompetent cervix
- Multiple gestation
- Polyhydramnios (uterine stretching)
- Trauma
- Obstetric conditions requiring pregnancy termination
- Maternal urinary tract infection

Associated Complications

Preterm newborns face complications related to immaturity of the central nervous system and other vital organs, making the already stressful extrauterine transition even more challenging (see Chap. 20). Subsequently, preterm newborns are at risk for numerous complications. Most of them receive care in a neonatal intensive care unit (NICU). If the birth facility does not have an NICU and preterm birth is expected, the laboring woman may be transferred to a facility with an NICU, if time permits. Otherwise, the newborn will be transported to the facility immediately after birth.

Birth Asphyxia. Preterm newborns may develop birth asphyxia from inadequate oxygen transfer during labor and birth. If a preterm newborn does not breathe spontaneously, the heart rate is below 100 beats per minute (bpm), or both, the health care team begins positive-pressure ventilations immediately. If the heart rate is below 60 bpm, they begin cardiopulmonary resuscitation (CPR) immediately. Central cyanosis and slow gasping respirations are indications to begin immediate rescue breathing. Intubation may be necessary to maintain a patent airway and to deliver more effective ventilations. A handheld manual resuscitation bag attached to an oxygen source may be required to deliver oxygen with assisted breaths.

The size of the endotracheal (ET) tube used for intubation demonstrates the tiny lumen of the preterm baby's airway. An ET tube of 2 to 2.5 mm is used for

(text continues on page 922)

A

Premature Infant

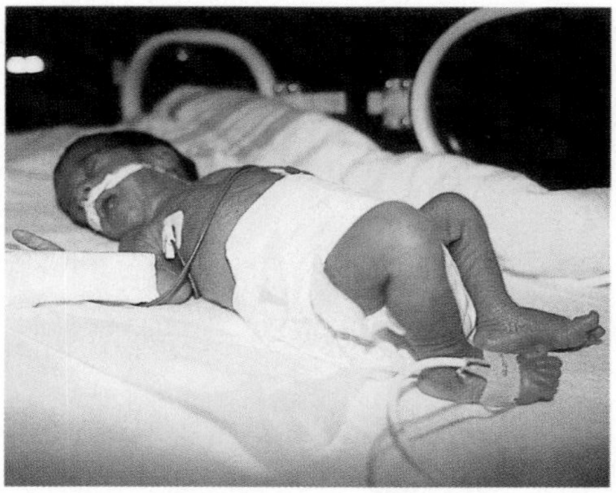

Full-term Infant

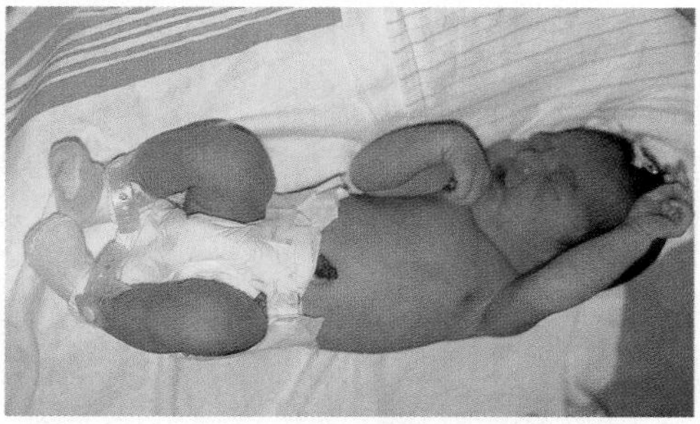

RESTING POSTURE *The premature infant is characterized by very little, if any, flexion in the upper extremities and only partial flexion of the lower extremities. The full-term infant exhibits flexion in all four extremities.*

B

Premature Infant, 28–32 Weeks

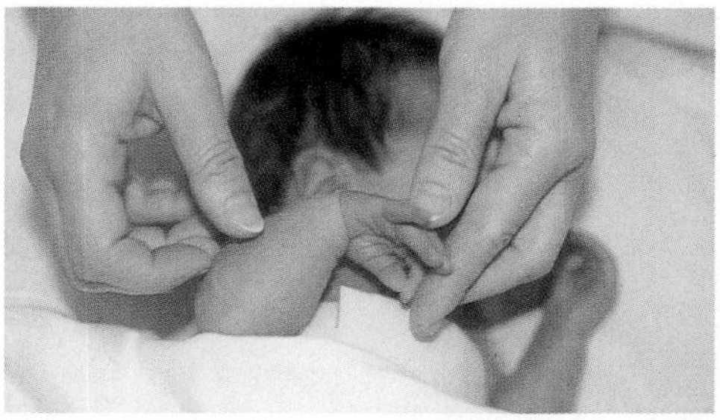

Full-term Infant

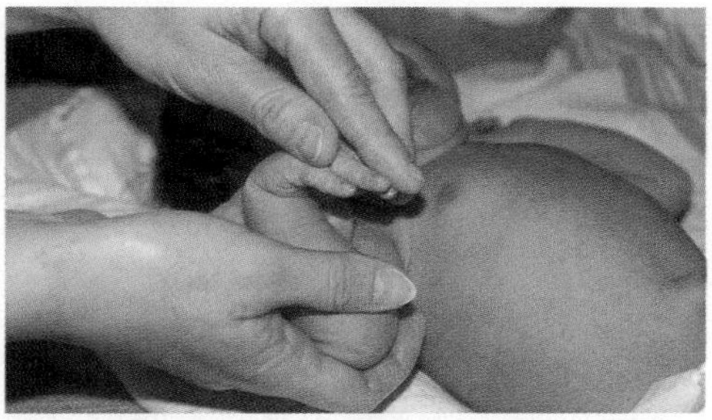

WRIST FLEXION *The wrist is flexed, applying enough pressure to get the hand as close to the forearm as possible. The angle between the hypothenar eminence and the ventral aspect of the forearm is measured. (Care must be taken not to rotate an infant's wrist.) The premature infant at 28–32 weeks' gestation will exhibit a 90° angle. With the full-term infant it is possible to flex the hand onto the arm.*

C

Premature Infant

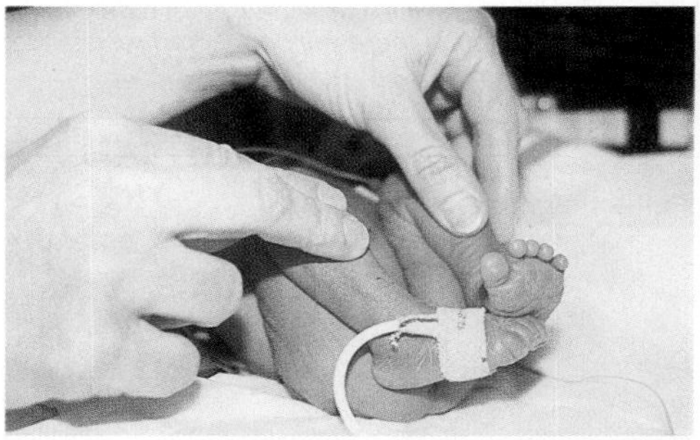

Full-term Infant

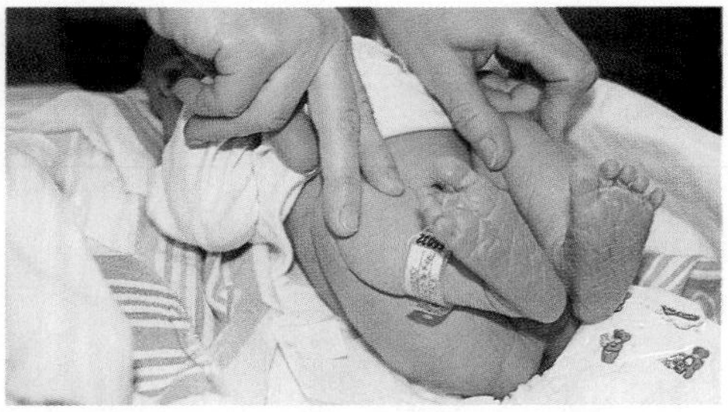

Response in Premature Infant

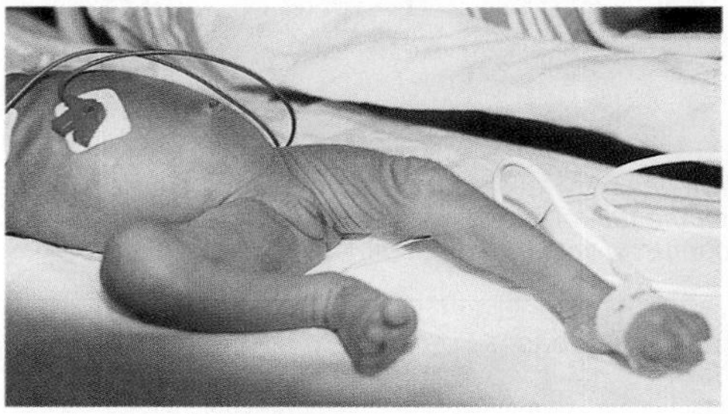

Response in Full-term Infant

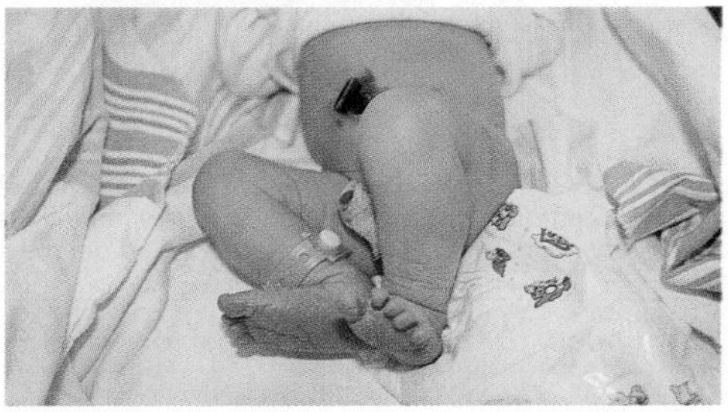

RECOIL OF EXTREMITIES *Place an infant supine. To test recoil of the legs (1) flex the legs and knees fully and hold for 5 seconds (shown in top photos), (2) extend the legs fully by pulling on the feet, (3) release. To test the arms, flex forearms and follow same procedure. In the premature infant response is minimal or absent (bottom left); in the full-term infant extremities return briskly to full flexion (bottom right).*

FIGURE 22.2 Physical and neuromuscular maturation in preterm and term newborns. (**A**) Resting posture. (**B**) Wrist flexion. (**C**) Recoil of extremities. *(Continued)*

D

Premature Infant | **Full-term Infant**

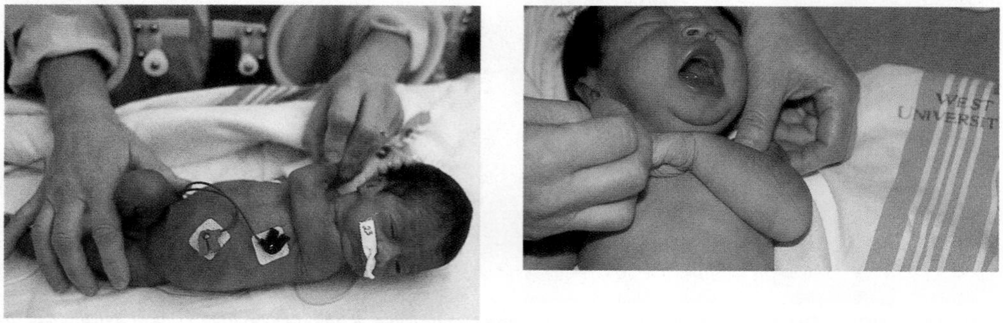

SCARF SIGN *Hold the baby supine, take the hand, and try to place it around the neck and above the opposite shoulder as far posteriorly as possible. Assist this maneuver by lifting the elbow across the body. See how far across the chest the elbow will go. In the premature infant the elbow will reach near or across the midline. In the full-term infant the elbow will not reach the midline.*

E

Premature Infant | **Full-term Infant**

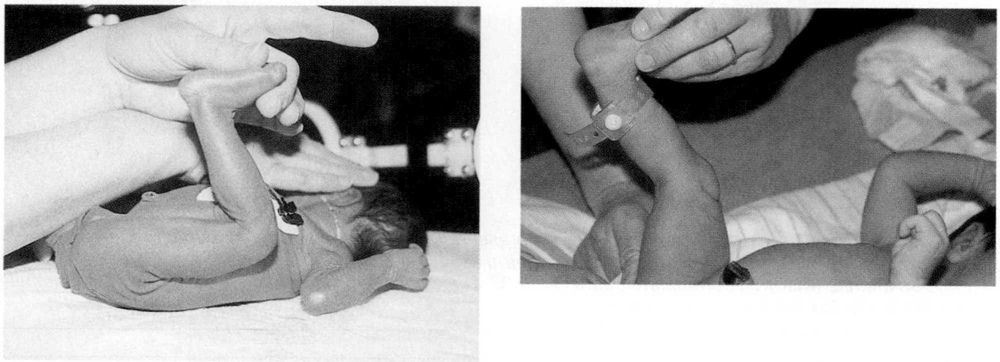

HEEL TO EAR *With the baby supine and the hips positioned flat on the bed, draw the baby's foot as near to the ear as it will go without forcing it. Observe the distance between the foot and head as well as the degree of extension at the knee. In the premature infant very little resistance will be met. In the full-term infant there will be marked resistance; it will be impossible to draw the baby's foot to the ear.*

F

Premature Infant | **Full-term Infant**

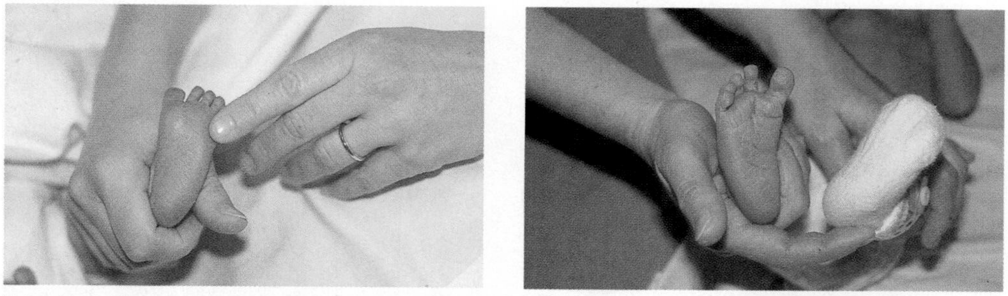

SOLE (PLANTAR) CREASES *The sole of the premature infant has very few or no creases. With the increasing gestation age, the number and depth of sole creases multiply, so that the full-term baby has creases involving the heel. (Wrinkles that occur after 24 hours of age can sometimes be confused with true creases.)*

FIGURE 22.2 *(Continued)* (**D**) Scarf sign. (**E**) Heel to ear. (**F**) Sole (plantar) creases.

G

Premature Infant | **Full-term Infant**

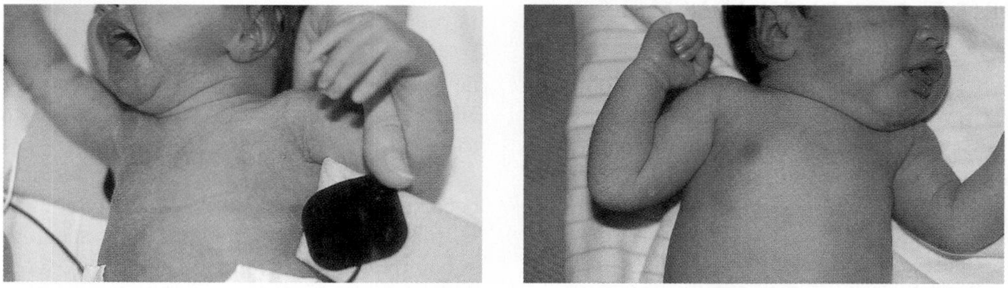

BREAST TISSUE *In infants younger than 34 weeks' gestation the areola and nipple are barely visible. After 34 weeks the areola becomes raised. Also, an infant of less than 36 weeks' gestation has no breast tissue. Breast tissue arises with increasing gestational age due to maternal hormonal stimulation. Thus, an infant of 39 to 40 weeks will have 5 to 6 mm of breast tissue, and this amount will increase with age.*

H

Premature Infant, 34–36 Weeks | **Full-term Infant**

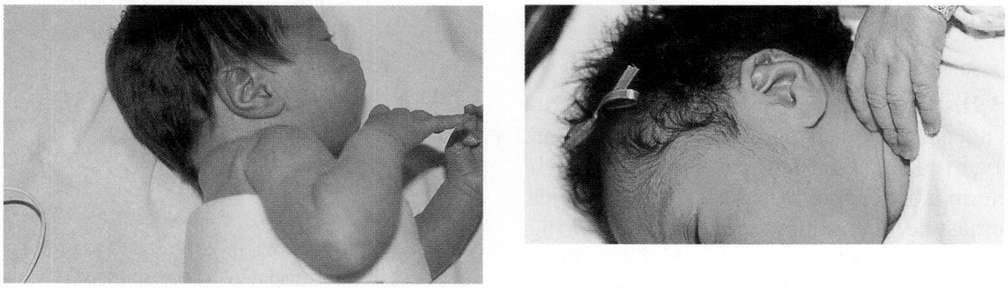

EARS *At fewer than 34 weeks' gestation infants have very flat, relatively shapeless ears. Shape develops over time so that an infant between 34 and 36 weeks has a slight incurving of the superior part of the ear; the term infant is characterized by incurving of two thirds of the pinna; and in an infant older than 39 weeks the incurving continues to the lobe. If the extremely premature infant's ear is folded over, it will stay folded. Cartilage begins to appear at approximately 32 weeks so that the ear returns slowly to its original position. In an infant of more than 40 weeks' gestation, there is enough ear cartilage so that the ear stands erect away from the head and returns quickly when folded. (When folding the ear over during examination be certain that the surrounding area is wiped clean or the ear may adhere to the vernix.)*

I

Premature Male | **Full-term Male**

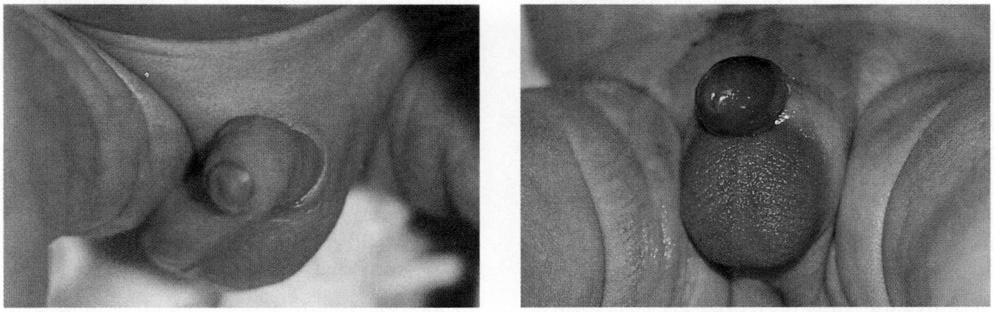

MALE GENITALIA *In the premature male the testes are very high in the inguinal canal and there are very few rugae on the scrotum. The full-term infant's testes are lower in the scrotum and many rugae have developed.*

J

Premature Female | **Full-term Female**

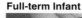

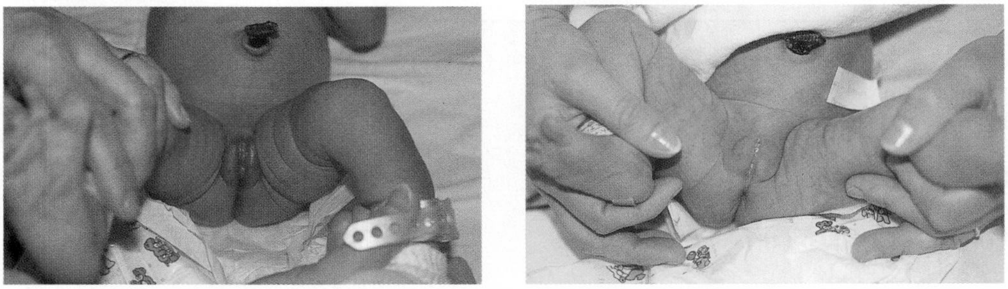

FEMALE GENITALIA *When the premature female is positioned on her back with hips abducted, the clitoris is very prominent and the labia majora are very small and widely separated. The labia minora and the clitoris are covered by the labia majora in the full-term infant.*

FIGURE 22.2 *(Continued)* (**G**) Breast tissue. (**H**) Ears. (**I**) Male genitalia. (**J**) Female genitalia.

VLBW newborns, whereas an ET tube of 3.5 to 4 mm is used for LBW newborns. Arterial blood gases are evaluated for oxygen and carbon dioxide concentrations and acid–base balance. The lowest possible concentration of oxygen is used to reduce the risk for oxygen toxicity while maintaining adequate oxygenation.

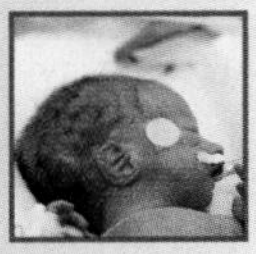

Think back to baby Mitchell from the chapter opener. Mitchell was intubated and placed on a ventilator. What size ET tube would the nurse expect to be used for care?

Respiratory Distress. The preterm newborn's most crucial need is adequate oxygenation. Respiratory support is the priority, even before birth in cases when it is obvious that preterm labor cannot be halted. Corticosteroids (eg, betamethasone) are administered to the laboring woman, which the placenta transfers to the fetus. They hasten fetal lung maturity and reduce the severity of respiratory illness. In addition to its respiratory benefits, antenatal corticosteroid therapy contributes to increased cardiac, renal, metabolic, and hematologic stability (Richardson et al., 1999). A new medication used to prevent prematurity from spontaneous preterm labor is 17-α-hydroxyprogesterone caproate. Researchers report that this drug helps reduce preterm births as well as minimize the need for supplemental oxygen in premature infants (Meis et al., 2003).

Respiratory distress may become apparent shortly after birth. Regardless of size, all preterm newborns are at risk for **respiratory distress syndrome** (RDS) related to deficiency of surfactant secondary to lung immaturity. Without adequate surfactant to reduce surface tension in the lungs and to promote alveolar stability, the alveoli tend to collapse with each expiration. Consequently, each breath requires the same high pressure as the initial breath at birth to inflate the lungs. The weak preterm newborn cannot sustain the work of breathing even using all accessory muscles and grunting, both of which attempt to keep the alveoli open.

Preterm newborns may receive an extract of naturally occurring surfactant at birth, which requires passage of an ET tube immediately after birth (Pharmacology Box 22.1). A commercial preparation of surfactant, such as Infasurf, Isosurf, or Surfanta, is then administered directly into the lungs through the ET tube. Then with a bag-breathing device connected to the ET tube, the surfactant is dispersed throughout the alveoli (Crowley, 2001). When surfactant is administered in this way at birth, the newborn is kept on a plane inclined by 30 degrees. Suctioning is avoided for 1 hour if possible to prevent inadvertent removal of surfactant before it can coat the alveoli. Auscultation of the lung fields of the newborn who has received ET surfactant typically reveals coarse rhonchi and crackles until the alveoli have absorbed the medication. The baby also may require mechanical ventilation (Fig. 22.3). Oxygen is administered at the lowest concentration possible to prevent damaging effects of oxygen on the preterm newborn's retina, called retinopathy of prematurity.

Retinopathy of Prematurity. Retinopathy of prematurity (ROP), formerly termed *retrolental fibroplasia,* results from administration of high oxygen concentrations that preterm newborns frequently require. Such high concentrations are toxic to the fragile retinal blood vessels of preterm infants, which begin to leak protein and tend to bleed (Porth, 2005). Negative effects include structural changes to the retinal tissue, tangling of retinal vessels, retinal detachment, and blindness (Hansen, 1998; Crowley, 2001).

The retinal vascular bed can sustain permanent damage and scarring when oxygen concentrations exceed 40%. Nevertheless, such concentrations may be required during resuscitation to ensure perfusion of the brain and vital organs. Monitoring oxygen saturation levels through evaluation of arterial blood gases and pulse oximetry is essential. In addition, referrals for eye examinations are indicated for all preterm newborns who have received oxygen therapy.

● PHARMACOLOGY 22.1 Surfactant (Survanta)

ACTION: Surfactant provides exogenous (naturally occurring) material to coat the alveoli, rapidly improving oxygenation and lung compliance.

PREGNANCY RISK CATEGORY: X

DOSAGE: 4 mL/kg intratracheally; four doses in first 48 hours of life

POSSIBLE ADVERSE EFFECTS: Transient bradycardia, rales

NURSING IMPLICATIONS

- Suction infant before administration.
- Assess infant's respiratory rate, rhythm, arterial blood gases, and color before administration.
- Ensure proper ET tube placement before dosing.
- Change infant's position during administration to encourage drug to flow to both lungs.
- Assess infant's respiratory rate, color, and arterial blood gases after administration.
- Do not suction ET tube for 1 hour after administration to avoid removing drug.

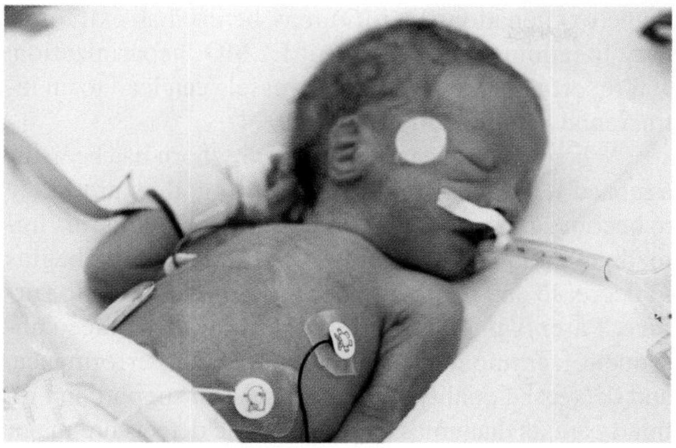

FIGURE 22.3 A preterm newborn receiving mechanical ventilation.

Bronchopulmonary Dysplasia. Infants often require continuous oxygen therapy through nasal cannula and bronchodilator therapy through nebulization. **Bronchopulmonary dysplasia (BPD)** is a chronic lung disease that results from immaturity and the use of long-term mechanical ventilation after the development of RDS (Ritchie, 2002). BPD predisposes the infant to respiratory infections and reactive airway disease.

Necessary referrals for continuing care include respiratory and home health care. The home care nurse monitors weekly oxygen saturation levels, which should remain at 94% to 95% (Bernbaum, 2000). Home chest percussion can be accomplished with an electric toothbrush that has gauze padding over the head of the apparatus. Upon discharge from the NICU, most preterm infants have apnea monitors in the home, and caregivers should be taught the basics of infant rescue breathing and CPR in the event that a need arises.

Feeding Problems. For preterm newborns, oral feedings may be delayed until sucking and swallowing reflexes are coordinated (usually at 32 to 34 weeks' gestation) (Jones et al., 2002). Before 32 weeks' gestation, newborns cannot suck, swallow, and breathe simultaneously and therefore are prone to aspiration (Anderson & Loughead, 2002). In addition, gastrointestinal immaturity poses problems and safety issues. For example, the underdeveloped esophageal sphincter predisposes the baby to painful gastroesophageal reflux. Stomach emptying is delayed; gut motility is diminished. Bile salts and pancreatic enzymes for digestion of enteral feedings are lacking.

To compound the feeding difficulties faced by preterm newborns, their nutritional needs actually are increased because birth interrupted fetal growth at its peak. Fluid needs are also greater than that of term newborns because of increased insensible losses through permeable skin surfaces and increased excretion related to renal inability to concentrate urine. If the preterm newborn does not receive fluid and nutritional support from the first day of life, dehydration and catabolism begin (Neu, 2002).

Anemia of Prematurity. Anemia of prematurity primarily results from the physiologic immaturity of the hematologic system, leading to diminished erythropoiesis. Frequent blood specimens needed for laboratory analysis can further exacerbate this condition.

Cold Stress. The preterm infant is susceptible to cold stress because of an inability to generate heat, increased heat loss, and impaired thermoregulation resulting from immaturity of the central nervous system. Brown fat deposits develop around vital organs late in gestation; the preterm infant lacks this protection against hypothermia (Hansen, 1998). Excessive heat loss also is attributable to the lack of insulating subcutaneous fat, a high body surface area–to–body mass ratio, and thin permeable skin with increased insensible fluid loss (Hansen, 1998). In term infants, positions that hold the extremities close to the body, such as full flexion, serve to prevent heat loss. The lack of flexion in preterm infants is demonstrated by a frog-like position with splayed extremities. Heat is readily lost to the environment through radiation.

Necrotizing Enterocolitis. Depending on gestational age, the preterm newborn's gastrointestinal tract has diminished gastric enzymes, decreased gut motility, weak esophageal sphincter tone, and delayed gastric emptying (Anderson & Loughead, 2002). When stressors such as infection, hypoxia, or other inflammatory mediators occur, gastrointestinal mucosal injury may lead to necrotizing enterocolitis (NEC) (Anderson & Loughead, 2002). NEC is an acute inflammatory bowel disorder associated with ischemia leading to bowel necrosis and perforation. With deficient oxygen, the mucus-secreting cells of the bowel are inactivated and bacteria invade the muscular layer of the bowel wall.

Because the premature newborn is susceptible to NEC, all efforts are made to halt preterm labor. Tocolytics such as ritodrine are used initially to reduce the frequency and intensity of uterine contractions (see Chap. 13). If given to prevent recurrent premature birth, 17-α-hydroxyprogesterone caproate has the added benefit of minimizing risks for NEC after birth (Meis et al., 2003). Breast milk feedings, especially with probiotics, protect the GI tract from injury and bacterial invasion, reducing the incidence and severity of NEC (Lin, et al., 2005).

If a baby shows the onset of symptoms of NEC, the nurse should withhold all oral or enteral feedings and notify the neonatologist or pediatrician immediately. Radiologic procedures such as flat-plate or abdominal computed tomography (CT) can confirm NEC. The nurse should administer and monitor total parenteral nutrition (TPN) until enteral feedings can be resumed. Surgical resection of the affected bowel segment and possibly the formation of an ostomy may be necessary when the intestine perforates or with peritonitis. The nurse should administer broad-spectrum antibiotics, IV fluids, and blood transfusion as prescribed. He or she should be vigilant and monitor continuously for changes in the newborn's condition because NEC is potentially life threatening. Risk for NEC is increased with persistent patent ductus arteriosus (PDA) following birth (Dollberg et al., 2005).

Persistent Patent Ductus Arteriosus. The ductus arteriosus, a fetal circulatory structure, bypasses the fetal lungs and normally closes at birth with the first cry (see Chap. 20). In preterm newborns, however, this structure may remain open (patent), especially in cases of RDS or when indomethacin, a tocolytic agent, was used to stop preterm labor (McConnell & Elixson, 2002). With persistent PDA, assessment findings reveal bounding pulses, increased pulse pressure from a low diastolic arterial pressure, and auscultation of a continuous murmur. An echocardiogram confirms the diagnosis; treatment is instituted to close the duct either pharmacologically with indomethacin or surgically with ligation. Because a secondary effect of indomethacin is vasoconstriction of the mesenteric blood vessels, this drug was thought to be implicated in bowel ischemia, contributing to NEC. Current research, however, does not support this finding. PDA independently contributes to NEC, unrelated to administration of indomethacin (Dollberg et al., 2005).

Intracranial Hemorrhage. The most common type of intracranial hemorrhage is bleeding within the brain ventricles, which usually develops in preterm infants who weigh less than 1500 g, are younger than 34 weeks' gestation, or both. The germinal matrix, a vascular embryonic lining of the ventricles that persists up to 35 weeks' gestation, increases susceptibility to bleeding under certain conditions. The most serious effects of intraventricular hemorrhage in this area are neurodevelopmental disability and death (Hardart et al., 2004).

Preterm infants at greatest risk for spontaneous intraventricular bleeding include those who have experienced additional stressors such as birth trauma, birth asphyxia, or RDS. When measures such as inhaled nitric oxide, high-frequency oscillatory ventilation, and exogenous surfactant cannot effectively relieve respiratory distress in a very preterm infant, extracorporeal membrane oxygenation (ECMO) may be used as extraordinary breathing support. Use of ECMO, heparinization, and reperfusion of the cerebral vessels can lead to an intracranial bleed (Hardart et al., 2004).

When parents learn that their newborn has been diagnosed with intraventricular bleeding, they are likely to become alarmed and extremely fearful about this immediate threat to well-being. Once the bleeding begins to decrease and resolve, other fears might begin to surface. Parents may worry that the infant will face subsequent learning disabilities, poor school performance, and decreased quality of life. Nurses can support and remind parents that unless the neurologic defects are major and irreversible, predictions about future developmental growth and adaptation depend on many variables, including family support, home environment, and the socioeconomic availability of resources. See Teaching Tips 22.1.

Postterm Newborns

Postterm newborns are born after 42 weeks' gestation (see Chap. 16). They develop problems when the aging placenta can no longer deliver adequate oxygen and nutrients. As a result, the fetus uses nutritional reserves, possibly catabolizing proteins for energy and survival. With placental insufficiency, the fetus receives poor oxygenation (hypoxemia) and nutrient transfer (starvation), which depletes glucose reserves normally stored in the liver. Hypoxia triggers increased production of red blood cells (polycythemia), which can pose serious problems (eg, thick viscous blood) when coupled with dehydration. Consequently, the baby may be predisposed to a debilitating or possibly fatal thrombotic event, such as stroke.

Newborn Characteristics

A postterm newborn typically looks lean, with an angular long body and little subcutaneous fat. This appearance is from depletion of the nutritional reserves developed during pregnancy leading to metabolism of body fats and protein.

Because the newborn is gestationally mature, plantar and palmar surfaces are deeply wrinkled. Hair is coarse and abundant. Nails are long and possibly meconium stained if there has been a history of fetal distress. The skin appears scaly and dry and also may be meconium

TEACHING TIPS 22.1 Empowering the Family of a Preterm Infant Recovering From an Intraventricular Bleed

The nurse should review with parents and caregivers the following tips for maximizing cerebral function in the stable infant following resolution of an intraventricular bleed:

- Visual stimulation
  - Present human faces in close proximity to the infant.
  - Use crib mobiles with colors, designs, and well-defined and distinctive patterns.
- Auditory stimulation
  - Regularly expose the newborn to voice interactions.
  - Play music around the infant.
- Motor stimulation
  - Assist the infant with patterning exercises to simulate crawling.

stained. Meconium in the amniotic fluid increases the risk for another serious complication: meconium aspiration. Based on biophysical profile, nonstress testing, and stress testing, health care providers may determine that placental insufficiency and resultant fetal hypoxemia contraindicate the stress of labor and vaginal birth. A cesarean birth may be deemed safest.

Associated Complications

A postterm newborn is at risk for complications primarily resulting from inadequate nutrition and hypoxemia. Examples include meconium aspiration syndrome (MAS), polycythemia, and hypoglycemia.

Meconium Aspiration Syndrome. Meconium may be aspirated in utero or with the newborn's first breath. In the presence of distress usually precipitated by hypoxemia, the fetus struggles, making respiratory efforts and bearing down with the abdominal musculature to expel meconium into the amniotic sac. Depending on the amount of meconium, the amniotic fluid can range from being lightly stained to turning thick, viscous, and opaque green (similar to pea soup). Because the fetus normally sucks and swallows amniotic fluid, it is common for newborn mouths and nasal passageways to be filled with it. When amniotic fluid is thick with tenacious meconium, the rush of air into the lungs with the first cry also transports these waste products, forming plugs in the lungs to reduce oxygen diffusion. The result can be pneumonia.

Risk for MAS may be identified intrapartally when rupture of the membranes reveals green amniotic fluid. With this finding, the health care team can intervene to minimize complications. Amnioinfusion with warmed normal saline can be used to dilute the "pea soup" meconium (see Chap. 16). Amnioinfusion drains the fluid from the maternal vagina onto an absorbent underpad. As additional fluid is instilled and drained, removal of meconium from the intrauterine cavity reduces the risk for MAS.

Additionally, health care personnel perform first nasal, then oral and pharyngeal, suction as soon as the fetal head emerges from the birth canal, usually while the fetal shoulders and thorax remain compressed (see Chap. 20). Deep tracheal suctioning is indicated before the first intake of breath. If personnel cannot accomplish satisfactory suction while the fetal body has yet to emerge, ET intubation may be necessary immediately at birth. Current neonatal resuscitation protocols require avoiding all stimulation of the newborn, including drying the skin, until vocal cords have been visualized and deep ET suction accomplished. Thirty seconds is the maximum time for suctioning before initiating ventilation (Kattwinkel, 2006).

MAS results in hypoxemia, as evidenced by tachypnea, retractions, and nasal flaring. Oxygen therapy is instituted to prevent blood from shunting away from the lungs secondary to increased pulmonary pressures. Continuous monitoring of respiratory status and vital signs is essential. Prophylactic antibiotic therapy and chest physiotherapy may be prescribed to prevent pneumonia.

Polycythemia. Dehydration and hemoconcentration in postterm newborns can result in polycythemia. Sluggish blood flow can predispose the newborn to thrombi, pulmonary emboli, and cerebrovascular accident (CVA). Neonatal nurses monitoring behavior, symmetry of movement, suck, cry, and Moro response may be the first to detect CVA. In such cases, after the airway is maintained, adequate hydration is the next priority because oxyhemoglobin travels on the red blood cell, and thick viscous blood can obstruct oxygen transport.

Hypoglycemia. Postterm newborns are at risk for hypoglycemia secondary to starvation and depletion of glycogen stores in utero. They require administration of fluids containing glucose. If a newborn is too weak or respiratory distress interferes with oral intake of sufficient fluids and calories, gavage feedings are indicated.

Clinical research has documented that several full-term, AGA newborns also develop hypoglycemia. See Research Highlight 20.2 in Chapter 20.

COLLABORATIVE CARE: COMPLICATIONS RELATED TO SIZE, GESTATIONAL AGE, OR BOTH

Newborns with complications related to size, gestational age, or both need astute assessment, early detection of problems, and prompt interventions. Typically, they require a multidisciplinary approach to meet their numerous and varied needs.

Assessment

Areas for and the process of assessment for newborns with size- or age-related complications are the same as for normal newborns (see Chap. 20). Certain areas, however, require close investigation to prevent or to minimize problems.

Respiratory Status

General respiratory assessments include initial and continuing appraisal of the motion of the chest wall and abdomen to check for inspiratory lag or asynchrony. The nurse should assess use of the nares and intercostal muscles (between the ribs) and note any undue effort manifested by xiphoid retraction or grunting sounds to increase intrathoracic pressure and to maintain alveolar stability during exhalation.

If complications compromise the ability to exchange oxygen and carbon dioxide, the nurse should assess for manifestations of respiratory insufficiency. Respiratory instability may progress to diminished respiratory effort that

● **TABLE 22.2 Common Skin Assessment Findings and Associated Complications**

FINDING	ASSOCIATED COMPLICATION
Reddish color	Preterm birth
Greenish tint	Meconium staining
Puffy and opaque	Infant of mother with diabetes
Bluish head/trunk	Deficient oxygen
Copious lanugo	Preterm birth
Scanty lanugo	Postterm birth
Yellow	Jaundice
Loose/wrinkled	Dehydration, postterm birth
Pallor	Hypoglycemia
Flushed face	Hyperglycemia
Bluish mottled extremities	Acrocyanosis, exposure to cold
Peeling/scaliness	Postterm birth

is unresponsive to stimulation, and eventually deteriorate to no respiratory effort whatsoever. Team members must promptly identify and remedy the cause of the respiratory distress before the newborn begins to decompensate and deteriorate. Using Assessment Tool 22.1, the nurse should evaluate the five criteria and assign each a value of 0, 1, or 2. A total of zero reflects no respiratory distress; a total of 2 to 4 indicates mild distress; a total of 5 or 6 signifies moderate distress; and totals of 7 or above indicate severe respiratory distress. The higher the number on the Silverman/Anderson tool, the greater the respiratory effort and energy expenditure, and the greater the incidence of eventual exhaustion, respiratory acidosis, and hypoxemia.

Special Concerns for Preterm Newborns

Tactile and thermal stimuli trigger respirations at birth. Additionally, chemoreceptors respond to low oxygen tension and elevated arterial carbon dioxide tension to stimulate the brain's respiratory center. Because preterm newborns lack lung and neuromuscular maturity to respond to birth with stable, effective respirations, the nurse should assess respiratory rate, depth, and regularity and document findings frequently. Rapid, irregular respirations are normal initially but should slow to 30 to 60 breaths per minute at rest. When stressed or stimulated excessively, the newborn will respond with rapid, irregular respirations. Tachypnea, tachycardia, and central cyanosis are indicators of poor tolerance to noxious stimuli or poor extrauterine transition. Unlike the acrocyanosis (mottled, bluish discoloration of extremities) seen in normal newborns, central cyanosis is seen in the head and trunk and indicates deficient oxygen and arterial desaturation.

Special Concerns for LGA Newborns

Newborns who experienced cesarean birth because of excessive size miss the beneficial mechanical stimulation of labor and vaginal birth, which compresses the chest to squeeze lung fluid from the alveoli and air passageways. Vaginal birth also stimulates chest wall recoil to facilitate the initial breath, which draws air into the partially cleared air passageways. The nurse should assess these infants for excessive mucus, regurgitation of mucus, or gagging efforts and diminished respiratory effort.

Skin

Newborn skin color may reflect various stages of fetal development and complications related to size, gestational age, or both. See Table 22.2.

Special Concerns for Postterm Newborn

Postterm newborns may have little vernix, leading to skin desquamation and peeling. Additionally, if the postterm newborn experienced intrauterine hypoxia from placental aging and deterioration, the skin may be stained greenish yellow from meconium in the amniotic fluid.

Special Concerns for LGA Newborns

When assessing an LGA newborn whose mother had diabetes, the nurse may observe opaque skin common with a full-term infant; however, excess body fat and fluid retention also may add a puffy edematous appearance. Hypoglycemia may give rise to pallor, whereas hyperglycemia would produce a flushed appearance.

Thermoregulation

Temperature control is an important goal for newborns with complications related to size, age, or both. The nurse may use invasive, noninvasive, or both methods of

● ASSESSMENT TOOL 22.1 Silverman/Anderson Tool for Assessing Respiratory Distress

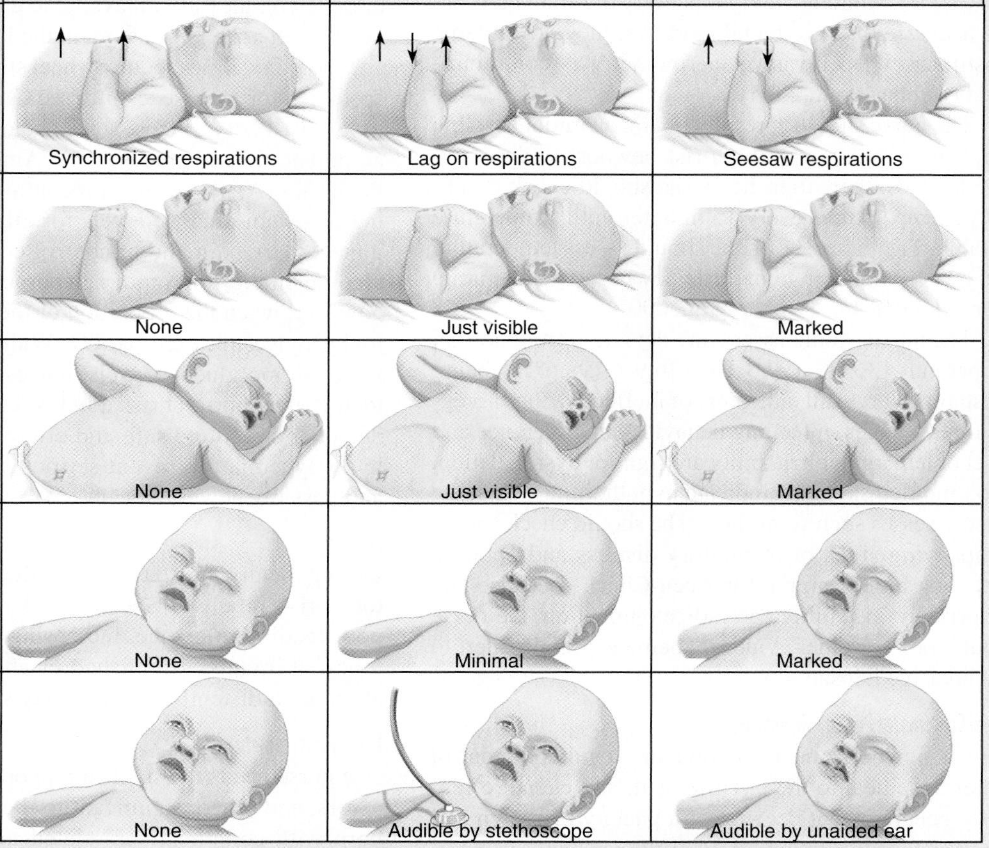

Feature observed	Score 0	Score 1	Score 2
Chest movement	Synchronized respirations	Lag on respirations	Seesaw respirations
Intercostal retraction	None	Just visible	Marked
Xiphoid retraction	None	Just visible	Marked
Nares dilation	None	Minimal	Marked
Expiratory grunt	None	Audible by stethoscope	Audible by unaided ear

(Used with permission from Silverman, W. A. & Anderson, D. H. [1956]. A controlled clinical trial of effects of water mist on obstructive respiratory signs, death rate, and necroscopy findings among premature infants. *Pediatrics, 17*[4], 1–9.)

temperature measurement. Two major disadvantages of rectal thermometry are increased risk for trauma and contamination from pathogens that could be life threatening to ELBW and VLBW preterm infants (Hebbar et al., 2005). Pulmonary artery and bladder thermistor catheters offer additional invasive routes for monitoring temperature in critically ill infants. Nevertheless, all invasive methods have risks (Hebbar et al., 2005). Noninvasive methods do not require contact with delicate, easily traumatized mucous membranes and include the axillary route and use of the temporal artery skin sensor. The latter method relies on the same infrared measurement technology as tympanic membrane thermometers used in pediatric care. Of the noninvasive methods, the axillary route has been identified as least accurate (Hebbar et al., 2005). Although temporal artery thermometers are less accurate than are rectal readings, they are suitable substitutes when invasive thermometry is contraindicated (Hebbar et al., 2005).

The nurse should carefully obtain an initial baseline rectal temperature on the high-risk newborn (unless contraindicated); thereafter, he or she should check noninvasive temperatures every 15 minutes until temperature is stable. Thereafter, he or she should assess temperature every 1 to 3 hours in nonfebrile newborns (temperature at or below 38°C) (Hebbar et al., 2005).

The nurse should assess any deviation from normal temperature [36.3°C (97.3°F) to 36.9°C (98.6°F)], being constantly alert to all indicators of ineffective thermoregulation. Changes in feeding behaviors and tolerance and onset of lethargy or irritability are signs of dysregulation. Cool, mottled skin may indicate hypothermia. When the nurse assesses such signs, he or she should check for accompanying signs of respiratory distress and obtain a heel stick blood sample for Accu-Check. Because any temperature instability can indicate infection, the nurse should look for other evidence, being especially alert to any invasive lines.

Special Concerns for Preterm Newborns

Preterm newborns have an immature regulatory control center, lose heat to the environment, and cannot effectively generate heat because of a paucity of brown and subcutaneous insulating fat. Poor flexion exposes maximum body surface area to the heat-lowering effects of conduction, radiation, and evaporation.

Special Concerns for Postterm Newborns

The postterm newborn also lacks subcutaneous insulating fat, having metabolized it along with muscle tissue in utero to compensate for decreased nutritional reserves. Phototherapy for newborns with jaundice may predispose them to iatrogenic hyperthermia resulting from heat given off by the fluorescent rays or the fiberoptic phototherapy blanket placed against the skin.

Glucose Levels

Identification of newborns at risk for hypoglycemia requires thorough review of the maternal history for such factors as a history of substance use, hypertension, and diabetes. The nurse should consider that a client may deny during the antepartal history use of illegal substances from fear of criminal prosecution or intervention by child protection agencies. Prenatal drug screening usually is performed during the first antepartal visit; nurses should refer women who are actively using drugs for substance abuse counseling.

SGA and preterm newborns also are at risk for hypoglycemia because they have decreased subcutaneous and brown fat and have been deprived of nutrients for growth. Subsequently, when glucose supplies are scarce or deficient, they use all available glucose for metabolic needs with none left to store in the liver as glycogen.

Some facilities require a heel stick to obtain a blood specimen for glucose testing (see Chap. 20). The laboratory must verify glucose levels below 40 mg/dL before administration of glucose. The American Academy of Pediatrics (AAP) no longer recommends routine screening of serum glucose levels for all newborns to avoid unnecessary pain and to control costs. The AAP does recommend testing of all newborns in a given nursery, however, when the proportion of them deemed "at risk" for hypoglycemia exceeds 50%. Without universal screening of serum glucose levels, nurses must be vigilant to identify newborns at risk quickly and accurately, and to detect and institute safe and effective management of hypoglycemia to prevent serious neurologic sequelae and possibly newborn death.

Feeding

During the first few days of life, the nurse should monitor at-risk infants for behavior changes (eg, lethargy), poor feeding tolerance, increasing gastric residuals in tube-fed infants, diminished or absent bowel sounds, abdominal distention, and bloody stools.

Family Assessment

The nurse needs to establish rapport with parents, caregivers, and others significant to the family of the newborn with complications related to size, gestation, or both. Once a trusting relationship is started, the nurse should use goal-directed communication to elicit information that will reveal the family's coping skills, strengths, and resources needed to adapt effectively.

The nurse may ask direct questions such as, "What were your feelings when you began preterm labor and realized that a premature birth was imminent?" Or the nurse may use shared observations such as: "You were holding so tightly to each other when you first came into the nursery to see your baby. It appeared that you were frightened by all the special equipment and lines." Discharge needs can be identified by asking questions such as "Who will be available to help you with infant care when you go home?" The nurse can inquire about transportation needs and finances if the infant is transferred to a distant hospital. The nurse specifically should assess any fears or concerns of family members that could compromise attachment, engrossment, and bonding with the infant.

The nurse should assess cultural, spiritual, and socioeconomic factors that affect family adaptation as well as beliefs about the health care delivery system. In that way, the nurse can be prepared to share a thorough but concise nursing assessment with other team members to effectively plan collaborative care that meets the unique needs of newborn and family.

The nurse should work with other team members to determine special equipment, supplies, or services needed at home (eg, oxygen, ventilator support, apnea monitor, special appliances for feeding). He or she should direct caregivers toward specific agencies for the recommended resources and collaborate with social service personnel. Home health agencies and nurses become invaluable for family members caring for newborns with complications. They may provide teaching, as well as physical and emotional support, and evaluate the effectiveness of supportive, preventive, and restorative care.

Select Potential Nursing Diagnoses

Nursing diagnoses appropriate for newborns with complications related to age, size, or both can be wide ranging. Some common examples include the following:

- **Impaired Gas Exchange** related to inadequate surfactant production
- **Ineffective Breathing Pattern** related to internal and external factors including cold stress, hypoglycemia, surfactant lack, and birth asphyxia
- **Ineffective Thermoregulation** related to immature central nervous system, inability to generate and conserve heat, excessive heat loss to the environment, and inadequate quantities of brown fat
- **Risk for Imbalanced Nutrition, Less Than Body Requirements** related to problems with ingestion, digestion, and metabolism
- **Risk for Infection** related to poorly developed immune system and invasive procedures
- **Risk for Disorganized Infant Behavior** related to noxious stressors required in the care of the high-risk infant (eg, frequent arterial sticks, arterial blood gases, intubation, mechanical ventilation)
- **Parental Anxiety** related to uncertain outcomes of a newborn with complications
- **Risk for Impaired Parenting** related to poor role transition secondary to added stressors
- **Risk for Caregiver Role Strain** related to fatigue and stress secondary to multiple needs of an ill newborn

Planning/Intervention

Numerous treatments appropriate for the newborn's specific circumstances may require the use of sophisticated technology and equipment. See Nursing Care Plan 22.1.

(text continues on page 934)

NURSING CARE PLAN 22.1

The Preterm Newborn

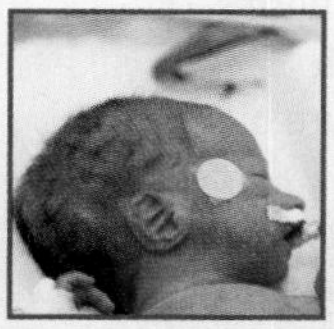

Recall Baby Mitchell, the preterm newborn described at the beginning of the chapter. Maternal history reveals two spontaneous abortions related to an incompetent cervix. With the pregnancy that produced Mitchell, cervical cerclage was performed.

Mitchell and his 34-year-old mother Alisha were febrile at Mitchell's birth. Both are now afebrile. Mitchell required ventilator support with 100% oxygen for the first 3 days of life before being weaned from the ventilator. He was extubated on day 5 and received oxygen therapy at 30%, which was gradually discontinued. Oxygen saturation levels on room air are now at 95% to 96%. He is to be weaned gradually from total parenteral nutrition and glucose-containing IV fluids. A nasogastric tube has been inserted to begin gavage feedings with his mother's breast milk with probiotics added, with the ultimate goal of progressing to oral feedings. Alisha states a desire to continue pumping breast milk to increase her supply in preparation for Mitchell's anticipated discharge home in 6 to 8 weeks.

Continued

NURSING CARE PLAN 22.1 ● The Preterm Newborn *(Continued)*

NURSING DIAGNOSIS

Risk for Imbalanced Nutrition, Less Than Body Requirements related to increased needs for nutrients, small stomach capacity, and immature gastrointestinal tract

EXPECTED OUTCOMES

- Mitchell will demonstrate steady weight gain appropriate to developmental age (minimum 20 to 30 g/day).
- Mitchell will demonstrate an ability to tolerate gavage feedings.

INTERVENTIONS	RATIONALES
Administer prescribed IV glucose, amino acids, and essential fatty acids (TPN), observing protocols for monitoring serum glucose, electrolytes, and urine specific gravity.	Glucose has a critical role in brain metabolism. Amino acids and proteins are required for growth. Fatty acids in the form of linoleic acid provide the major source of calories for energy. Monitoring glucose, electrolytes, and urine specific gravity provides valuable information about the therapeutic effectiveness of TPN and allows for early identification of potential complications.
Provide opportunity for non-nutritive sucking if suck reflex is present and respiratory distress is absent.	Non-nutritive sucking helps to satisfy the newborn's sucking need and promotes readiness for oral feedings. It also allows the newborn the opportunity to associate feelings of satiety and gastric fullness with the act of sucking.
Collaborate with pediatrician regarding timing, volume, and frequency of breast milk gavage feedings, with probiotics added twice daily to protect the bowel wall against NEC.	Timing and readiness are paramount to tolerance of feedings, which must be individualized to each newborn's physiologic condition. Early enteral feedings are withheld if the newborn has an ischemic condition (reducing perfusion to the gut). Gastrointestinal mucosal inflammation or injury also may have been mediated by infection such as that associated with PROM.
Confirm tube placement; once confirmed, begin gavage feedings as ordered.	A malpositioned feeding tube can lead to aspiration.
Weigh newborn every day at the same time each day using the same scale with the newborn wearing the same amount of clothing.	Weight is a reliable indicator of the newborn's overall condition, including nutritional status. It provides an objective measure of the effectiveness of therapy.
Assess newborn's tolerance to enteral feeding. ● Measure the abdominal circumference before each feed and record for reference to baseline. ● Check gastric residuals before each feed; measure and replace gastric contents. ● Subtract the amount of the gastric residual before and after the flush of the nasogastric tube from the total prescribed volume.	Assessment of feeding tolerance helps to evaluate effectiveness. Measuring abdominal circumference aids in identifying distention. Measuring gastric residuals provides information about the newborn's ability to absorb feedings; replacing residuals prevents fluid loss and electrolyte imbalances.

Continued

NURSING CARE PLAN 22.1 • The Preterm Newborn

INTERVENTIONS	RATIONALES
Assess urine output, recording the number and amount of voidings. Weigh each saturated diaper, subtracting dry weight of the diaper for output (1 mL urine=1 g, depending on renal maturity and ability of kidneys to concentrate urine). Monitor urine specific gravity.	Urine output and urine specific gravity are reliable indicators of renal function and hydration status. Accuracy in measurements is key.
Record the number, amount, and character of stools. Periodically check stools for occult blood.	Stool assessment provides important information about gastrointestinal tract function. Abdominal distention, increasing gastric residuals, and blood in the stools are classic signs of NEC.
Collaborate with pediatrician to progressively advance enteral feeding as TPN is decreased.	Feedings are individualized and progressed as the newborn develops. The expectation is that the newborn would be able to tolerate increased feedings.
As tolerated and ordered, gradually introduce oral feedings with breast milk through soft premature nipple or breast milk reservoir using gravity flow through a tiny soft tube allowing milk droplets into the newborn's mouth without sucking.	Excessive energy expenditure with the work of sucking negates the benefits of oral caloric intake by using the available calories for energy rather than for weight gain.
Hold the newborn upright with the head forward and chin tucked inward.	The chin-tuck maneuver minimizes the risk for aspiration.
Observe carefully for fatigue; discontinue oral feeding if newborn tires or feeding takes longer than 30 minutes; administer remainder of feeding by gavage.	Fatigue interferes with the newborn's ability to ingest the feeding and increases energy expenditure and oxygen demand.
Involve mother in feeding opportunities; provide teaching and support. Give praise, encouragement, and support to the mother pumping breast milk. Advise her of the value of breast milk in the infant's health and nutrition.	Pumping can be uncomfortable and requires considerable motivation to continue for a prolonged period when the newborn is too ill or weak to suckle.
Involve a lactation specialist to assist mother in obtaining a full-sized, hospital-grade breast pump and provide instructions. Initiate pumping within 6 to 8 hours postpartum. Help her double pump (both breasts) simultaneously for 15 minutes every 2 to 3 hours until a good supply of breast milk is obtained.	A lactation specialist can provide valuable information, support, and guidance to the mother about breastfeeding and maintaining her milk supply.
Encourage mother to pump once or twice during the night when prolactin levels are high.	The release of prolactin results in milk production and release in the breast.
Collaborate with a lactation specialist in teaching the mother how to store, transport, and prepare breast milk.	The woman can pump with privacy in the NICU while she provides "kangaroo care" (skin to skin physical contact to maintain warmth and colonize normal flora on the skin surface); however, not all feedings can be accomplished with freshly pumped breast milk because of the mother's need for rest. Breast milk must be stored in clean containers and refrigerated or frozen. Stored breast milk is warmed in a water bath rather than a microwave to prevent dangerous hot spots from causing burns.

Continued

NURSING CARE PLAN 22.1 ● The Preterm Newborn *(Continued)*

INTERVENTIONS	RATIONALES
Advise the mother to apply warm compresses and massage breasts before pumping; suggest the use of mental imaging of her baby; if necessary, suggest the use of oxytocin nasal spray if ordered to aid the let-down reflex (Spicer, 2001).	Warm compresses and massage promote the let-down reflex; mental imaging stimulates the release of oxytocin, which in turn aids in the let-down reflex.
Reinforce positive gains made by the newborn with gavage and progression to oral feedings	Positive reinforcement promotes continued participation and enhances feelings of self-esteem, thereby enhancing the chance for success.

EVALUATION

1. The newborn demonstrates increased body weight and is AGA by discharge.
2. The newborn ingests oral feedings of breast milk through premature nipple without evidence of difficulty swallowing or aspiration.

NURSING DIAGNOSES

- **Risk for Caregiver Role Strain** related to fatigue and stress secondary to added burdens of needs of preterm infant
- **Deficient Knowledge** related to multiple ongoing needs of preterm newborn

EXPECTED OUTCOMES

1. The mother and caregivers will identify possible areas of stress.
2. The mother and caregivers will list acceptable sources of support by which to reduce stress of caring for preterm newborn.
3. The mother and caregivers will identify the specific care measures required by her newborn.
4. The mother and caregivers will demonstrate beginning skills to care for the preterm newborn.

INTERVENTIONS	RATIONALES
Assess the client's level of understanding about needs of preterm newborn and required care.	Assessment provides a baseline to identify specific client needs and develop an individualized plan.
Discuss with client her concerns, feelings, and perceptions related to the preterm newborn and care measures during labor and birth.	Discussion provides opportunities to emphasize positive aspects of the current situation; verbalization of concerns aids in establishing sources of stress and problem areas that need to be addressed.
Communicate accurate facts and answer questions honestly. Reinforce factual information, emphasizing the uniqueness of each preterm newborn.	Open, honest communication promotes trust and helps to correct any misconceptions or misinformation. Facts help dispel unfounded fears, myths, or guilt feelings.

Continued

NURSING CARE PLAN 22.1 ● The Preterm Newborn

INTERVENTIONS	RATIONALES
Initiate a supportive approach for the breast-feeding mother of a premature infant.	A supportive approach fosters a trusting relationship and enhances the chances for success.
Teach the client what to expect relative to the preterm newborn's needs and care. Review expectations for growth and development.	An understanding of what to expect aids in reducing fear of the unknown.
Instruct the client in care measures, including necessary adaptations, such as use of premie nipple and small frequent feedings; also review measures for routine newborn care. Have the client return-demonstrate measures or skills as indicated.	Teaching enhances understanding. Return demonstration provides information for evaluating the success of teaching and aids in identifying areas needing additional education.
Encourage ample rest, including an afternoon nap, extra fluids (8 to 10 glasses per day), and balanced nutrition with extra protein. Advise mother to continue taking antepartal multivitamins.	Ample fluids and high-quality proteins are required to increase the quantity and quality of breast milk produced. Fatigue and anxiety can influence the breastfeeding experience negatively, which may hinder the let-down reflex. Adequate rest aids in meeting the demands of care.
Initiate a referral for social services and home care follow up. Investigate resources for help with household tasks. Encourage mother to use appropriate resources.	Social services can provide the family with additional resources for assistance and support. Home care follow-up provides additional opportunities for assessment and teaching as well as for determining the success of previous teaching.
Encourage participation in community support groups of parents with preterm newborns.	Participation in support groups allows for sharing and helps to diminish feelings of being overwhelmed and alone.
Maintain open lines of communication, including phone contact after discharge to inquire as to adjustment to full-time care of infant; allow verbalization of feelings and offer encouragement and tips for self and infant care as needed.	Follow-up communication aids in determining the transition to home, providing opportunities for positive reinforcement and identification of any areas that may develop into potential problems. Allowing the mother to verbalize feelings helps to alleviate stress and anxiety.

EVALUATION

1. The mother and caregivers identify acceptable resources by which to reduce their stress and strain, verbalizing an intent to use these resources as needed.
2. The mother and caregivers participate in developing a plan for home care with assistance from the health care team and community.
3. The mother and caregivers demonstrate safe and effective physical and developmental care, while verbalizing an understanding of the special needs of the preterm newborn.
4. The mother and caregivers create a plan for family adaptation to added time, energy, and fiscal resources and family responsibilities.

Outcomes are highly individualized. NIC/NOC Box 22.1 provides an overview of common interventions and outcome labels applied to newborns with size- or age-related complications. Some common outcomes may include the following:

- The newborn will maintain adequate oxygenation and respirations.
- The newborn will maintain a stable temperature.
- The newborn will ingest adequate nutrients.
- The newborn will remain free of infection.
- The newborn will respond appropriately to stimuli.
- The parents will demonstrate appropriate coping behaviors related to the newborn's status.
- The parents will exhibit positive responses to their newborn.
- The parents will participate in the care of their newborn.
- The parents will demonstrate competence in their ability to provide care for their newborn.
- The parents will verbalize measures to balance demands of caring for their newborn with other aspects of their life.

Oxygenation

When an infant demonstrates respiratory compromise (apnea, gasping respirations, heart rate below 100 bpm refractory to flow-by oxygen, persistent central cyanosis), the nurse should institute ventilation with oxygen immediately. Oxygen can be administered in various ways. Examples include the following:

- Flow-by oxygen: a mask placed in close proximity to the infant's face
- Oxygen hood: a hard clear material with a U-shaped cut out for the infant's neck and an inlet for oxygen
- Nasal cannula
- Continuous positive airway pressure (CPAP) (Fig. 22.4)

A self-inflating bag with a reservoir or flow-inflating device is acceptable for preterm infants as long as a disposable pressure manometer (DPM) limits the quantity of air given with this type of administration. The DPM is a clear hard plastic device that provides visual information about airway pressure in the newborn during ventilation. Excessive pressure is to be avoided to reduce the risk for pneumothorax. Recommended pressures are 20 cm for a preterm infant and 30 cm for a full-term infant. Method, flow rate, and percentage of oxygen administration are individualized. A Web site with short, informative videos for actual use of various methods of newborn oxygen administration and resuscitation is www.aap.org/nrp/educational_videos.html.

When newborns younger than 32 weeks' gestation require resuscitation, current guidelines (Kattwinkel, 2006) recommend blended oxygen (room air with 100%

NIC/NOC Box 22.1 Newborns With Complications

Common NIC Labels

- Airway Management
- Airway Suctioning
- Anticipatory Guidance
- Anxiety Reduction
- Attachment Promotion
- Bottle Feeding
- Coping Enhancement
- Developmental Care
- Enteral Tube Feeding
- Family Process Maintenance
- Fluid Monitoring
- Infant Care
- Infection Control
- Infection Protection
- Kangaroo Care
- Newborn Care
- Newborn Monitoring
- Non-nutritive Sucking
- Nutrition Management
- Nutrition Monitoring
- Nutrition Therapy
- Oxygen Therapy
- Pain Management
- Parent Education: Infant
- Parenting Promotion
- Positioning
- Respiratory Monitoring
- Resuscitation: Neonate
- Skin Surveillance
- Temperature Regulation
- Ventilation Assistance

Common NOC Labels

- Anxiety Control
- Coping
- Infection Status
- Nutritional Status
- Parent–Infant Attachment
- Parenting
- Preterm Infant Organization
- Respiratory Status: Airway Patency
- Respiratory Status: Gas Exchange
- Respiratory Status: Ventilation
- Thermoregulation: Neonate

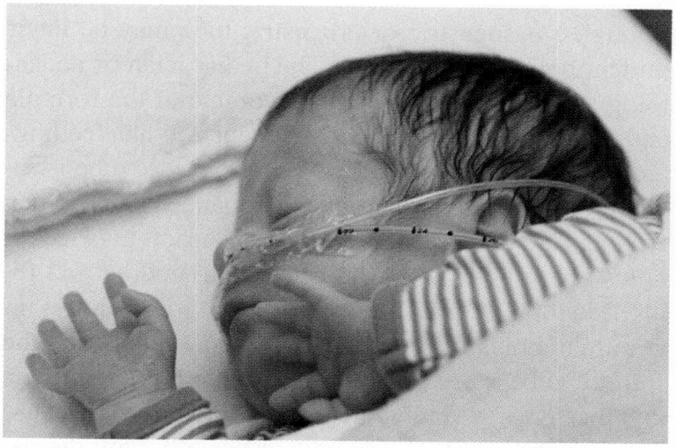

FIGURE 22.4 Delivery of oxygen therapy via nasal cannula in a preterm newborn.

O_2 mix) and use of an oximeter for adjustments to maintain oxygen saturations between 90% and 95%. The infant's heart rate is used as an indicator of effectiveness: if during resuscitation, heart rate does not rapidly accelerate above 100 bpm or there is no appreciable improvement in condition within 90 seconds of birth, the oxygen concentration is increased to 100%. A carbon dioxide monitor always should be used in conjunction with ET intubation to ensure tube placement not verified by heart rate acceleration following ET intubation. Oxygen administered by all sources must be warmed to avoid cold stress.

Effectiveness of oxygen administration with assisted ventilations result in the following outcomes:

- The newborn demonstrates improved color and no central cyanosis after 30 seconds of positive-pressure ventilations.
- The limp, flaccid newborn regains visible muscle tone.
- The newborn begins spontaneous breathing with oxygen.
- Saturation remains between 90% to 95%.

As the newborn matures or complications related to size resolve, team members wean him or her from invasive and more technical forms of oxygen administration. They deliver lesser concentrations of oxygen by nasal cannula. The two tiny prongs must be applied with the curve pointing downward (fitting the anatomy of the nares) and may be secured with small patches of paper or hypoallergenic tape to the cheek.

When a newborn requires extended oxygen delivery after discharge from the health care facility, the nurse should teach parents and other caregivers how to provide oxygen at home. Usual administration is by nasal cannula. The nurse must emphasize safety precautions. For example, candles and open gas flames must be avoided to prevent combustion. Smoking around infants must always be strictly avoided.

Thermoregulation

To prevent cold stress in preterm newborns, the nurse should immediately dry the newborn as it emerges from the mother to control a significant source of heat loss (Porth, 2005). He or she should promptly remove damp towels and cover any surface coming into contact with the infant (eg, x-ray plate) with a warmed receiving blanket. Oxygen, if indicated, is warmed and humidified.

Keeping the newborn in an open air, infrared radiant warmer equipped with a Servo control unit that communicates with a temperature probe placed on the skin can circumvent many avenues of heat loss. The radiant warmer comes on when the temperature drops below a preset range and automatically turns off if the temperature rises above the set range. A continuous digital reading is available. The nurse should document the temperature every 30 to 60 minutes initially, and then every 3 to 4 hours when the newborn is stable. Plexiglas shields surround the infant to block heat loss by convection. The nurse should continually monitor the functioning of all heat control mechanisms used to maintain a neutral thermal environment as well as the ambient temperature.

Resuscitation may not be mandated for all newborns having complications related to size, gestation, or both. Conditions that result in almost certain early death or rare survival pose ethical dilemmas for families and health care providers alike (AHA, AAP, 2005). Examples include gross immaturity and congenital conditions with high morbidity rates. Once a decision has been made to withhold resuscitation, or if resuscitation efforts have been unsuccessful, priority nursing considerations are to give consistent, quality care to the dying newborn and to show compassion and sensitivity to the wishes and needs of the family. Communication by and among all team members should reflect cultural and spiritual sensitivity.

Nurses may feel poorly prepared to deal with ethical issues arising from newborn complications related to size, gestation, or both. It is of tremendous benefit for novice nurses to volunteer to serve on hospital ethics committees and to take every opportunity for training and practice in advance of situations that require such skilled communications and sensitivity (See Ch. 1).

Nutrition

Term newborns have the necessary neuromuscular reflexes (root, suck, and swallow) and fully developed suck pads to ingest oral feedings without difficulty. The rhythm of intermittent feeding, internal feelings of hunger alternating with satiety, and a consistent caregiver provide the foundation for satisfying feeding behaviors. When newborns experience a problem with gestational age or size, oral feedings might need to be delayed. This is most common in SGA and preterm newborns.

Oral Feedings

When the newborn has adequate sucking and swallowing reflexes, gastrointestinal functioning, and energy levels, oral feedings are preferred. Breast milk, ideally from the newborn's mother rather than from a donor or milk bank (see Chap. 21), is most desirable, especially for preterm newborns. Preterm birth greatly affects the quality of maternal breast milk, increasing the lipids, proteins, sodium, chloride, iron, and immune globulins it contains to protect the baby against sepsis and NEC (Meier et al., 1999; Spicer, 2001). If human breast milk is unavailable, specialized formulas can supply needed extra calories (24 cal/oz rather than 20 cal/oz in regular formulas). These specialized formulas also are fortified with calcium, phosphorus, and iron to combat anemia of prematurity.

Commercially available "premie" nipples are shorter by ¼ to ½ inch and softer, making them easier for a preterm or weak LBW infant to compress. Frequency and amounts of feedings vary according to the newborn's size, age, and physical condition. Typically, a newborn near term can consume ¼ to ½ oz orally every 1 to 2 hours, whereas the very preterm newborn requires enteral feeding by orogastric or nasogastric tube because of absent or uncoordinated suck and swallow reflexes. During oral or enteral feeds, the nurse should observe the infant closely to evaluate tolerance. If heart rate or respiratory effort is increased, the nurse should stop the feeding to allow time for the baby to rest and recover. Oral and enteral feedings may be combined. The preterm infant who is neurologically mature enough for oral feedings may consume 8 mL of the prescribed ½-oz formula or breast milk before slowing or sleeping. He or she may take the remaining 6 mL by feeding tube, with the 1 mL flush calculated into the volume. If the infant continues to tolerate oral or enteral feedings, the nurse should increase the amount gradually according to metabolic needs (115 to 140 cal/kg/day of body weight), which are somewhat higher than that of full-term newborns.

Gavage Feedings

Gavage feedings are indicated for physiologically stable newborns who cannot ingest sufficient breast milk or formula orally to satisfy nutritive requirements (Nursing Procedure 22.1). Enteral feedings are withheld in cases of cardiovascular compromise (eg, respiratory distress, central cyanosis, tachypnea). Gestational or neurologic immaturity and birth conditions often necessitate gavage feedings, which require the insertion of a small-bore, soft, pliable feeding tube either through the nose or mouth and advanced into the stomach. Gavage feedings through a nasogastric or orogastric tube may be intermittent bolus or continuous. The pediatrician or neonatologist prescribes the type and volume of the formula and the tube flush volume and frequency. When feedings are continuous, the orogastric or nasogastric tube is secured with hypoallergenic tape and changed daily. When feedings are intermittent, the tube can be left in place for bolus feedings or removed after each feeding and reinserted for the next. The preterm infant who requires intermittent bolus feedings has a poor gag reflex, and the soft tiny tube causes less trauma with intermittent insertion than does the indwelling tube, which also can cause pressure and mucosal ischemia, especially with the nasogastric approach. Gastric residuals must be aspirated and measured every 2 hours when the feeding is continuous; the stomach contents are replaced unless there is a trend of increasing residuals or half the total hourly feed is aspirated. Gastric residuals are measured before each intermittent bolus feed, and gastric contents are replaced and the volume of gastric residual is deducted from the prescribed bolus feed.

Trophic Feedings

Trophic feedings, also called early or minimal enteral feedings, are given to stimulate the gut and to prime the gastrointestinal tract. Trophic feedings also prevent deterioration of the intestinal villi. They are not sufficient for meeting nutritional needs. Rather, they provide small-volume feedings (preferably breast milk or formula) to nourish the gut, promote intestinal maturation, and stimulate motility (Anderson & Loughead, 2002).

Non-nutritive Sucking

During the 8 to 10 weeks of alternative feedings that some preterm newborns require, many factors can contribute to feeding aversion and difficulties. Examples include unpleasant feelings associated with intubation or suction, IV feedings without oral stimulation, and decreased physical contact during feedings. Prolonged intubation also can alter the structure of the hard palate (Ritchie, 2002), making feeding motions difficult. For successful oral feedings, the newborn must create suction and then compress the nipple against the hard palate with anterior-posterior tongue movements. All these motions require neurologic maturity and practice because feeding is a learned behavior for preterm newborns. Thus, newborns with complications related to size or gestational age still need to suck, although this reflex may be inadequate.

Preterm infants can be observed sucking on feeding tubes that have been inserted orally rather than nasogastrically. This spontaneous behavior satisfies the need to suck and serves to increase readiness for oral feeding. An additional benefit of tube feeding is conservation of energy; however, when parents feeds a preterm infant

NURSING PROCEDURE 22.1

Administering a Gavage Feeding

PURPOSE

To provide nutrition to a physiologically stable newborn who cannot orally ingest sufficient breast milk or formula to satisfy normal nutritive requirements

ASSESSMENT AND PLANNING

- Check the newborn's medical record for frequency of feeding (continuous or intermittent), amount to give, and type (breast milk, formula, or specialized feeding).
- Assess the newborn's ability to suck and swallow.
- Inspect the nares and mouth for deformities that may contraindicate insertion of a tube into the mouth or nares.
- Assess parental knowledge of and previous exposure to this feeding method.
- Ensure that feeding is at room temperature. If necessary, remove feeding from refrigerator approximately 30 minutes before use; warm in a warm-water bath if indicated.
- Gather the necessary equipment:
  - 20 mL to 50 mL syringe or feeding solution container
  - Syringes for checking tube placement and flushing as appropriate (5 mL to 10 mL)
  - Appropriate-sized feeding tube depending on the size of the newborn (usually 5 or 8 French tube)
  - Feeding
  - Hypoallergenic tape
  - Stethoscope
  - pH paper
  - Water or water-soluble lubricant
  - Small rolled towel or blanket for positioning if appropriate
  - Clamp or cap for feeding tube (if tube is to remain in place)
  - Infusion pump (if a continuous feeding)

IMPLEMENTATION

1. Explain the procedure to the parents and answer any questions *to help allay their anxiety.*
2. Wash hands.
3. Position the newborn with the head slightly elevated. Measure the length of the catheter to be inserted from the tip of the nose to the earlobe and then to the midpoint of the area between the xiphoid process and umbilicus *to ensure that the tube reaches the stomach.* Mark the point with tape or indelible pen *to provide a reference point for insertion.*
4. Lubricate the feeding tube generously with sterile water *to ease passage of the tube and minimize the risk for trauma to the newborn's mucosa.*
5. Ensure that the newborn is positioned so that his or her head is slightly hyperflexed or in the "sniff" position. If necessary, use a rolled towel under the neck to help maintain this position. Insert the tube into one of the nares or through the mouth, directing the tube toward the back *to facilitate passage along the natural curvature of the area;* continue to pass the tube to the identified mark *to promote passage into the stomach.*
6. Check the position of the tube using two methods *to ensure proper placement in the stomach:*
   a. Attach a small syringe to the feeding tube and aspirate stomach contents, noting the amount, color, and consistency and return the fluid to the stomach *to prevent possible fluid and electrolyte imbalances.* If there is any question as to whether the fluid is stomach or respiratory fluid, test the fluid with pH paper. *Stomach fluid is acidic and has a pH of 1 to 3.*
   b. Attach a syringe filled with a small amount of air (up to 5 mL); instill air into the tube while auscultating the abdomen at the same time for gurgling or growling sounds *to identify accurate placement.*

Continued

NURSING PROCEDURE 22.1 CONTINUED

Administering a Gavage Feeding

7. Tape the tube in place *to secure it.* Measure and record the length of the tubing from where it exits the nose or mouth to the end of the tubing *for use as a reference to aid with future determinations of placement if tube remains inserted.*
8. Attach the syringe (with the barrel removed) or feeding solution container to the tube. Pour the specified amount of feeding into the syringe or container and allow the feeding to flow slowly into the tube by gravity. Adjust the height of the syringe or container to allow for a gentle slow flow of the feeding *to prevent too fast a flow, which could lead to regurgitation and aspiration.* Feeding time should range from 15 to 30 minutes.
9. If feeding does not flow from the syringe, reinsert the plunger and apply gentle pressure to initiate the flow and then allow the feeding to flow by gravity. Do not continue to push the entire feeding through the tube *to prevent excess pressure that could traumatize the mucosa and overdistend the stomach.*
10. If the tube is to be removed after the feeding, when the syringe or container empties, remove the tape while pinching the feeding tube to close it off and quickly, yet gently, remove the tube *to reduce the risk for irritation to the gastrointestinal tract and potential leakage of feeding into the trachea with withdrawal.*

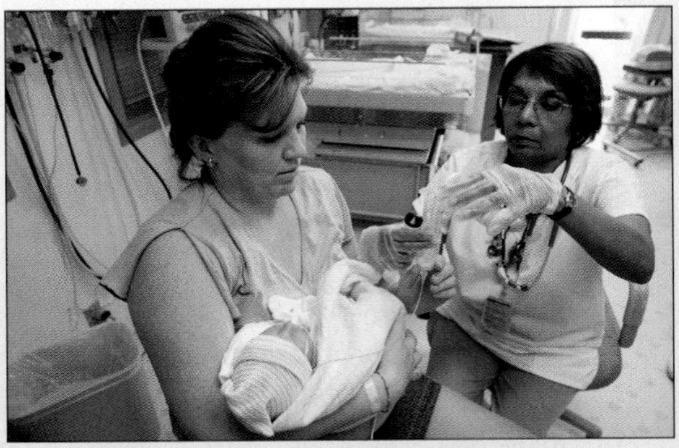

Step 8. Attaching the tube and feeding.

11. If the tube is to remain in place, as the syringe or container empties, flush the feeding tube with sterile water (approximately 1 to 5 mL) *to maintain tube patency* and then clamp or cap the tube *to prevent additional air from entering the stomach.*
12. Burp the newborn after the feeding if appropriate *to aid in air removal* or position the newborn on his or her right side with the head of the bed elevated approximately 30 degrees for 1 hour *to facilitate stomach emptying and reduce the risk for regurgitation and aspiration.*
13. Dispose of equipment and supplies as appropriate. Wash hands.
14. Record the time, amount of feeding, type of feeding, and how the newborn tolerated the feeding.

EVALUATION

- Feeding tube is inserted without injury to the newborn.
- Feeding tube is positioned in the stomach.
- The newborn received the feeding in the correct amount over 15 to 20 minutes without difficulty.
- The newborn tolerated the procedure well, without any episodes of regurgitation, vomiting, or signs and symptoms of aspiration.

AREAS FOR CONSIDERATION AND ADAPTATION

Lifespan Considerations

- Orogastric feedings are preferred for small infants because they are obligate nose breathers and insertion through the mouth is less disruptive and stressful. It also stimulates the sucking reflex. If continuous feedings are ordered, typically nasogastric feedings are used.
- If necessary, use a small rolled towel draped across the newborn's chest and secured under the shoulder *to help prevent inadvertent arm movement by the newborn.*

Continued

NURSING PROCEDURE 22.1

Administering a Gavage Feeding

- If appropriate, enlist the aid of an additional person, such as support person, parent, or other health care team member, *to help contain the newborn and prevent movement that could result in injury.*
- Encourage the parents to hold and swaddle their newborn during the feeding, just as if the newborn was being fed by the breast or bottle *to help promote a positive experience for the newborn.*
- Provide the newborn with non-nutritive sucking *to help satisfy the newborn's need to suck.*
- Always check gastric residuals before each intermittent feeding and reinstill the amount aspirated. Typically, the amount of residual aspirated is deducted from the prescribed amount of the planned feeding *to prevent overdistention.* Follow the agency's policy regarding residual amounts requiring notification of the health care provider.
- When administering continuous feedings, use an infusion pump *to regulate flow* and check residuals at specified intervals, such as every 4 hours *to evaluate the newborn's tolerance of the feeding.*
- Always check the placement of the tube before each intermittent feeding and at specified intervals during continuous feedings when the tubing remains in place.

Community-Based Considerations

- Keep in mind that infants may be discharged home with gavage feedings. Teach the parents or caregivers how to perform the feeding and have them return-demonstrate the procedure before discharge. Clean tap water, instead of sterile water, may be used to lubricate the tube for insertion and flushing.
- Reinforce the need for non-nutritive sucking opportunities and for cuddling and swaddling.
- Arrange for a home care follow-up to assist with the transition to the home. Enlist the aid of social services to help arrange the necessary supplies and equipment.
- Provide the family and caregivers with telephone numbers for use should a problem or difficulty arise.

orally and sees that the suck reflex is effective, it is difficult for them to understand the need for supplemental enteral feeding by tube. The nurse then must explain energy conservation and its relationship to weight gain. The work of sucking requires energy, and energy expenditure requires calories to support the physical effort of ingestion. The nurse can explain to the parents that a preterm or LBW infant has poorly developed suck pads, a small stomach capacity, and low capacity for activity. The baby is easily stressed by the need for frequent feedings beyond the capability to adapt. Allowing the infant to suck until sufficient calories are consumed to support growth and metabolism may overtax the preterm infant and actually result in overstressing him or her. Weight gain is less than expected when calculating total caloric intake because calories used for energy do not contribute to weight gain. An additional way to conserve energy in LBW infants is to prevent cold stress and to minimize heat loss through conduction, convection, evaporation, and radiation. Commercial knit premie caps are available, and some hospital auxiliary organizations provide hand-knit newborn caps that become keepsakes. If neither is available, the nurse can fashion a newborn cap from tubular cotton material called stockinette, which may be found in most hospitals. Scalp vessels bring blood and body warmth close to the skin surface; a cap can be used to reduce the energy expenditure required for thermoregulation.

Newborns who are too immature or sick to tolerate enteral feeding are fed parenterally but still require a pacifier for non-nutritive sucking, which satisfies a physiologic need as well as being a source of comfort (Fig. 22.5). The nurse can offer a commercial premie nipple, leaving the sterile covering over the rim that houses it. This measure prevents the newborn from sucking air and distending the abdomen. If the soft premie nipples available do not have a peel-away sterile covering on the back, the nurse can stuff the nipple with sterile gauze and occlude the nipple back with water-resistant or paper tape. The nurse should offer the pacifier in conjunction with enteral feedings so that the infant associates the feeling of a full stomach (satiety) with sucking.

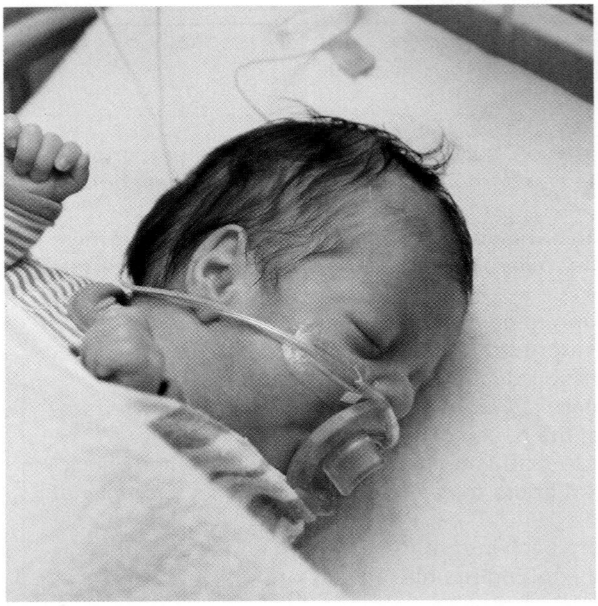

FIGURE 22.5 Non-nutritive sucking in a preterm baby.

Parenteral Nutrition

Historically, VLBW newborns are also very physiologically immature and cannot ingest and digest breast milk or formula by the enteral route. In such cases, the parenteral route is used to provide nutrition when the infant is stable enough. VLBW newborns also have a decreased tolerance to protein compared with other newborns. In the past, VLBW infants were not given parenteral amino acids early enough or in sufficient amounts to support their protein needs from a fear of protein intolerance and development of toxicity. Evidence-based nursing, however, demonstrates no complications in the VLBW newborn receiving amino acids parenterally up to 2.9 g/kg/day (Thureen et al., 1998).

Maintenance of Glucose Levels

Early and frequent oral feedings are the primary means by which the nurse acts to maintain glucose levels. If rooming-in is not an option, nursing infants should be taken to breast every 2 hours or on demand. When the newborn cannot ingest breast milk orally, the nurse should encourage the mother to pump milk for gavage feedings. Infants who cannot tolerate enteral feedings may require parenteral nutrition, such as those on ventilatory support or for whom enteral feeding is contraindicated (eg, NEC).

Because hypoglycemia can cause serious complications, the pediatrician may prescribe an initial feeding of glucose water to raise the blood glucose level quickly, followed by formula or breast milk to prevent rebound hypoglycemia. When the newborn cannot ingest or digest, glucose infusions should start immediately to support brain metabolism (Neu et al., 2002).

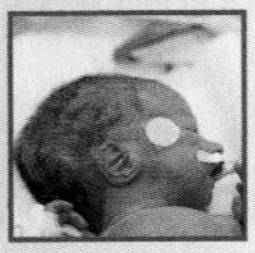

Baby Mitchell was placed on a ventilator. Which method(s) for providing nutrition would be most appropriate for him?

Attachment Promotion

Nurses can be instrumental in promoting family attachment when parents are separated from newborns in the NICU, the mother cannot breastfeed the baby, or both. When physical contact between parent and child is impossible, nurses can encourage parents to view their babies through the nursery window or isolette. Initially, they can give cues to promote identification. Nurses may wish to remark about any physical likeness of the child to parents or siblings and discuss the significance of naming the baby. Role-modeling attachment behaviors while parents watch also may be helpful.

When fetal illness or complication causes serious or irreversible disabilities, the nurse should allow family members to express anger, guilt, shame, remorse, or fear. Demonstrations of respect, caring, and empathy assist clients to assume their parental roles and to find meaning and purpose in whatever the future holds for the family. Primary caregivers need to discuss and thoroughly understand the implications for follow-up care and ongoing monitoring.

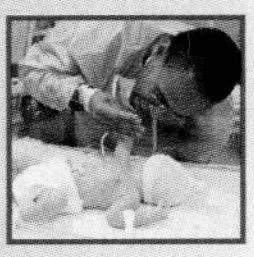

Think back to Madeline, the baby at the beginning of the chapter born with congenital cleft lip and palate. Madeline's mother, Danita, was visibly upset when she saw her baby. How could the nurse assist the family in promoting attachment?

Transcultural Awareness and Sensitivity

When newborn complications require intensive medical and nursing interventions, the family unit responds to the crisis based on cultural and religious beliefs. They can derive much comfort and stability from sensitive, caring nurses who demonstrate acceptance of and respect for practices they believe to be healing (Table 22.3). Differences in what is acceptable to families related to communication, personal space, voice tone, eye contact, and touch vary across cultural boundaries and even within cultures from different locales. Often, noncompliance or failure to agree to a prescribed treatment plan for a newborn experiencing a complication is related to parental cultural orientation. Culturally sensitive nurses are responsible for exploring beliefs, expectations, and desired practices.

TABLE 22.3 Cultural Practices in Newborn Care

ETHNIC OR CULTURAL BACKGROUND	CULTURAL BELIEF OR PRACTICE	NURSING IMPLICATIONS
Hispanic	Children and extended family are highly valued. The baby's father is the authority and decision maker; grandmothers are valued as child care experts. Modesty for a breastfeeding woman or a female infant exposed under the warmer is paramount. Male infant genitals may be exposed without embarrassment because of "macho" male sentiment (Colon, 2001; Steen & Anderson, 2002).	Present information with rationales to both parents but recognize the father as the final authority. Direct infant care teaching to the grandmother if present, never to the father. Provide a private place for breast pumping. Cover female genitals with cloth if unclothed during assessment.
Native American	Illness results from disharmony with nature. Depending on tribal variations, practices include healing rituals, smudging, and a medicine pouch worn around the neck. Parents believe strongly in home remedies/home cures (Davidhizar, 1999; Steen & Anderson, 2002).	Provide a place to conduct rituals without setting off smoke detectors or creating an unsafe environment. Welcome the Medicine man as a valued health resource. Negotiate with parents to pin medicine pouch to crib, advising other health care providers not to touch or open the pouch for inspection.
Hmong/Asian	Evil spirits cause illness. Strings tied on sick children protect them from evil spirits. Concern exists over the drawing of blood specimens because of the belief that blood is not replenished. Fever is treated with warm baths and swaddling. Shaman will be reluctant to come to hospital, but rather will want baby brought to him. Shaman conducts healing ceremony, burning incense, and making food offerings to ancestral spirit. Discussions of death in the baby's presence are avoided because they believe doing so will expose the infant to the bad spirit. Autopsy or organ donation prevents the body from being reborn intact (Steen & Anderson, 2002).	Provide teaching and explanations if the unstable infant cannot be safely transported to the shaman. Advocate for a place within the facility for the healing ceremony and burning of incense. If the oxygen source cannot safely be removed for the burning of incense, send blankets or garments worn by baby to the ceremony; allow the shaman to dress the infant in these garments after. Reassure family that only the smallest necessary blood samples will be taken. Speak only positive and optimistic words around the infant. Respect the family's postmortem desires. Coin rubbing may produce too much heat and friction for the skin of a preterm infant; ask parents to defer this practice with necessary explanations. Direct string tying away from IV sites.
Chinese	Illness and disease result from evil spirits/karma and are related to deeds in a former life. Yin and yang (hot and cold) must be balanced to attain inner harmony. Medical procedures and surgery interrupt internal harmony. Special amulets or charms with blessings from Buddha keep evil spirits away from a sick infant. Female family members are caregivers; a senior male family member is the designated decision maker. The word for death sounds like "four"; therefore, any room or crib numbered four is avoided. Fears and worries are personal and discussed only with close family members. Special days for medical interventions based on the Chinese calendar or folk history are better than others to ensure a good outcome (Chen & Rankin, 2002).	Establish trust through communication and caring acts. Obtain room reassignment for any number four. Show respect for family members and folk healer, making provisions to include them in care planning. Pin amulet to crib and communicate family wishes to keep amulet with infant at all times. Inquire about feelings and concerns in private, demonstrating caring. When possible, make provisions to reschedule surgery or special procedures on the optimal or desired days.
Appalachian families	A fatalistic perception of illness and death leads to a belief that outcomes are predestined and unchangeable (Davidhizar, 1999).	Check for adherence to immunization schedules and follow-up care. Explain rationale for all interventions. Be nonjudgmental when behavior is noncompliant while encouraging appropriate self-care and use of resources.
Muslim families	Children are highly valued and to be protected and nourished. Illness results from imbalance in heat or cold, wind currents, bad luck, or the evil eye. The child wears an amulet or blue stone to avoid the evil eye. Hope is maintained even when a condition is deemed terminal because Allah is in total control. When an infant is dying, his or her crib is turned to face Mecca (Steen & Anderson, 2002).	Provide a private place for prayer. Explain the purpose of the bilirubin light and the normalcy of the infant's body temperature. Protect from drafts during bathing. Allow the amulet to be kept in the crib if conditions prevent it being worn. Position the infant crib in the eastern direction as desired by family members.

The nursing care plan should incorporate and accommodate provisions for any belief system unless doing so may result in harm to the newborn. Nurses should provide explanations and determine what modifications to a particular desired practice would be acceptable to the caregivers. For example, if it is important to the parents to tie a red string around the newborn's limb or rub the baby with oil, the nurse can find ways to accommodate such requests without jeopardizing an IV site or the adherence of electrodes or temperature sensors to the skin of a newborn who requires monitoring (Colon, 2001).

Communication with the family is essential to learning what practices they deem important and what substitutions they accept. Reasonable cultural and religious provisions can be made without compromising treatment when the health care team demonstrates appropriate willingness to accommodate special needs. For example, some Native American tribes practice "smudging" to purify the body, which involves the burning of sweet grass by a *shaman.* The nurse can help the family find a place within the facility to perform smudging without compromising safety. He or she can promote and respect privacy unless the newborn's condition is too unstable for him or her to be away from an oxygen source or monitoring equipment during the 30-minute healing ceremony.

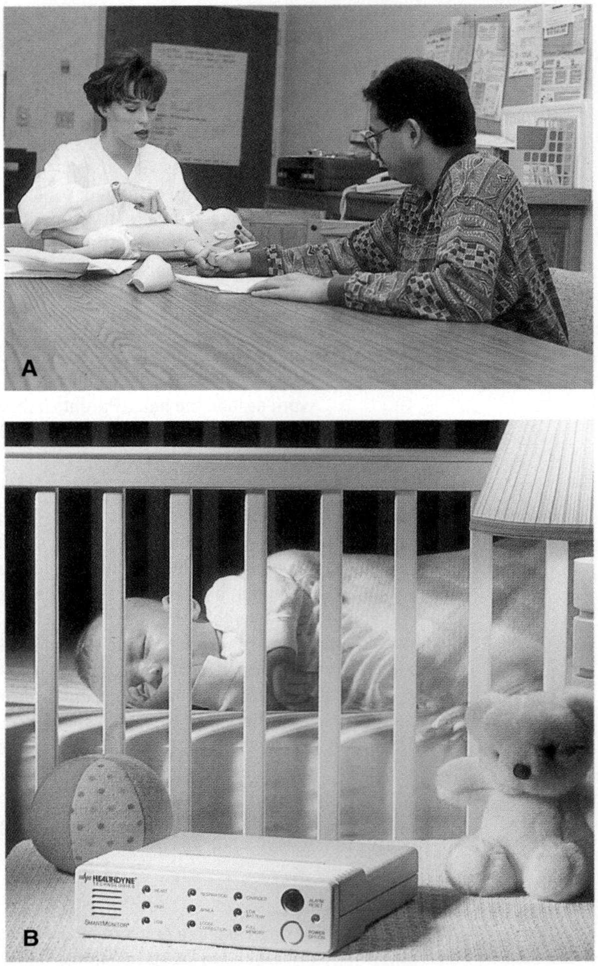

FIGURE 22.6 Parents of preterm babies usually must receive significant education before they can take their infants home with them for ongoing care. Topics commonly covered include (**A**) correct methods of administering infant CPR and (**B**) proper use of an apnea monitor at home.

Discharge Planning

In preparation for discharge, nurses should establish follow-up contact information with the parents, who are likely to feel anxious and overwhelmed by the total responsibility of care that they are assuming. Close relationships are common when health care providers work with preterm or ill newborns and their families during long hospitalizations. Families become attached to nurses and vice versa, which requires intervention to bridge the gap between critical care and parent care.

Discharge planning for the family of the newborn with ongoing complications related to size, gestation, or both must include teaching about the use of equipment such as apnea monitors, oxygen sources, and newborn resuscitation plus the obstructed airway maneuver for infants (Fig. 22.6). Parents may feel safe when caring for infants under nursing supervision, but be frightened by the prospect of independent care at home. Follow-up visits should focus on newborn weight gain and attainment of normal developmental milestones. The nurse should plot weight and length in two different colors: one to represent the percentile for actual chronologic age from birth date, and the other to reflect the percentile based on adjusted age using the expected term gestation age.

Long-term collaborative care requires referrals for hearing and vision screenings. The organ of Corti is sensitive to oxygen deficits; thus, deafness may result from any early hypoxemia that required resuscitation. Oxygen administration in high concentrations to raise oxygen saturation levels could lead to visual problems secondary to retinal bleeding and scarring. A pediatric ophthalmologist is necessary even without high concentrations of oxygen use because preterm newborns are more prone to strabismus and nearsightedness.

Evaluation

When a newborn has a complication related to size, gestational age, or both, the nurse should evaluate the effectiveness of care to promote nutrition. The underweight postterm newborn should demonstrate weight gain and increased urinary output as indicators of dietary well-being and hydration. Desired blood glucose levels are 40 to 60 mg/dL. The VLBW newborn should maintain a somewhat higher glucose concentration of 50 to 55 mg/dL (Neu et al., 2002).

Other indications of effective care include thermal stability and satisfactory extrauterine adaptation as evidenced by stable vital signs within normal ranges. Behaviorally, the newborn should demonstrate appropriate sleep–wake cycles and intact protective neurologic reflexes. No complications (eg, RDS, sepsis) reflect successful supportive and restorative management.

HYPERBILIRUBINEMIA

Hyperbilirubinemia refers to elevated serum bilirubin levels. The normal polycythemic state of the newborn accounts for nearly 80% of serum bilirubin, which results from the breakdown of damaged, dead, or dying red blood cells and subsequent hemoglobin metabolism. Metabolism of 1 g of hemoglobin can release as much as 35 mg of unconjugated bilirubin into the bloodstream. The unconjugated (indirect) bilirubin is transported to the liver, where it is chemically changed to conjugated (direct) bilirubin. The conjugated bilirubin then combines with bile and is deposited into the gastrointestinal tract for excretion in the stool. Intestinal flora acts on a smaller portion of conjugated bilirubin molecules, converting them to urobilinogen for urinary excretion. The chemical conversion of indirect to direct bilirubin, however, requires ample available glucose and serum albumin as well as adequate oxygenation (Hengst, 2002).

The typical manifestation of hyperbilirubinemia is yellow discoloration of the skin and tissues called *jaundice.* Many newborns experience mild, self-limiting *physiologic jaundice* (see Chap. 20) after the third day of life in formula-fed babies and later in breastfed babies. After the normal peak in breastfed newborns, the level slowly declines to normal (see Chap. 21). When hyperbilirubinemia persists or is untreated, the condition is termed *pathologic jaundice.* The following criteria lead to a diagnosis of pathologic jaundice:

- Bilirubin concentrations greater than 4 mg/dL in cord blood
- Total serum bilirubin levels increasing by more than 5 mg/dL over 24 hours or at a rate of 0.5 mg/dL or more over 4 to 8 hours
- Clinical jaundice within 24 hours of birth
- In a preterm newborn, serum bilirubin level above 10 mg/dL at any time
- In a term newborn, serum bilirubin level above 15 mg/dL at any time or clinical jaundice that persists for more than 10 days
- Visible jaundice that continues for more than 21 days in a preterm infant or 10 days in a term infant, unless the baby is breastfeeding (see Chap. 21) (Halamek & Stevenson, 2002)

Excessive indirect serum bilirubin may lead to neurotoxicity because bilirubin readily crosses the blood–brain barrier. Bilirubin deposited on the newborn's brain produces a condition called **kernicterus,** which can lead to serious neurologic sequelae, including permanent damage to the central nervous system, motor abnormalities, deafness, mental retardation, and seizures. Kernicterus also occasionally results in death (Gagnon et al., 2001).

Increasingly shorter postpartum hospital stays make identifying and monitoring newborns at risk for hyperbilirubinemia difficult. Jaundice and hyperbilirubinemia are responsible for most newborn readmissions to the hospital after early discharge (Reiser, 2001). The increased incidence of hyperbilirubinemia and an upward trend in cases of the less common kernicterus prompted the Joint Commission on Accreditation of Healthcare Organizations (JCAHO) to issue an alert to more than 5000 hospitals about this growing problem (Reiser, 2001).

COLLABORATIVE CARE: THE NEWBORN WITH HYPERBILIRUBINEMIA

Newborns require astute observation for jaundice and careful review of possible risk factors for hyperbilirubinemia. The nurse should collaborate with other team members to identify infants who may require follow-up after early discharge and to educate parents about jaundice and the normal time frame for its resolution. As client advocates, nurses should initiate collaborative therapeutic interventions as soon as they detect jaundice.

Assessment

Some newborns are at increased risk for hyperbilirubinemia because of prematurity, family history, ethnic background, birth trauma, and illness. Assessment Tool 22.2 provides a checklist for assessing a newborn's risk.

The nurse should correlate any onset of jaundice with the baby's age (in days of life and gestational) and feeding method (breast versus bottle) to differentiate between physiologic and pathologic jaundice. When assessing for signs of hyperbilirubinemia, the nurse should note the location of jaundice. Physiologic jaundice usually is most prominent on the tip of the nose, ear lobes, sclera, and upper trunk. The nurse must report any jaundice below the sternum and inspect the urine for a dark tea-colored appearance, which is indicative of urobilinogen. In addition, the nurse should assess the newborn's feeding behavior and alertness. He or she needs to report any dietary problems and lethargy immediately.

Select Potential Nursing Diagnoses

Many nursing diagnoses may be applicable to the newborn with hyperbilirubinemia. Common examples include the following:

- **Risk for Injury** related to increased serum bilirubin levels

ASSESSMENT TOOL 22.2 Checklist for Evaluating Hyperbilirubinemia Risks

- Is the baby of Asian, African, or Mediterranean descent? ____
- Did any of the baby's siblings have newborn jaundice? ____
- Was the baby born before the expected due date? ____
- Is the baby being exclusively breastfed? ____
- Did the baby experience birth trauma or bruising? ____
- Did the baby fail to pass meconium within the first 24 hours? ____
- Are fewer than 6 diapers saturated with urine per day? ____
- If present, does jaundice extend below the nipple line? ____
- Are medications given or passed through breast milk that impair bilirubin excretion (eg, Aspirin, acetaminophen, sulfa, alcohol, rifampin, erythromycin, corticosteroids, tetracycline)? ____
- Is there ABO or Rh mother–infant incompatibility? ____
- Does the newborn show signs of infection or sepsis? ____

A yes answer to any of these questions increases the risk for hyperbilirubinemia. ____

- **Risk for Impaired Skin Integrity** related to effects associated with phototherapy
- **Risk for Deficient Fluid Volume** related to increased insensible fluid losses related to phototherapy
- **Deficient Knowledge** (parental) related to use of phototherapy and necessary newborn care
- **Anxiety** (parental) related to newborn requiring treatment for hyperbilirubinemia

Planning/Intervention

Goals are individualized based on the severity of hyperbilirubinemia and proposed treatment. When planning care, prevention of common potential complications and monitoring the effectiveness of treatment are essential.

Bilirubin Level Monitoring

The newborn's bilirubin levels require close monitoring. Discharge from the facility will be delayed if an infant shows signs of significant hyperbilirubinemia. These include late passage of meconium stool, light tan-colored stools after milk ingestion, dark urine, poor feeding, and lethargy.

If jaundice is moderate (serum bilirubin levels of 12 to 15 mg/dL), the nurse should advise the mother to increase the frequency of feeding to 10 or more times per 24 hours while jaundice persists (Porter & Dennis, 2002). Supplements of water, glucose water, or both should be avoided because they reduce caloric intake and may lead to iatrogenic hyponatremia. If bilirubin levels are severe (greater than 15 mg/dL), the health care team may advise the mother to temporarily formula feed. The nurse should instruct the woman to pump breast milk as often as the newborn would have been fed to maintain production. Bilirubin levels related primarily to breastfeeding fall quickly. The woman may resume breastfeeding once the levels are within the normal range.

Monitoring of Intake and Output

The nurse should monitor and record the frequency and amount of each feeding. Often, the nursing mother voices anxiety about being unable to determine the actual quantity of breast milk the baby takes and the correlation between breastfeeding and jaundice, which can persist for weeks to months. The nurse should monitor the effectiveness of breastfeeding technique and reassure the mother that wet diapers are excellent indicators of a newborn's hydration status. Six to 10 wet diapers per 24 hours is acceptable. As the baby is excreting bilirubin (urobilinogen), the urine will be dark tea colored initially and gradually lighten. The nurse should monitor and record intake and output. He or she should use a gram scale to weigh wet diapers (1 g = 1 mL).

Phototherapy

Phototherapy involves exposing as much of the newborn's skin surface as possible to blue wavelengths of light to assist with the excretion of excess bilirubin. To prevent neurotoxicity, phototherapy is instituted when the total serum bilirubin level is at or above 15 ml/dL in infants 25 to 48 hours old, 18 mg/dL in infants 49 to 72 hours old, and 20 mg/dL in infants older than 72 hours (Porter & Dennis, 2002). An effective arrangement consists of four special blue bulbs with two daylight fluorescent tubes on either side (Fig. 22.7). To maximize conversion of bilirubin to the water-soluble form for excretion, the newborn may be placed on a fiberoptic pad as an additional modality for applying a light source. The fiberoptic pad may be less disturbing because it requires fewer position changes (Porter & Dennis, 2002).

FIGURE 22.7 Newborn receiving phototherapy.

The eyes of newborns receiving phototherapy must be protected from the light source. After manually closing each eye carefully, the nurse should apply small patches to each eye and secure them with a Velcro band around the oval circumference of the newborn's head (above the ears). The band should be snug and stay in place at all times while the newborn is under the lights. The nurse should remove eye pads when the infant is away from the UV light source for physical care and during transport to the mother's room for breastfeeding or at times of the day when the nonbreastfeeding newborn visits with parents. The nurse should change the eye pads each time he or she removes them and discard the Velcro straps with discontinuation of phototherapy.

Phototherapy can contribute to overheating and dehydration because it increases insensible fluid losses. Thus, the nurse should closely monitor newborn temperature and hydration. Some newborns develop a minor transient rash that requires no intervention (Akera & Ro, 2003). Diarrhea may necessitate oral administration of supplemental fluids. See Nursing Procedure 22.2.

Exchange Transfusion

Should jaundice fail to respond to intensive phototherapy, the team caring for the newborn may consider exchange transfusion. If the infant's family members are Jehovah's Witnesses, they may refuse blood and blood products. The nurse needs to assume a nonjudgmental and supportive role while keeping open lines of communication and continuing other therapeutic treatment modalities acceptable to this family.

When a newborn is to undergo exchange transfusion, the nurse first should positively identify the baby and obtain verification by a second licensed person who also verifies the blood product, blood type (donor and recipient), cross-match number, and expiration date. The nurse should ensure patency of the venous access, which is usually a catheter inserted into the umbilical vein. The physician prescribes the total amount of blood to be transfused as well as the volume (usually 2 to 10 mL) to withdraw and discard before the infusion of each replacement volume (2 to 10 mL) of compatible donor blood. Depending on how often the nurse withdraws and replaces blood to alternately administer the prescribed total volume, the transfusion may take 1 to 4 hours. Fresh blood from a compatible donor is required for infant transfusion because of the risk for electrolyte imbalance (calcium in particular) from the preservative (citrates) used in stored blood. The blood for each exchange should be administered at room temperature; the nurse can employ a commercial blood warmer when the remaining volume remains cold. Any blood outside of refrigeration for more than 4 hours must be discarded. The nurse should monitor the baby's vital signs closely and recheck indirect bilirubin levels after the infusion and for several subsequent days to ensure that they do not rise again.

Parental Education

Because of the increasing trend toward early discharge, nurses frequently need to instruct parents and caregivers in measures to monitor the progress of their newborns with complications. The nurse should teach parents to carefully inspect for onset of jaundice below the sternum or jaundice that develops, increases, or persists after discharge. If previously pale urine becomes dark or scant, the parent should notify a health care provider immediately. The caregivers also must monitor feeding behavior. Other indicators that parents should report promptly are lethargy, as evidenced by a sluggish newborn who fails to nurse vigorously, and excessive sleep.

Breastfeeding mothers are urged to consume sufficient fluids to support milk volume to enable frequent nursing; nonbreastfeeding mothers may offer water between feedings. Parents should check stools for excreted bile pigments as bilirubin levels decrease. Stools are greenish initially, becoming normal yellow-gold (depending on the type of liquid consumed) as bilirubin levels become normal.

Evaluation

The following outcome and discharge criteria ensure that treatment of hyperbilirubinemia has been effective:

- The newborn ingests sufficient formula or breast milk with supplemental water as needed to saturate five or more diapers per day.
- The newborn demonstrates intact skin with diminishing visible bilirubin pigment on the surface and in the excreta.
- Newborn behavior is appropriate to gestational age, with vigorous suck reflex and no irritability or lethargy.
- Parents and caregivers express confidence in their ability to monitor the newborn's health status relative to jaundice and state the intent to notify a health care provider promptly in the event of complications.

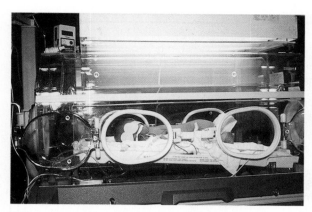

NURSING PROCEDURE 22.2
Performing Phototherapy

PURPOSE

To reduce serum bilirubin levels

ASSESSMENT AND PLANNING

- Assess parental knowledge of and previous exposure to the procedure.
- Inspect the newborn for signs and symptoms of jaundice.
- Evaluate test results of serum bilirubin levels.
- Assess overall newborn status, including vital signs, intake and output, and other parameters *to establish a baseline for future comparison.*
- Gather equipment
  - Light source (bilirubin lights or fiberoptic blanket or panel with protective covering)
  - Eye shields
- Check the light source for proper functioning.
- Review manufacturer's and agency's policy for light intensity and distance of lights from newborn.

IMPLEMENTATION

1. Explain the procedure to the parents; answer any questions they may have *to help alleviate fear and anxiety;* review the need for eye shields while the baby is under the lights *to protect the eyes;* reinforce the need to interact with the newborn; encourage parents to hold and cuddle baby when out of the lights and especially while feeding *to promote attachment.*
2. Set up bililights over the newborn's crib or isolette at the proper distance from the baby, according to agency policy *to ensure adequate exposure while minimizing risk for thermal injury.* If using a blanket or wrap, turn on the device.
3. Check the intensity of the lights with a photometer *to prevent injury to the newborn.*
4. Apply eye shields to the newborn's eyes, checking that the eyelids are closed before application *to prevent corneal injury.* Ensure a snug fit that occludes the eyes but not the nares. (Eye shields may or may not be needed if a blanket or wrap device is used. Check the manufacturer's instruction.) Place the newborn unclothed except for a small diaper under the lights *to maximize skin exposed to the lights while protecting the external genitalia.* If using a blanket or wrap, wrap the newborn in it.
5. Turn the newborn frequently while under the lights, approximately every 2 hours *to ensure exposure of all body parts, thereby promoting breakdown of bilirubin, preventing pressure areas, and providing stimulation.*
6. Monitor vital signs at least every 4 hours *to allow for early detection of complications.*
7. Assess intake and output; weigh diapers *to ensure accurate determination of output;* assess skin turgor and mucous membranes *to evaluate for possible dehydration secondary to increased insensible fluid losses.* Provide additional fluids as ordered *to prevent dehydration.*
8. Assess stool characteristics; change diapers frequently, and inspect perianal area closely for irritation or excoriation *because stools are often loose and may be irritating to the skin.*
9. Provide meticulous skin care *to prevent irritation and breakdown;* avoid the use of oily lubricants or skin lotions *to reduce the risk for intensifying the heat of the lamps leading to thermal injury.*
10. Assess serum bilirubin levels as ordered *to evaluate effectiveness of therapy.*
11. Replace eye shields frequently to prevent the risk for infection. Ensure that they are secured in the proper position *to prevent damage to the eyes and surrounding skin.*

Continued

NURSING PROCEDURE 22.2
Performing Phototherapy

12. Periodically, according to agency policy and manufacturer's instructions, monitor light intensity with a photometer *to reduce the risk for injury.*
13. Encourage parents to soothe and touch the newborn while under the lights; role-model soothing behaviors *to promote parental participation.* If using a blanket or wrap, encourage the parents to hold the newborn frequently *to promote bonding.*
14. Remove the newborn from the lights for feeding and periodically, but at least once every 8 hours, *to promote bonding and attachment;* remove eye shields while out of the bilirubin lights *to provide visual and sensory stimulation and allow for eye-to-eye contact between newborn and parents or caregivers.*
15. Arrange care activities *to promote comfort, reduce energy expenditure, and maximize time spent under the lights.*
16. Wash hands and document time therapy was started; type of therapy, including number of lights and type; light intensity; vital signs; use of eye shields; serum bilirubin levels; and newborn's status and response to therapy.

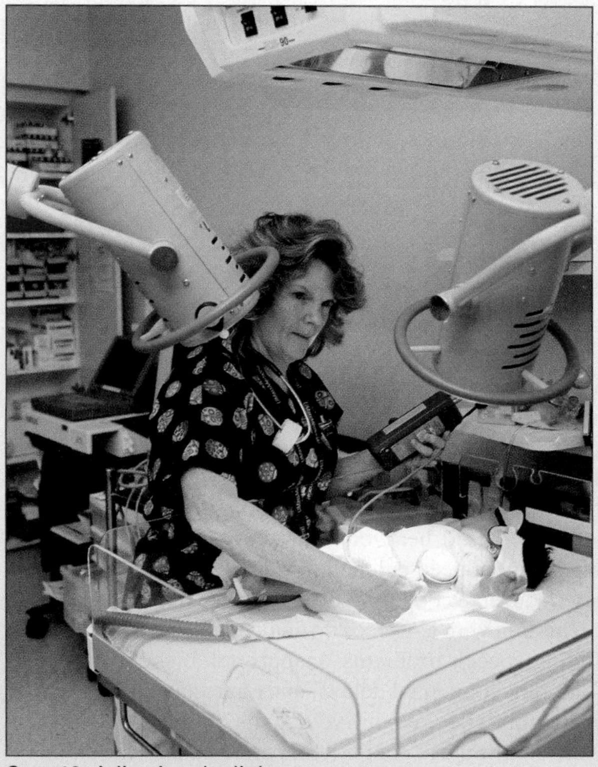
Step 12. Adjusting the lights.

EVALUATION

- Newborn tolerated therapy and remained free of complications and pain.
- Newborn's serum bilirubin levels demonstrated a gradual decrease to acceptable levels.
- Newborn and parents demonstrated positive attachment and bonding behaviors.

AREAS FOR ADAPTATION AND CONSIDERATION

Lifespan Considerations

- Bililights may be used in conjunction with a blanket or wrap device to enhance the effect when serum bilirubin levels continue to increase or are approaching critical levels.
- Document the newborn's ongoing status, including time spent out of the lights and parents' interaction with the newborn.

Community-Based Considerations

- Phototherapy may be provided in the home with conventional bililights or a blanket or wrap device. Often, a blanket or wrap device is chosen because of its ease of use.
- Ensure that parents understand how to administer phototherapy in the home; arrange for parents to provide a return demonstration of the procedure and care required.

Continued

NURSING PROCEDURE 22.2 CONTINUED

Performing Phototherap

- Arrange for home health care follow-up to assist with initiating therapy, provide ongoing education and assessment, obtain serial serum bilirubin levels, and offer support and guidance to the parents.
- Remind parents to ensure that they use a protective covering at all times with a blanket or wrap device to reduce the risk for injury to the newborn's fragile skin.
- Demonstrate to the parents how to record the necessary information about their newborn when receiving phototherapy, such as temperature, number of stools, and number of wet diapers. If appropriate, provide the parents with forms to use to record the data.

FETAL ALCOHOL SYNDROME

Fetal alcohol syndrome results from maternal use of alcohol during pregnancy. The characteristic craniofacial deformities of FAS are apparent at birth: a flat, thin upper lip; small eyes with short slits for openings (short palpebral fissures); and a flattened midface and profile with a short nose and low nasal bridge (Fig. 22.8). These features result from embryonic damage early in pregnancy. Decreased head circumference (microcephaly) results from reduced cerebellar brain cells later in pregnancy (Warren & Foudin, 2001).

Children with FAS face difficulties related to school, including speech problems, inappropriate social interactions, developmental delays, and aggressive behavior. Later in childhood, cognitive deficits and learning disabilities contribute to poor school performance. The child with FAS requires patience, nurturing, and special education; however, if parental substance abuse is ongoing, the chances that the child will receive appropriate care are at risk.

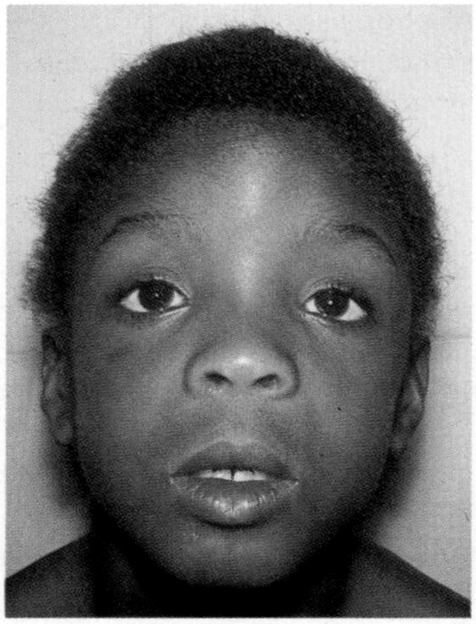

FIGURE 22.8 Facial characteristics of a child with fetal alcohol syndrome include short palpebral features, a wide and flattened groove in the midline of the upper lip, and thin lips.

Nurses direct care toward the newborn's immediate physical and psychosocial needs. If the mother continues to ingest alcohol to the point of intoxication, newborn care will be compromised, and the parent requires referral to community resources for alcohol addiction. In this event, social services must be contacted to evaluate safety issues (nurturing, feeding, risk for neglect) and possible placement of the child with foster care. Initially, the nurse should assess maternal–infant attachment and parental engrossment. Because of alcohol's effects and the characteristic appearance of the baby with FAS, parents may view the newborn negatively, rather than accepting him or her as a person to be nurtured and protected. Guilt may influence the parent–child relationship negatively, especially if the mother realizes the lifelong implications of impaired cognitive function. The nurse should role-model care by talking in a higher-pitched voice, making eye contact with the newborn, and demonstrating to the parents the baby's capabilities. He or she should show parents how to cuddle, feed and burp, diaper, and perform cord care for the baby. The nurse should discuss parameters for normal growth and development and encourage parents to stimulate the baby with bright-colored mobiles, talking, and singing. Praise for all demonstrations of nurturing care is essential. Team members must encourage follow-up care because these newborns will have ongoing special needs.

CONGENITAL ANOMALIES

The embryonic period is the time before organogenesis (formation of organs) (see Chap. 11). Three layers of primary cells (ectoderm, entoderm, and mesoderm) are the basis of all body structures and are susceptible to malformations. The ectoderm lines the amniotic cavity; the entoderm lines the yolk sac; the mesoderm arises in between.

Multiple congenital anomalies may arise from the same germ layer. In other words, when one congenital anomaly is present, other anomalies within that germ layer also are common. For example, the heart and kidneys both arise from the mesoderm; therefore, a newborn with a congenital heart defect also may have a kidney defect. The trachea and esophagus both form from the entodermic layer; thus, anomalies in both of these organs often occur together.

Genetic factors and teratogenic exposure are associated with congenital anomalies. Defects resulting from inherited traits usually involve only one germ layer. A virulent viral teratogen (eg, measles) can affect all germ layers and cause multiple anomalies. In a study of infants with congenital esophageal atresia, congenital heart disease was noted to be the most commonly associated defect (Leonard et al., 2001). Cardiac defects are also linked with omphaloceles and neural tube defects (Lockridge et al., 2002). When one major congenital anomaly is present, the nurse must be alert to other anomalies in various systems.

Nurses play a key role in educating women about factors associated with congenital anomalies. Because the embryonic heart begins beating only 24 days after conception, waiting until pregnancy is confirmed may be too late to begin teaching about the avoidance of teratogens. When pregnancies are planned, the nurse can influence quality of life significantly through early interventions, such as referrals to smoking cessation and alcohol abstinence programs and avoidance of workplace teratogens. If primary prevention is impossible, the nurse can be involved with early detection of congenital anomalies and begin instructing and preparing parents while the fetus is still in utero (Alderman, 2000). See Chapter 11 for more discussion.

Some congenital defects require emergency stabilization, possible transport to a distant facility, or corrective or palliative surgery. For example, anomalies involving the anterior abdominal wall and diaphragm pose serious complications and require immediate therapeutic intervention to avoid further damage and preventable complications. Table 22.4 identifies some common complications associated with congenital anomalies.

Having a newborn with a congenital anomaly is stressful to parents, especially when the problem is unexpected and families are not prepared. In some cases, a congenital anomaly is diagnosed prenatally, but its full effects are not realized until birth when it is actually visible or necessitates decisions and surgical consents.

TABLE 22.4 Incidence of Congenital Anomalies and Associated Newborn Complications

ANOMALY	INCIDENCE	ASSOCIATED COMPLICATIONS
Diaphragmatic hernia	1 in 3000	Respiratory distress at birth Poor prognosis with extensive pulmonary hypoplasia Chronic lung disease, feeding problems, gastroesophageal reflux diseases (GERD)
Spina bifida	1 in 1000	Trauma, infection secondary to break in the sac Nerve damage Motor and sensory impairment below the defect Bowel and bladder complications Latex allergy
Omphalocele	1 in 5000	Mechanical trauma, infection secondary to leak in the sac
Gastroschisis	1 in 10,000	Mechanical trauma to intestines Heat loss from exposure of internal organs to ambient temperature
Cleft lip	1 in 700 (general population; higher for Asian descent, lower for whites, lowest for African Americans)	Feeding difficulties, facial deformity
Cleft palate	1 in 700; Asians, 1 in 476; whites, 1 in 1000; African Americans, 1 in 2500	Feeding difficulties, frequent ear infections; impaired speech development, orthodontic problems
Esophageal atresia (EA)	1 in 3000	Alteration in nutrition/hydration requiring alternative route for food and fluids Aspiration from overflow of esophageal pouch
Tracheoesophageal fistula (TEF)	1 in 3000	Aspiration with sudden coughing, choking, and cyanosis
Developmental dysplasia of the hip (DDH)		Abnormal development of the affected hip; avascular necrosis of the femoral head if arterial blood flow is disrupted with osteoarthritis later in life
Subluxation	10 in 1000	
Dislocated	1 in 1000	

From Cleft Palate Foundation (2004): http://www.cleftline.org/aboutclp/; March of Dimes, http://www.modimes.org/professionals; March of Dimes Perinatal Data Center (2000), National Birth Defect Prevention Network (2000): http://www.nbdpn.org.

Congenital Heart Disease

Congenital heart disease (CHD) refers to a group of cardiac defects that change either the direction of blood flow or the normal structure and function of the heart chambers or great vessels. These anomalies range in severity from a single, common defect (ventricular septal defect [VSD]) to a syndrome of multiple defects. Antepartal diagnosis is possible through transvaginal four-chambered ultrasound.

Etiology

Several factors increase a newborn's risk for CHD (Box 22.4). Mortality rate depends on the severity of the lesion and newborn birth weight (Kecskes & Cartwright, 2002). Preterm and VLBW newborns are at increased risk for adverse outcomes and higher mortality (Kecskes & Cartwright, 2002).

Classification

Historically, CHD has been categorized as acyanotic (oxygenated blood is shunted left to right, placing added strain on the heart) or cyanotic (deoxygenated blood is shunted right to left and pumped into the systemic circulation); these terms are still in use. This classification system, however, may lead to an erroneous belief that a newborn having only oxygenated blood pumped forward into systemic circulation cannot become cyanotic, or that the newborn with a "cyanotic" heart defect is cyanotic at all times. Visible cyanosis is related directly to the amount of circulating oxyhemoglobin.

A more explanatory classification groups defects according to abnormalities involving inflow of blood to the lungs or outflow of blood from the heart, and the mixing of oxygen-saturated with desaturated blood in the heart or great vessels (Table 22.5). Ventricular and atrial septal defects and patent ductus arteriosus are examples of defects that increase pulmonary blood flow and thus can lead to pulmonary congestion and heart failure.

When blood outflow is obstructed from the right side of the heart en route to the lungs for oxygenation, back pressure builds, and desaturated blood is shunted from right to left through the foramen ovale (the fetal structure between the right and left atria to bypass fetal lungs). Cyanosis occurs when blood leaving the heart for the systemic circulation has not been routed through the lungs for oxygenation. Pulmonary stenosis is an example of an outflow defect. Blood outflow also can be obstructed from the left side of the heart with aortic stenosis or coarctation. Again, the obstructed outflow results in back pressure, forcing blood back into the pulmonary veins, resulting in pulmonary edema.

BOX 22.4 Risk Factors for Congenital Heart Disease

- Family history of congenital heart disease
- Maternal diabetes
- Maternal lupus erythematosus
- Living at high altitude
- First-trimester rubella exposure
- Maternal viral infections: cytomegalovirus, herpes, Coxsackie B
- Down syndrome (and other abnormal karyotypes)
- Preterm tocolysis with indomethacin (Indocin)
- Drug exposure: amphetamines, phenytoin, trimethadione, estrogen, progesterone, alcohol

Ventricular Septal Defect. VSD is the most common of all congenital cardiac anomalies. The defect can be small and relatively asymptomatic with possible spontaneous closure, or it may produce significant shunting of blood resulting in neonatal hypoxemia and congestive heart failure.

Tetralogy of Fallot. Tetralogy of Fallot consists of four defects: (1) VSD high in the ventricular septum, which allows for (2) the overriding aorta to be dextropositioned over the right and left ventricle; (3) stenosis of the pulmonary artery arising from the right ventricle; and (4) hypertrophy of the right heart secondary to the increased cardiac effort required to pump blood to the lungs. Depending on the severity of the defects and pump dysfunction, newborn survival may depend on patency of the ductus arteriosus to support pulmonary blood flow. In this case, prostaglandin E is used to keep the ductus arteriosus open (Westmoreland, 1999). Provisions for immediate intubation must be readily available if apnea occurs during prostaglandin infusion (McConnell & Elixson, 2002).

Patent Ductus Arteriosus. PDA occurs when the fetal structure connecting the aorta and pulmonary trunk remains open after birth. In utero, the ductus arteriosus allows blood oxygenated from the placenta to bypass the airless collapsed fetal lungs. This structure should functionally close within 48 hours after lung expansion with ambient air as a result of hormonal changes, increased arterial oxygen levels, and pressure changes in the lungs. By 1 to 3 months of age, anatomic closure of the ductus arteriosus should be attained (Westmoreland, 1999). With PDA, left-to-right shunting of oxygenated blood reroutes oxygenated blood to the pulmonary circuit, increasing workload on the heart. Congestive heart failure can develop.

Classic symptoms of PDA are "bounding pulses, a continuous murmur, and low diastolic arterial pressure" (McConnell & Elixson, 2002, p.17). Many newborns, however, especially those born preterm, present with only respiratory distress, tachypnea, and tachycardia, which may be confused with signs of sepsis. Echocardiography can confirm a diagnosis of PDA. The conservative approach for closure is indomethacin, unless drug-related

(text continues on page 955)

TABLE 22.5 Classifications of Congenital Heart Disease

HEART DEFECT	CYANOTIC VS. ACYANOTIC	BLOOD FLOW	COMMENTS	FIGURE
Ventricular septal defect (VSD)	Acyanotic	Because pressure is higher in the left side of the heart, oxygenated blood will be shunted from the left to the right ventricle to be recirculated to the lungs. This left to right shunting does not impair oxygenation of blood, but cardiac output is decreased, and cardiac workload is increased.	Size of defect dictates hemodynamic presentation. In 30% to 40% of cases, closure is spontaneous within the first 6 months. Surgical repair is required if infant exhibits failure to thrive, pulmonary hypertension, or right-to-left shunt greater than 2 to 1.	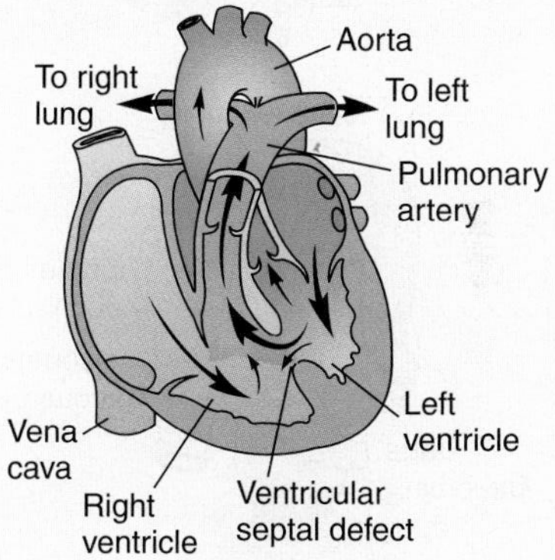
Atrial septal defect (ASD)	Acyanotic	Blood flow is inefficiently divided as some blood is directed back to the right atria to return to pulmonary circulation and some is directed forward into the left ventricle to be pumped into systemic circulation. The left-to-right shunting of blood decreases cardiac output and increases preload. Cyanosis is not typical because only oxygenated blood moves forward; however, congestion in the lungs can impair oxygenation and result in cyanosis.	Often symptomatic; 87% of secundum types close by 4 years. Primary and sinus types require surgery. Late sequelae include mitral valve prolapse, atrial fibrillation or flutter, and pulmonary hypertension. Congestive heart failure may develop from the increased work load on the heart.	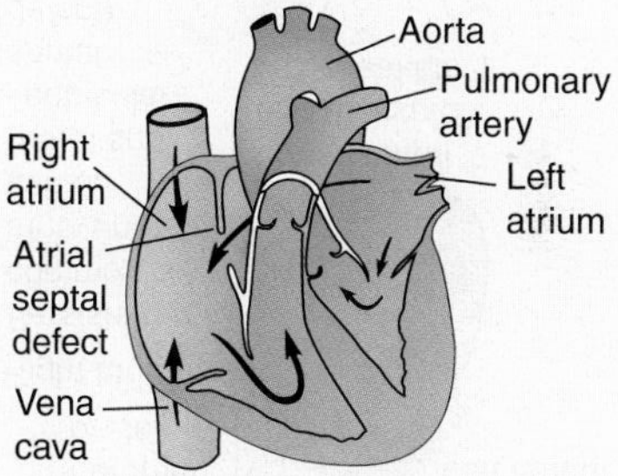

Continued

● **TABLE 22.5 Classifications of Congenital Heart Disease *(Continued)***

HEART DEFECT	CYANOTIC VS. ACYANOTIC	BLOOD FLOW	COMMENTS	FIGURE
Atrioventricular canal	Acyanotic	This defect allows oxygenated blood from the left atrium to flow backward into the right atrium. The abnormal tricuspid valve does not close properly to prevent backflow in the right atrium when the ventricle contracts. The ventricular septal defect produces left—to-right blood shunting, which mixes with deoxygenated blood in the right atrium.	Combination of the primum type of ASD, VSD, and common atrioventricular valve. Presentation similar to that of VSD. Palliative pulmonary artery banding in refractory congestive heart failure.	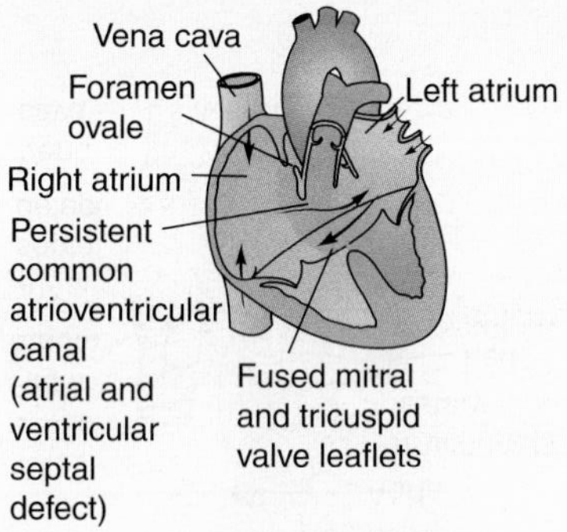
Pulmonary stenosis	Acyanotic	Forward blood flow by way of the pulmonary artery is impeded by narrowing of the lumen of the pulmonic valve or the artery just distal to the valve. Blood distends the right ventricle, leading to hypertrophy from excessive workload.	May be asymptomatic or result in severe congestive heart failure. Prostaglandin E_1 infusion at birth may be helpful. Valvular type may require balloon valvuloplasty.	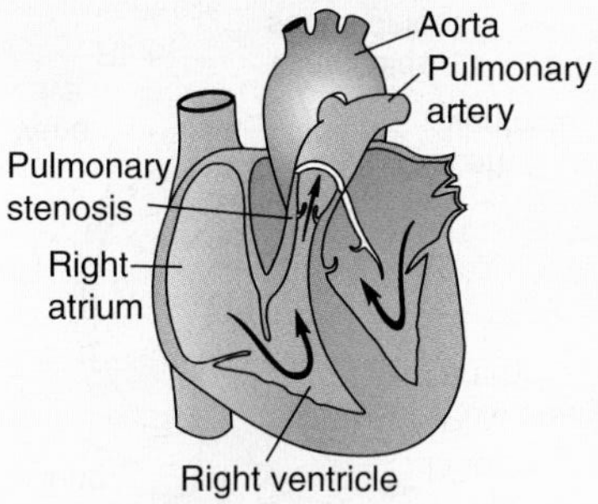
Patent ductus arteriosus (PDA)	Acyanotic	Aortic blood is shunted back into the pulmonary artery through the fetal structure (ductus arteriosus).	In preterm infants, spontaneous closure or indomethacin-induced closure. In term infants, spontaneous closure is less likely, and indomethacin is not helpful. Recurrent pneumonia may occur. Surgical ligation is usually required. No long-term sequelae if treated adequately.	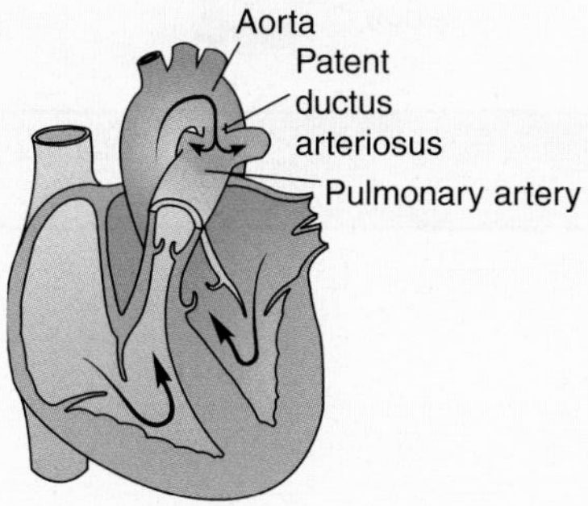

Aortic stenosis	Acyanotic	Narrowing or stricture of the aortic valve restricts forward blood flow from the left ventricle. Blood distends the left ventricle, leading to hypertrophy from excessive workload. Back pressure may result in distention of pulmonary veins and pulmonary edema.	May be asymptomatic. Valve replacement and anticoagulation may be required.	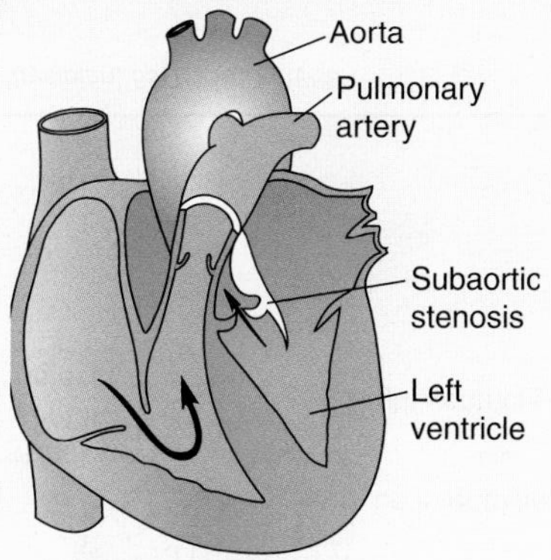
Coarctation of the aorta	Acyanotic	Because of kinking of the aorta, there is high pressure, turbulent blood flow proximal to the coarctation, and low pressure with decreased blood flow distal to the coarctation.	Up to 98% of cases occur at origin of left subclavian artery. Blood pressure is higher in arms than legs. Bounding pulses in arms and decreased pulses in legs.	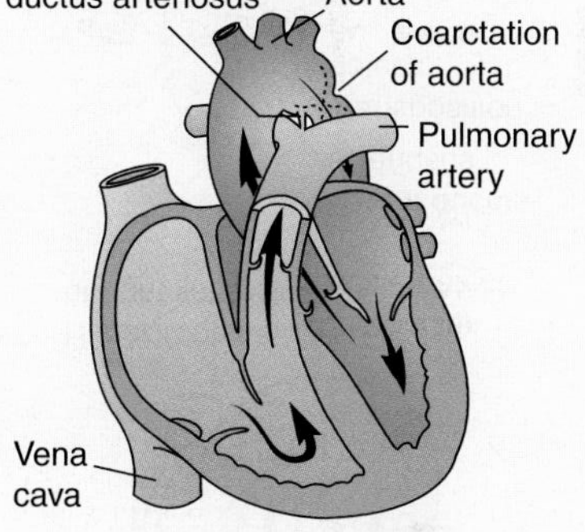

Continued

● **TABLE 22.5 Classifications of Congenital Heart Disease *(Continued)***

HEART DEFECT	CYANOTIC VS. ACYANOTIC	BLOOD FLOW	COMMENTS	FIGURE
Tetralogy of Fallot	Cyanotic	Because of pulmonary stenosis that restricts blood flow from the right heart into the pulmonary artery, and the VSD that is high in the ventricles and allows the aorta to override at the top of the VSD, blood from the right heart and left heart is pumped simultaneously forward via the aorta into the systemic circulation. The defect is classed as cyanotic because blood from the right heart is pumped forward into circulation bypassing oxygenation in the lungs.	Most common CHD beyond infancy. Defects include VSD, right ventricular hypertrophy, right outflow obstruction, and overriding aorta. Intermittent episodes of hyperpnea, irritability, cyanosis with decreased intensity of murmur. Palliative shunting may be necessary. Surgical repair required before age 4 years.	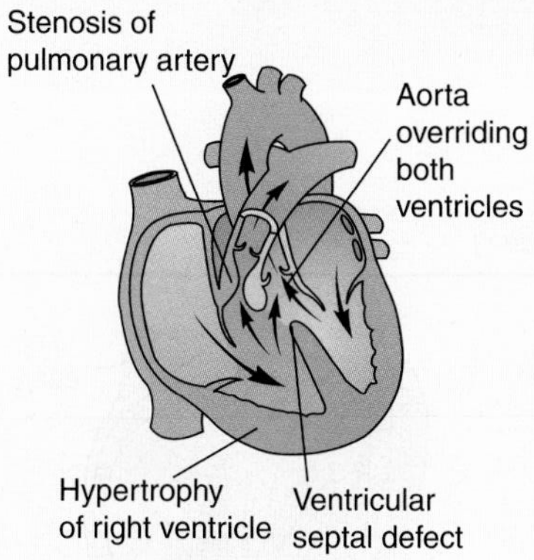
Transposition of the great arteries	Cyanotic	Deoxygenated blood from the right ventricle is pumped forward through the aorta, which arises from the right ventricle instead of the left. Blood is pumped to the lungs from the left ventricle through the pulmonary artery, which arises from the left rather than the right ventricle. The patent ductus that connects the aorta and pulmonary circulation allows some blood to be oxygenated and return to the left heart via the pulmonary veins to be shunted through the right atria through a defect in the atrial wall. This small amount of oxygenated blood can be moved forward into systemic circulation from the right ventricle and out the connecting aorta.	Transposition of pulmonary artery and aorta. Ductus dependent. Consider palliative balloon atrial septostomy, but definitive surgical switch of aorta and pulmonary artery required as soon as possible. Late complications include pulmonary stenosis, mitral regurgitation, aortic stenosis, coronary artery obstruction, ventricular dysfunction, and dysrhythmias.	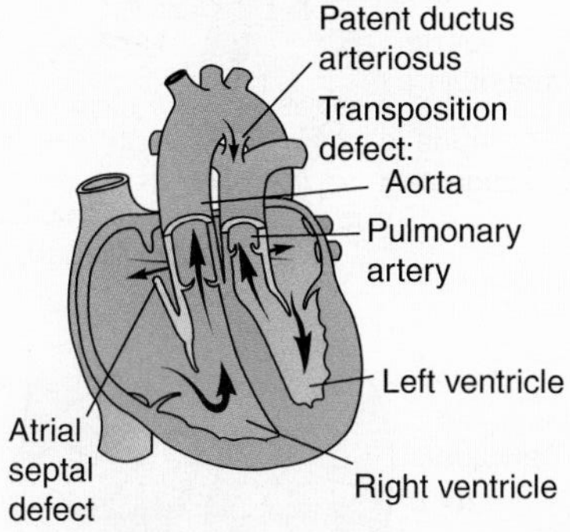

Text adapted from Saenz, R. B., Beebe, D. K., & Triplett, C. (1999). Caring for infants with congenital heart disease and their families. *American Family Physician, 59*(7), 1857–1868.

complications are considered too risky. An infant who is unresponsive to indomethacin requires surgical ligation (McConnell & Elixson, 2002).

When the foramen ovale (a fetal structure between the right and left atria) remains open in PDA, deoxygenated blood from the right atrium mixes with oxygenated blood in the left atrium. Indomethacin therapy is effective in the preterm newborn to effect closure.

Transposition of the Great Vessels. Oxygenated and deoxygenated blood mix when there is communication between the right and left heart chambers. The position of the great vessels can be switched, with the aorta (rather than the pulmonary artery) arising from the right side of the heart and the pulmonary artery (rather than the aorta) arising from the left side. The implication of this congenital defect is blood being moved forward into systemic circulation without first being routed to the lungs for oxygenation. This defect is called transposition of the great vessels and is incompatible with life. Immediate stabilization and surgical intervention are necessary. The ductus arteriosus and foramen ovale must remain open to allow oxygenated blood to be pumped to the systemic circulation to sustain life until surgical correction is accomplished. Prostaglandin E is administered to prevent normal closure of the ductus arteriosus, and the foramen ovale is enlarged by a balloon to create an artificial atrial septal defect.

Collaborative Management

Treatment parameters for the major types of CHD are presented in Table 22.6. A review of the antepartal record for factors that increase the risk for CHD is essential. The nurse also should be especially aware of the newborn's gestational age, respiratory status, and feeding behavior. In preterm newborns, PDA often is manifested by respiratory distress (McConnell & Elixson, 2002). If the laboring woman received indomethacin (Indocin) as a tocolytic agent, the risk for PDA in the newborn is doubled (McConnell & Elixson, 2002).

Many newborns with CHD appear normal in the first days or weeks of life and only begin to decompensate when stressed. The nurse should closely monitor for signs and symptoms associated with CHD (Box 22.5). He or she also should monitor bilateral pulses of the upper and lower extremities. When monitoring the newborn's response to oxygen therapy, the nurse should position the

TABLE 22.6 Nursing Interventions for Newborns with Congenital Heart Disease

INTERVENTION	SPECIFIC ACTIONS
Maintain adequate oxygenation.	Maintain patent airway. Assess need for intubation. If infant is to be transported and may require ventilatory support, intubate before transport.
Maintain IV access.	Provide needed peripheral IV (PIV) access. If infant is receiving prostaglandin E_1 through a PIV, maintain a second PIV or saline lock for backup access. Provide backup PIV or saline lock before transport or surgery. Maintain arterial line for blood gases, laboratory studies, and blood pressure monitoring. Ensure that IV tubing is clear of all air.
Decrease environmental causes of excess stimulation and oxygen consumption.	Maintain neutral thermal environment. Provide minimal stimulation by decreasing noise and light and clustering all care.
Provide optimal fluid balance.	Maintain strict intake and output, including precise documentation of all fluids the infant receives (eg, colloids, medications, medication flushes).
Administer medications.	Medications may be ordered to: ● Maintain patent ductus arteriosus ● Correct metabolic acidosis ● Provide inotropic support ● Prevent and treat congestive heart failure ● Prevent and treat infection ● Provide adequate volume ● Maintain sedation, decrease pain
Communicate with caregivers in transport teams and receiving hospital units.	Provide complete prenatal, delivery, and neonatal history of infant to caregivers along with present status. Give clear, understandable explanation of infant's condition. Arrange interpreter or chaplain services when appropriate.
Provide parental support.	Take infant to mother's room before transport if she has been unable to go to the nursery. Give parents telephone number of receiving unit or hospital along with directions. Contact social services if transportation or other support services may be needed.

Reprinted with permission from Westmoreland, D. (1999). Critical congenital cardiac defects in the newborn. *Journal of Perinatal & Neonatal Nursing, 12*(4), 85.

BOX 22.5 Signs and Symptoms Associated With Congenital Heart Disease

- Tachycardia > 200 beats/min
- Feeding difficulties; poor feeding; feeding times longer than 30 min
- Tachypnea; respiratory distress
- Diaphoresis
- Irritability
- Murmurs
- Pallor
- Cold extremities
- Cyanosis
- Hepatomegaly
- Recurrent pneumonia

pulse oximeter sensor device on the newborn's right hand and then on either foot, making note of any differences in oxygen saturation.

Newborns with CHD also may experience structural anomalies or diaphragmatic hernia, predisposing them to persistent pulmonary hypertension. Risk factors include meconium aspiration, RDS, heart anomalies with shunting, congenital diaphragmatic hernia, pneumonia, and sepsis. Depending on the severity of the hypoxemic respiratory failure, various treatments may be used: inhaled nitric oxide, high-frequency oscillatory ventilation, and extracorporeal membrane oxygenation (ECMO). ECMO may be used for respiratory failure of any origin.

Supportive nursing management for the newborn includes minimal handling to reduce energy expenditure and swaddling to provide containment and comfort. Noxious stimuli, such as when obtaining blood specimens for arterial blood gases or manipulating the newborn, tend to induce respiratory distress and cyanosis. The nurse preoxygenates and premedicates the newborn with a prescribed sedative before activities known to precipitate agitation (Lockridge et al., 2002).

Feeding is a stressor and may fatigue a seriously compromised newborn. Difficulties are associated with distress in the form of tachypnea, perspiring around the forehead and hairline during feeding, subcostal retractions, and feeding lasting more than 30 minutes. Using soft, smaller preterm nipples with enlarged holes can reduce the work of sucking (see the later section on feeding mechanisms for cleft lip and palate).

Depending on the severity of CHD, the newborn may be able to breastfeed and possibly demonstrate satisfactory weight gain. If weight gain is insufficient, breastfeeding must be supplemented with high-caloric formulas or enteral feedings through orogastric-nasogastric or gastrostomy-duodenal tubes. Often, nutritional intake is insufficient to meet the metabolic demands of congestive heart failure: tachycardia, increased oxygen consumption, and recurrent respiratory illness. Reduced nutritional intake also may be related to fatigue and the side effects of prescribed medication such as nausea, vomiting, and anorexia.

Because a diagnosis of CHD causes much distress for families, supportive interventions involve a collaborative culturally sensitive approach based on identified family needs. Caregiver role strain may be related to the demands of medical treatment and frequent transportation and visits to a distant facility with pediatric cardiology offices. These demands may be coupled with common stressors related to careers, care of other children, and housekeeping. The nurse must be aware of community resources, parental support groups, homemaker services, and respite care, giving appropriate referrals and recommendations according to the family needs. The availability of tele-echocardiography and pediatric cardiology through telemedicine can reduce medical expenses and improve time management when the family's community does not have immediate access to pediatric sonographers, pediatric cardiologists, or both (Sable et al., 2002).

The nurse supports positive coping by encouraging the family unit to focus on the newborn rather than the illness. Protectiveness must be balanced with normalcy. Caregivers can become so fearful of exposing the baby to infection sources that they isolate themselves with the infant. In becoming consumed with the care that the newborn with CHD requires, parents may ignore or neglect other siblings. Some defects are not always treated immediately in the newborn period. For example, sometimes surgery is delayed until an organ suitable for transplant is available. The effect that such delays can have on families may be devastating. In such instances, nurses can help the family cope by providing teaching about areas such as the best way to handle cyanotic episodes. Referrals to support groups, Web sites with other parents in similar situations, and other mechanisms for sharing common experiences also may be helpful.

QUOTE 22-1

"I was caring for a Chinese couple who expressed the belief that their newborn's congenital cardiac defect was linked to a problem with the baby's spirit, which was directly related to construction around their home during pregnancy. To be sensitive to their needs, I accommodated two desired changes that the family thought would alter the course of the baby's recovery: changing the baby's name (to rebuild internal harmony) and rescheduling the date of surgery to one specified by the Chinese folk healer as beneficial to postoperative healing. As a result, the family felt more at ease, experiencing less anxiety and more hope for a good outcome" (Chen & Rankin, 2002).

From a newborn nurse

Congenital Diaphragmatic Hernia

Congenital diaphragmatic hernia refers to the protrusion of abdominal contents (eg, a portion of the stomach or intestine) through an abnormality in the diaphragm (Fig. 22.9). It usually develops between 8 and 10 weeks' gestation when the pleuroperitoneal canals are fusing. As a result, the abdominal organs rise up through the defect and occupy space in the thoracic cavity. Intestinal organs may not actually invade the thoracic cavity, however, until later in pregnancy. Depending on the degree of pulmonary compression during the time when lung tissue should be developing, potentially fatal lung hypoplasia also may result.

Assessment Findings

If prenatal ultrasound identifies a congenital diaphragmatic hernia, birth in a facility with specialized care and a pediatric surgeon is advised (Lockridge et al., 2002). Fetal surgery has been possible for the past 20 years, but as of this writing, only two U.S. sites perform it (Farmer, 2003). Ten years ago at the University of California, San Francisco, fetal surgery was performed to repair a diaphragmatic hernia. After performing a maternal hysterotomy, the fetal torso was partially outside the uterus for this repair. The maternal risk at the time of surgery and future implications of possible uterine rupture coupled with the fetal outcome did not appear to be worth the risk to mother and fetus. This approach has been abandoned because outcomes were not improved over postnatal surgery, with the additional complications associated with maternal hysterotomy (Farmer, 2003). The National Institutes of Health are conducting clinical trials involving fetal bronchoscopic surgery. This procedure involves inserting a balloon to distend the fetal lungs. The only candidates for this procedure are those with very severe defects involving herniation of the liver through the diaphragm who would not survive long enough for extrauterine repair. Despite previous efforts at fetal surgical repair, currently the best time for surgery of congenital diaphragm is after birth of the newborn. This method is based on the risk to the mother and lack of improved outcomes obtained with fetal surgery (Farmer, 2003).

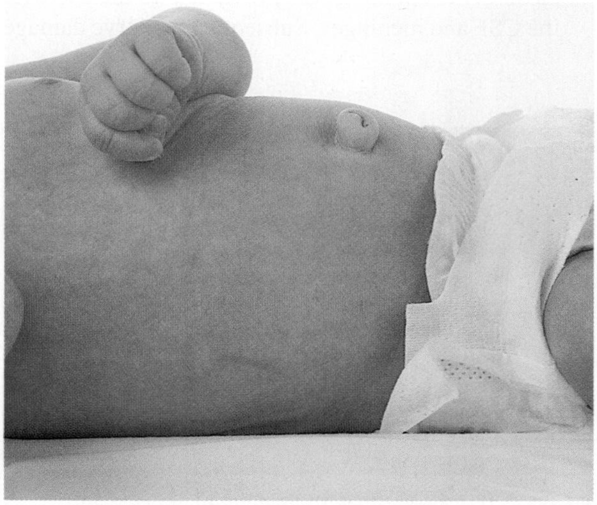

FIGURE 22.9 Congenital diaphragmatic hernia.

Collaborative Management

At birth, after determining the adequacy of oxygen exchange and ventilation, surgery is the only option and an immediate priority as soon as possible. The nurse is alert to signs of respiratory distress, which may be present with the first birth cry or develop hours or even days later depending on the size of the herniation. Resuscitation may be necessary at birth. Visualizing the newborn's respiratory effort and color provides immediate indicators of respiratory distress. Tachypnea, grunting, and intercostal retractions may be present because of impaired ventilatory exchange, which results from herniation of the stomach (normally in the abdominal cavity) into the thorax and displacing the lungs. Auscultation may reveal absent or decreased breath sounds and audible bowel sounds on the side of the chest with the herniation.

The nurse may detect an abnormal contour of the abdomen, chest, or both in the affected newborn. When appreciable loops of bowel are in the chest cavity rather than in the abdomen, the abdomen may appear flat or concave instead of rounded. A chest cavity filled with abdominal contents appears barrel shaped.

Administration of oxygen by hood or blow-by mask is indicated immediately. Increasing intrathoracic pressure with positive pressure bag-mask resuscitation may increase mediastinal shifting and can lead to pneumothorax; thus, this method should be avoided if at all possible (Lockridge et al., 2002). The nurse prepares the newborn for immediate nasogastric or orogastric intubation and decompression with gentle suction to prevent gastric distention and further restriction of respiratory excursion.

Pulse oximetry is used as a tool to monitor adequacy of respirations and ventilation. Maintaining the oxygen saturation above 90% determines the adequacy of oxygenation. The probe for pulse oximetry is positioned on the right hand of the newborn with the low limit alarm setting set at 89%. The umbilical cord should be left long to allow for cannulation and IV access. Because the infant will be NPO, IV fluids are administered to maintain hydration. Antibiotic therapy may be prescribed preoperatively because of the newborn's altered immune response (McKenney, 2001).

Parental anxiety and concern are extremely high when birth resuscitation is required. This anxiety is further compounded when plans are made for stabilization, possible transport to a tertiary care facility, or use of ECMO. Family-centered care requires honest, straightforward, positive communication, providing information and frequent updates regarding the newborn's condition and the plans for care.

Minimal handling of the newborn is indicated because of his or her increased oxygen needs related to stress and agitation. The nurse should promote attachment, however, by providing physical contact between the newborn and family as much as possible. Because of the relationship between cold stress and the development of acidosis, the newborn should be kept warm at all times. Swaddling promotes both comfort and warmth. The parents need instruction on how to hold the newborn upright, cupping the legs into a flexed position.

Neural Tube Defects

Neural tube defects (NTDs) refer to a group of anomalies involving the brain and spinal cord. Abnormal neural development may result in cephalic or spinal defects that range from mildly serious, to severe and disabling, to incompatible with life.

Types

NTDs include anencephaly, spina bifida, and encephalocele. Newborns with anencephaly have no cerebral hemispheres (Fig. 22.10). They may have functioning centers for cardiac and respiratory function because of an intact medulla oblongata. The condition is suspected antepartally with elevated levels of alpha-fetoprotein and confirmed diagnostically by sonogram. Parents usually are presented with the option to terminate the pregnancy because the fetus with only a brain stem will likely die soon after birth. Those with anencephaly who survive birth require long-term custodial care with no hope of independent living.

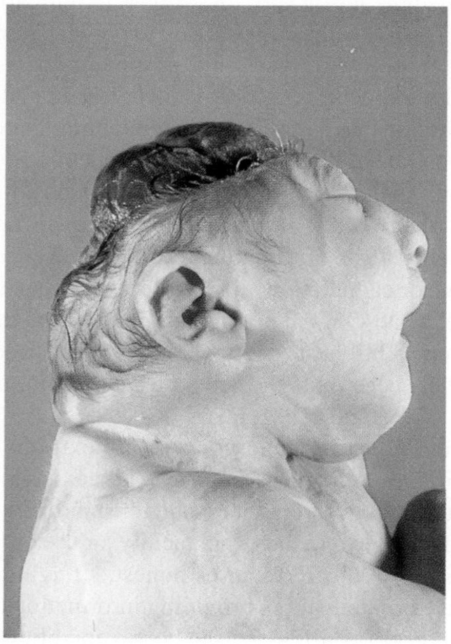

FIGURE 22.10 The newborn with anencephaly.

The most common NTD is **spina bifida,** which develops between 16 and 18 weeks' gestation at a rate of 1 per 1000 births. Spina bifida involves failure of the neural tube to close because of internal and external factors (Spina Bifida Association, 2003). It is not always fatal; however, it can be devastating to families because the baby has paralysis below the level of the defect and hydrocephaly that can lead to brain injury secondary to increased ICP. Because of quality-of-life issues, many women choose to terminate pregnancies with fetuses who have spina bifida. Others continue the pregnancy and assume care of the affected infant (Farmer, 2003).

Spina bifida can be manifested in one of three forms: spina bifida occulta, meningocele, or myelomeningocele (Fig. 22.11).

- *Spina bifida occulta* is not true spina bifida in that the neural tube is closed ("occulta" means hidden). It involves only the laminae of the vertebra, or the vertebral arch (Barker et al., 2002), and results in no sensory or motor deficits at birth. Nevertheless, neurologic deterioration may be gradual over time. Assessment reveals a dimple, thickening of the overlying skin, and possibly hair growth at the site.
- With **meningocele,** the neural tube fails to close, leaving an opening in the vertebral column with an external pouch containing cerebrospinal fluid (CSF). Meningocele is evident when the meninges (three-layered covering of the spinal cord) protrude through the congenital opening into a sac on the external surface of the back. The defect can occur anywhere along the spinal column but is most common in the lumbar area. Because the sac contains only CSF and meninges, there are no accompanying motor or sensory deficits. Although minor disabilities may occur later in life, nerve damage is rare (Spina Bifida Association, 2003).
- The most serious and disabling form of spina bifida is **myelomeningocele.** With failure of neural tube closure, the spinal nerves protrude into the sac with the CSF and meninges. Subsequently, nerve damage

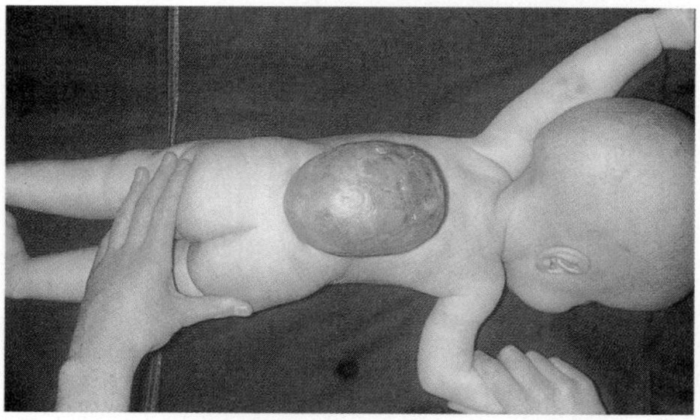

FIGURE 22.11 A newborn with myelomeningocele and hydrocephaly.

and severe motor and sensory disabilities can occur. **Hydrocephaly** (fluid collection in and surrounding the brain ventricles leading to an enlarged head) frequently accompanies myelomeningocele because herniation of brain tissue into the foramen magna prevents drainage of CSF while it is being manufactured continually in the brain (Barker et al., 2002).

Assessment Findings

Antepartal assessments include monitoring alpha-fetoprotein levels in women at risk: those with diabetes, elderly or very young gravidas, and those with a positive genetic history for spina bifida. Additional screening procedures may include magnetic resonance imaging (MRI) or CT scans (Barker et al., 2002). When spina bifida is diagnosed prenatally, treatment options include prenatal surgery to close the sac or cesarean birth to avoid trauma to the sac.

At birth, with the newborn prone, the nurse should visually inspect the spine from the base of the skull to the sacrum. He or she must document and report a dimpled indention over any area. An external mass is readily visible on inspection and appears as a glistening fluid-filled outpouching. The nurse must take extreme care to prevent trauma to a visible sac. The baby may need to undergo ultrasound evaluation for any neural tissue within the sac.

With a dressing protecting any visible sac in place (Lockridge et al., 2002), the nurse should assess and document the baby's neurologic reflexes (Babinski and leg recoil) below the defect and any mobility impairment or flaccidity. Assessment of bowel and bladder elimination patterns also provides clues to neurologic dysfunction. Lack of sphincter function leads to constant leakage of urine and stool (Barker et al., 2002).

The nurse should inspect the head for signs of hydrocephaly, which include an enlarged head with visible vessels. This enlargement, transmitted anteriorly, gives an appearance of an unusually high, wide, and protuberant forehead, which is called "bossing." The nurse should document a baseline head circumference at the level of the eyebrows to detect and evaluate the degree of bossing.

While the newborn is prone, the nurse should assess the skin for pressure areas, particularly on the knees and feet. A folded infant blanket under the groin area reduces strain on any lumbar lesion by keeping the hips slightly flexed.

Collaborative Management

Primary prevention of NTDs begins with optimal prepregnancy nutrition and folic acid supplementation (400 μg daily), which should continue throughout the first trimester (see Chaps. 2, 3, and 12). Newborns with spina bifida occulta typically require no treatment. For newborns with meningocele, surgery is initiated within 24 hours of birth to close and prevent any further damage or infection from a break in the sac. Preoperatively, the nurse should employ protective prone positioning, careful handling, and other measures to avoid trauma to the sac. Nurses have used padding around the lip and tape across the top of a small medicine cup fitted over the defect to secure the protective shield to the newborn's body. Any crack in the sac, no matter how minute, can be a portal of entry for organisms that can lead to possibly fatal meningitis. Thus, strict asepsis is a nursing priority at all times.

Fetal surgery to repair myelomeningocele is risky, although it has been performed. The most publicized of these surgeries involved a couple who refused a therapeutic abortion. The now famous surgeon successfully performed the fetal procedure in 1999 at Vanderbilt University Hospital. At the time of the repair, Samuel was 21 weeks' gestation. The child is alive and well as of this writing.

Before birth of the newborn, regardless of the type of defect, anxiety in parents and family members is common because of uncertain outcomes for both mother and baby. The nurse preparing the woman for a cesarean birth offers reassurance, information, and explanations regarding preoperative and postoperative expectations, including when she will be able to see her newborn (see Chap. 16). Ideally, transport of the newborn to surgery should occur after the woman is recovered fully from anesthesia and can view and touch him or her. If the newborn's father or another relative or support person indicates a desire to accompany the newborn to a distant facility with pediatric neurosurgical services, the nurse should investigate other people who can help the woman.

During initial airway management, the nurse should support the sac (if large) gently with a cupped, sterile, powder-free, nonlatex, gloved hand, lined with a nonadherent dressing material premoistened with normal saline. After careful transfer to the radiant warmer, he or she should place the newborn prone and apply a protective moist dressing to the sac according to the facility's protocol. For example, the Children's Hospital and Regional Medical Center of Seattle (Lockridge et al., 2002) lists steps for making a donut-shaped protective gauze dressing. The nurse can place a sterile small-bore feeding tube within the overlying gauze dressing to allow for the injection of 5 mL saline onto the inner dressing to maintain a sterile, occlusive, moist environment. He or she can then secure the entire dressing with 6-inch stretch mesh gauze.

Before and after surgery, the nurse should measure head circumference and compare the finding against the baseline measurement at birth. He or she should notify the primary physician or pediatric neurosurgeon of increasing circumference or deteriorating neurologic status.

Depending on the location and severity of the defect, complications following repair of spina bifida and placement of a ventriculoperitoneal shunt (if warranted by hydrocephaly), the nurse should reinforce with parents health care teaching and the possible need for neurology and physical therapy referrals for later mobility problems, as well as bladder and bowel training. Physical growth will require periodic shunt revisions. The nurse should teach caregivers to be alert to any behavioral changes, especially decreased level of consciousness, which could indicate increasing ICP from shunt malfunction.

Congenital Defects of the Abdominal Wall

Congenital defects of the abdominal wall typically include omphalocele and gastroschisis. **Omphalocele** results from a defect in the umbilical ring that allows abdominal contents contained within a peritoneal sac to protrude through the external abdominal surface at the base of the umbilical cord (Fig. 22.12). The less common **gastroschisis** also involves an opening in the anterior abdominal wall, usually to the right of the umbilical cord insertion (Kunz et al., 2005), through which eviscerated abdominal contents protrude. Because gastroschisis is a full-thickness defect of the abdominal wall and abdominal contents are *not* contained within a peritoneal sac, the internal abdominal contents are exposed to amniotic fluid. Amniotic fluid, composed largely of fetal urine and intestinal waste products, irritates the intestines and causes bowel thickening. When meconium is excreted into the amniotic fluid, a thick peel develops over the exposed intestines (Nichol et al., 2004). This is visible on prenatal ultrasound as matting of the bowel.

Incidence of other associated defects is high and may involve anomalies of the heart, gastrointestinal system, genitourinary system, and central nervous system. Unlike gastroschisis, omphalocele is linked to genetic and chromosomal syndromes. Risk factors include early maternal age, lower socioeconomic status, smoking, and use of over-the-counter preparations containing vasoactive properties such as pseudoephedrine (a common nasal decongestant). Findings also implicate the use of cyclooxygenase inhibitors and maternal substance abuse (Kunz et al., 2005).

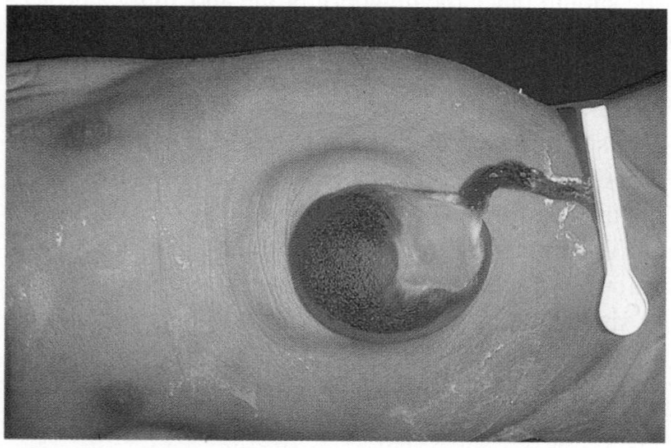

FIGURE 22.12 A newborn with the large and protruding sac characteristic of omphalocele.

Assessment Findings

Omphalocele and gastroschisis are readily visible at birth. When assessing omphalocele, the nurse should look for intactness of the peritoneal sac and evidence of organs visible within the sac. Usually the sac contains only the intestines, but sometimes the liver is there as well. The nurse also should document the size of the omphalocele, which can range from 2 to 12 cm.

Assessment of gastroschisis involves additional inspection (not manipulation) for twisting of intestines and changes in the color of the exposed intestines. The nurse should complete a thorough physical examination to evaluate for evidence of associated defects.

Collaborative Management

Any open abdominal defect predisposes the newborn to trauma of internal organs, infection, heat loss, and hypothermia. Timing and method of birth are related to fetal well-being, with best outcomes after 36 weeks' gestation (Ergun et al., 2005). Procedures start immediately after birth to stabilize the newborn and prepare for surgery. An elective cesarean birth may be planned to allow the newborn with known problems to emerge when pediatric surgical teams and intensive care beds are available; however, research findings do not support cesarean over vaginal birth in cases of the abdominal defect alone (Snyder & St. Peter, 2005). The high risk of stillbirth with gastroschisis (6% to 12%) also may be an indicator for cesarean birth when the pregnant woman reports decreased fetal movements. Follow-up ultrasound may demonstrate fetal gastric distention and a nonreactive nonstress test, indicating that the fetal heart does not accelerate as normal with movement felt by the pregnant woman (Nazir et al., 2005). A single surgery replaces internal contents (usually only intestines, but could be other organs as well, including the liver) back into the abdominal cavity. Because gastroschisis is not an isolated defect, highly likely cardiac lesions (eg, ASD, VSD) may require later surgery (Cachat et al., 2006).

Gentle handling is indicated to prevent trauma to the sac or exposed abdominal organs. Because newborns readily lose body heat to the environment through evaporation and radiation, the nurse should place the baby in a Servo-controlled open-air radiant warmer. If not readily available, the nurse should obtain a sterile bowel bag (usually available where abdominal surgeries are performed). Wearing sterile, nonlatex, powder-free gloves, the nurse should insert the newborn, feet first, into the bag. A high incidence of latex allergy in infants with congenital defects with organs on the outside of the body may be related to the frequency of exposure to latex materials (Barker et al., 2002); hence, all products in contact with the infant should be latex free. After containing the newborn within the sterile bag, the nurse should secure the drawstring tie on the bowel bag at the nipple level. This intervention helps to preserve warmth and protect against microbial contamination until transport and surgery can be accomplished.

The appearance of intestines outside the abdominal cavity can be a horrifying sight for parents. The nurse should assess their interpretation of what they have seen and explain the defect and measures being taken to ensure stabilization of the baby. When discussing surgery, the nurse should emphasize that the abdominal organs themselves are normal, and surgery to replace them into the abdominal cavity usually corrects the problem. If kinking or constriction have interrupted blood flow to the intestines, the nonviable intestines are surgically excised with anastomosis of the bowel and possibly a temporary ostomy.

Postoperatively, the newborn should be monitored for arterial hypertension, the cause of which is unknown and is more common with omphalocele (40% of cases) than with gastroschisis (10% of cases) (Cachet et al., 2006). Although such hypertension usually is transient, the newborn should be observed in a critical care setting for several days before antihypertensive therapy is begun. The nurse should be alert to signs of other postoperative complications such as sepsis, bowel obstruction, and NEC. Parenteral nutrition and fluids are indicated because oral feedings must be delayed until bowel function is well established (Snyder & St. Peter, 2005).

Cleft Lip and Cleft Palate

When embryonic structures of the upper lip, nose, and hard and soft palate fail to close and fuse, clefting results. Clefting may take many forms: complete or incomplete clefting of the lip only, either unilateral or bilateral, or in combination with complete or incomplete clefting of the palate (Fig. 22.13). **Oral–facial cleft** refers to defects involving both the lip and palate. Typically, when cleft lip occurs, the possibility of cleft palate also is increased. Infants having an isolated cleft palate (without cleft lip) are more prone to genetic syndromes accompanied by multiple other birth defects.

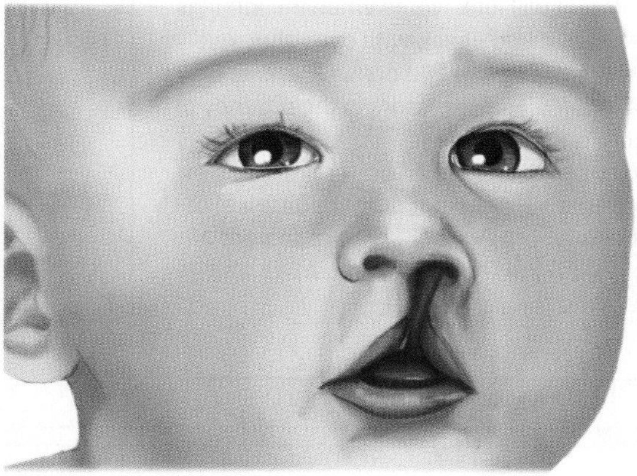

FIGURE 22.13 Cleft lip.

Etiology

The face and palate develop through embryonic cells that form the facial structures and separate the nasal passage from the oral cavity. These cells begin to coalesce, coming together from either side of the midline to the line that passes through the upper lip into each nostril. The hard palate likewise is formed by two shelves of tissue that grow from the sides and join together in the midline to separate the nasal and oral cavities (Crowley, 2001). Failure to fuse by the end of 7 to 8 weeks' gestation results in a congenital craniofacial defect at a rate of 1 in 2500 live births, with females affected more than males.

Incidence of cleft lip and palate varies among ethnic groups, but they are most prevalent in infants of Asian descent (see Table 22.4). These defects are least frequent in African American infants. Heredity and modifiable environmental factors are implicated, but the exact cause of craniofacial clefting is unknown (Uhlrich & Macklin, 2001). Research by the March of Dimes (2005) suggests that maternal smoking, alcohol consumption, and folic acid deficiency may be implicated; maternal use of antiseizure medications also may increase risks for cleft lip.

Assessment Findings

Defects involving the lip are apparent at birth, with a flattened nose and profile and clefts of the lip that extend into the nostrils. Palpating the hard palate with a gloved finger can easily reveal a large or a complete cleft palate. A small incomplete cleft palate may not be detected unless visualized with a light source.

Collaborative Management

Surgery is the primary treatment. Cleft lip can be repaired any time after birth. Many plastic surgeons use the "10 rule" (10 lbs, 10 weeks, 10 g/100 mL hemoglobin level) as a guideline for scheduling the operation. Unfortunately, this criterion denies younger babies the benefits of early repair, the most obvious being improved appearance (Sandberg et al., 2002). Additionally, early closure of the lip allows the infant to be able to create a suction for nursing. Advances in neonatal surgery and anesthesia have made safe repair possible at ages younger than 10 weeks. As the child grows, lip and nasal revisions may be necessary to improve appearance (Sandberg et al., 2002; Uhlrich & Mackin, 2001).

Repair of cleft palate may be delayed until 10 to 12 months of age to allow time for muscular growth. Surgery as early as possible during this time supports babbling and speech development. Later revisions to the palate may be necessary if speech is nasal (Sandberg et al., 2002). See Nursing Care Plan 22.2.

(text continues on page 964)

NURSING CARE PLAN 22.2

The Newborn With Cleft Lip and Palate

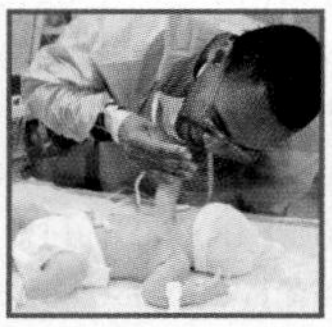

Recall Baby Madeline, described at the beginning of this chapter, who was born with a congenital cleft lip and palate. When taking a nursing history, Madeline's mother Danita denies any modifiable environmental risk factors during the pregnancy such as smoking or alcohol consumption. She reports that she took 400 mg of folic acid daily for an entire year before Madeline was conceived. Family history reveals two cousins born with craniofacial clefting deformities.

Baby Madeline appears healthy in every other way. Her mother continues to request verification that she has no other congenital defects. Neither parent has achieved a level of comfort with feeding. Danita and Louis decline the hospital's newborn photography plan, stating that they will wait to take photos after Baby Madeline's lip is "fixed."

NURSING DIAGNOSIS

Risk for Impaired Parenting related to difficulty with role transition secondary to added stressors of visible craniofacial defect

EXPECTED OUTCOMES

1. The parents will express their feelings of anger, grief, and guilt.
2. The parents will work together to nurture and protect their newborn.
3. The parents will verbalize positive remarks about the newborn and optimistic plans for repair of the craniofacial defect.
4. The parents will demonstrate progressive attachment and engrossment behaviors.

INTERVENTIONS	RATIONALES
Show before and after pictures of infants having craniofacial defects similar to Madeline's.	Photos evoke less emotion than an actual defect and can help to desensitize the real experience. Seeing "after" photos helps the parents to visualize past the defect toward the future.
Give updated reports about the newborn frequently, calling her by name and citing her positive behaviors. For example, "She likes to cuddle when you hold her close for bubbling"; "Madeline is such a good baby. She goes right to sleep after feeding!"	The newborn becomes more of a personality when behaviors are assigned to her.
Feed, diaper, and bring the newborn to visit during a quiet alert state when the baby is awake, but not hungry, wet, or crying.	The defect will look worse when the infant is red faced and upset, with eyes shut and mouth wide open and crying. Parents may face additional stressors in the urgency of comforting the infant.
Remain with the parents to hold the newborn while pointing out her positive traits. Point out positive normal characteristics such as eyes, long lashes, pretty hair, strong grasp, etc. Emphasize that the newborn is perfectly healthy in every other way.	Physical presence is a "buffer" and allows parents some space during appraisal of the newborn. Verbal encouragement and physical presence are supportive and provide reassurance.

Continued

NURSING CARE PLAN 22.2 ● The Newborn With Cleft Lip and Palate

INTERVENTIONS	RATIONALES
Smile while looking the newborn in the face to role-model attachment behaviors for the parents. Use the en face position and speak words of comfort and love in a soft voice. Hold and cuddle the newborn before handing her off to a parent.	Role modeling reinforces the normalcy of the newborn and affirms her value.
Encourage similar behaviors in the parents. Reinforce that it is okay to touch, stroke, or cuddle the newborn.	
Introduce parents to a support group or Internet site for contact with other parents of children with cleft lip and palate to share reactions and feelings as well as encouragement and support.	Group interactions with people who have had similar experiences can be an effective means by which to cope with similar stress reactions.

EVALUATION

1. The parents demonstrate acceptance of their newborn.
2. The parents show affection to their baby by such measures as kissing, holding, and looking directly at her.
3. The parents verbalize a realistic perception of the craniofacial defect and a plan for future care.

NURSING DIAGNOSIS

Risk for Imbalanced Nutrition: Less Than Body Requirements related to feeding difficulties associated with craniofacial defect

EXPECTED OUTCOMES

1. The parents will establish successful and satisfying feeding techniques.
2. The newborn will consume and retain 12 to 18 oz of formula or breast milk daily.
3. The newborn will produce sufficient urine to saturate 6 to 10 diapers per day.

INTERVENTIONS	RATIONALES
Collaborate with the nursing team to establish successful feeding techniques before introducing parents to the feeding behaviors.	Finding a successful feeding technique is a first step in teaching, avoiding the stress associated with trial and error.
Assist the parent to a comfortable, upright position; place the newborn in the parent's nondominant arm.	Sitting upright during feeding helps to prevent aspiration in the newborn. Use of the nondominant arm keeps the dominant hand available to manipulate the bottle and nipple for feeding.
Supply the parents with special equipment for feeding. Demonstrate how to place the elongated, soft, and easily compressed nipple into the newborn's mouth. Have the parents return-demonstrate.	Special nipples simplify feeding by closing off the cleft palate or being compressed easily by the existing portion of the palate. Demonstration is the optimal mode of teaching. Return demonstration indicates the extent of learning.

Continued

NURSING CARE PLAN 22.2 ● The Newborn With Cleft Lip and Palate *(Continued)*

INTERVENTIONS	RATIONALES
Teach the caregiver to sit the newborn upright on the lap, or to hold the newborn upright against the shoulder and to pat the back to burp or bubble the newborn after each ½ to 1 oz of liquid.	Typically, newborns swallow air with feeding, which may distend the stomach if unrelieved.
Monitor amount of breast milk or formula ingested. Assess daily weights and evaluate the number of wet diapers produced.	Monitoring intake and output provides an indication of hydration status. Weight gain is helpful in determining whether the newborn is receiving adequate calories for growth and development.

EVALUATION

1. The parents demonstrate feeding without difficulty, expressing confidence with feeding their newborn.
2. The newborn consumes and retains 2 to 3 oz of fluid with each feeding.
3. The newborn wets the established number of diapers.

QUOTE 22-2

"I was lucky that my baby's cleft lip was diagnosed in utero. The nurses worked with me to prepare me for what I would see and the feeding problems we were likely to encounter."

The mother of a child born with congenital clefting problems

Communication and Bonding Assistance. Therapeutic communication with the parents about the defect is essential immediately after birth. Even when they know about the problem in advance and have participated in antepartal interventions (eg, education, showing photos), parents and family members may be shocked when they actually see the extent of the problem. To help overcome a negative initial response, the nurse can introduce the defect as "correctable" and follow up by presenting the newborn as normal and healthy in all other ways. For example, the nurse might say: "Congratulations! You have a son with all the necessary equipment. This notch on the right side of his lip is called a cleft, a common defect that can be corrected. He needs to snuggle so that he can feel safe and warm before his first physical examination."

When preparing to introduce the newborn to the parents for the first visit, a keepsake picture can help promote a positive relationship by reinforcing that the baby is acceptable, valued, and lovable. After being bathed and dressed, the newborn is photographed dressed in a hospital garment with a brightly colored blanket background. Handprints and footprints can personalize the card to which the photo is attached. The nurse can reinforce the joy of new life and birth at every opportunity, such as when viewing the photo.

The nurse should role-model attachment behaviors in the presence of the parents and family unit. Looking into the newborn's face (en face position), smiling, enfolding, patting, and talking to the baby are all nurturing behaviors that reinforce the child's worth. While handing the newborn over to a parent, the nurse can emphasize the baby's positive characteristics by calling attention to thick curly hair or commenting on "whose big hands" the newborn inherited. The nurse should validate the mother's successful achievement of getting through childbirth and show empathy about any sad or uncomfortable feelings.

Feeding Assistance. Before a parent's first feeding sessions with the newborn, the nurse should review techniques known to work for the particular defect. A team approach and practice are helpful before the first feeding, which might be difficult. Various organizations offer tips and video instructions for new parents facing the challenge of feeding an infant with an oral–facial defect. Consultations with specialists who work with children with clefting disorders may be helpful.

Feeding tips should include basic guidelines of holding the infant upright, using special cleft palate nipples, and increasing the hole in a regular nipple to ensure a constant drip (Fig. 22.14). If a feeding takes longer than 30 minutes, parents can enlarge the hole by cutting an "X" into the distal end of the nipple. If the infant is receiving too much flow and appears to be struggling with the liquid, the size of the nipple hole is obviously too large.

By visualizing the hard palate, the nurse can determine the side of the oral cavity having the larger solid strip of hard palate. By offering a long soft nipple (Lamb's nipple) to the larger side directed toward the back of the oropharynx, the infant can simply compress the nipple between the flattened tongue and existing portion of hard palate to express milk without suction. The flanged nipple provides an attached covering that occludes the cleft in the hard palate and allows the infant to create suction. This device may be effective initially (although hard to use with very small infants); it must be resized as the infant grows. The nurse should advise the parents to burp the newborn frequently to control problems related to excess swallowed air.

Breastfeeding is possible with cleft lip because breast tissue can close off the cleft effectively. If the palate is widely separated, however, breastfeeding is difficult. The nurse can encourage mothers to pump breast milk and feed their babies through special nipples and appliances.

The nurse should encourage new parents not to be afraid and reassure them that nursing staff members are committed to helping them learn how to successfully feed their baby. Expressing confidence that the parent possesses the necessary skills to meet the challenges ahead fosters self-esteem. A satisfactory feeding should take no longer than 30 minutes; the infant should consume 2 to 3 oz of fluid. Weight gain and saturated diapers offer good indicators of sufficient nutritional intake.

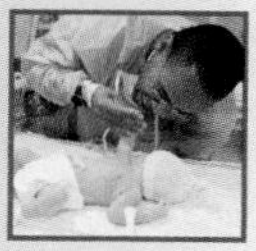

Remember Madeline, who had a congenital cleft lip and palate. Would she be a candidate for breastfeeding?

Parents should express comfort and satisfaction with infant feeding before discharge from the acute care setting. Should the primary caregiver feel insecure with feedings, social service referral for a home health nurse is indicated. The nurse also can be instrumental in introducing the family unit to community and on-line support groups and interactive chat sessions with other parents of infants with clefting defects. Additionally, the nurse should give the parents contact information for various manufacturers of specialized feeding devices.

Surgical Preparation and Support. In preparation for surgical repair, the parents and family meet with members of the craniofacial team who explain, inform, and prepare them for the infant's dramatic new look and oral capabilities (Box 22.6). The nurse should listen to fears and concerns and verify that parents correctly understand preoperative and postoperative events and care. Depending on the extent of repair, the operation should last approximately 3 hours (Sandberg et al., 2002). The nurse should relay frequent updates and reports from the operating room to the parents and ensure that the family has a comfortable area for waiting.

Postoperatively, the infant is likely to be somewhat fussy upon awakening from anesthesia. He or she should be quickly reunited with parents for comfort and nurturing. Feeding by breast or bottle (a primary comfort measure) is allowed immediately after surgery. Contrary to beliefs that led to previously rigid postoperative measures to protect the surgical site, feeding has not been proved to compromise the integrity of the suture line

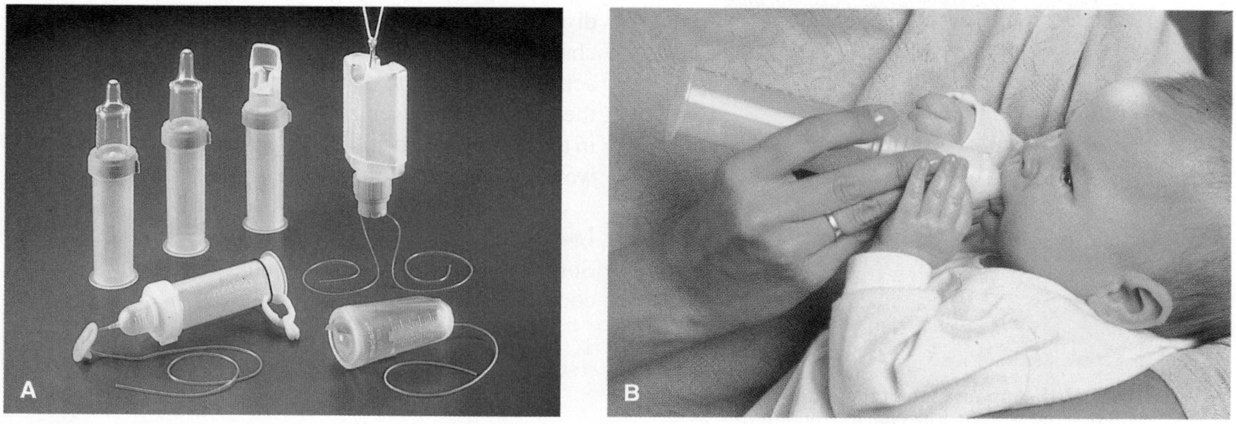

FIGURE 22.14 (**A**) Special nipples and feeding devices for the newborn with congenital cleft lip or palate. (**B**) Correct positioning for feeding the infant with clefting disorders.

BOX 22.6 Members of the Craniofacial Team

- Nurse
- Physician
- Dentist
- Orthodontist
- Prosthodontist
- Speech therapist
- Social worker
- Child psychologist
- Otolaryngologist
- Plastic surgeon
- Pediatric anesthesiologist

(Sandberg et al., 2002). The nurse should be alert to patency of small airways that swelling or secretions could easily obstruct. A splint-like appliance usually is applied in the operating room to prevent the child from stretching the upper lip when crying. The Logan bar (also called a Logan bow) helps protect the suture line and maintains approximation until healing by primary intention is established. Usually, the infant is discharged from the facility 1 to 2 days after surgery. By that time, the infant should be consuming and retaining the usual full feeding.

By the time that a cleft palate is repaired, the young child is eating solid foods (Fig. 22.15). Thus, all foods should be soft, similar to the consistency of whipped potatoes or applesauce. At the end of each feeding, several good swallows of clear tap water will effectively rinse food particles from the incision line. Because toddlers are known to explore their environment orally, elbow sleeve restraints and close monitoring may be necessary to deter thumb sucking or the placing of foreign objects in the mouth.

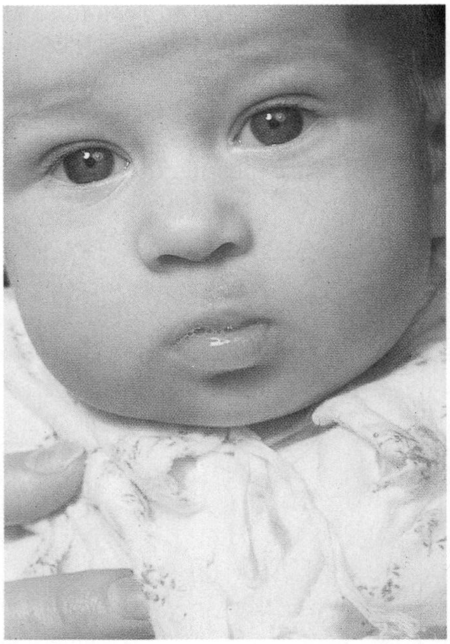

FIGURE 22.15 Appearance of the older infant who has undergone surgical correction of a cleft disorder.

Discharge Planning. Various members of the craniofacial team provide discharge instructions. An important directive is the need to monitor for signs of infection, including temperature above 101°F (rectal, axillary, or tympanic), erythema or drainage from the surgical site, or pain uncontrolled by acetaminophen. Infection can interfere with normal healing and may result in a less than optimal cosmetic result.

Esophageal and Tracheal Defects

Esophageal abnormalities develop early in utero. During the 4th to 5th gestational week, the foregut normally lengthens and separates into two distinct structures that eventually become the trachea and esophagus. Several variations of congenital anomalies are possible.

With **esophageal atresia (EA),** the esophageal passageway to the stomach is disrupted and closed off, ending in a blind pouch. The newborn may appear normal and healthy at birth with no visible abnormalities. When secretions or initial feedings drain into the blind pouch, an overflow may cause aspiration, coughing, and choking. Without surgery, the newborn has no means of ingesting fluid and receiving nutrition. Risks include aspiration and pneumonia.

A more immediately dangerous and potentially lethal **tracheoesophageal fistula** may compromise respiratory status at birth or soon afterward. With this defect, an abnormal connecting passageway (fistula) exists between the trachea and esophagus, created while these two structures were pulling apart to form two separate tubes. Because of the abnormality, fluid or food intended to pass from mouth to esophagus and onward to stomach may be diverted into the lungs. Likewise, air taken in by the trachea and intended for the lungs also may enter the stomach to cause gastric distention. Crying that compresses the abdominal musculature or having the head or chest in the dependent position may propel gastric contents upward into the fetal lung.

Types of Defects

Some varieties of tracheoesophageal fistula are more common than others.

1. In type A, the distal end of the esophagus is attached to the trunk of the trachea above the carina. The proximal end of the esophagus is a short stump that forms a blind pouch. Food and fluids have no route by which to enter

the stomach; with each inspiration, air from the trachea enters and distends the stomach. This route also allows gastric juice to enter the lungs through the fistula.

2. Type B is esophageal atresia only (without a corresponding fistula). The proximal esophagus ends in a blind pouch, and the distal esophagus is a closed stump not attached to the trachea. Because the stomach is not connected to the lung, gastric distention is not possible. The two ends of the esophagus are not joined; thus, there is no passageway for fluid or nutrition to enter the stomach. The blind pouch can fill with secretions or fluid that could overflow into the back of the oropharynx and be aspirated into the lung.
3. Type C is the rare "H-type" tracheoesophageal fistula, with an incidence of 1 in every 50,000 to 80,000 cases (Crabbe, 2003). It does not have accompanying esophageal atresia, but incomplete division of esophagus and trachea is apparent. The passageway from the oropharynx through the esophagus and into the stomach is patent. The fistula, which allows concomitant flow of oral fluid or tracheal air, usually is located high, near the second thoracic vertebra. This diagnosis is commonly missed because passage of a small-bore feeding tube at birth reveals a patent esophagus and aspiration of gastric fluid. Only when the esophagus is distended fully with diagnostic contrast media can the defect be visualized during a technique called the "pull-back" esophagogram (Butterworth et al., 2001). Obviously, during this procedure, care must be taken to avoid overflowing the contrast medium into the infant's lungs.
4. The type D defect can be rapidly fatal. Because the proximal esophagus is attached directly to the trachea, any oral feeding would go directly into the infant's lungs. The distal esophagus is closed off, and the stomach is flat and undistended. Gastric distention is impossible because the esophageal stump near the cardiac orifice of the stomach is not connected by way of fistula to the trachea.
5. Type E is a tracheoesophageal fistula with a connecting tracheal passageway to both the proximal and distal ends of the esophagus. Both fluid and air can enter the stomach and lung. This defect also can be rapidly fatal with the initial feeding of the newborn if the defect is not suspected and detected early.

See Figure 22.16.

Assessment Findings

With esophageal anomalies, the fetus cannot suck and swallow amniotic fluid. The clinic nurse monitoring antepartal measurements may notice increasing fundal height. Subsequent prenatal ultrasound may verify maternal polyhydramnios and no fetal fluid-filled stomach bubble (Brown & Nicolaides, 2000; Kalish et al., 2003). Brown and Nicolaides (2000) also described a high suspicion of esophageal atresia with tracheoesophageal fistula based on increased first-trimester fetal nuchal translucency. Antenatal recognition and in utero diagnosis of esophageal abnormalities may afford improved clinical outcomes based on measures to prevent aspiration pneumonia and early surgical correction (Brown & Nicolaides, 2000).

Symptoms at birth or shortly after vary in severity depending on the type of problem. Typically, the infant with the type A defect experiences noticeable abdominal distention because inhaled air with the birth cry goes directly into the stomach as well as the lungs. The flat stomach of the newborn before the birth cry immediately changes in contour, becoming rounded or convex with the first breath. With the newborn's head in a dependent position to facilitate normal drainage of oral secretions, the esophageal pouch may drain amniotic fluid and secretions that can be aspirated into the lung. Respiratory distress may develop. Conversely, the defect may not be noted until newborn nursery personnel detect indicators of tracheoesophageal atresia, fistula, or both. With esophageal atresia, an orogastric tube cannot be passed into the stomach. Rather, the tube coils into a blind esophageal pouch (Anuntaseree et al., 2002; Celayir & Erdogan, 2003).

Close observation of all newborns for cardinal symptoms of tracheoesophageal atresia and fistula is essential. Coughing, choking, and cyanosis with feeding are classic findings (Crabbe, 2003). Excessive salivation and drooling when in the side-lying position are additional indicators of esophageal atresia. Abdominal distention also is apparent when the distal segment of the esophagus is connected to the trachea. Crying (which compresses abdominal musculature) may result in cyanosis, yet when the oropharynx is suctioned, no secretions are present. Based on this assessment, the astute nurse should suspect aspiration of gastric contents into the lung. Because signs and symptoms may be intermittent and variable, a small trial feeding of sterile distilled water may be attempted to reproduce them under the watchful eye of the pediatrician, the pediatric gastroenterologist, or the thoracic surgeon (Crabbe, 2003; Patel et al., 2002). If test feeding by nasogastric tube produces no symptoms, yet the oral test feed is associated with choking, cyanosis, or aspiration, the H-type tracheoesophageal fistula is strongly suspected (Crabbe, 2003).

Misdiagnosis of esophageal fistula, especially the H type, results in frequent respiratory infections. Radiographic findings with such infants may reveal patchy infiltrates of the lungs from aspiration pneumonia and air in the bowel (Anuntaseree et al., 2002; Celayir & Erdogan, 2003).

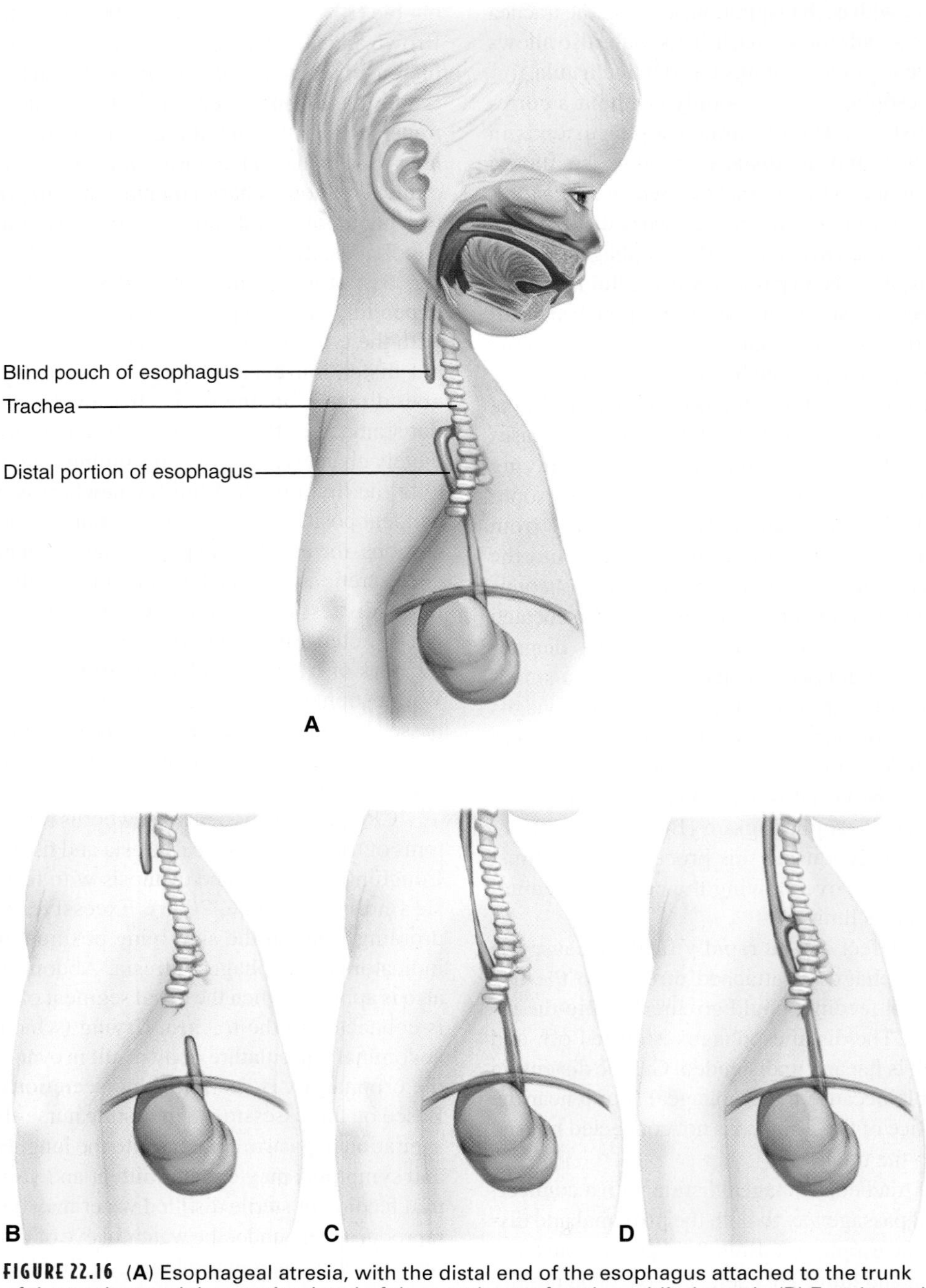

FIGURE 22.16 (**A**) Esophageal atresia, with the distal end of the esophagus attached to the trunk of the trachea and the proximal end of the esophagus forming a blind pouch. (**B**) Esophageal atresia without a corresponding fistula. (**C**) The rare "H-type" tracheoesophageal fistula. (**D**) Tracheoesophageal fistula with a connecting tracheal passageway to both the proximal and distal ends of the esophagus.

Collaborative Management

If a nurse suspects that a newborn has a tracheoesophageal fistula, he or she should allow nothing by mouth (NPO) and notify the pediatrician immediately. An additional priority is to position the infant prone with the head on a plane elevated to at least 30 degrees to prevent gastric reflux into the lungs. The nurse may pass a nasogastric tube if a test gavage feeding is prescribed and assist with supervised administration of the trial gavage. Suction equipment and an oxygen source must be available immediately in the event of respiratory distress secondary to aspiration. When the newborn is preterm and lacking necessary surfactant, RDS may complicate treatment. Positive-pressure ventilation usually is contraindicated with tracheoesophageal fistula because of the danger of abdominal distention. A neonatal cuffed ET tube, however, may be used to occlude the fistula and allow for mechanical ventilation (Greemberg et al., 1999).

While the newborn is NPO, the nurse should provide opportunities for non-nutritive sucking to promote comfort and security, as well as to help develop the oropharyngeal musculature. Hydration is maintained by IV fluids administered through the umbilical vein. Before corrective surgery, a gastrostomy tube may be inserted for decompression and to minimize gastric dilation and reflux (Greemberg et al., 1999). The nurse should monitor and maintain patency of the gastrostomy tube to gravity drainage. Underwater seal drainage may be used to prevent air from being sucked into the stomach with respirations, while allowing gas and gastric fluid to escape. With esophageal atresia, the blind pouch must be suctioned frequently using low intermittent pressure to prevent overflow mucus and aspiration. Pneumonia is a frequent postoperative complication because of the high risk for aspiration of gastric secretions and mucus into the trachea. Depending on the extent of surgery, the gastrostomy tube may be left in place postoperatively to provide an alternative feeding route while the internal suture lines heal. Oral feedings can resume when the integrity of the repair is intact, as documented with contrast studies.

Postoperatively, when any pneumonia is resolved and oral feeding is established, the nurse should monitor the newborn's eating behavior. Abnormal esophageal motility may result in residual dysphagia even after surgical correction (Crabbe, 2003). If surgery is delayed beyond infancy, the toddler may experience eating resistance, not having had earlier opportunities to enjoy oral feedings and to develop musculature used for ingestion and swallowing. Incidence of gastroesophageal reflux also is high following repair and may require further interventions for management (Crabbe, 2003; Konkin et al., 2003).

Imperforate Anus

Imperforate anus is the absence of an opening to the anus with failure of rectal descent (Fig. 22.17) (Quinn & Shannon, 2000). It occurs in approximately 1 in 5000 births, affecting more male than female infants. This congenital defect can be seen by the end of the embryonic period (7 to 8 weeks' gestation) and may vary in severity.

Assessment Findings

Nurses frequently discover imperforate anus during routine newborn assessment. Normally, the anus is midline and patent. An imperforate anus may be visible with stenosis, totally imperforate with no opening, or absent on the external surface. Anal defects are classified as either "low" or "high" depending on where the rectum stops anatomically. Radiographic studies can assist with classification by showing the level at which bowel gas patterns stop in relation to the pubococcygeal line and ischium (Quinn & Shannon, 2000).

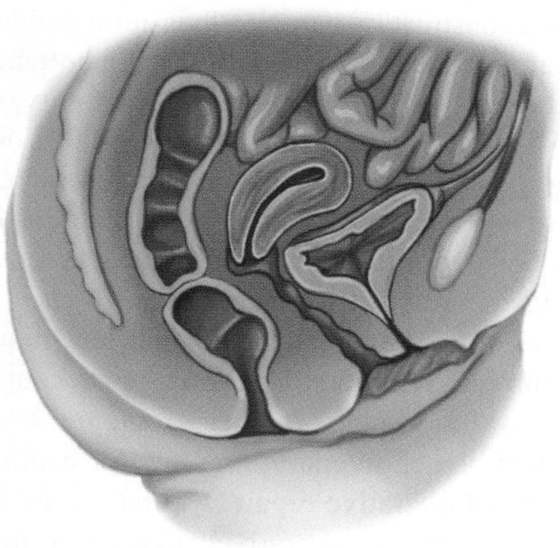

FIGURE 22.17 Imperforate anus.

During newborn assessment, the nurse should visualize the anus and verify patency by documenting passage of meconium within the first 24 hours of life. With trends toward earlier discharges from the hospital, however, some seemingly normal infants leave the health care facility before 24 hours of life have passed. Thus, nurses should advocate for protocols requiring newborns to remain in the facility until they pass meconium.

To test for reflex anal constriction, the nurse can stroke the anus lightly with a cotton-tipped applicator and observe for an anal "wink" verifying neurologic normalcy. With high defects, the rectum stops well above the muscle groups that make up the rectal sphincter (Quinn & Shannon, 2000). Lack of a wink reflex indicates that the newborn requires stool softeners and fiber for optimal bowel function.

Collaborative Management

Parents need to be informed of the congenital defect as soon as it is diagnosed because of the immediacy of elimination needs. The type of correction depends on the extent of the defect. High defects require immediate colostomy. Parents must be taught care of the ostomy site. Low defects are managed with anoplasty. If stenosis is the problem, a dilator may be used to prevent constriction of the new anus with instructions to continue regular dilation for several months. If innervation is damaged or lacking, constipation may occur in formula-fed infants; thus, breastfeeding is encouraged. Even after surgical correction, constipation may be a long-term problem, and parents are advised of the need for stool softeners and added fiber in the child's diet (National Library of Medicine & National Institutes of Health, 2003). Routine cleaning and diapering are adequate for the young infant. Protective ointments may be used if skin irritation is problematic; however, diapers should be checked regularly and changed promptly to prevent rash.

More complex anorectal anomalies may require extensive corrective surgery done in stages in conjunction with a colostomy, which provides a route for fecal elimination, and bowel diversion to allow for healing after completion of operative repair. A dilator may be used for several months postoperatively to keep the new anus from constricting during healing. The need for bowel habit training and dietary modifications may persist well into adolescence.

Skeletal Anomalies

Congenital skeletal anomalies typically involve the foot and ankle. *Talipes* refers to a congenital foot defect affecting the ankle, commonly called "club foot." Varieties of talipes are named according to the anatomic position of the deformity (inversion, eversion, or flexion). **Talipes equinovarus** is a combination of a downward and inward fixed position of flexion.

Etiology

Incidence of talipes equinovarus is 1 in 700 to 900 newborns. This anomaly affects boys more often than girls, with an increased frequency of hip subluxation in LGA infants (Lapunzina et al., 2002). Talipes is linked to heredity, and recent studies show a relationship between mothers who smoke and idiopathic talipes equinovarus (Skelly et al., 2002).

Assessment Findings

Visualization of the lower extremities at birth reveals talipes, which may be unilateral or bilateral. Testing the motion of the affected ankle reveals that the deformity is rigid and resists realignment, which differentiates talipes from the positional deformity seen in LGA newborns (Lapunzina et al., 2002).

Collaborative Management

Although talipes equinovarus is not life threatening, a twisted limb can be upsetting to parents. If untreated, it has the potential to be a major birth defect leading to permanent disability. Treatment usually is initiated soon after birth while the foot is malleable. It involves application of a cast to maintain corrected positioning of the foot (Fig. 22.18). Because of the infant's rapid growth, the foot needs to be manipulated and recasted first every few days, and later, every few weeks. Severe defects or those not responding to manipulation and casting may demand surgery.

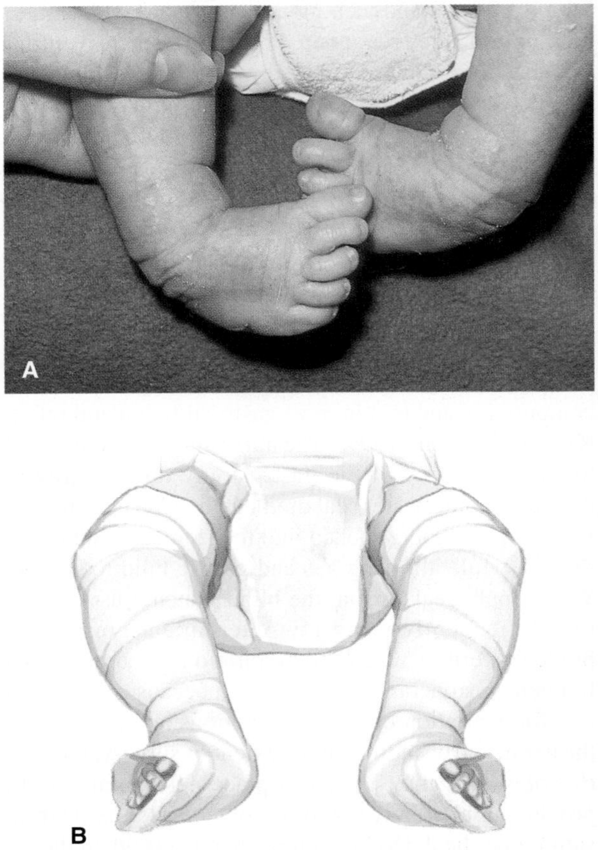

FIGURE 22.18 (**A**) Initial appearance of talipes equinovarus (clubfoot). (**B**) Application of the casts for treatment.

Once the foot has been correctly aligned, the child will need to perform a series of exercises and wear splints at night to maintain proper positioning. He or she also may require special shoes. Referral to a pediatric orthopedic specialist is indicated.

Parents need facts about the nature and treatment of the deformity. Nurses should be aware that relatives often experience grief upon seeing the defect. Giving information and listening empathetically always are indicated. Treatment usually takes months and requires frequent adjustments and applications of castings, splints, and appliances. Outpatient or clinic nurses usually are involved in assisting with such applications and evaluating the condition of the skin. Such follow-up visits provide opportunities for teaching parents and other caregivers how to evaluate the extremity, including checking the toes for warmth and color and assessing capillary refill, comparing findings bilaterally. Parents also should receive instructions in cast care, such as measures to ensure that the cast remains dry and to check for pressure, especially around the cast openings.

The nurse should verify parental understanding of the treatment plan and clarify explanations and instructions given by the orthopedist. Phone contact and follow-up between clinic visits provides encouragement and opportunities for family members to express concerns and ask questions.

Developmental Dysplasia of the Hip

Developmental dysplasia of the hip (DDH) refers to a group of hip abnormalities, ranging from a shallow acetabulum, to a stretched capsule with ligamentum teres, to complete dislocation. See Figure 22.19.

Acetabular dysplasia (also called preluxation), subluxation, and dislocation all stem from abnormalities during fetal development. Placental transfer of maternal hormones, intrauterine crowding, and breech presentation are prenatal factors that may lead to DDH. Frequency of hip subluxation is increased in LGA newborns (Lapunzina et al., 2002), perhaps because of a crowded intrauterine environment.

Assessment Findings

Following birth, nurses routinely assess all newborns (especially those who are LGA) for DDH. Visual inspection and a series of maneuvers should pinpoint indicators of the need for further diagnostic testing and referrals.

With the newborn lying on a firm surface, the nurse should grasp both ankles and manually extend both legs. This maneuver may reveal that one leg is slightly shorter than the other. With the baby still supine, the nurse can elicit the Galeazzi sign by flexing the infant's hips and knees while holding the feet on the examining table (Akera & Ro, 2003). The Galeazzi sign is positive if the nurse detects asymmetry upon visual comparison of the height of the knees. With the infant prone, the nurse visually should compare the skin folds from gluteal crease to knee, again comparing bilaterally.

Ortolani's maneuver is another method for detecting DDH. See Nursing Procedure 22.3. Diagnostic imaging will rule out false-positive clicks and confirm the diagnosis of DDH.

Nurses having contact with newborns and young infants should be alert for indicators of hip joint laxity that may not have been apparent at birth. Assessments should continue throughout health visits until the child is walking with an obviously normal gait.

Collaborative Management

Treatment should begin with diagnosis of the condition. The earlier treatment is initiated, the fewer complications the baby experiences, and the more favorable is the prognosis. The proximal femoral head must be centered in the acetabulum and then splinted with a device to keep the head of the femur in the reduced position. To maintain flexion of the knees and hips and abduction, the Pavlik harness commonly is used for infants up to 6 months old (Fig. 22.20). When worn continuously for 3 to 6 months, the Pavlik harness promotes muscle and cartilage development around the head of the femur for a stable hip.

If treatment is delayed and the infant develops adduction contractures, he or she needs more intensive therapy. Traction to slowly and gently stretch the hip to full abduction and hip spica casting to maintain reduction are then necessary. Spica casts must be removed and replaced to accommodate the child's growth. Older children must undergo open reduction.

Because of the lengthy nature of treatment, parents must understand the necessity and long-term implications of compliance with prescribed continuous splinting, as

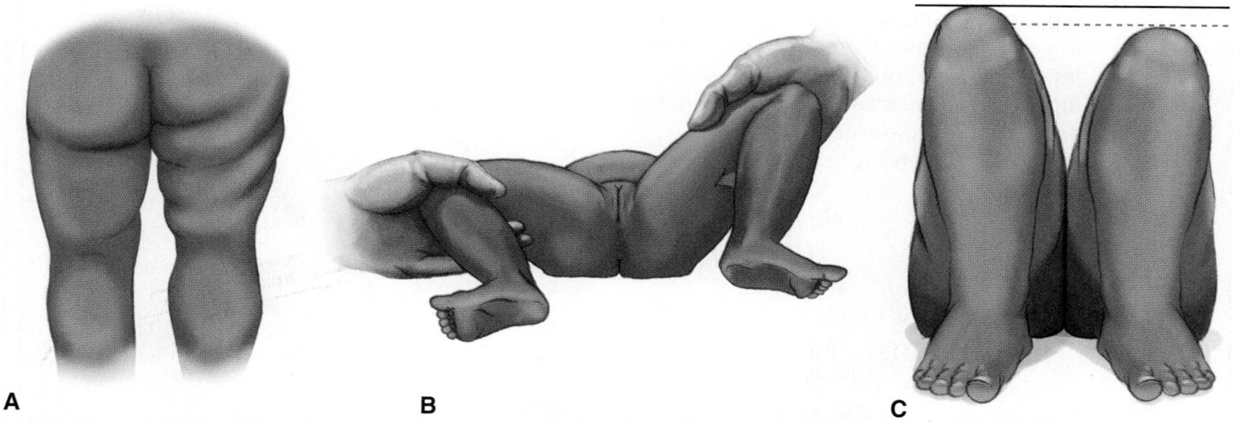

FIGURE 22.19 Developmental dysplasia of the hip is characterized by (**A**) asymmetric skin folds on the thighs or buttocks; (**B**) limited abduction of the hip; and (**C**) one leg appearing shorter than the other.

NURSING PROCEDURE 22.3

Performing Ortolani's and Barlow's Maneuvers

PURPOSE

To evaluate the newborn for evidence of developmental dysplasia of the hip (DDH)

ASSESSMENT AND PLANNING

- Review the newborn's medical record for factors that may predispose him or her to DDH.
- Question the parents about any past history of congenital problems, including those involving the leg.
- Assess parental knowledge of and previous exposure to the maneuvers.
- Inspect the newborn while he or she is supine for evidence of limb shortening on one side, and while he or she is prone for asymmetric gluteal and thigh folds.
- Flex both lower extremities at the knee and hip toward the abdomen; observe for differences in the height of the knees.
- Gather equipment
    - Flat, clean, warm surface

IMPLEMENTATION

1. Explain the maneuvers and their rationale to the parents *to help allay their anxiety.*
2. Wash hands; place the supine newborn on a firm, clean, warm surface *to facilitate testing and to minimize heat loss.*
3. Place hands on each lower extremity so that the middle finger is over the greater trochanter and the thumb is on the inner aspect of each thigh. Flex the knees and hips at a 90-degree angle toward the abdomen.
4. Abduct the hips while applying upward pressure *to determine if the head of the femur moves into the acetabulum;* listen or feel for a clicking or clucking sound, *which indicates a positive Ortolani's sign suggesting hip dislocation.*
5. Apply downward pressure while adducting the hips and maintaining knee flexion at 90 degrees. Note any feeling of the femoral head slipping out of the acetabulum, *which indicates a positive Barlow's sign suggesting dislocation.*
6. Return the newborn to a position of comfort.
7. Wash hands; document and report findings.

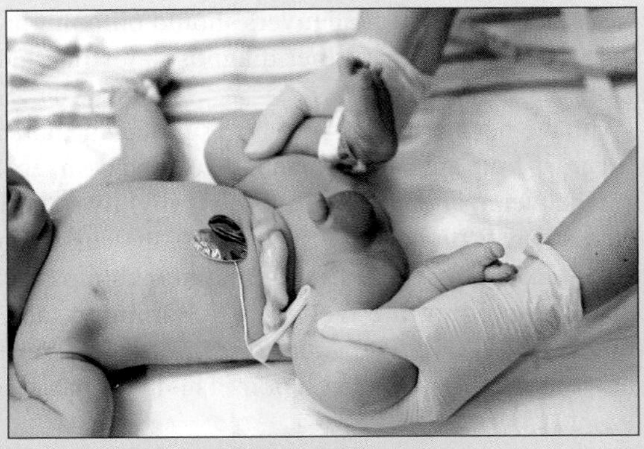

Step 4. Maneuver for Ortolani's sign.

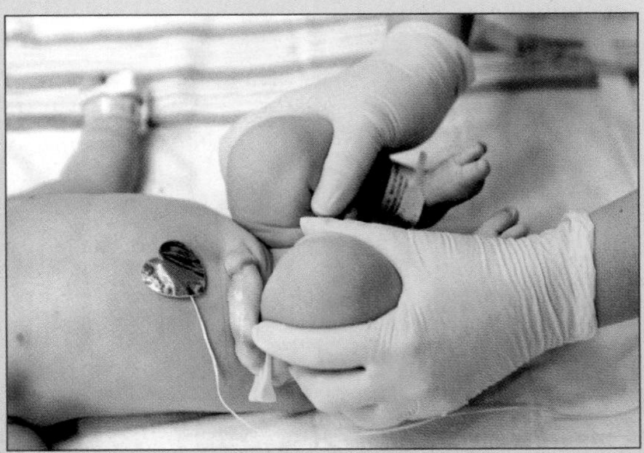

Step 5. Maneuver for Barlow's sign.

EVALUATION

- The newborn tolerated the maneuvers without difficulty or pain.
- The newborn exhibited no evidence of DDH.

Continued

NURSING PROCEDURE 22.3
Performing Ortolani's and Barlow's Maneuvers

AREAS FOR CONSIDERATION AND ADAPTATION
Lifespan Considerations
- Asymmetrical thigh folds may not be reliable indicators of DDH, because an uneven number of folds is a normal finding in some newborns.
- Perform these maneuvers very gently in the first few days after birth to prevent persistent dislocation from maneuvers done too vigorously.
- The earlier the condition is detected, the easier it is to correct; be aware that some newborns exhibit negative signs during initial assessment only to demonstrate evidence of DDH at a later health care visit.
- Inform parents of the need for follow-up testing to confirm the diagnosis.

well as the importance of maintaining hip flexion and abduction. For example, they will need extra time to bathe and dress the child because they will have to remove and reapply the harness or brace or work around the cast. Nurses should offer praise and encouragement to parents for their efforts. Parents should purchase clothing for the baby at least one size larger to accommodate hip abduction. Carrying the infant astride the hip, or holding the infant upright astride the leg of the caregiver may be comfortable.

Breastfeeding can be challenging when an infant has DDH. The woman can place pillows to her side to support the infant's trunk and legs behind her in a traditional football hold.

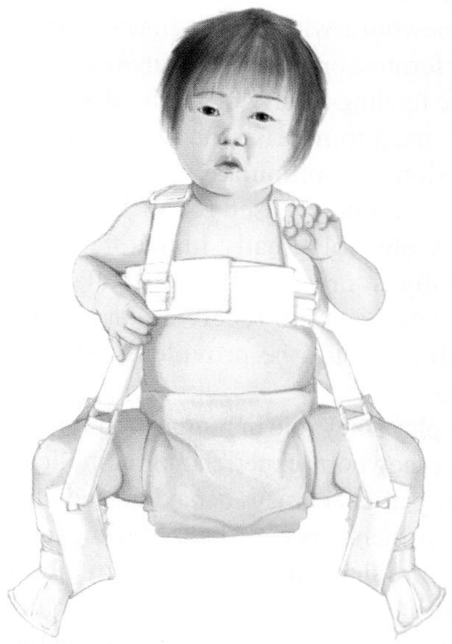

FIGURE 22.20 The Pavlik harness.

Commercial infant seats do not allow for hip abduction; rather, they force the infant into adduction. Thus, special infant seats and car restraint seats are necessary to fit the child's needs. When spica casting is necessary, the restraint device is modified to allow the infant's buttocks to rest on the edge of the seat with the cast extending over each side, secured with a chest strap and a center buckle. Orthopedic engineers design appliances according to specified needs.

Genitourinary Anomalies
Normally, the urethral opening is centered in the distal end of the penis in males, or midline below the clitoral hood in females. With hypospadias, the urethral opening is congenitally malpositioned dorsally on top of the penile shaft or ventrally underneath the surface of the penile shaft. Statistics related to frequency (1 in 150 to 300) are unreliable because hypospadias in females often remains undetected unless a girl or woman requires urethral catheterization, at which point health care providers have difficulty locating the urethral opening.

Hypospadias in males is apparent at birth during inspection of the penile shaft. It is not life threatening, but male children may be disturbed when the stream of urine sprays sideways. Additionally, a *chordee* (a fibrous band causing downward deflection of the penis) may lead to embarrassment and health-related concerns.

Treatment of hypospadias typically involves corrective surgery. Major associated risks include anesthesia, bleeding, and infection. Consultation with urology specialists also is indicated. Parents must understand the rationale for *not* circumcising the newborn male with hypospadias because the foreskin is an ideal tissue for graft that may be needed for the corrective repair. Practicing Jewish and Muslim families should investigate the possibility of having a ritual circumcision immediately before the corrective repair so that the foreskin can be harvested and used as necessary.

A nursery nurse who notes the obvious defect of hypospadias should document the location of the lesion (dorsal or ventral) and involvement of the glans penis, as well as any chordee. During examination of the newborn, the nurse should assess testicular descent by palpating and rolling the testicles gently between thumb and forefinger. Such examination is necessary because hypospadias is associated with cryptorchidism. In addition, the nurse should evaluate the newborn's urinary stream by applying a pediatric urine collection bag while the newborn remains undiapered.

Most new parents are interested in investigating their newborn to check that everything is "normal"—first counting fingers and toes, and later inspecting the genitals. When a newborn has obvious hypospadias, health care providers need to inform parents of the genital defect as soon as it is identified. The discussion may be distressing for the family, who might fear urologic, sexual, and psychological problems resulting from the defect. Nurses should provide information about the condition and measures to correct it, giving parents photos of children before and after surgical repair.

Questions to Ponder

1. How are the physical characteristics and potential complications of a preterm newborn similar to and yet different from those of a postterm newborn?
2. A Muslim couple requests that their newborn wear a protective amulet during phototherapy for hyperbilirubinemia.
   - Would wearing the amulet pose any health hazard to the newborn?
   - If wearing the amulet is contraindicated, what other options might be available to incorporate cultural and religious practices of the family?

SUMMARY

- Many different factors can present fetal risks and lead to newborn complications. Attempts to identify such risks begin as early as possible with genetic screening, health risk assessments, and early prenatal care and testing. Ongoing nursing assessments and evaluations during the first hours of life also help identify newborns at risk.
- Problems related to newborn size may be categorized as low birth weight (LBW), weight less than 5.5 lbs (2500 g); very low birth weight (VLBW), weight less than 1500 g; and extremely low birth weight (ELBW), weight of 1000 g or less.
- Newborns also may be classified by their expected size for weeks' gestation as average for gestational age (AGA; growth pattern is as expected for gestational age, and weight falls between the 10th and 90th percentile on an intrauterine growth chart); small for gestational age (SGA; weight below the 10th percentile on an intrauterine growth chart for the gestational age); and large for gestational age (LGA; weight about the 90th percentile on intrauterine growth charts for gestational age).
- A newborn born any time before the 38th week of gestation, independent of birth weight, is classified as preterm or premature. A newborn born after 42 weeks' gestation is classified as postterm.
- Key areas to assess for a newborn with complications related to size or gestational age include respiratory status, skin, thermoregulation, glucose levels, feeding, and family coping.
- Nurses need to establish rapport with parents, caregivers, and other significant family members to develop a trusting relationship. Using goal-directed communication is necessary to elicit information about the family's ability to cope with the complications, family strengths, and resources needed for effective adaptation.
- Oral feedings are preferred if the newborn has adequate sucking and swallowing reflexes, gastrointestinal functioning, and energy levels. Breast milk is most desirable, especially for preterm newborns. If not possible, specialized formulas containing 24 cal/oz and fortified with calcium, phosphorus, and iron can supply the needed extra calories. Special nipples, called "premie" nipples, are commercially available. They are shorter by ¼ to ½ inch and softer, making them easier to compress.
- Gavage feedings are indicated for the physiologically stable newborn who cannot ingest sufficient breast milk or formula orally to satisfy nutritive requirements. Trophic feedings (early or minimal enteral feedings) may be used to nourish the gut, promote intestinal maturation, and stimulate motility. Parenteral nutrition commonly is used for VLBW newborns who are very physiologically immature and cannot ingest or digest breast milk or formula by the enteral route. Any newborn receiving an alternative form of feeding should be provided with non-nutritive sucking.
- Nurses play a key role in promoting family attachment with the newborn experiencing complications. Role modeling of attachment behaviors and allowing time for family members to verbalize feelings are important.
- Hyperbilirubinemia (elevated serum bilirubin levels) is manifested by jaundice, a yellow discoloration of the skin and tissues. Mild, self-limiting jaundice (physio-

logic jaundice) develops approximately the third day after birth in formula-fed newborns and somewhat later in breast-fed newborns. When hyperbilirubinemia persists or remains untreated, pathologic jaundice occurs. Phototherapy is instituted when total serum bilirubin levels are at or above 15 mg/dL in newborns 25 to 48 hours old, 18 mg/dL in newborns 49 to 72 hours old, and 20 mg/dL in newborns older than 72 hours. Exchange transfusions may be used when jaundice does not respond to intensive phototherapy.

- Congenital heart disease refers to a group of cardiac defects that either change the direction of flow or change the normal structure and function of the heart chambers or great vessels. Ventricular septal defect is the most common of all congenital cardiac anomalies. Other defects include atrial septal defect, atrioventricular canal, pulmonary stenosis, patent ductus arteriosus, aortic stenosis, coarctation of the aorta, tetralogy of Fallot, and transposition of the great arteries.
- Congenital diaphragmatic hernia refers to the protrusion of abdominal contents through an abnormality in the diaphragm. As a result, abdominal contents rise up through the defect and occupy space in the thoracic cavity. Surgery is performed as soon after birth as possible.
- Neural tube defects (NTDs), a group of anomalies involving the brain and spinal cord, include anencephaly, spina bifida, and encephalocele. Spina bifida is the most common NTD and can be manifested in one of three forms: spina bifida occulta, meningocele, or myelomeningocele, the most serious and disabling form. Folic acid supplementation during pregnancy is a major primary prevention strategy.
- Congenital defects of the abdominal wall include omphalocele and gastroschisis. Gentle handling is essential to prevent trauma to the sac or exposed abdominal organs.
- Clefting, which occurs when the embryonic structures of the upper lip, nose, and hard and soft palate fail to close and fuse, may be complete or incomplete involving only the lip, unilateral or bilateral, or combined with complete or incomplete clefting of the palate. Surgery is the primary mode of treatment. Parents need much emotional support and teaching.
- Esophageal atresia involves a disruption in the esophageal passageway to the stomach, in which it is closed off and ends in a blind pouch. Without surgical intervention, the newborn has no way to ingest fluid and nutrition. Classic findings include coughing, choking, and cyanosis with feeding along with excessive salivation and drooling in the side-lying position. Tracheoesophageal fistula involves an abnormal opening between the trachea and esophagus that permits food and fluid to be diverted to the lungs, causing aspiration, and air from the trachea to enter the stomach, causing distention.
- Developmental dysplasia of the hip (DDH) refers to a group of hip abnormalities ranging from a shallow acetabulum, to a stretched capsule with ligamentum teres, to complete dislocation. A positive Galeazzi sign, Ortolani's maneuver, and Barlow's maneuver aid in determining DDH. Diagnostic imaging confirms the diagnosis.
- With hypospadias, the urethral opening may be located on the dorsal aspect (on top of the penile shaft) or ventrally (on the underneath surface of the penile shaft) instead of being positioned in the center in the distal end of the penile shaft or midline below the clitoral hood in females.

REVIEW QUESTIONS

1. Which of the following should the nurse expect to find when assessing a newborn at 42 weeks' gestation?
   A. Abundant lanugo
   B. Few plantar creases
   C. Dry, scaly skin
   D. Fused eyelids
2. Rupture of a client's membranes revealed thick, green-stained amniotic fluid. Which intervention should be the priority immediately following the birth of the newborn's head?
   A. Vigorously dry the newborn.
   B. Administer blow-by oxygen.
   C. Assess the apical heart rate.
   D. Perform suctioning.
3. When reviewing the medical record of an LGA newborn, which factor in the maternal history should the nurse identify as most likely associated with this condition?
   A. Exposure to rubella in the first trimester
   B. Diabetes
   C. Polyhydramnios
   D. Incompetent cervix
4. Which of the following serum bilirubin levels would lead the nurse to suspect that a preterm newborn has pathologic jaundice?
   A. 3 mg/dL
   B. 5 mg/dL
   C. 9 mg/dL
   D. 12 mg/dL
5. Which of the following would the nurse expect assessment findings in a newborn with fetal alcohol syndrome?
   A. Wide, broad upper lip
   B. Short nose
   C. High nasal bridge
   D. Large, protruding eyes

6. When planning the care for a newborn with hyperbilirubinemia who is to receive phototherapy, which intervention should the nurse be most likely to include?
   A. Applying small eye patches to each eye
   B. Keeping the newborn clothed in a T-shirt and diaper
   C. Turning the newborn every 6 to 8 hours
   D. Restricting fluids while the newborn is under the lights
7. Assessment of a newborn reveals absent breath sounds and audible bowel sounds with auscultation on the right side of the newborn's chest. The nurse interprets these findings as suggestive of
   A. congenital heart disease.
   B. respiratory distress syndrome.
   C. congenital diaphragmatic hernia.
   D. omphalocele.
8. Which of the following expected outcomes would be the highest priority when preparing a newborn with a cleft lip and palate for discharge?
   A. Extended family states that they will help to support the new family.
   B. Parents schedule a visit with the plastic surgeon for palate reconstruction.
   C. Parents demonstrate success with appropriate feeding techniques.
   D. Siblings exhibit beginning attachment behaviors with the newborn.
9. A nurse suspects that a newborn has a tracheoesophageal fistula. Which intervention would be most appropriate?
   A. Encourage the mother to breastfeed on demand.
   B. Place the baby prone, elevating the head 30 degrees.
   C. Institute positive-pressure ventilation.
   D. Prepare for insertion of a gastrostomy tube.
10. A female newborn diagnosed with developmental hip dysplasia is to be treated using a Pavlik harness. After teaching the parents about caring for the newborn, which statement by the parents indicates the need for additional teaching?
   A. "We'll make sure to schedule extra time in the morning to dress her."
   B. "She seems to like when I carry her astride on my hip."
   C. "We'll use the harness for 1 month and then she'll be fine."
   D. "We'll need to check out a special infant car seat for her to use."

REFERENCES

Akera, C., & Ro, S. (2003). Medical concerns in the neonatal period. *Clinics in Family Practice, 5*(2).

Alderman, C. (2000). Right from the start. *Nursing Standard, 15*(12), 16–18.

Anderson, D. M., & Loughead, J. L. (2002). Feeding the ill or preterm infant. *Neonatal Network 21*(7), 7–14.

Anuntaseree, W., Patrapinyokul, S., Suntorniohanakul, S., & Thongsuksal, P. (2002). Congenital bronchoesophageal fistula and tracheoesophageal fistula with esophageal atresia. *Pediatric Pulmonology, 33,* 162–164.

Askin D. F., & Diehl-Jones, W. L. (2003). The neonatal liver. Part III: Pathophysiology of liver dysfunction. *Neonatal Network—Journal of Neonatal Nursing, 22*(3) 5–15.

Ballard, J. L. (1999). New Ballard score expanded to include extremely premature infants. *Journal of Pediatrics, 119,* 417–423.

Barker, E., Saulino, M., & Caristo, A. M. (2002). Spina bifida. *RN, 65*(12), 33–38.

Blackwell, J. T. (2003). Clinical practice guidelines. Management of hyperbilirubinemia in the healthy term newborn. *Journal of the American Academy of Nurse Practitioners, 15*(5), 194–198.

Bernbaum, J. C. (2000). *Preterm infants in primary care: A guide to office management.* Columbus, OH: Ross Products Division, Abbott Laboratories.

Brown, J. P. (2001). Orthopaedic care of children with spina bifida: You've come a long way, baby! *Orthopaedic Nursing, 20*(4) 51–58.

Brown, R. N., & Nicolaides, K. H. (2000). Increased fetal nuchal translucency: Possible association with esophageal atresia. *Ultrasound in Obstetrics and Gynecology, 15,* 631–632.

Butterworth, S. A., Webber, E. M., & Jamieson, D. H. (2001). Pediatric surgical images: H-type tracheoesophageal fistula. *Journal of Pediatric Surgery, 36*(6), 958–959.

Cachat, F., Van Melle, G., McGahren, E. D., Reinberg, O., & Norwood, V. (2006). Arterial hypertension after surgical closure of omphalocele and gastroschisis. *Pediatric Nephrology, 21,* 225–229.

Catlin, A., & Carter, B. (2002). Creation of a neonatal end-of-life palliative care protocol. *Neonatal Network, Journal of Perinatology, 22*(3), 184–195.

Celayir, A. C., & Erdogan, E. (2003). Case reports: An infrequent cause of misdiagnosis in esophageal atresia. *Journal of Pediatric Surgery, 38*(9), 1389.

Chen, J. L., & Rankin, S. H. (2002). Using the resiliency model to deliver culturally sensitive care to Chinese families. *Journal of Pediatric Nursing, 17*(3), 157–166.

Colon, E. J. (2001). Culturally congruent care in the NICU. *AWHONN Lifelines, 5*(5), 60–64.

Cook, C. V., White, D., Svenson, L. W., Demianczuk, N. N., Bott, N., & Edwards, J. (2002). Where and to what extent is prevention of low birth weight possible? *Western Journal of Nursing Research, 24*(8), 887–904.

Cornblath, M., Hawdon, J. M., Williams, A. F., Synsley-Green, A., Ward-Platt, M. P., Schwartz, R., & Kalhan, S. C. (2000). Controversies regarding definition of neonatal hypoglycemia: Suggested operational thresholds. *Pediatrics, 105*(5), 1141–1145.

Cowett, R. M., & Loughead, J. L. (2002). Neonatal glucose metabolism: Differential diagnosis, evaluation, and treatment of hypoglycemia. *Neonatal Network—Journal of Neonatal Nursing, 21*(4), 9–19.

Cox, E. (2003). Synergy in practice: Caring for victims of intimate partner violence. *Critical Care Nursing Quarterly, 26*(4), 323–330.

Crabbe, D. C. G. (2003). Isolated tracheo-oesophageal fistula. *Paediatric Respiratory Reviews, 4,* 74–78.

Crowley, L. V. (2001). *An introduction to human disease: Pathology and pathophysiology correlations* (5th ed.). London: Jones & Bartlett Publishers.

Davidhizar, R. (1999). Assessing culturally diverse pediatric clients. *Pediatric Nursing, 25*(4), 371–378.

Dollberg, S., Lusky, A., & Reichman, B. (2005). Patent ductus arteriosus, indomethacin and necrotizing enterocolitis in very low birth weight infants: A population-based study. *Journal of Pediatric Gastroenterology and Nutrition, 40*(2), 184–188.

Eustace, L. W., Kang, D. H., & Coombs, D. (2003). Fetal alcohol syndrome: A growing concern for health care professionals. *Journal of Obstetric, Gynecologic, and Neonatal Nursing, 32* (2), 215–220.

Ergun, O., Barksdale, E., Ergun, F. S., Prosen, T., Qureshi, F. G., Reblock, K. R., Ford, H., & Hackam,, D. J. (2005). The timing of delivery of infants with gastroschisis influences outcome. *Journal of Pediatric Surgery, 40,* 424–428.

Farmer, D. (2003). Fetal surgery. *British Medical Journal, 326,* 461–462.

Gagnon, A. J., Waghorn, K., Jones, M. A., & Yang, H. (2001). Indicators nurses employ in deciding to test for hyperbilirubinemia. *Journal of Obstetric, Gynecologic, and Neonatal Nursing, 30*(6), 626–633.

Greemberg, L., Fisher, A., & Katz, A. (1999). Case report: Novel use of neonatal cuffed tracheal tube to occlude tracheo-oesophageal fistula. *Paediatric Anesthesia, 9,* 339–341.

Halamek, L., & Stevenson, D. (2002). Neonatal jaundice and liver disease. In A. Fanaroff & R. Martin (Eds.), *Neonatal–perinatal medicine: Diseases of the fetus and infant* (7th ed.). St. Louis: Mosby.

Hamberger, L. K., Guse, C., Boerger, J., Minsky, D., Pape, D., & Folsom, C. (2004). Evaluation of a health care provider training program to identify and help partner violence victims. *Journal of Family Violence, 19*(1), 1–11.

Hansen, M. (1998). *Pathophysiology: Foundations of disease and clinical intervention.* Philadelphia: W. B. Saunders.

Hardart, G. E., Hardart, M. K. M., & Arnold, J. H. (2004). Intracranial hemorrhage in premature neonates treated with extracorporeal membrane oxygenation correlates with conceptional age. *Journal of Pediatrics, 145*(2), 184–189.

Hay, W. W. (1999). Addressing hypoglycemia and hyperglycemia. *Pediatrics in Review, 20*(7), e4–e5.

Hebbar, K., Fortenberry, J. D., Rogers, K., Merritt, R., & Easley, K. (2005). Comparison of temporal artery thermometer to standard temperature measurements in pediatric intensive care unit patients.

Hengst, J. M. (2002). Direct hyperbilirubinemia: A case study of parenteral nutrition-induced cholestatic jaundice. *Neonatal Network—Journal of Neonatal Nursing, 21*(4), 57–69, 73–76.

Johnson, T. S. (2003). Hypoglycemia and the full-term newborn: How well does birth weight for gestational age predict risk? *Journal of Obstetric, Gynecologic, and Neonatal Nursing, 32*(1), 48–57.

Jones, M. W., Morgan, E., & Shelton, J. E. (2002). Dysphagia and oral feeding problems in the premature infant. *Neonatal Network—Journal of Neonatal Nursing, 21*(2), 51–57.

Kalish, R. B., Chasen, S. T., Rosenzweig, & Chervenak, F. A. (2003). Esophageal atresia and tracheoesophageal fistula: The impact of prenatal suspicion on neonatal outcome in a tertiary care center. *Journal of Perinatal Medicine, 31,* 111–114.

Kattwinkel, J. (Ed.) (2006). *Textbook of neonatal resuscitation* (5th ed.). Elk Grove Village, IL: American Academy of Pediatrics.

Kecskes, Z., & Cartwright, D. W. (2002). Poor outcome of very low birth weight babies with serious congenital heart disease. *Archives of Disease in Childhood—Fetal and Neonatal Edition, 87,* F31–F33. Available at: http://www.archdischild.com.

Kenner, C., Lott, J., & Flandermeyer, A. (1998). *Comprehensive neonatal nursing—A physiologic perspective* (2nd ed.). Philadelphia: W. B. Saunders.

Konkin, D. E., O'Hali, W. A., Webber, E. M., & Blair, G. (2003). Outcomes in esophageal atresia and tracheoesophageal fistula. *Journal of Pediatric Surgery, 38*(12), 1726–1729.

Kunz, L. H., Gilbert, W. M., & Towner, D. R. (2005). Increased incidence of cardiac anomalies in pregnancies complicated by gastroschisis. *American Journal of Obstetrics and Gynecology, 193,* 1248–1252.

Lapunzina, P., Lopez, J. S., Rittler, M., & Castilla, E. E. (2002). Risks of congenital anomalies in large for gestational age infants. *Journal of Pediatrics, 140*(2), 200–204.

Leonard, H., Barrett, A. M., Scott, J. E. S., & Wren, C. (2001). The influence of congenital heart disease on survival of infants with oesophageal atresia. *Archives of Disease in Childhood—Fetal and Neonatal Edition, 85,* F204–F206. Available at: http://www.archdischild.com.

Lin, H. C., Su, B. H., Chen, A. C., Tsai, C. H., Yeh, T. F., & Oh, W. (2005). Oral probiotics reduce the incidence and severity of necrotizing enterocolitis in very low birth weight infants. *Pediatrics, 115*(1), 1–4.

Lockridge, T., Caldwell, A. D., & Jason, P. (2002). Neonatal surgical emergencies: Stabilization and management. *Journal of Gynecologic and Neonatal Nursing, 31*(5), 328–339.

Lott, J. W. (2002). Concepts of altered health in children. In C. M. Porth (Ed.), *Pathophysiology: Concepts of altered health states* (6th ed., pp. 21–41). Philadelphia: Lippincott Williams & Wilkins.

Mainous, R. O. (2002). Infant massage as a component of developmental care: Past, present and future. *Holistic Nursing Practice, 17*(1), 1–7.

Maisels, M. J., Baltz, R. D., Bhutani, V. K., Newman, T. B., Rosenfeld, W., Stevenson, D. K., & Weinblatt, H. B. (2001). Neonatal jaundice and kernicterus. *Pediatrics, 108*(2).

March of Dimes. (2001). Birth defects and genetics: cleft lip and cleft palate. Retrieved January 9, 2006, from http://www.marchofdimes.com/pnhec/4439_1210asp.

Martin, S. L., Beaumont, J. L., & Kupper, L. L. (2003). Substance use before and during pregnancy links to intimate partner violence. *American Journal of Drug and Alcohol Abuse, 29*(3), 599–617.

McConnell, M. E., & Elixson, E. M. (2002). The neonate with suspected congenital heart disease. *Critical Care Nursing Quarterly, 25*(3), 17–25.

McKenney, W. M. (2001). Understanding the neonatal immune system: high risk for infection. *Neonatal Nursing, 21*(6), 35–47.

Meier, P., Brown, L., & Hurst, N. (1999). Breast feeding the preterm infant. In J. Riordan & K. Auerbach (Eds.), *Breast feeding and human lactation* (pp. 449–481). Sudbury, MA: Jones & Bartlett.

Meis, P. J., Klebanoff, M., Thom, E., Dombrowski, M. P., Sibai, B. Moawad, A. H., et al. (2003). Prevention of recurrent preterm delivery by 17 alpha hydroxyprogesterone caproate. *New England Journal of Medicine, 348*(24), 2379–2385.

Modricin-Talbott, M. A., Harrison, L. L., Groer, M. W., & Younger, S. (2003). The biobehavioral effects of gentle human touch on preterm infants. *Nursing Science Quarterly, 16*(1), 60–67.

Morelius, E., Lundh, U., & Nelson, N. (2002). Parental stress in relation to the severity of congenital heart disease in the offspring. *Pediatric Nursing, 28*(1), 28–34.

Montgomery, K. S. (2003). Nursing care for pregnant adolescents. *Journal of Obstetric, Gynecologic, and Neonatal Nursing, 32*(2), 249–257.

National Library of Medicine & National Institutes of Health. (2003, Feb. 10). Med-line plus health information: Imperforate anus repair. J. P. Dolan, M.D. Available at: http://www.nlm.nih.gov.

Nazir, M. A., Gimovsky, M. L., Vaydovsky, J., Kappy, K. A, & Polcaro, J. (2005). Fetal gastroschisis. *Journal of Reproductive Medicine, 50*(4), 287–290.

Neu, J. (2002). Aggressive nutritional support and nutritional adjuncts for premature and critically ill neonates. *Acta Pharmacologica Sinica.* Available at: http://www.ChinaPhar.com.

Newburn-Cook, C. V., White, D., Svenson, L. W., Demianczuk, N. N., Bott, N., & Edwards, J. (2002). Where and to what extent is prevention of low birth weight possible? *Western Journal of Nursing Research, 24*(8), 887–904.

Nichol, P. F., Hayman, A., Pryde, P. G., Go, L. L., & Lund, D. P. (2004). Meconium staining of amniotic fluid correlated with intestinal peel formation in gastroschisis. *Pediatric Surgery International, 20*(3), 211–214.

Patel, S. B., Ade-Ajayi, N., & Kiely, E. M. (2002). Oesophageal atresia: A simplified approach to early management. *Pediatric Surgery International, 18*(2–3): 87–89.

Porter, M. L., & Dennis, B. (2002). Hyperbilirubinemia in the term newborn. *American Family Physician, 65*(4), 606, 613–614.

Porth, C. M. (2005). *Pathophysiology: Concepts of altered health states* (7th ed.). Philadelphia: Lippincott Williams & Wilkins.

Pressler, J. L., Helm, J. M., Hepworth, J. T., & Wells, N. L. (2001). Behaviors of very preterm neonates as documented using NIDCAP observations. *Neonatal Network—Journal of Neonatal Nursing, 20*(8), 15–24.

Quinn, D., & Shannon, L. F. (2000). Radiology basics. Part V: Congenital anomalies of the gastrointestinal tract. *Neonatal Network—Journal of Neonatal Nursing, 19*(6), 50–51.

Reiser, D. (2001). Practice monographs. Hyperbilirubinemia: Exploring neonatal conditions related to bilirubin production. *AWHONN Lifelines, 5*(3), 55–61.

Richardson, D. K., Shah, B. L., Frantz, I. D. III, Bednarek, F., Rubin, L. P., & McCormick, M. C. (1999). Perinatal risk and severity of illness in newborns at 6 neonatal intensive care units. *American Journal of Public Health, 89*(4), 511–516.

Ritchie, S. K. (2002). Primary care of the premature infant discharged from the neonatal intensive care unit. *Maternal Child Nursing, 27*(2), 77–127.

Sable, C. A., Cummings, S. D., Pearson, G. D., Schratz, L. M., Cross, R. C., Quivers, E. S., Rudra, H., & Martin, G. R. (2002). Impact of telemedicine on the practice of pediatric cardiology in community hospitals. *Pediatrics, 109*(1).

Saenz, R. B., Beebe, D. K., & Triplett, C. (1999). Caring for infants with congenital heart disease and their families. *American Family Physician, 59*(7), 1857–1868.

Sandberg, D. J., Magee, W. P., & Denk, M. (2002). Neonatal cleft lip and cleft palate repair. *AORN Journal, 75*(3), 488, 490–499, 501, 503–504, 506–508.

Sirkin, A., Jalloh, T., & Lee, L. (2002). Selecting an accurate point-of-care testing system: Clinical and technical issues and implications in neonatal blood glucose monitoring. *Journal for Specialists in Pediatric Nursing, 33*(7), 104–112.

Skelly, A. C., Holt, V. L., Mosca, V. S., & Alderman, B. W. (2002). Talipes equinovarus and maternal smoking: A population-based case-control study in Washington state. *Teratology, 66*(2), 91–100.

Snyder, C. L., & St. Peter, S. D. (2005). Trends in mode of delivery for gastroschisis infants. *American Journal of Perinatology, 22*(7), 391–396.

Spicer, K. (2001). What every nurse need to know about breast pumping: instructing and supporting mothers of premature infants in the NICU. *Neonatal Network, 20*(4), 35–41.

Spina Bifida Association of America. (2003). Facts about spina bifida. Retrieved December 28, 2003, from http://www.sbaa.org/html/sbaa_facts.html.

Steen, S. E., & Anderson, B. A. (2002). Caring for children of other faiths. *Journal of Christian Nursing, 19*(2), 14–21.

Suarez, R. D., Grobman, W. A., & Parilla, B. V. (2001). Indomethacin tocolysis and intraventricular hemorrhage. *Obstetrics and Gynecology, 97,* 921–925.

Thureen, P. J., Anderson, A. H., Baron, K. A., Melara, D. L., Hay, W. W. Jr., & Fennessey, P. V. (1998). Protein balance in the first week of life in ventilated neonates receiving parenteral nutrition. *American Journal of Clinical Nutrition, 68,* 1128–1135.

Thomas, K. (2001). A critical neonate in the emergency department. *Journal of Emergency Nursing, 27*(2), 196–198.

Todd, S. J. T., LaSala, K. B., & Neil-Urban, S. (2001). An integrated approach to prenatal smoking cessation interventions. *Maternal Child Nursing, 25*(3), 185–190.

Tough, S. C., Newburn-Cook, C., Johnston, D. W., Svenson, L. W., Rose, S., & Belik, J. (2002). Delayed childbearing and its impact on population rate changes in lower birth weight, multiple birth, and preterm delivery. *Pediatrics, 109*(3), 399–403.

Tyson, J. E., & Saigal, S. (2005). Outcomes for extremely low-birth-weight infants. *Journal of the American Medical Association, 293*(3), 371–373.

Ulrich, K. S., & Mackin, A. L. (2001). Cleft lip and palate: Critical care extra. *American Journal of Nursing, 101*(3), 24AA–24HH.

Warren, K. R., & Foudin, L. L. (2001). Alcohol-related birth defects: the past, present, and future. *Alcohol Research and Health, 25*(3), 153–158.

Westmoreland, D. (1999). Critical congenital cardiac defects in the newborn. *Journal of Perinatal & Neonatal Nursing, 12*(4), 67–87.

Yariv, Y., Ben-Haroush, A., Chen, R., Rosenn, B., Hod, M., & Langer, O. (2004). Undiagnosed asymptomatic hypoglycemia. *Obstetrics & Gynecology, 104,* 88–93.

MENOPAUSE AND BEYOND

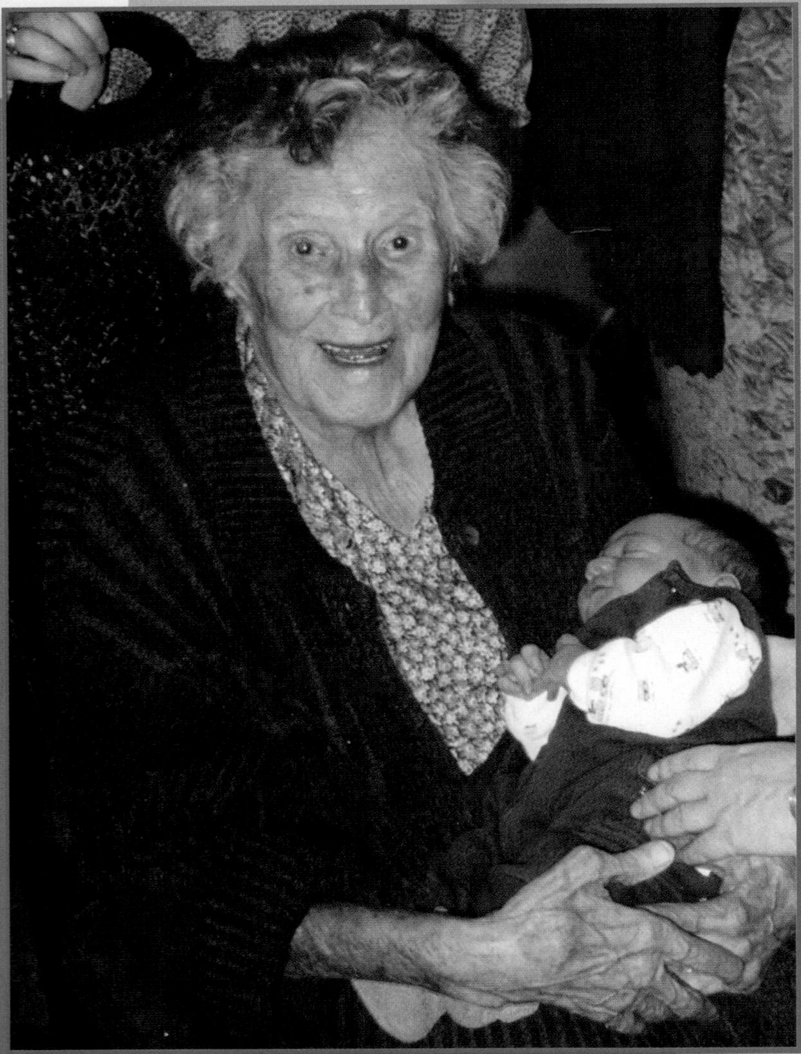

UNIT 6

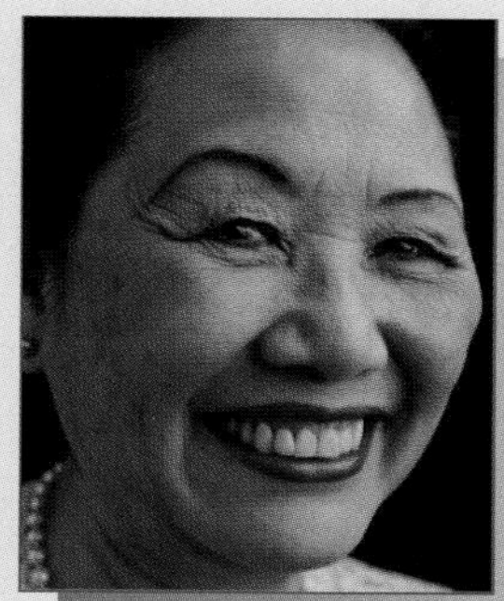
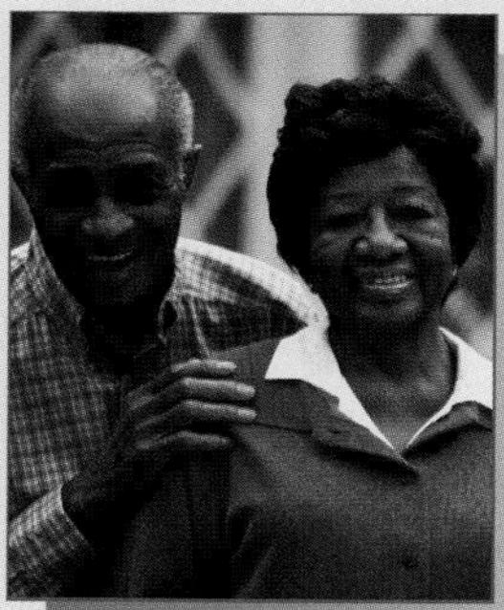
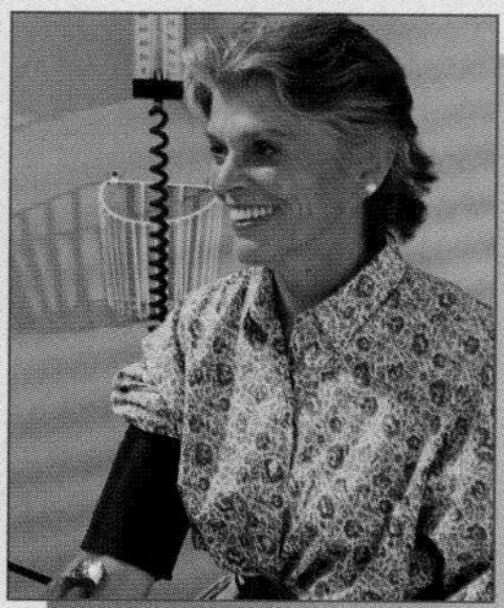
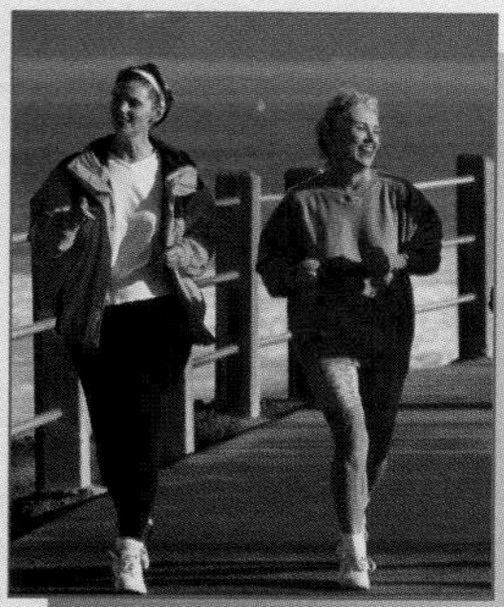

Women whose reproductive years are drawing to a close or have stopped completely make up the fastest-growing segment of the U.S. and Canadian populations. Appropriate, holistic care for such clients is a topic of growing importance for nurses and other health care providers, whose encounters with this segment of society are likely to increase significantly with time. This unit explores the needs, transitions, concerns, common abnormalities, and related care for perimenopausal, menopausal, and older women. It emphasizes the health risks and problems that naturally accompany age-related changes in female physiology, as well as the ways that today's women are diverging from previous generations as a result of social, economic, and political shifts. The inclusion of such content underscores the design and overall philosophy of this text, which is the importance of women's health across the entire lifespan, including, but not limited to, the context of childbearing.

CHAPTER 23

The Menopausal Experience

Susan A. Orshan

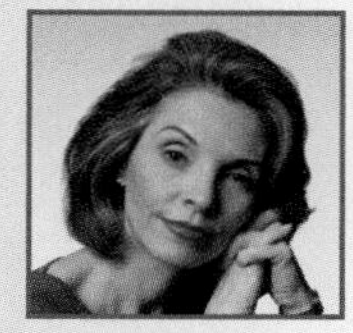

Fran, a 50-year-old married woman, comes to the clinic for a yearly examination. "I notice that I am having more frequent hot flashes," she says. "I wake up at night, drenched. They've really been disrupting my sleep." The client looks pale and tired. Further discussion reveals family transitions. "Both children now are living at college, and my husband is working a lot," Fran reports. "It's nice having more time for myself, but sometimes I feel lonely."

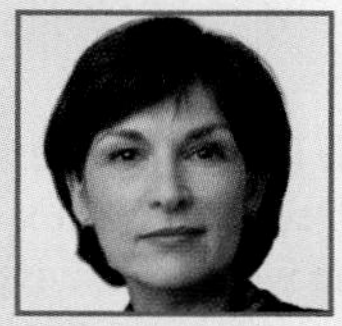

Carol, a 44-year-old white woman, experienced menopause 2 years ago. She has adjusted well and has tried to optimize her health by making positive lifestyle changes. Her health history includes cigarette smoking since age 18, which she quit 14 months ago. Carol was diagnosed recently with osteopenia. She states, "My mother had osteoporosis and broke her hip. That was a nightmare. I don't want that to happen to me."

You will learn more about Fran's and Carol's stories later. Nurses working with such clients need to understand the material in this chapter to manage care and address issues appropriately. Before beginning, consider the following points related to the above scenarios:

- Based on the information provided, what might be some short-term and long-term priorities for the nurse to establish with each client? Explain your answer.
- What physiologic events form the basis for Fran's symptoms? For Carol's?
- How are the menopausal experiences described above similar for each woman? How do they seem different?
- What further details would you expect the nurse to investigate with Fran? With Carol?
- What areas of health promotion, illness prevention, and teaching would the nurse need to address with each client?

LEARNING OBJECTIVES

On completion of this chapter, the reader should be able to:

- Discuss perimenopause and menopause from the view of health care providers.
- Explain client perspectives on menopause.
- Identify various sociocultural perspectives related to menopause.
- Describe physiologic changes inherent in the menopausal transition and their etiology.
- Identify common psychological adjustments in menopause.
- Summarize the components of assessment focused on menopausal-related changes.
- Discuss strategies to enhance the health and comfort of clients experiencing menopausal transition and their significant others.

KEY TERMS

andropause
climacteric
menopause
osteopenia
osteoporosis
perimenopause
premature ovarian failure

Almost half of a woman's life is spent after the natural cessation of menstruation known as **menopause.** In the United States, the average age of menopause is 51 to 53 years, with most women naturally experiencing this change between 40 and 58 years (Reynolds & Obermeyer, 2005; U.S. Department of Health and Human Services, 2005). The medical diagnosis of naturally occurring menopause is made retroactively: a woman who has not experienced menstruation for 12 consecutive months is regarded as being in menopause.

Perimenopause is the term given to the period immediately preceding menopause and continuing through the first 12 months of menopause, during which time ovarian hormones fluctuate, resulting in some effects commonly noted with this experience. The duration of perimenopause varies among women and may continue past menopause as estrogen sporadically fluctuates, resulting in postmenopausal vaginal bleeding (Buckler, 2005).

QUOTE 23-1

"Before we turned 40, my friends and I ignored our aches and pains, or figured they were the result of being active women. Now that we are in our 40s, we figure they mean that we are in perimenopause. Same pains, different meaning."

From a 45-year-old woman

How a woman views menopause reflects her personal, cultural, and societal perspectives (Deeks, 2004; Fu et al., 2003). In some cultures and for some women, menopause represents freedom—freedom from pregnancy, freedom to express wisdom, freedom to redefine themselves and their lives (Hvas, 2006) (Fig. 23.1). Their mothers or other significant older women may have shared their positive views of this change of life; thus, they also look forward to this new life event.

In other cultures and for other women, menopause is perceived as a taboo topic that represents loss—loss of youth, loss of attractiveness, loss of possibilities. These women may be ill prepared to handle the physiologic and accompanying psychological changes of perimenopause (Deeks & McCabe, 2004). With such a perspective, a woman in her 30s who experiences a hot flash or notices changes in her menstrual cycle may be at a loss to determine what is happening to her body. She may not connect these changes with the beginning of perimenopause and may be embarrassed to ask questions about her experience.

PHYSIOLOGIC BASIS OF NATURALLY OCCURRING PERIMENOPAUSE AND MENOPAUSE

During each normal menstrual cycle, the ovaries produce estrogen and progesterone in varying amounts in a rela-

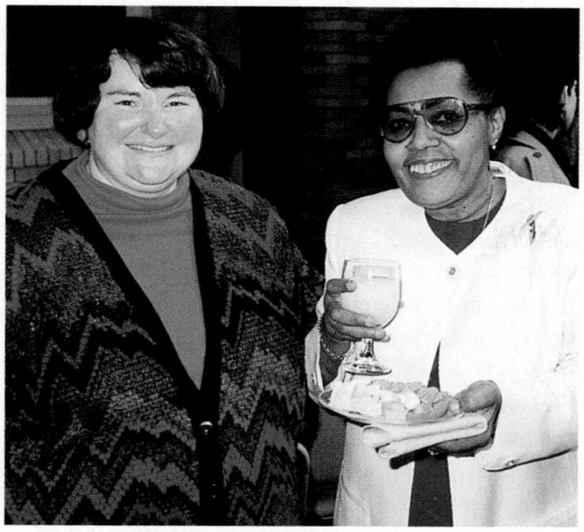

FIGURE 23.1 Many women welcome the menopause transition as providing freedom and opportunities not as available in earlier years more focused on childbearing and childrearing issues.

tively predictable pattern (see Chap. 6). Initially, estrogen is the dominant ovarian hormone, whereas progesterone is dominant in the second half of the cycle preceding menstruation. Fewer ovarian hormones during menstruation stimulate the anterior pituitary to secrete follicle-stimulating hormone (FSH), which in turn stimulates the ovarian follicle to mature and be released midcycle (*ovulation*). FSH decreases before ovulation. In turn, the anterior pituitary gland releases luteinizing hormone (LH) to stimulate the corpus luteum of the ruptured follicle to secrete progesterone and some estrogen. See Figure 23.2.

Follicular atresia, the breakdown of the follicles that would become ova, begins during the fetal period and continues until approximately the time of menopause, when almost all follicles are depleted (Broekmans et al., 2004). As the ovaries age, they secrete less estrogen and progesterone. The anterior pituitary gland responds by increasing secretion of FSH in an attempt to "jump-start" ovarian function, usually at approximately 37.5 years of age (although in women with premature ovarian failure [POF], this may occur in the teens or 20s) (Woad et al., 2006). Elevation in FSH increases the rate of follicular atresia, which may result in anovulatory cycles, thus decreasing fertility. This period of decreasing fertility is known as the **climacteric** and corresponds with perimenopause (American College of Obstetricians and Gynecologists [ACOG], 1995).

Approximately 6 months to 1 year before the onset of actual menopause, estrogen and progesterone secretion decrease more rapidly. Sporadic fluctuations in ovarian hormones resulting in postmenopausal bleeding, however, may continue for a few years past the cessation of menstruation (Buckler, 2005; van Voorhis, 2005).

The age at which menopause occurs naturally varies among women based on several factors. One study showed

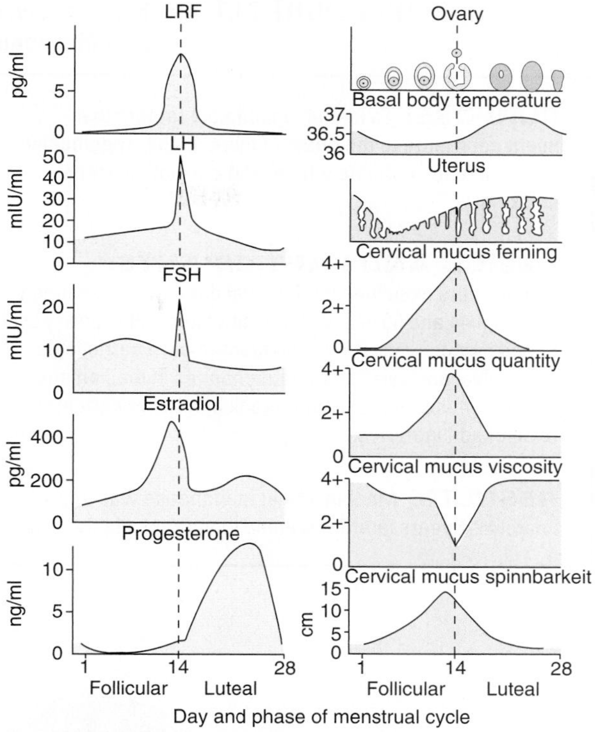

FIGURE 23.2 Hormonal and morphologic changes in the normal menstrual cycle.

significant associations between breastfeeding and alcohol consumption with early menopause (Dvornyk et al., 2006). Family history of early menopause; smoking history; overall number of lifetime ovulatory cycles, determined by such factors as early onset of menarche, not becoming pregnant, and not using oral contraceptives, which prevent ovulation; and socioeconomic status all influence the time of onset of menopause (Cramer & Xu, 1996; Hefler et al., 2006; Kinney et al., 2006; van Noord et al., 1997). See Research Highlight 23.1.

POTENTIAL CHANGES RELATED TO PERIMENOPAUSE AND MENOPAUSE

The degree to which a woman experiences the physiologic changes of perimenopause and menopause can vary greatly (Fig. 23.3). Even if two women experience similar changes, they may perceive those changes differently.

Menstrual Cycle

For most women, the first signs that they are entering perimenopause are changes in the length of their menstrual cycle and amount of flow. Cycle length may shorten 2 to 7 days as a result of a shortened follicular phase from increased FSH. Alternately, cycle length may increase from anovulatory cycles, along with a variation in flow amount and periodic midcycle spotting (Klein

RESEARCH HIGHLIGHT 23.1 Alcohol, Caffeine, and Smoking in Relation to Age at Menopause

PURPOSE: To identify modifiable factors that might contribute to the onset of menopause, specifically use of alcohol, caffeine intake, and current cigarette smoking

DESIGN AND PARTICIPANTS: Researchers examined longitudinal data from 494 women between 44 and 60 years of age, of whom 159 experienced menopause. They implemented parametric logistic survival analysis to estimate changes in median age at menopause for those who drank alcohol or caffeine or smoked cigarettes.

RESULTS: Median age at menopause was approximately 2.2 years later for women who drank alcohol 5 to 7 days per week than for women who did not drink alcohol. For those who drank at least 1 day per week, menopause was 1.3 years later. Caffeine intake was not associated with age at menopause. Current smoking of more than 13 cigarettes each day (6%) was linked with menopause approximately 3 years earlier than in women who smoked no or fewer than 13 cigarettes per day.

NURSING IMPLICATIONS: These results reflect a proestrogenic effect of moderate alcohol intake and an antiestrogenic effect of heavy cigarette smoking. To enjoy the benefits of estrogen for longer periods, women may wish to limit smoking and pursue interventions to assist with quitting or modifying this behavior.

Kinney, A., Kline, J., & Levin, B. (2006). *Maturitas, 54*(1), 27–38.

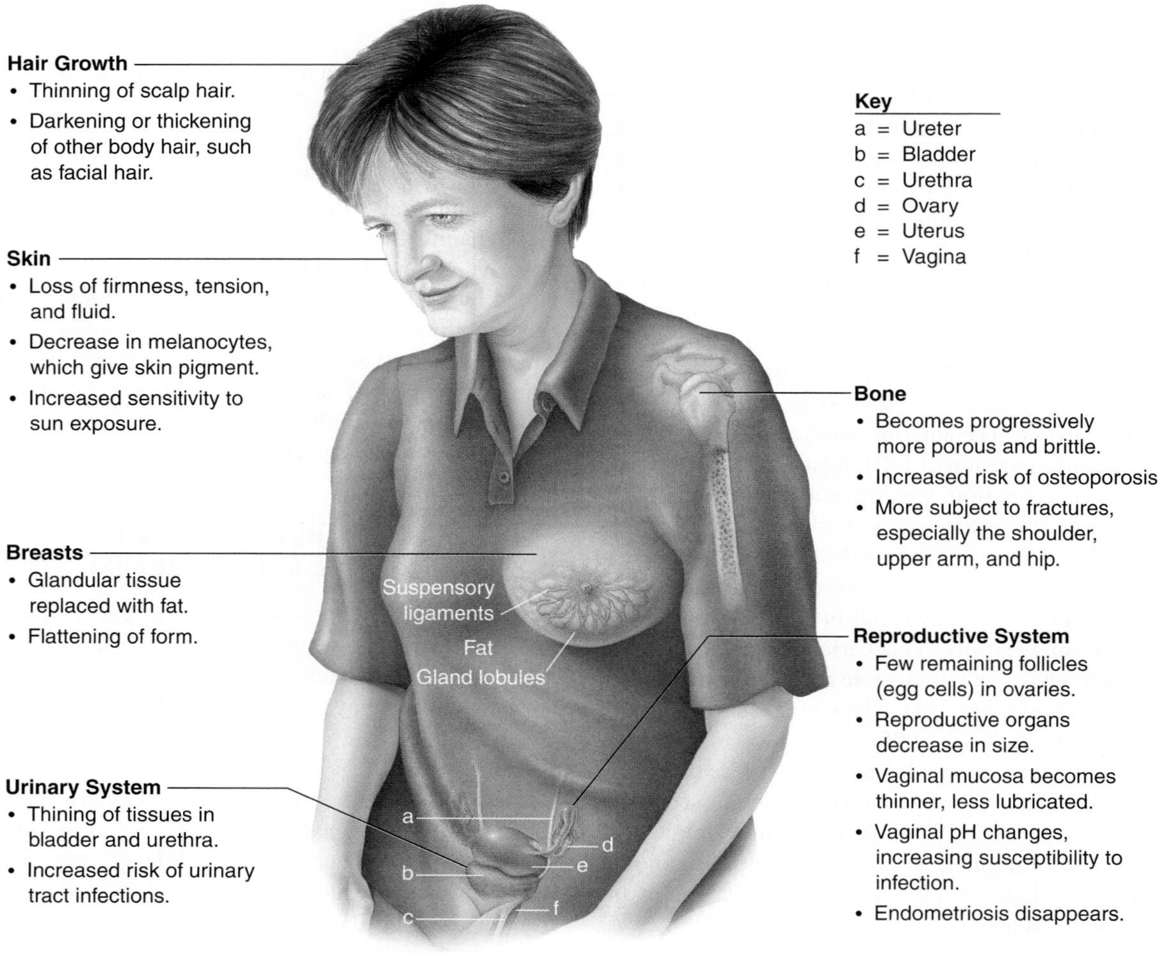
Hair Growth
• Thinning of scalp hair.
• Darkening or thickening of other body hair, such as facial hair.
Skin
• Loss of firmness, tension, and fluid.
• Decrease in melanocytes, which give skin pigment.
• Increased sensitivity to sun exposure.
Breasts
• Glandular tissue replaced with fat.
• Flattening of form.
Suspensory ligaments
Fat
Gland lobules
Urinary System
• Thining of tissues in bladder and urethra.
• Increased risk of urinary tract infections.
Key
a = Ureter
b = Bladder
c = Urethra
d = Ovary
e = Uterus
f = Vagina
Bone
• Becomes progressively more porous and brittle.
• Increased risk of osteoporosis
• More subject to fractures, especially the shoulder, upper arm, and hip.
Reproductive System
• Few remaining follicles (egg cells) in ovaries.
• Reproductive organs decrease in size.
• Vaginal mucosa becomes thinner, less lubricated.
• Vaginal pH changes, increasing susceptibility to infection.
• Endometriosis disappears.
a
b
c
d
e
f

FIGURE 23.3 Common physical changes associated with menopause.

& Soules, 1998; McVeigh, 2005; Mitchell et al., 2000; Santoro, 2005).

Vasomotor Symptoms

Approximately 65% to 80% of women in North America and Europe experience the "cardinal" vasomotor symptoms of menopause (hot flashes), sometimes accompanied by diaphoresis during the day, night, or both (Ratka et al., 2006). Such symptoms begin during perimenopause and may be related to decreased estrogen levels, although estrogen withdrawal alone does not account for them (Freedman, 2005). For example, some studies have shown a connection with cigarette smoking and increased incidence and intensity of hot flashes, regardless of estrogen levels (Gallichio et al., 2006; Whiteman et al., 2003). For most women, the hot flash mimics the red flush of embarrassment, appearing on the face, neck, and chest. It may last a few seconds to a few minutes, with an actual increase in skin temperature. For some women, it is accompanied by profuse diaphoresis. Many clients experience hot flashes at night, increasing the likelihood of sleep disturbances (Fig. 23.4).

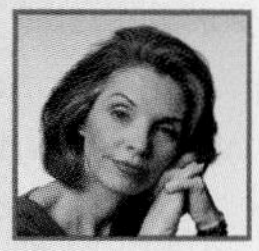

Think back to Fran, the woman at the beginning of the chapter experiencing hot flashes. How would the nurse gather additional information about Fran's problem?

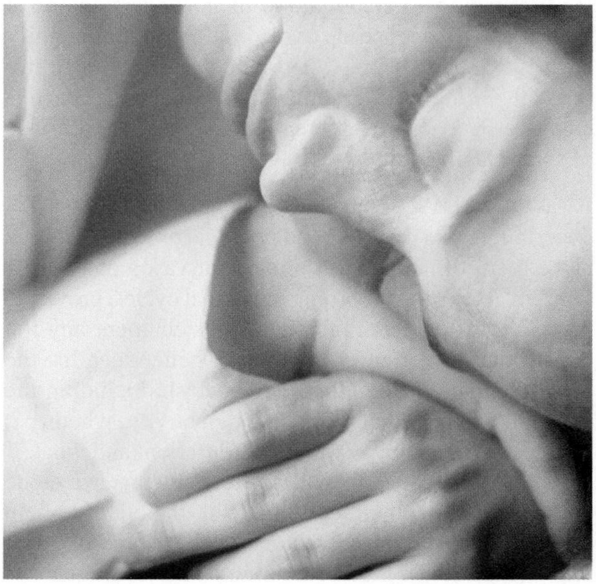

FIGURE 23.4 Vasomotor symptoms occurring during the night, commonly referred to as "night sweats," can contribute to sleep disturbances and subsequent fatigue and depression.

Genitourinary Symptoms

The urogenital tract is particularly sensitive to estrogen. During perimenopause and menopause, decreasing estrogen levels lead to thinning, and possible atrophy, of the vaginal mucosa; decreased vaginal lubrication; shortening of the vagina; increased vaginal pH (usually pH > 5); and uterine changes, along with thinning and laxity of the urinary structures, including the urethra and bladder (Ballagh, 2005; van Voorhis, 2005). These changes increase the client's risk for both urinary tract and vaginal infections.

Fertility

Women's fertility peaks at 24 years and then begins to decrease, with sharp declines between 35 and 40 years (Baird et al., 2005; Klein & Soules, 1998; Swanton & Child, 2005). Although follicular atresia is responsible for loss of actual oocytes, abnormalities related to meiosis in aging oocytes and decreased hormonal levels primarily are responsible for decreased fertility among women as they age (Klein & Soules, 1998). Nevertheless, fertility continues to be possible past 40 years. Pregnancy at this stage of life carries higher rates of complications, such as gestational diabetes, preeclampsia, and cesarean birth (see Chap. 12) (Baird et al., 2005; Jacobsson et al., 2004).

Mental Health Changes

For most clients during perimenopause and menopause, more is changing than just their hormones. Many women are experiencing major life events: the stress of family transitions, such as children becoming teenagers or leaving the house for college, divorce, widowhood, or caring for aging family members; career changes, including possible retirement; loss of fertility; and the perceived dual loss of youth and attractiveness (Deeks & McCabe, 2004; LeBoeuf & Carter, 1996; Mishra & Kuh, 2006). Clients most at risk for depression during this period are those who are sedentary and have been diagnosed previously with depression or who hold negative views of menopause (Avis et al., 1994; Dennerstein et al., 2004). Health care providers should keep in mind, however, that mental health changes in middle age may or may not be related to the hormonal changes of perimenopause and menopause (Nachtigall, 1998).

Women in midlife may experience hormone-related mood changes, irritability, lethargy, forgetfulness, nervousness, insomnia, and depression (Cohen et al., 2006; Frackiewicz & Cutler, 2000). Although these changes may be "labeled" during middle age as premenstrual syndrome, in reality they may be perimenopausal symptoms (Bachmann, 1994; Schmidt et al., 2004). It is not certain, however, whether these changes are the result of perimenopause, sleeping difficulties, or the life changes that occur when women reach their 30s or beyond.

Cardiovascular Disease

Coronary artery disease (CAD) is the number one cause of death among postmenopausal women (Hoyert et al., 2006). Estrogen protects women from CAD and myocardial infarction by increasing the ratio of high-density lipid (HDL) cholesterol to low-density lipid (LDL) cholesterol, increasing vasodilation and improving glucose metabolism. These changes result in a decrease of central abdominal adipose accumulation (Deroo & Korach, 2006). Once the protective mechanisms of estrogen have been diminished, LDL levels that were below those of men before the onset of menopause exceed those of men, and all the other cardiovascular benefits of estrogen are eliminated as well (Deroo & Korach, 2006). In fact, the rate of death from myocardial infarctions is greater in women than in men (Hoyert et al., 2006).

Osteopenia and Osteoporosis

Bone mass peaks between 30 and 35 years of age and decreases after that time, with losses accelerating in conjunction with estrogen deprivation at menopause (Deroo & Korach, 2006; Hobar, 2005). **Osteopenia,** a precursor to osteoporosis, is a condition in which bone density is reduced below that of the average woman of 35 years of age (Wild, 1998).

Osteoporosis includes both low bone mass density and microarchitectural deterioration of bone tissue, which leads to impaired skeletal integrity and fractures (Andrews et al., 2000). In the United States, 26% of women 65 years or older and 50% of women 85 years or older have osteoporosis. More than 1.5 million fractures annually are attributable to osteoporosis (Gass & Dawson-Hughes, 2006). See Chapters 2, 4, and 24.

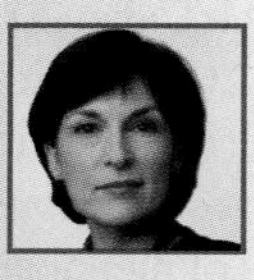

Consider Carol, the woman from the beginning of the chapter diagnosed with osteopenia. Would the nurse consider Carol to be at risk for fractures? What areas would be important for the nurse to assess?

Breast Cancer

Risks for breast cancer are related to many factors, including genetic, environmental, and lifestyle components (see Chap. 4). The amount of exposure to exogenous or endogenous estrogen (or both) increases a person's risk for developing breast cancer. In other words, a woman who experienced early menarche, late menopause, or both; never became pregnant; did not use oral contraceptives; or had some combination of these factors would be exposed to more estrogen through multiple ovulatory cycles than a woman who experienced late menarche, early menopause, or both and had multiple suppressed ovulatory cycles, either through pregnancy or oral contraceptive use. (See Chap. 4 for additional information.)

Other Alterations

Society tends to focus on hormonal changes occurring solely in women of "a certain age." The reality is that some women younger than 40 years, as well as men in midlife, also experience changes related to hormonal alterations. Young women may experience **premature ovarian failure** (POF) as a result of surgical or medical interventions, or for no apparent reason (Box 23.1). Men of "a certain age" also go through a hormonal change analogous to menopause, known as **andropause** (Box 23.2).

COLLABORATIVE CARE: MENOPAUSE

Assessment

A comprehensive assessment (Assessment Tool 23.1) of the client's experiences related to the menopause stage can facilitate informed decision making regarding any actions she may wish to take to promote a healthy lifestyle. Important areas of focus include menstruation, vasomotor symptoms, genitourinary problems, mental health, cardiovascular health, and musculoskeletal health.

Menstruation

The nurse should obtain the menstruation history, including the onset of menarche and any periods of amenorrhea or episodic cycle changes throughout the years. Providers may wish to encourage clients in perimenopause to keep a journal or diary recording their menstrual cycles, including the day of the month that menstruation begins and the number of days that the client bleeds. Developing such a diary can facilitate women's understanding of changes in the menstrual cycle and help them identify areas in which they may choose to change habits or initiate interventions. For some clients, this experience is empowering because it increases awareness and feelings of self-actualization.

Vasomotor Symptoms

Determining the presence and potential external etiology is the focus of nursing assessment for vasomotor symptoms. In addition to recording menstrual cycles, providers may choose to encourage clients to document any hot flashes they experience in a diary. A client can list the circumstances surrounding the hot flash, including the time, place, immediately preceding activity, whether it was accompanied by diaphoresis, duration, and what, if anything, alleviated the discomfort. In this way, the nurse can review the recordings with the client to help her identify precipitating factors to the vasomotor instability (Fig. 23.5). Again, although this technique has value in identifying physiologic patterns, it also empowers women to gain knowledge about their bodies, revealing ways in which they can control and improve health.

BOX 23.1 Premature Ovarian Failure

Between 1% and 5% of women younger than 40 years experience premature ovarian failure (POF), popularly known as premature menopause, decades before their peers become menopausal (Santoro, 2003; Woad et al., 2006). Induced POF occurs in women who undergo an oophorectomy or chemotherapy resulting in an abrupt loss of ovarian function. Other women have POF related to genetic alterations, such as fragile X or Turner's syndrome; enzyme deficiencies, such as galactosemia; autoimmune factors; or unknown causes (Santoro, 2003; Woad et al., 2006).

No characteristic menstrual history exists that would suggest the onset of idiopathic POF (Massin et al., 2006). Although family history appears to exist in some cases, it is by no means universal. In addition, discussions on menstruation may not be considered acceptable in some families, and therefore the histories may not be accurate.

Assessment for women experiencing or suspected of experiencing POF is the same as that of women with perimenopause or menopause. Once the assessment has been completed, serum follicle-stimulating hormone and luteinizing hormone levels will be needed to confirm the suspected medical diagnosis of POF (Bakalov & Nelson, 2005). Once the diagnosis is confirmed, symptom alleviation is achieved through the same strategies implemented for women with age-appropriate menopause.

Women with POF experience vasomotor instability and genitourinary effects, along with menstrual irregularities that will eventually lead to amenorrhea (obviously, women who have had a total hysterectomy will experience amenorrhea immediately). Additionally, risks for cardiovascular disease and osteoporosis are increased decades earlier than their age-appropriate menopausal peers (Bakalov & Nelson, 2005; Eastell, 2003).

While women with POF are experiencing menopausal symptoms and related decreased fertility, their peer group is focused on pregnancy issues. Although some clients with POF are fortunate enough to have a successful pregnancy on their own, most women who wish to become pregnant following a diagnosis of POF achieve pregnancy through medical interventions such as egg donation because their follicles are depleted (Corrigan et al., 2005; Mainini et al., 2003; Pandian et al., 2005; Vandborg & Lauszus, 2006).

Many of these women spend years dealing with their lack of support and the absence of a peer group that understands their unique situation—simultaneously experiencing infertility and menopausal symptoms (Groff et al., 2005; Orshan et al., 2001). For women with a known etiology of POF, there is the additional concern related to the etiology. There is a national support group for women with POF and their significant others (www.pofsupport.org), with local branches in many areas, to help women deal with this unique situation. However, this group cannot take away all of the isolation and pain experienced by these women in their interactions with a world that does not understand their situation.

BOX 23.2 Andropause

Men, as well as women, experience hormonal changes as they enter midlife. Men experience decreased levels of the testicular androgen hormone testosterone, with an ongoing decline of free testosterone levels after 40 years. Although this is a definite decrease, it is very gradual and does not result in a total cessation of exogenous hormones, as found with the loss of ovarian function in women (Vermeulen, 2000). Also, as with women, aging men experience overall changes related to both hormonal changes and life cycle events (Mooradian & Korenman, 2006).

Changes that are hormonal in origin include the following:

- Decreased sexual functioning, with decreased libido and erectile dysfunction (although changes may be secondary to medical conditions, such as diabetes mellitus) (Hafez & Hafez, 2004; Mooradian & Korenman, 2006)
- Alterations in adipose tissue distribution, including increased central and upper body fat (Gould et al., 2000)
- Regression of secondary sex characteristics, including decreased body hair (Hibberts et al., 1998; Vermeulen, 2000)
- Decreased bone mass, resulting in osteoporosis, although at a later age than in women (Hafez & Hafez, 2004; Vermeulen, 2000)
- Disturbances in vasomotor functioning, including hot flashes and diaphoresis (Gould et al., 2000; Vermeulen, 2000)
- Changes in cognitive and affective functioning, including decreased visual-spatial abilities, verbal fluency, sense of well-being, friendliness, and energy, and increased depression, anger, irritability, insomnia, nervousness, and forgetfulness (Burris, et al., 1992; Wang, et al., 1996; Tan, et al., 2004)

In addition, several psychological changes may be related to hormonal changes or to life cycle changes, including a shift in concern from career and social interests to family; increased need for affirmation and acceptance; increased awareness of mortality and death; and concerns about self-improvement and personal accomplishments (Mooradian & Korenman, 2006).

Many clients experience hot flashes immediately before and during the first few days of menstruation. Precipitating factors include hot temperatures, stress, alcohol, hot drinks, cigarette smoking, and spicy foods (Frackiewicz & Cutler, 2000; Sievert et al., 2006). Review of the diary could help to determine whether any of these or other factors are related to the hot flashes. If they do appear to be related, the client can take actions to avoid the precipitating factors or to limit the effects of the hot flash.

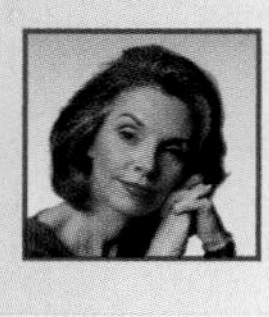

Remember Fran, the woman from the beginning of the chapter who was complaining of hot flashes. How might a diary help Fran?

ASSESSMENT TOOL 23.1 Guidelines for Perimenopause and Menopause

1. **Onset of Menarche:** "How old were you the first time that you got your period?"
2. **Characteristics of Cycle**
   Primary Inquiry: "Tell me about any changes in your menstrual cycle that you have noticed during the past 6 months."
   Follow-Up Questions:
   - "How many times in the past 6 months have you gotten your period?"
   - "How many days were there between the first day of one period (cycle) and the first day of the next period (cycle)?"
   - "How many pads/tampons did you use per day?"
   - "What color was the blood?"
   - "Were clots present?"
   - "What changes, if any, have there been in your period (cycle) compared with a few years ago?"
3. **Vasomotor Symptoms**
   Primary Inquiry: "Tell me about any hot flashes that you may have experienced in the last 6 months."
   Follow-Up Questions:
   - "Where do you first feel them?"
   - "Where do they spread to on your body?"
   - "When in your menstrual cycle are they most likely to occur?"
   - "What time of day/night do they occur most often?"
   - "If night, do they affect your rest?"
   - "Are they accompanied by sweating?"
   - "Are they more likely to occur if you are feeling warm, eat spicy foods, drink alcohol, or are feeling stressed?"
   - "What, if any, strategies have you found that decrease the frequency of hot flashes?"
   - "What, if any, strategies have you found that decrease the intensity of hot flashes?"
4. **Genitourinary Symptoms**
   Primary Inquiry: "Tell me about any changes you may have been experiencing regarding your urination (eg, passing water) during the past 6 months."
   Follow-Up Questions:
   - "Have you experienced any urinary leakage?"
   - "If yes, are any precipitating factors causing the leakage, such as coughing?"
   - "What actions have you taken to try and decrease the leakage?" (eg, Kegel exercises—recommended; decreasing fluid intake-not recommended)
   - "If so, have you found that they decrease the urine leakage?"
   - "Do you experience any pain when you urinate"?
   - "What is the color of your urine?"
5. **Sexuality Questions**
   Primary Inquiry: "Tell me about any changes you have been experiencing in your sexual activity during the past 6 months."
   Follow-Up Questions:
   - "During sexual intercourse, have you noticed that your vagina is taking longer to lubricate (become wet) or is not lubricating as much as it did a few years ago?"
   - "Have you experienced pain with sexual intercourse (dyspareunia)?"
   - "What action, if any, have you taken to decrease the pain with intercourse?" (eg, lubrication, hormone replacement therapy, meditation, relaxation techniques)
6. **Fertility**
   Primary Inquiry: "Tell me about your expectations/plans regarding your fertility at this time."
   Follow-Up Questions:
   - "Have you ever been pregnant?"
   - "If yes, how many times?"
   - "What were the outcomes?" (birth, spontaneous abortion, induced abortion)
   - "If no, what actions have you taken to prevent pregnancy?" (abstinence, type of family planning/contraception)
   - "Have you ever breastfed?"
   - "If so, how many children and for how long?"
   - "If you wish to become pregnant, have you begun to attempt to become pregnant?"
   - "How long have you been attempting to become pregnant?"
   - "Are you presently taking any medications to improve your fertility?"
   - "If yes, please name the medications."
7. **Mental Health Changes**
   Primary Inquiry: "Tell me about how your mood has been over the past 6 months."
   Follow-Up Questions:
   - "Have you experienced any recent changes in your mood, ability to feel happiness or joy, ability to remember things, sleep patterns, irritability, nervousness, or anxiety level?"
   - "If yes, in the past, have you ever felt or been diagnosed as depressed?"
   - "Did you ever experience any of these in the past?"
   - "If yes, which of the symptoms have you experienced and what was happening at that time in your life?"
   - "Have you experienced any recent changes in your life?" (family structure or role changes, career changes, change in perceived fertility status)

Continued

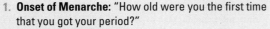

● ASSESSMENT TOOL 23.1 Guidelines for Perimenopause and Menopause

- "How do you feel about entering/being in midlife?"
- "Are you presently or have you previously taken any medications to help improve your mood or feelings about yourself?"

8. **Cardiovascular Disease**
   Primary Inquiry: "Tell me about the health of your heart during the past 6 months."
   Follow-Up Questions:
   - "Have you ever been diagnosed with any heart problems?"
   - "If yes, what is the name of the heart problem?"
   - "Do you presently, or have you previously, smoked cigarettes?"
   - "If yes, how many per day?"
   - "If you have stopped, when did you stop?"
   - "How often do you drink alcohol each week?"
   - "What is a typical daily diet?"
   - "Do exercise?"
   - "If yes, what type and how often?"
9. **Osteoporosis/Osteopenia**
   Primary Inquiry: "Tell me about the health of your bones during the past 6 months."
   Follow-Up Questions:
   - "Have you had a bone density scan?"
   - "If yes, when was your last scan?"
   - "What were the results?"
   - "Have you ever had a broken or fractured bone?"
   - "If yes, when?"
   - "What was the cause?"
   - "Do you presently take calcium supplements?" If yes, which one?
   - "If yes, when did you first start?"
   - "Are you taking any type of prescribed or nonprescribed herb or medication to promote bone strength?"
   - "What, if anything, are you doing to promote bone strength?"

   Note: The diet and exercise questions above are also directly related to this section.
10. **Breast Cancer**
    Primary Inquiry: "Tell me about the history of your breast health."
    Follow-Up Questions:
    - "Have you ever been diagnosed with breast cancer?"
    - "If yes, when was the diagnosis?"
    - "What treatment was initiated?"
    - "What is your present status?"
    - "Do you perform breast self-examination?"
    - "How often?"
    - "What were the findings?"
    - "When was the last time your breasts were examined by a health professional?"
    - "What were the findings?"
    - "When was your last mammogram?"
    - "What were the findings?"
    - "Are you presently taking any estrogen-containing preparations (eg, oral contraceptives, hormone replacement therapy)?"

Genitourinary Problems

Women in perimenopause frequently are not aware that this is the time they may begin to experience some genitourinary changes. Although the genital and urinary systems are related closely anatomically and physiologically, most women perceive them as two completely different areas. Assessment should reflect their beliefs as much as possible. Sensitivity during questioning is particularly important because many women are embarrassed when discussing issues of elimination and sexuality. Questions regarding the urinary tract may be easier for clients to respond to, so it may be best to begin genitourinary assessment focusing on this area, and then moving to questions related to the sexual organs.

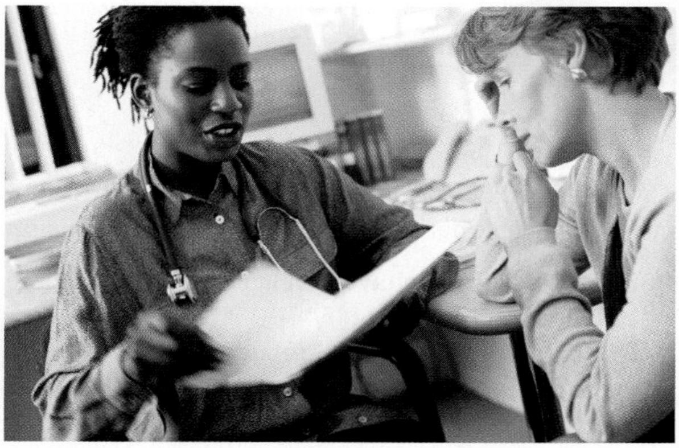

FIGURE 23.5 Reviewing journal findings with a client can help to identify patterns in menstrual cycle changes and vasomotor problems. Being able to understand and pinpoint these symptoms can help women feel more in control of anticipating and managing them.

The nurse should ask if the woman is experiencing urinary incontinence, urinary tract infections, or both. If responses are positive, the nurse needs to ask additional questions to determine more information about onset and severity.

Assessment of the genital tract focuses on questions about any vaginal infections and dyspareunia (Andrews et al., 2000). If dyspareunia is present, additional sexual information is necessary to determine its effects on the woman's life. Because few clients anticipate physiologic changes during perimenopause and menopause, they may perceive sexual difficulties as interpersonal, rather than physiologic (Bachmann, 1994).

This can lead to major changes in social support and sexual relationships.

Many women view the reality of decreasing fertility positively because they have either completed their families or decided not to have children. For the growing numbers of women trying to become pregnant during the later years of childbearing, however, issues surrounding fertility may be sensitive. Fertility assessment focuses on fertility history, including the outcome of any previous pregnancies, the client's present desires regarding pregnancy, and, if appropriate, what actions she is taking to achieve her desires—either contraception or fertility enhancement (see Chaps. 8 and 10). Assessing her knowledge base regarding her fertility choices (eg, birth control side effects, infertility treatments) should be initiated at this time.

Mental Health Status

Assessment of mental health status during perimenopause and menopause focuses on helping the nurse to gain insight into the client's past and present health. Together, the nurse and client need to identify personal, familial, and environmental factors that affect mental health and related coping mechanisms. Discussion of all the medications the client is presently taking should be included because some medications, including progestins (Wild, 1998) and other nonpsychological medications, may affect mental health.

Cardiovascular Health

Most women do not consider themselves at risk for cardiovascular disease (CVD) and may not understand the importance of assessment in this area. Some are frightened to learn that menopausal changes may increase their risk for developing CVD. The nurse should be prepared to provide support and education for clients before initiating cardiovascular assessment and examinations.

Thorough discussion of personal and familial risk factors for CVD is needed to assist the client to attain or maintain optimal cardiac health. Race is a significant factor in cardiovascular health risk. Among the different races and both sexes, African American women with diabetes are at highest risk for dying from myocardial infarction (Hoyert et al., 2006). Therefore, it is of particular importance that these women receive prompt and effective counseling regarding their cardiovascular risk.

For all clients, the nurse should identify knowledge concerning present cardiovascular status, along with personal and family history, risk factors, and beneficial activities. In addition, he or she should evaluate blood pressure, pulse, and serum total and HDL cholesterol levels to help develop a personalized, realistic plan of care (see Chap. 2).

Musculoskeletal Status

As discussed earlier in this chapter, decreased estrogen levels are partly responsible for the development of osteopenia and osteoporosis as women age (Andrews et al., 2000; Deroo & Korach, 2006). Additional factors that increase risk for musculoskeletal problems include early age at menopause, family history of osteoporosis, white or Asian race, small-boned stature, low body weight, nulliparity, sedentary lifestyle, smoking, excessive alcohol consumption, low sunlight exposure, high-fat diet, inadequate calcium intake throughout life, and excessive caffeine intake (Hobar, 2005).

Although risk factors for osteoporosis are the same for both African American and white women, African Americans have greater bone mass density at menopause and experience slower postmenopausal bone loss than do white women. Thus, African American women have approximately 50% the risk that white women have for developing osteoporosis (Hobar, 2005). Nevertheless, many African American women do sustain fractures and therefore need to receive the same education as non–African American women regarding osteopenia and osteoporosis.

The presence of osteopenia and osteoporosis can be determined through ultrasound or, more accurately, through dual energy x-ray absorptiometry (DEXA) scanning. Specific measurements of bone density are made at the lumbar spine, hip, distal radius, and ulna. If osteopenia or osteoporosis is diagnosed, medical conditions such as hyperthyroidism need to be ruled out to determine the appropriate treatment (Hobar, 2005). See Chapter 4 for more details.

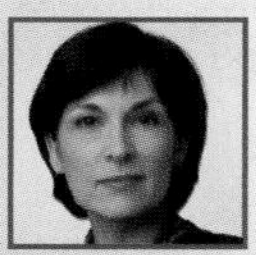

Carol has osteopenia. Based on the information at the beginning of the chapter, what risk factors are found in Carol's health history for osteopenia and osteoporosis?

Select Potential Nursing Diagnoses

The following are examples of NANDA diagnoses commonly applicable during perimenopause and menopause:

- **Health-Seeking Behaviors** related to perimenopause and menopause
- **Disturbed Body Image** related to alteration in menstruation
- **Ineffective Denial** related to pending loss of menstruation
- **Disturbed Sleep Pattern** related to body temperature fluctuations

- **Decisional Conflict** related to treatment options
- **Risk for Urge Urinary Incontinence** related to altered bladder capacity
- **Ineffective Sexuality Patterns** related to pain during intercourse
- **Situational Low Self-Esteem** related to urinary incontinence, altered sexual expression, or both
- **Effective Therapeutic Regimen** management related to seeking information
- **Deficient Knowledge** related to fertility issues during perimenopause
- **Anticipatory Grieving** related to decreased fertility
- **Impaired Adjustment** related to midlife changes
- **Risk for Powerlessness** related to midlife changes
- **Fatigue** related to depression, stress, or both
- **Ineffective Health Maintenance** related to lack of knowledge regarding changes in cardiovascular status
- **Deficient Knowledge** related to the hormonal effects on cardiovascular status
- **Health-Seeking Behaviors** related to potential alteration in bone integrity
- **Impaired Physical Mobility** related to alteration in bone integrity
- **Risk for Injury** related to loss of bone mass

Planning/Intervention

Nurses offer preparatory education to women in their 30s or younger, particularly if there appears to be an indication that that is needed. Once menstrual changes begin and the primary health care provider has ruled out pregnancy or other conditions that may cause irregularities (eg, endometrial cancer and leiomyomas [benign tumors]), the nurse should assure the woman that these changes are normal for her age. NIC/NOC Box 23.1 highlights some common nursing interventions and outcomes that may be appropriate for the woman approaching or experiencing menopause.

Some clients view the normal changes in the menstrual cycle as a positive sign that they are moving into the next phase of their life cycle. Others find the changes disruptive and uncomfortable. Nursing Care Plan 23.1 highlights the care of a woman experiencing physical and emotional changes related to menopause. For such clients, learning that these changes are a part of normal aging may help alleviate some of their concerns and help them to re-evaluate their perception of "normal."

Nurses need to provide anticipatory education to women and their partners so that they can correctly and promptly identify any changes that may be related to their changing physiology. Once such changes have been identified, health care providers can work with women to make informed decision making regarding the need for interventions.

NIC/NOC Box 23.1 Menopause

Common NIC Labels

- Coping Enhancement
- Exercise Promotion
- Fall Prevention
- Health Screening
- Risk Identification
- Role Enhancement
- Smoking Cessation Assistance
- Surveillance: Safety
- Teaching: Prescribed Diet
- Teaching: Prescribed Medication
- Teaching: Sexuality
- Weight Management

Common NOC Labels

- Health-Promoting Behaviors
- Health-Seeking Behaviors
- Knowledge: Health Behaviors
- Knowledge: Health Promotion
- Risk Control
- Risk Detection
- Safety Status: Falls Occurrence
- Safety Status: Physical Injury
- Self-Direction of Care

Pharmacologic Management

Pharmacologic preparations can alleviate many symptoms of perimenopause and menopause. Some of these medications are hormonal, whereas others fall within other drug classes. For example, providers may prescribe nonsteroidal anti-inflammatory medication for clients experiencing a greater menstrual flow than usual but for whom a change in cycle length is not a concern.

Hormone Replacement Therapy

Hormone replacement therapy (HRT), usually in the form of low-dose combined estrogen-progesterone oral contraceptives or progesterone-only pills, may be prescribed to regulate menstrual flow and cycles for eligible women (Table 23.1). During perimenopause, low-dose oral contraceptives provide the appropriate level of hormones to counteract the physiologic deprivation, while having the additional effect of providing contraception (see Chap. 8). For a client whose estrogen level is adequate but progesterone level is deficient, progesterone-only pills may be most appropriate. Using exogenous estrogen when it is not needed may cause breast tenderness and irregular bleeding (Frackiewicz & Cutler, 2000). The contraindications and side effects of both combined and progesterone-only oral contraceptives are the same with this age group as with younger women, as are the

NURSING CARE PLAN 23.1

The Woman Experiencing Menopausal Changes

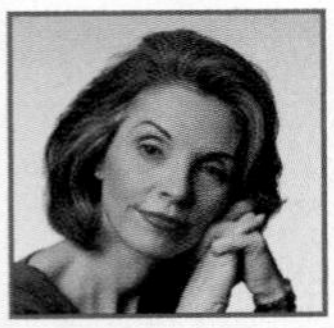

Fran, described at the start of this chapter, is experiencing hot flashes, sleep problems, and feelings of being alone. Further assessment reveals that her last menstrual period was 1 year ago. Since then, her hot flashes have increased to 3 to 4 times per week with diaphoresis. "It's been really upsetting. My children are gone. I'm tired all the time. I'm irritable and moody. I feel so unattractive and unwomanly now!"

NURSING DIAGNOSES

- **Risk for Powerlessness** related to physical and emotional changes associated with menopause
- **Impaired Adjustment** related to menopausal changes
- **Sleep Deprivation** related to increased hot flashes and diaphoresis at night

EXPECTED OUTCOMES

1. The client will identify physiologic and psychological changes accompanying menopause.
2. The client will state ways to increase control over symptoms.
3. The client will identify positive coping strategies.
4. The client will report at least two methods to promote sleep.

INTERVENTIONS	RATIONALES
Assess the client's knowledge about menopause and its accompanying physiologic and psychological changes.	Assessment provides a baseline from which to develop an individualized plan of care.
Review typical menopausal changes; correlate them with the client's current complaints.	Correlation aids in fostering better understanding on the client's part.
Investigate the meaning of menopause to the client and her feelings as a woman, mother, and wife.	Menopause means different things to different women. Some view menopause negatively, as a loss of youth and femininity; others may view it positively, as a time for new opportunities.
Remind the client that she is also experiencing other major life changes that reflect growth of her family.	Menopause is also a time of other major life events.
Discuss her concerns, feelings, and perceptions related to menopause and her family and how they are affecting her current situation.	Discussion provides opportunities to emphasize positive aspects; verbalization of concerns establishes sources of stress and problem areas to address.
Explain that many women experience hot flashes of varying intensity and frequency, commonly at night.	This knowledge can help the client feel less alone.
Have the client complete a diary detailing her experiences with hot flashes, including time, place, immediately preceding activity, whether it was accompanied by diaphoresis, how long it lasted, and what (if anything) alleviated the discomfort.	The diary can provide clues to possible precipitating factors that the client can then avoid.

Continued

NURSING CARE PLAN 23.1 ● The Woman Experiencing Menopausal Changes

INTERVENTIONS	RATIONALES
Assess the client's usual sleep routine; review measures to promote sleep.	Knowledge of habits aids in formulating appropriate suggestions.
Instruct the client to avoid daytime naps or to drink warm milk or take a warm bath before bedtime. Encourage a consistent routine before bedtime.	Avoiding daytime naps ensures that the client will be tired at bedtime. Warm milk contains L-tryptophan, a natural sleep aid. A warm bath helps promote relaxation. Consistency before bed aids in preparing for sleep.
Inquire about past methods used to cope with stressful situations; encourage the client to use methods that were successful; provide additional suggestions for ways to cope with the current situation.	Use of past successful methods enhances the chance of current success. Additional suggestions to deal with the current situation aid in relieving stress associated with outside variables and events and provide the client with various options, thereby promoting a greater feeling of control.
Assist the client to identify her own desires and goals.	Identification of the client's wishes is important in developing strategies appropriate for her.
Provide the client with accurate facts and communicate openly; answer questions honestly.	Open and honest communication promotes trust and helps correct any misconceptions or misinformation.
Review and reinforce the client's positive attributes about her self and her abilities.	Identification of positive attributes provides a foundation for enhancing self-esteem and aids in the realization that the client has an identity, is competent to care for herself, and is worthy of assistance.
Suggest participation in a support group.	Doing so promotes sharing, enhancing the realization that the client is not alone.
Arrange for referral to a mental health specialist if necessary.	A mental health specialist can assist with compromised coping mechanisms, depression, or a previous history of mental health problems.

EVALUATION

1. The client correlates events of menopause with current complaints.
2. The client identifies measures to adapt to changes.
3. The client demonstrates positive coping strategies.
4. The client reports an increase of at least one episode of nondisturbed sleep over 1 week.

nursing interventions. These are all discussed in detail in Chapter 8.

Once a client reaches menopause, she requires different levels of exogenous estrogen. For women with an intact uterus, oral or transdermal HRT containing both estrogen and progesterone may be prescribed. Estrogen without progesterone has been found to cause endometrial hyperplasia, which may lead to endometrial cancer (Frackiewicz & Cutler, 2000; Wild, 1998).

HRT can be either continuous or cyclic. Although clients following either regimen experience uterine bleeding initially, the cyclic form results in regular, monthly bleeding cycles, whereas women using the continuous form experience irregular bleeding.

For clients who have undergone a hysterectomy, estrogen replacement therapy (ERT) is appropriate. ERT may be administered orally, transdermally, vaginally, or through injections. The oral form protects the most

TABLE 23.1 Absolute and Potential Contraindications for Hormone Replacement Therapy

ABSOLUTE CONTRAINDICATIONS	POTENTIAL CONTRAINDICATIONS*
Undiagnosed abnormal vaginal bleeding	Breast cancer
Active/chronically severe hepatic disease	Active/recent (5 years) endometrial cancer
Active/recent thromboembolic disease	History of thromboembolic disease
	History of gallbladder disease
	Seizure disorders
	Migraine headaches

*In the presence of a potential contraindication, the decision to use hormone replacement therapy needs to be made by the woman and her primary care provider on an individual basis

Adapted from The North American Menopause Society. (2000). NAMS consensus opinion #3: A decision tree for the use of estrogen replacement therapy or hormone replacement therapy in postmenopausal women. *Menopause: The Journal of the North American Menopause Society, 7,* 76–86.

effectively against cardiovascular problems because of its beneficial effects on the liver and HDL cholesterol levels (Cutson & Meuleman, 2000). For women with liver concerns, transdermal administration may be preferable. Clients with vaginal changes may find that estrogen-containing cream alleviates some symptoms, including vaginal dryness.

In 2002, the Women's Health Initiative study reported that long-term use of HRT increased risks for breast cancer, cerebrovascular accident, and stroke (Writing Group, 2002). The potential risks posed by HRT has prompted many practitioners to move away from prescribing HRT for all women going through menopausal transitions and to focus more specifically on each client's particular circumstances. As of this writing, current practice is for the primary care provider to carefully evaluate the client's health history and work with her to make decisions relative to pharmacologic options. When making management decisions, the client and care provider need to consider the following points:

- The Women's Health Initiative does not recommend using HRT to prevent or to treat heart disease. Clients at risk for cardiovascular problems need a treatment approach focusing on lifestyle modifications, lipid-lowering agents, or both (Writing Group, 2002).
- Any clients taking HRT require the lowest possible dose. Most clients should not take HRT for more than 5 years.
- Alternatives to HRT include herbal therapies, selective estrogen receptor modulators, and bisphosphonates (see next discussion). Education related to these products would be individualized to the actual agent chosen.

Other adverse effects of HRT include breast tenderness, uterine bleeding, breast or endometrial cancer (depending on the type of HRT prescribed), thromboembolic disease, increased triglyceride levels, urinary tract infections, and gallbladder disease (Andrews et al., 2000; Cutson & Meuleman, 2000; Grodstein et al., 2004). Short-term common side effects of HRT include fluid retention, headaches, breast tenderness, nausea, and mood alterations.

Selective Estrogenic Receptor Modulators (SERMS)

SERMS, known as "designer estrogens," are estrogenic or antiestrogenic synthetic compounds that target specific organs, thereby avoiding some of the negative effects of estrogen (Lobo, 1999). The ideal SERM would have estrogenic-type activity in the brain, bone, cardiovascular system, and genitourinary system, and antiestrogenic activity in the breast and uterus. This SERM would decrease risks for cognitive impairment, Alzheimer's disease, osteoporosis, cardiovascular disease, breast cancer, and endometrial cancer.

Several SERMS are available to postmenopausal women. Raloxifene (Evista) is a benzothiophene approved by the U.S. Food and Drug Administration (FDA) for prophylactic treatment of osteoporosis (Karch, 2005). Although it is less effective than estrogen, it does not stimulate either the endometrial lining of the uterus or breast tissue, thus eliminating increased risks for cancers in these areas. Tamoxifen, a triphenylethylene, is prescribed frequently for clients following treatment of estrogen-sensitive breast cancer (Karch, 2005). Normally, clients recovering from breast cancer take tamoxifen for 5 years. With its antiestrogenic effect, tamoxifen may decrease the incidence of recurrent breast cancer; however, it does increase the risk for endometrial cancer.

Bisphosphonates

Bisphosphonates, such as alendronate (Fosamax), inhibit bone loss and increase bone mass density, decreasing fractures. Therapeutic treatment courses may be limited to 3 years to avoid osteomalacia (Cutson & Meuleman, 2000). For women experiencing osteopenia, the usual dosage is 5 mg/day; if osteoporosis is apparent, the dosage is usually double, at 10 mg/day (Karch, 2005). Nurses should make sure that the woman knows to take alendronate on an empty stomach. Clients should take the medication while upright and have nothing but water for the next 30 minutes (Karch, 2005). These measures decrease the risk for esophagitis and the main side effect, heartburn (Cutson & Meuleman, 2000).

Calcitonin

Calcitonin (Miacalcin) is a polypeptide hormone that increases bone mass density and decreases backbone fractures. Although there is an injectable form of calcitonin, a new intranasal form is being used, often with good results. The intranasal dose is 200 IU/day in postmenopausal women (Karch, 2005).

Complementary and Alternative Therapies

Nonpharmacologic strategies that have been successful in decreasing the effects of vasomotor symptoms include regular aerobic exercise, biofeedback, isoflavones (also known as dietary soy products), and black cohosh (Pepping, 1999). Many clients use herbal treatments to alleviate symptoms of perimenopause and menopause. Various sources have provided information about such herbal treatments, including Native American medicine, Eastern medicine, and many European cultures. Use of these remedies requires caution, however, because the herbal mixtures are not regulated and may have undesirable side effects. Furthermore, scientific support for claims about all herbal treatments is lacking.

Many herbal remedies are available; Complementary/Alternative Medicine Box 23.1 discusses a few of the more popular forms. For additional information, please refer to the References.

Infection Prevention and Sexual Comfort

Clients can avoid many of the potential difficulties related to genitourinary changes by implementing simple self-care actions. All clients can and should use such strategies to ensure optimal genitourinary health. For example, methods to decrease risk for infection include wearing cotton underwear and pantyhose with a cotton crotch, avoiding damp or tight-fitting clothing, voiding before and after sexual intercourse, and cleansing the perineum after defecating by wiping from front to back. Kegel exercises, which strengthen the pubococcygeal muscle, may help improve urinary continence (Frackiewicz & Cutler, 2000; Harvey, 2003; Hay-Smith & Dumoulin, 2006) and vaginal muscle tone. See Teaching Tips 23.1.

During this life stage, many women find that vaginal lubrication is decreased. Encouraging clients and their partners to increase time spent in foreplay during sexual encounters may help promote vaginal lubrication. Additionally, the client may wish to apply a water-based vaginal lubricant immediately before coitus. Doing so can help minimize problems with dyspareunia resulting from lack of vaginal lubrication. Of course, the nurse should be careful to follow-up on whether these measures solve the problem because ongoing pain or discomfort during intercourse may indicate a need for further physiologic or psychological intervention.

Fertility Control

QUOTE 23-2

"I love being in menopause! It is like being on my honeymoon again!"

A 55-year-old married woman

Many women welcome menopause because of its accompanying effects of absolving the chance of undesired or unintended pregnancy. Because the duration of perimenopause varies and pregnancy remains a possibility for many women well into their 40s, however, the client and, as appropriate, her partner need to make reproductive-control decisions to ensure support for their fertility choices. If a client desires to avoid pregnancy, the nurse should provide her with education regarding options for fertility control (see Chap. 8). Assuming that the client is in good health, these options are much the same as for younger women. Oral contraceptives may be prescribed as a low-dose form of HRT with the added benefit of pregnancy prevention.

Clients desiring pregnancy during this time of their lives need to be aware that chances of conception without intervention are not high. If such intervention is unsuccessful in helping a client achieve pregnancy with her own ova, oocyte donation may be a viable option. This and other measures to facilitate pregnancy are discussed in Chapter 10.

Stress Management and Coping

Reinforcing healthy coping mechanisms, and, if needed, helping clients develop additional coping strategies to deal with real and potential stresses related to perimenopause and menopause are of primary importance during this life phase. Clients with compromised coping mechanisms or a history of mental health alterations may benefit from a referral to a mental health specialist. Because previous episodes of depression appear to increase the likelihood of recurrence during this time, nurses should be aware of symptoms so that they can take appropriate actions immediately to alleviate or prevent depression in their clients (Dennerstein et al., 2004) (see Chap. 5).

Women experiencing insomnia may be exhibiting alterations in mental health that increased sleep will alleviate. For some women, avoiding daytime naps, drinking warm milk at bedtime (contains L-tryptophan), or taking a warm bath may promote relaxation and sleep. Stress management techniques, meditation, and regular exercise also may help. Support groups and psychological counseling may be appropriate for clients experiencing familial or career challenges, self-esteem issues, or both.

COMPLEMENTARY/ALTERNATIVE MEDICINE 23.1

Herbs for Menopausal Symptom Alleviation

- **Isoflavones:** Also called *phytoestrogens,* these include soy products and black cohosh (*Cimicifuga racemosa*). They are used to treat problems related to estrogen loss, such as vasomotor instability and vaginal dryness. For many clients, they are viable alternatives to prescription estrogen therapy, although their ability to decrease risks for osteoporosis and cardiovascular disease has not been established (Carroll, 2006; Frackiewicz & Cutler, 2000).
    - **Soy products** contain a natural form of dietary estrogen. Their isoflavones are much weaker than those of endogenous estrogen; however, studies have shown fewer vasomotor symptoms, decreased vaginal dryness and bone loss, and lower low-density lipoprotein and total cholesterol levels among clients who ingest soy products as part of their regular diet or as a dietary supplement (Cutson & Meuleman, 2000). Research findings on soy protein neither refute nor substantiate claims made by soy proponents (Andrews et al., 2000; Carroll, 2006). Recommended daily intake of soy is 45 g (Frackiewicz & Cutler, 2000). Sources include tofu, soy nuts, and soy milk. A new category of soy-fortified products is aimed at perimenopausal and menopausal women; it includes hot and cold cereals as well as over-the-counter nutritional supplements.
    - Native Americans and others have used **black cohosh** (*Cimicifuga racemosa*) for a wide variety of problems, including snakebite, malaria, and dysmenorrhea. It is one of the few herbal substances that has been pharmacologically standardized (Hardy, 2000). Its mechanism of action is uncertain (Kligler, 2003). The standardized form, Remifemin, has been the focus of clinical studies, the findings of which appear to support use for perimenopausal and menopausal symptoms. Some of these studies, however, lacked adequate control groups and included no long-term follow-up relative to effects (Carroll, 2006; Low Dog, 2005). Side effects of black cohosh include upset stomach, headache, weight gain, and syncope (Kligler, 2003). A flushed face, throbbing frontal headache, nausea, hypotension, and bradycardia are symptoms of overdose (Institute for Clinical Systems Improvement, 2000). Standard dosage of Remifemin is 40 mg/day (Cutson, et al, 2000). Because of the lack of data on the long-term effects of black cohosh, women may want to limit their duration of use of this herb to 6 months (Kronenberg & Fugh-Berman, 2002).
- **Yam:** Yam contains a precursor of progesterone known as diosgenin, which humans cannot convert to a usable form of progesterone. Wild yam cream is available over the counter; some women purchase it to alleviate symptoms of menopause. No evidence at this time, however, indicates that its use is an effective alternative to progesterone (Komesaroff et al., 2001). In fact, it should not be used in place of the progesterone component of hormone replacement therapy (Institute for Clinical Systems Improvement, 2000).
- **Dong Quai:** Dong Quai (*Angelica sinensis*), a coumarin, is a traditional Chinese herb with a reputation in the West as the "menopause herb." Although Western medicine uses Dong Quai as both a singular and compound element in herbal preparations, Chinese medicine limits its use to multiple-herb compounds. A carcinogenic agent in the essential oil of Dong Quai may or may not be significant in the available dosage preparations (Institute for Clinical Systems Improvement, 2000). Research focused on Dong Quai has not validated its use for menopausal symptoms (Low Dog, 2005). Dong Quai is contraindicated for women with menorrhagia or midcycle spotting and in those who also are taking blood-thinning medications (Learn & Higgins, 1999).

TEACHING TIPS 23.1 Kegel (Pelvic Floor) Exercises

The pubococcygeal or "PC" muscle helps to support the bladder and uterus in their proper position in the pelvis. Kegel exercises help to strengthen this important muscle of the pelvic floor. The technique is very simple:

- Kegel exercises can be done sitting, standing, or lying down. Only the person who is performing the exercise need know that it is being done. If the woman has trouble identifying the muscle, share with her that it is the muscle used to stop urinating as well as the muscle used to grip the penis during sexual intercourse.
- It is helpful for some clients to think of the PC muscle as an elevator. In the relaxed position, the muscle should be viewed as being at ground floor. The woman should slowly and consciously tighten the muscle past the first floor, second floor, third floor, and finally the penthouse.
- The muscle should stay at the penthouse for about 10 seconds, and then slowly descend down again to the ground floor.
- This should be repeated about 5 to 10 times, 3 or more times a day.

Pharmacologic intervention, including psychiatric medications for specific mental health alterations, may provide relief (see Chap. 5). Other women find that HRT promotes rest by alleviating hot flashes.

Information is conflicting regarding the influence of estrogen on the incidence of Alzheimer's disease among women. Proponents of the belief that estrogen decreases the incidence of Alzheimer's disease believe that HRT may be indicated for improvement of cognitive well-being (Wise, 2006).

St. John's wort (*Hypericum perforatum*) has been viewed as a "natural" method of treating depression and anxiety, but views on its efficacy are conflicting. St. John's wort has multiple known interactions with prescribed medications, including protease inhibitors used for HIV, cyclosporines, digoxins, β blockers, antidepressants, monoamine oxidase inhibitors, ephedra, and oral contraceptives (Karch, 2005; Williamson, 2006).

Cardiovascular Health

Education regarding the effects of perimenopause and menopause on cardiovascular health is important in helping women to understand the increased risks that accompany estrogen depletion. A healthy lifestyle is essential to maintaining or improving cardiovascular health.

Smoking is the most prevalent cause of mortality, followed by inactivity. Women who smoke heavily tend to experience menopause earlier than moderate smokers or nonsmokers (by 2 to 3 years) and therefore experience estrogen deprivation, along with all the negative effects related to lack of estrogen, for a longer time than nonsmokers (Kinney et al., 2006). Clients should be counseled to stop smoking and, if needed, referred to community support groups, over-the-counter medications, or a nurse practitioner or physician for appropriate medication to assist with smoking cessation.

Activity levels need to be evaluated and a safe, effective program of exercise initiated (Andrews et al., 2000). A referral to an exercise physiologist may be appropriate. A combination of aerobic and weight-bearing exercises helps decrease the risk for CAD, control postmenopausal lipoprotein levels, increase bone and muscle mass, aid sleep, and control weight. It also may decrease depression. Before assisting midlife and older adults in exercises, it is important to remind them of the precautions outlined in Teaching Tips 23.2.

Dietary intake is one of the most important influences over cardiovascular health. A well-balanced, low-fat diet is important in controlling cholesterol. After menopause, women are more likely to gain weight, creating additional strain on the heart (Gavaler & Rosenblum, 2003). To help prevent weight gain, clients need to be educated about changing caloric needs (see Chap. 3). Antioxidants, including vitamins C and E, may help prevent or reduce arterial LDL (Andrews et al., 2000). If the client has obesity, diabetes, hypertension, established cardiac problems, or a combination of these problems, a referral to a nutritionist may be appropriate because these medical conditions place her at even greater risk for cardiovascular problems.

Osteoporosis Prevention

Preventive care for osteopenia and osteoporosis is a lifestyle choice that optimally begins before perimenopause. A dietary intake high in calcium and regular participation in aerobic and weight-bearing exercise are important to preventing or limiting skeletal deterioration. Although clients can achieve higher bone mass density before menopause through exercise, once they are in menopause, exercise alone is not enough to maintain bone mass.

TEACHING TIPS 23.2 Exercise

- **Exercise should be pain free.** Remember, pain can emerge a few days after the exercise, so caution the exerciser to learn to listen to his or her body.
- **Keep breathing.** This can be crucial in an exerciser who has heart disease or hypertension.
- **Watch out for shoulder and neck tension.** Encourage the exerciser to inhale and, when exhaling, to exhale the stress from shoulders and neck.
- **Maintain good neck alignment.** Demonstrate how a small pillow or rolled-up towel can be placed behind the neck when in a supine position.
- **Hold weights with a neutral wrist.** Demonstrate the technique of holding a weight without bending the wrist backward.
- **Maintain normal spinal curves.** Demonstrate engaging abdominal muscles to protect the spine, rather than weaken the spine by altering its configuration.
- **Evaluate the exerciser's handgrip.** If the exerciser has a tendency to drop objects, encourage the use of a weight that can be strapped onto the exerciser's hand or wrist.
- **Avoid forward bending.** Share with the exerciser that bending increases the risk for spinal fracture.

Adapted from Daniels, D. (2000). *Exercises for osteoporosis.* New York: Hatherhleigh Press.

Following menopause, all women taking HRT should ingest 1200 mg/day of calcium. All women not taking HRT should ingest 1500 mg/day, along with 400 to 800 IU of vitamin D each day (Gold, 2005). Women also should continue to regularly participate in aerobic and weight-bearing exercises—the latter type may help to stimulate new bone formation (Beitz & Doren, 2004). Prescribed medications that can reverse or inhibit further bone loss include HRT; ERT; oral contraceptives; specific SERMS, such as raloxifene; and bisphosphonates, including alendronate (Fosamax). See Nursing Care Plan 23.2.

Evaluation

Evaluation varies according to the individualized plan and specific interventions. For all clients, increased understanding of expected changes is paramount. Once interventions have been initiated, they are deemed successful if the client experiences increased comfort and acceptance of the normal age-related changes. If the client and her health care provider choose an intervention or medication regimen, knowledge of expected outcomes, along with side effects and any danger signs, is imperative.

The client should understand the likelihood of becoming pregnant with a healthy fetus at this time and interventions that may be needed to facilitate or prevent conception. See Chapters 8 and 10 for the evaluation of interventions that may be initiated to control fertility.

Because of societal attitudes toward mental distress, evaluating mental health status and intervention success may be difficult. Determining the client's understanding of the etiology of mental health changes during this period is crucial, as is identifying her awareness of potential interventions. Any changes in mental health status need to be monitored continually, with further actions initiated as needed.

Evaluation of the client's diet, exercise regimen, and coping skills is necessary to assist her to achieve the most optimal cardiovascular health possible. Awareness of the client's knowledge level concerning the effects of osteopenia and osteoporosis is also of primary importance. Once such knowledge has been validated, the outcomes of actions or nonactions that the woman chooses to take can be determined.

Questions to Ponder

1. During an appointment with an infertility specialist, a 44-year-old woman with no viable follicles has been advised that if she and her husband wish to become pregnant, one of the most viable options is ova donation. During a counseling session with the nurse, the woman shares that her husband is very excited about the prospect, but that she is ambivalent because the child will not share her genetic traits, but those of her husband and a donor.
   - What are your personal feelings about facilitating a menopausal woman to become pregnant?
   - What additional information might be helpful for the nurse to have before responding?
   - What type of response may provide the woman with some comfort and support regarding her decision?

SUMMARY

- With aging, the ovaries secrete less estrogen and progesterone, resulting in increased secretion of FSH from the anterior pituitary, which increases the rate of follicular atresia. These developments lead to infertile anovulatory cycles and eventual depletion of ovarian follicles at approximately the time of menopause.
- Physiologic and psychological changes related to perimenopause and menopause are a combination of hormonal influences and lifestyle changes during midlife.
- The earliest signs of perimenopause include changes in menstruation cycle length and flow rate. Health care providers may encourage clients to keep a calendar that records the menstrual cycle and to use the findings to form a plan of care to manage changes.
- Vasomotor instability, including hot flashes and diaphoresis, most likely result from decreased endogenous estrogen.
- Genitourinary changes in menopause include atrophy of the vaginal lining, decreased vaginal lubrication, decreased libido, increased vaginal infections, and increased urinary urge incontinence and urinary tract infections.
- Fertility rapidly decreases throughout midlife; however, pregnancy continues to remain a possibility for many women well into their 40s.
- Mental health changes, including depression, irritability, lethargy, and forgetfulness, may be related to hormonal alterations of perimenopause and menopause or may be manifestations of life cycle events.
- Cardiovascular changes, particularly increased risks for cardiovascular disease and myocardial infarction, are related to the lipid and vascular alterations of estrogen depletion.
- Osteopenia and osteoporosis are particular concerns for white and Asian women, although women of African descent are also at risk. Decreased estrogen, along with familial and lifestyle factors, influence the risk for osteopenia and osteoporosis.
- Prescribed pharmacologic measures that can be used to combat the hormonal depletion of menopause include combined estrogen-progesterone therapy, estrogen replacement therapy, progesterone-only therapy, SERMS, bisphosphonates, and calcitonin.

NURSING CARE PLAN 23.2

The Menopausal Woman at Risk for Osteoporosis

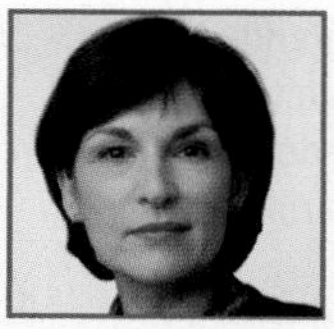

Carol is 44 years old and has been diagnosed with osteopenia, as described at the beginning of the chapter. Further assessment reveals that she exercises occasionally, going for short walks with friends 2 to 3 times per month. She says, "Since I stopped smoking, I've cut down my coffee intake to about 2 cups per day. I do use milk as my creamer in the coffee, though, and I try to eat a container of yogurt at least once a week." She denies any use of calcium supplements or herbal remedies. "I know I need to drink more milk, but I'm not a big fan. What else could I do?"

NURSING DIAGNOSES

- **Health-Seeking Behaviors** related to risk reduction and alteration in bone integrity
- **Risk for Injury** related to osteopenia and continued loss of bone mass

EXPECTED OUTCOMES

1. The client will identify measures to prevent or limit changes in bone integrity.
2. The client will verbalize ways to maintain safety to reduce the risk for fractures.

INTERVENTIONS	RATIONALES
Assess the client's knowledge of osteopenia and osteoporosis.	Assessment provides a baseline from which to develop an individualized plan.
Review the client's history for possible risk factors.	Risk factor identification is the first step in identifying areas that need intervention.
Question the client about food likes and dislikes; review high-calcium foods, encouraging her to eat those she prefers. Discuss foods high in vitamin D. Suggest the use of calcium-fortified foods.	Encouraging the client to select high-calcium foods that she prefers increases the chances for adherence. Vitamin D promotes calcium absorption and prevents further bone loss.
Encourage the client to reduce her intake of caffeinated beverages; suggest caffeine-free drinks and decaffeinated coffee.	Caffeine interferes with calcium absorption.
Offer positive reinforcement for smoking cessation.	Smoking increases risk for osteoporosis. Positive reinforcement fosters a sense of achievement, helping reduce the chance for relapse.
Review the client's daily routine.	Knowledge of her habits and routine aids in developing appropriate individualized suggestions that match the client's lifestyle.
Encourage the client to increase her activity level; suggest aerobic weight-bearing exercise 3 to 4 times each week for approximately 20 minutes each time; assist her to develop a workable plan based on her daily routine. If possible, encourage the client to exercise outdoors or to otherwise get 30 minutes of sunlight per day.	Aerobic weight-bearing exercise helps slow down bone loss. Weight-bearing exercise helps stimulate new bone formation. Sunlight provides vitamin D, which helps reduce bone loss.

Continued

NURSING CARE PLAN 23.2 ● The Menopausal Woman at Risk for Osteoporosis *(Continued)*

INTERVENTIONS	RATIONALES
Question the client about family, friends, or others who might join her in her activities.	Participation of others promotes sharing and provides encouragement for those involved.
Recommend that the client wear well-fitting supportive shoes when exercising; emphasize the need to warm up and cool down.	Proper footwear and warm-up and cool-down exercises are important to reduce the risk for injury.
Provide suggestions for safety measures in the home, such as avoiding throw rugs and loose extension cords that cross the room, having well-lit halls and stairs, using banisters or railings for support, and wearing shoes with nonskid soles.	Environmental safety measures reduce the risk for falls.
Advise the client to use an over-the-counter calcium supplement (1500 mg/day) with 400 to 800 IU of vitamin D if necessary.	Calcium supplementation is necessary to replace lost calcium and reduce bone loss.
Arrange for the client to have a follow-up DEXA scan 12 to 18 months from her first one.	Follow-up scanning is needed to evaluate bone mineral density and any progression of osteopenia to osteoporosis.

EVALUATION

1. The client demonstrates appropriate measures to reduce risk and minimize loss of bone mass.
2. The client remains injury free.

- Exercise, dietary intake, biofeedback, and prescribed HRT may be useful in improving vasomotor stability. Complementary treatments to alleviate the symptoms of perimenopause and menopause include isoflavones.
- Anticipatory education to limit or prevent genitourinary problems include teaching Kegel exercises, explaining the benefits of increasing sexual foreplay, and advising the client to use a vaginal lubricant before coitus.
- To prevent or facilitate pregnancy in women during this stage, providers must work with the client to identify her fertility choices and assist with providing contraception or, if needed, referrals for fertility promotion.
- Collaborative care related to mental health includes identification of potential issues, including insomnia and stress, and devising strategies to assist women in achieving mental health, based on the etiology of the changes.
- Beneficial lifestyle choices for cardiovascular health during this stage may include smoking cessation, exercise, and dietary changes. A well-balanced diet should contain calcium-rich foods and soy products. Relaxation and stress management are also vital.
- Assisting the client to prevent or control osteopenia and osteoporosis focuses on decreasing controllable risk factors (eg, smoking) and emphasizing the need for appropriate calcium and vitamin D supplementation.
- Premature ovarian failure occurs in women younger than 40 years of age who experience menopausal symptoms from either induced or naturally occurring ovarian failure. In addition, these women are simultaneously experiencing infertility at a time when many of their peers are experiencing parenthood, leading to potential psychosocial difficulties.
- Andropause is the term used to define the physiologic and psychological changes men begin to experience in midlife. As with women, completely differentiating life cycle changes from decreased hormone levels is difficult. Typical andropause changes include decreased bone mass, vasomotor disturbances, cognitive alterations, and decreased libido.

REVIEW QUESTIONS

1. A 40-year-old client asks the nurse, "When do you think I will go through menopause?" After completing an assessment, the nurse identifies which of the following factors as potentially increasing the woman's risk for early menopause?
   A. Menarche at age 14 years
   B. History of three previous pregnancies
   C. Use of oral contraceptives
   D. Breastfeeding her children
2. A 48-year-old woman comes to her gynecologist's office for a routine checkup. During the visit, she complains of hot flashes accompanied sporadically by excessive diaphoresis. The woman states that her menstrual cycle has remained static for the past 5 years, although before that time, the cycle was longer in length. She denies experiencing dyspareunia, altered libido, or urinary tract infections. To help determine an appropriate plan for this woman, which question should the nurse ask next?
   A. "How many days is your menstrual cycle now?"
   B. "Can you tell me a bit more about your hot flashes?"
   C. "Are you using a vaginal lubricant during intercourse?"
   D. "Do you ever eat any soy products?"
3. Which of these women would be at least risk for developing osteoporosis?
   A. A 45-year-old African American woman who exercises 3 times a week
   B. A 50-year-old white woman who works at a computer every day
   C. A 44-year-old Asian American woman who drinks 4 cups of tea per a day
   D. A 40-year-old white woman who has never been pregnant
4. Which suggestion if made by the nurse would be most appropriate for a menopausal client complaining of dyspareunia?
   A. Perform Kegel exercises 3 times per day
   B. Apply a water-soluble lubricant before intercourse
   C. Take a bisphosphonate such as alendronate (Fosamax)
   D. Wear cotton underwear and pantyhose with cotton crotch
5. When assessing a woman who is considering the use of estrogen replacement therapy, a history of which of the following would be of least concern?
   A. Hysterectomy
   B. Chronic severe liver disease
   C. Recent thromboembolism
   D. Breast cancer
6. The nurse is preparing a teaching plan for a local women's community group about menopause. Which of the following should the nurse be least likely to include in the teaching plan?
   A. The average age of menopause is about 51 to 52 years of age
   B. Men experience a change in hormonal levels with aging
   C. Levels of LDL drop with the onset of menopause
   D. Osteoporosis is a major cause of fractures after menopause
7. Which of the following assessment findings should lead the nurse to suspect that a client is experiencing a common adverse effect associated with her prescribed therapy with alendronate (Fosamax)?
   A. Fluid retention
   B. Heartburn
   C. Breast tenderness
   D. Mood alterations
8. A client states that she is taking a medication in the form of a nasal spray to reduce her risk for back fractures. Which medication is she most likely using?
   A. Calcitonin (Miacalcin)
   B. Raloxifene (Evista)
   C. Tamoxifen
   D. Atorvastatin (Lipitor)
9. Which of the following suggestions should the nurse include in a plan of care to promote the cardiovascular health of a menopausal woman?
   A. Limit the intake of vitamin C–containing foods
   B. Perform isometric exercises at least twice weekly
   C. Restrict intake to 1000 calories per day
   D. Eat foods high in polyunsaturated and monounsaturated fats
10. Nursing assessment of a healthy 27-year-old woman who is attending a gynecologic clinic reveals that, since the woman's healthy pregnancy 2 years earlier, she has had an irregular menstrual cycle, is experiencing periodic hot flashes, particularly at night, and complains of dyspareunia. Based on this information, the nurse should anticipate the need to next
    A. provide sexual counseling to the woman.
    B. suggest a referral to a mental health counselor.
    C. assess the woman's level of ovarian hormones.
    D. determine whether the woman is presently breastfeeding her child.

REFERENCES

American College of Obstetricians and Gynecologists (ACOG). (1995). Health maintenance for perimenopausal women. *ACOG Technical Bulletin, 210.*

Andrews, W. C., Weisman, C. S., Holleran, M. K., Johnson, C., Mort, E. A., O'Kane, M., et al. (2000). *Guidelines for counseling women on the management of menopause.* Retrieved June 2, 2006, from: http://www.jiwh.org/Resources/Guidelines%20for%20Menopause%2Epdf.

Avis, N. E., Brambilla, D., McKinlay, S. M., et al. (1994). A longitudinal analysis of the association between menopause and depression:

Results from the Massachusetts Women's Health Study. *Annals of Epidemiology, 4*(3), 214–220.

Bachmann, G. A. (1994). The changes before "the change": Strategies for the transition to the menopause. *Postgraduate Medicine, 95*(4), 113–115, 119–121, 124.

Baird, D. T., Collins, J., Egozcue, J., Evers, L. H., Gianaroli, L., Leridon, H., et al. (2005). Fertility and ageing. *Human Reproduction Update, 11*(3), 261–276.

Bakalov, V., & Nelson, L. M. (2005). Ovarian failure. [E-Medicine.] Retrieved June 8, 2006.

Ballagh, S. A. (2005). Vaginal hormone therapy for urogenital and menopausal symptoms. *Seminars in Reproductive Medicine, 23*(2), 126–140.

Beitz, R., & Doren, M. (2004). Physical activity and postmenopausal health. *Journal of the British Menopause Society, 10*(2), 70–74.

Broekmans, F. J., Faddy, M. J., Scheffer, G., & te Velde, E. R. (2004). Antral follicle counts are related to age at natural fertility loss and age at menopause. *Menopause, 11*(6 Pt. 1), 607–614.

Buckler, H. (2005). The menopause transition: Endocrine changes and clinical symptoms. *Journal of the British Menopause Society, 11*(2), 61–65.

Burris, A. S., Banks, S. M., Carter, C. S., Davidson, J. M., & Sherins, R. J. (1992). A long term prospective study of the physiologic and behavioural effects of hormone replacement in untreated hypogonadal men. *Journal of Andrology, 13*(4), 297–304.

Carroll, D. G. (2006). Nonhormonal therapies for hot flashes in menopause. *American Family Physician, 73*(3), 457–464.

Cohen, L. S., Soares, C. N., Vitonis, A. F., Otto, M. W., & Harlow, B. L. (2006). Risk for new onset of depression during the menopausal transition: The Harvard study of moods and cycles. *Archives of General Psychiatry, 63*(4), 385–390.

Corrigan, E. C., Raygada, M. J., Vanderhoof, V. H., & Nelson, L. M. (2005). A woman with spontaneous premature ovarian failure gives birth to a child with fragile X syndrome. *Fertility and Sterility, 84*(5), 1508.

Cramer, D. W., & Xu, H. (1996). Predicting age at menopause. *Maturitas, 23*(3), 319–326.

Cutson, T. M., & Meuleman, E. (2000). Managing menopause. *American Family Physician, 61*(5), 1391–1400.

Deeks, A. A. (2004). Is this menopause? Women in midlife—psychosocial issues. *Australian Family Physician, 33*(11), 889–893.

Deeks, A. A., & McCabe, M. P. (2004). Well-being and menopause: An investigation of purpose in life, self-acceptance and social role in premenopausal, perimenopausal and postmenopausal women. *Quality of Life Research, 13*(2), 389–398.

Dennerstein, L., Guthrie, J. R., Clark, M., Lehert, P., & Henderson, V. W. (2004). A population-based study of depressed mood in middle-aged, Australian-born women. *Menopause, 11*(5), 563–568.

Deroo, B. J., & Korach, K. S. (2006). Estrogen receptors and human disease. *Journal of Clinical Investigation, 116*(3), 561–570.

Dvornyk, V., Long, J. R., Liu, P. Y., Zhao, L. J., Shen, H., Recker, R. R., & Deng, H. W. (2006). Predictive factors for age at menopause in Caucasian females. *Maturitas, 54*(1), 19–26.

Eastell, R. (2003). Management of osteoporosis due to ovarian failure. *Medical Pediatric Oncology, 41*(3), 222–227.

Fu, S. Y., Anderson, D., & Courtney, M. (2003). Cross-cultural menopausal experience: Comparison of Australian and Taiwanese women. *Nursing and Health Sciences, 5*(1), 77–84.

Frackiewicz, E. J., & Cutler, N. R. (2000). Women's health care during the perimenopause. *Journal of the American Pharmacological Association, 40*(6), 800–811.

Freedman, R. R. (2005). Hot flashes: Behavioral treatments, mechanisms, and relation to sleep. *American Journal of Medicine, 118*(12 Suppl. 2), 124–130.

Gallicchio, L., Miller, S. R., Visvanathan, K., Lewis, L. M., Babus, J., Zacur, H., & Flaws, J. A. (2006). Cigarette smoking, estrogen levels, and hot flashes in midlife women. *Maturitas, 53*(2), 133–143.

Gass, M., & Dawson-Hughes, B. (2006). Preventing osteoporosis-related fractures: An overview. *American Journal of Medicine, 119*(4 Suppl. 1), S3–S11.

Gavaler, J. S., & Rosenblum, E. (2003). Predictors of postmenopausal body mass index and waist hip ratio in the Oklahoma postmenopausal health disparities study. *Journal of the American College of Nutrition, 22*(4), 269–276.

Gold, D. T. (2005). Elevated calcium requirements for women and unique approaches to improving calcium adherence. *Journal of Reproductive Medicine, 50*(11 Suppl.), 891–895.

Gould, D. C., Petty, R., & Jacobs, H. S. (2000). The male menopause—does it exist? *British Medical Journal, 320*(35), 858–860.

Grodstein, F., Lifford, K., Resnick, N. M., & Curhan, G. C. (2004). Postmenopausal hormone therapy and risk of developing urinary incontinence. *Obstetrics and Gynecology, 103*(2), 254–260.

Groff, A. A., Covington, S. N., Halverson, L. R., Fitzgerald, O. R., Vanderhoof, V., Calis, K., & Nelson, L. M. (2005). Assessing the emotional needs of women with spontaneous premature ovarian failure. *Fertility and Sterility, 83*(6), 1734–1741.

Hafez, B., & Hafez, E. S. (2004). Andropause: Endocrinology, erectile dysfunction, and prostate pathophysiology. *Archives of Andrology, 50*(2), 45–68.

Hardy, M. L. (2000). Herbs of special interest to women. *Journal of the American Pharmaceutical Association, 40*(2), 234–242.

Harvey, M. A. (2003). Pelvic floor exercises during and after pregnancy: A systematic review of their role in preventing pelvic floor dysfunction. *Journal of Obstetrics and Gynaecology in Canada, 25*(6), 451–453.

Hay-Smith, E. J., & Dumoulin, C. (2006). Pelvic floor muscle training versus no treatment, or inactive control treatments, for urinary incontinence in women. *Cochrane Database of Systematic Reviews, 25*(1): CD005654.

Hefler, L. A., Grimm, C., Bentz, E. K., Reinthaller, A., Heinze, G., & Tempfer, C. B. (2006). A model for predicting age at menopause in white women. *Fertility and Sterility, 85*(2), 451–454.

Hibberts, N. A., Howell, A. E., & Randall, V. A. (1998). Balding hair follicle dermal papilla cells contain higher levels of androgen receptors than those from non-balding scalp. *Journal of Endocrinology, 156,* 59.

Hobar, C. (2005). Osteoporosis. [E-Medicine]. Retrieved June 2, 2006, from http://www.emedicine.com/med/topic1693.htm.

Hoyert, D. L., Heron, M. P., Murphy, S. L., & Kung, H. (2006). *Deaths: Final data for 2003. National Vital Statistics Reports, 54*(13). Hyattsville, MD: National Center for Vital Statistics.

Hvas, L. (2006). Menopausal women's positive experience of growing older. *Maturitas, 54*(3), 245–251.

Institute for Clinical Systems Improvement. (2000). *Health Care Guidelines.*

Jacobsson, B., Ladfors, L., & Milsom, I. (2004). Advanced maternal age and adverse perinatal outcome. *Obstetrics and Gynecology, 104*(4), 727–733.

Karch, A. M. (2005). *2005 Lippincott's nursing drug guide.* Philadelphia: Lippincott Williams & Wilkins.

Kinney, A., Kline, J., & Levin, B. (2006). Alcohol, caffeine and smoking in relation to age at menopause. *Maturitas, 54*(1), 27–38.

Klein, N. A., & Soules, M. (1998). Endocrine changes of the perimenopause. *Clinical Obstetrics and Gynecology, 41*(4), 912–920.

Kligler, B. (2003). Black cohosh. *American Family Physician, 68*(1), 114–116.

Komesaroff, P. A., Black, C. V., Cable, V., & Sudhir, K. (2001). Effects of wild yam extract on menopausal symptoms, lipids and sex hormones in healthy menopausal women. *Climacterice, 4*(2), 144–150.

Kronenberg, F., & Fugh-Berman, A. (2002). Complementary and alternative medicine for menopausal symptoms: A review of randomized, controlled trials. *Annals of Internal Medicine, 137*(10), 805–813.

Learn, C. D., & Higgins, P. G. (1999). Harmonizing herbs. Managing menopause with help from Mother Earth. *AWHONN Lifelines, 3*(5), 39–43.

LeBoeuf, F. G., & Carter, S. G. (1996). Discomforts of the perimenopause. *Journal of Obstetric, Gynecologic, and Neonatal Nursing, 25*(2), 173–180.

Lobo, R. A. (1999). *Women's Health Clinical Management, Volume 1.* Available at: http://www.medscape.com.

Low Dog, T. (2005). Menopause: A review of botanical dietary supplements. *American Journal of Medicine, 118*(12 Suppl. 2), 98–108.

Mainini, G., Festa, B., Messalli, E. M., Torella, M., & Ragucci, A. (2003). Premature ovarian failure. Clinical evaluation of 32 cases. *Minerva Ginecologica, 55*(6), 525–529.

Massin, N., Czernichow, C., Thibaud, E., Kuttenn, F., Polak, M., & Touraine, P. (2006). Idiopathic premature ovarian failure in 63 young women. *Hormone Research, 65*(2), 89–95.

McVeigh, C. (2005). Perimenopause: More than hot flushes and night sweats for some Australian women. *Journal of Obstetric, Gynecologic, and Neonatal Nursing, 34*(1), 21–27.

Mishra, G., & Kuh, D. (2006). Perceived change in quality of life during the menopause. *Social Sciences and Medicine, 62*(1), 93–102.

Mitchell, E. S., Woods, N. F., & Mariella, A. (2000). Three stages of the menopausal transition from the Seattle midlife women's health study: Toward a more precise definition. *Menopause, 7*(5), 334–349.

Mooradian, A. D., & Korenman, S. G. (2006). Management of the cardinal features of andropause. *American Journal of Therapeutics, 13*(2), 145–160.

Nachtigall, L. E. (1998). The symptoms of perimenopause. *Clinical Obstetrics and Gynecology, 41*(4), 921–927.

Orshan, S. A., Furniss, K., Forst, C., & Santoro, N. (2001). The lived experience of premature ovarian failure. *Journal of Obstetric, Gynecologic, and Neonatal Nursing, 30*(2), 202–208.

Pandian, Z., Bhattacharya, S., Vale, L., & Tempelton, A. (2005). In vitro fertilization for unexplained subfertility. *Cochrane Database of Systematic Reviews, 18*(2), CD003357.

Pepping, J. (1999). Black cohosh: Cimicifuga racemosa. *American Journal of Health-System Pharmacy, 56,* 1400–1402.

Ratka, A., Miller, V., Brown, K., Raut, A., Cipher, D., Meczekalski, B., & Simpkins, J. W. (2006). Menopausal Vasomotor Symptoms (MVS) Survey for assessment of hot flashes. *Journal of Women's Health, 15*(1), 77–89.

Reynolds, R. F., & Obermeyer, C. M. (2005). Age at natural menopause in Spain and the United States: Results from the DAMES project. *American Journal of Human Biology, 17*(3), 331–340.

Santoro, N. (2005). The menopausal transition. *American Journal of Medicine, 118*(12 Suppl. 2), 8–13.

Santoro, N. (2003). Mechanisms of premature ovarian failure. *Annals of Endocrinology, 64*(2), 87–92.

Schmidt, P. J., Haq, N., & Rubinow, D. R. (2004). A longitudinal evaluation of the relationship between reproductive status and mood in perimenopausal women. *American Journal of Psychiatry, 161*(12), 2238–2244.

Sievert, L. L., Obermeyer, C. M., & Price, K. (2006). Determinants of hot flashes and night sweats. *Annals of Human Biology, 33*(1), 4–16.

Swanton, A., & Child, T. (2005). Reproduction and ovarian ageing. *Journal of the British Menopause Society, 11*(4), 126–131.

Tan, R. S., Pu, S. J., & Culberson, J. W. (2004). Role of androgens in mild cognitive impairment and possible interventions during andropause. *Medical Hypotheses, 62*(1), 14–18.

U.S. Department of Health and Human Services. (2005). Age page: Menopause. Retrieved May 2, 2006, from http://www.niapublications.org/agepages/menopause.asp.

Vandborg, M., & Lauszus, F. F. (2006). Premature ovarian failure and pregnancy. *Archives of Gynecology and Obstetrics, 273*(6), 387–388.

van Noord, P. A. H., Dubas, J. S., Dorland, M., Boersma, H., & te Velde, E. (1997). Age at natural menopause in a population-based screening cohort: The role of menarche, fecundity, and lifestyle factors. *Fertility and Sterility, 68*(1), 95–102.

Van Voorhis, B. J. (2005). Genitourinary symptoms in the menopausal transition. *American Journal of Medicine, 118*(12 Suppl. 2), 47–53.

Vermeulen, A. (2000). Andropause. *Maturitas, 34,* 5–15.

Wang, C., Alexander, G., Berman, N., Salehian, B., Davison, T., McDonald, V., et al. (1996). Testosterone replacement therapy improves mood in hypogonadal men: A clinical research centre study. *Journal of Clinical Endocrinology and Metabolism, 81,* 3578–3583.

Whiteman, M. K., Staropoli, C. A., Langenberg, P. W., McCarter, R. J., Kjerulff, K. H., & Flaws, J. A. (2003). Smoking, body mass, and hot flashes in midlife women. *Obstetrics and Gynecology, 101*(2), 264–272.

Wild, R. A. (1998). Risk factors: Assessment and preventive measures. *Clinical Obstetrics and Gynecology, 41*(4), 966–975.

Williamson, E. M. (2005). Interactions between herbal and conventional medicines. *Expert Opinion in Drug Safety,* 4(2), 355–378.

Wise, P. M. (2006). Estrogen therapy: Does it help or hurt the adult and aging brain? Insights derived from animal models. *Neuroscience, 138*(3), 831–855.

Woad, K. J., Watkins, W. J., Prendergast, D., & Shelling, A. N. (2006). The genetic basis of premature ovarian failure. *Australia and New Zealand Journal of Obstetrics and Gynaecology, 46*(3), 242–244.

Writing Group for the Women's Health Initiative Investigators. (2002). Risks and benefits of estrogen plus progestin in healthy postmenopausal women: Principal results from the Women's Health Initiative randomized controlled trial. *JAMA, 288*(3), 321–333.

Resources

Association of Women's Health, Obstetric, and Neonatal Nursing
2000 L Street, NW
Suite 740
Washington, DC 20026
202-261-2428
www.AWHONN.org

The North American Menopause Society
P.O. Box 94527
Cleveland, OH 94527
440-442-7550
www.menopause.org

Premature Ovarian Failure Support Group
P.O. Box 23643
Alexandria, VA 22304
www.pofsupport.org

CHAPTER 24

The Older Postmenopausal Woman

Susan Scanland and Christine Bradway

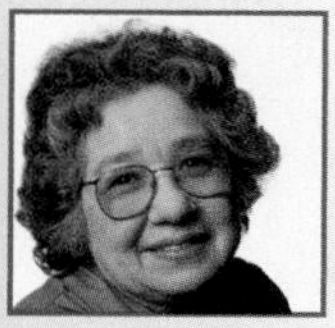

Ann, an independent and healthy 67-year-old, lives with her husband, daughter, and two grandchildren. She works part-time at the local library and is actively involved in volunteer activities. She enjoys gardening and tennis. During a routine checkup, Ann says to the nurse, "I need to discuss something. Lately, I've been having bladder problems. Sometimes when I sneeze or laugh, I leak. Once in awhile, when I'm walking home from the library, I have to rush inside to make it to the bathroom. I've been waking up at night needing to urinate. I've read a bit about this on the Internet, and I'm wondering if I have urinary incontinence."

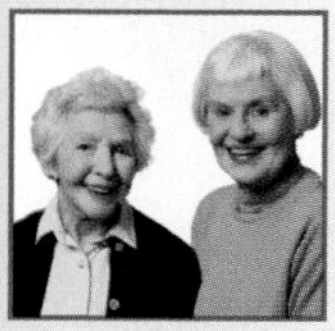

A home care nurse is working with Lena and Hannah, life partners of 25 years. Hannah, 71 years old, has dementia of the Alzheimer's type, late onset. Although Lena, 65 years old, can still care for Hannah at home, she has noticed that Hannah is becoming increasingly disengaged and forgetful. Lena is finding that most of her time is spent caring for Hannah and the house. At one point when they are alone, Lena says to the nurse, "I'd do anything for Hannah, but sometimes I feel so frustrated. The other day she tripped and fell and didn't seem to recognize me when I went to help her. I'm afraid she's going to wander from the house at night. I never thought this would happen to us."

You will learn more about these stories later in this chapter. Nurses working with such clients need to understand this chapter to manage care and address issues appropriately. Before beginning this chapter, consider the following points related to the above scenarios:

- What association might there be with these clients' problems and negative societal feelings and beliefs associated with aging? How can nurses help people understand the differences between normal aging and medical problems more common in older adults?
- Despite some clear differences, what things might the women in these scenarios have in common? What problems or circumstances are similar?
- Describe some specific strategies that the nurse can use to show sensitivity and compassion when working with these women.
- How can the nurse promote adaptation and adjustment for these clients?

LEARNING OBJECTIVES

On completion of this chapter, the reader should be able to:

- Facilitate effective communication with the older woman and her family or significant others.
- Elicit an informative health history from the older woman.
- Conduct a comprehensive assessment of the older woman, including lifestyle, medication, nutrition, function, social status, sexuality, safety and the environment, prevention and screening, sleep, and long-term health care wishes.
- Describe age-associated physiologic changes in each major body system, as well as in functional performance.
- Increase the ability to prevent, identify, and intervene in cases of inappropriate medication use and adverse drug reactions in older women.
- Identify women at high risk for common health conditions such as urinary incontinence, osteoporosis, falls, fractures, and immobility.
- Differentiate normal aging from cognitive and mental disorders such as depression, delirium, and dementia.
- Become familiar with nursing roles in home care, long-term care, and assisted living, with awareness of professional opportunities for registered and advanced practice nurses who specialize in gerontologic care.

KEY TERMS

actinic keratoses
activities of daily living (ADLs)
adverse drug reaction
ageism
agnosia
aphasia
apraxia
atypical presentation of illness
confabulation
cystocele
delirium
dyspareunia
dysphagia
dysthymia
elder mistreatment
fallaphobia
health care proxy
hyperthermia
hypothermia
isolated systolic hypertension (ISH)
myocardial ischemia
orthostatic (postural) hypotension
osteopenia
osteoporosis
pharmacodynamics
pharmacokinetics
polypharmacy
posterior vaginal wall prolapse
presbycardia
primary caregiver
primary health care provider
sleep phase advancement
syncope
xerostomia

Women are living longer than ever before. In 2002, women reaching 65 years old had an average life expectancy of an additional 19.5 years (U.S. Department of Health and Human Services [USDHHS] Administration on Aging [AoA], 2004). In 2000, women accounted for 58% of the U.S. population older than 65 years and 70% of the U.S. population older than 85 years (Federal Interagency Forum on Aging-Related Statistics, 2000). In 2003, there were 21 million older women and 14.9 million older men, or a sex ratio of 140 women for every 100 men. The female-to-male sex ratio increases with age, ranging from 115/100 for the age group 65 to 69 years old to a high of 226/100 for the age group 85 years and older (USDHHS AoA, 2004). Demographics in the 21st century will contribute to significant societal changes, with the aging population expected to double by 2050. The most rapid population growth is occurring in people older than 85 years. Between 1990 and 2000, their number increased more than 25% to more than 4 million (U.S. Census Bureau, 2000). Increasing numbers of older adults are living beyond 100 years, a group with health, emotional, and social needs previously unconsidered (Fig. 24.1).

Growth in the fields of gerontology and geriatrics has exploded, with fascinating clinical and research knowledge further promoting longevity and quality of life for older adults. Over the past 20 years, experts have chronologically defined age by numbers. For the future, experts predict that the focus will shift from describing aging in terms of predefined stages to focusing more on functional capacity and quality of life.

This chapter explores the unique needs of older postmenopausal women as they journey through the second half or last third of their lives. It focuses on functional status and its relationships to illness and common health conditions seen in older women. It describes assessment of various aspects of the older woman's lifestyle, circumstances, and environment for safety, appropriateness, and satisfaction. It analyzes common health conditions and medication use, interweaving their effects and uses in older women. Finally, the material addresses the nursing care of women across levels of function and setting, emphasizing "best practices" of gerontologic nursing care.

COMMUNICATING WITH THE OLDER WOMAN

Effective communication is essential to successful nursing care. Strong communication skills especially are important when dealing with older clients because of the multitude of factors that can affect communication adversely. For example, sensory impairments, effects of acute or chronic illness, medication effects, ageist attitudes on the part of the nurse, sociocultural factors, and a noisy or chaotic environment are all potential barriers to effective communication.

Using Interviewing Skills

Ageism is alive and well in a youth-oriented society, and health care providers may fall prey to this type of discrimination. Ageism causes negative attitudes toward and discriminatory behaviors against older adults. The term was coined by Robert Butler, MD, in 1961. Ageism includes prejudicial comments and inferior treatment from service providers, as well as discrimination through institutionalized practices and policies (American Psychological Association, 2006). For example, ageist beliefs may lead nurses to minimize a client's concerns simply because she is older, or to consider that the client is not "worth" investments of time or services. Nurses should examine their inner feelings to determine any traces of ageism.

QUOTE 24-1

"After I had fallen and broken my leg, one of the doctors was talking to me like I was a child. I was old enough to be her grandmother! It made so much of a difference when the nurses treated me with respect and like I was a normal person!"

From an 82-year-old client

Nurses are to be empathetic, genuine, objective, and nonpatronizing to clients. They should avoid using nicknames such as "honey," "doll," "sweetie," and "dear." These titles are condescending for older people who have lived full lives. Demeaning nicknames for older adults is called "elderspeak," and rates of elderspeak may be as high as 20% in long-term care settings (Jerrard, 2006). Listening is an extremely important skill, as is giving the

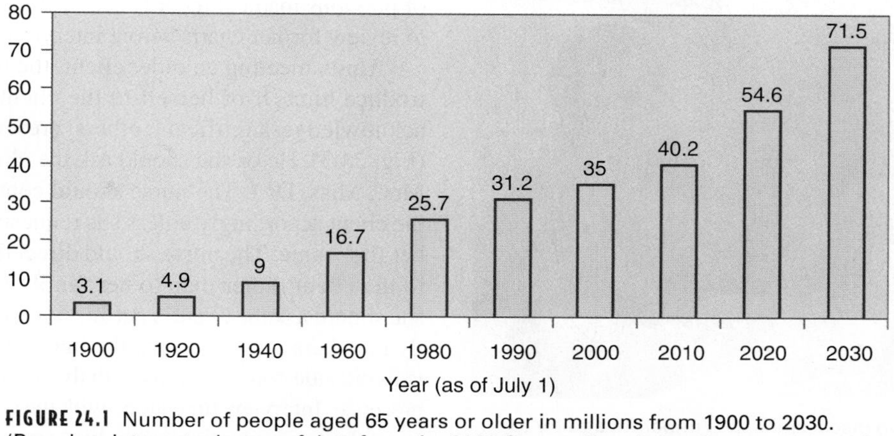

FIGURE 24.1 Number of people aged 65 years or older in millions from 1900 to 2030. (Based on Internet releases of data from the 2002 Current Population Survey of the U.S. Bureau of the Census.)

older person enough time to speak and express her concerns. Nurses also should keep interviews on target, however, to avoid going off on many tangents.

Standing taller than the interviewee may induce feelings of powerlessness and inferiority in her. For this reason, nurses should maintain eye-level contact with clients. If an older woman is in a wheelchair, the interviewer also should sit, facilitating direct eye contact (Fig. 24.2). Because hearing impairment is common in older adults, nurses should speak slowly to these clients in a normal tone of voice (Miller, 2004). They should not yell loudly because clients with hearing impairment often are sensitive to loud noises. Interviewers can purchase inexpensive amplifying devices to facilitate communication.

It is important not to interrupt or finish the client's thoughts or sentences even if she rambles. It is better to let the interviewee complete the thought. If the content is veering off-course, the nurse should acknowledge those remarks and return the interviewee to the main topic. It is effective at the interview's onset to let the client know exactly how much time is available and the specific goals of the interview. The nurse can then refer back to this information if the interview drifts off track. Using direct open-ended questions rather than inquiries that result in closed "yes" or "no" responses is important. An example of an open-ended question is, "Tell me about the pain in your hip." It is imperative that nurses assess nonverbal behaviors, which provide clues to internal emotions.

A quiet background facilitates communication. Examples of methods to enhance a quiet background include closing the door to the room, asking other people who are conversing to leave the room where the interview is being held, and shutting off the television or radio. Nurses also can augment understanding by using gestures, nonverbal language, and alternative communication techniques (eg, word board).

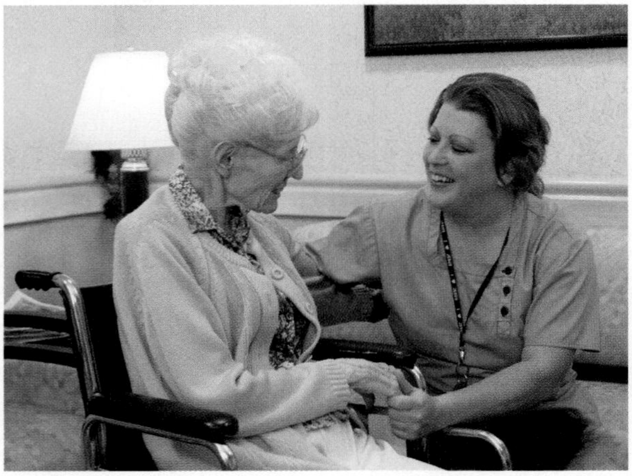

FIGURE 24.2 During discussions, it is imperative to try to maintain eye-level contact with clients, particularly those who require wheelchair assistance.

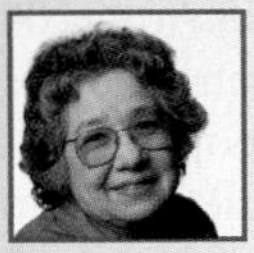

Consider Ann, the 67-year-old from the beginning of the chapter who reported having difficulty controlling her bladder. Describe how the nurse could facilitate an effective interview with Ann.

Obtaining a Health History

Taking a health history from an older person can be a challenging process. Many factors can affect the nurse's ability to obtain information. Often, older people have **atypical presentations of illness,** meaning that an illness presents without symptoms or with symptoms different from those that would occur in a young or middle-aged adult. An example is a "silent" myocardial infarction (MI), which may occur without symptoms, or present as confusion or dizziness in the older person, rather than with the classic chest pain found in a middle-aged person.

Older adults usually have at least one or more chronic, coexisting illnesses (Kane et al., 2004). Sometimes, it is difficult to sift through multiple symptoms when obtaining a history and determine what is clinically significant. The tendency in older clients is to underreport symptoms, contradicting conventional wisdom that older people overreport symptoms or suffer from excessive anxiety related to symptoms. For example, older women may "normalize" symptoms by attributing them to old age, underestimating their significance, and in turn, reducing the nurse's ability to identify and address important health issues. Some have suggested this behavior may result from denial regarding symptoms or not wanting to "bother" the health care provider.

Obtaining the history in an older person is more time consuming than with younger clients. The older adult has many years of past medical history to review. Many providers request that older clients complete an informal health status questionnaire before the office visit. Review of previous medical records is essential. It is timesaving to review former charts before interviewing a client.

Upon meeting an older client, the nurse should introduce himself or herself to the client first, and then acknowledge significant others present in the room (Fig. 24.3). He or she should ask the client her title (eg, Mrs., Miss, Dr.). The nurse should continue to address the client accordingly unless she requests to be called by her first name. The nurse should direct the conversation to the client rather than to her family members. He or she should ask the client's permission to have other family members present during the interview. It is essential to avoid side conversations with the family in the client's presence. Interview time alone with the client is important to explore confidential issues like sexuality, **elder mistreatment** (EM) (abuse, neglect, exploitation), or emo-

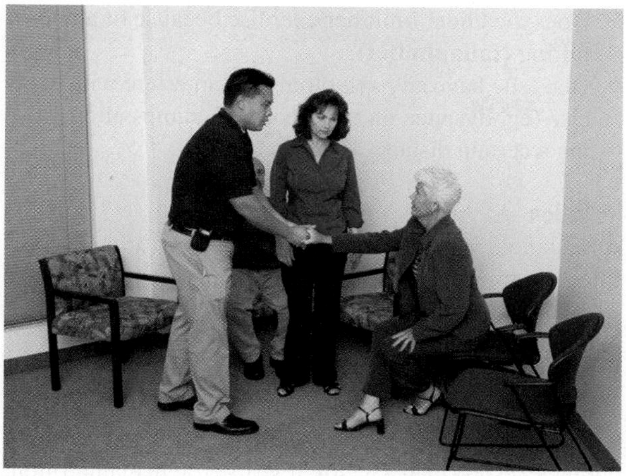

FIGURE 24.3 To convey respect and to establish a trusting and comfortable relationship, the nurse should introduce himself or herself to the client first and then acknowledge the presence of significant others who are with her.

tional concerns that the client may not want to share with the family. The nurse should ask the client her main concern, or why she is visiting today. Additionally, he or she should evaluate the family's main concern, relating it to the client's chief complaint.

The nurse should track the history of symptoms, including onset as well as changes over time. Discussing previous treatment successes and failures is important. The nurse should ask the client questions like, "What do you mean when you say that you are . . . ?" Quantifying fluctuating symptoms like pain (using a scale studied in older people; see Assessment Tool 24.3) is imperative, as is separating active and past problems and prioritizing the urgency of each current concern.

The nurse should inquire about symptoms related to common illnesses affecting elders. These include arthritis, hearing impairment, visual problems, and heart failure (HF). Usually, clients do not have just one concern but several simultaneous factors. Many complaints are the result of chronic illness, but the nurse must discern whether any complaints are caused by active or acute exacerbation of such chronic illness.

Addressing Barriers to Communication

In some situations, acute or chronic illnesses make communicating with an older adult difficult. Barriers to communication may occur if a person has experienced a stroke or a chronic neurologic illness. One example is Broca's expressive aphasia, in which the client has awkward articulation making simple phrases, even though the auditory system is preserved. Wernicke's aphasia results in fluent speech that is lacking in content. Speech apraxia can develop after a stroke or can result directly from a dementing process in the brain. Dysarthria results from inadequate control of speech caused by muscle weakness. It can develop with neuromuscular diseases or a stroke. It also can occur from muscle paralysis and lack of muscle coordination. Other speech barriers may be seen with Parkinson's disease, in which destruction of the basal ganglia affects speech, sometimes rendering speech completely inaudible. Neuronal degeneration of the frontal lobes also may affect speech quality. As a person progresses with dementia, the ability to understand abstractions becomes more impaired; it is more difficult for her to express herself through words. The person's vocabulary narrows, and she has difficulties choosing words. Other barriers to communication include overt laryngectomy and endotracheal intubation.

The nurse can address communication barriers by being sensitive to them and by addressing them with individualized interventions. Selected examples of nursing interventions to enhance communication are included in Box 24.1.

COMPREHENSIVE ASSESSMENT FOR THE OLDER WOMAN

This section addresses a comprehensive assessment of the older woman in several domains. Areas covered include lifestyle and habits, nutrition, medications, function, social issues, sexuality, safety and the environment, prevention and screening, sleep, and long-term health care wishes.

BOX 24.1 Interventions to Enhance Communication With Older Adults

- Take the time to introduce yourself to the client.
- Verbally exchange names and ask the woman what name she prefers to be called (eg, Ms. Dr., Mrs.) Use proper names, unless directed otherwise.
- Use a handshake, or touch when introduced. Be sensitive to cultural or gender differences that may indicate discomfort with the use of touch.
- Listen to what the older adult says.
- If at all possible, talk to the woman in a face-to-face position because this enhances verbal and nonverbal communication.
- As much as possible, remove physical barriers (eg, walker, bedside table) that compromise field of vision.
- Modify the environment to facilitate communication:
  - Provide a quiet setting
  - Eliminate competing noises (eg, turn off TV, radio)
  - Assure privacy
  - Optimize lighting by minimizing glare
- Introduce formal screening (eg, depression or cognitive testing) in a matter-of-fact manner. Explain the purpose and ask the client's permission to proceed.

From Miller, C. A. (2004). *Nursing for wellness in older adults. Theory and practice* (4th ed.). Philadelphia: Lippincott Williams & Wilkins.

Lifestyle

When considering the older woman's lifestyle, the nurse should assess health habits, particularly in the areas of smoking, alcohol use, and exercise.

Smoking and Tobacco Use

To conduct assessment of smoking and tobacco use, the nurse should ask the client the following questions:

- Does the woman smoke cigarettes or cigars?
- How many years has she smoked?
- What is the number of packs she has smoked over these years (to give a "pack/year" ratio)?
- Has the client ever attempted to stop smoking?
  - Has she used any nicotine products or Zyban (Wellbutrin) for smoking cessation?
  - Has she ever quit suddenly ("cold turkey")?
  - How long was she successful in nicotine abstinence?
  - What psychosocial, behavioral, or physical factors caused her to start smoking again?
- What is her rationale for continuing to smoke?
- Are other smokers in the household?
- Do her friends smoke?
- Does she frequent areas with multiple smokers?

Alcohol Use

Alcoholism is often a silent syndrome in older women. Typically, these clients underestimate or give false low reports of alcohol intake. Asking about alcohol intake is important: the amount and type of alcohol consumed daily, weekly, or monthly. Potentially harmful alcohol intake for women older than 65 years is considered more than one drink per day (Schmidt Luggen, 2006). Use of a screening instrument, such as the Ewing's (1984) CAGE mnemonic (see Chap. 2, Assessment Tool 2-2), can be extremely helpful as a first step in identifying and documenting alcohol abuse and dependence in older adults (Beullens & Aertgeerts, 2004). The Michigan Alcoholism Screening Test provides a variation of this tool specially targeted for older adults (Naegle, 2003; Schmidt Luggen, 2006) (Assessment Tool 24.1). In addition, questions about falls, dizziness, weight gain, and motor vehicle crashes can be subtle clues to alcohol misuse. Clinical Guidelines for alcohol disorders in older adults are available from the American Geriatrics Society (2003; www.americangeriatrics.org).

Exercise

It is important to find out what factors contribute to adherence or decreased participation in exercise for older women (Fig. 24.4). Questions to ask include the following:

- What are the woman's exercise patterns?
- What long-term exercise programs have been successful?
- Have there been any falls, accidents, or fractures related to exercise?
- Does the client limit her exercise because of a fear of falling (**fallaphobia**)?
- Does she have any symptoms that interfere with exercise (eg, dyspnea on exertion, calf cramps after walking a certain distance)?

Nutrition

Assessment of the older woman's nutrition is vital. The nurse should take a nutritional history by using the 24-hour food recall, asking the client, "What did you eat in the past 24 hours?" (see Chap. 3).

In addition to asking about a 24-hour food recall, the nurse also should check recent laboratory results to identify the older woman's serum albumin level. A serum albumin level less than 3.8 g/dL reveals protein malnutrition. Older adults with hypoalbuminemia have increased health care use and a higher mortality rate. Hospitalized elders with protein malnutrition have a longer length of stay, more complications, readmissions, and higher mortality (Jensen & Powers, 2002).

The prevention of **osteoporosis** should begin in a woman's younger years because maximal bone mass is achieved in the mid-30s (see Chap. 2). Determining the older woman's dietary calcium intake is crucial. In addition to calcium supplementation, the nurse should encourage women to eat foods high in calcium, including milk, cheese, yogurt, broccoli and other dark green vegetables, canned salmon or sardines, ice cream, and custard. Women who are lactose intolerant or cannot meet daily requirements for dietary calcium should be encouraged to use supplemental calcium or to shop for calcium-fortified foods (eg, orange juice, cereal, breads, waffles).

Dietary supplementation with elemental calcium (1200 mg/day) and vitamin D (800 IU/day) increases spine bone mineral density and reduces the risk for hip fractures and other nonvertebral fractures in older women (Rosen, 2005). The nurse also should assess the woman's dietary fiber content because many older adults become more sedentary and drink fewer fluids with aging, increasing the probability of constipation. If a client is taking medications with anticholinergic side effects, the likelihood of constipation increases dramatically. The nurse should assess the intake of high-fiber foods, such as cereals, whole grain breads, and fresh fruits and vegetables. He or she also should question the client's daily fluid intake. Most older women need to drink eight glasses of water per day. Many older people take in much less fluid because of declining age-related thirst mechanism. Immobility, with decreased ability to reach water sources, is often a cause of dehydration and constipation in older adults.

Other dietary areas the nurse should evaluate are caffeine intake and weight patterns, paying special attention to increases or decreases of more then 10 pounds in the past 5 years. Has there been a sudden weight loss? This could alert the provider to the possibility of a thyroid dis-

ASSESSMENT TOOL 24.1 Michigan Alcohol Screening Test

Please check "yes" or "no" for each question.

Question	Yes	No
1. Do you feel you are a normal drinker? ("normal"—drink as much or less than most other people)		
2. Have you ever awakened the morning after some drinking the night before and found that you could not remember a part of the evening?		
3. Does any near relative or close friend ever worry or complain about your drinking?		
4. Can you stop drinking without difficulty after one or two drinks?		
5. Do you ever feel guilty about your drinking?		
6. Have you ever attended a meeting of Alcoholics Anonymous (AA)?		
7. Have you ever gotten into physical fights when drinking?		
8. Has drinking ever created problems between you and a near relative or close friend?		
9. Has any family member or close friend gone to anyone for help about your drinking?		
10. Have you ever lost friends because of your drinking?		
11. Have you ever gotten into trouble at work because of drinking?		
12. Have you ever lost a job because of drinking?		
13. Have you ever neglected your obligations, your family, or your work for 2 days or more in a row because you were drinking?		
14. Do you drink before noon fairly often?		
15. Have you ever been told you have liver trouble such as cirrhosis?		
16. After heavy drinking, have you ever had delirium tremens (D.T.'s), severe shaking, visual or auditory (hearing) hallucinations?		
17. Have you ever gone to anyone for help about your drinking?		
18. Have you ever been hospitalized because of drinking?		
19. Has your drinking ever resulted in your being hospitalized in a psychiatric ward?		
20. Have you ever gone to any doctor, social worker, clergy, or mental health clinic for help with any emotional problem in which drinking was part of the problem?		
21. Have you been arrested more than once for driving under the influence of alcohol?		
22. Have you ever been arrested, even for a few hours, because of other behavior while drinking? (If *yes,* how many times?)		

SCORING

Give yourself one point for the following:

1.	No
2.	Yes
3.	Yes
4.	No
5.	Yes
6.	Yes
7. to **22.**	Yes

TOTALS

0 to 2:	No apparent problem
3 to 5:	Early or middle problem drinker
6 or more:	Problem drinker

order, depression, or cancer. What was the older woman's maximal height as an adult? This information is important to know in determining risk for osteoporosis. Older women may decrease several inches in height because of osteoporotic vertebral compression fractures. Does the person eat alone? Who prepares her meals? Who shops for groceries and how often? Can the older woman afford nutritional food? All these factors are an important part of the nutritional assessment.

Medications

Performing a thorough medication history when interviewing an older client is essential. People of all ages may be nonadherent with medication regimens for a wide

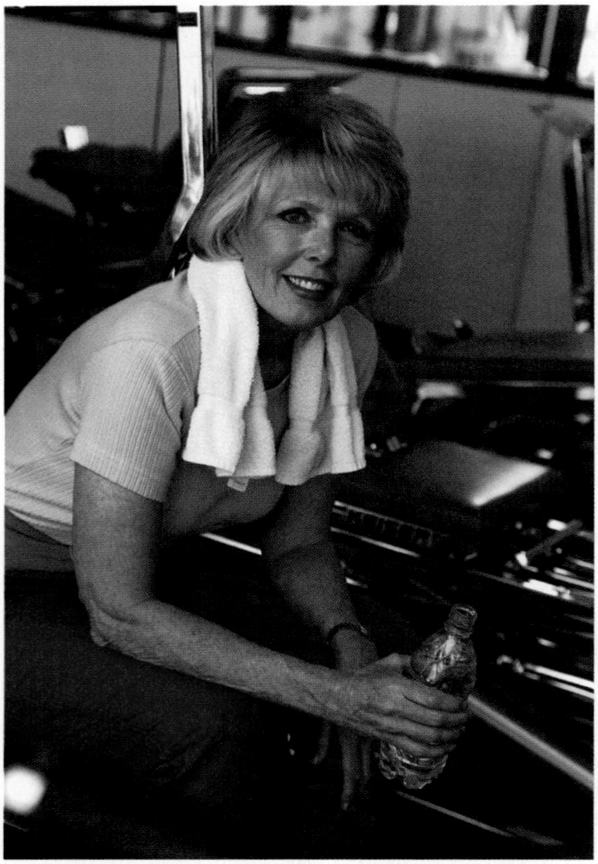

FIGURE 24.4 Exercise in older women can help maintain functional status, as well as contribute to overall health and well-being.

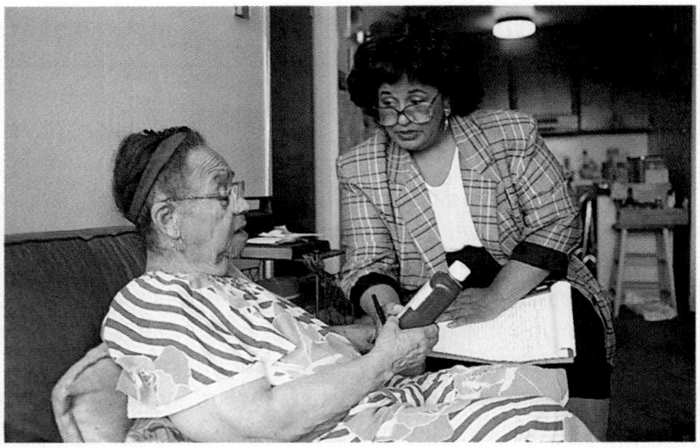

FIGURE 24.5 Adherence to medication regimens depends on several factors, including the client's cognitive capacity and family dynamics. (Photo © Kathy Sloane.)

variety of reasons (Fig. 24.5). A good way to elicit information about medication use is to ask questions nonjudgmentally and to give the older woman ample opportunities to discuss her understanding of over-the-counter and prescription medications. For example, the nurse could ask questions such as "What medications are you currently taking?," "How many times/days in the last week did you take (or forget to take) your pills?," "How do you think your medications are working for you?," and "Do you use any herbal, over-the-counter, or recreational drugs on a regular or occasional basis?"

The nurse should document the location and telephone number of the client's pharmacy and ask whether the pharmacy makes deliveries. Does the client use any other pharmacies? Does she have a prescription plan or participate in a specialized program for decreased medication payments based on income? Does the woman mail-order any medications from other countries or the Internet? Would any visual problems interfere with reading medication labels?

The nurse should review the client's history for any past experiences with, or current symptoms of, clinical depression. Depression may minimize the motivation necessary to follow a medication regimen. Additionally, the nurse should consider whether any confusion is present because dementia is a common cause of errors in self-administration of medication. The nurse should ask the older woman if she saves and reuses old prescriptions. Does she share medications with friends? How does she store and administer medications? Does she use a special medication container with the times of the day and days of the week? Does she have any history of allergic reactions to drugs (eg, documented rash, hives, anaphylaxis)? In an older woman, asking about the history of **adverse drug reactions** (ADRs) is equally important. ADRs are not allergic reactions; rather, they are defined as "unintended outcomes of a medication that occur because of the medication's chemical components" (Miller, 2004, p. 515). For example, an older woman may experience urinary incontinence (UI) as an adverse effect of a diuretic prescribed for the treatment of hypertension. Although ADRs are not unique to older adults, risk increases with age, primarily as a result of polypharmacy.

Ideally, the nurse should take the client's medication history through the "brown-bag" approach. In this scenario, the office receptionist, upon booking the appointment, asks the client to bring to the visit all her medications, including over-the-counter drugs, ointments, eye drops, herbs, and vitamins. In the home setting, the nurse can duplicate the brown-bag approach by assessing the client's medication cabinet with her permission. The nurse also inquires what medications other providers have prescribed. Is the **primary health care provider** coordinating medications prescribed by other specialists? The nurse specifically should ask the older woman about her use of eye drops, ointments, creams, and herbal drinks, foods, and supplements. Herbal preparations may interact with the multiple medications that many older adults consume. It is important to specifically ask about laxatives because some older clients forget to include them as medications.

The nurse also should evaluate storage issues. Keeping medications safe from grandchildren and others during child care or elder care responsibilities is essential to prevent accidental poisoning or overdosage.

Function

Functional assessment is an essential piece of a comprehensive geriatric assessment. In hospitalized elderly, functional status is a strong predictor of 90-day and 2-year mortality after discharge (Inouye et al., 1998). The ability of an older woman to function may affect her living arrangements, relationship with others, quality of life, and overall health. It is important for the nurse to assess and document baseline functional level when the older woman is well. Health care professionals can then use these findings for comparison if illnesses, ADRs, delirium, dementia, or depression change the client's level of function. They also can use the information gathered to communicate with one another about what constitutes baseline for the client on a daily basis. The main reason to assess function is to determine whether the older woman's living arrangements and social support match her functional needs. Knowing the woman's activity level has major implications for both her safety and quality of life.

Activities of Daily Living

Activities of daily living (ADLs) are those functions necessary for independent living. *Basic ADLs (BADLs)* include basic self-care tasks such as bathing, dressing, toileting, maintaining continence, feeding, and transferring. *Instrumental ADLs (IADLs)* are those activities that further enhance the client's ability to live independently. Examples include shopping for groceries; driving or using public transportation; using the telephone; preparing meals; doing housework, repair work, and laundry; taking medications, and handling finances. *Advanced ADLs (AADLs)* refer to the client's ability to fulfill societal, community, and family roles as well as participate in recreational or occupational tasks (Reuben, 2000) (Fig. 24.6).

When reviewing ADLs, the nurse should ask, "How do you . . . ?" for each component. Older adults needing assistance with BADLs usually require live-in assistance from family members or health care personnel or placement in long-term care facilities such as nursing homes. Elders with deficits in IADLs may live at home by themselves but are dependent on others to assist in completion of these tasks. Assisted-living facilities (ALFs) are rapidly growing in number to meet IADL and ADL needs of elders who do not require skilled or total nursing care. A woman's ability to complete AADLs depends on her ability to complete IADLs.

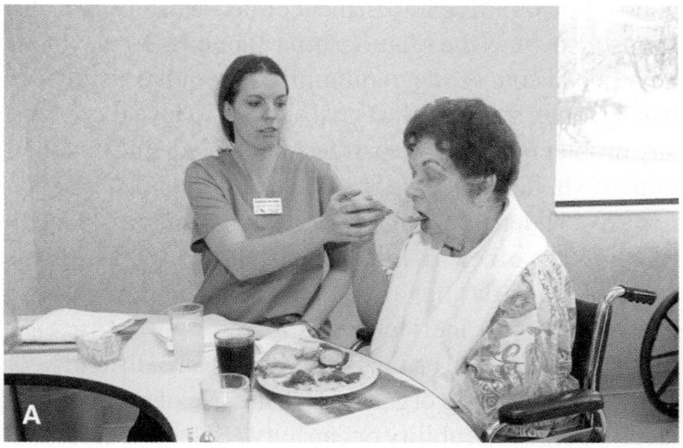
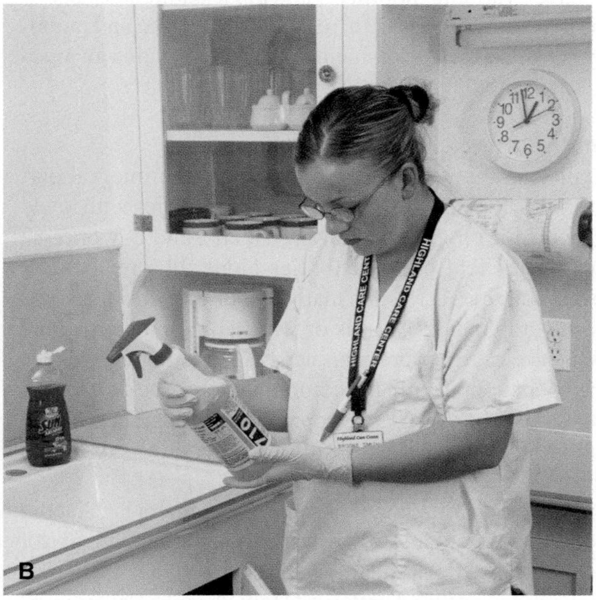
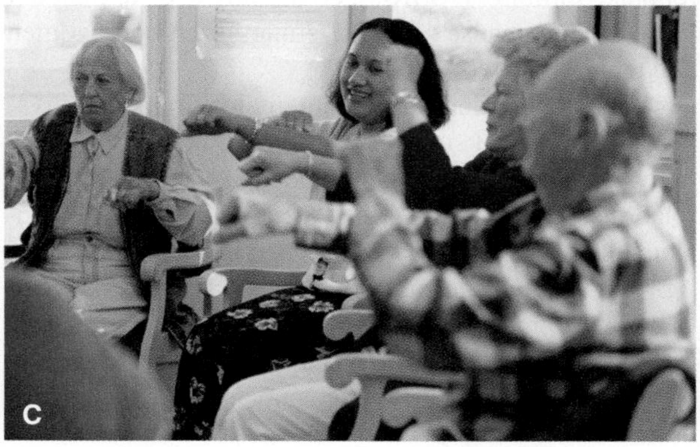

FIGURE 24.6 (**A**) Nurses may assist clients with such BADLs as feeding. (**B**) An example of assisting with IADLs may involve doing housework. (**C**) Nurses may help clients with AADLs through facilitating attendance at recreational or occupational tasks.

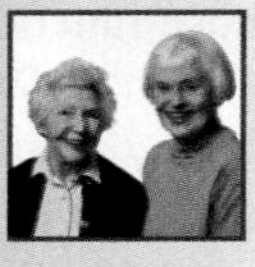

Recall Lena and Hannah, who were described at the beginning of the chapter. How would the nurse expect Lena's ability to complete ADLs to compare with that of Hannah?

Mobility

Performance-based testing of functional status should focus primarily on transfers, gait, and balance. The nurse should ask the client to stand from the seated position in a hard-backed chair while keeping her arms folded. Inability to complete this task suggests weakness of the lower extremities or quadriceps and is highly predictive of future disability. Once the client is standing, the nurse should observe her walking back and forth over a short distance, ideally with any usual walking aid. Abnormalities of gait include path deviation; diminished step height, length, or both; trips, slips, or near falls; and difficulty turning. The tasks of rising from the chair, walking 10 feet (3 meters), turning around and returning to the chair, turning, and then sitting back down in the chair (without using arms) make up the "Get Up and Go" test (Mathias et al., 1986; Podsiadlo & Richardson, 1991). People who take longer than 10 seconds to complete this sequence of maneuvers are at increased risk for falls (Gill, 2002). Those taking 10 to 19 seconds are considered "fairly mobile"; those taking 20 to 29 seconds are considered to have "variable mobility"; and those taking 30 seconds or more are considered "dependent" in balance and mobility (Gill, 2002). Assessment Tool 24.2 contains an algorithm to predict a client's risk for falls.

Social Aspects

Exploring the woman's relationships is an integral part of social assessment. How are her relationships with loved ones, children, grandchildren, friends, and coworkers? Does the client prefer activities alone, like reading, or group activities offered in many Senior Citizens' Centers? Is she employed? What is or was her main occupation? What are/were her previous activities and hobbies? Does the client volunteer in the community or serve on boards? Does she have child care responsibilities for grandchildren or caregiving responsibilities for other adults or elders (Fig. 24.7)?

Another component of social assessment is what the woman does on a 24-hour basis. Does she travel? If so, what distance does she travel? Is this a change from previous social or travel patterns? How does she get around? Can she make and reach appointments? What does she do for recreation and socialization? Changes in usual social activity patterns can indicate a subtle or acute change in physical or mental health.

The social assessment includes asking the older person whom she can depend on if she needs assistance or in an emergency. Women with functional impairment need regular, dependable assistance with IADLs and AADLs.

Research has shown a relationship between spiritual faith and level of health (Armer & Conn, 2001; Crowther et al., 2002). Therefore, it is important to assess the client's spirituality. Is the client active in an organized religion? Does she worship and participate in forgiveness and prayer? If not involved in organized religion, does she meditate or have a relationship with any type of Supreme Being? What are her views on life and death, and how are these related or unrelated to her spirituality?

QUOTE 24-2

"One of the hardest things about getting older and retiring has been the sense that I am removed from day-to-day activities. Sometimes, it just seems easier to stay at home and hope people will come to me, rather than pushing myself to get out there!"

An older woman talking about the challenges in staying active since she's retired

Sexuality

When assessing the sexuality and sexual needs of the older woman, the nurse may begin by asking the client if she is having any difficulty in this area that she would like to discuss. The nurse should ask whether the woman is currently in an intimate relationship with a person of the opposite or same sex (Fig. 24.8). Is there difficulty with intercourse as a result of any physical disability? Does the couple have a close relationship without intercourse? If cognitive impairment or depression exists in a spouse, how has the relationship changed? Do they need any special counseling to minimize or remove health care barriers interfering with sexual activity? Have there been any problems with male partners having erectile dysfunction? If so, has the male used any erectile aids, medications (eg, sildenafil [Viagra], vardenafil [Levitra], tadalafil [Cialis]), or other treatments? What has worked? It is important for the nurse to know what measures have been effective or ineffective.

Has the client or her partner had any difficulty or problems achieving orgasm? Has the use of medications affected orgasmic ability or capacity? Selective serotonin reuptake inhibitors (SSRIs), commonly used to treat depression, may cause sexual dysfunction in both women and men.

Is the client undergoing any major financial, physical, or emotional stressors? Is there a history of abuse in the relationship? If a person is not in a monogamous relationship for a long period, does she ever have unprotected intercourse? Does she engage in high-risk behaviors or have multiple partners? Is there a history of blood transfusion in the 1980s? Is there a history of sexually transmitted infections (STIs)? Has the woman ever been diagnosed with hepatitis, which may increase the risk for other STIs?

● ASSESSMENT TOOL 24.2 Algorithm for Fall Prevention in Older Adults

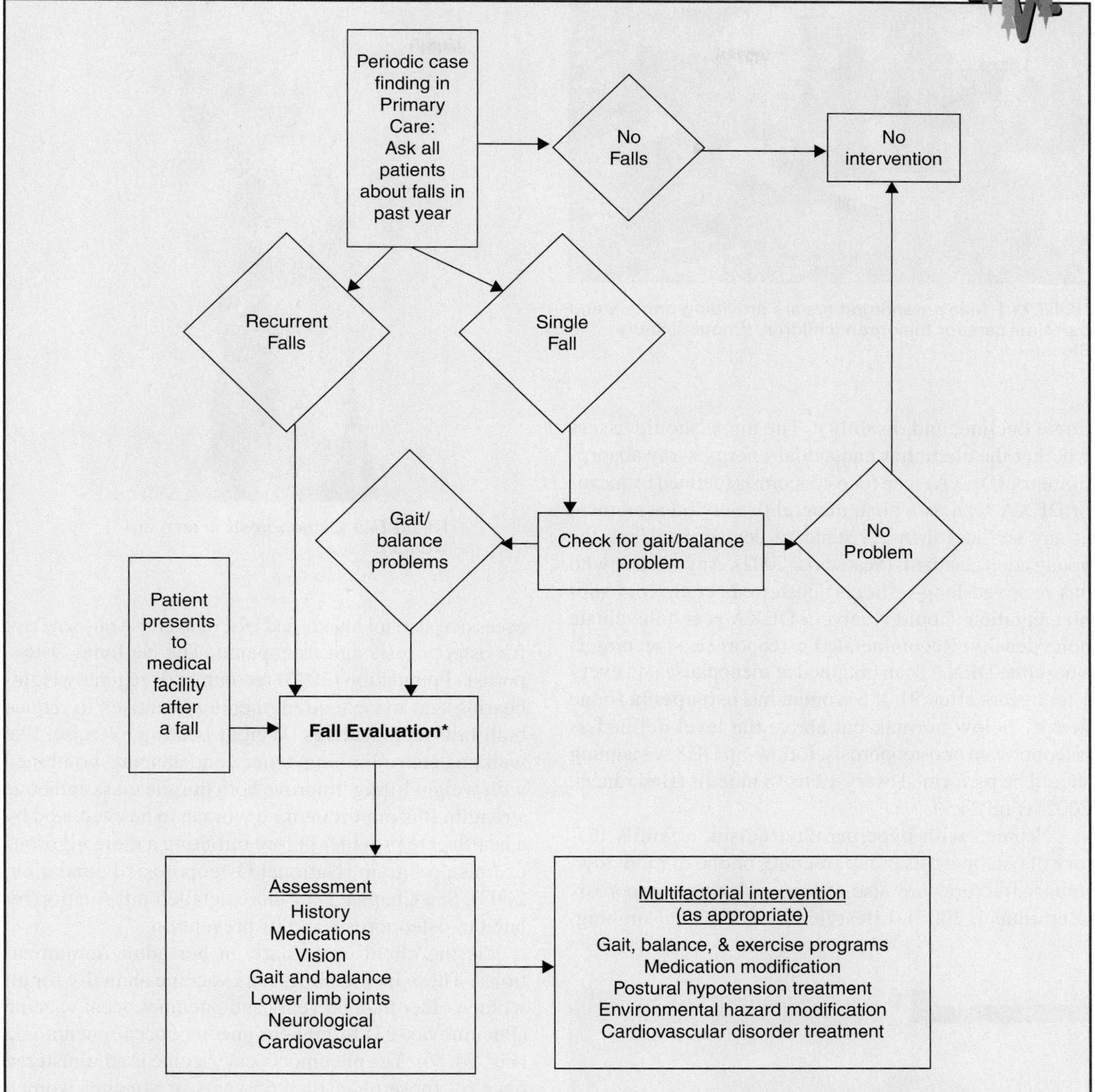

From American Geriatric Society, British Geriatrics Society, American Academy of Orthopaedic Surgeons. (2001). Guideline for the prevention of falls in older persons. *J Am Geriatr Soc, 49*(5), 664–672.

If the woman is a lesbian, has she had any problems in her relationship with her partner? Does her sexual orientation influence any health problems, relationship changes, or barriers to obtaining health care benefits and geriatric services? It is important for the nurse to understand additional factors that may create stress in a relationship. Significant changes and stress may occur if both women also have primary care giving responsibilities for aging parents or siblings. According to Cantor, Brennan, and Shippy (2004), 46% of lesbian, gay, bisexual, and transgender adults older than 50 years were currently providing or had provided caregiving for family members in the past 5 years, with 84% of the care recipients being parents.

Prevention and Screening

The nurse needs to motivate the postmenopausal woman to take an active role in preventing future illness, func-

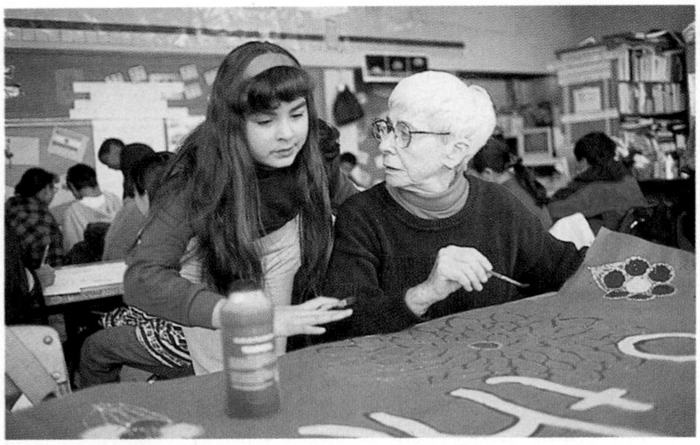

FIGURE 24.7 Many grandmothers are providing primary and part-time care for their grandchildren. (Photo © Kathy Sloane.)

tional decline, and disability. The nurse should assess whether the client has had a dual-energy x-ray absorptiometry (DEXA) scan for osteoporosis (defined by means of DEXA scan as a bone mineral density measurement at any site less then 2.5 standard deviations below the young adult standard; Prestwood, 2002). Any woman who has received long-term corticosteroids or thyroid supplementation should receive a DEXA scan to evaluate bone density. Recommended osteoporosis screening is a baseline DEXA scan obtained at menopause and every 1 to 2 years after 50. If a woman has **osteopenia** (bone density below normal, but above the level defined as osteoporosis) or osteoporosis, follow-up DEXA scanning should be performed every 12 to 18 months (Berarducci, 2002) (Fig. 24.9).

Women with hyperparathyroidism, a family history of osteoporosis or hip fracture, or one or more low-impact fractures are also at high risk for osteoporosis (Berarducci, 2002). Lifestyle issues such as smoking, excessive alcohol intake, and lack of exercise raise the risk for osteoporosis and osteopenia. The National Osteoporosis Foundation (2003) recommends regular weight-bearing and muscle-strengthening exercises to reduce both falls and fractures. Weight-bearing exercise, like walking, stair-climbing, tennis, and dancing, combined with weight lifting, improve both muscle mass and bone strength. It is important for a woman to be evaluated by a health care provider before initiating a more vigorous exercise program (National Osteoporosis Foundation, 2003). See Chapter 2 for more detailed information related to osteoporosis and its prevention.

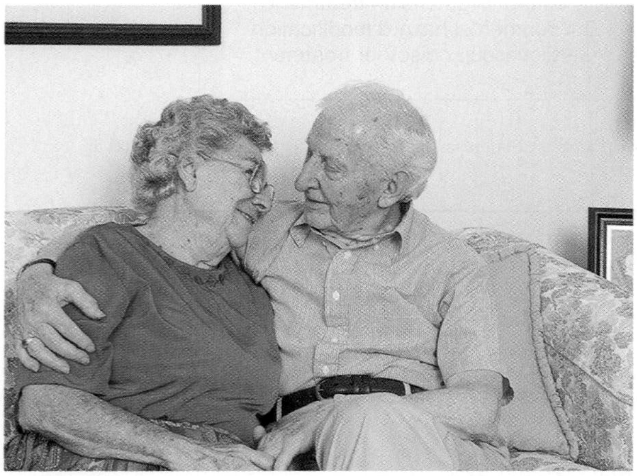

FIGURE 24.8 Sexual and romantic relationships continue into older adulthood; nurses need to assess the older woman's satisfaction with the quality of her sexual life.

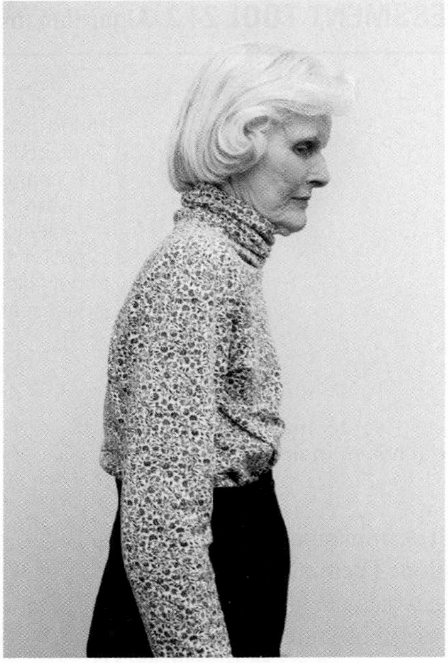

FIGURE 24.9 Osteoporosis in an older woman.

Is the client up to date on her adult immunizations? These include influenza vaccine annually for all women older than 65 years and pneumococcal vaccine (Pneumovax-23) to prevent pneumococcal pneumonia (Fig. 24.10). The pneumococcal vaccine is administered once for those older than 65 years or younger women with chronic illness. Revaccination is recommended every 7 to 10 years in high-risk clients (eg, women with a history of chronic obstructive lung disease [COPD]) (Bloom & Edelberg, 2002). The woman needs to receive a diphtheria-tetanus booster every 10 years. It is important to continue all immunizations as long as the person has some functional ability or if she would likely be treated for the illness that the immunization would prevent.

The nurse should determine whether the client is up to date with all cancer screening tests appropriate for age, functional status, and life expectancy. Incidence of cancer increases with age. Screenings recommended for older women include colonoscopy, fecal occult blood test-

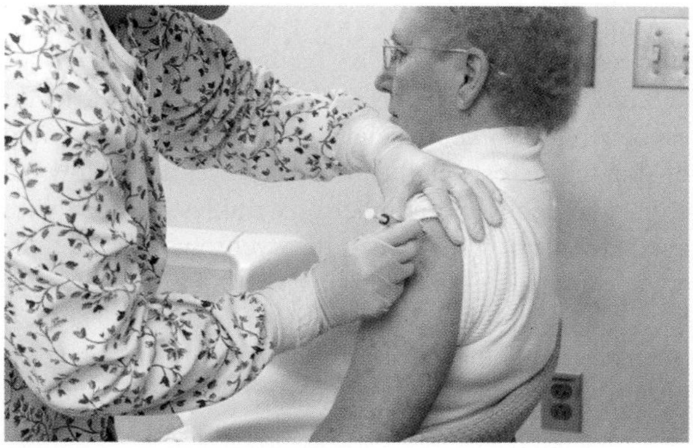

FIGURE 24.10 Regular immunizations for older clients are an essential health maintenance practice.

ing, rectal examination, mammogram, Pap test, and pelvic examination. There are exceptions to age-based routine screening, which include older women with a short life expectancy or whose multiple health problems or dementia would cause them to find screening burdensome. Screening needs to be individualized for each older woman, rather than simply age based (Goldstein et al., 2003).

Sleep

Sleep disorders are common in older women; thus, an accurate sleep history is vital. Does the client have difficulty falling or staying asleep? Symptoms to assess for include nocturia, pain, and shortness of breath. Does the spouse or significant other report any loud snoring, as with sleep apnea? Does the partner observe any periods when it seems that the client stops breathing or has coarse inspiratory noises? Does the client have early morning awakening and difficulty falling back to sleep? Clinical depression often presents with early morning awakening several hours before usual waking time. Anxiety may make it difficult to fall asleep because the person may ruminate over worries rather than relaxing. Dementia may cause reversal of the sleep–wake cycle. **Sleep phase advancement** occurs frequently in older adults, meaning that they go to bed and rise earlier than when they were younger.

Is the client spending more time than usual awake in bed? This is a common consequence of age-associated sleep changes. Does she take any medication to induce sleep? If so, is the medication a benzodiazepine or a newer nonbenzodiazepine sleep agent? How long has she been taking the drug? What is the dosage? How often does she use this? Has she noticed any daytime drowsiness that interferes with driving or operating other machinery? Has daytime fatigue contributed to any accidents or falls?

The nurse should inquire about sleep hygiene patterns. Does the client go to sleep and awaken the same time each day? Does she avoid activities such as television before going to bed? Does she avoid drinking large amounts of fluid, having caffeine, or exercising close to bedtime? How many episodes of nocturia does the person have each night? Can she return to sleep after voiding? Does she suffer from panic attacks during the night? Are any nightmares related to a traumatic event, such as sudden death of a spouse or child? Upon wakening during the night, does the client remain in bed or get out of bed for a diversional relaxing activity? Does she get any exercise during the day and sunlight exposure to improve the quality of her sleep? The Pittsburgh Sleep Quality Index is a useful instrument by which nurses can assess sleep disorders in their clients (Buysse et al., 1989). See Research Highlight 24.1 as well.

● RESEARCH HIGHLIGHT 24.1 The Use of Music to Promote Sleep in Older Women

Johnson, J. E. (2003). *Journal of Community Health Nursing, 20*(1), 27–35.

BACKGROUND: Several studies have shown that older adults, especially women, experience sleep-related difficulties. The most frequent complaint involves failure to initiate or maintain restful sleep. Various interventions to assist older women with this problem are available, including use of medications.

PURPOSE: The purpose of this study was to determine the effectiveness of music in assisting women to improve their sleep.

DESIGN: The study involved 52 women 70 years or older who had mentioned to their health care provider sleep problems at least 3 times per week for 6 months or more. The women in the study lived in their own homes and had not used any medications to enhance sleep within the 3 months of the study. Each woman chose music according to her taste, with data collected 10 nights before the use of music therapy, and then for 10 nights after the initiation of music therapy. The women kept a sleep log and were asked to rate their levels of sleep versus alertness on a scale from 1 (feeling alert) to 7 (struggling to stay awake).

RESULTS: Music therapy was successful in increasing sleepiness at bedtime, decreasing the time it took for participants to fall asleep, and decreasing the number of night awakenings.

NURSING IMPLICATIONS: Nurses should be aware that nonpharmacologic methods are available and can be successful for women struggling with sleep problems. This consideration may be especially important for older women already taking many medications.

Long-Term Health Care Wishes

The nurse needs to assess the woman's long-term wishes for health care. Has the client defined a Do Not Resuscitate order if she does not want to have cardiopulmonary resuscitation or aggressive life extension measures? Who is the power of attorney for health care? The power of attorney for health care should be determined when a person is competent. It is much more difficult for the family if this decision is not made. Is there a will for the woman's estate? Does she have an elder care attorney? Is the woman knowledgeable of estate planning to protect and maximize her assets for her heirs? County departments of aging often can obtain elder legal services for women who cannot afford to hire attorneys for elder care issues.

AGE-ASSOCIATED PHYSIOLOGIC CHANGES IN OLDER WOMEN

Physical aging is a universal phenomenon among living things. Every person has unique physiologic changes and a general health status based on multiple variables (Fig. 24.11). Such factors include genetics, family history, and lifestyle behaviors affecting health. Emotional, functional, and financial variables interplay in health outcomes, morbidity, and mortality. Patterns of physiologic changes in elders have been described over the past 20 years; however, it is important for the nurse to consider these in the context of the individual client. Aging does affect all body systems.

General Appearance

The recent popularity of cosmetic surgery, injections, and procedures has made age estimation more difficult, especially in women. Facial aging consists of loosening of skin turgor, especially around the eyes and below the chin. The depth and number of wrinkles increase with age, as do furrows between the eyebrows. Facial lines are accentuated with increasing years. Facial hair, eyebrows, and hair become more coarse and gray. The skin often has sun-damaged areas of darker pigmentation, and **actinic keratoses** (waxy-appearing nodules of various sizes). Tiny circular cherry angiomas are seen occasionally on the face and abdomen (Fig. 24.12).

Fair skinned, blue-eyed individuals are at highest risk for basal cell carcinoma; however, older women of all backgrounds are prone because this is the most common type of skin cancer. Basal cell carcinoma commonly presents on sun-exposed areas such as the face, ears, and neck. Basal cell carcinoma is circular, beginning as a small nodule with a central indentation. It gradually increases in size, with the circular (donut-shaped) border becoming more raised, having a translucent appearance. Squamous cell carcinoma and malignant melanoma also may occur in older adults (Fig. 24.13).

Gait Changes

General movement slows with advancing years, although there is considerable variance among older adults, depending on health status, level of activity, and amount of exercise. Gait speed declines. The center of gravity often

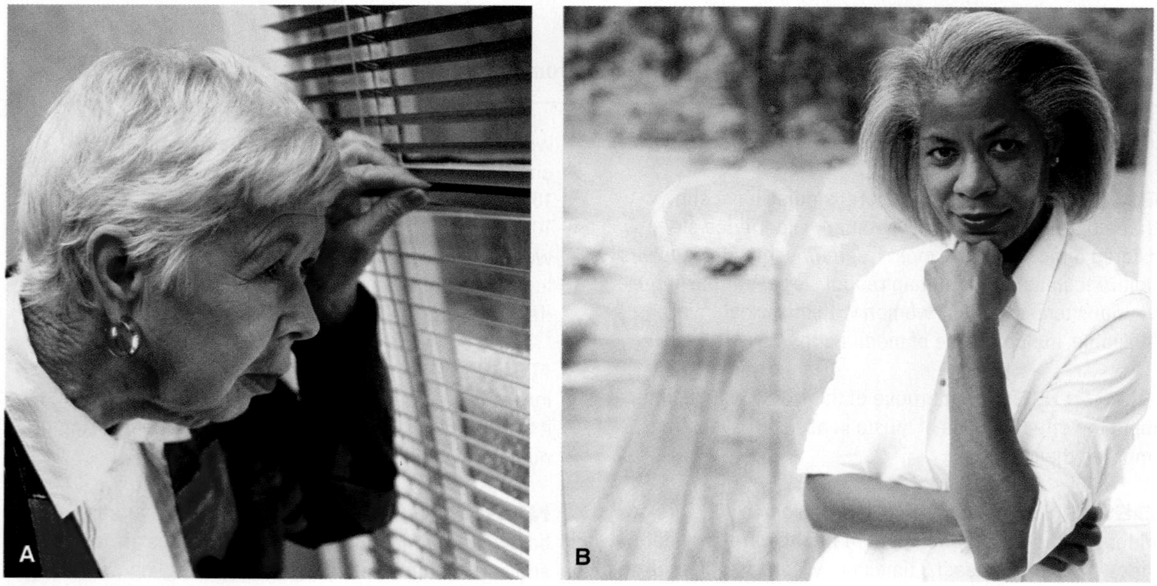

FIGURE 24.11 Both these women are 73 years old. The effects of aging vary based on many parameters, including genetics, ethnicity, general health, nutrition, stress, and other circumstances.

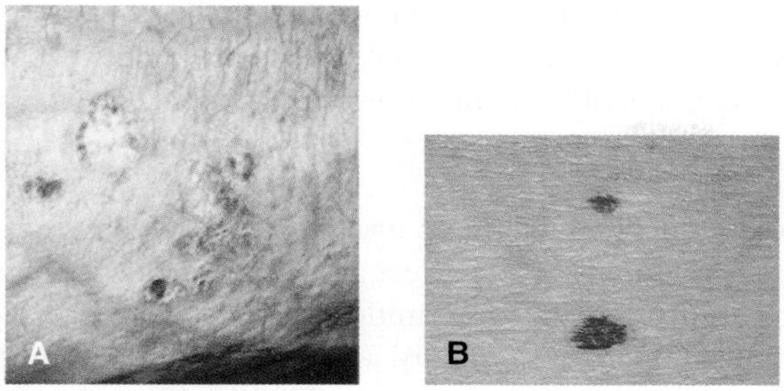

FIGURE 24.12 Skin changes in aging include (**A**) actinic keratoses and (**B**) cherry angiomas.

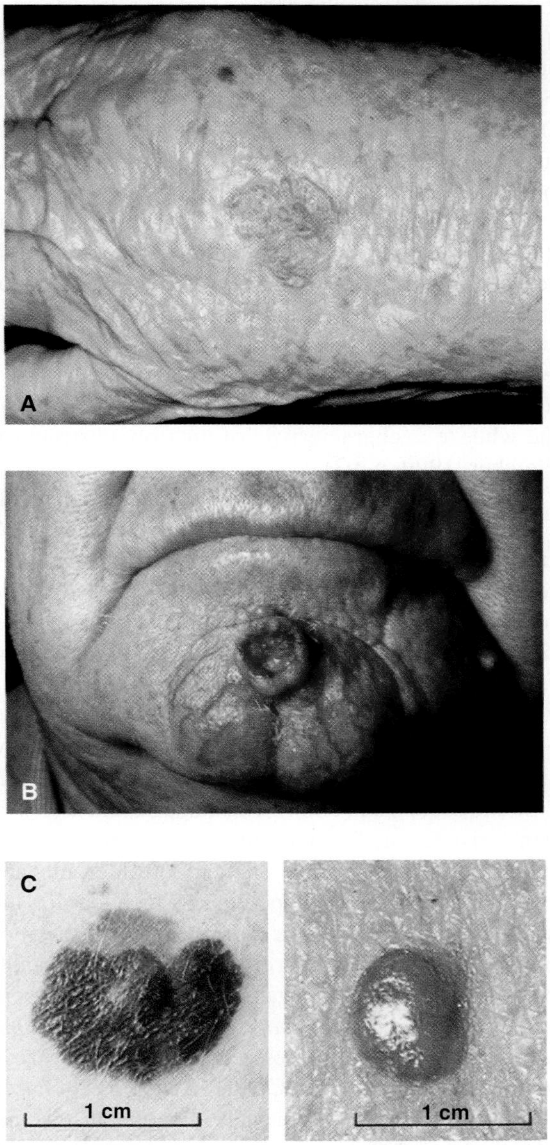

FIGURE 24.13 The incidence of skin cancer rises sharply for older adults. (**A**) Basal cell carcinoma. (**B**) Squamous cell carcinoma. (**C**) Malignant melanoma.

changes from straight vertical to more anterior from the base of support at the hips and below. Arm swing decreases slightly with age, as does the height of the gait swing. The foot does not clear the floor at a height that it does in younger people. Range of motion of the hips and knees frequently is limited because of osteoarthritis. Pain and foot deformities, especially hallux valgus (bunion), can alter the biomechanics of walking (Fig. 24.14).

Vital Signs

Alterations in vital signs require special attention. Infections in older adults often present without fever, so the nurse pays sharp attention to respiratory and pulse rates, as well as subtle cognitive changes. Use of a thermometer that records low temperatures is important because older adults are at increased risk for hypothermia as a result of age-associated thermoregulatory changes.

Proper measurement techniques are especially important. The nurse should measure blood pressure (BP) in both arms (during initial examination and periodically thereafter). Occlusive atherosclerotic disease of the subclavian or brachial artery often reduces systolic pressure in one arm. **Orthostatic (postural) hypotension** is common among older adults, particularly after meals (Applegate, 2003). Orthostatic hypotension is a risk factor for syncope, falls, fracture, morbidity, and mortality in older adults (Lipsitz, 2003). To assess for orthostatic hypotension, the nurse should take BP measurements while the client is sitting (after a 5-minute rest period) or in the supine position and then changing to a standing position. He or she should take the client's BP at or after 3 minutes in the standing position, with positive orthostasis defined as a systolic drop of 20 mm Hg or more or diastolic decrease of 10 mm Hg or more (Meyyazhagan & Messinger-Rapport, 2004). Symptoms such as lightheadedness, dizziness, or tachycardia also may accompany orthostatic hypotension.

Cardiovascular System

Cardiovascular disease (CVD) remains the leading killer of U.S. women and an important public health concern

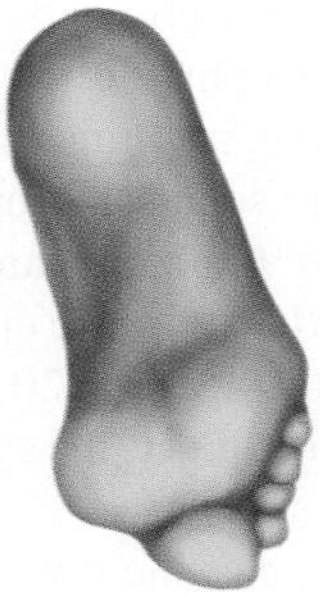

FIGURE 24.14 Bunions can cause gait abnormalities and other problems.

(Society for Women's Health Research, 2004). Historically, the rate of diagnostic accuracy in women with CVD has been less than in men because noninvasive tests may be less sensitive in women, studies have enrolled significantly fewer women than men, results have not traditionally been reported by gender, and for some, gender differences influence the clinical presentation of **myocardial ischemia** (decreased coronary blood flow) or acute MI (an infarct in the myocardium, usually caused by ischemia of a coronary artery) (Redberg & Shaw, 2003). For example, shortness of breath on exertion occurs more frequently than chest pain during an MI, or during periods of myocardial ischemia in elders. If pain occurs, it is less likely to be retrosternal (Aronow, 2003). The term "silent ischemia" or "silent MI" is used to describe ischemia or infarction without symptoms in older adults. Atypical presentations of ischemia or MI also may include the sudden onset of confusion, syncope, or a fall, and may occur without the classic symptoms of chest pain, dyspnea, and nausea common in younger and middle-aged people.

Another change in the cardiovascular system is an increased incidence of **isolated systolic hypertension (ISH),** defined as systolic BP greater than 140 mm Hg, accompanied by a diastolic BP less than 90 mm Hg. The cause is changes in the vascular media that result in increased intimal thickening and fibrosis. ISH is a significant risk factor for stroke in elders and needs aggressive assessment and treatment.

Blood vessels become less distensible with age, resulting in decreased vascular compliance and increased peripheral resistance. Smooth muscle vessel relaxation response also declines as a result of decreased β-adrenergic stimulation. Arterial wall cells change in size and shape, with irregularity in cell layering. The subendothelial layer increases thickness by greater connective tissue production and higher calcium and lipid deposits. Muscle layers thicken in the media (Burke & Laramie, 2000).

The heart itself undergoes numerous anatomic and physiologic changes associated with aging. Lipid deposits form along the sinoatrial node. The quantity of pacemaker cells decreases, which can lead to rhythm disturbances and arteriovenous block. Cardiac size has no significant change, with clinically insignificant minor left ventricular hypertrophy. Left ventricular compliance and relaxation decrease, resulting in increased atrial contraction. A fourth heart sound (S_4) may become audible as a result (Fletcher, 1999). More than 50% of older adults have a grade I/VI or II/VI systolic ejection murmur without radiation (Ebersole & Hess, 2001a). The most common murmur in older adults is the systolic aortic stenotic murmur.

Physiologically, cardiac output progressively decreases by approximately 1% per year, resulting in a limited cardiac reserve (**presbycardia**). Presbycardia becomes clinically significant when an older woman encounters physical or emotional stress, illness, or excitement. The tachycardic response found in younger people is blunted in older adults (Ebersole & Hess, 2001a).

Respiratory System

Age-associated anatomic and physiologic changes in the respiratory system affect an older woman's breathing ability. Skeletal deformities, the most notable being kyphosis, may accompany aging, but are much more accentuated with osteoporosis. The resulting increase in the chest's anterior-posterior diameter affects lung expansion. The chest wall stiffens as a result of kyphoscoliosis, calcification of intercostal cartilage, and arthritis in the costovertebral joints (Beers et al., 2006). Atrophy of the intercostal muscles occurs, as does a 25% decrease in diaphragmatic strength. The result is decreased forced vital capacity with forced expiratory volume in 1 second (FEV_1) decreases of 25 to 30 mL/year in nonsmokers and 60 to 70 mL/year in smokers (Ely, 2002). The barrel-chest shape makes auscultation of breath sounds more difficult and distant.

Dyspnea is a common complaint in older adults. In terms of the physical examination, "crackles are the most common physical finding, with contributing factors including atelectasis and age-related fibrotic changes in the lungs. The crackle is always an abnormal finding because the areas filled with fluid are not adequately exchanging air and are a potential source of infection. The wheeze is characteristic of air flow obstruction" (Fletcher, 1999, p. 93).

Ciliary function also is lost with age, which results in ineffective clearance of mucus from the airways. As a result, risk for lower respiratory tract infections increases. Aging of the respiratory system can lead to a decrease in the maximum volume of air that can be inhaled (*forced inspiratory volume*) and the maximum volume of air than can be expelled following maximum inhalation (*forced vital capacity*) (Miller, 2004).

Mortality from pneumonia is approximately five times greater in older adults than it is in younger adults (Bonomo & Johnson, 2004). The nurse should assess the client's risk factors for mortality with pneumonia, which include comorbidities, age 85 years or older, elevated serum creatinine level, hypotension, tachycardia, and hypothermia. *Streptococcal pneumoniae* is the most common causative organism of pneumonia in older adults; however, gram-negative organisms like *Haemophilus influenzae, Moraxella catarrhalis,* and *Klebsiella pneumoniae* are more frequent causes in clients in long-term care facilities and in those with COPD (Bonomo & Johnson, 2004). To prevent pneumonia, it is important that women older than 65 years receive the pneumococcal vaccine (Pneumovax-23).

Smoking increases risk for the development of COPD; thus, the nurse should encourage smoking cessation in older adults and assist them to set goals for quitting and enrolling in a smoking cessation program (Ely, 2002). Findings on physical examination that may indicate COPD include wheezing and dyspnea, with wheezing being the best predictor of limited air flow. Hyperresonance on percussion and a forced expiratory time greater than 9 seconds are common findings in clients with COPD or emphysema.

Nearly 50% of all asthma-related deaths occur in older adults (Ely, 2002). Asthma, an episodic reversible airway disease, causes inflammation and edema of the respiratory mucosa with excessive sputum production and bronchial spasm. Symptoms include wheezing, dyspnea, increased use of accessory muscles, intercostal muscle retractions, nasal flaring, diaphoresis, cyanosis, and tachypnea.

Gastrointestinal System

The normal gastrointestinal (GI) tract has the capacity for unimpaired absorption, digestion, and defecation. Anorexia usually has a defined etiology in older clients. The most frequent presentations are with clinical depression, side effects from medications, thyroid disorders, constipation, and cancer. Weight loss usually correlates with anorexia, which can decrease strength, functional status, and immunity.

Xerostomia, or dry mouth from decreased salivary secretions, is common in older adults and most often occurs as a result of medication side effects (Miller, 2004). In addition to xerostomia, older adults commonly suffer from several other oral health problems. Missing teeth, periodontal infections, or loose dentures will affect the ability to chew a solid diet. Estimates are that 40% of those older than 65 years are edentulous; other common findings include teeth-eroding surfaces, losing enamel, and changing degrees of root absorption (Eliopoulos, 2005; Linton, 1997). Oral health is important in older adults: the nurse should inquire about oral health and instruct women in measures to minimize or treat common oral health problems. Nursing measures include encouraging regular professional dental care, regular brushing and flossing, adequate fluid intake to prevent dehydration, regular medication review to identify drugs potentially causing or exacerbating xerostomia (eg, anticholinergic medications), and use of artificial saliva products as necessary to treat xerostomia.

Dysphagia (difficulty swallowing) can result from motility disorders, medications, vascular changes, strokes, and other neuromuscular disorders. Clients with impaired swallowing are at risk for aspiration pneumonia (Dziewas et al., 2004). The nurse should assess the client's history for dysphagia for solids, liquids, or both; he or she should observe for any dysphagia during meals.

A recent study (Srinivasan et al., 2004) found no differences in heartburn frequency between male and female respondents. Heartburn was significantly less common in participants older than 60 years than in young and middle-age respondents. The effects of heartburn on social activities in older clients were approximately 75% less than in young and middle-age people. Approximately 50% were aware of the term GERD (for gastroesophageal reflux disease). Few seniors were aware that swallowing difficulty, asthma, or hoarseness were possible symptoms of GERD. Malabsorption, not a normal aging change, is the most common small intestinal disorder in older adults. Lactose intolerance also may cause diarrhea in older women.

Diverticular disease occurs in 30% of older adults 60 years or older and in 65% of those 85 years or older (Triadafilopoulos, 2002). Diverticula are intestinal pouches that trap fecal material (Fig. 24.15). Diverticulosis occurs in elders at risk for constipation because of medications and decreased fiber and fluid intake. Usually asymptomatic, diverticulosis can cause constipation, bloating, distention, and discomfort. Acute inflammation causes diverticulitis (Eliopolous, 2005). With this condition, diverticula may rupture and bleed, causing blood to appear in the stool.

Genitourinary System

Women may encounter sexual difficulty during the postmenopausal phase of their lives. **Dyspareunia** (pain with intercourse) may occur with vaginal atrophy. This is the result of decreased vaginal lubrication related to estrogen deficiency. Libido in older women may be more related

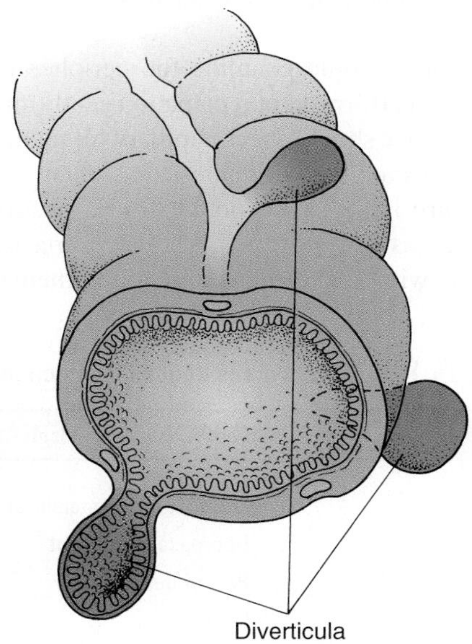

FIGURE 24.15 The formation of diverticulosis places older women at risk for constipation, bloating, distention, and discomfort. Acute inflammation causes diverticulitis, in which the diverticula may rupture and bleed.

to testosterone rather then estrogen. Chronic illnesses such as diabetes mellitus (DM), rheumatic disorders, breast cancer, and medications like antihistamines, antipsychotics, and antidepressants may cause negative changes in sexual function (Gentili et al., 2002). A smaller speculum may be helpful for vaginal examination in women with vaginal atrophy or a stenotic vaginal introitus. Clients with arthritic functional disabilities may benefit from use of the left lateral decubitus position for pelvic examinations. This can be done with the woman's knees flexed with greater flexion in the right hip.

Ovarian size decreases with aging. Palpable ovaries are abnormal in older women. This finding or increased uterine size needs evaluation for cancer (Davila, 2002). Women with uterine prolapse may have low back pain, fecal or urinary incontinence, or a palpable mass. The nurse should examine for anterior vaginal wall (**cystocele**) or **posterior vaginal wall prolapse** (enterocele or rectocele) (see Chaps. 4 and 19). Postmenopausal vaginal bleeding has many causes; this finding requires evaluation for carcinoma of the cervix, uterus, vulva, or ovaries (Davila, 2002).

Peripheral Vascular System

Clients with coronary or cerebrovascular atherosclerotic disease frequently have peripheral vascular disease (Table 24.1). The classic changes of intermittent claudication may be missed in older women who are not ambulatory. It is important to assess for jugular venous pulsation or distention with the client in the sitting position, especially for those with heart failure. Peripheral edema is common in venous insufficiency and heart failure.

The nurse should examine the peripheral arteries carefully and perform carotid palpation gently and unilaterally. The nurse should check capillary filling time in the client's toes by applying firm pressure to them. Full color should return in 3 to 5 seconds. Arterial insufficiency often appears as lower extremity pallor. Arterial occlusion may exhibit with severe pain, pallor, or erythema. Lower extremity assessment includes assessing venous return because decreased competence is common in older women. Mild or severe varicosities may be visible in the older woman's lower extremities. Erythema may result from cellulitis, dermatitis, or phlebitis. Decreased hair distribution in the lower extremities is frequent in arterial insufficiency and DM (Eliopolous, 2005; Flaherty et al., 2003).

The nurse should assess for any lower extremity ulcers. Venous insufficiency ulcers typically are large, medial, and irregular and often extend to the subcutaneous level. They frequently have "leaky" drainage. Arterial insufficiency ulcers tend to present laterally on the lower extremities.

Any client with DM needs regular pedal examinations by a nurse and a podiatrist, with evaluation for areas of pressure, breakdown, or necrosis to prevent amputation of a lower extremity (Fig. 24.16). Osteomyelitis of the bone is a frequent complication of diabetic foot ulcers and requires intensive intravenous therapy and infectious disease consultation, as well as vascular studies to prevent loss of the foot or lower leg.

Neurologic System

Amyloid plaques and tau protein neurofibrillary tangles can be identified in the brain of an older person. Brain weight, as well as appearance and configuration, may decrease with age. Slowing and decreased synaptic transmission may occur; however, these changes may have few effects on thinking and cognition. Age-associated changes in the structure and function of the neurologic system include slowed conduction of nerve impulses, a loss of neurons providing messages to and from the central nervous system, a decrease in available neurotransmitters, and a decrease in peripheral nerve functions (Hill-O'Neill & Shaughnessy, 2002).

Reaction time slows. Decreased baroreceptor function or cerebral blood flow can cause **syncope,** a loss of consciousness with less postural tone. Reflexes decrease, especially in the lower extremities. Obtaining

TABLE 24.1 Arterial Versus Venous Insufficiency

CHARACTERISTIC	CHRONIC ARTERIAL INSUFFICIENCY	CHRONIC VENOUS INSUFFICIENCY
Pain	Intermittent, especially at rest	None to aching on dependency
Pulses	Decreased or absent	Normal, although difficult to feel
Color	Pale or dusky red	Normal or cyanotic on dependency
Temperature	Cool	Normal
Edema	Absent or mild	Present, often marked
Skin changes	Thin, shiny, atrophic, with hair loss over feet and thick toenails	Brow around the ankles; possible skin thickening and scarring
Ulceration	Toes or trauma points on feet	Possibly at sides of ankle
Gangrene	May develop	Does not develop

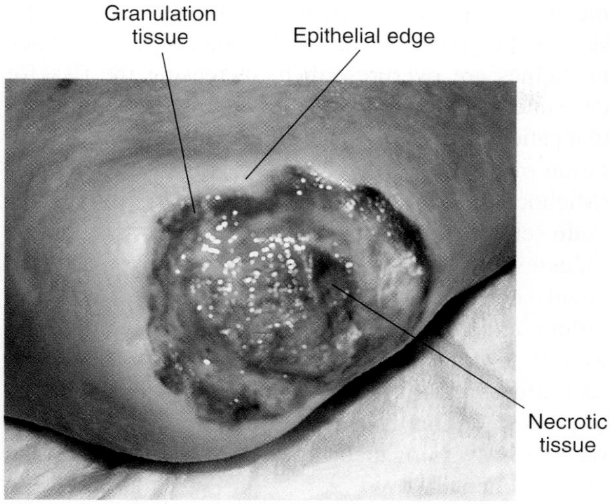

FIGURE 24.16 Older clients with immobility, diabetes, and other problems need regular skin assessments to prevent bed sores and related complications.

ankle reflexes in older adults is particularly difficult. Joints become more flexed with decreased muscle strength. Age-associated intention tremors increase with movement and are absent at rest.

Extremes in environmental temperatures pose risks for older women. **Hypothermia** occurs when the rectal temperature is 95°F (35°C) or below. Various factors are involved, including failure to vasoconstrict adequately on exposure to cold, decreased or absent shivering to generate heat, and failure of the metabolic rate to increase in response to cold (Ebersole & Hess, 2001b). Conversely, women may experience **hyperthermia.** Heat stroke, which causes death in many older adults, results from excessive heat storage with a decreased ability to rid the body of heat through evaporation, radiation, and conduction. Heat exhaustion, which may lead to heat stroke, exhibits with weakness, nausea, vomiting, diarrhea, increased bodily warmth, headache, and shortness of breath. This may proceed to delirium, psychosis, and loss of consciousness with increased systolic and decreased diastolic BP (increased pulse pressure), decreased cardiac output, and peripheral resistance, which may lead to death (Lugo-Amador, 2004).

Musculoskeletal System

Mobility is related to ability to perform ADLs and IADLs. Difficulty with mobility is commonly related to aging physiology and chronic illness. Inactivity leads to deconditioning of the musculoskeletal system, which has led health care professionals in recent years to emphasize the importance of continued exercise. A meta-analysis of studies on exercise in older adults showed that in 88% of cases, exercise improved muscle strength; 70% of cases showed improved aerobic capacity, and 63% showed improved range of motion and flexibility (Keysor & Jette, 2001).

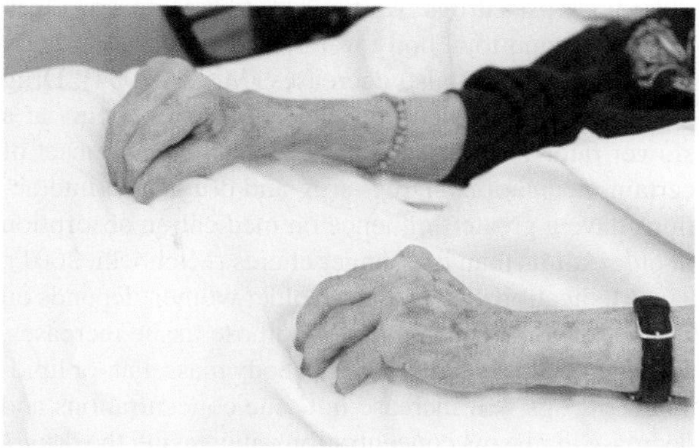

FIGURE 24.17 Rheumatoid arthritis in an older woman.

The nurse should assess the mobility status of the older woman regularly. Nursing assessment includes gait evaluation, unilateral favoring of an extremity, joint swelling, muscle atrophy, paralysis, or muscle weakness (Eliopolous, 2005). Observation of the older woman performing ADLs provides an ideal and practical musculoskeletal assessment. The nurse can do so in the office setting by observing the client ambulating, transferring into a chair or examination table, or rising from a wheelchair. It is important for the acute care and long-term care nurse to advance mobility as medically indicated. Significant bone loss can occur during periods of immobility.

Osteoarthritis (OA) is extremely common in older women, particularly in the knees, hips, feet, spine, and hands. The nurses should assess for OA by checking the client for decreased range of motion and crepitus of joints. Bony enlargement of the hands is present in the distal interphalangeal (Heberden's) and proximal interphalangeal (Bouchard's) nodes (Yurkow & Yudin, 2002).

Rheumatoid arthritis, characterized by bilateral symmetric inflammation of affected joints, usually affects the hands, wrists, knees, and feet (see Chap. 4). It often involves the metacarpal and proximal interphalangeal joints (Fig. 24.17). Swelling and tenderness occur, with decreased joint function. Hand deformities include ulnar deviation, swan neck deformity, and boutonniere lesions (Yurkow & Yudin, 2002).

AGING PHARMACOLOGY

People older than 65 years currently make up approximately 12% of the U.S. population yet consume 33% of all prescription drugs. By the year 2040, estimates are that the geriatric population will make up 25% of the total population but will be purchasing 50% of all prescription drugs (Semla & Rochon, 2002).

The field of aging **pharmacokinetics** examines how the older adult's body handles drugs. The field of aging **pharmacodynamics** examines the effect of drugs on the older person's body. Many factors influence how the older body uses drugs. Aging leads to a decrease in lean body mass and total body water, while increasing body fat. Renal function also decreases (Miller, 2004). Drug absorption is complete in older adults, but occurs at a slower rate. There may be a delay to the peak onset of certain medications. Drug–drug and drug–food interactions have a greater influence on medication absorption in older adults than in younger clients (Michocki, 2001).

Medication distribution in older women depends on several factors. The amount of adipose tissue increases, compared with a decrease in lean body mass. Fat- or lipid-soluble drugs will increase in tissue concentrations and decrease in plasma concentrations, increasing the drug's duration of effect in the body (Eliopoulos, 2005). Decreases in serum albumin levels can cause an increased amount of free active drug (Fulginiti et al., 2000).

Most drug metabolism occurs in the liver. The aging process leads to decreased hepatic blood flow, size, and mass (Semla & Rochon, 2002). Decreases in blood flow to the liver lead to less drug being delivered and metabolized by the liver (Fulginiti et al., 2000). Renal function decreases by 50% between 20 and 90 years, which affects drugs excreted by the kidneys. Thus, it takes these drugs longer to clear the body, resulting in prolonged half-lives. The result often is higher drug concentrations, especially in renally excreted medications like digoxin, diuretics, nonsteroidal anti-inflammatory drugs (NSAIDs), and captopril. Serum creatinine, which is used to reflect renal function in younger people, is not a reliable indicator of kidney function in older adults. This is because decreased muscle mass affects creatinine production in older adults, which may lead to false-normal serum creatinine results. Rather than relying on serum creatinine, the nurse calculates a more accurate estimation of renal function for older women by using the Cockroft and Gault (1976) equation:

$$(140 - \text{age}) \times \text{body weight (kg)} \div 72 \times \text{serum creatinine (mg/dL)} \times 0.85 = \text{mL (mL/min)}$$

Cardiac output, renal pathology, and state of hydration also affect aging pharmacokinetics and pharmacodynamics, as do chronic illnesses (Eliopolous, 2005).

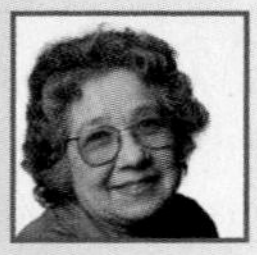

As part of evaluation, the nurse estimates 67-year-old Ann's renal function using the Cockroft and Gault equation. Ann weighs 165 lbs; her serum creatinine is 0.8 mg/dL. What would the nurse's estimation be?

The term **polypharmacy** has been used frequently in the past 15 years to describe the use of multiple drugs by the same client. Many older clients are using multiple medications prescribed by different health care professionals. Polypharmacy is undesirable, especially when medicines are overprescribed, increasing the risk for drug interactions. "Polypharmacy indicates that a particular patient receives too many drugs, drugs for a long duration of time, or drugs in exceedingly high dosages" (Michocki, 2001, p. 73). The current preferred term is "safe geriatric prescribing" because with certain chronic illnesses, multiple medications are necessary, as when clients need multiple agents for hypertension, heart failure, and DM. In such cases, these chronic illnesses usually require two or more medications to manage each illness. Fick and colleagues (2003) updated a list of potentially inappropriate medications to assist prescribers in avoiding medications known to cause ADRs in older clients.

An important general principle for safe prescribing is to begin dosage at the lowest dose available or to score the tablet in half if possible, adjusting to the lowest dose before increasing to the next level. Clinicians should taper doses upward slowly to observe the client for physical, biochemical, cognitive, functional, and behavioral changes.

QUOTE 24-3

"I have to take four different medications at various times during the day to treat different problems. Keeping track of all of them and the overall schedule is daunting, but my nurse is very helpful in assisting with this."

From an older client taking drugs for hypertension and arthritis, as well as calcium supplementation

COMMON CONDITIONS FOUND IN OLDER WOMEN

URINARY INCONTINENCE

UI affects approximately 17 million Americans and is five times more prevalent in women than in men (Wyman, 2004). It can cause morbidity, including cellulitis, pressure ulcers, urinary tract infections, falls, fractures, sleep deprivation, social withdrawal, depression, and sexual dysfunction. UI impairs quality of life, affecting emotional well-being, social function, and general health (DuBeau, 2002).

Types

Types of established UI include stress incontinence, urge incontinence, mixed incontinence, overflow incontinence, and functional incontinence:

- *Stress incontinence* is the loss of small amounts of urine without bladder contraction. It occurs when intrapelvic pressure increases with abdominal pressure. The urethral pressure is less then the bladder pressure.

Maneuvers that lead to increased intra-abdominal pressure (eg, sneezing, lifting, laughing, coughing, bending) can cause urinary leakage (Dowling-Castronovo & Bradway, 2003).

- *Urge incontinence* results from uninhibited bladder contractions or instability of detrusor (bladder smooth muscle) function. It is characterized by a strong urge to void immediately before urine is lost. Affected clients frequently report that they cannot get to the toilet before leakage or that they have "key in the lock" syndrome; that is, they lose urine on arriving home and unlocking the door. Moderate to large amounts of urine usually are lost. Many of these clients also report urinary frequency, symptoms of an overactive bladder (urinary frequency and urgency without incontinence), and nocturia (Dowling-Castronovo & Bradway, 2003).
- *Mixed incontinence* is a combination of stress and urge UI (Fantl et al., 1996). Mixed UI is frequently found in older women.
- *Overflow incontinence* results from detrusor underactivity, bladder outlet obstruction, or both. Urinary leakage is ongoing and low in volume. The postvoid residual urine is large. In women, the cause may be surgery for previous incontinence, cystocele, mechanical damage to the spine, or Parkinson's disease (DuBeau, 2002). Fecal impaction also may be the cause in an older woman.
- *Functional incontinence* stems from external factors like the client's inability to reach the toilet in time to void. It accompanies cognitive problems like dementia or delirium and also can be caused by a lack of personnel to assist clients in toileting. Another possible cause is any medication that slows psychomotor functioning, delaying time to get to the bathroom. Examples include central nervous system medications like hypnotics and tranquilizers. Antipsychotic medications, especially older, conventional neuroleptics with extrapyramidal side effects, may lead to drug-induced parkinsonism rigidity, which can significantly slow gait and functional ability to toilet.

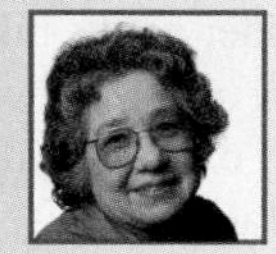

Remember Ann, the 67-year-old from the beginning of the chapter who is having bladder problems. Based on Ann's statements, which type of incontinence would the nurse suspect?

Etiology and Pathophysiology

In addition to the types of established UI, incontinence also can be caused by a transient condition, such as delirium, depression, urinary tract infection, atrophic vaginitis, and medications (eg, diuretics, anticholinergics, narcotics, and α-adrenergic agents); acute exacerbations of a chronic condition (eg, congestive heart failure presenting as nocturia and enuresis) or atypical presentation of a new condition (eg, the polyuria of DM can also cause UI); excessive fluid, resulting from oral intake above normal or cardiac overload; and constipation or stool impaction causing urinary outlet obstruction (Fantl et al., 1996; Ouslander, 2000). In most cases, transient causes of UI can be corrected (Fantl et al., 1996).

Assessment Findings

The workup for UI includes a urine dipstick to rule out the hyperglycemia of DM, protein, or hematuria, which could indicate renal pathology or cancer. If leukocytes are present on the dipstick, a urine culture and sensitivity should be performed. A postvoid residual volume measures the urine in the bladder after a completed void. This can be done by two methods. The easiest and most recent is use of a portable ultrasound device. The second method is urinary catheterization after voiding to measure the quantity of retained urine, with removal of the catheter after specimen collection. Postvoid residual readings above 200 mL are considered elevated; values between 50 and 200 mL require clinical judgment to determine results (Weiss, 2001).

A pelvic examination is necessary to assess for atrophic vaginitis, masses, prolapse, cystocele, rectocele, or enterocele. A rectal examination is needed to evaluate for fecal impaction or rectal masses.

Clients may keep bladder diaries for short periods (2 to 3 days) to determine the type of UI. Such a diary consists of a graph with 24 hours in the vertical column and assessment criteria along the horizontal column. Several examples of diaries are available (Fantl et al., 1996; National Institute of Diabetes and Digestive and Kidney Diseases, 1997); the nurse should choose the type that best fits the setting and population. For example, complex diaries provide a large amount of information but are not likely to be useful for women with moderate to severe cognitive impairment. Once completed, the nurse should review the bladder diary and use the information to assist with determining a diagnosis, and as a starting point for treatment. Typical areas of the bladder diary include the following:

- Did the client urinate in the toilet?
- When did episodes of UI occur?
- What was the associated activity at the time of leakage?
- Was an urge present?
- What was the type and amount of fluid intake?

Stress testing is done using the pad test when the bladder is full. The tester uses a gauze pad to measure urinary leakage after requesting that the client cough. Urinary leakage indicates stress incontinence. This is first done in the supine position; if results are negative, then the standing position is used. In the Marshall test, the examiner inserts his or her finger on either side of the client's urethra. He or she elevates the urethra and asks the client to cough. If a client leaks during the pad tests and has no leakage with the Marshall test, the possibility exists that her condition may improve with incontinence surgery (Weiss, 2001). Women with obvious pelvic or bladder prolapse require referral to a provider specializing in UI, such as an advanced practice continence nurse, urologist, gynecologist, or urogynecologist. A neurologic consult may be in order if a neurologic condition is the cause of the incontinence.

Urodynamic tests frequently done by specialists include urinometry, which measures urine flow with a disposable urine flow meter. Cystometrography produces pressure measurements within the bladder if the bladder is filled and also records intra-abdominal pressure with a rectal probe. Cystometrics are helpful to diagnose the detrusor overactivity and sphincter dysfunction. This is higher-level testing than the basic incontinence workup (Weiss, 2001).

Collaborative Management

Numerous treatment modalities are available for UI, depending on the type. Various surgical procedures and several medications can be useful in the management of UI; however, experts recommend that if possible, noninvasive, nonmedical therapies be used as first-line treatment strategies (Fantl et al., 1996). This section focuses on nonmedical therapies for the treatment of UI. NIC/NOC Box 24.1 highlights some of the nursing interventions and outcomes associated with urinary incontinence.

Elimination of bladder irritants, including alcohol, aspartame, and carbonated beverages, is important, especially for women suffering from urge UI or symptoms of an overactive bladder. Limiting fluid intake after 9 PM may reduce nighttime incontinence. Voiding pattern corrections also can assist in alleviating symptoms.

NIC/NOC Box 24.1 Urinary Incontinence

Common NIC Labels

- Pelvic Muscle Exercise
- Perineal Care
- Pessary Management
- Self-Care Assistance: Toileting
- Urinary Bladder Training
- Urinary Elimination Management
- Urinary Incontinence Care

Common NOC Labels

- Tissue Integrity: Skin and Mucous Membranes
- Urinary Continence
- Urinary Elimination

The nurse should encourage the client to empty her bladder completely with each void. Telling the client to pause when voiding is complete and to wait another minute to retry voiding again may help (Wyman, 1999). Scheduled voiding regimens are helpful for women with stress, urge, overflow, and functional UI. The nurse should evaluate the client's voiding schedule and inquire about episodes of UI. Using this information, he or she can suggest an individualized voiding schedule as a way to minimize or alleviate UI. For example, a woman with urge UI approximately every 3 hours may benefit from reorganizing her daily routine to include bathroom breaks every 2 to 2½ hours. Nursing Care Plan 24.1 provides information related to the care of a woman with urinary incontinence.

Prompted voiding is another nursing strategy whereby prescribed voiding schedules are adjusted to the client's voiding pattern. It is used for stress, urge, and functional incontinence, but not for overflow incontinence. Caregivers monitor the client's toileting and prompt her to void on a 2- to 3-hour schedule, as well as offering positive reinforcement for maintaining continence and attempting to void. This is helpful for cognitively or physically impaired clients; however, it requires significant commitment and effort on the part of the caregiver to be successful (Newman & Palmer, 2003).

Pelvic muscle exercises (PMEs) are used to treat stress, urge, and mixed UI (Wyman, 2003). The nurse should instruct women by explaining the purpose of the exercises, helping clients find the correct muscle to exercise, and instructing clients on the optimal technique and amount of PMEs for treating UI. See Chapter 23 for more information on these exercises.

FALLS AND FRACTURES

Control of posture by the central nervous system is determined by proprioception, sensory input, and vestibular input. Older adults have a righting reflex in which vestibular receptors detect any loss of stability. Muscles will oppose a postural sway. Younger adults correct weight shift at the hip, whereas older people use the feet instead of the hip to correct any shift in body posture. Older adults take a rapid step forward or backward to prevent being thrown off balance. They use protective reflexes by extending the arms to restore balance or to secure a surface.

Incidence of falls increases with age and varies according to where a person lives (ie, in the community, in a long-term care setting, or during an acute hospitalization). According to Kiel (2002), 30% to 40% of community-dwelling adults 65 years or older fall each year. Among those with a history of a fall in the previous year, the annual incidence of falls is close to 60%. In long-term care settings, approximately 50% of all residents fall each year.

NURSING CARE PLAN 24.1

The Older Client Experiencing Urinary Incontinence

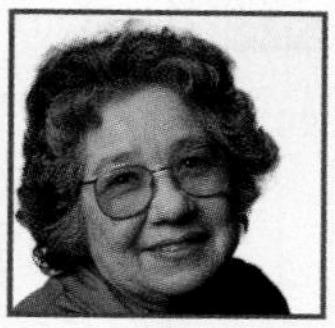

Remember Ann, the older woman struggling with bladder problems, described at the beginning of this chapter. Upon examination, the nurse finds that Ann's perineal area is slightly reddened and irritated. She states, "Sometimes I don't always make it to the bathroom. I've started to wear thin panty liners just in case."

NURSING DIAGNOSES

- **Stress Urinary Incontinence** related to age-associated changes in pelvic muscles and support structures and increased abdominal pressure
- **Deficient Knowledge** related to urinary incontinence
- **Urge Urinary Incontinence** related to bladder contractions.

EXPECTED OUTCOMES

1. The client will identify situations that affect urinary elimination.
2. The client will define urinary incontinence (UI) and possible contributing factors.
3. The client will report fewer episodes of stress and urge UI.

INTERVENTIONS	RATIONALES
Assess the client's knowledge base and current understanding about UI.	Assessment provides a baseline from which to develop an individualized teaching plan.
Assess for possible contributing factors to UI; review with the client possible factors that may lead to UI.	Atrophic vaginitis, medications, and acute or chronic conditions can lead to transient UI.
Question the client about any additional complaints related to urinary elimination, such as pain or burning. Obtain a urine dipstick and culture and sensitivity as ordered.	Hyperglycemia of diabetes or urinary tract infection can be a cause of UI.
Assist with obtaining a postvoid residual urine volume.	Elevated postvoid residual volumes require further evaluation.
Complete or assist with a pelvic examination.	Pelvic examination reveals clues to possible genitourinary conditions such as atrophic vaginitis, masses, uterine prolapse, cystocele, or rectocele that may lead to UI.
Instruct the client in how to keep a bladder diary for 2 to 3 days; review diary with the client.	Diary information provides additional information from which to determine a diagnosis and plan of care.
Prepare the client for testing, such as pad test or urodynamic tests.	Testing provides clues to the underlying cause of the client's UI.
Instruct the client to eliminate alcohol, aspartame, carbonated beverages, and smoking.	These substances are bladder irritants.
Suggest that the client limit her intake of fluids after dinner in the evening.	Limiting fluids after this time may help to reduce nighttime UI.
Encourage the client to empty her bladder completely with each voiding; assist her to set up a voiding schedule based on her lifestyle and activity level.	Complete bladder emptying reduces the risk for residual urine remaining in the bladder. Voiding schedules aid in minimizing and reducing episodes of UI.

Continued

NURSING CARE PLAN 24.1 ● The Older Client Experiencing Urinary Incontinence (*Continued*)

INTERVENTIONS	RATIONALES
Instruct the client in pelvic muscle exercises, including assistance with finding the correct muscles, optimal technique, and suggested number of times to perform the exercise (see Chap. 23).	Pelvic muscle exercises help to strengthen and tone these supportive muscles.

EVALUATION

1. The client identifies realistic measures to manage urinary elimination.
2. The client describes the underlying processes and factors involved in UI.
3. The client demonstrates an increase in control over urinary elimination.

NURSING DIAGNOSIS

Risk for Impaired Skin Integrity related to urinary leakage and incontinence

EXPECTED OUTCOMES

1. The client identifies measures to reduce risk for perineal irritation.
2. The client exhibits a reduction in perineal redness and irritation.

INTERVENTIONS	RATIONALES
Assess the client's current measures for perineal hygiene.	Assessment provides a baseline from which to develop an individualized plan of care.
Instruct the client to wash and dry the perineal area with mild soap and warm water after each voiding and bowel movement.	Cleansing after elimination reduces the risk for further irritation and possible infection.
Encourage the client to avoid perfumed soaps, lotions, or scented items, such as panty-liners.	Perfumes and scented items can further irritate the area.
Instruct the client to use cotton underwear.	Cotton allows air to circulate, decreasing the risk for perineal irritation.
Advise the client to keep the area as dry as possible; encourage her to change panty-liners frequently.	Increased moisture in the area can lead to further irritation and excoriation.

EVALUATION

1. The client exhibits a perineal area that is clean, dry, and intact without evidence of redness, irritation, or excoriation.
2. The client demonstrates measures to promote perineal hygiene.

Etiology and Pathophysiology

Falls may result from internal (intrinsic) or environmental (extrinsic) factors. Examples of intrinsic factors are delirium and dementia. Extrinsic factors include environmental hazards such as excessive bed height, inadequate lighting or assistive devices, loose carpets, full-length side rails, or an unfamiliar environment (American Medical Directors Association, 2003). Additional fall risk factors include gait and balance disorders, visual impairment, anticholinergic medications, postural hypotension, and syncope (Tinetti, 2003).

Complications

Complications resulting from falls are the leading cause of death from injury in men and women 65 years or older. Moreover, only approximately 50% of older people hospitalized because of a fall will be alive 1 year later (Kane et al., 2004). Other adverse outcomes of falls include the inability of nearly 50% of those who fall to get up without assistance following a fall.

Davidson and associates (2001) found that 1 to 2 years following a hip fracture, 27% of clients had persistent pain and 60% had decreased mobility that they attributed to the fracture. Whether a fall becomes a fracture depends on various factors, including bone mineral density, fall risk factors, the older adult's biomechanical protective responses, and the amount of local shock when hitting the surface.

Vertebral fractures in women may gradually cause a significant loss of height affecting stature. Paraspinal muscles shorten, and pain from muscle fatigue relating to postural maintenance occurs. Pain may become chronic, even after the vertebral fracture heals. Structural spinal changes affect the ribcage, pulmonary function, appetite, and weight (Old & Calvert, 2004). Kyphosis and a dowager's hump in the upper back may occur and further complicate gait, balance, and functional capacity, decreasing the woman's quality of life.

Another fall complication is fallaphobia, in which an older person becomes afraid to resume a previous level of ambulation because of a fear of falling. Fletcher and Hirdes (2004) identified an incidence of fallaphobia of 41.2% in frail home care elders. This fear can cause anxiety or panic. It is important for the nurse to identify fallaphobia. The nurse should watch to see whether the client clutches others while ambulating or transferring, maintains contact with environmental objects, or uses the wall to steady during ambulation (Gray-Miceli et al., 2005). The nurse then should intervene through consultation with physical therapy for physical strengthening, as well as instituting measures to decrease anxiety, such as offering psychological support (Fig. 24.18).

Assessment Findings

According to the American Geriatrics Society (2001), a fall evaluation is an assessment that includes the following:

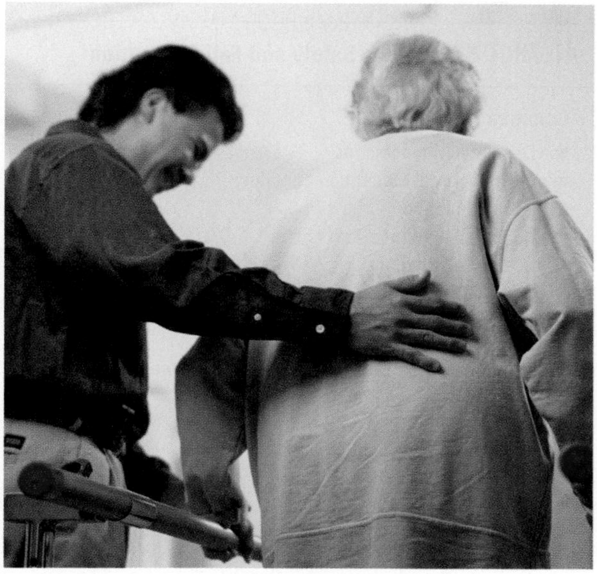

FIGURE 24.18 A physical therapist can assist clients having problems related to mobility.

- Examination of vision, gait and balance, and lower extremity joint function
- Examination of basic neurologic function, including mental status, muscle strength, lower extremity peripheral nerves, proprioception, reflexes, tests of cortical, extrapyramidal, and cerebellar function
- Assessment of basic cardiovascular status, including heart rate and rhythm, postural pulse, and blood pressure

In all settings, the nurse should assist the client to describe the circumstances related to a fall (Tideiksaar, 2002). Pertinent questions for the nursing history include those aimed at identifying the symptoms experienced at the time of the fall, the number of previous falls, fall location, activity and time of the fall, and any trauma (physical or psychological) suffered as a result (Tideiksaar, 2002). Mathias and associates' (1986) "Get Up and Go Test" is a good assessment of gait, balance, and postural control (see information given earlier in this chapter). Another excellent assessment of posture and stability is the chair rise test. The client rises from the chair with hands crossed over the chest, which should take less than 30 seconds to complete (Jones et al., 1999).

Collaborative Management

Strategies a nurse can use to prevent falls include recommending proper supportive footwear, a safe environment to minimize fall risks, physical therapy, and exercise to improve balance, strength, and flexibility. NIC/NOC Box 24.2 highlights some nursing interventions and outcomes related to safety measures and falls.

Tsang and Hui-Chan (2004) found that 4 weeks of intensive Tai Chi training was sufficient to improve balance

NIC/NOC Box 24.2 Safety and Fall Prevention

Common NIC Labels

- Dementia Management
- Environmental Management: Safety
- Health Education
- Home Maintenance Assistance
- Reality Orientation
- Surveillance: Safety

Common NOC Labels

- Safety Behavior: Home Physical Environment
- Safety Behavior: Personal
- Safety Status: Falls Occurrence
- Safety Status: Physical Injury

control in elderly subjects. Another important factor in decreasing the risk for falls is assessment of visual acuity and correction. It is also important that a physical therapist has professionally fit any adaptive device that an older woman uses (eg, cane, walker). Thin-soled well-fitting shoes are the best types of shoes to maximize proprioception and decrease the likelihood of a trip. These shoes should be flat. High heels in older women cause more instability because they decrease plantar flexion and effective gait. They also can catch on rugs, steps, or wooden decks. A podiatry consult is essential in older women with foot deformities because painful heels, bunions, or toes can affect both ambulation and balance. Orthotics worn inside the shoe can be customized to minimize the person's biomechanical abnormalities of gait and to prevent pressure areas in the feet. Foot hygiene, with proper podiatric nail care, will help prevent gait abnormalities and falls.

It is also important for the nurse to encourage clients to keep a fall diary. The client can do so for a short period (1 to 2 weeks) to find the precipitating factors before and during each fall episode. The client should note the date, time, and location of the fall, as well as the activity she was doing at the time of the fall along with related symptoms. Women at high risk for falling may want to consider hip protectors as one component of a multimodal approach to fall prevention (Resnick, 2004).

DELIRIUM

Delirium is a potentially fatal condition that is unrecognized in 32% to 66% of hospitalized older adults (Inouye, 1998). It has a 1-year mortality rate of 31.3% to 36.3% in elderly inpatients and nursing home residents (Laurila et al., 2004). Defined simply, **delirium** commonly appears as a state of agitated restlessness; however, people also can suffer from a hypoactive form of delirium with decreased activity as the hallmark feature. Delirium is a medical emergency for which health care providers must work diligently to identify the cause. Although the exact pathophysiologic mechanisms for delirium are unknown, older adults are at particularly high risk because anatomic deficits in the brain and imbalances in neurotransmitters controlling cognition, behavior, and mood are thought to be primarily responsible (Vanderbilt University Medical Center, 2004). Common contributing factors to delirium include infection, pain, cardiac or cerebrovascular events, ADRs, and metabolic abnormalities. Other causes include any acute event (eg, dehydration) or exacerbation of a chronic health problem (eg, anemia related to cancer), which can upset the older person's frail homeostatic balance.

The hallmark symptom of delirium is the inability to sustain, focus, or shift attention. There is an acute onset over hours to days, and a fluctuating course with clouding, altering consciousness, and somnolence, along with "dreamlike" experiences. The older adult with delirium experiences difficulty in following conversation or commands. Decision making is impaired, and persecutory delusions are common. Disorientation to time and place is likely. Perceptual abnormalities may progress to distortions, illusions, or hallucinations (Cole, 2004).

The Confusion Assessment Method (CAM) is a highly valid and reliable assessment for delirium (Inouye, 1998; Inouye, et al., 1990). It is frequently used in hospitals, but it can be applied across clinical settings. See Assessment Tool 24.3.

Another way to assess delirium is to perform digit span testing. The examiner recites one, two, or three numbers to the client at a rate of one digit per second. The client then repeats the numbers. The tester increases the numbers by one each time. People without cognitive impairment usually can remember seven digits forward and four digits backward. If a client has difficulty with this or spelling the word "world" backward, the likelihood of delirium is high.

The first and most important step in managing delirium is to identify the delirium and then to treat the causative factors. The nurse should work collaboratively with other members of the health care team to reach these goals. For example, the nurse should assess the client's current medications for any offending agents that may be causing or exacerbating the delirium (eg, sedatives, hypnotics, analgesics). Other nursing measures to treat delirium include early correction of dehydration, urinary tract infection, or pneumonia in a medically induced delirium. Environmental measures such as minimization of unnecessary stimuli and noise, use of hearing aids and eyeglasses, removal of indwelling urinary catheters and physical restraints, and early mobilization activities will assist hospitalized or bed-bound older adults with delirium (Kurlowicz, 2002; Vanderbilt University Medical Center, 2004).

● ASSESSMENT TOOL 24.3 Confusion Assessment Method (CAM), Shortened Version Worksheet

EVALUATOR: ______________________ DATE: ____________

I. ACUTE ONSET AND FLUCTUATING COURSE

BOX 1

a) Is there evidence of an acute change in mental status from the patient's baseline? No ______ Yes ______

b) Did the (abnormal) behavior fluctuate during the day, that is, tend to come and go or increase and decrease in severity? No ______ Yes ______

II. INATTENTION

Did the patient have difficulty focusing attention, for example, being easily distractible or having difficulty keeping track of what was being said? No ______ Yes ______

III. DISORGANIZED THINKING

BOX 2

Was the patient's thinking disorganized or incoherent, such as rambling or irrelevant conversation, unclear or illogical flow of ideas, or unpredictable switching from subject to subject? No ______ Yes ______

IV. ALTERED LEVEL OF CONSCIOUSNESS

Overall, how would you rate the patient's level of consciousness?

___ Alert (normal)

___ Vigilant (hyperalert)
___ Lethargic (drowsy, easily aroused)
___ Stupor (difficult to arouse)
___ Coma (unarousable)

Do any checks appear in this box? No ______ Yes ______

If all items in Box 1 are checked and at least one item in Box 2 is checked, a diagnosis of delirium is suggested.

Adapted from Inouye, S. K., et al. (1990). Clarifying confusion: The Confusion Assessment Method. A new method for detection of delirium. *Annals of Internal Medicine, 113,* 941–948.

DEMENTIA: ALZHEIMER'S DISEASE

Dementia has numerous causes, the most prevalent being Alzheimer's disease (AD), vascular dementia, and Lewy body dementia. AD affects 4 million people in the United States, a rate that will nearly quadruple to 14 million people by the year 2040 (Small, 2002). This progressive dementia is characterized by impaired cognition accompanied by alterations in personality and behavior and decreased functional status (Daly, 2001). AD is *not* part of normal aging but rather a form of neuropathology accompanied by neurotransmitter changes.

Assessment Findings

Onset of symptoms in AD is gradual, with manifestations of cognitive and functional decline occurring over months to years. The most important sign is cognitive loss; additional findings include forgetfulness, becoming lost in familiar areas, losing personal items consistently, experiencing difficulty with problem solving, changes in IADLs, personality changes, and occasionally mood changes (Kaye & Camicioli, 2000). Other problems related to AD include **aphasia,** which is disturbance in language not related to mechanical aspects of speech (Fig. 24.19); **apraxia,** which is failure to carry out motor tasks despite

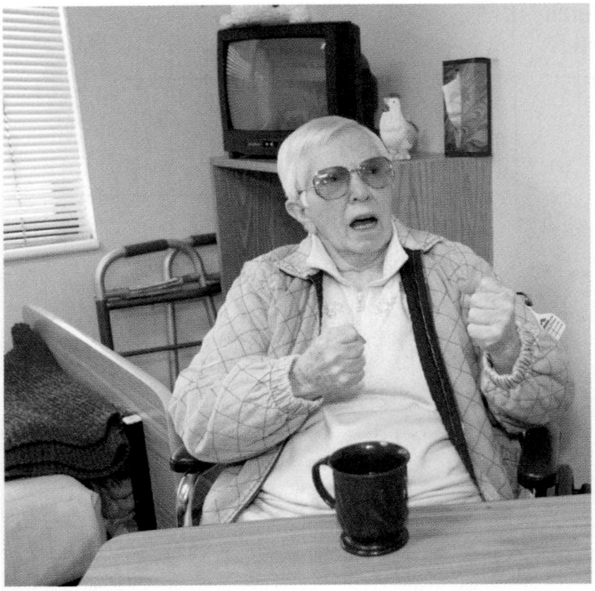

FIGURE 24.19 The communication problems associated with Alzheimer's disease can be particularly frustrating for clients.

intact motor and sensory function; and **agnosia,** which is failure to recognize or identify objects despite intact basic sensory function (Kaye & Camicioli, 2000).

AD progression causes additive neuronal destruction (Fig. 24.20). Behavioral symptoms such as agitation, insomnia, delusions, hallucinations, and wandering may occur. Paranoia and suspiciousness are common. Sleep cycle disruptions often develop with AD. Other behavioral problems, such as apathy, combativeness, hoarding behaviors, and physical or verbal aggression, manifest.

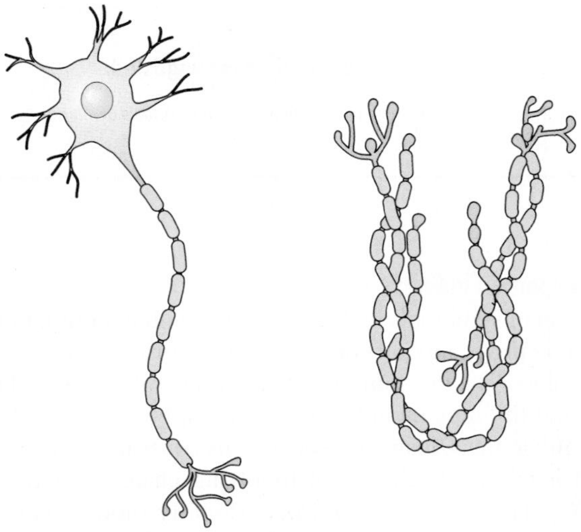

FIGURE 24.20 The brain neurons of clients with Alzheimer's disease are marked by tangles and plaques not found in the healthy brain.

Many older clients suffering from AD and other chronic cognitive impairments try to conceal their symptoms. **Confabulation** (telling imaginary stories to fill gaps in the memory of an event) is a common defense mechanism that many use when they realize they are dealing with early cognitive loss.

Safety assessment in women with the early stages of cognitive impairment includes the driving history and potential household dangers. Have there been any motor vehicle crashes or close calls? Does the spouse, partner, or others worry about the client's driving pattern? Was the woman ever lost for a significant time when driving the car? Have passengers compensated for any driving deficit (eg, telling the driver when to stop, when to turn)? Impaired cognition can also affect a woman's ability to take medication as prescribed, putting her at risk for underdosing and overdosing.

Diagnosis is based on a multifactorial process that includes laboratory and diagnostic workups to rule out other causes of cognitive impairment (eg, delirium, other neurologic disorders). The most important diagnostic clue is the history of cognitive loss, which the nurse gathers from the client, family members, or significant others. Other essential components of the dementia workup include a health history and physical examination.

The standard diagnostic workup for people experiencing cognitive impairment, as defined by the American Academy of Neurology (Knopman, et al., 2001), includes a complete blood count; a full chemistry panel; tests of vitamin B_{12} and thyroid function; and brain imaging (*ie,* noncontrast computed tomography [CT], magnetic resonance imaging [MRI]). Syphilis screening is mandatory only if the client has a high-risk sexual history or evidence of prior syphilis. Testing for HIV is appropriate if an older adult with cognitive impairment has a history of high-risk sexual practices.

The health history reveals forgetfulness, changes in IADLs, personality changes, and occasionally mood changes. The nurse should identify when symptoms began, functional losses since, the effects of these cognitive and functional changes, and alterations in social functioning and participation in occupational, volunteer, and recreational activities. The nurse also should ask about the existence of a family history of AD as one way to identify familial-onset AD (onset of AD symptoms before 65 years). The nurse should seek clues for decreased or guarded interactions with family members. He or she should use a delicate and calm approach when questioning the client about memory changes and cognitive loss. The client's statements may differ significantly from those of family members. The nurse should explore the family for history of depression or other psychiatric disorders, antidepressant medications that the client or family responded to, and a family history of Down syndrome.

The client must undergo a complete physical examination, with special attention given to the neurologic component to rule out focal deficits and other disorders presenting as delirium. The Mini-Mental State Examination (MMSE) is a cognitive test that clinicians use for initial screening assessment and longitudinal follow-up of cognitive status (Folstein et al., 1975). Thirty is a perfect score on the MMSE. Scores less than 24 usually indicate cognitive impairment requiring further evaluation and testing; however, educational level may alter the Folstein normal range. A rapid screening test for AD is the clock test, which evaluates visual spatial skills and executive functioning. Visual spatial skills become impaired early in AD. Using the clock test, the clinician asks the patient to draw a clock face and place the hands correctly at 2:50 or 11:10 (Gill, 2002). Errors with this task raise the likelihood of dementia and suggest the need for further evaluation and testing.

Collaborative Management

Initiation of cholinesterase inhibitors should occur as soon as a diagnosis of AD is reached. These medications (ie, donepezil [Aricept], rivastigmine [Exelon], and galantamine [Razadyne ER]) improve or slow the progression of losses in cognition and memory, functional status, and behaviors. Cholinesterase inhibitors are approved by the U.S. Food and Drug Administration (FDA) for mild to moderate AD, but effectiveness may continue into the late stage. Research studies are evaluating the effectiveness of these medications in other types of dementia (Doody et al., 2003). Early assessment for dementia is crucial because cholinesterase inhibitors are most effective when started early. The nurse should encourage the client to continue with therapy, or the client will lose the cognitive gain or stability that the medication provided. He or she should remind the client and caregiver that rivastigmine and galantamine must be taken with meals. Monthly titrations are essential to avoid nausea and vomiting as the dosage of the cholinesterase inhibitor is increased. NIC/NOC Box 24.3 highlights some common nursing interventions and outcomes for a patient with AD.

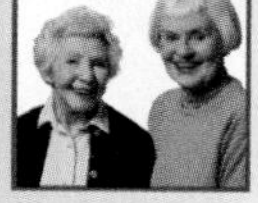

Think back to Lena and her partner, Hannah, described at the beginning of the chapter. Would cholinesterase inhibitors be appropriate for use with Hannah?

A new medication, memantine (Namenda), works on a different neurotransmitter system, the glutamate system. β-Amyloid in the Alzheimer's brain causes glutamate accumulation, with toxic effects to neurons. Memantine (Namenda) alters this process and prevents neuronal death and may be particularly effective in reducing clinical deterioration in individuals suffering from moderate to severe AD (Doody et al., 2003; Reisberg et al., 2003; Tariot et al., 2004; Winblad & Poritis 1999).

NIC/NOC Box 24.3 Alzheimer's Disease

Common NIC Labels

- Cognitive Restructuring
- Cognitive Stimulation
- Decision-Making Support
- Dementia Management
- Family Involvement Promotion
- Memory Training
- Mood Management
- Patient Rights Protection
- Reality Orientation
- Reminiscence Therapy

Common NOC Labels

- Cognitive Ability
- Cognitive Orientation
- Concentration
- Decision Making
- Distorted Thought Control
- Information Processing
- Memory

Other agents studied include NSAIDs and ginkgo biloba, neither of which has been shown effective in the treatment of mild to moderate dementia (Doody et al., 2003). Researchers currently are exploring the relationship between statin therapy and a lower incidence of AD. It is possible that statins, used for management of hypercholesterolemia, may prevent strokes leading to vascular dementia, which in turn, may play a role in the development of AD neurotoxicity.

Atypical antipsychotics have been studied for the management of AD to treat behavioral disturbances (eg, agitation, aggression, apathy, depression) that develop in the moderate to severe stages of the illness (Tariot, 2004). These medications are used as a last resort after behavioral and nonpharmacologic measures have failed. They are not FDA approved for psychosis of AD or other dementias. Research shows an increased risk for DM, cerebrovascular disease, and overall mortality (Schneider, 2006).

Nursing Care Plan 24.2 highlights the management of a client with AD and her caregiver.

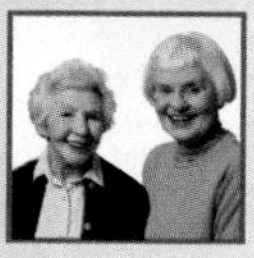

Lena is providing care to her partner, Hannah, who has AD. Suppose Lena asks, "I've heard that ginkgo biloba helps to improve memory. Would this help Hannah?" How should the nurse respond?

NURSING CARE PLAN 24.2

Clients Dealing With Dementia

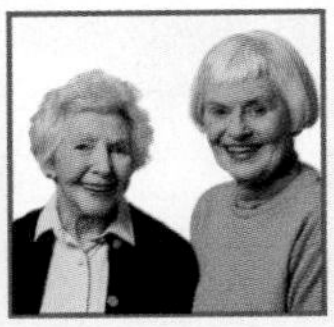

Think back to Lena, the woman caring for Hannah, her partner of 25 years who has Alzheimer's disease (AD). Lena tells the home care nurse, "I feel so frustrated sometimes, and tired. I think I'm just going to fall apart. But I can't leave Hannah."

NURSING DIAGNOSES

- **Caregiver Role Strain** related to being overwhelmed by responsibilities, fatigue, and depression
- **Risk for Injury** related to fatigue and partner's cognitive changes secondary to dementia
- **Ineffective Coping** related to demands of caring for ill partner
- **Deficient Knowledge** related to the care of a person experiencing cognitive decline

EXPECTED OUTCOMES

1. The client will experience fewer feelings of being overwhelmed.
2. The client will verbalize measures to aid in dealing with responsibilities.
3. The client will identify appropriate plans for needed relief.
4. The client and her partner will remain free of injury.
5. The client will identify appropriate methods for coping with and caring for the partner's decreasing health status.

INTERVENTIONS	RATIONALES
Assess the client's daily routine, including caregiving tasks necessary and the partner's ability to participate in care activities.	Assessment provides a baseline from which to develop an appropriate individualized plan of care. Information about the client's routine and partner's ability to participate provides clues to areas in which the family may need assistance.
Assess the client's strengths, limitations, and ability to manage caretaking activities.	Sleep deprivation, physical injury, and social isolation may occur if the client does not have the adequate resources and abilities.
Work with the client to develop a schedule of care that includes help from family and friends on a regular rotating basis.	Dividing caretaking responsibilities promotes physical endurance and emotional stability.
Develop a list of emergency contacts and their phone numbers.	An emergency contact list is important to allow for quick access to assistance in a crisis, thereby minimizing feelings of being overwhelmed.
In early stages recommend that the client and family attend to legal matters such as creating wills and preparing an advance directive. Suggest establishing *durable power of attorney* for health care, designating who may make decisions if the client becomes incompetent.	Dealing with legal matters before the client experiences severe cognitive changes is essential to ensure that the appropriate person has access to unencumbered funds and follows the partner's wishes regarding health care decisions.

Continued

NURSING CARE PLAN 24.2 ● Clients Dealing With Dementia

INTERVENTIONS	RATIONALES
Teach the client about measures to maintain partner's safety including: ● Maintaining consistency in routine ● Removing hazards, such as foot stools and small tables, from areas where the client walks, and keeping the areas well lit ● Ensuring that partner wears some type of medical alert identification ● Keeping a current photograph of the partner in the medical record	Consistency reduces confusion. Removing obstacles and slippery surfaces promotes safer ambulation. Adequate lighting reduces the risk for injury secondary to environmental hazards. Clients with AD are known to wander and not recall their current residence. Having the means to identify the client aids in search-and-rescue efforts.
Instruct the client in measures to promote partner's self-care including: ● Opening food containers and cutting food into bite-sized pieces in later stages ● Offering the partner fluids and snacks at 2-hour intervals while awake ● Ensuring scheduled toileting ● Providing partner with self-care devices such as comb and toothbrush and reviewing its use ● Modifying clothing with hook and loop fasteners or suspenders	Self-care promotes independence and self-esteem for the partner while alleviating some of the client's stress associated with caregiving. Minimal assistance facilitates self-care. Adequate fluid and food intake promotes adequate hydration and nutrition. Regular toileting reduces the potential for incontinence. Clients with AD commonly experience forgetfulness related to the names of items, their purpose, and their use. Clothing modifications promote independence in removal and donning.
Instruct the client in measures to promote communication with partner, such as using short simple explanations and directions, allowing time for the partner to answer, reducing environmental stimuli and noise, and keeping partner focused on one task at a time.	Clients with AD commonly experience problems in communication secondary to the decline in cognitive function.
Provide information about agencies that offer supportive services; initiate referral to agencies if appropriate. If necessary, arrange for additional help from a home care agency.	Additional support from outside agencies provides the client with assistance to deal with her and her partner's needs.
Assess for caregiver stress and depression	Caregivers often have difficulty balancing their personal and professional needs with caregiving demands, which can contribute to depression.

EVALUATION

1. The client seeks relief from caregiving responsibilities at least 1 or 2 days a week.
2. The client implements measures to deal with responsibilities.
3. The client and partner use appropriate measures to maintain safety.
4. The client uses appropriate strategies and techniques to deal with partner's declining health status.

DEPRESSION

According to Zerbe (1999), two thirds of women with major depression and **dysthymia** (depressed mood) remain undiagnosed (see Chap. 5). Depression often is underdiagnosed in the older population, in which it may occur as a unique syndrome, but more commonly accompanies another physical or mental disorder (Siegal et al., 2002).

Older adults with depression may have increased somatic complaints and increased risk factors for depression: female gender, disability, chronic illness, decreased financial or social resources, and past history (personal or family) of depression. Depressed mood increases the risk for dementia in elders, especially in cases of cognitive impairment (Siegal et al., 2002).

Many illnesses and chronic health conditions may cause or contribute to depression in older adults. These include neurologic problems like Parkinson's disease, stroke, and seizure disorders. Metabolic conditions like hypothyroidism and DM may cause depression in elders. Acute MI, COPD, cancer, and other systemic illnesses also may place older adults at increased risk for depression (Kurlowicz, 2002).

Assessment Findings

The most common assessment tool to evaluate depression in the elderly is the Geriatric Depression Scale (GDS) Short Form, which is a 15-item questionnaire evaluating life satisfaction, helplessness, hopelessness, and energy (Assessment Tool 24.4). A longer version is a 30-item scale, also called the GDS (Yesavage, 1988). A common mnemonic for nurses to use when assessing for depression is SIG E CAPS. These symptoms include the diagnostic criteria in the *Diagnostic and Statistical Manual of Mental Disorders* (DSM-IV-TR) (First et al., 2000):

- **S**leep
- **I**nterest
- **G**uilt
- **E**nergy
- **C**oncentration
- **A**ppetite
- **P**sychomotor changes
- **S**uicide

The elderly consume large amounts of prescriptive medications. Many pharmacologic agents may cause depression in elders (Kurlowicz, 2002). The nurse should complete a thorough medication review to determine whether any new symptoms of depression are associated with new or discontinued mediations.

It is important for nurses involved in home care or discharge planning to assess for the presence of guns in the older adult's home. Firearms have been the most successful method of suicide in both men and women (Adamek & Kaplan, 1996a, 1996b). Women who may be caring for a depressed significant other need to be counseled to have any firearms removed from the home or any location where the significant other may have access to guns.

Collaborative Management

Treatment of depression includes acute management to reverse the current episode and ongoing assessment and treatment to prevent a recurrence (Meyers, 2002). Several classifications of medications are used to treat depression. As discussed in Chapter 5, tricyclic antidepressants were used for many years; however, these medications have a higher side-effect and risk profile than the newer classes. The least anticholinergic of the tricyclics are nortriptyline (Pamelor) and desipramine (Norpramin). Clients taking these medications need to be monitored for ADRs including sedation, constipation, orthostatic hypotension, and complications of heart block (Meyers, 2002).

The SSRIs are equally effective as tricyclics, but have a lower rate of side effects and are better tolerated. This group includes escitalopram (Lexapro), citalopram (Celexa), sertraline (Zoloft), fluoxetine (Prozac), and paroxetine (Paxil). Despite a low side-effect profile, a small percentage of elders may develop hyponatremia, especially with high doses of SSRIs. Sexual dysfunction is common with this group of medications. Long-term use of SSRIs may cause weight gain. The nurse needs to be aware that SSRIs may displace warfarin (Coumadin) from protein binding sites, increasing warfarin's anticoagulant effects (Meyers, 2002).

Bupropion (Wellbutrin) is tolerated well with recommended doses and has a low risk for seizures at 0.4% (Meyers, 2002). Nevertheless, use should be avoided in older adults with an active or former seizure disorder. This is the same medication as Zyban, a smoking cessation medication. The nurse should ensure that both Wellbutrin and Zyban are not prescribed simultaneously.

Venlafaxine (Effexor) functions as an SSRI at lower doses and inhibits the reuptake of norepinephrine in higher doses, working on both neurotransmitter systems. Duloxetine (Cymbalta) targets both norepinephrine and serotonin at low doses. Venlafaxine, escitalopram, and paroxetine are three antidepressants that also have an FDA indication for generalized anxiety disorder. Mirtazapine (Remeron) is a norepinephrine antagonist. It is used frequently for depressed nursing home residents to increase appetite and weight gain.

Extreme care must be used with administration of monoamine oxidase inhibitors (MAOIs) in older women because orthostasis is a common side effect, increasing the risk for falls. Moreover, many food and drug interactions with MAOIs can cause a life-threatening hypertensive crisis. Any MAOIs used with an SSRI or meperidine (Demerol) can cause delirium, hyperthermia, and possibly a fatal serotonin syndrome (Fulginiti et al., 2000; Meyers, 2002).

● ASSESSMENT TOOL 24.4 Short Form: Geriatric Depression Scale

NAME ____________ AGE ________ SEX ________ DATE ________

WING ________ ROOM ________ PHYSICIAN ________ ASSESSOR ________

Scoring System

Answers indicating depression are highlighted. Each **bold faced** answer counts one (1) point.

1.	Are you basically satisfied with your life?	YES/**NO**
2.	Have you dropped any of your activities and interests?	**YES**/NO
3.	Do you feel that your life is empty?	**YES**/NO
4.	Do you often get bored?	**YES**/NO
5.	Are you in good spirits most of the time?	YES/**NO**
6.	Are you afraid that something bad is going to happen to you?	**YES**/NO
7.	Do you feel happy most of the time?	YES/**NO**
8.	Do you often feel helpless?	**YES**/NO
9.	Do you prefer to stay in your room/facility, rather than going out and doing new things?	**YES**/NO
10.	Do you feel you have more problems with memory than most?	**YES**/NO
11.	Do you think it is wonderful to be alive?	YES/**NO**
12.	Do you feel worthless the way you are now?	**YES**/NO
13.	Do you feel full of energy?	YES/**NO**
14.	Do you feel that your situation is hopeless?	**YES**/NO
15.	Do you think that most people are better off than you?	**YES**/NO

Score greater than 5 = Probable Depression **SCORE** ____

Notes/Current Medications: ________________

Instructions for Use:

1. Choose a quiet place, preferably the same location each time the test is administered.
2. The administration of this test should not be immediately after some mental trauma or unsteady period.
3. Speak in a soft pleasant tone.
4. Answer all questions by circling the answer (yes or no) to the question.
5. Add the total number of **BOLD FACED** answers circled and record that number in the "SCORE" box.
6. Scores totaling five (5) points or more indicate probable depression.

A 30-item version of the GDS is also available. Address inquiries regarding this scale to: Jerome A. Yesavage, M.D., Director, Psychiatric ICU, Veterans Administration Medical Center, 3801 Miranda Avenue, Palo Alto, CA 94304.

Electroconvulsive therapy has become popular in recent years. It is currently the standard treatment for late-life psychotic depression because these clients may not tolerate the doses of medications required to elicit a clinical antidepressant effect (Meyers, 2002).

PAIN

Pain is a frequent syndrome among older women with chronic health conditions. Pain often is undertreated, especially in nursing home residents who have dementia and cannot verbalize their pain. A verbally administered 0 to 10 scale is a good first choice for measuring pain intensity in most oriented older people (American Geriatrics Society, 2002). In this scenario, the clinician asks the client, "On a scale of 0 to 10, with 0 meaning no pain, and 10 meaning the worst pain possible, how much pain do you have now?" Other verbal descriptive scales, pain thermometers, and face pain scales have accepted validity for older adults; they may be more reliable for those with difficulty responding to the verbally administered 0 to 10 scale (American Geriatrics Society, 2002).

When taking the client's history for pain, the nurse should evaluate characteristics like intensity, frequency, character, location, duration, and precipitating, aggravating, and alleviating factors. The nurse should assess the level of pain within the context of the woman's functional status. He or she should document the effect of current pain on appetite, sleep, energy, mood, exercise, cognition, and sexual, social, and personal issues (Fig. 24.21). The nurse should evaluate the client's history of use of analgesics, previous and current medications, over-the-counter drugs, complementary/alternative therapies, and alcohol. He or she needs to note the effectiveness of previously tried treatments, including the client's satisfaction with current pain treatment. Clients with intact cognition can use a pain log or diary to assess intensity, use of medications, and response to treatments (American Geriatrics Society, 2002).

The physical examination for pain includes its location and any sites of pain radiation. The musculoskeletal and neurologic physical examinations must be thorough. Psychosocial evaluation includes the effects of pain on social, recreational, and occupational functioning. In clients with cognitive impairment, the nurse should assess for any new onset or exacerbation of delirium, dementia, or depression. The nurse carefully should look for nonverbal clues to pain and observe cognitively impaired clients during ambulation and transferring (Box 24.2).

Initiation of nonpharmacologic pain management can be an essential part of care. For example, referral to physical therapy and occupational therapy may be extremely helpful in preventing pain from muscular atrophy, immobility, or compromised muscle strength.

The American Geriatrics Society (2002) and the American College of Rheumatology (Schnitzer, 2002) have guidelines for pharmacologic pain management in older adults. Key recommendations include starting with acetaminophen for mild to moderate pain because of low cost, high efficacy, and low toxicity. Older adults at risk for gastrointestinal or renal complications may be prescribed cyclo-oxygenase II (COX II) inhibitors, which have less gastrointestinal toxicity than traditional NSAIDs. Guidelines also recommend opioid analgesics for severe pain or pain not controlled by NSAIDs, COX II medications, or both (American Geriatrics Society, 2002).

Chronic pain management includes avoiding the use of intermittent or "as needed" medication administration. Such delivery often leads to breakthrough pain and in-

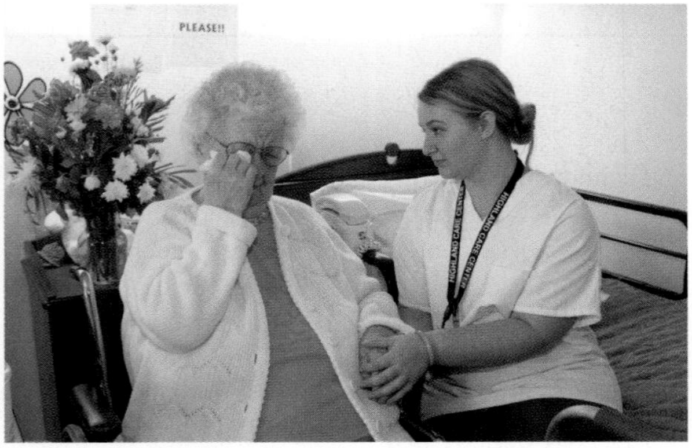

FIGURE 24.21 Discussing and documenting a client's pain and its effects are essential nursing interventions.

BOX 24.2 Common Pain Behaviors in Cognitively Impaired Elderly People

Facial Expressions
- Slight frown; sad, frightened face
- Grimacing, wrinkled forehead, closed or tightened eyes
- Any distorted expression
- Rapid blinking

Verbalizations, Vocalizations
- Sighing, moaning, groaning
- Grunting, chanting, calling out
- Noisy breathing
- Asking for help
- Verbal abuse

Body Movements
- Rigid, tense body posture, guarding
- Fidgeting
- Increased pacing, rocking
- Restricted movement
- Gait or mobility changes

Changes in Interpersonal Interactions
- Aggressive, combative, resisting care
- Decreased social interactions
- Socially inappropriate, disruptive
- Withdrawn

Changes in Activity Patterns or Routines
- Refusing food, appetite change
- Increase in rest periods
- Sleep, rest pattern changes
- Sudden cessation of common routines
- Increased wandering

Mental Status Changes
- Crying or tears
- Increased confusion
- Irritability or distress

Note some patients demonstrate little or no specific behavior associated with severe pain.

From American Geriatrics Society. (2002). Guidelines on the management of persistent pain in older persons. *Journal of the American Geriatrics Society, 50*(6), S205–S224.

adequate around-the-clock analgesia. This is especially a problem for clients with dementia or other conditions that compromise their ability to verbalize their level of pain and, in turn, receive adequate treatment.

Medications to avoid in older adults because of an increased risk for toxicity include indomethacin (Indocin), meclofenamate (Meclomen), piroxicam (Feldene), and tolmetin (Tolectin) (all NSAIDs). Opioids to avoid include meperidine (Demerol), propoxyphene (Darvon, Darvocet), and pentazocine (Talwin). Anticholinergics, especially amitriptyline (Elavil), should not be used. Because of better anticholinergic profiles, drugs with a lower anticholinergic profile (eg, desipramine [Norpramin]) are used occasionally in low doses for pain management; however, older women taking these drugs still require observation for anticholinergic side effects.

When managing pain in older adults, prevention of related constipation is an important nursing intervention. Constipation is a common side effect of opioids in older adults. A stool softener may be prescribed when initiating narcotic therapy. Another important measure is ensuring the client's safety in the environment. Sedative effects of pain medication may increase the risk for falls and confusion. Additionally, the nurse should evaluate the client for any problems with enuresis because pain medications may cause older adults to sleep through nocturnal urges to void.

The nurse assessing and reporting pain symptoms serves as a client advocate, helping to prevent suffering from undiagnosed and undertreated pain. The nurse should ensure that ongoing pain assessment, medication management, and nonpharmacologic pain management continue on a predetermined schedule, with appropriate documentation and reporting to the primary health care provider.

NURSING CARE OF THE HOMEBOUND WOMAN

Nursing agencies are the main sources of skilled nursing care for homebound older adults. The role of the home care nurse working with older women is complex, independent, and potentially rewarding. The nurse is in the unique position of assisting the woman to maximize function and maintain independence in the most desired setting: her own home. The role of the home health nurse has increased significantly in the past 20 years. Intravenous infusions, wound therapy, catheter care, and special nutritional supplementation devices are now routine home nursing interventions. The home care evaluation is vital because the nurse reports findings to the primary health care provider. Thus, the home health nurse often serves as the "telescope" for primary providers who cannot directly evaluate the home situation.

Observation of family dynamics and communication is integral to home assessment. The **primary caregiver** is a family member, significant other, or friend who assists the client to meet her functional needs. The primary caregiver can either live with the client or reside in his or her own home. In today's mobile society, the nurse often communicates from a distance with the primary caregiver or **health care proxy** (the person with medical decision-making abilities for the client if the client becomes mentally incapacitated).

The nurse should determine whether the client can accomplish ADLs with assistance from the primary caregiver. The caregiver may provide assistance with IADLs such as shopping, cooking, cleaning, laundry, and transportation for laboratory testing and physician or advanced practice nurse (APN) visits. The primary caregiver often organizes medications for the client, picks up prescriptions, pays bills, and handles other money management activities. The nurse needs to determine whether the primary caregiver's availability to assist with IADLs meets the client's functional needs.

QUOTE 24-4

"My mother had a live-in caregiver, so she was able to maintain her household. The caregiver and I really worked as a winning team. I think it made a big difference in my mother's quality of life."

A daughter talking about her now deceased mother's final years

Older women with more significant functional impairments need assistance with BADLs. Often in such cases, the primary caregiver assists with bathing, ambulating, transferring from various positions, and getting to the toilet. If the primary caregiver cannot meet these needs and the client experiences problems with personal hygiene or falls during transfers or trips to the bathroom, the client requires a higher level of nursing care (Fig. 24.22).

The nurse should connect clients lacking needed primary caregiver assistance with outside community agencies. To best do so, the nurse needs to be aware of the woman's insurance status, approximate income, and other financial resources (eg, investments, assets, retirement benefits, savings accounts, social security payments). Many community services are based on income eligibility and sliding scale status (fees charged based on the person's income). The visiting nurse needs to know whether her client has Medicare, Medical Assistance, or some other type of health care insurance because the type of reimbursement determines service eligibility (D'Angelo, 1999).

Home health nurses frequently work closely with the area Agency on Aging (AAA; call 1-800-677-1116 to find the nearest AAA). This state-based organization has chapters encompassing various counties and assigns

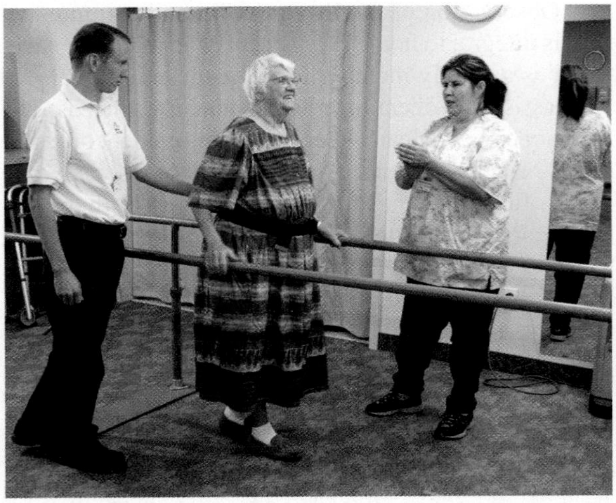

FIGURE 24.22 Clients who need assistance with ambulation, feeding, and other BADLs and who do not have adequate support from primary caregivers require a higher level of nursing intervention.

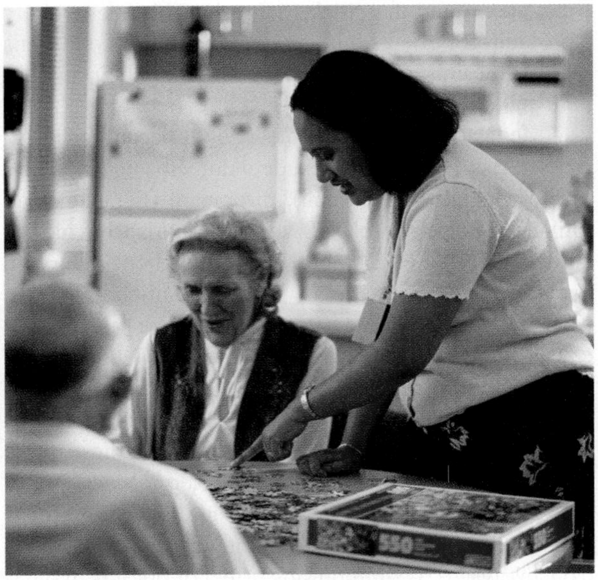

FIGURE 24.23 Senior citizen's centers provide a strong social and recreational outlet for older women and men.

case managers to clients eligible for service. These case managers connect older adults with legal and financial services. The area AAA has a Department of Adult Protective Services that investigates suspected cases of EM. Case managers also assist older adults to select alternative living arrangements. They investigate personal care homes, ALFs, and nursing home eligibility for clients who may no longer be capable of remaining at home (D'Angelo, 1999).

Other sources for community referrals include pharmacies that make home deliveries, "Meals on Wheels" or church-related food programs, and special transportation offered by the county or state (eg, wheelchair van, low-cost bus transportation to and from health care appointments). Ideally, the nurse is aware of any local optometrists, dentists, or podiatrists who make home visits. The nurse can recommend these providers to the primary health care provider or directly to families. Many states offer special visual and auditory support programs that supply adaptive devices to clients with sensory impairments. Some programs have related environmental counseling for older adults suffering from sensory deficits.

Senior citizen's centers offer historical, educational, and recreational trips, as well as specialized classes in such areas as painting, Tai Chi, and computers. The greatest advantage of senior citizen's centers is that they provide an outlet for older people to form new relationships and networks (Fig. 24.23).

Local libraries have bookmobiles. For clients with visual impairments, they supply books on audiocassette or compact disk for auditory reading enjoyment. Caregiver support groups have increased in availability and number and commonly are advertised on television bulletin boards and in local newspapers. Support groups can be general (eg, for chronic illness); there are also specific support groups, one of the most noteworthy being the Alzheimer's Association, which has local chapters in each state (www.alz.org; 1-800-272-3900). These support groups offer a network of informal support from other primary caregivers and clients suffering from illnesses.

The nurse should be aware of professional, scientifically based Internet sites related to specific disorders. Busy sons and daughters appreciate knowing where to access information on clinical illnesses or syndromes quickly. The nurse also should be familiar with local and regional health care providers who may have a special interest in AD, geriatric depression, and UI or other common conditions seen in older adults. He or she also needs to know of any gerontologic APNs, social workers, or psychologists specializing in geriatrics in the local area. The nurse can suggest consultation with such gerontologic specialists to the primary health care provider, or directly to the family members for discussion with the primary health care provider.

The home health nurse is knowledgeable regarding reputable home health product suppliers. These agencies often come to the client's home and measure for proper use of adaptive devices, such as canes, walkers, or wheelchairs. They offer emergency call systems to elderly people living alone at home. There are community programs that offer a phone check-in with elderly people living alone. These usually operate by calling the client directly; if there is no response, they will notify the predetermined next of kin or significant other. Programs offering telephone reminders for the client to take medications on time are available.

The home health nurse has a "golden" opportunity to observe family dynamics. It is important for the nurse to assess how family members are coping and assisting with loss of IADLs and ADLs in an older person. If involved with live-in or part-time caretaking, how are the primary caregivers coping? How has this task changed their family and work lives? Do the caregiver's siblings help share responsibilities? Does the primary caregiver have the physical and emotional ability, motivation, intelligence, time, and financial resources to implement and monitor the plan of care? Caregiving can be expensive and may be a financial stressor. Often, aged siblings care for a childless older woman. How is assisting the client affecting the primary caregiver's health and financial status? It is important for the nurse to assess this because he or she may be the connecting agent for financial and social assistance.

The nurse visiting the home also should assess for signs of potential caregiver burnout. Boling and Abbey (2000) note several signals: showing impatience with the cared-for person, discussing the caregiver's needs rather than the client's, and leaving the dependent person home unattended for long periods. Elder abuse, neglect, and exploitation (eg, EM) are terms commonly used to describe acts of commission or omission that result in harm or threatened harm to the health or welfare of an older adult (Flaherty et al., 2003). Risk factors for EM include cognitive impairment of the client, a family member, or both; dependency; and financial stress. Family history of substance abuse, mental illness, mental retardation, or abusive behavior also raises the risk (Fulmer, 2002). The nurse needs to privately and confidentially assess whether the older female has been hurt, hit, or sexually or financially exploited by a caregiver or other person. The nurse should be careful to follow the state laws for reporting EM through Adult Protective Services or the state agencies associated with aging services.

The nurse should assess older women for signs and symptoms of physical abuse by evaluating for weight loss, malnutrition, and dehydration. Personal hygiene may be neglected. The skin should be inspected for hematomas, bites, bruises, lacerations, or burns. Other signs of neglect include pressure ulcers, perineal rashes, and fecal impaction. Joint contractures may be present (Stiles et al., 2002). Evaluation of the potential abuser is also important; in situations of mistreatment, the abuser may appear hostile, blaming, and defensive (Welland, 2000). Signs of sexual abuse include bruises in the proximity of the sexual organs; vaginal or anal bleeding; genital infections or venereal disease; torn, bloody, or stained underwear; and reports of being raped or sexually assaulted (National Center for Elder Abuse, 2005).

NURSING CARE OF THE OLDER WOMAN IN OTHER ENVIRONMENTS

Assisted Living Facilities (ALFs) offer nursing care to older adults who need assistance with ADLs and are unsafe or uncomfortable living independently. These housing arrangements often exist within a larger health care campus. For example, a continuing care retirement community (CCRC) ensures lifetime use of various living options, such as independent apartments, ALFs (that provide help with IADLs and ADLs), and a long-term care facility (nursing home). Other examples of ALF options include high-rise or single apartment arrangements that provide some level of nursing care, but no independent apartments or long-term care facilities.

ALFs offer meals in a shared dining room (Fig. 24.24). Some ALFs also provide small kitchens in each resident's room or apartment. Transportation, cosmetology, laundry, and social and recreational activities are available in ALFs. Geriatricians and gerontologic APNs often provide primary health care and specialty services (eg, incontinence evaluation and management; geropsychiatric evaluations).

Long-term care (nursing home) facilities have different levels of nursing staff. They include nurse administrators and directors of nursing. The registered nurse assessment coordinator is responsible for data implementation into the minimum data set (MDS) form completed on people residing in long-term care facilities receiving reimbursement from Medicare, Medicaid, or both. Staff nurses are registered or licensed practical nurses that provide direct client care and oversee care given by nursing assistants. The nurses assess residents and plan their care, implement and evaluate care plans, and administer direct care, medications, and treatments (Lekan-Rutledge, 1997).

APNs working in long-term care settings include gerontologic clinical nurse specialists (CNSs), geronto-

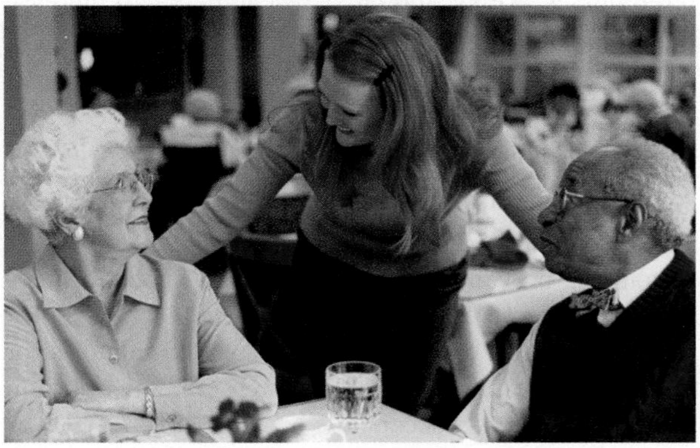

FIGURE 24.24 Shared social experiences, such as dining and recreation, are one of the strongest benefits of assisted living facilities for older clients.

logic nurse practitioners, and adult or family nurse practitioners. Wound care and ostomy nurses, continence nurse specialists, and CNSs with various specialty skills often provide nurse specialty consultation in the long-term care setting. Geropsychiatric or psychiatric clinical nurse specialists and geriatric or psychiatric nurse practitioners may be consulted in long-term care settings for management of depression and behavioral problems.

Care given in long-term care settings requires interdisciplinary collaboration. Nurses meet regularly with other team members to evaluate and make needed changes to the client's plan of care. Other team members include dieticians; physical, occupational, and speech therapists; psychologists; medical directors or attending physicians; APNs; and physician assistants. The consulting pharmacist is a valuable team member whom nurses can consult regarding medication use and drug interactions. He or she can help identify clients at high risk for ADRs. The recreational therapist is responsible for implementing socialization and structured activity programs during waking hours.

The Omnibus Budget Reconciliation Act (OBRA) of 1987 included regulatory requirements for long-term care facilities that participate in Medicare and Medicaid programs to be eligible for reimbursements. OBRA's emphasis is care outcomes. The MDS is a resident assessment form designed to facilitate ongoing outcome evaluations. The goal of OBRA was to ensure better quality of care in long-term care nursing facilities (Lekan-Rutledge, 1997).

Quality of care indicators (QI) measured on a regular basis include functional, psychosocial, nutritional, and hydration status. Other QIs include prevention of pressure ulcers, accidents, EM, infectious diseases, and UI, and appropriate medication use, especially of psychoactive drugs (Manard, 2002). The current nursing shortage has affected long-term care settings. Nurses of all education levels have the opportunity to specialize in long-term care. The need for gerontologic registered nurses, APNs, and nurse researchers will increase dramatically as the population older than 65 years doubles by 2050.

Questions to Ponder

1. How would you counsel a 55-year-old woman regarding prevention of common geriatric syndromes and ways to preserve her level of health?
2. Name several reasons why the rates of diagnosis for and treatment of dementia, depression, and delirium remain below an acceptable level of care.
3. You are an 85-year-old woman who has lived at home, in assisted living, and in a long-term nursing home setting. Describe the roles of nurses who have cared for you in each setting.

SUMMARY

- Twenty-first century nurses will care for aging baby boomers, who turn 65 in the year 2011. Demographic changes and trends affecting care of postmenopausal women include women continuing to outlive men; an unprecedented number of women older than 85 years, and a rapidly growing number of female centenarians. This translates to women living longer with one or multiple chronic illnesses.
- Data gathering and communicating with the postmenopausal woman require self-evaluation for ageist attitudes, allowing extra time for history taking, and excellent communication techniques to compensate for the deficiencies in vision, hearing, and cognition that some women experience in later years.
- Comprehensive assessment of the postmenopausal woman includes evaluation of lifestyle activities: tobacco and alcohol use, dietary and exercise patterns, and psychosocial adaptation to changes. These factors are evaluated in the context of personal and family medical history. A detailed medication history is vital because many older women experience adverse drug events that mimic common geriatric syndromes. Physiologic and physical examination findings are different from those in younger adults: all organ and body systems are affected by the aging process. The greatest indicator of the postmenopausal woman's health is her functional status, which tells the nurse of the woman's basic, instrumental, and advanced activities of daily living (ADLs). Fluctuations in ADLs often portray the cause or result of physical or mental illness, as well as cognitive decline. The social history is vital; as age or chronic illnesses increase, often the woman needs to expand utilization of her social support system. The nurse must realize sexual needs exist in women during the later phases of life and must assess and address them with respect and concern for the individual.
- Screening for osteoporosis is essential near the time of menopause because failure to identify and treat women with osteoporosis has a major impact on the quality of life during the later years. Sleep assessment is vital, as is educating the client regarding proper sleep hygiene. Postmenopausal women may be affected by hormonal changes, phase advancement, depression, anxiety, or cognitive changes, all which may alter sleep patterns and affect the woman's energy level and overall health.
- Geriatric syndromes (adverse drug events, urinary incontinence, falls, fractures, depression, and persistent pain) affect many women and have a major impact on quality of life. Unfortunately, these syndromes are often not aggressively assessed and treated. The nurse needs to understand the etiologies, thorough history, evaluation, and treatment of various types of uri-

nary incontinence: stress, urge, mixed, overflow, and functional incontinence. Falls need to be evaluated thoroughly with a specific falls history and physical evaluation across all settings. The nurse needs to identify extrinsic and intrinsic reasons for falls and use client education, exercise, physical therapy, proper footwear, and medication use. The nurse needs to use the assessment tools available for detection of delirium, depression, and dementia, as well as contributing causes. Early identification and prompt treatment of cognitive changes can reverse an acute confusional state or delay progression of a dementia like Alzheimer's disease. The nurse needs to understand the relationship of cognitive changes to functional changes for early identification and ongoing evaluation of these syndromes. Persistent pain is often underdiagnosed and undertreated. The nurse needs to assess pain thoroughly using standard pain tools and adequately document response to treatment. Cognitively impaired elderly women often present pain through nonverbal cues.

- The nurse working with elderly women must understand the levels of care that women may transition through in the later phase of their lives. Independent living with outpatient care, home care, assisted living, and long-term care offer various opportunities for nurses to work with elderly females. The nurse needs to assist the woman in planning health care and advanced directives for her later years. The nurse works with middle-aged or older women who serve as primary caregivers for parents, spouses, life partners, significant others, or siblings. It is essential that the nurse can support the caregiver–care recipient dyad to empower them as active members of the multidisciplinary health care team serving the postmenopausal female.

REVIEW QUESTIONS

1. When obtaining the health history from an older adult woman, which question would be most appropriate for the nurse to use?
   A. "Do you live with your son and daughter-in-law?"
   B. "How are you feeling today sweetie?"
   C. "What can you tell me about your shoulder pain?"
   D. "Are you having any pain right now?"
2. The nurse is assessing a 74-year-old female client's instrumental activities of daily living (IADLs). Which area should the nurse include in this assessment?
   A. Self-dressing
   B. Meal preparation
   C. Senior center activities
   D. Volunteer work
3. The nurse is preparing a presentation on osteoporosis for a local community women's group comprising women ranging in age from 50 to 75 years. As part of the presentation, the nurse should recommend that the women be screened for osteoporosis by DEXA scan at which of the following intervals?
   A. Every 6 months
   B. Every 1 to 2 years
   C. Every 3 to 4 years
   D. Every 5 to 10 years
4. When assessing an older female client, which of the following findings should the nurse consider most significant?
   A. Crackles on lung auscultation
   B. Decreased arm swing with walking
   C. Systolic blood pressure drop of 10 mm Hg on standing
   D. Decrease in forced vital capacity
5. Which of the following should the nurse need to keep in mind when administering medications to the older woman?
   A. A decrease in adipose tissue allows for an increase in the drug's duration of effect.
   B. Drug absorption is incomplete in the older adult woman, leading to erratic responses.
   C. The half-lives of drugs are shortened as a result of the decrease in renal function with age.
   D. The risk for adverse drug reactions is increased because of decreased serum albumin levels.
6. The home health care nurse arrives at the home of a 78-year-old female client who has had a surgical repair of her fractured hip. The nurse is developing a plan to reduce the client's risk for falling that focuses on extrinsic factors. Which areas should the nurse address? Select all that apply.
   A. Throw rugs in the kitchen
   B. Absence of grab bars in the shower
   C. Client's recent surgery on her hip
   D. Complaints of forgetfulness
   E. Electrical cord running across the living room
7. The physician prescribes a cholinesterase inhibitor for a woman with Alzheimer's disease (AD). Which drug should the nurse expect to administer?
   A. Memantine (Namenda)
   B. Vitamin E
   C. Donepezil (Aricept)
   D. Divalproex sodium (Depakote)
8. An older female client is diagnosed with depression and is to receive sertraline (Zoloft). The nurse teaches the client about possible side effects. Which of the following should the nurse include as most common?
   A. Sexual dysfunction
   B. Orthostasis
   C. Sedation
   D. Constipation
9. The nurse is discussing initiating pain management using medications with the family of an older adult female client with moderate pain. Which of the following should the nurse recommend?

A. Indomethacin (Indocin)
B. Piroxicam (Feldene)
C. Propoxyphene (Darvon)
D. Acetaminophen (Tylenol)

10. An 88-year-old female client is being cared for by her daughter in her daughter's home. The client has moderate dementia and needs assistance with bathing, dressing, and toileting. The daughter, a 65-year-old retired school teacher, lives with her 72-year-old husband. The husband, who had a stroke approximately 3 years ago, has some left-sided weakness and moderate osteoarthritis. The nurse making a home visit would most likely identify which nursing diagnosis as the priority?
A. Self-care deficit: bathing
B. Risk for caregiver role strain
C. Risk for injury
D. Impaired urinary elimination

REFERENCES

Adamek, M. E., & Kaplan, M. S. (1996a). Firearm suicide among older men. *Psychiatric Services, 47*(3), 304–306.

Adamek, M. E., & Kaplan, M. S. (1996b). The growing use of firearms by suicidal older women, 1979–1992: A research note. *Suicide & life-threatening behavior, 26*(1), 71–78.

American College of Rheumatology. (2000). Recommendations for the medical management of osteoarthritis of the hip and knee. *Arthritis & Rheumatism, 43,* 1905–1915.

American Geriatrics Society. (2003). *Clinical guidelines for alcohol use disorders in older adults.* Retrieved April 10, 2006, from http://www.americangeriatrics.org/products/positionpapers/alcohol.shtml.

American Geriatrics Society. (2001). Guideline for the prevention of falls in older persons. *Journal of the American Geriatrics Society, 49*(5), 667.

American Geriatrics Society. (2002). Guidelines on the management of persistent pain in older persons. *Journal of the American Geriatrics Society, 50*(6), S205–S224.

American Medical Directors Association. (2003). *Falls and fall risk.* Clinical Practice Guideline.

American Psychological Association. (2006). *Resolution on ageism.* Retrieved March 26, 2006, from http://www.apa.org/pi/aging/ageism.html.

Applegate, W. (2003). Hypertension. In *Merck manual of geriatrics on-line.* Retrieved July 10, 2003, from http://www.merck.com/pubs/mm_geriatrics/sec11/ch85.htm#ind11-085-5475.

Aronow, W. (2003). Coronary artery disease. In *Merck manual of geriatrics on-line.* Retrieved July 10, 2003, from http://www.merck.com/pubs/mm_geriatrics/sec11/ch88.htm#ind11-088-5612.

Armer, J. M., & Conn, V. S. (2001). Exploration of spirituality and health among diverse rural elderly individuals. *Journal of Gerontological Nursing, 27*(6), 28–37.

Beers, M. H., Jones, T. V., Berkwits, M., et al. (2006). Pulmonary disorders. *Merck manual of geriatrics* (2006). Retrieved March 26, 2006, from http://www.merck.com/mrkshared/mmg/home.jsp.

Berarducci, A. (2002). *Osteoporosis: Clinical issues, detection and treatment strategies.* Excel Continuing Education, Miami: American Academy of Nurse Practitioners Foundation.

Beullens, J., & Aertgeerts, B. (2004). Screening for alcohol abuse and dependence in older people using DSM criteria: A review. *Aging and Mental Health, 8*(1), 76–82.

Bloom, H., & Edelberg, H. K. (2002). Prevention. In E. L. Cobbs, E. H. Duthie, & J. B. Murphy (Eds.), *Geriatrics review syllabus: A core curriculum in geriatric medicine* (5th ed., pp. 61–67). Malden, MA: Blackwell Publishing for the American Geriatrics Society.

Boling, P. A., & Abbey, L. J. (2000). In-home assessment. In D. Osterweil, K. Brummel-Smith, & J. C. Beck (eds.), *Comprehensive geriatric assessment* (pp. 208–224). New York: McGraw-Hill.

Bonomo, R. A., & Johnson, M. A. (2004). Common infections. In C. S. Landefeld, R. M. Palmer, M. A. Johnson, C. B. Johnston, & W. L. Lyons (Eds.), *Current geriatric diagnosis and treatment* (pp. 348–358). New York: Lange Medical Books/McGraw-Hill.

Bradway, C., Hernly, S., & the NICHE Faculty. (1998). Urinary incontinence in older adults admitted to acute care. *Geriatric Nursing, 19*(2), 98–102.

Burke, M. M., & Laramie, J. A. (2000). The aging cardiovascular system. In M. M. Burke & J. A. Laramie (Eds.), *Primary care of the older adult: A multidisciplinary approach* (pp. 202–253). St. Louis: Mosby.

Buysse D. J., Reynolds C. F., III, & Monk, T. H. (1989). The Pittsburgh sleep quality index: A new instrument for psychiatric practice and research. *Psychiatric Practice and Research, 28*(2), 193–213.

Cantor, M. H., Brennan, M., & Shippy, R. A. (2004). *Caregiving among older lesbian, gay, trans-sexual and transgender New Yorkers.* New York: National Gay and Lesbian Task Force Policy Institute.

Cockcroft, D. W., & Gault, M. H. (1976). Prediction of creatinine clearance from serum creatinine. *Nephron, 16*(1), 31–41.

Cole, M. G. (2004). Delirium in elderly patients. *American Journal of Geriatric Psychiatry, 12*(1), 7–21.

Crowther, M. R., Parker, M. W., Achenbaum, W. A., Larimore, W. L., & Koenig, H. G. (2002). Rowe and Kahn's model of successful aging revisited: Positive spirituality—the forgotten factor. *Gerontologist, 42,* 613–620.

D'Angelo, A. M. (1999). Effectively managing the elderly client in the community. In. S. Zang & J. A. Allender (Eds.), *Home care of the elderly* (pp. 3–16). Philadelphia: Lippincott.

Daly, M. P. (2001). Dementia. In A. M. Adelman & M. P. Daly (Eds.), *20 Common problems in geriatrics* (pp. 237–260). New York: McGraw-Hill.

Davidson, C. W., Merrilees, M. J., Wilkinson, T. J., McKie, J. S., & Gilchrist, N. L. (2001). Hip fracture mortality and morbidity—can we do better? *New Zealand Medical Journal, 114*(1136), 329–332.

Davila, G. W. (2002). Gynecologic diseases and disorders. In E. L. Cobbs, E. H. Duthie, & J. B. Murphy (Eds.), *Geriatrics review syllabus: A core curriculum in geriatric medicine* (5th ed., pp. 350–356). Malden, MA: Blackwell Publishing for the American Geriatrics Society.

Doody, R. S., Grossberg, G. T., & Mintzer, J. E. (2003). Alzheimer's disease. Emerging non-cholinergic treatments. *Geriatrics (Supplement),* 3–15.

Dowling-Castronova, A., & Bradway, C. (2003). Urinary incontinence. In M. Mezey, T. Fulmer, I. Abraham, & D. Zwicker (Eds). *Geriatric nursing protocols for best practice* (2nd ed., pp. 83–98). New York: Springer.

DuBeau, C. E. (2002). Urinary incontinence. In E. L. Cobbs, E. H. Duthie, & J. B. Murphy (Eds.), *Geriatrics review syllabus: A core curriculum in geriatric medicine* (5th ed., pp. 139–148). Malden, MA: Blackwell Publishing for the American Geriatrics Society.

Dziewas, R., Ritter, M., Schilling, M., Konrad, C., Oelenberg, S., Nabavi, D. G., et al. (2004). Pneumonia in acute stroke patients fed by nasogastric tube. *Journal of Neurology and Neurosurgery and Psychiatry, 75,* 852–856.

Ebersole, P., & Hess, P. (2001a). Physical changes of aging. In P. Ebersole & P. Hess (Eds.), *Geriatric nursing and healthy aging* (pp. 88–105). St. Louis: Mosby.

Ebersole, P., & Hess, P. (2001b). Maintaining mobility and environmental safety. In P. Ebersole & P. Hess (Eds.), *Geriatric nursing and healthy aging* (pp. 460–479). St. Louis: Mosby.

Eliopoulos, C. (2005). *Gerontological nursing* (6th ed.). Philadelphia: Lippincott Williams & Wilkins.

Ely, E. W. (2002). Respiratory diseases and disorders. In E. L. Cobbs, E. H. Duthie, & J. B. Murphy (Eds.), *Geriatrics review syllabus: A core curriculum in geriatric medicine* (5th ed., pp. 316–321). Malden, MA: Blackwell Publishing for the American Geriatrics Society.

Ewing, J. A. (1984). Detecting alcoholism: The CAGE questionnaire. *Journal of the American Medical Association,* 252, 1905–1907.

Fantl, A., Newman, D. K., Colling, J., et al. (1996). *Urinary incontinence in adults: Acute and chronic management.* AHCPR Publication No. 96-0682. Rockville, MD: Agency for Health Care Policy and Research, U.S. Department of Health and Human Services.

Federal Interagency Forum on Aging-Related Statistics. (2000). *Older Americans 2000: Key indicators of well-being.* Federal Interagency Forum on Aging-Related Statistics. Washington, DC: U.S. Government Printing Office.

Fick, D. M., Cooper J. W., Wade, W. E., et al. (2003). Updating the Beers criteria for potentially inappropriate medication use in older adults. *Archives of Internal Medicine, 163*(22), 2716–2724.

First, M. B., Frances, A., & Pincus, H. A. (2000). *DSM-IV-TR handbook of differential diagnosis.* Arlington, VA: American Psychiatric Publishing.

Flaherty, E., Fulmer, T. T., & Mezey, M. (Eds.) (2003). *Geriatric nursing review syllabus.* New York: American Geriatrics Society.

Fletcher, K. R. (1999). Physical and laboratory assessment. In J. K. Stone, J. F. Wyman & S. A. Salisbury (Eds.), *Clinical gerontological nursing. A guide to advanced practice* (pp. 85–111). Philadelphia: W. B. Saunders.

Fletcher, P. C., & Hirdes, J. P. (2004). Restriction in activity associated with fear of falling among community-based seniors using home care services. *Age and Ageing, 33*(3), 273–279.

Folstein, M. F., Folstein, S., & McHugh, P. R. (1975). Mini-mental state, MMSE: A practical method for grading the cognitive state of patients for clinicians. *Journal of Psychiatric Research, 12*(3), 189–198.

Fulginiti, T. P., Messer, P. S., & Musolf Neri, L. (2000). *Handbook of geriatric drug therapy:* Springhouse, PA: Springhouse Corporation.

Fulmer, T. (2002). Elder mistreatment. In E. L. Cobbs, E. H. Duthie, & J. B. Murphy (Eds.), *Geriatrics review syllabus: A core curriculum in geriatric medicine* (5th ed., pp. 54–60). Malden, MA: Blackwell Publishing for the American Geriatrics Society.

Gentili, A., Kuno, H., & Mulligan, T. (2002). Disorders of sexual function. In E. L. Cobbs, E. H. Duthie, & J. B. Murphy (eds.), *Geriatrics review syllabus: A core curriculum in geriatric medicine* (5th ed., pp. 356–362). Malden, MA: Blackwell Publishing for the American Geriatrics Society.

Gill, T. M. (2002). Assessment: Approach to the elderly patient. In E. L. Cobbs, E. H. Duthie, & J. B. Murphy (Eds.), *Geriatrics review syllabus: A core curriculum in geriatric medicine* (5th ed., pp. 49–53). Malden, MA: Blackwell Publishing for the American Geriatrics Society.

Goldstein, M. K., Sachs, G. A., & Mouton, C. P. (2003). Health screening decisions for older adults: AGS position paper. *Journal of the American Geriatrics Society, 51*(2), 270–271.

Gravenstein, S., & Davidson, H. E. (2001). *A pocket guide to dementia and associated behavioral symptoms.* Norfolk, VA: Insight Therapeutics LLC.

Gray-Miceli, D., Johnson, J., & Strumpf, N. (2005). A stepwise approach to a comprehensive post-fall assessment. *Annals of Long-Term Care: Clinical Care and Aging, 13*(12), 16–24.

Hill-O'Neill, K. A., & Shaughnessy, M. (2002). Dizziness and stroke. In V. T. Cotter & N. E. Strumpf (Eds.), *Advanced practice nursing with older adults* (pp. 163–181). New York: McGraw-Hill.

Inouye, S. K. (1998). Delirium in hospitalized older patients: Recognition and risk factors. *Journal of Geriatric Psychiatry and Neurology, 11,* 118–125.

Inouye, S. K., Peduzzi, P. N., & Robinson, J. T. (1998). Importance of functional measures in predicting mortality among older hospitalized patients. *Journal of the American Medical Association, 279*(15), 1197–1193.

Inouye, S. K., Van Dyck, C. H., Alessi, C. A., Balkin, S., Siegal, A. P., & Horwitz, R. I. (1990). Clarifying confusion: The confusion assessment method. A new method for detection of delirium. *Annals of Internal Medicine, 113,* 941–948.

Jensen, G. L., & Powers, J. S. (2002). Malnutrition. In E. L. Cobbs, E. H. Duthie, & J. B. Murphy (Eds.), *Geriatrics review syllabus: A core curriculum in geriatric medicine* (5th ed., pp. 191–198). Malden, MA: Blackwell Publishing for the American Geriatrics Society.

Jerrard, J. (2006). Eliminate elderspeak and restore dignity. *Caring for the Ages, 14.*

Jones, C. J., Rikli, R. E., & Beam, W. C. (1999). A 30-s chair-stand test as a measure of lower body strength in community-residing older adults. *Research Quarterly Exercise and Sport, 70*(2), 113–119.

Kane, R. L., Ouslander, J. G., & Abrass, I. B. (2004). *Essentials of clinical geriatrics.* New York: McGraw-Hill.

Kaye, J., & Camicioli, R. (2000). Dementia. In D. Osterweil, K. Brummel-Smith & J. C. Beck (Eds.), *Comprehensive geriatric assessment* (pp. 507–554). St. Louis: McGraw-Hill.

Keysor, J., & Jette, A. (2001). Have we oversold the benefit of late-life exercise? *Journal of Gerontology Medical Sciences, 65*(7), 412–423.

Kiel, B. P. (2002). Falls. In E. L. Cobbs, E. H. Duthie, & J. B. Murphy (Eds.), *Geriatrics review syllabus: A core curriculum in geriatric medicine* (5th ed., pp. 148–149). Malden, MA: Blackwell Publishing for the American Geriatrics Society.

Knopman, D. S., DeKosky, S. T., & Cummings, J. L. (2001). The practice parameter diagnosis of dementia and evidence based review. *Neurology, 56,* 1143–1153.

Kurlowicz, L. H. (2002). Delirium and depression. In V. T. Cotter & N. E. Strumpf, *Advanced practice nursing with older adults* (pp. 141–162). New York: McGraw-Hill.

Laurila, J. V., Pitkala, K. H., Strandberg, T. E., & Tilvis, R. S. (2004). Impact of different diagnostic criteria on prognosis of delirium: A prospective study. *Dementia and Geriatric Cognitive Disorders, 18*(3–4), 240–244.

Lekan-Rutledge, D. (1997). Gerontological nursing in long-term care facilities. In M. A. Matteson, E. S. McConnell, & A. D. Linton (Eds.), *Gerontological nursing concepts and practice* (2nd ed., pp. 930–965). Philadelphia: W. B. Saunders.

Linton, A. D. (1997). Age-related changes in the gastrointestinal system. In M. A. Matteson, E. S. McConnell, & A. D. Linton (Eds.), *Gerontological nursing concepts and practice* (2nd ed., pp. 316–335). Philadelphia: W. B. Saunders.

Lipsitz, L. A. (2003). Syncope. In *Merck manual of geriatrics on-line.* Retrieved July 10, 2003, from http://www.merck.com/pubs/mm_geriatrics/sec2/ch18.htm#ind02-018-1155.

Lugo-Amador, N. M. (2004). Heat-related illness. *Emergency Medicine Clinics of North America, 22* (2), 315–327.

Manard, B. (2002). *Nursing home quality indicators: Their uses and limitations.* Washington, DC: AARP Policy Institute. Retrieved March 27, 2006, from http://assets.aarp.org/rgcenter/health/2002_16_homes.pdf.

Mathias, S., Nayak, U. S. L., & Isaacs, B. (1986). Balance in elderly patients: The "get up and go" test. *Archives of Physical Medicine Rehabilitation 67,* 387–389.

Meyers, B. S. (2002). Depression and other mood disorders. In E. L. Cobbs, E. H. Duthie, & J. B. Murphy (Eds.), *Geriatrics review syllabus: A core curriculum in geriatric medicine* (5th ed., pp. 219–227). Malden, MA: Blackwell Publishing for the American Geriatrics Society.

Meyyazhagan, S., & Messinger-Rapport, B. J. (2004). Hypertension. In C. S. Landefeld, R. M. Palmer, M. A. Johnson, C. B. Johnston, & W. L. Lyons. *Current geriatric diagnosis and treatment* (pp. 183–190). New York: Lange Medical Books/McGraw-Hill.

Michocki, R. J. (2001). Polypharmacy and principles of drug therapy. In A. M. Adelman & M. T. Daly (Eds.), *20 Common problems in geriatrics* (pp. 69–81). New York: McGraw-Hill.

Miller, C. A. (2004). *Nursing for wellness in older adults. Theory and practice* (4th ed.). Philadelphia: Lippincott Williams & Wilkins.

Naegle, M. A. (2003). Alcohol use screening and instrument. Retrieved March 27, 2006, from http://72.14.203.104/search?q=cache:ocpphqQ02KMJ:www.hartfordign.org/publications/trythis/issue17.pdf+geriatric+version+of+Michigan+screening+alcohol+test&hl=en&gl=us&ct=clnk&cd=1.

National Center on Elder Abuse. (2005). Sexual abuse. Retrieved March 25, 2006, from http://www.elderabusecenter.org/default.cfm?p=basics.cfm.

National Institute of Diabetes and Digestive and Kidney Diseases. (1997). *Your daily bladder diary.* Bethesda, MD: National Kidney and Urologic Diseases Information Clearinghouse, National Institutes of Health.

National Osteoporosis Foundation. (2003). *Clinical guidelines.* Retrieved July 10, 2003, from http://www.nof.org.

Newman, D. K., & Palmer, M. H. (Eds.) (2003). The state of the science on urinary incontinence. *American Journal of Nursing, 3,* 1–58.

Old, J. L., & Calvert, M. (2004). Vertebral compression fractures in the elderly. *American Family Physician, 69*(1), 111–119.

Ouslander, J. G. (2000). Urinary incontinence. In D. Osterweil, K. Brummel-Smith & J. C. Beck (Eds.), *Comprehensive geriatric assessment* (pp. 555–572). New York: McGraw-Hill.

Podsiadlo, D., & Richardson, S. (1991). The timed "Up and Go": A test of basic functional mobility for frail elderly persons. *Journal of the American Geriatrics Society, 38,* 142–148.

Prestwood, K. M. (2002). Osteoporosis and osteomalacia. In E. L. Cobbs, E. H. Duthie, & J. B. Murphy (Eds.), *Geriatrics review syllabus: A core curriculum in geriatric medicine* (5th ed., pp. 181–190). Malden, MA: Blackwell Publishing for the American Geriatrics Society.

Redberg, R. R., & Shaw, L. J. (2003). Diagnosis of coronary artery disease in women. *Progress in Cardiovascular Diseases, 46*(3), 239–258.

Reisberg, B., Doody, R., Stoffler, A., Schmitt, F., Ferris, S., Mobius, H. J., & the Memantine Study Group (2003). Memantine in moderate to severe Alzheimer's disease. *New England Journal of Medicine, 348,* 1333–1341.

Resnick, B. (2004). Research review: Prevention of hip fractures by external hip protectors: A randomized controlled trial. *Geriatric Nursing, 25*(3), 184–185.

Reuben, D. B. (2000). Multidimensional assessment in the community. In D. Osterweil, K. Brummel-Smith, & J. C. Beck (Eds.), *Comprehensive geriatric assessment* (pp. 173–186). New York: McGraw-Hill.

Rosen, C. J. (2005). Postmenopausal osteoporosis. *New England Journal of Medicine, 353,* 595–603.

Schmidt Luggen, A. (2006). Alcohol and the older adult: The good, the bad and the risky. *Advance for Nurse Practitioners, 14*(1), 47–52.

Schneider, L. S. (2006). Efficacy and adverse effects of atypical antipsychotics for dementia: Meta-analysis of randomized, placebo-controlled trials. *American Journal of Geriatric Psychiatry, 14*(3), 191–210.

Schnitzer, T. J. (2002). Update of ACR guidelines for osteoarthritis: Role of the coxibs. *Journal of Pain and Symptom Management, 23*(4), S24–30, S31–4.

Semla, T. P., & Rochon, P. A. (2002). Pharmacotherapy. In E. L. Cobbs, E. H. Duthie, & J. B. Murphy (Eds.), *Geriatrics review syllabus: A core curriculum in geriatric medicine* (5th ed., pp. 37–44). Malden, MA: Blackwell Publishing for the American Geriatrics Society.

Siegal, A. P., Kennedy, G. J., & Alexopoulos, G. S. (2002). Compendium on issues in geriatric depression. *Clinical Geriatrics.* Plainsboro, NJ: MultiMedia Health Care/Freedom, LLC.

Small, G. W. (2002). Dementia. In E. L. Cobbs, E. H. Duthie, & J. B. Murphy (Eds.), *Geriatrics review syllabus: A core curriculum in geriatric medicine* (5th ed., pp. 117–124). Malden, MA: Blackwell Publishing for the American Geriatrics Society.

Society for Women's Health Research. (2004). Report findings affirm health of women hinges on reform of clinical research. Retrieved August 11, 2004, from http://www.eurekalert.org.

Srinivasan, R., Tutuian R., Schoenfeld, P., et al. (2004). Profile of GERD in the adult population of a northeast urban community. *Journal of Clinical Gastroenterology, 38*(8), 651–657.

Stiles, M. M., Koren, C., & Walsh, K. (2002). Identifying elder abuse in the primary care setting. *Clinical Geriatrics, 10*(7), 33–41.

Tariot, P. N. (2004). Clinical effectiveness of atypical antipsychotics in dementia. *Journal of Clinical Psychiatry, 65*(S11), 3–4.

Tariot, P. N., Farlow, M. R., Grossberg, G. T., Graham, S. M., McDonald, S., & Gergel, I. (2004). Memantine treatment in patients with moderate to severe Alzheimer disease already receiving donepezil. *Journal of the American Medical Association, 291*(3), 317–324.

Tideiksaar, R. (2002). Clinical assessment and evaluation. In R. Tideiksaar (Ed.), *Falls in older people: prevention and management* (3rd ed, pp. 41–57). Baltimore: Health Professions Press, Inc.

Tinetti, M. (2003). Preventing falls in elderly persons. *New England Journal of Medicine, 348*(1) 42–49.

Triadafilopoulos, G. (2002). Gastrointestinal diseases and disorders. In E. L. Cobbs, E. H. Duthie, & J. B. Murphy (Eds.), *Geriatrics review syllabus: A core curriculum in geriatric medicine* (5th ed., pp. 327–331). Mahen, MA: Blackwell Publishing for the American Geriatrics Society.

Tsang, W. W., & Hui-Chan, C. W. (2004). Effect of 4- and 8-week intensive Tai Chi training on balance control in the elderly. *Medicine and Science in Sports and Exercise, 36*(4), 648–657.

U.S. Census Bureau. (2002). *Demographic trends in the 20th century* (Census 2000 Special Reports, Series CENSR-4). Washington, DC: U.S. Government Printing Office.

U.S. Department of Health and Human Services Administration on Aging (Online) (USDHHS-AoA). (2004). *A profile of older Americans.* Retrieved March 27, 2006, from http://www.aoa.gov/prof/Statistics/profile/2004/2004profile.doc.

Vanderbilt University Medical Center. (2004). Brain dysfunction in critically ill patients. Retrieved August 12, 2004, from http://www.icudelirium.org.

Volpato, S., Leveille, S. G., Blaum, C., Fried, L. P., & Guralnik, J. M. (2005). Risk factors for falls in older disabled women with diabetes: The Women's Health and Aging study. *Journal of Gerontology: Medical Sciences, 60A,* 1539–1545.

Weiss, B. D. (2001). Urinary incontinence. In A. M. Adelman & M. P. Daly (Eds.), *Common problems in geriatrics* (pp. 85–115). New York: McGraw-Hill.

Welland, D. (2000). Abuse of older persons: An overview. *Holistic Nursing Practices, 14*(4), 40–50.

Winblad, B., & Poritis, N. (1999). Memantine in severe dementia: Results of the M-best study (benefit and efficacy in severely demented patients during treatment with memantine). *International Journal of Geriatric Psychiatry, 14,* 135–146.

Wyman, J. F. (1999). Urinary incontinence. In J. T. Stone, J. F. Wyman, & S. A. Salisbury (Eds.), *Gerontological nursing: A guide to advanced practice* (pp. 203–235). Philadelphia: W. B. Saunders.

Wyman, J. F. (2003). Treatment of urinary incontinence in men and older women. *American Journal of Nursing, 3*(Suppl.), 26–35.

Wyman, J. F. (2004). Stress urinary incontinence: An update. *American Journal for Nurse Practitioners,* Special supplement, May.

Yesavage, J. A. (1988). Geriatric depression scale. *Psychopharmacology Bulletin, 24,* 709.

Yurkow, J., & Yudin, J. (2002). Musculoskeletal problems. In V. Cotter & N. Strumpf (Eds.), *Advanced practice nursing with older adults* (pp. 229–283). New York: McGraw-Hill.

Zerbe, K. J. (1999). *Mental health in primary care.* Philadelphia: W. B. Saunders.

APPENDIX A

Women's Health and Emergency/ Disaster Preparedness

Lisa Bernardo

Disasters are situations that (1) disrupt essential services such as housing, transportation, communications, sanitation, water, and health care; (2) require responses from people outside the affected community; and (3) pose unforeseen, serious, and immediate public health threats (Gebbie & Qureshi, 2002). They can be natural or man-made.

Natural disasters result from ecological threats or disruptions that exceed the adjustment capacity of the affected community (Lechat, 1979). Examples include large fires or floods, hurricanes, and earthquakes. Natural disasters can lead to mass casualties and epidemics, potentially involving entire regions. Related health concerns involve obtaining shelter, food, and clothing; controlling the spread of diseases; and treating injuries.

Man-made disasters are clearly caused by human action. Examples include war, armed conflict, overwhelming environmental contamination, and significant technological catastrophe. Mass casualties, epidemics, quarantines, or decontaminations can result. Man-made disasters can involve nuclear, biologic, or chemical agents. *Terrorism,* a form of man-made disaster, involves the tactical use of efficient, highly lethal weapons for strategic purposes (Maniscalco & Christen, 2001). It aims to accomplish objectives through violence and may rely on radiologic, biologic, chemical, or explosive weaponry. Usually, women and children are not specifically the targets of man-made disasters. They can be involved, however, as members of an affected community or as a consequence of actions by others.

GENERAL EMERGENCY PREPAREDNESS FOR PREGNANT WOMEN AND CHILDREN

The recent devastation left by the Asian tsunami and Hurricane Katrina serve as grim reminders of the need for not only preparedness but also recovery and long-term rebuilding (Homeland Security Council, 2006). *Emergency preparedness* means the planning for materials and responses needed in an unexpected event. Numerous agencies have recommendations (Appendix Table 1).

Emergency preparedness should be part of every family's home (Appendix Table 2). Pregnant women should incorporate their own special needs when planning for emergencies. Women go into labor, babies are born, and life events continue despite public health crises.

Nurses, midwives, nurse practitioners, and women's health experts can collaborate with community agencies to prepare hospitals, shelters, and other venues for the needs of pregnant and lactating women, newborns, and families. These professionals draw on their knowledge, skills, and abilities to provide safe passage for families during dire circumstances using minimal interventions to achieve positive outcomes (Keeney, 2004a). They are adept at addressing public health issues related to women and children (Keeney, 2004b).

APPENDIX TABLE 1 Agencies and Websites for Emergency Preparedness Information

AGENCY	WEBSITE
American Academy of Pediatrics	www.aap.org
Association of Maternal and Child Health Programs	www.amchp.org
American Red Cross	www.arc.org
Emergency Medical Services for Children	www.ems-c.org
Federal Emergency Management Agency	www.fema.gov/kids/
Maternal-Child Health Bureau	www.mch.gov
Office of Homeland Security	www.ready.gov
International Committee of the Red Cross	www.icrc.org
International Federation of Red Cross and Red Crescent Societies	www.ifrc.org
International Critical Incident Stress Foundation	www.icisf.org
National Center for Post Traumatic Stress Disorder	www.ncptsd.org
Doulas of North America	www.dona.org
National Center for Pediatric Emergency Preparedness	www.ncdp.mailman.columbia.edu/program_**pediatric**.htm
Metropolitan Medical Response System	www.mmrs.fema.gov

APPENDIX TABLE 2 Example of an Emergency Preparedness Plan Checklist

Emergency Phone Numbers:

Police__________ **Fire**__________ **EMS**__________ **Poison Control**__________

Utility Phone Numbers:

Gas__________ **Electric**__________ **Water/sewage**__________

Physician Phone Numbers:

Primary Care Physician__________ **Pediatrician**__________ **Obstetrician**__________

GENERAL HOUSEHOLD	YES	NO	SUGGESTIONS
I have three meeting places where I could meet my family should we become separated: (1) one near my home, such as a neighbor's; (2) one 1 to 2 miles away in case it is not safe to return home; (3) one 3 or more miles away should I need to evacuate my neighborhood.			
I and all my family members have the phone number of an out of area or out of state relative whom we can call to give information of our whereabouts.			
I know the location of and how to use the shut off valves for water, gas, and electricity.			
My homeowner's or renter's insurance policy is up to date and consistent with disasters common in my geographic location (e.g., floods).			
I have some cash or traveler's checks in my home, should I need to evacuate.			
I have a resource with whom I could leave my pet(s) should I need to evacuate to a shelter.			
Special arrangements have been made for people in my home with disabilities.			
Special arrangements have been made for children or elderly in my home who may need care if I am required to stay at work.			
Emergency Supply Kit			
I have a disaster supply kit that contains food, water, and essential supplies for at least 3 days.			
I have extra food and water should I be confined to home for up to 2 weeks (pregnant women and newborns need double the water of adults).			

Continued

APPENDIX TABLE 2 Example of an Emergency Preparedness Plan Checklist

GENERAL HOUSEHOLD	YES	NO	SUGGESTIONS
I have a small emergency preparedness supply kit in my car that also includes flares, jumper cables, and seasonal supplies.			
I have food and water for my pet(s).			
I have foods for people in my home with special dietary needs, such as formula, baby foods, etc.			
I have prescription medication for storage (check with a physician for samples or contact the pharmacist for shelf life).			
I have extra supplies for contact lens care, hearing aids, etc.			
I have additional supplies for newborns, infants, and young children such as a breast pump, diapers, clothing, comfort toys, clothing, etc.			
I have a non-prescription emergency drug supply in my disaster kit that includes			
● Aspirin and non-aspirin pain reliever			
● Antidiarrhea medication			
● Antacid			
● Laxative			
● Vitamins (prenatal vitamins)			
I have a non-prescription emergency drug supply in my disaster kit for infants and children:			
● Infant acetaminophen			
● Child acetaminophen			
● Child ibuprofen			
● Vitamins			
Emergency Supplies			
I have a the following available in my home:			
Portable, battery-powered radio or TV and extra batteries			
Flashlight and extra batteries			
Matches in a waterproof container			
Duct tape/scissors			
Plastic sheeting			
Whistle			
Small canister, A-B-C type fire extinguisher			
Leather work gloves			
Paper, pens, and pencils			
Battery-operated travel alarm clock			
I have the following kitchen items:			
Manual can opener			
Mess kits or paper cups, plates, and plastic utensils			
All-purpose knife			
Household liquid bleach to treat drinking water and disinfect items			
Sugar, salt, pepper			
Aluminum foil and plastic wrap			
Re-sealing plastic bags			
Small cooking stove with extra fuel			
Moist hand wipes			
I have the following clothes for myself (and for children or elderly, if applicable):			
Jacket or coat			
Long pants			

Continued

● **APPENDIX TABLE 2** **Example of an Emergency Preparedness Plan Checklist *(Continued)***

GENERAL HOUSEHOLD	YES	NO	SUGGESTIONS
Long sleeve shirt			
Sturdy shoes			
Hat and gloves			
Sleeping bag			
I have the following sanitation supplies:			
Toilet paper			
Personal hygiene (toothbrush, toothpaste, soap)			
Feminine supplies			
Plastic garbage bags			
Plastic bucket with tight lid			
Other items you would add to your list?			
___			
___			
___			
___			
___			

During an emergency response, maintaining family integrity is of utmost importance. In shelters and designated relief areas, pregnant and nursing women, children, and their families should be kept together in a warm, safe space. Using evidence-based interventions to promote bonding (e.g., kangaroo care, infant sucking, skin-to-skin contact) can reduce stress for the mother and promote security for the infant (White-Traut, 2004).

Should a public health emergency require mass public immunization, pregnant women and children reporting to the clinic should receive the same standard of care as others. Clinic personnel should refer women identifying themselves as pregnant to the Pregnant Station, where such clients will be asked the names of their obstetric providers and given counseling (Votava, 2003). Sometimes, recommended chemoprophylaxis following a biologic exposure will not be administered to pregnant women because of potential teratogenic effects or because the substance is not licensed for use in pregnancy. Pregnant women may have to forgo prophylaxis or treatment and continue through the clinic to receive treatment for other children and relatives. Thus, any plans for chemoprophylaxis must address specific guidelines for the appropriate treatment of pregnant women (Jamieson et al., 2005).

SPECIFIC THREATS TO PREGNANT WOMEN AND CHILDREN AND APPROPRIATE RESPONSES

Little is known about how potential bioterrorist agents may affect pregnant women and fetuses. During uncertain times, women may have questions related to information they hear from news reports and other sources. Nurses, midwives, and women's health experts should be prepared to answer questions honestly and to the best of their abilities, relative to the information available. The Centers for Disease Control and Prevention (CDC, www.cdc.gov) have the most current information on bioterrorism and other public health emergencies. Obstetricians and other practitioners should understand the process or procedure for reporting suspicious disease presentations, in both inpatient and outpatient settings, to proper state and federal health authorities (Jamieson et al., 2004).

Nuclear and Radiologic Agents

Release of nuclear and radiologic materials can be intentional or unintentional. A *simple radiological device* releases radioactive material in a highly populated area (e.g., sports arena, airport, train station) to irradiate humans (Edsall, 2003). A *radiological dispersal device* releases radioactive material through an explosive in a populated area; the affected people and first responders sustain physical trauma and radiation exposure (Edsall, 2003). A *nuclear reactor sabotage,* though highly unlikely, could occur through the disabling of a nuclear reactor's cooling system (Edsall, 2003). An *improvised nuclear device* is the detonation of a homemade "bomb" to release substantial radiation (weapons grade plutonium or uranium) with subsequent fallout (Edsall, 2003). The detonation of a *nuclear weapon,* while extremely remote, would cause high mortality and long-term radiation contamination.

Radioactive materials enter the body through inhalation, ingestion, absorption, or puncture/injection (open wounds or cuts) (Office for Domestic Preparedness, 2005). Irradiation occurs through exposure, contamination, and incorporation.

- With *exposure,* the body is exposed to radiation; while the person can be seriously injured, he or she is **neither radioactive nor contaminated** and can be treated according to the severity of the problem (Edsall, 2003; Office for Domestic Preparedness, 2005). Exposure is similar to receiving X-rays or solar energy (Office for Domestic Preparedness, 2005). No decontamination is necessary.
- *Contamination* can be internal or external. With *internal contamination,* a person inhales, ingests, or absorbs solid, liquid, or gas radiation particles (Edsall, 2003). With *external contamination,* a person comes into contact with solid or liquid radioactive materials in the atmosphere, contaminating their exposed skin surfaces and clothes (Edsall, 2003; Office for Domestic Preparedness, 2005). External exposure to the radiation continues for as long as the person remains in contact with the radioactive material (Office for Domestic Preparedness, 2005). Removal of affected clothing results in 90% decontamination (Jarrett, 1999; Walter, 2005). The person rarely has enough radioactive material on the body to create a dangerous situation for responders (Office for Domestic Preparedness, 2005).
- *Incorporation* is uptake of radioactive material into organs, tissues, and cells (Edsall, 2003; Office for Domestic Preparedness, 2005). It occurs only with internal contamination (Edsall, 2003). The person with incorporation presents a minimal risk to responders, but he or she also may be externally contaminated (Office for Domestic Preparedness, 2005).

A dose of radiation is measured as a rad (radiation absorbed dose) and defined as the deposition of 0.01 joule of energy in one kilogram of tissue (Edsall, 2003). The Gray (Gy) unit is an international measuring system whereby 100 rad equals 1 Gy (Edsall, 2003). Gray units (Gy) measure radiation doses and identify cellular response to radiation exposure; such response is either an early or late effect (Skorga et al., 2003).

Radiation illness depends on the radiation dose involved, as well as the affected person's pre-existing health, age, and sex (Skorga et al., 2003). Children, older adults, men, and people with chronic illness are more likely to have negative outcomes following high-dose radiation (Skorga et al., 2003). Long-term effects of high-dose radiation include amenorrhea, sterility, disturbances in blood cell formation, cataracts, premature aging, and cancer (Skorga et al., 2003). Tissues and organs especially sensitive to radiation include lymph tissue, bone marrow, skin, intestines, kidneys, and reproductive organs (Skorga et al., 2003). Leukemia and cancers of the skin, breast, lung, and thyroid are common outcomes (Skorga et al., 2003).

Radioactive materials affect the growing fetus. Pregnant women may ingest radioactive nuclides, such as those emitted from nuclear power plants, through food and water (Mangano et al., 2003). Inside the body, these nuclides release alpha, beta, and gamma radiation, causing damage to developing fetal cells (Mangano et al., 2003). When damaged cells cannot repair themselves, malignancy may result. Mangano et al. (2003) conducted an epidemiologic study on cancer incidence in children residing near 103 operating U.S. nuclear reactors. Findings suggest that 11% of cancers in those participants younger than 10 years are linked to radioactive emissions. Further study is needed to determine additional contributing factors.

Exposure to radiation from diagnostic tests or occupational exposures within regulatory limits will not cause untoward fetal health effects (CDC, 2005a). Exposure following bioterrorism, however, may pose maternal and fetal health hazards. The CDC (2005a) stratify health outcomes following radiation during blastogenesis, organogenesis, and fetogenesis. For instance, an acute radiation dose less than 0.05 Gy (5 rads) has no detectable noncancer health effects to organisms in any stage of development. An exposure of 0.05 to 0.5 Gy (5–50 rads) results in a slightly increased risk of major malformations and growth retardation during organogenesis and possible growth retardation, reduced IQ, and severe mental retardation during fetogenesis (CDC, 2005a). A radiation dosage above 0.50 Gy (50 rads) can cause acute radiation syndrome in the mother, depending on the whole-body dose. Fetal outcomes such as major malformations, neurologic and motor deficiencies, growth retardation, reduced IQ, severe mental retardation, and growth retardation are likely (CDC, 2005a). Miscarriage also is a possibility. Therefore, any pregnant woman exposed to more than 0.25 Gy of radiation should also have the fetal dose estimated (Waselenko et al., 2004). The fetal radiation dose may be lower, except in cases of radioiodine exposure, because the fetal thyroid gland uptakes more iodine than the adult thyroid gland (Waselenko et al., 2004). While the lifetime cancer risks from prenatal radiation exposure are unknown, the CDC (2005a) suggest that they are probably slightly higher than such risks from radiation exposure in childhood.

Treatment

Geiger counters are used to detect radioactive contamination or radiologic materials. Dose-rate meters measure the level of exposure to ionizing radiation.

Advanced life support protocols always take precedence over radiation concerns. In cases of external and internal contamination, EMS personnel must wear protective clothing and gloves, in accordance with agency policies and procedures; when entering highly contaminated areas, they must wear respirators. They can perform surface decontamination in cases in which the affected person has no or minimal physical injuries; in cases of life-threatening injuries, the client must be stabilized before responders perform surface decontamination (Mettler & Voelz, 2002).

The best treatment for the fetus is to care for the mother. Pregnant women should receive the same treatment as nonpregnant women (Waselenko et al., 2004). A health physicist and maternal-fetal specialist should be consulted; risks and benefits of any therapy should be carefully explained to the woman prior to initiation (Waselenko et al., 2004). Understandably, pregnant women will require special counseling to facilitate coping (CDC, 2005b).

Protecting the thyroid from radioiodine exposure is critical for pregnant women and children. Prior to or following exposure to radioiodine, potassium iodide (KI) should be administered to prevent absorption of radioactive iodine and thus prevent thyroid cancer (Skorga et al., 2003). The fetal thyroid gland usually does not begin to function until the 12th week of gestation (Waselenko et al., 2004). Pregnant women in their second and third trimesters should receive KI to protect both the maternal and fetal thyroids (Waselenko et al., 2004). Note that KI protects against exposure *only* to Iodine 131; it does *not* protect against other types of radiation.

Many states have distributed KI tablets to residents living within 10 miles of their nuclear power plants. KI is prepared in tablets, making it easy to store. To be effective, a person must take KI shortly before or within several hours of exposure (Mettler & Voelz, 2002). State health department officials would announce when residents should take KI tablets in the event of a community emergency.

Infants and young children cannot swallow tablets. When dissolved in water, the fluid of KI is too salty to drink (Food and Drug Administration, 2002). To disguise the taste, parents can crush and mix the tablet with raspberry syrup, low-fat chocolate milk, orange juice, or flat soda (cola) (Pelsor et al., 2002). Nurses or parents can crush one 130-mg KI tablet into small pieces, add 4 teaspoonfuls of water, and then add 4 teaspoons of one of the aforementioned fluids (Food and Drug Administration, 2002). Each teaspoon contains 16.25 mg of KI. This mixture will keep up to 7 days in the refrigerator (Food and Drug Administration, 2002). The recommended daily dose for KI in children 4 to 18 years is 65 mg (4 teaspoonfuls); for children 1 month through 3 years, 32 mg (2 teaspoonfuls); and for infants younger than 1 month, 16 mg (1 teaspoonful) (Food and Drug Administration, 2002). Daily dosing should continue until risk of exposure has passed, other measures (eg, evacuation, control of the food and milk supply) have been implemented successfully, or both (Food and Drug Administration, 2001). Overall, the benefits of KI exceed the risks of overdosing, especially in children; however, particular attention to dose and duration of treatment should be afforded for infants and pregnant women (Food and Drug Administration, 2001). Pregnant or lactating women exposed to 5 Gy or more should receive 130 mg of KI daily (one tablet) (FDA, 2001). Neonates ideally should receive the lowest dose (16 mg) of KI tablets (either whole or fractions) or fresh saturated KI solution, which may be diluted in milk, formula, or water and the appropriate volume administered (FDA, 2001).

Pregnant women should be given KI for maternal and fetal protection. Because of the risk of blocking fetal thyroid function with excess stable iodine, repeat dosing of pregnant women with KI should be avoided. Lactating females should be given KI, as for other young adults, and potentially to reduce the radioiodine content of breast milk, but not as method of delivery of KI to infants, who should get their KI directly. As for direct administration of KI, stable iodine as a component of breast milk may also pose a risk of hypothyroidism in nursing neonates. Therefore, repeat dosing with KI should be avoided in lactating mothers, except during continuing severe contamination. If repeat maternal dosing is necessary, the nursing neonate should be monitored for potential hypothyroidism by measurement of TSH (and FT4, if indicated), and thyroid hormone therapy may be initiated.

Following exposure to cesium-137 and thallium, Prussian blue is administered. This substance enhances excretion of radioactive agents in the stool, thereby decreasing internal radiation exposure (Chung & Shannon, 2005). Dosage for Prussian blue is 3 to 10 g/day by mouth (0.21–0.32 g/kg/day) (Columbia University Mailman School of Public Health National Center for Disaster Preparedness, 2005). Complications and side effects from the radiation exposure will require the standard treatment.

Following exposure to plutonium, curium, and americium, chelation with pentetate calcium trisodium (Ca DTPA), pentetate zinc trisodium (Zn-DTPA), or dimercapto-propane-1-sulfonic acid (DMPS) can be administered (Chung & Shannon, 2005). Ca-DTPA and Zn-DTPA chelate with metals and are excreted in the urine (Chung & Shannon, 2005). These medications are administered by inhalation or intravenously at 14 mg/kg, up to 1 g (Chung & Shannon, 2005).

Protection of Nurses and Health Care Professionals

If not completed in the prehospital setting, decontamination is performed according to hospital and local emergency services guidelines. Only personnel trained to perform decontamination and fitted with personal protective equipment should participate. Clients may have concomitant explosion injuries, which are treated first with standard advanced trauma life support measures. Pregnant women may be hospitalized or sent home, depending on their level of exposure, concomitant injuries, health condition, and due date.

Nurses and physicians counseling pregnant women exposed to radiation should review current CDC guidelines and offer social and spiritual support. A CDC fact sheet for pregnant women entitled "Possible Health Effects of Radiation Exposure on Unborn Babies" can be found in English and Spanish at http://www.bt.cdc.gov/radiation/prenatal.asp.

Biological Agents

Numerous biological agents can affect the health of pregnant women, fetuses, and newborns. Two agents likely to be used in bioterrorist attacks are smallpox and anthrax.

Smallpox

Smallpox (*variola* virus) is a highly contagious disease that has been internationally eradicated but may be disseminated by unscrupulous people with access to the causative virus remaining through supposedly defunct bioweapons programs. The CDC classify smallpox, anthrax, plague, and tularemia as Category A biologic agents. Such agents (1) are easily disseminated or transmitted person to person; (2) cause high mortality with potential for major public health effects; (3) might cause public panic and social disruption; and (4) require special action for public health preparedness (Greenfield et al., 2002).

Smallpox has no known cure. Variola infects humans, the only natural reservoirs, through transmission into the respiratory tract, open lesions, conjunctivae, and placenta (Veenema, 2003; Heyman, 2004). The course of the disease is as follows (Veenema, 2003; Heyman, 2004):

- *Incubation period:* The live virus enters the body in droplets, spreads to the lymph nodes, and replicates for 3 to 4 days. The client is asymptomatic.
- *Prodromal period:* Approximately 7 to 14 days after exposure, the virus multiplies in the lymphatic tissues. The client develops fever, malaise, headache, vomiting, abdominal pain, and perhaps erythema. If he or she dies, the cause is toxemia. Infected leukocytes collect in small blood vessels in the upper respiratory tract and dermis, producing lesions that appear in the mouth approximately 24 hours before they show up on the skin. These lesions ulcerate easily, and live virus is shed into the saliva, making the person highly infectious.
- *Manifestation period:* Approximately 14 days after infection, fever may decrease or remain elevated. Scabs form around day 22. Smallpox lesions appear in crops over 1 to 2 days, beginning on the face and distal extremities (centrifugal distribution). The rash is macular at first, then becomes papular, and finally becomes pustular, crusting and forming scabs.
- *Outcome period:* Smallpox primarily affects the dermis and immune system; exposed clients tend to develop immunity to the disease.

Pregnant women are more susceptible to complications and death from smallpox than are other adults. White et al. (2002) and Constantin et al. (2003) reviewed the literature on smallpox infections in pregnant women, most of which was from the early 1900s when the disease was active. Their reviews found that pregnant women were more susceptible to hemorrhagic smallpox, characterized by fever, backache, a diffuse coppery red rash, and a rapid decline in health (White et al., 2002; Constantin et al., 2003). Within 24 hours of symptom onset, conditions noted included spontaneous ecchymoses; epistaxis; bleeding gums; an intense, erythematous rash; and subconjunctival hemorrhage. Death usually resulted from sepsis.

Fetuses exposed to maternal smallpox contracted congenital variola, the incidence of which ranged from 9% to 60% (White et al., 2002). Congenital variola appears as a giant dermal pox and diffuse necrotic lesions of the viscera and placenta. White et al. (2002) analyzed numerous case and cluster reports of babies born during smallpox epidemics and concluded that the nature of vertical smallpox transmission is unpredictable. Constantin et al. (2003) concluded that smallpox is more severe in pregnant women compared to nonpregnant women and men. They found high rates of abortions, stillbirths, and preterm births in pregnant women infected with smallpox. No evidence of teratogenicity of the *variola* virus has been reported.

Treatment. A pregnant woman seeking treatment for suspected or confirmed smallpox immediately should be put in isolation. Nurses caring for her should have received the voluntary smallpox vaccination (see below). They must monitor the client for disease progression; maintain fluid and electrolyte balance; initiate comfort measures; and offer emotional support. They need to monitor fetal health and look for signs of premature labor or miscarriage.

During labor and birth, isolation precautions would be necessary. The newborn may or may not have the disease, depending on when the mother contracted smallpox. Health care providers should monitor the newborn for signs of the disease and keep the baby isolated from other newborns. White et al. (2002) reported that infants born to mothers with smallpox developed the disease up to 56 days after birth. Therefore, it would be anticipated that an infant born to a woman with smallpox would remain hospitalized in isolation for at least 14 days.

During a suspected or confirmed smallpox outbreak, nurses will be informed of isolation and quarantine procedures in accordance with state public health authorities, state emergency management agencies, and the CDC. If a diagnosis of smallpox is confirmed, vaccination and 17 days of quarantine are mandatory (Suarez & Hankins, 2002). Vaccination within 2 to 3 days of initial exposure to smallpox almost completely protects against the disease and reduces symptomatology (Suarez & Hankins, 2002).

Prevention. Administration of the smallpox vaccine is a primary care prevention measure to protect the public. Nevertheless, administration during pregnancy is controversial, because the pregnant woman's immune system is depressed and the smallpox vaccine is a live virus (Dryvax). Furthermore, the risk of fetal vaccinia, a rare and serious infection, is increased (Anonymous, 2003; Jamieson et al., 2005). No prenatal test is available to diagnose fetal vaccinia. Thus, risks versus benefits of administering the vaccine need to be balanced when considering the woman's position as a susceptible host (James, 2005).

Current recommendations are for smallpox vaccine not to be administered routinely to pregnant women (Heyman, 2004). The vaccine should be administered to pregnant women during a bioterrorism incident in which they have been definitely exposed to the virus, such as face-to-face, household, or close-proximity contact with a person with confirmed smallpox (Advisory Committee on Immunization Practices, 2001).

Between November 5, 2001 and April 24, 2003, 60,000 women of childbearing age (18 to 44 years) were vaccinated against smallpox; they were U.S. military personnel, civilian health care and public health workers, and clinical research study volunteers (Anonymous, 2003). Of these women, 103 inadvertently received the smallpox vaccine while pregnant or conceived within 4 weeks of vaccination (Anonymous, 2003). Efforts to decrease the chances of prenatal exposure to the vaccine include improved education programs prior to administration. In response to the unanticipated vaccination of pregnant women, two programs have been initiated. The first is a collaborative effort by the CDC, state health departments, and U.S. Food and Drug Administration to identify the immunized women. The second, established by the CDC, is the National Smallpox Vaccine in Pregnancy Registry, which will follow women during their pregnancies and track the infants after birth. The women will be monitored, and outcomes will be reported by trimester (CDC, 2003). Nurses can refer women who received the smallpox vaccine while or before they knew they were pregnant to the Registry by contacting the CDC at 404-639-8253 or 877-554-4625.

Protection of Nurses and Health Care Professionals. Because routine U.S. smallpox vaccination ceased in 1972, most people are not currently immunized against it. Debate continues about the immune response to smallpox among those vaccinated before 1972. Some believe adequate protection from smallpox persists, while others promote revaccination.

Between 2002 and 2003, the CDC, through state health departments, initiated a voluntary smallpox vaccination program for nurses, first responders, and health care professionals. The purpose was to create a pool of vaccinated workers who could care for people infected with smallpox. While it is unlikely that nurses employed in maternity settings would be requested to receive the vaccine, they may be called on to manage or provide care for infected pregnant women or newborns. Nurses must be aware of the side effects and contraindications to taking the smallpox vaccine prior to its administration.

Nurses caring for clients with smallpox should wear personal protective equipment to prevent disease transmission. Removal of contaminated bedding and bodily fluids should follow state health department guidelines.

Anthrax

Anthrax (*Bacillus anthracis*) is a Gram-positive spore-forming bacterium. The reservoir for *B. anthracis* is soil, where it can persist for decades (Greenfield et al., 2002). Anthrax is a zoonotic disease (transmitted from infected animals to humans). While immunization of cattle, sheep, goats, and horses in the United States generally prevents anthrax, outbreaks do occur in wild animals, particularly deer (Greenfield et al., 2002). Anthrax is transmitted to humans via contaminated flesh, blood excreta, hair, wool, hides, and manufactured products (Greenfield et al., 2002). The three types are cutaneous, inhalation, and gastrointestinal/oropharyngeal. The last U.S. case of naturally occurring inhalation anthrax was 1976; the last case of natural cutaneous anthrax was in 2000. In 2006, a male contracted cutaneous anthrax from a goat hide he used to make a drum; he was treated for exposure.

In 2001, an anthrax attack occurred through the postal system in which envelopes containing anthrax spores were delivered to unsuspecting individuals. Twenty-two people were infected, with 11 confirmed cases of inhalational anthrax, 7 confirmed cases of cutaneous anthrax, and 4 suspected cases of cutaneous anthrax (Greenfield et al., 2002). Among the victims was a 7 month old who contracted cutaneous anthrax at his mother's workplace (Freedman et al., 2002). The baby was hospitalized for 17 days; his symptoms resolved successfully 30 days after admission (Freedman et al., 2002). Others died in this attack, the perpetrator of which is still at large.

Treatment. Anthrax in pregnant women is uncommon, with few cases in the literature. In one report, two pregnant women who contracted anthrax were treated successfully, and both gave birth to preterm infants who were infection-free (Kadanali et al., 2003). Pregnant women exposed to anthrax should be referred to their obstetric care provider and an infectious disease specialist (James, 2005). While human-to-human transmission of anthrax is weak, nurses treating infected clients should use standard barrier isolation precautions (Kare et al., 2002). People coming into direct contact with suspected anthrax-infected substances should wash all exposed skin and clothing with soap and water and receive prophylactic antibiotics until the substance is identified (Kare et al., 2002). Should laboratory testing confirm anthrax, the nurse must notify the state health department and CDC.

Antibiotics to treat anthrax include ciprofloxacin, doxycycline, and penicillin; prophylaxis is given for 60 days (Kare et al., 2002). This period is necessary because anthrax spores may remain in the lungs for 60 days. Ciprofloxacin or doxycycline should be the initial treatment of localized cutaneous anthrax in infants and children (CDC, 2001). For children younger than 2 years, initial treatment of cutaneous anthrax is intravenous; combination therapy with additional antimicrobials should be considered (CDC, 2001). Because amoxicillin is known to be safe for infants, it is an option for treatment in breastfeeding mothers when *B. anthracis* is known to be penicillin-susceptible and there is no contraindication to maternal amoxicillin use (CDC, 2001).

Doxycycline and fluoroquinolones (ciprofloxacin) should be used as first-line agents in the treatment of anthrax, despite permanent tooth discoloration and cartilage atrophy, until antibiotic susceptibility testing can be performed (Kare et al., 2002). The dosage of ciprofloxacin is 500 mg twice a day for 60 days for asymptomatic pregnant women (CDC, 2001b; ACOG Committee on Obstetric Practice, 2002). If the *B. anthracis* strain is penicillin-sensitive, exposed asymptomatic pregnant women can consider prophylactic therapy with amoxicillin, 500 mg three times a day for 60 days (CDC, 2001b). Doxycycline should be used cautiously in asymptomatic pregnant women and should only be used when there are contraindications to the other antimicrobial medications (CDC, 2001b; ACOG Committee on Obstetric Practice, 2002). Pregnant women receiving doxycycline should receive liver function tests periodically (James, 2005). Breastfeeding mothers who need to take ciprofloxacin or doxycycline should consider expressing and discarding their breast milk, which allows for the resumption of breast feeding once the treatment is completed (CDC, 2001a). Decisions about treatment regimens, breastfeeding, and other maternal-child issues should be determined by the mother and her obstetric care professional, in consultation with infectious disease experts. Women receiving prophylactic treatment who become pregnant should continue taking the medication and consult their obstetrician or health care professional on how to proceed (CDC, 2001b).

Ciprofloxacin use during pregnancy is unlikely to result in fetal malformations, although data are inconclusive (CDC, 2001b). Doxycycline, a tetracycline, carries risks to fetal development of dental staining of the primary teeth, possible depressed bone growth, and defective dental enamel; rarely, hepatic necrosis has been reported in pregnant women taking this drug (CDC, 2001b; James, 2005). Penicillins are generally considered safe for use during pregnancy and have no associated risk for fetal malformation (CDC, 2001b).

Protection of Nurses and Health Care Professionals. The first U.S. anthrax vaccine (BioThrax) was licensed in 1970 and is given to active military and reserve personnel older than 18 years (Kare et al., 2002; AAP, 2003). Its use is limited to laboratory workers and military personnel who may be repeatedly exposed to *B. anthracis* (AAP, 2003). The vaccine also is administered to those with a high incidence of occupational exposure: park rangers, sheepherders, and tanners. It is not used in pregnant women or children. Nurses can protect themselves by using universal precautions when caring for anthrax-infected clients, because anthrax is not a communicable disease.

Chemical Exposures

Pregnant women may be exposed to chemical agents intentionally or unintentionally. Such exposure can harm the mother, fetus, or both. *Nerve agents* inhibit acetylcholinesterase at neural junctions in the cholinergic nervous system (Lynch & Thomas, 2004). When acetylcholinesterase is unavailable to break down acetylcholine, the nervous system becomes overstimulated. Signs and symptoms are **s**alivation, **l**acrimation, **u**rination, **d**efecation, **g**astrointestinal upset, and **e**mesis (SLUDGE). They depend on the amount of the agent and the route of exposure (i.e., inhalation versus cutaneous).

Treatment

Standard surface decontamination may be undertaken, depending on the route of exposure. Definitive treatment following nerve agent exposure is administration of atropine and 2-PAM (pralidoxime). Health care professionals should seek consultation from the woman's obstetric health provider and a toxicologist once the antidotes are administered and the client is stable. Few data are available on the effects of nerve agent or other chemical exposures and their treatment in pregnant women (Bailey, 1997). Caution should be used when breastfeeding following nerve agent exposure (Rotenberg & Newmark, 2003). Despite nerve agents not being highly lipophilic, a small dermal exposure may not result in signs and symptoms for a few hours (Rotenberg & Newmark, 2003). Therefore, nursing mothers should pump and discard their breast milk until toxicologists and public health specialists have deemed it safe to resume nursing (Rotenberg & Newmark, 2003).

Protection of Nurses and Health Care Professionals

Nurses undertaking surface decontamination receive specialized training and wear decontamination-specific personal protective equipment. Once decontamination is completed, the care of pregnant women continues as outlined above. A very high air flow volume in any room where these clients are treated is essential to avoid staff exposure to secondary off gassing of the chemical agent.

REFERENCES

ACOG Committee on Obstetric Practice. (2002). Management of asymptomatic pregnant or lactating women exposed to anthrax. *Obstetrics & Gynecology, 99*(2), 366–368.

Advisory Committee on Immunization Practices. (2001). Vaccinia (smallpox) vaccine: Recommendations of the Advisory Committee on Immunization Practices (ACIP). *Morbidity and Mortality Weekly Report, 50*(RR10), 1–25.

American Academy of Pediatrics, 2003. (2003). Summaries of infectious diseases. In: L. Pickering (Ed.), *Red book: 2003 report of the committee on infectious diseases* (26th ed., pp. 196–199). Elk Grove, IL: Author.

Anonymous. (2003). Pregnant pause: Vaccinia given despite screening. *Bioterrorism Watch,* July/August, 30–32.

Bailey, B. (1997). Organophosphate poisoning in pregnancy. *Annals of Emergency Medicine, 29*(2), 299.

Centers for Disease Control and Prevention. (2001a). Notice to readers: Update: Interim recommendations for antimicrobial prophylaxis for children and breastfeeding mothers and treatment of children with anthrax. *Morbidity and Mortality Weekly Report, 50*(45), 1014–1016.

Centers for Disease Control and Prevention. (2001b). Updated recommendations for antimicrobial prophylaxis among asymptomatic pregnant women after exposure to *Bacillus anthracis. Morbidity and Mortality Weekly Report, 50,* 960.

Centers for Disease Control and Prevention. (2003). Notice to readers: National smallpox vaccine in pregnancy registry. *Morbidity and Mortality Weekly Review, 52*(12), 256.

Centers for Disease Control and Prevention. (2005a). Prenatal radiation exposure: A fact sheet for physicians. Retrieved April 2, 2006, http://www.bt.cdc.gov/radiation/prenatalphysician.asp.

Centers for Disease Control and Prevention (2005b). Radiological terrorism. Emergency management pocket guide for clinicians. Retrieved March 4, 2006, www.bt.cdc.gov/radiation/pocket.asp

Chung, S., & Shannon, M. (2005). Hospital planning for acts of terrorism and other public health emergencies involving children. *Archives of Diseases in Children 90,* 1300–1307.

Columbia University Mailman School of Public Health National Center for Disaster Preparedness. Pediatric preparedness for disasters and terrorism: A national consensus conference.

Constantin, C., Martinelli, A., Foster, S., Bonney, E. & Strickland, O. (2003). Smallpox: A disease of the past? Consideration for midwives. *Journal of Midwifery and Women's Health, 48,* 258–267.

Edsall, K. (2003). Radiological and nuclear incidents and terrorism. In F. Walter (Ed.), *Advanced Hazmat Life Support Provider Manual* (3rd ed., pp. 361–388). Tucson, AZ: Arizona Board of Regents for the University of Arizona.

Food and Drug Administration. (2001). Guidance: Potassium iodide as a thyroid blocking agent in radiation emergencies. U.S. Department of Health and Human Services, Food and Drug Administration, Center for Drug Evaluation and Research. Accessed April 2, 2006, www.fda.gov/cder/guidance/4825fnl.pdf

Food and Drug Administration. (2002). Home preparation procedure for emergency administration of potassium iodide tablets to infants and small children. Accessed from the World Wide Web, April 3, 2006. http://www.fda.gov/cder/drugprepare/kiprep130mg.htm

Freedman, A., Afonja, O., Chang, M., Mostashari, F., Blaser, M., Perez-Perez, G., et al. (2002). Cutaneous anthrax associated with microangiopathic hemolytic anemia and coagulopathy in a 7-month-old infant. *Journal of the American Medical Association, 287*(7), 869–874.

Gebbie, K., & Qureshi, K. (2002). Emergency and disaster preparedness: Core competencies for nurses: What every nurse should but may not know. *American Journal of Nursing, 102*(1), 46–51.

Greenfield, R., Drevets, D., Machado, L., Voskuhl, G., Cornea, P., & Bronze, M. (2002). Bacterial pathogens as biological weapons and agents of bioterrorism. *American Journal of Medical Sciences, 323*(6), 299–315.

Heyman, D. (2004). *Control of communicable diseases manual* (18th ed). Washington, DC: American Public Health Association.

Homeland Security Council. (2006). *National strategy for pandemic influenza: Implementation plan and briefing book.* Washington, DC: Author.

James, D. (2005). Terrorism and the pregnant woman. *Journal of Perinatal and Neonatal Nursing, 19*(3), 226–237.

Jamieson, D., Cono, J., Richards, C., & Treadwell, T. (2004). The role of the obstetrician-gynecologist in emerging infectious diseases: Monkeypox and pregnancy. *Obstetrics & Gynecology, 103*(4), 754–756.

Jamieson, D., Jernigan, D., Ellis, J., & Treadwell, T. (2005). Emerging infections and pregnancy: West Nile virus, monkeypox, severe acute respiratory syndrome, and bioterrorism. *Clinics in Perinatology, 32,* 765–776.

Jarrett, D. (1999). *Medical management of radiological casualties.* Bethesda, MD: Military Medical Operations Office, Armed Forces Radiobiology Research Institute.

Kadanali, A., Tasyaran, M., & Kadanali, S. (2003). Anthrax during pregnancy: Case reports and review. *Clinical Infectious Diseases, 36,* 1343–1346.

Kare, J., Roham, T., & Hardin, E. (2002). Plague and anthrax: Ancient diseases, modern warfare. *Topics in Emergency Medicine, 24*(3), 77–87.

Keeney, G. (2004a). Disasters happen: Would you know what you can do? *Journal of Midwifery & Women's Health, 49*(4), S1.

Keeney, G. (2004b). Disaster preparedness: What do we do now? *Journal of Midwifery & Women's Health, 49*(4), S2–6.

Lechat, M. (1979). Disasters and public health. *Bulletin of the World Health Organization, 57*(1), 11–17.

Lynch, E., & Thomas, T. (2004). Pediatric considerations in chemical exposures. Are we prepared? *Pediatric Emergency Care, 20*(3), 198–205.

Mangano, J., Sherman, J., Chang, C., Dave, A., Feinberg, E., & Frimer, M. (2003). Elevated childhood cancer incidence proximate to U.S. nuclear power plants. *Archives of Environmental Health, 58*(2), 74–82.

Maniscalco, P., & Christen, H. (2001). *Understanding terrorism and managing the consequences.* Upper Saddle River, NJ: Prentice Hall.

Mettler, F., & Voelz, G. (2002). Current concepts: Major radiation exposure—What to expect and how to respond. *New England Journal of Medicine, 346*(20), 1554–1561.

Office for Domestic Preparedness. (2005). *Weapons of mass destruction (WMD) Awareness Level WMD Training, Student Manual AWR-160.* Washington, DC: U.S. Department of Homeland Security.

Pelsor, F., Sadrieh, N., & Machado, S. (2002). Palatability evaluations of potassium iodide solid dosage tablets ground and mixed in drinks. Rockville, MD: U.S. Food and Drug Administration.

Rotenberg, J., & Newmark, J. (2003). Nerve agent attacks on children: Diagnosis and management. *Pediatrics, 112,* 648–658.

Skorga, P., Persell, D., Arangie, P., Gilbert-Palmer, D., Winters, R., Stokes, E. & Young, C. (2003). Caring for victims of nuclear and radiological terrorism. *Nurse Practitioner, 28*(2), 24–41.

Suarez, V., & Hankins, G. (2002). Smallpox and pregnancy: From eradicated disease to bioterrorist threat. *Obstetrics and Gynecology, 100*(1), 87–93.

Veenema, T. (2003). Diagnosis, management, and containment of smallpox infections. *Disaster Management and Response, 1*(1), 1–6.

Votava, K. (2003). Design and implementation of mass immunization and prophylactic antibiotics clinics. In T. Veenema (Ed.), *Disaster nursing and emergency preparedness for chemical, biological and radiological terrorism and other hazards* (pp. 400–417). New York: Springer Publishing Co.

Waselenko, J., MacVittie, T., Blakely, W., Pesik, N., Wiley, A., Dickerson, W., et al. (2004). Medical management of the acute radiation syndrome: Recommendations of the strategic national stockpile radiation working group. *Annals of Internal Medicine, 140*(12), 1037–1051.

White, S., Henretig, F., & Dukes, R. (2002). Medical management of vulnerable populations and co-morbid conditions of victims of bioterrorism. *Emergency Medicine Clinics of North America, 20*(2), 365–392.

White-Traut, R. (2004). Providing a nurturing environment for infants in adverse situations: Multisensory strategies for newborn care. *Journal of Midwifery & Women's Health, 49*(4), S36–41.

APPENDIX B

Answers to Case-Based Questions

CHAPTER 1

1. The nurse should investigate options such as having her husband or the children assume some responsibility for planning and cooking healthy meals. (If Elaine's youngest is in middle school, these children are old enough to provide such assistance.) Elaine also might consider making and freezing extra nutritious meals on the weekends and simply reheating them (or having her family do so) on the nights she works. The nurse also should encourage the client to discuss with her husband the need for him to help with house duties now that she is working outside the home.
2. Georgia's family support systems seem challenging. She cannot rely on her parents and seems dependent on her older female relatives for assistance. These women are likely to have limited resources for appropriate nutrition and healthcare.
3. The nurse should schedule the appointment at a time that is convenient and does not compromise work attendance for the client. Also, he or she should emphasize that while another appointment may cost money, monitoring and checking health now may wind up being a long-term financial savings if doing so helps prevent chronic and expensive problems such as hypertension or depression.
4. The nurse should respect the client's wish for confidentiality while emphasizing the importance of going to regular prenatal appointments, eating and resting adequately, and taking prenatal vitamins if the client is considering maintaining the pregnancy. He or she should refer the client to community resources that might be able to help provide some assistance.
5. The nurse may be concerned about the family's reaction to the pregnancy. The relatives may be resistant to supporting another person in their household. They may try to influence the client's decisions relative to the pregnancy.
6. The nurse can examine the parameters of the study with the client to see if she does qualify for participation. He or she should explore with the client whether the additional money that might come from the study is worth the risk in postponing medication. The nurse also needs to consider whether the study really might positively influence the client's problem for which medication was prescribed and whether Elaine's participation could be a potentially effective intervention.

CHAPTER 2

1. Renee has voiced concern about being at a healthy weight. The nurse needs to explore whether Renee's beliefs about what actually is a healthy weight are accurate. In addition, the nurse should evaluate the client's commitment to making and adhering to a plan, especially in light of her statement about being so busy.
2. 136 pounds divided by 2.2 is 61.8 kg. 5′5″ = 65 inches, which divided by 39.4 is 1.65 m. 1.65 m squared equals 2.72 m. 61.8 kg divided by 2.72 equals 22.7 (Jill's BMI).
3. Renee may prefer exercises that can include her son. For example, she might take brisk walks while pushing her son in a stroller. She could join a community facility that offers baby-sitting while clients exercise. Alternatively, Renee could arrange for someone to watch her son at night while she attends a local gym.
4. Linda is experiencing menopause. Most bone loss occurs within the first 5 to 7 years after cessation of menstruation. Linda works 50 hours a week and spends most of that time sitting at a computer. Inactivity thus

may be a risk factor. She also reports that she doesn't like milk, so low calcium intake may be a risk factor.

5. Linda can eat low-fat yogurt or cheese. She also can consume soy-based beverages with added calcium, calcium-fortified breakfast cereals and fruit juices, and dark green leafy vegetables. If necessary, she also can take calcium supplements.
6. In addition to the information normally gathered during a health assessment, the nurse needs to obtain a thorough reproductive history because this is Jill's first reproductive health visit. Critical information includes age at menarche, menstrual history (cycle frequency, duration, and typical flow), and any signs and symptoms of premenstrual syndrome. Also, the nurse should evaluate Jill's sexual activity, use of safer-sex practices, and method of contraception (as well as her awareness of various types). Another important measure would be to evaluate Jill's knowledge about fertility and sexually transmitted infections.
7. Linda might apply a water-soluble lubricant (e.g., K-Y jelly) before or during sexual intercourse. She and her partner also might extend foreplay to enhance lubrication.
8. Linda should undergo a yearly mammogram. She should undergo a Pap smear and pelvic examination annually with the option of every 1 to 3 years after three consecutive normal results, as long as she has minimal or no risk factors for cervical cancer. The nurse also should encourage her to perform monthly breast self-examinations.

CHAPTER 3

1. Sheila might be at risk for inadequate protein, vitamin B12, iron, and zinc.
2. Betsy's BMI is 18.
3. A weight gain of 15 to 25 lbs is recommended for clients with a pre-pregnancy BMI of 27 (see Table 3-6). Sheila is in her third trimester. Thus, her weight should be 159 to 169 lbs.
4. Appropriate suggestions include other dairy products such as yogurt, cheese, and ice cream. Nondairy products that are high in calcium include green leafy vegetables (e.g., kale, broccoli), sesame seeds, tofu, and calcium-fortified juices and breads.
5. Betsy's statement reflects self-focus, a key aspect of adolescent development. The nurse should determine the exact meaning of the statement and work to correct any misinformation.
6. The nurse should begin by exploring what foods Betsy dislikes and her concerns about becoming "fat." Lack of knowledge about sound nutritional intake may promote the ingestion of empty calories and unhealthy foods, such as those high in saturated fat or low in vitamins and minerals. Next, the nurse should address Betsy's typical dietary intake, possibly using a 24-hour recall, to gather data about the types and amounts of food that the client eats. Results can help the nurse target areas for additional instruction. A third key area is to assess Betsy's food preferences, which will help nurse and client develop an individualized nutritional plan that promotes Betsy's sense of autonomy and contributes to her participation.

CHAPTER 4

1. Vaginal discharge with itching and irritation might indicate an STI. The nurse should further investigate whether Lela has dysuria, pelvic pain, intermenstrual bleeding, or other general symptoms of STIs. He or she also should ask about the amount and characteristics of the discharge and obtain cultures for diagnostic evaluation of the exact cause.
2. The nurse needs to find out the color of the vaginal discharge, which is gray/white or watery with BV. The nurse also should ask about any odor of the discharge, which with BV is fishy and especially noticeable after intercourse. To confirm a diagnosis of BV, a specimen of vaginal fluid needs to be obtained and examined for a pH greater than 4.5 with evidence of BV organisms.
3. Jade has a family history of breast cancer; no information is given about other genetic risks. Her reproductive history reveals pregnancy at 19 years and menarche at 11 years. Studies show that women who experience their first full-term pregnancy before 22 years are at decreased risk, whereas women who experience menarche before 12 years appear to be at increased risk. Jade is African American; although risk of breast cancer is lower for this group than for whites, mortality rates have remained constant. Jade's inconsistent physical activity may be a risk, because increased exercise has been associated with a decreased risk for breast cancer.
4. Jade's statements imply lack of understanding of the causes of and risks associated with breast cancer. A priority nursing diagnosis for her is "Deficient Knowledge."

CHAPTER 5

1. Maria would be at Erikson's stage of "intimacy vs isolation," and thus would be concerned with developing mature attachments and making commitments. Her decisions during this stage can have far-reaching consequences into midlife.
2. Maria's statements reflect hopelessness and desperation. Factors placing her at risk for self-harm include

the many demands on her time and attention, isolation associated with a language barrier, low self-esteem, and sense of shame about her Hispanic background. The nurse should complete a suicide assessment and refer Maria for mental health services.

3. Gladys is easily distracted and seems to be responding to something or someone other than the nurse. Her behavior may suggest a response to auditory hallucinations. Also, Gladys verbalizes that voices may be coming from the fetus. Although she says it would be unusual, she thinks that it could happen. Thus, she is manifesting false beliefs.
4. Maria thinks she is responsible for the abuse and is making excuses for her husband's behavior. Her statements indicate that she is in the enduring phase.
5. The nurse should investigate Gladys's comment closely. Alcohol use/abuse during pregnancy poses numerous fetal risks and may be contributing to the client's auditory hallucinations. Further investigation (e.g., with the CAGE questionnaire) would help identify Gladys's patterns of alcohol use. Once he or she has more information, the nurse can initiate interventions, such as teaching about the fetal effects of maternal alcohol use and initiating referrals for support in assisting Gladys to stop drinking.
6. Akathisia refers to continuous observable restlessness. Gladys may exhibit such behaviors as fidgety movements, arm or leg swinging, pacing, inability to stand or sit still for more than a few minutes, and foot-to-foot rocking when standing.

CHAPTER 6

1. Gender identity is reflected in a person's sense of maleness or femaleness, as well as in his or her acceptance and internalization of the roles of that gender. Kendra's appearance and dress suggest acceptance of her "femaleness." The initial information indicates that she is comfortable with her gender role.
2. Rochelle's concerns are common for many parents of teens. The nurse should respond calmly, paying particular attention to the meaning behind Rochelle's statements. First, the nurse should determine any specific concerns or fears. For example, is Rochelle afraid that Kendra may become pregnant or develop an STI? Once Rochelle has pinpointed her worries, the nurse needs to address them. He or she should explain that many teens are preoccupied with sexual issues and developments related to changes in hormones, appearance, and body functions. The nurse could mention that dating prepares adolescents for mature relationships and helps them improve their social skills. Throughout the discussion, the nurse should reinforce that teens are striving for identity, self-confidence, self-esteem, and trust in preparation for future mature relationships.
3. The nurse should review whether the client has indeed experienced menopause and when this happened. He or she should ask Patti whether sexual problems coincided with changes in menstrual function and if the couple took any measures at the time to address the difficulties.
4. The nurse should shift the focus of assessment from exploration of the client's age and physiology to a discussion of how long she has been attracted to other women and how sure she feels about her sexual orientation. The nurse could then refer the client to appropriate resources for assistance in working through her feelings, accepting her identity, and figuring out her future relative to her marriage and sexual orientation.

CHAPTER 7

1. The couple is preparing for their new role as parents. Pregnancy affects each partner, as well as the overall family unit. Olivia expresses anxiety by stating that she is "overwhelmed." Possibly she is concerned about being a good mother; maybe she worries about how the baby will change her lifestyle. She also notes changes in Tyler's behavior. He also may be anxious about potential changes in responsibilities, or he may be struggling to cope with his wife's feelings. Many changes are occurring even before the baby is born.
2. Once the baby arrives, the family system must establish new balance. The couple's emotional reactions to each other may increase anxiety to a degree that might have been less intense with more communication. The addition of the child creates a triangle, with husband and wife forming independent relationships with the child and each family member assuming different roles in the triangle as the child ages.
3. The duration of fertility treatments varies widely. Because the Jewish faith so highly values children, the couple may have continued treatments until an adoptable child was available. Or they may have wanted to exhaust all possibility of conceiving a biological child who was genetically connected to the faith and culture of their ancestors before choosing adoption.
4. The birth mother is grieving and needs the opportunity to hold and spend time with the baby, acquainting herself with the newborn before beginning to accept her loss. Although she has initially relinquished the newborn to Jacob and Rachel, the birth mother can still change her mind. Therefore, during this interaction, the nurse should be alert for statements or behaviors that might indicate that the birth mother is unsure of or felt coerced into making the decision.

CHAPTER 8

1. The nurse should determine exactly what Veena means. If Veena says that she wants to be responsible for what is used and how, then a diaphragm may be appropriate. The nurse also should explore how comfortable Veena is with touching herself and whether she has the manual dexterity to apply spermicide to the diaphragm, as well as to insert and remove it.
2. The nurse should explore options with the client that provide hormonal contraception but do not need as much maintenance as daily-dose methods require. Examples may include the contraceptive patch or Depo-Provera.
3. The nurse should explore Kenya's reasons for choosing NFP. She may have misconceptions that need to be corrected. In addition, the nurse should assess Kenya's knowledge about her menstrual cycle and period of fertility. A major area of focus is the client's menstrual history, including information about menarche, cycle length, and regularity. Because some methods of NFP involve checking cervical mucus, the nurse should determine how comfortable Kenya is with touching her genitals to do so. The nurse also should discuss the possibility of including Darrell in future sessions to ensure that both partners understand that success with NFP requires the couple to abstain from intercourse during fertile days.
4. The nurse should perform a thorough health history that reviews full medical, sexual, family, and social details. Information about lifestyle, financial status, plans for future pregnancy, and involvement from a partner is crucial to helping Veena make an informed decision. Additionally, the nurse should gather information about any cultural, religious, or personal beliefs that may influence Veena's options. He or she should investigate exactly what the client knows about the various types of contraception, being alert to any misconceptions. Doing so helps to form the basis for an appropriate contraceptive education plan.

CHAPTER 9

1. The nurse would need to question the client further about her religious beliefs to determine their degree of influence. In addition, he or she needs to gather other information to better understand which elements are most important to the client in making decisions about the future of the pregnancy to develop a culturally appropriate and individualized plan of care.
2. Multiple factors were probably involved. The fetus had severe physical and congenital abnormalities that likely would have required advanced care throughout the child's life. Providing such care may have caused physical, emotional, and financial stressors that were too numerous for Gina to have felt she could handle.
3. The gestation would be in the first trimester. Thus, the abortion method may be vacuum aspiration, methotrexate and misoprostol, or mefipristone and misoprostol.
4. Gina most likely underwent dilatation and evacuation because prenatal testing (amniocentesis) was not done until 16 weeks' gestation (second trimester).

CHAPTER 10

1. Stacy is verbalizing a common myth related to infertility. The nurse should clearly and tactfully explain that infertility is a medical condition with a wide range of causes. Also, he or she should further investigate whether cultural or religious beliefs are influencing the client.
2. In some cases, a definitive cause of infertility cannot be determined. The best response is to address Ted's concerns honestly and openly, making sure to approach the topic empathetically. In addition, the nurse should explore what coping methods the couple has used, reinforce positive strategies, and provide ongoing support. They may benefit from participation in support groups or from community resources and counseling.
3. The nurse should clarify what Stacy means by "the doctors couldn't find anything wrong." Did both Stacy and her ex-husband undergo fertility testing? If so, what types of testing were performed? If fertility testing was not completed, then the nurse should ask how the couple and doctors concluded that nothing was wrong.
4. Through laparoscopy, examiners can explore the internal organs to identify problems such as adhesions, structural abnormalities, and endometrial implants that may be the cause of infertility. Additionally, dye instilled through laparoscopy can reveal tubal patency, the shape of the uterine cavity, and, any defects that could interfere with embryonic implantation or development.
5. The most appropriate recommendation is gamete intrafallopian transfer (GIFT), in which eggs are retrieved, but then eggs fertilized with sperm are deposited directly into the fallopian tubes. Thus, fertilization occurs within the woman, not in a laboratory. Additionally, it deposits all eggs, leaving none available for cryopreservation or destruction.

CHAPTER 11

1. Based on Table 11-4, a fetus between 13 to 16 weeks can weigh 60 to 200 g, which is roughly $\frac{1}{10}$ lb (0.132 lbs) to $\frac{1}{2}$ lb (0.44 lbs), or 2 to 7 oz.
2. Using the typical obstetrical standard of 40 weeks, the pregnancy embryologically would be at 10 weeks' gestation. This would be the fetal period of development.

3. Down syndrome is a *trisomy,* a common form of aneuploidy, which is characterized by the addition or deletion of one or more (but fewer than 23) chromosomes.
4. A pedigree would provide additional information about the family members with the chronic conditions of concern. The nurse could then better understand how close these relatives are to the client to better evaluate risks. The client also mentions a distant cousin with a problem, which may be a "family secret" needing more investigation.
5. The client's advanced maternal age makes her a suitable candidate for maternal serum marker screening, which may identify trisomy disorders and neural tube defects.

CHAPTER 12

1. Pregnant teens face numerous challenges. Nurses working with them need to assess physical and psychosocial status. Adolescents need adequate nutrition, sleep, and rest to promote growth and development. Needs for nutrition, sleep, and rest also increase during pregnancy. Thus, dietary intake and activity/rest patterns would be key areas of concern. In addition, adolescents are striving for identity and a sense of independence. Pregnancy, however, causes changes in identity and compounds a client's need for outside support. The nurse should examine the teen's current living situation and the physical, psychological, and social support available from family, the father of the child and possibly his family, friends, and the community.
2. Striae gravidarum indicate small ruptures in the skin's connective layer. These marks appear with each pregnancy; although they may fade, they never disappear completely. Because Millie has been pregnant twice before, she most likely would have stretch marks. As her current pregnancy progresses, she probably will develop more striae gravidarum.
3. By 12 weeks' gestation, the client most likely would have a softened cervix (Goddell's sign); a dark violet coloration of her cervix, vagina, and vulva (Chadwick's sign); and a softened lower part of the uterus (Hegar's sign). Additionally, uterine enlargement will probably be noticeable, because Millie is a multigravida. The fundus should be palpable just above the symphysis pubis. Lastly, her serum hCG level should be elevated.
4. According to the information originally presented, this is Millie's third pregnancy and both of her children were born at term. Therefore, her history of past pregnancies would be 3-2-0-0-2. According to the changed history, she had a spontaneous abortion and a living child born prematurely. Therefore, this past pregnancy history would be documented as 3-1-1-1-2.

CHAPTER 13

1. Each of Harriet's three children has specific needs, so child care could be a source of stress. If Harriet works outside the home, the family's financial situation could be compromised. Harriet, too, may experience increased anxiety over the fetus. She may feel isolated or that she is missing out on normal activities. All these elements can alter family dynamics and relationships.
2. Selena has a history of giving birth to a large baby; a family history of diabetes, most likely type 2; and advanced maternal age. She belongs to an ethnic group considered high risk.
3. The nurse needs to explain the differences between gestational and type 2 diabetes and how treatment plans are individualized for each client. He or she should review the effects of pregnancy on glucose control and the need to closely monitor glucose levels to ensure healthy maternal and fetal outcomes.
4. Harriet has two main risk factors: multiparity and hypertension in previous pregnancies.
5. Risks include abruptio placentae, acute renal failure, pulmonary edema, cerebral hemorrhage, pre-eclampsia, eclampsia, and intrauterine growth restriction.

CHAPTER 14

1. Belinda needs information about the labor process and measures used to control labor pain. She and her husband need to understand the different approaches to labor and birth that are available so that they can make an informed decision that best meets their preferences.
2. Belinda mentions hearing negative information about labor. Such stories may be based on personal experiences or traditional ideas about childbirth. Belinda's desire for an epidural reflects ideas associated with obstetric anesthesia that began in the late 1800s and early 1900s.
3. If Clarice's and Joel's son is struggling with the idea of a new baby, sibling education classes might help. Also, prenatal education programs for the entire family and hospital/birthing facility tours can promote sharing and sibling participation. Moreover, Clarice and Joel may benefit from a refresher program that reviews the birth experience to refresh their skills and knowledge.

CHAPTER 15

1. Tyrese reports increased urination and decreased abdominal tightness, both of which suggest lightening. She mentions a backache, which may be from mild and early uterine contractions, pressure on the sacroiliac

joint from the effects of relaxin, or both. The nurse needs more data about these symptoms. First, he or she should explore if Tyrese has any burning or pain with the urinary frequency to rule out a possible urinary tract infection. Also, the nurse should measure fundal height to determine if the fetus has indeed "dropped." He or she should inspect Tyrese's abdomen for change in shape, which would indicate that the uterus has moved forward. The nurse should ask for details about the backache, specifically its frequency, duration, intensity, and accompanying symptoms. A backache that fluctuates regularly, increases in intensity, or is accompanied by pelvic pressure or cramping suggests labor. Other assessments would include evaluation for cervical dilatation and effacement.

2. Cervical dilatation = 1; cervical effacement = 1; station = 1; cervical consistency = 2; cervical position = 1. The total score would be 6.
3. With occiput posterior positioning, labor tends to be prolonged. The mother usually has increased back pain, especially because the fetal head usually is not well flexed. The nurse would need to assess for back pain and have the client rate her pain to institute measures of comfort.
4. Increased stress could affect the progress of labor. Worry can increase anxiety, possibly compounding pain perception and leading to a need for additional relief measures.
5. The FHR pattern described is variable decelerations, which usually are associated with compression of the umbilical cord. The nurse should immediately change Yolanda's position and then reassess FHR to determine if the change corrected the problem. The nurse may need to change the client's position again and reassess to ensure that the pattern has returned to baseline.
6. Because Yolanda reports moderate contractions with a frequency of every 7 to 8 minutes and a duration of approximately 45 to 60 seconds, she is most likely in the first stage of labor.
7. The nurse should expect the contractions to increase in intensity, frequency, and duration. The client most likely will begin to complain of rectal pressure and the need to push or bear down once cervical dilation is completed.

CHAPTER 16

1. This is Carlotta's first pregnancy, so she may be anxious, uncertain, or fearful about the unknown. In addition, she expresses concerns about pain and hoping that she will not need an epidural. Her post-term status may be another source of stress. Her boyfriend's presence can be helpful. Depending on how labor progresses, both of them may need additional support.
2. Frequent maternal position changes (e.g., getting on the hands and knees, side-lying, sitting, walking, using a birthing ball) may help open the pelvis further to promote fetal turning. Throughout, team members must provide pain-relief measures and support so that the woman changes positions safely and without discomfort.
3. Carlotta is post-term, with subsequent increased risks for fetal morbidity and mortality. Examples include inadequate fetal nutrition and oxygenation secondary to decreased placental function and increased risk for meconium staining (and aspiration).
4. This Bishop's score is 9, which indicates a cervix favorable and suitable for induction. A score of 8 or more indicates an increased likelihood of a successful vaginal birth.
5. Carlotta is to receive 2 milliunits per minute; in 1 hour (60 minutes) she would receive 120 milliunits. There are 10 milliunits in one milliliter, so 120 milliunits would be in 12 milliliters.

CHAPTER 17

1. Marnie's contractions reflect the latent phase of the first stage of labor. Her cervix most likely is beginning to dilate, and her perineal tissue is starting to stretch. As she moves to the active phase of the first stage, contraction frequency and intensity will increase significantly. Marnie probably will experience more pain from continued perineal stretching as the cervix dilates and becomes effaced. At the transition phase, contractions will peak in intensity, occur frequently, and last longer. The intensity of the pain associated with contractions may lead to increased anxiety, irritability, and feelings of loss of control, possibly compounding her pain level.
2. Contributing factors would include the extent of pain with each previous labor, the duration of these prior experiences, the speed and effectiveness of actions to control past pain, measures used for relief, support from others (e.g., staff, husband, family), coping methods used and their effectiveness, cultural background and beliefs about labor pain, and any concomitant stressors.
3. Promethazine causes drowsiness and sedation for 2 to 8 hours; it has been 3 hours since it was administered. Thus, ambulation might place the client at risk for injury. The nurse should ask whether the client is experiencing any drowsiness or sedation. In addition, he or she should check the client's vital signs. If the client's condition is stable, the nurse might place the head of the bed upright to see how the client tolerates the position change. Next, the nurse might have the client dangle her legs at the side of the bed. If the client remains stable, then the nurse might try ambulating with

the client to the bathroom, staying with her at all times to prevent injury.

4. The nurse should explain that it may take 2 to 3 days for Marnie to excrete 95% of the meperidine. Breast-feeding women may have residual amounts of this drug in their breast milk up to 56 hours after administration of a 50 mg dose. The mother can transfer the meperidine in her system to the newborn through the breast milk. Because the newborn liver is immature and cannot readily metabolize the medication, the baby who has received meperidine tends to exhibit problems with latching on and sleepiness.
5. The FACES pain rating scale probably would be best. The client could easily point to the face depicting her pain level, thus avoiding any miscommunication because of the language barrier.
6. Key measures to treat postdural headache involve hydration. The nurse should encourage the client to increase intake of water and caffeinated beverages. An IV infusion of Lactated Ringer's solution at 150 ccs/hr may help replace the lost cerebrospinal fluid. The nurse should encourage consumption of caffeine because it causes cerebral vasoconstriction. The client should be placed on bed rest. Analgesics may be beneficial, but this measure is not always effective.

CHAPTER 18

1. Nadia's estrogen and progesterone levels should decrease dramatically. Subsequently, her prolactin level should be greatly increased, which would allow her to produce milk for nursing.
2. Jody is being seen on her sixth postpartum day. Using the rule that uterine involution progresses 1 cm each day, the nurse would expect to palpate the fundus approximately 6 cm below the umbilicus. In addition, Jody should have lochia serosa (pale pink color).
3. The nurse's should teach Chelsea about Nadia's physiologic and psychological changes at this time. He or she should explain what to expect for her partner, the baby, and herself. The nurse should emphasize how Chelsea can best promote Nadia's and her own adaptation to the parental role. Suggestions may focus on aiding Nadia to obtain adequate rest and sleep and ways that support people can assist both women during this transition.
4. The nurse should begin by explaining how hormonal changes help prepare the breasts for nursing. Next, he or she should reassure Jody that while her breasts have filled with milk, lack of newborn stimulation eventually will cause milk production to stop, easing discomfort. Until then, Jody can take measures to ease pain, such as wearing a supportive bra and applying cool compresses to the breasts. The nurse should remind Jody to avoid nipple and breast stimulation.
5. The most common cause of a fundus displaced from midline and above its intended position is a distended bladder. First, the nurse should palpate the bladder for distention. Then, he or she should check whether Nadia has voided; if not, the nurse should encourage her to do so. If Nadia cannot void, she may require catheterization. If a distended bladder is not the cause, the nurse should anticipate the need for uterine massage.

CHAPTER 19

1. Factors placing Rosanna at increased risk for postpartum hemorrhage include multiparity, prolonged labor, and labor augmentation with oxytocin. In addition, she may have a distended bladder because she has not yet voided, which interferes with uterine contraction and further compounds her risk for hemorrhage.
2. The nurse needs to weigh a dry perineal pad and the dry protective pad. Then, he or she should weigh each pad soaked with blood. The nurse should then subtract the dry pad weight from the soaked pad weight for each. Finally, the nurse should add the two amounts to arrive at a total estimated blood loss.
3. This finding is highly suggestive of a distended bladder, which interferes with uterine involution. The nurse should assess the bladder for distention and initiate measures to promote voiding. If possible, he or she can help Rosanna to the bathroom to void on the toilet. Promoting the normal sitting position for urination may be all that is necessary. In addition, the nurse can employ other techniques to stimulate voiding, such as turning on the faucet so that the client hears the sound of running water, placing Rosanna's hand in a basin of warm water, and running warm water over her perineum. If the client still cannot void, the nurse should notify the health care provider because bimanual compression may be necessary. Also, the nurse should anticipate the need for catheterization to relieve the urinary distention.
4. The nurse needs to question Leslie about the pattern of her fever, including times of day when it is highest. Fever associated with endometritis typically peaks in the evening and has irregular spikes. In addition, the nurse should ask what the client means about her incision being very sore. Is the site itself sore? Is the client having abdominal pain in the area of the incision? Is she experiencing tenderness when she touches the area? Abdominal pain and tenderness on palpation suggest endometritis. The nurse also should question Leslie about vaginal drainage, including amount, color, and, most importantly, odor. The drainage of endometritis is usually malodorous.
5. Typical signs and symptoms of an infected incision include redness, swelling, induration, and warmth. In addition, the edges of the wound may be beginning to

separate. Serosanguinous or purulent drainage may be oozing from the area. Palpation of the site would reveal tenderness and potentially fluid accumulation that may drain as serosanguinous or purulent.

CHAPTER 20

1. Apgar scores of 5 at 1 minute and 6 at 5 minutes suggest that Thomas may be having some problems with the extrauterine transition. Subsequently, the nurse should continue assigning scores every 5 minutes up to 20 minutes. Depending on the newborn's status, the nurse also should anticipate the need for resuscitative measures.
2. The nurse should teach the mother to use mild nonmedicated soaps for bathing the newborn. Perfumed soaps can be absorbed percutaneously; if alkaline, they can alter the pH of the newborn's skin and thus compromise its protective function.
3. Circumcision places the newborn at risk for bleeding. Therefore, the nurse should ensure that William has received vitamin K prior to the procedure to reduce his risk for bleeding.
4. Thomas is most likely losing heat through convection. Although he is clothed, he is lying uncovered on a bed, probably near a doorway. If the bed is near a window on the exterior wall, he might lose heat via radiation.
5. The nurse should approach Thomas calmly and use the bulb syringe to suction his mouth and nose to prevent aspiration. While clearing his airways, the nurse should explain to his mother what is happening and the rationale for the actions used, while at the same time reassuring her that such choking can happen normally in newborns. The nurse also needs to teach the mother how to use the bulb syringe and to help her gain confidence in her ability to care for her son. Follow-up guidance, reassurance, and support are also important.
6. The first intervention is to ensure that the parents, primarily the father, clearly understand the procedure. The nurse should thoroughly explain the risks and benefits of circumcision and explore the parents' reasons for choosing it. Second, the nurse should investigate the father's specific concerns about the procedure. Additionally, the nurse should teach measures used to promote comfort and manage pain. Finally, the nurse should review specific actions that the parents can use to provide comfort after the procedure, such as swaddling and holding William.

CHAPTER 21

1. Lindsay's cesarean birth may or may not have been anticipated. If unanticipated, she may be experiencing feelings of inadequacy over not giving birth vaginally. Additionally, the effects of the surgery and the increased demands of caring for a newborn may have left her overly tired. The nurse should investigate the support available to Lindsay, such as from a partner or other family members. Lack of support would further compound her difficulties.
2. Breastfeeding would not be advised if Joelle had a herpes simplex virus lesion on her breast. In this case, the nurse should instruct Joelle to temporarily pump and discard breast milk until the lesion healed. Once healed, she could then resume breastfeeding.
3. At 6 weeks postpartum, Lindsay is producing mature human milk.
4. Lindsay's incision site may be contributing to discomfort with specific feeding positions. Women who underwent cesarean births may find the football hold and sidelying position comfortable for nursing. The side-lying position also would allow Lindsay to rest during feedings. An alternative would be the over-the-shoulder position with the mother lying down.
5. A breastfed infant typically eats 8 to 12 times over 24 hours. The nurse should instruct Joelle to look for satiety cues, such as the infant falling off the breast, pushing the nipple from the mouth, or stopping sucking. A general timeframe for the length of breastfeeding sessions is 20 to 30 minutes on the first breast (or until infant demonstrates satiety cues) and then offering the other breast. Complete emptying of at least one breast is recommended. Other guidelines suggest 10 to 15 minutes per feeding during the first few days to promote small frequent sessions without fatiguing the mother. Other indicators of successful breastfeeding include 6 to 8 wet diapers over 24 hours (by days 4 to 7 of life) and 3 to 4 stools per day (by day 3 of life).

CHAPTER 22

1. Mitchell, born at 30 weeks' gestation, would be classified as preterm. His birth weight was 3lbs, 8oz (1590 g); therefore, he would be classified as low birth weight (LBW).
2. Mitchell is LBW and thus would most likely need an endotracheal tube of 3.5 to 4 mm.
3. Because Mitchell is intubated and on a ventilator, he most likely would require enteral or parenteral nutrition. He also needs measures to assist him with nonnutritive sucking.
4. The nurse should allow Danita to express her feelings while demonstrating ongoing respect for all family members. Open and empathetic communication is essential. The nurse can point out the baby's family-related characteristics, such as Madeline having Danita's nose or eyes. In addition, the nurse should emphasize normal newborn characteristics (e.g., alertness, strong grasp). Additionally, the nurse should encourage Danita to touch, stroke, and hold Madeline

to facilitate closeness. Throughout interactions, the nurse plays a key role in teaching Danita and Louie about the correctability of the defect.

5. Breastfeeding is possible when a newborn has a cleft lip because breast tissue can close off the cleft effectively. In cases of cleft palate, the ability to conduct breastfeeding depends on the degree of separation of the palate. If the palate is widely separated, breastfeeding would be difficult. In this case, the nurse would encourage Danita to pump her breasts for milk and then to feed it to Madeline through special nipples or appliances as appropriate.

CHAPTER 23

1. The nurse should ask open-ended questions to elicit more information about the hot flashes. Asking Fran to describe her symptoms would be an appropriate way to start. Because the client states that she is experiencing hot flashes more often, the nurse should determine what she means specifically. For example, the nurse should ask about the frequency of episodes each week and if they occur during the day, at night, or both. The nurse also should question where the client first senses the hot flashes, if any factors seem to precipitate them (e.g., stress, alcohol consumption, spicy food intake), and what, if anything, relieves them.
2. Osteopenia is a precursor to osteoporosis, so Carol is at risk for fractures. The nurse should review three major areas: nutritional information for calcium intake; medication history for use of calcium supplements, prescribed or nonprescribed herbs or medications, or both to promote bone strength; and activity and exercise patterns.
3. A diary might help Fran to identify the pattern of and precipitating factors for hot flashes. In addition, writing in a journal might increase her sense of control over the situation. If precipitating factors are obvious, then the client and nurse could develop a plan to help minimize occurrences. Diary keeping also provides an opportunity for Fran to learn about the changes in her body. Moreover, the diary can act as a means to evaluate how successful the plan is.
4. Carol's risk factors for osteopenia and osteoporosis include Caucasian race, early age at menopause, family history of osteoporosis, and smoking.

CHAPTER 24

1. The nurse should be empathetic, genuine, objective, and nonpatronizing. The client's chief concern is the elimination problem, which is a sensitive and private topic. Thus, the nurse should close the examining room door or curtain during history taking. The nurse also should not attribute the problem to the client's age without further inquiry. He or she should use open-ended questions to gather specifics. Observing nonverbal behaviors as the client describes the problem can provide clues about her emotional status.
2. Lena, the primary caregiver, should be able to complete BADLs. She might need assistance in completing IADLs (e.g., grocery shopping, doing household repairs), because of the time she spends caring for Hannah. Lena's ability to complete AADLs probably is constrained severely based on her statements about the time spent assisting Hannah and managing the home. Hannah needs assistance with BADLs, and her ability to perform IADLs and AADLs would be curtailed severely because of her cognitive changes and the need for Lena to provide for her care.
3. The nurse should divide 165 lbs by 2.2 to arrive at weight in kg, which is 75 kg. Then, the nurse should complete the following equation:

$$(140 - 67) \times 75 \text{ kg} \div (72 \times 0.8 \times 0.85)$$

$$73 \times 75 \text{ kg} \div 48.96$$

$$5475 \times 48.96 = 111.8 \text{ mL/min}$$

4. Ann reports urine leakage when she coughs or sneezes, which suggests stress incontinence. She also reports needing to rush to the bathroom, suggesting urge incontinence. Therefore, the nurse should suspect mixed incontinence.
5. Cholinesterase inhibitors are appropriate for clients with moderate to severe AD, such as Hannah. In addition, the nurse should determine the onset of Hannah's AD, because these drugs are most effective when started early.
6. Studies have not shown use of ginkgo biloba as effective for mild to moderate AD. Therefore, the nurse would caution Lena against its use for Hannah.

APPENDIX C

Answers and Rationales for End-of-Chapter Review Questions

CHAPTER 2

1. **B.** Studies show that women are more likely to exercise consistently with a companion. Clients can become discouraged with exercise if they focus on long-term goals, because results can be slow. Ideally, people should vary aerobic, flexibility, and weight-bearing exercises.
2. **D.** Clients are most likely to continue exercises that reflect their preferences. Metabolic rate and nutrient intake would not form the basis for a program. The client also may not want to change her appearance.
3. **A.** Regular alcohol consumption can decrease bone density, which may lead to osteoporosis. Protein is not a prevention or management strategy for osteoporosis, nor is how the client divides exercise. Weight-bearing exercise helps prevent osteoporosis.
4. **D.** Of the items presented, fresh orange juice has the most calcium.
5. **C.** Menopause decreases risk for iron-deficiency anemia, which is a natural potential complication of the monthly blood loss of menstruation. The other clients are still menstruating.
6. **C.** Diabetes can potentially alter normal vaginal pH and flora, creating an environment favorable to yeast overgrowth. Osteoporosis, lactation, and postpartum status are not common risk factors for yeast infection.
7. **C.** Ideally, the first Pap smear is performed before a woman is sexually active. Regularly participating in low-impact aerobic exercise, consuming calcium daily, and consistently performing monthly breast self-examinations are correct health-promotion strategies.
8. **D.** HPV is the most frequent virus linked to cervical cancer.
9. **A.** Research has shown no link between oral contraceptives and cervical cancer. Identified risk factors for cervical cancer include early sexual intercourse, multiple partners, and smoking.
10. **D.** At the end of each menstrual cycle, the breasts have the least fluid and hormonal influences, which makes performing BSE comfortable and also enhances accuracy. Fluid and hormonal fluctuations in the breasts are more problematic at the other times.

CHAPTER 3

1. **D.** Women of normal pre-pregnancy weight should gain 25 to 35 lbs over three trimesters. Gaining 16 lbs per trimester is more than recommended, while 15 to 20 total lbs is insufficient. The client should consume foods she enjoys as part of a healthy, balanced pregnancy diet.
2. **A.** Folic acid supplementation can help prevent neural tube defects if maternal stores are adequate before the client conceives. Supplementation needs to be ongoing. Adequacy of stores of folic acid is not related to the menstrual cycle. Waiting until the client has missed a period or pregnancy has been confirmed is too late to initiate preventive supplementation.
3. **B.** The Food Guide Pyramid is a source for suggesting selections from various food groups to help design

a balanced diet. It is not a retrospective tool for analysis of actual food consumption.

4. **A.** Frequent nursing can stimulate the milk supply. Supplemental feedings may confuse the baby, disrupting breastfeeding. Switching to formula feeding should not be the first strategy if the woman wants to continue nursing. Caffeinated beverages can interfere with milk production.
5. **A.** These micronutrients may be deficient in women using IUDs.
6. **C.** Clients trying to control total cholesterol level should consume approximately 30% of total daily calories from fat.
7. **A**
8. **D.** This client is postmenopausal and no longer losing iron during monthly menstruation.
9. **A.** Vegan diets may be low in nutrients found in meat: B12, iron, and zinc.

CHAPTER 4

1. **D.** Although joint pain is common with SLE, inflammation and swelling of multiple joints are more common with rheumatoid arthritis. With SLE, a butterfly-shaped facial rash is common. Diagnostic tests may show an abnormal C-reactive protein level, an elevated erythrocyte sedimentation rate, and a positive antinuclear antibody titer.
2. **C.** Chlamydia can reside in the cervix for many years, damaging the fallopian tubes. Resulting pelvic inflammatory disease may cause fertility problems. Although early mild symptoms may include purulent vaginal discharge with urination, the infection often is asymptomatic. Painless ulcer formation suggests syphilis. Chlamydia is not treated with penicillin.
3. **A.** A T-4 cell count at or below 200/mm^3 indicates AIDS.
4. **D.** Genital herpes is caused by a virus; thus, an antiviral agent such as acyclovir (Zovirax) would be the most likely treatment. Azithromycin, ofloxacin, and metronidazole are commonly used medications for bacterial STIs.
5. **B.** Most breast cancers start in the upper quadrant and spread to the axillary lymph nodes. More women die from lung cancer than breast cancer each year. Many who develop breast cancer have no risk factors other than aging. Risks are increased for women older than 60 years.
6. **A.** Numbness or tingling on the chest wall and inner arm is normal for up to 1 year after surgery; it does not need to be reported. Clients should not carry or lift anything more than 15 lbs. Blood pressure measurements, infusions, and injections are contraindicated in the involved arm. Sleeping on or wearing tight garments around the affected arm could impair circulation.
7. **B.** The client is seeking information; therefore, explaining the underlying hormonal contribution is most appropriate. Telling her that she probably has an infection is incorrect and nontherapeutic. Advising her that menstrual cramps are normal and asking if she needs a prescription are inappropriate because these responses ignore the client's need for information.
8. **D.** Menorrhagia and frequent vaginal bleeding are common symptoms of leiomyomas. High fever and pain on cervical movement suggest pelvic inflammatory disease. Dysmenorrhea and irregular vaginal bleeding are common with endometriosis. Abnormal bleeding in menopause with pelvic pain suggests endometrial cancer.
9. **A.** Routine Pap testing is the best method for detecting cervical dysplasia and preventing cancer. CA-125 testing is used to screen for ovarian cancer. Condoms are preventive against STIs. Perineal hygiene is important for health but not preventive against cervical dysplasia.
10. **C.** Antibiotics are prescribed for 7 to 10 days to treat cystitis. The client should complete the entire prescription to fully eradicate the bacteria. Urinating after intercourse helps reduce the risk of infection. Recurrences need prompt and thorough treatment to prevent upper UTIs. Cranberry juice has been found to decrease recurrent UTIs, especially in older women.

CHAPTER 5

1. **C.** While exercise can help with stress management, the duration the client suggests may be ineffective. The other measures may assist with stress management.
2. **B.** The first step is to make sure that the client recognizes she is being abused. Only after the client has expressed awareness of the abuse can the nurse assist her with escape, new housing, and documentation of injuries for future litigation.
3. **C.** The client needs to admit her problem and develop a realistic body image. Until then, other interventions will be largely ineffective.
4. **A.** Psychoactive drugs treat mental illness but may have teratogenic effects, depending on their levels of risk. They act not only on target sites, but on other parts of the body. While these drugs are effective, many are considered unsafe or potentially unsafe in pregnancy.
5. **C.** The client's stoic behaviors reflect an effort to regain control. Her response may be normal for her and not necessarily indicative of another problem. Whether she is handling the situation well and is concerned about her physical injuries are subjective issues.
6. **B.** The nurse should ensure that he or she understands the client's specific issue by restating it in similar

words. The client is not focusing on health insurance or other life changes. Giving opinions about how the client has managed money is a value judgment, which is not therapeutic.

7. **C.** Any suggestive statements need further exploration about potential for suicide so that the nurse can take action to protect the client's safety. The family's feelings are secondary, as is the client's career. How long the client has felt this way is less important than protecting safety.
8. **C.** Ongoing fatigue is a primary symptom of postpartum depression.
9. **C.** Neglect of hygiene is an indicator of depression. Cleanliness and attention to dress may indicate that the client's mood is improving. While a strong social support network is helpful, it will not directly reflect effectiveness of interventions unless there is evidence that the client is interacting with members of this group regularly. Eating healthy and regularly exercising are good health promotion activities, but usually are not direct indicators of a client's mood.
10. **A.** The most important aspect of care for the client with schizophrenia is ensuring that she takes her medications and receives ongoing treatment to monitor for relapses. Relying on the client's reports about voices and powers may be problematic if the client is neglecting her treatment plan. Many clients with schizophrenia have difficulty functioning adequately for long enough to sustain employment or to participate in the community.

CHAPTER 6

1. **D.** Many parents confuse sexual orientation with gender identity. They may question whether small children who adopt behaviors associated with the opposite sex are homosexual.
2. **B.** Children of preschool age commonly adopt behaviors of the opposite sex without the activity being related to sexual orientation or preferences.
3. **C.** Focusing on legal limitations allows the nurse to remain neutral about the client's religious practice while ensuring that he or she does not support any behavior that could result in a crime.
4. A
5. **C.** Menopause is the absence of menstrual cycles for 12 months or more. Nevertheless, Mary may still become pregnant if she has continued to ovulate.
6. **C.** Short stature is commonly associated with premature testosterone production and secretion.
7. **A.** Several medications can lead to problems with erectile function. While understanding the partner's view of the problem may be necessary, the first step should be pinpointing the cause of the problem. Exercise and sexual practices should not have an influence on erectility.
8. **B.** Teens need to know how to protect themselves against STIs. Providing birth control to a teen who does not want to engage in sexual activity might lead to confusion. Many homosexuals are aware of their orientation before adolescence. Forcing children to discuss sexual issues can lead to communication problems.

CHAPTER 7

1. **B.**
2. **C.**
3. **A.** Family processes focus on roles and decision making. Illnesses, discipline, and recreation are tied to family functions.
4. **B.** Open discussion of problems reflects healthy family communication. Third-party interpretations, refusing to share internal views, and discrepancies between words and feelings are signs of dysfunctional communication.
5. **B.** Each person moves toward differentiation when he or she begins to separate thinking from feeling to form independent opinions, rather than relying on those of people close to him or her.
6. **A.** The nurse cannot guide clients toward solutions without adequate information. He or she should avoid taking sides, even if one argument is more logical than another. Giving suggestions before fully understanding the situation is a mistake. Leaving the family alone is not helpful.
7. **D.** Closed adoption means that no contact occurs between birth and adoptive parents. Rights and circumstances in open adoptions vary. Children in closed adoptions sometimes learn about their biologic parents later in life. Parental satisfaction with adoption is not solely tied to type.
8. D

CHAPTER 8

1. **B.** COCs affect the clotting mechanism, thereby increasing the risk of thromboembolic events. Fibrocystic breast changes and irritable bowel syndrome are not contraindications. Smokers older than 35 years should not use COCs because of their increased risk of myocardial infarction.
2. D
3. D
4. **B.** A reservoir should remain at the tip of the condom to collect ejaculate. The man should put on the condom as soon as the penis is erect, because some fluid may leak before ejaculation. He should remove the condom carefully while the penis remains erect to avoid spilling the contents. A new condom for each sexual act prevents breakage/leakage.

5. **A.** Studies have found an *increased* risk of HIV transmission with spermicide use.
6. **C.** COCs will not prevent STIs.
7. **B**
8. **A.** Methods that contain estrogen, such as COCs, the vaginal contraceptive ring, and the contraceptive patch, are not suggested for breastfeeding women.
9. **B.** Use of a diaphragm during menstruation may increase risk of toxic shock syndrome. The woman should leave the diaphragm in place for 6 to 8 hours after intercourse. With repeated acts of intercourse, the client should leave the diaphragm in place and insert more spermicide into the vagina. The woman should replace her diaphragm every 2 years or if the device is leaking.
10. **B**

CHAPTER 9

1. **C.** Nurses should not share personal beliefs with clients, even when asked, because doing so may influence a client's independent decision making. Many nurses who believe abortion is unacceptable work successfully in women's health.
2. **A**
3. **C.** Judaism permits abortion when continuing a pregnancy would endanger the woman's life or affect physical or emotional health adversely. It views the fetus as part of the woman's body from 40 days after conception until delivery of the presenting part.
4. **A.** The nurse should first identify his or her own beliefs and biases about abortion. Nurses are obligated to discuss with clients the full range of options available to them with respectful attitudes for all possibilities. Nurses should never imply or make it evident that they find one option more acceptable than another. In addition, the nurse must ensure that the client has the necessary information to make an independent decision.
5. **C.** Vacuum aspiration involves administration of a local anesthetic followed by insertion into the cervix of a thin plastic catheter attached to suction or syringe for evacuation of the contents.
6. **C.** Discharge teaching should include information about notifying the health care provider if elevated temperature, excessive cramping or tenderness, or excessive bleeding develops. Other teaching should cover avoiding the use of tampons and sexual activity while she is actively bleeding, expecting bleeding similar to that of a heavy menstrual period, and expecting menses to resume 4 to 6 weeks after the procedure. Strong narcotic analgesics should not be necessary.
7. **D.** The client should receive RhoGAM to prevent Rh isoimmunization.

CHAPTER 10

1. **D.** Infertility evaluations begin with a normal health assessment and progress in invasiveness as necessary. The other methods come after a health history and physical examination.
2. **D.** Some cases of infertility cannot be explained through testing. While testing can be stressful, it is more important for the nurse to ensure that clients understand they may not receive answers. Encouraging clients to continue with testing is inappropriate. While review of each test is helpful, this is not the best response.
3. **B.** Ferning is the only response that indicates ovulation.
4. **B.** Men should deliver the ejaculate to the laboratory within a specified time. The container does not need to be sterile. It should be kept at body temperature. The client does not need to avoid ejaculating for 3 days prior to providing a specimen.
5. **B.** Clients who are trying to conceive should expect ovulation once their basal body temperature begins to rise after being at its lowest point within that cycle.
6. **B.** Studies have not shown a link between previous induced abortions and infertility. The client does not mention a history of spontaneous abortion. No evidence supports the idea of infertility being linked to guilt or remorse about past events.
7. **C.** Cigarette smoking has been liked with impaired fertility.
8. **A.** Impaired fecundity is the term used when a woman can become pregnant but cannot continue the gestation to a point of viability.
9. **A.** Of the options listed, obesity is a potential risk factor for infertility.
10. **B.** Infertility medications are taken by women, not men.

CHAPTER 11

1. **D.** Through physical examination, the health care provider would be able to identify the client's exhibited characteristics. Pedigree, chromosome analysis, and DNA analysis all would focus on "hidden" genetic or molecular components of the person's makeup.
2. **C**
3. **B**
4. **C**
5. **A.** Finding out if chromosomal abnormalities contributed to previous pregnancy losses is the first step in determining the client's risk for recurrent miscarriage.
6. **A.** False positive results on maternal serum alphafetoprotein screening (MSAFP) are most commonly related to misdated pregnancies.

7. **C.** Caucasians are at increased risk for cystic fibrosis. A client without a family history of this problem could still be a carrier. Preventive care would involve screening for carrier status.
8. **C**
9. **A.** The nonstress test checks for problems with uteroplacental sufficiency, which would indicate the need for an immediate birth.
10. **B.** Of these options, reviewing screening tests performed is the most important priority.

CHAPTER 12

1. **B.** Women older than 35 years tend to be aware of their increased risk for miscarriage and often express related concerns. Nothing in the information presented suggests that the client fears the unknown, may not want to be pregnant, or is experiencing changes in her mental health.
2. **B.** The nurse should review with each client aspects of culture and religion of importance to the client. Some people do not follow all the traditions of their culture or faith. An interpreter would be needed only if the client does not understand English. Although the client is Muslim, she may not observe Friday as a religious day. Nothing indicates that additional time is needed.
3. **B.** Urinary frequency usually occurs in the first and third trimesters, when the uterus and fetal head (once lightening occurs) put pressure on the bladder. Urinary frequency at other times may indicate infection, which may predispose the client to pyelonephritis and preterm labor. Nasal stuffiness is a normal finding, resulting from elevated estrogen levels. Tingling in the breasts is normal as they enlarge and vascularity increases. Darkened spots on the nose and cheeks result from increased circulating hormones. Such spots usually fade after childbirth.
4. **D.** Ultrasound can detect movement of the fetal heart as early as the 7th week. This positive sign of pregnancy has no other possible cause. The woman will not be able to feel the fetus move until 18 to 20 weeks' gestation, which will delay the reassurance she seems to need now. Until a positive sign is confirmed, no evidence proves definitely that she is pregnant. A positive result on a pregnancy test may be caused by reasons other than pregnancy.
5. **B.** G is the client's total pregnancies, including the current one (4). T is the number of infants born at 37 or more weeks' gestation (1). P is the number of infants born after 20 weeks' but before completion of 37 weeks' gestation (2). A is the number of pregnancies that ended in spontaneous or therapeutic abortion (1). L is the number of children currently alive (3).
6. **C.** Naegele's rule begins with the first day of the last normal period, subtracts 3 months (September 2), and adds 7 days (September 9). The EDD is September 9.
7. **A.** Low heels will assist with varicose veins. The client should not massage the area. Pregnant women should not indiscriminately increase exercise. Varicose veins may not disappear after birth.
8. **A.** While these symptoms are normal for the stage of pregnancy, the nurse should investigate each to ensure that they are not the result of other, more serious, causes.
9. **B.** Emptying a cat's litter box predisposes a pregnant woman to toxoplasmosis, which can lead to spontaneous abortion if contracted in the first trimester or to congenital infection in the newborn if contracted in the last trimester. There is no problem with close contact with dogs or cats; the only precaution is avoidance of changing the cat's litter box.
10. **A.** These findings would result in a score of 10 on the biophysical profile, indicating a healthy fetus. The fetus has demonstrated activity by stretching, flexing arms and legs, and moving. Nothing indicates sleep, need for immediate birth, or fetal compromise.

CHAPTER 13

1. **C.** The risk of asthma exacerbation during pregnancy is related directly to asthma severity. The most common exacerbation period in pregnancy is from gestational weeks 24 to 36.
2. **A.** Women with chronic hemolytic anemia may appear jaundiced from hemolysis of RBCs. They may suffer from gallstones (cholelithiasis) and splenomegaly. Severe bone pain is associated with acute sickle cell crisis.
3. **D.** During labor, the pregnant woman with HIV may receive antibiotic therapy at least 4 hours before birth to protect the fetus/newborn. Intravenous retroviral therapy also may be used. Procedures such as rupturing the membranes and using internal electronic fetal monitoring are avoided to reduce the risk of vertical transmission. Cesarean birth is under investigation as a way to decrease perinatal HIV transmission.
4. **B.** Hypotonia is associated with congenital rubella syndrome. Fetal effects of parvovirus include anemia, fetal non-immune hydrops, and fetal death in the second or third trimester.
5. **A.** The woman is describing common findings associated with pyelonephritis. The temperature typically spikes and then returns to normal or even progresses to hypothermia. Acute renal failure is manifested by signs and symptoms such as fluid imbalances, changes in vital signs, malaise, irritation, and disorientation. Gestational hypertension is indicated by blood pressure greater than or equal to 140/90 mm Hg

or diastolic pressure greater than or equal to 90 mm Hg with or without proteinuria. Hypoglycemia would be indicated by decreased blood glucose levels, hunger, weakness, dizziness, confusion, headache, diaphoresis, and irritability.

6. **C.** Self-blood glucose monitoring typically involves testing a blood sample, obtained by fingerstick, with a glucose meter. Usually, the pregnant client needs to monitor her blood glucose level four times a day (prandial and pre-prandial) and record the results on a written log to allow for easing tracking of patterns. Testing is not limited to one sample a day before breakfast. Eating a light snack or administering insulin before testing would interfere with test accuracy.
7. **C.** Although the nurse might refer the client to a local shelter or give her information about such resources, this action is the lowest priority.
8. **D.** Oral fluid intake would not be allowed until the client has not vomited for 48 hours.
9. **B.** Often the first indication of magnesium toxicity is absence of deep tendon reflexes, such as the knee-jerk reflex. Muscle weakness is a possible side effect of magnesium therapy, whereas flaccid paralysis occurs with toxicity. Seizures suggest eclampsia. A respiratory rate of 18 breaths per minute is within normal parameters.
10. **D.** A complete molar pregnancy is a form of gestational trophoblastic disease, in which trophoblastic villi abnormally proliferate and degenerate. Although gestational tissue is found, the pregnancy is not viable. The statement about an umbilical cord indicates that the client needs more teaching about GTD. Complete molar pregnancy increases the risk for choriocarcinoma, a dangerous and rapidly spreading malignancy. After dilatation and curettage for GTD, the client must undergo follow-up testing of her hCG levels for 1 year to evaluate for malignancy. Because of the cancer risk, the client must be careful to avoid pregnancy for 1 year after GTD.

CHAPTER 14

1. **A.** Control in birth is a major benchmark for the mother's satisfaction and ability to move past the experience and provide for her newborn. Use of nonpharmacologic pain-relief methods, extent of childbirth education, and past childbirth experiences all influence who controls the decision about how a woman gives birth.
2. **C.** For colonial women, attending births before their own pregnancies was their childbirth education. Most births were attended by midwives, not physicians. Mothers typically spent 3 to 4 weeks after birth lying in, not before. Births were usually spaced 15 to 20 months apart.
3. **D**
4. **B.** Psychoprophylaxis emphasizes strategies such as controlled breathing, abdominal stroking, and pressure application to prevent pain rather than the use of chemicals to remove it. The Dick-Read method focuses on breaking the fear-tension-pain cycle by creating healthy bodies and attitudes able to deal with the strong physical sensations of labor and birth.
5. **D.** Early 20th century prenatal classes typically focused on maternal hygiene, nutrition, and baby care. Focus on the partner did not evolve until the 1970s.
6. **B.** Hypnobirthing consists of a series of techniques that the laboring woman uses to decrease pain and emotional stress without drugs. The Dick-Read method focuses on physical exercises, relaxation, and breathing to break the fear-tension-pain cycle. Lamaze is a psychoprophylactic method emphasizing controlled breathing, abdominal stroking, and pressure application. Birthing from Within involves the use of mind-focusing practices.
7. **B.** A doula provides continuous support to the woman before, during, and after childbirth. A hypnotherapist is specially trained in breathing, relaxation techniques, and hypnosis. Boot Camp for New Dads involves mentors teaching new fathers about supporting mothers during labor and newborn care. A nurse midwife is educated in nursing and midwifery and possesses evidence of certification according to the requirements of the American College of Nurse-Midwives.
8. **C.** The La Leche League involves members sharing information and experiences about breastfeeding while offering one another support on this and other parenting choices.
9. **D.** The time of conscious decision making to become a parent is when holistic, health promoting, and empowering childbirth education should begin.
10. **A.** Natural childbirth research focused on the concept that pain could be deconditioned and that a new response to pain could be created. Use of antiseptics made hospitals safer for childbirth. Maternal survival was the focus of determining childbirth success during colonial times. During the 1700s and 1800s, a change was steady from female to male birth attendants.

CHAPTER 15

1. **B.** The pelvis or buttocks of the fetus lying over the pelvic inlet indicates this as the presenting part and would be documented as a breech presentation. With a cephalic presentation, the head is the presenting part; a shoulder presentation indicates that the shoulder is the presenting part. Transverse refers to fetal lie.
2. **A.** A presenting part that has descended to a level at or past the pelvic inlet is said to be engaged. Float-

ing indicates that the presenting part has not yet entered the true pelvis. A −1 station indicates that the presenting part is 1 cm above the ischial spines. Crowning refers to the appearance of the fetal head at the perineum.

3. **D.** The most effective way to assess the intensity of contractions is to palpate the uterine fundus for tightening. Auscultating with a Doppler ultrasound would provide information about fetal heart rate. Although observing the client's facial expression and asking her to rate intensity would help determine her pain, this information would not be as effective as actual palpation.
4. **B.** Duration is the time from the beginning to the end of a single contraction. Frequency is the time from the beginning of one contraction to the beginning of the next contraction. Acme refers to the peak of a contraction. Intensity refers to the strength of the contraction.
5. **D.** After spontaneous rupture of membranes, umbilical cord prolapse is possible, so the nurse should first assess FHR for indicative changes. If FHR remains stable, then the nurse should do the Nitrazine paper test to ensure that the leakage was indeed amniotic fluid. The nurse should then assist with cleaning perineum and notify the primary care provider.
6. **B.** Before auscultating FHR, the nurse first determines the location of the fetal back, where the strongest heart sounds are transmitted. Because the fetal back is toward the mother's left side and the fetus is vertex, auscultation should begin in the left lower quadrant.
7. **A.** An FHR that slows during the peak of a contraction and then returns to baseline indicates an early deceleration. It is considered a normal physiologic response. Uteroplacental insufficiency and uterine hyperstimulation would lead to late decelerations, in which the FHR would decrease after the peak of a contraction and end with the contraction. Umbilical cord compression would be demonstrated by variable decelerations.
8. **B.** A doula is a professionally trained supportive companion who focuses on supporting the laboring woman through each contraction. The doula's focus is the client, not the primary care provider or partner. The doula may provide information to assist the woman in making decisions or support the woman's choices but not make decisions for her.
9. **A.** The characteristics presented are found with the latent phase of the first stage of labor. During the transition phase, cervical dilatation and effacement are complete with relatively strong contractions and beginning urges to bear down. The second stage is characterized by the strong urge to push as the fetus moves through the birth canal, perineal bulging, and ultimately birth. The third stage involves separation and expulsion of the placenta.
10. **C.** An episiotomy is a surgical incision of the perineum to enlarge the outlet. An amniotomy is artificial rupturing of the membranes. Labor augmentation involves the use of medication to enhance contractions. Effacement refers to the thinning of the cervical tissue.

CHAPTER 16

1. **D.** Oxytocin would likely be contraindicated because it could further exacerbate hypertonic uterine contractions, interfering with fetal oxygenation. Intravenous fluid therapy is appropriate to maintain hydration and electrolyte balance. Intramuscular morphine may be used to inhibit the uncoordinated contraction pattern. A short-acting barbiturate may be ordered to promote rest.
2. **C.** Both before and after ECV, the client should undergo a non-stress test to evaluate fetal well-being. An ultrasound may be used before ECV to determine nuchal cord and adequate amniotic fluid volume, which would increase the chances of success with ECV. An emergency cesarean birth may be done instead of or in addition to ECV if fetal or maternal distress or complications occur during the procedure. McRobert's maneuver is used for shoulder dystocia.
3. **A.** The woman whose fetus is in the OP position typically has back pain with contractions. She may describe her labor primarily as back pain. Fetal heart sounds may be auscultated at the umbilicus or laterally, rather than in the lower abdominal quadrants. Palpating the fetal back may be difficult with OP positioning. In a breech presentation, the buttocks are the presenting part.
4. **D.** To treat shoulder dystocia, the first step is McRobert's maneuver (hyperflexion of the client's legs into a knee-chest position). Next, team members would apply gentle suprapubic pressure. This would be followed by assisting the woman into the knee-chest position, and then using the Woods screen rotational maneuver.
5. **B.** Tocolytic therapy generally is used when preterm labor has been definitively diagnosed, gestational age is greater than 20 weeks but less than 36 weeks, fetal weight is estimated as less than 2500 g, and the fetal lung profile shows signs of immaturity. Preterm labor is diagnosed with regular uterine contractions and rupture of membranes.
6. **D.** The Bishop's scoring method assigns a score of 0 to 3 for each of five factors: cervical dilation, cervical length, station, consistency, and position. A total of 8 or more indicates a cervix suitable for induction, which increases the likelihood of a successful vaginal birth.

7. **A.** A battledore placenta is not considered clinically significant. In velamentous placenta, the umbilical vessels course unprotected for long distances through the membranes to insert into the placental margin. If they pass over the internal cervical os, they are at risk for compression by the presenting fetal part. This type also is at risk of tearing when the membranes rupture. In circumvallate placenta, the membranes fold back on the fetal surface of the placenta, exposing part of the umbilical cord. Such exposure increases the risk of hemorrhage both before and after birth. In succenturiate placenta, one or more small accessory lobes develop in the membranes at a distance from the main placenta. Connecting vessels may tear during birth or with rupture of the membranes. After placental expulsion, retention of one or more lobes in the uterus can cause maternal postpartum hemorrhage.
8. **C.** With umbilical cord prolapse, interventions focus on relieving pressure of the fetal presenting part on the cord. The knee-chest, Trendelenburg, or Sims lateral position is effective in achieving this.
9. **B.** When oxytocin is being administered, the goal is for contractions to occur every 2 to 3 minutes, lasting 45 to 60 seconds. Resting tone should not exceed 20 mm Hg; contraction intensity should not be above 60 mm Hg.
10. **A.** A transverse incision is made in the thinnest and least active portion of the uterus, thus minimizing blood loss. The area is easiest to repair, decreasing the chances of uterine rupture with subsequent pregnancies. Suturing occurs in two layers, which seals off the incision and helps to prevent lochia from entering the peritoneal cavity. A classic or vertical incision allows rapid access to the fetus if complications develop. It also allows for the birth of a fetus in breech presentation younger than 34 weeks. Closure requires three layers of absorbable sutures. Unfortunately, a classic incision requires cutting into the full thickness of the uterine corpus.

CHAPTER 17

1. **B.** Malignant hyperthermia is a hypermetabolic response to common inhalation anesthetics (e.g., halothane) and depolarizing muscle relaxants (e.g., anectine) used with general anesthesia.
2. **D.** Clients can receive inadvertent spinal anesthesia during epidural insertion if the needle pierces the spinal column. The hole created by the needle allows spinal fluid leakage. Severe headaches can occur with initial ambulation because of the sudden shift in spinal fluid volume.
3. **C.** While all the interventions help with relaxation and pain management, giving nalbuphine and promethazine would produce the most optimal pain relief at this time. Secobarbital is usually given early in labor; however, this drug provides rest and sedation only. Nonpharmacologic methods may be inadequate to relieve pain. It is too early to administer epidural anesthesia.
4. **A.** Somatic pain is a deeper pain associated with the later phases of the first stage and with the second stage of labor.
5. **A**
6. **C.** The FLACC score is for use with unconscious clients and thus must rely on subjective observation, not self-report. The Wong-Baker Faces Pain Scale is an objective reporting mechanism.
7. **D.** The area of injection described is the epidural space outside the spinal column.
8. **B.** It can take 2 to 3 days for the body to excrete 95% of meperidine. Demerol that remains during this time is excreted in breast milk, causing the breastfed newborn to be sleepy and have problems with latching.
9. **C.** The client is experiencing hypotension from the epidural. The most immediate response is to increase IV fluids and to give oxygen by face mask. The nurse should try to rectify the problem with increased IV fluids and oxygen therapy before calling the anesthesiologist. Ephedrine is the last action if the others fail to rectify the problem.

CHAPTER 18

1. **A.** Although urinary overflow can be seen as frequency, the amounts voided are smaller than the 500 mL this client is voiding. Diuresis in the first week postpartum is normal. Although frequency is a symptom of a urinary tract infection, no other assessment data suggest this problem. Trauma to the pelvic muscles usually manifests as urinary retention, not frequency.
2. **D.** The fundus should be at or 2 to 3 fingerbreadths below the umbilicus during the fourth stage of labor. A fundus above the umbilicus may be the result of uterine blood clots, retained placental fragments, or a full bladder. Each condition predisposes the woman to postpartum hemorrhage. Moderate rubra at this time is normal, as is a decreased pulse rate. Abdominal pains are commonly related to breastfeeding.
3. **C.** Normal hemoglobin is 12 to 16 g/dl. For several days after birth, this value fluctuates near pregnancy level and then rises. The WBC normally is elevated (25,000 to 30,000/μL) during the postpartum period. Normal hematocrit values are 0.37 to 0.47. Normal serum iron is 80 to 159.
4. **B.** Although lochia will increase if the uterus is atonic, these developments may not occur simultaneously. If the nurse cannot feel the fundus in the

abdomen, it is atonic and requires massage for contraction. Oxytocin may be ordered, but administration should be a secondary action on the second day and implemented only if fundal massage does not result in uterine contraction. The second day postpartum is too early for the fundus to be so low in the abdomen.

5. **D.** Menstruation may return normally in women who are breastfeeding any time from 8 weeks to 18 months. Menstruation may return in women who do not breastfeed as early as 6 weeks. Although women who breastfeed may have menstruation return as early as 6 to 8 weeks, stating that it can be expected may cause increased anxiety if it occurs later.
6. **B.** Warm compresses facilitate vasodilation, provide comfort, and assist with the movement of blood and milk. Lanolin ointment is appropriate for painful nipples. Cool compresses facilitate vasoconstriction, which decreases milk production. Expression of milk may contribute to engorgement because the breasts produce milk in relation to demand.
7. **C.** Postpartum depression has no absolute set of symptoms; each case is unique. Bipolar disorder is more common with postpartum psychosis than with postpartum depression. Shortness of breath and sensations of smothering are associated with anxiety disorders. It is important for the safety of both mother and baby that the nurse asks questions that may be considered sensitive (e.g., if she has had any thoughts of harming herself or her baby).
8. **B.** How the client became pregnant is irrelevant. Her partner is part of her family, and the nurse should include her in all aspects of care. Acting as though nothing is different about the client may lead the woman to feel that her sexual orientation is being minimized or negated. The nurse may choose to ask the woman if she wishes the nurse to tell anyone else about her sexual orientation; however, the nurse should not do so without the client's consent.
9. **C.** Implementing teaching every time the nurse is with the client is overwhelming. Postpartum women often have difficulty taking in a lot of new material. It is better to determine and to focus on essential information.
10. **B.** Women may experience difficulty voiding up to 14 hours postpartum. A full bladder can displace the fundus upward and contribute to uterine atony, which may be the cause of the increased flow. If assessment of the bladder reveals that it is not distended, then the nurse should massage the boggy uterus. The nurse can take these actions without notifying a physician. No evidence suggests clots. The nurse may administer oxytocin to stimulate uterine contraction; however, he or she should implement the other steps first.

CHAPTER 19

1. **C.** Urinary catheterization would increase risk for urinary tract infection, not endometritis. Premature rupture of membranes, prolonged labor, cesarean birth, multiple vaginal examinations, placement of intrauterine catheters or fetal scalp electrodes, and manual removal of the placenta are known risk factors that may introduce bacterial organisms into the uterine cavity.
2. **B.** Bleeding from a genital laceration typically is bright red and appears to spurt. Dark red steady bleeding and a boggy uterus suggest uterine atony. Purulent lochia suggests uterine infection.
3. **D.** Postpartum hemorrhage is blood loss greater than 500 mL (454 g) during or after the third stage of labor. A total pad weight of 675 g would be considered postpartum hemorrhage.
4. **C.** A vulvar hematoma presents as a tense fluctuant mass with ecchymosis on the vulvar area. Signs of uterine prolapse are dysmenorrhea, irregular periods, low back pain, infertility, recurrent vaginal infections, urinary incontinence, dyspareunia, varicose veins, and aching legs. Parametritis is the extension of a uterine infection into the broad ligament, manifested by prolonged fever, lateral extension of abdominal pain, rebound tenderness, and a firm tender mass in one or both adnexa. Uterine inversion refers to dropping of the fundus into the endometrial cavity, possibly extending beyond the cervical os. Findings include a nonpalpable fundus, profuse bleeding, and obvious alterations during abdominal examination.
5. **B.** The priority is to restore circulating volume through intravenous fluid therapy, thereby helping to restore and maintain hemodynamic stability. Although late postpartum hemorrhage and intrauterine infection are highly correlated, this is not the priority. Surgical curettage is performed only when nonsurgical interventions are ineffective. Applying ice to the perineum may promote vasoconstriction to that area, but it is used only in the first 24 hours after birth.
6. **B.** Limiting the frequency of urination can lead to urinary stasis and UTIs. Instead, the woman should empty her bladder frequently. Other behaviors to prevent UTIs include a high fluid intake to flush the bladder, good perineal hygiene, and a front to back wiping motion before and after voiding or bowel movements.
7. **C.** The nurse should encourage breastfeeding to ensure emptying, thereby preventing milk stasis.
8. **D.** Deep vein thrombosis is characterized by unilateral leg pain, swelling, warmth, calf tenderness on ambulation, inequality in size of the lower extremities, enlargement and warmth of the vein over the

site of the thrombus, and positive Homans' sign. Dyspnea, sudden chest pain, and hemoptysis are indicative of a pulmonary embolism.

9. **A.** The main medical therapy for a client with peripartum cardiomyopathy is angiotensin-converting enzyme (ACE) inhibitors. Although anticoagulant therapy may be ordered to reduce the risk of thrombotic and embolic complications, it is not the main treatment. NSAIDs are used to treat mild to moderate pain and superficial thrombophlebitis. Cephalosporin antibiotics are often used to treat mastitis.
10. **C.** This finding is most likely with postpartum depression. Hallucinations, delusions, and confusion are associated with postpartum psychosis.

CHAPTER 20

1. **C.** Blood vessels in the fetal lungs are tightly constricted; blood pressure is high (high pulmonary vascular resistance). The systemic blood pressure in the fetus is low (low systemic vascular resistance).
2. **A.** Gestational age, sex, muscle tone, weight, length, and head circumference are important to note, but not as essential as color, respirations, and heart rate. Temperature is not measured in the first minute of life.
3. **C.** Central cyanosis denotes lack of oxygen to the tissues and necessitates supplemental oxygen. Acrocyanosis and circumoral cyanosis usually are normal in the first 24 hours of life. Jaundice is a yellowish color to the skin or sclera indicating excess bilirubin in the blood.
4. **B.** Apgar scores reflect the newborn's response to the extrauterine environment and resuscitative efforts, which are not delayed until Apgar scores are determined. Apgar scores are assigned at 1 and 5 minutes of age; if the 5-minute score is not at least 7, additional scores are assigned every 5 minutes thereafter up to 20 minutes of age. The Apgar score, particularly at 1 minute, is not sufficient evidence on which to base neurologic outcome.
5. **A.** These are some symptoms of hypoglycemia, although it is important to remember that some infants with hypoglycemia are asymptomatic.
6. **B.** Duskiness (central cyanosis) indicates lack of oxygen to the tissues. Because the baby is pink when crying (and breathing through the mouth), the nurse should suspect nasal or upper airway obstruction (the airway may be blocked when the baby quiets and closes the mouth).
7. **A.** These are the normal expected parameters for a newborn's initial voiding and stooling.
8. **A.** This is the only correct answer. None of the other statements is accurate.
9. **B.** Infants should be placed supine for sleeping to reduce risk for SIDS.
10. **A.** Although signs of newborn illness can be vague, major indicators of sepsis are respiratory distress and temperature instability. Newborns manifest temperature instability more often than fever as a sign of illness; soft frequent stools (not diarrhea) do not indicate illness in a newborn. Newborns have a reduced capacity to sweat and do not shiver, except as a late response to hypothermia. Periodic breathing is normal in the newborn. Nevus simplex is a "stork bite mark," a commonly found vascular birthmark.

CHAPTER 21

1. A
2. **C.** Weight loss is not obligatory for breast-feeding mothers. Breast-fed babies usually gain weight at a slower rate than do bottle-fed babies. Maternal-child bonding can (and should) occur regardless of chosen feeding type.
3. **B.** The mother is forcing the infant to finish each bottle, which is causing emesis from too great a volume of feeding.
4. **D.** Information about what the baby eats can help the nurse to assess the adequacy of the fluid intake.
5. **A.** Heating a feeding under warm, running water allows for quick, even heating without the risk of hot spots that can occur with use of the microwave.
6. **D.** A woman should pump for a minimum of five times per day for a total of at least 100 minutes in a 24-hour period.
7. **A.** A breast-fed baby needs to eat 8 to 12 times in a 24-hour period.
8. **B.** A palpable breast lump in a lactating woman with warmth at the site likely indicates a plugged milk duct.
9. **B.** 358 ml/d / 2.98 kg = 120 ml/kg/d, 120 ml/kg/d × 0.67 Cal/ml = 80 Cal/kg/d

CHAPTER 22

1. **C.** A post-term newborn most likely would exhibit dry scaly skin. Lanugo is absent; plantar creases are deep and numerous. Abundant lanugo and few plantar creases are typical findings in preterm newborns. If the newborn is very preterm, the eyelids may be fused.
2. **D.** Green, thick, stained amniotic fluid suggests meconium, which places the newborn at risk for meconium aspiration syndrome (MAS). As soon as the fetal head emerges from the birth canal, nasal, then oral and pharyngeal suctioning is done. Deep tracheal suctioning is indicated before the newborn

takes the first breath. All stimulation of the newborn, including drying the skin, must be delayed until the vocal cords have been visualized and deep endotracheal suctioning has been done. Other interventions such as administering blow-by oxygen and assessing apical heart rate would be accomplished later, once the airway is cleared of meconium.

3. **B.** Risk factors associated with LGA newborns include maternal history of diabetes, excessive pregnancy weight gain, high maternal birth weight, previous LGA infant, maternal pregravid obesity, multiparity, and fetal exposure to high estrogen levels. Exposure to rubella in the first trimester is associated with congenital heart disease. Polyhydramnios and incompetent cervix are associated with preterm birth.
4. **D**
5. **B.** Characteristics of FAS include a short nose; a flat, thin upper lip; small eyes with short slits for openings; a flattened midface and profile; and a low nasal bridge.
6. **A.** Small patches on both eyes protect them from the phototherapy lights. During phototherapy, the newborn should be unclothed to expose the maximum surface area of skin. The nurse needs to turn the newborn frequently, not just every 6 to 8 hours, to maximize exposure. Dehydration is possible with phototherapy because of increased insensible fluid loss. Additional fluids most likely will be necessary.
7. **C.** Congenital diaphragmatic hernia refers to an abnormality that allows the abdominal contents to rise up and protrude through the defect and occupy space in the thoracic cavity. Auscultation reveals absent or decreased breath sounds and audible bowel sounds on the side with the herniation. Common manifestations of congenital heart disease include tachycardia, tachypnea, poor or prolonged feeding, pallor, cold extremities, murmurs, and irritability. Manifestations of respiratory distress syndrome include rapid, irregular respirations, tachycardia, and central cyanosis. An omphalocele is a sac containing abdominal contents that protrudes through the external abdominal surface at the base of the umbilical cord.
8. **C.** The highest priority is for the newborn to receive adequate nutrition, which requires adaptive techniques because of the craniofacial defect. An outcome in which parents demonstrate success with feeding is most important. Support from extended family members, a scheduled visit to the surgeon, and sibling attachment are important, but are not as high priorities.
9. **B.** The nurse should position the newborn prone and elevate the head at least 30 degrees to prevent gastric reflux into the lung. In addition, the nurse should give the newborn nothing by mouth and notify the pediatrician immediately. The nurse may pass a nasogastric tube if a test gavage feeding is prescribed. A gastrostomy tube would not be used.
10. **C.** Treatment for DDH typically is lengthy. The parent's statement about using the harness for 1 month indicates a need for more instruction. Parents often need extra time to remove and reapply the harness during bathing and dressing the newborn. Carrying the newborn astride the hip or holding her upright on the leg can be helpful for her caregivers. Commercial infant seats do not allow for hip abduction; therefore, special infant seats and car restraints are necessary.

CHAPTER 23

1. **D.** Although age of menopause varies among women, factors correlated with it include breastfeeding, alcohol consumption, family history of early menopause, smoking history, early onset of menarche, never becoming pregnant, and never using oral contraceptives.
2. **B.** The nurse needs to gather more information about the client's chief complaint (hot flashes). The nurse can best obtain answers by using open-ended questions. Asking about the client's menstrual cycle is not directly related to her chief complaint. Inquiring about the use of a vaginal lubricant presumes that the client is experiencing vaginal dryness or dyspareunia, which she has not described. Although soy products have been associated with decreased vasomotor symptoms, this question would be more appropriate once the nurse has gathered additional information.
3. **A.** Although risk factors are the same for both African-American and Caucasian women, African Americans have greater bone mass density at menopause and experience slower postmenopausal bone loss than Caucasian women do. African-American women have approximately 50% the risk that Caucasian women have for osteoporosis. Other risk factors for osteopenia and osteoporosis include Asian race, family history of osteoporosis, early age at menopause, small-boned stature, low body weight, nulliparity, sedentary lifestyle, smoking, excessive alcohol consumption, low sunlight exposure, high-fat diet, inadequate calcium intake throughout life, and excessive caffeine intake.
4. **B.** Dyspareunia is related to a decrease in or lack of vaginal lubrication. Using a water-based lubricant immediately before coitus and increasing sexual foreplay may help promote vaginal lubrication. Kegel exercises would help manage urinary incontinence.

A biphosphate would be useful in preventing osteoporosis. Wearing cotton underwear and panty hose with a cotton crotch helps to reduce the risk of infection.

5. **A.** Estrogen replacement therapy is appropriate for women who have undergone a hysterectomy. HRT is absolutely contraindicated in women who have active or chronic severe hepatic disease, active or recent thromboembolic disease, and undiagnosed abnormal vaginal bleeding. HRT is potentially contraindicated in women with breast cancer, active or recent (within 5 years) endometrial cancer, history of thromboembolic disease, history of gallbladder disease, seizure disorders, and migraine headaches.
6. **C.** With menopause, loss of estrogen protection leads to increased LDL levels, exceeding those of men. In addition, women lose other cardiovascular benefits of estrogen. The average age of menopause is 51.4 years. Men, like women, experience hormonal changes with aging. Osteoporosis is a leading cause of impaired skeletal integrity and fractures after menopause.
7. **B.** A common adverse effect of alendronate (Fosamax) is heartburn. Fluid retention, breast tenderness, and mood alterations are common adverse effects associated with HRT.
8. **A.** Calcitonin (Miacalcin), available in injectable and intranasal forms, increases bone mass density and decreases backbone fractures. Raloxifene (Evista) is an oral selective estrogenic receptor modulator approved for prophylactic treatment of osteoporosis. Tamoxifen may be prescribed to prevent breast cancer recurrence. Atorvastatin is an antihyperlipemic agent.
9. **D.** The nurse should encourage clients to eat foods high in polyunsaturated and monounsaturated fats, while reducing intake of foods with saturated and trans fats. Antioxidants, such as vitamins C and E, may help prevent or reduce arterial LDLs. Aerobic exercise is important for cardiovascular health. Restricting intake to 1000 cal/day is not appropriate. Although the client may need to decrease her caloric intake, it still needs to be balanced and individualized according to her specific needs and circumstances.
10. **C.** Assessing ovarian hormone levels is key to determining if the client is experiencing premature ovarian failure. Once the nurse has obtained these levels, he or she can plan further interventions. Referrals for counseling depend on the situation. Breastfeeding is not relevant.

CHAPTER 24

1. **C.** When communicating with older adults, nurses should use direct, open-ended questions to elicit information. Asking about shoulder pain allows the client to describe her feelings in her own words. Asking the client about her living situation and if she is having pain right now are direct questions that could be important; however, they would elicit only "yes" or "no" answers, limiting the client's responses. Although asking a general lead-in question about how the client is feeling would be appropriate, calling her "sweetie" would be patronizing and incorrect.
2. **B.** IADLs further enhance the client's ability to live independently. They include such things as preparing meals, shopping for groceries, driving, doing housework, and handling finances. Ability to dress oneself is an example of a BADL. Participation in senior center activities and volunteer work are examples of AADLs.
3. **B.** Osteoporosis screening is recommended as follows: baseline DEXA scan at menopause and every 1 to 2 years after age 50 years. If the woman has osteopenia or osteoporosis, she should undergo follow-up DEXA scanning every 12 to 18 months.
4. **A.** Crackles, the most common physical finding in older adults, are always abnormal because they indicate inadequate air exchange, which is a potential source of infection. Decreased arm swing with walking is a normal age-associated change. A decrease in systolic blood pressure of 20 mm Hg or more or in diastolic blood pressure of 10 mm Hg or more indicates orthostasis. Decreases in forced vital capacity of 25 to 30 mL per year are age-associated respiratory system changes resulting from atrophy of the intercostal muscles and decreased diaphragmatic strength.
5. **D.** Decreased serum albumin levels can lead to an increased amount of free active drug, which subsequently leads to more adverse drug reactions and toxic effects. Adipose tissue increases, not decreases; as a result, fat/lipid-soluble drugs have increased tissue and decreased plasma concentrations. The result is a longer duration of effect by the drug on the body. Drug absorption in the older adult is complete but at a slower rate. Renal function decreases in older adults. Drugs excreted by the kidneys take longer to clear the body; thus, their half-lives are prolonged.
6. **A, B, and E.** Extrinsic factors are environmental hazards. Examples may include throw rugs; clutter; missing grab bars or rails in the bathroom, tub, or shower; exposed wires or cords; carpet holes or folds; poorly placed light switches; lack of a raised toilet seat; and no use of slip-resistant materials or surfaces on a floor, tub, or shower. The client's recent hip surgery and complaints of forgetfulness would be considered intrinsic (internal) factors.
7. **C.** Donepezil (Aricept), rivastigmine (Exelon), and galantamine (Reminyl) are examples of choli-

nesterase inhibitors used to treat AD. Memantine (Namenda) works on the glutamate neurotransmitter system. Vitamin E is used with cholinesterase inhibitors and memantine to help delay the progression of moderately severe cases of AD. Divalproex (Depakote), an anticonvulsant, has been shown to reduce impulsivity and agitation in clients with AD.

8. **A.** The most common side effect associated with sertraline (Zoloft), a selective serotonin reuptake inhibitor (SSRI), is sexual dysfunction.

9. **D.** For the client with mild to moderate pain, the American Geriatrics Society and American College of Rheumatology recommend starting with acetaminophen because of its low cost, high efficacy, and low toxicity. The other drugs should be avoided in older adults because of their increased risks for toxicity.

10. **B.** Based on the scenario, the client's daughter is most likely taking care of both her husband and her mother. The mother requires assistance with BADLs. The husband probably needs help because of his history of cerebrovascular accident, weakness, and osteoarthritis. Thus, the daughter would be at risk for caregiver role strain.

Breathing Instructions for Labor and Childbirth

Cleansing Breathing. This breathing is like the "bread of a sandwich," done at the beginning and end of each contraction. The breathing "filler" varies with the strength of the contraction. At the beginning and end of each contraction, take in a long breath through the nose; exhale out the mouth. Inhalation should be as long as exhalation.

Slow-paced Breathing. This is exactly as the name describes—breathing done when the client is not having a contraction and is relaxed and calm. Slow-paced breathing helps relax the muscles, thus increasing uterine contraction and moving oxygen-rich blood to the uterus and fetus. After a cleansing breath, continue to breathe very slowly and deeply, directly into the uterus. The pace should be half as fast as normal breathing. Once the contraction ends, repeat the cleansing breath and visualize something relaxing.

Modified-paced Breathing. When slow-paced breathing no longer effectively allows the client to stay "on top" of the contraction, **modified-paced breathing** should begin. The pace is about twice as fast as normal breathing. It is similar to running a race. You start slow; as you gain momentum, you pick up speed. As speed increases, breathing rate increases and becomes shallower. After a cleansing breath, breathe with the contraction, increasing the rate with the contraction intensity. Breathing is focused mainly on the lungs, not the uterus, because you need to increase your breathing rate. To do so, you need to make the breaths shallower. Focus your breathing on expanding the lungs and therefore increasing the oxygen available to the fetus. Finish with a cleansing breath.

Some people find difficulty with modified-paced breathing because they breathe so quickly (hyperventilate) that they become dizzy and may feel faint. If this happens, place your hand (or a bag) over your nose and mouth. Breathing will automatically slow because you will be inhaling carbon dioxide that you just exhaled. Another way to stop hyperventilating is to focus on your coach's face and to breathe in time with him or her.

Patterned-paced Breathing. This pattern requires more concentration than the previous "fillers." It is more effective against hyperventilation and will help decrease the chance of inadvertently pushing before your body is ready. Naturally, start with a cleansing breath; then follow this pattern: inhale, exhale, inhale, blow. Force the blow from pursed lips. Repeat until the contraction ends, and then complete with a cleansing breath. If you feel the urge to push, which may happen at the height of the contraction and indicates that the fetus has moved down in your pelvis, repeat the blowing without inhaling or exhaling. Once the urge to push has passed, restart the original pattern: inhale, exhale, inhale, blow. Complete with a cleansing breath.

Remember that just because the fetus is low in the pelvis, it does not mean that the cervix is open enough to facilitate birth. Do not to push until it has been determined via manual vaginal examination that the cervix is dilated enough to allow the fetus to pass through.

Glossary

Abortion: Termination of pregnancy before the fetus can exist independently outside the uterus.

Abstinence: Not engaging in vaginal intercourse.

Acceleration: An increase of at least 15 beats per minute over the baseline fetal heart rate that lasts at least 15 seconds, often associated with fetal activity.

Acid mantle: State of the fetal/newborn skin in which the surface pH is lower than 5 and acts as a bacteriostatic barrier.

Acme: The peak of a uterine contraction.

Acrocyanosis: Bluish discoloration normally found in the newborn soles and palms.

Actinic keratoses: Waxy-appearing skin nodules that vary in size.

Active labor: The second part of the first stage of labor, with cervical dilatation from 4 to 7 cm.

Activities of daily living (ADLs): Functions necessary for independent living.

Adolescence: Developmental stage beginning with puberty and lasting another 8 to 10 years.

Adolescent pregnancy: Pregnancy occurring between menarche and 19 years of age.

Adverse drug reaction: An unintended outcome of a medication.

Afterbirth: The expelled placenta and membranes following birth of a baby.

Afterpains: Postpartum uterine contractions.

Ageism: Stereotypes or prejudices applied to older adults, purely on the basis of their age.

Agency adoption: Adoption through a licensed organization that does all necessary legal, administrative, and social work to ensure efficient handling of processes in children's best interests.

Agnosia: Failure to recognize or identify objects despite intact basic sensory function.

Allele: The different compositions for a gene at a specific location on a chromosome; each gene has two or more distinct DNA compositions.

Alternative therapies: Treatment modalities used in place of traditional methods.

Ambulatory epidural pump: A drug delivery system that dispenses a preset intravenous dose of a narcotic agent into the client during epidural anesthesia.

Amenorrhea: Absence or suppression of menstruation.

Amnioinfusion: Infusion of a volume of warmed, sterile, Ringer's lactate solution or normal saline through a catheter to increase amniotic fluid volume, thus improving fetal and placental oxygenation, helping to cushion the umbilical cord, and diluting any meconium.

Amniotic fluid embolism: An embolism that results when a tear in the amnion and chorion provides a mechanism by which amniotic fluid can enter the maternal circulation and reach the pulmonary capillaries.

Amniotomy: Artificial rupture of the membranes using an amniohook.

Analgesia: Use of medication to decrease or alter the normal sensation of pain.

Androgen: Any steroid hormone with masculinizing effects.

Androgyny: The concept that both sexes exhibit the best qualities of both masculine and feminine stereotypes.

Andropause: Decrease in androgen production (specifically testosterone) that occurs in men during midlife or beyond, resulting in physical and psychological changes.

Anesthesia: Use of medication to provide partial or complete loss of sensation with or without loss of consciousness.

Anorexia nervosa: An eating disorder characterized by disturbed body image, extreme fear about being fat, and emaciation.

Antiphospholipid syndrome: An autoimmune disease characterized by the presence of antiphospholipid antibodies and at least one clinical manifestation, with venous or arterial thrombosis and recurrent fetal loss being the most common.

Apgar score: A standard tool used to assess and document the infant's response to birth by rating at 1 minute and 5 minutes after birth the baby's appearance (color), pulse (heart rate), grimace (reflex irritability), activity (muscle tone), and respiration (respiratory effort).

Aphasia: A language disturbance not related to mechanical aspects of speech.

Apnea: Temporary cessation of breathing.

Approach cues: Newborn behaviors that indicate a readiness to interact with the environment.

Apraxia: Failure to carry out motor tasks despite intact motor and sensory function.

Arrest disorder: Dystocia that develops during active labor and is characterized by a prolonged deceleration phase (at least 3 hours in a nullipara and 1 hour in a multipara); secondary arrest of cervical dilation (none for more than 2 hours); arrest of the descent of the fetal head (more than 60 minutes in a nullipara and 30 minutes in a multipara); and failure of the descent of the fetal head (none during the first stage, deceleration phase, or second stage).

Assisted hatching: Direct injection of a single sperm into an ovum, with microscopic holes drilled in the zona pellucida to facilitate fertilization.

Assisted reproductive technologies: All fertility procedures in which ova and sperm are artificially handled.

Association: Presentation of a recurring cluster of anomalies known to not be associated with a syndrome or sequence.

Attachments: Those significant relationships between an infant/child and his or her caregivers.

Attitude: The relationship of the fetal parts to one another. Attitudes are described as being in a state of flexion or extension.

Atypical presentation of illness: An illness that presents either without symptoms or with symptoms different from typical.

Augmentation of labor: Artificial stimulation of labor that began spontaneously but has progressed ineffectively.

Average for gestational age (AGA): Designation given when a newborn's weight falls between the 10th and 90th percentiles for gestational age.

Avoidance cues: Time-out signals indicating a newborn is tired or overstimulated and needs a break from interaction.

Bacterial vaginosis: An infection that develops when harmful vaginal bacteria increase and outnumber normal vaginal flora.

Ballard Gestational Age Assessment Tool: A scale of six physical and six neuromuscular criteria to estimate gestational ages.

Baseline bradycardia: A baseline fetal heart rate less than 120 bpm.

Baseline tachycardia: A baseline fetal heart rate greater than 160 bpm.

Baseline variability: The rhythm or beat-to-beat interval changes in the fetal heart rate. Long-term variability refers to oscillations or undulations of the baseline fetal heart rate.

Benign: Noncancerous; does not invade nearby tissue or spread to other parts of the body.

Bilateral tubal ligation: Procedures that interrupt the patency of or block the fallopian tubes to prevent pregnancy.

Bingeing: Consumption of large amounts of calories in short periods.

Bilirubin: A yellow pigment formed from hemoglobin as a byproduct of red blood cell breakdown.

Bisexual: Having an attraction to or sexual relationships with the same sex and the opposite sex.

Bishop score: A system for rating the readiness of the cervix for labor based on assessment of cervical position, consistency, effacement, and dilatation, as well as the fetal station.

Blastomere: The individual undifferentiated cell(s) of a dividing embryo prior to the formation of a blastocyst.

Blended family: A family that brings children from previous relationships into the family of a married couple.

Bloody show: Pinkish-tinged vaginal discharge, often mixed with mucus, caused by rupture of capillaries in the cervix as it begins to efface and dilate.

Body mass index (BMI): A calculated measure of weight in relation to height.

Boggy uterus: A uterus that has not contracted adequately; also called *atonic uterus.*

Bone-density scan: One of various screening tests used to monitor bone mineral density and fracture risk in menopausal women and those with risk factors for osteoporosis.

Bradycardia: In a newborn, a persistent resting apical heart rate below 100 beats/min.

Braxton-Hicks contractions: Intermittent uterine contractions throughout pregnancy beginning approximately the fourth month; they may be painful or painless; also called "false labor."

BRCA1: A gene on chromosome 17 that normally helps to suppress cell growth. An altered gene results in higher risk for breast, ovarian, or prostate cancer.

BRCA2: A gene on chromosome 13 that normally helps suppress cell growth. An altered gene results in higher risk for breast, ovarian, or prostate cancer.

Breakthrough bleeding (BTB): Vaginal bleeding at times other than menses.

Breast reconstruction: Surgery to rebuild a breast's shape after a mastectomy.

Breast self-examination (BSE): A method for women to check their own breasts for lumps and changes by physical examination.

Breech presentation: A fetus whose presenting part is the buttocks.

Bregma: The area of the fetal head that includes the anterior fontanel.

Brick dust spots: Pink stains that may normally appear in the urine of both male and female newborns as a result of uric acid crystals.

Bronchopulmonary dysplasia (BDP): A chronic lung disease that results from prematurity and long-term mechanical ventilation after the development of respiratory distress syndrome.

Brown adipose tissue (BAT): Highly vascular brown fat found around the scapulae, kidneys, adrenal glands, head, neck, heart, great vessels, and axillary regions of the term newborn, which generates more energy than any other body tissue and increases local temperature.

Bulimia nervosa: An eating disorder characterized by the consumption of extreme amounts of food with subsequent behaviors to eliminate the excess calories.

Candidiasis: Infection that develops from overgrowth of *Candida albicans* (also called a *yeast infection*).

Carcinoma in situ: Cervical cancer that involves only the cells in which it began.

Cephalopelvic disproportion: A term used when the size or shape of the fetal head or the maternal pelvis does not allow passage of the fetus through the maternal pelvis.

Cerclage: Suturing of the cervix, sometimes used to manage cervical insufficiency.

Certified nurse-midwife (CNM): An individual educated in nursing and midwifery, who has evidence of certification according to the requirements of the American College of Nurse-Midwives.

Cervical cap: A firm rubber cap with a rim sized to fit over the cervix to prevent pregnancy.

Cervical dysplasia: A benign condition that involves abnormal changes in the cervical cells.

Cervical insufficiency: A condition in which the cervix dilates painlessly before gestation has progressed normally.

Cervical ripening: The process of physical softening and stretching of the cervix in preparation for labor and birth that may be accomplished through natural or artificial means.

Cervical stenosis: Narrowing or closing of the cervical os.

Chadwick's sign: Violet-bluish color of the vagina and cervix that results from secretion of estrogen increasing vascularity to these areas during pregnancy.

Chloasma: Darkened pigmentation of the face, usually across the nose and cheeks, which sometimes occurs during pregnancy; also called *melasma* or the "*mask of pregnancy.*"

Chromosome: A threadlike strand of DNA, RNA, and proteins in the nucleus of animal and plant cells that carries genes and transmits hereditary information.

Chronic sorrow: The continuous re-living of the unexpected or undesired loss of a person, expectation, or goal, resulting in the expression of sadness, anger, and guilt.

Circumcision: Surgical removal of the foreskin from the end of the penis.

Circumoral cyanosis: Blue discoloration around the newborn's mouth, which is normal for the first 24 hours of life and then requires evaluation.

Client-controlled analgesia: A drug delivery system that dispenses a preset intravenous dose of a narcotic agent when the client pushes a button attached via an electric cord to a device.

Clinical breast examination: Observation and palpation of the breast by an experienced clinician to find any change that the woman herself missed during self-examination.

Climacteric: Period of decreasing fertility that corresponds with perimenopause.

Closed adoption: Adoption with no contact between the birth and adoptive parents.

Coenzyme: A small organic molecule that increases enzyme activity.

Cofactor: A small inorganic or organic substance that works with enzymes to promote chemical reactions.

Colic: Unconsolable crying in an infant for which no physical cause can be found, which lasts more than 3 hours a day, occurs at least 3 days a week, and continues for at least 3 weeks.

Colostrum: The initial breast secretion produced during pregnancy and for the first several days postpartum; it is rich in nutrients and contains immunity transferred passively to the infant.

Colposcopy: Use of a lighted magnifying instrument to examine the vagina and cervix.

Combined oral contraceptives (COCs): Pills containing estrogen and progestin that, when taken daily, prevent pregnancy by inhibiting ovulation and thickening cervical mucus.

Complementary proteins: Two or more proteins that, when combined, supply all essential amino acids, but alone lack at least one essential amino acid.

Complementary therapies: Nontraditional therapies that can interface with traditional medical and surgical therapies.

Complete protein: A dietary protein that contains all essential amino acids in proportions similar to those required by humans.

Conception: The uniting of male sperm with a female ovum.

Condylomata: Genital warts usually found on the external genitalia that result from infection with human papillomavirus.

Confabulation: Telling imaginary stories to fill in gaps in the memory of an event.

Congenital diaphragmatic hernia: Protrusion of abdominal contents through an abnormality in the diaphragm.

Conization: Surgery to remove a cone-shaped piece of tissue from the cervix and cervical canal. When used as a diagnostic tool it is called *cone biopsy.*

Constriction rings: Rare rings in the uterus that usually conform to a fetal depression and do not extend all the way around the uterus. The area of spasm is thick, but the lower uterine segment does not become stretched or thinned.

Contraception: Any method used to prevent pregnancy.

Contraceptive sponge: A soft device sold over the counter that fits over a woman's cervix and releases spermicide to prevent fertilization.

Contraction: Intermittent tightening of the uterine muscles during labor, which accomplishes cervical effacement and dilation and facilitates fetal descent through the pelvis.

Contraction duration: The length of a uterine contraction, measured from the beginning to the end of the contraction and recorded in seconds.

Contraction frequency: Measurement of the interval of labor contractions, lasting from the beginning of one contraction to the beginning of the next, and recorded in minutes.

Contraction intensity: The increase in uterine pressure during a contraction.

Cord prolapse: Term used when a portion of the umbilical cord falls in front of, lies beside, or hangs below the fetal presenting part.

Corpus luteum: A mass that forms from granulation cells and fluid and secretes progesterone and estrogen during the secretory phase of the menstrual cycle.

Couplet care: A model of care in which mother and baby are treated as a unit; also called *mother–baby care.*

Critical thinking: A higher level, complex thought process through which competent, comprehensive decision-making and problem-solving can result in informed, intelligent choices.

Crowning: Encircling of the widest part of the fetal head by the vaginal opening before birth.

Cultural competence: Attaining cultural knowledge, having an open attitude, and implementing appropriate clinical skills.

Cultural identity: Religion, rites of passage, language, dietary habits, and leisure activities.

Cultural relativism: The belief that the behaviors and practices of people should be judged only from the context of their cultural system.

Cystitis: Inflammation of the bladder.

Cystocele: Abnormal downward protrusion of the bladder into the anterior vaginal wall.

Deep venous thrombosis (DVT): A condition involving the deep veins of the legs associated with obstruction and clot formation.

Deceleration: A deviation of the fetal heart rate below baseline that persists for at least 10 to 15 seconds but for less than 2 minutes.

Deformation: The result of a mechanical event that abnormally molds an otherwise healthy tissue. It is often reversible after birth.

Delirium: A medical emergency marked by agitated restlessness or decreased activity.

Denominator: The arbitrarily chosen landmark on the fetal presenting part used to describe position.

Developmental dysplasia of the hip (DDH): A group of hip abnormalities, ranging from a shallow acetabulum, to a stretched capsule with ligamentum teres, to complete dislocation.

Diabetes mellitus: A chronic disorder of carbohydrate metabolism in which the blood glucose level is continuously above normal. It results from a relative or absolute lack of insulin.

Diaphragm: A flexible latex ring covered with a latex dome inserted into the vagina to cover the cervix and prevent pregnancy.

Diastasis: Separation of the recti abdominis muscles along the median line.

Differentiation of self: How much a person separates himself or herself from family members.

Dilation: The opening of the cervical canal, measured from 0 to 10 cm.

Disruption: A change in the morphology of a structure after its formation.

Disseminated intravascular coagulopathy: A disorder in which many defects in the coagulation cascade result in inappropriate clotting throughout the body.

Dizygotic twins: Also called *fraternal twins;* the result of separate sperm independently fertilizing two or more oocytes within a single menstrual cycle.

Dominant: The need for only one copy of an allele to express an associated trait or gene product. This single copy may be from either the mother or father.

Doula: A Greek word meaning *woman's servant.* In labor, it refers to a supportive companion professionally trained to provide continuous support to a woman throughout the process.

Ductus arteriosus: A fetal circulatory structure that connects the pulmonary artery and descending aorta, causing most of the blood to detour the fetal lungs.

Dysfunctional uterine bleeding: Abnormal or irregular bleeding not related to pregnancy, infection, or tumor.

Dysmenorrhea: Painful menstruation.

Dysmorphology: Field of study that evaluates fetuses, stillborns, infants, children, and adults with or suspected to have a disorder associated with a malformation, deformation, or disruption in their development.

Dyspareunia: Pain with intercourse, which may develop as a result of vaginal atrophy.

Dysphagia: Difficulty swallowing.

Dysthymic disorder: Persistent depressed mood without the severity of major depression.

Dystocia: Abnormal or dysfunctional labor.

Early deceleration: A decrease in fetal heart rate that begins and ends at the same time as the uterine contraction, causing a consistent U-shaped waveform that mirrors the contraction on an electronic fetal monitor; thought to be caused by compression of the fetal head.

Early labor: The first phase of first-stage labor, with the cervix dilating from 0 to 3 cm; also called the *latent phase.*

Early postpartum hemorrhage: Excessive bleeding within 24 hours of birth.

Eclampsia: Life-threatening problem that develops as a consequence of uncontrolled hypertension in pregnancy, with convulsions, twitching, and tonic-clonic contractions.

Ecomap: Device that illustrates a family's relationship to a larger community.

Ectopic pregnancy: Implantation of the products of conception anywhere other than the uterus.

Effacement: Thinning or flattening of the edge of the cervical os, measured from 0% to 100%.

Elder mistreatment: Acts of abuse, neglect, or exploitation against older adults.

Electronic fetal monitoring (EFM): Continuous recording of the fetal heart rate and uterine contractions by an electronic fetal monitor using external or internal modes.

Endometriosis: A disorder in which endometrial tissue normally found in the uterus escapes through the fallopian tubes into the pelvic cavity.

Engagement: Entry of the widest part of the fetal presenting part at the maternal pelvic inlet, with the presenting part at 0 station.

Engorgement: Swelling of breast tissue caused by congestion and increased vascularity.

Enterocele: Bulging of the bowel through the posterior cul-de-sac and vaginal wall.

Epidural anesthesia block: Injection of local anesthetic agents into the epidural space between the dura mater and the ligamentum flavum between the fourth and fifth lumbar vertebrae via a small tube inserted into the client's back by an anesthesiologist.

Epidural blood patch: Injection of 10 to 15 ml of autologous blood into the epidural space, which then forms a clot that covers a tear or hole in the dura mater around the spinal cord to prevent further leakage of spinal fluid.

Episiotomy: A surgical incision of the perineum made just prior to the birth of a baby.

Esophageal atresia: A congenital disorder in which the esophageal passageway to the stomach is disrupted and closed off, ending in a blind pouch.

Estrogen: A predominant female hormone.

Ethically based practice: Integration of formal and informal ethical principles and beliefs in the practice of nursing.

Evidence-based decision making: A continuous interactive process involving the explicit, conscientious, and judicious consideration of the best available evidence.

Evidence-based health care: Decisions that affect the care of clients taken with appropriate weight accorded to all valid, relevant information.

Evidence-based practice: The conscientious, explicit, and judicious use of current best evidence in making decisions about the care of individual clients.

Extended family: A child living with at least one parent and at least one other person who is not part of the nuclear family.

Extended kin network: Two or more households in close proximity to each other that share social support, responsibility, goods, and services.

External cephalic version: A procedure in which a fetus is turned in utero from noncephalic (usually breech) to cephalic presentation.

Failure to progress: Labor in which the cervix does not dilate normally despite normal uterine contractions and no cephalopelvic disproportion.

Fallaphobia: Fear of falling.

Family: A group of individuals bound together by commitment and affection with relationships that last from several years to the lifespan of the members.

Female condom: A polyurethane sheath inserted into the vagina to prevent pregnancy.

Female genital mutilation: Any procedure that involves partial or total removal of the external female genitalia or any other injury to female genital organs for nontherapeutic reasons.

Fertility awareness methods: Methods (including calendar, basal body temperature, and cervical mucous tracking) that determine ovulation and are used with a barrier method or withdrawal during the fertile time to prevent pregnancy.

Fertility rate: Ratio of births to the number of women in their childbearing years within a specific group.

Fetal alcohol syndrome: Characteristic deformities that result from maternal use of alcohol during pregnancy.

Fibroadenoma: A painless solid breast mass or lump with well-defined borders that is usually mobile and generally noncancerous.

First stage of labor: Labor from the onset of regular contractions to 10 cm of cervical dilatation; this stage is further divided into early, active, and transition phases.

Fontanelles: Soft spots at the top (anterior) and back (posterior) of the fetal head, covered with strong connective tissue where the unfused bones of the fetal skull intersect at the suture lines.

Foramen ovale: A fetal circulatory structure that allows blood to pump directly from the right to the left ventricle.

Forceps: Stainless-steel instruments that can fit around the head of the fetus to help pull him or her through the vaginal outlet.

Foremilk: Breast milk delivered during the first 5 to 10 minutes of a feeding.

Fortified: Term used to indicate that a nutrient has been added to a food.

Fourth stage of labor: The period from delivery of the placenta until 1 hour after birth.

Free-flow oxygen: Oxygen higher than 21% that blows passively through oxygen tubing, an oxygen mask, or the mask of a flow-inflating oxygen bag.

Functional residual capacity: State in which the newborn's first breaths are deep enough to displace the liquid in the airways and to retain some air in the alveoli so that subsequent breaths are less difficult.

Fundus: The uppermost portion of the uterus, above the point of insertion of the fallopian tubes.

Gamete intrafallopian transfer (GIFT): Transfer of ovum and sperm to the fallopian tube for fertilization.

Gametogenesis: The postpuberty process by which germ cells yield mature gametes.

Gastroesophageal reflux (GER): In newborns, occasional burps, emesis, or nonregurgitant reflux associated with failure to thrive, irritability with feeding, anemia, hematemesis, pneumonia, and apnea.

Gastroschisis: A congenital opening in the anterior abdominal wall, usually to the right of the umbilical cord insertion, through which eviscerated abdominal contents protrude.

Gender constancy: Understanding that gender does not change despite external alterations.

Gender identity: A person's sense of maleness or femaleness, acceptance of the role of that gender, and internalization of the gender and gender role.

Gender role development: The process by which children come to know and accept the social implications of their sex.

General anesthesia: The use of short-acting intravenous sedation followed by endotracheal intubation and the use of inhalation anesthetics, rendering the client unconscious.

Genes: The basic units of heredity located along the DNA of each chromosome.

Genetic counseling: A process of information gathering, clinical and laboratory evaluation, and information sharing about the occurrence of or risk for a genetic disorder.

Genetics: The field of study that investigates variations within the human genome.

Genital herpes: A chronic lifelong sexually transmitted infection caused by the herpes simplex virus.

Genogram: A device that uses visual links and other symbols to depict family relationships.

Genotype: The specific sequence for each gene in a person's own unique genetic code.

Gestational diabetes: Glucose intolerance of varying severity first occurring or diagnosed during pregnancy.

Gestational trophoblastic disease: Abnormal proliferation and degeneration of the trophoblastic villi.

Glycemic index: A measure of how quickly and how high blood sugar increases after a certain food is eaten.

Goodell's sign: Softening of the cervix that develops during the second month of pregnancy; caused by increased vascularity, hypertrophy, and hyperplasia in the area.

Health: Total physical, psychological, and social well-being.

Health care proxy: The person who has medical decision-making abilities for the client if she becomes mentally incapacitated.

Health promotion: A process that enables people to address cultural, social, and political factors to increase control over and to improve their health.

Hegar's sign: Softening of the isthmus, the area between the cervix and the body of the uterus, that occurs approximately the 6th to 8th week of gestation.

HELLP: The acronym used to describe a syndrome consisting of hemolysis, elevated liver enzymes, and low platelet count.

Hematoma: A localized collection of blood that results from bleeding into the connective tissue beneath the vaginal mucosa or vulvar skin as a consequence of tissue injury or trauma.

Hemorrhoids: Rectal varicose veins that may protrude from the anus or be hidden internally.

Hepatitis: Inflammation of the liver resulting from different viruses.

Hermaphroditism: A condition in which a person has both ovarian and testicular tissue.

High-risk pregnancy: A pregnancy in which the life or health of the fetus, mother, or both is vulnerable because of a medical or obstetric condition.

Hindmilk: Breast milk at the end of a feeding session, which is high in fat and calories.

Holistic: Philosophy of care that views the whole as greater than the sum of the parts. In family care, the view that a woman is not only having a baby but also meeting challenges of need fulfillment, integration, adaptation, and role fulfillment.

Homan's sign: An assessment for thrombus formation in which the foot is dorsiflexed to check for sharp pain in the posterior calf (a positive Homans' sign).

Hydrocephalus: Excess accumulation of cerebrospinal fluid in the brain ventricles and subsequent cranial enlargement.

Hyperbilirubinemia: Elevated serum bilirubin level.

Hyperemesis gravidarum: Excessive vomiting causing weight loss greater than 5% of prepregnancy weight together with dehydration, electrolyte imbalance, and ketosis.

Hyperstimulation: Either a series of single contractions lasting 2 minutes or more or a contraction frequency of five or more in 10 minutes. Contractions of normal duration within 1 minute of each other would also be included.

Hyperthermia: Heat stroke and heat exhaustion resulting from excessive heat storage with a decreased ability to rid the body of heat through evaporation, radiation, and conduction.

Hypertonic uterine contractions: Contractions in which the uterine midsegment contracts with more force than the fundus or the impulses in each upper uterine corner are not synchronized.

Hypnobirthing: A series of relaxation techniques used to help laboring mothers to decrease pain and emotional stress of childbirth without the use of drugs.

Hypofibrinogenemia: A low level of fibrinogen, a necessary protein in the clotting cascade. The condition may be congenital or acquired.

Hypoglycemia: In newborns, a plasma glucose concentration less than 45 mg/dl for term and preterm infants.

Hypothermia: Rectal temperature of 95°F (35°C) or below.

Hypotonic uterine contractions: Contractions that have no basal tone, are infrequent, and fail to dilate the cervix satisfactorily.

Hypoxia: Abnormally low oxygen concentration in tissues.

Hysterectomy: Surgical removal of the uterus.

Intracytoplasmic sperm injection (ICSI): Injection of one sperm directly into the ovum for fertilization, with transfer of the resultant embryo to the uterus.

Impaired fecundity: Inability to carry a pregnancy to a live birth.

Imperforate anus: Congenital absence of an opening to the anus with failure of rectal descent.

Incompetent cervix: A condition in which the cervix dilates painlessly before gestation has progressed normally; also called *cervical insufficiency.*

Incomplete proteins: Foods lacking one or more of the nine indispensable amino acids.

Indirect bilirubin: Bilirubin bound to circulating albumin in the bloodstream that has not yet been metabolized in the liver; also called *unconjugated bilirubin.*

Induced abortion: Pregnancy termination that does not occur spontaneously.

Induction of labor: Artificial stimulation of labor prior to its natural onset.

Infant formula: Substance patterned after the composition of breast milk or the outcomes of the postprandial breast-fed infant and given to babies as a feeding source.

Infant mortality: Rate of deaths in the first year of life.

Infertility: Inability to achieve pregnancy after 1 year of appropriately timed, unprotected intercourse.

Inflammatory breast cancer: A rare type of breast cancer in which cells block the lymph vessels in the skin and breast.

Informed consent: The verbal or written process by which a health client or prospective research subject is informed of the risks/benefits, personal rights, and other additional pertinent information, regarding participating in either an intervention or a research study.

Informed decision making and consent: The process followed to provide and assist people in a socioculturally appropriate manner to choose a plan of care based on full disclosure of the science and known benefits, risks, limitations, and human and financial resource costs associated with available interventions for that care.

Inner strength: The capacity to build oneself through a developmental process that positively moves a person through challenging events.

International adoption: Adoption in which the adoptive parent(s) and child are from two different countries.

Intracytoplasmic sperm injection (ICSI): Process in which an ovum and sperm are retrieved and fertilized in a laboratory, the sperm are introduced directly into the cytoplasm of the ovum, and the results are transferred to a woman's uterus for implantation and development.

Intrauterine device (IUD): A plastic T-shaped device placed into the uterine cavity to provide contraception by preventing fertilization and implantation.

Intrauterine growth restriction (IUGR): A condition in which the fetus is small and undernourished for gestational age.

In vitro fertilization (IVF): Process in which an ovum and sperm are retrieved and fertilized in a laboratory, then transferred to a woman's uterus for implantation and development.

Involution: The process of uterine contraction and shrinking that follows birth.

Isolated systolic hypertension (ISH): Systolic blood pressure greater than 170 mm Hg, accompanied by a diastolic blood pressure less than 90 mm Hg, caused by changes in the vascular media that result in increased intimal thickening and fibrosis.

Jaundice: Yellowish discoloration of the skin that results from elevated bilirubin levels.

Kegel's exercises: Strengthening exercises in which a woman alternately contracts and relaxes her perineal muscles (as though stopping urination) to help strengthen them.

Kernicterus: Bilirubin deposited on the newborn's brain, which can lead to serious neurologic sequelae.

Labor: The series of events by which the products of conception are expelled from the mother's body.

Lactational amenorrhea method: Prevention of pregnancy during the first 6 postpartum months through breastfeeding exclusively.

Laminaria tents: Small cones of dried seaweed that, when exposed to moisture, expand.

Lanugo: Fine hair on the cheeks, shoulders, forehead, and pinna of ears in newborns.

Laparoscopy: Pelvic examination with an instrument inserted through a small incision in the abdominal wall.

Large for gestational age (LGA): Designation given when a newborn weighs more than the 90th percentile for gestation.

Late deceleration: A deceleration of the fetal heart rate that begins after the peak and finishes after the end of the contraction; it is associated with compromised uteroplacental perfusion.

Late postpartum hemorrhage: Excessive vaginal bleeding after the first 24 hours of birth.

Learned hopelessness: A behavioral theory that posits that negative thought patterns, as often observed in depressed and suicidal people, are learned.

Leiomyoma (fibroid tumor): A benign mass of muscle and fibrous connective tissue in the uterus.

Leopold's maneuvers: A systematic approach of external palpation used to determine fetal position and presentation.

Leukorrhea: Asymptomatic, normal mucous discharge from the vagina and cervix throughout pregnancy.

Lie: The relationship of the fetal long axis (spine) to the maternal long axis (spine).

Lightening: A lay term describing settlement of the fetal presenting part into the maternal pelvis.

Linea nigra: A dark line that appears from the sternum to the pubis in some pregnant women, caused by increased secretion of the pituitary melanin-stimulating hormone.

Local anesthesia: Direct administration of an anesthetic agent into tissues to induce the absence of sensation in a small area of the body.

Lochia: Vaginal flow that occurs following birth.

Lochia alba: Whitish or yellowish lochia that usually lasts from postpartum day 10 to postpartum weeks 5 to 6.

Lochia rubra: Dark red lochia that usually lasts immediately after childbirth until postpartum day 3 or 4.

Lochia serosa: Pink lochia that usually lasts from postpartum day 3 or 4 until postpartum day 10.

Low birth weight (LBW): Designation when a newborn weighs less than 2500 grams (5.5 pounds).

Lymphedema: A collection of excess fluid in tissue resulting in swelling.

Macronutrients: Nutrients that provide energy: carbohydrate, fat, and protein.

Macrosomia: Term used to indicate an infant whose birth weight is 9 lbs (4000 g) or more; also called a *high birth weight infant.*

Male condom: A flexible sheath of latex, sheep intestine, or polyurethane that covers the penis to contain the contents of ejaculate.

Malformation: The complete or partial absence of a fetal structure.

Malposition: Presentation by the fetal head such that the diameter of the skull in relation to the maternal pelvis is greater than normal.

Malpresentation: Any fetal presentation other than vertex.

Mammogram: A soft tissue x-ray of the breast that may be used to evaluate a lump or to screen for signs of breast cancer.

Mastalgia: Pain in the breasts, associated with cyclical hormonal changes or trauma.

Mastectomy: Surgery to remove the breast or as much of the breast tissue as possible.

Mastitis: Inflammation of the breast tissue.

Masturbation: Self-manipulation of the genitals for sexual pleasure.

Maternal morbidity: A condition outside of normal pregnancy, labor, and birth that negatively affects a woman's health during those times; reported in terms of 1000 live births.

Maternal mortality: Deaths during or within 1 year after the end of pregnancy that result from 1) complications of pregnancy itself; 2) a chain of events initiated by pregnancy; or 3) aggravation of an unrelated condition by the physiologic effects of pregnancy-related deaths.

Mature human milk: Milk that contains more lactose and fat than does colostrum and begins approximately 2 weeks postpartum, lasting until 7 to 8 months of lactation.

Mechanisms of labor: The movements the fetus must accomplish to negotiate passage through the maternal pelvis and be born, including engagement, descent, flexion, internal rotation, extension, restitution, external rotation, and expulsion; also called *cardinal movements.*

Meconium: The newborn's first stool.

Meiosis: The process of cell division used solely by germ cells to produce gametes with 23 chromosomes, half the normal complement of 46 chromosomes.

Menarche: The beginning of menstruation and the ability of the female to reproduce.

Meningocele: Failure of the neural tube to close, leaving an opening in the vertebral column with an external pouch containing cerebrospinal fluid.

Menopause: Amenorrhea for 12 consecutive months; it is diagnosed retroactively and experienced concurrently with the last year of perimenopause.

Menorrhagia: Irregular vaginal bleeding that is excessive in flow and length.

Menstrual cycle: Cycle lasting an average of 28 days during which the woman's body prepares an internal environment for conceiving and housing a pregnancy.

Menstrual phase: The menstrual cycle from days 1 to 4 during which the endometrial lining that developed in anticipation of a fertilized ovum is sloughed off as bloody vaginal discharge.

Mental health literacy: Knowledge and beliefs about mental disorders that help the person to recognize, manage, and prevent the disorders.

Metabolic rate: A measure of energy production, or how fast the body burns calories.

Metalloenzyme: An enzyme whose structure contains one or more minerals.

Mid-arm circumference: A measure of skeletal muscle mass in which the examiner uses a tape measure to encircle the client's nondominant arm at the midpoint of the upper arm between shoulder and elbow.

Midwife: A person who, having been regularly admitted to a midwifery educational program duly recognized in the country of location, has successfully completed the required course of studies in midwifery and has acquired the requisite qualifications to be registered, legally licensed, or both to practice midwifery.

Milk bank: An agency that collects donor human milk, verifies its safety, and distributes it on request.

Minority sexual orientation: Sexual orientation other than heterosexual.

Miscarriage: A pregnancy lost before 20 weeks' gestation.

Mitosis: Cell division whereby a single cell replicates itself and forms two new cells.

Molding: The elongated shaping of the fetal head as it moves through the bony pelvis during labor and birth; caused by the normal overriding of the unfused fetal cranial bones.

Monozygotic twins: Also called *identical twins;* the result of an alteration in the normal development of a zygote, which causes the zygote to split and grow into two genetically identical beings.

Montgomery's tubercles: Elevated sebaceous glands of the areola that appear during middle to late pregnancy. They secrete a protective lipid substance during lactation.

Morning sickness: Nausea and vomiting that is usually limited to the first trimester of pregnancy, although it may continue beyond this.

Morula: The dividing embryo that contains 16 or more blastomeres prior to cell differentiation.

Mother-Friendly Childbirth™ Initiative: A document that defines mother-friendly services in hospitals, birth centers, and home birth practices as those that promote birth as a normal, natural, and healthy process; empower women to develop confidence in their ability to give birth and care for their babies; give women autonomy to make informed choices about the care they and their baby receive; do no harm by applying only medically necessary interventions; and take responsibility for the quality of care provided, based on the needs of the mother and child.

Multifactorial disorder: A disorder that results from the interaction of multiple genes with environmental factors.

Multigravida: A woman who has been pregnant prior to the current pregnancy.

Multiparity: A woman who has had two or more births at greater than 20 weeks' gestation.

Multiple pregnancy: Gestation with two or more fetuses.

Mutations: Inheritable and permanent alterations in the DNA sequence of a gene.

Myelomeningocele: Failure of the neural tube to close with protrusion of the spinal nerves into the sac with the cerebrospinal fluid and meninges.

Myocardial ischemia: Decreased coronary blood flow.

Nagele's rule: Method of estimating the expected date of delivery by subtracting 3 months and adding 7 days to the first day of the woman's last normal menstrual period.

Narcotic agonist-antagonists: Analgesic agents that stimulate opiate receptors, resulting in pain relief, and block specific opiate receptors, alleviating maternal and respiratory depression.

Narcotic antagonist: A drug used primarily to treat narcotic-induced respiratory depression.

Natural family planning: Methods (including calendar, basal body temperature, and cervical mucous tracking) that determine ovulation and rely upon abstinence during the fertile time to prevent pregnancy.

Neutral thermal environment (NTE): An environmental goal for all newborns, in which heat production and oxygen consumption are minimized so that body temperature stays normal without requiring physiologic mechanisms that increase metabolic rate and oxygen consumption.

Nociceptive stimuli: Stimuli of such intensity that they may cause tissue damage.

Nocturnal emission: Ejaculation of semen during sleep in males.

Nonshivering thermogenesis (NST): The main source of heat production in the newborn, triggered at a mean skin temperature of 35–36°C (95–96.8°F), in which thermal receptors transmit impulses to the hypothalamus, which stimulates the sympathetic nervous system and causes norepinephrine release in brown adipose tissue.

Normal birth: Birth with the aim of care to achieve a healthy mother and child with the least possible level of intervention that is compatible with safety.

Nucleotide: The building block of DNA and RNA composed of a base, sugar, and protein.

Nursing supplementer: A device that contains breast milk or formula and delivers the feeding by a tube placed near the mother's nipple and into the infant's mouth.

Nutrient density: A variable used to assess the quality of a food choice.

Nutritional assessment: The summative evaluation of factors that affect nutritional status, including general state of health, educational background, socioeconomic issues, weight history, and current body mass index (BMI).

Nutritional screening: A review of key factors related to nutritional status, such as recent weight loss, diagnoses that warrant closer attention, and acute gastrointestinal problems.

Obesity: Body mass index of 30 or more. In pregnancy it can also be determined by a pre-pregnancy or pregnancy weight of more than 200 lbs., or being 110% of ideal body weight at the first prenatal visit.

Occipitoposterior (OP) position: Fetal position in which the fetal occiput is found in the posterior part of the maternal pelvis.

Occiput: Head.

Oligohydramnios: Amniotic fluid less than 300 mL or an amniotic fluid index of 5 cm or less.

Omphalocele: A congenital defect in the umbilical ring that allows abdominal contents contained within a peritoneal sac to protrude through the external abdominal surface at the base of the umbilical cord.

Oocyte: The female gamete (egg) that contains half of a child's genetic material, received from his or her biologic mother.

Open adoption: Adoption in which the biological parent(s), adoptee, and adoptive parent(s) have an ongoing association, ranging from sharing pictures or letters to ongoing visitation.

Operculum: Mucus plug during pregnancy and helps protect the uterus against infection.

Oral–facial cleft: Congenital defect of both the lip and palate.

Orthostatic (postural) hypotension: A drop in systolic blood pressure of 20 mm Hg or more, or a drop in diastolic blood pressure of 10 mm Hg when rising from a sitting position.

Osteopenia: Bone density below normal, but above the level of defined osteoporosis.

Osteoporosis: Low bone mass density and microarchitectural deterioration of bone tissue, which increases risk/incidence of skeletal fractures and breaks.

Ovulation: Rupture of a mature follicle and release of its ovum.

Pain threshold: The point at which a sensation is physically perceived as painful.

Pain tolerance: The maximum amount of pain that a person is willing to endure.

Pap smear: A screening test to detect cancer of the uterus by which cells are scraped from the cervix and examined under a microscope.

Para: The number of births a woman has had after the 20th week of gestation.

Pathologic retraction ring: An exaggeration of the normal physiologic retraction ring found at the junction of the upper and lower uterine segments.

Pelvic inflammatory disease: Infection of the uterus, fallopian tubes, and adjacent pelvic structures not associated with pregnancy or surgery.

Pelvic inlet: The upper border of the true pelvis; also called the *pelvic brim* or *linea terminalis.*

Pelvic outlet: The lower border of the true pelvis.

Pelvic relaxation: Term denoting congenital or acquired weakness of pelvic support structures.

Perimenopause: Period preceding menopause and continuing through the first 12 months of menopause, when ovarian hormones fluctuate, resulting in some of the effects of menopause and possibly postmenopausal vaginal bleeding.

Periodic breathing: Pauses in newborn breathing of less than 15 seconds.

Peripartum cardiomyopathy (PPCM): Congestive heart failure in the last month of gestation through 5 months postpartum in a woman with no previous cardiac disease.

Peritonitis: A potentially life-threatening infection of the peritoneum or abdominal cavity.

Pharmacodynamics: The effect of drugs on the older person's body.

Pharmacokinetics: How the older adult's body handles drugs.

Phenotype: The type and extent of clinical manifestation of a gene by a person.

Phototherapy: Exposing as much of the newborn's skin surface as possible to blue wavelengths of light to assist with the excretion of excess bilirubin.

Physiologic jaundice: Normal visible jaundice in a newborn whose bilirubin levels have reached a total serum value of 5 to 7 mg/dl in the first few days after birth.

Phytochemicals: Plant-based nutrients that may have protective properties.

Pica: Eating or craving non-food substances, such as starch, clay, dirt, or ice.

Piper forceps: A special type of forceps used in breech presentations with an aftercoming head.

Placenta previa: A placenta implanted in the lower uterine segment near or over the internal cervical os.

Placental abruption: Premature separation of a normally implanted placenta from the uterine wall; also called *abruptio placentae.*

Plugged milk duct: A tender hot breast lump resulting from accumulated milk or dead cells.

Polycystic ovarian syndrome: A common cause of ovarian dysfunction and imbalanced hormones, with symptoms including obesity, hirsutism, menstrual problems, and infertility.

Polypharmacy: Use of multiple drugs by the same client.

Position: The relationship of a landmark on the presenting part of the fetus to the front, back, or side of the maternal pelvis.

Postmenopause: The phase of a woman's life marked by at least 1 year of complete cessation of menses.

Postpartum blues: Also called "maternity blues," a mild mood condition following childbirth marked by tearfulness, emotional variability, irritability, and anxiety.

Postpartum depression: An episode of depression within the first 4 weeks after childbirth.

Postpartum hemorrhage: Blood loss greater than 500 ml during or after the third stage of labor.

Post-term: Gestation that has reached 42 weeks from the first day of the last menstrual period in the woman with a 28-day menstrual cycle.

Precipitous labor: Labor that lasts less than 3 hours, caused by uterine contractions that are more frequent, intense, or both than normal.

Pre-eclampsia: Hypertension after 20 weeks' gestation with proteinuria.

Premature ovarian failure: Failure of the ovaries to produce hormones in a woman younger than 40 years of age.

Premenstrual syndrome: Regular premenstrual physical or emotional symptoms that interfere with daily living and functioning at home and work.

Presbycardia: Limited cardiac reserve.

Presentation: The part of the fetal body that appears at the pelvic outlet first; also called the *presenting part.*

Presenting part: The part of the fetal body that appears at the pelvic outlet first; also called *presentation.*

Preterm: Designation given when birth occurs before 37 completed weeks of pregnancy; also called *premature.*

Preterm labor: Uterine contractions between 20 to 37 weeks' gestation that cause progressive cervical changes (dilatation, effacement, or both).

Preterm premature rupture of membranes (pPROM): Spontaneous rupture of the amniotic membrane prior to 37 weeks of gestation.

Primary caregiver: A family member, significant other, or friend who assists the client to meet her functional needs.

Primary health care provider: Health care provider responsible for handling first contact into the health care system who provides a continuum of care, evaluation, management, health maintenance, and appropriate referrals.

Primary infertility: Complete inability in a man or a woman to conceive.

Primigravida: A woman whose current pregnancy is her first.

Private adoption: Adoption without involvement from a licensed agency.

Prodromal labor: A period of regular or irregular contractions toward the end of pregnancy that does not result in progressive cervical dilatation.

Proliferative phase: The menstrual cycle from days 5 to 13, during which hormonal secretions stimulate the growth of various follicles and thickening of the endometrial lining in preparation for housing a fertilized ovum.

Protein hydrolysate: Formulas containing short peptide chains and free amino acids from the casein or whey component of cow milk for the protein source.

Protraction disorder: A classification of dysfunctional labor characterized by delayed cervical dilation and slowed descent of the fetal head.

Pseudohermaphroditism: A condition in which the appearance of the outer genitalia fails to match the internal sex organs.

Pseudomenses/pseudomenstruation: Small amounts of bloody mucus discharged from the vagina of female newborns as a consequence of the withdrawal of maternal hormones.

Psychoprophylaxis: Emphasis on the prevention of pain by psychological strategies rather than removing pain by chemical means.

Puberty: The point at which reproduction becomes physically possible (8 to 14 years of age).

Puerperal infection: Temperature of 100.4°F (38.0°C) or greater on any two of the first 10 days following childbirth, exclusive of the first 24 hours.

Puerperium: The period from birth until 42 days postpartum.

Pulmonary embolism: A rare complication of deep vein thrombosis in which a portion of the clot breaks free and is carried through the circulatory system until it lodges in the pulmonary artery, where it occludes the vessel and obstructs pulmonary blood flow.

Quickening: Fetal movements felt by the mother herself at approximately 18 to 20 weeks' gestation in a primigravida, or 16 to 18 weeks' gestation in the multigravida.

Radiant warmer: A mattress on a cart, with a heat source above it, used to warm the newborn or to prevent cooling during procedures that require exposure.

Recessive: The need for two copies of the same allele form to be present for a trait or gene product to be expressed.

Rectocele: Abnormal protrusion of the anterior rectal wall into the vaginal wall.

Referred pain: Pain felt at a site different from that of an injured or diseased organ or part of the body, such as pain in the abdomen that is felt in the back, flank, or thighs.

Retinopathy of prematurity (RPS): A condition in preterm newborns resulting from the administration of high oxygen concentrations that they frequently require, which causes the fragile retinal blood to leak protein and bleed.

Retractions: An abnormal finding in newborns when they suck the ribs or sternum inward with inhalation because of use of accessory muscles during respiratory distress.

Rheumatoid arthritis: Symmetrical inflammation of the joints.

Risk factor: An action or behavior that increases a person's risk to develop a condition.

Rites of passage: Traditions, often ceremonious, that mark specific milestones in a human life.

Rooting reflex: A reflex in newborns by which they open their mouths and turn their heads in search of a nipple, or suck on their fingers or hands to indicate they are preparing for a feeding.

Second stage of labor: The period of labor from 10 cm of cervical dilatation to the birth of the baby; also called *expulsion.*

Secondary infertility: Inability to conceive when one or both parties have conceived previously.

Secretory phase: The menstrual cycle from days 15 to 28 during which progesterone dominates and enhances the menstrual lining in case implantation should take place.

Sedative hypnotics: Agents that reduce anxiety and induce sleep.

Self-management: Decisions and actions a person takes regarding health and quality of life.

Sequence: A cluster of anomalies that stem from a single major defect in fetal development.

Sex compatibility: Comfort with a certain sex.

Sex linked: Term used in relation to the genes located on the X and Y sex chromosomes, the 23rd pair, which determine gender.

Sexually transmitted infections (STIs)/sexually transmitted diseases (STDs): Infections transmitted through sexual contact, including vaginal, oral, or anal intercourse.

Shoulder dystocia: Failure of the fetal shoulders to traverse the pelvis spontaneously after birth of the fetal head.

Sickle cell crisis: Exacerbations of sickling in clients with sickle cell disease.

Sickle cell disease: An autosomal recessive disorder that results in serious, chronic, incurable hemolytic anemia.

Single-parent family: A family headed by an adult not currently living with a spouse.

Sleep phase advancement: A sleep pattern in which older adults go to bed and rise earlier than when they were younger.

Small for gestational age (SGA): Designation given when an infant's weight for gestational age falls below the 10th percentile.

Somatic pain: Deep pain resulting from the stretching of tissues.

Spermatid: The male gamete (sperm) that contains half of a child's genetic material, received from his or her father.

Spina bifida: Failure of the neural tube to close because of internal and external factors, with paralysis occurring below the level of the defect and hydrocephaly that can lead to brain injury.

Spinal anesthesia: Injection of a local anesthetic through the third, fourth, or fifth lumbar vertebrae into the subarachnoid space where the medication mixes with cerebrospinal fluid.

Spontaneous rupture of membranes (SROM): The natural breaking of the bag of waters, or amniotic sac, either before or during labor.

Station: The relationship of the presenting part of the fetus to an imaginary line drawn at the level of the ischial spines within the maternal pelvis.

Stigma: Being in a reduced form or holding a lesser status because of an attribute that differentiates one from other people.

Stillbirth: A pregnancy of more than 20 weeks' gestation that ends in fetal death.

Striae gravidarum: Pink or reddish streaks that appear on the sides and lower abdomen as a result of stretching of the connective layer of skin; commonly referred to as "*stretch marks.*"

Subinvolution: A condition in which normal postpartal involution of the uterus is slowed or stopped and accompanied by prolonged lochial discharge or excessive uterine bleeding.

Sudden Infant Death Syndrome (SIDS): The sudden death of an infant younger than 1 year, which remains unexplained after a thorough case investigation, including performance of a complete autopsy, examination of the death scene, and review of the clinical history.

Superficial venous thrombosis: Inflammation, clot formation, and resulting flow obstruction that is confined to the superficial saphenous venous system; also called *phlebitis.*

Supine postural hypotension syndrome: Hypotension and dizziness that occur when a pregnant woman lies on her back, resulting from compression of the vena cava against the spine.

Surfactant: A substance made of phospholipids and proteins secreted onto the alveolar surface, which causes retention of air in the lungs, decreasing surface tension at the air–liquid interface and promoting normal lung function.

Syncope: Loss of consciousness with decreased postural tone.

Syndrome: The clustering of multiple separate anomalies known to be primary outcomes of a single adverse event.

System: A unit in which the whole is greater than the sum of its parts.

Systemic lupus erythematosus: A chronic inflammatory disorder of the connective tissue with effects ranging from mild to severe.

Tachycardia: In a newborn, a resting apical heart rate of 180 to 200 beats/min.

Tachypnea: In a newborn, a resting respiratory rate greater than 60 breaths/min.

Talipes equinovarus: A congenital defect in which the foot has a downward and inward fixed position of flexion.

Teratogen: Any biologic, physical, chemical, or radiologic agent that causes structural or functional damage to a fetus.

Term: Designation used for an infant born between 38 and 42 weeks' gestation.

Testosterone: The dominant male hormone.

Therapeutic abortion: Pregnancy termination done to reduce health risks in the mother.

Third stage of labor: Separation and expulsion of the afterbirth.

Thromboembolic disorder: The formation of a blood clot or clots inside a blood vessel caused by inflammation or partial obstruction of the vessel.

Thrush: An oral yeast infection, commonly colonized as *Candida albicans* or *Candida parapsilosis.*

Total bilirubin: The sum of indirect and direct bilirubin values.

Tracheoesophageal fistula: A congenital defect in which an abnormal connecting passageway exists between the trachea and esophagus. Fluid or food intended to pass from mouth to esophagus and onward to stomach may thus be diverted into the lungs. Likewise, air taken in by the trachea and intended for the lungs also may enter the stomach to cause gastric distention.

Traditional nuclear family: Married parents with biologic children and no other people living in the household.

Transitional milk: Milk produced at approximately 7 to 10 days of lactation that serves as a bridge between colostrum and mature breast milk; it has increased lactose, fat, and calories, but fewer immunoglobulins and total proteins than does colostrum.

Transition phase: The last part of first-stage labor with cervical dilatation between 8 to 10 cm.

Triangle: A three-person system, the smallest available to form a stable relationship.

Trichomoniasis: A sexually transmitted infection caused by the protozoan parasite *Trichomonas vaginitis.*

Trimester: A period of approximately 3 months; especially any of three periods of approximately 3 months each into which a human pregnancy is divided.

Twilight sleep: Delivery of a combination of morphine sulfate and inhaled scopolamine hydrobromide to relieve labor pain and produce amnesia for labor and birth.

Two-parent family: Children living with a parent who is married with his or her spouse present.

Typical use failure rate: The number of women who become pregnant during their first year of use of a contraceptive method, which includes women who use the method correctly and those who use it incorrectly.

Ultrasound: A diagnostic test that uses sound waves to form a picture.

Unconjugated bilirubin: Bilirubin bound to circulating albumin in the bloodstream that has not yet been metabolized in the liver; also called *indirect bilirubin.*

Urethrocele: Bulging of the urethra into the vaginal wall.

Uterine atony: Failure of the uterus to contract adequately.

Uterine displacement: Deviation of the normal placement of the uterus.

Uterine inversion: Dropping of the uterine fundus into the endometrial cavity, possibly beyond the external cervical os.

Uterine prolapse: Descent of the uterus into the vaginal canal.

Uterine rupture: Separation of the uterine wall with or without fetal expulsion.

Vacuum extractor: A cup-shaped device attached to a suction pump and applied to the fetal head to remove it from the vaginal outlet.

Vaginal birth after cesarean (VBAC): The term used for a vaginal birth to a woman who has undergone at least one previous cesarean birth.

Variable deceleration: A rapid decrease in the fetal heart rate followed by a rapid return to baseline during or between contractions (with a characteristic V shape).

Variation: The life cycle outcome of each person's unique response to nature (genetic code) and nurture (environment), beginning before conception and ending with death.

Vasectomy: Interrupting the vas deferens through ligation and cautery to prevent pregnancy.

Vegan: A vegetarian who eats and uses no meat or meat products, such as eggs or milk.

Vernix caseosa: A normal greasy yellow-white substance that covers the newborn skin.

Vertex: The top portion of the fetal head between the anterior and posterior fontanelles.

Very low birthweight: Designation assigned when a newborn weighs less than 1500 grams (3⅓ pounds).

Viability: The point at which vital organs are able to support life of a fetus outside the uterus.

Visceral pain: Poorly localized pain that usually originates in body organs; occurs in response to stretching, distention, inflammation, or ischemia of the organ.

Witch's milk: Colloquial term for the milky substance discharged from the female newborn's breasts as a result of the influence of maternal hormones.

Withdrawal: Also called *coitus interruptus,* the complete removal of the penis from the vagina before ejaculation to prevent conception.

Women's health: The health care of nonpregnant women across the lifespan with a focus on health issues distinct and of specific concern to women.

Xerostomia: Dry mouth from decreased salivary secretions.

Zygote: The fertilized oocyte prior to the first cellular division and development of the embryo.

Zygote intrafallopian transfer (ZIFT): Fertilization in a laboratory with transfer of the resultant zygote to the woman's fallopian tube.

INDEX

Note: Pages followed by b indicate boxed material; those followed by f indicate figures; those followed by t indicate tables.

C

T

ASSESSMENT TOOLS

COMPLEMENTARY/ ALTERNATIVE MEDICINE

NIC/NOC BOXES

NURSING CARE PLANS